UNIT I Foundations of Critical Care Nursing

UNIT II Cardiovascular Alterations

UNIT III Pulmonary Alterations

UNIT IV Neurologic Alterations

UNIT V Kidney Alterations

UNIT VI Gastrointestinal Alterations

UNIT VII Endocrine Alterations

UNIT VIII Multisystem Alterations

UNIT IX Special Populations

APPENDIXES

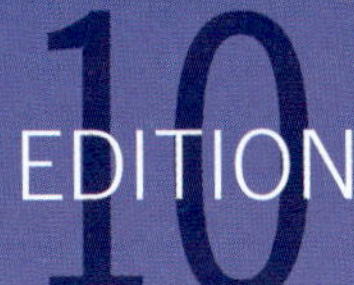

CRITICAL CARE NURSING

DIAGNOSIS AND MANAGEMENT

Linda D. Urden[†]**, DNSc, RN, CNS, FAAN**
Professor Emeritus
Hahn School of Nursing and Health Science
University of San Diego
San Diego, California

Kathleen M. Stacy, PhD, RN, APRN-CNS, CCNS, FCNS
Critical Care Clinical Nurse Specialist
Clinical Professor
Hahn School of Nursing and Health Science
University of San Diego
San Diego, California

Mary E. Lough, PhD, RN, CNS, FCCM, FAHA, FCNS, FAAN
Implementation Scientist, Clinical Nurse Specialist
Center for Professional Practice
Stanford Health Care
Stanford, California

Clinical Associate Professor
Primary Care and Population Health
Department of Medicine
Stanford University
Stanford, California

Clinical Professor
Department of Physiological Nursing
University of California at San Francisco
San Francisco, California

Kimberly Sanchez, PhD, RN, CCRN, ACCNS-AG
Nurse Scientist
Clinical Nurse Specialist
Nursing
Keck Medical Center of USC
Los Angeles, California

[†]Deceased. Dr. Urden passed away during the late publication stages of the 10th edition.

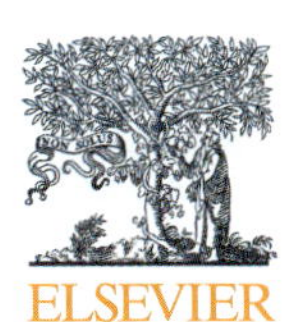
ELSEVIER

Elsevier
3251 Riverport Lane
St. Louis, Missouri 63043

CRITICAL CARE NURSING: DIAGNOSIS AND MANAGEMENT, TENTH EDITION ISBN: 978-0-443-11581-3

Notice

Practitioners and researchers must always rely on their own experience and knowledge in evaluating and using any information, methods, compounds, or experiments described herein. Because of rapid advances in the medical sciences, in particular, independent verification of diagnoses and drug dosages should be made. To the fullest extent of the law, no responsibility is assumed by Elsevier, authors, editors, or contributors for any injury and/or damage to persons or property as a matter of product liability, negligence or otherwise, or from any use or operation of any methods, products, instructions, or ideas contained in the material herein.

Executive Content Strategist: Lee Henderson
Director, Content Development: Laurie K. Gower
Content Development Specialist: Brooke Kannady
Publishing Services Manager: Deepthi Unni
Project Manager: Nayagi Anandan
Design Direction: Renee Duenow

Printed in India

Last digit is the print number: 9 8 7 6 5 4 3 2 1

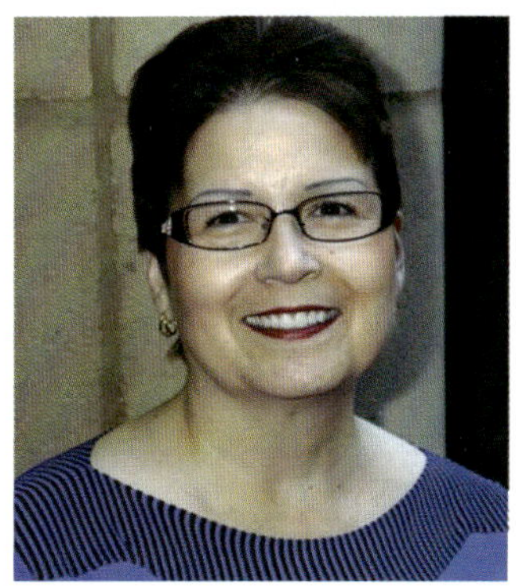

Linda D. Urden
1948 – 2024

This book is dedicated to the memory of our colleague and friend, Dr. Linda Urden, a founding editor and author of this text. Dr. Urden's pioneering work and unwavering commitment to nursing have inspired generations of nurses through 10 editions. May this book stand as a testament to her enduring impact on nursing, a field she transformed with wisdom, passion, and unyielding compassion. Though no longer with us, her words remind us of the profound impact one person can have on the lives of many. Dr. Urden's vision for nursing transcended boundaries, creating a legacy that will endure as long as there are nurses caring for critically ill patients.

To Linda D. Johnson, RN, BSN,
my first friend and mentor in critical care for all her wisdom, expertise, and support for me through the years. She left us way too soon and will always be remembered with love and affection.
LDU

To my granddaughter, KK. May you grow up in a safer and healthier world.
KMS

To all the critical care nurses throughout the world. Thank you for your dedication every day.
MEL

Para mi Ma y mi Pa. Gracias por enseñarme que todo es posible en la vida.
Ma, siempre estarás conmigo, guiándome, aconsejándome, y dándome la abundancia de tu amor.
Thank you to the nurses who mentored me in all stages of my career and those from whom I continue to learn. May this text guide current and future nurses.
KS

ABOUT THE AUTHORS

Linda D. Urden, DNSc, RN, CNS, NE-BC, FAAN

Linda Urden received her diploma in nursing from Barnes Hospital School of Nursing, St. Louis, Missouri; her BSN from Pepperdine University, Malibu, California; her MN, Cardiovascular Clinical Nurse Specialist, from UCLA; and her DNSc from the University of San Diego. Dr. Urden held a variety of clinical and administrative positions, with accountabilities for quality, evidence-based practice, research, education, advanced practice, and academia. In her various positions, she strove to create cultures that are sensitive to differentiated practice and ensure healthy work environments, supporting excellence in nursing practice. In addition to this text, Dr. Urden coauthored nine editions of *Priorities in Critical Care Nursing*. Other publications were in the areas of ethics, research, outcomes measurement, management and care delivery redesign, executive decision support databases, collaborative practice models, clinical nurse specialist outcomes, and Magnet environments. Her research integrated clinical, fiscal, quality, and behavioral outcomes of care delivery and services.

Kathleen M. Stacy, PhD, RN, APRN-CNS, CCNS, FCNS

Kathleen Stacy has been a nurse for more than 45 years, the majority of which she has spent working in critical care. She graduated in 1978 with a BS in nursing from the State University of New York at Plattsburgh, in 1989 with an MS in critical care nursing from San Diego State University, and in 2010 with a PhD in nursing from the University of San Diego. She has held a variety of positions, including staff nurse, clinical educator, outcomes manager, nurse manager, and clinical nurse specialist. Currently Dr. Stacy is a clinical professor at the Hahn School of Nursing and Health Science at the University of San Diego. She is the past program manager of the clinical nurse specialist concentration. Dr. Stacy is actively engaged in the ongoing process of curriculum transformation, refining educational frameworks to enhance learning experiences and meet the evolving needs of students and stakeholders alike. In addition to this text, Dr. Stacy has coauthored eight editions of *Priorities in Critical Care Nursing*.

Mary E. Lough, PhD, RN, CNS, FCCM, FAHA, FCNS, FAAN

Mary E. Lough is a critical care nurse with experience as a staff nurse, educator, clinical nurse specialist, and nurse scientist in critical care. She received her BSN from the University of Manchester in England and her MS and PhD from the University of California, San Francisco (UCSF). Dr. Lough is an implementation scientist at Stanford Health Care in Stanford, California and she currently facilitates an evidence-based practice/implementation science fellowship for clinical nurses. Dr. Lough holds a clinical faculty position in the medical school at Stanford University. She is a Clinical Professor in the Department of Physiological Nursing at her alma mater, UCSF. Dr. Lough is a fellow in the Society of Critical Care Medicine (SCCM), the American Heart Association (AHA), the National Association of Clinical Nurse Specialists (NACNS), and the American Academy of Nursing (AAN). Dr. Lough has co-authored nine editions of *Critical Care Nursing: Diagnosis and Management*, nine editions of *Priorities in Critical Care Nursing*, and has published many other articles, research papers, and books. She greatly appreciates the benefits of a clinically grounded textbook because when she began her career as a critical care nurse so little information was available.

Kimberly Sanchez, PhD, RN, CCRN, ACCNS-AG

Kimberly Sanchez is a nurse scientist and clinical nurse specialist with nursing practice expertise in the adult-gerontology population and clinical expertise in the health care needs of critically ill patients. Dr. Sanchez received her Doctor of Philosophy in Nursing Science and her Master of Science in Nursing from the University of San Diego and her Bachelor of Science in Nursing from Mount St. Mary's College in Los Angeles. She is double credentialed as a clinical nurse specialist and in critical care nursing by the American Association of Critical-Care Nurses. As a clinical nurse specialist, Dr. Sanchez assesses and evaluates health care practices and processes to improve health care delivery and outcomes; leads and mentors others on evidence-based practice changes; provides clinical expertise; upholds nursing practice; and initiates systems innovations. As a nurse scientist, Dr. Sanchez conducts nursing research and mentors nurses on the conduct of research within the hospital. Her research interests focus on independent nursing functions and patient outcomes. In addition to this text, Dr. Sanchez coauthored the 9th edition of *Priorities in Critical Care Nursing*.

CONTRIBUTORS

Ellen Arce, MSN, RN, CCRN
Transplant Coordinator
Lung Transplant
Stanford Health Care
Palo Alto, California
Chapter 35 Organ Donation and Transplantation

Daniel L. Arellano, PhD, RN, ACNP-BC, FNP-BC, CCRN, CEN, CFRN, EMT-P, FCCM, FAANP
Advanced Practice Nurse
Critical Care
University of Texas MD Anderson Cancer Center
Houston, Texas;
Assistant Professor of Nursing–Clinical Undergraduate Studies
University of Texas Health Science Center at Houston Cizik School of Nursing
Houston, Texas
Chapter 14 Cardiovascular Therapeutic Management

Sarah J. Berger, MS, RN, CNS, ACCNS-AG, CCRN
Clinical Nurse Specialist
Adult Critical Care
UCSF Medical Center
San Francisco, California
Chapter 12 Cardiovascular Diagnostic Procedures

Janine Wong Berta, MS, RD-AP, CNSC
Clinical Nutrition Supervisor
Clinical Nutrition
Stanford Health Care
Palo Alto, California;
Instructor
Nutrition, Food Science, and Packaging
San Jose State University
San Jose, California
Chapter 6 Nutrition Alterations and Management

Darlene Burke, PhD, MS, MA, RN, CCRN-K, CNE
Owner/Consultant
Professional Source Nurse Consulting
Carlsbad, California;
Associate Faculty
Nursing and Allied Health
Mira Costa College
Oceanside, California
Chapter 16 Pulmonary Clinical Assessment
Chapter 17 Pulmonary Diagnostic Procedures

Natalie Brianna de Haas-Rowland, MSN, RN, CCNS, CCRN-CSC-CMC
Clinical Nurse Specialist
Nursing
Keck Medical Center of USC
Los Angeles, California
Chapter 4 Facilitating Care Transitions

Caroline Etland, PhD, RN
Associate Faculty
Hahn School of Nursing
University of San Diego
San Diego, California;
Clinical Nurse Specialist
Caster Institute for Nursing Excellence
Sharp Healthcare
San Diego, California
Chapter 9 Palliative and End-of-Life Care

Corey Fry, DNP, ACNP-BC, CSC
Assistant Professor
Anesthesiology and Perioperative Medicine
Oregon Health and Science University
Portland, Oregon
Chapter 13 Cardiovascular Disorders

Céiline Géilinas, PhD, RN, FCAN
Professor
Ingram School of Nursing
McGill University
Montreal, Quebec, Canada;
Senior Researcher
Centre for Nursing Research
Jewish General Hospital
Montreal, Quebec, Canada
Chapter 7 Pain and Pain Management

Brandi Holcomb, DNP, APRN, AGACNP-BC, CCRN
Advanced Practice Clinician
Cardiothoracic Surgery
Christus Trinity Mother Frances Health System
Tyler, Texas;
Clinical Faculty, Graduate School of Nursing
University of Texas at El Paso
El Paso, Texas
Chapter 14 Cardiovascular Therapeutic Management

Misty Jenkins, ACNP-BC
Acute Care Nurse Practitioner
Pulmonary Critical Care
Ochsner Medical Center
New Orleans, Louisiana
Chapter 39 The Older Adult Patient

Allison M. Lang, MSN, CRNP, AGACNP-BC
Nurse Practitioner
Neurosurgery
Thomas Jefferson University Hospital
Philadelphia, Pennsylvania
Chapter 22 Neurologic Disorders and Therapeutic Management

Amy Larsen, MS, RN, CNS, ACCNS-AG, CCRN, SCRN
Clinical Nurse Specialist
Adult Critical Care
UCSF Medical Center
San Francisco, California
Chapter 12 Cardiovascular Diagnostic Procedures

Roy Lee, PharmD, BCPS
Heart, Lung, & Heart-Lung Transplant Pharmacist
Cardiothoracic Transplant and Pharmacy
Stanford Health Care
Stanford, California
Chapter 35 Organ Donation and Transplantation

Cynthia A. Lewis, MS, RN, APRN-CNS, CPN
Clinical Nurse Specialist
Medical Unit
Rady Children's Hospital San Diego
San Diego, California
Chapter 38 The Pediatric Patient

Juliana Liu, MSN, RN, ANP-BC
Nurse Practitioner, Program Manager
Adult Pulmonary Hypertension Service
Stanford Healthcare
Stanford, California
Chapter 13 Cardiovascular Disorders

Mary E. Lough, PhD, RN, CNS, FCCM, FAHA, FCNS, FAAN
Implementation Scientist, Clinical Nurse Specialist
Center for Professional Practice
Stanford Health Care
Stanford, California

Clinical Associate Professor
Primary Care and Population Health
Department of Medicine
Stanford University
Stanford, California

Clinical Professor
Department of Physiological Nursing
University of California at San Francisco
San Francisco, California
Chapter 3 Genetic Issues
Chapter 8 Sedation, Agitation, and Delirium Management
Chapter 10 Cardiovascular Anatomy and Physiology
Chapter 11 Cardiovascular Clinical Assessment
Chapter 12 Cardiovascular Diagnostic Procedures
Chapter 13 Cardiovascular Disorders
Chapter 14 Cardiovascular Therapeutic Management
Chapter 29 Endocrine Anatomy and Physiology
Chapter 30 Endocrine Clinical Assessment and Diagnostic Procedures
Chapter 31 Endocrine Disorders and Therapeutic Management

Lauren Malinowksi-Falk, MSN, CRNP, AGACNP-BC
Nurse Practitioner
Farber Hospitalist
Thomas Jefferson University Hospital
Philadelphia, Pennsylvania
Chapter 21 Neurologic Clinical Assessment and Diagnostic Procedures

Lisa Mancuso, BSN, RN, CCRN, CLCP, LNCC
Owner, Independent Contractor
Mancuso Medical Legal Consulting
Holliston, Massachusetts;
Program Director
Consult Division
OnPoint Legal Nurse Consulting
Philadelphia, Pennsylvania
Chapter 2 Ethical and Legal Issues

Eugene Emil Mondor, MN, RN, BScN, CNS, CNCC(C)
Clinical Nurse Specialist
Adult Critical Care
Royal Alexandra Hospital
Edmonton, Alberta, Canada
Chapter 32 Trauma

Robyn Myers, MSN, RN
Pediatric Nurse Practitioner
Pediatric General Surgery
Washington University/St. Louis Children's Hospital
St. Louis, Missouri
Chapter 34 Burns

Gabriela Oro, DNP, MSN, AGACNP-BC
Heart Transplant and MCS Nurse Practitioner
Heart Transplant and MCS Program
Stanford Health Care
Stanford, California
Chapter 35 Organ Donation and Transplantation

Tara J. Redwantz, BSN, RN, FNP-BC
Abdominal Transplant Kidney and Liver Transplant Surgery
Ochsner Health System
New Orleans, Louisiana
Chapter 35 Organ Donation and Transplantation

Kimberly Sanchez, PhD, RN, CCRN, ACCNS-AG
Nurse Scientist
Clinical Nurse Specialist
Nursing
Keck Medical Center of USC
Los Angeles, California
Chapter 4 Facilitating Care Transitions
Chapter 6 Nutrition Alterations and Management
Chapter 23 Kidney Anatomy and Physiology
Chapter 24 Kidney Clinical Assessment and Diagnostic Procedures
Chapter 25 Kidney Disorders and Therapeutic Management
Chapter 26 Gastrointestinal Anatomy and Physiology
Chapter 27 Gastrointestinal Clinical Assessment and Diagnostic Procedures
Chapter 28 Gastrointestinal Disorders and Therapeutic Management
Chapter 33 Sepsis, Shock, and Multiple Organ Dysfunction Syndrome
Chapter 37 The Obstetric Patient

Cass Piper Sandoval, MS, RN, CNS, CCRN, CCNS
Clinical Nurse Specialist
Department of Adult Cardiovascular Critical Care
UCSF Health
San Francisco, California
Chapter 12 Cardiovascular Diagnostic Procedures

Carol J. Scotto, PhD, RN
Assistant Professor
Nursing
Ursuline College
Pepper Pike, Ohio
Chapter 5 Psychosocial and Spiritual Considerations

Jennifer Seigel, MSN, RN, CPNP, CWCN
Washington University School of Medicine
Pediatric Surgery/Pediatric Acute Wound Service (PAWS)
St. Louis Children's Hospital
St. Louis, Missouri
Chapter 34 Burns

Teresa Jane Shafer, MSN, RN, CPTC
Transplantation Consultant
Organ Transplantation
Teresa Shafer Consulting LLC
Benbrook, Texas
Chapter 35 Organ Donation and Transplantation

Kathleen M. Stacy, PhD, RN, APRN-CNS, CCNS, FCNS
Critical Care Clinical Nurse Specialist
Clinical Professor
Hahn School of Nursing and Health Science
University of San Diego
San Diego, California
Chapter 15 Pulmonary Anatomy and Physiology
Chapter 18 Pulmonary Disorders
Chapter 19 Pulmonary Therapeutic Management
Chapter 20 Neurologic Anatomy and Physiology
Chapter 29 Endocrine Anatomy and Physiology
Chapter 30 Endocrine Clinical Assessment and Diagnostic Procedures

Carol Ann Suarez, MSN, APRN, ACNS-BC, FNP
Clinical Nurse Specialist
Pulmonary/Trauma Intermediate Care Units
Palomar Medical Center
Mission Viejo, California;
Clinical Faculty
Health and Human Services–Nursing
California State University San Marcos
San Marcos, California
Chapter 36 Hematologic and Oncologic Emergencies

Nikki Taylor, MS, BSN, RN, AGCNS-BC
Clinical Nurse Specialist
Cardiac/Thoracic Surgery, Cardiovascular Moderate Care
University of Michigan Health System
Ann Arbor, Michigan;
Adjunct Clinical Instructor
School of Nursing
University of Michigan
Ann Arbor, Michigan
Chapter 14 Cardiovascular Therapeutic Management

Linda D. Urden, DNSc, RN, CNS, NE-BC, FAAN
Professor Emerita
Hahn School of Nursing and Health Sciences
University of San Diego
San Diego, California
Chapter 1 Critical Care Nursing Practice

Melissa Voltz, BSBA, MSN, RN, FNP-C
Nurse Practitioner
Urology
Ochsner Medical Center
New Orleans, Louisiana
Chapter 35 Organ Donation and Transplantation

Karen Wilkinson, MN, ARNP, LNCC, CLNCP
Owner
Legal Nurse Consulting
Wilkinson Legal Nurse Consulting
Seattle, Washington;
Director of Education
American Association of Legal Nurse Consulting
Chicago, Illinois
Chapter 2 Ethical and Legal Issues

Schawnte P. Williams-Taylor, BSN, RN, MBA, MS, CPTC
Vice President, Family Engagement and Donation Services
Organ Procurement Administration
LifeGift
Houston, Texas
Chapter 35 Organ Donation and Transplantation

Carrie M. Wilson, MSN, RN
Pediatric Nurse Practitioner
Pediatric General Surgery
Washington University
St. Louis, Missouri
Chapter 34 Burns

Kathrine Anne Winnie, DNP, RN, CCRN, AGCNS-BC
Clinical Nurse Specialist
Nursing
Keck Medical Center of USC
Los Angeles, California
Chapter 4 Facilitating Care Transitions
Chapter 23 Kidney Anatomy and Physiology
Chapter 24 Kidney Clinical Assessment and Diagnostic Procedures
Chapter 25 Kidney Disorders and Therapeutic Management
Chapter 26 Gastrointestinal Anatomy and Physiology
Chapter 27 Gastrointestinal Clinical Assessment and Diagnostic Procedures
Chapter 28 Gastrointestinal Disorders and Therapeutic Management
Chapter 33 Sepsis, Shock, and Multiple Organ Dysfunction Syndrome
Chapter 37 The Obstetric Patient

Fiona Winterbottom, DNP, RN
Clinical Nurse Specialist
Critical Care
Ochsner Medical Center
New Orleans, Louisiana
Chapter 39 The Older Adult Patient

PREFACE

We extend our deepest gratitude to the multitude of students and nurses whose contributions have made the preceding nine editions of this book a resounding success. Their support reaffirms our dedication to celebrating the remarkable efforts of critical care nurses and to advocating for evidence-based nursing practices within the intricate critical care setting. Actively seeking input from users of past editions, we enthusiastically integrated their valuable feedback on format, content, and organization. With this tenth edition, we proudly present a comprehensive resource tailored to the needs of critical care nurses, thoughtfully organized for clarity and understanding.

ORGANIZATION

The book is structured into nine units and three appendices, each centered around variations in dimensions of human functioning across biopsychosocial realms.

- Unit I, "Foundations of Critical Care Nursing," is the cornerstone of practice. It addresses fundamental principles applicable to critically ill patients regardless of their physiological alterations.
  - While chapters can be explored in any order, we recommend commencing with Chapter 1, "Critical Care Nursing Practice," as it elucidates the fundamental assumptions underpinning the book's entirety.
  - Chapter 2, "Ethical and Legal Issues," offers insights into navigating daily ethical dilemmas in critical care and provides essential knowledge on issues with potential legal ramifications.
  - In Chapter 3, "Genetic Issues," readers delve into the biological foundations of genetics, exploring various genetic and genomic studies alongside examples of genetic diseases and pharmacogenetic syndromes prevalent in critical care.
  - Chapter 4, "Facilitating Care Transitions," sheds light on the critical process of patient movement across care settings, procedural departments, and discharge to different facilities. It covers hand-off communication protocols, procedural details, and crucial patient and family education principles.
  - Chapter 5, "Psychosocial and Spiritual Considerations," examines the theoretical underpinnings and nursing strategies for addressing alterations in self-concept, spiritual practices, and coping mechanisms.
  - Chapter 6, "Nutrition Alterations and Management," provides comprehensive insights into the nutritional requirements of critically ill patients, offering tailored recommendations for various disorders.
  - Chapter 7, "Pain and Pain Management," explores pain and its management in critically ill patients.
  - Chapter 8, "Sedation, Agitation, and Delirium Management," delves into the intricacies of managing sedation, agitation, and delirium.
  - Lastly, Chapter 9, "Palliative and End-of-Life Care," outlines specialized approaches for addressing the unique needs of patients nearing the end of life, emphasizing palliative care principles.
- Unit II, "Cardiovascular Alterations," and Unit III, "Pulmonary Alterations," are meticulously structured, each comprising the following chapters:
  - Anatomy and Physiology
  - Clinical Assessment
  - Diagnostic Procedures
  - Disorders
  - Therapeutic Management

  This systematic arrangement facilitates swift access to information for students and clinicians while allowing instructors to tailor teaching approaches by assigning chapters according to individual student requirements.
- Similarly, Unit IV, "Neurologic Alterations," Unit V, "Kidney Alterations," Unit VI, "Gastrointestinal Alterations," and Unit VII, "Endocrine Alterations," adhere to a parallel organizational pattern:
  - Anatomy and Physiology
  - Clinical Assessment and Diagnostic Procedures
  - Disorders and Therapeutic Management

  These four units merge clinical assessment parameters and diagnostic procedures into one chapter, while disorders and therapeutic management are consolidated into another chapter.
- Unit VIII, "Multisystem Alterations," focuses on disorders impacting multiple body systems, necessitating a distinct discussion category. This unit comprises five chapters: "Trauma," "Sepsis, Shock, and Multiple Organ Dysfunction Syndrome," "Burns," "Organ Donation and Transplantation," and "Hematologic and Oncologic Emergencies."
- Unit IX, "Special Populations," addresses the unique needs of critically ill obstetric, pediatric, and geriatric patients in the critical care unit.
- Appendix A, "Patient Care Management Plans," provides organized access to patient care management plans alphabetically arranged by diagnosis, facilitating ease of use for students and practitioners.
- Appendix B, "Physiologic Formulas for Critical Care," presents commonly encountered hemodynamic, pulmonary, and other critical care calculations in easily understandable formulas. It also offers recommendations for nutrition supplements.
- Finally, Appendix C lists the most common laboratory tests expressed in Système International (SI) units, predominantly used in Canada. Conventional units utilized in the United States are presented in parentheses for reference.

SPECIAL FEATURES

A prominent theme throughout the book underscores evidence-based nursing interventions tied to patient diagnoses, highlighting the robustness of critical care nursing practice. Whenever feasible, evidence-based critical care practices are seamlessly integrated into nursing interventions. Several features to facilitate critical care nursing practice are found throughout the book:

- **Case Studies** enrich student learning and foster critical thinking by illustrating the clinical trajectory of patients experiencing the history, clinical assessment, diagnostic procedures, and diagnoses discussed in the corresponding unit or chapter. Each Case Study includes critical thinking questions to stimulate discussion, with answers available on the Evolve website as a supplemental resource for instructors.

- **Data Collection** boxes within the clinical assessment chapters contain essential information integral to the patient's history.
- **Diagnosis and Patient Care Management** boxes succinctly summarize diagnoses associated with specific disorders, referencing the corresponding patient care management plans in Appendix A.
- **Patient and Family Education Plan** boxes, positioned within the disorders chapters, outline key topics to be covered in patient and family education sessions, which prepare patients for discharge.
- **Pharmacologic Management** tables in the therapeutic management chapters outline common medications and any special considerations relevant to treating various disorders presented in the text.
- **Patient-Centered Critical Care** boxes are strategically placed throughout the chapters, highlighting the evolving landscape of critical care with a greater emphasis on patient and family involvement. These boxes feature evidence-based discussions on topics such as family meetings, patient diaries, family attending rounds, debriefing after a code, creating a calming environment, early mobility, pet visitation, transition of care, older adult patients, 24/7 visitation, and music therapy.
- In addition to the previously discussed boxes, other boxes found throughout the book include the following:
    - **Quality** boxes examine improvements to enhance the quality and safety of health care systems and individual patient outcomes.
    - **Patient Safety** boxes promote and reinforce principles, practices, and strategies pertinent to ensuring patients' safety and well-being in the critical care setting.
    - **Evidence-Based Practice** boxes contain essential information, guidelines, and evidence-based recommendations focused on minimizing risks, preventing errors, and optimizing patient outcomes.
    - **Team Work and Collaboration** boxes discuss functioning effectively within nursing and interprofessional teams, fostering open communication, mutual respect, and shared decision making to achieve quality patient care.
    - **Patient-Centered Care** boxes explore situations that illustrate providing compassionate and coordinated care based on respect for patients' preferences, values, and needs.

NEW TO THIS EDITION

- This edition introduces **Social Determinants of Health (SDOH)** boxes, which delve into discussions on specific determinants of health and offer insights into future research and policy recommendations. These SDOH boxes are strategically placed throughout the book to enrich the reader's understanding of SDOH and its impact on critically ill patients.
- Another notable addition to this edition is the **Supporting the Well-Being of Nurses** boxes. In alignment with a consensus study report by the National Academy of Medicine, a pivotal objective is leveraging nursing capacity and expertise to promote health equity. Essential to achieving this goal is the support of nursing well-being. Numerous models have been proposed and endorsed by professional organizations. This edition introduces a model and elucidates its components through vignettes scattered across the chapters, highlighting the importance of nurturing nursing well-being.
- **Disorder Summary** figures have also been added to this edition and are interspersed throughout the disorders chapters to enhance student comprehension of complex medical conditions. These figures encapsulate key information under sections such as "Clinical and Diagnostic Assessments," "Signs," and "Nursing Interventions," streamlining the learning process.
- Lastly, **Informatics** boxes have been added to this edition and are found throughout the book. These boxes explore using information and technology to communicate, manage knowledge, mitigate error, and support decision making in nursing practice.

Critical Care Nursing: Diagnosis and Management, 10th Edition, represents our continued commitment to bringing you the finest in all things a textbook can offer: the best and brightest contributing and consulting authors, the latest scientific research befitting the current state of health care and nursing, an organizational format that exercises diagnostic reasoning skills and is logical and consistent, and outstanding artwork and illustrations that enhance student learning. We pledge our continued commitment to excellence in critical care education.

Linda D. Urden
Kathleen M. Stacy
Mary E. Lough
Kimberly Sanchez

ACKNOWLEDGMENTS

A project of this book's magnitude is never merely the work of its authors. The concerted talent, hard work, and inspiration of a multitude of people have produced *Critical Care Nursing: Diagnosis and Management*, 10th edition and have helped to make it the state-of-the-science text. A "tradition of publishing excellence" has been evident throughout our partnership with Elsevier. We deeply appreciate the assistance of Lee Henderson, Executive Content Strategist, and Brooke Kannady, Content Development Specialist, who have helped us document and refine our ideas and transform this book into a reality. Their creativity, expertise, availability, and generosity of time and resources have been invaluable to us throughout this endeavor. We are also grateful to Nayagi Anandan, Project Manager, for her scrupulous attention to detail, and to designer Renee Duenow for her expertise.

Finally, we wish to thank the authors who contributed work to the first nine editions. Without the foundation they provided, a 10th edition would not have been born. We continue to be proud of our partnership with Elsevier, the teamwork and mutual respect among the four co-editors, and the final published book.

Linda D. Urden
Kathleen M. Stacy
Mary E. Lough
Kimberly Sanchez

CONTENTS

1

Critical Care Nursing Practice

Linda D. Urden

http://evolve.elsevier.com/Urden/CriticalCareNursing

This chapter provides an overview of the evolution of critical care nursing and describes the trends and current issues affecting critical care nurses and interdisciplinary teams. The information in this chapter serves as the framework for the remainder of the book in the areas of professional nursing practice and accountability, decision making, patient care management, holistic care, cultural sensitivity and competency, interdisciplinary collaboration, evidence-based practice (EBP), quality, and safety. Additionally, the importance of the effect of social determinants of health on patients in critical care is highlighted throughout the book. Lastly, we emphasize the stressors that face critical care nurses and how resources and supports can be established by peers, organizations, and nurses themselves.

HISTORY OF CRITICAL CARE

Critical care evolved from the recognition that the needs of patients with acute, life-threatening illness or injury could be better met if the patients were organized in distinct areas of the hospital. In the 1800s, Florence Nightingale described the advantages of placing patients recovering from surgery in a separate area of the hospital.

During World War II, shock wards were established to care for critically injured patients. The 1950s brought the new technology of mechanical ventilation and the need to group patients receiving this new therapy in one location, thus the first specialty ICU: respiratory. By the late 1960s, most U.S. hospitals had at least one ICU. The Society of Critical Care Medicine (SCCM) was established in 1970 and has become the driving force for critical care practice guidelines, education, and interdisciplinary collaborative initiatives. SCCM is the largest nonprofit medical organization dedicated to promoting excellence in the practice of critical care.[1]

Critical care nursing was organized as a specialty less than 60 years ago; before that time, critical care nursing was practiced wherever there were critically ill patients. The development of new medical interventions and technology prompted recognition that nursing was important in monitoring and observation of critically ill patients. Physicians depended on nurses to watch for critical changes in the condition of patients in the physicians' absence, and they sometimes depended on the nurses to initiate emergency medical treatment.

As sophisticated technology began to support more elaborate medical interventions, hospitals began to organize separate units to make more efficient use of equipment and specially trained staff. Postoperative care, once provided by private duty nurses on general nursing wards throughout the hospital, was moved into recovery rooms where nurses with specialized knowledge regarding anesthesia recovery provided the patient care.

The nursing shortage after World War II forced the grouping of postoperative patients into designated recovery areas so that appropriate monitoring and care could be provided. The technologies and combat experiences of health care providers during the wars of the 20th century also provided an impetus for specialized medical and nursing care in the civilian setting. Medical and surgical ICUs segregated the most critically ill patients in locations where they could be cared for by nurses with specialized knowledge in those areas of care. By the 1960s, nurses had begun to consolidate their knowledge and practice into focused areas such as coronary care, nephrology, and intensive care. In the hospital units established for patients needing such specialized care, nurses assumed many functions and responsibilities formerly reserved for physicians, and they assumed a new authority by virtue of their knowledge and expertise.

Contemporary Critical Care

Modern critical care is provided to patients by a multidisciplinary team of health care professionals who have in-depth education and expertise in the specialty field of critical care. The team consists of physician intensivists, specialty physicians, nurses, advanced practice nurses (APNs) such as clinical nurse specialists (CNSs) and nurse practitioners (NPs), and other specialty clinicians: pharmacists, respiratory therapy practitioners, other specialized therapists, social workers, and clergy. Critical care is provided in specialized units or departments, and importance is placed on the continuum of care, with an efficient and as seamless as possible transition of care from one setting to another (see Chapter 4).

Critical care patients are at high risk for actual or potential life-threatening health problems. Patients who are more critically ill require more intensive and vigilant nursing care. These nurses practice in various settings: adult, pediatric, and neonatal critical care units; step-down, telemetry, progressive, or transitional care units; interventional radiology departments; and postoperative recovery units. Nurses are knowledge workers

BOX 1.1 Examples of Expanded Registered Nurse Roles in Critical Care

- Charge nurse
- Supervisor, shift relief supervisor
- Preceptor
- Dialysis nurse, other specialty nurse
- Trauma team nurse
- Rapid Response Team member
- Shared Governance Committee member—other committee member, depending on how the unit is organized
- Mentor
- Unit greeter
- Unit newsletter editor
- Educator
- Quality/safety nurse
- Infection monitor nurse
- Academic liaison

because they are highly vigilant and use their intelligence and cognition to go past tasks and quickly pull together multiple data to make decisions regarding subtle or deteriorating conditions. They work with both technical and theoretical knowledge.

The designation of progressive care units (also known as *step-down, telemetry*, and *subacute*, to name a few) is considered part of the continuum of critical care. Prior to this, patients who were placed on these units would have been exclusively in critical care units. However, with the use of additional technology and monitoring capabilities, newer care delivery models, and additional nurse education, these units are considered the best environment for patients who do not need intensive monitoring with highly technologic monitoring. The patients are less complex, are more stable, have a decreased need for physiologic monitoring, and have more self-care capabilities. They can serve as a bridge between critical care units and medical-surgical units while providing high-quality and cost-effective care at the same time.[2] Additionally, these progressive units can be found throughout the acute care setting, leaving critical care unit beds for patients who need the highest level of care and monitoring.

Critical Care Nursing Roles

Nurses provide and contribute to the care of critically ill patients in a variety of roles. The most prevalent role for the professional registered nurse (RN) is that of direct care provider. Other nursing roles may be delineated requiring additional education and competencies that are designed to meet the needs of the patient population and management of unit management. For example, some role responsibilities that are important for acute care and critical care nurses to facilitate patient care and support unit functions are found in Box 1.1.

Expanded-Role Nursing Positions

Nurses in expanded-role nursing positions interact with critical care patients, families, and the health care team. Nurse care coordinators work closely with the care providers to ensure appropriate, timely care and services and to promote continuity of care from one setting to another. Other nurse clinicians, such as patient educators, cardiac rehabilitation specialists, physician office nurses, and infection control specialists, also contribute to care. The specific types of expanded-role nursing positions are determined by patient needs and individual organizational resources.

Advanced Practice Nurses

APNs have met educational and clinical requirements beyond the basic nursing educational requirements for all nurses. The most commonly seen APNs in critical care areas are the CNS and the NP or acute care nurse practitioner (ACNP). APNs have a broad depth of knowledge and expertise in their specialty area and manage complex clinical and systems issues. The organizational system and existing resources of an institution determine what roles may be needed and how the roles function.

CNSs serve in specialty roles that use their clinical, teaching, research, leadership, and consultative abilities. They work in direct clinical roles and systems or administrative roles and in various other settings in the health care system. CNSs work closely with all members of the health care team, mentor staff, lead quality teams, and consult on complex patients. They are instrumental in ensuring that care is evidence based and that safety programs are in place. CNSs may be organized by specialty, such as cardiovascular care, or by function, such as cardiac rehabilitation. CNSs also may be designated as care coordinators for specific patient populations.

NPs and ACNPs manage direct clinical care of a group of patients and have various levels of prescriptive authority, depending on the state and practice area in which they work. They also provide care consistency, interact with families, plan for patient discharge, and provide teaching to patients, families, and other members of the health care team.[2]

SOCIAL DETERMINANTS OF HEALTH (SDOH)

SDOH Domains

Healthy People 2030[3] is the fifth iteration of the Healthy People initiative and builds on knowledge gains on the past four decades to address the most critical public health priorities and challenges in the United States for the next 10 years. Healthy People defines health disparity as a health difference that is closely linked with social, economic, and/or environmental disadvantage. Health disparities adversely affect group of people who have systematically experienced greater obstacles to health based on their racial or ethnic group, religion, socioeconomic status, gender, age, mental health, cognitive, sensory, or physical disability; sexual orientation or gender identity; geographic location; or other characteristics linked to discrimination or exclusion.[3]

Social Determinants of Health are the conditions in the environments where people are born, live, work, play, worship, and age that affect a wide range of health, functioning, and quality-of-life outcomes and risks.[4] These domains are categorized into five areas—see Box 1.2.

SDOH have major impacts on health, quality of life and well-being in all people.

Disparities Among People

Note the following resulting disparities among peoples[4]:

- Literacy skills, language
- Education, job opportunities, income
- Polluted water and air
- Safe housing, neighborhoods, and transportation
- Racism, discrimination, violence
- Access to nutritious foods
- Physical activity opportunities
- Community networks

Inequities Among People[5,6]

- People who don't have access to grocery stores/healthy foods are less likely to have good nutrition, which raises their risk of health conditions like heart disease, diabetes, obesity, and lower life expectancy
- In the United States, 1 in 10 people live in poverty and many can't afford healthy food, health care, and housing
- People with disabilities, injuries, or conditions like arthritis may be especially limited in their ability to work and focus on their health
- Children from low-income families, those with disabilities, and those who experience discrimination like bullying are more likely to struggle with math and reading, less likely to graduate high school, and more likely to have heart disease and health problems
- People without insurance are less likely to have primary care providers and they may not be able to afford the health care services and medications they need or necessary screenings

SDOH Goal

One important overall SDOH goal is to increase the proportion of adults who get recommended evidence-based preventative health care.[7] This statistic has remained relatively stable with no detectable change since the last measurement. However, the target was set at a higher number; this is an example of an indicator that does not directly impact in the ICU but does ultimately influence through overall health to an illness that could cause a person to end up in critical care.

So what can the clinician in critical care do to address SDOHs? It starts with recognition of the initial factors. Knowing that there are issues in a certain domain that can be addressed in the critical care unit may be all that can be done at the time. However, an assessment with referral to the next level of care provider or case manager/social worker or external placement if the patient is being discharged to another care facility.

As can be identified in the brief discussion in this chapter, SDOHs are larger issues, multifactorial and complex, and are not be resolved easily or perhaps ever by this point in the person's life. Recognition and perhaps some other community resources need to be brought into a person's unique situation so that there can be some interventions established to focus on priority areas of importance.

A new feature created for this book edition focuses on SDOHs with discussions of the specific determinant of health, clinical interventions for inpatient care, and future research and policy recommendations. These SDOH boxes are interspersed throughout the book. For example, refer to the Hospitalized Patients With Underlying Substance Abuse box.

SOCIAL DETERMINANTS OF HEALTH

Hospitalized Patients With Underlying Substance Abuse

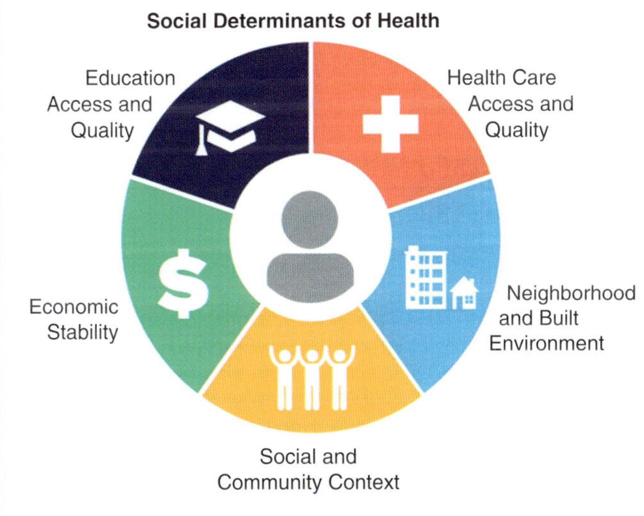

The escalating opioid crisis affects all health care sectors and settings nationally. This crisis was proclaimed to be an epidemic and a public health emergency in 2019 by the United States Department of Health and Human Services. They reported that an alarming 11.5 million persons (all genders and ages) misused prescription medications.[1]

An astounding 20% to 50% of those admitted to hospitals possess substance abuse disorders.[2] Additionally, hospitalized patients have increased comorbidities and health care costs and greater risk for readmissions.[3] Those who require ICU care have longer ICU stays, higher APACHE II scores, and higher mortality.[4] Researchers in one study indicated that substance abuse admissions into the ICU use about 25% of resources.[4]

Caring for these patients is frustrating for nursing staff as there are additional needs related to the addictive disease that are beyond the admitted diagnosis treatment regimen. Recognition of withdrawal symptoms such as the following is essential: increased agitation, tachycardia, chills, flushing, muscle aches, rhinorrhea, tremors, sweating, anxiety, insomnia, diarrhea, nausea, and vomiting.[5] Recommendations for care of patients with addiction include the following:

- Start with compassion[5]
- Collect a detailed history of both medical and substance use
- Conduct thorough admission assessment regarding issues surrounding use of addictive substances
- Complete appraisal of both prescription and street medications
- Document the patient's health care provider(s) and supports regarding addiction
- Include family/significant other into care and discharge planning
- Utilize a collaborative approach in the plan of care[5]
- Carefully consider implications for integration of abused medications into the plan of care
- Prior to discharge, assess treatment readiness[5]
- Educate (for discharge) on harm reduction practices, i.e., educate on safe practices with continued substance abuse practices[5]
- Upon discharge, provide information on local resources[5]

References

1. United States Department of Health and Human Services. *What is the U.S. opiod epidemic?*, 2019. https:hhs.gov/opiods/about-the-epidemic/index.html.
2. Neville K, Roan N. Challenges in nursing practice: Nurses' perceptions in caring for hospitalized medical-surgical with substance abuse/dependence. *JONA*. 2014;44(6):339346.
3. Thompson HM, Hill K, Jadhav R, Webb TA, Pollack M, Karnik N. The substance use intervention team: A preliminary analysis of a population-level strategy to address the opiod crisis at an academic medical center. *J Addict Med*. 2019;13(6):440–463.
4. Westerhausen D, Perkins AJ, Conley J, Kahn BA, Farber M. Burden of substance abuse related admissions to the medical ICU. *Chest*. 2020;157(1):61–66.
5. Riley K, Evans MM, Worozbyt K, Kowalchik K. Caring for an opioid addicted patient in a medical-surgical setting: best practice recommendations. *Medsurg Nurs*. 2019 28(2):4–7.

Illustration from Healthy People 2030, U.S. Department of Health and Human Services, Office of Disease Prevention and Health Promotion. Retrieved September 8, 2022, from https://health.gov/healthypeople/objectives-and-data/social-determinants-health.

BOX 1.2 Social Determinants of Health (SDOH)

Social determinants of health are the conditions in the environments where people are born, live, work, play, worship, and age that affect a wide range of health functioning and quality-of-life outcomes and risks.

Economic Stability

In the U.S., 1 in 10 people live in poverty and many people can't afford things like healthy food, health care, and housing. Healthy People 2030 focuses on helping more people achieve economic stability.

Education Access and Quality

People with higher levels of education are more likely to be healthier and live longer. Healthy People 2030 focuses on providing high-quality educational opportunities for children and adolescents—and on helping do well in school.

Health Care Access and Quality

Many people in the United States don't get the health care services they need. Healthy People 2030 focuses on improving health by helping people get timely, high-quality health care services.

Neighborhood and Built Environment

The neighborhoods people live in have a major impact on their health and well-being. Healthy People 2030 focuses on improving health and safety in the places where people live, work, play, learn, and play.

Social and Community Context

People's relationships and interactions with family, friends, co-workers, and community members can have a major impact on their health and well-being. Healthy People 2030 focuses on helping people get the social support they need in the places where they work, live, learn, and play.

Adapted from Social Determinants of Heath. Healthy People 2030. U.S. Department of Health and Human Services, Office of Disease Prevention and Health Promotion. From https://odphp.health.gov/healthypeople/objectives-and-data/social-determinants-health.

CRITICAL CARE PROFESSIONAL ACCOUNTABILITY

Critical Care Professional Organizations

Society of Critical Care Medicine (SCCM)

Professional organizations support critical care practitioners by providing numerous resources and networks. SCCM is a multidisciplinary, multispecialty, international organization. The mission of SCCM is to secure the highest quality, cost-efficient care for all critically ill patients. Their numerous publications and educational opportunities provide cutting-edge critical care information to critical care practitioners.[1]

American Association of Critical Care Nurses (AACN)

The nursing specialty organization most closely associated with critical care nurses is AACN. Created in 1969, it is the world's largest specialty nursing organization. AACN is focused on "creating a healthcare system driven by the needs of patients and their families, where acute and critical care nurses make their optimal contribution."[2]

AACN serves its members through a national organization and many local chapters. The top priority of the organization is education of critical care nurses via national, regional, local, and online opportunities. AACN publishes numerous materials, journals, EBP summaries, practice alerts, linkages between critical care nurses, and job postings related to the specialty. It also provides multiple clinical tools to support critical care patient and nursing practice. AACN is at the forefront of setting professional standards of care. See Chapter 2 and Box 2.7 for discussion of nursing standards and specific delineation of critical care nursing standards.

The *AACN Certification Corporation* was created in the 1970s and is a separate company that develops and administers many critical care specialty certification examinations for RNs. The examinations are provided in specialties such as neonatal care, pediatric care, critical care, progressive care, "virtual" critical care unit, and remote monitoring (e-ICU).

There are also certifications for APNs. According to the Certification Corporation, certification is considered one method to maintain high quality of care and to protect consumers of care and services: "Achieving board certification demonstrates to patients, employers and the public that a nurse's knowledge reflects national standards and a deep commitment to patient safety."[2] Evidence shows that there are more positive outcomes when care is delivered by health care providers who are certified in their specialty. More than 120,000 acute and critical care nurses currently hold AACN certification in one of the specialties.[2]

AACN also recognizes critical care and acute care units that provide a high level of care in a healthy work environment through its *Beacon Award for Excellence*.[2] It reflects on a unit with a supportive overall environment with teamwork and collaboration that is distinguished by lower turnover and higher morale.

These criteria must be met: (1) leadership structures, (2) appropriate staffing and engagement, (3) effective communication and knowledge management and learning development, (4) EBP and processes, and (5) outcome measures. The award is given at three levels that reflect significant improvement on the path to excellence: bronze, silver, and gold.

A unit that receives this award has demonstrated exceptional clinical outcomes and overall patient and staff satisfaction. According to the AACN 2023 Annual Report, there were 193 critical care designated Beacon units at that time.[2]

EVIDENCE-BASED NURSING PRACTICE

Factors Driving EBP

Much of early medical and nursing practice was based on nonscientific traditions and intuition. These traditions and rituals, which were based on folklore, gut instinct, trial and error, and personal preference, were often passed down from one generation of practitioners to the next. Some examples of critical care nursing practice based on nonscientific traditions include Trendelenburg positioning for hypotension, use of rectal tubes to manage fecal incontinence, gastric residual volume and aspiration risk, accuracy of assessment of body temperature, and suctioning artificial airways every 2 hours.

Multiple changes and increased health care costs have led to an increased presence of managed care, pay for performance, and regulations with punitive financial actions toward health care organizations that do not meet established thresholds. This has resulted in a greater emphasis on demonstrating the effectiveness of treatments and practices on outcomes.

Emphasis is on greater efficiency, cost effectiveness, quality of life, and patient satisfaction engagement. It has become essential for nurses to use the best data available to make patient care decisions and carry out appropriate nursing interventions.

Tools to Assist Nurses With Adoption of Scientific Evidence

By using an approach employing a scientific basis, with its ability to explain and predict, nurses can provide research-based interventions with consistent, positive outcomes. The content of this book is research based, with the most current, cutting-edge research abstracted and placed throughout the chapters as appropriate to topical discussions.

The increasingly complex and changing health care system presents many challenges to creating an EBP. Appropriate research studies must be designed to answer clinical questions, and research findings must be used to make necessary changes for implementation in practice. Multiple EBP and research utilization models exist to guide practitioners in the use of existing research findings and will not be discussed here.

Evidence-based nursing practice considers the best research evidence on the care topic, clinical expertise of the nurse, and patient preferences. Bourgault stated that there is a need to bridge the gap between appropriate, scientifically sound research to clinical practice. When there is not research evidence to support a practice, nursing uses critical thinking and clinical judgment on which to base a practice decision.[8]

It is essential that critical care nurses are current with the latest evidence to guide their practice and ensure that they implement the most current procedures to ensure the best possible outcomes for those to whom they provide care. AACN has promulgated several EBP summaries in the form of a *practice alert* to facilitate this care. Being an evidence-based clinician is now the standard, not the exception, and strategies must be in place so that this can occur in everyone's practice. Tools must be in place to make sure that EBP is accessible to all clinicians in a timely manner and that all are informed of the latest literature.[9]

These alerts are short directives that can be used as a quick reference for practice areas. They are succinct, supported by evidence, and address both nursing and multidisciplinary activities. Each alert is organized into five areas and includes 1) scope and impact of the problem, 2) expected outcome, 3) supporting evidence, 4) implementation/organizational support for the practice, 5) and references. Examples of Practice Alerts are listed in Box 1.3.

Diagnosis and Patient Care Management

It is crucial that nurses document their observations, nursing diagnosis of patient conditions, and interventions that they carry out to address these issues. Nurses use their knowledge, critical thinking, and ability to link physiologic data with patient symptomology to diagnose actual or potential health problems.

The ability to capture these components is important to demonstrate the effectiveness of professional nursing practice on outcomes, including clinical, financial, and organizational indicators. In order to accomplish this, there must be a consistent methodology that includes common terms that will provide classifications across a variety of patient conditions and settings.

The classification that will be used for this book is the *International Classification for Nursing Practice* (ICNP). ICNP is a collaborative project coordinated under the International Council of Nurses (ICN). There are three elements of ICNP: (1) nursing phenomena, sometimes referred to as nursing diagnosis; (2) nursing interventions; and (3) nursing outcomes.[10] ICNP data-based information is collected in two areas: nursing intervention statements and nursing diagnosis and outcome statements across the continuum of care.

Catalogs have been created in both areas and are meant to be used as reference tools to document care that reflects their practice. The tools are intended to be useful at the point of care and do not replace nursing clinical judgment and decision-making.[11–13] *Diagnosis and Patient Care Management* boxes that reflect related patient conditions are found throughout the book and are designated with the () icon. For example, see Box 22.7. Also see Appendix A Patient Care Management Plans.

It is essential that nurses are skillful in clinical reasoning and clinical judgment to address the complexities of health care. Traditionally, the educational approach for nurses has been promoting linear thinking and memorization of health care data such as physiologic values, symptomology, definitions of conditions, and lists of possible related disorders. This no longer meets the needs of nurses who need to quickly assimilate multiple data points to design the most evidence-based, accurate, and timely plan of care.

In addition to critical thinking skills, it requires organizational skills and analysis of the information and application of previously learned knowledge. Throughout this book is a *new feature that* succinctly summarizes the disorder and further organized into three distinct components: 1) clinical and diagnostic assessments, 2) cardinal signs, and 3) nursing interventions. This model facilitates the nurse to rather quickly integrate all of the relevant facts into one prominently highlighted summary of key data to create an action plan. For example, see Box 18.1.

BOX 1.3 Evidence-based Practice

Sampling of AACN Practice Alerts

- Manual Prone Positioning in Adults: Reducing the Risk of Harm Through Evidence-Based Practices (February 2023)
- Prevention of CAUTI in Adults (last reviewed April 2022)
- Obtaining Accurate Noninvasive Blood Pressure Measurement in Adults (last reviewed May 2021)
- PA/CVP Monitoring in Adults (last reviewed July 2021)
- Managing Alarms in Acute Care Across the Life Span: Electrocardiography and Pulse Oximetry (April 2018) (December 2018)
- Accurate Dysrhythmia Monitoring in Adults (updated May 2018)
- Ensuring Accurate S-T Segment Monitoring (updated May 2018)
- Prevention of Aspiration in Adults (updated May 2018)
- Managing Alarms in Acute Care Across the Life Span (April 2018)
- Assessing Pain in Critically Ill Adults (December 2018)

American Association of Critical-Care Nurses. Practice Alerts. AACN website. March 1, 2020. Accessed March 7, 2024.https://www.aacn.org/clinical-resources/practice-alerts

HOLISTIC CRITICAL CARE NURSING

Caring

The high technology-driven critical care environment is fast paced and directed toward monitoring and treating life-threatening changes in patients' conditions. For this reason, the priority for care is using technology and treatments necessary for maintaining stability in the physiologic functioning of the patient. Great emphasis is placed on technical skills and professional competence and responsiveness to critical emergencies.

In this fast-paced, highly technologic health care environment, there is concern that diminished emphasis on the caring component of nursing may occur. Nowhere is this more evident than in areas in which critical care nursing is practiced. Keeping the *care* in nursing care is one of our biggest challenges.

The critical care nurse must be able to deliver high-quality care skillfully, using all appropriate technologies, while incorporating psychosocial and other holistic approaches as appropriate to the patient and his or her condition.

The caring aspect between nurses and patients is most fundamental to the relationship and to the health care experience. Non-caring is indicated by physical and emotional absence, inhumane and belittling interactions, and lack of recognition of the patient's uniqueness. Holistic care focuses on human integrity and stresses that the body, the mind, and the spirit are interdependent and inseparable. All aspects need to be considered in planning and delivering care.

Patient-Centered Care

The differences between nurses' and patients' perceptions of caring point to the importance of establishing individualized care that recognizes the uniqueness of each patient's preferences, condition, and physiologic and psychosocial status. It is clearly understood by care providers that a patient's physical condition progresses in predictable stages, depending on the presence or absence of comorbid condition

What is not understood as distinctly is the effect of psychosocial issues on the healing process. For this reason, special consideration must be given to determining the unique interventions that can positively affect each person and help the patient progress toward the desired outcomes.

An important aspect in the care delivery to and recovery of critically ill patients is the personal support of family members and significant others. The value of patient-centered and family-centered care should not be underestimated. It is important for families to be included in care decisions and to be encouraged to participate in the care of the patient as appropriate to the patient's personal needs and physiologic stability. This important aspect is represented in the Patient-Centered Critical Care boxes throughout the book.

PATIENT-CENTERED CRITICAL CARE

Creating a Calm Environment in Critical Care

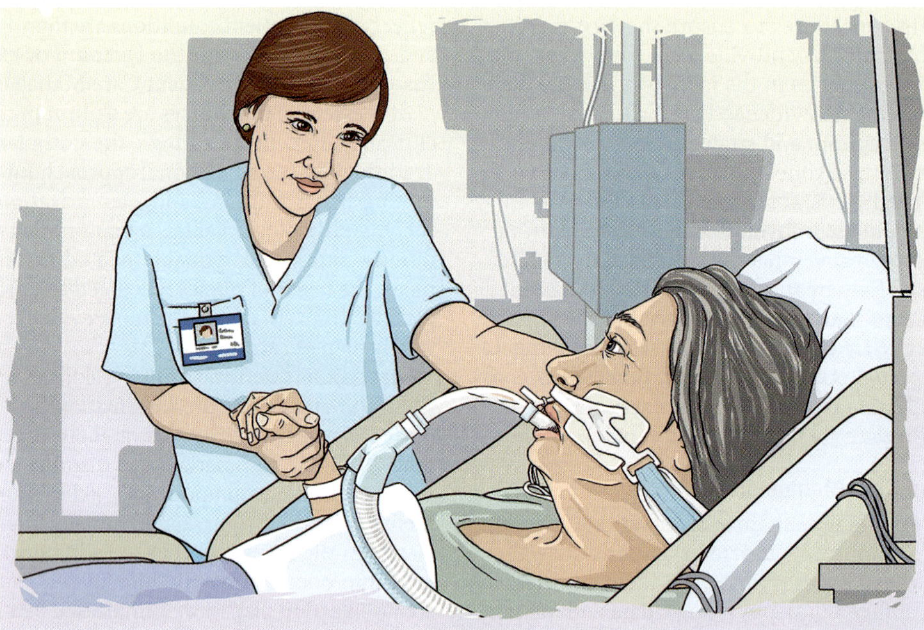

The critical care unit is a stressful environment for patients and for their family members—with the understanding that family is whomever the patient designates to be at their bedside. The critical care unit is also stressful because of the number of alarms, 24/7 routines, unfamiliar environment, and often an uncertain prognosis.

Amid a multitude of clinical tasks, nurses create a connection with their patients by explaining what is happening, preserving patient dignity, holding a hand when needed, and providing exceptional care.

The critical care unit can be frightening for patients and families. It may be the first time that they have experienced such a complex and fast-paced care setting, with unfamiliar noises, strange smells, and multiple machines, each with its own alarm. Many clinicians quickly come and go, using unfamiliar terms as they speak with each other and with patients and families.

All of this is confusing and overwhelming for patients and families who may perceive that they are a bother to the clinicians and do not ask questions or seek clarifications. It is incumbent on health care professionals to ensure that these issues be minimized and that patients and families are well informed and feel safe and included in all aspects required decisions about their treatments and care. Humanizing the critical care unit is an imperative.

The culture of adult critical care units is changing to become more patient centered and family focused. Older hospitals and critical care units were built to be convenient for the nurses, doctors, and other health care staff. Modern critical care units have spaces for family members and families to be present at the hospital without a schedule, sometimes called *open visiting.*

In many hospitals, a family member is encouraged to sleep in a family area in the patient's room and to attend morning rounds. Many innovations are being used to help patients recover, including use of patient diaries, pet therapy, and music. Early mobility means patients are out of bed more quickly even if still on a ventilator.

Much greater emphasis is placed on communication with the patient and family about prognosis, either at the bedside or in a conference room. Communication builds trust and knowledge. When possible, the patient and family are included in the bedside report and in hand-off between units. For health care professionals there is also more emphasis on effective communication and on professionals working as a team, whether at bedside rounds or debriefing after a code.

Cultural Care

The increasing diversity of the nation brings opportunities and challenges for health care providers, systems, and policy makers to deliver culturally competent services. Cultural competence is defined as "the ability of providers and organizations to effectively deliver health care services that meet the social, cultural, and linguistic needs of the patients."[14]

A culturally competent health care system can help improve health care outcomes and quality of care and can contribute to the elimination of racial and health disparities. Racial and ethnic minorities have higher morbidity and mortality from chronic diseases. These people do not have a regular doctor and are less likely to seek preventative health services or management of chronic conditions. Language and communication barriers are problematic for them, and there are lower levels of literacy. Lack of cultural competence may lead to patient dissatisfaction.

This is not new in health care, but it is gaining emphasis and importance as the world becomes more accessible to all as the result of increasing technologies and interfaces with places and peoples.

Diversity includes not only ethnic sensitivity but also sensitivity and openness to differences in lifestyles, opinions, values, and beliefs. Significant differences exist among the cultural beliefs and practices of racial and ethnic minority groups and the level of their acculturation into mainstream American culture.

Cultural competence is one way to ensure that individual differences related to culture are incorporated into the plan of care. Nurses must possess knowledge about biocultural, psychosocial, and linguistic differences in diverse populations to make accurate assessments. Interventions must be tailored to the uniqueness of each patient and family. See Box 1.4 for nursing practice cultural and linguistic competencies.[15]

COMPLEMENTARY AND ALTERNATIVE THERAPIES

The two terms *alternative* and *complementary* have been in the mainstream for several years. *Alternative* therapy denotes that a specific therapy is an option or alternative to what is considered conventional treatment of a condition or state. The term *complementary* was proposed to describe therapies that can be used to complement or support conventional treatments.

Acknowledging the rise in complementary health practitioners, the AACN has published thoughtful guidelines for consideration by the critical care nurse when implementing complementary therapies in the critical care patient care areas.[16,17]

This section includes a brief discussion about nontraditional complementary therapies that are used in critical care areas.

Mindfulness

Mindfulness is a newer technique that has gained popularity due to its ability to be practiced in a myriad of settings, with no financial outlay or special equipment, etc. Interest in it has increased exponentially over the past three decades. It is a process of "openly attending, with one's awareness, to one's experience in the present moment,"[18] contrary to the regular day experiences in which our minds wander to various topics and thoughts.

Randomized controlled studies have reported positive impact on stress, depression, chronic pain, anxiety, and addiction. Using the technique, is a time when one focuses on sensations, mental images, emotions, perceptual experiences, mental talk. It is also a time when one can be open and be curious, detached, and inviting and newness.[18]

Although this may or may not be something that can actually be practiced in the ICU, it may be introduced to family members and patients, with resources to have upon transfer on discharge home for a later time. It may also be something that patients already use and can incorporate it into their ICU routine while in the unit with nursing support.

The remaining techniques to be discussed are more "assistive," or "hands-on," in nature with nurse or family member, etc.

Massage

Back massage, previously practiced as part of routine care of patients, has been eliminated for various reasons, including time constraints, greater use of technology, and increasing complexity of care requirements. However, there is a scientific basis for concluding that massage offers positive effects on physiologic and psychologic outcomes, even if minimal.

A review of the literature revealed that the most common effect of massage was reduction in chronic low back pain. There was also a short-term positive effect on short-term neck and shoulder pain. Only a small number of studies have looked at massage for headache and results have not been consistent.[19]

Even though research has not clearly demonstrated significant positive findings regarding massage, it would appear that patient comfort and pain relief—no matter how small—could be a marker and satisfier to indicate that massage could be a nursing intervention to patients who desire a massage.

Animal-Assisted Intervention

Animal-assisted intervention (AAI) is a relatively new term but the practice was actually established over 100 years ago in Belgium. AAI is defined as a "goal-oriented and structured process that intentionally comprises animal-human interactions to provide therapeutic advantages to humans."[20] Research has demonstrated positive outcomes with interactions of animals and geriatric population in the areas of positive social behaviors, reduced mood disturbances, increased weight gain, and agitation.[20,21] Additionally, strong satisfaction for the program was reported by the patient, family members, and clinicians.[21]

In critical care, working with an animal can remove the sense of isolation and instill a reality; exercise with specific ROM activities; increase attention span; and reduce stress, pain, fatigue, and anxiety. It also appears to provide an increased energy for recovery from their illness or surgery.[20,21]

BOX 1.4 Cultural and Linguistic Competencies

International Council of Nurses, Reviewed and Revised 2013

- Developing an awareness of one's own culture without letting it have an undue influence on those from other backgrounds
- Demonstrating knowledge and understanding of different cultures
- Accepting that there may be differences between the cultural beliefs and values of the health care provider and the client
- Accepting and respecting cultural differences to be congruent with the client's culture and expectations
- Providing culturally appropriate care so as to deliver the best possible client outcomes
- Adapting care to be congruent with the client's culture and expectations

https://icn.ch/sites/default/files/2013-4/B03_Cultural_Linguistic_Competence.pdf

The use of animals has increased as an adjunct to healing in the care of patients of all ages in various settings. Pet visitation programs have been created in various health care delivery settings, including acute care, long-term care, and hospice. In the acute care setting, animals are brought in to provide additional solace and comfort for patients who are critically or terminally ill.

Fish aquariums are used in patient areas and family areas because they humanize the surroundings. Scientific evidence indicates that animal-assisted therapy results in positive patient outcomes in the areas of attention, mobility, and orientation. Other reports have shown improved communication and mood in patients.

Music Therapy

According to the American Music Therapy Association (AMTA), music therapy is the "clinical and evidence-based use of music interventions to accomplish individualized goals within a therapeutic relationship by a credentialed professional."[22] Music therapy interventions can address a variety of health care and educational goals and many benefit physical, emotional, cognitive, and social needs. It is administered by a credentialed professional who has completed an approved music therapy program. It includes creating, singing, and moving and/or listening to music.

According to the AMTA, research has demonstrated music therapy effectiveness using music therapy in communication, overall physical rehabilitation, movement, motivation, support for patients and families, and an outlet for expression of feelings. The AMTA reports that the research base in music is growing stronger.

One study reported significant decreases in respiratory rate, heart rate, and self-reported anxiety and pain.[23] A recent study published in 2023 by Golino and colleagues described that live music therapy significantly reduced agitation and heart rate in adult patients receiving mechanical ventilation.[24] Offering music to a patient or family member is a low-tech intervention that may be beneficial in decreasing pain, anxiety, blocking the noise, and "passing the time" in the ICU setting for patients. It is truly a nursing intervention and one that can be easy to implement.

TECHNOLOGY IN CRITICAL CARE

Growth in technologies has been seen throughout health care, especially in critical care settings. All providers are challenged to learn new equipment, monitoring devices, and related therapies that contribute to care and services.[25] Technology can automate existing processes such as transitioning from manual procedures to electronic pumps to deliver intravenous fluids.

Technology can also augment or add value to the work.

An example of augmentation is the evolving electronic health record (EHR) that was originally designed to capture data for clinical decision making and to increase the efficiency of health care providers. There are complexities inherent in providing a "user-friendly" EHR.[26]

A tremendous amount of data can be translated into meaningful information with which to make decisions. For this reason, it is important that critical care nurses are involved in the selection, trial, education, and evaluation of any health care informatics technologies that are being considered for their practice areas. Nurse informaticists, CNSs, NPs, specialty nurses, educators, and managers are also essential in the selection processes so that all aspects are considered.[27]

New Technologies and Products

One area for involvement of critical care nurses is in assessing new technologies and products that come into the system. There are often numerous avenues through which products enter, such as product fairs, individual physicians, vendors, and supply departments. It is important that all proposed new products are overseen by a central committee or group that establishes criteria by which to select, pilot, evaluate, adopt, and communicate about the new product.[26]

Criteria that can be used in the initial assessment of proposed products include:

1. clinical relevance
2. integration with existing supplies and equipment
3. cost
4. scope of adoption
5. required education for the changeover (if a replacement), and
6. safety

This type of process ensures consistency and the same standards regarding product selection across the organization.

Tele-ICU

A more recent opportunity for critical care nurses is working in a role that encompasses the Tele-ICU. Tele-ICU is defined as "a collaborative interprofessional care model focused on critically ill patients that is enabled by leveraging audio, video, data and other technologies to engage critical care experts in patient care, along with clinicians at collaborating sites. Services may be expanded to include other acute and progressive care patients."[28]

Telemedicine was initially employed in outpatient areas, remote rural geographic locations, and areas where there was a dearth of medical providers. At the present time, Tele-ICUs are used in areas when there are limited resources on site. Experts (critical care nurses, critical care CNSs, NPs, and critical care physician intensivists, among others) are in a central distant site. Technologies relay continuous surveillance with monitoring information and communication among care providers. Each Tele-ICU varies in size and geographic setting as well as location within the hospital. A key component of each is the availability of back-up experts for the local medical providers.

Practice Work Environment Standards are used as the basis for nursing practice (see discussion later in this chapter). Critical care nurses use artificial intelligence (AI) to enhance monitoring, improve clinical decision-making, and establish their plan of care for the patients. However, it is also crucial that they use their expertise and knowledge to detect potential errors prior to implementing an incorrect order.[29]

Williams and colleagues reported research findings in which Tele-ICU nurses' intentional use of advanced technology, rather than the technology itself, supports and enhances proactive Tele-ICU practice to prevent failure to rescue.[30] Although there were limitations in this study—small number of subjects and not generalizable outside of the specialty unit—it does have interesting findings.

Teamwork and organization across all geographic settings are essential and add complexity to the Tele-ICU care model.[30] AACN has promulgated *TeleICU Nursing Practice Recommendations* that are organized into essential elements for (1) Tele-ICU nurses, (2) TeleICU nurse leaders, (3) TeleICU nurses and nurse leaders, and (4) TeleICU health care organizations.[30]

The AACN *Healthy Work Environment* (HWE) model is used as the basis for nursing practice for Tele-ICU nursing practice (refer to later in this chapter for an in-depth discussion of the HWE.

INTERPROFESSIONAL COLLABORATIVE PRACTICE

It is more important than ever to create and enhance partnerships, because the resulting interdependence and collaboration among disciplines is essential to achieving positive patient outcomes.

Interprofessional Collaborative Practice

The Interprofessional Education Collaborative (IPEC) updated the *Core Competencies for Interprofessional Collaborative Practice* in 2023. IPEC sponsors included associations of nursing, dentistry, medicine, osteopathy, public health, and pharmacy. Their goal was to establish a set of competencies to serve as a framework for professional socialization of health care professionals. They also intended to assess the relevance of the competencies and develop an action plan for implementation.[31]

These competencies are especially important at the present time as we move forward with health care refinancing, quality initiatives, and explore innovative care delivery models using the skill sets of all health care providers in the most effective and efficient manner. Box 1.5 delineates the four interprofessional collaborative core competencies.

Schwab and colleagues reported that a rapid in-person multidisciplinary mortality review in the ICU, conducted weekly, identified deaths that were preventable. The intent was to learn from the quality improvement project so that interventions could be used in the future. They found that even though the death rates and preventable outcomes were low in number, they did learn from the reviews, which lead to systemic changes and better outcomes in future patient.[32]

In a more resent study, Pun et al.[33] studied interprofessional team collaboration and work environment health in 68 U.S. ICUs. Teamwork and work environment were rated positively, with the highest score being "partnership/shared decision-making." However, scores differed among the team: rehab therapists, pharmacists, RNs, and RTs were lower than physicians.

Work environment health and teamwork were rated by all as good but not excellent. The authors concluded that care coordination and meaningful recognition can be improved.[33] It appears that teamwork and collaboration is a complex and multifactorial complex and one that needs to be studied within a systems framework that will capture all of the features of such an intricate concept. One special type of collaborative team is described in the next section.

Rapid Response Teams (RRTs)

RRTs were created to address deteriorating patients in noncritical care areas of the hospital who were not surrounded by resources to handle direct emergency situations. Set criteria were established that nurses caring for those patients who met the criteria could "call" an RRT and a team would respond immediately to the patient and resolve the situation with standing protocol to avoid a more critical situation, or stabilize the patient for transfer into the ICU. The intent is to quickly respond to the medical condition and stabilize to avoid greater deterioration. See Box 1.6 for further details.

Interdisciplinary Care Management Models and Tools

Several models of care delivery and care management are used in health care. An overview of the various terms and models is presented in this chapter, but readers are encouraged to seek additional resources and consultation for a more in-depth explanation of the models.

Care Management

Care management is a system of integrated processes designed to enable, support, and coordinate patient care throughout the continuum of health care services. Care management takes place in many different settings; care is delivered by various professional health care team members and nonlicensed providers, as appropriate.

BOX 1.5 Core Competencies for Interprofessional Collaborative Practice

There are four main competency areas:

Values and Ethics: Work with team members to maintain a climate of shared values, ethical conduct, and mutual respect.

Roles and Responsibilities: Use the knowledge of one's own role and team members' expertise to address individual and population health outcomes.

Communication: Communicate in a responsive, responsible, respectful, and compassionate manner with team members.

Teams and Teamwork: Apply values and principles of the science of teamwork to adapt one's own role in a variety of team settings.

Coordination of care and services may be done by the health care staff or the insurance or payer staff. Care management must be patient focused, continuum driven, and results oriented, and it must employ a team approach. Another term associated with this model of care is *disease state management*, which connotes the process of managing a population's health over a lifetime. However, in disease state management, there is a focus on managing complex and chronic disease states such as diabetes or heart failure over the entire continuum.

Case Management

Case management is the process of overseeing the care of patients and organizing services in collaboration with the patient's physician or primary health care provider. The case manager may be a nurse, allied health care provider, or primary care provider.

Case managers may be assigned to a specific population group (e.g., cardiovascular surgery, orthopedic, cancer, geriatric) and facilitate effective coordination of care services as patients move in and out of different settings. Ideally, the case manager oversees the care of the patient across the continuum of care.

Care Management Tools

Many quality improvement tools are available to providers for care management. The three evidence-based tools addressed in this chapter are clinical algorithm, practice guideline, and protocol. All these tools may be embedded in the EHR.

Algorithm

An *algorithm* is a stepwise decision-making flowchart for a specific care process or processes. Algorithms guide the clinician through the "if, then" decision-making process, addressing patient responses to particular treatments. Well-known examples of algorithms are the advanced cardiac life support algorithms published by the American Heart Association. Weaning, medication selection, medication titration, individual practitioner variance, and appropriate patient placement algorithms have been developed to give practitioners additional standardized decision-making abilities.

Practice Guideline

A *practice guideline* is usually created by an expert panel and developed by a professional organization (e.g., AACN, SCCM, *American College of Cardiology*, and government agencies such as the *Agency for Health Care Research and Quality*). Practice guidelines are generally written in text prose style rather than in the flowchart format of algorithms.

For example, SCCM appointed an international committee to establish *Guidelines for the Management of Sepsis and Septic Shock* (2021). They recommended future research and development of tools to translate research findings into practice.[34] Another interdisciplinary team was convened by SCCM to create the *Clinical Practice Guidelines for the Rapid Sequence Intubation in the Critically Ill Adult Patient*.[35]

A *protocol* is a common tool in research studies. Protocols are more directive and rigid than guidelines, and providers are not supposed to vary from a protocol. Patients are screened carefully for specific entry criteria before being started on a protocol. There are many national research protocols, such as for cancer and chemotherapy studies.

Protocols are helpful when built-in alerts signal the provider to potentially serious problems. Computerization of protocols assists providers in being more proactive regarding dangerous medication interactions, abnormal laboratory values, and other untoward effects that are preprogrammed into the computer.

Order Set

An *order set* consists of preprinted provider orders that are used to expedite the order process after a standard has been validated through analytic review of practice and research. Order sets complement and increase compliance with existing practice standards. They can also be used to represent an algorithm or protocol in order format.

Managing and Tracking Outcome Variances

The EHR provides a repository in which data can be collected consistently and accurately for tracking patient care outcomes. All variances must be addressed and managed in a timely manner by the health care team members. All the previously described tools provide methods to track variances. Whether variance coding is included in the EHR or is tracked by another quality improvement method, individual and aggregate data must be assessed and analyzed. This provides excellent data by which to identify systems issues and to make revisions in procedures and care management.

Except for protocols, which are more rigid and research based, algorithms and guidelines can be used according to the practitioner's discretion. Tracking variances from the expected standard is one method to determine the utility of the tools in particular settings and patient populations. There must be a link between the care management system and the quality improvement program so that changes can be made as appropriate to positively affect the outcomes of care and services.

QUALITY, SAFETY, AND REGULATORY ISSUES IN CRITICAL CARE

Quality and Safety Issues

Patient safety has become a major focus of attention by health care consumers, providers of care, and administrators of health care institutions. The definitions of medical errors and approaches to resolving patient safety issues often differ among nurses, physicians, administrators, and other health care providers. Subsequently through its use of expert panels, the *Institute of Medicine* (IOM) has published numerous other important reports related to quality, safety, and the nursing environment.

In the critical care environment, patients are particularly vulnerable because of their compromised physiologic status, multiple technologic and pharmacologic interventions, and multiple care providers who frequently work at a fast pace. Medication administration is one of the most error-prone nursing interventions for critical care nurses.

BOX 1.6 Safety

Rapid Response Team (RRT)

Inpatients often show signs of clinical deterioration for several hours prior to arrest, and more than 20,000 annual cases of in-hospital arrest could be prevented if clinical deterioration can be detected early on.[1–3]

It is critical that nurses play an integral part in the identification and intervention should clinical deterioration arise

Early identification of deterioration can trigger appropriate management, thereby reducing the need for higher acuity care, reducing length of hospitalization and admission costs, thus improving survival.[4]

The RRT is composed of a multidisciplinary team that extends critical care services throughout the hospital in the noncritical care setting.[3–11]

The most common model of the RRT is a critical care nurse–led model, with some models including physicians, respiratory therapists[12] and advanced practice providers such as nurse practitioners[13] and CNSs.

Research has demonstrated that RRTs have decreased overall mortality, length of stay, and unnecessary transfer to the critical care unit.[14]

Many RRTs have emergency standing orders or protocols, so it is important to understand the level of intervention they can provide.

Examples of standing orders that RRTs can initiate include establishing emergent intravenous access, administration of medications such as naloxone for oversedation, and even lab and diagnostic orders such as electrolytes, arterial blood gases, chest x-ray, and electrocardiograms.[15]

RRTs are capable of providing critical care without boundaries, and some models even support following up on patients discharged from the critical care unit, proactively evaluate high-risk patients, and provide education and act as a liaison between the primary nurse and multidisciplinary teams.[16]

The role of the primary nurse during RRT activation is very crucial. The primary nurse knows a wealth of information about the patient, including diagnosis, treatments, physiologic status, and rationale (trigger) for calling the RRT.

References

1. Smith GB, Prytherch DR, Schmidt P, et al. Hospital-wide physiological surveillance: A new approach to the early identification and management of the sick patient. *Resuscitation*. 2006;71(1):19–28.
2. Beaumont K, Luettel D, Thomson R. Deterioration in hospital patients: early signs and appropriate actions. *Nurs Stand*. 2008;23(1):43–48.
3. Padilla RM, Urden LD, Stacy KM. Nurses' perceptions of barriers to rapid response system activation: A systematic review. *Dimens Crit Care Nurs*. 2018;37(5):259–271.
4. Vincent JL, et al. Improving detection of patient deterioration in the general hospital war environment. *Eur J Anaesthesiol*. 2018;35(5):325–333. https://doi.org/10.1097/EJA.0000000000000798.
5. Stolldorf DP, Jones CB. Deployment of rapid response teams by 31 hospitals in a statewide collaborative. *Jt Comm J Qual Patient Saf*. 2015;41(4):186–191. https://doi.org/10.1016/s1553-7250(15)41024-4.
6. Kohn LT, Corrigan J, Donaldson MS. *To Err Is Human: Building a Safer Health System*. Washington, DC: National Academy Press; 2000.
7. Institute of Medicine. *Crossing the Quality Chasm: a New Health System for the 21st Century*. Washington, DC: National Academy Press; 2001.
8. Berwick DM, Calkins DR, McCannon CJ, et al. The 100,000 Lives Campaign: setting a goal and a deadline for improving health care quality. *JAMA*. 2006;295(3):324–327. https://doi.org/10.1001/jama.295.3.324.
9. Society for Rapid Response Systems. About Rapid Response Systems: Making Hospitals Safer. <https://rapidresponsesystems.org/?page_id=1074>; Accessed January 2020.
10. Agency for Healthcare Research and Quality. Rapid Response Systems. <https://psnet.ahrq.gov/primer/rapid-response-systems>; Accessed January 2020.
13. Morse KJ, Warshawsky D, Moore JM, et al. A new role for the ACNP: the rapid response team leader. *Crit Care Nurs Q*. 2006;29(2):137–146.
12. Jenkins SD, Lindsey PL. Clinical nurse specialists as leaders in rapid response. *Clin Nurse Spec: J Adv Nurs Pract*. 2010;24(1):24–30. https://doi.org/10.1097/NUR.0b013e3181c4abe9.
13. DeVita MA, Bellomo R, Hillman K. Findings of the first consensus conference on medical emergency teams. *Crit Care Med*. 2006;34(9):2463–2478.
14. Bellomo R, Goldsmith D, Uchino S, et al. Prospective controlled trial of effect of medical emergency team on postoperative morbidity and mortality rates. *Crit Care Med*. 2004;32(4):916–921.
15. Institute for Clinical Systems Improvement. Rapid Response Team Sample Order Set. <http://www.ihi.org/resources/Pages/Tools/RapidResponseTeamSampleOrderSet.aspx>; Accessed February 2020.
16. Good VS, Kirkwood PL. *Advanced Critical Care Nursing. Unit 1: The Evolving Critical Care Environment*. 2nd ed. St Louis: Elsevier; 2017.

The hectic, fast-paced environment where unplanned events are the norm can lead to medication errors. Many medication errors are related to system failures, with distraction as a major factor. Various interventions have been created to decrease medication errors. When an injury or inappropriate care occurs, it is crucial that health care professionals promptly explain how the injury or mistake occurred and the short-term or long-term effects on the patient and family.

The patient and family should be informed that the factors involved in the injury will be investigated so that steps can be taken to reduce or prevent the likelihood of similar injury to other patients.

It has been shown that intimidating and disruptive clinician behaviors can lead to errors and preventable adverse patient outcomes.

These behaviors include verbal outbursts, physical threats, and more passive behaviors such as refusing to carry out a task or procedure. These types of expressions are not rare in health care organizations.

Hawkins and Morse[36] recently reported finding from their ethnographic secondary analysis and revealed three interesting themes of practice of nursing work. The first was "chasing a standard of care" in which the nurses were attempting to meet both internal and external standards, but never quite achieved the desired changes. There were forced reorganization and shifting priorities, exhibited by med schedules and patient turnover, thus needing to prioritize meds and renegotiate routines.

The second these was "prioritizing practice" that was characterized with patient turnover, admissions, and meds—again. The third category was "re-negotiating routines" that was related to prerequisites of care, provision of care, and provision of care.

Adding all of these up, no wonder the result is many times stress, cognitive overload, and a perceived indifference surrounding medication safety. The study authors stated that the "rich description identified characteristics of the nurses' work as cyclical, chaotic, and complex shattering studies that explained nurses' work as linear."[36]

If these behaviors go unaddressed, it can lead to extreme dissatisfaction, depression, and turnover. There also may be systems issues that lead to or perpetuate these situations, such as push for increased productivity, financial constraints, fear of litigation, and embedded hierarchies in the organization.

Technologies are both a solution to error-prone procedures and functions and another potential cause for error. Consider barcode medication administration procedures, multiple bedside testing devices, computerized medical records, bedside monitoring, computerized physician order entry, and many other technologies now in development. Each can be a great assistance to the clinician, but each must be monitored for effectiveness and accuracy to ensure the best in outcomes as intended for specific use

Quality and Safety Regulations

There are numerous regulations governing health care, including local, state, national, Medicare/Medicaid, and payer requirements. In this chapter, key regulations and accreditation standards affecting most critical care areas are discussed.

The Joint Commission (TJC) is an independent, not-for-profit organization that certifies more than 19,000 health care organizations in the United States. Its goal is to evaluate these health care entities using their preestablished standards of performance to ensure that high levels of care are provided in these entities. It establishes *National Patient Safety Goals* (NPSGs) annually[37] that are to be implemented in health care organizations (Box 1.7).

TJC has also mandated a "Do Not Use" List. This list consists of abbreviations that may be confused with other similar ones. For example, do not use "U" or "u" for unit; instead, write out "unit." Another example is do not use "IU"; instead write out "International Unit." Refer to TJC for a complete "Do Not Use" List.[38]

BOX 1.7 Joint Commission 2023 Hospital National Patient Safety Goals

- Use medications safely
- Use alarms safely
- Prevent infection
- Improve health care
- Identify patient safety risk
- Use medications safely
- Prevent mistakes in surgery
- Use alarms safely
- Prevent infection
- Identify patient safety risk

https://www.jointcommission.org/-/media/thj/documents/standards/national-patient-safety-goals/2023/hop-npsg-simplified-2023-july.pdf

The Safe Medical Devices Act requires that hospitals report serious or potentially serious device-related injuries or illness of patients or employees to the manufacturer of the device and to the *U.S. Food and Drug Administration* (FDA) if a death has occurred. In addition, implantable devices must be documented and tracked. This reporting serves as an early warning system so that the FDA can obtain information on device problems. Failure to comply with the act results in civil action.[39]

The FDA requires that a drug company place a boxed warning on the labeling of a prescription drug or in literature describing it. This boxed warning (also known as a "*black box warning*") signifies that medical studies indicate that the drug carries a significant risk of serious or life-threatening adverse effects.[40] Examples include warfarin, celecoxib (Celebrex), rosiglitazone (Avandia), and ciprofloxacin (Cipro). Alerts are published as soon as a drug is found to meet the criteria. Providers are to use caution when prescribing the medications and to consider alternative medications that have fewer adverse effects.

Quality and Safety Resources

The Institute for Safe Medication Practices (ISMP) is a not-for-profit organization dedicated to medication error prevention and safe medication use. It has numerous tools to assist care providers, including newsletters, education programs, safety alerts, consulting, patient education materials, and error-reporting systems. One newsletter is devoted specifically to nurses. It offers a very comprehensive array of tools.[41]

The Institute for Healthcare Improvement (IHI) is an interdisciplinary organization focused on quality that also offers many tools and resources, including educational materials, conferences, case studies, publications, white papers, and quality measure tools. IHI developed the "bundle" concept, which consists of EBPs on specific high-risk quality issues as determined by a multidisciplinary group. IHI publishes many bundles, such as central line, ventilator, and sepsis bundles.[42] The *National Quality Forum* (NQF) is another not-for-profit organization that facilitates consensus building with multiple partners to establish national priorities and goals for performance improvement. They also establish common definitions and consistent measurement. In addition, their goal is that all health care providers and stakeholders are educated regarding quality, priorities, and outcomes.[43]

The *Healthcare Information and Management Systems Society* (HIMSS) is an interdisciplinary organization focused on patient safety and quality of care. This organization specifically focuses on integration of patient safety tools and practices to enhance communication, quality, efficiency, productivity, and clinical support systems.

CHALLENGES FACING NURSES

In 2023, registered nurses were ranked the most honest and ethical professional for the 21st year, among a group of physicians, pharmacists, and high school teachers. The second highest-rated profession was physicians, rated 17% behind nurses.[45] Since the COVID pandemic, nursing has been more in the limelight with a much greater understanding of exactly what nursing entails, the difficulties, the stresses, the ongoing education that is required, and the family and social commitments that are missed due to career requirements. These next sections will discuss challenges and opportunities for nurses as we move forward with our various careers.

Compassion Fatigue

When a person is physically, emotionally, and spiritually exhausted from caring for others, they cannot bring their best to patients and the rest of the health care team. In varying degrees, it impacts everyone who cares for people who are suffering or who have experienced trauma. According to Vaughn, nurses who experience compassion fatigue find little to no pleasure in their work and often struggle to get through their day. It can directly compromise their job performance.[46] Causes for this vary, but include stress, sustained exposure to traumatic work events, emotional and physical job demands, and lack of control over work environment.[47] See Box 1.8 for symptoms of compassion fatigue.

To avoid the extremes of either becoming overly involved in patients' suffering or detaching from them, nurses can use self-care activities to maintain balance. Nurses are encouraged to use *self-reflection* when feeling overwhelmed and consider the source of their feelings. There are often multiple causes for feeling overwhelmed, such as sadness about a particular patient, overwork, lateral hostility at work, and disruptions in one's personal life.

Reflection is an important first step, because without awareness, it is difficult to identify possible solutions. Talking with friends, a spiritual care provider, or a close colleague can help the nurse recognize grief and reflect on the meaning of work. Mindfulness is another technique (described earlier in this chapter for patients) that can also be used by nurses.

Monitor Alert and Alarm Fatigue

Alarm fatigue occurs when busy nurses are exposed to numerous frequent safety alerts and become desensitized as the result of listening to them. This desensitization can lead to longer response times or to missing important alarms. Physiological alarms are the most frequent device alarm used to monitor patient status in the hospital setting. The cause of "overexuberant" alerts and alarms is multifactorial and therefore most challenging to resolve.[48]

Incivility

It seems contra-intuitive that nursing—a caring, compassion, and empathetic profession— would have incivility and bullying behaviors among its members. Unfortunately, however, they do exist. According to the American Nurses Association (ANA), *incivility* can take the form of rude and discourteous actions, of gossiping and spreading rumors, and of refusing to assist a co-worker. All of those impact the dignity of the co-worker and violate professional standards of respect. Also included may be name-calling, expressing public criticism, and using a condescending tone to the co-worker.[49]

Bullying

Bullying is characterized by repeated, unwanted, harmful actions intended to humiliate, offend, and cause distress to the recipient. These actions harm, undermine, and degrade the other person and occur with greater frequency and intensity than those incivility actions. These actions may include hostile remarks, threats, verbal attacks, taunts, intimidation, and withholding of support.[49]

BOX 1.8 Compassion Fatigue Symptoms

Physical
- Exhaustion
- Fatigue
- Headaches
- Muscle aches and pains

Mental of Emotional
- Anxiety
- Apathy
- Depression
- Forgetfulness

Workplace Performance
- Depersonalization or lack of connection to patients
- Difficulty concentrations
- Increased errors or impaired work performance
- Lack of empathy towards patients

From Loera S, Howell M, Mulligan P, Busch D. Prevent compassion fatigue through self-compassion. *Amer Nurs J.* 2022;17(9)28–31.

Workplace Violence (WPV)

The *National Institute for Occupational Safety and Health* (NIOSH) defines *WPV* as an act or threat ranging from verbal abuse to physical assault towards individuals at their place of work while on duty.[50] Of the four types of WPV, client-on-worker violence is the most common in healthcare settings, with nurses being at highest risk for WPV when compared to other healthcare professions.[51] "Client" includes the patient, their family, and their visitors.[50]

Other types of WPV are criminal intent, worker-on-worker, and personal relationship.[50]

One study was reported in the literature that examined the impact of workplace violence exposure on types of mental health of nurses. The finding showed that mental health issues increased with cumulative exposure and that they were two to three times more likely to report high levels of posttraumatic stress disorder (PTSD), anxiety, depression, and burnout compared to their counterparts with no exposure to violence.[52]

Kim and colleagues described findings of a study that improvement in hospital strategies aimed at patient safety culture, including team cohesion with handoffs and transitions, could positively influence a reduction in WPV and burnout among health care workers.[53,54]

Risk Factors for Client-on-Worker Violence

There are clinical, environmental, organizational, and socioeconomic risk factors for *client-on-WPV*.[50] Substance abuse, history of violence, cognitive impairment, and dissatisfaction with medical management (e.g., pain control) are some clinical risk factors for violence. The absence of visitor screening, reduced security presence, poor facility design, and unsecured furniture are some environmental risk factors for violence.

Reduced staffing, time-consuming reporting procedures, and relaxed policies on violence prevention are some organizational risk factors for violence. Neighborhood demographics (e.g., poverty, crime) are socioeconomic risk factors for violence.[50] The ANA has reported that bullying and incivility can adversely affect the quality of patient care and outcomes, contribute to the development of psychological conditions, and reduce the RN's level of job satisfaction and organizational commitment.[54] See Box 1.9, *ANA Statement on Incivility, Bullying, and Workplace Violence.*

SUPPORTING HEALTH AND EQUITY OF THE NATION

The Future of Nursing 2020-2030, Charting a Path to Achieve Health Equity was updated and published in 2021. As nurses represent the largest health care professionals to interact with people of all backgrounds, they live and work in a variety of settings in health, education, and communities.[55]

> *The report recommends that all relevant state, federal, and private organizations enable nurses to practice to the full extent of their education and training by removing practice barriers that prevent them from: more fully addressing social needs and social determinants of health: and by improving health care access, quality, and value.*

According to a consensus study report prepared by the National Academy of Medicine, the ultimate goal is "the achievement of health equity in the United States built on strengthened nursing capacity and expertise."[55] See Box 1.10 for the role of nurses in advancing health equity.

The report concludes that nurses are "bridge builders and collaborators who connect with people, communities and organizations to promote health and well-being."[55]

It also points to the recent pandemic as the impetus that has proven nursing's adeptness at being able to face significant new challenges and "sparked" overdue conversations regarding difficult topics, racism among them. The report ends with this crucial statement for the future of nursing: *"Policy makers and system leaders should seize this moment to support, strengthen, and transform the largest segment of the health care workforce so nurses can help chart our country's course to good health and well-being for all."*[55]

SUPPORTING THE WELL-BEING OF NURSES

One of the recommendations from the above-mentioned report was supporting the well-being of nurses. There are many models in the literature and those that have been promulgated by

SUPPORTING NURSE WELL-BEING

I was fortunate to be hired as a new graduate RN into the medical ICU where I have worked for three years. The unit was designated as an AACN Beacon unit last year and we are also a Magnet™ hospital. Thus, we have a great supportive environment that is well recognized as providing excellence in care by both other health care providers as well as our community. I learn something new every day during our intra-professional rounds and by either consultation or through formal educational offerings given by our clinical nurse specialist. However even with all of those opportunities, I felt a little bored and thought there was something missing. My friend talked about becoming AACN certified and asked me and three other nurses to consider joining her in this effort. After we gave it greater consideration and discovered more about the certification process, we decided to not only "go for it," but also take a prep course and study together. After all, there is safety in numbers and it will be easier for the three of us to keep each other motivated and on track. So, after this is accomplished, I will probably explore graduate study opportunities!

The above vignette shows how one person lost perspective on further growth and was "lost" in the status quo. After introspection and seeking out friends for new potential opportunities, the certification strategy opened up the mind to something new that could "jump-start" the intellectual process again. Intellectual wellness is an active quest of obtaining an optimal intellectual state. It is not how intelligent one is—which is the traditional way of thinking. Intellectual wellness recognizes abilities and finding ways to expand knowledge and skills. It includes being open as well as exposing oneself to new ideas, perspectives, people, and beliefs. In addition to personal and professional development, cultural involvement, community involvement, and personal hobbies can promote intellectual wellness. Creativity is also a key to intellectual wellness. Engaging in mentally stimulating activities may also reduce cognitive impairment and thus lower the risk of dementia and Alzheimer disease.

Consider the following to maintain intellectual wellness:

- Seek out educational opportunities for professional growth: certification; clinical inservices; academic advancement; journal CEU offerings
- Actively participate in your professional organizations
- Travel—near or far; take short trips in your own community to places you have never been before; participate in a travel medical trip; take a cruise, train ride
- Visit local museums—of all kinds
- Attend a play, opera, or ballet
- Play mind-stimulating games: crossword puzzles, Sudoku, Risk, Clue, etc.
- Participate in community activities; try something new: cooking class; exercise group; book club; hiking group; community-organized trip
- Read—anything; seek out a new genre to expand your knowledge base
- Volunteer—you will be very welcome
- Learn a new language
- Paint, needlepoint, scrapbook, garden, take up photography; try a musical instrument
- Watch documentaries, both of your interest and something for which you know nothing
- Take classes on topics you know nothing about

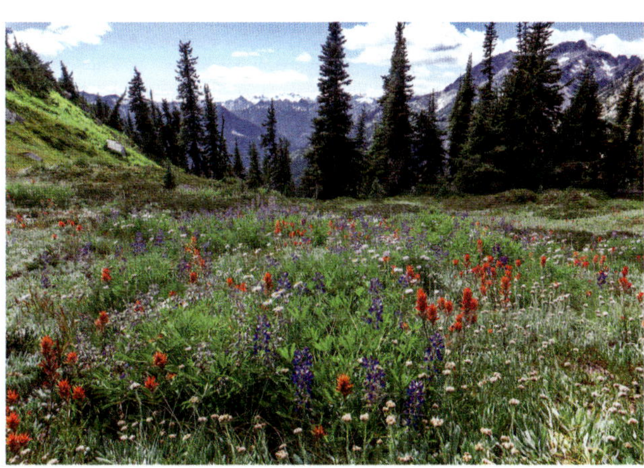

Every now and then one's mind is stretched by a new idea or sensation, and never shrinks back to its former dimensions...
Oliver Wendell Holmes, Sr.

BOX 1.9 ANA Statement on Civility, Bullying and Workplace Violence

Recommendations for Registered Nurses (RNs): Incivility and Bullying

- RNs must make a commitment to—and accept responsibility for—establishing and promoting healthy interpersonal relationships with one another and with all members of the health care team.
- RNs must be cognizant of their own interactions, including actions taken and not taken and communication with others.
- RNs should establish an agreed-upon code word or signal to seek support when feeling threatened.
- Use clear communication verbally, nonverbally, and in writing (including social media).
- Treat others with respect, dignity, collegiality, and kindness.
- Consider how personal words and actions affect others.
- Avoid gossip and spreading rumors; rely on facts and not conjecture.
- Collaborate and share information where appropriate.
- Offer assistance when needed, and, if refused, accept refusal gracefully.
- Take responsibility or be accountable for one's own actions.
- Recognize that abuse of power or authority is never acceptable.
- Speak directly to the person with whom one has an issue.
- Demonstrate openness to other points of view, perspectives, experiences, and ideas.
- Be polite and respectful, and apologize when indicated.
- Encourage, support, and mentor others, including new nurses and experienced nurses.
- Listen to others with interest and respect.

Recommendations for Nurses: Workplace Violence

- Understand the importance of using situational awareness to identify the potential for violence before it occurs.
- For example, question the presence and purpose of all unknown individuals in the work environment.
- Learn the importance of paying attention to one's surroundings and of being vigilant in unfamiliar surroundings. Learn how to assess the work environment and individuals within it for potential threat or danger. Learn to recognize cues that suggest a potential threat, a danger, or an impending crisis situation.
- Be aware of and know how to use environmental controls to both prevent and reduce violent incidents.
- Continually incorporate personal health and wellness strategies that will minimize workplace stressors.
  - Provide and be open to receiving constructive, timely, and respectful feedback from colleagues, health care consumers, family members.
  - Participate in the implementation of the comprehensive workplace violence program.
  - Use crisis intervention and management strategies to assess, plan, and intervene in order to reduce the potential for workplace violence.
  - Use existing environmental controls (visitor access, panic buttons, etc.).
  - Use the approved reporting system.

    Report concerns about weaknesses in the system in order to improve processes and communication.

    Engage in evaluation and continued improvement of the workplace violence prevention program.

    Participate, as appropriate, in postincident meetings.

    Refer bystanders, surviving colleagues, and family members to grief and bereavement counseling or other appropriate health services following the injury, death, murder, or suicide of an employee or patient.

    Express sympathy and provide support to bystanders and survivors after a colleague or patient is injured or dies during a violent workplace incident.

BOX 1.10 Role of Nurses in Advancing Health Equity

- Acting now to improve the health and well-being of the nation
- Lifting barriers to expand the contributions of nursing
- Designing better payment models
- Strengthening nursing education
- Valuing community and public health nursing
- Fostering nurses' roles as leaders and advocates
- Preparing nursed to respond to disasters
- Supporting the health and well-being of nurses

BOX 1.11 Dimensions of Wellness

1. Physical Wellness

   Physical wellness includes healthy eating, proactively taking care of health issues that arise, and maintaining healthy daily practices.
2. Career Wellness

   Engaging in work that provides personal satisfaction and enrichment and is consistent with your values, goals, and lifestyle will keep you professionally healthy.
3. Social Wellness

   Building a network of support based on interdependence, mutual respect, and trust with your friends, family, and coworkers leads to social wellness.
4. Creative Wellness

   Creative wellness means valuing and participating in a diverse range of arts and cultural experiences to understand and appreciate your surrounding world.
5. Environmental Wellness

   Being environmentally well means recognizing the responsibility to preserve, protect, and improve the environment and appreciate your connection to nature.
6. Spiritual Wellness

   Spiritual wellness includes being open to exploring your own beliefs and respecting others' beliefs.
7. Emotional Wellness

   Emotional wellness is being able to identify, express, and manage your full range of feelings.
8. Financial Wellness

   Financial wellness includes being fully aware of your financial status and budget, and the ability to manage your financial goals.
9. Intellectual

   An intellectually well person values lifelong learning, develops moral reasoning, fosters critical thinking, expands world view, and engages in education for the pursuit of knowledge.

our professional nursing organizations (ANA, AACN, ENA, to name a few). Also, many frameworks have come from academia with similar topics and categories.

The model we have selected for this book is that created by Dr. Melnyk and colleagues at Ohio State University.[56,57] The model consists of nine dimensions—refer to Box 1.11. A new feature in this book is our creation of vignettes addressing each of the nine dimensions of wellness that are scattered throughout the book. Each one consists of a nurse describing experience related to the specific wellness dimension followed by an overview of the category and considerations for personal interventions, as needed. For example, see the Supporting the Well-Being of Nurses box.

HEALTHY WORK ENVIRONMENT (HWE)

The health care environment is stressful; increasing challenges in the areas of financial constraints, regulatory requirements, consumer scrutiny, quickly changing technologies and treatment regimens, and workforce diversity contribute daily to conflicts and difficulties. In this environment, it is essential to offer support for health care providers that can mitigate these challenges and ensure a healthy place to work.

There is an increasing amount of evidence that unhealthy work environments lead to medical errors, suboptimal safety monitoring, ineffective communication among health care providers, and increased conflict and stress among care providers. Synthesis of research in the area of work environment has demonstrated that a combination of leadership styles and characteristics contributes to the development and sustainability of HWEs.

AACN has formulated standards for establishing and sustaining HWEs. The intent of the standards is to promote creation of environments that have a positive impact on nursing and patient outcomes. Evidence-based and relationship-centered principles were used to create the standards of professional performance. A summary of the six standards is provided in Box 1.12

Fig. 1.1 illustrates the interdependence of each standard and the ultimate impact on optimal patient outcomes and clinical excellence. Blake described using the HWE standards as a blueprint to implement the model on their organization's road to excellence.[58]

Kester et al. reported findings from a study in which they examined HWE before and 2 years after implementation of the model. There was improvement in staff satisfaction, turnover, and average tenure demonstrating improved retention.[59] Everyone

BOX 1.12 Healthy Work Environment Standards

Standard I: Skilled Communication

Nurses must be as proficient in communication skills as they are in clinical skills.

Standard II: True Collaboration

Nurses must be relentless in pursuing and fostering true collaboration.

Standard III: Effective Decision Making

Nurses must be valued and committed partners in making policy, directing and evaluating clinical care, and leading organizational operations.

Standard IV: Appropriate Staffing

Staffing must ensure the effective match between patient needs and nurse competencies.

Standard V: Meaningful Recognition

Nurses must be recognized and must recognize others for the value each brings to the work of the organization.

Standard VI: Authentic Leadership

Nurse leaders must fully embrace the imperative of a healthy work environment, authentically live it, and engage others in its achievement.

From American Association of Critical-Care Nurses (AACN). *Standards for Establishing and Sustaining Healthy Work Environments. A Journey to Excellence.* 2nd ed. AACN; 2016.

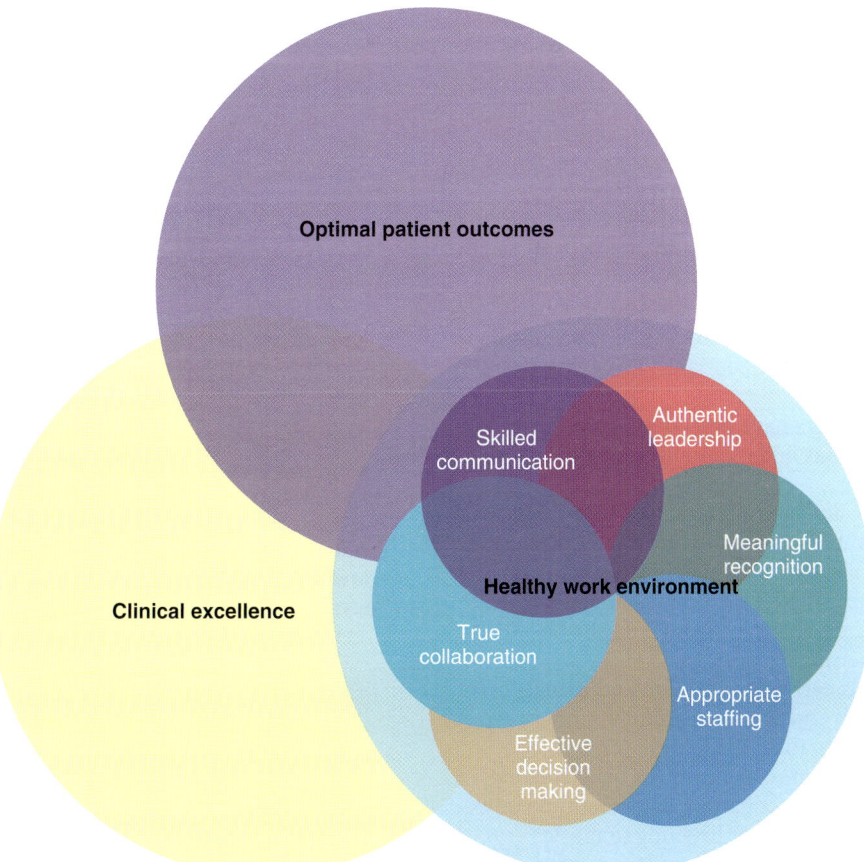

FIG. 1.1 Interdependence of Healthy Work Environment, Clinical Excellence, and Optimal Patient Outcomes. (From American Association of Critical-Care Nurses. *Standards for Establishing and Sustaining Healthy Work Environments.* 2nd ed. AACN; 2016.)

has a role in creating and sustaining the HWE. Although managers have a major role in establishing the culture, staff members greatly affect the culture by mentoring new staff members, role modeling behaviors, and leading interdisciplinary teams.

In addition to the HWE standards,[60] AACN has multiple other resources that can be used to gain a greater depth of knowledge, implementation, and evaluation of the unit environment. An important first step is to assess the unit baseline work environment status. AACN has created a research-based valid and reliable survey for interprofessional administration. This is an important first step to creating a work plan and time frame toward a HWE.

KEY POINTS

- Health disparities adversely affect group of people who have systematically experienced greater obstacles to health based on their racial or ethnic group, religion, socioeconomic status, gender, age, mental health, cognitive, sensory, or physical disability; sexual orientation or gender identity; geographic location; or other characteristics linked to discrimination or exclusion.
- It is essential for nurses to use the best data available to make patient care decisions and to carry out the appropriate interventions.
- Everyone has a role in creating and sustaining the HWE.
- In addition to establishing a common language to describe nursing practice across settings and clinical populations, ICNP provides the ability to compare care and project trends in nursing treatments and interventions.
- The critical care nurse must be able to deliver high-quality care skillfully, using all appropriate technologies, while incorporating psychosocial and other holistic approaches as appropriate to the time and condition of the patient.
- Nurses must possess knowledge about biocultural, psychosocial, and linguistic differences in diverse populations to make accurate assessments and plan interventions.
- Although nursing has independent and dependent nursing actions, it is essential that an interdependence with all health care providers is actualized.
- It is more important than ever to create and enhance partnerships, because the resulting interdependence and collaboration among disciplines is essential to achieving positive patient outcomes.
- Multiple quality indicators have been developed for critical care; nurses are pivotal in quality monitoring and improvement.
- *AACN Practice Alerts* are succinct, evidence-based directives for critical care nurses and other health care providers to ensure that the most current evidence is used to provide safe care.
- The rapid response team (RRT) is a multidisciplinary team that extends critical care services throughout the hospital in the noncritical care setting.
- The goal of the RRT is early identification and management of clinical deterioration and averting cardiopulmonary arrest or unintended transfer to the critical care unit.
- Nurses can promote emotional health by participating in calming activities, such as meditation, daily gratitude reflections, deep breathing, walking, or listening to music.
- Bullying and is characterized by repeated, unwanted, harmful actions intended to humiliate and cause distress to the recipient.
- Bullying and incivility are never sanctioned in any setting and must be addressed and stopped.
- HWEs are essential for establishing collaborative, trusting, and safe environments for the delivery of patient care.
- Nurse wellness consists of nine components: intellectual, spiritual, physical, psychological, social, financial, emotional, career, environmental.
- Cultural competence is defined as "the ability of providers and organizations to effectively deliver health care services that meet the social, cultural, and linguistic needs of the patients."

Visit the Evolve site at http://evolve.elsevier.com/Urden/CriticalCareNursing for additional study materials.

REFERENCES

1. Society of Critical Care Medicine. About SCCM: history of critical care. http://www.sccm.org. Accessed November 18, 2024.
2. American Association of Critical Care Nurses. About AACN. https://aacn.org/about-aacn. Accessed November 18, 2024.
3. Healthy People 2030. https://health.gov/our-work/national-health-initiatives/healty-people/healthy-people-2030; Accessed November 18, 2024.
4. Social Determinants of Health-Healthy People 2030. https://health.gov/healthypeople/priority-areas/social-determinants-health. Accessed November 18, 2024.
5. Health Care Access and Quality. https://health.gov/healthypeople/objectives-and-data/browse-objectives/health-care-access-and-quality. Accessed November 18, 2024.
6. Health Care. https://health.gov/healthypeople/objectives-and-data/browse-objectives/health-care. Accessed November 18, 2024.
7. Increase the Proportion of Adults Who Get Recommended Evidence-Based Preventative Health Care. https://odphp.health.gov/healthypeople/objectives-and-data/browse-objectives/health-care-access-and-quality/increase-proportion-adults-who-get-recommended-evidence-based-preventive-health-care-ahs-08. Accessed November 18, 2024.
8. Bourgault AM. Bridging evidence-based practice and research. *Crit Care Nurse.* 2018;38(6):10. https://doi.org/10.4037/ccn2018278.
9. Makic MBF, Svoboda E. Staying informed of best evidence to guide practice. *AACN Adv Crit Care.* 2023;34(1):63–66. https://doi.org/10.4037/aacnacc2023372.
10. International Classification for Nursing Practice (ICNP). https://www.icn.ch/how-we-do-it/projects/ehealth-icnptm/about-icnp. Accessed November 18, 2024.
11. Upvall MJ, Bourgault AM, Pigon C, Swartzman CA. Exemplars illustrating de-implementation of tradition-based practices. *Crit Care Nurse.* 2019;39(6):64. https://doi.org/10.4037/ccn2019534.
12. International Classification for Nursing Practice (ICNP). Nursing diagnosis and outcome statements. https://www.ICN.org; 2019. Accessed October 24, 2023.
13. International Classification for Nursing Practice (ICNP). Nursing intervention statements. 2019. https://www.icn.org; Accessed October 24, 2023.
14. Health Policy Institute, Georgetown University. Cultural competence in health care: is it important for people with chronic conditions? https://hpi.georgetown.edu/cultural/. Accessed November 18, 2024.
15. International Council of Nurses. *Cultural and Linguistic Competence Position Statement.* Adopted; 2007. reviewed 2013. https://icn.ch. Accessed October 26, 2023.
16. Kramlich D. Strategies for acute and critical care nurses implementing complementary therapies requested by patients and family members. *Crit Care Nurs.* 2016;36(6):52–58. https://doi.org/10.4037/ccn2016974.
17. Kramlich D. Complementary health practitioners in the acute and critical care setting: nursing considerations. *Crit Care Nurs.* 2017;37(3):60–65. https://doi.org/10.40037/ccn2017181.

18. Creswell JD. Mindfulness interventions. *Annu Rev Psychol.* 2016;68:491–516. https://doi.org/10.1146/annurev-psych-042716-051139.
19. U.S. Department Health and Human Services National Institutes of Health. Massage therapy for health: what the science says. https://www.nccih:nih.gov/health/providers/digest/massage-therapy-for-health-science. Accessed October 26, 2023.
20. Malik J. Animal-assisted interventions in intensive care delirium: a literature review. *AACN Adv Crit Care* 32(4): 391-397) 2121. https://doi.org/10.4037/aacnacc2021707.
21. Lovell T, Ranse K. Animal-assistive activities in the intensive care unit: a scoping review. *Intensive Crit Care Nurs* 73(12). https://doi.org/10.1016/j.1ccn.2022.103304.
22. American Music Therapy Association. Definition and quotes about music therapy. https://www.musictherapy.org/. Accessed October 24, 2023.
23. Golino AJ, Leone R, Gollenberg A, et al. Impact of an active music therapy intervention on intensive care patients. *Amer J Crit Care.* 2019;28(1):48. https://doi.org/10.4037/ajcc2019792.
24. Golino AJ, Leone R, Gollenberg A, et al. Receptive therapy for patients receiving mechanical ventilation in the intensive care unit. *Amer J Crit Care.* 2023;32(2):109–115. https://doi.org/10.4037/ajcc2023499.
25. Harrington L. Going digital: what does it really mean for nursing? *AACN Adv Crit Care.* 2016;4(27):358. https://doi.org/10.4037/aacnacc2016263.
26. Lavoie-Tremblay M, O'Connor P, Lavigne GL, et al. Effective strategies to spread redesigning care processes among healthcare teams. *J Nurse Scholarship.* May 2015. https://doi.org/10.1111/jnu.12141.
27. Anderson RJ, Sparbel K, Barr RN, Doerschug K, Corbridge S. Electronic health record tool to promote team communication and early patient mobility in the intensive care unit. *Crit Care Nurs.* 2018;38(6):23–34. https://doi.org/10.4037/ccn2018813.
28. American Association of Critical Care Nurses. *AACN Tele-Critical Care Nursing Practice: An Expert Consensus Statement Supporting Acute, Progressive and Critical Care*; 2022. https://www.aacn.org. Accessed October 26, 2023.
29. Alderden JG, Johnny JD. Artificial intelligence and the critical care nurse. *Crit Care Nurs.* 2023;43(5):7–8. https://doi.org/10.4037/ccn2023755.
30. Williams LMS, Nemeth LS, Johnson E, Armaignac DL, Magwood GS. Telemedicine intensive care unit nursing interventions to prevent failure to rescue. *Amer J Crit Care.* 2019;28(1):64–75. https://doi.org/10.4037/ajcc2019577.
31. Interprofessional Education Collaborative. (2023). *IPEC Core Competencies for Interprofessional Collaborative Practice: Version 3.* Washington, DC: Interprofessional Education Collaborative. https://www.ipecollaborative.org/ipec-core-competencies. Accessed November 19, 2024.
32. Schwab KE, Simon W, Yamamoto M, et al. Rapid mortality review in the intensive care unit: an in-person, multidisciplinary improvement initiative. *Amer J Crit Care.* 2021;30(2):e32–e39. https:/doi.org/10.4037/ajcc2021829.
33. Pun BT, Jun J, Tan A, et al. Interprofessional team collaboration and work environment health in 68 US intensive care units. *Amer J Crit Care.* 2022;31(6):443–451. https://doi.org/10.4037/ajcc2022546.
34. Evans L, Rhodes A, Alhazzani W, et al. Executive Summary: surviving sepsis campaign (SSC): international guidelines for the management and treatment of sepsis and septic shock 2021. *Crit Care Med.* 2021;49(11):1974–1982. https://doi.org/10.1097/CCM.00000000005357. www.ccmjournal.
35. Acquisto NM, Mosier JM, Bittner EA, et al. Society of medicine clinical practice guidelines for rapid sequence intubation in the critically ill adult patient: executive summary. *Crit Care Med.* 2023;51(10):1408–1410. www.ccmjournal.org. doi:0.097/ccm.00000000000005999.
36. Hawkins SF, Morse JM. Untenable expectations: nurses' work in the context of medication administration, error, and the organization. *Global Qual Nurs Res.* 2022;9(1–17). https://doi.org/10.1177/23333936221131779.
37. The Joint Commission. National Patient Safety Goals, 2025. https://www.jointcommission.org/standards/national-patient-safety-goals/hospital-national-patient-safety-goals/. Accessed November 18, 2024.
38. The Joint Commission. *Facts about the official* "Do Not Use" List. http://www.jointcommission.org. Accessed October 24, 2023.
39. Medical Device Reporting (MDR). http://www.fda.gov/MedicalDevices/Safety/ReportaProblem/default.htm. Accessed October 24, 2023.
40. US Department Health and Human Services, Food and Drug Administration: warnings for Industry: warnings and precautions, contraindications, contraindications, and boxed warning sections of labeling for human prescriptive drug and biological products-content and format; October 2011.
41. Institute for Safe Medication Practices. About ISMP. http://www.ISMP.org. Accessed October 24, 2023.
42. Institute for Healthcare Improvement. Using bundles to improve health care quality. http://www.ihi.org. Accessed 16.02.20.
43. National Quality Forum. About NQF. http://www.NQF.org. Accessed October 26, 2023
44. Healthcare Information and Management Systems Society. Patient safety and quality outcomes. http://www.HIMSS.org. Accessed October 26, 2023.
45. ANA Enterprise News (no author). Nurses ranked most honest and ethical professionals for 21st year. *Am Nurse J.* March; 18(3): 31.
46. Vaughn N. Nursing Compassion fatigue and burnout vs moral inquiry. *Nurse.com Blog. February.* 2023;9. https://www.nurse.com/blog/nursing-compassion-fatigue-and-burnout-vs-burnout-vs-moral-inquiry/.
47. Tripathi SK, Mulkey DC. Implementing brief mindfulness-based interventions to reduce compassion fatigue. *Crit Care Nurs.* 2023;43(5):32–38. https://doi.org/10.4037/ccn2023745.
48. Reducing the safety hazards of monitor alert and alert fatigue. https://psnet.ahrq.gov/perspective/reducing-safety-hazards-monitor-alert-and-alarm-fatigue. Assessed October 26, 2023
49. American Nurses Association. Position statement on incivility, bullying, and workplace violence, 2015. Accessed October 26, 2023.
50. Centers for Disease Control and Prevention, The National Institute for Occupational Safety and Health Occupational Violence at https://www.cdc.gov/niosh/topics/violence/default.html. Accessed October 26, 2023.
51. The Joint Commission prevention of workplace violence. https://www.jointcommission.org/patient-safety-topics/workplace-violence-prevention/
52. Havaei F. Does the type of exposure to workplace violence matter to nurses' mental health? *Healthcare.* 2021;41(1):9. https://www.doi.org/10.3390/healthcare9010041.
53. Kim S, Kitzmiller R, Baernholdt M, Lynn MR, Jones CB, et al. Patient Safety Culture: the impact on workplace violence and health worker burnout. *Workplace Health Safety.* 2023;(2):78–88. https://doi.org/10.1177/21650799221126364.
54. American Nurses Association. Issue Brief: Reporting Incidents of Workplace Violence, 2019. https://www.nursingworld.org. Accessed October 26, 2023.
55. The Future of Nursing 2020-2030. *Charting a Path to Achieve Health Equity Consensus Study Report Highlights.* Prepared by the National Academy of Medicine; 2021. https://nationalacademies.org. Accessed October 15, 2023.
56. Melnyck, BK., Neale S, editors. *Dimensions of Wellness:evidence-Based Tactics for Optimizing Your Health and Well-Being.* The Ohio State University.
57. Melnyck BK, Nealy S. 9 Dimensions of wellness. *Amer Nurs Today.* 2018;13(1):10–11.
58. Blake N, Sandoval R, Sangalang R, Reyes J, Anderson K, Hunt D, et al. A hospital's roadmap for improving nursing excellence using AACN's Healthy Work Environment Standards. *AACN Adv Crit Care.* 2022;33(2):208–211. https://doi.org/10.4037/aacnacc2022632.
59. Kester K, Pena H, Shuford C, et al. Implementing AACN's healthy work environment framework in an intensive care unit. *Amer J Crit Care.* 2021;30(6):426–433. https://doi.org/10.4037/ajcc2021108.
60. American Association of Critical-Care Nurses. AACN *Standards for Establishing and Sustaining Healthy Work Environments. A Journey to Excellence.* 2nd ed. http://www.aacn.org. Accessed November 4, 2023.

2

Ethical and Legal Issues

Lisa Mancuso and Karen Wilkinson

ETHICAL ISSUES

Local, state, and federal legal systems and ethics overlap in many areas and affect health care in a range of matters, from a lawsuit between private parties to enforcement actions brought by government agencies against individuals or health systems. Understanding the law as it applies to nursing care and nursing ethics/principles will guide nursing actions essential to providing compassionate, competent, quality nursing care.

This chapter provides an overview of ethical principles and professional nursing ethics. It highlights some laws and legal procedures that are prominent in nursing practice. Some of the laws and legal systems that figure prominently in nursing practice include (1) administrative law (illustrated by the regulation of the profession by state boards of nursing [BONs]), (2) tort law (illustrated through negligence lawsuits against nurses for their actions or inactions), (3) constitutional law (illustrated through a discussion of the legal rights of patients to accept or refuse treatment), and (4) federal and state health care statutory laws (illustrated through self-determination laws and select federal laws).

Day-to-day decisions in critical care fall within the realm of ethics; each act can show or fail to show respect for the person or patient. The daily practice of critical care nursing involves ethical decision making and frequently involves ethical problems. Ethical problems occur when there are potential alternative actions for a patient, and those actions conflict; individuals may be uncertain about the thing to do.

The practice of nursing is influenced by and sometimes governed by the law. Legal systems operate at the local, state, and federal levels. These systems affect health care in a range of matters, from a lawsuit between private parties to enforcement actions brought by government agencies against individuals or health systems.

Understanding professional nursing ethics and ethical principles with the ability to use a decision-making model to guide nursing actions is essential to providing compassionate, competent, quality nursing care.

Critical care nurses will find that law and ethics overlap in many areas, and the issues may become so intertwined that it becomes difficult to separate the two. Both have similar goals, except there is no enforcement system for ethical guidelines.

Some of the laws and legal systems that figure prominently in nursing practice include (1) administrative law (illustrated by the regulation of the profession by state BONs), (2) tort law (illustrated through negligence lawsuits against nurses for their actions or inactions), (3) constitutional law (illustrated through a discussion of the legal rights of patients to accept or refuse treatment), and (4) federal and state health care statutory laws (illustrated through self-determination laws and select federal laws).

Morals Versus Ethics

Morals are traditions of belief about right or wrong human behavior. Informed by individual and group values, morality consists of standards of conduct that include moral principles, rules, virtues, rights, and responsibilities.

Morals, Ethics, and Ethical Problems

Moral norms form the basis for proper action and provide a framework for evaluating behavior through a system of ethics.[1,2] *Ethics* is a generic term for the reasoned inquiry and understanding of a moral life, in other words, a systematic examination of morality. Different theories or systems of ethics identify which moral norms (or rules) should be used and prioritized to evaluate whether conduct is ethical.[1,2]

Applied ethics, of which health care ethics is a branch, is the attempt to use moral norms to evaluate conduct and to resolve particular ethical problems in context.[1] The extreme situations at the end of life or beginning of life garner most of the attention around health care ethics; however, day-to-day nursing decisions and actions also implicate ethics.[3] Day-to-day nursing decisions fall within the realm of ethics if they (1) pertain to things within the nurse's control and (2) show respect or fail to show respect for patients (or their loved ones).[4]

Therefore, most nursing decisions and interactions with patients fall within the realm of ethics.

Most of the time, there is a right thing to do, and it can be done without conflict or resulting harm. Rainer et al. found that the most common ethical problems identified by nurses involved end-of-life care, conflicts with physicians, organizational restraints, conflicts with patients' families, and conflicts between required interventions and patients' privacy and dignity.[27]

Ethical problems (also called *ethical* or *moral dilemmas*) occur only when there is some conflict surrounding an ethical decision.[4] An ethical problem exists if a person is morally obligated or appears to be obligated to two or more conflicting potential courses of action. The result is that both something right and something wrong will occur.[1,2]

There are three kinds of ethical problems: cognitive, social, and volitional. In nursing, cognitive problems arise when the nurse is genuinely uncertain about the right thing to do. Social problems occur when there is disagreement among health care team members, family members, or other stakeholders about

PATIENT-CENTERED CRITICAL CARE

Creating a Calm Environment in Critical Care

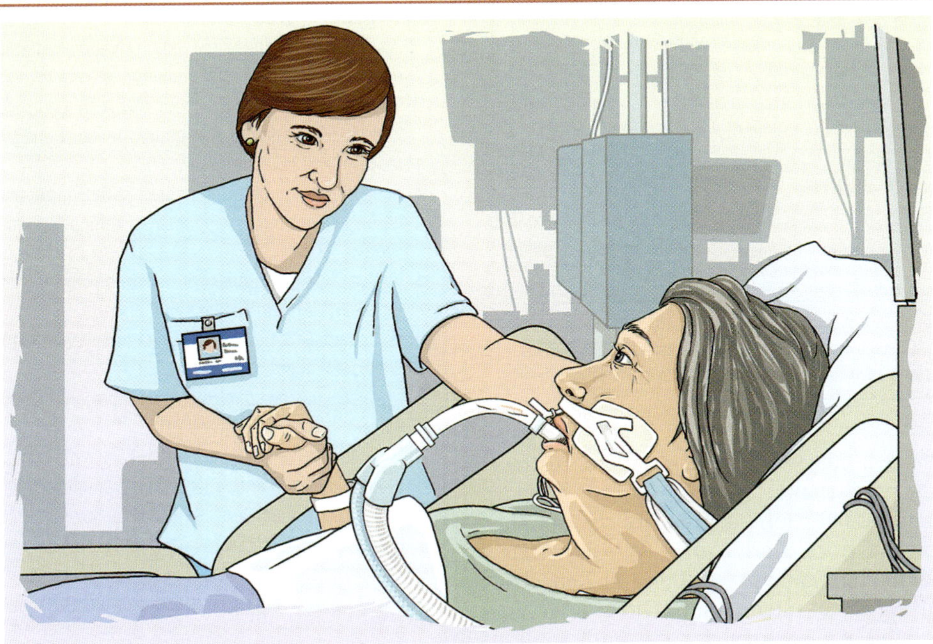

The critical care unit is a stressful environment for patients and for their family members—with the understanding that family is whomever the patient designates to be at their bedside. The critical care unit is also stressful because of the number of alarms, 24/7 routines, unfamiliar environment, and often an uncertain prognosis.

Amid a multitude of clinical tasks, nurses create a connection with their patients by explaining what is happening, preserving patient dignity, holding a hand when that is needed, and providing exceptional care.

the right thing to do. Volitional problems occur when a nurse knows the right thing to do but does not know if they will do it or can do it, usually because of power imbalances or organizational pressures. Volitional problems are often associated with moral distress.

Nurses, Moral Distress, and Moral Courage

Nurses work within a system in constant flux. Health care is a highly regulated, complicated industry, and health care organizations are complex systems with varying authority structures and power dynamics. As the most constant health professional presence at the bedside, critical care nurses navigate the complexities in health care in a high-stakes, high-stress environment while also managing (1) frontline patient care, including emergency situations; (2) increasingly innovative and highly technical care delivery; (3) financial and staffing constraints; and (4) emotional and behavioral responses from patients and families, coworkers, and themselves. These direct care, organizational, and structural pressures amplify a complex moral environment with frequent ethical dilemmas.[3]

These pressures can exacerbate the nurse's feelings of powerlessness and lack of control and contribute to detachment from the ethical impact of day-to-day decisions, compassion fatigue, and burnout.

Moral distress is widely discussed in the literature as a serious problem for nurses. Jameton[5] first described moral distress as distress that occurs when the nurse knows the correct thing to do but is prevented from acting on it.[4] This overlaps with volitional ethical problems: The nurse knows the ethically appropriate action but feels unable to act consistently with that course or acts inconsistently, and therefore unethically, because of one or more barriers.[4,6]

These barriers can include the medical plan of care, workplace dynamics, levels of nurse empowerment, organizational rules, imbalanced power dynamics, interpersonal conflict, or individual psychosocial processes. High levels of moral distress often signal unit or system-wide issues.[7]

Moral distress has two components: (1) initial distress, which occurs contemporaneously with the situation creating the distress; and (2) reactive distress (or moral residue), which includes lingering feelings about one's failure to act and is associated with long-term consequences to the nurse.[7]

These consequences are significant, including compassion fatigue and burnout, precisely because "moral distress involves the violation of one's core moral values, can erode personal integrity, and may undermine moral identity."[7]

In critical care, moral distress arises most frequently from using technology at the end of life, particularly when it is seen as medically nonbeneficial (or futile). It also occurs when surrogate decision makers refuse consent for care that nurses perceive as in the patient's best interest or when nurses have difficulty accessing resources to reduce patient suffering.

These and other situations may cause nurses to act in ways that are contrary to personal and professional values in the initial moral distress phase. Significant emotional and physical stress and resulting feelings of loss of personal integrity and professional dissatisfaction are common in the moral residue or reactive distress phase of moral distress. Over time, relationships with coworkers and patients and the quality of care are negatively affected. Personal relationships and family life may

BOX 2.1 American Association of Critical-Care Nurses Position Statement

Moral Distress in Times of Crisis

"Moral distress is a complex, challenging problem with damaging repercussions that are often ignored in healthcare work environments. This problem is exacerbated in times of crisis. AACN asserts that every institution must implement readily accessible resources to identify and mitigate the harmful effects of moral distress. In addition, nurses must not hesitate to seek professional ethical support and other types of counseling when experiencing moral distress or feeling a loss of personal integrity. Skilled communication is necessary to ensure that institutional leaders and frontline nurses are allies during times of crisis."

American Association of Critical-Care Nurses. AACN Position Statement: Moral Distress in Times of Crisis. AACN website. March 1, 2020. Accessed March 7, 2024. https://www.aacn.org/policy-and-advocacy/aacnposition-statement-moral-distress-in-times-of-crisis.

also be negatively affected; nurses experiencing moral distress may resign or leave the profession.[3,7,8]

Tools to address and resolve moral distress are critical. The American Association of Critical-Care Nurses (AACN), *Statement on Moral Distress in Times of Crisis* (see Box 2.1). Reflective debriefing is a promising direct intervention. Direct interventions are believed to assist the nurse to more confidently analyze the ethical issues involved, identify the underlying conflicts, and engage instead of discounting emotions to empower them in future decision making.[7]

Indirect interventions focus on separate issues that may indirectly reduce moral distress, such as efforts to improve nurses' comfort levels with dying or specialized ethics training programs. General interventions are aimed at institutional-level issues that contribute to moral distress, such as nurse-physician relationships.

When interventions to reduce moral distress are effective, they build moral resilience.[7] Box 2.2 contains a list of actions that nurses can take individually to address moral distress and build moral resilience.

Rushton defines *moral resilience* as "the capacity of an individual to sustain or restore their integrity in response to moral complexity, confusion, distress, or setbacks."[7] The capacity to develop and improve moral resilience has been identified as critical to reducing moral distress and enhancing ethical competence. The capacity to develop and improve moral resilience has been identified as critical to reducing moral distress and enhancing ethical competence.

The American Nurses Association (ANA) provides an excellent overview of the concept in *A Call to Action: Exploring Moral Resilience Toward a Culture of Ethical Practice*.[9] Nurses who are morally resilient likely feel empowered to exercise moral courage, and moral courage may prevent moral distress in the first instance.[10]

Moral courage is defined by Hu et al. as "courage or inner strength a person has when acting in ethical conflicts according to ethical principles and one's own values and beliefs, even at the risk of negative outcomes for the acting individual."[11] Moral courage is compromised by situations in which nurses are not free to advocate for themselves, for their patients, and for practices and policies that serve the ends of caregiving.

Abdeen et al. identified the attributes of courageous nurses: true presence, moral integrity, responsibility, honesty, advocacy, commitment and perseverance, and personal sacrifice.[12] These attributes can only manifest in an organizational environment that supports moral courage. Organizations can do this through

BOX 2.2 Recommendations to Foster Individual Moral Resilience

Individual Nurse's Actions

1. Adopt ANA Healthy Nurse Healthy Nation™ strategies to support your general well-being as a foundation for cultivating moral resilience.
2. Read, review, and implement the ANA Code of Ethics for Nurses with Interpretive Statements to gain knowledge and strengthen ethical competence.
3. Seek opportunities to learn how to recognize, analyze, and take ethically grounded action in response to ethical complexity, disagreement, or conflict.
4. Cultivate self-awareness to recognize and respond to your symptoms of moral suffering, including moral distress.
5. Pursue educational opportunities to cultivate mindfulness, ethical competence, and moral resilience.
6. Develop your personal plan to support well-being and build moral resilience.
7. Become involved and initiate workplace efforts to address the root causes of moral distress and other forms of moral suffering.
8. Develop and practice skills in communication, mindfulness, conflict transformation, and interprofessional collaboration.
9. Identify and use personal resources within your organization or community, such as ethics committees, peer to peer support, employee assistance program

From American Nurses Association. A Call to Action: Exploring Moral Resilience Toward a Culture of Ethical Practice. Accessed May 29, 2023. www.nursingworld.org/~4907b6/globalassets/docs/ana/ana-call-to-action--exploring-moral-resilience-final.pdf.

policies and practices that support ethical competence, allow for diverse opinions, foster peer support, and support continued inquiry.

Virtues

Virtues are habits of character or learned behaviors that predispose individuals to behave ethically. In addition to courage, the virtues commonly expected of nurses include knowledge, wisdom, patience, compassion, and honesty. In contrast to personality traits or actions, virtues focus on the nurse's character or ways of being a moral person.[1,8]

An often overlooked but critical virtue for all health care professionals is humility. The virtue of humility encompasses several other practices, including self-knowledge, reflection, perspective taking, and intellectual honesty (admitting what you do not know and seeking help).[2] The virtue of caring may be particularly important for nursing; some have distinguished between caring *about* the patient and caring *for* the patient as two kinds of embodied virtues in nursing.[13] Practicing these virtues can better prepare nurses to act in an ethically appropriate and professional manner.

PRINCIPLES OF HEALTH CARE ETHICS

In health care, certain principles—descriptive and prescriptive rules that provide a basis for ethical reasoning and actions—are standard norms applied when analyzing ethical issues.[14]

Ethical Principles

These principles are used in this chapter and explained in Table 2.1.

When principles conflict, the nurse and other stakeholders must carefully justify privileging one principle over another.

TABLE 2.1 Principles of Health Care Ethics

Principle	Description
Respect for Persons/ Autonomy	The principle of respect for persons requires nurses to respect the patient's inherent dignity and capacity for rational choice; this includes the obligation to honor the patient's right to autonomy, which is the right to determine what is done to or for them without coercion or undue interference from others.[1,10] Autonomy is also the foundation of informed consent's legal and ethical requirements. It includes the right of patients with the decision making capacity to refuse some or all treatments.[1,10]
Beneficence/ Nonmaleficence	The ethical principles of beneficence and nonmaleficence require actions that maximize good and minimize harm to the patient, often in a delicate balance. The principle of beneficence presupposes compassion and requires the promotion of others' well-being through positive action and the desire to do good.[1,19] Nonmaleficence dictates that nurses prevent and minimize harm and correct harmful situations.[19] Benefits must be maximized, and harms must be minimized.
Justice	The principle of justice means an equitable distribution of social benefits and burdens in society.[1,19] The most common example of the principle of justice is the allocation of the limited resource of organs for transplant. Another is access to health care, an issue of social justice, although it is not a constitutional right in the United States.
Fidelity	The moral principle of fidelity involves the notions of loyalty, faithfulness, and honoring of commitments.[1] Patients and families must be able to trust and have faith in the therapeutic relationship between the provider, nurse, and other health care members. The health care team must ensure that the trust relationship is not threatened or obligations are not left unfulfilled.[1,10]
Veracity	The principle of telling the truth is veracity and is the basis of trust in the health care provider–patient relationship.[1,19] Veracity allows for the formulation of meaningful treatment goals and expectations based on truth and autonomy. Nurses must tell the truth to their patients so as not to give them knowingly false reassurance or damage their credibility with patients. Veracity can be violated by deliberately not telling the truth or withholding all or part of the truth.

Justification requires those involved to carefully describe the reasons for their actions and specify why the individual circumstances in the context of the patient's situation warrant overriding one or more principles in favor of others.[1]

For example, imagine caring for an 80-year-old patient with a long history of insulin-dependent diabetes mellitus with an unhealed, chronically infected lower limb wound for which amputation is recommended. The patient has the capacity, has very few social supports, lives alone, and refuses consent to the surgery. The goals of care that the patient has identified include living as happily and pain free as possible for however long she might live.

This is a classic conflict between autonomy (honoring the patient's wishes) and beneficence (advancing the course of action most likely to benefit the patient medically). Justification would include an analysis in context. For example, there is a general rule to honor the patient's autonomy, which is especially strong when there is no emergency. Forcing a patient with a life-limiting condition and limited social support to undergo an unwanted amputation is likely to cause more pain and a loss of independence and harm underlying health care provider–patient relationships.

Thus, a specified rule of respecting the chronically ill patient's autonomy to refuse treatment that may treat a problem but undermine the goals of care emerges.

Providers also make daily decisions in which underlying principles conflict. However, there is no ethical problem because all stakeholders agree with the right action, and that action can be taken. In these instances, a principle is adhered to while others are overridden, but a conscious analysis is not always undertaken.

Nonetheless, justification and specification are occurring on some level.[8] For example, drawing arterial blood gases (ABGs) carries risks and harms the patient by puncturing the skin and causing pain; therefore, the action is contrary to the principle of nonmaleficence (avoiding harm). However, the action is taken based on a desire to benefit the patient's respiratory status by allowing interventions tailored to the patient's current ventilation and oxygenation status. Thus, the principle of nonmaleficence is overridden by the principle of beneficence. That action is justified because the information (ABG results) will allow for adjustments to respiratory care for the patient in that specific circumstance.

Conflicting Principles, Paternalism, and Medical Futility

Conflict between principles is common and usually does not lead to an ethical problem. For example, suppose a patient is unconscious and needs emergency surgery for suspected peritonitis secondary to appendicitis and rupture. Surgery does harm to the patient and carries the potential for further harm to the patient in terms of risks; however, the benefits of surgery outweigh the need to avoid harm because of the known general clinical effectiveness of the intervention and the lack of reasonable, less harmful alternatives. In addition, the potential for further harm in the absence of surgical intervention is very high in terms of sepsis and possible death.

On balance, surgery honors beneficence. Because the patient is unconscious and cannot consent, autonomy is overridden. However, this is justified because time is of the essence, and delay would increase the likelihood of harm in this particular situation. It is justifiable to override autonomy in this situation because of the competing reality of death in a patient with a treatable condition. This is an ethical resolution of conflicting principles.

Principles can also be resolved in an unethical way. Two common examples of the unethical resolution of conflicting principles are paternalism and continuation of nonbeneficial care (medical futility), which are explained further in Table 2.2.

Paternalism is an example of an unethical resolution of conflicting principles of beneficence and autonomy. Nurses must guard against their own paternalism in critical care and practice the virtues of humility through careful self-reflection. Postoperative care, designed to assist the patient with achieving a quick recovery, is a good example. Encouraging the patient to turn, cough, and deep breathe and increasing the patient's activity through dangling, sitting in a chair, and ambulating all promote beneficence and nonmaleficence.

TABLE 2.2 Unethical Resolution of Conflicting Principles

Paternalism	Paternalism exists when the nurse or physician makes a decision for the patient without consulting the patient or by disregarding the patient's preferences. Fast-paced and high-pressure health care environments may lead less thoughtful providers to impose their recommendations on patients implicitly or explicitly.[14]
Medical Futility	*Medical futility* has been defined in countless ways; many prefer the terms *medically ineffective* or *nonbeneficial care.* In general, futility means that the treatments, especially aggressive critical care, do not meet the underlying care goals (i.e., the treatment harms the patient in some way without countervailing justification, such as a benefit for the patient's overall condition). This usually occurs when there is a conflict between beneficence, nonmaleficence, and sometimes autonomy.[14]

However, forcing this activity over the patient's objection or threatening the patient into compliance is paternalistic. Nurses are obligated to address underlying reasons for refusal, such as pain and sleep deprivation, and offer the patient options. Open and effective communication can lead to a resolution that benefits the patient and is not paternalistic.

Physiologic or scientific futility is when the intervention cannot treat the problem.[10,15] The classic example of physiologic futility is administering antibiotics for a viral infection. Quantitative or probabilistic futility refers to outcomes based on statistical evidence when there is a lack of generalizable research and conflicting thresholds for treatments to be considered futile.[10]

Ethical futility is treatment that would not serve the patient's underlying interests, values, and preferences.[15] Perhaps a helpful way to think about futility in the context of critical care is as an unethical balance of the principles of beneficence and nonmaleficence (doing harm with no balancing or overriding benefit) or as paternalism (imposing the provider's idea of benefits contrary to the values and preferences of the patient). It can also occur when providers continue nonbeneficial care because a patient's surrogate wants "everything done" (i.e., deference to autonomy despite no benefit and continued harm).

In critical care, futility is most often discussed in the context of end-of-life interventions. This is a pervasive ethical problem in the United States. According to Jamie et al.,[16] "Death is not necessarily a medical failure; a bad death is not only a medical failure but also an ethical breakdown."

Too many people in the United States experience a bad death. In general, providers fail to discuss death with patients, fail to refer to programs such as hospice or even palliative care appropriately, and persist in aggressively treating patients in high-tech settings far past the appropriate time. Moral distress is widespread among nurses who feel compelled to provide continued, painful, invasive care that will not benefit the patient or is contrary to the patient's wishes.[17]

Critical care nurses are at the forefront of this reality and can educate patients and families about options, clarify the realities associated with coding patients, and work with health care colleagues to foster thoughtfulness about the goals of care. Communication and problem-solving skills are essential to preventing conflicting goals and providing nonbeneficial care at the end of life.

PROFESSIONAL NURSING ETHICS AND THE *NURSING CODE OF ETHICS*

A professional code of ethics forms the framework for any profession. It is based on three elements: (1) the professional code of ethics, (2) the purpose of the profession, and (3) the standards of practice of the professional.[18]

The code of ethics developed by the profession delineates its values and relationships with and among members of the profession and society. The need for the profession and its inherent promise to provide certain duties form a contract between nursing and society. The professional standards describe the specifics of practice in various settings and subspecialties. Nursing professionals must stay consistent with their values and ethics and maintain an ethical environment wherever nursing care and services are performed.[18–20]

The *ANA Code of Ethics for Nurses*, updated in 2015,[19] is the guide used by the nursing profession, as it gives a voice to who we are as nurses at our very core and provides the primary source of ethical guidance for the nursing profession. This reflects our fundamental values and ideals as individual nurses and professional group members. The nursing code of ethics contains nine statements and directives for ethical nursing behavior.[20] Further delineation of each of the provisions, along with in-depth discussion and examples of application, can be found on the ANA website, https://www.nursingworld.org/practice-policy/nursing-excellence/ethics/code-of-ethics-for-nurses/

Situational and Organizational Ethical Decision Making in Critical Care

As discussed earlier, the critical care nurse encounters ethical issues daily. Usberg et al.[21] studied nurses involved in ethical problems, their early indicators and risk factors, nurse actions, and outcomes. These studies derived risk factors for patients, families, health care providers, and health care organizations.

Additionally, they delineated several early indicators for ethical dilemmas (Box 2.2). Research has indicated that screening critically ill patients periodically may help identify ethical conflicts earlier.[6] Specific actions for nursing leaders to address ethically complex situations and facilitate resolution include fostering open and early communication, providing robust ethics education, and promoting interdisciplinary practice (see Box 2.3).[10]

Health care organizations and authors have emphasized that responding to individual ethical issues is not enough; there must be a proactive program with a systematic approach to address ethical situations.[22,23] Preventive programs should identify, prioritize, and address concerns about ethics at an organizational level. Over time, measurable outcomes should demonstrate reduced disparities between current and ideal practices.[24]

Neglect of ethical problems or inadequate processes or resolution at the individual or systems level results in harm to more than patients; this often results in poor staff morale, moral distress, increased operational and legal costs, negative public relations, and loss of trust in the profession. Because nurses are on the frontline of health care ethics, especially in the critical care setting, they have a unique and essential role in resolving ethical problems. Box 2.4 lists resources related to ethics.

The Nurse's Role in Addressing Discrimination: Protecting and Promoting Inclusive Strategies

Various social determinants (social class, gender, race/ethnicity, socioeconomic status, disability, age, geographic

BOX 2.3 Early Indicators for Ethical Dilemmas

- Signs of patient suffering (prolonged, unrelieved pain)
- Signs of unrealistic expectations (unwavering belief in patient recovery)
- Signs of nurses' moral distress (believe treatment not helpful, causes suffering)
- Signs of conflict (disagreement, different opinions)
- Signs of poor communication (avoidance of end of life and other difficult topics)
- Signs of ethics violations (disrespect for autonomy, disregard of right to information)

From Pavlish CL, Hellyer JH, Brown-Saltzman K, Miers AG, Squire K. Screening situations for risk of ethical conflicts: a pilot study. *Am J Crit Care.* 2015;24(3):248–256.

location, sexual orientation, and gender identity, among others) contribute (either alone or in concert) to the generation of inequalities, discrimination, marginalization, and social exclusion, all of which have complex effects on people's health and well-being. Because nurses interact with all health care staff, they are in the position to oversee patient experiences and lead efforts to educate staff in the fundamentals of providing respectful care to all patients with cultural humility.

Health disparities and discrimination continue to exist and can be found in the critical care setting. This can affect patients' health. Critical care nurses and the profession as a whole must address discriminatory practices that are either intentional or unintentional. Given the impact of unintentional discrimination based on attitudes and stereotyping, the critical care nurse must examine their biases and prejudices for indications of discriminatory actions.

The ANA states that all nurses must recognize the potential impact of unconscious bias and practices contributing to discrimination and actively seek opportunities to promote the inclusion of all people in providing quality health care while eradicating disparities.[25] The ANA recommends the implementation of the activities listed in Box 2.5.

Frameworks for Resolving Ethical Problems

Ethical problems are ubiquitous in critical care and often related to conflicts surrounding the use of technology, including the withdrawal of technology. As mentioned earlier, ethical problems in critical care occur when there is (1) conflict between the right action and the ability to take it, (2) uncertainty about the right action, or (3) conflict about which of several right actions is most ethical.[16]

Dealing with an ethical problem requires the individuals involved to pause, expand group consciousness about the issue, validate assumptions, look for patterns of thoughts or behaviors, and effectively facilitate reflection and inquiry before making any decision.[19]

A model or framework should be used to organize the relevant concerns, examine the issues, and generate possible solutions to facilitate the ethical decision-making process. Numerous ethical decision-making models exist in the literature.[1,4,10,13,22] Jonsen et al.[13] have elucidated a logical and well-accepted model along the lines of the systematic format that practicing physicians have been taught and have practiced for a long time (Chief Complaint, History of Present Illness, Past History, Pertinent Family and Social History, Review of Systems, Physical Examination, and Laboratory and Imaging Studies). The model includes the following:

- Clinical assessment (identifying medical problems, treatment options, and goals of care)
- Patient (finding and clarifying patient preferences on treatment options and goals of care)
- Quality of life (QOL) (effects of medical problems, interventions, and treatment on patient's QOL with awareness of individual biases on what constitutes an acceptable QOL)

BOX 2.4 Internet Resources

Ethical Issues

- American Journal of Bioethics: www.bioethics.net
  - Bioethics news and blog
- American Nurses Association (ANA): www.nursingworld.org
  - Code of Ethics for Nurses: www.nursingworld.org/practice-policy/nursing-excellence/ethics/code-of-ethics-for-nurses/
  - Multiple position statements on ethical issues in nursing
    - Ethical Considerations for Local and Global Volunteerism
    - The Nurse's Role When a Patient Requests Medical Aid in Dying
    - The Nurse's Role in Addressing Discrimination: Protecting and Promoting Inclusive Strategies in Practice Settings, Policy, and Advocacy
    - Ethical Responsibility to Manage Pain and the Suffering it Causes
    - Interdisciplinary Guidelines for Care of Women Presenting to the Emergency Department with Pregnancy Loss
    - Nursing Advocacy for LGBTQ Populations
    - Nonpunitive Treatment of Pregnant and Breast-Feeding Women with Substance Use Disorders
    - Nutrition and Hydration at the End of Life
    - Capital Punishment and Nurses' Participation in Capital Punishment
    - Nurses' Roles and Responsibilities in Providing Care and Support at the End of Life
    - The Nurse's Role in Ethics and Human Rights: Protecting and Promoting Individual Worth, Dignity, and Human Rights In Practice Settings
    - Therapeutic Use of Marijuana and Related Cannabinoids Position Statement
    - Nursing Care and Do Not Resuscitate (DNR) and Allow Natural Death Decisions
    - Reduction of Patient Restraint and Seclusion in Health Care Settings
- American Society for Bioethics and the Humanities (ASBH): www.asbh.org
  - Not-for-profit organization committed to education and research in clinical ethics
  - Core Competencies for Clinical Ethics Consultants
  - Health Care Ethics Consultant Certification Program
  - Code of Ethics for Clinical Ethicists
  - Nursing ethics interest group (affinity group)
- Catholic Health Care Association of the United States: www.chausa.org/ethics/overview
  - Catholic health care facilities are the largest group of nonprofit health care facilities in the United States. Nurses working in Catholic health care must understand the additional ethical norms applicable, including the Ethical and Religious Directives for Catholic Health Care, in delivering care and resolving problems
- The Hastings Center: www.thehastingscenter.org
  - Independent, nonpartisan, nonprofit bioethics research institute
  - Provides educational resources and conferences, publications, and ethics consultation
- United States Department of Veterans Affairs National Center for Ethics in Health Care: https://www.ethics.va.gov/

BOX 2.5 ANA Position Statement Addressing Discrimination

- Intentional or blatant discriminatory practices must not be tolerated and must be immediately addressed.
- Nurses must engage in a period of self-reflection regarding their personal and professional values regarding civility, mutual respect, and inclusiveness, and resolve any potential conflicts in ways that ensure patient safety and promote the best interests of the patient.
- Nurses must seek out and support nursing practice environments that embrace inclusive strategies and promote civility and mutual respect regarding patients, coworkers, and members of the community.
- Nurses must advocate for policies that are inclusive and promote civility and human rights for all health care workers, patients, and others within the organization and community.
- Nurses must encourage all health care agencies to adopt and aggressively maintain policies, procedures, and practices that embrace inclusiveness, promote civility and mutual respect, contain methods for reporting violations, and require interventions to avoid recurrence.
- Nurses must work both within the profession and with other health care professionals, social workers, clergy, and advocacy organizations to create diverse, inclusive communities that promote, protect, and sustain high-quality, effective, efficient, and safe health care practices.
- Nurses in all environments and at all levels must embrace the concepts of justice and caring, diversity and inclusiveness, and civility and mutual respect as guiding principles within the provision of health care.
- Nurse researchers must support and conduct research that is inclusive in nature, including diverse populations and their health care needs.
- Nurse managers, supervisors, and administrators must assess policies to ensure support of inclusiveness, civility, and mutual respect, acknowledging that the lack of such policies may result in environments that fail to sustain high-quality, effective, efficient, and safe health care practices.
- Nurse educators must promote a diverse workforce by developing education practices to attract and retain students from all backgrounds. An increased number of diverse nurses in the workforce will begin to reflect the diversity of the overall population in the United States.
- Nurses must embrace a patient-centered approach responsive to the individual cultural needs and concerns of their patients and families.

From ANA Position Statement: The Nurse's Role in Addressing Discrimination: Protecting and Promoting Inclusive Strategies in Practice Settings, Policy, and Advocacy. Accessed June 8, 2023. www.nursingworld.org/~4ab207/globalassets/practiceandpolicy/nursing-excellence/ana-position-statements/social-causes-and-health-care/the-nurses-role-in-addressing-discrimination.pdf.

- Context (many factors that include family, cultural, spiritual, religious, economic, and legal)

Using this model, the nurse and medical providers can identify the conflicting principles, ascertain by weighing and balancing what should prevail, and turn to ethics literature and expert opinion when in doubt. To illustrate the use of this model, consider the following straightforward example.

An older adult woman with chronic obstructive pulmonary disease (COPD) on continuous oxygen for the past 2 years with shortness of breath with minimal exertion is admitted with COVID-19, sepsis, and respiratory failure. She has a previous history of two admissions to the ICU requiring intubation and mechanical ventilation. She is on a ventilator, receiving artificial nutrition through an oral gastric tube, intravenous fluids and vasopressors, and numerous antibiotics for pneumonia.

The patient does not have the capacity and does not have an advance directive. The patient's only child, an adult daughter, speaks to the team via teleconference and states her mother would not want to remain on the ventilator and requests that it be withdrawn. The treating physician believes that weaning the patient from the ventilator may be possible after the pneumonia is treated. The initial question is whether withdrawing the ventilator is ethically appropriate.

There is evidence of physiological futility (multisystem organ failure in the setting of preexisting end-stage COPD, and medical interventions would not reverse the decline). It is appropriate then to discuss the patient's condition with her family, with the goal of discontinuing life-sustaining interventions.

This discussion should be done with sensitivity, compassion, and empathy with the goal of involving the palliative care team for care to alleviate her symptoms and support the daughter and family until her death and beyond in their grief. The goals of care and communication with the family is complicated by the visitation restrictions in place due to the pandemic.

STRATEGIES FOR THE PROMOTION OF ETHICAL DECISION MAKING

The complexity of health care and ethical dilemmas encountered frequently in clinical practice demand the establishment of expertise in clinical ethics and mechanisms and processes for resolution.

Clinical ethics (also known as *health care ethics* or *bioethics*) arose directly from dilemmas in critical care situations, such as the availability of artificial cardiopulmonary support, dialysis, and organ transplantation in the past 40 years. Clinical ethics is now an established, interdisciplinary profession, and hospitals almost always have resources available to mitigate and resolve ethical problems.

Institutional Ethicists, Ethics Committees, and Ethics Consultation Services

Almost every hospital has an institutional ethics committee (IEC), and many have ethics consultation services or individual professional ethicists assigned to hospitals. IECs arose in response to ethical and legal dilemmas in the 1960s and 1970s. In some states, the law requires them, and they are strongly encouraged as part of accreditation by The Joint Commission as part of the requirement that hospitals have mechanisms for addressing ethical issues in patient care.

IECs were initially envisioned to provide education and foster ethical approaches to systemic and organizational issues. IECs still function this way at some facilities when individual ethicists or consultation services exist to assist providers and families at the bedside with ethical dilemmas. At others, IECs serve primarily as consultation services to assist with individual ethical problems.

Many facilities have specialized or subdivided IECs based on clinical service. Regardless of the person, service, or committee involved, every hospital should have one or more ways to assist with ethical problems at the bedside (ethics consultations). Ethics consultations can provide the various stakeholders with an informed "outside" perspective and use professional expertise to assist with resolution. Recommendations issued in response to ethics consultations are general guidance rather than mandates.

Ethics Rounds and Conferences

At hospitals with individual ethicists or consultation services, ethicists often round with other providers on each patient in critical care. Without this more structured approach, nurses may consider developing a standard method of conducting ethics rounds with the assistance of their facility's ethicist or a member of the IEC.

Ethics rounds can increase the early identification of risk factors for emerging ethical problems and allow for proactive resolution. An individual patient ethics conference may be scheduled to include appropriate stakeholders or a multidisciplinary group to discuss unit issues.

LEGAL ISSUES

Generally speaking, the law concerns minimum standards rather than best practices or even ethical practices. In other words, a practice that meets legal criteria is often far less than what meets ethical criteria or criteria for best practices. Nursing licensure is one example; licensure is a legal tool to protect the public. Holding a nursing license indicates only that a nurse has demonstrated the minimum basic competencies to practice as an entry-level nurse. Licensure does not set best practices.

Effective nursing is about more than minimal competencies. The National Council of State Boards of Nursing (NCSBN) is an organization that works to develop policy and consistent standards throughout the state licensing boards. The NCSBN defines nursing as (1) a scientific process founded on a professional body of knowledge, (2) a learned profession based on an understanding of the human condition across the life span and the relationship of a patient with others and within the environment, and (3) an art dedicated to caring for others.[51]

The following information about the law will assist nurses in navigating the increasingly complex and rapidly evolving health care system: (1) the basic foundations of law; (2) the differences between legal thresholds and quality and scope of practice; (3) the ways laws affect practice; and (4) and the ability of nurses to influence health law and policy.

ADMINISTRATIVE LAW: PROFESSIONAL REGULATION

Boards of Nursing and Nurse Practice Acts

For most nurses, the first professional interaction with a legal system is through the licensure process. The ability to practice as a licensed professional nurse is a privilege granted by the state. It is a function of each state's authority to promote and protect the health and welfare of its citizens.

State BONs are administrative bodies created by—and operate under—state nursing practice acts (NPAs). NPAs are state laws (statutes) written and passed by state lawmakers and signed by the governor. NPAs set out somewhat general standards for safe practice. BONs develop more specific rules (or regulations) for interpreting and enforcing the NPAs.

This process of empowering agencies is generally the same at the state and federal levels. Administrative agencies, such as BONs, are created and granted power under statutes written and passed by legislatures and signed by the governor (in the case of state law) or the president (in the case of federal law). Administrative agencies develop, propose, amend, and enforce specific regulations in their areas.

These regulations are developed or amended through a process of rulemaking that includes notice to and feedback from the public before finalization. Rulemaking allows agencies to adapt to changes in carrying out the statute without requiring the legislature to create or amend laws, which is usually a longer, less agile process.

For example, NPAs statutes might establish that nurses must have formal education in nursing before being licensed. The BON would then have regulations that explain what formal education means, such as degree and institutional accreditation requirements and the consequences to candidates for inaccurate representations about their education. In other words, BONs are responsible for "the interpretation and enforcement of the provisions" of NPAs.[26] The work of BONs is just one example of an administrative system but is the most relevant because BONs control the ability to practice.

Functions of Boards of Nursing

The regulation of nursing practice is intended to protect the health and safety of state citizens by (1) regulating the conditions of licensure, (2) regulating the scope of practice, (3) establishing a framework of standards of nursing practice, (4) removing incompetent or unsafe practitioners through disciplinary actions, and (5) prohibiting unlicensed persons from providing services reserved for licensed individuals. In addition, the regulation of nursing can enhance the professional status and the public's trust in nurses.

Scope of Practice

BONs maintain expectations for and limits of nursing practice in each state through the licensure of nurses and through challenges to nonnurses engaged in professional activities that intrude on the nursing scope of practice. *Scope of practice* generally refers to the broad range of activities nurses perform and manage in delivering care that "require education and training consistent with professional standards commensurate with the RN's education, demonstrated competencies, and experience."[27]

Scope of practice is framed broadly to account for the many professional nursing settings and roles and also to account for activities that are reserved for professional nurses and activities that may be delegated with appropriate supervision.

Scope of practice provisions are also intended to prevent unlicensed professionals from providing services reserved for licensed professionals. The absolute outside limits of the scope of practice are sometimes challenging to define and are occasionally the subject of disciplinary actions by BONs or other professional licensure boards.

The outcomes of these disciplinary actions are sometimes appealed to state courts. In some cases, these challenges arise from other professional licensing boards, such as state medical boards, in response to circumstances within their state. Several important legal cases have demonstrated the importance of the scope of practice. In *Sermchief v Gonzales*,[28] the Supreme Court of Missouri heard a case involving two nurses working with several rural Missouri physicians to provide women's health care services.

The nurses engaged in health counseling, routine pelvic examinations, testing such as Pap smears, and community education under standing orders from physicians. Quality of care was not an issue; all parties agreed the nurses provided excellent care and the patients were satisfied. The issue was whether they were practicing within the scope of nursing practice or were infringing on the scope of medical practice (practicing medicine without a license). The court held in favor of the nurses because their work was within the boundaries of the NPA in existence at the time and within the limits of the physicians' orders.

Standards of Practice

BONs typically develop state standards of nursing practice through rulemaking. The NCSBN publishes Model Rules for BONs to use as an example of appropriate standards.[51] These standards of practice communicate the expectations of safe and effective nursing practice within the scope of practice. State standards of practice also assist BONs in evaluating the ongoing practice of nursing. "The NPA may require safe practice, whereas the rules may specify a plan for safe practice."[29] Thus, to fully understand the expectations for and limitations of nursing in a particular state, it is necessary to review the BON's NPA and the regulations (also known as *rules).*

Nursing Practice Act

The NCSBN also publishes a Model Nursing Act (Model Act) and Model Administrative Rules (Model Rules) as example NPAs and regulations for individual states to adopt in part or entirely as their own NPA and BON regulations.[29] Actual state laws governing professional nursing practice vary from state to state in the degree to which they have adopted all or part of the current or previous model acts and rules. Nonetheless, the Model Act scope of practice provisions (Box 2.6) help illustrate the registered nurse's scope of practice.

In addition to standards developed by BONs, many specialty nursing organizations have developed standards of practice. The BON standards establish broad expectations of safety and efficacy, whereas specialty standards are aimed at fostering excellence in the specialized field.

An example of specialty standards is those developed by the AACN.[30] The AACN standards are presented in Box 2.7. These specialty standards help establish and measure quality care, and they often reflect a consensus opinion of experts in the particular specialty of appropriate nursing care.

Nursing Standards of Care

The extent to which specialty standards are introduced in a legal context varies widely from state to state. Of note, the legal term of the *standard of care* is not the same as the standards of practice. In some cases, specialty standards of practice or care have been introduced in court to help establish a legal standard of care, but not all courts will consider these. The legal standard of care and the use of specialty standards are discussed further in the following section on tort law.

BOX 2.6 Scope of Practice (Activities of Professional Nurses)

Model Nursing Act (Model Statutory Law)

The practice of registered nursing shall include:

1. Providing comprehensive nursing assessment of the health status of patients.
2. Collaborating with health care team to develop and coordinate an integrated patient-centered health care plan.
3. Developing the comprehensive patient-centered health care plan, including (a) applying knowledge based on the biological, psychological, and social aspects of the patient's condition; (b) participating in and establishing patient diagnoses; (c) setting goals to meet identified health care needs; and (d) prescribing nursing interventions.
4. Implementing nursing care through the execution of independent nursing strategies and the provision of regimens requested, ordered, or prescribed by authorized health care providers.
5. Evaluating responses to interventions and the effectiveness of the plan of care.
6. Provides education by (a) designing and implementing teaching plans based on patient needs or patient population; (b) teaching the theory and practice of nursing; and (c) educating others as appropriate.
7. Delegating nursing interventions to implement the plan of care while maintaining accountability of the outcome.
8. Delegates to another only those nursing measures for which that delegate has the necessary skills and competence to accomplish safely.
9. Assigning nursing interventions to implement the plan of care.
10. Providing for the maintenance of safe and effective nursing care rendered directly or indirectly.
11. Advocating the best interest of patients.
12. Communicating and collaborating with other health care providers in the management of health care and the implementation of the total health care regimen within and across care settings.
13. Managing, supervising, and evaluating the practice of nursing.
14. Teaching the theory and practice of nursing.
15. Participating in development of health care policies, procedures, and systems.
16. Wearing identification that clearly identifies the nurse as an RN when providing direct patient care, unless wearing identification creates a safety or health risk for either the nurse or the patient.
17. Other acts that require education and training consistent with professional standards as prescribed by the BON and commensurate with the RN's education, demonstrated competencies, and experience.

BON, State board of nursing; *RN*, registered nurse.
Modified from National Council of the State Boards of Nursing (NCSBN). *NCSBN Model Act.* NCSBN; 2012, revised 2021.

Tort Law: Negligence and Professional Malpractice, Intentional Torts

Tort Law

Many civil lawsuits for injuries fall under the legal heading of torts. Torts are civil lawsuits based on negligent actions, inactions, or intentional acts, such as assault, battery, or defamation. For the lay public, the standard for behavior for negligence is based on reasonableness or what a reasonably prudent person would do under the circumstances. This is also known as ordinary negligence.

In a professional capacity, individuals are judged on their professional standard of care. Nurses caring for acutely and critically ill patients may be alleged to have acted or failed to act in a manner inconsistent with the professional standard of care as part of a lawsuit that focuses in whole or in part on the alleged failure. This is professional malpractice or negligence law applied to professional behavior.

There are many types of cases based in tort law, but this chapter focuses on negligence and professional malpractice, the intentional torts of assault and battery. These laws will also be illustrated in specific clinical circumstances. These include respiratory management of acutely and critically ill patients and liability associated with blood transfusions, infection control, and informed consent.

Ordinary Negligence

Generally speaking, the standard for negligence is failing to meet the standard of care, which is what a reasonably prudent

BOX 2.7 Standards of Care for Acute and Critical Care Nursing

Standard 1: Assessment

The nurse obtains comprehensive data pertinent to the situation and/or patient's health.

Competencies

1. Collects data from the patient, family, other health care providers, and the community, as appropriate, to develop a holistic picture of the patient's needs or conditions
2. Prioritizes data collection based on patient characteristics related to the immediate condition and anticipated needs
3. Uses valid evidence-based assessment techniques, instruments, and tools
4. Documents relevant data in a clear and retrievable format

Standard 2: Diagnosis

The nurse analyzes and synthesizes data from the assessment in determining diagnoses or conditions relevant to care.

Competencies

1. Derives diagnoses and relevant conditions from the assessment data
2. Validates diagnoses with the patient, family, and other health care providers
3. Documents diagnoses and relevant conditions in a clear and retrievable format

Standard 3: Outcomes Identification

The nurse identifies optimal outcomes for the patient.

Competencies

1. Identifies outcomes from assessments and diagnoses in collaboration with the patient, family, and interprofessional team
2. Identifies preferences and values in formulating appropriate outcomes that meet diversity and cultural needs in collaboration with the patient, family, and interprofessional team
3. Considers associated risks, benefits, best available evidence, clinical expertise, and essential costs when formulating outcomes, to avoid placing unnecessary financial burdens on the patient and/or family
4. Modifies outcomes based on changes in a patient's condition or situation
5. Documents identified outcomes as measurable goals in a clear and retrievable format

Standard 4: Planning

The nurse caring for the patient develops a plan that prescribes strategies and alternatives to attain outcomes.

Competencies

1. Uses clinical judgment and inquiry in developing an individualized plan using best evidence
2. Collaborates with the patient, family, and interprofessional team to develop the plan
3. Establishes priorities and continuity of care within the plan (transfer of information/handoffs)
4. Includes strategies for health promotion/education and prevention of complications or injury
5. Considers associated risks, benefits, best evidence, clinical expertise, resources, and cost when developing the plan
6. Documents and provides handoff of the plan in a clear and retrievable manner

Standard 5: Implementation

The nurse caring for the patient implements the plan.

Competencies

1. Employs strategies to promote and maintain a safe environment
2. Coordinates implementation of the plan with the patient, family, and interprofessional team
3. Intervenes to prevent and minimize complications and alleviate suffering
4. Facilitates learning for patients, families, and the community
5. Provides age and developmentally appropriate care with respect to diversity
6. Documents implementation in a clear and retrievable format

Standard 6: Evaluation

The nurse evaluates processes and progress toward attainment of goals and outcomes.

Competencies

1. Conducts systematic and ongoing evaluations using evidence-based techniques, tools, and instruments
2. Collaborates with the patient, family, and interprofessional team in the evaluation process
3. Revises the assessment, diagnoses, outcomes identification, plan, and interventions based on information gained during the evaluation process
4. Documents the results of evaluations in a clear and retrievable format

Modified from American Association of Critical-Care Nurses. *AACN Scope and Standards for Progressive and Critical Care Nursing Practice.* AACN; 2019.

person would do under the same or similar circumstances. There are four criteria or for all negligence cases, duty, breach, causation, and harm:

- The nurse has a duty to deliver care based on professional standards.
- A breach of that duty occurs when the duty has not meet those standards.
- Causation becomes evident when negative outcomes occur.
- Harm is identified to the person that has monetary value.

All four elements must be satisfied for a case to go forward. For example, suppose a grocery store employee mops the floor but fails to block off the area or put up a "wet floor" sign, and a customer walks in the area, falls and breaks a hip, and is left with hospital bills and lost wages. The grocery store has a duty to its customers to behave as a reasonably prudent grocery store under the circumstances, which would include providing a reasonably safe environment and warning customers regarding areas of danger.

Failing to warn customers is a breach of that duty because the store failed to act as a reasonably prudent store under the circumstances. Because the customer had no warning, she walked on the wet floor, fell, and suffered the harm of a broken hip. The customer would not have sustained the broken hip if the area had been blocked off. Finally, there are monetary damages in the form of hospital bills and lost wages. This is an example of ordinary negligence in which any person could make a determination of what is reasonable in a given circumstance. A juror need not hear from a professional to determine what is reasonably prudent practice for the grocery store (standard for nonnegligent behavior) in this case.

Negligence in the professional health care context differs in that expert testimony is needed to establish what a reasonably prudent practitioner would do under the circumstances (the standard of care). These cases are referred to as *professional negligence or professional malpractice.*

Professional Malpractice

Although negligence claims apply to anyone, malpractice requires the alleged wrongdoer to have special standing as a professional. In civil cases alleging wrongdoing by health care professionals, the terms *malpractice* and professional *negligence* are used interchangeably. Malpractice is a negligence action applied to a professional, as the court in *Candler General Hospital Inc. v McNorrill* explained.[31]

Suppose a nurse's actions or inactions are inconsistent with the standard of care, causing harm to the patient. In that case, the nurse (and usually the nurse's employer) is subject to liability in professional negligence (meaning they may be ordered to pay the patient for that harm.) Just as in ordinary negligence, the person bringing the lawsuit (plaintiff) must prove the elements of negligence. In the health care context, the patient-plaintiffs (person[s] bringing the lawsuit) must prove

- that the nurse had a duty to care for the patient,
- that the nurse breached that duty by deviating from the standard of care, and
- that the breach actually caused the
- harm that would not have occurred in the absence of negligence.

These four elements are described further in Table 2.3. The legal standard of care for nurses is established by expert testimony of a nurse in a similar practice area. It is generally "the care that an ordinarily prudent *nurse* would perform under the same circumstances." In the case of specialized nurses, the standard of care is measured against the "learning, care, and skill normally possessed and exercised by practitioners of that specialty under the same or similar circumstances."[32]

The standard of care determination focuses more on the accepted practice of competent nurses rather than the best practice of excellent nurses (which may be reflected in some specialty standards of practice). In addition to expert testimony, courts may rely on multiple types of evidence to establish the standard of care. (See Table 2.3.)

Duty

Once a nurse-patient relationship is established, the nurse assumes the duty to provide care within the standard of care. This duty cannot be waived or overridden by the instructions of a physician or hospital administrator. *Lunsford v Board of Nurse Examiners*[33] illustrates this principle. In this case, Donald Floyd arrived at an emergency department (ED) in Texas complaining of chest pain and pressure that radiated down his left arm. Mr. Floyd was accompanied by Ms. Farrell, who asked a physician sitting at the nurses' station to examine Mr. Floyd. The physician told Ms. Farrell that Nurse Lunsford would interview Mr. Floyd before he would see a physician.

The physician then instructed Nurse Lunsford to transfer Mr. Floyd to a neighboring hospital located 24 miles away because the equipment that would likely be needed to treat Mr. Floyd was already in use by another patient. Nurse Lunsford then interviewed Mr. Floyd and suspected cardiac involvement. Because of the transfer instruction that she received from the physician, Nurse Lunsford instructed Ms. Farrell to drive Mr. Floyd to the neighboring hospital and to speed and drive with her flashers on.

Reportedly, Nurse Lunsford also asked Ms. Farrell if she knew cardiopulmonary resuscitation and suggested that she might need to perform cardiopulmonary resuscitation at some point on the way. Within approximately 5 miles of the Harlingen ED, Mr. Floyd died as a result of cardiac arrest in Ms. Farrell's car.

An administrative complaint was subsequently filed with the Texas Board of Nurse Examiners, alleging negligence and challenging Nurse Lunsford's nursing licensure. After a hearing on the matter, the Texas Board of Nurse Examiners suspended the license of Nurse Lunsford for 1 year. Nurse Lunsford appealed the decision, and the court determined that Nurse Lunsford and other nurses who are similarly situated have a duty to (1) evaluate the status of persons who are ill and seeking professional help and (2) implement care needed to stabilize a patient's condition and to prevent complications.

TABLE 2.3 Elements for Professional Malpractice[32]

Element	Description
Duty	• Duty to the injured party is the first element of a malpractice case and is established through the existence of the nurse-patient relationship. Nurses assume a duty to the patient to provide care consistent with the standard of care when the nurse-patient relationship is established. Case law recognizes the nurse-patient relationship as a separate and distinct relationship from the doctor-patient relationship. • It is a prerequisite for determining whether a nurse owes the patient a duty to provide care in accordance with the requisite standard of care. If a nurse shows that they (1) were not assigned to that particular patient on the date that the negligence allegedly occurred or (2) were not working on the day or at the time the negligence allegedly occurred, there was no relationship and, therefore, no duty. Because no duty is imposed on the nurse, negligence allegations will fail.
Breach	• Breach is the failure to act consistently within applicable standards of care. For a nurse to be found negligent, the patient-plaintiff must establish that the nurse had a duty to provide care and failed to provide care consistent with those standards. Moreover, the nurse's failure, or breach, must have caused the damages about which the patient-plaintiff seeks redress. A breach of duty does not exist if the standard of care is met.
Harm Caused by the Breach	• Patient-plaintiffs must prove that the nurse breached their duty to the patient and that the breach caused the patient to sustain injuries or damages for which they seek monetary remuneration. Causation of the harm is pivotal in civil cases filed against nurses. If patient-plaintiffs fail to establish that some act or omission directly resulted in the harm or if something else can be shown to have caused the harm, recovery will be denied.
Damages	• Damages are the monetary value or cost of the injury suffered. For liability to be imposed against a nurse caring for an acutely or critically ill patient, that patient must prove that something the nurse did or failed to do was inconsistent with the standard of care and the inconsistency caused harm or injury with a monetary value. Patient-plaintiffs in a malpractice case can usually point to additional medical bills associated with their injuries to satisfy this element.

According to the Texas Court of Appeals, Nurse Lunsford failed to act reasonably and breached her duty to Mr. Floyd when she failed to (1) assess him, (2) inform the physician of the life-threatening nature of his condition, and (3) take appropriate action to stabilize him and prevent his death. The court also pointed out that hospital policy or physician orders do not relieve nurses of their duty to patients.

Breach

In *Sparks v St. Luke's Regional Medical Center*,[34] the family of Thomas Sparks sued St. Luke's Regional Medical Center and treating physicians, alleging that their negligence resulted in Thomas Sparks sustaining brain damage after he was extubated. The case reached the Idaho Supreme Court. The court concluded that although Mr. Sparks suffered severe harm, no breach of duty existed, and the evidence established the standard of care for extubation and subsequent hospital care was met.

The *Sparks* case demonstrated that courts often consider many sources of evidence in determining the standard of care. These may include applicable NPAs; specialty practice standards; job descriptions; organizational policies, procedures, protocols, and pathways; and other reference sources, including case law, journal articles, textbooks, and other manuscripts.

Actions that are consistent with professional practice standards may be used as evidence that the nurse did not breach their duty to patients. Even if not used as evidence for the standard of care, these standards guide quality nursing care. Nurses caring for acutely and critically ill patients should practice per the practice specialty standards issued by the AACN. These standards provide guidance for nurses and increasingly offer definitive guidance in courtrooms.

For example, in *Newsom v Lake Charles Memorial Hospital*,[35] the court used AACN standards along with expert testimony to evaluate the action of critical care nurses caring for a patient who died shortly after the removal of an intraaortic balloon pump. Viewing the totality of the circumstances, the court determined that the hospital, through its nurses, was negligent in properly alerting the patient's physician of a 60-point drop in systolic blood pressure and failing to monitor the patient for bleeding closely.

Documents or policies specific to the nurse's employer or practice setting may also be used to inform the appropriate standard of care. For example, a nurse's job description or employment contract may contain provisions requiring a nurse to act or refrain from acting in a specific manner and within a specific period. Failure to adhere to those provisions could give rise to negligent causes of action wherein the patient-plaintiff asserts that the nurse failed to act in accordance with their job description or employment contract.

Accordingly, job descriptions and employment contracts should reflect the standard of care and articulate reasonable behavior expectations. Nurses caring for acutely and critically ill patients must act in a manner consistent with organizational policies, procedures, protocols, and clinical pathways. Failure to do so may result in liability if a patient is harmed because of the failure. For example, in *Teffeteller v University of Minnesota*,[36] a nurse's failure to follow an institutional protocol resulted in liability after a critically ill pediatric patient died of opioid toxicity.

Harm Caused by the Breach

McMullen v Ohio State University Hospitals[37] dealt with the causation issue and was ultimately decided by the Ohio Supreme Court. In *McMullen*, an intubated patient on mechanical ventilation experienced oxygen desaturation and hypotension and exhibited cyanosis and dyspnea. The nurse also reported an audible "squeak," which was thought to be a cuff leak on the endotracheal tube. The nurse believed the patient was dying and paged the on-call physicians "stat." However, the nurse removed the patient's endotracheal tube before the physicians arrived. It took over 20 minutes to successfully reintubate the patient; the patient never regained consciousness and died 7 days later.

The patient's estate brought a wrongful death cause of action against the Ohio State University Hospitals based on the nurse's negligence in removing the endotracheal tube (thereby causing the loss of an airway). After appeals to the Ohio Supreme Court, the court held the nurse's actions caused the harm because the removal of the patient's endotracheal tube in an uncontrolled environment was negligent and set into motion a chain of events that directly caused the patient to die of anoxic brain injury.

Damages

The number of nurses being named defendants in these cases is increasing, especially for advanced practice nurses. Nurses caring for acutely and critically ill patients need to carefully consider whether to purchase professional liability insurance and, if so, the necessary amount and type of coverage. Most institutions will provide some level of malpractice insurance coverage for nurses, but the amount and circumstances under which each nurse is covered are important considerations. In addition, institutional policies will generally not cover actions against nurses brought by the state BON.

Professional Malpractice and the Nursing Process

Malpractice claims may be premised on care delivered at any point from the moment a nurse-patient relationship is established to patient discharge. What constitutes reasonable care has been the focus of many cases filed against health care professionals and the hospitals in which they practice. For nurses, there seems to be an emerging trend. Suppose the nurse reasonably executes every component of the nursing process by assessing, planning, implementing, and evaluating the care per the requisite standard of care. In that case, reasonable care will have been provided. However, if the nurse fails with regard to a single component of the nursing process, care provided to an acutely or critically ill patient may be deemed insufficient, unreasonable, and negligent. The following cases are examples of malpractice resulting from failures in particular stages of the nursing process.

Assessment Failure: Failure to Assess and Analyze the Level of Care Needed by the Patient

Nurses caring for acutely and critically ill patients have a duty to assess and analyze the level of care their patients need. Where a nurse allegedly fails to fulfill this responsibility, liability for negligence may be threatened. *Brandon HMA, Inc. v Bradshaw*[38] demonstrates how courts handle failure to assess and analyze the level of care required.

In *Brandon*, Dawn Bradshaw sustained permanent injuries because of negligence by the nursing staff during her hospitalization for bacterial pneumonia. After a chest tube was inserted, nurses failed to assess or take vital signs on Ms. Bradshaw for 4 hours and 30 minutes. When Ms. Bradshaw was finally assessed, she was nauseated, disoriented, sweating profusely, and unable to follow verbal commands. Approximately 10 minutes later, she experienced cardiac arrest. Although Ms. Bradshaw was resuscitated, she sustained a brain injury from anoxia. She was discharged to a rehabilitation facility specializing in the treatment of brain injury.

The case was tried before a jury; the jury agreed that Ms. Bradshaw sustained permanent, severe brain damage related to oxygen deprivation because of the nursing staff's negligence. The nurse's failure to assess Ms. Bradshaw made it impossible to intervene earlier to prevent the cardiac arrest and, therefore, her oxygen deprivation. The jury awarded Ms. Bradshaw $9 million in damages.

To withstand allegations of failure to assess and analyze, it is essential for nurses not only to assess and analyze the level of care needed by patients but also to document their assessment findings and all actions taken to care for patients properly. Failure to assess and analyze the situation and to document the assessment findings, the interventions, and the patient's response to those interventions exposes the nurse and, as in the *Brandon* case, the hospital to liability for negligence. See Informatics Box 2.8 regarding nurses' overreliance on technology.

Assessment Failure: Failure to Assess and Clarify the Patient's Condition

Upon assuming care, nurses are responsible for obtaining appropriate and complete information on a patient's condition. This includes adequately assessing the patient and clarifying and reporting any discrepancies. A case from Alabama illustrates these responsibilities. In *Brookwood Health Services v Borden*,[39] Mr. Borden developed severe back and leg pain and new-onset numbness in his legs at home a few days after a lumbar laminectomy.

After a phone consultation with his surgeon, Mr. Borden was taken to the ED, where he exhibited some motor deficits to his toes and ankles; he could lift his legs off the bed and was continent. Computed tomography scan revealed a small hematoma. Mr. Borden was admitted to the hospital around midnight under his surgeon's care with orders that included neurovascular checks every 2 hours and an order to "call admitting physician for any questions, problems, change of status, or for further orders."

The nurse receiving Mr. Borden on the unit, Nurse Tolbert, assessed him at 12:15 a.m. and documented that he was wet from incontinence, could not move his legs, and had weak pedal pulses. Nurse Tolbert did not notify the physician or check his ED records. At trial, Nurse Tolbert said she had received an oral report from an ED nurse and that his condition was consistent with that report. However, she did not document that report.

The day nurse received a report from Tolbert and documented an assessment at 7:00 a.m. consistent with Tolbert's. Mr. Borden's physician discovered the change in his condition a few hours later and ordered an emergency computed tomography scan that revealed a large hematoma compressing the cauda equina that required emergency surgery. Mr. Borden was left permanently disabled with chronic pain, incontinence, significant mobility problems, and impotence.

Based on the nurse's failure to adequately assess Mr. Borden; consider his present status in light of his clinical history (e.g., he was walking and continent less than 8 hours earlier); and clarify Mr. Borden's status via discussion with Mr. Borden, the ED record, or the physician, Mr. Borden sued the hospital for negligence that resulted in his permanent disability that may have been prevented with earlier intervention and emergency surgery.

BOX 2.8 Informatics

Overreliance on Technology by Nurses

- There can be no question that technology has advanced and enhanced health care treatments and outcomes over the years.
- Artificial intelligence, data input, algorithm, decision making and analysis can take the place and time of busy clinicians in assisting medical issues to resolution.
- However, the expertise of clinicians and critical thinking processes behind every action, algorithm, and decision must be perfectly matched with that of the expert clinicians.
- The reality is technology is fallible. If technology is fallible, how much should nurses rely on it?[1]
- As health care continues to grow and expand, we are seeing more technologies connected physically to patients for monitoring; delivering various treatments and medications; and providing specimen testing, both continually and at intervals.
- Artificial intelligence is rapidly advancing into health care, which is scary to many people, not knowing its full impact outside of health care let alone what it might be capable of with humans and data dealing with health and disease.
- Technology is "intended to be beneficial to your nursing practice. It should be designed so that it not only supports your practice but also makes it safer." [2, p15]
- Nurses are at the frontlines of new technology for patient care that is coming rapidly and sometimes even without much notice. According to Harrington, nurses are not the only health care clinicians who can rely too much on technology.
- Additionally, there is a variation in how nurses trust technology, their levels of experience, workload, amount of fatigue, and other factors that can influence the extent to which they actually rely on the technology at any given point in time.[1]
- Harrington made the following recommendations for nursing practice to increase awareness of the limitations of technology, including the following:
  1. "Hospitals and health care systems purchasing nurse-facing technologies should carefully examine published research on reliability performed by vendors and researchers.
  2. Training on nurse-facing technologies should include:
     a. The purpose of the technology in achieving specific patient-centered goals
     b. The role of technology in patient safety
     c. How the technology supports nurses physical and mental tasks
     d. Automation bias and automation complacency so that not too much trust is placed in the technology
     e. How nurses can monitor technology as a part of patient care processes"[1, p.86]
- It is important for nurses to adapt their practice as time moves forward, always questioning if something does "not seem just right" or that sixth sense nursing feeling that things don't match up.
- Refer to Harrington's article for more detailed recommendations for practice and technology. She concluded her article with these wise statements: "Nursing expertise in today's technology-intensive practice environment requires us to change how we think; it does not replace our need to think. We need to expand our nursing expertise to include knowledge of how technology influences our practice and our role in making that influence a positive one and avoiding negative consequences."[1, p.85]

The jury awarded him $5 million in damages. The Alabama Supreme Court ultimately changed that award based on the failure of Mr. Borden's attorney to present adequate expert testimony of the nursing standard of care; however, the facts of the case serve as an example of how nursing vigilance or lack thereof can severely affect a patient's life and lead to liability.

Planning Failure: Failure to Appropriately Diagnose

Nurses caring for acutely and critically ill patients must plan effective courses of treatment, and such a course of treatment depends on a proper diagnosis. Historically, failure to diagnose cases have been filed against physicians rather than nurses. However, nurses who identify patient signs and symptoms may find themselves the target of a failure to diagnose case. They must be aware that liability may be imposed if the plan of care is based on an erroneous or missed diagnosis if nursing staff fails to document or notify providers of findings.

Implementation Failure: Failure to Communicate Patient Findings in a Timely Manner

Nurses caring for acutely and critically ill patients must promptly communicate troublesome patient findings. Failure to properly communicate patient findings can be devastating for patients and can be the reason that patients file malpractice causes of action. *Denesia v St. Elizabeth Community Health Center*[40] exemplifies how courts handle these kinds of cases. In *Denesia*, it was alleged that the death of patient Lucille Denesia was the result of the failure of the nursing staff to appropriately notify the physician in a timely manner of an alarmingly high partial thromboplastin time (PTT) and change in patient status indicative of a neurologic compromise.

Ms. Denesia was admitted to the hospital with a suspected embolic stroke secondary to her history of atrial fibrillation. To prevent further emboli, anticoagulation therapy, including heparin injection, a heparin drip, and oral warfarin (Coumadin), was ordered, along with a PTT level 4 hours after initiation. The PTT level was obtained at 4:00 p.m. and 5:30 p.m. The laboratory notified the nurse that the level was 200 seconds (far beyond the therapeutic range). The nurse reported placing a call to the physician's answering service, but she did not follow up.

Shortly after 6:30 p.m., the nurse noted a 6-second arrhythmia, and Ms. Denesia was vomiting with headache pain. The nurse called Ms. Denesia's cardiologist but did not document her conversation and could not recall the details; the cardiologist contended that she reported only the arrhythmia, not the PTT level or status change. Approximately 75 minutes later, the nurse spoke with the primary treating physician; again, she did not document the conversation and could not remember what she had told him.

The primary treating physician testified that he was not informed of the PTT result but ordered the intravenous infusion of heparin to be reduced. Over the next several hours, Ms. Denesia had multiple vomiting episodes despite repeated administration of antinausea medication. She slept for a few hours but awoke with vomiting followed by lethargy, motor weakness, and other symptoms of neurologic compromise. The primary physician was notified; he discontinued the heparin and transferred the patient to the critical care unit. Ms. Denesia lapsed into a coma and died of a massive cerebral hemorrhage.

The case was appealed to the Supreme Court of Nebraska, where the justices ordered that the case be retried, but the parties settled before a retrial; the outcome is unavailable. The case provides a cautionary tale on the importance of monitoring patient status, communicating changes, and documenting those communications. For nurses caring for acutely and critically ill patients, it is imperative that interactions with physicians, whether in person or over the telephone, be documented, including the information conveyed during those interactions. This litigation might have been avoided if the nurse had taken the time to document what she told the cardiologist and the primary treating physician.

Implementation Failure: Failure to Take Appropriate Action

Cases from across the United States continue to affirm that it is the nurse's responsibility to take affirmative action when action is indicated. *Garcia v United States*[41] is one such case. In *Garcia*, Candido Garcia was admitted to a Veterans Administration Medical Center to remove chronic subdural hematomas with the insertion of Jackson-Pratt drains and revision of a ventriculoperitoneal shunt. He arrived at the unit around 6:25 p.m. His nurse briefly assessed him and went to lunch. Around 7:00 p.m., his daughter reported that her father was making strange hand movements, snorting noises, and emitting white bubbles from his mouth. Mr. Garcia's wife also noted the changes and reported the occurrence to another nurse on the ward, who dismissed her concerns.

At around 7:30 p.m., Mr. Garcia's nurse returned from lunch and found him unconscious and red blood in his surgical drains. The nurse did not document actions taken to alert Mr. Garcia's physicians, and his physicians reported they received a routine page shortly before 8:00 p.m. They, therefore, did not see Mr. Garcia until 8:15 p.m. Although he underwent an emergency craniotomy for bleeding, the delay in obtaining proper medical assistance resulted in a severe long-term disability; he had quadriplegia, required a tracheostomy, and had cognitive impairments. The hospital was liable for negligence based on the inaction of the nurses, and Mr. Garcia was awarded more than $2.3 million in damages. In reaching its decision, the court found that the nursing staff should have recognized the emergency nature of the situation and taken proper steps to notify the attending physician.

Failure to take appropriate action in cases involving acutely and critically ill patients has included not only issues regarding physician notification but also failure to follow physician orders,[42,43] failure to treat properly,[44] and failure to administer medication appropriately.[45–48] To avoid allegations of failure to take appropriate action, nurses caring for acutely and critically ill patients must recognize the signs and symptoms of complications and patient compromise. Nurses must also ensure that those signs and symptoms are communicated to the physician in a timely manner and take other affirmative action that is authorized and appropriate. Patient findings, interventions and actions taken, and patient responses to interventions must be documented.

Implementation Failure: Failure to Document

Nurses caring for acutely and critically ill patients are required not only to take appropriate action but also to accurately document their findings, interventions performed, and patients' responses to interventions. Failure to thoroughly and accurately document any aspect of care gives rise to negligence causes of action.

Haney v Alexander,[48] a case from North Carolina, demonstrates how courts and juries deal with a nurse's failure to document properly. In *Haney*, a nurse caring for a patient experiencing atrial fibrillation failed to take, record, and communicate all the patient's vital signs and failed to properly document medication orders and administration, leading to a double dose. Shortly after the second dose of medication, the patient was found dead.

The court of appeals concluded that the nurse was negligent in several respects, including failure to document vital signs, medication orders, and medication administration, and that the nurse's negligence contributed to the patient's death. The *Haney* case and many other cases discussed so far illustrate the consequences of inadequate documentation of care delivered, communications with other team members, interventions and actions taken, and the patient's response to interventions and actions. Failure to thoroughly document prevents nurses from defending their actions in the event they are accused of professional malpractice.

Implementation Failure: Failure to Preserve Patient Privacy

Nurses have a legal duty to preserve patient privacy and confidentiality. State and federal statutes and case law affirms this duty. For example, in *Randi A.J. v Long Island Surgical Center*,[44] the patient was awarded more than $300,000 in damages after a nurse disclosed her confidential information to the patient's mother; furthermore, the patient had given the surgical center specific instructions not to call her home, as she wished to keep her information private. The nurse's failure to preserve the patient's privacy and the facility's lack of a procedure or policy for preserving privacy resulted in their liability.

In addition, nurses' actions could expose their employers to severe penalties from the federal government for violations of federal laws, such as the Health Insurance Portability and Accountability Act (HIPAA).[49]

Nurses can ensure that the privacy of acutely and critically ill patients is protected by following patient directives and institutional policies and procedures, which should comply with state and federal privacy laws. Nurses must also avoid any discussions about specific patients with anyone except other health care professionals involved in the patient's care. Discussions about specific patients are never appropriate in public areas, such as elevators, cafeterias, gift shops, and parking lots.

Evaluation Failure: Failure to Act as a Patient Advocate

From admission to discharge, nurses have a duty to act as a patient advocate. For nurses caring for acutely and critically ill patients, this duty imposes the responsibility to evaluate the care being given to patients. The landmark failure to advocate case was *Darling v Charleston Community Memorial Hospital*,[50] a case that was decided by the Illinois Supreme Court. Dorrence Darling II was an 18-year-old athlete treated at Charleston Community Memorial Hospital after a leg fracture. Mr. Darling's fractured leg was placed in a plaster cast and in traction.

Shortly after the cast was applied, he began to complain of new, severe pain in the casted leg, and his toes protruding from the cast became swollen and discolored; later, the toes were cold and insensitive to tactile stimulation. Over the next 3 days, the physician cut small notches in the cast around the toes, cut 3 inches off the cast from the foot, and finally used a saw to split the sides of the cast and, in the process, cut both sides of Mr. Darling's broken leg.

The nursing staff noted blood, drainage, and a terrible odor by this time. At no point did the nurses advocate for more aggressive treatment or a second opinion or notify the hospital administration. Mr. Darling was transferred to another hospital 14 days after his admission. Eventually, he required a below-the-knee amputation because of the severe necrotic tissue secondary to circulatory compromise from improper casting.

A jury found the hospital liable for Mr. Darling's injuries through the negligent actions of the nursing staff and the physician. The case was appealed to the Illinois Supreme Court, which upheld the verdict, stating that the nursing staff failed to assess circulation properly, failed to recognize that circulatory compromise was occurring promptly, and therefore failed to prevent the irreversible effects of prolonged inadequate circulation. Had they recognized the significance of the symptoms, the nursing staff could have exercised their duty to inform hospital authorities so that appropriate action could be taken. Because they failed to act as a patient advocate, Dorrence lost his leg, and the hospital was liable for their failure.

The courts continue to hold that all nurses, including nurses caring for acutely and critically ill patients, have a nondelegatable duty to act as patient advocates. Failure to act as a patient advocate exposes the nurse and the hospital to substantial liability and, more importantly, exposes patients to life-altering and life-ending complications that could have been avoided. Advocating for the patient means taking concerns up the chain of command. Simply documenting concerns is insufficient to protect the nurse from liability.

Somewhat different, yet similar, is the case of *Rowe v Sisters of Pallottine*.[51] Mr. Rowe was seen in an ED after a motorcycle accident. He reported pain in his left knee, numbness, and an absent pulse was noted in his left foot. The ED physician discharged Mr. Rowe with instructions to return if his symptoms worsened.

The nurse caring for Mr. Rowe repeatedly assessed Mr. Rowe, questioned the physician's decision to discharge Mr. Rowe, and extensively documented her concerns in the nursing notes, especially regarding the lack of a pulse. She also informed Mr. Rowe's parents, who were with him, that there was no pulse in the foot. At trial, she explained her documentation as an effort to "cover herself."

Nonetheless, the jury awarded Mr. Rowe nearly $1 million, partly based on the nurse's negligence in failing to advocate for the patient properly. The nurses had breached the standard of care by not adequately advocating for the patient when he was discharged with unexplained and unaddressed symptoms. The court explained that nurses were obligated to take their concerns up the chain of command.

Wrongful Death

Wrongful death cases are a variation of negligence action in which the harm is the individual's death. Similar to ordinary negligence, wrongful death claims can also be brought against nonprofessionals.

However, in the professional health care context, these claims are identical to professional negligence cases except that the harm caused by the professionals is the death of the patient, and the plaintiff is the survivor of the patient, such as a spouse or adult child.

For families and health care professionals, wrongful death cases are among the most traumatic. In these cases, the life-and-death nature of the health care experience is exposed. In reviewing these kinds of cases, one learns that what is at issue is rarely the use, misuse, or malfunction of sophisticated, cutting-edge technology or the miscalculation of a complex formula.

On the contrary, a review of wrongful death cases suggests that the alleged failures are typically foundational matters of patient care and critical thinking. For instance, failure to thoroughly assess a patient, to take vital signs, to properly administer medication, or to administer portable oxygen to a patient with respiratory compromise has been the focus of most of the wrongful death cases discussed in this chapter.

To avoid wrongful death liability, nurses caring for acutely and critically ill patients must remain vigilant, recognize the signs and symptoms of complications and compromise, and take affirmative action to advocate for the patient's best interest.

Negligent Informed Consent

Negligent informed consent is a special cause of action in negligence that evolved as paternalism in health care was being rejected in favor of honoring patient autonomy. The foundational case in this area is *Canterbury v Spence*.[52] In Canterbury, a 19-year-old typist underwent a laminectomy for ongoing back pain. Before the surgery, he was told that he would need to undergo a laminectomy only to correct what the doctor suspected was a ruptured disc.

The patient's mother inquired whether the operation was serious, to which the doctor replied, "Not any more than any other operation." After the operation, the patient suffered ascending paralysis, necessitating emergency surgery. Years later, the patient had ongoing hemiparesis and bowel and bladder incontinence.

The court announced a new negligence action for failure to obtain informed consent and explained that informed consent legally requires the provider to disclose the following: (1) the nature and purpose of the proposed treatment, (2) the alternatives to that treatment (including doing nothing), (3) the benefits of the treatment, and (4) the material risks of the treatment. To succeed, a plaintiff must show that (1) the consent process was deficient, (2) the patient relied on that deficient consent process, and (3) the patient would not have undergone the procedure if the consent process had been adequate.

Assault and Battery

Assault and battery are examples of intentional torts (rather than negligence) frequently brought against health care providers. Although they are often used together, they are actually two separate torts.[53]

Assault is any intentional act that creates imminent apprehension of harmful or offensive contact with the plaintiff. With assault, no actual contact is necessary. Battery is any intentional act that brings about actual harmful or offensive contact with the plaintiff. *Harmful* means physical harm, whereas *offensive* means contact that a reasonable person would consider offensive under the circumstances.

In health care cases, patient consent is a defense to these claims. Consent can be general or limited in scope. Assault may be alleged if a patient was aware that they would be touched in a manner not authorized by informed consent. For example, the act of telling a patient that they will be restrained may be assault.

Battery occurs if the health care professional touches the patient in an unauthorized manner. The act of restraining a patient without consent is battery. Another defense to assault and battery is an emergency situation. Thus, cutting a patient's throat to create an emergency tracheostomy to create an airway may be justified, whereas cutting a patient's neck on the wrong side in opposition to the informed consent may be battery. It did not matter that the surgery was performed competently and, in fact, benefited the patient. Every patient has a right to say what is done with their body, and allowing battery actions acknowledges individual dignity and autonomy.

CONSTITUTIONAL LAW: PATIENT DECISION MAKING

U.S. Constitutional Right for Self-Determination (14th Amendment)

Patient autonomy or self-determination is a right guaranteed by state law and the U.S. Constitution under the 14th Amendment. The right of competent adult patients to refuse treatment is well established.

This right has evolved from the laws of informed consent, the laws of assault and battery (the right to be free from fear of harm and unwanted touching), and historic legal rights granted to individuals to say what is done with their own bodies. The U.S. Supreme Court described this as the right to "possession and control of his own person, free from all restraint or interference of others, unless by clear and unquestionable authority of law."[54]

Patients with Decision-Making Capacity

Decision-making capacity means a person has the ability to (1) take in and understand information, (2) process the information in accordance with their own personal values and goals, (3) make a decision based on the information, and (4) communicate the decision. A person does not lack decision-making capacity merely because the decision is at odds with what others would decide, even if it seems foolish.[1] A person with decision-making capacity is often described as having capacity or as competent.

In the health care setting, a *competent adult* patient has the right to refuse even life-sustaining treatment for any reason without regard for that individual's motivations. *Bouvia v Superior Court*[56] is representative of this principle. In *Bouvia*, a young woman with significant mobility disabilities refused to eat, and the facility in which she resided placed a nasogastric tube in Ms. Bouvia against her will out of concern that she was starving to death.

The facility also subjected her to countless competency and psychiatric evaluations, all indicating she was fully competent (or had decision-making capacity). Ms. Bouvia sued the facility, asking the court to issue an order preventing them from treating her against her will. The facility countered by arguing that Ms. Bouvia should not be allowed to accept their treatment of her in some respects (basic skin care, mobility, wound care, and pain medications) and refuse it in others (force feedings).

The court strongly disagreed with the facility and held, on constitutional grounds, that because she was a competent adult who understood the consequences of her decisions, she was free to consent to some but not all treatments and that she could not be compelled to accept food.

It is now well settled that competent adult patients may refuse treatment (in all or part) for any reason or no reason at all. U.S. law values individual autonomy to such a degree that a competent patient's wishes can rarely be legally overruled. However, no constitutional right is absolute, and there are legal frameworks for determining when a competing state interest may outweigh an individual right.

For example, the right to refuse treatment or restrictions on movement can, in extreme situations, be overcome by the state's interest in the health and safety of citizens. Mandatory quarantine after exposure to lethal infections, such as Ebola, is one such example. In the typical health care setting, there is little legal justification to override the wishes of a competent patient to *refuse* medical treatment. The reverse is not true: Patients have no constitutional right to demand treatment.

Critical care nurses are involved in many instances of refusal of treatment or the decision to withdraw or withhold possible treatment. This situation is difficult regardless of whether the patient has decision-making capacity, and nurses need to remember that there are times when the legal rights of patients and what feels like the "right thing to do" will match and times when these will seem at odds. Health care decisions become most complex when patients lose the capacity to make their own decisions.

These decisions can also be problematic for patients who were never competent to make their own decisions. Navigating the law surrounding the right to refuse treatment in patients who do not have decision-making capacity is much more legally complicated than for patients with decision-making capacity.

Patients Without Decision-Making Capacity

Patients without decision-making capacity include previously competent individuals (individuals who reached adulthood but lost competence because of illness or injury), individuals who were never competent (individuals born with severe to profound cognitive disabilities), individuals who are not yet competent (primarily children younger than the age of majority), and individuals with fluctuating competence (e.g., individuals with cyclic disorders, such as the manic phase of bipolar disorder, that can seriously impair decision making).

The law allows for others to stand in their place as surrogate decision makers. The law also imposes standards of judgment for surrogate decision makers to guide and evaluate decisions.

Numerous legal mechanisms exist that can simplify the legal issues surrounding decision making for patients without decision-making capacity. The ethical and emotional issues are much more nuanced. State laws may specify categories of individuals who may make decisions for patients who have lost capacity (often called *statutory surrogates*). State probate laws allow for the appointment of a guardian to make some or all decisions for individuals who have more sustained loss of capacity.

Adults who have capacity can plan for decisions and appoint decision makers to direct their future care through advance directives (statements of wishes in future situations or the appointment of a future decision maker in the event they should lose capacity). These include, but are not limited to, living wills, individual directives, and durable powers of attorney. The legal requirements and analyses are more stringent for decisions that may directly affect life, including decisions to forgo or withdraw treatment at the end of life.

Never and Not Yet Competent Patients

Competent adults can refuse treatment for any reason, even if others believe it is in opposition to their best interests. However, the law imposes a best interest standard for patients who are not yet competent (i.e., children) and patients who were never competent. The standard is self-explanatory; parents and legal guardians of children have a legal obligation to make informed decisions based on the best interests of the patient. As a child matures, there are increased legal obligations to involve the patient in health care decision making based on what is developmentally appropriate in each situation.

Occasionally the judgment of a parent or guardian will inevitably clash with that of the provider or the maturing child. Every effort should be made by the nurse and the extended health care team to facilitate discussion, understanding, and resolution without resorting to the courts. However, there are procedures in every state to petition the court on an emergent basis to evaluate and rule on what is in the patient's best interest. A common example in critical care involves courts requesting an override of parents refusing blood administration to their children based on religious objections. Courts should consider the situation's totality in making such a determination. Factors such as the likelihood of success in ordering such an intervention, the degree of invasion involved, the patient's prognosis, and any expressed wishes of the child are all considered.

Previously Competent Patients

Most legal decisions involve decisions to withdraw or forgo life-sustaining treatment in patients without decisional capacity and who have not specified their wishes before losing capacity. The rapid advancement of medical care coupled with the emergence of critical care units and associated technologies—such as mechanical ventilation, vasopressors and inotropic agents, and resuscitation techniques in the second half of the 20th century brought new challenges. For the first time, hospitals were keeping patients alive with technology without a legal discontinuation framework.

The courts began hearing these challenges in the late 1960s; several highly publicized cases starting in the 1970s concerned the withdrawal of treatment in young women who previously had capacity. In each of these cases, the patient had sustained devastating neurologic injury, and a legal challenge was presented to their families' ability to refuse continued treatment, including nutrition and hydration.[56–58] In each case, the same family members were entrusted for years to make medical decisions for complex and life-threatening procedures on behalf of the patients, but the request to withdraw care was met with years of struggle in the legal system. This was partly because of a state's right to establish high standards for evidence of what the patient would have wanted before allowing withdrawal.

In addition to affirming the state's ability to set high evidence standards in favor of preserving life, these cases established that in the absence of specific directions from the patient, surrogate decision makers should make a substituted judgment standard. This means that decision makers must base their decisions on the patient's known preferences and values before they lost capacity and use their best judgment in deciding what the patient would have wanted (in light of those values and preferences).

The surrogate decision maker's judgment about what should be done may differ from what they determine the patient would have wanted. They must abandon personal values and preferences and instead assume the preferences and values of the patient in making the decision. This is an enormous responsibility and a difficult task. The agony already associated with these difficult decisions can be lessened to the extent that patients can make their wishes known in advance.

These decisions, beginning with *In re Quinlan*,[36] initiated the slow process of state-by-state legislation to provide competent adults with a way to direct their care in the event of future incapacity legally. Today, there is a wide variety of state law–based procedures for individuals with decision-making capacity to direct their future care through documents and the appointment of surrogate decision makers in the event they should lose capacity. Each state has resources on the available options for residents.

Advance Directives

Patients themselves can provide clear direction by preparing statements (usually required to be in writing) in advance that specify their wishes. *Advance directive* is a generic term meaning all statements of future health care wishes in the event of incapacity. These statements include the living will and the durable power of attorney for health care.

The *living will* specifies that if certain circumstances occur, such as terminal illness, the patient will decline specific treatments, such as cardiopulmonary resuscitation and mechanical ventilation. It has proven to be of limited value because it only covers some treatments; for example, in some states, nutritional support may not be declined through a living will.

Living wills are more useful if the patient has a life-limiting condition and can use the living will to express their wishes in light of the anticipated course of their condition. Advance directives vary by state but are generally legally binding documents that allow individuals to specify various preferences, including naming people they want to serve as their decision makers, particular treatments they want to avoid, and circumstances in which they wish to avoid them. The *durable power of attorney for health care or health care proxy* is a directive through which a patient designates an "agent," someone who will make decisions for the patient if the patient becomes unable to do so. The agent is obligated to use the patient's values and preferences to make the decision the patient would make if they were able to do so. This is the most helpful tool if the agent is selected carefully and understands the associated responsibilities. This is a challenging task, and individuals are urged to consider their choice of agent carefully.

Each state has requirements for advance directives and the form they must take to be valid and legally enforceable. Once a patient creates an advance directive in their own state, other states will honor it under the full faith and credit doctrine. Nurses may care for critically ill patients in one state who have executed an advance directive in another. The fact that it was drafted in another state does not negate its validity.

The Patient Self-Determination Act of 1990 is an example of a federal statute that affects practice.[54] The Act was a response to medicine's ability to keep people alive with advanced technology and the decision-making difficulties that arose in response. It was designed to encourage competent patients to consider what they would want in the event of serious illness and to encourage them to complete advance directives.

The Act requires most health care institutions to provide patients at the time of admission written information about their rights under state law to make medical decisions, including the right to refuse treatment and the right to formulate advance directives. The Act also makes it illegal for a facility to require advance directives or discriminate against patients based on their advance directive or lack thereof.

Providers must have written policies and procedures (1) to inform all adult patients at initiation of treatment of their right to execute an advance directive and of the provider's policies on the implementation of that right, (2) to document in the medical record whether an individual has executed an advance directive, (3) *not* to condition care and treatment or otherwise discriminate on the basis of whether a patient has executed an advance directive, (4) to comply with state laws on advance directives, and (5) to provide information and education to staff and the community on advance directives.

Futile (or Nonbeneficial) Treatment and Orders Not to Resuscitate

Especially in critical care, nurses face situations where continued aggressive treatment is extremely unlikely to benefit the patient. This may mean that supportive care and comfort are the best actions for the patient's well-being.

All critical care nurses will observe and deliver care at some point that feels useless, unnecessary, and even harmful and painful to the patient. Nurses play an incredibly valuable role in the health care team by advocating for the best interest of the patient in a holistic way. Nurses may be responsible for reminding the team of the "big picture" and the need to provide quality of life and compassionate care to the patient.

Many providers have reported feeling obligated to continue treating patients in the absence of any reasonable chance of improvement. There is no legal obligation to provide care that is not, in the provider's judgment, reasonably calculated to improve the patient's condition or symptoms. Nurses sometimes face situations where the patient (or the patient's family or surrogate decision maker) wants to stop treatment, but the treating physician is opposed.

At other times, the entire health care team believes that aggressive treatment is no longer appropriate, but the family resists. Although patients have a legal right to refuse treatment, there is no corresponding right to receive treatment. To deal with these situations, most institutions have futility policies for discontinuing nonbeneficial care. Some states have laws to deal with these situations designed to facilitate communication between providers and patients, with procedures for resolution.

A section of the Texas Advance Directives Act, often deemed the *Texas Futile Care Law*,[58] creates a specific process for providers withdrawing or refusing to provide futile care, even over the patient's objections. Do not resuscitate (DNR) orders are the oldest form of effectuating a patient's wishes to refuse future medical treatment. However, they historically were the purview of the physician alone rather than an order communicating the patient's and providers' shared decisions.

As part of some institutional futility policies, unilateral DNR orders (which the physician orders without the patient's agreement) are permitted but should be rarely used. Furthermore, state laws vary as to the permissibility of the practice. Institutional DNR policies should be well established and tested after decades of implementation. Policies that address orders to withhold or withdraw treatment should exist in all critical care units, and nurses should be familiar with those policies. The policies should include the patient's diagnosis, prognosis, and consent if competent or the surrogate decision maker's consent if the patient is not competent.

Any conflict with advance directives or family member opinion should also be documented. DNR orders often require a second practitioner's concurrence and should require periodic review. Most importantly, they should be specific and clear. Nurses caring for patients with DNR orders should precisely understand what that means regarding appropriate intervention.

Other orders to withhold or withdraw treatment may involve any intervention, including mechanical ventilation, oxygen, intravenous vasoactive agents or other medications, serial laboratory tests, imaging tests, pulmonary artery catheters, and other invasive monitoring. The legal and ethical implications of these orders must be carefully considered on an individual basis. Hospital policies should exist to guide the withdrawal of care considering state and federal legal constraints. In addition, hospital ethicists and ethics committees can play a valuable role in providers negotiating these decisions' complexities.

Brain Death

Since 2013, new legal issues surrounding brain death have emerged that have relevance for critical care nurses. Patients are legally dead by the *irreversible cessation* of either (1) the cardiopulmonary system or (2) the entire brain, including the brainstem. Death is pronounced in accordance with acceptable medical standards. Typically, the determination of death by neurologic criteria is done in accordance with hospital policy and follows the guidelines set out by the American Academy of Neurology.[59–61]

It is crucial that critical care nurses understand the difference between catastrophic neurologic injury and brain death, which means that examinations have been conducted in accordance with guidelines and the patient has no function of the brain or brainstem. Nurses are responsible for correctly using this terminology, especially when communicating with the patient's family members. Once testing consistent with brain death is confirmed, the patient is declared dead, and either the patient is prepared for the allocation of organs or all mechanical support is removed because they are *legally dead*. This is not the same as withdrawing care for terminally ill but still alive patients.

Some states, such as California and New York, allow for a short delay in removing equipment to accommodate family concerns, typically interpreted as 24 hours. Only New Jersey allows families to refuse a declaration of brain death based on religious objections. However, California, New York, and Illinois state provisions require "reasonable accommodation" for religious beliefs.[44,54,59,60]

However, local judges have increasingly granted orders on behalf of patient families to temporarily prevent hospitals from removing mechanical ventilation and other supportive interventions. These orders typically allow for second opinions and additional testing to confirm death by irreversible cessation of total brain function, including the brainstem. In some cases, they have turned into protracted legal battles, as in the case of Jahi McMath,[61] a girl who was on mechanical ventilation for years after a legal declaration of death based on neurologic criteria.

In addition, recent research suggests that not all institutional policies are consistent with following evidence-based guidelines in making a determination of death.[61] Critical care nurses are essential in these efforts, and they must understand the physical condition the patient must be in for testing to commence and serve as an advocate with the physician in ensuring testing is conducted appropriately. For example, the patient's partial pressure of carbon dioxide levels and temperature must be normalized, and certain medications must be absent or at low levels before testing.

LEGAL ISSUES LOOKING FORWARD

This chapter could not begin to cover the labyrinth of legal issues affecting nursing practice. Each year brings new developments in legislation, case law, and administrative law that can change nursing practice. Most recently, the Patient Protection and Affordable Care Act of 2010 (ACA)[62] instituted sweeping changes in areas ranging from eligibility for health care coverage to funding of medical and nursing research to numerous workplace programs that are intended to enhance the supply of advanced practice nurses.

Of particular interest to nurses, many aspects of the ACA enhance the value and reimbursement of advanced practice registered nurses. There are several government and private organization websites with excellent information on health care law. See Box 2.9.

BOX 2.9 Internet Resources

Legal Issues

- American Association of Legal Nurse Consultants: www.aalnc.org
- American Association of Nurse Attorneys: www.TAANA.org
- American College of Legal Medicine: www.ACLM.org
- American Health Care Lawyers Association: www.healthlawyers.org
- American Society of Law and Medicine: www.ASLME.org
- Health Care Law Resources and Information: www.findlaw.org
- Health and Human Resources: https://www.hhs.gov/

CASE STUDY 2.1 Ethical Dilemma Regarding Ventilatory Support

Brief Patient History

Mr. X is a 67-year-old obese man. He has a 2-year history of emphysema (100 packs/year history of tobacco abuse in the past) with two recent hospitalizations for pneumonia that required ventilatory support. Mr. X states that he does not want to be placed on a ventilator again but does not want to suffer either. He was involved in a motor vehicle accident and sustained blunt trauma to the trunk and lower extremities, with bilateral femur fractures. Although his condition is critical, he is expected to recover. Mr. X received morphine 5 mg by intravenous push in the emergency department, with minimal pain relief; however, he has experienced new-onset confusion. Mr. X's spouse and children express concern about the risk of respiratory depression from pain medication. They state that they would rather Mr. X experience pain than have him placed on the ventilator again.

Focused Clinical Assessment

Mr. X is admitted to the critical care unit from the emergency department with blood transfusions in progress. Buck's traction (5 lb) has been applied to both lower extremities. He is awake, alert, and oriented to person, time, place, and situation. Mr. X is breathing through his mouth, taking shallow breaths. He complains of right upper quadrant abdominal pain when taking a deep breath. His skin is warm and dry. Mr. X is able to move his toes on command, and lower extremity sensation to touch is intact; however, he is complaining of severe bilateral lower extremity pain with restlessness.

Diagnostic Procedures

Arterial blood gas values are as follows: PaO_2, 55 mm Hg; $PaCO_2$, 28 mm Hg; pH, 7.35; HCO_3^-, 24 mEq/L; O_2 saturation, 88%. Hematocrit is 24%, and hemoglobin is 8 g/dL. Patient reports pain is 10 on the Baker-Wong Faces Scale; Riker Sedation-Agitation Scale score = 5.

Medical Diagnosis

Mr. X is diagnosed with a hepatic hematoma and bilateral femur fractures from a motor vehicle accident.

Questions

1. What major outcomes do you expect to achieve for this patient?
2. What problems or risks must be managed to achieve these outcomes?
3. What interventions could be initiated to monitor, prevent, manage, or eliminate the problems and risks identified?
4. What interventions could be initiated to promote optimal functioning, safety, and well-being of the patient?
5. What technology can be used to monitor this patient and prevent complications?
6. What other interprofessional team members are needed to assist with the management of this patient?
7. What possible learning needs would you anticipate for this patient?
8. What cultural and age-related factors might have a bearing on the patient's plan of care?
9. Does he have an advance directive that further explains his wishes?
   a. Has he previously appointed a surrogate decision maker in the event of his incapacity?
   b. Who are the stakeholders involved?
   c. What ethical principles are in conflict here? Are other relevant legal norms involved?
   d. What are the options? How do they play out in the short term and long term?
   e. How would you resolve this problem?

CASE STUDY 2.2 Patient With Legal Issues

Brief Patient History

Mr. A is an 87-year-old man. He has a history of aortic stenosis; however, he has been relatively healthy until recent episodes of syncope. Mr. A lives in an assisted living facility because of forgetfulness but was independent in activities of daily living before this hospitalization.

Focused Clinical Assessment

Mr. A was admitted to the critical care unit yesterday after undergoing aortic valvuloplasty. Mr. A has not received any opioids or benzodiazepines since the interventional procedure yesterday. The night nurse reported that Mr. A was confused to place when awakened during the night but commented that this is normal for an 87-year-old.

This morning, Mr. A was oriented to person, time, place, and situation. He is easily aroused but dozes off and on when unstimulated. Although Mr. A is able to follow simple commands, he requires repeated instructions. The nurse failed to document or report the patient's mental status change or abnormal serum electrolyte findings to the physician.

Diagnostic Procedures

Mr. A's baseline vital signs were as follows: blood pressure of 110/62 mm Hg, heart rate of 82 beats/min (sinus rhythm), respiratory rate of 18 breaths/min, and temperature of 98.4°F. The chest radiograph is normal; oxygen saturation (pulse oximetry) is 96% on room air. Results from serum electrolyte analysis include the following: sodium of 120 mmol/L, potassium of 4.1 mmol/L, chloride of 95 mmol/L, carbon dioxide of 25 mEq/L, blood urea nitrogen of 60 mg/dL, and creatinine of 2 mg/dL.

Medical Diagnosis

Mr. A is diagnosed with delirium secondary to hyponatremia.

Questions

1. What major outcomes do you expect to achieve for this patient?
2. What problems or risks must be managed to achieve these outcomes?
3. What interventions must be initiated to monitor, prevent, manage, or eliminate the problems and risks identified?
4. What interventions should be initiated to promote optimal functioning, safety, and well-being of the patient?
5. What technology can be used to monitor this patient and prevent complications?
6. What other interprofessional team members are needed to assist you with the management of this patient?
7. What possible learning needs would you anticipate for this patient?
8. What cultural and age-related factors might have a bearing on the patient's plan of care?

KEY POINTS

- Day-to-day decisions in critical care fall within the realm of ethics; each act can show or fail to show respect for the person or patient. The daily practice of critical care nursing involves ethical decision making and frequently involves ethical problems.
- Ethical problems occur when there are potential alternative actions for a patient, and those actions conflict; individuals may be uncertain about the right thing to do, or there may be disagreement among team members about the right thing to do.
- Moral distress occurs when a nurse feels unable to act in an ethical manner because of the medical plan of care, organizational restraints, workplace dynamics, or other barriers.
- Ethical principles help guide practice, but often one action simultaneously honors one principle while overriding another. Overriding a principle must be justified in the context of the situation.
- By using an ethical decision-making framework, nurses and other stakeholders can arrive at a decision that considers and honors the patient's values and preferences and is consistent with ethical principles and the nurse's professional code of nursing ethics.
- All facilities have professional ethics resources available to nurses and providers; these include IECs, individual clinical ethicists, and clinical ethics consultation services.
- Nursing is (1) a scientific process founded on a professional body of knowledge, (2) a learned profession based on an understanding of the human condition across the life span and the relationship of a patient with others and within the environment, and (3) an art dedicated to caring for others.
- The ability to practice professional nursing is a privilege granted by state law and, under the direction of BONs, state administrative agencies charged with protecting the health and welfare of state citizens by limiting nursing practice to qualified individuals who have demonstrated at least minimal competencies.
- Nursing scope of practice is defined by state NPAs. Standards of practice are delineated by BONs and are used as a basic measure of safe and effective nursing practice.
- Standards of practice and standards of professional performance, such as those promulgated by the AACN, further delineate expectations of nurses in providing quality nursing care and may help inform the standard of care in the legal context.
- Common legal theories based in civil litigation include professional negligence, wrongful death, and assault and battery. Nurses have a duty to their patients to provide care that is consistent with what a reasonably prudent nurse in the same situation would provide. This is the legal standard of care.
- Taking affirmative action that is responsive to the patient's condition and documenting those actions can diminish the risk of liability.
- Thorough documentation of nursing actions taken to protect or advocate for the patient is essential.
- Nurses can minimize the risk of liability by remaining true to the professional obligations to advocate for the best interests of the patient; attending to the patient's status, including carefully listening to and acting on patient reports or changes in status; documenting all of these issues; and taking unresolved or unexplained concerns up the chain of command.
- A competent patient has a constitutional right to refuse treatment, including lifesaving treatment, for any reason at all.
- States may require additional procedural protections when a decision maker wishes to withdraw care from patients who are not competent.
- Judicial intervention in decision making is an option but should be seen as a last resort. Interdisciplinary cooperation, discussion, and collaboration between providers and decision makers should be fully explored first.
- Providers of health care must comply with requirements relating to patients' advance directives.
- Any orders to withdraw or withhold treatment, including DNR orders, should be entered into the patient's medical record with full documentation by the responsible physician about the patient's prognosis and the patient's agreement or, alternatively, the family's consensus. These should be done in compliance with institutional policy.

- Brain death has a very specific clinical and legal meaning. Declaration of death by neurologic criteria requires examination in accordance with evidence-based medical standards, and hospital policies should comport with these standards. Critical care nurses should be familiar with these standards.

Internet resources related to legal content may be found in Box 2.9.

Visit the Evolve site at http://evolve.elsevier.com/Urden/CriticalCareNursing for additional study materials.

REFERENCES

1. Beauchamp TL, Childress JF. *Principles of Biomedical Ethics*. 8th ed. Oxford: Oxford University Press; 2019.
2. Furrow B, Greaney TL, Johnson SH, et al. *Bioethics: Health Care Law and Ethics*. 8th ed. Eagan MN: West Publishing; 2018.
3. Rainer J, Schneider JK, Lorenz RA. Ethical dilemmas in nursing: an integrative review. *J Clin Nurs*. 2018;27:19–20.
4. DuBois JA. *Framework for Analyzing Ethics Cases, Ethics in Mental Health Research*. New York: Oxford Press; 2008. Accessed August 15, 2019.
5. Jameton A. *Nursing Practice: The Ethical Issues*. Englewood Cliffs, NJ: Prentice-Hall; 1984.
6. Giannetta N, Villa G, Bonetti L, et al. Moral distress scores of nurses working in intensive care units for adults using Corley's Scale: a systematic review. *Int J Environ Res Public Health*. 2022;19(10640).
7. Rushton, C. Transforming moral suffering by cultivating moral resilience and ethical practice. Am J Crit Care. 32(3): 156.
8. Kalani Z, Barkhordari-Sharifabad M, Chehelmard N. Correlation between moral distress and clinical competence in COVID-19 ICU nurses. *BMC Nursing*. 2023;22:107.
9. American Nurses Association, A Call to Action: Exploring moral resilience toward a culture of ethical practice, www.nursing world.org/B4907b6/globalassets/docs/ana/ana-call-to-action-exploringmoral-resilience-final.pdf. Accessed 29.05.23.
10. Wocial L. Resilience as an incomplete strategy for coping with moral distress in critical care nurses. *Critical Care Nurse*. 2020;40(6):62–66.
11. Hu K, Liu J, Zhu L, Zhou Y. Clinical nurses' moral courage and related factors: an empowerment perspective. *BMC Nursing*. 2022;21:321.
12. Abdeen MA, Atia NM. Ethical work climate, moral courage, moral distress and organizational citizenship behavior among nurses. *Int J Nurs Educ*. 2020;12(3):104–110.
13. Jonsen AR, Siegler M, Winslade WJ. *Clinical Ethics: A Practical Approach to Ethical Decisions in Clinical Medicine*. 9th ed. New York: McGraw Hill; 2022.
14. Buka P. *Essential Law and Ethics in Nursing*. 3rd ed. New York: Routledge; 2020.
15. Altaker KW, Howie-Esquivel J, Cataldo JK. Relationships among palliative care, ethical climate, empowerment, and moral distress in intensive care unit nurses. *Am J Crit Care*. 2018;27(4).
16. Lo JJ, Graves N, Chee JH, Hildon ZJ. A systematic review defining nonbeneficial and inappropriate end-of-life treatment in patients with non-cancer diagnoses: theoretical development for multi-stakeholder intervention design in acute care settings. *BMC Palliative Care*. 2022;21(1):195.
17. Shaw JA, Sethi N, Block BL. Five things every clinician should know about AI ethics in intensive care. *Intensive Care Med*. 2021;47:157–159.
18. Momennasab M, Homayoon Z, Torabizadeh C. Critical care nurses' adherence to ethical codes and its association with spiritual well-being and moral sensitivity. *Crit Care Res Pract*. 2023:8248948. Accessed May 23, 2023.
19. American Nurses Association. *Code of Ethics for Nurses with Interpretative Statements*; 2015. https://www.nursingworld.org/practice-policy/nursing-excellence/ethics/code-of-ethics-for-nurses/coe-view-only/.
20. Winland-Brown J, Lachman VD, Swanson EO. The new code of ethics for nurses with interpretative statements (2015): practical clinical application, part 1. *Medsurg Nurs*. 2015;24(4):268.
21. Usberg G, Uibu E, Urban R, Kangasniemi M. Ethical conflicts in nursing: an interview study. *Nurs Ethics*. 2021;28(2):230–241. https://doi.org/10.1177/0969733020945751.
22. Gilvari T, Abbaszadeh A, Borhani F, Mohamadi P, Saberi N. Relationship of the hospital ethical climate with nurses' attitude to interprofessional collaboration. *JCDR*. 2019;13(11):16–19.
23. Meyer EC, Carnevale FA, Lillehei C, Uveges MK. Widening the ethical lens in critical care settings. *AACN Adv Crit Care*. 2020;31(2):210–220.
24. Chen E. Ethics in the ICU: Negotiating requests for inappropriate treatments. *Critical Care Alert*. 2021;29(3):1–5.
25. ANA Position Statement: The Nurse's Role in Addressing Discrimination: Protecting and Promoting Inclusive Strategies in Practice Settings, Policy, and Advocacy. *Online J Issues Nurs*. 2019;24(3). https://doi.org/10.3912/OJIN.Vol24No03PoSCol01.
26. National Council of the State Boards of Nursing (NCSBN). *NCSBN Model Act*. Chicago, IL: NCSBN; 2012. revised 2021.
27. National Council of the State Boards of Nursing (NCSBN). *NCSBN Model Nursing Practice Act and Model Nursing Administrative Rules*. Chicago, IL: NCSBN; 2021.
28. *Sermchief v Gonzales, 660 SW2d 683* (Mo 1983).
29. Russell KA. Nurse practice acts guide and govern: Update 2017. *J Nurs Regul*. 2017;8(3):18–23.
30. American Association of Critical-Care Nurses (AACN). *AACN Scope and Standards for Progressive and Critical Care Nursing Practice*. Aliso Viejo, CA: AACN; 2019.
31. *Candler General Hospital Inc. v McNorrill, 354 SE2d 872* (Ga. 1987).
32. Dowie I. Understanding the standard of care required by nurses. *Nurs Stand*. 2020;35(4):29–34.
33. *Lunsford v Board of Nurse Examiners, 648 SW2d 391* (Tx. App. 1983).
34. *Sparks v St. Luke's Regional Medical Center, 768 P.2d 768* (Idaho 1989).
35. *Newsome v Lake Charles Hospital, 954 So. 2d 380* (La Ct. App. 2007).
36. *Teffeteller v University of Minnesota, 645 NW2d 420* (Minn. 2002).
37. *McMullen v Ohio State University Hospitals, 725 NE2d 1117* (Ohio 2002).
38. *Brandon HMA, Inc. v Bradshaw, 809 So.2d 611* (Miss. 2001).
39. *Brookwood Health Services v Bordon, Sup. Ct. Alabama* (2015).
40. *Denesia v St. Elizabeth Community Health Center, 454 NW2d 294* (Neb. 1990).
41. *Garcia v United States, 697 F.Supp. 1570* (Colo. 1988).
42. *Keyser v Garner, 922 P.2d 409* (Idaho 1996).
43. *Long v Methodist Hospital of Indiana, 699 NE2d 1164* (Ind. 1998).
44. *Randi A. J. v Long Island Health Care, 842 N.Y.S.2d 558* (N.Y. App. 2007).
45. *Ginsberg v St. Michaels Hospital, 678 A.2d 271* (N.J. 1996).
46. *Richardson v Miller, 44 SW3d 1* (Tenn. 2000).
47. *Lattimore v. Dickey, 23 Cal.App.4th 959, 968* (2015).
48. *Haney v Alexander, 323 SE2d 430* (1984).
49. *The Health Insurance Portability and Accountability Act of 1996 (HIPAA), Public Law 104–191, enacted on August 21,* 1996
50. *Darling v Charleston Comm. Mem. Hosp., 211 NE2d 614* (Ill. 1965).
51. *Rowe v Sisters of Saint Pallottine Missionary Society, 560 S.E.2d 491* (2007).
52. Resilience and ethical practice. *Am J Crit Care Nurs*. 32(3):156.
53. *Canteburry v. Spence, 150 U.S. App. D.C. 263, 464 F.2d 772* (1972)
54. Restatement of torts (2nd), American law institute. §§. 1965;13:21.
55. Patient self determination act, omnibus budget reconciliation act of 1990. *Pub.L.* 1990:101–508.
56. *Bouvia v Superior Court, 179 Cal. App. 3d 1127, 225 Cal. Rptr. 297, 1986 Cal. App. LEXIS 1467* (Cal. App. 2d Dist. 1986).
57. *Owensboro Mercy Health System v Payne, 24 SW3d 675* (Ky. 1999).
58. *Uniform Determination of Death Act* (1981).
59. *Texas Advance Directives Act, Texas Health and Safety Code, Section 166* (1999).
60. Truog RD, Krishnamurthy K, Tasker RC. Brain death-Moving beyond consistency in the diagnostic criteria. *JAMA*. 2020;324(11):1045–1047.
61. Lyons K. Jahi McMath's family takes brain-death lawsuit to federal court. *SF Gate*. 2015.
62. Rady M. The capacity for consciousness and the clinical diagnosis of brain death: are we using the correct gold standard? *Can J Anaesth*; 68(10): 1576–1577.
63. *Patient Protection and Affordable Care Act and Reconciliation Act*; 2010.
64. Harrington L. Nurses overreliance on fallible technology. *Adv Crit Car*. 2023;34(2):84–87. https://.org/10.4037/aacnancc2023526.
65. Harrington L. The RaDonda Vaught case: a critical conversation on nursing practice and technology. *Adv Crit Car*. 2023;34(1):11–15. https://doi.org/10.4037/aacnacc2023873.

3

Genetic Issues

Mary E. Lough

http://evolve.elsevier.com/Urden/CriticalCareNursing

The field of genetics and genomics continues to expand. Given the exponential growth of information, and the decreasing costs of genomic sequencing with the promise of *precision medicine*, knowledge about this field is essential for all health care professionals.[1,2]

This chapter includes an overview of the biologic basis of genomics; a description of the different types of genetic and genomic studies; some examples of genetic diseases and pharmacogenetic syndromes; social, ethical, and legal concerns; and discussion of genetic and genomic competencies for nurses. A list of genetic and genomic terms is provided at the end of the chapter.

GENETICS AND GENOMICS

Genetics is the study of heredity, particularly as it relates to the ability of individual genes to transfer heritable physical characteristics. *Genes* are specific sequences of deoxyribonucleic acid (DNA) located on chromosomes within the nucleus of each cell (Fig. 3.1). Genes contain the blueprint for protein production that results in the physical characteristics of every individual. Early pioneering work in human genetics focused on single-gene variants that are rare in the population but have a large effect on a specific individual and follow classic inheritance patterns. Approximately 7000 rare disorders have been identified.[3] Although single-gene conditions are relatively rare in the population, cumulatively they affect approximately 30 million people in the United States and over 300 million people worldwide.[3] Single-gene disorders include Huntington disease, Tourette syndrome, cystic fibrosis, and Duchenne muscular dystrophy. In single-gene variant disorders, the influence of genetics is strong, and the environmental effects are very weak.

Genomics refers to the study of all the genetic material within the cell and encompasses the environmental interaction and effect on biologic and physical characteristics. Thus, genomics is a much larger and more complex area of study. The *genome* is the complete set of DNA in an organism. Each human nucleated somatic cell contains a copy of the complete genome. The exceptions are reproductive cells (oocytes and sperm), which contain only one-half of the paired chromosomes, and red blood cells, because they do not have a nucleus. The human genome contains 20,000 to 25,000 protein-coding genes, which represent less than 2% of the total genome.[4]

Many disease conditions that are commonly seen in the modern world result from a confluence of environmental and genomic influences. These are described as *complex traits* or *polygenic* conditions. Furthermore, environmental conditions can alter the expression of different genes and consequently enhance the signs and symptoms associated with a disease. This represents a field of research known as *epigenetics*. Coronary artery disease is an example of a widespread disease that has both a strong environmental component (diet, obesity, diabetes, smoking) and a genomic effect that alters the risk of developing the condition.[5,6] Whole genome sequencing methods and genome-wide association studies (GWAS) are employed to examine multiple genes simultaneously. As the cost of genomic sequencing decreases, this will increasingly be a viable clinical option.[7] Nowhere is the genomic influence more evident than in pharmacogenomics, or the unique individual response to medications (environmental interaction with medications) based on gene expression (genomic interaction with medications).[8]

GENETIC AND GENOMIC STRUCTURE AND FUNCTION

Chromosomes

The nucleus inside each human cell contains each person's full genetic blueprint of 23 pairs of chromosomes—22 pairs of autosomes and 1 pair of sex chromosomes—making a total of 46.[5] A number system is used to identify each chromosome. The chromosomes are traditionally arranged in order of size, starting with the largest (chromosome 1) to the smallest (chromosome 22), with the sex chromosomes placed last or to the side. A schematic of this chromosome arrangement to show the variation in size is shown in Fig. 3.2A; the chromosomes are not arranged this way inside the cell. A *karyotype* is the arrangement of human chromosomes from largest to smallest, as shown in the sequence in Fig. 3.2B.

Each chromosome consists of an unbroken strand of DNA. To fit all this genetic material inside the cell nucleus, the DNA is tightly coiled inside the chromosomes in a hierarchical order of compact structures. A specialized class of proteins called *histones* organizes the double-stranded DNA into what looks like a set of tightly coiled springs (see Fig. 3.1).

Each somatic chromosome, also called an *autosome*, is made of two strands, called *chromatids*, which are joined near the center (see Fig. 3.1). This central region is called the *centromere*, and the ends of the chromatids are called *telomeres*. The segments of the chromosome separated by the centromere are called *arms*. The shorter arm of each chromosome is called *p* (for *petit*, or small), and the longer arm is called *q*. Differential staining of chromosomes produces alternating dark and light transverse

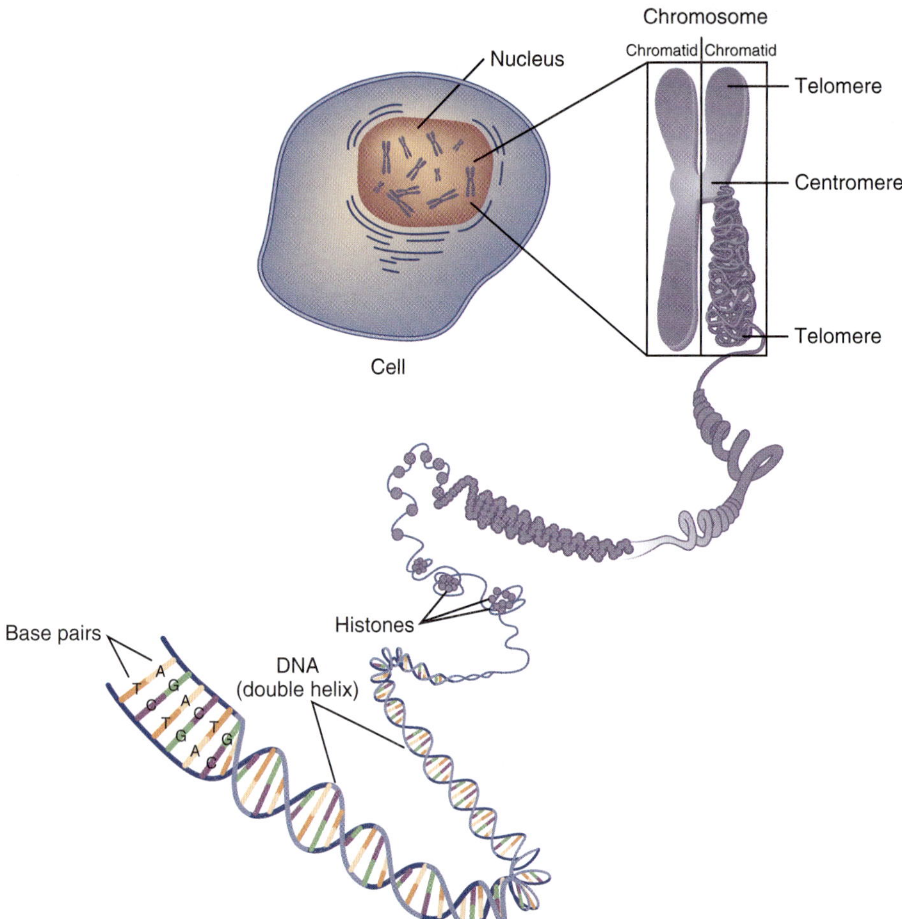

FIG. 3.1 Chromosomes Are Tightly Packed With DNA and Reside in the Nucleus of the Cell.

bands. The bands are labeled p1, p2, p3, and so forth on the p arm and q1, q2, q3, and so forth on the q arm, counted from the centromere toward the telomeres.

The p and q labels and bands are used to specify the location of specific DNA sections on the chromosome. There are also subbands within the major bands. This series of letters and numbers is the equivalent of an address for the location of a gene on a chromosome. For example, the cystic fibrosis gene *CFTR* (cystic fibrosis transmembrane conductance regulator) is located at 7q31.2, which indicates it is on chromosome 7, q arm, band 3, subband 1, and subsubband 2.[9]

DNA and the Double Helix

DNA is foundational to genetics. Within the nucleus of the cell within each chromosome, DNA is arranged like a ladder, with two long strands of subunits twisted around each other to form the double-stranded three-dimensional helix.

The subunits within each DNA strand are called *nucleotides* or *bases*, and they are combined in pairs to form the rungs of the DNA ladder. Four nucleotide bases comprise the "letters" in the genetic DNA "alphabet."

- Adenine (A)
- Thymine (T)
- Guanine (G)
- Cytosine (C)

Each nucleotide base is attached to a phosphorylated molecule of the five-carbon sugar deoxyribose that forms the backbone of the DNA chain and can be visualized as the two sides of a ladder that twists like a corkscrew (Fig. 3.3). A helix is described as spiral shape around a center line that can rotate rightward or leftward, and in DNA it is a double helix. The bases in the double helix are sized and paired so that G can only pair with C, and only T can pair with A, to achieve a consistent distance across the width of the DNA strand. These can be paired as:

- G-C
- T-A
- C-G
- A-T

The combinations are known as *base pairs* (see Fig. 3.3). There are approximately 3 billion bases in the human genome, based on findings from the Human Genome Project.[4]

The two DNA strands are orientated in opposite directions. Each DNA strand has a specific direction that is labeled as the 3′ end or the 5′ end (pronounced 3 prime and 5 prime) (see Fig. 3.3). Because the DNA strands face in opposite directions, the 3′ end of one strand is always matched to the 5′ end of the other strand. This fact becomes important for replication (discussed next). The 3′ end is described as the *leading strand*, because new nucleotides can be added only at the 3′ end.

DNA Replication

Before a cell divides, it needs to make a second copy of the entire DNA content within the cell. This process is called *DNA replication*. Sections of the DNA double helix separate longitudinally,

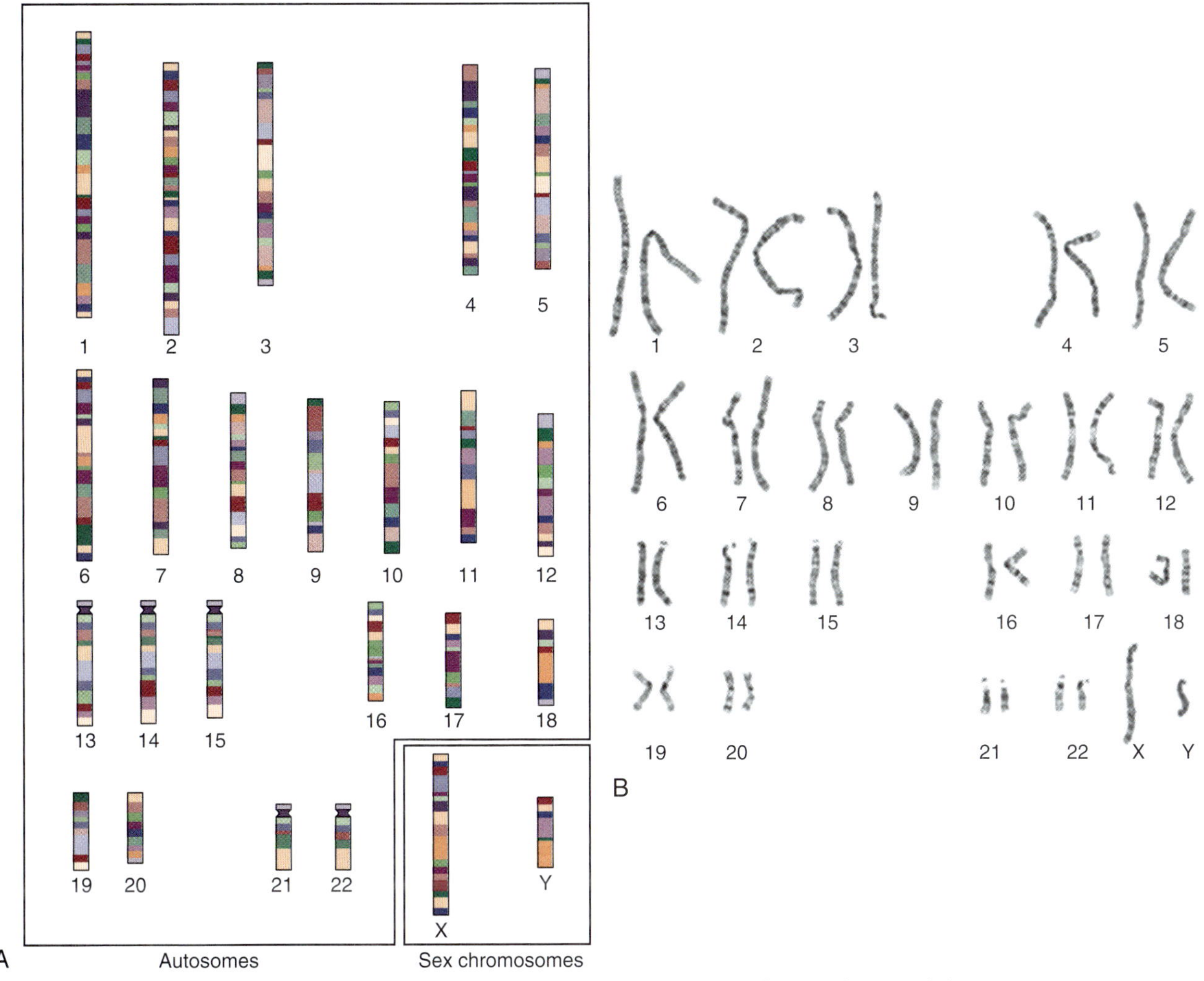

FIG. 3.2 (A) Schematic of standard chromosomal arrangement used for classification of chromosomes by number, arranged from the largest (chromosome 1) to the smallest (chromosome 22). Chromosomes 1 to 22 are known as autosomes. Autosomal chromosomes are present in two identical copies, which are the same in men and women. The sex chromosomes are X (female) and Y (male). (B) This is a male karyotype because the sex chromosome arrangement is XY. The striped bands that appear on the chromosomes are achieved by use of specialized staining techniques.

creating openings between base pairs, known as *replication bubbles*, and mirror-image copies are made from the original strands. Stated another way, each of the two original DNA strands provide a template that will be copied. The originals are called the *parent strands*, and the mirror-image copies are described as the *daughter strands*.

In Fig. 3.4, the parent strand is colored blue with the 5′ and 3′ ends of each parent strand labeled. The daughter strands are colored red. The replication process is facilitated by *DNA polymerase*, an enzyme that lengthens the DNA strand by the addition of new nucleotide bases at the 3′ end of the daughter strand (see Fig. 3.4). After DNA replication is accomplished, the cell uses a sophisticated mechanism for identifying and fixing errors in the replicated strand.[10] Following this procedure, the cell is ready to divide, and each new cell will contain a copy of the original DNA code.

DNA Alphabet

The nucleotides A, T, C, and G can be thought of as "letters" of a genetic alphabet that are combined into three-letter "words" that are transcribed (written) from DNA into ribonucleic acid (RNA). These three-letter "words" are each translated into 1 of 20 amino acids, used to make the polypeptide chains that constitute proteins. This process may be briefly written as DNA → RNA → protein.[5,11]

Transcription

The purpose of DNA transcription is to make an RNA strand without compromising the original genetic material. The DNA strand with the genetic code that is being transcribed is labeled as the *sense* strand, or sometimes as the *coding strand*. A new mirror-image RNA strand is constructed by the process of transcription. The new RNA strand is known by various names (RNA transcript, RNA antisense strand). The new RNA antisense strand is the mirror image of the DNA sense strand (Fig. 3.5).

To visualize how the process of transcription works, it may be helpful to study Fig. 3.5 and locate the names of the different strands; the DNA strand is colored blue, and the RNA strand is colored green.

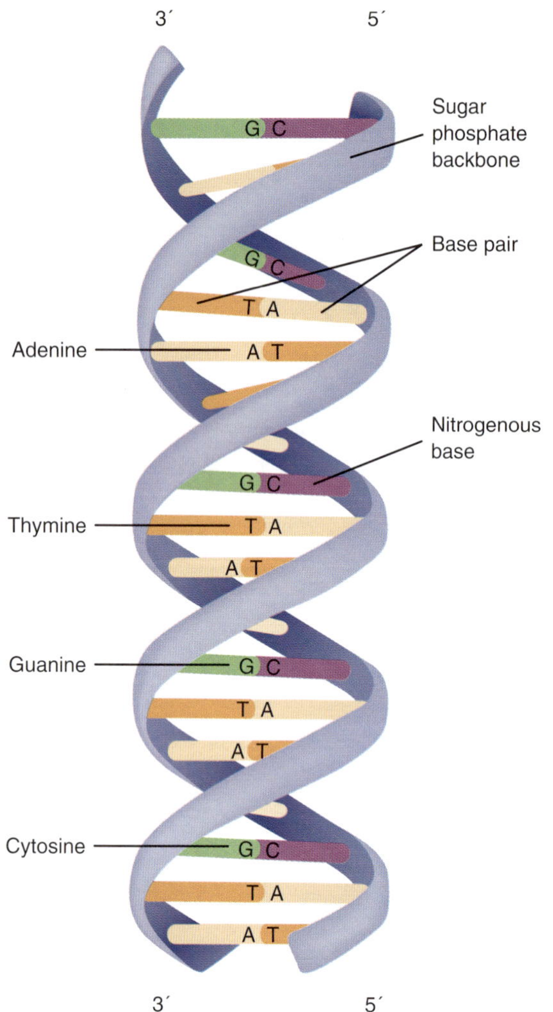

FIG. 3.3 Deoxyribonucleic Acid (DNA) Double Helix.

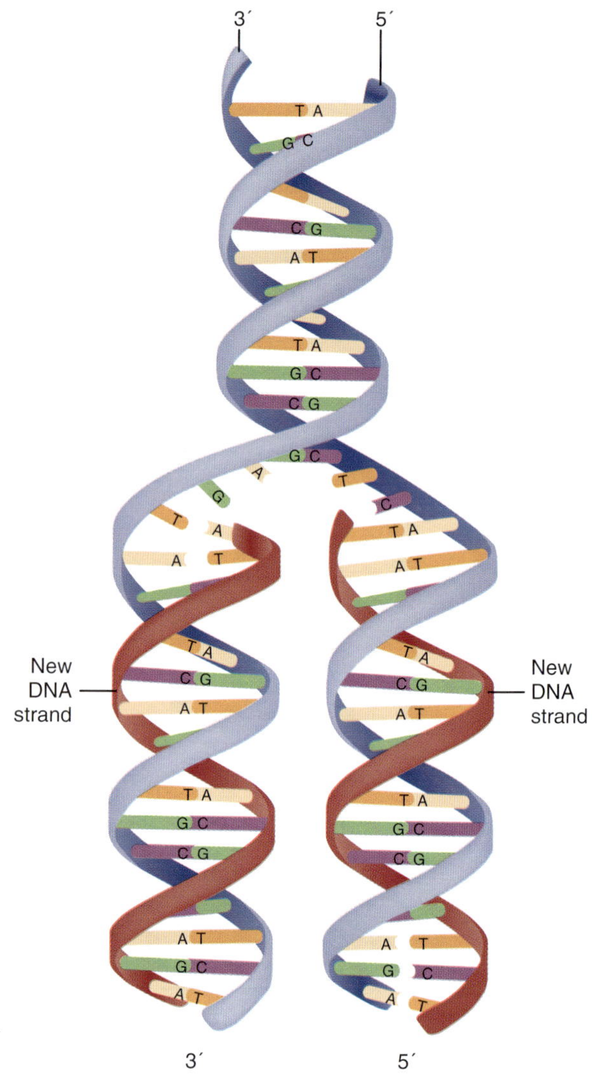

FIG. 3.4 DNA Replication Occurs Before Cell Divides. The template is provided by the original DNA strand (colored *blue*). The mirror-image DNA strand (colored *red*) is adding nucleotides to elongate the new DNA strand.

When RNA is transcribed one significant change occurs. The adenosine (A) DNA base is paired with a new base called uracil (U) in the RNA transcript (see Fig. 3.5). Each RNA strand has a 3′ end (called three-prime and conceptualized as a head) and a 5′ end (called five-prime and conceptualized as a tail). The growing RNA strand adds bases only at the 3′ end. The RNA strand, called *messenger RNA*, then leaves the nucleus of the cell, and the next action takes place in the cytoplasm.

Translation

The purpose of DNA translation is to create amino acid chains. The RNA bases, or "three-letter words" called *codons* (Table 3.1), are used to specify an amino acid. The three-base RNA codons are designed to code for 1 of 20 amino acids. Some codons signal to stop the sequence; these termination sequences are UAA, UAG, and UGA. The three-letter codons are not unique; for example, both UAU and UUC code for the amino acid phenylalanine. Most amino acids can be made from more than one codon. This can be appreciated by an examination of the list of three-letter codons, the corresponding three-letter amino acid abbreviation, the single-letter abbreviation, and the name of the amino acid in Table 3.1. The process by which proteins are made from instructions encoded in DNA is called *gene expression*.

Only a brief review of how DNA contributes to the genetic code is possible in this chapter. The volume of information that underpins genetics and genomics reflects the work of many scientists who performed research to advance this knowledge, and it may take some individual study or additional classes to fully master the content.[11]

Telomeres

Telomeres are the biologic structures that protect the ends of the DNA strands at the end of the chromasome.[12] Telomeres are often likened to the protective plastic caps placed on the ends of shoelaces to stop the laces unraveling (see Fig. 3.1). These are not static structures, because telomeres shorten over a lifetime and with illness. The significance of telomere shortening in inflammatory health conditions, cancer and ageing, are active areas of research.[13–16]

Genetic Variation

Genetic variation is common to all species, including humans. Genetic diversity is beneficial because this facilitates biological adaption and resilience. In contrast, low genetic diversity occurs when a population has a limited gene pool. Genetically,

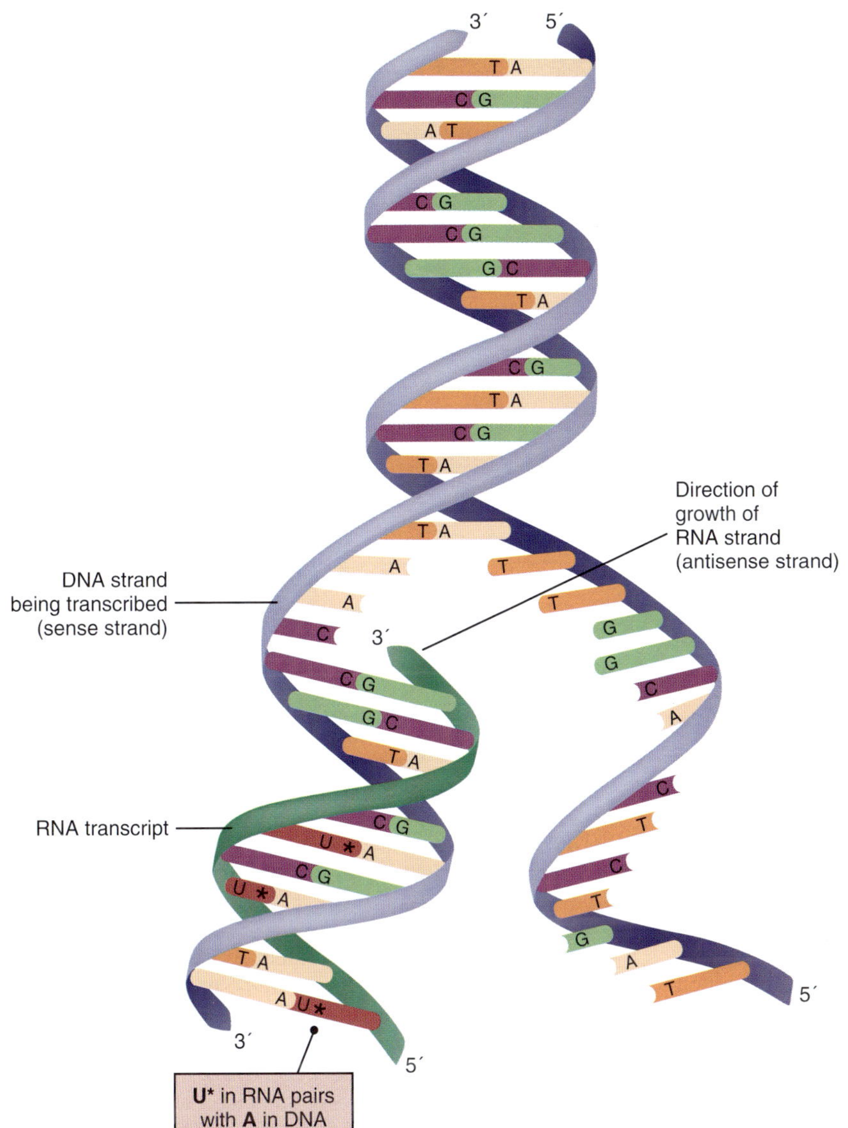

FIG. 3.5 DNA Transcription and Production of Complementary RNA Strand. The template DNA strand is colored *blue*. The RNA nucleotide uracil (*U*) pairs with the DNA nucleotide adenine (*A*) in the growing RNA strand (colored *green*).

variation means that individuals do not have the same nucleotides (A, C, T, G) in the same positions on the DNA strand.

Nucleotide differences result in the expression of different proteins and physical traits. Many nucleotide changes produce no visible external alteration, although those that have health-related consequences are of great interest to clinicians, patients, and researchers. Genetic variation can result from a variety of changes. It can be a single-letter substitution of one nucleotide base for another that can produce an inappropriate stop codon or produce a codon for a different amino acid. The amino acid codes are shown in Table 3.1.

Genetic material in the chromosome can also be deleted (Fig. 3.6A), new information from another chromosome can be inserted (Fig. 3.6B), or a tandem repeat (multiple repeats of the same sequence) may produce duplicate genetic material within the chromosome (Fig. 3.6C). *Translocation* of genetic material describes a process in which chromosomes break and genetic material is moved from one chromosome to another. For example, the Philadelphia chromosome, or Philadelphia translocation, is a specific chromosomal abnormality associated with chronic myelogenous leukemia (CML).[17] It results from a reciprocal translocation between chromosomes 9 and 22, in which parts of these two chromosomes switch places, producing the oncogenic Philadelphia chromosome and development of dysregulated tyrosine kinase.[17]

Mutation

The term *genetic mutation* refers to a change in the DNA genetic sequence that can be inherited, often this is a clinically recognizable condition. The inheritance may also be described as a polymorphism. In genetics, the word *mutation* does not imply a negative connotation of being more deadly than other genetic changes.

Single Nucleotide Polymorphisms

When a genetic variant occurs frequently and is present in 1% or more of the population, it is described as a *genetic polymorphism*. The most common change is the substitution of one

TABLE 3.1 The Genetic Code: Amino Acids[a]

First nucleotide in codon	Second nucleotide in codon																Third nucleotide
	U				A				C				G				
U	UUU	Phe	F	*Phenylalanine*	CUC	Ser	S	*Serine*	UAU	Tyr	Y	*Tyrosine*	UGU	Cys	C	*Cysteine*	U
	UUC	Phe	F	*Phenylalanine*	UUC	Ser	S	*Serine*	UAC	Tyr	Y	*Tyrosine*	UGC	Cys	C	*Cysteine*	C
	UUA	Leu	L	*Leucine*	UCA	Ser	S	*Serine*	UAA	Termination	UGA	Termination					A
	UUG	Leu	L	*Leucine*	UCG	Ser	S	*Serine*	UAG	Termination	UGG	Trp	W	*Tryptophan*			G
C	CUU	Leu	L	*Leucine*	CCU	Pro	P	*Proline*	CAU	His	H	*Histidine*	CGU	Arg	R	*Arginine*	U
	CUC	Leu	L	*Leucine*	CCC	Pro	P	*Proline*	CAU	His	H	*Histidine*	CGC	Arg	R	*Arginine*	C
	CUA	Leu	L	*Leucine*	CCA	Pro	P	*Proline*	CAA	Gln	Q	*Glutamine*	CGA	Arg	R	*Arginine*	A
	CUG	Leu	L	*Leucine*	CCG	Pro	P	*Proline*	CAG	Gln	Q	*Glutamine*	CGG	Arg	R	*Arginine*	G
A	AUU	Ile	I	*Isoleucine*	ACU	Thr	T	*Threonine*	AAU	Asn	N	*Asparagine*	AGU	ser	S	*Serine*	U
	AUC	Ile	I	*Isoleucine*	ACC	Thr	T	*Threonine*	AAC	Asn	N	*Asparagine*	AGC	ser	S	*Serine*	C
	AUA	Ile	I	*Isoleucine*	ACA	Thr	T	*Threonine*	AAA	Lys	K	*Lysine*	AGA	Arg	R	*Arginine*	A
	AUG	Met	M	*Methionine*	ACG	Thr	T	*Threonine*	AAG	Lys	K	*Lysine*	AGG	Arg	R	*Arginine*	G
G	GUU	Val	V	*Valine*	GCU	Ala	A	*Alanine*	CAU	Asp	D	*Aspartic acid*	GGU	Gly	G	*Glycine*	U
	GUC	Val	V	*Valine*	GCC	Ala	A	*Alanine*	GAC	Asp	D	*Aspartic acid*	GGC	Gly	G	*Glycine*	C
	GUA	Val	V	*Valine*	GCA	Ala	A	*Alanine*	GAA	Gl u	E	*Glutamic acid*	GGA	Gly	G	*Glycine*	A
	GUG	Val	V	*Valine*	GCG	Ala	A	*Alanine*	GAG	Gl u	E	*Glutamic acid*	GGG	Gly	G	*Glycine*	G

Third nucleotide in codon

[a]Amino acids are the building blocks of proteins. The 20 amino acids are constructed from information contained in the DNA blueprint that is translated and transcribed by RNA. This transfer of information from DNA to amino acids is called the genetic code. Triple sets of bases (codons) are transcribed into the 20 amino acids. There are 64 possible combinations of codons, and several codons code for the same amino acids. The amino acids are connected in long polypeptide chains that form proteins. Three combinations signal the end of a protein chain: UAA, UAG, and UGA. Each three-letter codon also has a single-letter abbreviation, which is shown in the table.

single-nucleotide base. A single-letter switch is known as a *single nucleotide polymorphism* (SNP; pronounced "snip") (Fig. 3.7). This is significant when the SNP occurs in a region of DNA that codes for an amino acid. If the SNP change alters the amino acid product that is produced, it is called a *nonsynonymous SNP*, or *missense SNP*. If a nonsynonymous SNP occurs in a coding region, it may affect protein structure and lead to alterations in phenotype (disease manifestation). An example is the G-to-A coding SNP at the 1691 site of the factor V gene associated with blood coagulation.[18] This polymorphism leads to the substitution of an arginine (A) by glutamine (G) at amino acid position 506, which alters one of the cleavage sites for activated protein C. Factor Va inactivation is slowed down because the cleavage site is atypical. This change in one amino acid reduces the anticoagulant activity of factor V, induces a hypercoagulable state, and consequently increases risk of deep vein thrombosis (DVT) (see Box 3.1).

Approximately 5% of the population carries one copy of the factor V allele (heterozygous) who inherited an allele from only one parent, has an increased lifetime risk of venous thrombosis, that is threefold to fivefold compared to the nonaffected population.[19] A person with two copies of the factor V allele (homozygous) who inherited two alleles, one from each parent, has a 10-fold increased lifetime risk of venous thrombosis compared to the general population.[19] Factor V thrombophilia is one of several genetically inherited conditions that increase the risk of venous thrombosis.[19]

Alleles

Another name for a variant of a gene that occurs at a single locus is an *allele*. Allele symbols consist of the gene symbol, an asterisk, and the italicized allele designation. For example, the apolipoprotein E gene (*APOE*) has three major alleles (*APOE2, APOE3, APOE4*), and each allele codes for a different isoform of the ApoE protein.[20,21] *APOE4* expression is associated with both early-onset and late-onset Alzheimer disease (LOAD) and is dependent on which of the *APOE* alleles are expressed. In practical terms, a person with one *APOE4* allele has a risk of developing Alzheimer disease approximately 5 years earlier; a person with two copies of the *APOE4* allele has a risk of developing Alzheimer disease approximately 10 years earlier. Conversely, the average onset of Alzheimer disease is delayed by 5 years if a person has one copy of the *APOE2* allele.[22,23]

Not all changes in the DNA sequence have deleterious effects. Most SNPs have no effect because they are *synonymous SNPs*, variants that code for the same amino acid (see Table 3.1), or because they are located in a noncoding genomic region.

GENETIC INHERITANCE

All genetic and genomic disorders do not have the same cause. The categories of disorders are chromosome disorders, single-gene disorders, complex gene and multifactorial disorders, and mitochondrial disorders. Many genetic disorders are inherited, but other genetic changes appear spontaneously in the genome. These may be caused by errors of DNA transcription and sometimes can be passed to future generations in some disorders.

Chromosome Disorders

In chromosome disorders, the entire chromosome or very large segments of the chromosome are damaged, missing, duplicated, or otherwise altered. Down syndrome (trisomy 21), in which

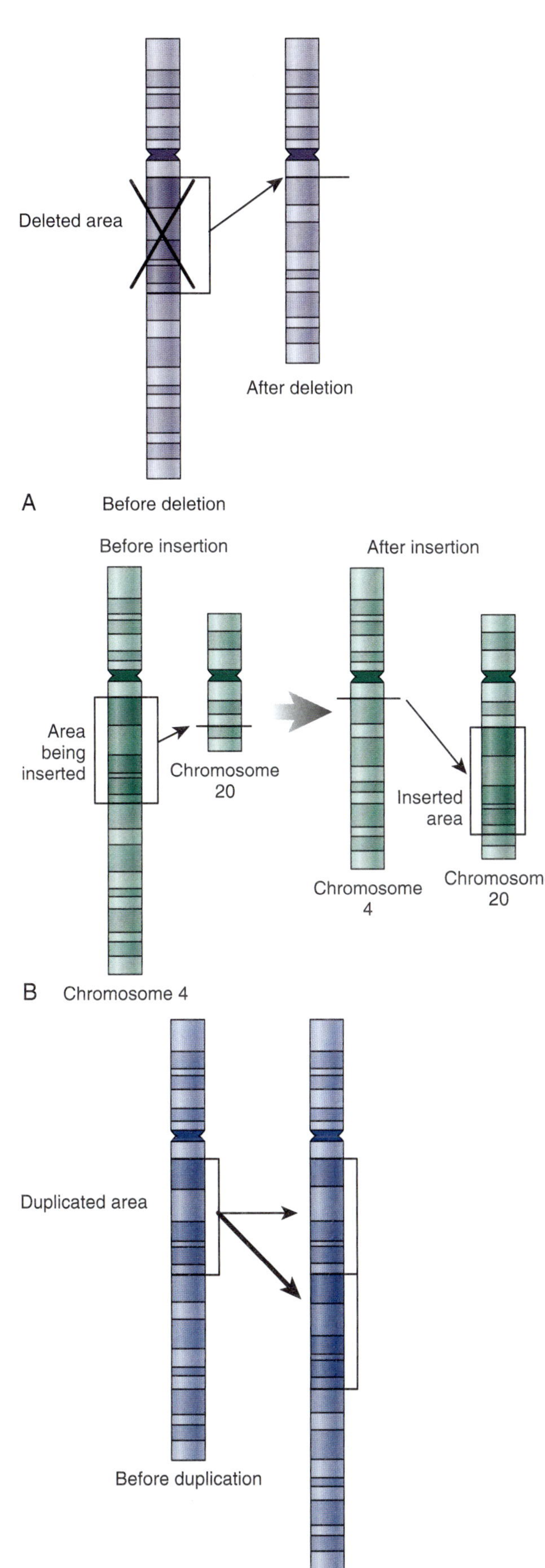

FIG. 3.6 (A) Deletion of chromosomal genetic material. (B) Insertion of genetic material from one chromosome to another. (C) Duplication of chromosomal genetic material.

there is an extra copy of chromosome 21, is an example of a chromosome disorder.

Single-Gene Disorders

In single-gene disorders, a single gene is altered. Single-gene disorders can result from inheritance of one dominant gene or two recessive genes. Cystic fibrosis, sickle cell disease, hemophilia A and B, and Marfan syndrome are examples of single-gene disorders. Single-gene disorders may also be described as monogenetic or mendelian gene disorders. Single-gene disorders are rare in the population and often have significant physical effects.[5]

Complex Gene and Gene-Environment Disorders

In some disorders, many genes interact to produce the condition, or there must be an interaction between vulnerable genes and the environment. Cardiovascular atherosclerotic diseases and type 2 diabetes are examples of complex gene disorders that result from an interaction of genetic and environmental factors.[5] Pharmacogenetic syndromes, resulting from the interactions of genes and medications, are also in this category.

Mitochondrial Disorders

Some diseases are caused by alterations in mitochondrial DNA. Mitochondrial DNA is totally different and separate from the double-helix DNA found in the nucleus. Mitochondrial DNA has a circular chromosome that is located inside the mitochondria that are intracellular organelles found in the cytoplasm.[24]

Mitochondrial DNA is transferred to offspring by maternal transmission only because mitochondria are preserved in oocytes but are destroyed in sperm during fertilization. Mitochondrial genetic diseases are associated with disorders of enzyme function that disrupt mitochondrial energy production. Tissues and organs that have high-energy requirements such as skeletal muscles, the heart, and the central nervous system are most often affected.[24–26]

Genotype and Phenotype

Genotype. The *genotype* refers to the genetic makeup at a particular locus or location on a specific chromosome within the genome; this conceptually resembles a unique street address.

Phenotype. The *phenotype* refers to the signs and symptoms that are clinically associated with a particular genetic condition; this is conceptually not unlike the defining characteristics of the house, or apartment.

Copy Number Variation

Copy number variation (CNV) adds another level of variation to the human genome. CNV describes structural changes of DNA, larger than 1 kilobase, that include insertions, deletions, and inversions. The effect of CNVs on frequently seen diseases appears to be negligible, but when rare DNA loci associated with a disease state are inserted, the "dose" of affected DNA can alter disease expression. Examples include familial Parkinson disease, and schizophrenia. CNVs either can be associated with a mendelian gene inheritance or can appear de novo, as a new variant, in the genome.

GENETIC HISTORY AND FAMILY PEDIGREE

One of the tools used to determine whether a disease has a genetic component is construction of a family pedigree.[27] For clinicians, it is important to develop the skills to ask questions

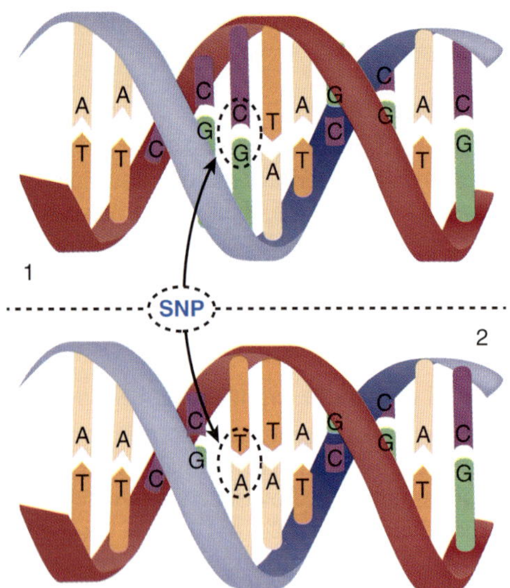

FIG. 3.7 Single Nucleotide Polymorphism (SNP) Where One Nucleotide Base Letter is Replaced by a Different Base Letter.

to elucidate which family members are affected and which are unaffected and then to identify the standardized symbols used in the construction of a pedigree.[27] The use of a legend to explain what the symbols mean prevents misinterpretation and allows for the recent addition of new symbols to reflect sex and gender diversity.[28] The *proband* is the name given to the first person diagnosed in the family pedigree.[27]

Homozygous Versus Heterozygous

All persons inherit genetic material from their father and mother. If an individual inherits two identical genes at a specific locus (genetic address) from both parents, the person is described as homozygous for that gene. This has consequences if the gene is associated with a disease.

- **Homozygous.** If the genes from each parent are the same at a locus, the person is described as homozygous for that gene. Generally, if the inherited genes (alleles) are associated with a disease, a person who is homozygous will have signs and symptoms.
- **Heterozygous.** If the genes from each parent differ at a locus, the person is described as heterozygous for that gene. If the inherited gene (allele) is associated with a disease, a person who is heterozygous will typically not have signs of a disease, because the nonaffected allele will be functional and take over.

BOX 3.1 Genetic Conditions in Critical Care: Deep Vein Thrombosis and Factor V Leiden

Clinical Presentation

- Carriers of the coagulation factor V Leiden polymorphism are at increased risk for venous thromboembolism, identified by deep vein thrombosis (DVT) or pulmonary embolism. The phenotype (clinical signs and symptoms) is defined by an increased incidence of blood clots. Factor V Leiden thrombophilia is suspected in individuals with a history of DVT or pulmonary embolism and in people with first-degree family members who have experienced recurrent thromboemboli. Assessment is warranted for women who experience DVT during pregnancy or DVT while on oral contraceptives or hormone replacement therapy (HRT). Factor V Leiden is found in up to 25% of patients with venous thromboembolism and in 50% of patients with familial thrombophilia.[18]

Genetic Evidence

- The factor V (*F5*) gene is located on chromosome 1 on the long arm at position 23 (1q23). Factor V Leiden polymorphism refers to the specific G-to-A substitution at nucleotide 1691 in the coagulation factor V gene (genotype). This causes a single amino acid replacement at position 506 from arginine to glutamine. The resultant nonfunctional gene protein is called factor V Leiden.[18]

Normal factor V circulates in plasma as an inactive cofactor. Activation by thrombin results in the formation of factor Va, which serves as a cofactor in the conversion of prothrombin to thrombin. To express its anticoagulant function, normal factor Va must be cleaved by activated protein C (APC) at arginine in the 506 position and then at other sites within the factor Va molecule. Factor Va Leiden cannot be cleaved by APC because there is a glutamine at the 506 position. Therefore, factor Va Leiden is inactivated more slowly than normal factor Va. This leaves more factor Va available within the prothrombin complex, which increases coagulation with ongoing generation of thrombin.

The term *Leiden* in the name refers to the town in the Netherlands where the gene was initially discovered. Factor V Leiden is also the most common cause of APC resistance, which may additively increase the risk of thrombosis.

Gene-Environment Interactions

- The standard risk factors for DVT also apply to patients with factor V Leiden. The risk for DVT is increased by smoking, obesity, immobility, and trauma. Several additional genetic defects in the factor V gene have been identified as possible risk factors for thrombosis. One study identified seven other SNPs associated with DVT occurrence. Individuals with two or more genetic risk factors (gene-gene interactions) are at much higher risk for DVT.[18] Studies to evaluate this risk are ongoing.

Inheritance

- The factor V Leiden allele is inherited in an autosomal dominant pattern.[18] This means a person needs only one copy (allele) of the factor V Leiden gene (heterozygous) to have a threefold to eightfold increased risk for DVT.[18] People who are homozygous have two copies of the variant gene (one from each parent) and have a 10-fold to 80-fold increased risk of DVT.[18]

Who Should Undergo Genetic Testing?

- Genetic testing is reserved for individuals in high-risk groups who have experienced a first DVT before age 60 years; individuals who have experienced a first, unprovoked (no environmental stimuli) DVT at any age; and individuals with a history of recurrent DVT. There is no recommendation to test asymptomatic family members unless they have additional risk factors.[18]

To test for factor V Leiden, the first step is to do an APC resistance assay. If the blood test shows APC resistance, it is likely the person carries the factor V Leiden variant, and genetic testing is undertaken as a secondary analysis.[18]

Direct-to-Consumer Testing?

With direct-to-consumer testing, the opportunity to obtain personalized information about genes and related medical conditions is remarkably easy. A survey of 2354 participants, who had received information about their Factor V Leiden status, and their Factor II Prothrombin variant status from 23andMe, Inc., provided more information.[83] Most participants described that they were satisfied to have this information, whether they were negative (n = 1110) or positive (n = 1224) for the prothrombotic alleles, and most perceived that this knowledge was helpful in their discussions with health care providers.[83]

Modes of Inheritance

One of the keys to understanding genetics is to understand the vocabulary. All humans have 23 pairs of chromosomes. One pair is sex linked: XX for a woman and XY for a man. The other 22 chromosomes are called *autosomes;* the term *autosomal inheritance* is derived from this word. Examples of three pedigrees that illustrate single-gene inheritance patterns and the symbols used to construct a pedigree are shown in Fig. 3.8 with examples described in the following sections.

Autosomal Dominant Inheritance

Autosomal dominant inheritance is described as a dominant pattern because only one copy of an affected gene is required to transmit the condition. The person has inherited one affected gene from one parent and one healthy gene from the other parent and is described as heterozygous for that gene. Typically, the disease appears in every generation. Each child of an affected parent has a 50% chance of inheriting the condition, depending on whether a parent has transmitted the affected gene. Male and female offspring are equally likely to inherit and transmit the condition (see Fig. 3.8A). Examples of conditions with autosomal dominant inheritance patterns include familial hypercholesterolemia, Marfan syndrome, and hypertrophic cardiomyopathy.[29]

Autosomal Recessive Inheritance

With an autosomal recessive pattern of inheritance, the disease or condition manifests only if the person has received an affected gene from both parents. The parents each carry the gene but are not themselves affected. The parents are heterozygous because they have one copy of a normally functioning gene and one copy of an affected gene. Any of their children has a 25% chance to inherit in these combinations: one normal and one affected gene (heterozygous carrier), two normal genes (unaffected), or two affected genes (homozygous affected). Persons who are homozygous for the gene associated with the disease always are affected, which means they demonstrate the phenotype of the disease (see Fig. 3.8B). In autosomal recessive inheritance, the phenotype associated with the condition is seen more often in siblings (sibships) than in the parents. Conditions associated with autosomal recessive inheritance include cystic fibrosis and sickle cell disease.

Sex-Linked Inheritance

Traits controlled by genes located on the sex chromosomes are sex linked. Red-green color blindness and hemophilia are examples of X-linked conditions.[5] Women always have two X chromosomes (XX), one from the mother and one from the father. Even if the mother carried an affected *F8* gene, the gene on the unaffected X chromosome from the father confers the ability to make the coagulation factor, and female offspring avoid hemophilia. However, male (XY) offspring inherit one X chromosome from their mother and one Y chromosome from their father. If the mother's X chromosome carries the affected *F8* gene, the male offspring is unable to make sufficient factor VIII and manifests the bleeding disorder known as hemophilia A. The same inheritance pattern occurs with an affected *F9* gene that cannot produce coagulation factor IX, resulting in hemophilia B. Both conditions can result in life-threatening bleeding.

In an X-linked disorder, each son has a 50% chance of having hemophilia, and each daughter has a 50% chance of being a carrier. In a family pedigree, the absence of direct male-to-male transmission makes this condition identifiable as an X-linked disorder. Hemophilia A is an example of a single-gene disorder. Fig. 3.8C illustrates an X-linked family pedigree for hemophilia A; a man who is affected (generation I) may pass the X-linked *F8* gene only to his daughters (generation II), who may pass the gene to sons who will be affected or to daughters who will be carriers (generation III). A girl will be affected only if she receives an affected X-linked gene from both her father and her mother, as occurs in generation IV.

Hemophilia A and Hemophilia B. Hemophilia A and B both have a single-gene X-linked recessive inheritance pattern. Hemophilia results from inadequate production of essential clotting factor proteins, resulting in bleeding that is not controlled by normal clotting processes.[30]

- **Hemophilia A.** The *F8* gene codes for the protein that makes coagulation factor VIII and is located on the X chromosome. Inadequate factor VIII is associated with hemophilia A. See Fig. 3.8C for a recessive inheritance pedigree example.
- **Hemophilia B.** The *F9* gene codes for the protein that makes coagulation factor IX and is located on the X chromosome. Inadequate factor IX is associated with hemophilia B.

At the present time, hemophilia is treated by replacement clotting factors. Researchers are investigating gene therapy as a potential cure for hemophilia A and B.

OBTAINING GENETICS AND GENOMICS INFORMATION

Genetic information can be collected in many ways and for many purposes, including research, health improvement, and increasingly by law enforcement. All the methods described below may be used to link the phenotype, genotype, and environment. Methods can be descriptive (interviewing family members), epidemiologic (following a cohort of patients with a known condition), collecting biologic samples (blood test, buccal swab), and involve genetic sequencing and analysis.

Genetic Epidemiology and Phenotypes

A phenotype is the physical expression of a trait or disease. Before a gene can be mapped (genotyped), it is essential to have a reliable phenotype that can be consistently measured, although this is not a one-to-one relationship in many cases.[31] One of the challenges in applying genetics to the critical care environment is that the genotype is stable, but the phenotype is dynamic. Phenotypes are different at different stages of a disease and are influenced by medications, environmental factors, and gene-gene interactions. It is helpful to discuss the methods used outside of the critical care unit as a way of understanding the challenges in the application of genomics in this arena.

Family-Based Genetic Studies

In genetic epidemiologic research of a rare disease, it can be a challenge to find enough people to study. One method is to work with large, extended families, known as *kinships*, which have several family members affected with the disease. Genetic testing is done to construct a genetic linkage map of the area close to the polymorphic gene found in that family. Family-based studies can identify a significant phenotype-genotype relationship. Subsequently, it is important to do studies of other groups to determine whether the original finding is unique to the kinship or can be generalized to people outside the family.

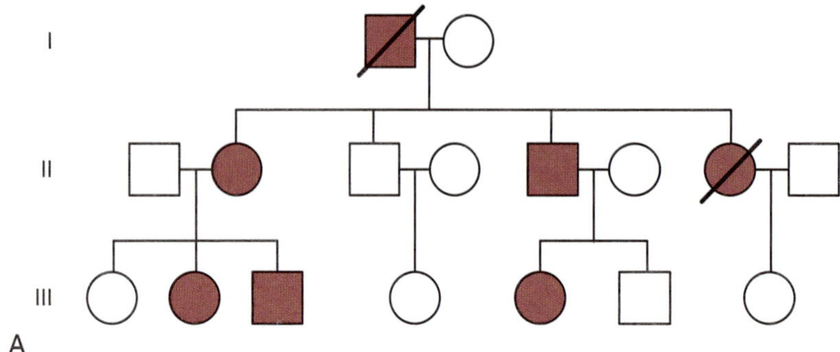

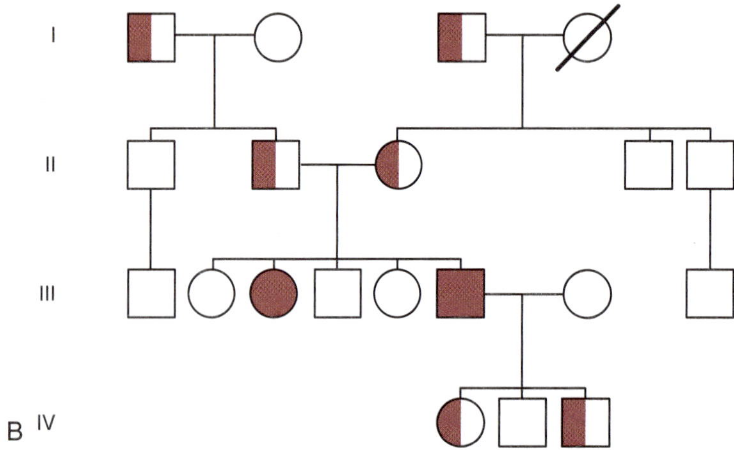

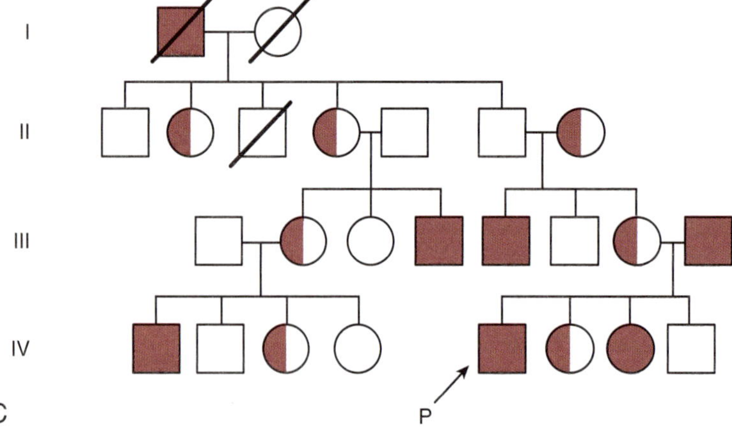

FIG. 3.8 (A) Pedigree of a dominant mode of inheritance. (B) Pedigree of a recessive mode of inheritance. (C) Pedigree of an X-linked mode of inheritance. See text for further information.

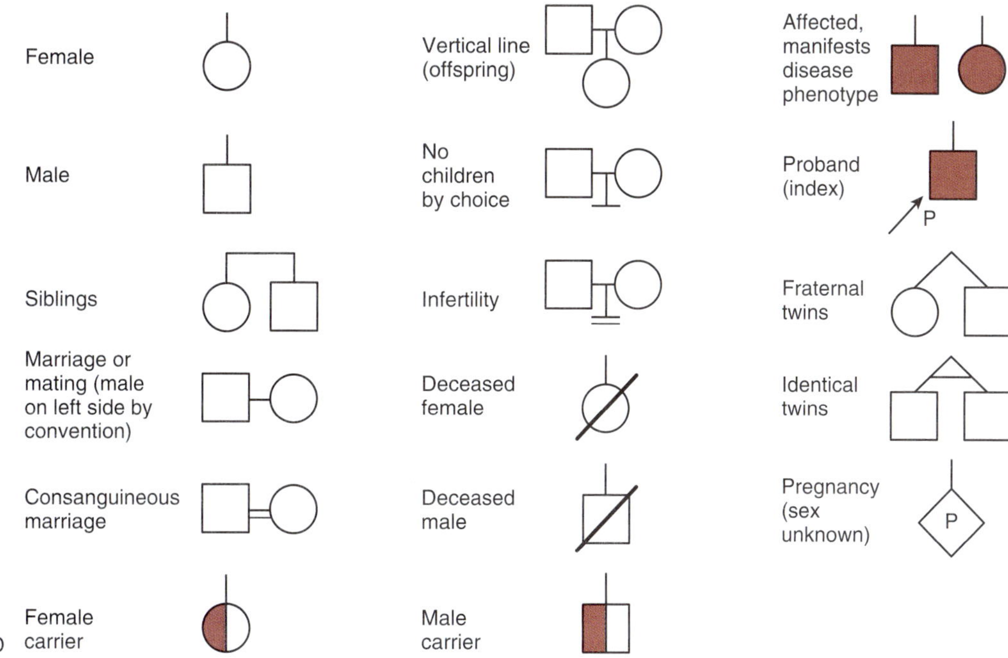

FIG. 3.8, cont'd (D) Symbols used to construct a pedigree.

Genetic Association Studies

Genetic association studies recruit a diverse group of individuals to determine whether a trait is universal or found only in selected groups. Genetic studies can be conducted in isolated populations, or in highly mixed groups. Several national biobanks have been established to study genetic associations within specific countries.[32] It is important to collect information about ancestral and racial heritage to enable linkage of phenotypic and genotypic data. Diverse populations are sometimes called *admixed populations*, indicating that many different heritage groups have been included in the mix of people. The purpose of these different kinds of studies is to make a clear phenotype-genotype match and to identify which genetic conditions are associated with ancestral groups and which genetic conditions are universal.

Case-Control Studies

In case-control studies, individuals are identified with the phenotypic and genotypic traits of a disease (cases). These cases are then matched to nonrelated control subjects by age, race, sex, and sometimes other associated disease factors.

Candidate Gene Studies

Candidate gene studies usually are exploratory studies in which a gene is suspected as a contributor to a phenotype or disease. Unrelated individuals with the phenotype are then tested for presence of the gene. These studies are usually smaller, and there is a strong biologic rationale for investigating the association between genotype and phenotype.

Genome-Wide Association Studies

GWAS examine the breadth of the human genome and typically use very large samples. The intent is to use genetic microarray technology and statistical computational power to find SNPs associated with a disease. Some GWAS are conducted with the intent of finding additional genes. However, one of the strengths of the GWAS model is that it does not have to begin with a biologic model in mind as long as the disease of interest is sufficiently common in the population. By testing thousands of SNPs, the researchers may find associations that have not been detected by other methods. The classic example was a GWAS of 14,000 individuals (cases) with 3000 shared controls genotyped to find SNPs associated with seven common diseases.[33] Significant new SNPs were found for five of seven diseases: type 1 diabetes, type 2 diabetes, rheumatoid arthritis, Crohn disease, and coronary artery disease.[33] New GWAS are published every month, and the *National Human Genome Research Institute* maintains an online catalog of published studies that can be searched by disease trait, chromosomal region, gene, or SNP.[34]

GENOME MAPPING PROJECTS

Knowledge about the human genome has expanded by purposefully increasing the diversity of collection and sequencing studies. A few key genomic projects are listed to describe some of the methods used, although this is only a fraction of all the work that has been done to understand the human genome.

Human Genome Project

The Human Genome Project is an international collaborative project that began in 1990 with the goal of making a map of all the human genes (the genome). The initial genome sequence was published in 2003. Although the initial human genome map was created from the DNA of only a few people,[4] it provided the foundation for future work. A complete sequence of a human genome, without gaps, was recently completed,[35] although neither does this sequence capture the variation in all human populations.[36]

One major finding from the initial human genome was that the number of genes possessed by humans was not as large as expected. The number of protein-coding genes in the chromosome is estimated to be between 20,000 and 25,000.[4] Although researchers were initially surprised that the gene number was not higher, it is now known that many posttranscriptional alterations occur that actively change the protein product. The ongoing research agenda is to understand all these additional sequence elements as described in the following sections. Many of the outcomes are publicly available as listed below.

ENCODE Project

The *EN*Cyclopedia *O*f *D*NA *E*lements (ENCODE) is a research-based public database of cell and tissue research, which identifies human genes and the proteins and other biologic products that are encoded by these genes.[37–39] The ENCODE project originated in 2003 and is ongoing.[38]

Exome Sequencing Project

Exons are the sections of DNA that code for proteins. The Exome Sequencing Project searches for more information about single-gene disorders, sometimes called *mendelian gene disorders*, or *monogenetic disorders*.[40] Sickle cell disease and cystic fibrosis are both examples of single-gene disorders. Whole exome sequencing has the potential to find more disease-causing mutations because 85% of known mutations are within the exon regions.

Human Proteome Project

The goal of the *Human Proteome Project* is to catalog all protein-coding genes.[41,42] Proteins have been described as "machines of life"[42] because proteins are central to structural and biochemical functions in the human body. The process of protein manufacture is diagrammed as follows: DNA (exon or protein-coding gene) → messenger RNA → transfer RNA → 3 nucleotide amino acid (codon) → chain of amino acids → protein. Changes in this process can be associated with disease states. The *Human Protein Atlas* is an online resource that documents the proteome.[43]

Many protein-coding genes are very specific, including genes that function during one phase of life (in utero) and are silenced after birth. Other genes have multiple variants that alter the protein shape, and consequently alter function and phenotype. For the gene (*7q31.2*) that encodes the CFTR protein, over 2000 variants have been found, related to multiple phenotypes for cystic fibrosis.[44]

Human Microbiome Project

In the healthy human body, microbial cells vastly outnumber human cells, sometimes being described as our second genome.[45] The human body is host to many microbial communities (human microbiome) located on the skin and in the nose, mouth, and gastrointestinal and urogenital tracts. The spectrum of these microbial communities was previously almost entirely unknown. The *Human Microbiome Project* was designed to identify the core human microbiome and to determine whether changes in the human microbiome can be correlated with changes in human health.[45] The human microbiome project is highly relevant to critical care because so many patients experience antibiotic-associated disruption of the gastrointestinal tract and diarrhea from infection with *Clostridioides difficile* (*Clostridium difficile or C. diff*).[46] The interaction of host bacteria, pathologic bacteria, the critical care environment, and pharmacogenetics has the potential to bring novel insights to current understanding of critical illness.

GENETIC DIVERSITY

Increasing the diversity in the representation of genetic data is extremely important. The initial human genome sequence was from a few individuals of European ancestry and the goal since has been to gather information from diverse ancestries and to understand the biology of how genes influence health and disease worldwide.[47–49]

The oldest human genetic lineages originate from the continent of Africa. The migration waves of humans out of Africa toward northern latitudes resulted in loss of genetic diversity because the genetic pool of the groups that migrated was smaller. Several studies have shown higher levels of nucleotide and haplotype diversity of nuclear and mitochondrial genomes in Africans compared with non-Africans.[50,51]

Diversity, Haplotype Blocks, and Linkage Disequilibrium

Recombination of different sections of the chromosome is one genetic mechanism that increases diversity. This was demonstrated in the International HapMap Project, an early project designed to increase the ancestral diversity of genetic samples. HapMap created a database of over 3 million SNPs representing several ancestrally diverse populations.[52] Genetically, the HapMap displays short linear sections of genetic loci on the same chromosome known as haplotypes or haplotype blocks. Loci are grouped as a haplotype if they are close to each other on a chromosome and are inherited as a linear group. Genetic epidemiologists call this grouped pattern *linkage disequilibrium*.[53] In other words, because the loci are linked by shared ancestry, genetic information is inherited in genetic "chunks" or "blocks" rather than as individual genes.

The mixing of sections of different chromosomes that are inherited from each parent is called *recombination*.[53] The resultant linked genetic loci are called haplotypes. The edges of the haplotypes are conceptualized as areas where minimal ancestral relationship remains. In the human genome, thousands of recombination areas result in significant change over time as illustrated by the hypothetical example of how a haplotype could theoretically change over the span of 1000 generations, from African ancestral chromosomes to modern chromosomes (Fig. 3.9). The biologic rationale for recombination is to increase genetic diversity.

Increasingly genetic databases are being created in Africa, Asia, South America, and other continents that were not included in the first wave of genetic discoveries.[47,54] An expanded genetic pool allows for both discovery of novel variants[54] and the study of universal diseases such as type 2 diabetes.[55–57]

GENETICS IN CRITICAL CARE

The next step in the genomics revolution will be to connect the growing amounts of research data to clinical interventions that may help patients. The areas of clinical practice that have received the most genetic attention are thrombophilia, hemophilia, cancer, cardiovascular disease, and pharmacogenomics.

Thrombosis Genetics

The likelihood of DVTs and other thromboses is increased if a patient carries a variant allele for a gene that codes for any of the blood clotting factors.

Factor V Leiden and Thrombosis

For patients with factor V Leiden, a substitution of glutamine (G) for arginine (A) at position 506 alters one of the cleavage

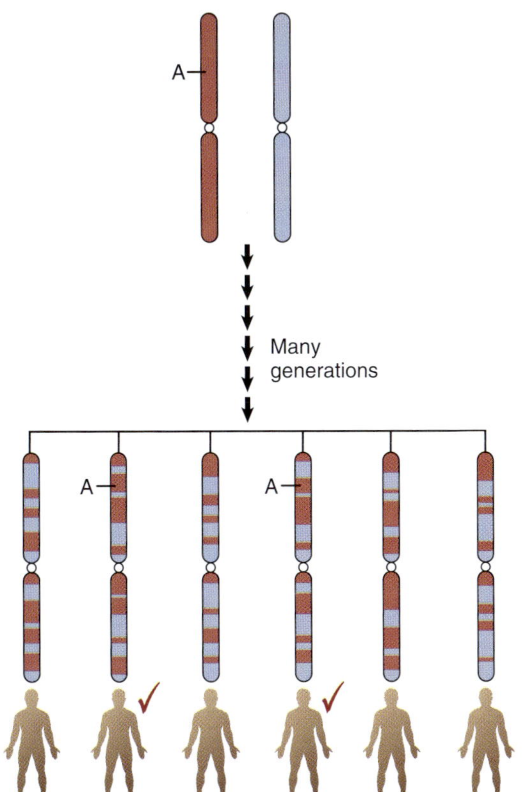

FIG. 3.9 Effect of Recombination on Ancestral Chromosomes. A gene is labeled *A* on the red ancestral chromosome. It is an example of a gene that has been conserved in modern chromosomes in one-third of cases. The gene (*A*) is associated with a specific phenotype or trait (shown as a checkmark). Because of recombination of chromosomes over thousands of generations, two-thirds of modern chromosomes no longer carry this gene.

sites for *Activated Protein C* (APC). This slows factor Va inactivation and blood is more likely to clot. In the critical care setting this increases risk of DVT and pulmonary embolus (see Box 3.1). Factor V Leiden is the most common inherited thrombophilia.

Prothrombin Gene Mutation and Thrombosis

A mutation in the gene that codes for the production of prothrombin (coagulation factor II) causes an overproduction of prothrombin, which increases clot formation and increases risk of any venous thrombosis, from DVT to pulmonary embolism.[58] This is the second more common inherited thrombophilia. In procoagulant gene mutations, gene-environment interactions are especially important when the forced immobility (environment) due to illness meets excess prothrombin (gene), increasing the risk of thromboses. For women with this mutation, pregnancy also increases the risk of a thrombosis developing.[59]

Cancer Genetics

Cancer genetics are described as *somatic,* which means "related to the body." Somatic mutations are changes within a specific group of body tissues that are not heritable. Somatic changes often are related to changes in genetic markers associated with cancer.[60]

The Cancer Genome Atlas

There is strong evidence that many forms of cancer are caused by epigenetic alterations; one mechanism is the addition of methyl groups to specific genes to block their effect, a process sometimes referred to as *gene silencing*. Epigenetic changes can disrupt the normal balance in cell proliferation, cell survival, and cell differentiation. The *Cancer Genome Atlas* (TCGA) project was established to accelerate understanding of the molecular basis of human cancers.[61] The large-scale genome sequencing techniques, first developed in the Human Genome Project, are used to sequence genes associated with lethal and common cancers. The goal is to document all cancer genetic changes from chromosomal rearrangements to DNA mutations to epigenetic changes (chemical modifications of DNA that can turn genes on or off without altering the DNA sequence). The cancer atlas findings have shown that targeting specialized biologic pathways in many lethal cancers may be more important than focusing on single genes.

CARDIOVASCULAR GENETICS

Genetic markers are now included in many cardiovascular research studies to improve understanding of the genomic and environmental factors that underpin cardiovascular disease.

Long QT Syndrome

Long QT syndrome (LQTS) is a hereditary cardiac channelopathy with many different genotypes and a phenotype that manifests as a prolongation of the corrected QT interval (QTc) on the electrocardiogram (ECG).[62–64] More than 80% of cases of LQTS are caused by three gene mutations.[62–64] Affected individuals have an increased risk of sudden cardiac death (SCD) (Box 3.2). Not all patients who have the LQTS genotype are aware of their condition, and not all have a prolonged QTc at rest. In the critical care unit, these patients are at high risk of gene-environment, or gene-medication, interactions that can lengthen the QTc interval and entrain polymorphic ventricular tachycardia, also known as *torsades de pointes*; see discussion on torsades de pointes in Chapter 12. Acquired LQT is much more common, caused by hypokalemia or medications, and the combination can create a gene-electrolyte or gene-medication interaction that is highly proarrhythmic.[62–64]

Familial Inherited Cardiomyopathies

The spectrum of cardiomyopathy genotypes and phenotypes is diverse. Some are single-gene disorders (inherited), and some are complex trait disorders with a strong environmental component, such as coronary artery disease.

Noninherited cardiomyopathy from ischemic or valvular heart disease is described in Chapter 13.

Hypertrophic Cardiomyopathy

Hypertrophic cardiomyopathy is the most frequently encountered inherited cardiomyopathy. It is a single gene disorder, with predominantly autosomal dominant inheritance.[65] Two genes, *MYH7* and *MYBPC3*, that encode for cardiac sarcomere proteins account for 40% of cases.[65] Inheritance of either one of the causative gene mutations increases risk for the condition. The risk of dysrhythmias and SCD is high for patients who manifest a hypertrophic phenotype.[66] To identify other members of the family who may be affected, it is recommended to construct a three-generation pedigree and perform genetic testing.

BOX 3.2 Genetic Conditions in Critical Care: Long QT Syndrome

Clinical Presentation

- Long QT syndrome (LQTS) is a cardiac genetic disorder associated with prolongation of the QT interval. This is defined as a corrected QT interval (QTc) longer than 500 msec on a resting ECG. LQTS is estimated to affect 1 in 2000 individuals and is one of the causes of sudden cardiac death (SCD).[62–64]

Patients are frequently identified following a syncopal episode, a life-threatening dysrhythmia such as torsades de pointes, or an aborted SCD.[86] Treatment regimens include beta-blockers.[86] For patients with LQTS who are at high risk of cardiac arrest, insertion of a pacemaker/internal cardioverter defibrillator is warranted.[86]

Critically ill patients with undiagnosed LQTS are vulnerable to additional prolongation of the QT interval from various medications. The American Heart Association recommends monitoring of the QTc interval. See Chapter 12 for more explanation about the QTc interval.

Genetic Evidence

- Several genes have been identified for LQTS but over 80% of LQTS is associated with three genes.[62–64] All encode protein components of the cardiac ion channels and modulate ionic flow. This is why LQTS disorders are often described as "channelopathies."
- In children, this may be described as congenital LQTS.[87] Additionally, several LQTS genes are associated with other conditions in addition to the cardiac manifestations.[86] The three gene-channelopathies described below are only associated with cardiac electrocardiographic dysrhythmias.

Phenotype	Gene	Cardiac Channel	Stimuli	Dysrhythmia Syncopal Events[86]	Sudden Cardiac Death Risk[86]	Function
LQTS1	*KCNQ1*	Potassium	Exercise Emotion	63%	6%–8%	Encodes a potassium channel protein, active in phase 3 of the cardiac action potential
LQTS2	*KCNH2*	Potassium	Auditory Exercise	46%	6%–8%	Encodes a potassium channel protein that normally terminates the cardiac action potential
LQTS3	*SCN5A*	Sodium	Sleep	18%	6%–8%	Encodes a sodium channel protein, active in phase 0 of the cardiac action potential

Gene-Environment Interactions

- Gene-environment interactions are significant for patients with LQTS and vary by genotype and by individual.

Inheritance

- LQTS1, LQTS2, and LQTS3 all have an autosomal dominant pattern of inheritance.[86] Not all individuals have the same phenotype, even with the same genotype. This is thought to be related to the influence of additional genes acting in concert with the primary gene to alter the cardiac action potential to cause QTc prolongation.

Who Should Undergo Genetic Testing?

- Clinical genetic testing is available for LQTS. Genetic testing is very helpful in families of patients with LQTS.[87] If the family member has a prolonged QTc interval, the reasonable assumption during the cardiac and genetic work-up is that they have the mutation. It is also important to test family members with a normal QTc interval, as up to 25% have "concealed" LQTS, meaning they have a normal QTc interval on resting ECG.[86] This is because of a genetic concept termed *penetrance*, in which the same gene does not have the same phenotypic effect on everyone who is affected. If a person carries the genetic mutation but has a normal QTc interval at rest, they may still be vulnerable during exercise, physiologic stress, electrolyte imbalance, or if prescribed a medication that prolongs the QTc interval.

Dilated Cardiomyopathy

Familial dilated cardiomyopathy is associated with mutations in multiple genes; 51 genes have been implicated, and 19 genes have strong links with dilated cardiomyopathy.[67] Most have an autosomal dominant mode of inheritance. The phenotype is left ventricular enlargement with systolic dysfunction, often with affected family members. Phenotype presentation is variable, even in patients with a known causative gene.

Arrhythmogenic Right Ventricular Cardiomyopathy

Arrhythmogenic right ventricular cardiomyopathy (ARVC) or dysplasia (ARVD) is a rare genetic disorder where the myocardium is progressively replaced by fatty/fibrous tissue and this is associated with lethal dysrhythmias. ARVC inheritance has been associated with 16 genes that encode for cardiac dermasome proteins.[68,69] Autosomal dominant inheritance appears to be most frequent per family pedigree charts.[68]

PHARMACOGENETICS

Pharmacogenetics is the study of gene-medication interactions.[8] Pharmacogenetics is likely to be the most visible effect of genetics encountered in the adult critical care unit, particularly in relation to the cytochrome P450 (CYP450) family of enzymes involved in medication metabolism.

Cytochrome P450 and Medication Metabolism

The CYP450 enzymes are a superfamily of heme-containing enzymes that are vital for medication metabolism. The CYP450 family contains 57 functional genes that code for enzymes involved in medication metabolism. The isoenzymes *CYP3A4* and *CYP3A5* metabolize approximately 50% of medications, and they constitute approximately 60% of the total hepatic CYP450 enzyme content.[70] The metabolism of more than 90% of the most clinically important medications can be accounted for by seven CYP isoenzymes: 3A4, 3A5, 1A2, 2C9, 2C19, 2D6, and 2E1.[70] *CYP3A4* can be used to understand what the abbreviations represent.[70]

- *CYP* represents the symbol for all cytochrome P450 proteins
- *3* denotes the gene family
- *A* designates the subfamily
- *4* represents the individual gene

The FDA now requires that new medications undergo testing for interactions with the CYP450 pathway before release.[71]

Warfarin

Warfarin (Coumadin) was, until recently, a frequently prescribed anticoagulant for patients with atrial fibrillation, mechanical cardiac valves, and thrombotic disorders. Variants in the CYP450 enzyme *CYP2C9* gene and in the vitamin K epoxide reductase complex subunit 1 gene (*VKORC1*) contribute to the considerable dose variation seen with this anticoagulant.[72] The vitamin K epoxide reductase (VKOR) enzyme activates the vitamin K–dependent clotting factors (II, VII, IX, X). Warfarin is used to inhibit the VKOR complex to prevent clot formation.

Warfarin dose variability between patients to achieve a therapeutic international normalized ratio (INR) ranges from 10% to 45%, depending on *CYP2C9* and *VKORC1* polymorphisms. Genetic testing is not currently recommended for everyone who takes warfarin. Laboratory tests to detect the *CYP2C9* and *VKORC1* variants are available at specialized reference laboratories. The FDA added a warning label on the package to alert clinicians about *CYP2C9* and *VKORC1* polymorphism interactions and their effects on warfarin dosing. These genetic interactions, plus the option of newer anticoagulant medications, mean that warfarin is prescribed less frequently today.

Malignant Hyperthermia

Malignant hyperthermia is a rare inherited genetic disorder that negatively affects skeletal muscle on exposure to volatile anesthetics and depolarizing muscle relaxants. It may be unexpectedly discovered during general anesthesia. In malignant hyperthermia, calcium is released from the muscle sarcoplasmic reticulum and induces life-threatening muscle contracture with skeletal muscle rigidity, increased carbon dioxide production, acidosis, and elevated temperature. The first causative gene to be identified was the ryanodine receptor 1 gene (*RYR1*) located at chromosome 19q13.1.[73] The *RYR1* gene encodes for a ryanodine receptor that releases stored calcium from the sarcoplasmic reticulum in muscle.[73–76] Malignant hyperthermia is described in more detail in Box 3.3.

GENE EDITING—CRISPR-Cas9 TECHNOLOGY

Gene editing, once the realm of science fiction, is now feasible for any sequenced genome. The technology, known as *CRISPR-Cas9*, which stands for "*c*lustered *r*egularly *i*nterspaced *s*hort *p*alindromic *r*epeat" (Cas9), has revolutionized the field of gene editing in the biologic sciences. The Cas9 enzyme creates breaks at a target site of double-stranded DNA. The gene can then be disabled, or a new gene with a different function can be inserted at the site. This technology has the potential to offer a cure for diseases caused by a single gene, such as Huntington disease, and hemophilia. This research has now progressed from animal models to human trials. CRISPR has opened a new era in genetic treatment options, and one of the first research breakthroughs is for sickle cell disease.[77,78]

BOX 3.3 Genetic Conditions in Critical Care: Malignant Hyperthermia

Clinical Presentation

- Malignant hyperthermia is a pharmacogenetic syndrome. It is a disorder of skeletal muscle calcium regulation. On exposure to volatile anesthetics and depolarizing muscle relaxants, susceptible patients experience life-threatening symptoms, including sustained muscle contracture with skeletal muscle rigidity, which causes metabolic acidosis, tachycardia, and fever. Early physiologic warning signs include rigidity of the masseter muscle and a sudden rise end-tidal carbon dioxide level ($ETCO_2$). The symptoms result from a dysregulated abnormally high release of intracellular calcium in skeletal muscle.[73–76]

Genetic Evidence

- Genetic linkage studies associated the malignant hyperthermia phenotype with the ryanodine receptor 1 gene (*RYR1*) at chromosome 19q13.1 in affected families.[88] Calcium transport from muscle sarcoplasmic reticulum through the ryanodine receptor into the sarcoplasm occurs during muscular excitation and contraction. The *RYR1* gene is highly polymorphic, with more than 400 variants, of which 31 mutations are known to cause the condition.[88] The presence of any of these mutations is diagnostic for malignant hyperthermia susceptibility. Genetic testing by muscle biopsy is available to identify causative *RYR1* gene mutations.[73–76]

Gene-Environment Interactions

- Malignant hyperthermia is an example of a gene-medication-environment interaction. It is not an allergy, and it occurs under the specific environmental condition of general anesthesia with inhalation anesthetics (e.g., chloroform, desflurane, enflurane, halothane, isoflurane, methoxyflurane, sevoflurane, trichloroethylene) and depolarizing muscle relaxants (e.g., succinylcholine).[73,88]

Inheritance

- Malignant hyperthermia is inherited in an autosomal dominant pattern. This means that only one affected allele is needed to have the condition and that children of an affected person have a 50% chance of inheriting the mutated *RYR1* gene.

Who Should Undergo Genetic Testing?

- Malignant hyperthermia crisis under general anesthesia is rare. The genetic test for *RYR1* is not recommended as a general screening test. Genetic testing is recommended only for individuals who have experienced a malignant hyperthermia crisis, individuals who are first-degree relatives of a person with known malignant hyperthermia, or individuals who have had a positive result from a muscle biopsy.[75,76] The value of the genetic test is that when a mutation is discovered, family members with the same mutation are considered susceptible to malignant hyperthermia and can avoid a diagnostic muscle biopsy. The major advantage of being aware of the diagnosis is that high-risk anesthetics can be avoided for general anesthesia in individuals susceptible to malignant hyperthermia.

Sickle Cell Disease CRISPR Gene Editing

In December 2023 the U.S. Food and Drug Administration (FDA) approved the first gene editing treatment for sickle cell disease using CRISPR Technology. The drug is called exa-cel (Casgevy) and was developed by Vertex Pharmaceuticals and CRISPR Therapeutics. Briefly the process is:

- Stem cells are removed from the affected patient's bone marrow.

- The cells are grown in the laboratory (outside the body) and will undergo gene editing using CRISPR Cas9 to deactivate *BCL11A* in the bone marrow stem cells.[77,78]
- The gene editing turns off the genetic switch that normally causes fetal hemoglobin to stop being produced after birth. As a result, fetal hemoglobin will now be produced.
- High-dose chemotherapy is administered to depress the patient's own bone marrow.
- The gene-edited cells are returned to the patient in a series of blood transfusions to replenish the bone marrow with the gene-edited cells.

The reason to promote fetal hemoglobin production is because it has a normal spherical shape. The sickle cell mutation in gene *HBB*, located on chromosome 11p15.5, only affects adult hemoglobin, and fetal hemoglobin is unaffected. By increasing the amount of fetal hemoglobin (by reversing the genetic fetal to adult hemoglobin switch *BCL11A*) there will be more spherical red blood cells to carry oxygen and prevent clumping of the sickled cells.

The clinical goal of the treatment is to prevent sickled cells from linking together and blocking small blood vessels. This therapy is in its infancy, and the FDA has requested follow-up for 15 years to assess for long-term effectiveness, side effects, complications, and to determine if it is truly a cure for sickle cell disease. Other gene-based based therapies are in research and development.

GENETICS, GENOMICS, AND NURSING

As genetics and genomics exert more influence in clinical practice, there will be implications for the knowledge base of nurses and other professionals in health care. The learning curve may be steep. The addition of genetics also introduces new ethical and legal dilemmas into health care discussions. Genetics and genomics will have a big effect on how health and illness are conceptualized in the future. Genetics and genomics are already required content for baccalaureate nursing education, and this knowledge is now recommended for nurses with graduate degrees.[81] Essential competencies for nursing practice have been developed by the American Nurses Association, and examples are listed in Table 3.2.[82]

It is always demanding to embrace a new model of health care delivery, and that is the challenge for all health care professionals in the coming decades. The tsunami of genetic information that is now flowing into research journals will rapidly make its way into clinical practice, including into critical care. This flood of new and relevant information will mandate that nurses understand genetic terms, incorporate genetic pedigree information into the history and physical examination, and have knowledge about pharmacogenetic interventions. Genetics and genomics constitute a complex area of study, made more so by the rapid evolution of scientific knowledge. One way to begin

SOCIAL DETERMINANTS OF HEALTH

Health Disparities Associated with Sickle Cell Disease

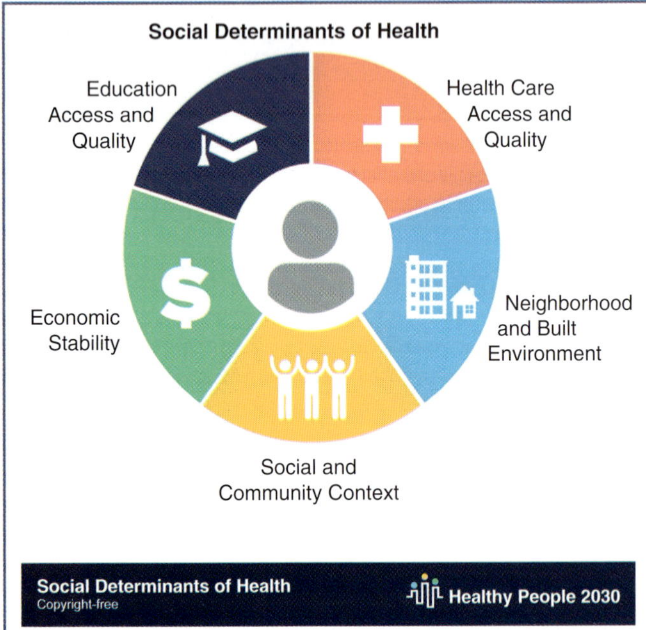

Sickle cell disease (SCD) is a genetic blood disorder that primarily affects individuals of African, African American, Mediterranean, Middle Eastern, and South Asian descent. Historically, individuals with SCD, particularly those from minority and marginalized communities, have faced health care disparities.[80] These disparities include limited access to specialized care, delayed diagnosis, and unequal access to treatments and clinical trials. While the underlying cause of sickle cell anemia is genetic, social factors can influence the management and outcomes of individuals with this condition.

- Access to quality health care, including insurance coverage, proximity to health care facilities, and the availability of specialists, can significantly impact the management of the disease.
- Socioeconomic factors such as income, education, and employment status can influence a person's ability to access health care and afford necessary treatments and medications. Lower socioeconomic status may lead to delayed or inadequate care.
- Discrimination and social stigma related to sickle cell disease can affect a person's mental health and quality of life. Negative stereotypes or misconceptions about the disorder can create barriers to social and health care interactions.
- Understanding the disease and how to manage it is crucial for individuals with sickle cell anemia. Low health literacy and limited access to educational resources can hinder self-care and adherence to treatment plans.
- Environmental conditions, such as exposure to extreme temperatures and air pollution, can trigger sickle cell crises and worsen symptoms. Living in areas with a high disease prevalence can also impact an individual's social support network.
- Individuals with SCD and their families may benefit from genetic counseling to understand the inheritance pattern and make informed family planning decisions. Access to such services can vary based on location and resources.
- Ensuring diversity in clinical trials and research studies related to SCD is critical. Historically, minority populations have been underrepresented in clinical trials, leading to a lack of effective evidence-based treatments for all patient groups.

Addressing these issues is essential to improve the quality of life and health outcomes for individuals with sickle cell anemia. Health care policies, community programs, and advocacy efforts play a role in addressing these factors and reducing health disparities associated with the disease.[79,80]

Reference

1. Porter JS, Heitzer AM, Crosby LE, Hankins JS. Social determinants of health: The next frontier for improving care and outcomes in sickle cell disease. *Lancet Haematol.* 2023;10(8):e571–e573. https://doi.org/10.1016/S2352-3026(23)00185-0.

Illustration from Healthy People 2030, U.S. Department of Health and Human Services, Office of Disease Prevention and Health Promotion. Retrieved September 8, 2022, from https://health.gov/healthypeople/objectives-and-data/social-determinants-health.

TABLE 3.2 Essential Genetics and Genomics Competencies for Nurses

Domain	Competencies of the Registered Nurse
Professional Responsibilities	
Competent nursing incorporating genetic and genomic knowledge and skills	Recognizes when one's own attitudes and values related to genetic and genomic science may affect care provided to patients Advocates for patients' access to desired genetic or genomic services and resources, including support groups Examines competency of practice on a regular basis, identifying areas of strength and areas in which professional development related to genetics and genomics would be beneficial Incorporates genetic and genomic technologies and information into registered nurse practice Demonstrates in practice the importance of tailoring genetic and genomic information and services to patients based on their culture, religion, knowledge level, literacy, and preferred language Advocates for the rights of all patients for autonomous, informed genetic and genomic-related decision making and voluntary action
Professional Practice and Assessment	
Application and integration of knowledge	Demonstrates an understanding of the relationship of genetics or genomics to health, prevention, screening, diagnostics, prognostics, selection of treatment, and monitoring of treatment effectiveness Demonstrates an ability to elicit a minimum of three generations of family health history information Constructs a pedigree from collected family history information using standardized symbols and terminology Collects personal, health, and developmental histories that consider genetic, environmental, and genomic influences and risks Conducts comprehensive health and physical assessments that incorporate knowledge about genetic, environmental, and genomic influences and risk factors Critically analyzes the history and physical assessment findings for genetic, environmental, and genomic influences and risk factors Assesses patients' knowledge, perceptions, and responses to genetic and genomic information Develops plan of care that incorporates genetic and genomic assessment information
Identification of needed information	Identifies patients who may benefit from specific genetic and genomic information or services based on assessment data Identifies credible, accurate, appropriate, and current genetic and genomic information, resources, services, and technologies specific to given patients Identifies ethical, ethnic or ancestral, cultural, religious, legal, fiscal, and societal issues related to genetic and genomic information and technologies Defines issues that undermine the rights of all patients for autonomous, informed genetic- and genomic-related decision making and voluntary action
Assistance with referrals	Facilitates referrals for specialized genetic and genomic services for patients, as needed
Provision of education, care, and support	Provides patients with interpretation of selective genetic and genomic information or services Provides patients with credible, accurate, appropriate, and current genetic and genomic information, resources, services, and technologies that facilitate decision making Uses health promotion and disease prevention practices that consider genetic and genomic influences on risk with personal and environmental risk factors Incorporates knowledge of genetic or genomic risk factors (e.g., patient with a genetic predisposition for high cholesterol levels who can benefit from a change in lifestyle to decrease the likelihood that the genotype will be expressed) Uses genetic- and genomic-based interventions and information to improve patients' outcomes Collaborates with health care providers in providing genetic and genomic health care Collaborates with insurance providers or payers to facilitate reimbursement for genetic and genomic health care services Performs interventions and treatments appropriate to patients' genetic and genomic health care needs Evaluates effect and effectiveness of genetic and genomic technology, information, interventions, and treatments on patients' outcomes

From Consensus Panel on Genetic/Genomic Nursing Competencies. *Essentials of Genetic and Genomic Nursing: Competencies, Curricula Guidelines, and Outcome Indicators.* 3rd ed. American Nurses Association; 2009.

is to look at some of the free, Internet-based, interactive educational tutorials listed in Box 3.4 at the end of this chapter and to become familiar with the genetic and genomic vocabulary in the key terms list at the end of the chapter.

Ethical and Legal Issues in Genetics and Genomics

A paramount concern in the genomic era is to protect the privacy of individuals' unique genetic information. Many countries have established biobanks as repositories of genetic material, and many tissue samples are stored in medical center tissue banks. Because all of the individual's genome is contained within the cell, genomic identity or susceptibility to diseases can easily be determined from a small sample. It is essential to ensure that ethical and legal protections keep pace with technical innovation. Key issues are who *owns* the genetic material and *consent* as to who has access to the genetic information. Debate about

BOX 3.4 Internet Resources

Genomic Databases and References

- National Human Genome Resource Institute (NHGRI): https://www.genome.gov
- Genome-wide association studies (GWAS) catalog maintained by NHGRI: http://www.genome.gov/gwastudies/
- GeneReviews: https://www.ncbi.nlm.nih.gov/books/NBK1116/
- The Cancer Genome Atlas (TCGA): http://cancergenome.nih.gov/

Malignant Hyperthermia

- European Malignant Hyperthermia Group: http://www.emhg.org
- Malignant Hyperthermia Association of the United States: http://www.mhaus.org
- OMIM, ryanodine receptor 1 gene (*RYR1*): http://omim.org/entry/180901

Sickle Cell Disease

- Centers for Disease Control and Prevention (CDC): Sickle Cells Disease: www.cdc.gov/ncbddd/sicklecell/index.html
- Sickle Cell Disease Association of America (SCSAA): www.sicklecelldisease.org/
- CDC and SCDAA sickle cell trait toolkit: www.cdc.gov/ncbddd/sicklecell/toolkit.html

Organizations

- International Society of Nurses in Genetics (ISONG): http://www.isong.org/

Tutorials and Education

- DNA Learning Center, Cold Spring Harbor Laboratory: http://www.dnalc.org/home.html
- Educational materials about genetics and genomics from NHGRI: http://www.genome.gov/Education/

these issues is expected to continue as new advances push the technical limits of what can be discovered from a few drops of blood, a muscle biopsy sample, or a cheek swab.

Direct-to-Consumer Tests

A new frontier in genomics is the ability of any individual to voluntarily undergo genetic testing. Several private companies advertise this service on the Internet. Patients send a sample of their DNA—usually a swab from the inside of the cheek (buccal swab)—to check for selected genetic risks. Other websites offer paternity testing from buccal swabs of the child and father. Many countries are now enacting laws to ensure individuals' genomic information is protected. Genetic counselors caution that the results may be hard to understand or misleading for some individuals, but clearly this information is of great interest to many people.[83]

Genetic Information Nondiscrimination Act

The Genetic Information Nondiscrimination Act (GINA) of 2008 is an essential piece of legislation designed to prevent abuse of genetic information in employment and health insurance decisions in the United States.[84] The purpose of GINA is to protect individuals who may have the gene for a disorder—but do not manifest the phenotype—from being penalized. Some people who may be at risk for a genetic disorder may not undergo testing because they fear that a positive result would affect their employability. GINA also mandates that genetic information about individuals and their families have the same protections as health information.

It is important that clinicians understand that the GINA legislation does not cover all categories of insurance. It offers no protection against discrimination for life insurance, disability insurance, or long-term care insurance.[85] The GINA legislation does not cover members of the military, individuals covered by the US Department of Veterans Affairs, or individuals covered by the Indian Health Service.[85] The GINA legislation was designed to protect individuals with a genetic predisposition who did not have signs, symptoms, or disability. The Americans With Disabilities Act (ADA) provides protections against discrimination for individuals who have disabilities.[85] Nonetheless, the details of both GINA and ADA continue to be challenged through the legal system.[85]

HUMAN GENETICS KEY TERMS

Allele: One of several alternative gene variants that can exist at a single locus (location) on a chromosome. The term *allele* may also be used when referring to SNP variants. The most frequently found allele in a population is called the *wild-type allele.*

Candidate gene: A gene that is believed to cause or contribute to a disease. This term is typically used when the gene will be included in a research study.

Chromosomes: Structures made of DNA and proteins and located in the nuclei of cells. Chromosomes come in pairs, and a normal human cell contains 46 chromosomes: 22 pairs of autosomes and a pair of sex chromosomes. Chromosomes are composed of genes, regulatory sequences, and noncoding DNA segments.

Codon: Three-sequence nucleotide bases that code for an amino acid.

CRISPR-Cas9: **C**lustered **r**egularly **i**nterspaced **s**hort **p**alindromic **r**epeat (Cas9) is a molecular gene-editing tool.

DNA: Deoxyribonucleic acid is made up of four nucleotide bases: adenine (A), guanine (G), cytosine (C), and thymine (T). DNA is heritable genetic information that resides in chromosomes inside each cell nucleus.

Epigenetic: Chemical modifications of DNA that can turn genes on or off without altering the DNA sequence. Epigenetic changes are not heritable.

Gene: A unit of inheritance; a working subunit of DNA. Each of the 20,000 to 25,000 genes in the body contains the code for a specific product, typically a protein such as an enzyme, and other specific tissue cells.

Gene expression: The process by which the coded information of a gene is translated into the structures present and operating in the cell, such as proteins or RNA.

Gene map: A description of the relative positions of genes on a chromosome and the distance between them.

Genetic linkage maps: DNA maps that assign relative chromosomal locations to genetic locations—either genes for known traits or distinctive sequences of DNA—on the basis of how frequently they are inherited together.

Genetics: The scientific study of heredity, which is how particular qualities or traits are transmitted from parents to offspring. Traditionally, the focus has been on individual genes and their effect on uncommon single-gene disorders. At the present time, the study of genetics also involves multigene disorders and gene-environment interactions.

Genomics: The expansive study of all the genes in the human genome, including gene-gene interactions, gene interactions with the environment, and the influence of other psychosocial and cultural factors.

Genotype: The genetic code sequence carried by an individual.

Haplotype: Closely linked loci on a chromosome. Haplotype blocks denote chromosomal regions where SNPs are in strong linkage disequilibrium, and they are mapped in the HapMap Project database.

HapMap Project: A map of haplotype blocks that researchers use when searching for candidate genes. Haplotypes are cataloged according to racial and ethnic group in the HapMap database.

Heterozygous: Possessing two different sequences (alleles) of a particular gene, with one inherited from each parent.

Homozygous: Possessing two identical sequences of a particular gene, with one inherited from each parent.

Linkage: The association of genes or markers that lie very near each other on a chromosome. Linked genes and markers tend to be inherited together.

Linkage analysis: A gene-mapping technique that finds patterns of heredity in large, high-risk families to locate a disease-causing gene mutation by identifying traits that are coinherited with the gene.

Linkage disequilibrium: The nonrandom association between alleles at different loci. These alleles at loci occur together on the same section of a chromosome more often than would be predicted by chance alone. This technique has been used to determine which genes are linked and inherited together.

Locus, loci: The place on a chromosome where a specific gene is located, similar in concept to a street address for the gene. The singular term is *locus*, and the plural is *loci.*

Mendelian diseases: Single-gene disorders that appear in families in dominant or recessive inheritance patterns.

Mutation: A change, deletion, or rearrangement in an individual's DNA sequence that may lead to the synthesis of an altered protein or the inability to produce the protein at all.

Nucleotide: A building block of DNA or RNA that consists of one nitrogenous base, one phosphate molecule, and one glucose molecule.

Pedigree: A graphic multigenerational family health history that uses standardized symbols.

Pharmacogenomics: The study of genetically determined responses to medications, genetic variation in medication metabolizing enzymes, and consequent alteration in medication effectiveness across the genome.

Phenotype: The observable manifestation of a genetic trait that results from a specific genotype or gene-environment interaction. These are physical characteristics, such as the signs and symptoms associated with a disease.

Polymorphism: A common variation in the sequence of DNA that occurs in more than 1% of the population. The most frequent sequence is referred to as the *wild type*, and less common variants are called *polymorphisms.*

Proband: The first person diagnosed with a condition in a family pedigree. An arrow in the family pedigree identifies the proband.

Single nucleotide polymorphism (SNP): A change in the DNA nucleotide sequence caused by replacement of a single nucleotide base. If the change of nucleotide results in a different protein product, it is called a *nonsynonymous SNP.* If the protein product is not changed, it is called a *synonymous SNP.*

Somatic cells: All body cells except the reproductive cells.

Telomeres: Repetitive sequences of DNA that protect the ends of the chromosome.

Transcription: The process used by DNA to code for messenger RNA.

Translation: The process used by RNA to code for a protein.

Whole exome sequencing: Sequencing of protein-coding regions of DNA.

KEY POINTS

- DNA is arranged inside the nucleus of the cell. DNA resembles a ladder with two long strands twisted around each other to form a double-stranded helix made up of nucleotide base pairs. There are 20,000 to 25,000 genes in the human genome.
- Coagulation-related conditions that have a genetic component include factor V Leiden thrombosis and hemophilia A and B.
- Pharmacogenetic syndromes represent medication-gene interactions; examples include malignant hyperthermia secondary to *RYR1* polymorphisms, and warfarin dosage affected by *CYP2C9* and *VKORC1* polymorphisms.
- Cardiac conditions that have a genetic component include hypertrophic cardiomyopathy and LQTS.
- The GINA legislation in the United States is designed to prevent the use of an individual's genetic risk profile in employment and insurance decisions.
- Genetic and genomic competency is recommended for all RNs.

Visit the Evolve site at http://evolve.elsevier.com/Urden/CriticalCareNursing for additional study materials.

REFERENCES

1. Kurnat-Thoma E, Fu MR, Henderson WA, et al. Current status and future directions of U.S. genomic nursing health care policy. *Nurs Outlook.* 2021;69(3):471–488. https://doi.org/10.1016/j.outlook.2020.12.006.
2. National Human Genome Research Institute. Discipline-Specific Genomic Competencies. https://www.genome.gov/For-Health-Professionals/Provider-Genomics-Education-Resources/Competencies. Accessed May 5, 2024.
3. Marwaha S, Knowles JW, Ashley EA. A guide for the diagnosis of rare and undiagnosed disease: beyond the exome. *Genome Med.* 2022;14(1):23. https://doi.org/10.1186/s13073-022-01026-w.
4. International Human Genome Sequencing Consortium. Finishing the euchromatic sequence of the human genome. *Nature.* 2004;431(7011):931–945. https://doi.org/10.1038/nature03001.
5. Musunuru K, Hickey KT, Al-Khatib SM, et al. Basic concepts and potential applications of genetics and genomics for cardiovascular and stroke clinicians: a scientific statement from the American Heart Association. *Circ Cardiovasc Genet.* 2015;8(1):216–242. https://doi.org/10.1161/HCG.0000000000000020.
6. Hartiala JA, Hilser JR, Biswas S, Lusis AJ, Allayee H. Gene-environment interactions for cardiovascular disease. *Curr Atheroscler Rep.* 2021;23(12):75. https://doi.org/10.1007/s11883-021-00974-9.
7. Uffelmann E, Huang QQ, Munung NS, et al. Genome-wide association studies. *Nat Rev Methods Primers.* 2021;1(1):59. https://doi.org/10.1038/s43586-021-00056-9.
8. Roden DM, McLeod HL, Relling MV, et al. Pharmacogenomics. *Lancet.* 2019;394(10197):521–532. https://doi.org/10.1016/S0140-6736(19)31276-0.
9. Brennan ML, Schrijver I. Cystic fibrosis: a review of associated phenotypes, use of molecular diagnostic approaches, genetic characteristics, progress, and dilemmas. *J Mol Diagn.* 2016;18(1):3–14. https://doi.org/10.1016/j.jmoldx.2015.06.010.

10. Odell ID, Wallace SS, Pederson DS. Rules of engagement for base excision repair in chromatin. *J Cell Physiol.* 2013;228(2):258–266. https://doi.org/10.1002/jcp.24134.
11. Cold Spring Harbor Laboratory. DNA from the Beginning – an animated primer of 75 experiments that made modern genetics. http://www.dnaftb.org/. Accessed May 5, 2024.
12. Armanios M. The role of telomeres in human disease. *Annu Rev Genom Hum Genet.* 2022;23(1):363–381. https://doi.org/10.1146/annurev-genom-010422-091101.
13. Bühring J, Hecker M, Fitzner B, Zettl UK. Systematic review of studies on telomere length in patients with multiple sclerosis. *Aging Dis.* 2021;12(5):1272–1286. https://doi.org/10.14336/AD.2021.0106.
14. Liu S, Nong W, Ji L, et al. The regulatory feedback of inflammatory signaling and telomere/telomerase complex dysfunction in chronic inflammatory diseases. *Exp Gerontol.* 2023;174:112132. https://doi.org/10.1016/j.exger.2023.112132.
15. Lansdorp PM. Telomeres, telomerase and cancer. *Arch Med Res.* 2022;53(8):741–746. https://doi.org/10.1016/j.arcmed.2022.10.004.
16. Rossiello F, Jurk D, Passos JF, d'Adda Di Fagagna F. Telomere dysfunction in ageing and age-related diseases. *Nat Cell Biol.* 2022;24(2):135–147. https://doi.org/10.1038/s41556-022-00842-x.
17. Soverini S, Bassan R, Lion T. Treatment and monitoring of Philadelphia chromosome-positive leukemia patients: recent advances and remaining challenges. *J Hematol Oncol.* 2019;12(1):39. https://doi.org/10.1186/s13045-019-0729-2.
18. Kujovich JL. Factor V leiden thrombophilia. *Genet Med.* 2011;13(1):1–16. https://doi.org/10.1097/GIM.0b013e3181faa0f2.
19. MacCallum P, Bowles L, Keeling D. Diagnosis and management of heritable thrombophilias. *BMJ.* 2014;349:g4387. https://doi.org/10.1136/bmj.g4387.
20. Belloy ME, Napolioni V, Greicius MD. A quarter century of APOE and Alzheimer's disease: progress to date and the path forward. *Neuron.* 2019;101(5):820–838. https://doi.org/10.1016/j.neuron.2019.01.056.
21. Abondio P, Sazzini M, Garagnani P, et al. The genetic variability of APOE in different human populations and its implications for longevity. *Genes.* 2019;10(3):222. https://doi.org/10.3390/genes10030222.
22. Yu JT, Tan L, Hardy J. Apolipoprotein E in Alzheimer's disease: an update. *Annu Rev Neurosci.* 2014;37:79–100. https://doi.org/10.1146/annurev-neuro-071013-014300.
23. Yang LG, March ZM, Stephenson RA, Narayan PS. Apolipoprotein E in lipid metabolism and neurodegenerative disease. *Trends Endocrinol Metabol.* 2023;34(8):430–445. https://doi.org/10.1016/j.tem.2023.05.002.
24. Sharma N, Pasala MS, Prakash A. Mitochondrial DNA: Epigenetics and environment. *Environ Mol Mutagen.* 2019;60(8):668–682. https://doi.org/10.1002/em.22319.
25. Russell OM, Gorman GS, Lightowlers RN, Turnbull DM. Mitochondrial diseases: hope for the future. *Cell.* 2020;181(1):168–188. https://doi.org/10.1016/j.cell.2020.02.051.
26. Alqahtani T, Deore SL, Kide AA, et al. Mitochondrial dysfunction and oxidative stress in Alzheimer's disease, and Parkinson's disease, Huntington's disease and Amyotrophic Lateral Sclerosis – an updated review. *Mitochondrion.* 2023;71:83–92. https://doi.org/10.1016/j.mito.2023.05.007.
27. Bennett RL, French KS, Resta RG, Doyle DL. Standardized human pedigree nomenclature: update and assessment of the recommendations of the national society of genetic counselors. *J Genet Counsel.* 2008;17(5):424–433. https://doi.org/10.1007/s10897-008-9169-9.
28. Bennett RL, French KS, Resta RG, Austin J. Practice resource–focused revision: standardized pedigree nomenclature update centered on sex and gender inclusivity: a practice resource of the National Society of Genetic Counselors. *J Genet Counsel.* 2022;31(6):1238–1248. https://doi.org/10.1002/jgc4.1621.
29. McNally EM, Mestroni L. Dilated cardiomyopathy: genetic determinants and mechanisms. *Circ Res.* 2017;121(7):731–748. https://doi.org/10.1161/CIRCRESAHA.116.309396.
30. Karch C, Masser–Frye D, Limjoco J, et al. The odds and implications of coinheritance of hemophilia A and B. *Res Pract Thromb Haemost.* 2020;4(5):931–935. https://doi.org/10.1002/rth2.12345.
31. Fisch GS. Whither the genotype-phenotype relationship? An historical and methodological appraisal. *Am J Med Genet.* 2017;175(3):343–353. https://doi.org/10.1002/ajmg.c.31571.
32. Kurki MI, Karjalainen J, Palta P, et al. FinnGen provides genetic insights from a well-phenotyped isolated population. *Nature.* 2023;613(7944):508–518. https://doi.org/10.1038/s41586-022-05473-8.
33. The Wellcome Trust Case Control Consortium, Management Committee, Burton PR, et al. Genome-wide association study of 14,000 cases of seven common diseases and 3,000 shared controls. *Nature.* 2007;447(7145):661–678. https://doi.org/10.1038/nature05911.
34. Sollis E, Mosaku A, Abid A, et al. The NHGRI-EBI GWAS Catalog: knowledgebase and deposition resource. *Nucleic Acids Res.* 2023;51(D1):D977–D985. https://doi.org/10.1093/nar/gkac1010.
35. Nurk S, Koren S, Rhie A, et al. The complete sequence of a human genome. *Science.* 2022;376(6588):44–53. https://doi.org/10.1126/science.abj6987.
36. Lovell JT, Grimwood J. The first complete human genome. *Nature.* 2022;606(7914):468–469. https://doi.org/10.1038/d41586-022-01368-w.
37. The Encyclopedia of DNA Elements (ENCODE). https://www.genome.gov/Funded-Programs-Projects/ENCODE-Project-ENCyclopedia-Of-DNA-Elements. Accessed May 5, 2024.
38. ENCODE Encyclopedia, Version 4: Genomic annotations – ENCODE. https://www.encodeproject.org/data/annotations/. Accessed May 5, 2024.
39. The ENCODE Project Consortium, Abascal F, Acosta R, et al. Expanded encyclopaedias of DNA elements in the human and mouse genomes. *Nature.* 2020;583(7818):699–710. https://doi.org/10.1038/s41586-020-2493-4.
40. Ewans LJ, Minoche AE, Schofield D, et al. Whole exome and genome sequencing in mendelian disorders: a diagnostic and health economic analysis. *Eur J Hum Genet.* 2022;30(10):1121–1131. https://doi.org/10.1038/s41431-022-01162-2.
41. Adhikari S, Nice EC, Deutsch EW, et al. A high-stringency blueprint of the human proteome. *Nat Commun.* 2020;11(1):5301. https://doi.org/10.1038/s41467-020-19045-9.
42. Roehrl MH, Roehrl VB, Wang JY. Proteome-based pathology: the next frontier in precision medicine. *Expert Rev Precis Med Drug Dev.* 2021;6(1):1–4. https://doi.org/10.1080/23808993.2021.1854611.
43. The Human Protein Atlas. Accessed May 5, 2024. https://www.proteinatlas.org/.
44. Hanssens LS, Duchateau J, Casimir GJ. CFTR protein: not just a chloride channel? *Cells.* 2021;10(11):2844. https://doi.org/10.3390/cells10112844.
45. The Integrative HMP (iHMP) Research Network Consortium. The integrative human microbiome project. *Nature.* 2019;569(7758):641–648. https://doi.org/10.1038/s41586-019-1238-8.
46. Gonzales-Luna AJ, Carlson TJ, Garey KW. Gut microbiota changes associated with Clostridioides difficile infection and its various treatment strategies. *Gut Microb.* 2023;15(1):2223345. https://doi.org/10.1080/19490976.2023.2223345.
47. Fatumo S, Chikowore T, Choudhury A, Ayub M, Martin AR, Kuchenbaecker K. A roadmap to increase diversity in genomic studies. *Nat Med.* 2022;28(2):243–250. https://doi.org/10.1038/s41591-021-01672-4.
48. Wang T, Antonacci-Fulton L, Howe K, et al. The Human Pangenome Project: a global resource to map genomic diversity. *Nature.* 2022;604(7906):437–446. https://doi.org/10.1038/s41586-022-04601-8.
49. Liao WW, Asri M, Ebler J, et al. A draft human pangenome reference. *Nature.* 2023;617(7960):312–324. https://doi.org/10.1038/s41586-023-05896-x.
50. Tishkoff SA, Williams SM. Genetic analysis of African populations: human evolution and complex disease. *Nat Rev Genet.* 2002;3(8):611–621. https://doi.org/10.1038/nrg865.
51. Maier PA, Runfeldt G, Estes RJ, Vilar MG. African mitochondrial haplogroup L7: a 100,000-year-old maternal human lineage discovered through reassessment and new sequencing. *Sci Rep.* 2022;12(1):10747. https://doi.org/10.1038/s41598-022-13856-0.
52. International HapMap Consortium, Frazer KA, Ballinger DG, et al. A second generation human haplotype map of over 3.1 million SNPs. *Nature.* 2007;449(7164):851–861. https://doi.org/10.1038/nature06258.

53. Sved JA, Hill WG. One hundred years of linkage disequilibrium. *Genetics.* 2018;209(3):629–636. https://doi.org/10.1534/genetics.118.300642.
54. Wonkam A, Munung NS, Dandara C, Esoh KK, Hanchard NA, Landoure G. Five priorities of African genomics research: the next frontier. *Annu Rev Genom Hum Genet.* 2022;23(1):499–521. https://doi.org/10.1146/annurev-genom-111521-102452.
55. Mahajan A, Spracklen CN, Zhang W, et al. Multi-ancestry genetic study of type 2 diabetes highlights the power of diverse populations for discovery and translation. *Nat Genet.* 2022;54(5):560–572. https://doi.org/10.1038/s41588-022-01058-3.
56. Spracklen CN, Sim X. Progress in defining the genetic contribution to type 2 diabetes in individuals of East Asian ancestry. *Curr Diab Rep.* 2021;21(6):17. https://doi.org/10.1007/s11892-021-01388-2.
57. Ke C, Narayan KMV, Chan JCN, Jha P, Shah BR. Pathophysiology, phenotypes and management of type 2 diabetes mellitus in Indian and Chinese populations. *Nat Rev Endocrinol.* 2022;18(7):413–432. https://doi.org/10.1038/s41574-022-00669-4.
58. Elkattawy S, Alyacoub R, Singh KS, Fichadiya H, Kessler W. Prothrombin G20210A gene mutation-induced recurrent deep vein thrombosis and pulmonary embolism: case report and literature review. *J Investig Med High Impact Case Rep.* 2022;10:232470962110584. https://doi.org/10.1177/23247096211058486.
59. Nikolaeva MG, Momot AP, Zainulina MS, Yasafova NN, Taranenko IA. Pregnancy complications in G20210A mutation carriers associated with high prothrombin activity. *Thrombosis J.* 2021;19(1):41. https://doi.org/10.1186/s12959-021-00289-4.
60. Akdemir KC, Le VT, Kim JM, et al. Somatic mutation distributions in cancer genomes vary with three-dimensional chromatin structure. *Nat Genet.* 2020;52(11):1178–1188. https://doi.org/10.1038/s41588-020-0708-0.
61. The Cancer Genome Atlas (TCGA). https://www.genome.gov/Funded-Programs-Projects/Cancer-Genome-Atlas. Accessed May 5, 2024.
62. Adler A, Novelli V, Amin AS, et al. An international, multicentered, evidence-based reappraisal of genes reported to cause congenital long QT syndrome. *Circulation.* 2020;141(6):418–428. https://doi.org/10.1161/CIRCULATIONAHA.119.043132.
63. Wilde AAM, Amin AS, Postema PG. Diagnosis, management and therapeutic strategies for congenital long QT syndrome. *Heart.* 2022;108(5):332–338. https://doi.org/10.1136/heartjnl-2020-318259.
64. Shah SR, Park K, Alweis R. Long QT syndrome: a comprehensive review of the literature and current evidence. *Curr Probl Cardiol.* 2019;44(3):92–106. https://doi.org/10.1016/j.cpcardiol.2018.04.002.
65. Marian AJ. Molecular genetic basis of hypertrophic cardiomyopathy. *Circ Res.* 2021;128(10):1533–1553. https://doi.org/10.1161/CIRCRESAHA.121.318346.
66. Writing Committee Members, Ommen SR, Mital S, et al. 2020 AHA/ACC guideline for the diagnosis and treatment of patients with hypertrophic cardiomyopathy: a report of the American College of Cardiology/American Heart Association Joint Committee on Clinical Practice Guidelines. *Circulation.* 2020;142(25). https://doi.org/10.1161/CIR.0000000000000937.
67. Jordan E, Peterson L, Ai T, et al. Evidence-based assessment of genes in dilated cardiomyopathy. *Circulation.* 2021;144(1):7–19. https://doi.org/10.1161/CIRCULATIONAHA.120.053033.
68. Van Lint FHM, Murray B, Tichnell C, et al. Arrhythmogenic right ventricular cardiomyopathy-associated desmosomal variants are rarely de novo: segregation and haplotype analysis of a multinational cohort. *Circ Genom Precis Med.* 2019;12(8):e002467. https://doi.org/10.1161/CIRCGEN.119.002467.
69. Gandjbakhch E, Redheuil A, Pousset F, Charron P, Frank R. Clinical diagnosis, imaging, and genetics of Arrhythmogenic right ventricular cardiomyopathy/dysplasia: JACC state-of-the-art review. *J Am Coll Cardiol.* 2018;72(7):784–804. https://doi.org/10.1016/j.jacc.2018.05.065.
70. Mann HJ. Drug-associated disease: cytochrome P450 interactions. *Crit Care Clin.* 2006;22(2):329–345. https://doi.org/10.1016/j.ccc.2006.02.004.
71. Cicali EJ, Smith DM, Duong BQ, Kovar LG, Cavallari LH, Johnson JA. A scoping review of the evidence behind cytochrome P450 2D6 isoenzyme inhibitor classifications. *Clin Pharma Ther.* 2020;108(1):116–125. https://doi.org/10.1002/cpt.1768.
72. Johnson JA, Gong L, Whirl-Carrillo M, et al. Clinical pharmacogenetics implementation consortium guidelines for CYP2C9 and VKORC1 genotypes and warfarin dosing. *Clin Pharmacol Ther.* 2011;90(4):625–629. https://doi.org/10.1038/clpt.2011.185.
73. Frassanito L, Sbaraglia F, Piersanti A, et al. Real evidence and misconceptions about malignant hyperthermia in children: a narrative review. *JCM.* 2023;12(12):3869. https://doi.org/10.3390/jcm12123869.
74. Bin X, Wang B, Tang Z. Malignant hyperthermia: a killer if ignored. *J Perianesth Nurs.* 2022;37(4):435–444. https://doi.org/10.1016/j.jopan.2021.08.018.
75. Hopkins PM, Girard T, Dalay S, et al. Malignant hyperthermia 2020: guideline from the Association of Anaesthetists. *Anaesthesia.* 2021;76(5):655–664. https://doi.org/10.1111/anae.15317.
76. Rüffert H, Bastian B, Bendixen D, et al. Consensus guidelines on perioperative management of malignant hyperthermia suspected or susceptible patients from the European Malignant Hyperthermia Group. *Br J Anaesth.* 2021;126(1):120–130. https://doi.org/10.1016/j.bja.2020.09.029.
77. Frangoul H, Altshuler D, Cappellini MD, et al. CRISPR-Cas9 gene editing for sickle cell disease and β-thalassemia. *N Engl J Med.* 2021;384(3):252–260. https://doi.org/10.1056/NEJMoa2031054.
78. Sharma A, Boelens JJ, Cancio M, et al. CRISPR-Cas9 editing of the *HBG1* and *HBG2* promoters to treat sickle cell disease. *N Engl J Med.* 2023;389(9):820–832. https://doi.org/10.1056/NEJMoa2215643.
79. Social Determinants of Health – Healthy People 2030 | health.gov. Accessed May 5, 2024. https://health.gov/healthypeople/priority-areas/social-determinants-health.
80. Porter JS, Heitzer AM, Crosby LE, Hankins JS. Social determinants of health: the next frontier for improving care and outcomes in sickle cell disease. *Lancet Haematol.* 2023;10(8):e571–e573. https://doi.org/10.1016/S2352-3026(23)00185-0.
81. Greco KE, Tinley S, Seibert D. Development of the essential genetic and genomic competencies for nurses with graduate degrees. *Annu Rev Nurs Res.* 2011;29:173–190. https://doi.org/10.1891/0739-6686.29.173.
82. Jenkins J. *American Nurses Association: Essentials of Genetic and Genomic Nursing Competencies, Curricula Guidelines and Outcome Indicators.* 2nd ed. American Nurses Association; International Society of Nurses in Genetics; 2009.
83. Elson SL, Furlotte NA, Hromatka BS, et al. Direct–to–consumer genetic testing for factor V Leiden and prothrombin 20210G>A: the consumer experience. *Mol Genet Genomic Med.* 2020;8(11):e1468. https://doi.org/10.1002/mgg3.1468.
84. Health law – genetics – congress restricts use of genetic information by insurers and employers. Genetic Information Nondiscrimination Act of 2008, Pub. L. No. 110-233, 122 Stat. 881 (to be codified in scattered sections of 26, 29, and 42 U.S.C.). *Harv Law Rev.* 2009;122(3):1038–1045.
85. Suter SM. GINA at 10 years: the battle over 'genetic information' continues in court. *J Law Biosci.* 2018;5(3):495–526. https://doi.org/10.1093/jlb/lsz002.
86. Alders M. Long QT syndrome – GeneReviews® – NCBI bookshelf. Published February 8 https://www.ncbi.nlm.nih.gov/books//NBK1129/; 2018. Accessed May 5, 2024.
87. Krahn AD, Laksman Z, Sy RW, et al. Congenital long QT syndrome. *JACC Clin Electrophysiol.* 2022;8(5):687–706. https://doi.org/10.1016/j.jacep.2022.02.017.
88. Rosenberg H, Pollock N, Schiemann A, Bulger T, Stowell K. Malignant hyperthermia: a review. *Orphanet J Rare Dis.* 2015;10:93. https://doi.org/10.1186/s13023-015-0310-1.

4

Facilitating Care Transitions

Kimberly Sanchez, Kathrine Anne Winnie, and Natalie B. de Haas-Rowland

http://evolve.elsevier.com/Urden/CriticalCareNursing

Transferring patients between health care professionals or to different levels of care has been an evolving topic of concern in the health care community. Numerous risks are associated with transitions in care, including complications and negative outcomes.[1] Specifically, patients transitioning from a critical care setting are at high risk of clinical deterioration.[2] This chapter describes care transitions and outlines potential locations and levels of care that precede or follow admission to a critical care area. This chapter further presents core components and special considerations of care transitions. Lastly, this chapter introduces transition models or programs.

CARE TRANSITIONS

Care transitions have been defined as changes in the setting where care is delivered[3] or as changes to the extent of health care services provided, including the degree of monitoring, assessing, planning, intervening, and evaluating.[4] Care transitions to and from critical care are determined by the severity of illness and intensity of services, with patients transitioning into critical care for advanced monitoring and technologies and from critical care when these requirements lessen.[5]

In some cases, patients transition between two critical care areas when specialized monitoring and technologies are needed. Transitions of care may be temporary, such as when a patient is transferred to the operating room and then returns to their previous location, or transitions may be permanent, such as the transfer of a patient to hospice for end-of-life care.[6] Care transitions can be described by location and intensity of care provided. See Table 4.1 for transitional locations and levels of care.

The delivery of quality care during care transitions is attained through the health care team sharing the same goal for the patient, communicating sufficient breadth and depth of the patient's condition, understanding the role expectations of each other, minimizing safety risks by developing and carrying out an organized plan of care between different locations/levels of care, and ensuring patients and families remain informed and an integral part of the entire process. Fragmented care transitions negatively affect patients, families, health care professionals, and health care systems.[20] General examples include a lack of patient and caregiver engagement, poor continuity of care, insufficient patient knowledge regarding symptom management, lack of coordination of services, poor communication between the care team and patient/family, mismanaged chronic health conditions, and poor communication of treatment regimens.[21] Specifically, The Joint Commission (TJC) estimates that 80% of medical errors have some element of communication breakdown as the cause or as a contributing factor,[22] emphasizing the importance of avoiding communication-related events between health care providers, units, or facilities. Quality care transitions require a multifaceted approach that accounts for core components and patient-specific considerations.

CORE COMPONENTS TO ANY CARE TRANSITION

Quality outcomes are achieved when components of care transitions include management of complex health issues and medications, engagement and education of patients and caregivers, accountability of the health care team, continuity of care, and appropriate coordination of physical transport.[21] The management of complex conditions includes identifying high-risk patients, anticipating and planning for their needs, managing coexisting chronic conditions, ensuring the medication regimen is based on evidence, and recognizing other health and social risks to decrease readmissions or prevent extended hospital lengths of stay.[21] Engagement of the patient in developing shared goals and participating in shared decision making is a natural evolution when the health care team connects with the patient, builds a trusting relationship, and understands what is important to their patient.[21] Caregiver engagement is fostered through similar efforts made by the health care team.[21] Emotional distress should be addressed with appropriate interventions to support well-being.[21] Patients and families need to feel cared for and confident about care transitions, to feel clear about who is accountable for their care, and to feel prepared for and capable of implementing care plans.[23] During care transitions, the health care team should be timely and consistent when completing role responsibilities and trust the plan of care to promote care continuity.[21] Negative outcomes can be mitigated by incorporating core components to all care transitions.

Management of Complex Health Issues and Medications

Recognition of patients at risk for poor outcomes is a strategy for managing complex health issues.[21] Patients with multiple chronic conditions, cognitive deficits, history of mental health issues, and frequent hospitalizations; those unable to independently perform activities of daily living; and older adults have been identified as being at high risk for complications in care transitions.[24] Once risk has been recognized, transitional care interventions for those patients are prioritized to reduce threats to safety and improve outcomes. Patient management is initiated with the assessment of health issues and, when necessary, early treatment of chronic conditions and symptoms. Routinely reviewing the appropriateness of ordered medications and dosages can prevent errors.[21]

TABLE 4.1 Transitional Locations and Levels of Care

Acute Care Description	
Other critical care area	Provides specialized monitoring and/or technology, advanced cardiopulmonary life support, and stabilization or management of complex acute injury and/or illness.[7] Transferring between critical care areas may be necessary to provide specific specialty care (e.g., stroke management),[8] when patients and their families prefer a hospital closer to home, or when type of insurance dictates facility used.
Step-down area	Provides intermediates services for unstable patients who no longer require critical care services or have deteriorated in telemetry or medical-surgical areas.[8,9]
Telemetry area	Provides stable patients with continuous electrocardiographic monitoring and/or interventions of greater intensity than those provided in medical-surgical areas.[8,10]
Medical-surgical area	Provides general medical and surgical care for stable patients with a wide variety of illnesses.[11]
Long-term acute care hospital (LTAC or LTACH) or long-term care hospital (LTCH)	Provides stable patients with time and services to address more than one chronic condition before returning home, usually necessitating a hospitalization longer than 25 days.[12]
Postacute Care	
Inpatient rehabilitation area	Provides nursing services along with physical, occupational, and/or speech therapy after discharge from the acute phase of hospitalization with the goal of restoring optimal function before returning home. Patients admitted to a rehabilitation area must be able to tolerate and benefit from 3 hours of therapy each day at least 5 days per week.[12,13]
Subacute care area	Provides nursing and rehabilitation services after discharge from an acute hospitalization of 3 or more days before returning home. Patients admitted to a subacute care area require fewer hours of therapy per day than an inpatient rehabilitation area and more intense skilled care than a skilled nursing facility.[13,14]
Assisted living area	Provides a combination of housing, assistance with daily activities, and supportive wellness activities, which may or may not include health care services, with the goal of maximizing independence.[15]
Additional Services Provided in Various Settings (e.g., standalone facilities or within facilities or home)	
Skilled care	Service provided daily by licensed professionals.[14] Skilled nursing care may include wound care treatments, intravenous therapy, and injections.
Palliative care	Provides relief from the symptoms of serious illness rather than focusing on the underlying disease process.[16]
Hospice care	Provides comprehensive medical and social support services throughout the dying process. Hospice services are normally rendered when life expectancy is less than 6 months.[16,17]
Custodial care (i.e., long-term care services)	Provides assistance with activities of daily living and does not require skilled care services.[14]
Additional Locations Within a Health Care Facility	
Operating room	Where surgical procedures are performed and require an aseptic field.[18]
Procedural area	Where procedures are performed without requiring an aseptic field (e.g., interventional radiology).[18]
Emergency department	Provides 24-hour unscheduled medical care for patients experiencing trauma, acute illnesses, or other emergent conditions.[19]

Medication Reconciliation

According to TJC,[25] medication reconciliation is the process by which a provider compares a patient's current medication regimen to new medications that are ordered for the patient and resolves any discrepancies. In one review of the literature, 88% of medication errors on admission included high-risk medications such as anticoagulants or medications for seizure prophylaxis.[26] A careful medication reconciliation should address duplications, omissions, possible interactions between medications, and the need to continue current medications. The most common error noted is that of omission.[27] Medication discrepancies may result in patient harm or poor outcomes, and it is for this reason that the medication reconciliation process is one of TJC's National Patient Safety Goals (NPSG) with five critical elements for performance.

The latest NPSG elements for performance include:

- Providers will obtain information on the medications the patient is taking immediately before admission.
- The hospital will define which information should be collected, which should include medication name, dose, route, frequency, and purpose. Information collected is documented in a list or similar format to facilitate medication management while in the hospital and after discharge. The hospital must also define which admission settings require a medication reconciliation to be performed, including the emergency department, primary care offices, outpatient radiology, or ambulatory surgery.
- Providers will compare the medication information that the patient provided with the new medications ordered for the patient to identify and resolve discrepancies. Possible discrepancies may include omissions (not restarting medications from home that should be continued), duplications (prescribing the same medication, possibly in a different form or dose, without discontinuing the home route or dose of the medication), contraindications, unclear information, and any other changes.
- The patient or family will be provided with written information on the medications the patient is prescribed when he or she is discharged from the hospital or outpatient encounter.
- The patient or family will be provided information about the importance of managing their medication information after he or she is discharged from the hospital or at the end of an outpatient encounter. Information about safe medication management may include providing an updated list of medications to the primary care provider, taking medications as

prescribed, and carrying an updated medication list always in case of an emergency.

The importance of medication reconciliation during care transitions can be highlighted when considering special populations such as older adults or patients with certain disease processes, such as Parkinson disease. Patients with Parkinson disease are especially vulnerable during care transitions, because missed, late, omitted, or inappropriate medications (such as those which interact with Parkinson disease medications) can directly result in complications, especially confusion, falls, and aspiration, all of which have a significant effect on length of stay and patient outcomes.[28] Only 33% of the patients with Parkinson disease who are hospitalized in the United States return home after hospitalization. Approximately 63% are discharged to some type of facility, and 3.9% die while hospitalized, even though Parkinson disease is often not the admitting diagnosis. This is just one example of the detrimental effects of not completing a thorough medication reconciliation on admission, transfer, and discharge.

Each point of reconciliation presents its own set of challenges or barriers. Successful performance of a thorough medication reconciliation can be affected by several factors: interfacility/intrafacility process variation, lack of agreement or understanding of each profession's role in the reconciliation process, and dependence on the patient's ability to provide accurate medication information.[27] The importance of patient and family knowledge and motivation to maintain an updated list of all medications cannot be understated. It contributes to difficulties encountered by hospital providers and staff when taking medication histories.

The introduction and expansion of the use of technology in the health care setting have brought its own set of challenges, including inadequate design, poor usability, and lack of evidence for user satisfaction. Although health information technology has seen vast growth and advancement since the introduction of medication reconciliation as a National Patient Safety Goal in 2005, there is still a great deal of variability in how it is used. Interoperability, or the ability for electronic systems to "talk" to one another, may facilitate the medication reconciliation process (Box 4.1). The use of technology may leave underserved areas struggling to keep up with systems if there is limited funding.

Current literature regarding medication reconciliation is focused on admission and discharge reconciliation. These are both crucial points in the patient's hospital course, especially in terms of medication reconciliation. However, it is important to note that errors also occur when patients are transferred to different levels of care. Institute for Safe Medication Practices[29] illustrates several examples of medication errors caused by failure in the medication reconciliation process throughout the continuum of care. Approximately 50% of patients who transferred out of the critical care unit to a lower level of care experienced an actual medication error during the care transition.[30] The most frequent error noted was the inappropriate continuation of medications after transferring out of critical care. Although the study revealed that most of these errors did not result in patient harm, it clearly demonstrated that errors are frequent and that more research is needed to understand the effect of medication errors related to intrafacility transfer between different levels of care.

BOX 4.1 Informatics

Interoperability and Medication Reconciliation

Interoperability in health care refers to the ability of different health care information systems and software applications to communicate, exchange data, and use that data cohesively. Medication reconciliation is a systematic process of comparing a patient's current list of medications with any newly prescribed medications to identify discrepancies and ensure safe and appropriate medication use. This process is crucial during care transitions, such as hospital admissions, discharges, or transfers between health care settings. In medication reconciliation, interoperability ensures that relevant patient medication information can be shared seamlessly among health care systems, such as electronic health records (EHRs), pharmacies, and primary care practices. Here are some examples of how interoperability facilitates medication reconciliation:

- It allows health care practitioners to access a comprehensive medication history for a patient, including medications prescribed by different practitioners and filled at various pharmacies.
- It ensures all practitioners can access the most current information regarding patient medication regimen changes as they can be updated in real-time.
- It helps identify and resolve discrepancies in medication lists, reducing the risk of medication errors and adverse drug events.
- It facilitates communication between different health care settings, ensuring that the medication reconciliation process is comprehensive and that all relevant providers are informed.

In summary, interoperability and medication reconciliation are interconnected in the health care system. Interoperability ensures the seamless exchange of medication information, while medication reconciliation uses this information to verify and reconcile a patient's medication list, ultimately promoting patient safety and quality of care. These processes are critical in preventing medication-related errors and improving patient outcomes.

Patient and Family Education

Timing of Education

Patients transitioning between settings, services, providers, and levels of care receive a large amount of new information in a relatively short period, and it may be difficult to prioritize the multitude of learning needs that are required during a period of critical illness. This can lead to potential knowledge deficits during the high-risk transition period. Learning needs during care transitions can be separated into three different categories to help set teaching priorities (Table 4.2). Education during the initial contact or first hours of critical illness should be directed toward the reduction of immediate stress, anxiety, and fear rather than future lifestyle alterations or rehabilitation needs. Interventions during this time are targeted to address the immediate plan of care and promote comfort and familiarity with the environment and equipment. Education after immediate critical needs are addressed and throughout the continuum of care should reinforce routine care, promote involvement in the plan of care, ensure understanding of medication regimens and disease processes, and support self-management strategies with the anticipation of discharge from the setting or level of care. Education during a care transition should focus on informing patients and families of the rationale for a change in level of care, what to expect after the care transition, and who to contact should questions regarding the plan of care arise. Education provided should optimize learning by taking into consideration the changing learning needs of patients and families in anticipation of and during care transitions.

Education Strategies and Evaluation

Nurses are in a unique position to facilitate and evaluate learning as they continuously interact with patients and families, discussing their progress, updating them on treatment plans, and describing procedures. Every patient and family interaction can

TABLE 4.2 Patient and Family Educational Needs in Critical Care

Category	Educational Needs
Initial contact during immediate critical needs	• Address immediate plan of care (e.g., next 24 hours): procedures, diagnostic testing, treatments, and interventions • Provide orientation to the environment: call light, bed controls, contact information, visitation • Review what to expect in the environment and what the patient may look like (e.g., invasive tubes, drains, and lines) • Explain rationale for equipment (e.g., monitors, machines, and pumps) • Promote patient-centered activities: talk to patient, hold the patient's hand, promote rest and participation in plan of care
Continuous care after immediate critical needs are addressed	• Outline day-to-day routine: degree of monitoring and assessments, frequency of interventions, timing of medication administration, timing of diagnostic testing, timing of and roles represented during interprofessional rounds, timing of and involvement in shift changes, visitation • Address involvement in plan of care: developing daily goals, monitoring progress, preparing for anticipated treatments, acknowledging accomplishments (e.g., attainment of previously established daily goals) • Explain medication regimen: rationale for administration, anticipated effects, potential side effects to report to the health care team • Communicate potential sensations or discomforts of any procedures (e.g., chest tube removal, catheter removals) • Discuss disease process: what it is, how it will affect life, need for advance directive, and symptoms to report to health care team • Review self-management strategies and anticipated discharge needs
Transition to a different setting or level of care	Sending setting or level of care • Explain the need to transfer to, from, or between critical care area(s) • Communicate when the transfer will occur • Outline what to expect in the different setting or level of care • Name the new caregiver(s) and provider(s) • Provide directions on receiving unit location and contact information Receiving setting or level of care • Reinforce need to transfer to, from, or between critical care area(s) • Provide orientation to the environment • Outline routine care: meal deliveries, shift changes, interprofessional rounding, diagnostic testing • Communicate expectations about self-care and activities of daily living while maintaining safety

be thought of as a brief education encounter; however, providing education to critically ill patients may be ineffective because of the impaired cognition and comprehension that commonly accompany critical illness. The nurse must leverage every teachable moment and take advantage of the patient's readiness and willingness to learn without providing an overload of information that will then be easily forgotten. Nurses must recognize that learning does not usually take place in one session. Patients may be able to remember only two to three pieces of information in one education session, and a method such as teach-back may be needed to verify comprehension.[31] In verifying comprehension, the patient or family is asked to teach-back the information given and receive additional education if they are unable. These steps of asking the patient or family, gauging comprehension, and providing additional education are then repeated with the intent that the patient will be able to teach-back the content. When educating patients and families, nurses need to use teaching strategies and consider individual learning styles to facilitate the transfer of information.

Patient- and Family-Centered Education

Nurses and health care providers should respect and respond to patient and family preferences, needs, and values when providing education to increase patient and family preparation for the transition process. Families of critically ill patients report their greatest need is for information as they experience gaps in care and emotional distress, anxiety, and fear during transitions. Preexisting and newly diagnosed chronic conditions increase the amount and complexity of information needed by patients and families. Additionally, patient teaching regarding new home medication regimens, therapies, and treatment goals may initially be on hold as the medical team adjusts the plan based on the patient's condition. Patient and caregiver education needs to be directed to specific patient goals or concerns and be relevant to the plan of care.[21] When the values of the patient and family guide clinical decisions, they are better able to cope with care transitions, have reduced anxiety and stress, and experience shorter length of stay.[32] Nurses and other health care team members need to consider the informational and emotional support needs of patients and families. Patient-centered education regarding critical care experiences is recommended to meet these needs.

Health Care Team Member Accountability

Interprofessional teams are made up of individuals from different professions and occupations with varied and specialized knowledge, skills, and approaches to providing care who communicate and work together as colleagues, to provide quality, individualized care for patients.[33] The purpose of the interprofessional health care team is to enhance patient outcomes through collaboration, communication, shared decision making, and shared goal setting.[34] Interprofessional team members offer recommendations specific to their scope of practice, participate in goal setting, and provide input on safety and quality issues.[34]

Common members of the interprofessional team in critical care areas include patients, families, nurses, providers, pharmacists, respiratory care practitioners, social workers, dietitians, physical therapists, occupational therapists, speech therapists, case managers, clergy, and representatives from other professions or occupations. During care transitions extending throughout the continuity of care from inpatient to outpatient settings, a specific individual may be tasked with additional responsibilities varying from performing supplemental assessments and interventions,[21] providing follow-up phone calls or home visits,[35] and coordinating care.[35] In some instances, this specific individual is an advanced practice nurse, such as a clinical nurse specialist or nurse practitioner,[21,35] a registered nurse or social worker,[35] or other health care (e.g., transitions navigator) or non–health care team members (e.g., care coordinator). Interprofessional teams work together and maintain mutual accountability for meeting team goals.[34] See Chapter 1 for further discussion regarding teamwork and collaboration.

Handoff

Nurses and other health care team members maintain professional responsibility for patients for limited periods and are also responsible for transferring that responsibility during a care transition.[6] When a transfer of care is performed, the involved caregivers participate in a handoff process in which the sender will communicate sufficient breadth and depth of information to assist the receiver in safely and effectively performing patient care responsibilities. The sender should always encourage the receiver to ask questions and clarify discussion points.[22] Transitions from the operating room to critical care are unique, in that multiple members of the health care team will be giving handoff at the same time.[6] To reduce the fragmented approach to care, the operating room nurse, critical care nurse, critical care provider, anesthesia provider, and surgeon should participate in one comprehensive postoperative handoff that addresses all aspects of the surgical case performed and the updated plan of care.[6] Team training focusing on effective communication may be necessary if the group handoff process is new to the organization.[6] A comprehensive process for handoff is important[22] to maintain and transfer responsibility among and between health care team members.[6]

Standardizing Handoffs. Using standardized elements and available documentation while providing verbal handoff communication at the bedside is preferred[22] and has been shown to improve the handoff process by reducing omissions of relevant information.[36] Standardized elements may be compiled in checklist, template, or script format and often incorporate a mnemonic such a SBAR (situation, background, assessment, and recommendation) or I-PASS (illness severity, patient summary, action list, situation awareness and contingency plans, and synthesis by the receiver)[6,22] to prompt the sharing of important information. Although the current plan of care, treatment goals, medical and psychosocial history, and current medications should be incorporated into and reviewed during the handoff process, other content to be shared may vary based on the patient's severity of illness and the intensity of services required.[22] Each care setting, level of care, or workgroup may adjust their standardized tool to fit the needs of their work area.[22] A standardized handoff communication process for transitions should be followed to reduce communication failures or misunderstandings that could lead to safety events.[22]

Barriers to Handoff Communication. Barriers to successful handoff communication during care transitions include time constraints, frequent interruptions, and distraction.[6,36] Irrespective of time constraints, handoff should be prioritized to reduce negative outcomes that may result from fragmented care. Interruptions during handoff report may be best addressed by setting the expectation that only patient-specific discussions will occur during handoff report, nonurgent issues will be addressed later, and urgent tasks are completed before beginning the handoff process.[22] Distractions will be avoided by focusing attention[36] on the information being provided and not concurrently performing patient care activities while participating in the handoff process. Barriers should not deter nurse and other health care team members from actively engaging in handoff communication.

Continuity of Care

Planning for care transitions includes a robust consideration of patient and family needs for the next phase of their care. Many times, this plan of care outlines the need for ensuring comprehension and implementation of self-management strategies, ordering and delivering necessary supplies, scheduling of additional services and follow-up appointments,[26] and evaluating the risks for mortality and readmission.[8] However, this plan is dependent on where the patient is on the continuum of care. The successful implementation of a patient's plan of care is also dependent on health care team members' knowledge, ability, and willingness to execute the plan as mutually agreed on to attain a shared patient goal.

National guidelines and institution-specific policies on critical care admission and discharge criteria assist nurses and other health care team members in anticipating the needs of patients and families. Guidelines on the appropriateness of admission to and discharge from critical care areas include physiologic parameters and/or monitoring requirements to facilitate care transitions.[8,37] These guidelines may also provide recommendations on how to prioritize admissions and discharges or what resources might be needed when planning admissions and discharges.[8] Institutional policies may outline the specific needs of their patient populations having considered their critical care and/or organizational resources.[8] As seen in Table 4.1, locations and levels of care differ in the services they provide, with critical care areas encompassing specialized—often life-supporting—monitoring and/or technology to custodial care, encompassing activities of daily living and the delivery of skilled care services. Differentiating care settings and understanding the extent of the services they provide informs the plan of care and expected care transitions of critically ill patients.

Coordination of Physical Transport

Critically ill patients may require transport for several reasons during hospitalization. Transport may be conducted within the facility for tests, procedures, or to different levels of care. Patients are at higher risk for adverse events during transport.[38] Because there are varying definitions of the term *adverse event*, the reported incidence varies widely from 1.7% to 75.7%. Commonly noted patient-centric adverse events during transport included physiologic alterations such as hypotension, increased oxygen requirements or decreased oxygen saturation, temperature alterations, patient discomfort, tissue damage, and anxiety or agitation. Nonpatient-specific adverse events include equipment malfunctions such as battery failure, depletion of portable oxygen supplies,[39] tangling of lines, and accidental dislodgement of catheters or drains. In addition, patients who are transported to procedural or testing areas may be more difficult for staff to visualize and monitor closely, such as in a magnetic resonance imaging (MRI) suite, putting the patient at further risk for adverse events or complications.

PATIENT-CENTERED CRITICAL CARE

Transitions of Care and Handoff Communication

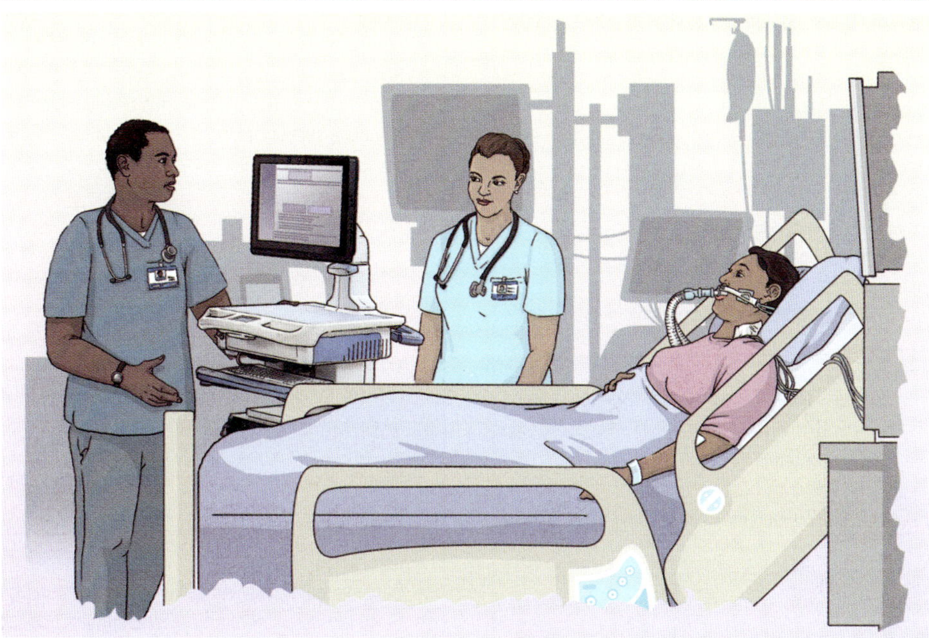

Each day there are many handoffs between nurses for breaks or at the end of shift. Each handoff provides an opportunity to demonstrate a transfer of trust. A brief verbal description of the background and plan of care can assure the patient and family that vital information will not be lost, and that all of the nurses on the unit are skilled practitioners and communicators.

If the patient needs to go back to the operating room urgently or have an urgent diagnostic procedure, the handoff is essential to ensure high-quality, safe care in all settings.

At a point when the patient's condition is no longer critical, transfer out of the unit is often the next step. Patients and families may have anxieties about the move from the intensive care unit to another level of care. Acknowledging the concerns about a different nurse-to-patient ratio and using the same principles of transfer of trust can help alleviate anxiety, as can setting expectations that because the patient has made progress medically, increasing independence is normal and expected.

Another reason to communicate clearly with the patient, family, and the receiving unit is to avoid lapses in treatment that may precipitate readmission back to critical care. A transfer of trust and vital information is important to reassure the patient that the same treatments will continue seamlessly toward discharge to home.

There are necessary components of safe protocols for transporting critically ill patients.[39] Protocols should include pretransport communication and coordination, a list of necessary equipment, monitoring guidelines, expected documentation, required transport personnel, and training. In addition to these, a risk analysis should be conducted for each transport. In a study of 502 transports, the highest incidence of adverse events occurred in patients with the highest acuity, emphasizing the need for a thorough evaluation of the patient's clinical status before transport.[40] Before patient transport, an analysis should be conducted to determine whether the benefit of the transport outweighs the risk. One study of patients with neurologic injuries noted that only 5.5% of computed tomography scans conducted resulted in a new surgical intervention.[38] The care team should always evaluate the availability of bedside testing before transporting the patient out of the critical care unit for testing.

It is recommended that a checklist be used when the decision is made to transport a patient.[38,41] The use of a checklist ensures that all appropriate safety measures are in place, thus reducing the risk of adverse events. The use of a checklist can also assist in identifying transports that may be considered higher risk. A comprehensive checklist should include physiologic red flags, such as high ventilator support requirements, unstable cervical fractures, or new or increasing vasopressor requirements, which can prompt the care team to consider additional safety measures for transport, such as the addition of a physician to the transport team for patients who are at higher likelihood of deterioration during transport. See Box 4.2 regarding physiologic red flags.

The latest Critical Care Medicine Guidelines for Transport[42] recommend that at least two personnel accompany all critical care patients during transport. At least one team member should be a critical care nurse. The second team member may be a respiratory therapist or technician. In many institutions, a respiratory therapist must accompany patients who are mechanically ventilated during transport. The checklist should also incorporate a list of necessary equipment for safe transport and ensure that test-specific items such as the completion of an MRI safety screening or establishing working intravenous access for contrast administration are met before patient transport.

Critical care patients must receive the same physiologic monitoring during transport as in the critical care unit. Necessary

BOX 4.2 Safety

Physiologic Red Flags

- High ventilatory requirements reflecting difficulty oxygenating adequately and/or ventilated patient
- Examples:
- Fraction of inspired oxygen (FiO_2) >60%
- Positive end-expiratory pressure (PEEP) >10 cm H_2O, plateau pressure >30 cm H_2O
- Pressure limiting despite sedation
- Inverse ratio ventilation, high-frequency oscillatory ventilation
- Dependence on noninvasive ventilation without battery power
- Multiple chest tubes and/or unable to tolerate being off suction
- Hemodynamically unstable cardiac rhythm despite antiarrhythmic therapy
- Transvenous pacemaker with poor capture
- Dependence on intraaortic balloon pump
- Labile blood pressure requiring frequent fluid boluses or titration of infusions
- Bleeding patient with ongoing resuscitation
- Retractable intracranial pressure requiring frequent intervention
- Patient with abdominal compartment syndrome (unless going to operating room for decompression laparotomy)
- Open abdomen with exposed viscera
- Continuous renal replacement therapy
- Unstable cervical spine fracture

Data from Day D. Keeping patients safe during intrahospital transport. *Crit Care Nurse.* 2010;30(4):18–32. doi:10.4037/ccn2010446; Comeau OY, Armendariz-Batiste J, Woodby SA. Safety first! Using a checklist for intrafacility transport of adult intensive care patients. *Crit Care Nurse.* 2015;35(5):16–25. doi:10.4037/ccn2015991; and Parmentier-Decrucq E, Poissy J, Favory R, Nseir S, Onimus T, Guerry MJ, Durocher A, Mathieu D. Adverse events during intrahospital transport of critically ill patients: incidence and risk factors. *Ann Intensive Care.* 2013;3(1):10. doi:10.1186/2110-5820-3-10.

BOX 4.3 Safety

Basic Transport Equipment

Airway

- Airway: oral/nasal airways
- Sedation
- Intubation tray with various sizes of endotracheal tubes
- Complete suction setup (at least 1) with adequate tubing length, Yankauer device

Breathing

- Oxygen saturation pulse oximeter
- Oxygen delivery devices: nasal cannula, Venturi high-flow mask, nonrebreather mask
- Bag valve mask (anesthesia bag/self-inflating bag), fitted with positive end-expiratory pressure valve
- Full oxygen tank with enough supply for flow requirements plus 30 min
- Oxygen wall source at destination with flowmeter and adequate tubing length
- Ventilator capable of matching intensive care unit ventilator settings

Circulation

- Cardiac monitor
- Defibrillator with pacing capacity and defibrillator/pacing pads
- Blood pressure cuff of proper size; stethoscope
- Supplies to establish intravenous access
- Isotonic crystalloid intravenous fluid with big-bore tubing to establish "code line"
- Standard resuscitation drugs: epinephrine, atropine, amiodarone with filter
- Adequate supply of vasoactive medications, analgesia to meet patient's anticipated needs (with orders/protocols to cover administration)
- Temperature probe or thermometer
- Location of nearest code cart; move cart closer if patient's acuity necessitates

Data from Day D. Keeping patients safe during intrahospital transport. *Crit Care Nurse.* 2010;30(4):18–32. doi:10.4037/ccn2010446. Permission obtained to use table directly.

equipment and medications required for safe transport can be divided into three categories: airway, breathing, and circulation (Box 4.3). When a patient is placed on different equipment for transport, such as switching from a bedside monitor to a portable monitor, it is recommended that the patient be monitored on the new equipment for a short period before beginning transport to ensure all equipment is in working order. Monitoring and alarm parameters must also be checked, and patient-specific alarms settings must be programmed before transport.

Consideration should also be given to the availability of monitoring at the receiving destination. At a minimum, the destination should have an oxygen source, suction, accessible electrical outlets, monitors with the same monitoring capabilities as critical care unit monitors, and a code cart.[39] In addition to standard electrocardiogram, pulse oximetry and end-tidal CO_2 monitoring, critically ill patients often have additional monitoring parameters and equipment that have specific safety considerations. See Box 4.4 for special equipment considerations when transporting patients. Box 4.5 describes issues to consider when transporting isolation patients.

The availability of basic emergency medications should be considered before every transport. In addition to emergency medications, the transport team should ensure that enough quantities of all continuously infusing medications are available while the patient is receiving care outside of the critical care unit. It is recommended that premedication be discussed during planning.[40] Based on the incidence of adverse events studied during transport, optimizing the patient's fluid status and reducing nausea before transport may prevent adverse events (hypotension and nausea/vomiting).[40] Ensure that other important pretransport medications are considered, including analgesics and antianxiety medications, because these medications may not be readily available at the receiving destination. Lastly, if a patient will be in a procedural or diagnostic area for an extended period, any antibiotic medication that is scheduled during the off-unit time should be readily available and administered per provider orders.

A complete handoff report, including a review of the current medication list, should take place if the transport will involve transfer of care to a new primary caregiver, such as transporting a critical care patient to the operating room. Evidence supports critically ill patients receiving the same level of care and supervision during intrahospital transport as they receive in the critical care unit. During intrahospital transport, lapses in documentation of basic information, such as vital signs, is common. Implementation of a tool to facilitate documentation during transport should be considered to bridge this gap in documentation.[47] Posttransport, any complications or unexpected events should be documented according to facility guidelines.[38]

BOX 4.4 Safety

Special Equipment Considerations for Transport

Urinary catheter: To reduce the risk of catheter-associated urinary tract infections (CAUTI), empty the urinary catheter drainage bag before transport[43] and avoid placing urinary catheter drainage bag on the gurney or bed during transport. Maintain the collection bag below the level of the bladder.[44] Ensure that the urinary catheter is secured to the patient's thigh to minimize the risk of trauma or dislodgement during transport.

Chest tubes: Take precautions to ensure that chest tubes are not dislodged during transport. Ensure that the chest tube drainage system is kept below the level of the chest to prevent backflow if the patient's chest tube is to water seal. Do not clamp chest tubes during transport. Portable suction should be used for patients with pneumothoraxes with large air leaks, high ventilatory requirements, or high chest tube output. Patients without these complications are typically safe to transport without suction until they arrive at the receiving destination, but a brief trial on water seal is recommended before transport.[39]

Pulmonary arterial lines: Pulmonary arterial lines must be continuously monitored during transport to ensure immediate identification of migration to the right ventricle, which may cause arrhythmias, and migration to the continuous wedge position, which may cause pulmonary artery infarct or perforation.[39]

Arterial lines: Arterial lines should be continuously monitored to ensure identification of arterial catheter dislodgement, which may result in significant blood loss.[42]

External ventricular drainage device (EVD)/lumbar drain: All patients with an EVD should have intracranial pressure (ICP) monitoring during transport. Traditionally, routine clamping of EVDs and lumbar drains has been recommended during transport to avoid complications associated with the overdrainage of cerebrospinal fluid (CSF). However, more recent literature suggests that routine clamping of EVDs and lumbar drains during transport may lead to elevated ICP or CSF measurements during transport, increasing the risk for further cerebrovascular injury. It is recommended that a trial be performed before transport to assess patient tolerance of a clamped EVD or lumbar drain before the decision to clamp the drain during transport.[45]

ECMO: Extracorporeal Life Support Organization (ELSO) provides guidelines for the intrahospital transport of patients undergoing extracorporeal membrane oxygenation (ECMO). https://www.elso.org/default.aspx

BOX 4.5 Safety

Transporting Isolation Patients[46]

Contact Precautions

- Use personal protective equipment (PPE) appropriately, including gloves and gown. Wear a gown and gloves for all interactions that may involve contact with the patient or the patient's environment. Donning PPE upon room entry and properly discarding before exiting the patient room are done to contain pathogens.
- Limit transport and movement of patients outside of the room to medically necessary purposes. When transport or movement is necessary, cover or contain the infected or colonized areas of the patient's body. Remove and dispose of contaminated PPE and perform hand hygiene before transporting patients on Contact Precautions. Don clean PPE to handle the patient at the transport location.

Droplet Precautions

- Limit transport and movement of patients outside of the room to medically necessary purposes. If transport or movement outside of the room is necessary, instruct patient to wear a mask and follow respiratory hygiene/cough etiquette.

Airborne Precautions

- Limit transport and movement of patients outside of the room to medically necessary purposes. If transport or movement outside an airborne infection isolation room (AIIR) is necessary, instruct patients to wear a surgical mask, if possible, and observe respiratory hygiene/cough etiquette. Health care personnel transporting patients who are on airborne precautions do not need to wear a mask or respirator during transport if the patient is wearing a mask and infectious skin lesions are covered.

SPECIAL CONSIDERATIONS DURING CARE TRANSITIONS

Changes in Baseline Physical and Cognitive Function

Frailty is an age- or disease-related state in which physiologic reserves have decreased, increasing a patient's risk for morbidity and mortality when exposed to internal or external stressors.[48] Up to 40% of frail patients experience prolonged lengths of stay in hospitals and higher readmissions from physical and cognitive complications compared with patients of the same age who are not frail.[48] When admitted to critical care areas, frail patients are at an increased risk of in-hospital deaths and reduced likelihood of survival after discharge.[48] The contributing factors of frailty should be addressed by an interprofessional team with the goal to restore optimal physical and cognitive function. Cognitive complications such as delirium are further addressed in Chapter 8.

Older Adults

As individuals age, cognitive, physiologic, and psychologic changes occur that must be considered during care transitions. Decisions regarding critical care admission or discharge of adults over the age of 80 must be inclusive of comorbidities, severity of illness, baseline functional status, and preferences—and not be based on age alone.[8] See Chapter 39 for detailed information on best practices when providing care for the older adult patient.

Racial and Ethnic Disparities

Black and Hispanic individuals are more likely to be admitted to the hospital compared with non-Hispanic white individuals.[49] Black patients with chronic conditions such as diabetes, hypertension, and asthma are three to five times more likely to be admitted to the hospital compared with non-Hispanic white patients.[49] Hispanic patients with the same chronic conditions are two to three times more likely to be admitted to the hospital compared with non-Hispanic white patients.[49] Once hospitalized, non-Hispanic white patients are 1.23 times more likely to receive referrals to home health care services than Hispanic patients after controlling for gender, insurance type, age, and length of stay.[50] Not having insurance was linked more to the observed disparities than was being Hispanic and should be considered when planning care transitions for this population.[50] Both black and Hispanic patients had higher rates of preventable hospitalizations compared with non-Hispanic white individuals.[49] Asians, on the other hand, have lower rates of preventable hospitalizations compared with non-Hispanic white individuals.[49]

Rural Communities

The Affordable Care Act aims to transition health care in the United States from a model of episodic care that is offered during periods of acute illness or exacerbation to preventive care supported by early identification of disease and earlier intervention.[51,52] Successful transitions of care reduce fragmentations, episodic care, and concomitant hospital readmissions.[35,53–56] Transitional care models that endeavor to prevent acute episodes of illness are expected and have demonstrated improved patient outcomes and cost containment.[26]

Americans living in rural areas experience numerous health care challenges, including a lack of specialty services, board-certified intensivists, and other resources.[57] Compared with the urban population, those living in rural areas are at greater risk of dying from heart disease, cancer, stroke, chronic lower respiratory disease, and unintentional injuries. Obesity, tobacco use, and suicide rates are also higher in rural areas. Access to chronic care management is hindered by the lack of local primary care providers, poverty, and difficulty accessing health care professionals because of distance, terrain, and adverse weather. Follow-up visits may be poorly attended.[58]

The transfer of patients to larger tertiary care centers with advanced critical care services is common, resulting in frequent care transitions. Telecritical care has been used in rural areas to support hospitals that lack intensivist staffing, to reduce transfers, and to standardize care. Telemedicine is a solution for the lack of specialists in rural areas and has been employed for advanced neurologic assessments performed by neurosurgeons, pain consults, dysphagia screening, and providing patient education for stroke and heart failure patients. Policies developed to support urban health care systems may not address the issues prevalent in rural areas, but when programs do include the use of care coordination services, a designated individual is an asset in preventing duplication of services, connecting the patient with community resources, and assisting the patient in managing chronic conditions. See Chapter 1 for further discussion of telemedicine.

End of Life

Providing care at the end of life is an important and complex component of acute and critical care nursing. See Chapter 9 for detailed information on best practices in end-of-life and hospice care.

MODELS OR PROGRAMS FOR CARE TRANSITIONS

Approximately 18% of Medicare patients are readmitted to the hospital within 30 days of discharge at a cost of $15 to $17 billion per year.[59] The current inefficient care delivery system combined with poor management of care transitions is not only a serious financial burden, but it also leads to poor patient

SOCIAL DETERMINANTS OF HEALTH

Increasing the Health Literacy of the Population

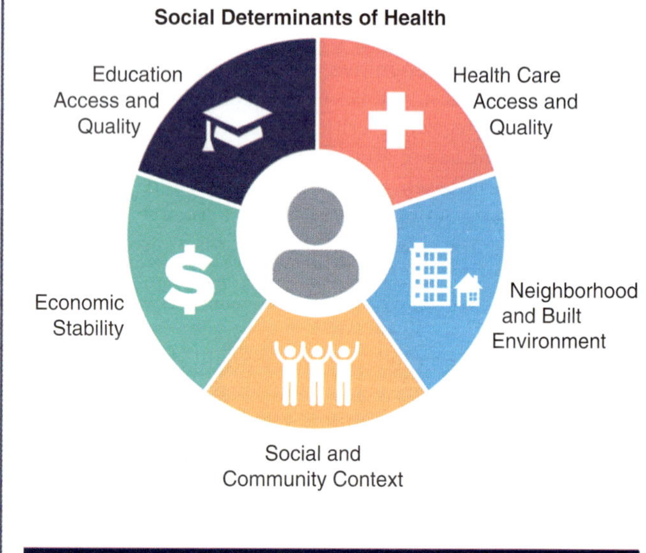

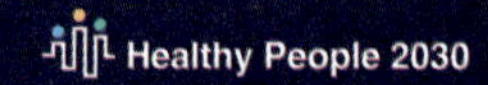

Health literacy is the ability of individuals to obtain, process, understand, appraise, and use basic health information for decision making and action planning that will impact their health status.[1,2] Limited health literacy contributes to reduced knowledge of medication regimens and reduced knowledge and skills for managing disease processes.[1] Limited health literacy disproportionally affects the older adult, people with disabilities, people of lower socioeconomic status, ethnic minorities, people with limited English proficiency, and people with limited education.[1] The practices and policies limiting access to quality education places people with low health literacy at an increased risk for poorer health and the development of chronic disease, resulting in a twofold higher mortality rate compared to people with adequate health literacy.[1] Limited health literacy has contributed to increased health care costs, totaling more than $100 billion annually.[1]

Improving health literacy may mediate the social determinants of health that contribute to health disparities.[2] Efforts should focus on interventions to improve health literacy but not substitute the need to address underlying inequities in the distribution of power, resources, and opportunity.[2] Practical strategies to improve health literacy are limited but organizations, such as public libraries, are exploring innovating ways to engage the community and prioritize health literacy.[3] Further research is needed to establish evidence-based interventions to improve health literacy.[4]

References

1. Schillinger D. The intersections between social determinants of health, health literacy, and health disparities. *Stud Health Technol Inform.* 2020;269:22–41. https://doi.org/10.3233/SHTI200020.
2. Nutbeam D, Lloyd JE. Understanding and responding to health literacy as a social determent of health. *Annu Rev Public Health.* 2021;42:159–173. https://doi.org/10.1146/annurev-publhealth-090419-102529.
3. Sacramento public library and healthy people: prioritizing health literacy to meet community members' needs. U.S. Department of Health and Human Services; 2022. https://health.gov/news/202210/sacramento-public-library-and-healthy-people-prioritizing-health-literacy-meet-community-members-needs. Accessed September 16, 2023.
4. Increase the health literacy of the population – HC/HIT-R01. Health People 2030. https://health.gov/healthypeople/objectives-and-data/browse-objectives/health-communication/increase-health-literacy-population-hchit-r01. Accessed September 16, 2023.

Illustration from Healthy People 2030, U.S. Department of Health and Human Services, Office of Disease Prevention and Health Promotion. Retrieved September 8, 2022, from https://health.gov/healthypeople/objectives-and-data/social-determinants-health.

outcomes, patient dissatisfaction, and inappropriate use of emergency rooms and other outpatient services.[60] According to the Medicare Payment Advisory Commission (MedPAC), approximately 12% of these readmissions are potentially avoidable. A 10% reduction in the rate of readmissions could save Medicare $1 billion.[61] To reduce readmissions, the Centers for Medicare & Medicaid Services introduced the Hospital Readmissions Reduction Program (HRRP) in 2012, which reduces Medicare fee-for-service payments to hospitals with excessive readmission rates.[62] The following conditions and procedures are included in this program:

- Acute myocardial infarction (AMI)
- Chronic obstructive pulmonary disease (COPD)
- Heart failure (HF)
- Pneumonia
- Coronary artery bypass graft (CABG) surgery
- Elective primary total hip arthroplasty and/or total knee arthroplasty (THA/TKA)

As part of continued efforts to ensure that patients are able to make informed decisions about their care, starting in early 2020 all HRRP information is available to the public on Hospital Compare,[62] a website that provides consumers information about how well hospitals provide care. Readmission to the critical care unit is less common than hospital readmission; however, between 4% and 10% of critical care patients are readmitted to the critical care unit within 72 hours of discharge. Patients who are readmitted to the critical care unit have a 21% increased risk of mortality than those who do not.[63] To effectively reduce readmissions and improve patient outcomes, it is imperative that hospital systems adopt an evidence-based transitions of care model.[26] Models or programs for care transitions provide interprofessional, multimodal interventions to improve patient outcomes; decrease readmissions; and reduce hospital costs.[64] See Box 4.6 for a summary of select models or programs for care transitions.

ADDITIONAL RESOURCES

Refer to Box 4.7 for internet resources related to facilitating care transitions.

KEY POINTS

Care transitions have been defined as changes in the setting where care is delivered or as changes to the extent of health care services provided.

- The delivery of quality care during care transitions is attained through:
  - The health care team sharing the same goal for the patient,
  - Communicating sufficient breadth and depth of the patient's condition,
  - Understanding the role expectations of each other,
  - Minimizing safety risks by developing and carrying out an organized plan of care between different locations/levels of care, and
  - Ensuring patients and families remain informed and an integral part of the entire process.
- Management of complex health issues and medications
  - Recognize patients at high risk for poor outcomes and prioritize interventions to reduce threats to safety and improve outcomes.

BOX 4.6 SELECT MODELS OR PROGRAMS FOR CARE TRANSITIONS

Transitional Care Model (TCM): The *transitional care model* is the most comprehensive hospital-to-home care transition model or program and is used to improve care of at-risk older adults. An advanced practice nurse (e.g., clinical nurse specialist or nurse practitioner) acts as the transitional care nurse (TCN) and works across the health care continuum. In both the inpatient and outpatient setting, the TCN is a part of the interprofessional team and collaborates on the development and implementation of the plan of care. Assessment of learning needs, education, telephone check-ins, home visits, and accompanying the patient to medical appointments are all a part of the service.[26]

Project RED (Re-Engineering Discharge): The Project RED (Re-Engineering Discharge) program uses a nursing discharge advocate to perform education and prepare for discharge. Medication reconciliation, coordination of postdischarge appointments, and a postdischarge summary are all part of the role of the nursing discharge advocate. Additional components of Project RED include developing patient care plans, assessing patient and family knowledge of the care plan, and communicating with the primary care provider.[26]

Project BOOST (Better Outcomes for Older adults through Safe Transitions): The Project BOOST (Better Outcomes for Older adults through Safe Transitions) program facilitates older adults being discharged from the hospital to home. Unlike other transition programs, Project BOOST focuses on assisting organizations with developing processes to improve care transition. Project BOOST provides mentorship and program development support to hospitals and assists with removing implementation barriers the organization may encounter. Project BOOST representatives use telephone calls to support organizations and their coordination of patient care.[26]

Care Transitions Intervention (CTI): The Care Transitions Intervention (CTI) program is structured around four pillars: medication self-management, patient-kept records, indicators of deterioration, and follow-up. Transition coaches in the CTI program are advanced practice nurses, registered nurses, or social workers. The patient and caregiver are persuaded to take ownership of their medical care. This is done by having patients manage their medications, maintain a patient-kept health record, and monitor indicators of deterioration. The patients are equipped to evaluate if their condition is getting worse or if they have experienced a harmful medication event. Additionally, the transition coach engages the patient, performing follow-up at the patient's home and through telephone calls.

Coordinated-Transitional Care Program: Although the Coordinated-Transitional Care Program was for hospital-to-community transitions, the program differed from the others as it was exclusively for veterans. Most supportive activities took place in the hospital before discharge, and the interventions were centered around discharge rounds and medication reconciliation. Medication education was performed by a pharmacist at discharge and nurses or case managers performed follow-up phone calls. Outcome measures demonstrate the value in transitions programs, with programs inclusive of multiple interventions showing the largest benefit.[26]

BOX 4.7 Internet Resources

Facilitating Care Transitions

- Case Management Society of America: https://www.cmsa.org/
- Institute for Healthcare Improvement: www.ihi.org/knowledge/Pages/Tools/HowtoGuideImprovingTransitionstoReduceAvoidableRehospitalizations.aspx
- The Care Transitions Program: https://caretransitions.org/
- The National Transitions of Care Coalition: https://www.ntocc.org/

- Medication reconciliation is the process by which a provider compares a patient's current medication regimen to new medications that are ordered for the patient and resolves any discrepancies to avoid errors of omission during care transitions.
- Patient and family education
  - During care transitions, patients receive a large amount of new information in a relatively short period. Learning needs are to be prioritized to avoid potential knowledge deficits during the high-risk transition period.
  - Nurses and other health care team members need to consider the informational and emotional support needs of patients and families. Patient-centered education regarding critical care experiences is recommended to meet these needs.
- Health care team member accountability
  - Interprofessional teams are made up of individuals from different professions and occupations with varied and specialized knowledge, skills, and approaches to providing care who communicate and work together as colleagues to provide quality, individualized care for patients.
  - Nurses and other health care team members maintain professional responsibility for patients for limited periods and are also responsible for transferring that responsibility during a care transition. Using standardized elements and available documentation while providing verbal handoff communication at the bedside is preferred and has been shown to improve the handoff process by reducing omissions of relevant information.
- Continuity of care
  - Planning for care transitions includes a robust consideration of patient and family needs for the next phase of the patient's care.
  - National guidelines and institution-specific policies on critical care admission and discharge criteria assist nurses and other health care team members in anticipating the needs of patients and families.
- Coordination of physical transport
  - Critically ill patients may require transport for several reasons during hospitalization. Coordinate physical transport of patients while monitoring the patient's physiologic response to transport, ensuring proper equipment is available and used and preventing the transmission of infection.
- Special considerations during care transitions exist for patients:
  - With changes in their baseline physical and cognitive function,
  - Who are older adults,
  - Belonging to disparate racial and ethnic groups,
  - Living in rural communities, and/or
  - Reaching the end of their lives.
  - Models or programs for care transitions provide interprofessional, multimodal interventions to improve patient outcomes, decrease readmissions, and reduce hospital costs.

Visit the Evolve site at http://evolve.elsevier.com/Urden/CriticalCareNursing for additional study materials.

CASE STUDY 4.1 Facilitating Care Transitions in Critical Care

The patient is a 59-year old Hispanic man with nonalcoholic cirrhosis/end-stage liver disease and does not qualify for a liver transplant. He is oriented to person, place, and situation, with periods of confusion caused by worsening encephalopathy. He is in critical care for continuous renal replacement therapy (CRRT) due to a labile blood pressure and not tolerating hemodialysis and for monitoring for a recurrent gastrointestinal bleed. He is scheduled for a transjugular intrahepatic portosystemic shunt (TIPS) procedure in 2 days. The plan is for the patient to return home 3 days postoperatively if he is tolerating intermittent hemodialysis. His wife will perform custodial care, but she is hesitant because he has fallen twice at home and she has made several comments about how the hospital just wants to rush him out every time. The patient has commented that he has not been included in decisions about his care, and he does not want to be rushed home when he is too much work for his wife.

Orders

NPO
Blood pressure measurements every 15 minutes
CRRT: Remove 50 mL/h
Laboratory testing: CBC every 12 hours, BMP every 6 hours while on CRRT

Medications

- Lactulose 20 g/30 mL every 6 hours and titrate to three to four bowel movements per day
- Norepinephrine infusion to keep mean arterial pressure >65 (currently not infusing)
- Albumin 25% 100 mL intravenously every 12 hours

Questions

1. What major outcomes do you expect to achieve for this patient?
2. What problems or risks must be managed to achieve these outcomes?
3. What interventions could be initiated to monitor, prevent, manage, or eliminate the problems and risks identified?
4. What interventions could be initiated to promote optimal functioning, safety, and well-being of the patient?
5. What technology can be used to monitor this patient and prevent complications?
6. What other interprofessional team members are needed to assist with the management of this patient?
7. What possible learning needs would you anticipate for this patient?
8. What cultural and age-related factors might have a bearing on the patient's plan of care?

BMP, Basic metabolic panel; *CBC*, complete blood count; *CRRT*, continuous renal replacement therapies; *NPO*, nothing by mouth.

REFERENCES

1. Shahsavari H, Zarei M, Mamaghani A. Transitional care: concept analysis using Rogers' evolutionary approach. *Int J Nurs Stud*. 2019;99:103387. https://doi.org/10.1016/j.ijnurstu.2019.103387.
2. Hoffman RL, Saucier J, Dasani S, et al. Development and implementation of a risk identification tool to facilitate critical care. *Int J Qual Health Care*. 2017;29(3):412–419. https://doi.org/10.1093/intqhc/mzx032.
3. Coffey A, Mulcaby H, Savage E, et al. Transitional care interventions: relevance for nursing in the community. *Public Health Nurs*. 2017;34(5):454–460. https://doi.org/10.1111/phn.12324.
4. Definitions of transitional care. National Association of Clinical Nurse Specialists; 2023. https://nacns.org/professional-resources/toolkits-and-reports/transitions-of-care/definitions-of-transitional-care/. Accessed September 16, 2023.
5. Stacy K. Progressive care units: different but the same. *Crit Care Nurse*. 2011;31(3):77–83. https://doi.org/10.4037/ccn2011644.
6. Rhudy L. Handoff from operating room to intensive care unit: specific pathways to decrease patient adverse events. *Nurs Clin North Am*. 2019;54(3):335–345. https://doi.org/10.1016/j.cnur.2019.04.003.
7. Critical care statistics. Society of Critical Care Medicine. https://www.sccm.org/Communications/Critical-Care-Statistics. Accessed September 16, 2023.
8. Nates JL, Nunnally M, Kleinpell R, et al. ICU admission, discharge, and triage guidelines: a framework to enhance clinical operations, development of institutional policies, and further research. *Crit Care Med*. 2016;44(8):1553–1602. https://doi.org/10.1097/CCM.0000000000001856.
9. Prin M, Wunsch H. The role of stepdown beds in hospital care. *Am J Respir Crit Care Med*. 2014;190(11):1210–1216. https://doi.org/10.1164/rccm.201406-1117PP.
10. Chen EH, Hollander JE. When do patients need admission to a telemetry bed? *J Emerg Med*. 2007;33(1):53–60. https://doi.org/10.1016/j.jemermed.2007.01.017.
11. What is medical-surgical nursing? Academy of Medical-Surgical Nurses. https://amsn.org/About-AMSN/What-Is-Med-Surg-Nursing; 2023. Accessed September 16, 2023.
12. Centers for MedicareMedicaid Services. What are long-term care hospitals? https://www.medicare.gov/pubs/pdf/11347-Long-Term-Care-Hospitals.pdf; 2019. Accessed September 16, 2023.
13. Stefanacci RG. Admission criteria for facility-based post-acute services. *Population Health Learning Network*. 2015. https://www.hmpgloballearningnetwork.com/site/altc/articles/admission-criteria-facility-based-post-acute-services. Accessed September 16, 2023.
14. The Commission for Case Management Certification. Glossary of terms. n.d. https://ccmcertification.org/sites/ccmc/files/docs/2022/CCMC-22-GlossaryUpdate-Final%20Final%20with%20CM%20def%20update.pdf. Accessed September 16, 2023.
15. What is assisted living. National Centers for Assisted Living; 2023. https://www.ahcancal.org/ncal/about/assistedliving/Pages/What-is-Assisted-Living.aspx. Accessed September 16, 2023.
16. Buss MK, Rock LK, McCarthy EP. Understanding palliative care and hospice: a review for primary care providers. *Mayo Clin Proc*. 2017;92(2):280–286. https://doi.org/10.1016/j.mayocp.2016.11.007.
17. Bonebrake D, Culver C, Call K, Ward-Smith P. Clinically differentiating palliative care and hospice. *Clin J Oncol Nurs*. 2010;14(3):273–275. https://doi.org/10.1188/10.CJON.273-275.
18. Burlingame B. Operating room requirements for 2014 and beyond. Facility Guidelines Institute Guidelines. 2014. https://www.fgiguidelines.org/wp-content/uploads/2015/10/FGI_Update_ORs_140915.pdf. Accessed September 16, 2023.
19. Emergency Department Performance Measures and Benchmarking Summit. The Consensus Statement. https://qualityindicators.ahrq.gov/Downloads/Resources/Publications/2006/EDPerformanceMeasures-ConsensusStatement.pdf. Accessed September 16, 2023.
20. Reducing care fragmentation: a toolkit for coordinating care. California Healthcare Foundation. https://www.act-center.org/application/files/7016/3112/2157/Toolkit_Reducing_Care_Fragmentation.pdf. Accessed September 16, 2023.
21. Naylor MD, Shaid EC, Carpenter D, et al. Components of comprehensive and effective transitional care. *J Am Geriatr Soc*. 2017;65(6):1119–1125. https://doi.org/10.1111/jgs.14782.
22. Jewell JA, Committee on Hospital Care. Standardization of inpatient handoff communication. *Pediatrics*. 2016;138(5):e20162681. https://doi.org/10.1542/peds.2016-2681.
23. Mitchell SE, Laurens V, Weigel GM, et al. Care transitions from patient and caregiver perspectives. *Ann Fam Med*. 2018;16(3):225–231. https://doi.org/10.1370/afm.2222.
24. Hirschman K, Shaid E, McCAuley K, Pauly M, Naylor MD. Continuity of care: the transitional care model. *Online J Issues Nurs*. 2015;20(3):1.
25. The Joint Commission. National Patient Safety Goals®; 2023. https://www.jointcommission.org/-/media/tjc/documents/standards/national-patient-safety-goals/2023/npsg_chapter_hap_jul2023.pdf. Accessed September 16, 2023.
26. Rochester-Eyeguokan CD, Pincus KJ, Patel RS, Reitz SJ. The current landscape of transitions of care practice models: a scoping review. *Pharmacotherapy*. 2016;36(1):117–133. https://doi.org/10.1002/phar.1685.
27. Rungvivatjarus T, Kuelbs CL, Miller L, et al. Medication reconciliation improvement utilizing process redesign and clinical decision support. *Joint Comm J Qual Patient Saf*. 2020;46(1):27–36. https://doi.org/10.1016/j.jcjq.2019.09.001.
28. Ellis DM, Hickey S, Prieto P, et al. Medication safety of patients with Parkinson's disease during care transitions: educating nursing students. *Nurs Educ Perspect*. 2019;40(6):E22–E24. https://doi.org/10.1097/01.NEP.0000000000000532.
29. Institute for Safe Medication Practices. Building a case for medication reconciliation. *ISMP Med Saf Alert*. 2005;10(8). https://www.medscape.com/viewarticle/505420. Accessed September 16, 2023.
30. Tully AP, Hammond DA, Li C, Jarrell AS, Kruer RM. Evaluation of medication errors at the transition of care from an ICU to non-ICU location. *Crit Care Med*. 2019;47(4):543–549. https://doi.org/10.1097/CCM.0000000000003633.
31. Use the teach-back method: tool #5. Agency for Healthcare Research and Quality. Content last reviewed September 2020. https://www.ahrq.gov/health-literacy/quality-resources/tools/literacy-toolkit/healthlittoolkit2-tool5.html. Accessed September 16, 2023.
32. Backman C, Chartrand J, Dingwall O, Shea B. Effectiveness of a person- and family-centered care transition interventions: a systematic review protocol. *Syst Rev*. 2017;6(1):158. https://doi.org/10.1186/s13643-017-0554-z.
33. Institute of Medicine (US) Committee on the Health Professions Education Summit. *Health Professions Education: A Bridge to Quality*. Washington, DC: National Academies Press; 2003. https://www.ncbi.nlm.nih.gov/books/NBK221528/. Accessed September 16, 2023.
34. Franklin CM, Bernhardt JM, Lopez RP, Long-Middleton ER, Davis S. Interprofessional teamwork and collaboration between community health workers and healthcare teams: an integrative review. *Health Ser Res Manag Epidemiol*. 2015;2:2333392815573312. https://doi.org/10.1177/2333392815573312.
35. Enderlin CA, McLeskey N, Rooker JL, et al. Review of current conceptual models and frameworks to guide transitions of care in older adults. *Geriatr Nurs*. 2013;34(1):47–52. https://doi.org/10.1016/j.gerinurse.2012.08.003.
36. Rhudy LM, Johston MR, Kreckle CA, et al. Change-of-shift nursing handoff interruptions: implications for evidence-based practice. *Worldviews Nurs*. 2019;16(5):362–370. https://doi.org/10.1111/wvn.12390.
37. Nasraway SA, Cohen IL, Dennis RC, et al. Guidelines on admission and discharge for adult intermediate care units. American College of Critical Care Medicine of the Society of Critical Care Medicine. *Crit Care Med*. 1998;26(3):607–610. https://doi.org/10.1097/00003246-199803000-00039.
38. Comeau OY, Armendariz-Batiste J, Woodby SA. Safety first! Using a checklist for intrafacility transport of adult intensive care patients. *Crit Care Nurse*. 2015;35(5):16–25. https://doi.org/10.4037/ccn2015991.
39. Day D. Keeping patients safe during intrahospital transport. *Crit Care Nurse*. 2010;30(4):18–32. https://doi.org/10.4037/ccn2010446.

40. Jones HM, Zychowicz ME, Champagne M, Thornlow DK. Intrahospital transport of the critically ill patient: a standardized evaluation plan. *Dimens Crit Care Nurs*. 2016;35(3):133–146. https://doi.org/10.1097/DCC.0000000000000176.
41. Williams P, Karuppiah S, Greentree K, Darvall J. A checklist for intrahospital transport of critically ill patients improves compliance with transportation safety guidelines. *Aust Crit Care*. 2020;33(1):20–24. https://doi.org/10.1016/j.aucc.2019.02.004.
42. Warren J, Fromm RE, Orr RA, Rotello LC, Horst M, American College of Critical Care Medicine. Guidelines for the inter- and intrahospital transport of critically ill patients. *Crit Care Med*. 2004;32(1):256–262. https://doi.org/10.1097/01.CCM.0000104917.39204.0A.
43. Newman DK. Indications – indwelling catheters. *UroToday*. 2023. https://www.urotoday.com/urinary-catheters-home/indwelling-catheters/description/indications.html#:~:text=Urinary%20catheters%20have%20various%20medical,IUC%20may%20have%20a%20role. Accessed September 16, 2023.
44. Gould CV, Umscheid C, Agarwal RK, Kuntz G, Pegues DA, The Healthcare Infection Control Practices Committee. Guideline for prevention of catheter-associated urinary tract infections 2009. Healthcare Infection Control Practices Advisory Committee. Content last updated June 2019. https://www.cdc.gov/infectioncontrol/pdf/guidelines/cauti-guidelines-H.pdf. Accessed September 16, 2023.
45. Chaikittisilpa N, Lele AV, Lyons VH, et al. Risk of routinely clamping external ventricular drains for intrahospital transport in neurocritically ill cerebrovascular patients. *Neurocritical Care*. 2017;26(2):196–204. https://doi.org/10.1007/s12028-016-0308-0.
46. Transmission-based precautions. Centers for Disease Control and Prevention; 2016. https://www.cdc.gov/infectioncontrol/basics/transmission-based-precautions.html. Accessed September 16, 2023.
47. Jardena RL, Quirke S. Improving safety and documentation in intrahospital transport: development of an intrahospital transport tool for critically ill patients. *Intensive Crit Care Nurs*. 2010;26(2):101–107. https://doi.org/10.1016/j.iccn.2009.12.007.
48. Gibson JA, Crowe S. Frailty in critical care: examining implications for clinical practices. *Crit Care Nurs*. 2018;38(3):29–35. https://doi.org/10.4037/ccn2018336.
49. Russo CA, Andrews RM, Coffey RM. Racial and ethnic disparities in potentially preventable hospitalizations, 2003. Healthcare Cost and Utilization Project: Statistical Brief #10. https://hcup-us.ahrq.gov/reports/statbriefs/sb10.pdf; 2006. Accessed September 16, 2023.
50. Crist JD, Koerner KM, Hepworth JT, et al. Differences in transitional care provided to Mexican American and non-Hispanic white older adults. *J Transcult Nurs*. 2017;28(2):159–167. https://doi.org/10.1177/1043659615613420.
51. Care coordination. Agency for Healthcare Research and Quality. Priorities in focus – care coordination. Content last reviewed August 2018. https://www.ahrq.gov/ncepcr/care/coordination.html. Accessed September 16, 2023.
52. Baldwin KM, Black D, Hammond S. Developing a rural transitional care community case management program using clinical nurse specialists. *Clin Nurse Spec*. 2014;28(3):147–155. https://doi.org/10.1097/NUR.0000000000000044.
53. Ahmed OI, Rak DJ. Hospital readmission among participants in a transitional case management program. *Am J Manag Care*. 2010;16(10):778–783.
54. Naylor MD, Aiken LH, Kurtzman ET, Olds DM, Hirshman KB. The care span: the importance of transitional care in achieving health reform. *Health Aff*. 2011;30(4):746–754. https://doi.org/10.1377/hlthaff.2011.0041.
55. Shu CC, Hsu NC, Lin YF, Wang JY, Lin JW, Ko WJ. Integrated postdischarge transitional care in a hospitalist system to improve discharge outcomes: an experimental study. *BMC Med*. 2011;9:96. https://doi.org/10.1186/1741-7015-9-96.
56. Smith SB, Alexander JW. Nursing perception of patient transitions from hospitals to home with home health. *Prof Case Manage*. 2012;17(4):175–185. https://doi.org/10.1097/NCM.0b013e31825297e8.
57. Goedika CC, Moecklia J, Cram PM, Reisingerab HS. Introduction of Tele-ICU in rural hospitals: changing organizational culture to harness benefits. *Intensive Crit Care Nurs*. 2017;40:51–56. https://doi.org/10.1016/j.iccn.2016.10.001.
58. *Reinventing Rural Health Care: A Case Study of Seven Upper Midwest States*. Bipartisan Policy Center; 2018. https://bipartisanpolicy.org/wp-content/uploads/2018/01/BPC-Health-Reinventing-Rural-Health-Care-1.pdf. Accessed September 16, 2023.
59. Graham KL, Auerbach AD, Schnipper JL, et al. Preventability of early versus late hospital readmissions in a national cohort of general medicine patients. *Ann Intern Med*. 2018;168(11):766–774. https://doi.org/10.7326/M17-172460.
60. Delisle DR. Care transitions programs: a review of hospitalbased programs targeted to reduce readmissions. *Prof Case Manag*. 2013;18(6):273–283. https://doi.org/10.1097/NCM.0b013e31829d9cf3.
61. McIlvennan CK, Eapen ZJ, Allen AA. Hospital readmissions reduction program. *Circulation*. 2020;131(20):1796–1803.
62. *Hospital Readmissions Reduction Program (HRRP)*. Centers for Medicare & Medicaid Services; 2023. https://www.cms.gov/Medicare/Medicare-Fee-for-Service-Payment/AcuteInpatientPPS/Readmissions-Reduction-Program. Accessed September 16, 2023.
63. Woldhek AL, Rijkenberg S, Bosman R, van der Voort P. Readmission of ICU patients: a quality indicator? *J Crit Care*. 2017;38:328–334. https://doi.org/10.1016/j.jcrc.2016.12.001.
64. Kamermayer AK, Leasure AR, Anderson L. The effectiveness of transitions-of-care interventions in reducing hospital readmissions and mortality. A systematic review. *Dimens Crit Care Nurs*. 2017;36(6):311–316. https://doi.org/10.1097/DCC.0000000000000266.

5

Psychosocial and Spiritual Considerations

Carrie J. Scotto

http://evolve.elsevier.com/Urden/CriticalCareNursing

A 42-year-old woman with significant injuries is admitted to the critical care unit. She had been driving to an athletic event with her family when their car was hit head-on by a truck driven by an intoxicated driver. Her husband and young son were killed instantly. Although her airbag deployed, she sustained a severe concussion. Shattered glass resulted in skin cuts and a deep laceration in her cheek.

Patients are admitted to critical care units when they require urgent physical care. Survival and recovery are dependent on the use of technical interventions carried out by a skilled critical care team. However, when a person is seriously ill or injured, it is not only the body that suffers. Critical illness and injury impact the whole person—body, mind, and spirit. In the case of the woman in the preceding paragraph, the psychological impact of the trauma and her loss will become apparent. Anger toward the impaired driver, guilt over surviving, and profound depression may ensue. She may experience spiritual distress and hopelessness.

Due to the multifaceted impact of illness and injury on a human being, a holistic approach is essential to foster the most optimal recovery. Psychological and spiritual variables have significant impact on outcomes in physically compromised, vulnerable patients. Psychosocial interventions have the potential to support a patient's hope, energy, and the will to survive.

Critical care nurses provide psychosocial care by communicating with compassion and understanding, practicing dignity-enhancing care, supporting patient coping and self-control, and engaging the patient's spiritual resources. Additionally psychosocial care extends to the family and significant others. Those close to the patient provide support resources, but they are also vulnerable in the face of acute, uncertain events. Critical care nurses recognize that, while often challenging and stressful, acute events have the potential to elicit patient strengths and trigger a readiness for psychological and spiritual well-being.

This chapter focuses on psychosocial, psychiatric, and spiritual challenges experienced by critically ill patients. We explore nursing care related to psychological, social, and spiritual health. Holistic nursing interventions that help patients and family members cope effectively and thrive during a stressful experience are emphasized.

The term *stress* is often used to indicate a negative experience or internal tension. Yet an acute stress response is an essential and protective reaction to a stressor, designed to mobilize the body's response to threats for the purpose of survival. The stress response is described in detail in Unit VII Endocrine Alterations.

STRESSORS IN CRITICAL CARE

Stressors faced by critical care patients are numerous and represent all aspects of the human condition. Normal life patterns are disrupted, and patients experience alterations in social roles, job status, and finances. They are in strange, frightening, and restrictive environments. Critically ill patients experience distressing physical reactions, lack of control, fear of medical equipment, loss of meaning, and relationship disturbances during and after treatment in a critical care unit. Box 5.1 identifies stressors faced by critical care patients.

Coping With Stress and Illness

The stressors of critical illness are so numerous and severe that patients and families can become overwhelmed. Stress-related problems include anxiety, fear, low self-esteem, hopelessness, powerlessness, spiritual distress, and ineffective coping. These problems can quickly drain the resources of the patient and significant others. The most important nursing response to patients at risk for overwhelming stress is to reduce or eliminate the stressors that they experience. See Appendix A, Patient Care Management Plan: Stress Overload.

Coping Mechanisms

Coping mechanisms are intentional processes used to adjust, adapt, and successfully meet life stressors. Each patient's response to stress is unique and depends on a variety of environmental factors and individual differences, including cognitive variables, the person's place in the life cycle, the degree of social support, and the person's perception of the nature of the stressor or loss.[1]

If patients are coping effectively, they appear relatively comfortable with self and others, form valid appraisal of stressors, make decisions consistent with personal preferences and values, and have access to needed resources. Effective coping mechanisms help a person maintain a perception of an acceptable degree of control and empowers them to take necessary actions, share concerns, use healthy denial, and manage troublesome life challenges and uncertainties.

Most people have a repertoire of coping mechanisms to manage stressful situations and life challenges. Coping mechanisms are learned and practiced over a lifetime and are based on the person's sense of the effectiveness of any given strategy for adapting to the stressor.[1]

A person's coping mechanisms may or may not be effective. Their usefulness depends on the nature and seriousness of the challenge, the person's prior experience with a similar situation, or the extent to which the coping mechanism can be used in a given situation.

BOX 5.1 Common Stressors for Patients in Critical Care Units

- Pain, discomfort, and physical restrictions
- Unfamiliar environments with excessive light, noises, alarms, and distressing events
- Loss of ability to express oneself verbally when intubated
- Unfamiliar bodily sensations resulting from bed rest, medications, surgery, or symptoms
- Threat of death
- Lack of sleep
- Loss of autonomy and control over one's body, environment, privacy, and daily activities
- Boredom broken only by brief visits, threatening stimuli, and procedural touch
- Separation from family, friends, and meaningful social roles and work
- Loss of dignity, embarrassing exposures, and a sense of vulnerability
- Worry about finances, potential job loss, and stress on loved ones
- Uncertainty about future and fear of permanent residual health deficits
- Unanswered spiritual questions and concerns about meaning of the events and life

Individual Response to Stressors Depends on:

- Individual's perception of stressors
- Acute or chronic nature of stressors
- Cumulative effect of multiple stressors
- Effectiveness of the individual's usual coping strategies and style
- Degree of social support

For example, a person may ordinarily cope with a distressing situation by careful problem analysis, information gathering, talking things over, and getting some refreshing sleep. Those coping methods may not work during acute illness in critical care environments. This decreased coping may be due to such factors as the inability to speak or process information, sleep disruption, diminished access to resources, and limited time to make decisions.

Ineffective coping is defined as the impairment of a person's adaptive behaviors and problem-solving abilities when meeting life's demands and necessary roles.

Manifestations of ineffective coping in critical illness include verbalization of an inability to cope, anxiety, and being unable to meet basic needs. The patient exhibits inappropriate use of defense mechanisms and has diminished problem-solving abilities. The patient may display apathy or destructive behavior toward self and others.

Promoting Optimal Coping

A goal of expert psychosocial-spiritual care is to promote patient and family flourishing, empowering them to experience as much control and predictability as possible. As noted earlier, coping is a dynamic process involving cognitive and behavioral efforts to manage specific internal or external demands that are perceived to exceed the person's resources. The key to effective coping is to encourage the use of the best mix of strategies appropriate for a given situation.

Most adults cope by relying on their previously developed conscious and unconscious coping strategies and defense mechanisms, which are automatically triggered in a stressful situation. Teaching new coping skills to people who are experiencing acute psychological stress may be unrealistic. However, by using active listening skills and initiating conversations with patients and family members, the nurse can identify the coping resources, skills, and preferences that may be most helpful.

Defense Mechanisms. Defense mechanisms are automatic coping styles that protect people from anxiety. Adaptive defense mechanisms are considered to be healthy. Using defensive mechanisms maladaptively occurs when one or more defense mechanism is used to excess, especially with immature defense mechanisms. They are used in response to an internal or external stressor and may be evident when patients or family members feel out of control and unable to cope.

Regression and Denial. Two common defense mechanisms especially evident in critical care settings are regression and denial. Regression is an unconscious defense mechanism. It is characterized as reverting to an earlier developmental level in response to stress. A simple example of regression is when a five-year-old begins to suck her thumb when the new baby arrives.

In terms of patients, regression often occurs when patients give up former roles, autonomy, and privacy. This type of regression is natural as patients relinquish control and rely on others for the most basic needs. The need to stay in control and resist the care that others provide could jeopardize a patient's outcome. Too much regression may result in patients relinquishing all control and responsibility for themselves and becoming excessively dependent on others. Behaviors such as complaining, moaning, clinging to staff, and excessive emotion can interfere with recovery. Excessive regression may also negatively impact nurse-patient relationships.

Recognizing that regression and dependence are part of the critically ill/injured experience helps to engender empathetic responses to patient regression. Although regressive behaviors can be frustrating to caregivers, confrontations or reprimands should be avoided. Threatening responses from staff may worsen a situation in which the patient is already struggling with the loss of dependence, autonomy, and self-worth.

Denial is conscious and unconscious attempts to escape unpleasant or anxiety-provoking thoughts, needs, feelings, and wishes by ignoring their existence.[1] Critically ill patients or their family members may use denial as a defense mechanism to protect against and manage an overwhelming sense of threat brought on by illness, injury, or impending death. Denial may be healthy and protective, allowing people to accept realities gradually. It allows the unconscious mind time to absorb and process distressing information.

Unhealthy denial is using it excessively and persistently. Too much denial prevents people from acting when they need to. For example, a person could ignore a persistent cough and blood-tinged sputum, resulting in a dangerous delay of care or foregoing it completely.

Family members and significant others are also affected by denial. If they are unable to cope with a loved one's serious, irreversible illness, they may only focus on a full recovery. They resist having realistic discussions concerning goals of care, insist on repeated resuscitation attempts, or invest in home remodeling in anticipation of a homecoming. They may regard caregivers who try to discuss anything other than a full recovery as being negative or untrustworthy people.

Nurses may find it particularly difficult to communicate with people who seem to be using denial to their own detriment. It may seem to the caregiver that the person would cope better by facing the realities of a situation and by taking the steps needed to go on with life. Family members and significant others may have firm or fixed denial. In this case, they are best supported by caregivers who recognize the protectiveness of denial.

With time they may exhibit cues that indicate a readiness to accept the reality of their situation and a need for further support and education. See Appendix A, Nursing Management Plan: Impaired Family Coping.

Anxiety

Anxiety is a normal subjective human response to a perceived or actual threat, which can range from a vague, generalized feeling of discomfort to a state of panic and loss of control. Feelings of anxiety are common in critically ill patients but are often undetected by care providers.[2] Anxiety and agitation in critical care patients can complicate patient recovery secondary to unplanned extubating, episodes of shortness of breath, and behavioral changes.[3]

The physiologic effects of anxiety can produce negative effects in critically ill patients by activating the sympathetic nervous system. Anxiety in patients is manifested in four levels of anxiety: mild, moderate, severe, and panic.

The first two levels of anxiety tend to be adaptive. Mild anxiety is characterized by a heightened sense of awareness and a sharp focus. Physical symptoms may include slight discomfort, restlessness, irritability, or mild tension-relieving behaviors (e.g., nail biting, foot or finger tapping, fidgeting).

Moderate anxiety results in a sharper focus on specific details to the exclusion of other peripheral details. Learning is more difficult in this level of anxiety, but it is possible. Sympathetic nervous system symptoms such as an increased pulse, respiratory rate, and perspiration along with mild somatic symptoms such as gastric discomfort, headache, and urinary urgency. Voice tremors and shaking may be noticed.

When anxiety becomes severe, the perceptual field is greatly reduced. The person may focus on one detail or many scattered details. Learning and problem solving are not possible, and the person may seem dazed and confused. Behavior is automatic and aimed at reducing the anxiety. Somatic symptoms such as headache, nausea, dizziness, and insomnia may increase. Patients in severe levels of anxiety may have a pounding heart, hyperventilation, and a sense of doom.

Panic is the most extreme level of anxiety. In this state, behavior is markedly dysregulated, and processing the environment is impossible. Extreme behaviors such as running, shouting, screaming, or full withdrawal may occur. Hallucinations or false sensory perceptions may be present. Physical behavior is erratic, uncoordinated, and impulsive. Acute panic may lead to exhaustion.

Critical care nurses most often rely on behavioral indicators, such as agitation and restlessness, and physiologic parameters, such as increased heart rate and blood pressure, to gauge anxiety.[3] Behavioral or vital sign changes do not provide consistently reliable indicators of anxiety and may lead to underestimation of the extent of anxiety in critical care patients. Using valid scales for evaluating patients' self-perceived anxiety levels can be helpful in determining the level and extent of anxiety. See Appendix A, Patient Care Management Plan: Anxiety.

AI (Artificial Intelligence) has been making significant advancements in health care and has the potential to revolutionize various aspects of the industry. See Box 5.2.

BOX 5.2 Informatics

Artificial Intelligence in Health Care

Here are key areas where AI is being utilized in health care:

- Diagnosis:
  - AI algorithms can analyze medical data, such as images, laboratory results, and patient records, to assist practitioners with diagnosing diseases such as cancer, cardiac disease, and neurological disorders.
- Medical Imaging Interpretation:
  - AI can detect subtle patterns and anomalies in radiologic imaging, aiding radiologists in diagnosing diseases more accurately and quickly.
- Medication Development:
  - AI can predict the effectiveness and safety of medications, optimizing the development process.
- Personalized Treatment:
  - AI can analyze patient data to recommend personalized treatment plans based on a patient's genetic makeup, medical history, and other factors, leading to more effective and targeted treatments.
- Natural Language Processing (NLP):
  - NLP allows computers to understand and generate human language, which can be used to transcribe medical records, extract information from clinical notes, and facilitate practitioner-patient communication.
- Virtual Health Assistants:
  - AI-powered chatbots and virtual assistants provide patients with medical information, answer basic health care questions, schedule appointments, and offer medication reminders.
- Remote Patient Monitoring:
  - AI-enabled devices can track patient vital signs and health metrics remotely, allowing health care practitioners to monitor patients with chronic conditions and intervene if necessary.
- Predictive Analytics:
  - AI can analyze historical patient data to predict disease outbreaks, patient admission rates, and resource requirements, helping health care organizations plan and allocate resources more effectively.
- Robotic Surgery:
  - AI-assisted robots can perform surgery with precision, aiding surgeons in complex procedures and minimizing the risk of human error.
- Epidemiology and Public Health:
  - AI can analyze large datasets to track disease outbreaks, monitor public health trends, and inform public health interventions.

While AI offers numerous benefits to health care, challenges remain, including data privacy concerns, regulatory hurdles, ethical considerations, and the need for rigorous validation of AI algorithms. Striking a balance between innovation and patient safety is crucial as AI transforms healthcare practices.[1]

Reference

Chen M, Decary M. Artificial intelligence in healthcare: an essential guide for health leaders. *Health Manage Forum.* 2020;33(1):10–18. https://do.org/10.1177/08404704.

Alterations in Self-Concept

The stressors imposed by serious illness, trauma, and surgical procedures can cause disturbances in the patient's self-concept. Self-concept is a perception of one's own behavior, abilities, and unique characteristics. It develops as a result of a person's experiences, interactions with others and the environment, and how those interactions are valued. Self-concept evolves over the lifespan. Patients admitted to critical care settings may experience self-concept challenges as their self-perceptions shift according to circumstances.

Patients in critical care units have little time to adjust to their altered health status, and they may be unable to clearly understand the implications of the situation. Self-concept also includes body image, self-esteem, and personal identity.

Body Image Disturbance

The physical body is central to an individual's self-concept. Body image is the mental picture we have of our bodies and its physical functioning at a given time. Body image includes attitudes and feelings about one's appearance, abilities, and gender. Body image evolves over time. It is influenced by interpersonal and environmental interactions and emotional experiences and aspirations both past and present.

Bodily sensations in a state of illness are often unfamiliar and may not make sense to the patient, which creates a cascade of stress responses.[4] Patients in critical care units experience prolonged confinement to the bed, position disorientation, sensory deprivation, muscle atrophy, metabolic pattern alteration, mechanical ventilation, pain, profound weakness, nutritional alterations, and medication-induced physical symptoms.

Disturbances in body image in critical care arise when the person fails to perceive or adapt to the changes that are imposed by the situation. In some instances, the individuals may feel betrayed by a body that no longer seems under control. Body image issues often emerge and resolve over time. Critical care nurses can help patients recognize temporary changes in body appearance and function. They can also help patients understand and cope with changes that are permanent. See Appendix A, Patient Care Management Plan: Disturbed Body Image.

Low Self-Esteem

Self-esteem refers to how well one's behavior correlates with a sense of the ideal self and is closely linked to one's sense of self-worth. Having a strong self-esteem helps a person deal with maturational and situational life crises more easily. The effect of self-esteem on a patient's energy and recovery is significant. Illness robs a person of perspective, often leading to a situational low self-esteem and feelings of powerlessness, helplessness, and depression. Low self-esteem impairs one's ability to adapt.

A patient may refuse to participate in self-care, exhibit self-destructive behavior, or become passive, asking no questions and permitting others to make all decisions. A comprehensive approach to recovery includes the provision of ongoing supportive measures designed to help patients promote and maintain self-esteem. See Appendix A, Patient Care Management Plan: Situational Low Self-Esteem.

Disturbed Personal Identity

Disturbed personal identity is the inability of a person to differentiate the self as a unique and separate human being from others within a social environment. The sense of depersonalization that accompanies identity disturbance results in high levels of anxiety. Personal identity disturbance can result from the effects of psychoactive medications; biochemical imbalances in the brain; and organic brain disorders, dementia, traumatic brain injury, amnesia, or delirium.

A careful nursing assessment, including the use of psychiatric or neurologic consultation, is essential in cases of identity disturbance. Disorientation and confusion—common in patients in critical care settings—are influenced by several factors, including the severity of the physical problem, chemical imbalances, sensory overload or deprivation, and previous illness or health care experiences. See Appendix A, Patient Care Management: Disturbed Personal Identity.

Compromised Dignity

A sense of human dignity is the foundation for self-concept. A sense of dignity includes a person's positive self-regard, an ability to invest in one's own life, and feeling valued by others.

During a critical health care stay, patients are subjected to intense physical, psychological, and lifestyle scrutiny.[5]

They are literally and figuratively exposed at a highly vulnerable moment. Patients in acute care settings must, by necessity, give up the things that give them a sense of self: clothing, daily habits, and privacy. Their bodies are frequently uncovered to people who assess them for pathology and irregularities.

Often patients cannot communicate their preferences or give permission for assessments, tests, or interventions. Family members and other support people have restricted access to patients and are unable to speak on the patient's behalf.

The critical care environment has its own culture that influences the behaviors of the health care providers. The cultural rules of critical care environments include objectification of the person for more precise physiologic management, disempowerment, distancing the self from the experience of others, and indifference.

The authority of the medical model can supersede patient experiences, interpretations, and meanings.[6] Although health care providers do not intend to humiliate patients, they become accustomed to the cultural attitudes and circumstances that diminish patients' dignity.

Enhancing Dignity

When people are treated with dignity and respect, they are put in the best position to recover their health and well-being. The practice of care that enhances a patient's dignity is anchored in authentic human presence, the giving of one's whole attention and being to another person in a given moment.

When authentically present, a nurse goes beyond scientific information and is attuned to a patient's needs, experiences, and emotions in a way that facilitates healing.[7]

SUPPORTING NURSE WELL-BEING

Spiritual Well-Being

The past month in the med ICU had been the most difficult since the Covid crisis at its peak: several deaths of younger people, unusually short staffing, and personal family emergencies. I had worked many extra shifts and was totally exhausted physically and mentally. I have my dream job in the ICU and love my co-workers and have an understanding and supporting supervisor. But I was questioning if I wanted to continue in this environment, or even if I wanted to stay in nursing. Fortunately, I had a one-week vacation scheduled and was encouraged by both my friends and supervisor to take the time. I drove up the coast by myself and had a lot of time to reflect and think about the future—what did I really want to do, what did I enjoy doing, what needed to change, how I could modify my life to fit into my future plans? During this time, I was able to really reconnect with me and how I wanted to proceed. The crowning touch was watching a spectacular sunset over the ocean—it solidified everything!

The above example demonstrates how one person had become spiritually disconnected with their spiritual self—values, goals, meaning, and purpose—in life. By taking time to focus and examine all aspects of their personal and professional life, peace and harmony was established. Spiritual wellness is the ability to develop congruency and consistency between beliefs and practices that gives one a sense of meaning and purpose. It may or may not center around specific religious traditions and needs to be tended so that one does not lose direction and focus to one's center and purpose. Consider the following actions to maintain spiritual wellness.

- Explore what you believe is your sense of meaning and purpose.
- Take time every day to "decompress," even if a few minutes, in the shower or bath, preparing meals, pruning flowers, folding clothes, meditation, prayer, etc.
- Create and practice affirmations consistently.
- Participate in activities to "give back" to the community, profession, family, friends.
- Create structured activities to mark life passages—yours, and family/friends.
- Connect/reconnect with *positive* persons who share your values and goals.
- Consider becoming an active advocate for causes/activities that speak to your inner and spiritual self.

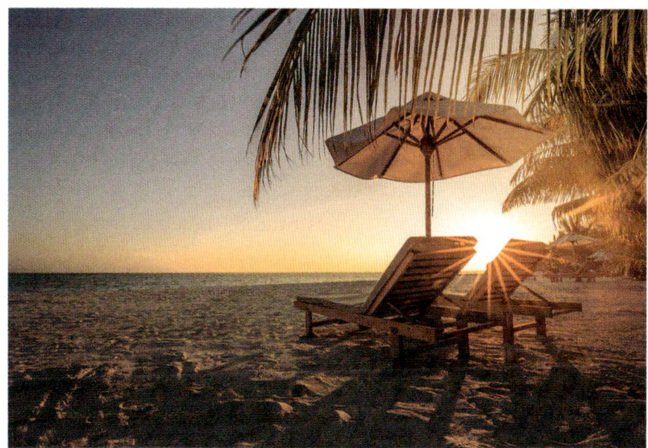

(Copyright © istock.com/daniciobota)

You're a spiritual person having a human experience. You're not a human being having a spiritual experience...

Deepak Chopra

Dignity-enhancing perspectives include recognition of a patient's need to maintain a continuity of the self, roles, and legacy. Dignity-enhancing care has four components: attitude, behaviors, compassion, and dialogue. A nurse's first step in providing dignity-conserving care involves reflecting on personal attitudes and assumptions about other people and their situations. Attitudes, worldviews, and beliefs about a patient or family member influence your openness and ability to develop a trusting relationship.

Dignity-enhancing care is manifest in behaviors. Attending to the patient's physical appearance affirms the person's self-esteem and a healthy body image. Cleanliness and absence of body odors give patients a sense of worth. When providing physical care, provide privacy, respect social boundaries, and ask permission before touching when possible. Validate the patient by respecting personal preferences.

Simply spending time with patients as they share their life stories helps the nurse know the patient better and facilitates the development of patient-centered interventions. Calling them by their preferred names or titles helps to reinforce the patient's self-concept and identity. Obtain the patient's permission to include others in private conversations.[8]

Supporting and maintaining dignity and privacy is a basic role of nurses. In the critical care setting, nurses practicing dignity-conserving care seek to identify sources of threats to dignity inherent in health care contexts, including the level of a person's independence and symptoms of distress.[5] Caregivers who are more aware of their own feelings and humanity are less likely to be aware of the patients' concerns and avoid unintentionally minimizing patients' emotions and experiences.[5,6]

Powerlessness

A person's control of the use of time, space, and resources is compromised in the critical care unit as basic issues such as the choice of clothing are restricted. Patients cannot decide who enters the room, who provides personal care, or who intrudes with painful treatments.

People who are critically ill are more likely to experience powerlessness due to their poor health, the structured care environment, a loss of interpersonal interactions with their usual support system, an inability to maintain cultural or religious practices, or a helpless coping style. The degree of powerlessness a person experiences depends on a perceived sense of control, the type of loss that was experienced, and the availability of social support.

Powerlessness can be manifested by a refusal to participate in decision making, disengagement from the plan of care, expressions of self-doubt, or a seeming lack of interest in recovery. Poor interactions with health care providers who are perceived as imposing restrictions can make the situation worse. Patients may react aggressively, may try bargaining, or may refuse to comply with diagnostic and treatment regimens. Patients may become apathetic regarding areas of life over which they still maintain some influence because so much control has been taken from them. See Appendix A, Patient Care Management Plan: Powerlessness.

Supporting Self-Control in Powerlessness in Critically Ill Patients

One of the most effective ways to decrease the stress of being in a critical care environment is giving patients as much control over their care and the environment as possible. Allow patients to make decisions as they are able, such as how and when to administer personal hygiene, diet preferences, and the timing of nursing interventions. Inform patients and family members about daily activities, tests, or therapies; their purpose; and anticipated effects.

Critical care patients are often unable to see or turn around to witness what is going on in their environments. During treatments and procedures, provide the patient with explanations, brief discussions on what to expect, the anticipated time of a procedure, and descriptions of what is happening during an intervention. On one hand, the patient for whom control is important should be helped to maintain control in as many areas in life as possible. On the other hand, a patient must be given the opportunity to not exercise control if having too many choices provokes even greater stress.

Spiritual Responses

Many of the psychosocial issues already discussed in this chapter are rooted in the spiritual dimension of life, an area with the deepest importance for many people. The spiritual dimension encompasses the elements of life that provide meaning, purpose, hope, and connectedness to others and a higher power.[9]

Spiritual Distress

Spiritual distress is a disruption in the life principle that defines a person and transcends the biologic and psychosocial nature.[10] Physical or psychiatric illness, prolonged pain, and suffering can challenge a person's spirituality. Separation from religious or spiritual practices and rituals, coupled with pain, may bring about spiritual distress for both patients and their families.

Patients experiencing spiritual distress may question the meaning of suffering and death in relation to their personal belief system. They may wonder why the illness or injury has happened to them or may believe that a higher power has failed them in the time of greatest need. Some people may question their existence, verbalize a wish to die, or express anger. Unresolved spiritual distress may lead to a sense of hopelessness and an unwillingness to consent to further treatment.[11]

Hopelessness

Hopelessness is a subjective state in which an individual sees extremely limited or no alternatives and is unable to mobilize energy. Feelings of hopelessness can greatly hinder recovery.[12] Conditions that increase a person's risk for feeling hopeless include a loss of dignity, long-term stress, loss of self-esteem, spiritual distress, and isolation, all of which can occur in a critical care experience. Patients who feel hopeless may be less involved in their recovery, withdraw from the support of others, and lack the energy and initiative to engage in increasing degrees of self-care.[13]

Engaging Spiritual Resources. Providing effective spiritual care is an essential aspect for patient recovery in critical care units. Spiritual support helps patients restore and maintain the integrity of their body, mind, and spirit.[10,14] Researchers report greater healing, inner peace, acceptance of reality, spiritual growth, and enhanced resiliency among other benefits of spiritual support.[10,11,14]

Hope is a spiritual process arising out of a sense of being meaningfully connected to oneself, others, and powers greater than the self.[13] With hope, a person is able to transition from a state of vulnerability to a point of being able to live as fully as possible.[10] The need for hope is stimulated by a demand to adapt or change in unexpected situations, as is the case for people who are critically ill.[12,13]

When people have hope and belief in their goals, they are empowered to engage in their own recovery. Although hope has a future orientation, it also affects people in the present. An element of hope must be maintained for survival[15] and is an essential component in the successful treatment of illness.[12,13]

A time of crisis can lead to a time of positive spiritual renewal and readiness for an enhanced spiritual life. Spiritual and religious beliefs and practices often give patients and family members some measure of acceptance of an illness, a sense of mastery and control, strength to endure the stressors of illness, and a source of hope and trust beyond what medical interventions can provide.

Transformative spiritual care strategies are particularly helpful in times of crisis and uncertainty. When faced with significant life challenges, people need resources to transcend their circumstances and know that no matter what happens, they will endure. Spiritual resources include faith in a higher power, support communities, a sense of hope and meaning in life, and religious practices.

The nurse plays a pivotal, potentially inspirational role to engender hope in patients through spiritual support. Nursing interventions that engender hope can be quite simple, quiet, and informal. Listening to patients' concerns, being present, enhancing dignity, and developing caring and trusting relationships with patients give hope. People hope for different things over the course of an illness. Listen for shifts in what patients hope for, explore their view of the situation, and help identify ways to meet their desired goals.[11]

Although distinctions between spiritual and religious concerns are important to recognize, many people find spiritual strength in their adherence to a particular religious tradition. They get inspiration to endure, hope, comfort, assurance, and confidence from the texts, rituals, and beliefs of their faith communities. Facilitate patient access to religious rituals, prayer, and scripture reading as hope-sustaining activities, and help patients make connections to their spiritual or cultural communities.

Collaborate with the hospital's spiritual care department when you sense that a person has unmet or unaddressed spiritual questions or needs. Often a professional spiritual care provider is the best person to assess spiritual needs and plan helpful interventions.

Spiritual and religious leaders can also provide valuable insights when discussing ethical decisions that may have implications for the person's values and beliefs. Religious, spiritual, or philosophic practices can also directly inform diet, hygiene practices, and rituals surrounding birth, death, and medical interventions. See Appendix A, Patient Care Management: Impaired Spiritual Status.

PROVIDING SUPPORT

Providing Holistic Care

Critical care nurses possess sophisticated knowledge of anatomy and physiology, the pathophysiology of disease processes, and appropriate nursing interventions. In addition, nurses who practice holistic critical care also need the knowledge, wisdom, and skills to interpret the internal human responses to experiences of serious illness or injury.

Attention to the whole patient is the goal of nursing care and is vitally important for critical care patients, families, and nurses. Nightingale[16] believed that it was "unthinkable to consider sick humans as mere bodies who could be treated in isolation from their minds and spirits." Essential skills that underlie nursing interventions for psychosocial care include using communication patterns based on compassion and care, practicing dignity-enhancing care, supporting patient coping, using a family-centered focus, and engaging spiritual resources.

Psychosocial Support

Although physical care is essential to preserving life, psychosocial interventions are not only life affirming but are also life sustaining. Feeling alone, marginalized, and powerless may result in losing the will to live and cause increased physical compromise and decline.

Fortunately, despite the fast-paced environment of critical care settings, the relatively small nurse-to-patient ratio may provide the time necessary for emotional and spiritual support. This type of support can even be provided while providing physical care. The following paragraphs summarize essential psychosocial interventions.

Caring Communication

Caring and compassionate verbal and nonverbal communication is essential in the critical care environment. Challenges to caring communication for seriously ill patients are listed in Box 5.3. None of the most common challenges are related to technical issues of medical management. Instead, the top challenges are focused on communication. Patients and family members rank their needs for communication with health care providers as one of the most important aspects of feeling cared for in the critical care setting, especially regarding patients who are unable to speak.[17–19]

Interviews with patients after critical care revealed that they believed that a nurse's caring attitude led to more positive memories of their experience. Patients also reported less stress when they perceived nurses to be caring, warm, and competent, and when nurses demonstrated respect.[20]

BOX 5.3 Patient-Centered Care

Challenges for Caring Communication

- Inadequate communication between the critical care team and family members
- Insufficient staff knowledge of effective communication
- Unrealistic family and provider expectations
- Family disagreements
- Lack of advance directives
- Voiceless patients
- Suboptimal space for having meaningful conversations.

Patients interpret a nurse's expression of empathy and physical contact as evidence of caring and support.[21]

Sharing concerns with a caring and understanding listener can relieve emotional or spiritual distress. Patients are consoled knowing that they are not alone when they sense that someone knows and cares about their feelings and experiences. Although patients may share concerns with family members, they may be reluctant to burden them and may find that talking to a nurse feels emotionally safer.

A patient who copes by talking to others will benefit from a nurse who recognizes when the patient needs to talk and who knows how to listen.[19,21]

Strong critical care nurses initiate and engage in difficult conversations. Most patients need to talk about their fears and prefer conversations that balance their need for honesty with their need to maintain hope.[19] Yet, it is important to note that cultural differences affect the role of directness in communicating with patients and family members. People in Western and American cultures expect and value honesty and truth telling in difficult situations. Patients and family members from other cultures may have taboos surrounding what should be discussed regarding the diagnosis and prognosis in serious illness.[21]

Careful medical and nursing assessments, use of family and team conferences, and enlisting the assistance of a spiritual counselor lead to more effective crisis and decision-making conversations. Box 5.4 contains strategies for communicating with patients and family members in critical care settings. See also Appendix A, Patient Care Management Plan: Impaired Verbal Communication.

Promoting Trust

Effective verbal and nonverbal communication is essential for the development of trust in a nurse-patient relationship. Trust manifests itself in the belief of critical care patients that the people they depend on will get them through the illness and will be able to manage complications. A patient needs to trust the nurse's competence in the physical and technical aspects of care and rely on what the nurse says.

Patients are profound observers of their caregivers and read them well. Trust and hope are decreased when inaccurate information is given or nurses do not follow through on what they say.

Communicating With Compassion

Compassion refers to the awareness of another person's suffering coupled with a sincere intention to alleviate emotional and

BOX 5.4 Patient-Centered Care

Strategies for Communicating With Patients and Family Members

- Be patient. What is routine for caregivers can be stressful and new to patients and family members.
- Repeat information as many times as necessary. Stress reduces concentration, memory, and comprehension, especially in unfamiliar situations.
- Assess patient and family knowledge level and prior experience with critical care.
- Use understandable language and define medical terms without talking down.
- Ask clarifying questions to help validate understanding.
- Use a welcoming, open communication style. Critical care units can feel intimidating to people unfamiliar with the environment.
- Offer frequent updates regarding the patient's condition, even if not asked.
- Engage in conversations of meaning with patients and family members, even if brief. Often critical care conversations are reduced to conveying only technical aspects of care.
- Honor privacy and provide space for family conferences.
- Speak to patients, even if they are unconscious. This conveys caring to family, and words may comfort the patient even if there is no response.
- Use communication boards or other devices with patients who are unable to speak.
- Give patients time to respond and ask questions they can answer easily.
- Speak slowly and look at patients when communicating. Gestures, lip movements, and facial expressions convey important messages.

physical distress. In compassion, caregivers are able to identify with another person and recognize a shared humanity. Showing compassion can be simple, in acts of consideration, kindness, or a simple touch.

Critical care nurses frequently touch people in the completion of procedures and caregiving activities. Keeping in mind individual and cultural differences, nurses include nonprocedural touch in their care. The use of touch intended to communicate care and comfort can be an important part of patient healing and interpersonal connection.

At the most basic level, patients and family members need timely updates, explanations, repetition of unfamiliar information, and thorough information sharing.[22] At a deeper level, patients need to feel that they are heard by their caregivers and know that their personhood is valued and respected.[23–25]

Complementary and Alternative Therapies

Integrative health care practices involve a blending of allopathic medical health care methods with patient-identified complementary therapies.[26] The type of complementary or integrative therapies used depends on a patient's preferences, coping style, physical capabilities, and personality type.

Music therapy, relaxation, guided imagery, therapeutic massage, visualization, prayer, biofeedback, and mindfulness meditation are potentially useful for critically ill patients. Significant decreases in anxiety and symptom distress have been attributed to the simple act of touch. Although more research is needed to support the value of complementary therapies on selected outcomes in critically ill hospitalized patients, early studies support their potential as therapeutic nursing interventions (also see Chapter 1).

Environmental Support

People are continuous with their environments. Alterations in the physical environment of critical care units can provide a sense of calm, enhance patient coping, and facilitate healing.[26] Nurses can make changes in care environments to give patients a greater sense of comfort and familiarity while they are in the unit.

Critical care areas are bright, loud, and busy. Close patient doors, turn off unnecessary equipment, and limit conversation at workstations. Music can promote relaxation in critical care areas when used during waking hours and with patient consent. Allow for natural sunlight if possible, and position patients so that they can see out of windows, which helps maintain orientation to time.

Familiarize patient rooms by displaying photographs, cards, drawings, and favored items. Sleep deprivation is a serious concern in critical care environments. Plan care activities to limit nighttime interruptions and collaborate with laboratory and other staff to decrease sleep interruptions.[26] The use of earplugs during sleeping hours has been shown to improve patients' subjective experience of sleep.[27]

FAMILY-CENTERED CARE

Family-centered care, an AACN practice standard for critical care, formalizes the patient and family as the unit of care. Family-centered care is based on the belief that patients and families should participate in decisions together and that patients need their families for love, understanding, and support while coping with critical illness.[29]

The nurse's observable support of family members at the bedside gives the patient comfort. The patient determines who counts as family. Biologic or legal issues notwithstanding, it is the nature of the patient's relationships that determines the extent of interaction with others.

The elements essential to family-centered care include respect, collaboration, and support.

Research demonstrates that family members of critical care patients want understandable information that is given in a timely manner. They want reassurance that their loved one is being monitored and is receiving the best care possible. Family members also need to be allowed access to their loved ones.[28,30] Some family members are reassured by helping with caregiving if this is acceptable to the patient.

Family members are particularly sensitive to a nurse's words and actions, making it essential that the nurse convey understanding and acceptance. The critical care nurse can observe the quality of the patient-family interaction and formulate interventions that will aid the family in supporting the patient.[30] The critical care nurse provides interventions aimed at supporting family members throughout the patient's stay in the unit.

Visitation Policies

Although practices vary among critical care units, a more relaxed visitation policy humanizes the environment and facilitates healing. The AACN recommends unrestricted visiting for hospitalized patients. Giving family members access to their loved ones enhances patient and family satisfaction and improves safety of care.

Family members have insight into the patient's behaviors and preferences, especially with patients who are unable to communicate. Interacting with family members reduces patient anxiety and enhances a sense of control.[31,32] Including patients and family members in critical care interdisciplinary rounds has been shown to improve perceptions of accessibility and communication.[32]

Recent research[33,34] indicates that although some hospitals have open visitation policies, these are often applied in a case-by-case basis. Nurses report concerns about interference with care delivery, sanitation, patient fatigue, and security as reasons to restrict visiting. Tailoring visitation to best care for the patient and availability of the visitors in recommended.[34]

COMORBID PSYCHIATRIC DISORDERS

The incidence of psychiatric conditions following a critical care unit stay ranges from 1% to 62%.[35] These psychiatric conditions include posttraumatic stress disorder, major depressive disorder, and anxiety disorders.[36] In addition, these conditions often co-occur. When symptoms disorder are present, there is a 65% chance that one of the other two disorders will co-occur.

SOCIAL DETERMINANTS OF HEALTH

Hospitalized Patients With Underlying Mental Health Issues

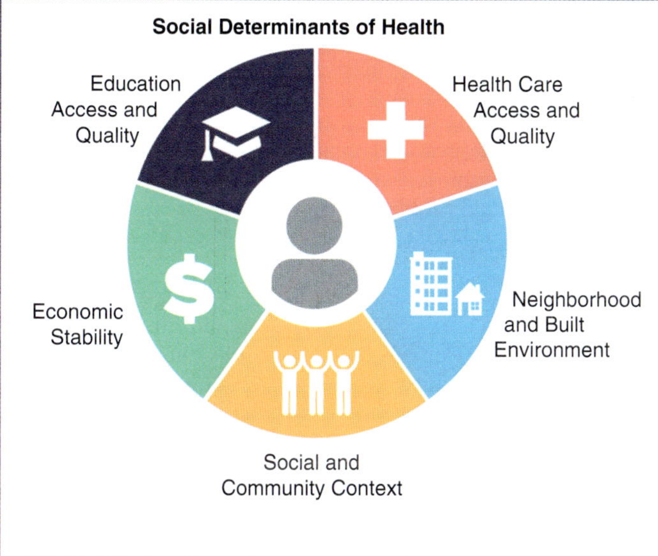

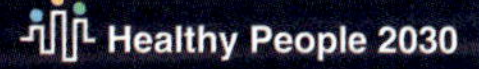

According to the Centers for Disease Control (CDC), mental health includes our emotional, psychological, and social well-being, and it affects how we think, feel, and act. It also helps determine how we handle stress, relate to others, and make health choices. Thus, it really impacts every aspect of our life throughout all of our life stages. More than 50% of persons will be diagnosed with a mental illness or disorder at some point in their lifetime, and 1 in 25 Americans lives with a serious mental illness such as schizophrenia, bipolar disorder, or major depression.[1]

According to researchers, there is an association between serious mental illness (SMI) and worse general health.[2] Persons with SMI have more comorbidities than those without mental health issues, experience a higher mortality rate, and have a lower life expectancy rate. About half of those persons have medical comorbid conditions, and as many as 35% have undiagnosed medical comorbid conditions. Thus, a very few do not have conditions in addition to their SMI. The leading comorbidities are urinary, digestive, neoplastic, pulmonary, and circulatory.[1]

The Healthcare Cost and Utilization Project (HCUP) reported nearly 7.7 million (21.7%) of inpatient patients stays consisted of mental and substance abuse secondary diagnoses in 2016.[1] Inpatient stays comprising these diagnoses were more likely to be through the emergency department and costs and lengths of stay were greater than those without these diagnoses.[1]

Several factors must be considered when caring for critically ill patients with underlying mental health issues[2]:

- Gather detailed history of medical background.
- Document patient's mental health provider(s) and supports.
- Seek additional or clarifying information from the family/significant others.
- Conduct thorough admission assessment regarding mental health issues, diagnosis(es), medications, treatment regimes.
- Document patient's mental health provider(s) and other medical supports.
- Seek additional information or clarifying information from the family/significant others.
- Complete admission assessment regarding mental health issues, diagnosis(es), medications, treatment regimes.

References

1. Agency for Healthcare Research and Quality. https://hcup-us.ahrq.gov>reports>statbriefs.
2. Riley K, Evans MM, Worozbyt K, Kowalchik K. Caring for opiod addicted patient in a medical-surgical setting: best practice recommendations. *MedSurg Nurs.* 2019;28(2):4–7.

Illustration from Healthy People 2030, U.S. Department of Health and Human Services, Office of Disease Prevention and Health Promotion. Retrieved September 8, 2022, from https://health.gov/healthypeople/objectives-and-data/social-determinants-health.

The risk factors for the development of psychiatric conditions include previous psychiatric conditions, lower education level, being female, preexisting psychiatric conditions, and the use of analgesia and sedation. Common comorbid conditions include alcohol withdrawal, major depressive disorder, posttraumatic stress disorder (PTSD), and post–intensive care syndrome (PICS).

Major Depressive Disorder

An estimated 20% to 40% of people discharged from the critical care unit will suffer from major depression.[37] Symptoms of a depressive disorder must last 2 weeks for a diagnosis to be made. Diagnostic criteria for major depressive disorder include are found in Box 5.5.

Certain attributes make a person at greater risk for this disorder.[38] Perceived helplessness, or lack of control over the situation, is a significant predictor. Recalling, thinking, and obsessing about traumatic experiences in the critical care unit can also set the stage for depression.

Major depressive disorder carries deadly consequences. People with depressive symptoms are 47% more likely to die during the first 2 years after discharge from critical care settings than those without.[38] Increased risk of death has not been found in post–critical care unit sufferers of posttraumatic stress disorder or anxiety.

Posttraumatic Stress Disorder

Experiencing one or more traumatic events may trigger symptoms of PTSD. Nearly 25% of people surviving a critical illness and an intensive care unit stay subsequently exhibit symptoms of PTSD.[39] Posttraumatic stress reactions involve a wide range of responses that are listed in Box 5.6. Significant others are also at risk for developing posttraumatic stress reactions. Prolonged periods of uncertainty, anxious waiting, disrupted sleep patterns, financial concerns, witnessing emergency interventions, and confronting fears of loss and death are profoundly unsettling. Although posttraumatic reactions may not be evident for weeks to months after an event, critical care nurses should be aware of the potential for complications of critical care unit stays.[40]

The COVID-19 pandemic has brought increased awareness of PTSD after critical treatment.[41] Care providers can take steps to manage or eliminate as many stressors as possible and encourage realistic discussions of the patient's experiences by explaining events carefully. Talking openly about recovery timelines and the gradual process of regaining strength, or about the process of terminal illness and final choices, will help reduce the fear of the unknown.

The process of identifying PTSD risk and symptoms is complex and multidimensional. The American Psychiatric Association's online assessment measures (see Box 5.6) provides tools for PTSD screening for both children and adults.

BOX 5.5 Symptoms of Major Depressive Disorder

- A depressed mood most of the time
- Lack of interest in usual activities
- Significant weight loss or weight gain
- Insomnia or hypersomnia
- Psychomotor agitation or retardation
- Fatigue or loss of energy
- Feelings of guilt and worthlessness
- Difficulty thinking, concentrating, or making decisions
- Suicidal ideation

BOX 5.6 Elements of Assessment for PTSD

- Flashbacks, feeling as if a stressful experience from the past is happening all over again
- Feeling very emotionally upset when something reminded you of a stressful experience
- Trying to avoid thoughts, feelings, or physical sensations that reminded you of a stressful experience
- Thinking that a stressful event happened because you or someone else (who didn't directly harm you) did something wrong or didn't do everything possible to prevent it, or because of something about you
- Having a very negative emotional state (for example, you were experiencing lots of fear, anger, guilt, shame, or horror) after a stressful experience
- Losing interest in activities you used to enjoy before having a stressful experience
- Being "super alert," on guard, or constantly on the lookout for danger
- Feeling jumpy or easily startled when you hear an unexpected noise

Post–Intensive Care Syndrome

Advances in critical care treatment have saved countless lives. However, survival is often followed by profound physical, cognitive, and mental health impairment known as PICS.

Sixty-four percent of ICU survivors experience at least one symptom of PICS, and 56% have persistent symptoms 12 months later.[42] A third of survivors will not return to their previous employment.[43] These impairments are the result of the length and severity of the physical illness or injury, the necessary treatments, and the resources and resiliency of the patient. Significant others may also experience cognitive impairment and psychologic distress after the discharge or death of a loved one in critical care.[44]

Symptoms include physical impairments such as weight loss, muscle weakness, neurological dysfunction, and fatigue. Cognitive impairments include global cognitive decline, impaired executive function, and ICU delirium. Mental health impairments include depression, anxiety, and delusion. Diagnosis is accomplished by initial screening that leads to specific evaluations for identified problem areas.[45]

Prevention and Management of PICS

Two of the most important factors in preventing PICS are minimizing sedation and facilitating early mobilization during critical care stays.[43] Evaluation for signs and symptoms of PICS is an important role of critical care nurses. Even in the most critical patients, initiating rehabilitation services as early as 24 to 48 hours after admission is known to optimize outcomes. See Box 5.7.

Refer to Box 5.8 for internet resources related to psychosocial and spiritual resources.

BOX 5.7 Interventions to Mitigate PICS[49,50]

- Bedside report: Allows family members and patients to listen to change-of-shift reports, ask questions, and make suggestions for care.
- Five minutes at the bedside: At the beginning of the shift, nurses sit for 5 minutes to listen to patients and families, provide emotional support and information, and set goals.
- Communication boards: Boards in patients' rooms can convey goals and identify tests or procedures for the day.
- Hourly rounding: When nurses make rounds on patients and families every hour, they can offer updates and respond to questions.
- Narrating care: While delivering patient care, nurses can explain and talk about what they are doing.
- Informal and formal education: Empowers patients and family members and increases coping strategies. Written content is helpful to reinforce learning.
- Patient and family diaries: Diaries document the patient's condition, treatments, and education. Diaries reinforce real memories rather than imagined ones.
- Family participation in care: Patients want to hear about life outside the critical care unit. Family members can share this information while helping with hygiene, range-of-motion exercises, and feedings. This participation will be helpful as the patient makes the transition to home care.

Note: Holistic ICU aftercare programs to address the chronic problems of PICS are being developed but are not yet available as a standard of care.

BOX 5.8 Internet Resources

Psychosocial and Spiritual Considerations

The experiences and needs of families of comatose patients after cardiac arrest and severe neurotrauma.

https://journals.lww.com/ccejournal/Fulltext/2022/03000/The_Experiences_and_Needs_of_Families_of_Comatose.10.aspx

Critical Care Nurses' Experiences with Spiritual Care: The SPIRIT Study: https://aacnjournals.org/ajcconline/article-abstract/27/3/212/4199/Critical-Care-NursesExperiences-With-Spiritual?redirectedFrom=fulltext

Improving the patient experience by focusing on spiritual care: http://acphospitalist.org/archives/2016/06/spiritual-care.htm

Intensive Care: A Guide for Patients and Families:

Patient Communicator App: https://www.sccm.org/MyICUCare/THRIVE/Patient-and-Family-Resources/Patient-and-Family

Pediatric Post Intensive Care Syndrome and the Family: https://www.sccm.org/MyICUCare/Resources/Intensive-Care-A-Guide-for-Patients-and-Relatives

Post Intensive Care Support Group: https://www.facebook.com/groups/227842144513131/

Spiritual Support: https://intermountainhealthcare.org/services/hospice-palliative-care/services/spiritual-support/

Ten Relaxation Techniques That Zap Stress Fast: https://www.webmd.com/balance/guide/blissing-out-10-relaxation-techniques-reduce-stress-spot#1

CASE STUDY 5.1 Patient With Psychosocial Needs

Brief Patient History

Sophia is a 17-year-old woman who took an acetaminophen (Tylenol) overdose after her boyfriend broke up with her. She states that she did not want to kill herself but just wanted to scare her boyfriend. She was unaware of the serious threat that acetaminophen posed to the liver. Sophia is embarrassed by the need for a psychiatric evaluation and is terrified by the potential for severe liver damage and even death.

Focused Clinical Assessment

Sophia is admitted to the critical care unit from the emergency department in stable condition. She is awake, alert, and oriented to person, time, place, and situation. She is irritable, withdrawn, and wants to be left alone. Her parents stay at her bedside. They share with the nurse their intense feelings of fear, confusion, and uncertainty concerning their daughter's serious psychiatric and physical condition.

Diagnostic Procedures

A psychiatric evaluation was completed, with the recommendation that Sophia receive inpatient psychiatric care when medically stable.

Medical Diagnosis

Sophia is diagnosed with acetaminophen toxicity and risk for hepatic failure along with suicidal behavior disorder.

Questions

1. What major outcomes do you expect to achieve for this patient?
2. What problems or risks must be managed to achieve these outcomes?
3. What interventions must be initiated to monitor, prevent, manage, or eliminate the problems and risks identified?
4. What interventions should be initiated to promote optimal functioning, safety, and well-being of the patient?
5. What possible learning needs do you anticipate for this patient?
6. What cultural and age-related factors may have a bearing on the patient's plan of care?
7. What technology can be used to monitor the patient and prevent complications?
8. What other interprofessional team members are needed to assist with the management of this patient?

KEY POINTS

- Because of the multifaceted effect of illness and injury on a human being, a holistic approach is essential to foster an optimal recovery.
- Coping mechanisms are useful in dealing with stressors.
- Two common coping mechanisms that are often used to excess in critical care environments are regression (reverting to a less independent state) and denial (pathologic avoidance of a real problem).
- Anxiety can be observed behaviorally, elicited verbally, and measured with standardized assessment tools.
- Critical care environments may result in the self-concept disturbances of disturbed body image, low self-esteem, and personal identity disturbances.
- Compromised dignity, powerlessness, spiritual distress, and hopelessness are issues common to critical care settings.
- Although physiologic care is essential to life, psychosocial interventions are also life-sustaining by providing and supporting security, trust, dignity, compassion, coping, self-control, and spirituality.
- Environmental support by critical care nurses is aimed at reducing noise and bright lights and limiting nighttime disruptions.
- The use of natural light, soothing music, and familiar items such as photographs may increase the patient's orientation and feeling off.
- Comorbid psychiatric disorders may result in critical care stays. Addressing these disorders and their potential side effects is part of critical care nursing.
- Up to 62% of critical care survivors experience posttraumatic stress disorder (PTSD), major depressive disorder, and anxiety disorders.
- Post–intensive care syndrome (PICS) is identified as profound physical, cognitive, and mental health impairment that occurs after leaving intensive care.
- PICS can be mitigated by a number of interventions while in intensive care and requires complex follow-up care. Family members may also be affected.

REFERENCES

1. Halter M, ed. *Varcarolis' Foundations of Psychiatric Mental Health Nursing: A Clinical Approach.* 9th ed. St. Louis: Elsevier; 2022.
2. Perpina-Galvan J, Richart-Martinez M. Scales for evaluating self perceived anxiety levels in patients admitted to intensive care units: a review. *Am J Crit Care.* 2009;18(6):571.
3. Jaber S, et al. A prospective study of agitation in a medicalsurgical ICU: incidence, risk factors, and outcomes. *Chest.* 2005;128(4):2749.
4. Fredriksen S, Ringsberg K. Living the situation stress-experiences among intensive care patients. *Intensive Crit Care Nurs.* 2007;23:124.
5. Husum T, Legernes E, Pederden R. "A plea for recognition": Users experience of humiliation during health care. *Intl J Law and Psychiatry.* 2018;62:148–153. https://doi.org/10.1016/j.ijlp.2018.11.004.
6. Malterud K, Hollnagel H. Avoiding humiliations in the clinical encounter. *Scand J Prim Health Care.* 2007;25:69. https://doi.org/10.1080/02813430701237721.
7. Newman M. *Transforming Presence: The Difference That Nursing Makes.* Philadelphia, PA: FA Davis; 2008.
8. Tilsley A, et al. Identifying intensive care staff cultural, spiritual, and ethical beliefs to successfully implement a dying pathway: a two stage mixed methods sequential design. *Aust Crit Care.* 2015;28(1):38.
9. Timmins F, Kelly J. Spiritual assessment in intensive and cardiac care nursing. *Nurs Crit Care.* 2008;13(3). 124–13.

10. Burkhart L, Hogan N. An experiential theory of spiritual care in nursing practice. *Qual Hlth Res.* 2008;18(7):928–938. https://doi.org/10.1177/1049732308318027.
11. Caldeira T. Understanding spirituality and spiritual care in nursing. *Nsg Stnd.* 2015;31(10):50–57. Doi: 107748/ns.2017.e10311.
12. Baalen C, Grypdonck M, Van Hecke A, Verhaeghe S. Hope dies last: a qualitative study into the meaning of hope for people with cancer in palliative care. *Eur J of Cancer Care.* 2016;25:570–579. https://doi.org/10.1111/ecc.12500.
13. Hammer K, Mogensen O, Hall E. The meaning of hope in nursing research: a meta-analysis. *Scand J Caring Sci.* 2009;23:549–557. https://doi.org/10.1111/j.1471-6712.2008.00635.x.
14. Ramezani M, Ahmadi F, Mohammadi E, Kazemnejad A. Spiritual care in nursing: a concept analysis. *Intnl Nsg Review.* 2014;61:211–219.
15. Haraldsson L, Lennart C, Conlon L, Henricson M. The experience of ICU patients during follow up sessions: a qualitative study. *Intensive Crit Care Nurs.* 2012;40(7):2033.
16. Nightingale F. *Notes on Nursing: What It Is and What It Is Not.* New York, NY: D. Appleton and Company; 1860.
17. Happ M, et al. Nurse-patient communication interactions in the intensive care unit. *Am J Crit Care Nurs.* 2011;20(2):e28.
18. Stajduha K, et al. Patient perceptions of helpful communication in the context of advanced cancer. *J Clin Nurs.* 2010;19:2039.
19. Lowey S. Communication between the nurse and family caregiver in end-of-life care: a review of the literature. *J Hosp Pall Nursing.* 2008;10(1):35.
20. Grossbach I. Promoting effective communication for patients receiving mechanical ventilation. *Crit Care Nurs.* 2011;31(3):46.
21. Scheunermann L, et al. How clinicians discuss critically ill patients' preferences and values with surrogates: an empirical analysis. *Crit Care Med.* 2015;43(4):757–764.
22. Pecanac K, King B. Nurse-family communication during and after family meetings in the intensive care unit. *J Nsg Scholar.* 2019;51(2):129–137. https://doi.org/10.1111/jnu.12459.
23. Garg S. Patients family satisfaction in intensive care unit: a leap forward. *Indian J Crit Care Med.* 2022;26(2):161–164.
24. Gutierrez K. Experiences and needs of families regarding prognostic communication in a intensive care unit: supporting families at the end of life. *Crit Care Nsg Q.* 2012;35(3):299–313. https://doi.org/10.1097/CNQobo13e31825ee0d.
25. Schubart J, Wojnat M, Dillard J, et al. ICU family communication and health care professionals: a qualitative analysis of perspectives. *Intensive and CritCare Nsg.* 2015;31:315–321. https://doi.org/10.1016/j/iccn.2015/02.003.
26. Bazuin D, Cardon K. Creating healing intensive care unit environments: physical and psychological considerations in designing critical care areas. *Crit Care Nurs.* 2011;24(4):259.
27. Scotto C, et al. Earplugs improve patients' subjective experience of sleep in critical care. *Crit Care Nurs.* 2009;14(4):180–184.
28. Nolan K, Waren N. Meeting the needs of family members of ICU patients. *Crit Care Nurs Q.* 2014;37(4):393–406.
29. Davidson E, Aslakson A, Long C, et al. Guidelines for family-centered care in the neonatal, pediatric, and adult ICU. *Crit Care Med.* 2017;45(1):103–128.
30. Institute for Patient-and Family-Centered Care. *What Is PFCC? Patient-and Family-Centered Care.* 2018. http://www.ipfcc.org/about/pfcc.html. Accessed June 1, 2023.
31. Hart A, Hardin S, Townsend A, Mahrle-Henson A. Critical care visitation. *Dim Nsg Res.* 2013;32(6):289–299. https://doi.org/10.1097/01.DCC.0000434515.58265.7d.
32. Jacobowski N, et al. Communication in critical care: family rounds in the intensive care unit. *Am J Crit Care.* 2010;19(5):421.
33. Fike G, Smith-Stoner M, Blue D, Alhan A. Current trends and practices of intensive care unit visitation. *J Doc Nsg Prac.* 2018;11(2):168–174. https://doi.org/10.1891/2380-9418.11.2.169.
34. Milner K, Goncalves S, Marmo S. Is open visitation really open in adult intensive care units in the United States? *Amer J Crit Care.* 2020;29(3):221–225. https://doi.org/10.4037/ajcc2020331.
35. Rawal G, Yadav S, Kumar R. Post-intensive care syndrome: an overview. *J Transl Int Med.* 2017;5(2):90–92.
36. Hatch R, et al. Anxiety, depression, and post-traumatic stress disorder after critical illness: a UK-wide prospective cohort study. *Critical Care.* 2018;22:310. https://doi.org/10.1186/s13054-018-2223-6.
37. Wintermann G, et al. Predictors of major depressive disorder following intensive care of chronically critically ill patients. *Crit Care Res Prac.* 2018. https://doi.org/10.1155/2018/1586736.
38. Rabiee A, Nikayin S, Hashem M, et al. Depressive symptoms after critical illness: a systematic review and meta-analysis. *Crit Care Med.* 2016;44:1744–1753.
39. Battle E, James K, Bromfield T, Temblett P. Predictors of posttraumatic stress disorder following critical illness: a mixed methods study. *J of Intensive Care Soc.* 2017;18(4):289–293. https://doi.org/10.1177/1751143717713853. 2017.
40. Warlan H, Howland L. Posttraumatic stress syndrome associated with stays in the intensive care unit: importance of nurses' involvement. *Crit Care Ns.* 2015;30(3):44–53.46.
41. Miori S, Sanna A, Lassola S, et al. Incidence, risk factors, and consequences of post-traumatic stress disorder symptoms in survivors of COVID-19-ralted ARDS. *Int J Envirn Res Public Health.* 2023;2:5504. https://doi.org/10.3390/ijerph20085504.
42. Hiser S, Fatima A, Ali M, Needham D. Post-intensive care syndrome (PICS): recent updates. *J Intensive Care.* 2023;11(23). https://doi.org/10.1186/s40560-023-00670-7.
43. Lee M, Jiyeon K, Jeong Y. Risk factors for post-intensive care syndrome: a systematic review and meta-analysis. *Aust Crit Care.* 2019;33:287–294. https://doi.org/10.1016/jaucc201910.004.
44. Dunn H, Balas M, Hetland B. Krupp. Post-intensive care syndrome: a review for the primary care NP. *The Ns Practioner.* 2022;47(11):15–22.
45. Twibell K, Petty A, Olynger A, Abebe S. Families and post-intensive care syndrome. *American Nurse Today.* 2018;13(4). https://www.americannursetoday.com/familiespost-intensive-care-syndrome/.

6

Nutrition Alterations and Management

Janine Wong Berta and Kimberly Sanchez

http://evolve.elsevier.com/Urden/CriticalCareNursing

Nutrition support is an essential component of providing comprehensive care to critically ill patients. Malnutrition can be related to any essential nutrient or nutrients. A serious type of malnutrition found frequently among hospitalized patients is protein-calorie malnutrition (PCM). Malnutrition is associated with a variety of adverse outcomes, including wound dehiscence, infections, pressure injuries, respiratory failure requiring ventilation, longer hospital stays, and death. A nutrition screening must be conducted on every patient, and a more thorough nutrition assessment is completed by a registered dietitian nutritionist (RD or RDN) or by a nutrition care specialist (e.g., nurse or provider with specialized expertise in nutrition) on any patient screened to be nutritionally at risk. This chapter provides an overview of nutrient metabolism, nutrition status assessment, malnutrition, nutrition support, and refeeding syndrome. Additionally, nutrition for each of the system alterations is discussed along with nursing management.

NUTRIENT METABOLISM

Nutrients are chemical substances found in foods that are needed for human life, growth, maintenance, and repair of body tissues. The main nutrients in foods are carbohydrates, proteins, fats, vitamins, minerals, and water. The process by which nutrients are used at the cellular level is known as *metabolism*. The energy-yielding nutrients or macronutrients are carbohydrates, proteins, and fats. For proper metabolic functioning, adequate amounts of micronutrients, such as vitamins, minerals (including electrolytes), and trace elements, also must be supplied to the human body. The functions, digestion, and metabolism of energy-yielding nutrients are described in Table 6.1.

FOCUSED ASSESSMENT OF NUTRITION STATUS

It is common practice to perform a nutrition screening on every patient within 24 hours of admission to an acute care hospital and it is recommended practice that this screening occur at least within 48 hours of admission.[1] A patient questionnaire, nursing admission form, or the provider's admission note usually provides enough screening information to determine whether the patient is at nutrition risk (Box 6.1). Patients nutritionally at risk need a thorough nutrition assessment by a dietician, who will perform a continuous cycle of assessment, diagnosis, intervention, and monitoring though reassessments in order to facilitate the nutrition care plan.[2]

A focused nutrition assessment involves collection of four types of information: (1) diet and pertinent health history; (2) clinical signs and physical manifestations; (3) anthropometric measurements; and (4) laboratory studies. This information provides a basis for (1) identifying patients who are malnourished or at risk of malnutrition (Box 6.1); (2) determining the nutrition needs of individual patients; and (3) selecting the most appropriate methods of nutrition support for patients with or at risk of developing nutrition deficits.

Assessment information must be evaluated in the context of the patient's overall clinical situation. Nutrition status and intervention efficacy are better evaluated if assessment information is collected serially and trended over time rather than obtaining this information in only one assessment. Whenever possible, data should be measured in place of patient self-report or family provided information. In addition, an interprofessional team approach to nutrition assessment is key to ensuring the best quality of care from screening for nutrition risk to providing and evaluating nutrition interventions. Effective team communication ensures that at-risk patients receive timely nutrition support and interventions that will improve clinical outcomes.

Diet and Pertinent Health History

Information about dietary intake and significant variations in weight is a vital part of the nutrition history. Dietary intake can be evaluated in several ways, including a 24-hour diet recall, a diet record, or a diet history. The 24-hour diet recall of all food and beverage intake is easily and quickly performed, but it may not reflect the patient's usual intake and has limited usefulness. The diet record, a listing of the type and amount of all foods and beverages consumed for some period (usually 3 days), is useful for evaluating the adequacy of the patient's intake. However, such a record reveals little about the patient's habitual intake before the illness or injury. The diet history consists of a detailed interview about the patient's usual intake, along with social, familial, cultural, economic, educational, and health-related factors that may affect intake. While all of these assessment methods are useful for general nutrition assessment, in the critical care setting, habitual intake and behaviors matter less as many patients are artificially fed. The most pertinent nutritional history to obtain is focused on recent intake and weight changes to determine how nutritionally depleted a patient is on presentation, to assess for malnutrition and refeeding risk. Food allergies and intolerances are also important pieces of information to obtain to ensure that artificial nutrition will not provoke a reaction. Other information to include in a nutrition history is listed in Box 6.2.

TABLE 6.1 Energy-Yielding Nutrients

Nutrient	Energy	Primary Function	Molecular Digestion	Metabolic Reactions	Storage
Carbohydrate (CHO)	4 kcal/g	Glucose provides the energy needed to maintain cellular functions, including transport across cell membranes, secretion of specific hormones, muscle contraction, and synthesis of new substances. Most of the energy produced from carbohydrate metabolism is used to form adenosine triphosphate, the principal form of immediately available energy within all body cells.	CHO are broken down into glucose, fructose, and galactose within the digestive tract and absorbed. Fructose and galactose are then converted into glucose for metabolism.	*Glycolysis* is the process of breaking down glucose to produce adenosine triphosphate. *Gluconeogenesis* is the process of manufacturing glucose from nonglucose precursors. This process is carried out primarily in the liver and, to a lesser extent, the kidneys.	Glucose is stored as glycogen, primarily in the liver and muscle cells.
Protein	4 kcal/g	Proteins provide the structural basis of all lean body mass, such as the vital organs and skeletal muscle. Proteins are important for visceral (cellular) functions, such as initiation of chemical reactions (e.g., hormones, enzymes), transportation of other substances (e.g., apoproteins, albumin), preservation of immune function (e.g., antibodies), and maintenance of osmotic pressure (e.g., albumin) and blood neutrality (e.g., buffers). Some amino acids are used as energy.	Proteins, which consist of chains of hundreds or thousands of amino acids, are broken down into amino acids and *dipeptides* or *tripeptides* (chains of two or three amino acids, respectively) that can be absorbed across the intestinal wall.	*Protein turnover* is the continuous three-step process in which proteins are synthesized, broken down into amino acids, and then resynthesized into new protein. In an injured or undernourished individual, many of the amino acids released by tissue breakdown may be used for *gluconeogenesis,* leading to the undesirable breakdown of lean body mass. The amine group is essential for protein synthesis, but the nonamine portion of the molecule (ketoacid) is used in gluconeogenesis. If a ketoacid is used for gluconeogenesis, the amine group can be excreted in the urine as ammonia or urea.	Proteins make up the lean body mass, which consists primarily of skeletal muscle and visceral organ. Proteins from throughout the body may be mobilized to be used for gluconeogenesis in times of undernutrition.
Lipid	9 kcal/g	Lipids, primarily in the form of triglycerides, provide a stored source of energy. Lipids are also involved in functions such as the maintenance of cell membranes and the manufacture of prostaglandins.	Lipids are partially broken down (hydrolyzed) in the digestive tract to form monoglycerides and diglycerides. Bile salts emulsify with fatty acids and monoglycerides into micelles that cross the intestinal absorptive surface. Inside the intestinal cells, monoglycerides and long-chain fatty acids form triglycerides and are surrounded by phospholipids to form *chylomicron.* Chylomicrons are transported from the intestine through the lymphatic system, then to the blood circulation to be delivered to the liver or other tissues. Chylomicrons are broken down outside the cell with the aid of lipoprotein lipase and enter the cell as fatty acids and glycerol. Short-chain fatty acids (less than 8 carbon atoms long) and medium-chain fatty acids (8 to 12 carbon atoms long) are water soluble and can be absorbed without hydrolysis or formation into a chylomicron.	*Lipolysis* is the breakdown of intracellular triglycerides, which provides fatty acids for energy production and glycerol for *gluconeogenesis.* *Ketogenesis* is the process of breaking down fatty acids into ketones (β-hydroxybutyrate, acetoacetate, and acetone). In the absence of glucose, fatty acid breakdown and ketone production are increased. Ketogenesis occurs in the liver. Ketones can be directly oxidized by the brain and skeletal muscle and used for energy.	Triglycerides are stored in the adipose tissue.

BOX 6.1 Patients Who Are at Risk for Malnutrition

Adults Who Experience Any of the Following
- Involuntary loss or gain of a significant amount of weight (>10% of usual body weight in 6 months, >5% in 1 month), even if the weight achieved by loss or gain is appropriate for height
- Chronic disease
- Chronic use of a modified diet
- Increased metabolic requirements
- Illness or surgery that may interfere with nutrition intake
- Inadequate nutrient intake for >7 days
- Regular use of three or more medications
- Food insecurity

BOX 6.2 DATA COLLECTION

Nutritional History

Inadequate Intake of Nutrients
- Alcohol or polysubstance abuse
- Anorexia, severe or prolonged nausea, or vomiting
- Confusion
- Poor dentition
- Food insecurity
- Fatigue
- Depression
- Multiple or prolonged hospitalization

Inadequate Digestion or Absorption of Nutrients
- Previous gastrointestinal surgeries, especially gastrectomy, jejunoileal bypass, and ileal resection
- Pancreatic diseases
- Inflammatory or malabsorptive bowel diseases

Increased Nutrient Losses
- Severe diarrhea or vomiting
- Fistulas, draining abscesses, wounds, pressure injuries
- Peritoneal dialysis or hemodialysis

Increased Nutrient Requirements
- Fever
- Surgery, trauma, burns, infection
- Cancer (pancreatic, lung, gastric, esophageal)
- Physiologic demands (pregnancy, lactation, growth)

Clinical Signs and Physical Manifestations

A thorough nutrition-focused physical examination (NFPE) is an essential part of a nutrition assessment. The NFPE should be performed by a trained clinician specializing in nutrition. The comprehensive NFPE moves from head to toe, evaluating the fat and muscle stores, signs of nutrient deficiencies in the hair, skin, nails, mouth, edema, and in some settings, functional status with a hand grip dynamometer. The NFPE should be repeated regularly to track changes in nutritional status.[3] If an NFPE is not completed, visual observation from any provider is often adequate to identify overt wasting. Common findings that may indicate an altered nutrition state are listed in Box 6.3.

As part of a comprehensive assessment, a dietitian or specialized nutrition clinician who is trained in NFPE should perform these exams and obtain anthropometric measurements.[3]

BOX 6.3 Clinical Manifestations of Nutrition Alterations

Manifestations That May Indicate Protein-Calorie Malnutrition
- Hair loss; dull, dry, brittle hair; change in color, banding
- Loss of subcutaneous tissue; muscle wasting
- Poor wound healing; pressure injuries
- Hepatomegaly
- Edema
- Decline in functional status

Manifestations Often Present in Vitamin and Mineral Deficiencies
- Hair: Corkscrew hair, alopecia, dull, dry hair
- Eyes: Pale or red and inflamed conjunctiva, angular blepharitis, night blindness, angular palpebritis, sticky eyelids, Bitot's spots, ophthalmoplegia
- Mouth: Soreness, burning, angular stomatitis, cheilitis, beefy red tongue, glossitis, purplish/magenta tongue, gingivitis, hypogeusia, dysgeusia
- Nails: Koilonychia, splinter hemorrhage, brittle, soft, dry, weak/thin, central ridges
- Skin: Slow wound healing, pressure injuries, seborrheic dermatitis, petechiae, purpura, xerosis, perifollicular hemorrhage, dry, pellagra

Manifestations Often Observed With Excessive Vitamin Intake
- Angular stomatitis or cheilitis, yellow or orange pigmentation
- Cutaneous flushing

From Mordarski B. *Nutrition Focused Physical Exam Pocket Guide.* 3rd ed. Academy of Nutrition and Dietetics; 2022.

Anthropometric Measurements

Height and current weight are essential anthropometric measurements, and they should be measured rather than obtained through a patient or family report. The most important reason for obtaining anthropometric measurements is to be able to detect changes in the measurements over time (e.g., track response to nutrition therapy). A simple calculation may be used for interpreting appropriateness of weight or height for adults and older adolescents: body mass index (BMI).

$$BMI = Weight \div Height^2$$

For this calculation, weight is measured in kilograms, and height is measured in meters. BMI values are independent of age and sex and are used for assessing health risk. The BMI can be classified as shown in Table 6.2.

During critical illness, changes in anthropometric measures such as weight are more likely to reflect changes in body water and its distribution. Good judgment must be used in interpreting anthropometric data. For example, edema may mask significant weight loss. Despite these limitations, weight remains an important measure of nutrition status, and any recent weight change must be evaluated.

Laboratory Studies

A wide range of laboratory tests can provide information about nutrition status but must be interpreted within the context of the patient's overall clinical condition. No diagnostic tests for evaluation of nutrition are perfect, and care must be taken in interpreting the results of the tests. For example, albumin and prealbumin were once thought to reflect nutritional status;

TABLE 6.2 Adult Body Mass Index Classifications

Classification	BMI (kg/m²)
Underweight	<18.5
Normal	18.5–24.99
Overweight	25–29.99
Obese class I	30–34.99
Obese class II	35–39.99
Obese class III	≥40

BMI, Body mass index; *kg*, kilogram; *m*, meter.

however, both are negative acute phase reactants and therefore serum values are associated with inflammation rather than nutritional status.[4]

Evaluating Nutrition Assessment Findings

A key part of the nutrition assessment process is using gathered patient information to estimate nutrient—specifically calorie or energy—needs. In the inpatient setting, working with the dietitian, estimated energy needs can be measured or calculated as described subsequently.

Determining Nutrition Needs

Various methods can be used in clinical practice to estimate caloric requirements. *Indirect calorimetry*, a method by which energy expenditure is calculated from oxygen consumption (VO_2) and carbon dioxide production (VCO_2), is the most accurate method for determining caloric needs.[5] Indirect calorimetry is useful in patients suspected to have a high metabolic rate or for which a validated equation does not exist. The test can be performed on ventilated and nonventilated patients. Some ventilators are constructed so that they can perform indirect calorimetry. However, for most patients, indirect calorimetry requires the use of a metabolic cart, which is not available in all institutions. To maintain accuracy and reliability of measurement, several testing criteria must be met, including a fraction of inspired oxygen (FiO_2) < 60% for ventilated patients, no supplemental O_2 for nonventilated patients, and stable and quiet conditions to achieve steady state.[6]

Although indirect calorimetry is considered the most accurate method to determine energy expenditure, its availability is limited. In lieu of a measurement, a variety of formulas have been developed that estimate energy expenditure; however, the accuracy of these formulas compared to indirect calorimetry is highly variable.[6–10] Table 6.3 provides a rough estimate of caloric needs so that the interprofessional team can quickly determine whether patients are being seriously underfed or overfed. Estimates of protein needs are provided in Table 6.4. Commonly used formulas for critically ill patients can be found in Appendix B.

The goal of nutrition assessment is to obtain the most accurate estimate of nutritional requirements. Underfeeding and overfeeding must be avoided during critical illness. Overfeeding results in excessive production of carbon dioxide, which can be a burden in a patient with pulmonary compromise. Overfeeding increases fat stores, which can contribute to insulin resistance and hyperglycemia. Hyperglycemia is associated with several adverse outcomes.[1]

TABLE 6.3 Estimating Energy Needs Based on Patient Characteristics

Patient Characteristics	Estimated Caloric Needs
BMI <30 kg/m² Sedentary activity or no injury Relatively inactive individual without regular aerobic exercise; patient without severe injury or sepsis	25–30 kcal/kg*/day
BMI <30 kg/m² Moderate activity or injury Individual obtaining regular aerobic exercise plus routine activities; patient with trauma or sepsis	30–35 kcal/kg*/day
BMI <30 kg/m² Very active or severe injury Manual laborer or athlete in very active training; patient with major burns or trauma	40 kcal/kg*/day
BMI 30–49.99 kg/m² Obese	11–14 kcal/kg/day Using *ideal* body weight
BMI ≥50 kg/m² Obese	22–25 kcal/kg/day Using *actual* body weight

*The weight used for this calculation should be dry weight or usual body weight if patients are following aggressive volume resuscitation or have edema or anasarca.
BMI, Body mass index; *kcal*, kilocalorie; *kg*, kilogram; *m*, meter.

TABLE 6.4 Estimating Protein Needs

Patient Characteristics	Estimated Protein Needs
BMI <30 kg/m²	1.2–2 g/kg/day Using *actual* body weight
BMI <30 kg/m² With burns or multitrauma	1.5–2 g/kg/day Using *actual* body weight
BMI 30–39.99 kg/m²	2 g/kg/day Using *ideal* body weight
BMI ≥40 kg/m²	2.5 g/kg/day Using *ideal* body weight

Note: Protein recommendations should be reevaluated based on nitrogen balance studies with the goal of achieving nitrogen equilibrium. Nitrogen balance studies are the most accurate way to assess protein needs.

MALNUTRITION

The prevalence of malnutrition in the critical care unit ranges from 38% to 68%.[11] Iatrogenic malnutrition develops in approximately one-third of patients who were well nourished upon admission.[12] Although illness or injury is a major factor contributing to development of malnutrition, other possible contributing factors are lack of communication among the nurses, providers, and dietitians responsible for the care of these patients; frequent diagnostic testing and procedures, which lead to interruption in feeding; medications and other therapies that cause anorexia, nausea, or vomiting and thus interfere with food intake; insufficient monitoring of nutrient intake; and inadequate use of supplements, tube feedings, or parenteral nutrition to maintain nutrition status.

Nutrition status tends to deteriorate during hospitalization unless appropriate nutrition support is started early and continually reassessed. Malnutrition in hospitalized patients is associated with a wide variety of adverse outcomes, including higher incidences of complications, increased mortality rates, lengths of stay, readmissions, hospital costs, infections, and risk of death.[13–16] It is rare for a patient to exhibit a lack of only one nutrient. Nutrition deficiencies usually are combined, with the patient lacking adequate amounts of protein, calories, and possibly vitamins and minerals.

Etiology-Based Approach in Defining Malnutrition

The Academy of Nutrition and Dietetics (AND) and the American Society for Parenteral and Enteral Nutrition (ASPEN) jointly released a consensus statement outlining recommendations for the identification and documentation of adult malnutrition in clinical practice.[17] The statement proposes an etiology-based approach in defining malnutrition that considers the role of inflammation. The three etiology-based malnutrition definitions for patients who have been identified as having compromised intake or loss of body mass are (1) starvation-related malnutrition without inflammation (e.g., pure chronic starvation, anorexia nervosa); (2) chronic disease–related malnutrition with mild to moderate degree of inflammation (e.g., organ failure, pancreatic cancer, sarcopenic obesity); and (3) acute disease–related or injury-related malnutrition with marked inflammatory response (e.g., major infection, burns) (Fig. 6.1).[17]

Two or more of the following six characteristics are currently recommended for the diagnosis of adult malnutrition: insufficient energy intake, weight loss, loss of subcutaneous fat, loss of muscle mass, localized or generalized fluid accumulation that may sometimes mask weight loss, and reduced grip strength[17] (Table 6.5). It is recommended that these characteristics be examined as a part of nutrition assessment and if identified should be documented at baseline and at frequent intervals during reassessments throughout the patient's hospital stay.

Phenotypic and Etiologic Based Approach in Defining Malnutrition

Despite the development of the AND-ASPEN etiology-based malnutrition criteria, the demand for a globally accepted consensus definition of malnutrition persisted. The Global Leadership Initiative on Malnutrition (GLIM) subsequently released a two-step approach for diagnosing malnutrition which includes phenotypic criteria (nonvolitional weight loss, low BMI, and reduced muscle mass) and etiologic criteria (reduced food intake or assimilation, and inflammation or disease burden). At least one criterion from each category is necessary to diagnose malnutrition. From there the severity of malnutrition is further graded into moderate or severe based on the phenotypic criteria (Table 6.6).[18] Validation of these criteria is ongoing.

Protein-Calorie Malnutrition

Malnutrition results from the lack of intake of necessary nutrients or improper absorption and distribution, as well as from excessive intake of some nutrients. Malnutrition can be related to any essential nutrient or nutrients, but a serious type of malnutrition found frequently among hospitalized patients is PCM. Poor intake or impaired absorption of protein and energy from carbohydrate and fat worsens the debilitation that may occur in response to critical illness. In PCM, the body proteins are broken down for gluconeogenesis, reducing the supply of amino acids needed for maintenance of body proteins and healing. Malnutrition can be caused by simple starvation—the inadequate intake of nutrients (e.g., in a patient with anorexia related to cancer). It also can result from an injury that increases the metabolic rate beyond the supply of nutrients (hypermetabolism). In a seriously ill patient, if malnutrition occurs, usually it is the result of the combined effects of starvation and hypermetabolism. See Fig. 6.2 for a summary of key concepts related to PCM.

Metabolic Response to Starvation and Stress

To understand the development of malnutrition in the hospitalized patient, the nurse must understand the metabolic response

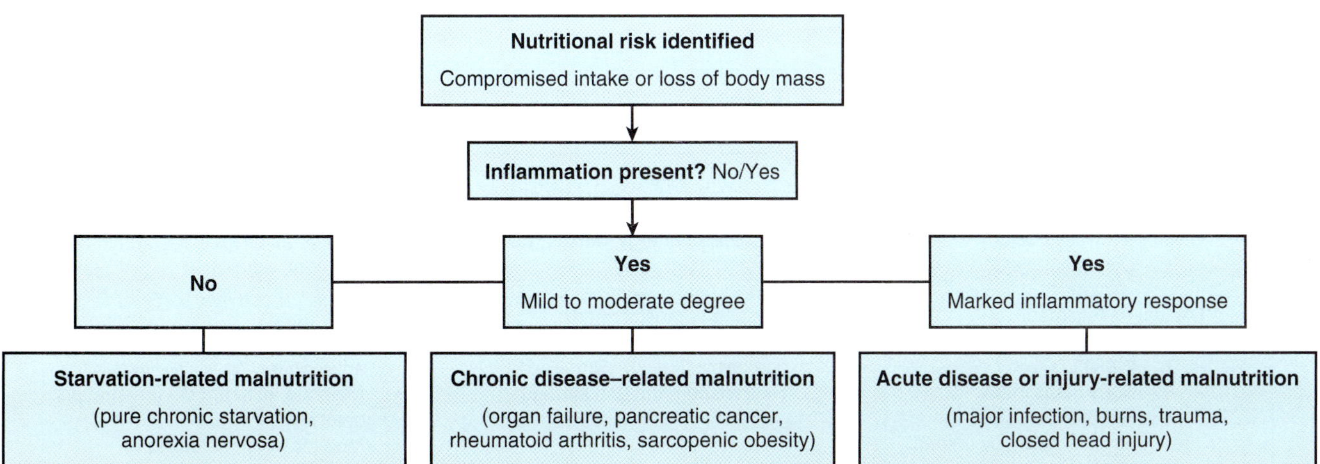

FIG. 6.1 Etiology-Based Malnutrition Definitions, Incorporating the Role of Inflammation in Disease-Related Malnutrition. (From White JV, Guenter P, Jensen G, Malone A, Schofield M; Academy of Nutrition and Dietetics Malnutrition Work Group; A.S.P.E.N. Malnutrition Task Force; A.S.P.E.N. Board of Directors. Consensus statement of the Academy of Nutrition and Dietetics/American Society for Parenteral and Enteral Nutrition. Characteristics recommended for the identification and documentation of adult malnutrition (undernutrition). *J Acad Nutr Diet.* 2012;112(5):730–738. https://doi.org/10.1016/j.jand.2012.03.012)

TABLE 6.5 Malnutrition Diagnosis

Clinical Characteristic	Malnutrition in the Context of Acute Illness or Injury: Nonsevere (Moderate) Malnutrition	Malnutrition in the Context of Acute Illness or Injury: Severe Malnutrition	Malnutrition in the Context of Chronic Illness: Nonsevere (Moderate) Malnutrition	Malnutrition in the Context of Chronic Illness: Severe Malnutrition	Malnutrition in the Context of Social or Environmental Circumstances: Nonsevere (Moderate) Malnutrition	Malnutrition in the Context of Social or Environmental Circumstances: Severe Malnutrition
Energy intake	<75% of estimated energy requirement for >7 days	<50% of estimated energy requirement for >5 days	<75% of estimated energy requirement for >1 month	<75% of estimated energy requirement for >1 month	<75% of estimated energy requirement for >3 months	<50% of estimated energy requirement for >1 month
Weight loss	1%–2% over 1 week 5% over 1 month 7.5% over 3 months	>2% over 1 week >5% over 1 month >7.5% over 3 months	5% over 1 month 7.5% over 3 months 10% over 6 months 20% over 1 year	>5% over 1 month >7.5% over 3 months >10% over 6 months >20% over 1 year	5% over 1 month 7.5% over 3 months 10% over 6 months 20% over 1 year	>5% over 1 month >7.5% over 3 months >10% over 6 months >20% over 1 year
Body fat loss	Mild	Moderate	Mild	Severe	Mild	Severe
Muscle mass loss	Mild	Moderate	Mild	Severe	Mild	Severe
Fluid accumulation	Mild	Moderate to severe	Mild	Severe	Mild	Severe
Reduced grip strength	Not applicable	Measurably reduced	Not applicable	Measurably reduced	Not applicable	Measurably reduced

A minimum of two of the six characteristics is recommended for diagnosis of either severe or nonsevere malnutrition.

TABLE 6.6 Global Leadership Initiative on Malnutrition (GLIM) Criteria for Diagnosing Malnutrition

	Phenotypic Criteria: Weight Loss (%)	Phenotypic Criteria: Low BMI	Phenotypic Criteria: Reduced Muscle Mass	Etiologic Criteria: Reduced Food Intake or Assimilation	Etiologic Criteria: Acute Disease/Injury or Chronic Disease Related
Moderate grade	5%–10% in the past 6 months or 10%–20% beyond 6 months	<20 if <70 years <22 if ≥70 years	Mild to moderate deficit measured by validated body composition measuring techniques	<50% of ER >1 week or Any reduction for > 2 weeks or Any chronic GI condition that adversely impacts food assimilation or absorption	Acute disease/injury or chronic disease related
Severe grade	>10% within the past 6 months or >20% beyond 6 months	<18.5 if < 70 years <20 if ≥ 70 years	Severe deficit measured by validated body composition measuring techniques		

Protein-Calorie Malnutrition

Clinical and Diagnostic Assessments

- History and Risk Factors
  - Dietary intake and weight history
- Clinical Assessment
  - Height
  - Weight
  - Body mass index
  - Nutrition-focused physical exam by trained clinician specializing in nutrition
- Diagnostic Procedures
  - Handgrip strength may be measured with a handgrip dynamometer

Signs

- Decreased energy intake
- Unintentional weight loss
- Wasting of fat mass
- Wasting of muscle mass
- Accumulation of fluid (e.g., edema)
- Decreased hand grip strength

Nursing Interventions

- Screen all patients for nutrition risk upon admission
- Administer nutrition therapy as prescribed
- Promote oral intake when appropriate
- Maintain accurate documentation of intake
- Monitor weight, stooling patterns, tolerance to nutrition interventions
- Manage symptoms interfering with nutrition tolerance
- Communicate progress and barriers with the dietitian and multidisciplinary care team

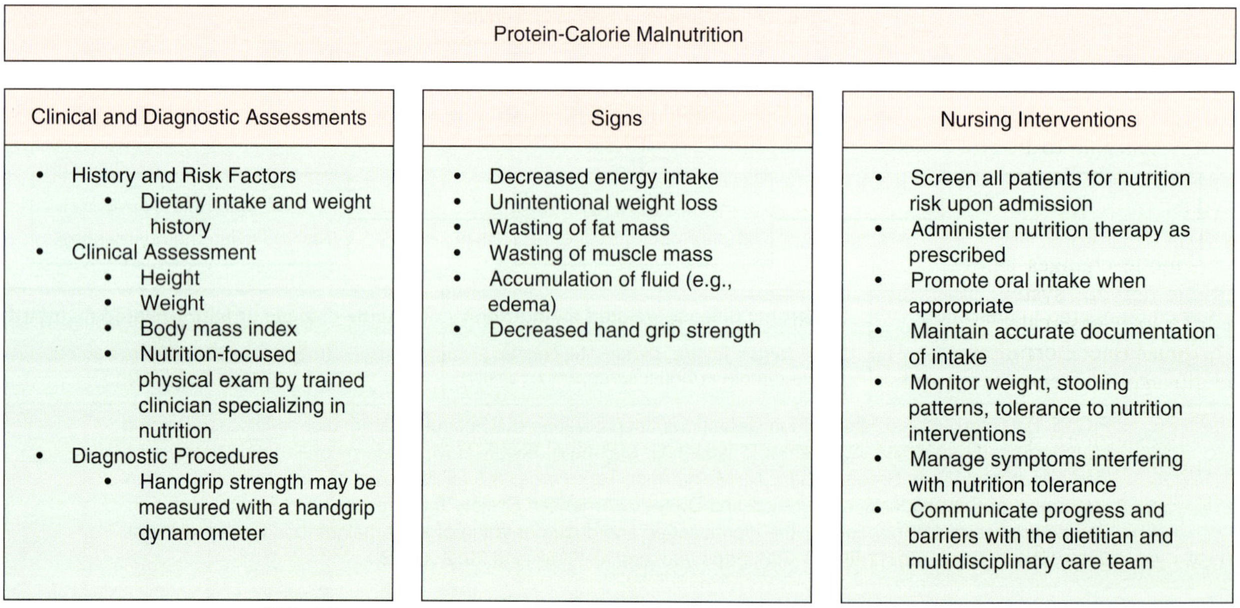

FIG. 6.2 Summary of Key Concepts Related to "Protein-Calorie Malnutrition."

to starvation and physiologic stress. Changes in endocrine status and metabolism together determine the onset and extent of malnutrition. Nutrition imbalance occurs when the demand for nutrients is greater than the exogenous nutrient supply. The major difference between a person who is starved and one who is starved and injured is that the latter has an increased reliance on tissue protein breakdown to provide precursors for glucose production to meet increased energy demands. Although carbohydrate and fat metabolism are also affected, the main concern is about protein metabolism and homeostasis.

The body relies on its protein stores to provide substrates for gluconeogenesis because glucose becomes the major fuel source. This mobilization of substrates occurs at the expense of body tissue and function at a time when the needs for protein synthesis (e.g., wound healing, acute-phase proteins) also are high. Hyperglycemia results from the effects of increased catecholamines, glucocorticoids, and glucagon. Loss of protein results in a negative nitrogen balance and weight loss. Catabolism may be unresponsive to nutrient intake.

Gluconeogenesis

During an acute, nonstressed fast, blood levels of glucose and insulin fall, and glucagon levels rise. Glucagon stimulates the liver to release glucose from its glycogen reserves, which become exhausted within a few hours. Glucagon also stimulates gluconeogenesis, and skeletal muscle provides a large amount of the substrates required for gluconeogenesis. As fasting progresses, fat becomes the primary source of fuel, and the blood ketone levels begin to increase. After the circulating ketone level rises, the brain is able to use ketones for 70% of its energy, decreasing the total body's reliance on glucose as an energy source. As gluconeogenesis from protein precursors decreases, protein breakdown and nitrogen excretion also slow. Some tissues, such as red blood cells, the renal medulla, and 30% of brain cells, are obligatory glucose users, and they continue to require a small amount of amino acids for gluconeogenesis. However, endogenous protein stores are spared from use for gluconeogenesis to a major extent, and protein homeostasis is partially restored.

Hypermetabolism

Critically ill patients are at risk for a combination of starvation and the physiologic stress resulting from injury, trauma, major surgery, or sepsis. Starvation occurs because the person must have nothing by mouth (NPO) for surgical procedures, is unable to eat because of disease-related factors, or is too hemodynamically unstable to be fed. The physiologic stress causes an increased metabolic rate (hypermetabolism) that results in increased oxygen consumption and energy expenditure.

The hypermetabolic process results from increased catabolic hormone changes caused by the stressful event. The sympathetic nervous system is stimulated, causing the adrenal medulla to release catecholamines (epinephrine and norepinephrine). Other hormones released in response to stress include glucagon, adrenocorticotropic hormone, antidiuretic hormone, and glucocorticoids and mineralocorticoids (e.g., cortisol, aldosterone). Cytokines are peptide messengers secreted by macrophages as part of the inflammatory response, and they serve as hormonal regulators of the immune system. Cytokine levels increase in response to sepsis and trauma. Important cytokines include tumor necrosis factor, cachectin, interleukin-1, and interleukin-6. All these hormonal changes cause nutrient substrates, primarily amino acids, to move from peripheral tissues (e.g., skeletal muscle) to the liver for gluconeogenesis.

ORAL INTAKE

Swallow Evaluation for Oral Intake

Completing a swallow evaluation prior to initiating oral intake is important to prevent aspiration.[19] Swallow evaluations include screening protocols and possibly instrumental assessments.[19]

Screening Protocols

Screening protocols identify patients who are high risk for dysphagia.[19] These protocols may start with indications and contraindications, water or multiconsistency swallowing procedures, and observation of signs of aspiration (e.g., coughing, throat clearing, drooling, stridor, hoarse voice).[19] In water swallowing screening protocols, the patient is asked to swallow different volumes of water from a teaspoon and/or cup.[19] In multiconsistency swallowing screening protocols, the patient is asked to swallow a combination of liquid, nectar-like, pudding-like, and/or solid consistencies.[19] Unfortunately, these screening protocols are limited as the patient would have to display overt signs of aspiration to inform if oral intake is appropriate.[19] Patients who have subclinical signs of aspiration (e.g., no cough) may need additional, instrumental assessments.[19]

Instrumental Assessments

Instrumental assessment of swallowing with ultrasound, video fluoroscopy, or fiberoptic endoscopy requires training for the health care professional who will be performing these assessments.[20]

Ultrasound. Ultrasound may be used to evaluate swallow-related muscles and swallowing function.[20] When completing a swallow evaluation via ultrasound, the tongue, pharynx, larynx, esophagus, and hyoid bone should be observed.[20] Food or liquid residue and aspiration may be visualized as the ultrasound allows for static and dynamic imaging.[20] A swallow assessment with an ultrasound allows for the least invasive method of evaluating swallowing function compared to video fluoroscopy or fiberoptic endoscopy and is becoming more widely researched for clinical practice.[20]

Video fluoroscopic swallow studies. Video fluoroscopic swallow studies (VFSSs) are more accurate in identifying dysphagia compared to screening protocols because they provide a direct and dynamic visualization of all the phases of swallowing.[20,21] VFSSs are also known as modified bariums swallow study because a barium sulfate preparation is mixed into multiconsistency food or liquid, allowing for a fluoroscopic analysis.[21] Some patient considerations for this assessment include the exposure to radiation,[20,21] the potential for poor positioning of the patient when swallowing the barium preparation that may result in abnormal swallowing,[21] and the patient stability to be transported to radiology for the examination.[20]

Fiberoptic endoscopic evaluation of swallow. Fiberoptic endoscopic evaluation of swallow (FEES) studies are also more accurate in identifying dysphagia compared to screening protocols because they provide direct visualization of the

SUPPORTING NURSE WELL-BEING

Social Wellness—Personal

After working in the ICU for over 5 years, I decided to go back to school to obtain a graduate degree. I started school and continued to work my three scheduled shifts a week. My first semester in graduate school was easy to manage with my work schedule and social calendar. Starting my second semester in graduate school, I needed to complete clinical hours in addition to my classes. I still kept my full-time, three-day-a week schedule during this time. I had been keeping up with some of my social activities, like casual get-togethers, movie outings, and dinner events. This was also an eventful time in my friends' lives—I received invitations for their bridal or baby showers, their weddings or their child's birthday party, and their promotion parties. I was starting to feel overwhelmed by my professional and personal commitments. I wanted to focus on my schooling, but I also wanted to celebrate my friends' accomplishments as they so often have mine. I had to start declining invitations. I missed the casual get-togethers, birthdays, and celebratory events leading up to weddings. I was starting to think, 'Am I a bad friend?'

The above vignette shows how one person is affected by the need to fulfill social commitments. Social wellness is not gauged by one's presence or absence at gatherings. Additionally, social interactions that become obligations lose their luster and therapeutic benefits. Social relationships and activities shouldn't be a stressor, but a contributor to health. Social wellness is having a network of people who are interdependent and share mutual trust and respect, allowing for an awareness of and sensitivity to fluctuating life circumstances. Open conversations about one's life during different phases may help feeling supported and maintain social connectedness even if physically absent for a defined time frame. Conversely, these open conversations communicate times in one's life when the physical presence of one's social network is needed to get through difficult times. In either case, the communication among one's social network is intentional, and the response of social support is genuine. The social aspect of life becomes a refuge from other stressors and adds to one's mental health.

Consider the following to maintain social wellness:

- Evaluate your current social interactions: How do you contribute to your social network? What feelings are evoked from interacting within your social network?
- Determine your social needs.
- Actively communicate and be intentional in that social communication.
- Be genuine during and open to life circumstances.
- Embrace your need for space or interaction among your friends.
- Consider professional resources should you face continued barriers to achieving or maintaining social wellness.

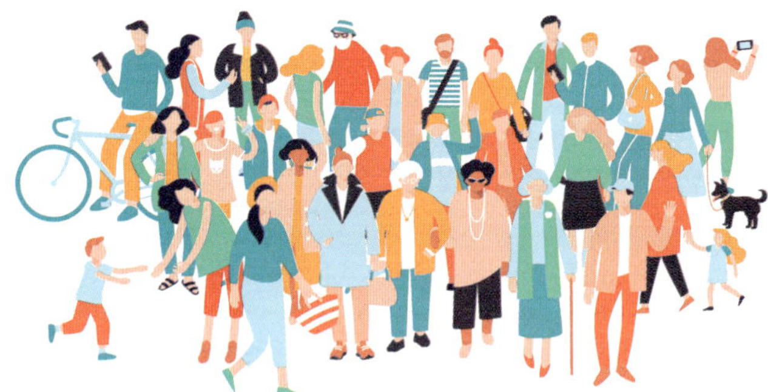

(Copyright © iStock.com/bluebearry.)

We are like islands in the sea, separate on the surface but connected in the deep...

-William James

glottis.[21] In a FEES study, a flexible fiberoptic laryngoscope is passed through the nose into the hypopharynx to visualize swallowing of different food consistencies and assess patient's tolerance of different swallowing maneuvers.[21] The FEES study is a beneficial bedside procedure as it is does not require patient transport and it also is beneficial as it limits the patient's exposure to radiation, but because of the position of the laryngoscope in the hypopharynx, the other phases of swallowing (preparatory, oral, and esophageal) are not visualized as in the VFSS.[21] Patient considerations for this assessment include management of pain from insertion of the probe in the nasal cavity.[19]

Oral Supplementation

Oral supplementation may be necessary for patients who can eat and have normal digestion and absorption but cannot consume enough regular foods to meet caloric and protein needs. Patients with mild to moderate anorexia, burns, or trauma sometimes fall into this category. To improve intake and tolerance of supplements, the critical care nurse can take several steps, as follows:

1. Collaborate with the dietitian to choose appropriate products and allow the patient to participate in the selection process, if possible. Milkshakes, smoothies, and commercial supplements provide an easily tolerated, dense source of calories, and protein. However, lactose intolerance is common among adults. Individuals with this problem require commercial lactose-free supplements, beverages prepared with lactose-free milk or milk alternatives, or lactase enzyme taken with milk products.
2. Offer to serve commercial supplements well chilled or on ice, which improves palatability.
3. Advise patients to sip commercial supplements slowly, consuming no more than 240 mL over 30 to 45 minutes. These products contain easily digestible carbohydrates. If formulas are consumed too quickly, rapid hydrolysis of the carbohydrate in the duodenum can contribute to dumping syndrome, characterized by abdominal cramping, weakness, tachycardia, and diarrhea.
4. Record all supplement intake separately on the intake-and-output sheet so that it can be differentiated from intake of water and other liquids.

ENTERAL AND PARENTERAL NUTRITION SUPPORT

Nutrition support is the provision of specially formulated or delivered enteral or parenteral nutrients to maintain or restore optimal nutrition status.[1] It is an essential adjunct in the prevention and management of malnutrition in critically ill patients. The goal of nutrition support therapy is to provide enough support for body requirements, which may minimize complications and promote positive clinical outcomes.[1] Evidence-based nutrition guidelines for critically ill adults who require a stay of more than 3 days in the critical care unit were published by The Society of Critical Care Medicine and ASPEN. The publication is based on an extensive review of 480 articles and a subsequent update was published providing recommendations on five foundational questions regarding calorie and protein targets and use of enteral and parenteral nutrition. The interprofessional team is encouraged to become familiar with these evidence-based guidelines.[1,22]

When possible, the enteral route is the preferred method of feeding over parenteral nutrition. The proposed advantages of enteral nutrition over parenteral nutrition include lower cost and better maintenance of gut integrity and function.[1] There has been a longstanding association between parenteral nutrition and infection risk; however, these associations in the literature predate the advances of central line bundles, attention to glycemic control, and avoidance of overfeeding. The latest ASPEN guidelines clarify that the use of either feeding modality in the first week of critical illness will not impact infection risk or mortality.[22]

Critical care nurses must have a broad understanding of nutrition support, including the indications for nutrition support, evaluation of feeding delivery and tolerance, and the prevention and management of associated complications.

Enteral Nutrition

Enteral nutrition or tube feedings are used for patients who have at least some digestive and absorptive capability but are unable or unwilling to consume enough by mouth. The GI tract plays an important role in maintaining immunologic defenses, which is why nutrition by the enteral route is thought to be physiologically beneficial. Some of the intrinsic mechanisms in the GI tract to prevent infections include neutrophils; the normal acidic gastric pH; motility, which limits GI tract colonization by pathogenic bacteria; the normal gut microflora, which inhibit growth of or destroy some pathogenic organisms; rapid desquamation and regeneration of intestinal epithelial cells; the layer of mucus secreted by GI tract cells; and bile, which detoxifies endotoxin in the intestine and delivers immunoglobulin A to the intestine. A second line of defense against invasion of intestinal bacteria is the gut-associated lymphoid tissue. The systemic immune defenses in the GI tract are stimulated by the presence of food within it. Providing enteral nutrition maintains all of the normal functions of the GI tract stated earlier, thereby serving to maintain gut integrity, modulate the stress and systemic immune response, and abate disease severity.[1,23]

Patients who are experiencing severe stress that greatly increases their nutrition needs (caused by major surgery, burns, or trauma) often benefit from tube feedings. A variety of commercial enteral feeding products are available, some of which are designed to meet the specialized needs of critically ill patients. Immune-modulating formulas containing glutamine, arginine, nucleic acids, eicosapentaenoic acid (EPA), and docosahexaenoic acid (DHA) are recommended for trauma and postsurgical patients; however, use of most other specialty formulas is not evidence based.[1] Enteral formula types and the nutrition indications for each are listed in Table 6.7.

Immune-enhancing formulas have emerged as a means to protect and stimulate the immune system. Some enterally delivered nutrients that may benefit critically ill patients include the amino acids glutamine and arginine, the omega-3 (n-3) fatty acids, and nucleic acids.[24] Glutamine is the major fuel of the small intestinal cells. It is considered a nonessential amino acid, but it becomes conditionally essential in illness. Arginine is involved in protein synthesis and is a precursor of nitric oxide, a molecule that stimulates vasodilation. The omega-3 fatty acids, derived primarily from fish oils, are involved in synthesis of eicosanoids (molecules with hormone-like activity)—prostaglandins, prostacyclin, and leukotrienes—and may modulate the inflammatory response.[24]

Early enteral nutrition, administered with the first 24 to 48 hours of critical illness, has been shown to reduce infections, hospital length of stay, and mortality. Current guidelines support the early initiation of nutrition support in critically ill patients who will be unable to meet their nutrient needs orally.[1] To avoid complications associated with intestinal ischemia and infarction, enteral nutrition must be initiated only after fluid resuscitation and adequate perfusion have been achieved.[1] Patients who need high doses of vasoactive medication infusions are at high risk for intestinal ischemia, and enteral feeding should be started cautiously and with a low fiber formula.[25,26]

Enteral Feeding Access

Achievement of enteral access is the cornerstone of enteral nutrition therapy. Several techniques can be used to facilitate enteral access. These include surgical methods, bedside methods, fluoroscopy, endoscopy, electromagnetic signaling, camera equipped, ultrasound guided, and air insufflation.[27] Use of an electromagnetically guided feeding tube placement device has allowed nurses and other qualified practitioners to place and confirm postpyloric feeding tubes at the bedside and obviated the need for additional radiographic confirmation.[28,29]

After the tube is placed, the correct location must be confirmed before feedings are started and regularly throughout the course of enteral feedings. Radiographs are the most accurate way of assessing tube placement, but repeated radiographs are costly and can expose the patient to excessive radiation. After correct placement has been confirmed, marking the exit site of the tube to check for movement is helpful. Alternative methods for confirming tube placement have been researched that attempt to verify placement in the stomach or small intestine; however, radiography remains the gold standard, whereas use of electromagnetic confirmation is being validated in a variety of patient populations.[30–32]

Location and Type of Feeding Tube

Choosing an enteral feeding route should take into consideration several factors including duration of therapy, function of all parts of the gastrointestinal (GI) tract, aspiration risk, GI tolerance, and social and economic factors.[1,30] Nasal intubation is the simplest and most commonly used route for enteral access. This method allows access to the stomach, duodenum, or jejunum. Tube enterostomy—a gastrostomy or jejunostomy—is used primarily for long-term feedings (4–6 weeks or more) and when obstruction makes the nasoenteral route inaccessible. A conventional gastrostomy or jejunostomy is often

TABLE 6.7 Enteral Formulas

Formula Type	Nutrition Uses	Clinical Examples	Examples of Commercial Products (Manufacturer)
Formulas Used When GI Tract Is Fully Functional			
Polymeric (standard): Contains whole proteins (10%–15% of calories), long-chain triglycerides (25%–40% of calories), and glucose polymers or oligosaccharides (50%–60% of calories); comes with or without fiber	Inability to ingest food Inability to consume enough to meet needs	Oral or esophageal cancer Coma, stroke Anorexia resulting from chronic illness Burns or trauma	Ensure (Abbott) Osmolite (Abbott) Jevity (Abbott) Boost (Nestlé) Nutren (Nestlé) Fibersource (Nestlé) Isosource (Nestlé)
High-protein: Same as polymeric except protein provides about 25% of calories	Same as polymeric plus mild catabolism and protein deficits	Trauma or burns Sepsis	Promote (Abbott) Replete (Nestlé)
Concentrated: Same as polymeric except concentrated to 2 calories/mL	Same as polymeric but fluid restriction needed	Heart failure Neurosurgery COPD Liver disease	TwoCal HN (Abbott) Nutren 2.0 (Nestlé)
Formulas Used When GI Function Is Impaired			
Elemental or predigested: Contains hydrolyzed (partially digested) protein, peptides (short chains of amino acids) and/or amino acids, little fat (<10% of calories) or high MCT, and glucose polymers or oligosaccharides	Impaired digestion and/or absorption	Radiation enteritis Inflammatory bowel disease	Vital (Abbott) Peptamen (Nestlé) Vivonex (Nestlé)
Diets for Specific Disease States[a]			
Renal failure: Concentrated in calories; low sodium, potassium, magnesium, phosphorus, and vitamins A and D; low protein for renal insufficiency; higher protein formulas for dialyzed patients	Renal insufficiency Dialysis	Predialysis Hemodialysis or peritoneal dialysis	Nepro (Abbott) Suplena (Abbott) Novasource Renal (Nestlé)
Pulmonary dysfunction: Low carbohydrate, high fat, concentrated in calories	Respiratory insufficiency	Ventilator dependence	Pulmocare (Abbott) Nutren Pulmonary (Nestlé)
Glucose intolerance: High fat, low carbohydrate (most contain fiber and fructose)	Glucose intolerance	Individuals with diabetes mellitus whose blood sugar is poorly controlled with standard formulas	Glucerna (Abbott) Diabetisource (Nestlé) Glytrol (Nestlé)
Critical care, wound healing: High protein; most contain MCT to improve fat absorption; some have increased zinc and vitamin C for wound healing; some are high in antioxidants (vitamin E, beta-carotene); some are enriched with arginine, glutamine, or omega-3 fatty acids	Critical illness	Severe trauma Perisurgical	Pivot (Abbott) Impact (Nestlé)

[a]There is little evidence supporting the use of disease-specific formulas.

BCAA, Branched chain–enriched amino acid; *COPD*, chronic obstructive pulmonary disease; *GI*, gastrointestinal; *MCT*, medium-chain triglyceride.

performed at the time of other abdominal surgery. The percutaneous endoscopic gastrostomy tube has become extremely popular because it can be inserted at the bedside without the use of general anesthetics. Percutaneous endoscopic jejunostomy tubes are also used. Fig. 6.3 shows the locations of tube feeding sites.

Critically ill patients may not tolerate early enteral feeding because of impaired gastric motility, ileus, or medications administered in the early phase of illness. Traditionally, postpyloric feeding has been favored in the critical care setting.[1] Postpyloric feedings have demonstrated an advantage over intragastric feedings with improved GI tolerance, lower incidence of aspiration and pneumonia, and shorter critical care unit and hospital LOS.[33] However, recent literature shows that in patients with preserved GI function, gastric bolus or intermittent feeding may reduce incidence of aspiration and have comparable tolerance.[34,35]

One challenge in comparing the superiority of gastric versus postpyloric feeding is the lack of a standard definition of enteral feeding intolerance. There is little evidence to support a correlation between gastric residual volume (GRV) and tolerance to feedings, gastric emptying, and potential aspiration, and therefore, monitoring of GRV is no longer recommended as part of routine nursing care. When GRV is monitored, enteral feeding should not be held unless the GRV exceeds 500 mL.[1] Prokinetic agents, including metoclopramide and erythromycin, have been used to improve gastric motility and promote early enteral nutrition in critically ill patients.[1,28]

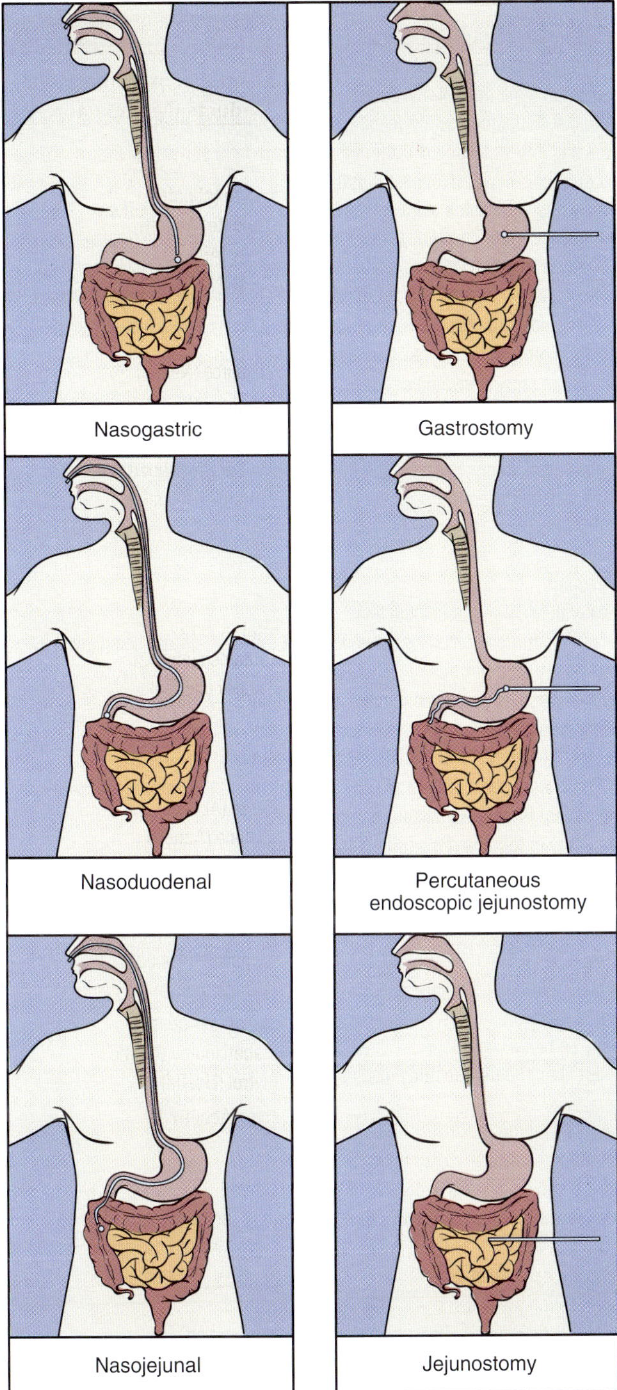

FIG. 6.3 Tube Feeding Sites.

Assessment and Prevention of Feeding Tube Complications

Nursing care of patients receiving enteral nutrition involves prevention and management of complications associated with the use of feeding tubes. Patient care management of these problems is summarized in Box 6.4. The skin around the feeding tube should be cleaned at least daily, and the tape around the tube should be replaced whenever loosened or soiled. Secure taping helps prevent movement of the tube, which may irritate the nares or oral mucosa or result in accidental dislodgment. The tube must be taped in the dependent position to prevent unnecessary pressure and prevent necrosis. Commercially available attachment devices may be used to avoid inadvertent dislodgment.

Enterostomy sites should be cleansed daily with mild soap and water. Tubes should be maintained according to manufacturer instructions.[27,29] Drainage at the enterostomy site should be addressed promptly depending on the type of drainage.[29] Buried bumper syndrome may occur when the gastrostomy device disk, or bumper, is pulled tight against the abdominal wall. To prevent this, it is necessary to minimize tension on the disk.[29] The tube may also become dislodged. When this occurs in a stoma tract that is not mature, peritonitis can result and therefore dislodgement is an urgent issue and tubes should be replaced immediately.[29]

Aspiration. Pulmonary aspiration of enteral formulas and subsequent pneumonia is a serious complication of enteral feeding in critically ill patients. Risk factors for aspiration include sedation, use of paralytics, supine positioning, improperly positioned feeding tubes, mechanical ventilation, reflux and vomiting, and advanced age.[29] To reduce the risk of pulmonary aspiration of formula during enteral feeding, the nurse must keep the head of the bed elevated unless contraindicated; temporarily stop feedings when the patient must be supine for prolonged periods; keep the cuff of the endotracheal tube inflated as appropriate during enteral feeding, if applicable; and be alert to any increase in nausea or abdominal distention and address with prokinetic agents.[29]

Two bedside methods have been used in the past to detect pulmonary aspiration of enteral feeding. One is the addition of blue dye to the enteral formula and observation of the patient for any dye-tinged tracheal secretions, and the other is glucose testing of tracheal secretions to detect the presence of the glucose-containing enteral formula.[36–38] There is no established protocol for blue dye testing. Although it has been used routinely in clinical practice for several years, there is no evidence to support its efficacy or safety. It lacks sensitivity and specificity in ruling out aspiration. Numerous clinical reports of systemic absorption of blue dye and adverse outcomes have been described.[37,38] The glucose oxidase method may cause false-positive reactions if blood is present. It has a low sensitivity when low-glucose formulas are used, and it has questionable specificity.[36] Glucose oxidase testing and blue food coloring are not recommended as appropriate methods for detecting aspiration of enteral feedings.[37,39]

Diarrhea and constipation. Diarrhea is common in patients receiving enteral nutrition, with an incidence of 2% to 95%.[34] No single definition has been established for diarrhea; however, a suggested definition is stool volume ≥750 mL or three to five bowel movements in 24 hours.[40] Diarrhea in enterally fed critically ill patients has many factors. Common causes include medications, malabsorption, primary diseases of the GI tract, infection, and bacterial overgrowth.[29,40] Osmotic diarrhea caused by the administration of hyperosmotic elixir medications straight into the small bowel is often mistaken for enteral feeding intolerance. While the cause of diarrhea is being determined, nurses must provide adequate fluid and electrolyte replacement and maintain skin integrity. Constipation is a complication of enteral feeding that may result from dehydration, bed rest, opioid administration, or lack of adequate fiber in enteral formulas.[29] However, providing fiber in hemodynamically unstable patients is not recommended.[26] Bowel movements

BOX 6.4 Safety

Patient Care Management of Enteral Tube Feeding Complications

Complication	Contributing Factors	Prevention or Correction
Pulmonary aspiration (signs and symptoms include tachypnea, shortness of breath, hypoxia, and infiltrate on chest radiographs)	Feeding tube positioned in esophagus or respiratory tract Regurgitation of formula	Confirm proper tube placement before administering any feeding Check tube placement at least every 4–8 h during continuous feedings Elevate the head to 30–45 degrees during feedings unless contraindicated Consider giving feeding into small bowel rather than stomach in high-risk patients If artificial airway in place, keep cuff inflated during feeding Metoclopramide may improve gastric emptying and decrease risk of regurgitation Evaluate feeding tolerance every 2 h initially, then less frequently as condition becomes stable Intolerance may be manifested by bloating, abdominal distention and pain, lack of stool and flatus, diminished or absent bowel sounds, tense abdomen, increased tympany, nausea and vomiting, gastric residual volume >500 mL, although a high residual volume in the absence of other abnormal findings may not be grounds for stopping feedings (measuring residual volume is not recommended as routine practice) If intolerance is suspected, abdominal radiographs may be obtained to check for distended gastric bubble, distended loops of bowel, or air-fluid levels
Diarrhea	Medications with GI side effects (e.g., antibiotics, digitalis, laxatives, magnesium-containing antacids, quinidine, caffeine)	Evaluate the patient's medications to determine their potential for causing diarrhea, and consult the pharmacist if necessary
	Predisposing illness (e.g., short bowel syndrome, inflammatory bowel disease)	Use continuous feedings Consider a formula with MCT and/or soluble fiber
	Hypertonic formula or medications (liquid formulations), which can cause dumping syndrome	Evaluate formula administration procedures to ensure that feedings are not being given by bolus infusion Administer formula continuously or by slow intermittent infusion Dilute enteral medications well
	Bacterial contamination of formula	Use scrupulously clean technique in administering tube feedings Prepare formula with sterile water if there are any concerns about the safety of the water supply or if the patient is seriously immunocompromised Keep opened containers of formula refrigerated, and discard them within 24 h; discard enteral feeding containers and administration sets every 24 h Hang formula no more than 4–8 h unless it comes prepackaged in sterile administration sets
	Fecal impaction with seepage of liquid stool around impaction	Perform a digital rectal examination to rule out impaction; see guidelines for prevention of constipation below
Constipation	Low-fiber formula, creating little fecal bulk, lack of fiber	Consider using a fiber-containing formula Ensure fluid intake is adequate Stool softeners may be beneficial
	Poor GI motility (gastroparesis, various GI disease states, critical illness)	Use formula without fiber and treat motility medically
	Medications with GI side effects (e.g., opioid pain medications)	Ensure fluid intake is adequate Stool softeners may be beneficial
Tube occlusion	Medications administered by tube that physically plug the tube or coagulate the formula, causing it to clog the tube	If medications must be given by tube, avoid use of crushed tablets Consult with the pharmacist to determine whether medications can be dispensed as elixirs or suspensions Dilute elixirs to prevent osmotic diarrhea Ensure crushed medication, when used, are adequately pulverized Irrigate tube with water before and after administering any medication Never add any medication to formula unless the two are known to be compatible
	Stagnant formula Sedimentation of formula	Irrigate tube every 4–8 h during continuous feedings and after every intermittent feeding If residuals are measured, flush tube thoroughly before drawing the residual and after returning formula to the stomach because gastric juices left in tube may cause precipitation of formula Instilling pancreatic enzymes into tube can remove or prevent some occlusions
Gastric retention	Delayed gastric emptying related to head trauma, sepsis, diabetic or uremic gastroparesis, electrolyte balance, or other illness	The cause must be corrected if possible Consult with the provider about use of postpyloric feedings or prokinetic agents to stimulate gastric emptying Encourage the patient to lie in the right lateral position frequently, unless contraindicated
Mesenteric ischemia	High dose vasopressor agents, impaired splanchnic blood flow	Prevention is paramount due to the high associated mortality Consult with provider and dietitian regarding appropriateness of initiating/continuing enteral feeding with concurrent use of vasopressors Use fiber-free formula and lower fat formula Hold enteral feeding if hemodynamic status worsens

GI, Gastrointestinal; *MCT*, medium-chain triglyceride; *h*, hour; *mL*, milliliter.

From Mueller CM. *The ASPEN Adult Nutrition Support Core Curriculum*. 3rd ed. American Society for Parenteral and Enteral Nutrition; 2017.

should be assessed daily. The nurse must ensure adequate fluid, promote optimal mobility, and administer laxatives and stool softeners as necessary.

Feeding tube occlusion. Tube occlusion may also occur as a result of stagnant formula, inadequately crushed pills, or medication interactions with formula. Enteral infusion pumps should be used, and tubes should be flushed before feeding infusions are paused, medications are infused, or gastric residuals are checked. Liquid medications or elixirs should be used when possible to avoid tube occlusion with pill fragments, but these should be diluted with water because elixirs are often very hypertonic and can contribute to osmotic diarrhea. However, the volume of fluid required to adequately dilute a hyperosmotic elixir is often beyond what many patients can tolerate in a single flush; therefore, crushed tablets may be the better option. The risk of tube occlusion versus the risk of diarrhea from hyperosmotic elixirs must be balanced and evaluated on a patient-by-patient basis. The use of pancreatic enzymes in the feeding tube may be successful in removing a clog after it has formed.[41]

Regular irrigation helps prevent feeding tube occlusion. Usually, irrigation with 20 to 30 mL of warm water every 3 to 4 hours during continuous feedings and before and after intermittent feedings and medication administration can maintain patency.[1] The volume of irrigant may have to be reduced for fluid restriction. Automatic enteral flush pumps are also available. Although cranberry juice or cola beverages are sometimes used in an effort to reduce the incidence of tube occlusion, water is the preferred irrigant because it has been shown to be superior in maintaining tube patency.[42] Beverages high in sugar or acidity may actually lead to more occlusions by binding to the inside of the tube, compromising the integrity of the structural integrity of the tube or causing precipitation of the proteins in the enteral formula.

Formula Delivery

Careful attention to administration of tube feedings can prevent many complications. Very clean or aseptic technique in the handling and administration of the formula can help prevent bacterial contamination and a resultant infection. Open system formula delivery uses cartons of formula transferred to a feeding container. Wash hands before opening, hang enough formula for just 8 hours of infusion, and do not add new formula to formula that is already hanging. Closed systems that use a prefilled sterile container that can be spiked with the enteral tube are also available.[29,42]

Tube feedings may be administered in four different feeding modalities: continuous, cyclic, intermittent, or bolus. *Continuous* feeding infuses enteral formula with a pump over 24 hours. It is preferred for the most unstable critically ill patients. *Cyclic* feeding infuses formula with a pump in less than 24 hours. Nocturnal cyclic feeding is a typical modality for patients transitioning to oral feedings but not yet able to consume their entire nutrient needs from diet. *Intermittent* feeding provides a larger volume of formula over a shorter period of time, usually 20 to 60 minutes, 4 to 6 times per day, via a pump. *Bolus* feedings similarly provide a large volume of formula, 4 to 6 times per day, but unlike intermittent feeding, is administered via syringe over 10 minutes or less.[43] Bolus feedings are typically reserved for gastric enteral access, as the stomach is able to expand to accommodate the rapidly infused formula volume. Intermittent and bolus feedings mimic the normal pattern of eating and therefore derive the most natural physiologic response to feeding. Bolus feedings administered into the small bowel, which is not able to expand in the same manner as the stomach, are likely to cause distention, vomiting, and dumping syndrome with diarrhea.[29,43] If rapid infusion of bolus feeding is not well tolerated, nurses can gradually drip intermittent feedings, with each feeding lasting 20 to 30 minutes or longer, to promote optimal assimilation.

Evaluating Enteral Nutritional Intake

Critically ill patients have so many needs for care that it is easy to overlook the importance of nutrition. Many studies have shown that critically ill patients receive considerably less enteral nutrition than required, as low as 33% of the prescribed volume.[26] This is a complication unique to enteral nutrition and is not observed with total parenteral nutrition (TPN). The discrepancy in nutrition intake has a variety of causes, including process-related factors (critical care unit–related interruptions, real or perceived intolerance, and provider attitudes).[26] The enteral delivery practices in the critical care unit and clinicians' concerns about aspiration may lead to inappropriate and prolonged interruptions in enteral feeding.

Volume-based feeding is a nursing-driven, evidence-based feeding protocol that aims to achieve a daily goal volume of enteral formula infusion as opposed to running feedings at a continuous rate. This allows the nurse to adjust the rate of feeding to make up for feeding interruptions to achieve the daily goal volume. Volume-based feeding is often combined with more aggressive feeding interventions, such as faster feeding initiation, use of prokinetics, and supplemental protein modulars. Volume-based feeding has been shown to increase nutritional delivery by approximately 10% to 12% without adversely affecting glycemic control or feeding tolerance.[44,45]

Preventing Tubing and Catheter Misconnections

Tubing and catheter misconnection errors have gained the attention of The Joint Commission and the U.S. Food and Drug Administration (FDA).[46,47] Examples of misconnection errors include misconnecting an enteric feeding tube into an intravenous catheter or injection of an intravenous fluid into a tracheostomy cuff inflation tube. These misconnection errors are potentially life threatening, and new tubing connectors, known as ENFit, prevent enteral to intravenous connection and were developed in response and rolled out globally.[48,49]

Parenteral Nutrition

Parenteral nutrition refers to the delivery of all nutrients by the intravenous route. It is used when the GI tract is not functional or when nutrition needs cannot be met solely through the GI tract. Candidates for parenteral nutrition include patients who have severely impaired absorption (e.g., short bowel syndrome, collagen vascular diseases such as scleroderma or Ehlers-Danlos syndrome, radiation enteritis), intestinal obstruction, peritonitis, or prolonged ileus. Some postoperative, trauma, or burn patients may need parenteral nutrition to supplement the nutrient intake that they are able to tolerate by the enteral route.

Types of Parenteral Nutrition

TPN involves administration of highly concentrated dextrose, amino acids, fats, electrolytes, vitamins and trace elements, providing a rich source of calories capable of meeting nearly all nutritional requirements for most patients. These highly concentrated solutions are hyperosmolar and must be delivered through a central vein. Peripheral parenteral nutrition (PPN) is a more dilute solution with a recommended maximum osmolality of 900 mOsm/L that may be delivered safely through a peripheral vein.[50] PPN solution delivers nutrition support in a large volume that cannot be tolerated by patients who require fluid restriction. It provides short-term nutrition support for a few days to less than 2 weeks and, due to the restricted osmolality, may not cover 100% of nutrient needs in some cases. Regardless of the route of administration, TPN and PPN solutions are highly complex and may include over 40 ingredients. Parenteral nutrition is considered a high alert medication.[51]

Parenteral nutrition may be packaged with lipid emulsions included or separated from the rest of the solution. Parenteral nutrition with lipid emulsions hung separately is referred to as 2 in 1, whereas parenteral nutrition with all components in one bag is referred to as 3 in 1.

Lipid emulsion. Lipids or fat emulsions provide calories for energy and prevent essential fatty acid deficiency. In contrast to dextrose–amino acid solutions, intravenous lipid emulsions provide a rich environment for the growth of bacteria and fungi, including *Candida albicans*. Historically, 0.22-micron filters were used to filter out possible precipitates from the parenteral nutrition solution, but lipid emulsions cannot be filtered through an in-line 0.22-micron filter because some particles in the emulsions have larger diameters than this. The effectiveness of 0.22-micron filters has not been compared to 1.2-micron filters which do allow flow of lipid emulsions while capturing *Candida albicans*. Therefore, recent recommendations have suggested sole use of a 1.2-micron filter to eliminate confusion and promote compliance with a single filter set-up.[52] Lipid emulsions are handled with strict asepsis, and they must be discarded within 12 to 24 hours of hanging.[53]

Nursing Management of Potential Complications

Nursing management of patients receiving TPN should focus on prevention and correction of complications. Nursing management of TPN complications is described in Box 6.5.

Metabolic complications associated with parenteral nutrition include glucose intolerance and electrolyte imbalance. Insulin can be added to the TPN solution or can be infused as a separate drip to control glucose levels. Rapid cessation of TPN may lead to rebound hypoglycemia; therefore, tapering the infusion at least 1 hour is a common practice.[51] Serum electrolytes are obtained prior to starting TPN. During critical illness, levels should be monitored and corrected daily and then weekly or twice weekly after the patient is more stable.

Because TPN requires an indwelling catheter in a central vein, potential complications such as air embolism, pneumothorax, deep vein thrombosis (DVT), and infection are possible. Air embolism may result from insertion or catheter disconnections. A pneumothorax may develop from the insertion of the central venous catheter. Patients requiring multiple intravenous therapies and frequent blood sampling usually have multilumen central venous catheters, and TPN is often infused through these catheters. These multilumen catheters have been associated with increased DVT and infection incidence.[54] See detailed information on the prevention of central venous catheter–related bloodstream infections in Chapter 12.

Monitoring and Evaluation of Nutrition Support

An interprofessional approach is required in evaluating the effects of nutrition support on clinical outcomes. Assessment of response to nutrition support is an ongoing process that involves physical examination, anthropometric measurements, and biochemical evaluation. Daily monitoring of nutrition intake is an important aspect of critical care and is a key element in preventing problems associated with underfeeding and overfeeding. Daily weights and the maintenance of accurate intake-and-output records are crucial for evaluating nutrition progress and the state of hydration in the patient receiving nutrition support. Monitoring serum levels of electrolytes, calcium, phosphorus, and magnesium is necessary to assess fluid balance and tolerance to nutritional intake. Blood urea nitrogen and creatinine levels may reflect the adequacy of renal function to handle nutrition support. Blood glucose is an indicator of the patient's tolerance of the carbohydrate load but may be altered by other medical processes. Serum triglyceride concentrations (in patients receiving intravenous lipid emulsions) reflect the ability of the tissues to metabolize the lipids. Liver function tests reflect hepatic tolerance to parenteral nutrition as the liver is susceptible to injury if parenteral nutrition is not properly dosed or used long term; however, it can also be altered by other medical processes.

REFEEDING SYNDROME

Refeeding syndrome is a potentially lethal condition characterized by generalized fluid and electrolyte imbalance. It occurs as a potential complication after initiation of oral, enteral, or parenteral nutrition in malnourished patients. During chronic starvation, several compensatory metabolic changes occur leading to an overall depletion of total body electrolytes and vitamin deficiencies, but preservation of serum levels may be present, masking initial risk for refeeding syndrome. The reintroduction of carbohydrates leads to increased insulin production. This increases intracellular demand for phosphorus, potassium, magnesium, vitamins, and minerals.[55] These metabolic demands result in severe shifts from the extracellular compartment. Increased insulin levels also result in fluid retention. Severe hypophosphatemia, hypokalemia, and hypomagnesemia result in altered cardiac, GI, and neurologic function. In particular, hypophosphatemia causes a decrease in 2,3-diphosphoglycerate and limits the many reactions that require adenosine triphosphate. Hypophosphatemia and other electrolyte deficiencies may lead to respiratory failure, acute heart failure, and dysrhythmias.

It is important to anticipate refeeding syndrome in patients who may be at risk. Patients with chronic malnutrition or underfeeding, chronic alcoholism, or anorexia nervosa and patients maintained NPO for several days with evidence of stress are at risk for refeeding syndrome.[55] The ASPEN consensus criteria for identifying adult patients at risk for refeeding syndrome are listed in Box 6.6. In high-risk patients, nutrition support should be started cautiously at 33% of required calories and slowly advanced over 3 to 6 days as tolerated with concurrent daily supplementation of 100 mg thiamine and multivitamin. Close monitoring of serum electrolytes before and during feeding is essential. Normal values do not always reflect total body stores. Correction of preexisting electrolyte imbalances is necessary before initiation of feeding. Continued monitoring and supplementation with electrolytes and vitamins are necessary throughout the first week of nutrition support.[55]

BOX 6.5 **Safety**

Nursing Management of Total Parenteral Nutrition Complications

Complication	Clinical Manifestations	Prevention or Correction
Hyperglycemia	Thirst, headache, lethargy, increased urinary output	Administer TPN within 10% of ordered rate Monitor blood glucose level at least daily until stable The patient may require insulin added to TPN if hyperglycemia is persistent Sudden appearance of hyperglycemia in a patient who was previously tolerating the same glucose load may indicate the onset of sepsis
Hypoglycemia	Diaphoresis, shakiness, confusion, loss of consciousness	Infuse TPN within 10% of ordered rate Monitor blood glucose until stable If hypoglycemia is present, administer oral carbohydrate If the patient is unconscious or oral intake is contraindicated, the provider may order an IV bolus of dextrose
Hypertriglyceridemia	Serum triglyceride concentrations elevated (especially serious if >400 mg/dL); serum may appear turbid	Monitor serum triglycerides at baseline, 6 h after lipid infusion, and at least three times weekly until stable in patients receiving lipid emulsions Reduce lipid provision in consultation with the dietitian
Catheter-related sepsis	Fever, chills, glucose intolerance, positive blood culture	Use aseptic technique when handling catheter, IV tubing, and TPN solutions Hang a bag of TPN no longer than 24 h and lipid emulsion no longer than 12–24 h Use an in-line 1.2-micron filter with TPN to remove microorganisms Avoid drawing blood, infusing blood or blood products, piggybacking other IV solutions into TPN IV tubing, or attaching manometers or transducers through the TPN infusion line, if possible If catheter-related sepsis is suspected, remove the catheter, and administer antibiotics as ordered
Air embolism	Sudden chest pain, dyspnea, headache, confusion	Maintain occlusion when catheter is not in use If air embolism is suspected, clamp catheter lumens, place the patient in left lateral decubitus and Trendelenburg positions (to trap air in the apex of the right ventricle, away from the outflow tract), and administer oxygen and CPR as needed Immediately notify provider, who may attempt to aspirate air from the heart If pneumothorax is suspected, assist with needle aspiration or chest tube insertion, if necessary
Central venous thrombosis	Edema of neck, shoulder, pain in ipsilateral arm and neck; tight feeling in throat, prominent venous pattern over anterior chest	If thrombosis is confirmed, administer anticoagulants and antibiotics as ordered
Catheter occlusion or semiocclusion	No flow or sluggish flow through the catheter	Prevent with 0.9% normal saline flush between all medications and infusions Ensure external clamps and kinks are opened. Pinch off syndrome requires removal of the catheter

CPR, Cardiopulmonary resuscitation; *IV*, intravenous; *tPA*, tissue plasminogen activator; *TPN*, total parenteral nutrition.
From Cook LS. Infusion-related air embolism. *J Infus Nurs* 2013;36(1):26–36. https://doi.org/10.1097/NAN.0b013e318279a804 and Mueller CM. *The ASPEN Adult Nutrition Support Core Curriculum.* 3rd ed. American Society for Parenteral and Enteral Nutrition; 2017.

NUTRITIONAL CONSIDERATIONS FOR ALTERATIONS IN BODY SYSTEMS

Nutrition-related assessment findings vary widely depending on the type of disorder present. Some common assessment findings are listed in Table 6.8. A nutrition assessment provides the nurse and other members of the health care team the information necessary to plan the patient's nutrition care and education.

Nutrition and Cardiovascular Alterations

Diet and cardiovascular disease may interact in various ways. Excessive nutrient intake—manifested by overweight or obesity and a diet rich in cholesterol and saturated fat—is a risk factor for development of arteriosclerotic heart disease. However, the consequences of chronic myocardial insufficiency can include malnutrition. The major nutrition concerns relate to appropriateness of body weight and the levels of serum lipids and blood pressure.

Myocardial Infarction

Short-term interventions. In the early period after a myocardial infarction, nutrition interventions and education are designed to reduce angina, cardiac workload, and risk of dysrhythmia. Meal size, caffeine intake, and food temperatures are some dietary factors that are of concern. Small, frequent snacks are preferable to larger meals for patients with severe myocardial compromise or postprandial angina.

If caffeine is included in the diet, its effects should be monitored. Because caffeine is a stimulant, it may increase heart rate and myocardial oxygen demand. In the United States and in most industrial nations, coffee is the richest source of caffeine in the diet, with approximately 150 mg of

TABLE 6.9 Metabolic Syndrome Definition[a]

Risk Factor	Defining Level
Elevated Waist Circumference	
Men	≥40 inches (≥102 cm)
Women	≥35 inches (≥88 cm)
Elevated triglycerides	≥150 mg/dL (≥1.7 mmol/L) *or* on medication treatment for elevated triglycerides
Reduced HDL Cholesterol	
Men	<40 mg/dL (<1.03 mmol/L)
Women	<50 mg/dL (<1.3 mmol/L) *or* on medication treatment for reduced HDL cholesterol
Fasting hypertriglyceridemia	≥100 mg/dL
Elevated blood pressure	≥130 mm Hg systolic or ≥85 mm Hg diastolic *or* on antihypertensive medication treatment in a patient with a history of hypertension

[a]Metabolic syndrome is diagnosed when three of five of the listed risk factors are present.
HDL, High-density lipoprotein.

Nutrition and Pulmonary Alterations

Malnutrition has extremely adverse effects on respiratory function, decreasing surfactant production, diaphragmatic mass, vital capacity, and immunocompetence. Patients with acute respiratory disorders find it difficult to consume adequate oral nutrients and can rapidly become malnourished. Individuals who have an acute illness superimposed on chronic respiratory problems are also at high risk. Up to half of patients with chronic obstructive pulmonary disease have malnutrition, and weight loss is a key component of malnutrition.[65] However, patients with undernutrition and end-stage chronic obstructive pulmonary disease often cannot tolerate the increase in metabolic demand that occurs during refeeding. They also are at significant risk for development of cor pulmonale and may fail to tolerate the fluid required for delivery of enteral or parenteral nutrition support. Prevention of severe nutrition deficits, rather than correction of deficits after they have occurred, is important in nutrition management of these patients (see Chapter 19 for information on pulmonary disorders).

Patients with respiratory compromise are especially vulnerable to the effects of fluid volume excess and must be assessed continually for this complication, particularly during enteral and parenteral feeding.

Prevent or Correct Undernutrition and Underweight

The nurse and dietitian work together to encourage oral intake in undernourished or potentially undernourished patients who are capable of eating. Small, frequent feedings are especially important, because a very full stomach can interfere with diaphragmatic movement. Mouth care should be provided before meals and snacks to clear the palate of the taste of sputum and medications. Administering bronchodilators with food can help reduce the gastric irritation caused by these medications.

Many patients require enteral tube feeding because of anorexia, dyspnea, debilitation, or need for ventilatory support. It is especially important for the nurse to be alert to the risk of pulmonary aspiration in a patient with an artificial airway (Box 6.4).

Avoid Overfeeding

Overfeeding of total calories can impair pulmonary function. Carbon dioxide (CO_2) is a metabolic byproduct of carbohydrate and lipids. The volume of carbon dioxide produced (VCO_2) increases when excessive calories are artificially provided. This is unlikely to be significant in a patient who is eating foods. Instead, it is an iatrogenic complication of excessive infusion of enteral or parenteral nutrition. Excessive calorie intake can increase in the partial pressure of carbon dioxide in arterial blood ($PaCO_2$) sufficiently to make it difficult to wean a patient from the ventilator. A balanced regimen with lipids and carbohydrates providing the nonprotein calories is optimal for a patient with respiratory compromise, and the patient needs to be reassessed continually to ensure that caloric intake is not excessive.[1]

Excessive lipid intake can impair capillary gas exchange in the lungs, although this is not usually sufficient to produce an increase $PaCO_2$ or decrease in the partial pressure of oxygen in the arterial blood (PaO_2).[66] However, a patient with severe respiratory alteration may be further compromised by lipid overdose. If lipid intake is maintained at no more than 1 g/kg per day, lipid excess is rarely a problem. Serum triglyceride levels greater than 400 mg/dL may indicate inadequate lipid clearance and a need to decrease the lipid dosage.

Prevent Fluid Volume Excess

Pulmonary edema and failure of the right side of the heart, which may be precipitated by fluid volume excess, further worsen the status of a patient with respiratory compromise. Maintaining careful intake and output records allows for accurate assessment of fluid balance. Usually, the patient requires no more than 35 to 40 mL/kg per day of fluid. For a patient receiving nutrition support, fluid intake can be reduced by using concentrated TPN, by using tube feeding formulas that provide at least 1.5 to 2 calories/mL (the dietitian can recommend appropriate formulas), and by choosing oral supplements that are low in fluid. Additionally, powdered glucose polymers or powdered protein products can be used to increase caloric intake without increasing volume. The nurse plays a valuable role in continually reassessing the patient's state of hydration and recommending changes in fluid intake.

Nutrition and Neurologic Alterations

Because neurologic disorders such as stroke and closed head injury tend to be long-term problems, good nutrition care is necessary to prevent nutrition deficits and promote well-being.

Oral Feedings

Patients with dysphagia or weakness of the swallowing musculature often experience the greatest difficulty in swallowing foods that are dry or thin liquids, such as water, that are difficult to control. For these patients, the nurse, the dietitian, and the speech language pathologist can work together to plan suitable meals and evaluate patient acceptance and tolerance.

Soft, moist foods are usually easier to swallow than dry foods. An upright sitting position is preferable during meals, if possible, to allow gravity to facilitate effective swallowing. Water and other thin liquids may be especially difficult for a person with swallowing dysfunction to manage. Beverages may be thickened with commercial thickening products, with infant cereal, or with yogurt if the patient has difficulty swallowing thin fluids. Fruit nectars may be better tolerated than thinner juices.

The patient should not be rushed while eating, because this may increase the risk of pulmonary aspiration. Providing small amounts of food at frequent intervals rather than larger amounts only at mealtimes may help the patient feel less need to hurry. Suction equipment should be kept available in case aspiration occurs. Dysphagia is frustrating and frightening for the patient and requires much understanding and patience by the family and caregivers.

Tube Feedings

Patients who are unconscious or unable to eat because of severe dysphagia or weakness require tube feedings. Prompt initiation of nutrition support must be a priority in patients with neurologic impairments. Needs for protein and calories are increased by infection and fever, as may occur in a patient with encephalitis or meningitis. Needs for protein, calories, zinc, and vitamin C are increased during wound healing, as occurs in trauma patients and patients with pressure injuries.

Patients with neurologic deficits are at increased risk for certain complications (particularly pulmonary aspiration) during tube feeding and require especially careful nursing management. Patients of most concern are (1) patients with an impaired gag reflex, such as some patients with cerebrovascular accident; (2) patients with delayed gastric emptying, such as patients in the early period after spinal cord injury; and (3) patients likely to experience seizures. Interventions to prevent pulmonary aspiration are listed in Box 6.4.

Hyperglycemia is a common complication in patients receiving corticosteroids. Regular monitoring of blood glucose levels is an important part of care of such patients. They may require insulin to control hyperglycemia.

Prompt use of nutrition support is especially important for patients with head injuries, because head injury causes marked catabolism and hypermetabolism, even in patients who receive barbiturates, which should decrease metabolic demands. Patients with head injury rapidly exhaust glycogen stores and begin to use body proteins to meet energy needs, a process that can quickly lead to PCM. Cortisol, epinephrine, and norepinephrine levels increase leading to increase the metabolic rate and caloric demands, causing mobilization of body fat and proteins to meet the increased energy needs. Patients with head injury undergo an inflammatory response and may be febrile, creating increased needs for protein and calories. Improvement in outcome and reduction in complications have been observed in patients with head injury who receive adequate nutrition support early in the hospital course.[67,68]

Prevention of Overweight and Obesity

Many stable patients with neurologic disorders are less active than their healthy counterparts and require fewer calories. They may become overweight or obese if given normal amounts of calories for their age and sex. Within 1 or 2 months after spinal cord injury, substantial amounts of muscle atrophy and loss of body mass begin to occur as a result of denervation and disuse. However, the caloric needs of this population vary greatly,[69] likely depending on the extent of injury and clinical course. Indirect calorimetry should be used where available, weight trends should be considered within the context of the injury, and a nutrition-focused physical exam should be done with regard to the functional capabilities of each patient.

Patients with dysphagia or extreme swallowing musculature weakness may rely on very soft, easy-to-chew foods that are usually more dense in calories than bulky, high-fiber foods. They also may gain unneeded weight that will hamper their care and impede mobility. For these reasons, nutrition education of the patient with a spinal cord injury and family should include instruction about prevention of undesirable weight gain.

Nutrition and Kidney Alterations

Providing adequate nutrition care for patients with renal disease can be extremely challenging. Although renal disturbances and their treatments can markedly increase needs for nutrients, necessary restrictions in intake of fluid, protein, phosphorus, and potassium make delivery of adequate calories, vitamins, and minerals difficult. A thorough nutrition assessment provides the basis for successful nutrition management in patients with renal disease.

Nutrition needs of patients with renal disease are complex. The goal of nutrition intervention is to balance adequate calories, protein, vitamins, and minerals, while avoiding excesses of protein, fluid, electrolytes, and other nutrients with potential toxicity (see Chapter 25 for information on kidney disorders).

Protein

The kidney is responsible for excreting nitrogen from amino acids or proteins in the form of urea. When urinary excretion of urea is impaired in renal failure, blood urea nitrogen increases. Excessive protein intake may worsen uremia. However, patients with renal failure often have other physiologic stresses that increase protein or amino acid needs, such as losses because of dialysis, wounds, and fistulas; use of corticosteroid medications that exert a catabolic effect; increased endogenous secretion of catecholamines, corticosteroids, and glucagon, all of which can cause or aggravate catabolism; metabolic acidosis, which stimulates protein breakdown; and catabolic conditions such as trauma, surgery, and sepsis.[70] Patients with acute kidney injury need adequate amounts of protein to prevent malnutrition and other complications.[71]

Patients with stable acute kidney injury without evidence of fluid overload or electrolyte or acid-base disturbances can often be managed conservatively without dialysis. However, when renal function worsens, some form of renal replacement therapy is required to maintain homeostasis and prevent metabolic complications. During hemodialysis, amino acids are freely filtered and lost, but proteins such as albumin and immunoglobulin are not. Proteins and amino acids are removed during peritoneal dialysis, creating a greater nutrition requirement for protein.[72] Protein needs may be higher, depending on the level of stress. To limit catabolism, patients with acute kidney injury on dialysis therapy should receive approximately 1.3 to 1.5 g of protein/kg per day (with a maximum of 2.0 g of protein/kg per day), depending on catabolic rate, renal function, and dialysis losses.[1,72]

Fluid

A patient with renal insufficiency usually does not require a fluid restriction until urine output begins to diminish. Patients receiving hemodialysis are limited to a fluid intake resulting in a

SOCIAL DETERMINANTS OF HEALTH

Reducing Household Food Insecurity and Hunger

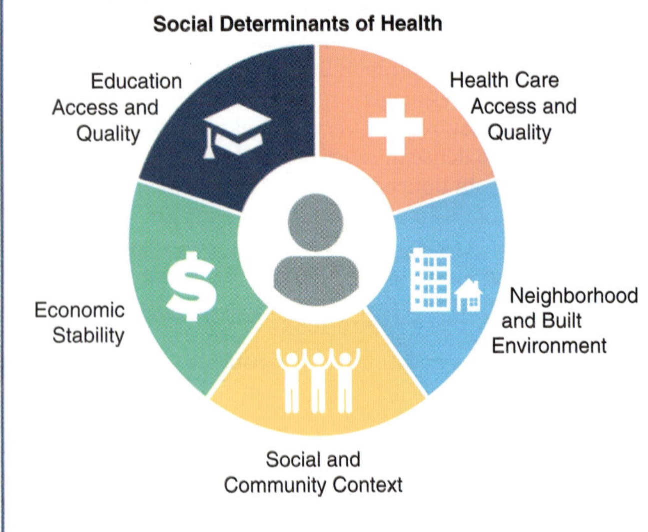

Social Determinants of Health
Copyright-free

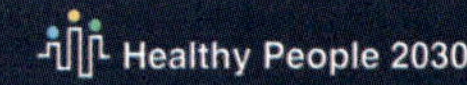

The United States Department of Agriculture categorizes food insecurity into two types: (1) low food security and (2) very low food security.[1] An individual with low food security reports reduced quality, variety, and desirability of their diet.[1] An individual with very low food security reports disrupted eating patterns and reduced food intake.[1] Food insecurity is an economic and social condition of limited or uncertain access to appropriate food.[1] Hunger is a physiological condition that may result from food insecurity.[1] In 2021, the prevalence of food insecurity reported by households was about 10%.[1] Of those households, over 90% reported indicators of food insecurity (e.g., worried food would run out, food did not last, could not afford a balanced meal, cut or skipped a meal), about 50% reported feeling hungry but did not eat and lost weight, and 30% had not eaten in the whole day because of the lack of money for food.[1] Food insecurity disproportionally affects single-mother households,[2] households with incomes below the poverty line,[2] and persons from racial and ethnic minorities.[3]

The practices and policies limiting access to affordable and nutritious food place people with food insecurity at an increased risk for poorer health and the development of chronic disease.[3]

Improving access, affordability, and quality of food options in communities may mediate the social determinants of health that contribute to food insecurity and hunger.[3] Efforts should focus on interventions to improve food security but not substitute the need to address underlying inequities in the distribution of resources.[3] Current strategies to promote food security are focused on developing local community health programs, utilizing federal supplemental programs, and changing local and federal policies.[3] Further research is needed to address the issues related to food insecurity and hunger.[3]

References

1. U.S. Department of Agriculture. *Definitions of Food Security.* 2022. https://www.ers.usda.gov/topics/food-nutrition-assistance/food-security-in-the-u-s/definitions-of-food-security/. Accessed October 3, 2023.
2. U.S. Department of Agriculture. *Food Security and Nutrition Assistance.* 2023. https://www.ers.usda.gov/data-products/ag-and-food-statistics-charting-the-essentials/food-security-and-nutrition-assistance/. Accessed October 3, 2023.
3. National Institute on Minority Health and Health Disparities. *Food Accessibility, Insecurity, and Health Outcomes.* 2023. https://www.nimhd.nih.gov/resources/understanding-health-disparities/food-accessibility-insecurity-and-health-outcomes.html. Accessed October 3, 2023.

Illustration from Healthy People 2030, U.S. Department of Health and Human Services, Office of Disease Prevention and Health Promotion. Retrieved September 8, 2022, from https://health.gov/healthypeople/objectives-and-data/social-determinants-health.

gain of no more than 0.45 kg (1 lb) per day on the days between dialysis. This generally means a daily intake of 500 to 750 mL plus the volume lost in urine. Enteral formulas containing 1.5 to 2 calories/mL or more provide a concentrated source of calories for tube-fed patients who require fluid restriction. Intravenous lipids, particularly 20% emulsions, can be used to supply concentrated calories for the patient receiving TPN.

Energy (Calories)

Energy needs are not increased by renal failure, but adequate calories must be provided to avoid catabolism.[70,72] It is essential that the renal patient receive an adequate number of calories to prevent catabolism of body tissues to meet energy needs. Catabolism reduces muscle mass and other functional body tissues, and it releases nitrogen that must be excreted by the kidney. Adults with renal insufficiency need approximately 30 to 35 calories/kg per day to prevent catabolism and ensure that all protein consumed is used for anabolism rather than to meet energy needs.[72] After renal transplantation, when the patient usually receives large doses of corticosteroids, it is especially important to ensure that caloric intake is adequate (usually 25 to 35 calories/kg per day) to prevent undue catabolism.

Glucose in the peritoneal dialysate may be a significant source of calories and a contributing factor in hypertriglyceridemia. Approximately 45% to 70% of the glucose instilled during peritoneal dialysis to serve as an osmotic agent may be absorbed, and this must be considered part of the patient's carbohydrate intake.[73] The glucose monohydrate dextrose, used in intravenous and dialysate solutions, supplies 3.4 kcal/g. If the patient receives 4.25% glucose (4.25 g glucose/100 mL solution) in the dialysate, they receive:

$$42.5\,\text{g}\frac{\text{dextrose}}{\text{L}}\text{dialysate}\times 3.4\frac{\text{kcal}}{\text{g}}\text{dextrose}\times 0.7$$
$$=1010\frac{\text{kcal}}{\text{L}}\text{dialysate}$$

To help control hypertriglyceridemia, only approximately 30% to 35% of the patient's calories should come from carbohydrates, including glucose from the dialysate. The major portion of dietary carbohydrate should come from complex carbohydrates.

Consuming at least 20 to 25 g of fiber daily can help control triglyceride levels. Sources of dietary fiber include cooked dried beans and peas (5 to 7 g fiber/0.5 cup); cereals containing whole grains (not 100% bran); berries, apples, oranges, pears, corn, and peas (3 to 5 g/serving); whole-grain breads; and most fruits and vegetables other than those listed previously (1 to 2 g/serving). Wheat bran is a good source of fiber (5 to 10 g/oz), but it is also a good source of phosphorus and may cause renal failure to progress more rapidly. For tube-fed patients, a formula containing dietary fiber can be chosen. To help control hypertriglyceridemia and to provide concentrated calories in minimal fluid, fat may need to supply 40% of the patient's calories.

Hypercholesterolemia is commonly found in patients with renal failure, and unsaturated fats and oils (corn, soybean, sunflower, safflower, cottonseed, canola, and olive) are preferred over saturated fats (primarily from meats and dairy products), which tend to raise cholesterol levels. The necessary restriction of meat, milk, and other protein foods in the diet helps lower intake of cholesterol and saturated fat. Intravenous lipids and the long-chain fats found in most commercial enteral formulas are primarily polyunsaturated.

Other Nutrients

Certain nutrients such as potassium and phosphorus are restricted because they are excreted by the kidney. The patient has no specific requirement for the fat-soluble vitamins A, E, and K because they are not removed in appreciable amounts by dialysis, and restriction generally prevents development of toxicity. Patients with end-stage renal disease may have decreased clearance of vitamin A, and levels should be monitored. The needs for several water-soluble vitamins and trace minerals are increased in dialysis patients because they are small enough to pass freely through the dialysis filter. Vitamins and minerals should be supplemented as necessary.[72]

Nutrition and Gastrointestinal Alterations

Because the GI tract is inherently related to nutrition, impairment of the GI tract and its accessory organs has a major effect on nutrition. Two of the most serious GI-related illnesses seen among critically ill patients are hepatic failure and pancreatitis, and the following discussion focuses on these disorders (see Chapter 28).

Hepatic Failure

The liver is the most important metabolic organ. It is responsible for over 500 metabolic pathways including carbohydrate, fat, and protein metabolism; vitamin storage and activation; and detoxification of waste products. Liver failure is associated with a wide spectrum of metabolic alterations. Because the diseased liver has impaired ability to deactivate hormones, levels of circulating glucagon, epinephrine, and cortisol are elevated. These hormones promote catabolism of body tissues and cause glycogen stores to be exhausted. Release of lipids from their storage depots is accelerated, but the liver has decreased ability to metabolize them for energy. Moreover, inadequate production of bile salts by the liver results in malabsorption of fat from the diet. Body proteins are used for energy sources, producing tissue wasting. The damaged liver cannot clear ammonia from the circulation adequately, and ammonia accumulates in the brain. The ammonia may contribute to the encephalopathic symptoms and to brain edema. Aggressive treatment with lactulose is considered first-line therapy in the management of acute hepatic encephalopathy.[74]

Monitoring fluid and electrolyte status. Ascites and edema are caused by a combination of factors. Oncotic pressure in the plasma decreases because of the reduction of production of albumin and other plasma proteins by the diseased liver, increased portal pressure caused by obstruction, and renal sodium retention from secondary hyperaldosteronism. To control the fluid retention, restriction of sodium (usually 2000 mg) and fluid (≤1500 mL daily) usually is necessary in conjunction with the administration of diuretics. Patients are weighed daily to evaluate the success of treatment. Physical status and laboratory data must be closely monitored for deficiencies of potassium; phosphorus; zinc; and vitamins A, D, K, thiamine, folate, and pyridoxine.[74]

Provision of a nutritious diet and evaluation of response to dietary protein. PCM and nutrition deficiencies are common in patients with liver failure. The causes of malnutrition are complex and usually are related to decreased intake, malabsorption, maldigestion, and abnormal nutrient metabolism. Nutrition intervention is individualized and based on these metabolic changes, but generally patients with liver disease will have higher calorie and protein targets depending on the severity of disease and comorbid conditions.[74] Protein restriction, which could lead to PCM, is not recommended as a management strategy for patients with liver disease.[1,74]

Anorexia may interfere with oral intake, and the nurse may need to provide much encouragement to the patient to ensure intake of an adequate diet. Prospective calorie counts may need to be instituted to provide objective evidence of oral intake. Small, frequent feedings are usually better tolerated by an anorexic patient than three large meals daily. If patients are unable to meet their caloric needs, they may require oral supplements or enteral feeding. Small-bore nasoenteric feeding tubes can be used safely without increasing risk of variceal bleeding.[74] TPN should be reserved for patients who are absolutely unable to tolerate enteral feeding.[1,74] Diarrhea from concurrent administration of lactulose should not be confused with feeding intolerance.

A diet adequate in calories is provided to help prevent catabolism and to prevent the use of dietary protein for energy needs.[74] In cases of malabsorption, medium-chain triglycerides may be used to meet caloric needs. Pancreatic enzymes may also be considered for malabsorption problems.

Branched chain–enriched amino acid (BCAA)–enriched products have been developed for enteral and parenteral nutrition of patients with hepatic disease. However, no substantial evidence exists showing that BCAAs are superior to standard formulas in regard to nitrogen balance or as treatment for encephalopathy.[1,74] A patient who undergoes successful liver transplantation is usually able to tolerate a regular diet with few restrictions. Intake during the postoperative period must be adequate to support nutrition repletion and healing; however, many patients requiring liver transplant also have PCM and may require even more protein and calories. Immunosuppressant therapy (corticosteroids and cyclosporine or tacrolimus) contributes to glucose intolerance. Dietary measures to control glucose intolerance include (1) obtaining approximately 30% of dietary calories from fat, (2) emphasizing complex sources of carbohydrates, and (3) eating several small meals daily. Moderate exercise often helps improve glucose tolerance.

Pancreatitis

The pancreas is an exocrine and endocrine gland required for normal digestion and metabolism of proteins, carbohydrates, and fats. Acute pancreatitis is an inflammatory process that occurs as a result of autodigestion of the pancreas by enzymes normally secreted by that organ. Food intake stimulates pancreatic secretion, increasing the damage to the pancreas and the pain associated with the disorder. Patients usually present with abdominal pain and tenderness and with elevations of pancreatic enzymes. Patients with the mild form of acute pancreatitis do not require nutrition support and generally resume oral feeding within 7 days.[1] Chronic pancreatitis may develop, and it is characterized by fibrosis of pancreatic cells. This results in loss of exocrine and endocrine function because of the destruction of acinar and islet cells. The loss of exocrine function leads to malabsorption and steatorrhea. In chronic pancreatitis, the loss of endocrine function results in impaired glucose tolerance.[75]

Prevention of further damage to the pancreas and preventing nutrition deficits. Effective nutrition management is a key treatment for patients with acute pancreatitis or exacerbations of chronic pancreatitis. The concern that feeding may stimulate the production of digestive enzymes and perpetuate tissue damage has led to the widespread use of TPN and bowel rest. Evidence suggest that for patients with severe pancreatitis, providing enteral nutrition support is more beneficial than prolonged bowel rest and provision of TPN.[1,75] The results of randomized studies comparing TPN with enteral nutrition indicate that enteral nutrition is preferable to TPN in patients with severe acute pancreatitis, reducing rates of mortality and multiple organ failure.[75] Enteral nutrition can be administered via the nasogastric route with a standard polymeric formula in most patients. Nasojejunal feeding and or peptide-based formulas are modifications that can be used for patients who fail standard enteral nutrition therapy.[1,75] Patients unable to tolerate enteral nutrition should receive TPN, and some patients may require a combination of enteral nutrition and TPN to meet nutrition requirements.[1,75]

When oral intake is possible, an unrestricted diet should be provided while allowing the patient to self-regulate intake to their tolerance.[1] For patients with signs and symptoms of exocrine pancreatic insufficiency, pancreatic enzyme replacement therapy is indicated.[75] Guidelines for the treatment of diabetes (discussed later) are appropriate for the care of patients with glucose intolerance or diabetes related to pancreatitis.

Nutrition and Endocrine Alterations

Endocrine alterations have far-reaching effects on all body systems and affect nutrition status in a variety of ways. One of the most common endocrine problems in the general population and among critically ill patients is diabetes mellitus (see Chapter 31).

Because of the prevalence of patients with non-insulin-dependent diabetes mellitus (type 2 diabetes) among the hospitalized population and the association of type 2 diabetes with overweight, the nutrition problems most commonly identified in patients with endocrine alterations are overweight and obesity. Hyperglycemia and hyperlipidemia are other common findings in patients with diabetes.

Nutrition Support and Blood Glucose Control

Patients with insulin-dependent diabetes mellitus (type 1 diabetes) or endocrine dysfunction caused by pancreatitis often have weight loss and malnutrition as a result of tissue catabolism because they cannot use dietary carbohydrates to meet energy needs. Although patients with type 2 diabetes are more likely to be overweight than underweight, they also may become malnourished as a result of chronic or acute infections, trauma, major surgery, or other illnesses. Nutrition support should not be neglected because a patient is obese, as PCM can develop in these patients. When a patient is not expected to be able to eat for at least 5 to 7 days or inadequate intake persists for that period, initiation of tube feedings or TPN is indicated. No disease process benefits from starvation, and development or progression of nutrition deficits may contribute to complications such as pressure injuries, pulmonary or urinary tract infections, and sepsis, which prolong hospitalization, increase the costs of care, and may result in death.

Blood glucose control is especially important in the care of surgical patients, with higher glucose levels contributing to poor wound healing and longer lengths of stay.[76] Poorly controlled diabetes reduces immune function by impairing granulocyte adherence, chemotaxis, and phagocytosis.

To maintain tight control of blood glucose, glucose levels are monitored regularly, usually several times a day, until the patient is stable. Patients unable to tolerate oral diets or enteral feeding may require TPN to meet nutrition requirements during acute illness. Regular insulin added to the solution is a common method of managing hyperglycemia in the patient receiving TPN. The dosage required may be larger than the patient's usual dose, because some of the insulin adheres to glass bottles and plastic bags or administration sets. Multiple injections or, preferably, a continuous infusion of regular insulin may be used to maintain tight control of blood glucose in the enterally fed patient. The following glucose goals are recommended: 140 to 180 mg/dL in critically ill patients or a tighter range of 110 to 140 mg/dL in patients with acute cardiac ischemia or an acute neurological event.[76]

Gastroparesis occurs in about 10% of patients with diabetes.[77] In patients receiving enteral tube feedings, the postpyloric route (through a nasoduodenal, nasojejunal, or jejunostomy tube) may be the most effective, because gastroparesis may limit tolerance of intragastric tube feedings. Postpyloric feedings are given continuously, because dumping syndrome and poor absorption may occur if feedings are given rapidly into the small bowel. Continuous enteral infusions are associated with improved control of blood glucose. Fiber-enriched formulas may slow the absorption of the carbohydrate, producing a more delayed and sustained glycemic response. Most standard formulas contain balanced proportions of carbohydrate, protein, and fats appropriate for diabetic patients.

Severe Vomiting or Diarrhea in Patients With Type 1 Diabetes Mellitus

When insulin-dependent patients experience vomiting and diarrhea severe enough to interfere significantly with oral intake or result in excessive fluid and electrolyte losses, adequate carbohydrates and fluids must be supplied. Nausea and vomiting should be treated with antiemetic medication. Delayed gastric emptying is common in diabetes and may improve with administration of prokinetic agents.[77] Small amounts of food or liquids taken every 15 to 20 minutes usually are the best tolerated by a patient with nausea and vomiting. Foods and beverages containing approximately 15 g of carbohydrate include ½ cup of regular gelatin, ½ cup of custard, ¾ cup of regular ginger ale, ½ cup of a regular soft drink, and ½ cup of orange or apple juice. Blood glucose levels should be monitored at least every 2 to 4 hours.

Nutrition Education in Diabetes

Self-monitoring of blood glucose is essential in maintaining diabetic control, and nutrition is considered the most critical component of diabetes care in achieving blood glucose goals.[78] Meals are based on heart-healthy diet principles, according to which saturated fat and cholesterol are limited and protein accounts for 15% to 20% of total calories.[79] Most carbohydrate foods should be whole grains, fruits, vegetables, and low-fat milk.[79] Evidence-based medical nutrition therapy supports hospitals implementing a consistent carbohydrate meal plan for diabetic patients.[79] The meal plan is based on the amount of carbohydrate that is consistent from meal to meal each day. Although exact calorie levels are not specified, a typical daily menu provides approximately 1500 to 2000 calories with a range of three to five carbohydrate foods at each meal, each containing 15 g of carbohydrate.

Careful monitoring of dietary intake and blood glucose levels is essential during critical illness to meet nutrition needs and maintain glucose control. Avoidance of overfeeding limits hyperglycemia and associated complications. Insulin can be adjusted to maintain blood glucose control based on frequent monitoring. Intensive insulin therapy has been shown to reduce mortality rates for critically ill surgical patients.[76] It is vital for the dietitian to work closely with the interprofessional team to determine feeding methods; appropriate enteral formulas; and the amounts of protein, lipid, and carbohydrate supplied in parenteral nutrition.

Nutrition and Surgery

Enhanced recovery after surgery (ERAS) describes the culmination of individual evidence-based practices into streamlined care protocols during the perioperative period. Several sets of guidelines have been published for a variety of elective surgical procedures. These protocols include presurgical, intraoperative, and postsurgical practices that involve the entire interprofessional team. Successful implementation of these guidelines has led to substantial improvement in recovery time, reduced hospital length of stay, and reduced postsurgical complications.

Preoperative Nutrition Optimization

Identifying and correcting malnutrition can mitigate the risk of morbidity and mortality that is associated with preoperative malnutrition. Patients should be screened for malnutrition at the time of diagnosis using a validated screening tool such as the Perioperative Nutrition Screening Score.[80] Patients identified at risk for malnutrition should be referred to the dietitian for individualized interventions to correct malnutrition before surgery.

Preoperative Nutrition Preparation

Patients should be allowed to consume a light meal up to 6 hours before surgery and clear liquids up to 2 hours before surgery. Administration of an oral maltodextrin beverage the evening before surgery and 2 to 3 hours before anesthesia has been demonstrated to improve postoperative insulin sensitivity, decrease protein catabolism, and maintain muscle strength. Caution should be taken when administering high-carbohydrate beverages to patients with diabetes and/or gastroparesis.[81,82]

Postoperative Nutrition Interventions

The goals of postoperative ERAS interventions include timely return of bowel function, normoglycemia, and adequate nutritional intake. Postoperative nausea and vomiting affect 50% and 30%, respectively, of all surgical patients and may result in dehydration and delayed achievement of nutritional goals. All surgical patients should be considered for prophylactic antiemetic therapy. Routine use of nasogastric decompression should be avoided. An oral diet can be initiated immediately after surgery, and patients should be allowed to choose regular foods. Early postoperative oral feeding has been associated with decreased length of stay.[80-82] Allowing patients a choice in their meal selection can help optimize GI tolerance to oral intake, as patients in the postoperative period do not tend to have an appetite for high-fat or high-fiber foods and are rarely able to overconsume calories. Standard oral nutrition supplements can be used to augment intake. Oral immunonutrition supplements are also available but evidence as to their efficacy over a standard oral supplement is not yet clear.[80,81]

For patients who require tube feeding, enteral nutrition can be started along the same timeline as an oral diet. Several other aspects of ERAS protocols are aimed at improving insulin sensitivity and reducing hyperglycemia in the postoperative period, but blood glucose monitoring and insulin should be used to ensure normoglycemia.

EVOLUTION OF NUTRITION SCIENCE

As with all aspects of health sciences, nutrition knowledge and the evidence base for clinical practice are constantly evolving. Nutrition research in particular is very challenging, and often published consensus reviews and guidelines can only provide recommendations for clinical practice based on low-quality evidence. Heterogeneity of patient population, multiple confounding variables on meaningful outcomes, and the practical challenges associated with providing well-controlled nutrition interventions in research trials are some of the challenges with developing a robust evidence base for the practice of medical nutrition therapy. Many of the major trials on nutrition interventions in critical care have used mortality as a primary outcome. However, detecting an effect of nutrition therapy on mortality in the current context of critical care advances would require trials in the tens of thousands; therefore, more attention should be given to other patient-centered outcomes such as functional status.[83]

ADDITIONAL RESOURCES

Refer to Box 6.7 for Internet resources related to nutrition alterations and management.

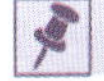

BOX 6.7 Internet Resources

Nutrition Alterations and Management

- Academy of Nutrition and Dietetics: https://www.eatright.org/
- American Society for Parenteral and Enteral Nutrition: http://www.nutritioncare.org/
- Malnutrition Quality Improvement Initiative: http://malnutritionquality.org/
- European Society for Clinical Nutrition and Metabolism: https://www.espen.org
- ERAS Society: http://erassociety.org

CASE STUDY 6.1 Patient With Nutrition Alterations

Brief Patient History

Mrs. W is a 72-year-old person with moderate dementia, atrial fibrillation, and hypertension. Mrs. W lives at home with 24-hour caregivers. Mrs. W has a prior medical history of transient ischemia attack, recurrent urinary tract infection, sepsis, and medication noncompliance. Mrs. W presents to the emergency department with left-sided facial droop, left-sided paralysis, and slurred speech. Mrs. W was found in this condition upon waking by her caregivers and brought immediately to the emergency department.

Diagnostic Procedures

Mrs. W is 5 feet 2 inches tall and weighs 95 lb. Vital signs are as follows: blood pressure of 115/95 mm Hg, heart rate of 107 beats/min (sinus rhythm), respiratory rate of 18 breaths/min, and temperature of 98.2°F. A computed tomography scan reveals a right middle cerebral artery ischemic stroke. Mrs. W underwent successful thrombectomy.

Clinical Assessment

Mrs. W is admitted to the critical care unit for neurologic monitoring. Mrs. W is dysarthric and remains weak on the left side. A speech therapist evaluates and determines that the patient is not safe to swallow. Artificial feeding is recommended, the family is amenable to a short-term trial of tube feeding. The dietitian is consulted and recommends continuous tube feeding with a standard, fiber-containing formula.

Questions

1. What major outcomes do you expect to achieve for this patient?
2. What problems or risks must be managed to achieve these outcomes?
3. What interventions could be initiated to monitor, prevent, manage, or eliminate the problems and risks identified?
4. What interventions could be initiated to promote optimal functioning, safety, and well-being of the patient?
5. What technology can be used to monitor this patient and prevent complications?
6. What other interprofessional team members are needed to assist with the management of this patient?
7. What possible learning needs would you anticipate for this patient?
8. What cultural and age-related factors might have a bearing on the patient's plan of care?

KEY POINTS

Nutrient Metabolism

- The major purposes of metabolism of the energy-yielding nutrients are the production of energy and the formation and preservation of lean body mass.

Focused Assessment of Nutrition Status

- Nutrition screening should be conducted on every patient, and a more thorough nutrition assessment should be completed by a dietitian on any patient screened to be nutritionally at risk.

Malnutrition

- Malnutrition can be related to any essential nutrient or nutrients, but a serious type of malnutrition found frequently among hospitalized patients is protein-calorie malnutrition.
- Malnutrition is associated with various adverse outcomes, including wound dehiscence, pressure injuries, infections, respiratory failure requiring ventilation, longer hospital stays, readmission, and death.

Oral Intake

- Completing a swallow evaluation prior to initiating oral intake is important to prevent aspiration.
- Swallow evaluations include screening protocols and possibly instrumental assessments with ultrasound, video fluoroscopy, or fiberoptic endoscopy.
- Oral supplementation may be necessary for patients who can eat and have normal digestion and absorption.

Enteral and Nutritional Nutrition Support

- Whenever possible, the enteral route is the preferred method of feeding because of lower cost, better maintenance of gut integrity, and decreased hospital stay.
- Early enteral nutrition (within the first 24 to 48 hours of critical illness) reduces septic complications and improves feeding tolerance in critically ill patients.
- It is essential to check tube placement before feedings and regularly throughout the course of enteral feedings.

Refeeding Syndrome

- Refeeding syndrome is a potentially lethal condition characterized by generalized fluid and electrolyte imbalance. Patients should be screened for refeeding syndrome before initiating nutrition support.
- Patients with chronic malnutrition or underfeeding, chronic alcoholism, or anorexia nervosa and patients maintained NPO for several days with evidence of stress are at risk for refeeding syndrome.

Nutritional Considerations for Alterations in Body Systems

- Nutrition-related assessment findings vary widely depending on the type of disorder present.
- In the early period after a myocardial infarction, interventions are aimed at reducing angina, cardiac workload, and the risk of dysrhythmia; meal size, caffeine intake, and food temperatures are monitored closely.
- Because of anorexia, dyspnea, debilitation, or the need for ventilatory support, many patients with pulmonary alterations require enteral tube feeding.
- Patients with dysphagia or weakness of the swallowing musculature often experience the greatest difficulty in swallowing foods that are dry or thin liquids, such as water, which are difficult to control. Beverages may be thickened with commercial thickening products, infant cereal, or yogurt; fruit nectars may be better tolerated than fruit juices.
- The nutritional goal in patients with kidney disease is to balance adequate calories, protein, vitamins, and minerals while avoiding excesses of proteins, fluid, electrolytes, and other nutrients with potential toxicities.
- Causes of malnutrition in liver failure are complex and related to decreased intake, malabsorption, maldigestion, and abnormal nutrient metabolism.
- In a patient with pancreatitis, enteral feeding is ideally delivered past the ligament of Treitz, which will not stimulate the production of digestive enzymes; however, gastric feeding is also acceptable.
- One of the most common endocrine problems in the general population and among critically ill patients is diabetes.
- Patients should be allowed to consume a light meal up to 6 hours before surgery and clear liquids up to 2 hours before surgery. An oral carbohydrate beverage should be

administered the evening before surgery and 2 to 3 hours before anesthesia. An oral diet can be initiated within 4 hours of surgery, and patients should be allowed to choose regular foods.

Visit the Evolve site at http://evolve.elsevier.com/Urden/CriticalCareNursing for additional study materials.

REFERENCES

1. McClave SA, Taylor BE, Martindale RG, Society of Critical Care Medicine; American Society for Parenteral and Enteral Nutrition, et al. Guidelines for the provision and assessment of nutrition support therapy in the adult critically ill patient: Society of Critical Care Medicine (SCCM) and American Society for Parenteral and Enteral Nutrition (A.S.P.E.N.). *JPEN J Parenter Enteral Nutr*. 2016;40(2):159–211. https://doi.org/10.1177/0148607115621863.
2. Ukleja A, Gilbert K, Mogensen KM, et al. Task Force on Standards for Nutrition Support: Adult Hospitalized Patients, the American Society for
3. Hamilton C. *Nutrition-Focused Physical Exam: An Illustrated Handbook*. 2nd ed. American Society of Parenteral and Enteral Nutrition; 2016.
4. Evans DC, Corkins MR, Malone A, et al. The use of visceral proteins as nutrition markers: an ASPEN position paper. *Nutr Clin Pract*. 2021;36(1):22–28. https://doi.org/10.1002/ncp.10588.
5. Singer P, Singer J. Clinical guide for the use of metabolic carts: indirect calorimetry—no longer the orphan of energy estimation. *Nutr Clin Pract*. 2016;31(1):30–38. https://doi.org/10.1177/0884533615622536.
6. Siobal MS, Baltz JE, Wright J. A guide to the nutritional assessment and treatment of the critically ill patient. 2nd ed. *Respiratory Care*. 2021. https://www.aarc.org/wp-content/uploads/2014/11/nutrition_guide.pdf. Accessed September 28, 2023.
7. Frankenfield DC, Ashcraft CM. Toward the development of predictive equations for resting metabolic rate in acutely ill spontaneously breathing patients. *JPEN J Parenter Enteral Nutr*. 2017;41(7):1155–1161. https://doi.org/10.1177/0148607116657647.
8. Parker EA, Feinberg TM, Wappel S, Verceles AC. Considerations when using predictive equations to estimate energy needs among older, hospitalized patients: a narrative review. *Curr Nutr Rep*. 2017;6(2):102–110. https://doi.org/10.1007/s13668-017-0196-8.
9. Dickerson RN, Patel JJ, McClain CJ. Protein and calorie requirements associated with the presence of obesity. *Nutr Clin Pract*. 2017;32(1_suppl):86S–93S. https://doi.org/10.1177/0884533617691745.
10. Tignanelli CJ, Andrews AG, Sieloff KM, et al. Are predictive energy expenditure equations in ventilated surgery patients accurate? *J Intensive Care Med*. 2019;34(5):426–431. https://doi.org/10.1177/0885066617702077.
11. Lew CCH, Yandell R, Fraser RJL, Chua AP, Chong MFF, Miller M. Association between malnutrition and clinical outcomes in the intensive care unit: a systematic review [Formula: see text]. *JPEN J Parenter Enteral Nutr*. 2017;41(5):744–758. https://doi.org/10.1177/0148607115625638.
12. Sharma K, Mogensen KM, Robinson MK. Pathophysiology of critical illness and role of nutrition. *Nutr Clin Pract*. 2019;34(1):12–22. https://doi.org/10.1002/ncp.10232.
13. Guenter P, Abdelhadi R, Anthony P, et al. Malnutrition diagnoses and associated outcomes in hospitalized patients: United States, 2018. *Nutr Clin Pract*. 2021;36(5):957–969. https://doi.org/10.1002/ncp.10771.
14. Hudson L, Chittams J, Griffith C, Compher C. Malnutrition identified by Academy of Nutrition and Dietetics/American Society for Parenteral and Enteral Nutrition is associated with more 30-day readmissions, greater hospital mortality, and longer hospital stays: a retrospective analysis of nutrition assessment data in a major medical center. *JPEN J Parenter Enteral Nutr*. 2018;42(5):892–897. https://doi.org/10.1002/jpen.1021.
15. Lew CCH, Yandell R, Fraser RJL, Chua AP, Chong MFF, Miller M. Association between malnutrition and clinical outcomes in the intensive care unit: a systematic review [Formula: see text]. *JPEN J Parenter Enteral Nutr*. 2017;41(5):744–758. https://doi.org/10.1177/0148607115625638.
16. Mogensen KM, Malone A, Becker P, et al. Malnutrition Committee of the American Society for Parenteral and Enteral Nutrition (ASPEN). Academy of Nutrition and Dietetics/American Society for Parenteral and Enteral Nutrition consensus malnutrition characteristics: usability and association with outcomes. *Nutr Clin Pract*. 2019;34(5):657–665. https://doi.org/10.1002/ncp.10310.
17. White JV, Guenter P, Jensen G, Malone A, Schofield M, Academy Malnutrition Work Group, A.S.P.E.N. Malnutrition Task Force, A.S.P.E.N. Board of Directors. Consensus statement: Academy of Nutrition and Dietetics and American Society for Parenteral and Enteral Nutrition: characteristics recommended for the identification and documentation of adult malnutrition (undernutrition). *JPEN J Parenter Enteral Nutr*. 2012;36(3):275–283. https://doi.org/10.1177/0148607112440285.
18. Cederholm T, Jensen GL, Correia MITD, GLIM Core Leadership Committee, GLIM Working Group, et al. GLIM criteria for the diagnosis of malnutrition – a consensus report from the global clinical nutrition community. *Clin Nutr*. 2019;38(1):1–9. https://doi.org/10.1016/j.clnu.2018.08.002.
19. Labeit B, Michou E, Hamdy S, et al. The assessment of dysphagia after stroke: state of the art and future directions. *Lancet Neurol*. 2023;22(9):858–870. https://doi.org/10.1016/S1474-4422(23)00153-9.
20. Maeda K, Nagasaka M, Nagano A, et al. Ultrasonography for eating and swallowing assessment: a narrative review of integrated insights for noninvasive clinical practice. *Nutrients*. 2023;15(16):3560. https://doi.org/10.3390/nu15163560.
21. Lawlor CM, Choi SS. Videofluoroscopic swallow study and fiberoptic endoscopic evaluation of swallow, which is superior? *Laryngoscope*. 2023;133(10):2445–2446. https://doi.org/10.1002/lary.30755.
22. Compher C, Bingham AL, McCall M, et al. Guidelines for the provision of nutrition support therapy in the adult critically ill patient: the American Society for Parenteral and Enteral Nutrition. *JPEN J Parenter Enteral Nutr*. 2022;46(1):12–41. https://doi.org/10.1002/jpen.2267.
23. Liu Y, Zhao W, Chen W, et al. Effects of early enteral nutrition on immune function and prognosis of patients with sepsis on mechanical ventilation. *J Intensive Care Med*. 2020;35(10):1053–1061. https://doi.org/10.1177/0885066618809893.
24. Church A, Zoeller S. Enteral nutrition product formulations: a review of available products and indications for use. *Nutr Clin Pract*. 2023;38(2):277–300. https://doi.org/10.1002/ncp.10960.
25. Yang S, Wu X, Yu W, Li J. Early enteral nutrition in critically ill patients with hemodynamic instability: an evidence-based review and practical advice. *Nutr Clin Pract*. 2014;29(1):90–96. https://doi.org/10.1177/0884533613516167.
26. Bechtold ML, Brown PM, Escuro A, ASPEN Enteral Nutrition Committee, et al. When is enteral nutrition indicated? *JPEN J Parenter Enteral Nutr*. 2022;46(7):1470–1496. https://doi.org/10.1002/jpen.2364.
27. Reddick CA, Greaves JR, Flaherty JE, Callihan LE, Larimer CH, Allen SA. Choosing wisely: enteral feeding tube selection, placement, and considerations before and beyond the procedure room. *Nutr Clin Pract*. 2023;38(2):216–239. https://doi.org/10.1002/ncp.10959.
28. Neyens RR, Hill ML, Huber MR, Chalela JA. Prokinetic agents with enteral nutrition. In: Rajendram R, Preedy VR, Patel VB, eds. *Diet and Nutrition in Critical Care*. New York, NY: Springer; 2015:1323–1332.
29. Malone A, Carney LN, Carrera AL, Mays A. *ASPEN Enteral Nutrition Handbook*. 2nd ed. Silver Spring, MD: American Society for Parenteral and Enteral Nutrition; 2019.
30. Powers J, Luebbehusen M, Aguirre L, et al. Improved safety and efficacy of small-bore feeding tube confirmation using an electromagnetic placement device. *Nutr Clin Pract*. 2018;33(2):268–273. https://doi.org/10.1002/ncp.10062.
31. Carter M, Roberts S, Carson JA. Small-bowel feeding tube placement at bedside: electronic medical device placement and x-ray agreement. *Nutr Clin Pract*. 2018;33(2):274–280. https://doi.org/10.1002/ncp.10072.
32. Lash K, Oppel R, Hasse J. Successful placement of nasointestinal feeding tubes using an electromagnetic sensor-guided enteral access system in patients with left ventricular assist devices. *Nutr Clin Pract*. 2018;33(2):281–285. https://doi.org/10.1002/ncp.10065.
33. Liu Y, Wang Y, Zhang B, Wang J, Sun L, Xiao Q. Gastric-tube versus post-pyloric feeding in critical patients: a systematic review and meta-analysis

of pulmonary aspiration- and nutrition-related outcomes. *Eur J Clin Nutr.* 2021;75(9):1337–1348. https://doi.org/10.1038/s41430-021-00860-2.
34. Bolgeo T, Di Matteo R, Gallione C, et al. Intragastric prepyloric enteral nutrition, bolus vs continuous in the adult patient: a systematic review and meta-analysis. *Nutr Clin Pract.* 2022;37(4):762–772. https://doi.org/10.1002/ncp.10836.
35. Thong D, Halim Z, Chia J, Chua F, Wong A. Systematic review and meta-analysis of the effectiveness of continuous vs intermittent enteral nutrition in critically ill adults. *JPEN J Parenter Enteral Nutr.* 2022;46(6):1243–1257. https://doi.org/10.1002/jpen.2324.
36. Metheny NA, Mills AC, Stewart BJ. Monitoring for intolerance to gastric tube feedings: a national survey. *Am J Crit Care.* 2012;21(2):e33–e40. https://doi.org/10.4037/ajcc2012647.
37. Maloney JP, Ryan TA. Detection of aspiration in enterally fed patients: a requiem for bedside monitors of aspiration. *JPEN J Parenter Enteral Nutr.* 2002;26(6 Suppl):S34–S41; discussion S41-S42. https://doi.org/10.1177/014860710202600606.
38. Lucarelli MR, Shirk MB, Julian MW, Crouser ED. Toxicity of food Drug and cosmetic blue No. 1 dye in critically ill patients. *Chest.* 2004;125(2):793–795. https://doi.org/10.1378/chest.125.2.793.
39. McClave SA, DeMeo MT, DeLegge MH, et al. North American summit on aspiration in the critically ill patient: consensus statement. *JPEN J Parenter Enteral Nutr.* 2002;26(6 Suppl):S80–S85. https://doi.org/10.1177/014860710202600613.
40. Pitta MR, Campos FM, Monteiro AG, Cunha AGF, Porto JD, Gomes RR. Tutorial on diarrhea and enteral nutrition: a comprehensive step-by-step approach. *JPEN J Parenter Enteral Nutr.* 2019;43(8):1008–1019. https://doi.org/10.1002/jpen.1674.
41. Stumpf JL, Kurian RM, Vuong J, Dang K, Kraft MD. Efficacy of a Creon delayed-release pancreatic enzyme protocol for clearing occluded enteral feeding tubes. *Ann Pharmacother.* 2014;48(4):483–487. https://doi.org/10.1177/1060028013515435.
42. Bankhead R, Boullata JB, Brantley S, et al. A.S.P.E.N. Board of Directors. A.S.P.E.N. enteral nutrition practice recommendations. *JPEN J Parenter Enteral Nutr.* 2009;33(2):122–167. https://doi.org/10.1177/0148607108330314.
43. Ichimaru S. Methods of enteral nutrition administration in critically ill patients: continuous, cyclic, intermittent, and bolus feeding. *Nutr Clin Pract.* 2018;33(6):790–795. https://doi.org/10.1002/ncp.10105.
44. Roberts S, Brody R, Rawal S, Byham-Gray L. Volume-based vs rate-based enteral nutrition in the intensive care unit: impact on nutrition delivery and glycemic control. *JPEN J Parenter Enteral Nutr.* 2019;43(3):365–375. https://doi.org/10.1002/jpen.1428.
45. McClave SA, Saad MA, Esterle M, et al. Volume-based feeding in the critically ill patient. *JPEN J Parenter Enteral Nutr.* 2015;39(6):707–712. https://doi.org/10.1177/0148607114540004.
46. Medical device connectors. US Food and Drug Administration; 2018. https://www.fda.gov/MedicalDevices/ProductsandMedicalProcedures/GeneralHospitalDevicesandSupplies/TubingandLuerMisconnections/default.htm#misconnections. Accessed October 2, 2023.
47. Sentinel event alert 36. Tubing misconnections a persistent and potentially deadly occurrence. The Joint Commission; 2016. https://www.jointcommission.org/resources/sentinel-event/sentinel-event-alert-newsletters/sentinel-event-alert-53-managing-risk-during-transition-to-new-iso-tubing-connector-standards/. Accessed October 2, 2023.
48. Sentinel event alert 53: managing risk during transition to new ISO tubing connector standards. The Joint Commission; 2023. https://www.jointcommission.org/resources/sentinel-event/sentinel-event-alert-newsletters/sentinel-event-alert-53-managing-risk-during-transition-to-new-iso-tubing-connector-standards/. Accessed October 2, 2023.
49. Implementing the ENFit initiative for preventing enteral tubing misconnections. ECRI; 2017. https://www.ecri.org/components/HDJournal/Pages/ENFit-for-Preventing-Enteral-Tubing-Misconnections.aspx. Accessed October 2, 2023.
50. Boullata JI, Gilbert K, Sacks G, et al. American Society for Parenteral and Enteral Nutrition. A.S.P.E.N. clinical guidelines. Parenteral nutrition ordering, order review, compounding, labeling, and dispensing. *JPEN J Parenter Enteral Nutr.* 2014;38(3):334–377. https://doi.org/10.1177/0148607114521833.
51. Ayers P, Adams S, Boullata J, et al. American Society for Parenteral and Enteral Nutrition. A.S.P.E.N. parenteral nutrition safety consensus recommendations. *JPEN J Parenter Enteral Nutr.* 2014;38(3):296–333. https://doi.org/10.1177/0148607113511992.
52. Worthington P, Gura KM, Kraft MD, Nishikawa R, Guenter P, Sacks GS, ASPEN PN Safety Committee. Update on the use of filters for parenteral nutrition: an ASPEN position paper. *Nutr Clin Pract.* 2021;36(1):29–39. https://doi.org/10.1002/ncp.10587.
53. Mirtallo JM, Ayers P, Boullata J, et al. ASPEN lipid injectable emulsion safety recommendations, part 1: background and adult considerations. *Nutr Clin Pract.* 2020;35(5):769–782. https://doi.org/10.1002/ncp.10496.
54. Ayers P, et al. Parenteral nutrition access devices. In: Ayers P, Bobo ES, Hunt RT, Mays AA, Worthington PH, eds. *ASPEN Parenteral Nutrition Handbook.* 3rd ed. Silver Spring, MD: American Society for Parenteral and Enteral Nutrition; 2020.
55. da Silva JSV, Seres DS, Sabino K, et al. Parenteral Nutrition Safety and Clinical Practice Committees. American Society for Parenteral and Enteral Nutrition. ASPEN consensus recommendations for refeeding syndrome. *Nutr Clin Pract.* 2020;35(2):178–195. https://doi.org/10.1002/ncp.10474.
56. Adult nutrition care – nutrition intervention. *Nutrition Care Manual*; 2023. https://www.nutritioncaremanual.org/adult-nutrition-care. Accessed October 3, 2023.
57. The American Heart Association diet and lifestyle recommendations. American Heart Association; 2023. https://www.heart.org/en/healthy-living/healthy-eating/eat-smart/nutrition-basics/aha-diet-and-lifestyle-recommendations. Accessed October 3, 2023.
58. Grundy SM, Stone NJ, Bailey AL, et al. 2018 AHA/ACC/AACVPR/AAPA/ABC/ACPM/ADA/AGS/APhA/ASPC/NLA/PCNA guideline on the management of blood cholesterol: a report of the American College of Cardiology/American Heart Association Task Force on Clinical Practice Guidelines. *Circulation.* 2019;139(25):e1082–e1143. https://doi.org/10.1161/CIR.0000000000000625.
59. Fahed G, Aoun L, Bou Zerdan M, et al. Metabolic syndrome: updates on pathophysiology and management in 2021. *Int J Mol Sci.* 2022;23(2):786. https://doi.org/10.3390/ijms23020786.
60. Ebbing M, Bleie Ø, Ueland PM, et al. Mortality and cardiovascular events in patients treated with homocysteine-lowering B vitamins after coronary angiography: a randomized controlled trial. *JAMA.* 2008;300(7):795–804. https://doi.org/10.1001/jama.300.7.795.
61. Filippou CD, Tsioufis CP, Thomopoulos CG, et al. Dietary Approaches to Stop Hypertension (DASH) diet and blood pressure reduction in adults with and without hypertension: a systematic review and meta-analysis of randomized controlled trials. *Adv Nutr.* 2020;11(5):1150–1160. https://doi.org/10.1093/advances/nmaa041.
62. Adult nutrition care – nutrient prescription. *Nutrition Care Manual.* 2023. https://www.nutritioncaremanual.org/adult-nutrition-care. Accessed October 3, 2023.
63. Directo D, Lee SR. Cancer cachexia: underlying mechanisms and potential therapeutic interventions. *Metabolites.* 2023;13(9):1024. https://doi.org/10.3390/metabo13091024.
64. Christensen HM, Kistorp C, Schou M, et al. Prevalence of cachexia in chronic heart failure and characteristics of body composition and metabolic status. *Endocrine.* 2013;43(3):626–634. https://doi.org/10.1007/s12020-012-9836-3.
65. Yde SK, Mikkelsen S, Brath MSG, Holst M. Unintentional weight loss is reflected in worse one-year clinical outcomes among COPD outpatients. *Clin Nutr.* 2023;42(11):2173–2180. https://doi.org/10.1016/j.clnu.2023.09.012.
66. Boisramé-Helms J, Toti F, Hasselmann M, Meziani F. Lipid emulsions for parenteral nutrition in critical illness. *Prog Lipid Res.* 2015;60:1–16. https://doi.org/10.1016/j.plipres.2015.08.002.
67. Şimşek T, Şimşek HU, Cantürk NZ. Response to trauma and metabolic changes: posttraumatic metabolism. *Ulus Cerrahi Derg.* 2014;30(3):153–159. https://doi.org/10.5152/UCD.2014.2653.
68. Wang X, Dong Y, Han X, Qi XQ, Huang CG, Hou LJ. Nutritional support for patients sustaining traumatic brain injury: a systematic review and meta-analysis of prospective studies. *PLoS One.* 2013;8(3):e58838. https://doi.org/10.1371/journal.pone.0058838.

69. Nevin AN, Steenson J, Vivanit A, Hickman IJ. Investigation of measured and predicted resting energy needs in adults after spinal cord injury: a systematic review. *Spinal Cord*. 2016;54(4):248–253. https://doi.org/10.1038/sc.2015.193.
70. Ikizler TA, Cano NJ, Franch H, et al. International Society of Renal Nutrition and Metabolism. Prevention and treatment of protein energy wasting in chronic kidney disease patients: a consensus statement by the International Society of Renal Nutrition and Metabolism. *Kidney Int*. 2013;84(6):1096–1107. https://doi.org/10.1038/ki.2013.147.
71. Piccoli GB, Cederholm T, Avesani CM, et al. Nutritional status and the risk of malnutrition in older adults with chronic kidney disease – implications for low protein intake and nutritional care: a critical review endorsed by ERN-ERA and ESPEN. *Clin Nutr*. 2023;42(4):443–457. https://doi.org/10.1016/j.clnu.2023.01.018.
72. Fiaccadori E, Sabatino A, Barazzoni R, et al. ESPEN guideline on clinical nutrition in hospitalized patients with acute or chronic kidney disease. *Clin Nutr*. 2021;40(4):1644–1668. https://doi.org/10.1016/j.clnu.2021.01.028.
73. Wen Y, Guo Q, Yang X, et al. High glucose concentrations in peritoneal dialysate are associated with all-cause and cardiovascular disease mortality in continuous ambulatory peritoneal dialysis patients. *Perit Dial Int*. 2015;35(1):70–77. https://doi.org/10.3747/pdi.2013.00083.
74. Bischoff SC, Bernal W, Dasarathy S, et al. ESPEN practical guideline: clinical nutrition in liver disease. *Clin Nutr*. 2020;39(12):3533–3562. https://doi.org/10.1016/j.clnu.2020.09.001.
75. Arvanitakis M, Ockenga J, Bezmarevic M, et al. ESPEN guideline on clinical nutrition in acute and chronic pancreatitis. *Clin Nutr*. 2020;39(3):612–631. https://doi.org/10.1016/j.clnu.2020.01.004.
76. Silva-Perez LJ, Benitez-Lopez MA, Varon J, Surani S. Management of critically ill patients with diabetes. *World J Diabetes*. 2017;8(3):89–96. https://doi.org/10.4239/wjd.v8.i3.89.
77. Li L, Wang L, Long R, Song L, Yue R. Prevalence of gastroparesis in diabetic patients: a systematic review and meta-analysis. *Sci Rep*. 2023;13(1):14015.
78. Samson SL, Vellanki P, Blonde L, et al. American Association of Clinical Endocrinology consensus statement: comprehensive type 2 diabetes management algorithm – 2023 update [published correction appears in *Endocr Pract*. 2023 Sep;29(9):746]. *Endocr Pract*. 2023;29(5):305–340. https://doi.org/10.1016/j.eprac.2023.02.001.
79. Evert AB, Boucher JL, Cypress M, et al. Nutrition therapy recommendations for the management of adults with diabetes. *Diabetes Care*. 2014;37(Suppl 1):S120–S143. https://doi.org/10.2337/dc14-S120.
80. Noorian S, Kwaan MR, Jaffe N, Yaceczko SD, Chau LW. Perioperative nutrition for gastrointestinal surgery: on the cutting edge. *Nutr Clin Pract*. 2023;38(3):539–556. https://doi.org/10.1002/ncp.10970.
81. Weimann A, Braga M, Carli F, et al. ESPEN practical guideline: clinical nutrition in surgery. *Clin Nutr*. 2021;40(7):4745–4761. https://doi.org/10.1016/j.clnu.2021.03.031.
82. Gustafsson UO, Scott MJ, Hubner M, et al. Guidelines for perioperative care in elective colorectal surgery: Enhanced Recovery after Surgery (ERAS®) Society recommendations: 2018. *World J Surg*. 2019;43(3):659–695. https://doi.org/10.1007/s00268-018-4844-y.
83. Fetterplace K, Ridley EJ, Beach L, et al. Quantifying response to nutrition therapy during critical illness: implications for clinical practice and research? A narrative review. *JPEN J Parenter Enteral Nutr*. 2021;45(2):251–266. https://doi.org/10.1002/jpen.1949.

7

Pain and Pain Management

Céline Gélinas

http://evolve.elsevier.com/Urden/CriticalCareNursing

Most, if not all, patients will experience some degree of pain during their stay in the critical care unit, and the prevalence of moderate to severe pain in this population is high (>50%)[1] and disturbingly similar to that described two decades ago.[2] Acute pain is an important risk factor for the chronic pain development, and chronic pain after discharge from the critical care unit is high with prevalence ranging from 28% to 77%, which can negatively affect daily functioning and quality of life.[3] Therefore, adequate management of pain is crucial and should be rethought considering the context of the opioid crisis in North America.[4,5] Pain treatment should not rely on opioids solely and must be based on a multimodal approach including nonopioids and nonpharmacologic interventions.[6,7] This chapter discusses common challenges related to pain assessment and evidence-based tools as well as approaches for optimal and safe pain management.

PAIN

Appropriate pain assessment is the foundation of effective pain treatment. Because pain is recognized as a personal experience, the patient's self-report is considered the reference standard measure for pain and should be obtained as often as possible.[8] In critical care, many factors, such as the administration of sedative agents, the use of mechanical ventilation, altered levels of consciousness, and delirium, may affect communication with patients.[9] These obstacles make pain assessment more complex. Nevertheless, except for being unable to speak, many mechanically ventilated patients can communicate that they are in pain by using head nodding, using hand motions, or seeking attention with other movements.[9] In such a situation, various communication methods are available and should be used to facilitate the self-report of symptoms in mechanically ventilated patients.[10]

Self-report pain intensity scales have been used with postoperative mechanically ventilated patients who were asked to point on the scale.[1] With a greater degree of critical illness, providing a pain intensity self-report becomes more difficult because it requires concentration and energy. When the patient is unable to communicate in any way, behavioral assessment tools are alternative pain reference measures to use as described in clinical guidelines and recommendations developed in North America.[6,11-13] Pain is frequently encountered in critical care, and there is increased emphasis on the professional responsibility to provide effective and safe management of pain. The critical care nurse must understand the mechanisms, assessment process, and appropriate therapeutic interventions for managing pain.

Definition and Description of Pain

According to the updated definition by the *International Association for Study on Pain* (IASP), pain is described as an unpleasant sensory and emotional experience associated with, or resembling that associated with, actual or potential tissue damage.[8] Therefore, pain is always a personal experience that is influenced by biological, psychological, and social factors. Williams and Craig[14] have also highlighted that pain is a distressing experience associated with sensory, emotional, cognitive, and social/behavioral components. In summary, pain is a personal and multidimensional experience. The patient's self-report is the reference standard measure of pain that should be obtained whenever possible and respected.[8,15] However, in the critical care context, many patients are unable to self-report their pain. Anand and Craig[16] have proposed an alternative definition for nonverbal patients, in this case infants, but the same principle applies to any nonverbal population, stating that changes in behaviors caused by pain are valuable forms of self-report and should be considered as alternative measures of pain. The IASP has also acknowledged that the inability to communicate verbally does not negate the possibility that an individual is experiencing pain and should receive appropriate pain management.[8] Pain assessment must be designed to conform to the communication capabilities of the patient.

Components of Pain

The experience of pain includes several components:[14,17]

- The sensory component is the perception of many characteristics of pain such as intensity, location, and quality.
- The emotional component includes negative emotions such as unpleasantness, distress, and anticipation that may be associated with the experience of pain. Anxiety and fear can also be related to the experience of pain.
- The cognitive component refers to the interpretation or the meaning of pain by the person who is experiencing it.
- The behavioral component includes the behaviors used by the person to express, avoid, or control pain.
- The physiologic component refers to nociception and the stress response.

Types of Pain

Pain can be acute or chronic, with different sensations related to the origin of the pain: nociceptive, neuropathic, or nociplastic.[8] A patient may present with different types of pain simultaneously, which refers to mixed pain.[18]

Acute Pain

Acute pain has a short duration, it usually corresponds to the healing process, and it should not exceed 3 months.[19] It implies tissue damage that is usually from an identifiable cause. If undertreated, acute pain may bring a prolonged stress response and lead to permanent damage to the patient's nervous system. In such a situation, acute pain can become chronic.

Chronic Pain

Chronic pain persists or recurs for more than 3 months after the healing process from the tissue damage, and it may or may not be associated with an illness.[19] Chronic pain may develop from acute pain that is poorly managed and involves complex physiological mechanisms. Both acute and chronic pain can have a nociceptive, neuropathic, or nociplastic origin.

Nociceptive Pain

Nociceptive pain arises from activation of nociceptors, and it can be somatic or visceral.[8,20] Somatic pain involves superficial tissues such as the skin, muscles, joints, and bones. Its location is well defined. Visceral pain involves organs such as the heart, stomach, and liver. Its location is diffuse, and it can be referred to a different location in the body. Not all organs are sensitive to pain, and some can be damaged extensively without the patient feeling anything. For example, many diseases of the liver, lungs, or kidneys are completely painless, and the only symptoms felt are symptoms derived from the abnormal functioning of these organs. Relatively minor lesions in viscera such as the stomach, the bladder, or the ureters can produce excruciating pain, as these organs are abundantly innervated by sensory neurons that signal harmful events.[21]

Neuropathic Pain

Neuropathic pain arises from a lesion or disease affecting the somatosensory system.[8] The origin of neuropathic pain may be peripheral or central. Neuralgia and neuropathy are examples related to peripheral neuropathic pain, which implies damage of the peripheral somatosensory system. Central neuropathic pain involves the central somatosensory cortex and can be experienced by patients after a cerebral stroke or a brain injury. Neuropathic pain can be difficult to manage and frequently requires a multimodal approach (i.e., combinations of several pharmacologic or nonpharmacologic treatments).[20]

Nociplastic Pain

Nociplastic pain has emerged in the IASP terminology of pain. This type of pain arises from an alteration of the nociceptive function, despite no clear evidence of tissue damage causing the activation of nociceptors or evidence for disease or lesion of the somatosensory system causing the pain.[8,17] Fibromyalgia, irritable bowel syndrome, and complex regional pain syndrome are examples of nociplastic pain.[22]

PHYSIOLOGY OF PAIN

Physiologic mechanisms of pain integrate many pain components. In transduction, stimuli are sources of pain that trigger the liberation of neurotransmitters. In transmission, diffusion of the action potential along the spinal column may lead to muscle rigidity—a reflex activity that can be observed as a behavioral indicator associated with pain. Muscle rigidity may also influence respiratory rate and amplitude, leading to hypoventilation. In perception, the patient's self-report of emotional, cognitive, and sensory information can be obtained, and behavioral responses to pain may also be observed. Finally, in modulation, pain sensation may be attenuated by ascending and descending mechanisms.

Nociception

Nociception represents the neural processes of encoding and processing noxious stimuli necessary, but not sufficient, for pain.[8] Pain results from the integration of the nociceptive signal into specific cortical areas of the brain associated with higher mental processes and consciousness. In other words, pain is the conscious experience that emerges from nociception.

Four processes are involved in nociception:[20]

1. Transduction
2. Transmission
3. Perception
4. Modulation

The four processes are shown in Fig. 7.1, with pain assessment integrated with nociception.

Transduction

Transduction refers to mechanical (e.g., surgical incision), thermal (e.g., burn), or chemical (e.g., toxic substance) stimuli that damage tissues. In critical care, many nociceptive stimuli exist, including the patient's acute illness or condition, invasive technology used for the patient, and multiple interventions and standard care procedures that have to be done. These stimuli, also called stressors, stimulate the liberation of many chemical substances, such as prostaglandins, bradykinin, serotonin, histamine, glutamate, and substance P. These neurotransmitters stimulate peripheral nociceptive receptors and initiate nociceptive transmission.

Transmission

As a result of transduction, an action potential is produced and is transmitted by nociceptive nerve fibers in the spinal cord that reach higher centers of the brain. This is called transmission, and it represents the second process of nociception. The principal nociceptive fibers are the A-delta (Aδ) and C fibers. Large-diameter, myelinated Aδ fibers that transmit well-localized, sharp pain which often leads to reflex withdrawal. Small-diameter, unmyelinated C fibers transmit diffuse, dull, aching pain. These fibers transmit the noxious sensation from the periphery through the dorsal root of the spinal cord. With the liberation of substance P, these fibers then synapse with ascending spinothalamic fibers to the central nervous system (CNS). These spinothalamic fibers are clustered into two specific pathways: neospinothalamic (NS) and paleospinothalamic (PS) pathways. Generally, the Aδ fibers transmit the pain sensation to the brain within the NS pathway, and the C fibers use the PS pathway.[23]

Through synapsing of nociceptive fibers with motor fibers in the spinal cord, muscle rigidity can appear because of a reflex activity.[24] Muscle rigidity is a behavioral indicator associated with pain.[25] It can contribute to immobility and decrease diaphragmatic excursion. This can lead to hypoventilation and hypoxemia. Hypoxemia can be detected by a pulse oximeter (SpO_2) and by monitoring of arterial partial pressure of oxygen (PaO_2). The interaction of a ventilated patient with the machine (e.g., activation of alarms, fighting the ventilator) also may indicate the presence of pain.[26]

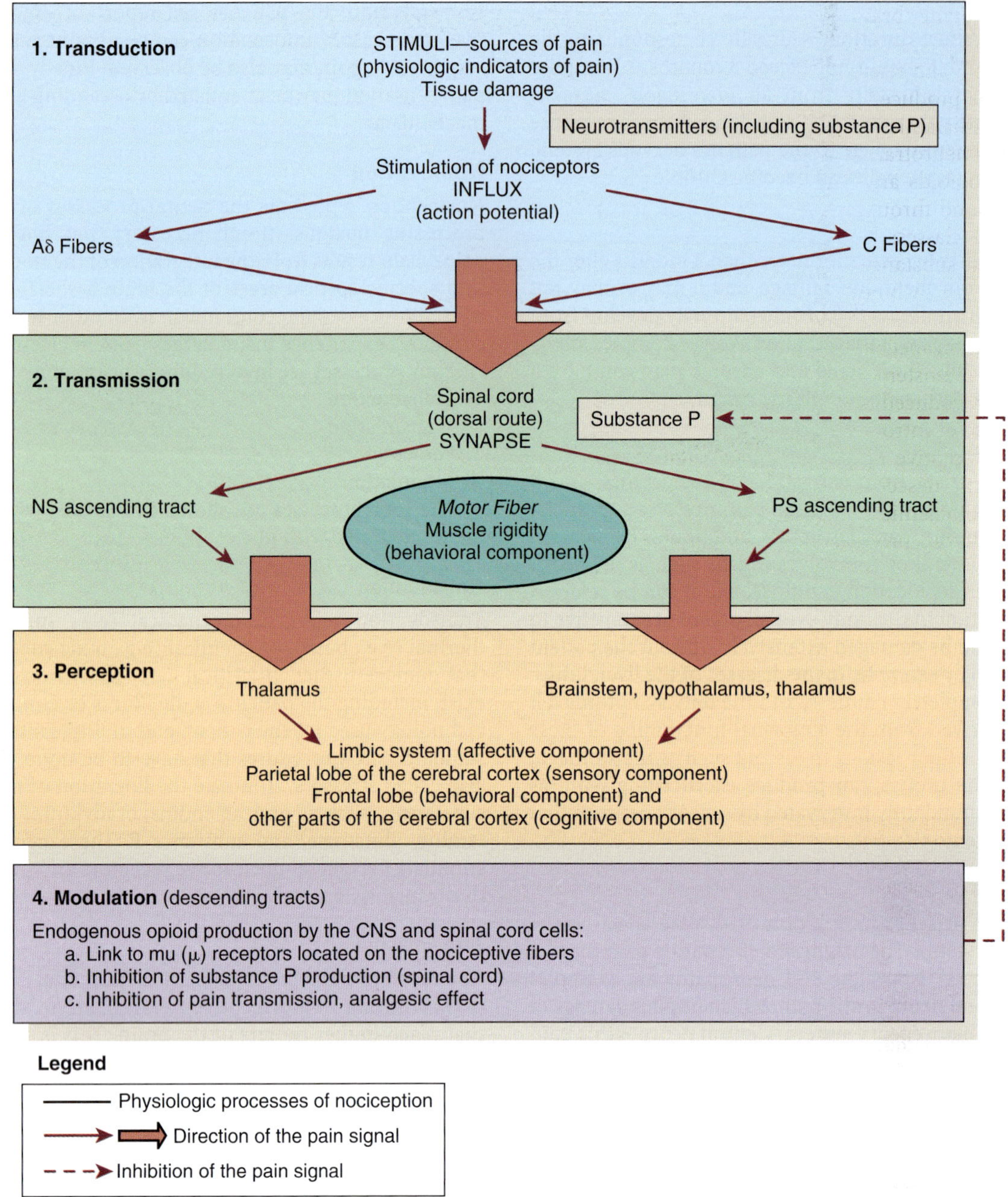

FIG. 7.1 Integration of Pain Assessment in the Four Processes of Nociception. *CNS*, Central nervous system; *NS*, neospinothalamic pathway; *PS*, paleospinothalamic pathway. (Courtesy Céline Gélinas, Ingram School of Nursing, McGill University, Canada.)

Perception

The nociceptive message is transmitted by the spinothalamic pathways to centers in the brain, where it is perceived as pain. Pain sensation transmitted by the NS pathway reaches the thalamus, and the pain sensation transmitted by the PS pathway reaches the brainstem, hypothalamus, and thalamus.[23] These parts of the CNS contribute to the initial perception of pain. Projections to the limbic system and the frontal cortex allow expression of the emotional component of pain.[27] Projections to the sensory cortex located in the parietal lobe allow the patient to describe the sensory characteristics of pain, such as location, intensity, and quality.[27,28] The cognitive component of pain involves many parts of the cerebral cortex and is complex. These three components (emotional, cognitive, and sensory) represent the personal interpretation of pain. Parallel to this perception process, certain facial expressions and body movements are behavioral indicators of pain occurring because of pain fiber projections to the motor cortex in the frontal lobe.

Modulation

Modulation is a process by which noxious stimuli that travel from the nociceptive receptors to the CNS may be enhanced or inhibited. Pain can be modulated by ascending and descending mechanisms. A typical example of ascending pain modulation is rubbing an injury site, which activates large A-beta (Aβ) fibers related to touch in the periphery. Stimulation of these fibers activates inhibitory interneurons in the dorsal horn of the spinal cord, preventing nociceptive signal transmission from the periphery to the higher brain regions. The physiologic basis of this mechanism of pain modulation was elucidated by Melzack and Wall in 1965[29] and refers to the gate control theory. Analgesia may also be produced at the level of the spinal cord and brainstem (spinothalamic pathway) via the release of endogenous opioids and neurotransmitters.

Endogenous opioids are naturally occurring morphinelike pentapeptides found throughout the nervous system and exist in three general classes: beta-endorphins, enkephalins, and dynorphins. These substances block neuronal activity related to nociceptive impulses by binding to opioid mu (μ) receptor sites in the central and peripheral nervous systems.[23] In the ascending pain-modulation mechanism, endogenous opioids may be produced in the brainstem, and the dorsal horn or exogenous opioids may be introduced by administration of an opioid analgesic. The released or introduced opioids bind to the mu-opioid receptors on nociceptive nerve fibers, blocking the release of substance P. In the descending pain modulation mechanism, the efferent spinothalamic nerve fibers that descend from the brain can inhibit the propagation of the nociceptive signal by triggering the release of endogenous opioids in the brainstem and in the spinal cord. Serotonin and norepinephrine are important inhibitory neurotransmitters that act in the CNS. These substances are also released by the descending fibers of the descending spinothalamic pathway.[30] The use of distraction, relaxation, and imagery techniques can facilitate the release of endogenous opioids and has been shown to reduce the overall pain experience.[31]

Biologic Stress Response

A biologic stress response may be activated by pain, an obvious stressor. This stress response involves the nervous, endocrine, and immune systems in the hypothalamic–pituitary–adrenal axis.[32] The biologic stress response includes a short-term direct response, a midterm response, and a long-term indirect response. All the indicators identified within the biologic stress response are not specific to pain because they can be attributed to other distress conditions, homeostatic changes, and medications.[12] Biologic stress mechanisms are depicted in Fig. 7.2.

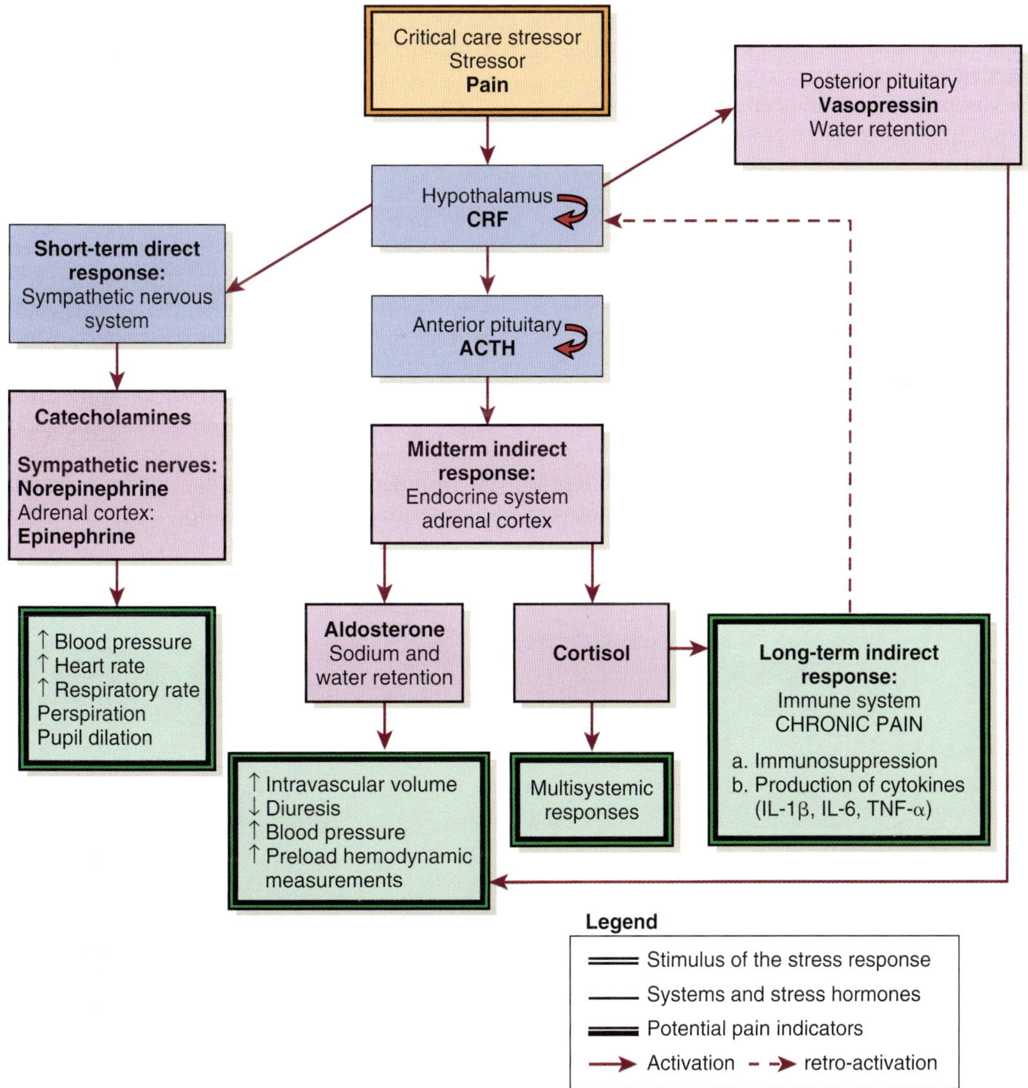

FIG. 7.2 Integration of Potential Physiologic Pain Indicators in the Biologic Stress Response. *ACTH*, Adrenocorticotropic hormone; *CRF*, corticotropin-releasing factor; *IL*, interleukin; *TNF*, tumor necrosis factor. (Courtesy Céline Gélinas, Ingram School of Nursing, McGill University, Canada.)

Short-Term Direct Response

In the presence of a stressor such as pain, the hypothalamus releases corticotropin-releasing factor, which activates the sympathetic nervous system (SNS). Norepinephrine is then released from the terminals of sympathetic nerves, and epinephrine is released from the adrenal cortex. This mechanism constitutes the short-term direct stress response. The effects of these stress hormones allow observation of physiologic responses associated with activation of SNS. For example, increased blood pressure, increased heart rate, and increased respiratory rate are common signs of acute stress and may be associated with pain.[9] Pupil dilation also can be observed.[33,34]

If pain persists over time, or injuries are located in the bladder or the intestines, the parasympathetic nervous system may be dominant. The blood pressure and heart rate may decrease rather than increase. The absence of pain-related indicators related to the activation of the SNS does not imply an absence of pain sensation.[35]

Midterm Indirect Response

At midterm, the corticotropin-releasing factor released from the hypothalamus stimulates the anterior pituitary to release adrenocorticotropic hormone and the posterior pituitary to release vasopressin, the antidiuretic hormone. Adrenocorticotropic hormone activates the adrenal cortex to release aldosterone and cortisol. Vasopressin and aldosterone increase sodium and water retention. This increases intravascular volume and decreases diuresis and increases blood pressure and cardiac preload. Cortisol also may contribute to systemic responses such as infection and hyperglycemia.

At midterm, pain may be associated with decreased diuresis, increased blood pressure, increased central venous pressure, and increased pulmonary artery occlusion pressure. However, changes in these parameters are not specific to pain, and their associations with pain are not supported by empiric data.

Long-Term Indirect Response

The stress hormones, specifically cortisol, have a long-term influence on the immune system in two ways: immunosuppression and release of cytokines.[36] Cytokines may prolong by retroactivation the release of cortisol, which may exacerbate tissue damage, contributing to the chronic pain process.[37]

COMMUNICATION FRAMEWORK FOR PAIN ASSESSMENT

As previously stated, self-report of pain is not always possible to obtain in critically ill patients, as many of them may be unable to self-report during their stay in the critical care unit. When the patient is unable to self-report, the expression of pain can be examined from the perspective of the communications model of pain.[38] The foundation of this model is that observational measures capture behaviors that are less subject to voluntary control and more automatic compared with self-report measures that depend on higher mental processes. Consequently, observational measures should be used to assess pain when the individual's self-report is unavailable, as is often the case in critically ill patients.

This communication A → B → C model conceptualizes pain as an internal state (Fig. 7.3)

- Is encoded in particular features of expressive behaviors
- Allows observers (in this case nurses) to draw inferences
- Is about the nature of the sender's (i.e., the patient) experience

More specifically, when an individual is exposed to a nociceptive stimulus known to be painful, information about real or potential tissue damage is transmitted and processed centrally into the brain. The processing of a nociceptive stimulus can be modulated by intrapersonal or contextual factors influencing the way information is integrated and consequently how pain is experienced in each individual. In critical care, intrapersonal factors that could potentially influence the processing of a nociceptive stimulus include the patient's sociodemographic characteristics, severity of critical illness or injury, level of sedation, and level of consciousness. Similarly, examples of contextual factors specific to the critical care unit environment that could influence the patient's pain experience include mechanical ventilation and administration of sedative

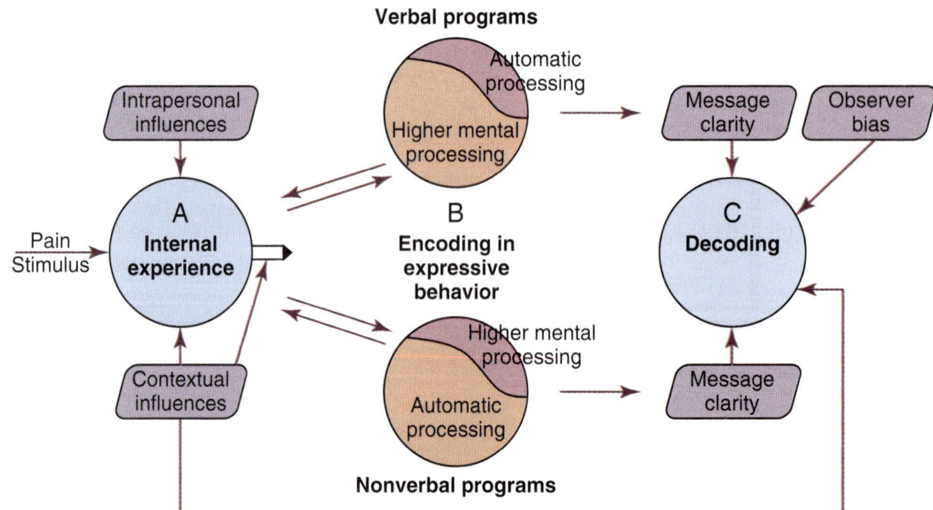

FIG. 7.3 Communications Model of Pain. (Redrawn from Hadjistavropoulos T, Craig KD. A theoretical framework for understanding self-report and observational measures of pain: a communications model. *Behav Res Ther.* 2002;40:551.)

and opioid agents. Taking into account the various intrapersonal and contextual factors, critically ill patients may express their pain through different patterns of verbal and nonverbal expressive modalities. The depicted pattern depends largely on the degree of impairment in the cortical areas of the brain associated with consciousness. Although some patients with a mild alteration of the level of consciousness may still have the capacity to self-report or express their pain with voluntary behaviors (e.g., pointing to the pain site), others with a severe alteration of the level of consciousness might respond to pain only through behavioral and autonomic reactions such as reflex or fluctuations in physiologic signs. Whether patients are able to express their pain through self-report, behavioral or autonomic reactions undoubtedly affects the clarity of the message and the capacity of nurses to identify the specific nature of patients' pain. Because behaviors are difficult to decode, educational training of nurses is necessary to support them in developing the competence of adequately assessing pain behaviors using observational measures.

PAIN ASSESSMENT

Pain assessment is an integral part of nursing care. Assessment is a prerequisite for adequate pain control and relief. As stated earlier, pain is a personal, multidimensional concept that requires comprehensive assessment. Many factors may alter verbal communication in critically ill patients, making pain assessment more challenging. This situation should not discourage nurses from assessing pain in these vulnerable patients, because acute pain is a stressor that can exacerbate their condition.

Pain assessment has two major components: (1) nonobservable, or personal, and (2) observable, or objective. The complexity of pain assessment requires the use of multiple strategies by critical care nurses. In the following sections, patient, health professional, and organizational barriers to pain assessment and management are addressed, and recommendations are proposed.

Personal Component of Pain Assessment

Pain is known as a personal experience. The personal component of pain assessment refers to the patient's self-report about their sensorial, emotional, and cognitive experience of pain. Because it is considered the reference standard measure of pain, the patient's self-report must be obtained whenever possible.[12,39] A simple yes or no (presence versus absence of pain) should be considered a valid self-report. Mechanical ventilation should not be a barrier for nurses to document patients' self-reports of pain. Many mechanically ventilated patients can communicate that they have pain or can use pain scales by pointing to numbers or symbols on the scale. Attempts should be made to obtain a self-report before concluding that a patient is unable to self-report.[12] More importantly, sufficient time should be allowed for the patient to respond with each attempt.[12,39]

If sedation and cognition levels allow the patient to give more information about pain, a multidimensional primary assessment can be documented. Multidimensional pain assessment tools that include the sensorial, emotional, and cognitive components are available, such as:

- Brief Pain Inventory[40]
- Initial Pain Assessment Tool[20]
- Short-form McGill Pain Questionnaire[41]

However, because of the administration of sedative and analgesic agents in mechanically ventilated patients, the tool must be short enough to be completed. The short-form McGill Pain Questionnaire takes a few minutes to complete and has been used to assess mechanically ventilated patients who were in a stable condition.[2] A comprehensive pain assessment is indicated on admission or when a new pain occurs, otherwise regular monitoring of pain intensity is common practice.

The patient's self-report of pain can also be obtained by questioning the patient using the mnemonic PQRSTUV:[42]

P: Provocative and palliative or aggravating factors
Q: Quality
R: Region or location, radiation
S: Severity and other symptoms
T: Timing
U: Understanding
V: Values

P: Provocative and Palliative or Aggravating Factors

The **P** in the mnemonic indicates what provokes or causes the patient's pain, what were they or their body doing when the pain occurred, and what makes the pain worse or better. For example, deep breathing intensifying chest pain in the case of pericarditis is an illustration of an aggravating factor. Moderating factors that reduce or alleviate pain or discomfort are also important findings and may include resting to diminish burning chest pain that causes angina. Knowledge of any intensifying or alleviating conditions can contribute to the patient's plan of care throughout the continuum of care.

Q: Quality

The **Q** in the mnemonic refers to the quality of the pain or the pain sensation that the patient is experiencing. The patient may describe the pain as dull, aching, sharp, burning, or stabbing. This information provides the nurse with data regarding the type of pain the patient is experiencing (e.g., somatic or visceral). The differentiation between types of pain may contribute to the determination of cause and management. A patient who has had open-heart surgery may complain of chest pain that is shooting or burning.[43] This information can lead the nurse to investigate for cutaneous or bone injuries from a sternotomy. Another patient may describe a sharp thoracic pain that may lead the nurse to consider visceral pain from a pulmonary embolism. A description of pain is important because it provides a baseline account, allowing the critical care nurse to monitor changes in the type of pain, which may indicate a change in the underlying pathology.

R: Region or Location, Radiation

R usually is easy for the patient to identify, although visceral pain is more difficult for the patient to localize.[20] If the patient has difficulty naming the location or is mechanically ventilated, ask the patient to point to the location on their body or on a simple anatomic drawing.[44]

S: Severity and Other Symptoms

S, the severity or intensity of pain, is a measurement that has undergone much investigation. Many pain intensity scales are available, including the descriptive and numeric pain rating scales that are often used in the critical care environment (Fig. 7.4). Many critical care units use a specific pain intensity scale. The use of a single tool provides consistency of assessment and

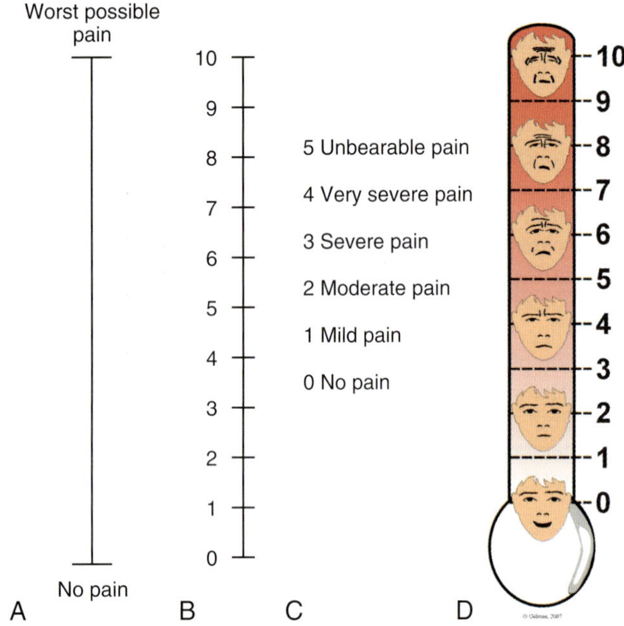

FIG. 7.4 Pain Intensity Scales (Vertical Format). Visual analog scale (VAS). (B) Numeric Rating Scale (NRS). (C) Descriptive rating scale (DRS). (D) Faces Pain Thermometer. (Courtesy Céline Gélinas, Ingram School of Nursing, McGill University, Canada.)

documentation. A visual numeric format of a 0-to-10 self-report scale (e.g., Numeric Rating Scale, Thermometer) has been found to be the most feasible in critically ill adults.[6,45] Asking the patient to grade their pain on a scale of 0 to 10 using a visual format is a consistent method and aids the nurse in objectifying the personal aspect of the patient's pain. However, the patient's tool preference should be considered.

The **S** in the mnemonic also refers to other symptoms accompanying the patient's pain experience, such as shortness of breath, nausea, and fatigue. Anxiety and fear are common emotions associated with pain.

T: Timing

The **T** in the mnemonic refers to documenting the onset, duration, and frequency of pain. This information can help determine whether the origin of the pain is acute or chronic. The duration of pain can indicate the severity of the problem. For example, chest pain of less than 15 minutes' duration may be angina, and chest pain lasting more than 15 minutes may indicate a myocardial infarction.

U: Understanding

The **U** in the mnemonic is the patient's perception of the problem or cognitive experience of pain. Patients with known cardiac problems can tell the nurse whether their pain is the same as what they experienced during the myocardial infarction. Patients with a cerebral hemorrhage often describe experiencing the worst headache they have ever had.

V: Values

The **V** refers to values and preferences for pain treatment, which may guide the nurse and the medical team regarding the care and treatment plan in alignment with the patient's decisions.

Because of the patient's change in communication, lack of concentration, and the life-or-death immediacy of most actions in the critical care environment, pain assessment is often reduced to minimal information. Begin by asking, "Do you have pain?" The use of a simple yes or no question allows the patient to answer verbally or to indicate their response by nodding the head or by other signs. It is easier for mechanically ventilated patients to communicate with nurses in this way because they cannot express themselves verbally.

Observable or Objective Component of Pain Assessment

When the patient's self-report is impossible to obtain, nurses can rely on the observation of behavioral indicators, which are strongly emphasized in clinical recommendations and guidelines for pain management in nonverbal patients.[6,11–13] Fluctuations in vital signs should never be used alone but rather considered as a cue to begin further assessment for pain with valid methods.[6,11–13]

Pain-related behaviors have been described in critically ill patients and were studied in the AACN Thunder Project II[46] and in the *Europain* study.[1] Behaviors including facial expressions, muscle rigidity, and vocalization were associated with self-reported pain and were significant predictors of pain intensity and pain distress. Several behavioral scales have been developed for assessing pain in critically ill nonverbal adult patients.[47] The clinical guidelines of the Society of Critical Care Medicine (SCCM) recommend both the Behavioral Pain Scale (BPS)[48] and its version for the nonintubated patient (BPS-NI)[49] and the Critical-Care Pain Observation Tool (CPOT)[50] for clinical use in critically ill adult patients unable to self-report.[6] The implementation of these scales in critical care units has led to enhanced nursing practices of pain assessment and management and improved patient outcomes, including decreases in mechanical ventilation duration, infection rates, and adverse events.[51]

Behavioral Pain Scale

The BPS for the intubated patient[48] and its adapted version for the nonintubated patient (BPS-NI)[49] are shown in Table 7.1, and their use has been validated in various critical care patient groups in different countries.[47] Both versions of the tool have shown high interrater reliability with trained critical care nurses and other health professionals. The validity of the use of the BPS and BPS-NI has been supported by the association of significantly higher BPS scores during nociceptive procedures known to be painful (e.g., turning, endotracheal suctioning, peripheral venous cannulation) compared with rest or nonnociceptive procedures (e.g., arterial catheter dressing change, compression stocking applications, eye care). Positive associations were also found between BPS/BPS-NI score and patients' self-report of pain intensity during nociceptive procedures. A cut-off score greater than 5 for the presence of pain was established with the BPS.[47] The BPS can be used quickly, and most clinicians were satisfied with its ease of use.[52]

Critical-Care Pain Observation Tool

The CPOT[50] shown in Table 7.2 was tested widely in various critical care patient groups in multiple countries.[47] Similarly to the BPS/BPS-NI, good interrater reliability of CPOT scores was achieved with trained critical care nurses. Validity of the CPOT use was supported with significantly higher CPOT scores during nociceptive procedures (e.g., turning with or without other care, endotracheal suctioning, chest tube removal) compared with rest or nonnociceptive procedures (e.g., taking blood pressure, central catheter dressing change). Positive associations were

TABLE 7.1 Behavioral Pain Scale and Non-Intubated Version

Item	Description	Score
Facial expression	Relaxed	1
	Partially tightened (e.g., brow lowering)	2
	Fully tightened (e.g., eyelid closing)	3
	Grimacing	4
Upper limbs	No movement	1
	Partially bent	2
	Fully bent with finger flexion	3
	Permanently retracted	4
Compliance with ventilation	Tolerating movement	1
	Coughing but tolerating ventilation for most of the time	2
	Fighting ventilator	3
	Unable to control ventilation	4
OR		
Vocalization	No pain vocalization	1
	Moaning not frequent (≤3/min) or not prolonged (≤3 seconds)	2
	Moaning frequent (>3/min) or prolonged (>3 seconds)	3
	Howling or verbal complaint including "Ow! Ouch!" or breath holding	4
Total		**3–12**

Modified from Payen JF, et al. Assessing pain in critically ill sedated patients by using a behavioral pain scale. *Crit Care Med.* 2001;29(12):2258.

TABLE 7.2 Critical-Care Pain Observation Tool and Neuro Version

Item	CPOT Description	CPOT-Neuro Description	Score
Facial expression 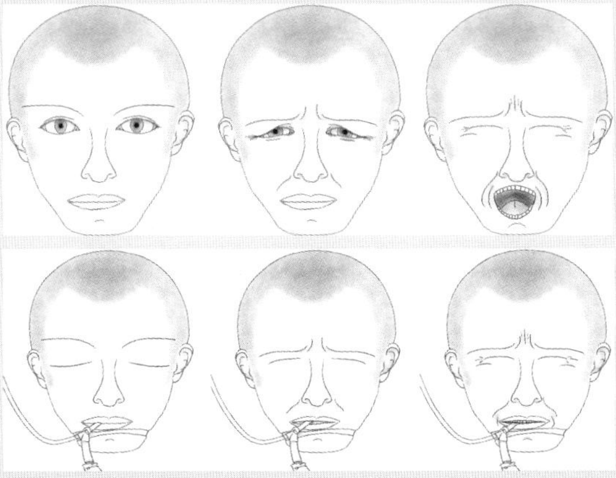	Relaxed/Neutral (no facial muscle tension)	Relaxed/Neutral (no facial muscle tension)	0
	Tense (brow lowering, orbit tightening, mild contraction around nose and mouth may be observed)	Brow lowering	1
	Grimacing (brow lowering, eyes tightly closed, mouth opening or biting the endotracheal tube)	Contraction of upper face or Grimacing (upper face contraction: brow lowering and eye tightening) (grimace: brow lowering, eyes tightly closed, mouth opening or biting the endotracheal tube)	2
	N/A		
Body movements	Absence of movements or normal position (does not move at all or movements not aimed toward the pain site or not made for the purpose of protection)	Absence of movements (does not move at all)	0
	Protection (slow, cautious movements, touching or rubbing the pain site, seeking attention through movements)	Nonpurposeful movements (slow, cautious movements, limb flexion not aimed at reaching pain site)	1
	Restlessness/agitation (pulling tube, attempting to sit up, moving limbs/thrashing, not following commands, striking at staff, trying to climb out of bed)	Purposeful movements and/or restlessness/agitation (purposeful movements: trying to reach pr touching/rubbing pain site, withdrawing) (restlessness/agitation: refer to description of CPOT)	2

Continued

TABLE 7.2 **Critical-Care Pain Observation Tool and Neuro Version—cont'd**

Item	CPOT Description	CPOT-Neuro Description	Score
Compliance with the ventilator (intubated patients)	Tolerating ventilator or movement (alarms not activated, easy ventilation)	Tolerating ventilator (alarms not activated, easy ventilation)	0
	Coughing but tolerating (coughing, alarms are activated but stop spontaneously)	Activating alarms Coughing, alarms may be activated but stop spontaneously	1
	Fighting ventilator (asynchrony: blocking ventilation, alarms frequently activated)	Fighting ventilator (asynchrony: blocking ventilation, alarms frequently activated)	2
OR			
Vocalization (nonintubated patient)	Talking in normal tone or no sound	Talking in normal tone or no sound	0
	Sighing, moaning	Sighing, moaning	1
	Crying out, sobbing	Verbal complaints of pain, crying out	2
Muscle tension	Relaxed (no resistance to passive movements)	Relaxed (no resistance to passive movements)	0
	Tense/Rigid (resistance to passive movements)	Tense/Rigid (resistance to passive movements)	1
	Very tense/Very rigid (strong resistance to passive movements , incapacity to complete them, clenched fists)	N/A	2
Total			**8**

The patient must be observed at rest for 1 minute to obtain a baseline value of the CPOT/CPOT-Neuro. Then the patient should be observed during standard care procedures (e.g., turning, wound care) to detect any changes in the patient's behaviors.

Observation of patient at rest (baseline).

The nurse looks at the patient's face and body to note any visible reactions for an observation period of 1 minute. The nurse gives a score for all items except for muscle tension. At the end of the 1-minute period, the nurse holds the patient's arm in both hands. The nurse places one hand at the elbow and uses the other one to hold the patient's hand. Then the nurse performs a passive flexion and extension of the upper limb and feels any resistance the patient may exhibit. If the movements are performed easily, the patient is found to be relaxed with no resistance (score 0). If the movements can still be performed but with more strength, then it is concluded that the patient is showing resistance to movements (score 1). If the nurse cannot complete the movements, strong resistance is felt (score 2 on CPOT scale only). The patient may also clench their fists. The maximum score for muscle tension is 1 on the CPOT-Neuro.

Observation of patient during a standard care procedure.

While performing a procedure known to be painful, the nurse looks at the patient's face to note any reactions such as brow lowering or grimacing. These reactions may be brief or can last longer. For the scoring of the CPOT-Neuro, the nurse also looks for tearing or face flushing. The nurse also looks out for body movements. For instance, the nurse looks for protective movements such as the patient trying to reach or touching the pain site (e.g., surgical incision, injury site). In the mechanically ventilated patient, the nurse pays attention to alarms and if they stop spontaneously or require a nursing intervention (e.g., reassurance, administering medication). According to muscle tension, the nurse can feel if the patient is resisting against the movement.

The patient should be evaluated before and at the peak effect of an analgesic agent to assess whether the treatment was effective in relieving pain.

The patient should be attributed the highest score observed during the observation period.

The patient should be attributed a score for each behavior included in the CPOT/CPOT-Neuro. Muscle tension should be evaluated last, because it may lead to behavioral reactions not necessarily related to pain but more to the actual stimulation. According to compliance with the ventilator, the nurse must check that the endotracheal tube is well positioned and for the presence of secretions, which could lead to higher scores for this item.

Figure of facial expressions courtesy Céline Gélinas, Ingram School of Nursing, McGill University, Canada.

Modified from Gélinas C, Fillion L, Puntillo KA, Viens C, Fortier M. Validation of the Critical-Care Pain Observation Tool (CPOT) in adult patients. *Am J Crit Care.* 2006;15:420.

And Gélinas C, Bérubé M, Puntillo KA, et al. Validation of the Critical-Care Pain Observation Tool-Neuro for the assessment of pain in brain-injured adults in the intensive care unit: A prospective cohort study. *BMC Critical Care.* 2021;25:142.

found between the CPOT scores and the patient's self-report of pain intensity during nociceptive procedures. A cut-off score greater than 2 for the presence of pain was established with the CPOT.[47] Feasibility and clinical utility of the CPOT were positively evaluated by critical care nurses, which was sustained at 12 months after implementation of the tool.[53] Nurses agreed that the CPOT was quick enough to be used in the critical care unit, simple to understand, easy to complete, and helpful for nursing practice (see Table 7.2).

An adapted version of the tool has been made available for use in critically ill adults with a brain injury and alteration of consciousness. In fact, this critical care group was found to exhibit different behavioral responses to pain. For example, instead of grimacing, brain-injured patients with altered levels of consciousness seemed to react mostly by lowering their eyebrows, showing face flushing, tearing, and exhibiting limb flexion when exposed to pain.[54,55] Such findings highlighted the need to adapt the CPOT for this vulnerable critical care group and is called the CPOT-Neuro.[56] The CPOT-Neuro includes five items (i.e., facial expressions, autonomic responses, body movements, muscle rigidity, and ventilator compliance for intubated patients or vocalization for nonintubated patients). The total score from 0 to 8 remains the same as for the CPOT and a similar cut-off score greater than 2 was found.[56] Most nurses agreed that the CPOT-Neuro was feasible to use and relevant for clinical practice.[57]

Use of Cut-off Scores

A cut-off score refers to the score on a specific scale associated with the best probability of correctly ruling in or ruling out a patient with a specific condition—in this case, pain. The use of a cut-off score with behavioral pain scales can help identify when pain is highly likely to be present and guide nurses

BOX 7.1 Case Example of Using a Cut-Off Score With the Critical-Care Pain Observation Tool (CPOT)

A patient is admitted to the critical care unit after cardiac surgery. He is mechanically ventilated and too drowsy to communicate effectively with the nurse using signs (e.g., head nodding or pointing on a communication board). However, he seems to be uncomfortable, as he becomes agitated each time he is touched. The nurse in charge is puzzled about the need to administer an analgesic or a sedative—both prescribed on the postoperative care protocol. She first assesses for the presence of pain and gets a score of 4 out of 8 on the CPOT as the patient grimaces and attempts to sit in the bed. Considering that a CPOT score higher than 2 strongly suggests the presence of pain, the nurse gives a dose of subcutaneous analgesic. The patient has a relaxed face and is cautiously moving his hand from time to time toward the surgical wound on his chest 30 minutes after the administration of the analgesic. The CPOT score is now 1 out of 8, indicating pain relief, as it dropped from 4 to 1 (i.e., more than 2 points).

in determining whether an intervention to alleviate pain is required. Also, a cut-off score can help evaluate the effectiveness of pain management interventions. Cut-off scores are established using a criterion (i.e., a reference standard in the field). As mentioned previously, in the case of pain, the patient's self-report is known as the reference standard criterion.

Behavioral pain scores should be interpreted differently from the patient's self-report pain intensity scores. Although they both represent pain scores, they are measuring different dimensions of pain that are interrelated. More specifically, behavioral scores based on the nurse's observations are associated with the behavioral dimension of pain, and the patient's self-report of pain intensity relates to the sensory dimension of pain.[14] Although self-reported pain intensity scores and behavioral pain scores move in the same direction (i.e., when one score increases, the other score increases as well), they are not equal scores.[11,12] Therefore, it is important to know that behavioral pain scales only allow the detection of the presence versus absence of pain. Box 7.1 provides a case example showing how a cut-off score can be used in practice.

Limitations Related to the Use of Behavioral Pain Scales

Behavioral pain scales have been validated for pain assessment in critically ill patients, but they have some limitations. They are impossible to monitor in patients unable to respond behaviorally to pain, such as patients with paralysis or under the effects of neuromuscular blocking agents. Also, behavioral responses may be blurred with the administration of high doses of sedative agents. Minimal behavioral responses to painful procedures were found in unconscious, mechanically ventilated, critically ill adults who were more heavily sedated compared with conscious patients.[25]

When selecting a scale, nurses should make sure that it has been tested in a patient population and context in which they plan to use it. A scale can be shown to be valid only with a specific group of people and in a given context.[58] In addition to the use of a validated behavioral pain scale, nurses should consult family members to better understand the patient's pain behaviors and their specific reactions at rest and during activity, or procedures should be documented in the chart.[11–13]

Physiologic Indicators

When patients cannot react behaviorally to pain, the only possible clues left for the detection of pain are physiologic indicators. Vital signs (i.e., blood pressure, heart rate, respiratory rate) have received some attention; however, their validity in the pain assessment process is not supported. Although vital signs generally increase during painful procedures, they have also been found to decrease or to remain stable. Moreover, vital signs are not consistently related to the patient's self-report of pain, and they are not predictive of pain.[59]

In the American Society for Pain Management Nursing (ASPMN) recommendations[12] and the SCCM guidelines,[6] it is stated that vital signs should not be considered as primary indicators of pain because they can be attributed to other distress conditions, homeostatic changes, and medications. Instead, changes in vital signs should be considered a cue to begin further assessment of pain with appropriate tools.[6,11,12]

Besides vital signs, the pupil dilation reflex (PDR) was associated with pain scores in surgical critical care patients,[33] but contradictory findings have been found, especially in brain-injured critical care patients.[32,34] PDR may be influenced by factors other than pain, such as the administration of high doses of opioids and brain injury.

Other innovative technology may have some potential. The Analgesia Nociception Index (which is based on heart rate variability) and the Nociception Level Index (which is based on multiple parameters related to heart rate, heart rate variability, galvanic skin response, and peripheral temperature) have been shown to be useful in detecting nociceptive procedures and pain scores in critically ill adults,[60–62] but more research is needed.

Challenges to Pain Assessment and Management

Communication

The most obvious patient barrier to the assessment of pain in critical care patients is an alteration in the ability to communicate. A patient who is mechanically ventilated cannot verbalize a description of the pain. If the patient can communicate in any way, such as by head nodding or pointing, they may report the pain in that manner. If writing is possible, the patient may be able to describe the pain in detail. With patients unable to self-report, the nurse relies on validated behavioral pain scales such as the BPS/BPS-NI[48,49] and the CPOT[50] to assess the presence of pain.[6,11,12]

The patient's family can contribute in the assessment of pain. The family is intimately knowledgeable of the patient's behavioral responses to pain[63,64] and can assist the nurse in identifying clues. Referring to a behavioral tool such as the CPOT has been found to support them in confirming their observations of the patient's pain behaviors.[65] An adapted version of the CPOT for family members (CPOT-Fam) has also been recently developed.[66] A family member's impression of a patient's pain should be considered in the pain assessment process of a critically ill patient.[6,11,12]

Altered Level of Consciousness and Unconsciousness

A patient who either is unconscious or has an altered level of consciousness presents a dilemma for all clinicians. Because pain relies on cortical response to provide recognition, the belief that the patient with a brain injury altering higher cortical function has no perception of pain may persist. Conversely, the inability to interpret the nociceptive transmission does not negate the transmission. Interviews by Lawrence[67] with 100 patients who recalled their experiences from a time when they were unconscious revealed that 25% of them could hear, understand, and respond emotionally to what was being said.

Experts recommend assuming that patients who are unconscious or with an altered level of consciousness have pain and that they be treated the same way as conscious patients are treated when they are exposed to sources of pain.[12] It has been demonstrated that behavioral indicators of pain can be observed in reaction to a painful procedure in critically ill patients, no matter their level of consciousness or ability to self-report.[24,25] Moreover, it has been shown that some cortical activation related to pain perception is still present in unconscious patients in a neurovegetative state.[68] Knowing this, the critical care nurse can initiate a discussion with the other members of the health care team to formulate a plan of care for the patient's comfort.

Older Adult Patients

Many older adult patients do not complain much about pain. Misconceptions such as believing that pain is a normal consequence of aging or being afraid to disturb the health care team are barriers to pain expression for older adults.[20] Cognitive deficits present additional pain assessment barriers. Many older adult patients with mild to moderate cognitive impairments and even some with severe impairment can use pain intensity scales.[69] Vertical pain intensity scales are more easily understood by this group of patients (see Fig. 7.4).[69] Older patients with cognitive deficits should receive repeated instructions and be given sufficient time to respond.

When the self-report of pain is impossible to obtain, direct observation of pain-related behaviors is highly recommended in this population.[12,69] More than 25 behavioral tools have been developed for older patients with cognitive deficits.[70] The Pain Assessment Checklist for Seniors with Limited Ability to Communicate (PACSLAC)[71] and the Pain Assessment in Advanced Dementia (PAINAD)[72] are recommended by experts.[69,73] Only the PAINAD has been tested for use in a critical care context, but the vocalization item is not applicable to mechanically ventilated patients, and further validation studies are required.[47]

Delirious Patients

Delirium is a form of transient cognitive impairment that is highly prevalent in critically ill patients.[6] Not much evidence is available on pain assessment tools that are valid for use in this specific patient population. The BPS-NI was initially tested in 30 critically ill patients with 84% being positive for delirium.[49] Higher BPS-NI scores were found during turning compared with rest and catheter dressing change supporting its ability to discriminate between nociceptive and nonnociceptive procedures. Findings with the CPOT in 40 delirious critically ill patients were similar. Higher CPOT scores were found during nociceptive procedures (e.g., repositioning, endotracheal suctioning, and dressing change of a wound) compared with a nonnociceptive procedure (e.g., taking blood pressure).[74] Further testing of behavioral pain scales is encouraged to provide clinicians with valid tools for use in this challenging clientele. Adequate pain management is also important, because pain is a modifiable factor of delirium.[6] See Chapter 8 for more detailed discussion of the patient with delirium.

Cultural Influences

Another barrier to accurate pain assessment is cultural influences on pain and pain reporting.[75] Cultural influences are compounded when the patient speaks a language other than that of the health team members. To facilitate communication, the use of a pain intensity scale in the patient's language is vital. The 0-to-10 numeric pain scales have been translated into many different languages.[20]

Although this chapter does not address specific cultural groups and their typical responses to pain, a few best practice statements can be made.

- When assessing a patient from a cultural group different from your own, it should not be assumed the patient will have a specific response to pain or exhibit a particular behavior because of their culture. Patients have individual responses to pain. The health care practitioner may wrongfully assign or expect behaviors that a patient will not exhibit.
- Ask about role of pain in the life of the patient. The nurse must communicate with the patient or the family to ascertain what that role is.
- Some cultures believe that God's test or punishment takes the form of pain. Persons with these cultural backgrounds do not necessarily believe that the pain should be relieved.
- Some cultures perceive pain as being associated with an imbalance in life. Persons from these cultures believe they need to manipulate the environment to restore balance to control pain.[75]

The complexities and intricacies of cultural beliefs require more extensive discussion than is possible here. It is important for the nurse to support, whenever possible, the special beliefs and needs of the patient and their family to provide the most therapeutic environment for healing to occur.

Opioid-Related Tolerance and Physical Dependence

Tolerance is defined as a diminution of opioid effects over time. Physical dependence and tolerance to opioids may develop if the medication is given over a long period.

Opioid-Related Iatrogenic Withdrawal Syndrome

Physical dependence is manifested by withdrawal symptoms when opioids used alone or with benzodiazepines are abruptly stopped. This is known as *iatrogenic withdrawal syndrome* (IWS). Patients at higher risk of IWS are current opioid users and those who are opioid-naïve (i.e., never used or not used in the past week) and received opioids during a prolonged critical care unit hospitalization.

Signs and symptoms of IWS are multisystemic, including central nervous system irritability (e.g., restlessness, insomnia), sympathetic nervous system activation (e.g., diaphoresis, lacrimation, piloerection, yawning), and gastrointestinal system (e.g., diarrhea, nausea, and vomiting).[76,77] These signs and symptoms are not specific to IWS and can occur in many other clinical conditions. Criteria in the *Diagnostic and Statistical Manual of Mental Disorders* 5th edition (DSM-5) established to identify IWS include the following:[76]

- Reduction or discontinuation of opioids after high or prolonged use
- Development of three or more manifestations of IWS
- Determination that manifestations are not related to other clinical conditions[76]

Withdrawal may be avoided by weaning the patient from the opioid slowly to allow the brain to reestablish neurochemical balance in the absence of the opioid.[20] Preventive strategies may also be used and are aimed at minimizing the use of opioids. Practice guidelines promote the use of nonpharmacologic interventions (e.g., massage, music therapy, relaxation techniques) and of nonopioids.[6]

Opioid Use Disorder and Opioid Misuse

In a national report analyzing data from 2009 to 2015 in the United States, critical care admissions for opioid overdoses increased over the study period by 34%, from 44 per 10,000 to 59 per 10,000 admissions. The mortality rate of critical care admissions related to opioid overdoses increased and reached 10% in 2015.[5] Opioid use disorder and opioid misuse have rapidly escalated in North America in the last decade and are important determinants of the opioid crisis.

Opioid use disorder (previously known as opioid addiction) is defined as a problematic pattern of opioid use that leads to serious impairment or distress.[76] In alignment with the definition of medication misuse,[78] opioid misuse can be described as the use of opioids in a manner other than as directed by a physician, such as use in higher doses, more frequent doses, or longer than indicated or using someone else's medication. Guidelines recommend a reduction of opioid prescription for chronic pain,[79] and this is also in alignment with the PADIS (pain, agitation, delirium, immobility, and sleep disruption) guidelines recommending the use of a multimodal analgesia approach with low doses of opioids when appropriate.[6] Tools are available to assist the nurse in assessing the patient's level of risk of opioid use disorder and opioid misuse. Some of the tools that are recommended in guidelines include:

- Screener and Opioid Assessment for Patients with Pain (SOAPP-R)[80]
- Opioid Risk Tool for Opioid Use Disorder (ORT-OUD)[81]
- Opioid Compliance Checklist (OCC)[82]

Medication use and opioid risk assessment should be performed by the critical care nurse at admission and before discharge to ensure that appropriate and safe follow-up is provided to the patient.[83]

Health Organization Responsibilities in Pain Management

Effective and safe pain management must be a priority for the health care organization. Every organization must analyze its pain management issues and practices and provide education about pain and pain management to staff. Pain must be assessed in all critically ill patients, regardless of their clinical condition or their level of consciousness. The implementation of pain assessment tools is essential so that the health care team can establish a common language of communication that can facilitate interprofessional collaboration.[84] The use of a pain flow sheet allows ongoing pain assessment and complete documentation of pain management in the critical care setting.

There is an increased commitment to clinical practice guidelines and standards for pain assessment and management by organizations such as The Joint Commission (https://www.jointcommission.org) has considerable influence in health care institutions. In addition, strategies to enhance collaboration among health care professionals may include interdisciplinary care rounds or case reviews. Patients have the right to be consulted about their pain care plan and should be involved in making decisions. The organization must continually evaluate outcomes and work to improve the quality of pain management.

PAIN MANAGEMENT

The management of pain in a critically ill patient is as multidimensional as its assessment and is a multidisciplinary team effort. A multimodal analgesic approach based on pharmacologic and nonpharmacologic interventions should be adopted to achieve optimal pain management while using the lowest effective doses of opioids when appropriate.[6] Pain management decisions should be based on pain assessment findings, and reassessment of pain at the peak effect of analgesics determines the effectiveness of analgesia. A pain management algorithm using the 0-to-10 NRS and CPOT is provided in Fig. 7.5. The algorithm includes regular pain assessments at rest and during standard care procedures. When a low pain score is obtained (i.e., NRS = 1–3, CPOT = 1–2), a nonopioid analgesic and/or nonpharmacologic interventions may be used. When a significant pain score is detected (i.e., NRS >3, CPOT >2), the administration of a nonopioid and/or low dose of opioid may be considered, and subsequent reassessment of pain (ideally at the peak effect of the opioid or within 1 hour of administration) is necessary to determine the effectiveness of

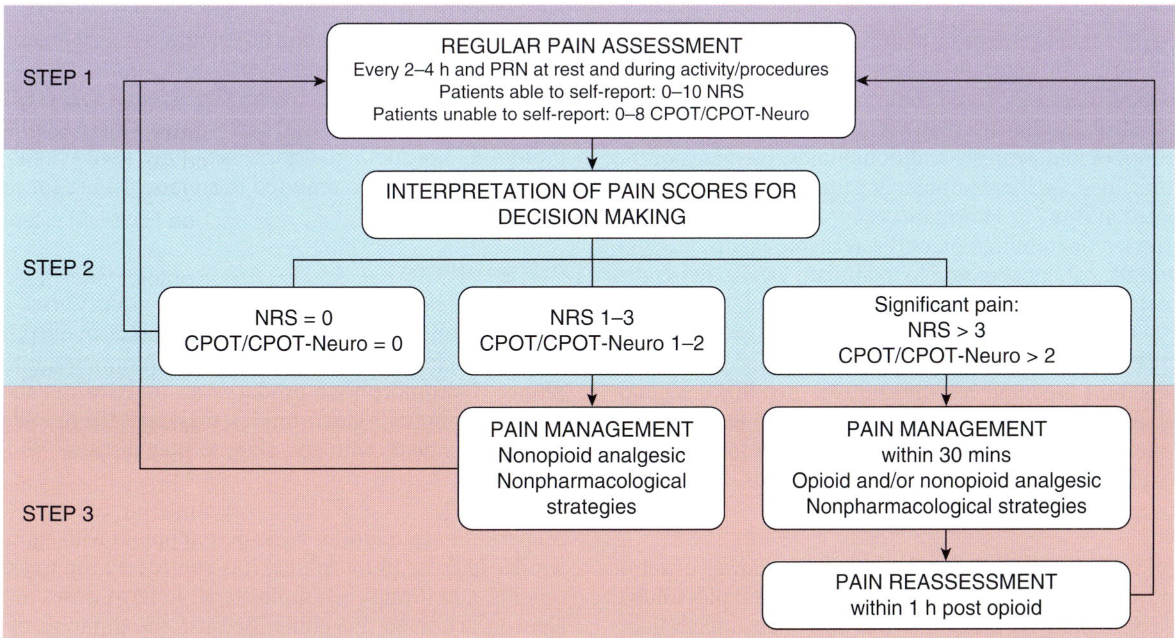

FIG. 7.5 Pain Management Algorithm with Numeric Rating Scale (NRS) and Critical-Care Pain Observation Tool (CPOT). (Redrawn from Gélinas C. Pain assessment in the critically ill adult: recent evidence and new trends. *Intensive Crit Care Nurs.* 2016;34:4.)

BOX 7.2 Summary of Pain Management Guidelines[6]

- Patients in critical care routinely experience pain at rest and during procedures, including regular activities (e.g., endotracheal suctioning, turning) and discrete procedures (e.g., tube or drain removal, arterial catheter insertion).
- Perform routine pain assessment in all patients.
- In patients who are able to self-report their level of pain, use a 0 to 10 numerical rating scale, either verbally or visually.
- The BPS/BPS-NI (scale 3–12) and CPOT* (scale 0–8) are the most valid and reliable behavioral pain scales. A BPS/BPS-NI >5 or a CPOT >2 indicates that the patient has significant pain.
- When the patient is unable to self-report, the family can be involved in their loved one's pain assessment process if they feel comfortable doing so.
- Vital signs should be used only as a cue for further pain assessment using appropriate and validated methods such as the patient's self-report (whenever possible) or a behavioral scale (i.e., BPS/BPS-NI, CPOT).
- An assessment-driven, protocol-based, stepwise approach for pain and sedation management in critically ill adults is recommended.
- A multimodal analgesic approach to pain management is encouraged.
- Adjuvants to opioid therapy include acetaminophen, ketamine (in postsurgical critical care patients), and neuropathic pain medication (e.g., gabapentin, carbamazepine, pregabalin) for neuropathic pain management or after cardiovascular surgery.
- The lowest effective dose of an opioid may be used for procedural pain management, and NSAIDs may be used for discrete and infrequent procedures (e.g., chest tube removal).
- Massage, music, relaxation techniques, and ice therapy are effective and feasible nonpharmacologic interventions for procedural and/or nonprocedural pain management.

*CPOT-Neuro is an adaptation of the CPOT scale for critically ill patients with a brain injury which has shown similar psychometric properties and with same cutoff score >2.[56]

analgesia. Effectiveness of analgesia is considered if a reduction in greater than 3 points on the NRS[85] or greater than 2 on the CPOT[86] or a score of 0 on either scale is achieved.

Pharmacologic Management of Pain

Pharmacologic management of pain has infinite variety in the critical care unit. Although this chapter is not an in-depth discussion of pharmacology, some commonly administered agents are discussed. Pain pharmacology is divided into two categories of action, opioid agonists and nonopioids. Elements of the PADIS guidelines[6] for the treatment of pain in critically ill adults are presented in Box 7.2. How pain is approached and managed is a progression or combination of the available agents, the type of pain, and the patient response to treatment. Fig. 7.6 illustrates the analgesic action sites in relation to nociception.

Opioid Analgesics

The opioids most used and recommended as first-line analgesics are the agonists. These opioids bind to mu receptors (transmission process) (see Fig. 7.6), which appear to be responsible for pain relief. Additional pharmacologic information is presented in Table 7.3.

Morphine

Because of its water solubility, morphine has a slower onset of action and a longer duration compared with the lipid-soluble opioids (e.g., fentanyl). Morphine has two main metabolites: morphine-3-glucuronide (M3G, inactive) and morphine-6-glucuronide (M6G, active). M6G is responsible for the analgesic effect but may accumulate and cause excessive sedation in patients with kidney failure or hepatic dysfunction. Therefore, the use of lower doses and close monitoring of side effects is recommended.[87,88] Morphine is available in a variety of delivery methods. It is the standard by which all other opioids are measured. It is also the agent that most closely mimics the endogenous opioids in the human pain modulation system.

Morphine is indicated for severe pain. It has additional actions that are helpful for managing other symptoms. Morphine dilates peripheral veins and arteries, making it useful in reducing myocardial workload. Morphine is also viewed as an antianxiety agent because of the calming effect it produces.

Many side effects have been reported with the use of morphine (see Table 7.3). The hypotensive effect can be particularly problematic in a patient who is hypovolemic. The vasodilation effect is potentiated in volume-depleted patients, and the hemodynamic status must be carefully monitored. Volume resuscitation restores blood pressure in the event of a prolonged hypotensive response.

Fentanyl

Fentanyl is a synthetic opioid preferred for critically ill patients with hemodynamic instability or morphine allergy. It is a lipid-soluble agent that has a more rapid onset than morphine and a shorter duration. The metabolites of fentanyl are largely inactive and nontoxic, which makes it an effective and safe opioid in the critical care setting. Fentanyl and hydromorphone are preferred in hemodynamically unstable patients and in patients with impaired kidney function.[87,88] It is available in intravenous, intraspinal, and transdermal forms. The transdermal form is commonly referred to as the "Duragesic patch" or the "72-hour patch."

When fentanyl is given by rapid administration and at higher doses, it has been associated with the additional hazard of bradycardia and rigidity in the chest wall muscles.[87] The use of transdermal fentanyl is rarely indicated in critically ill patients. The customary use of the "fentanyl patch" is for patients experiencing chronic pain or cancer pain; in critical care, it is used for patients who require extended pain control. Transdermal delivery requires 12 to 16 hours for onset of action, and the patch has a duration of action of 72 hours.[20] If this delivery method is used, the patient will require other opioid management until the transdermal fentanyl takes effect.

Fentanyl is also available in a sublingual form. Although it is rarely used in the critical care setting where the IV route is preferred. The sublingual form is mainly used for cancer pain, and more evidence is required to support its use for noncancer pain in critical care.[89]

Hydromorphone

Hydromorphone is a semisynthetic opioid. Onset of action and duration are similar to morphine.[20] It is an effective opioid with multiple routes of delivery and is more potent than morphine. Hydromorphone produces an inactive metabolite (i.e., hydromorphone-3-glucuronide), making it the opioid of choice for use in patients with end-stage kidney disease.[87,88]

Meperidine

Meperidine (Demerol) is a less potent opioid with agonist effects similar to those of morphine. It is considered the weakest of the opioids, and it must be administered in large doses to be equivalent in action to morphine. Because the duration of action is short, dosing is frequent. A major concern with this medication is the metabolite *normeperidine*, which is a CNS neurotoxic agent. At high doses in patients with kidney failure or liver dysfunction

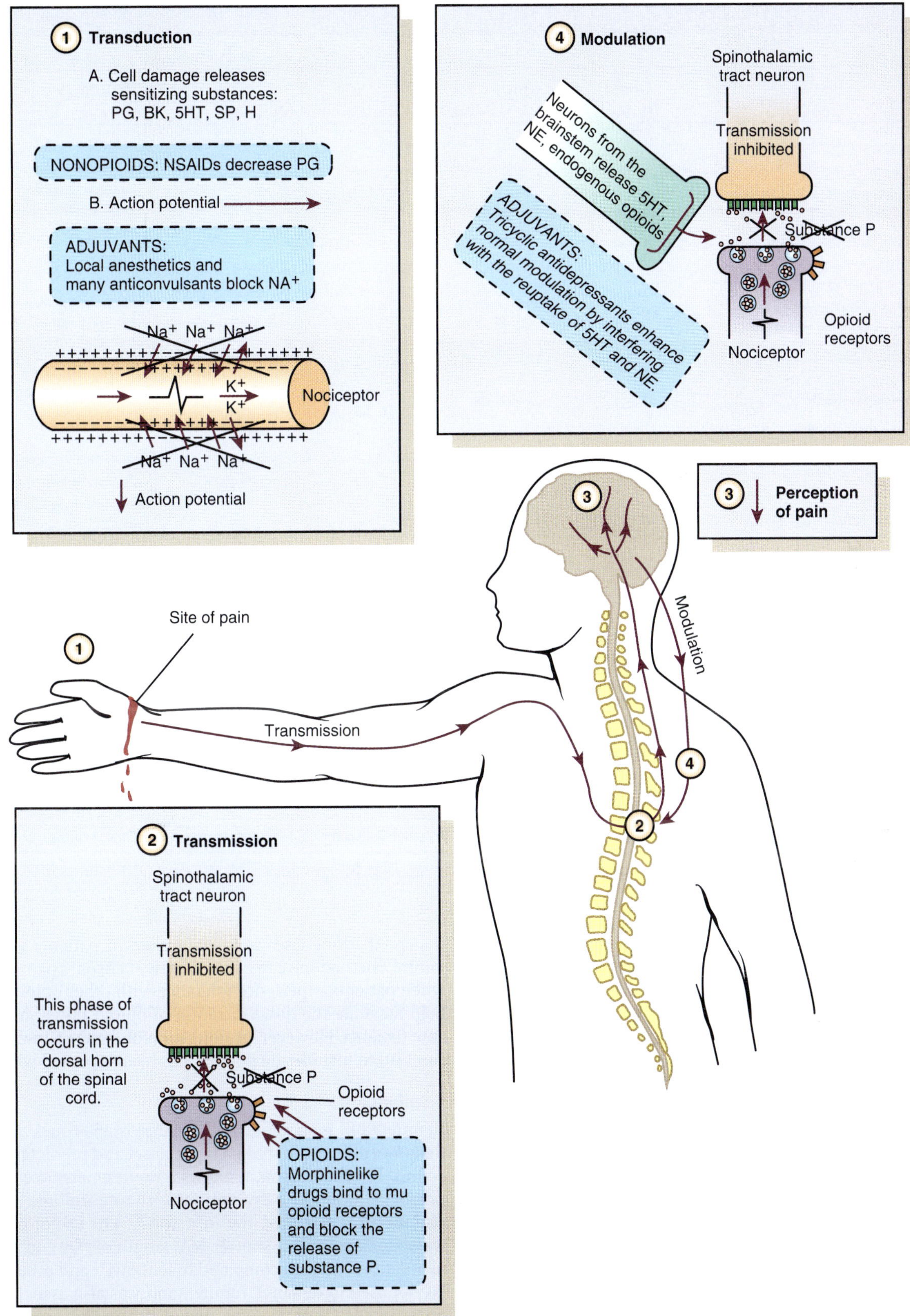

FIG. 7.6 Nociception and Analgesic Action Sites. *BK*, Bradykinin; *H*, histamine; *PG*, prostaglandins; *SP*, substance P; *5HT*, serotonin. (From McCaffery M, Pasero C. *Pain: Clinical Manual for Nursing Practice*. 2nd ed. Mosby; 1999.)

TABLE 7.3 PHARMACOLOGIC MANAGEMENT

Pain

Medication	Dosage	Onset (min)	Duration (h)	Available Routes	Properties	Side Effects and Comments
Morphine	1–4 mg IV bolus	5–10	3–4	PO, SL, R, IV, IM, SC, EA, IA	Analgesia, antianxiety	Standard for comparison Side effects: sedation, respiratory depression, euphoria or dysphoria, hypotension, nausea, vomiting, pruritus, constipation, urinary retention 1–10 mg/h IV infusion M6G can accumulate in patients with renal failure or hepatic dysfunction
Fentanyl	25–100 mcg IV bolus 25–200 mcg/h IV infusion	1–5	0.5–4	OTFC, IV, IM, TD, EA, IA	Analgesia, antianxiety	Same side effects as morphine Rigidity with high doses
Hydromorphone (Dilaudid)	0.2–1 mg IV bolus 0.2–2 mg/h IV infusion	5	3–4	PO, R, IV, IM, SC, EA, IA	Analgesia, antianxiety	Same side effects as morphine
Codeine	15–30 mg IM, SC	10–20	3–4	PO, IM, SC	Analgesia (mild to moderate pain)	Lacks potency (unpredictable absorption; not all patients convert it to active form to achieve analgesia) Most common side effects: light-headedness, dizziness, shortness of breath, sedation, nausea, vomiting
Acetaminophen	325–1000 mg maximum of 4 g/day	20–30	4–6	PO, R	Analgesia, antipyretic	Rare side effects Hepatotoxicity
Ketorolac (Toradol)	15–30 mg IV	<10	6–8	PO, IM, IV	Analgesia, minimum antiinflammatory effect	Short-term use (<5 days) Side effects: gastric ulceration, bleeding, exacerbation of renal insufficiency Use with care in older adult and renal failure patients

EA, Epidural analgesia; *IA*, intrathecal analgesia; *IM*, intramuscular; *IV*, intravenous; *M6G*, morphine-6-glucuronide; *OTFC*, oral transmucosal fentanyl citrate; *PO*, oral; *R*, rectal; *SC*, subcutaneous; *SL*, sublingual; *TD*, transdermal.

or in older adults, it may induce CNS toxicity, including irritability, muscle spasticity, tremors, agitation, and seizures.[20] Although meperidine is useful in short-term specific conditions (e.g., treating postoperative shivering),[90] it should not be used routinely for analgesia in the critical care unit.[88]

Codeine

Codeine has limited use in the management of severe pain. It is rarely used in the critical care unit. It provides analgesia for mild to moderate pain, and it is usually compounded with a nonopioid (e.g., acetaminophen). To be active, codeine must be metabolized in the liver to morphine.[20] Codeine is available only through oral, intramuscular, and subcutaneous routes, and its absorption can be reduced in a critical care patient by altered gastrointestinal motility and decreased tissue perfusion.

Methadone

Methadone is a synthetic opioid with morphine-like properties but less sedation. It is longer acting than morphine and has a long half-life; this makes it difficult to titrate in critical care patients. Methadone lacks active metabolites, and routes other than the kidney eliminate 60% of the medication. This means that methadone does not accumulate in patients with kidney failure. Methadone can be used to treat chronic pain syndromes when patients experience tolerance with other opioids and may help facilitate the down-titration of opioid infusions in critical care patients. However, prolongation of the Q–T interval, which can lead to torsades de pointes, has been reported with its use.[88]

Remifentanil

Remifentanil is an agonist opioid that is 250 times more potent than morphine, and it has a rapid onset and predictable offset of action. For this reason, it allows a rapid emergence from sedation, facilitating the evaluation of the neurologic state of the patient after stopping the infusion.[88] The use of remifentanil was associated with a shorter ICU length of stay and mechanical ventilation duration compared to fentanyl[91] and other opioids.[92] As opposed to fentanyl, remifentanil was also associated with a lower incidence of postoperative delirium.[93]

Sufentanil

Sufentanil is an agonist opioid that is 7 to 13 times more potent than fentanyl and 500 to 1000 times more potent than morphine. It has more pronounced sedation properties than fentanyl and other opioids. Patients given sufentanil require minimal sedative agent doses to achieve an adequate sedation level. It has a rapid distribution and a high clearance rate, preventing accumulation when given for a long period.[94] Sufentanil has a longer emergence from sedation compared with remifentanil, but it has a longer analgesic effect after its administration is stopped.[95] Similarly to remifentanil, sufentanil was associated with a shorter mechanical ventilation duration compared to fentanyl.[91]

Preventing and Treating Opioid-Induced Respiratory Depression

Respiratory depression is the most life-threatening opioid side effect. Although no universal definition of respiratory depression exists, it is usually described in terms of decreased respiratory rate (fewer than 8 or 10 breaths/min), decreased SpO_2 levels, or elevated end-tidal carbon dioxide ($ETCO_2$) levels.[96] A change in the patient's level of consciousness or an increase in sedation normally precedes respiratory depression.

Many risk factors for opioid-induced respiratory depression have been identified. Patients at risk include those with advanced age; obesity; sleep apnea; impaired renal, pulmonary, hepatic, or cardiac functioning; patients in whom pain is controlled after a period of poor control; opioid-naïve patients (i.e., receiving opioids for less than a week); patients with concurrent use of CNS depressants; and those at postoperative day 1.[97] The risk of respiratory depression increases when other medications with CNS depressant effects (e.g., benzodiazepines, antiemetics, neuroleptics, antihistamines) are concomitantly administered.

Monitoring Opioid Analgesia

Guidelines on monitoring for patients receiving opioid analgesia were revised by ASPMN.[97] In addition to assessing pain intensity as a targeted outcome of analgesia, regular sedation and respiratory assessments should be done. Valid and reliable sedation scales developed for use in critically ill patients should be employed (see Table 8.1 in Chapter 8). Respirations should be evaluated over 1 minute and qualified according to rate, rhythm, and depth of chest excursion. Technology-supported monitoring (e.g., continuous pulse oximetry and capnography) can be useful in high-risk patients. Snoring is a warning sign. It can be a sign of respiratory depression associated with airway obstruction by the tongue, leading to hypoxemia and possibly to cardiorespiratory arrest.[20,97] More vigilant monitoring should be performed when patients may be at greater risk, such as during the first 24 hours after surgery or after an increase in the dose of an opioid or a change in opioid agent or route of administration.

Opioid Reversal

Critical respiratory depression can be readily reversed with administration of the opioid antagonist naloxone.[20] The usual dose is 0.4 mg, which is mixed with 10 mL of normal saline (for a concentration of 0.04 mg/mL). Naloxone is normally given intravenously very slowly (0.5 mL over 2 minutes) while the patient is carefully monitored for reversal of the respiratory signs. Naloxone administration can be discontinued as soon as the patient is responsive to physical stimulation and able to take deep breaths. However, the medication should be kept nearby. Because the duration of naloxone is shorter than most opioids, another dose may be needed 30 minutes after the first dose. The nurse must monitor sedation and respiratory status and remind the patient to breathe deeply every 1 to 2 minutes until he or she becomes more alert. The benefits of reversing respiratory depression with naloxone must be carefully weighed against the risk of a sudden onset of pain and the difficulty achieving pain relief. To prevent this from occurring, it is important to provide a nonopioid medication for pain relief. Moreover, the use of naloxone is not recommended after prolonged analgesia because it can induce withdrawal and may cause nausea and cardiovascular complications (e.g., dysrhythmias).

Nonopioid Analgesics

In the PADIS guidelines, the use of nonopioids or adjuvants in combination with an opioid is recommended to reduce opioid requirements and opioid-related side effects.[6] This strategy provides greater analgesic effect through action at the peripheral and central levels. Pharmacologic information is presented in Table 7.3.

Sedative With Analgesic Properties: Dexmedetomidine

Dexmedetomidine (Precedex) is a short-acting alpha-2 agonist that is indicated for short-term sedation of mechanically ventilated patients in the critical care unit. Its mechanism of action is unique and differs from the mechanism of action of other commonly used sedatives in critical care. Compared with midazolam (Versed) or lorazepam (Ativan), whose hypnotic effects act mainly on the limbic system, the cortex, or both, the effect of dexmedetomidine is in the locus caeruleus section of the brainstem. As a result, patients receiving dexmedetomidine intravenous infusions are calm and sleepy, yet remain easily arousable. For this reason, dexmedetomidine is ideal for mild to moderate sedation, often referred to as conscious sedation. Refer to Chapter 8 for details on dosage and administration.

Dexmedetomidine also possesses an analgesic property. The analgesic effects of dexmedetomidine are principally due to spinal antinociception via binding to nonnoradrenergic receptors (heteroreceptors) located on the dorsal horn neurons of the spinal cord. Dexmedetomidine has been found to decrease pain intensity and opioid requirements in the postoperative recovery of adults.[98] It has also been associated with a reduced risk of delirium in mechanically ventilated adults in the critical care setting. However, it is not without undesirable effects. Inhibition of noradrenergic receptors in the brainstem and the spinal cord often causes hypotension and bradycardia. The use of dexmedetomidine is suggested over other sedative agents when the desirable effects such as a reduction in delirium risk are valued over undesirable effects.[99]

Acetaminophen

Acetaminophen is an analgesic used to treat mild to moderate pain and is a suggested adjunct to an opioid for pain management in critically ill adults.[6,100] It inhibits the synthesis of neurotransmitter prostaglandins in the CNS, and this is why it does not have antiinflammatory properties.[20] Acetaminophen is metabolized by two pathways:

- Major (nontoxic metabolite)
- Minor (toxic metabolite that is rapidly converted into a nontoxic form by glutathione). In an acetaminophen overdose, a larger amount is processed by the minor pathway, which results in a larger quantity of toxic metabolites and may cause damage to the liver. Within therapeutic doses, side effects are rare. The total daily dose should not exceed 4 g in 24 hours. The nurse must consider other products containing acetaminophen that the patient may receive when calculating the

total daily dose of acetaminophen. Special care must be taken for patients with liver dysfunction, malnutrition, or a history of excess alcohol consumption; total dose of acetaminophen in these patients should not exceed 2 g/day.[20]

Nonsteroidal Antiinflammatory Drugs

The use of nonsteroidal antiinflammatory drugs (NSAIDs) in combination with opioids is indicated in patients with acute musculoskeletal and soft tissue inflammation.[20] The use of an NSAID is suggested as an alternative for pain management during discrete and infrequent procedures in critically ill adults.[6] The addition of NSAIDs to opioids in postoperative pain management plan was associated with a reduction in daily opioid doses and pain scores in critical care patients.[101]

The mechanism of action of NSAIDs is to block the action of cyclooxygenase (COX), the enzyme that converts arachidonic acid to prostaglandins. COX has two forms: COX-1 and COX-2. The production of prostaglandins (transduction process) is inhibited by blocking the action of COX (see Fig. 7.6). NSAIDs can be grouped as

- First-generation: COX-1 and COX-2 inhibitors such as aspirin, ibuprofen, naproxen, and ketorolac
- Second-generation: COX-2 inhibitors such as celecoxib

The inhibition of COX-1 is thought to be responsible for many of the side effects of NSAIDs, such as gastric ulceration, bleeding as a result of platelet inhibition, and acute kidney injury (AKI). In contrast, the inhibition of COX-2 is responsible for the suppression of pain and inflammation.[20] Second-generation NSAIDs are associated with minimal risks of serious adverse effects, but their role in critically ill patients is unknown.

Ketorolac

Ketorolac is the most appropriate NSAID for use in the critical care setting. Not all critically ill patients are candidates for ketorolac therapy because of its side effects. Caution is advised for using ketorolac in older adults or in patients with kidney dysfunction because of their slower clearance rates. Because ketorolac is an NSAID, monitoring for clumping of platelets is of primary importance. Laboratory data should be evaluated for an increase in bleeding time, and the patient should be assessed for any signs of abnormal bleeding. Moreover, prolonged use of ketorolac for more than 5 days was associated with an increase in kidney failure and bleeding. It is important to consider the concurrent use of opioids and NSAIDs to effect pain modification at both areas of transmission. This combination of agents often significantly reduces the amount of opioids required for effective pain management.[101]

Ketamine

Low-dose ketamine is suggested as an adjunct to opioid therapy in postsurgical critical care adult patients.[6,100] Ketamine is a dissociative anesthetic agent that has analgesic properties. It was traditionally used intravenously for procedural pain in burn patients. It is also available in enteral routes. Compared with opioids, ketamine has the benefit of sparing the respiratory drive, but it has many side effects related to the release of catecholamines and the emergence of delirium. For this reason, ketamine is not recommended for routine therapy in critically ill patients. Before ketamine is administered, the dissociative state should be explained to the patient. *Dissociative state* refers to the feelings of separateness from the environment, loss of control, hallucinations, and vivid dreams. The use of benzodiazepines (e.g., midazolam) can reduce the incidence of this unpleasant effect.[20]

Lidocaine

Lidocaine is another anesthetic that can be used for procedural and acute pain or for some patients with chronic neuropathic pain.[20] When used locally, anesthetics act through the transduction process (see Fig. 7.6). The routine use of intravenous (IV) lidocaine is not suggested for pain management in critically ill adults.[6]

Anticonvulsants

Anticonvulsants (e.g., carbamazepine, gabapentin, pregabalin) are first-line analgesics for lancing neuropathic pain. Their use with opioids is recommended for neuropathic pain management in critically ill adults and is suggested for use in adults after cardiovascular surgery.[6] Use of anticonvulsants has been associated with a reduction in pain scores and opioid doses in critical care patients.[100] Even if the specific mechanism for pain relief is unknown, analgesia probably results from the suppression of sodium ion (Na+) discharges, reducing the neuronal hyperexcitability (action potential) in the transduction process (see Fig. 7.6).[20]

Antidepressants

Antidepressants are also considered as analgesics in various chronic pain syndromes such as headache, fibromyalgia, low back pain, neuropathy, central pain, and cancer pain. The analgesic dose is often lower than the dose required to treat depression. Antidepressant adjuvant analgesics are usually divided into two main groups: tricyclic antidepressants (e.g., amitriptyline, imipramine, desipramine) and biogenic amine reuptake inhibitors (e.g., venlafaxine, paroxetine, sertraline). The mechanism of analgesia most widely accepted is the ability of antidepressants to block the reuptake of neurotransmitters serotonin and norepinephrine in the CNS.[20] This increases the activity of the modulation process (see Fig. 7.6).

Delivery Methods

The most common route for medication administration is the intravenous route by means of continuous infusion, bolus administration, or patient-controlled analgesia (PCA). Traditionally, the choice has been intravenous bolus administration. The benefits of this method are the rapid onset of action and the ease of titration. The major disadvantage is the increase and decrease of the serum level of the opioid, leading to periods of pain control with periods of breakthrough pain.

Continuous infusion of opioids with an infusion pump provides constant blood levels of the ordered opioid; this promotes a consistent level of comfort. It is a particularly helpful method of administration during sleep because the patient awakens with an adequate level of pain relief. It is important that the patient be given the loading dose that relieves the pain and raises the circulating dose of the medication. After the basal rate is established, the patient maintains a steady state of pain control unless there is additional pain from a procedure, an activity, or a change in the patient's condition. In this situation, physician orders to administer additional boluses of opioid need to be available.

Patient-Controlled Analgesia

PCA is a method of medication delivery that uses the intravenous route and an infusion pump. It allows the patient to self-administer small doses of analgesics. Different opioids can be used, but the most extensively used is morphine. This method of medication delivery allows the patient to control the level of

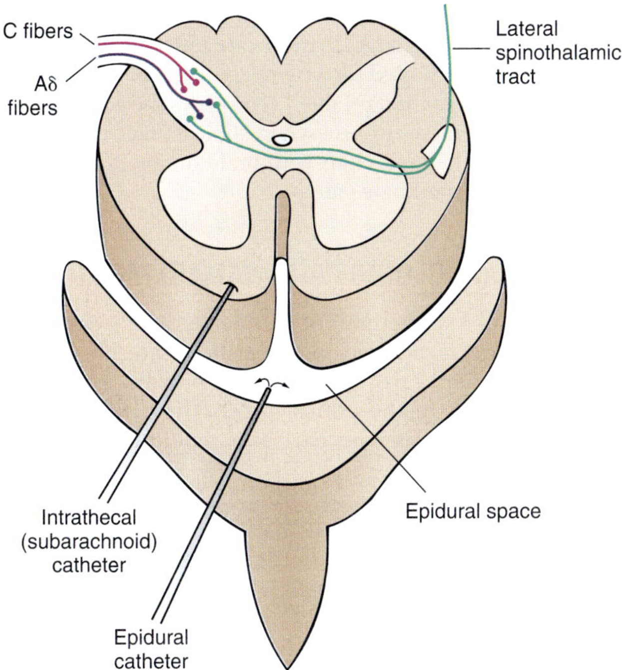

FIG. 7.7 Intraspinal Catheter Placement in a Spinal Cord Cross-Section.

pain and sedation and to avoid the peaks and valleys of intermittent dosing by the health care professional. The patient can self-administer a bolus of medication the moment the pain begins, acting preemptively.

Certain patients are not candidates for PCA. Patients with alterations in the level of consciousness or mentation are unable to understand the use of the equipment. Very elderly patients and patients with kidney or liver dysfunction may require careful screening for PCA.

Allowing the patient to self-administer opioid doses does not diminish the role of the critical care nurse in pain management. The nurse advises about necessary changes to the prescription and continues to monitor the effects of the medication and doses. The patient is closely monitored during the first 2 hours of therapy and after every change in the prescription. If the patient's pain does not respond within the first 2 hours of therapy, a total reassessment of the pain state is essential. The nurse monitors the number of boluses the patient delivers. If the patient is pressing the button to bolus medication more often than the prescription, the dose may be insufficient to maintain pain control. Naloxone must be readily available to reverse opioid-induced respiratory depression. Ideally, a patient undergoing an elective procedure requiring opioid analgesia postoperatively is instructed in the use of PCA during preoperative teaching. This allows the patient to become comfortable with the concept of self-medication before use.

Intraspinal Pain Control

Intraspinal anesthesia uses the concept that the spinal cord is the primary link in nociceptive transmission. The goal is to mimic the body's endogenous opioid pain modification system by interfering with the transmission of pain and providing an opioid receptor binding agent directly into the spinal cord. The hemodynamic status of the patient changes very little.

Intraspinal anesthesia is particularly appropriate for pain in the thorax, upper abdomen, and lower extremities. The two intraspinal routes are intrathecal and epidural (Fig. 7.7). Regardless of the route, the effects of the opioid agonist used are similar, and assessment parameters are the same as those used for other routes.

Intrathecal Analgesia

Intrathecal (subarachnoid) opioids are placed directly into the cerebrospinal fluid and attach to spinal cord receptor sites. Opioids introduced at this site act quickly at the dorsal horn. The dural sheath is punctured, eliminating the barrier for pathogens between the environment and the cerebrospinal fluid. This creates the risk of serious infections. The intrathecal route is usually reserved for intraoperative use. Single-bolus dosing provides short-term relief for short-lived pain (the pain of labor and delivery is well managed using this regimen). Side effects of intrathecal pain control include postdural puncture headache and infection.

Epidural Analgesia

Epidural analgesia is commonly used in the critical care unit after major abdominal surgery, nephrectomy, thoracotomy, and major orthopedic procedures. Certain conditions preclude the use of this pain control method, including systemic infection, anticoagulation, and increased intracranial pressure. Epidural delivery of opioids provides longer lasting pain relief with less dosing of opioids. When delivered into the epidural space, 5 mg of morphine may be effective for 6 to 24 hours compared with 3 to 4 hours when delivered intravenously. Opioids infused in the epidural space are more unpredictable than opioids administered intrathecally. The epidural space is filled with fatty tissue and is external to the dura mater. The fatty tissue interferes with uptake, and the dura mater acts as a barrier to diffusion, making diffusion rate difficult to predict.

The type of medication used determines the rapidity of medication diffusion. Hydrophilic medications (e.g., morphine) are water soluble and penetrate the dura mater slowly, giving them a longer onset and duration of action. Lipophilic medications (e.g., fentanyl) are lipid soluble; they penetrate the dura rapidly and have a rapid onset of action and a shorter duration of action.

The dura mater acts as a physical barrier and causes delay in diffusion of the medication. Compared with the intrathecal route, it allows more medication to be absorbed in the systemic circulation, requiring greater doses for pain relief. Medications delivered epidurally may be administered by bolus or by continuous infusion. Epidural analgesia is being used more often in the critical care environment, and it requires careful monitoring.

The nurse must assess the patient for respiratory depression. This phenomenon may occur early in the therapy or within 24 hours after initiation. The epidural catheter also puts the patient at risk for infection. The efficiency of this pain control method and the increased mobility of the patient do not diminish the nurse's responsibility to monitor and evaluate the outcomes of the pain management protocol in use.

Equianalgesia

When a modification of opioid is considered, the nurse must be aware of equianalgesic dosages. In doing any conversion, the goal is to provide equal analgesic effects with the new agents. This concept is referred to as *equianalgesia*. Morphine is the standard for the conversion of opioids. Prescribed dosages must consider the patient's age and health status.[20] The critical care nurse must have access to a chart on the unit for easy referral to administer the correct dosages of opioids to critically ill patients. Because of the variety of agents and routes, professional pain

BOX 7.3 Guide to Using Equianalgesic Charts

- Equianalgesic means approximately the same pain relief.
- The equianalgesic chart is a guideline. Doses and intervals between doses are titrated according to the individual's response.
- The equianalgesic chart is helpful when switching from one medication to another or when switching from one route of administration to another.
- Dosages in the equianalgesic chart for moderate to severe pain are not necessarily starting doses. The doses suggest a ratio for comparing the analgesia of one medication with another.
- For older patients, initially reduce the recommended adult opioid dose for moderate to severe pain by 25% to 50%.
- The longer the patient has been receiving opioids, the more conservative the starting dose of a *new* opioid should be.

organizations have developed equianalgesia charts for use by health care professionals. All critical care units need to have an equianalgesic chart posted for easy reference. Box 7.3 presents a guide to using these charts. Table 7.4 provides the equianalgesic dose for different medications used in clinical practice. Table 7.5 presents an equianalgesic chart with oral nonopioid and opioid doses for mild to moderate pain.

NONPHARMACOLOGIC PAIN MANAGEMENT

Although numerous methods of pain management other than medications are mentioned in the critical care literature,[102] only a few studies have been done to provide evidence of their effectiveness in the critical care setting.[7,103] Nonpharmacologic interventions are part of a multimodal analgesic

TABLE 7.4 Equianalgesic Chart Approximate Equivalent Doses of Opioids for Moderate to Severe Pain

Analgesic	Parenteral (IM, SC, IV) Route (mg)[a,b]	PO Route (mg)[a]	Comments
Mu Opioid Agonists			
Morphine	10	30	Standard for comparison; multiple routes of administration; available in immediate-release and controlled-release formulations; active metabolite M6G can accumulate with repeated dosing in renal failure
Codeine	130	200 NR	IM has unpredictable absorption and high side effect profile; use PO for mild to moderate pain; usually compounded with nonopioid (e.g., Tylenol No. 3)
Fentanyl	100 mcg/h parenterally and transdermally ≅ 4 mg/h morphine parenterally; 1 mcg/h transdermally ≅ 2 mg/24 h morphine PO	—	Short half-life, but at steady state, slow elimination from tissues can lead to prolonged half-life (up to 12 h); start opioid-naïve patients on no more than 25 mcg/h transdermally; transdermal fentanyl NR for acute pain management; available by oral transmucosal route
Hydromorphone (Dilaudid)	1.5	7.5	Useful alternative to morphine; no evidence that metabolites are clinically relevant; shorter duration than morphine; available in high-potency parenteral formulation (10 mg/mL) useful for SC infusion; 3 mg rectal ≅ 650 mg aspirin PO; with repeated dosing (e.g., PCA), it is more likely than 2–3 mg parenteral hydromorphone = 10 mg parenteral morphine
Levorphanol (Levo-Dromoran)	2	4	Longer acting than morphine when given repeatedly; long half-life can lead to accumulation within 2–3 days of repeated dosing
Meperidine	75	300 NR	No longer preferred as first-line opioid for management of acute or chronic pain because of potential toxicity from accumulation of metabolite, normeperidine; normeperidine has 15–20 h half-life and is not reversed by naloxone; NR in elderly patients or patients with impaired renal function; NR by continuous IV infusion
Oxycodone	—	20	Used for moderate pain when combined with nonopioid (e.g., Percocet, Tylox); available as single entity in immediate-release and controlled-release formulations (e.g., OxyContin); can be used similar to PO morphine for severe pain
Oxymorphone (Numorphan)	1	10 rectal	Used for moderate to severe pain; no PO formulation
Agonist-Antagonist Opioids[c]			
Buprenorphine (Buprenex)	0.4	—	Not readily reversed by naloxone; NR for laboring patients
Butorphanol (Stadol)	2	—	Available in nasal spray
Dezocine (Dalgan)	10	—	
Nalbuphine (Nubain)	10	—	
Pentazocine (Talwin)	30	50	

[a]Duration of analgesia is dose dependent; the higher the dose, usually the longer the duration.

[b]IV boluses may be used to produce analgesia that lasts approximately as long as IM or SC doses. However, of all routes of administration, IV produces the highest peak concentration of the medication, and the peak concentration is associated with the highest level of toxicity (e.g., sedation). To decrease the peak effect and reduce the level of toxicity, IV boluses may be administered more slowly (e.g., 10 mg of morphine over a 15-min period), or smaller doses may be administered more often (e.g., 5 mg of morphine every 1–1.5 h).

[c]Not recommended for severe, escalating pain. If used in combination with mu agonists, may reverse analgesia and precipitate withdrawal in opioid-dependent patients.

FDA, U.S. Food and Drug Administration; *IM*, intramuscular; *IV*, intravenous; *M6G*, morphine-6-glucuronide; *NR*, not recommended; *PCA*, patient-controlled analgesia; *PO*, per os (by mouth); *PRN*, pro re nata (as needed); *SC*, subcutaneous.

From Pasero C, McCaffery M. *Pain Assessment and Pharmacologic Management*. Elsevier; 2011.

TABLE 7.5 Equianalgesic Chart Approximate Equivalent Doses of PO Nonopioids and Opioids for Mild to Moderate Pain

Analgesic	PO Dosage (mg)
Nonopioids	
Acetaminophen	650
Aspirin (ASA)	650
Opioids[a]	
Codeine	32–60
Hydrocodone[b]	5
Meperidine (Demerol)	50
Oxycodone[c]	3–5
Propoxyphene (Darvon)	65–100

[a]Often combined with acetaminophen; avoid exceeding maximum total daily dose of acetaminophen (4000 mg/day).
[b]Combined with acetaminophen (e.g., Vicodin, Lortab).
[c]Combined with acetaminophen (e.g., Percocet, Tylox); also available alone as controlled-release OxyContin and immediate-release formulations.
ASA, Acetylsalicylic acid; *PO*, per os (oral).
Selected references for more information: McCaffery M, Pasero C. Acetaminophen and NSAIDS: adult dosing information. In: Pasero C, McCaffery M. *Pain Assessment and Pharmacologic Management.* Mosby; 2011: 211. American Pain Society (APS). *Principles of Analgesic Use in the Treatment of Acute Pain and Cancer Pain.* 3rd ed. APS; 1992. Kaiko R, et al. Analgesic efficacy of controlled-release (CR) oxycodone and CR morphine. *Clin Pharmacol Ther.* 1996;59:130.
Modified from Pasero C, McCaffery M. *Pain Assessment and Pharmacologic Management.* Elsevier; 2011.

approach, and they are often used in combination with pharmacologic interventions to optimize pain relief. Many nonpharmacologic interventions including massage, ice therapy, music, and relaxation techniques are suggested in the PADIS guidelines for procedural and/or nonprocedural pain management and are part of the ICU Liberation Bundle because they are simple and safe to use.[6,7] It is crucial that nurses be provided with the appropriate training and equipment required to apply nonpharmacologic interventions for pain management in critically ill patients.

The key to success with any of these interventions is a comprehensive understanding of their mechanism of action so that the therapy matches the needs of the patient. Most of the following interventions require the patient's cooperation. There must be some commitment to the treatment on the part of the patient, and the family may be involved also.[104]

Physical Techniques

Stimulating other non–pain sensory fibers (Aβ) in the periphery modifies pain transmission. These fibers are stimulated by thermal changes, as in simple massage and ice therapy.

Massage

The effect of massage on pain relief was mainly tested in postoperative critical care patients following cardiac surgery. A systematic review and meta-analysis of 12 randomized controlled trials (RCTs) revealed that massage was effective in reducing postoperative pain in critical care cardiac surgery patients compared with usual care or sham massage (e.g., hand holding).[105] Duration of massage (10–30 minutes), frequency (single or repeated administration), and body area (back, feet and hands, or only hands) varied across RCTs. Massage can be administered by nurses following minimal training (3–6 hours).

BOX 7.4 Internet Resources

Pain and Pain Management

- American Society for Pain Management Nursing (ASPMN): http://www.aspmn.org/
- Canadian Pain Society (CPS): https://www.canadianpainsociety.ca/
- International Association for the Study on Pain (IASP): https://www.iasp-pain.org/
- Joint Commission: https://www.jointcommission.org/
- Society of Critical Care Medicine (SCCM): https://www.sccm.org/

Ice Therapy

Ice therapy applied for 15 to 20 minutes was found to be helpful to reduce procedural pain (e.g., chest tube removal) when used in combination with an analgesia in critically ill patients.[106] RCTs were conducted in cardiac surgery critical care patients, and the panel felt this intervention could be generalizable to other procedures.[6]

Cognitive-Behavioral Techniques

Using the cortical interpretation of pain as the foundation, several interventions can reduce the patient's pain report, including cognitive-behavioral techniques such as relaxation and music.

Deep Breathing and Relaxation

Breathing techniques were mainly studied and were found to reduce procedural pain (chest tube removal) when timed with an opioid in cardiac surgery critical care patients.[6] Relaxation decreases oxygen consumption and muscle tone, and it can decrease heart rate and blood pressure. Relaxation gives the patient a sense of control over the pain and reduces muscle tension and anxiety. Deep-breathing exercises can be as simple as teaching the patient to inhale slowly through the nose and to exhale through pursed lips.[107]

Music

Music is a commonly used intervention for relaxation. In a systematic review and meta-analysis of 18 RCTs, the administration of 20 to 30 minutes of music has been found to be effective in reducing pain in critically ill adults.[108] The music should be supplied by a small set of headphones, although some patients may prefer not to use them. It is important to educate the patient and family regarding the role of music in relaxation and pain control and to provide music of the patient's choice.[108] The family of the patient unable to self-report may assist the nurse in the selection of music based on the patient's preferences, and music delivery.[104]

Bundle Interventions

A bundling of interventions includes the combination of interventions. The ABCDE care bundle has been implemented in ICUs with improved interprofessional collaboration and care coordination and positive patient outcomes.[109,110] Another randomized controlled trial (RCT) testing three modalities (i.e., relaxation, massage, and music) showed a decrease in the incidence and pain scores of critically ill patients.[111] Bundled interventions follow the same schedule and require the same resources as those of single interventions.

CASE STUDY 7.1 Patient With Pain

Brief Patient History

Ms. Peterson is a 47-year-old female admitted to the intensive care unit (ICU) following a fall of several meters which resulted in a brain injury (subdural hemorrhage), with thoracic and orthopedic trauma on the left side. Past medical history includes type 2 diabetes mellitus with neuropathy of both lower limbs. Her chronic pain is effectively managed with daily doses of gabapentin. Ms. Peterson was intubated and mechanically ventilated due to an altered level of consciousness and deteriorating respiratory parameters. She is receiving IV infusions of fentanyl (1 mcg/kg/h) and propofol (0.5 mg/kg/h). Fentanyl bolus can be administered for breakthrough pain. Regular doses of acetaminophen are also prescribed.

Clinical Assessment

Ms. Peterson is unable to self-report with an altered level of consciousness (Glasgow Coma Scale score of 9) and moderately sedated (Richmond Agitation Sedation Scale score of –3). During bed turning procedures, she grimaces, activates the alarms of the ventilator, tries to reach her thorax with her intact arm, and resists to movements. At the last turning procedure, the nurse observed tears. Family members are concerned that their mother will suffer more pain in addition to the challenges she has with the management of her chronic pain. They also mention that their mother really likes to listen to music, that it helps her to relax and provides her comfort.

Diagnostic Procedures

CPOT-Neuro scores during turning procedures are 4 and above.
RASS scores fluctuate between –2 and –3.

Medical Diagnosis

The diagnosis is acute pain from polytrauma superimposed on chronic neuropathic pain involving both lower extremities.

Questions

1. What type(s) of pain is Ms. Peterson most likely to suffer from considering her clinical condition and past medical history? Relate type(s) of pain to their source or cause.
2. What is the best method for pain assessment according to the person's capacity to communicate?
3. At what frequency should pain be assessed?
4. What preventive intervention would be appropriate to consider prior to a standard care procedure known to be painful such as turning?
5. How can the effectiveness of analgesia be assessed? (Hint: see Algorithm in Fig. 7.5.)
6. Describe a pain management plan for Ms. M. that aligns with a multimodal analgesia approach and her pain condition.
7. What is the role of family members in pain assessment and pain management? As a nurse, how can you support the family members in the pain assessment/management process?

ADDITIONAL RESOURCES

See Box 7.4 for Internet resources related to pain and pain management.

KEY POINTS

- Pain in a critically ill patient is difficult to assess and manage. There are many sources of pain in the critical care setting, and the effects of unrelieved acute pain can have a significant effect on the patient's recovery.
- When possible, the patient's self-report of pain must be obtained. A simple yes or no communicated by head nodding from a mechanically ventilated patient is considered a valid self-report of pain.
- When the patient's self-report is unavailable, behavioral scales are alternative measures of pain assessment; standardized tools (e.g., BPS/BPS-NI, CPOT/CPOT-Neuro) have been developed for assessment of pain in nonverbal critically ill patients.
- The critical care nurse must collaborate with the multidisciplinary team to ensure that a plan of care for management of the patient's pain is developed. A multimodal analgesic approach should be prioritized to reduce the use of opioids and to optimize pain relief and patient safety. To fully participate, the nurse must have extensive knowledge of nonpharmacologic and pharmacologic interventions designed to achieve effective pain relief.

Visit the Evolve site at http://evolve.elsevier.com/Urden/CriticalCareNursing for additional study materials.

REFERENCES

1. Puntillo KA, Max A, Timsit JF, et al. Determinants of procedural pain intensity in the intensive care unit: the Europain® study. *Am J Respir Crit Care Med*. 2014;189(1):39–47. https://doi.org/10.1164/rccm.201306-1174OC.
2. Puntillo KA, White C, Morris AB, et al. Patients' perceptions and responses to procedural pain: results from Thunder Project *II*. *Am J Crit Care*. 10(4):238–251.
3. Mäkinen OJ, Bäcklund ME, Liisanantti J, Peltomaa M, Karlsson S, Kalliomäki ML. Persistent pain in intensive care survivors: a systematic review. *Br J Anaesth*. 2020;125(2):149–158. https://doi.org/10.1016/j.bja.2020.04.084.
4. Belzak L, Halverson J. The opioid crisis in Canada: a national perspective. *Health Promot Chronic Dis Prev Can*. 2018;38(6):224–233. https://doi.org/10.1016/j.bja.2020.04.084.
5. Stevens JP, Wall MJ, Novack L, Marshall J, Hsu DJ, Howell MD. The critical care crisis of opioid overdoses in the United States. *Ann Am Thorac Soc*. 2017;14(12):1803–1809. https://doi.org/10.1513/AnnalsATS.201701-022OC.
6. Devlin JW, Skrobik Y, Gélinas C, et al. Clinical practice guidelines for the prevention and management of pain, agitation/sedation, delirium, immobility, and sleep disruption in adult patients in the ICU. *Crit Care Med*. 2018;46(9):e825–e873. https://doi.org/10.1097/CCM.0000000000003299.
7. Martorella G. Characteristics of nonpharmacological interventions for pain management in the ICU: a scoping review. *AACN Adv Crit Care*. 2019;30(4):388–397. https://doi.org/10.4037/aacnacc2019281.
8. International Association for the Study of Pain. IASP Terminology. https://www.iasp-pain.org/resources/terminology/; 2020. Accessed September 19, 2023 Accessed.
9. Gélinas C. Pain assessment in the critically ill adult: recent evidence and new trends. Intensive *Crit Care Nurse*. 34:1–11. https://doi.org/10.4037/aacnacc2019281.
10. Karlsen MMW, Ølnes MA, Heyn LG. Communication with patients in intensive care units: a scoping review. *Nurs Crit Care*. 2018;24(3):115–131. https://doi.org/10.4037/ajcc2011989.
11. AACN Practice Alert. Assessing pain in critically ill adults. *Crit Care Nurs*. 2018;38(6):e13–e16. https://doi.org/10.4037/ccn2018781.
12. Herr K, Coyne PJ, Ely E, Gélinas C, Manworren RCB. Pain assessment in the patient unable to self-report: clinical practice recommendations in support of the ASPMN 2019 position statement. *Pain Manag Nurs*. 2019;20(5):404–417. https://doi.org/10.4037/ajcc2018271.

13. Herr K, Coyne PJ, Ely E, Gélinas C, Manworren RCB. ASPMN 2019 Position Statement: pain assessment in the patient unable to self-report. *Pain Manag Nurs*. 2019;20(5):402–403. https://doi.org/10.1016/j.pmn.2019.07.007.
14. Williams AC, Craig KD. Updating the definition of pain. *Pain*. 2016;157(11):2420–2423. https://doi.org/10.1097/j.pain.0000000000000613.
15. McCaffery M. *Nursing Management of the Patient With Pain*. 2nd ed. Philadelphia: Lippincott; 1979.
16. Anand KJ, Craig KD. New perspectives on the definition of pain. *Pain*. 1996;67(1):3–6. https://doi.org/10.1016/0304-3959(96)03135-1.
17. Raja SN, Carr DB, Cohen M, et al. The revised International Association for the Study of Pain definition of pain: Concepts, challenges, and compromises. *Pain*. 2020;161(9):1976–1982. https://doi.org/10.1097/j.pain.0000000000001939.
18. Freynhagen R, Parada HA, Calderon-Ospina CA, et al. Current understanding of the mixed pain concept: a brief narrative review. *Curr Med Res Opin*. 2019;35(6):1011–1018. https://doi.org/10.1080/03007995.2018.1552042.
19. World Health Organization (WHO). International Classification of Diseases 11th revision (ICM-11): The Global Standard for Diagnostic Health Information. World Health Organization [online]. https://icd.who.int/en Accessed on September 19, 2023.
20. Pasero C, McCaffery M. *Pain assessment and pharmacologic management*. St. Louis: Elsevier/Mosby; 2011.
21. Cervero F, Laird JM. Visceral pain. *Lancet*. 1999;353(9170):2145–2148. https://doi.org/10.1016/S0140-6736(99)01306-9.
22. Fitzcharles MA, Cohen SP, Clauw DJ, Littlejohn G, Usui C, Häuser W. Nociplastic pain: towards an understanding of prevalent pain conditions. *Lancet*. 2021;397:2098–2110.23. https://doi.org/10.1016/S0140-6736(21)00392-5.
23. Melzack R, Wall PD. *The challenge of pain*. 2nd ed. London, England: Penguin Books; 1996. Updated.
24. Carr DB, Goudas LC. Acute pain. *Lancet*. 1999;353(9169):2051–2058. https://doi.org/10.1016/S0140-6736(99)03313-9.
25. Gélinas C, Puntillo KA, Levin P, Azoulay E. The behavior pain assessment tool for critically ill adults: a validation study in 28 countries. *PAIN*. 2017;158(5):811–821. https://doi.org/10.1097/j.pain.0000000000000834.
26. Gélinas C, Arbour C. Behavioral and physiologic indicators during a nociceptive procedure in conscious and unconscious mechanically ventilated adults: similar or different? *J Crit Care*. 2009;24(4):617. https://doi.org/10.1016/j.jcrc.2009.01.013. 628.e627.
27. Rainville P. Brain mechanisms of pain affect and pain modulation. *Curr Opin Neurobiol*. 2002;12(2):195–204. https://doi.org/10.1016/s0959-4388(02)00313-6.
28. Derbyshire SW, Osborn J. Modeling pain circuits: how imaging may modify perception. *Neuroimaging Clin N Am*. 2007;17(4):485–493. https://doi.org/10.1016/j.nic.2007.09.004.
29. Melzack R, Wall PD. Pain mechanisms: a new theory. *Science*. 1965;150(3699):971–979. https://doi.org/10.1126/science.150.3699.971.
30. Marks DM, Shah MJ, Patkar AA, Masand PS, Park GY, Pae CU. Serotonin-norepinephrine reuptake inhibitors for pain control: premise and promise. *Curr Neuropharmacol*. 2009;7(4):331–336. https://doi.org/10.2174/157015909790031201.
31. Lorenz J, Minoshima S, Casey KL. Keeping pain out of mind: the role of the dorsolateral prefrontal cortex in pain modulation. *Brain*. 2003;126(Pt 5):1079–1091. https://doi.org/10.1093/brain/awg102.
32. Rogers JL. *McCance & Huether's Pathophysiology: The biologic basis for disease in adults and children*. 9th ed. St-Louis: Elsevier; 2024.
33. Bernard C, Delmas V, Duflos C, et al. Assessing pain in critically ill brain-injured patients: a psychometric comparison of 3 pain scales and videopupillometry. *PAIN*. 2019;160(11):2535–2543. https://doi.org/10.1097/j.pain.0000000000001637.
34. Vinclair M, Schilte C, Roudaud F, et al. Using Pupillary Pain Index to Assess Nociception in Sedated Critically Ill Patients. *Anesth Analg*. 2019;129(6):1540–1546. https://doi.org/10.1213/ANE.0000000000004173.
35. Puntillo KA, Miaskowski C, Kehrle K, Stannard D, Gleeson S, Nye P. Relationship between behavioral and physiological indicators of pain, critical care patients' self-reports of pain, and opioid administration. *Crit Care Med*. 1997;25(7):1159–1166. https://doi.org/10.1097/00003246-199707000-00017.
36. Rabin BS, Cohen S, Ganguli R, Lysle DT, Cunnick JE. Bidirectional interaction between the central nervous system and the immune system. *Crit Rev Immunol*. 1989;9(4):279–312.
37. Melzack R. Pain and stress: a new perspective. In: Gatchel RJ, Turk DC, eds. *Psychosocial Factors in Pain: Critical Perspectives*. New York: Guilford Press; 1999.
38. Hadjistavropoulos T, Craig KD. A theoretical framework for understanding self-report and observational measures of pain: A communications model. *Behav Res Ther*. 2002;40(5):551–570. https://doi.org/10.1016/s0005-7967(01)00072-9.
39. Chanques G, Gélinas C. Monitoring pain in the intensive care unit (ICU). *Intensive Care Med*. 2022;48:1508–1511. https://doi.org/10.1007/s00134-022-06807-w.
40. Daut RL, Cleeland CS. The prevalence and severity of pain in cancer. *Cancer*. 1982;50(9):1913–1918. https://doi.org/10.1002/1097-0142(19821101)50:9<1913::aid-cncr2820500944>3.0.co;2-r.
41. Melzack R. The short-form McGill Pain Questionnaire. *Pain*. 1987;30(2):191–197. https://doi.org/10.1016/0304-3959(87)91074-8.
42. Jarvis C, Eckhardt A. *Physical examination & health assessment*. 9th ed. St. Louis: Elsevier; 2023.
43. Gélinas C. Management of pain in cardiac surgery ICU patients: have we improved over time? *Intensive Crit Care Nurs*. 2007;23(5):298–303. https://doi.org/10.1016/j.iccn.2007.03.002.
44. Puntillo KA. Pain management. In: Schell HM, Puntillo KA, eds. *Critical care nursing secrets*. 2nd ed. Philadelphia: Mosby; 2012.
45. Chanques G, Viel E, Constantin JM, et al. The measurement of pain in intensive care unit: comparison of 5 self-report intensity scales. *Pain*. 2010;151(3):711–721. https://doi.org/10.1016/j.pain.2010.08.039.
46. Puntillo KA, Morris AB, Thompson CL, Stanik-Hutt J, White CA, Wild LR. Pain behaviors observed during six common procedures: results from Thunder Project II. *Crit Care Med*. 2004;32(2):421–427. https://doi.org/10.1097/01.CCM.0000108875.35298.D2.
47. Gélinas C, Joffe AM, Szumita PM, et al. A psychometric analysis update of behavioral pain assessment tools in noncommunicative, critically ill adults. *AACN Advanced Crit Care*. 2019;30(4):365–387. https://doi.org/10.4037/aacnacc2019952.
48. Payen JF, Bru O, Bosson JL, et al. Assessing pain in critically ill sedated patients by using a behavioral pain scale. *Crit Care Med*. 2001;29(12):2258–2263. https://doi.org/10.1097/00003246-200112000-00004.
49. Chanques G, Payen JF, Mercier G, et al. Assessing pain in nonintubated critically ill patients unable to self report: an adaptation of the Behavioral Pain Scale. *Intensive Care Med*. 2009;35(12):2060–2067. https://doi.org/10.1007/s00134-009-1590-5.
50. Gélinas C, Fillion L, Puntillo KA, Viens C, Fortier M. Validation of the Critical-Care Pain Observation Tool in adult patients. *Am J Crit Care*. 2006;15(4):420–427.
51. Georgiou E, Hadjibalassi M, Lambrinou E, Andreou P, Papathanassoglou ED. The impact of pain assessment on critically ill patients' outcomes: a systematic review. *Biomed Res Int*. 2015;2015:503830. https://doi.org/10.1155/2015/503830.
52. Chanques G, Pohlman A, Kress JP, et al. Psychometric comparison of three behavioural scales for the assessment of pain in critically ill patients unable to self-report. *Crit Care*. 2014;18(5):R160. https://doi.org/10.1186/cc14000.
53. Gélinas C, Ross M, Boitor M, Desjardins S, Vaillant F, Michaud C. Nurses' evaluations of the CPOT use at 12-month post-implementation in the intensive care unit. *Nurs Crit Care*. 2014;19(6):272–280. https://doi.org/10.1111/nicc.12084.
54. Gélinas C, Boitor M, Puntillo KA, et al. Behaviors indicative of pain in brain-injured adult patients with different levels of consciousness in the intensive care unit. *J Pain Symptom Manage*. 2019;57(4):761–773. https://doi.org/10.1016/j.jpainsymman.2018.12.333.

55. Roulin MJ, Ramelet AS. Behavioral changes in brain-injured critical care adults with different levels of consciousness during nociceptive stimulation: an observational study. *Intensive Care Med*. 2014;40:1115–1123. https://doi.org/10.1007/s00134-014-3380-y.
56. Gélinas C, Bérubé M, Puntillo KA, et al. Validation of the Critical-Care Pain Observation Tool-Neuro for the assessment of pain in brain-injured adults in the intensive care unit: A prospective cohort study. *BMC Critical Care*. 2021;25:142. https://doi.org/10.1186/s13054-021-03561-1.
57. Richard-Lalonde M, Bérubé M, Williams V, Bernard F, Tsoller D, Gélinas C. Nurses' Evaluations of the Feasibility and Clinical Utility of the Use of the Critical-Care Pain Observation Tool-Neuro in Critically Ill Brain-Injured Patients. *Science of Nursing and Health Practices*. 2019;2(2): Article 2.
58. Streiner DL, Norman GR, Cairney J. *Health measurement scales: a practical guide to their development and use*. 6th ed. Oxford: Oxford University Press; 2024.
59. Shahiri ST, Gélinas C. The validity of vital signs for pain assessment in critically ill adults. *Pain Manag Nurs*. 2023;24(3):318–328. https://doi.org/10.1016/j.pmn.2023.01.004.
60. Chanques G, Tarri T, Ride A, et al. Analgesia nociception index for the assessment of pain in critically ill patients: a diagnostic accuracy study. *Br J Anaesth*. 2017;119(4):812–820. https://doi.org/10.1093/bja/aex210.
61. Gélinas C, Shahiri TS, Richard-Lalonde M, et al. Exploration of a Multi-Parameter Technology for Pain Assessment in Postoperative Patients After Cardiac Surgery in the Intensive Care Unit: The Nociception Level Index (NOL)™. *J Pain Res*. 2021;14:3723–3731. https://doi.org/10.2147/JPR.S332845.
62. Shahiri S, Richard-Lalonde M, Richebé P, Gélinas C. Exploration of the Nociception Level (NOLt) Index for pain assessment during endotracheal suctioning in mechanically ventilated patients in the intensive care unit: An observational and feasibility study. *Pain Manag Nurs*. 2020;21(5):428–434. https://doi.org/10.1016/j.pmn.2020.02.067.
63. Vanderbyl B, Gélinas C. Family perspectives of traumatically brain injured patient pain behaviors in the intensive care unit. *Pain Manage Nurs*. 2017;18(4):202–213. https://doi.org/10.1016/j.pmn.2017.04.005.
64. Richard-Lalonde M, Boitor M, Mohand-Said S, Gélinas C. Family members' perceptions of pain behaviors and pain management of adult patients unable to self-report in the intensive care unit: A qualitative descriptive study. *Canadian J Pain*. 2018;2(1):315e323. https://doi.org/10.1080/24740527.2018.1544458.
65. Mohand-Saïd S, Richard-Lalonde M, Boitor M, Gélinas C. Family members' experiences with observing pain behaviors using the Critical-Care Pain Observation Tool. *Pain Manage Nurs*. 2019;20(5):455–461. https://doi.org/10.1016/j.pmn.2018.11.001.
66. Shahid A, Sept BG, Owen VS, et al. Preliminary clinical testing to inform development of the Critical-Care Pain Observation Tool for families (CPOT-Fam). *Can J Pain*. 2023;7(2):2235399. https://doi.org/10.1080/24740527.2023.2235399.
67. Lawrence M. The unconscious experience. *Am J Crit Care*. 1995;4:227–232.
68. Laureys S, et al. Cortical processing of noxious somatosensory stimuli in the persistent vegetative state. *Neuroimage*. 2002;17:732–741.
69. Hadjistavropoulos T, Herr K, Prkachin KM, et al. Pain assessment in elderly adults with dementia. *Lancet Neurol*. 2014;13:1216–1227. https://doi.org/10.1016/S1474-4422(14)70103-6.
70. Lichtner V, Dowding D, Esterhuizen P, et al. Pain assessment for people with dementia: a systematic review of systematic reviews of pain assessment tools. *BMC Geriatr*. 2014;14:138. https://doi.org/10.1186/1471-2318-14-13871.
71. Fuchs-Labelle S, Hadjistavropoulos T. Development and preliminary validation of the Pain Assessment Checklist for Seniors with Limited Ability to Communicate (PACSLAC). *Pain Manag Nurs*. 2004;5:37–49. https://doi.org/10.1016/j.pmn.2003.10.001.
72. Warden V, Hurley AC, Volicer L. Development and psychometric evaluation of the Pain Assessment in Advanced Dementia (PAINAD) scale. *J Am Med Dir Assoc*. 2003;4:9–15. https://doi.org/10.1097/01.JAM.0000043422.31640.F7.
73. Herr K, Bursch H, Ersek M, et al. Use of pain-behavioral assessment tools in the nursing home: expert consensus recommendations for practice. *J Gerontol Nurs*. 2010;36:18–29. https://doi.org/10.3928/00989134-20100108-04.
74. Kanji S, MacPhee H, Singh A, et al. Validation of the critical care pain observation tool in critically ill patients with delirium: a prospective cohort study. *Crit Care Med*. 2016;44(5):943–947. https://doi.org/10.1097/CCM.0000000000001522.
74. Davidhizar R, Giger JN. A review of the literature on care of clients in pain who are culturally diverse. *Int Nurs Rev*. 2004;51:47–55. https://doi.org/10.1111/j.1466-7657.2003.00208.x.
75. Cammarano WB, Pittet JF, Weitz S, Schlobohm RM, Marks JD. Acute withdrawal syndrome related to the administration of analgesic and sedative medications in adult intensive care unit patients. *Crit Care Med*. 1998;26(4):676–684. https://doi.org/10.1097/00003246-199804000-00015.
76. American Psychiatric Association. *Diagnostic and statistical manual of mental disorders (DSM-5)*. 5th ed. Washington, DC: American Psychiatric Publishing; 2013.
77. Arroyo-Novoa M, Figueroa-Ramos MI, Puntillo KA. Opioid and benzodiazepine iatrogenic withdrawal syndrome in patients in the intensive care unit. *AACN Adv Crit Care*. 2019;30(4):353–364. https://doi.org/10.4037/aacnacc2019267.
78. Centers for Disease Control and Prevention. Illicit drug use. https://www.cdc.gov/nchs/hus/sources-definitions/illicit-drug-use.htm. Accessed June 30, 2024 Accessed on.
79. Dowell D, Haegerich TM, Chou R. CDC guidelines for prescribing opioids for chronic pain - United States. *MMWR Recomm Rep*. 2016;65(RR-1):1–49.
80. Butler SF, Budman SH, Fernandez K, Jamison RN. Validation of a screener and opioid assessment measure for patients with chronic pain. *Pain*. 2004;112:65–75. https://doi.org/10.1016/j.pain.2004.07.026.
81. Cheatle MD, Compton PA, Dhingra L, Wasser TE, O'Brien CP. Development of the revised opioid risk tool to predict opioid use disorder in patients with chronic non-malignant pain. *J Pain*. 2019;20(7):842–851. https://doi.org/10.1016/j.jpain.2019.01.011.
82. Jamison RN, Martel MO, Huang C-C, Jurcik D, Edwards RR. Efficacy of the opioid compliance checklist to monitor chronic pain patients receiving opioid therapy in primary care. *J Pain*. 2016;17(4):414–423. https://doi.org/10.1016/j.jpain.2015.12.004.
83. Marie StB. Assessing patients' risk for opioid use disorder. AACN *Adv Crit Care*. 30(4):343–352. https://doi.org/10.4037/aacnacc2019931.
84. Rose L. Interprofessional collaboration in the ICU: how to define? *Nurs Crit Care*. 2011;16:5–10. https://doi.org/10.1111/j.1478-5153.2010.00398.x.
85. Cepeda MS, Africano JM, Polo R, Alcala R, Carr DB. What decline in pain intensity is meaningful to patients with acute pain? *Pain*. 2003;105(1-2):151–157. https://doi.org/10.1016/s0304-3959(03)00176-3.
86. Gélinas C, Arbour C, Michaud C, Vaillant F, Desjardins S. Implementation of the Critical-Care Pain Observation Tool on pain assessment/management nursing practices in an intensive care unit with nonverbal critically ill adults: a before and after study. *Int J Nurs Stud*. 2011;48(12):1495–1504. https://doi.org/10.1016/j.ijnurstu.2011.03.012.
87. Devlin JW, Szumita PM. Analgesia-first sedation and nonopioid multimodal analgesia in the intensive care unit. In: Rajendram R, Patel VB, Preedy VR, Martin CR, eds. *Features and Assessments of Pain*. Elsevier Inc.; 2022:57–68. https://doi.org/10.1016/B978-0-12-818988-7.00018-2. Chapter 6.
88. Panahi Y, Dehcheshmeh HS, Mojtahedzadeh M, Joneidi–-Jafari N, Johnston TP, Sahebkar A. Analgesic and sedative agents used in the intensive care unit: A review. *J Cell Biochem*. 2018;119:8684–8693.
89. Miner JR. Sublingual analgesia: a promising proposal for the treatment of pain. *Expert Opin Drug Deliv*. 2020;17(2):123–126. https://doi.org/10.1080/17425247.2020.1714588.
90. Ashley E, Given J. Pain management in the critically ill. *Br J Perioper Nurs*. 2008;18:504. https://doi.org/10.1177/175045890801801106.
91. Wang W, He O, Wang M, et al. Associations of Fentanyl, Sufentanil, and Remifentanil With Length of Stay and Mortality Among Mechanically Ventilated Patients: A Registry-Based Cohort Study. *Front Pharmacol*. 2022;13:858531. https://doi.org/10.3389/fphar.2022.858531.

92. Yang S, Zhao H, Wang H, Zhang H, An Y. Comparison between remifentanil and other opioids in adult critically ill patients: A systematic review and meta-analysis. *Medicine*. 2021;100(38):e27275. https://doi.org/10.1097/MD.0000000000027275.
93. Radtke FM, Franck M, Lorenz M, et al. Remifentanyl reduces the incidence of postoperative delirium. *J Int Med Res*. 2010;38:1225. https://doi.org/10.1177/147323001003800403.
94. Ethuin F, Boudaoud S, Leblanc I, et al. Pharmacokinetics of long-term sufentanyl infusion for sedation in ICU patients. *Intensive Care Med*. 2003;29:1916–1920. https://doi.org/10.1007/s00134-003-1920-y.
95. Soltész S, Biedler A, Silomon M, Schöpflin I, Molter GP. Recovery after remifentanyl and sufentanyl for analgesia and sedation of mechanically ventilated patients after trauma or major surgery. *Br J Anaesth*. 2001;86:763–768. https://doi.org/10.1093/bja/86.6.763.
96. Jarzyna D, Jungquist CR, Pasero C, et al. American Society for Pain Management Nursing guidelines on monitoring for opioid-induced sedation and respiratory depression. *Pain Manage Nurs*. 2011;12(3):118–145. https://doi.org/10.1016/j.pmn.2011.06.008.
97. Jungquist CR, Willens JS, Dunwoody DR, Klingman KJ, Polomano RC. American Society for Pain Management nursing guidelines on monitoring for opioid-induced advancing sedation and respiratory depression: revisions. *Pain Manage Nurs*. 2020;21(1):7–25. https://doi.org/10.1016/j.pmn.2019.06.007.
98. Wang X, Liu N, Chen J, et al. Effect of Intravenous Dexmedetomidine During General Anesthesia on Acute Postoperative Pain in Adults: A Systematic Review and Meta-Analysis of Randomized Controlled Trials. *Clin J Pain*. 2018;34(12):1180–1191. https://doi.org/10.1097/AJP.0000000000000630.
99. Møller MH, Alhazzani W, Lewis K, et al. Use of dexmedetomidine for sedation in mechanically ventilated adult ICU patients: a rapid practice guideline. *Intensive Care Med*. 2022;48:801–810. https://doi.org/10.1007/s00134-022-06660-x.
100. Wheeler K, Grilli R, Centofanti JC, et al. Adjuvant analgesic use in the critically ill: A systematic review and meta-analysis. *Crit Care Explor*. 2020;2(7):e0157. https://doi.org/10.1097/CCE.0000000000000157.
101. Ma CH, Tworek KB, Kung JY, et al. Systemic Nonsteroidal Anti-Inflammatories for Analgesia in Postoperative Critical Care Patients: A Systematic Review and MetaAnalysis of Randomized Control Trials. *Critical Care Explor*. 2023;5(7):e0938. https://doi.org/10.1097/CCE.0000000000000938.
102. Faigeles B, Howie-Esquivel J, Miaskowski C, et al. Predictors and use of nonpharmacologic interventions for procedural pain associated with turning among hospitalized adults. *Pain Manag Nurs*. 2013;14(2):85–93. https://doi.org/10.1016/j.pmn.2010.02.004.
103. Nordness MF, Hayhurst CJ, Pandharipande P. Current Perspectives on the Assessment and Management of Pain in the Intensive Care Unit. *J Pain Res*. 2021;14:1733–1744. https://doi.org/10.2147/JPR.S256406.
104. Gosselin E, Richard-Lalonde M. Role of Family members in pain management in adult critical care. *AACN Adv Crit Care*. 2019;30(4):398–410. https://doi.org/10.4037/aacnacc2019275.
105. Boitor M, Gélinas C, Richard-Lalonde M, Thombs BD. The effect of massage on acute postoperative pain in critically and acutely ill adults post-thoracic surgery: systematic review and meta-analysis of randomized controlled trials. *Heart Lung*. 2017;46:339–346. https://doi.org/10.1016/j.hrtlng.2017.05.005.
106. Lu HY, Lin MY, Tsai PS, Chiu HY, Fang SC. Effectiveness of Cold Therapy for Pain and Anxiety Associated with Chest Tube Removal: A Systematic Review and Meta-Analysis of Randomized Controlled Trials. *Pain Manage Nurs*. 2024;25:34–45. https://doi.org/10.1016/j.pmn.2023.04.016.
107. Friesner SA, Curry DM, Moddeman GR. Comparison of two pain management strategies during chest tube removal: relaxation exercise with opioids and opioids alone. *Heart Lung*. 2006;35:269–276. https://doi.org/10.1016/j.hrtlng.2005.10.005.
108. Richard-Lalonde M, Gélinas C, Boitor M, et al. The effect of music on pain in the adult intensive care unit: a systematic review of randomized controlled trials. *J Pain Symptom Manage*. 2020;59(6):1304–1309.e6. https://doi.org/10.1016/j.jpainsymman.2019.12.359.
109. Balas MC, Burke WJ, Gannon D, et al. Implementing the Awakening and Breathing Coordination, Delirium Monitoring/Management, and Early Exercise/Mobility Bundle into Everyday Care: Opportunities, Challenges, and Lessons Learned for Implementing the ICU Pain, Agitation, and Delirium Guidelines. *Crit Care Med*. 2013;41(9):S116–S127.106. https://doi.org/10.1097/CCM.0b013e3182a17064.
110. Pun BT, Balas MC, Barnes-Daly MA, et al. Caring for Critically Ill Patients with the ABCDEF Bundle: Results of the ICU Liberation Collaborative in Over 15,000 Adults. *Crit Care Med*. 2019;47(1):3–14. https://doi.org/10.1097/CCM.0000000000003482.
111. Papathanassoglou EDE, Hadjibalassi M, Miltiadous P, et al. Effects of an integrative nursing intervention on pain in critically ill patients: a pilot clinical trial. *Am J Crit Care*. 2018;27(3):172–185. https://doi.org/10.4037/ajcc2018271.

8

Sedation, Agitation, and Delirium Management

Mary E. Lough

http://evolve.elsevier.com/Urden/CriticalCareNursing

SEDATION

One of the challenges facing clinicians is how to provide a therapeutic healing environment for patients in the alarm-filled, emergency-focused critical care unit. Many critical care patients demonstrate agitation and discomfort caused by painful procedures, invasive tubes, sleep deprivation, fear, anxiety, and physiologic stress. Sedative medications are used to manage discomfort, including having a plan to avoid oversedation. Clinical practice guidelines have been developed by the Society of Critical Care Medicine (SCCM) to improve management of sedation, agitation, delirium, sleep, mobility, and rehabilitation in critically ill patients.[1,2]

Sedation and Agitation Assessment Scales

The use of a validated scale is recommended to standardize assessments of agitation and sedation in a critically ill adult.[1] Two scales are recommended in the current guidelines (Table 8.1).[1]

- The Richmond Agitation-Sedation Scale (RASS)[3,4]
- The Sedation-Agitation Scale (SAS)[5]

Because individuals do not metabolize sedative medications at the same rate, the use of a standardized scale ensures that continuous infusions of sedatives such as propofol or dexmedetomidine are titrated to a specific measurable outcome. Collaboratively, the critical care team is required to assign the sedation level goal that is most appropriate for each individual patient and reassess frequently. The current guidelines recommend light sedation for critically ill patients receiving mechanical ventilation.[1]

Pain Assessment Scales

The first step in the assessment of an agitated patient is to rule out any sensations of pain.[1] Clinical assessment is more challenging when the patient is obtunded or has an artificial airway in place. If the patient can communicate, the verbal pain scale of 0 to 10 is very useful. If the patient is intubated and cannot vocalize, pain assessment becomes considerably more complex.[6] Two validated behavioral pain scales are recommended for pain assessment, especially nonverbal assessment in critically ill adults:[1]

- The Behavioral Pain Scale (BPS)
- The Critical-Care Pain Observation Scale (CPOT)

These pain scales are shown in Table 7.1 (BPS) and Table 7.2 (CPOT) in Chapter 7. Preemptive analgesia should be provided before painful procedures.[1] The SCCM guidelines recommend that all critically ill, intubated, mechanically ventilated patients have stated goals for analgesia and sedation.[1] The next step is to determine the minimum level of sedation required for an individual patient.[1] Research to determine the optimal level of sedation in critical illness is ongoing to achieve optimal patient outcomes with the least complications.[7,8]

Levels of Sedation

The purpose of using standardized sedation levels in critical care is to provide consistency of patient assessment by all members of the critical care team. Several different tools are available, and although there is a variety of scoring systems, all assess the same spectrum of patient-response behaviors.

In addition to the clinical setting, depth of sedation may be described using the general descriptive terms defined by the American Association of Anesthesiologists (Box 8.1).[9]

- *Light sedation* (minimal sedation) refers to pharmacologic relief of anxiety (anxiolysis) so that the patient is alert and can respond to verbal commands (approximates RASS 0 or may be written as −1 to +1, and SAS 4).[1,3,5,9]
- *Moderate sedation* describes pharmacologic depression of patient consciousness where the patient can respond to verbal commands. This is also described as *procedural sedation*, or *conscious sedation*, as no artificial airway is required. This may be the target level when tubes or lines are to be inserted (approximates RASS −2 to −3; and SAS 3 to 4).[1,3,5,9]
- *Deep sedation* describes pharmacologic depression of patient consciousness to where the patient cannot maintain an open airway and is difficult to arouse (approximates RASS −4 to −5 and SAS 2).[1,3,5,9]
- *General anesthesia* describes pharmacologic depression of patient consciousness using multiple medications, administered by a physician anesthesiologist or a nurse anesthetist (approximates RASS −5 and SAS 1).[1,3,5,9]

When the patient has a depressed level of consciousness because of sedation (moderate, deep, or general anesthesia), vigilant monitoring of cardiac and respiratory function and vital signs is required. To ensure patient safety, qualified clinicians to monitor and recover the patient must always be present. The clinician administering the sedative medication must be qualified to manage the patient appropriate to their area of practice, licensure, and training.

Pharmacologic Management of Sedation

Achievement of the lightest possible sedation to provide comfort for an alert patient is now the expected standard in critical care.[10] To achieve this goal, it is necessary for all members of the clinical team to be familiar with the pharmacokinetics

TABLE 8.1 Sedation Scales

Score	Description	Definition
Richmond Agitation-Sedation Scale (RASS)[a,b]		
+4	Combative	Overtly combative, violent, immediate danger to staff
+3	Very agitated	Pulls or removes tube(s) or catheter(s); aggressive
+2	Agitated	Frequent nonpurposeful movement; fights ventilator
+1	Restless	Anxious but movements not aggressive or vigorous
0	Alert and calm	
−1	Drowsy	Not fully alert, but has sustained awakening (eye opening/eye contact) to voice (>10 s)
−2	Light sedation	Briefly awakens with eye contact to voice (<10 s)
−3	Moderate sedation	Movement or eye opening to voice (but no eye contact)
−4	Deep sedation	No response to voice, but movement or eye opening to physical stimulation
−5	Unresponsive	No response to voice or physical stimulation
Sedation-Agitation Scale (SAS)[c]		
7	Dangerously agitated	Pulls at ETT, tries to remove catheters, climbs over bed rail, strikes at staff, thrashes side to side
6	Very agitated	Does not calm despite frequent verbal reminding of limits, requires physical restraints, bites ETT
5	Agitated	Anxious or mildly agitated, attempts to sit up, calms down to verbal instructions
4	Calm and cooperative	Calm, awakens easily, follows commands
3	Sedated	Difficult to arouse, awakens to verbal stimuli or gentle shaking but drifts off again; follows simple commands
2	Very sedated	Arouses to physical stimuli but does not communicate or follow commands; may move spontaneously
1	Unarousable	Minimal or no response to noxious stimuli; does not communicate or follow commands

[a]Sessler CN, Gosnell MS, Grap MJ, et al. The Richmond Agitation-Sedation Scale: validity and reliability in adult intensive care unit patients. *Am J Respir Crit Care Med.* 2002;166:1338–1344.
[b]Ely EW, Truman B, Shintani A, et al. Monitoring sedation status over time in ICU patients: reliability and validity of the Richmond Agitation-Sedation Scale (RASS). *JAMA.* 2003;289:2983–2991.
[c]Riker RR, Picard JT, Fraser GL. Prospective evaluation of the Sedation-Agitation Scale for adult critically ill patients. *Crit Care Med.* 1999;27:1325–1329.
ETT, Endotracheal tube.

of frequently used categories of sedatives. Additionally, if the patient is experiencing pain, analgesia must be administered in addition to any sedative agents (see Chapter 7).[1] Sedative medications include benzodiazepines, sedative-hypnotic agents such as propofol, and the central alpha agonist dexmedetomidine (Table 8.2). Dexmedetomidine-based and propofol-based sedative regimens are the current recommendations for sedation of mechanically ventilated adult patients.[1]

BOX 8.1 Evidence-Based Practice

Levels of Sedation

Light Sedation (Minimal Sedation, Anxiolysis)

Medication-induced state during which patients respond normally to verbal commands. Although cognitive function and coordination may be impaired, ventilatory and cardiovascular functions are unaffected.

Moderate Sedation With Analgesia (Conscious Sedation, Procedural Sedation)

Medication-induced depression of consciousness during which patients respond purposefully to verbal commands, alone or accompanied by light tactile stimulation. No interventions are required to maintain a patent airway, and spontaneous ventilation is adequate. Cardiovascular function is usually maintained.

Deep Sedation and Analgesia

Medication-induced depression of consciousness during which patients cannot be easily aroused but respond purposefully after repeated or painful stimulation. The ability to maintain ventilatory function independently is impaired. Patients require assistance in maintaining a patent airway, and spontaneous ventilation may be inadequate. Cardiovascular function is usually maintained.

General Anesthesia

Medication-induced loss of consciousness during which patients are not arousable, even by painful stimulation. The ability to maintain ventilatory function independently is impaired, and assistance to maintain a patent airway is required. Positive pressure ventilation may be required because of depressed spontaneous ventilation or medication-induced depression of neuromuscular function. Cardiovascular function may be impaired.

Data from the American Association of Anesthesiologists. Continuum of depth of sedation: definition of general anesthesia and levels of sedation/analgesia. 1999; revised 2014. https://www.asahq.org/standards-and-guidelines?q=moderate%20sedation.

All sedatives are to be administered to a specific target level identified by a RASS or SAS level appropriate to the patient's clinical condition. A target level is specified every day and reevaluated whenever there is a change in sedation dosage or patient condition. One likely sedation goal is that the patient is awake and calm, specified as a target sedation level of RASS 0 or SAS 4. This describes a patient who follows simple verbal commands without agitation and who can sustain eye contact for at least 10 seconds, as described in Table 8.1.

When the intent is to provide deep sedation for a critical illness, the target sedation level is specified as RASS −4 to −5 or SAS 1 to 2. These target values describe a mechanically ventilated patient who is not responsive to a spoken voice and who does not respond purposefully to physical stimulation. If this is not the clinically intended level of consciousness, sedative infusions should be turned down or turned off. If deep sedation or neuromuscular blockade is prescribed, a frontal electrocochleogram monitor is recommended to evaluate deeper sedation levels because of the absence of patient responsiveness at RASS −5 or SAS 1.[1]

Benzodiazepines

Benzodiazepines have powerful amnesic properties that inhibit reception of new sensory information. Benzodiazepines do not confer analgesia. The benzodiazepines most often used are diazepam (Valium), midazolam (Versed), and lorazepam

TABLE 8.2 PHARMACOLOGIC MANAGEMENT

Sedation

Medication	Dosage	Action	Special Considerations
Benzodiazepines			
Diazepam	Loading dose IV: 5–10 mg/kg slowly Intermittent maintenance dose IV: 0.03–0.1 mg/kg every 30 min–6 h as needed	Anxiolysis Amnesia Sedation	Onset: 2–5 min after IV administration Side effects: hypotension, respiratory depression Half-life: long (20–120 h); active metabolites also contribute to prolonged sedative effect. Tolerance: physical tolerance develops with prolonged use, and higher doses of medication are required to achieve same effect over time; slow wean required from diazepam after continuous prolonged use; no active metabolites. Phlebitis occurs with peripheral IV administration.
Lorazepam	Loading dose IV: 0.02–0.04 mg/kg (≤2 mg) slowly Intermittent maintenance IV every 2–6 h: 0.02–0.6 mg/kg slowly Continuous IV maintenance infusion: 0.01–0.1 mg/kg/h (≤10 mg/h)	Anxiolysis Amnesia Sedation	Onset: 15–20 min after IV administration Side effects: hypotension, respiratory depression, propylene glycol–related acidosis, nephrotoxicity Half-life: relatively long (8–15 h) Tolerance: physical tolerance develops with use, and higher medication dosage is required to achieve same effect over time; slow wean required from lorazepam after continuous prolonged use. Solvent-related acidosis and kidney failure occur at high doses.
Midazolam	Loading dose IV: 0.01–0.05 mg/kg slowly over several minutes Continuous IV maintenance infusion: 0.02–0.1 mg/kg/h	Anxiolysis Amnesia Sedation	Onset: 2–5 min after IV administration Side effects: hypotension, respiratory depression Half-life: 3–11 h; sedative effect is prolonged when midazolam infusion has continued for many days, owing to presence of active sedative metabolites; sedative effect is also prolonged in kidney failure. Tolerance: physical tolerance develops with prolonged use, and higher medication dosages are required to achieve same effect over time; slow wean required from midazolam after prolonged use.
Sedative-Hypnotics			
Propofol	Loading dose IV: 5 mcg/kg/min over 5 min Continuous IV maintenance infusion: 5–50 mcg/kg/min	Anxiolysis Amnesia Sedation	Onset: very rapid onset (1–2 min) after IV administration Side effects: hypotension, respiratory depression (patient must be intubated and mechanically ventilated to eliminate this complication), pain at injection site if administered via peripheral IV line; pancreatitis; hypertriglyceridemia, propofol-related infusion syndrome, allergic reactions Half-life: 1–2 min when used as short-term agent; with prolonged continuous IV infusion, half-life extends to 50 ± 18.6 h. Effective short-term anesthetic agent, useful for rapid "wake-up" of patients for assessment; if continuous infusion is used for many days, emergence from sedation can take hours or days; sedative effect depends on dose administered, depth of sedation, and length of time sedated. Change IV infusion tubing every 6–12 h. Requires dedicated IV catheter and tubing (do not mix with other medications). Monitor serum triglyceride levels.
Central Alpha-Adrenergic Receptor Agonists			
Dexmedetomidine	Loading dose IV: 1 mcg/kg over 10 min Continuous IV maintenance infusion: 0.2–0.7 mcg/kg/h	Anxiolysis Analgesia Sedation	Onset: 5–10 min Side effects: Bradycardia, hypotension, loss of airway reflexes Half-life: 1.8–3.1 h No active metabolites Intermittent bolus dosing is not recommended. Maintenance infusion is adjusted to achieve desired level of sedation.

IV, Intravenous.

Data from Barr J, Fraser GL, Puntillo K, et al. Clinical practice guidelines for the management of pain, agitation, and delirium in adult patients in the intensive care unit. *Crit Care Med.* 2013;41:263–306.

(Ativan). However, benzodiazepines are no longer recommended for sedation of mechanically ventilated critically ill adults because benzodiazepine-based sedative regimens are associated with longer duration of mechanical ventilation and delirium.[10,11]

The major unwanted side effects associated with benzodiazepines are delirium, dose-related respiratory depression, and hypotension. If needed, flumazenil (Romazicon) is the antidote used to reverse benzodiazepine overdose in symptomatic patients. Flumazenil should be used with caution in patients with benzodiazepine dependence, because rapid withdrawal can induce seizures and other adverse side effects.[11,12]

Sedative-Hypnotic Agents—Propofol

Propofol is a powerful sedative and respiratory depressant used for sedation in mechanically ventilated patients in critical care.[13] It is immediately identifiable by its white milky appearance, and it is always dispensed in a glass container. At high doses (greater than 100 to 200 mcg/kg per minute), propofol is intended to produce a state of general anesthesia in the operating room. In the critical care unit, propofol is prescribed as a continuous infusion at lower doses (5 to 50 mcg/kg per minute) to induce sedation in critically ill patients. Because propofol is lipid soluble, it quickly crosses cell membranes, including the cells that compose the blood-brain barrier. This allows rapid onset of sedation (30 to 60 seconds) with subsequent loss of consciousness.[13,14] In addition to a rapid onset of action, propofol has a very short half-life with initial use (2 to 4 minutes), is rapidly eliminated from the body (30 to 60 minutes), and does not have active metabolites.[14] The short half-life makes propofol an ideal sedative when a patient will need to be quickly awakened for a spontaneous awakening trial and spontaneous breathing trial or to assess neurologic status. Propofol is clinically effective because it can be titrated down, or turned off, when a patient is mechanically ventilated, and may decrease time to extubation.

Propofol is not an analgesic. Therefore, it is important to add an opiate to ensure adequate pain control. Nor is propofol a reliable amnesic, and patients sedated with only propofol can have vivid recollections of their experiences. If amnesia is required during a procedure, a short-acting opiate such as fentanyl can be administered.

The risk of complications increases with prolonged administration of propofol at doses greater than 5 mg/kg/hour for longer than 48 hours.[13] The term *propofol-related infusion syndrome* describes metabolic acidosis, muscular weakness, rhabdomyolysis, myoglobinuria, acute kidney injury, and cardiovascular dysrhythmias. This condition has a mortality of 50% (48% in adults, 52% in children) based on published case reports.[15]

A rare benign effect of propofol infusion is green urine.[13] Urine discoloration occurs when the patient's liver cannot metabolize all of the propofol, and the remainder is excreted via the kidney. Propofol is not nephrotoxic, and the urine returns to a normal color when the medication is stopped. Secondary side effects related to the fat-emulsion carrier include hyperlipidemia, hypertriglyceridemia, and acute pancreatitis. Serum triglycerides should be measured on all patients who receive propofol for longer than 48 hours. Propofol should not be administered to patients with known allergies to soy or eggs, because the intralipid carrier contains soybean oil, glycerol, and egg-lecetin.[13]

Propofol is a lipid-based emulsion, a medium highly conducive to bacterial growth.[16,17] For this reason, the manufacturer and the Centers for Disease Control and Prevention (CDC) recommend that the tubing be changed every 12 hours to prevent catheter-related infections.[17,18] Use of aseptic technique is mandatory to prevent infection.[17,18] Nursing vigilance is required to monitor sedation levels and to be alert for the rare but significant risk of propofol-related complications. Table 8.2 provides additional information.

Central Alpha Agonists—Dexmedetomidine

Two central alpha-adrenergic agonists with sedative properties are available. Dexmedetomidine (Precedex) is prescribed as a continuous infusion. Clonidine (Catapres) is a skin patch and may be prescribed for patients experiencing *alcohol withdrawal syndrome* (AWS; see later discussion in this chapter).

Dexmedetomidine is an alpha-2 agonist that is approved by the U.S. Food and Drug Administration for use as a short-term sedative (less than 24 hours) in mechanically ventilated patients. Sedation occurs when the medication activates post-synaptic alpha-2 receptors in the central nervous system in the brain. This activation inhibits norepinephrine release and blocks sympathetic nervous system fight-or-flight functions, leading to sedation. Sympathetic nervous system inhibition may cause hypotension and bradycardia. Analgesic effects occur because dexmedetomidine binds to alpha-2 receptors in the spinal cord. These unique mechanisms of action allow patients to be lightly sedated, and also to be interactive, which aligns with the most recent sedation guidelines.[1] In a recently published clinical trial, there was no difference in the duration of delirium, or days of mechanical ventilation, between patients receiving dexmedetomidine and patients receiving propofol.[19]

Dexmedetomidine is administered with a loading dose of 1 mcg/kg over 10 minutes, followed by a continuous infusion of 0.4 mcg/kg (range 0.2 to 0.7 mcg/kg per hour).[20] Dexmedetomidine has a short half-life (6 minutes) and is eliminated from the body in approximately 2 hours. Elimination from the body is dramatically slowed if the patient has liver failure (see Table 8.2).

Many patients have other sedatives or opiates infusing in addition to dexmedetomidine, and the combination may potentiate the overall sedative effect. Monitoring of sedation level, blood pressure, heart rate, respiratory rate, and pulse oximetry is required. Dexmedetomidine confers sedation and analgesic effects without respiratory depression. Consequently, patients can be extubated while still on a dexmedetomidine infusion. This can be helpful for patients who are anxious during ventilator weaning.

Daily Sedation Interruption

One strategy to avoid the pitfalls of sedative dependence and withdrawal is to turn off the sedative infusions once each day. The goals of sedation interruption are to allow for clinical assessment without sedatives infusing and to use a protocol to safely lower the sedative infusion dose. This intervention has been given several names, including *sedation vacation* and *spontaneous awakening trial (SAT)*.[1] At a scheduled time, all continuously infusing sedatives are stopped. Sometimes analgesics are also stopped, depending on the hospital's protocol. The patient is allowed to regain consciousness for clinical assessment using a standardized instrument such as RASS or SAS (see Table 8.1).[19] The patient is carefully monitored, and when awareness is attained, an assessment of level of consciousness and neurologic function is performed. It is essential that a protocol be in place for the nurse to restart the sedatives if the patient experiences either a deleterious change in vital signs (high/low blood pressure or heart rate) or becomes highly agitated, pulling at lines or tubes and endangering their safety. In many protocols, when the sedative medications are restarted, a lower dose is used to avoid dependence.

A typical protocol is to schedule the daily sedative interruption in the morning, conduct a clinical assessment and spontaneous breathing trial, then restart the sedative and opiate infusions at 50% of the previous morning dose and adjust upward until the desired sedation goal is achieved.

Other protocols forgo infusions and use intermittent intravenous push for "as-needed" sedatives and analgesics to manage pain and sedation. Another approach is to maintain the patient at a lighter level of sedation all the time rather than specifying specific times to stop the sedatives.

An important nursing responsibility is to prevent the patient from coming to harm during sedative or analgesic medication withdrawal (Table 8.3). If the patient is seriously agitated, it is vital to consult with the physician and pharmacist to establish an effective treatment plan that allows safe weaning from sedative medications (see Table 8.1).

Agitation

Agitation describes hyperactive patient movements that range in intensity from slight restless hand and body movements to pulling out lines and tubes or physical aggression and self-harm. Some common causes of agitation include pain, anxiety, delirium, hypoxia, ventilator dyssynchrony, neurologic injury, uncomfortable position, full bladder, sleep deprivation, alcohol withdrawal, sepsis, medication reaction, and organ failure. In the past, when a patient showed physical signs of agitation, a benzodiazepine sedative (lorazepam or midazolam) was quickly administered to reduce the patient's mental awareness and hyperactivity (see Table 8.2). However, because benzodiazepines have been associated with a higher incidence of delirium, these medications are no longer recommended.[1]

Agitation is assessed using a validated scale such as SAS or RASS (see Table 8.1). Standardized assessment scales allow clinicians to identify agitation in its milder forms and to potentially ameliorate the patient's symptoms. The goal is to treat the cause of the agitation rather than to overmedicate. When patients are dangerously agitated (SAS +7), are combative (RASS +4), or could endanger themselves or others, immediate sedation is warranted. In these extreme situations, a benzodiazepine may be administered.[20]

TABLE 8.3 Signs and Symptoms of Sedative or Analgesic Medication Withdrawal[a]

System	Opiate Withdrawal	Benzodiazepine Withdrawal[b]
Neurologic	Delirium, tremors, seizures	Agitation, anxiety, delirium, tremors, myoclonus, headache, seizures, fatigue, paresthesias, sleep disturbances
Sensory	Dilation of pupils, teary eyes, irritability, increased sensitivity to pain, sweating, yawning	Increased sensitivity to light/sound, sweating
Musculoskeletal	Cramps, muscle aches	Muscle cramps
Gastrointestinal	Vomiting, diarrhea	Nausea, diarrhea
Respiratory	Tachypnea	Tachypnea

[a]Data on propofol are limited, but withdrawal symptoms after prolonged use are similar to withdrawal symptoms of benzodiazepines.
[b]Not all symptoms are seen in all patients.

DELIRIUM

Delirium is a global impairment of cognitive processes, usually of sudden onset, coupled with disorientation, impaired short-term memory, altered sensory perceptions (i.e., hallucinations), abnormal thought processes, and inappropriate behavior. Routine monitoring for delirium is recommended.[1] Delirium is more prevalent than generally recognized; it is difficult to diagnose in a critically ill patient and represents acute brain dysfunction caused by sepsis, critical illness, or dysfunction of other vital organs. Greater than 50% of patients in critical care areas experience delirium.[21] Delirium increases hospital stay and mortality rates for patients who are mechanically ventilated.

When patients are agitated, restless, and pulling at tubes and lines, they are often identified as being delirious. In this scenario, delirium may be colloquially described as *ICU psychosis* or *sundowner syndrome*. However, a delirious patient is not always agitated, and it is much more difficult to detect delirium when a patient is physically calm.

Specific scoring instruments are available to assess delirium, and two have been validated for use with mechanically ventilated critical care patients:[1]

- The *Confusion Assessment Method for the Intensive Care Unit* (CAM-ICU) (Figs. 8.1 and 8.2)[22,23]
- The *Intensive Care Delirium Screening Checklist* (ICDSC) (Fig. 8.3)[24,25]

Both of these delirium tools are used in tandem with the RASS to exclude patients in coma.[3,4] Coma is a known risk factor

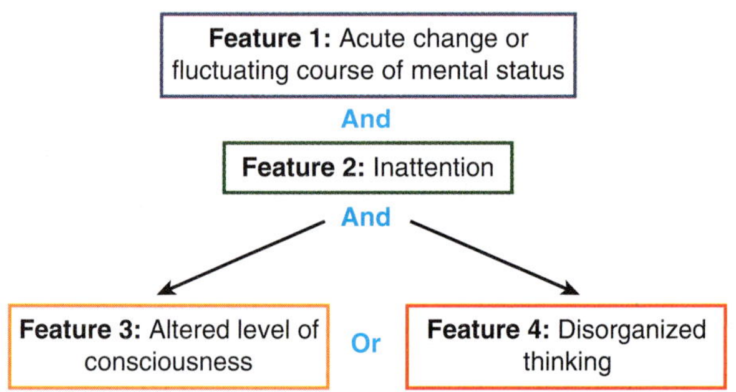

FIG. 8.1 Confusion Assessment Method for the Intensive Care Unit (CAM-ICU). Delirium is defined as positive in Feature 1 *and* Feature 2 and *either* Feature 3 *or* Feature 4. (Copyright 2002, E. Wesley Ely, MD, MPH, and Vanderbilt University. All rights reserved.)

for development of delirium. Both CAM-ICU and ICDSC provide a structured format to evaluate delirium for verbal patients and for nonverbal and mechanically ventilated patients.[26–28]

Pharmacologic Management of Delirium

Pharmacologic treatment of delirium is challenging.[1] The neuroleptic medication haloperidol (Haldol) has traditionally been administered to treat hyperactive delirium. More recent studies have shown that haloperidol or other atypical antipsychotics do not reduce the incidence or the duration of delirium.[1,21] An additional challenge with haloperidol is that it prolongs the Q-Tc interval, increasing the patient's risk of the ventricular dysrhythmia *torsades de pointes*.[20]

Sedative medications to avoid when possible include the benzodiazepines midazolam and lorazepam, as these have a strong association with delirium, especially at higher doses.[21] Morphine used in conjunction with benzodiazepines also has shown an increased risk for delirium.[21]

No sedative medication has yet been identified that prevents delirium. Novel antipsychotic medications have not proven to be helpful.[29] Nor have the sedative medications propofol or

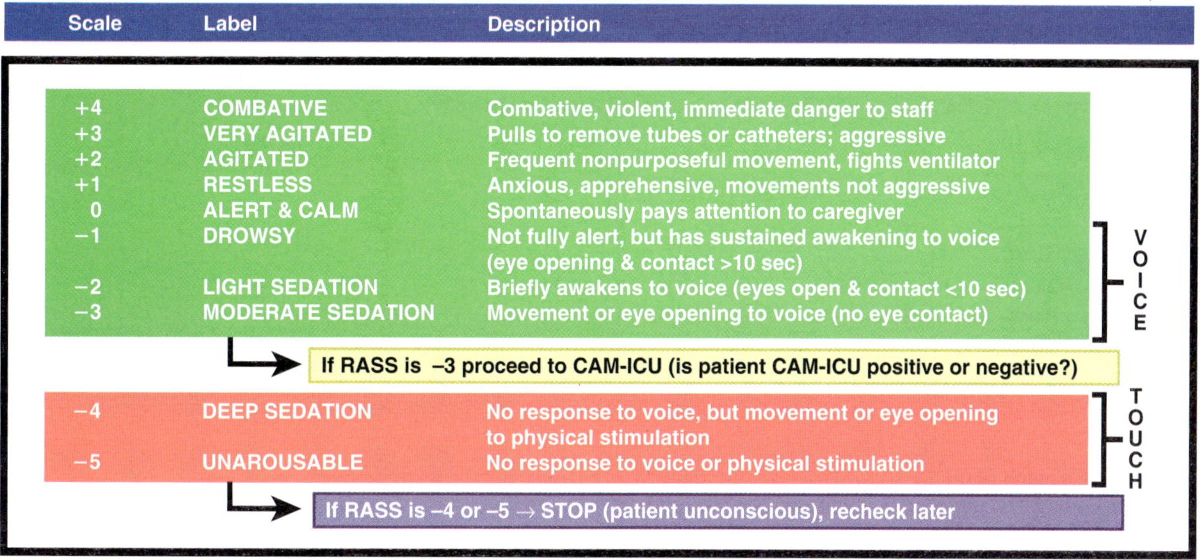

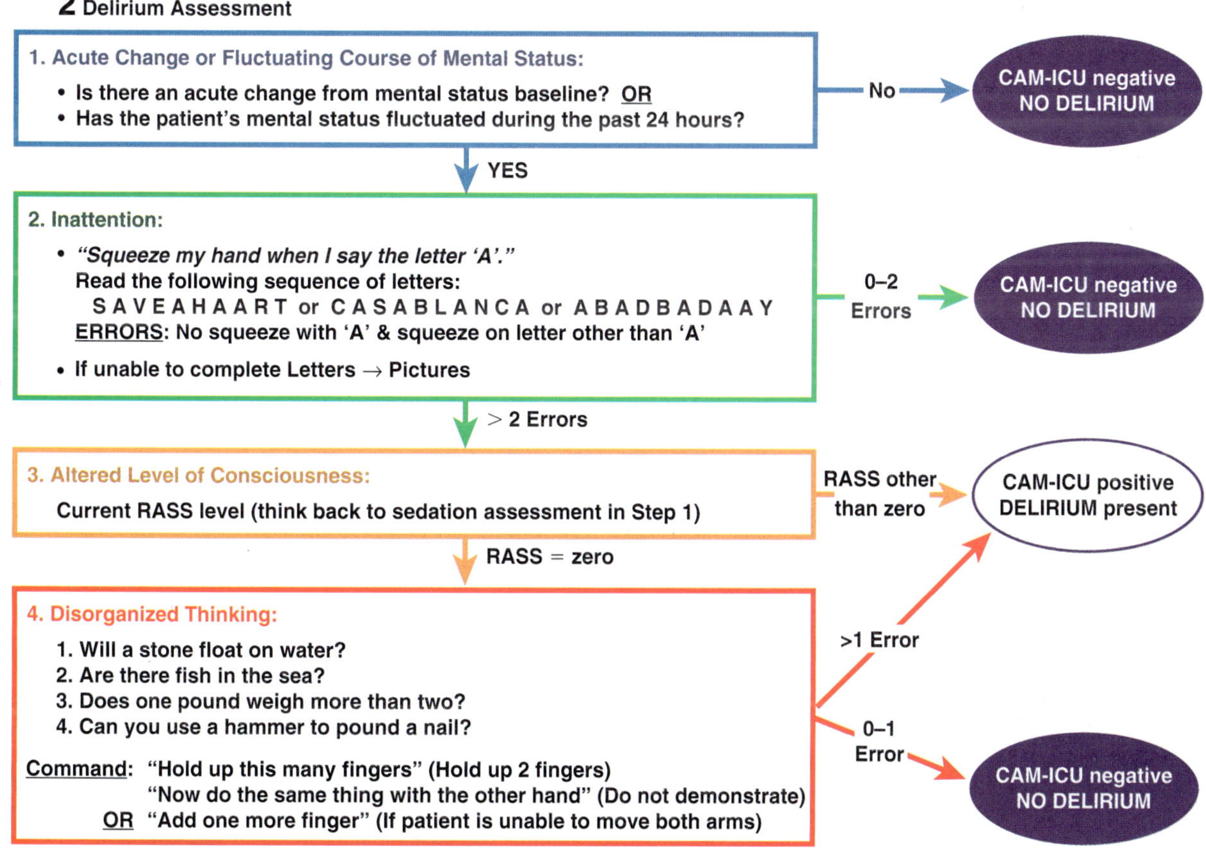

FIG. 8.2 Confusion Assessment Method for the Intensive Care Unit (CAM-ICU) Delirium Assessment. Step 1: Sedation Assessment; Step 2: Delirium Assessment. *RASS*, Richmond Agitation Sedation Scale. (Copyright 2002, E. Wesley Ely, MD, MPH, and Vanderbilt University. All rights reserved.)

The Intensive Care Delirium Screening Checklist (ICDSC)

1. Altered level of consciousness

(A) No response or (B) the need for vigorous stimulation in order to obtain any response signified a severe alteration in the level of consciousness precluding evaluation. If there is coma (A) or stupor (B) most of the time period, then a dash (—) is entered and there is no further evaluation for that period.
(C) Drowsiness or response to a mild to moderate stimulation implies an altered level of consciousness and scores 1 point.
(D) Wakefulness or sleeping state that could easily be aroused is considered normal and scores zero points.
(E) Hypervigilance is rated as an abnormal level of consciousness and scores 1 point.

2. Inattention

Difficulty in following a conversation or instruction, easily distracted by external stimuli, or difficulty in shifting focus scores 1 point.

3. Disorientation

Any obvious mistake in time, place, or person scores 1 point.

4. Hallucination, delusion, or psychosis

The unequivocal clinical manifestation of hallucination or of behavior probably due to hallucination (eg, trying to catch a nonexistent object) or delusion or gross impairment in reality testing scores 1 point.

5. Psychomotor agitation or retardation

Hyperactivity requiring the use of additional sedative drugs or restraints in order to control potential danger (eg, pulling out IV lines, hitting staff), hypoactivity, or clinically noticeable psychomotor slowing scores 1 point.

6. Inappropriate speech or mood

Inappropriate, disorganized, or incoherent speech or inappropriate mood related to events or situation scores 1 point.

7. Sleep/wake cycle disturbance

Sleeping less than four hours, waking frequently at night (do not consider wakefulness initiated by medical staff or loud environment), or sleeping during most of the day scores 1 point.

8. Symptom fluctuation

Fluctuation of the manifestation of any item or symptom over 24 hours (eg, from one shift to another) scores 1 point.

How to Calculate a Score for the ICDSC*

Patient Evaluation	Day 1	Day 2	Day 3	Day 4	Day 5
Altered level of consciousness (A-E)*					
Inattention					
Disorientation					
Hallucination, delusion, psychosis					
Psychomotor agitation or retardation					
Inappropriate speech or mood					
Sleep-wake cycle disturbance					
Symptom fluctuation					
Total Score (0-8)					

*Level of Consciousness	Score
A: no response	–
B: response to intense and repeated stimulation (loud voice and pain)	–
C: response to mild or moderate stimulation	1
D: normal wakefulness	0
E: exaggerated response to normal stimulation	1
If **A** or **B**, do not complete patient evaluation for the period.	

Scoring System

The scale is completed based on information collected from each 8-hour shift or from the previous 24 hours. Obvious manifestation of an item = 1 point. No manifestation of an item or no assessment possible = 0 points. The score of each item is entered in the corresponding space and is 0 or 1. A total score of ≥4 on any given day has a 99% sensitivity for correlation with a psychiatric diagnosis of delirium.

FIG. 8.3 Intensive Care Delirium Screening Checklist (ICDSC). *The ICDSC is also used in tandem with the Richmond Agitation-Sedation Scale (RASS) (see Table 8.1) to assess sedation-agitation in addition to delirium. (From Bergeron N, Dubois MJ, Dunmont M, Dial S, Skrobik Y. Intensive Care Delirium Screening Checklist: evaluation of a new screening tool. *Intensive Care Med.* 2001;27:859–864.)

dexmedetomidine demonstrated a reduction in delirium incidence or duration.[10,19] Because there is no pharmacologic resolution for delirium, the use of the lightest level of sedation that is tolerable for the patient is recommended.[1]

Interventions to Prevent Delirium

In mechanically ventilated patients, the interventions used to decrease delirium include using light sedation, scheduling a daily sedative interruption (awakening), scheduling a spontaneous breathing trial, daily delirium monitoring, and early mobility.[1] Early mobility may prevent the muscle weakness that accompanies long periods of bed rest during critical illness and may reduce the cognitive complications associated with prolonged illness that many patients experience.[1]

Sleep protocols are used in many critical care units to increase the opportunity for patients to sleep at night. The protocols include dimming lights at night, ensuring there are periods of time when tubes are not manipulated, providing earplugs or eye masks, and clustering nursing care interventions to provide uninterrupted rest periods.

Physical restraints are often used in critical care units to avoid patient self-removal of lines or tubes. However, to prevent unpleasant patient memories of being restrained, avoidance of physical restraint is recommended in current delirium management guidelines.[1]

Post–Intensive Care Unit Syndrome

Many patients experience depression and cognitive changes or cognitive decline after surviving a critical illness. This condition is named *post–intensive care syndrome* (PICS). Some patients have preexisting conditions that increase their risk, including advanced age and prior cognitive impairment.[21] The PICS risk factors are similar to the risks for delirium,[21] and both delirium and a prolonged critical illness are risk factors for PICS.[30] At this time the interventions to reduce delirium are the same as those to reduce PICS.[21] More research is ongoing in this area.

Patient Diaries

Writing a patient diary has been used as an intervention to try to reduce PICS. The diary is written in everyday language and completed by the critical care team (nurses, doctors, respiratory therapists, rehabilitation therapists, and others) and family members. Later, the diary can be used to answer questions such as, "What happened when I was attached to the breathing machine?" and "How long was I unconscious?" There is no evidence that creating a patient diary reduces delirium or PICS; however, the diary can provide a practical mechanism to later describe the many events the patient cannot remember.[31] Expectations must be tempered with the knowledge that in survivors of critical illness, the use of a diary did not prevent posttraumatic stress disorder (PTSD) symptoms.[32,33]

ALCOHOL WITHDRAWAL SYNDROME AND DELIRIUM TREMENS

Critically ill patients who are alcohol dependent and were drinking before hospital admission are at risk of severe AWS.[34–36] Severe AWS is associated with an increased risk of delirium, hallucinations, seizures, need for mechanical ventilation, and death. When hyperactive agitated delirium is caused by alcohol withdrawal, it is termed *delirium tremens* (DT).[35] After hospital admission, approximately 50% of alcohol-dependent patients experience AWS-related symptoms as their blood alcohol concentration decreases.[35] Fewer than 5% of patients with AWS experience severe complications such as delirium or a seizure.[35]

Alcohol Use Screening Tools

There are several screening tools to identify alcohol dependence and severity of alcohol withdrawal.[37] Two tools that are widely used are listed here.

- The *Alcohol Use Disorders Identification Test* (AUDIT) is used to identify alcohol dependence, see Table 32.1 in Chapter 32.[35]
- The *Clinical Institute Withdrawal Assessment of Alcohol Scale* (revised) (CIWA-Ar)[37,38] is used to assess the severity of alcohol withdrawal.[37,38]

Pharmacologic Management of Alcohol Withdrawal

Management of alcohol withdrawal involves close monitoring for escalation of signs and symptoms, including agitation, tremor, anxiety, and sweating, before the patient experiences severe complications such as hallucinations and seizures. Administration of long-acting medications to control symptoms may be listed in a hospital protocol. For example, a CIWA-Ar score >10 necessitates pharmacologic intervention.[37] The medications include intravenous benzodiazepines, phenobarbital, and adjunctive sedative medications, with variations depending on the local protocols being used.

Often benzodiazepines are administered in response to increased signs of agitation associated with DTs, with dosage guided by a clinical protocol. This is known as an *AWS symptom-triggered* approach.[34,35]

Benzodiazepines are the first-line of treatment in AWS, typically diazepam or lorazepam.[37] These have a long half-life and high lipid solubility. Lipid-soluble medications quickly cross the blood-brain barrier and enter the central nervous system to produce a sedative effect.

Phenobarbital is being studied for treatment of AWS in critical care.[39–41] Additionally, nonbenzodiazepine adjunctive medications may be added, including dexmedetomidine, clonidine, propofol, ketamine, barbiturates, and haloperidol, depending on hospital protocols.[36] Multivitamins, including thiamine (vitamin B_1), are administered prophylactically to prevent additional neurologic sequelae.[34] Oral or intravenous alcohol should never be administered to treat AWS.[37]

Delirium related to alcohol withdrawal is managed pharmacologically in a very different way from delirium from other causes. Long-acting medications, phenobarbital, or benzodiazepines are the medications used in AWS. In contrast, long-acting benzodiazepines are contraindicated for treatment of delirium from non–alcohol-related causes.[1]

COLLABORATIVE MANAGEMENT

Collaborative management of anxiety, agitation, sedation, and delirium is a responsibility shared by all members of the health care team, as indicated by the clinical practice guidelines summarized in Box 8.2. Recognition of the problem is the first step toward a solution to establish a more effective standard of patient care in management of sedation, analgesia, and delirium.

ADDITIONAL RESOURCES

See Box 8.3 for Internet resources related to sedation, agitation, and delirium management.

CASE STUDY 8.1 Patient With Delirium

Brief Patient History

Mr. K is a 42-year-old Asian man who is in your city on a business trip. He is transported to your facility from his hotel because of a witnessed grand mal seizure. Paramedics administered lorazepam in the field. Mr. K's wife reports by phone that he is in good health and that she is not aware that he takes any medications regularly. She states that he recently quit drinking alcohol because of pressure from the family. She also comments that she thinks he takes alprazolam to calm his nerves once in a while.

Focused Clinical Assessment

Mr. K is admitted to the critical care unit from the emergency department with hypertension, restlessness, mental confusion, paranoid ideations with rambling speech, and visual and auditory hallucinations. Mr. K's skin is warm and moist. Intravenous administration of thiamine, folic acid, multivitamins, and magnesium was begun in the emergency department. Physician orders were written for lorazepam every 6 hours and clonidine every 4 hours as needed for delirium-related symptoms.

Diagnostic Procedures

Mr. K's baseline vital signs are as follows: blood pressure of 190/92 mm Hg, heart rate of 130 beats/min (sinus tachycardia), respiratory rate of 26 breaths/min, and temperature of 98.8°F. Pulse oximetry oxygen saturation is 90% on 4 L/min oxygen using a nasal cannula. Assessment of delirium with the Confusion Assessment Method indicates the presence of acute and fluctuating change in mental status, inattention, and disorganized thinking. The Sedation-Agitation Scale score is 5. Serum and urine toxicology studies are negative for ethyl alcohol, cannabis, and opioids; urine is strongly positive for benzodiazepines. Sodium level is 135 mmol/L, potassium level is 4.3 mmol/L, chloride level is 84 mmol/L, carbon dioxide level is 26 mEq/L, calcium level is 8 mg/dL, magnesium level is 2.0 mg/dL, and gamma-glutamyl transferase level is 80 units/L.

Medical Diagnosis

Mr. K is diagnosed with delirium tremens caused by alcohol and benzodiazepine withdrawal.

Questions

1. What major outcomes do you expect to achieve for this patient?
2. What problems or risks must be managed to achieve these outcomes?
3. What interventions must be initiated to monitor, prevent, manage, or eliminate the problems and risks identified?
4. What interventions should be initiated to promote optimal functioning, safety, and well-being of the patient?
5. What technology can be used to monitor this patient and prevent complications?
6. What other interprofessional team members are needed to assist with the management of this patient?
7. What possible learning needs do you anticipate for this patient?
8. What cultural and age-related factors may have a bearing on the patient's plan of care?

BOX 8.2 Evidence-Based Practice

Summary of Guidelines for Assessment and Treatment of Agitation and Delirium

- Detection and treatment of pain, agitation, and delirium should be reassessed frequently.
- Patients should be awake and able to purposely follow commands to participate in their care unless a clinical indication for deeper sedation exists.

Agitation

- Agitation in critically ill patients may result from inadequately treated pain, anxiety, delirium, or ventilator dyssynchrony.
- Depth and quality of sedation should be routinely assessed in all critical care patients.
- RASS and SAS are the most valid and reliable scales for assessing quality and depth of sedation in critically ill patients.
- Target lightest possible level of sedation and/or use daily sedative interruption.
- Use sedation protocols and checklists to facilitate sedation management.
- Suggest using analgesia-first sedation for intubated and mechanically ventilated critically ill patients.
- Use either propofol or dexmedetomidine, rather than benzodiazepines for sedation in mechanically ventilated adult patients.

Delirium

- Delirium assessment should be routinely performed in all critically ill patients.
- CAM-ICU and ICDSC delirium monitoring tools are the most valid and reliable scales to assess delirium in mechanically ventilated patients.
- Mobilize critical care patients as early as possible to reduce incidence and duration of delirium and to improve functional outcomes.
- Promote sleep in critically ill patients by controlling light and noise, clustering patient care activities, and decreasing stimuli at night.
- Avoid use of antipsychotics in patients who are at risk for torsades de pointes.
- Avoid use of benzodiazepines in critically ill patients with delirium unrelated to alcohol/benzodiazepine withdrawal.

CSM-ICU, Confusion Assessment Method for the Intensive Care Unit; *ICDSC*, Intensive Care Delirium Screening Checklist; *RASS*, Richmond Agitation-Sedation Scale; *SAS*, Sedation-Agitation Scale.

Data from Devlin JW, Skrobik Y, Gélinas C, et al. Clinical practice guidelines for the prevention and management of pain, agitation/sedation, delirium, immobility, and sleep disruption in adult patients in the ICU. *Crit Care Med.* 2018;46(9):e825–e873.

BOX 8.3 Internet Resources

Sedation, Agitation, and Delirium Management

- Delirium/Sedation: https://www.icudelirium.org/
- Pain Agitation Delirium Guidelines: https://www.sccm.org/Research/Guidelines
- The Joint Commission: https://www.jointcommission.org/en/resources/for-consumers/speak-up-campaigns/anesthesia-and-sedation

KEY POINTS

- Use a validated sedation-agitation assessment scale (RASS or SAS) and titrate sedation medications to achieve the lightest possible level of sedation to prevent immobility-associated problems and delirium.
- Benzodiazepines are not recommended for routine sedation of mechanically ventilated adult patients.
- Dexmedetomidine and propofol are recommended for sedation of mechanically ventilated adult patients.
- Daily interruption of sedation and a spontaneous breathing trial are recommended for patients who are mechanically ventilated.
- Delirium can be hypoactive (withdrawn) or hyperactive (with agitation) and is a common complication of critical illness.

- Use a validated delirium assessment instrument (CAM-ICU or ICDSC) to identify delirium.
- Pharmacologic management of delirium most commonly includes treatment with haloperidol.
- Nonpharmacologic interventions to prevent delirium include provision of adequate sleep and early mobility.
- Use a validated alcohol withdrawal syndrome (AWS) assessment instrument (CIWA-Ar) to identify alcohol withdrawal severity.
- Delirium tremens (DTs) is a complication of AWS.
- The benzodiazepines diazepam (Valium) and lorazepam (Ativan) are used in the treatment of delirium tremens.

Visit the Evolve site at http://evolve.elsevier.com/Urden/CriticalCareNursing for additional study materials.

REFERENCES

1. Devlin JW, Skrobik Y, Gélinas C, et al. Clinical practice guidelines for the prevention and management of pain, agitation/sedation, delirium, immobility, and sleep disruption in adult patients in the ICU. *Crit Care Med*. 2018;46(9):e825–e873. https://doi.org/10.1097/CCM.0000000000003299.
2. Page V, McKenzie C. Sedation in the intensive care unit. *Curr Anesthesiol Rep*. 2021;11(2):92–100. https://doi.org/10.1007/s40140-021-00446-5.
3. Sessler CN, Gosnell MS, Grap MJ, et al. The Richmond Agitation-Sedation Scale: validity and reliability in adult intensive care unit patients. *Am J Respir Crit Care Med*. 2002;166(10):1338–1344. https://doi.org/10.1164/rccm.2107138.
4. Ely EW, Truman B, Shintani A, et al. Monitoring sedation status over time in ICU patients: reliability and validity of the Richmond Agitation-Sedation Scale (RASS). *JAMA*. 2003;289(22):2983–2991. https://doi.org/10.1001/jama.289.22.2983.
5. Riker RR. Prospective evaluation of the Sedation-Agitation Scale for adult critically ill patients. 27(7):1325–1329.
6. Chanques G, Constantin JM, Devlin JW, et al. Analgesia and sedation in patients with ARDS. *Intensive Care Med*. 2020;46(12):2342–2356. https://doi.org/10.1007/s00134-020-06307-9.
7. Olsen HT, Nedergaard HK, Strøm T, et al. Nonsedation or light sedation in critically ill, mechanically ventilated patients. *N Engl J Med*. 2020;382(12):1103–1111. https://doi.org/10.1056/NEJMoa1906759.
8. Shehabi Y, Bellomo R, Kadiman S, et al. Sedation intensity in the first 48 hours of mechanical ventilation and 180-day mortality: a multinational prospective longitudinal cohort study. *Crit Care Med*. 2018;46(6):850–859. https://doi.org/10.1097/CCM.0000000000003071.
9. American Association of Anesthesiologists. Statement on Continuum of Depth of Sedation: Definition of General Anesthesia and Levels of Sedation/Analgesia. https://www.asahq.org/standards-and-practice-parameters/statement-on-continuum-of-depth-of-sedation-definition-of-general-anesthesia-and-levels-of-sedation-analgesia. Accessed September 13, 2023.
10. Stollings JL, Balas MC, Chanques G. Evolution of sedation management in the intensive care unit (ICU). *Intensive Care Med*. 2022;48(11):1625–1628. https://doi.org/10.1007/s00134-022-06806-x.
11. Penninga EI, Graudal N, Ladekarl MB, Jürgens G. Adverse events associated with flumazenil treatment for the management of suspected benzodiazepine intoxication—a systematic review with meta-analyses of randomised trials. *Basic Clin Pharmacol Toxicol*. 2016;118(1):37–44. https://doi.org/10.1111/bcpt.12434.
12. Schult RF, Omar D, Wiegand TJ, Gordetsky RM, Acquisto NM. Experience with lower dose flumazenil at an academic medical center. *Am J Emerg Med*. 2021;49:399–401. https://doi.org/10.1016/j.ajem.2021.02.002.
13. Sahinovic MM, Struys MMRF, Absalom AR. Clinical pharmacokinetics and pharmacodynamics of propofol. *Clin Pharmacokinet*. 2018;57(12):1539–1558. https://doi.org/10.1007/s40262-018-0672-3.
14. Dinis-Oliveira RJ. Metabolic profiles of propofol and fospropofol: clinical and forensic interpretative aspects. *Biomed Res Int*. 2018;2018:6852857. https://doi.org/10.1155/2018/6852857.
15. Hemphill S, McMenamin L, Bellamy MC, Hopkins PM. Propofol infusion syndrome: a structured literature review and analysis of published case reports. *Br J Anaesth*. 2019;122(4):448–459. https://doi.org/10.1016/j.bja.2018.12.025.
16. Zorrilla-Vaca A, Arevalo JJ, Escandón-Vargas K, Soltanifar D, Mirski MA. Infectious disease risk associated with contaminated propofol anesthesia, 1989-2014(1). *Emerg Infect Dis*. 2016;22(6):981–992. https://doi.org/10.3201/eid2206.150376.
17. Regier BA, Meyer TA, McAllister RK. Propofol 2%: understanding a new concentration of a well-known medication. *Proc (Bayl Univ Med Cent)*. 2021;34(5):642–643. https://doi.org/10.1080/08998280.2021.1937009.
18. Adler AC. Propofol: review of potential risks during administration. *AANA J*. 2017;85(2):104–107.
19. Hughes CG, Mailloux PT, Devlin JW, et al. Dexmedetomidine or propofol for sedation in mechanically ventilated adults with sepsis. *N Engl J Med*. 2021;384(15):1424–1436. https://doi.org/10.1056/NEJMoa2024922.
20. Barr J, Fraser GL, Puntillo K, et al. Clinical practice guidelines for the management of pain, agitation, and delirium in adult patients in the intensive care unit. *Crit Care Med*. 2013;41(1):263–306. https://doi.org/10.1097/CCM.0b013e3182783b72.
21. Mart MF, Williams Roberson S, Salas B, Pandharipande PP, Ely EW. Prevention and management of delirium in the intensive care unit. *Semin Respir Crit Care Med*. 2021;42(1):112–126. https://doi.org/10.1055/s-0040-1710572.
22. Ely EW, Inouye SK, Bernard GR, et al. Delirium in mechanically ventilated patients: validity and reliability of the confusion assessment method for the intensive care unit (CAM-ICU). *JAMA*. 2001;286(21):2703–2710. https://doi.org/10.1001/jama.286.21.2703.
23. Ely EW, Margolin R, Francis J, et al. Evaluation of delirium in critically ill patients: validation of the confusion assessment method for the intensive care unit (CAM-ICU). *Crit Care Med*. 2001;29(7):1370–1379. https://doi.org/10.1097/00003246-200107000-00012.
24. Bergeron N, Dubois MJ, Dumont M, Dial S, Skrobik Y. Intensive care delirium screening checklist: evaluation of a new screening tool. *Intensive Care Med*. 2001;27(5):859–864. https://doi.org/10.1007/s001340100909.
25. Ouimet S, Riker R, Bergeron N, Cossette M, Kavanagh B, Skrobik Y. Subsyndromal delirium in the ICU: evidence for a disease spectrum. *Intensive Care Med*. 2007;33(6):1007–1013. https://doi.org/10.1007/s00134-007-0618-y.
26. Gélinas C, Bérubé M, Chevrier A, et al. Delirium assessment tools for use in critically ill adults: a psychometric analysis and systematic review. *Crit Care Nurse*. 2018;38(1):38–49. https://doi.org/10.4037/ccn2018633.
27. Krewulak KD, Rosgen BK, Ely EW, Stelfox HT, Fiest KM. The CAM-ICU-7 and ICDSC as measures of delirium severity in critically ill adult patients. *PLoS One*. 2020;15(11):e0242378. https://doi.org/10.1371/journal.pone.0242378.
28. Chen TJ, Chung YW, Chang HCR, et al. Diagnostic accuracy of the CAM-ICU and ICDSC in detecting intensive care unit delirium: a bivariate meta-analysis. *Int J Nurs Stud*. 2021;113:103782. https://doi.org/10.1016/j.ijnurstu.2020.103782.
29. Girard TD, Exline MC, Carson SS, et al. Haloperidol and ziprasidone for treatment of delirium in critical illness. *N Engl J Med*. 2018;379(26):2506–2516. https://doi.org/10.1056/NEJMoa1808217.
30. Lee M, Kang J, Jeong YJ. Risk factors for post-intensive care syndrome: a systematic review and meta-analysis. *Aust Crit Care*. 2020;33(3):287–294. https://doi.org/10.1016/j.aucc.2019.10.004.
31. Ullman AJ, Aitken LM, Rattray J, et al. Diaries for recovery from critical illness. *Cochrane Database Syst Rev*. 2014;2014(12):CD010468. https://doi.org/10.1002/14651858.CD010468.pub2.
32. Garrouste-Orgeas M, Flahault C, Vinatier I, et al. Effect of an ICU diary on posttraumatic stress disorder symptoms among patients receiving mechanical ventilation: a randomized clinical trial. *JAMA*. 2019;322(3):229–239. https://doi.org/10.1001/jama.2019.9058.
33. Sayde GE, Stefanescu A, Conrad E, Nielsen N, Hammer R. Implementing an intensive care unit (ICU) diary program at a large academic medical

center: results from a randomized control trial evaluating psychological morbidity associated with critical illness. *Gen Hosp Psychiatry.* 2020;66:96–102. https://doi.org/10.1016/j.genhosppsych.2020.06.017.
34. Dixit D, Endicott J, Burry L, et al. Management of acute alcohol withdrawal syndrome in critically ill patients. *Pharmacotherapy.* 2016;36(7):797–822. https://doi.org/10.1002/phar.1770.
35. Schuckit MA. Recognition and management of withdrawal delirium (delirium tremens). *N Engl J Med.* 2014;371(22):2109–2113. https://doi.org/10.1056/NEJMra1407298.
36. Foertsch MJ, Winter JB, Rhoades AG, Martin LT, Droege CA, Ernst NE. Recognition, assessment, and pharmacotherapeutic treatment of alcohol withdrawal syndrome in the intensive care unit. *Crit Care Nurs Q.* 2019;42(1):12–29. https://doi.org/10.1097/CNQ.0000000000000233.
37. American Association of Addiction Medicine. The ASAM Clinical Practice Guideline on Alcohol Withdrawal Management. Published 2020. https://www.asam.org/quality-care/clinical-guidelines/alcohol-withdrawal-management-guideline. Accessed September 20, 2023.
38. Sen S, Grgurich P, Tulolo A, et al. A symptom-triggered benzodiazepine protocol utilizing SAS and CIWA-Ar scoring for the treatment of alcohol withdrawal syndrome in the critically ill. *Ann Pharmacother.* 2017;51(2):101–110. https://doi.org/10.1177/1060028016672036.
39. Hawa F, Gilbert L, Gilbert B, et al. Phenobarbital versus lorazepam for management of alcohol withdrawal syndrome: a retrospective cohort study. *Cureus.* 2021;13(2):e13282. https://doi.org/10.7759/cureus.13282.
40. Oks M, Cleven KL, Healy L, et al. The safety and utility of phenobarbital use for the treatment of severe alcohol withdrawal syndrome in the medical intensive care unit. *J Intensive Care Med.* 2020;35(9):844–850. https://doi.org/10.1177/0885066618783947.
41. Tidwell WP, Thomas TL, Pouliot JD, Canonico AE, Webber AJ. Treatment of alcohol withdrawal syndrome: phenobarbital vs CIWA-Ar protocol. *Am J Crit Care.* 2018;27(6):454–460. https://doi.org/10.4037/ajcc2018745.

Palliative and End-of-Life Care

Caroline Etland

http://evolve.elsevier.com/Urden/CriticalCareNursing

Palliative care and end-of-life care are crucial aspects of health care aimed at improving the quality of life for individuals with serious or life-limiting illnesses and supporting them and their families during challenging times. While both are related to caring for individuals nearing the end of their lives, there are distinct differences. Palliative care is specialized medical care focused on providing relief from the symptoms and stress of a serious illness. It's appropriate at any age and any stage of a serious illness, and it can be provided alongside curative treatment. The goal is to improve the quality of life for both the patient and their family. End-of-life care is a specific type of care for individuals who are in the final stages of a terminal illness or are nearing the end of their life. The focus shifts from attempting to cure the illness to ensuring the person is as comfortable and pain free as possible. Both concepts are discussed in this chapter.

END-OF-LIFE CHALLENGES

End-of-life care in hospitals has improved in the past two decades. Still, many opportunities for improvement exist, particularly concerning earlier identification of patients' wishes and avoidance of nonbeneficial treatment. To respond to this need, the academic preparation of the interprofessional team regarding end-of-life care has increased due to new evidence and regulatory mandates.[1–3]

Language

Increasing the complexity of these challenges, our clinical culture and professional training emphasize saving lives, and the language that describes the end of life uses negative terminology, such as forgoing life-sustaining treatments, do not resuscitate (DNR), and withdrawing care. The phrase withdrawal of care should never be used, as it can cause families to think there will be no comfort measures or assistance provided after a decision is made to discontinue mechanical ventilation and other life-sustaining treatments.[4] A more accurate term is withdrawal of treatment. Equally important is the cultural shift toward more accurate language in health care and popular literature to describe end-of-life decision making and medical interventions, such as allow natural death instead of do not attempt resuscitation and withholding of nonbeneficial treatment in place of futile care.[5] This shift toward more realistic descriptors reflects extensive research in health care, especially palliative care, and the effectiveness of goals-of-care discussions with patients with serious illnesses before crisis events. As trends in health care change, more evidence regarding the timing and effectiveness of supportive care will be incorporated into treatment protocols and care plans.

Barriers

More attention is being given to the quality of the end-of-life experience of patients with serious illnesses, particularly patients who become critically ill. Research studies suggest that medical care for patients with advanced illness is characterized by inadequately treated physical distress, fragmented care systems, poor communication between physicians, patients, and families, and enormous strains on family caregivers and support systems.[6–8] In addition to health care system barriers to good end-of-life care, mainstream media has significantly influenced misconceptions about the success rate of medical interventions in seriously ill patients.

A familiar media presentation of life and death in the hospital is a critical event in a patient who is resuscitated and immediately awakens with full capacity. In reality, treatment options are usually explained in rapid technical language, followed by a frightening question, "Do you want us to keep going?" or "Tell us what you want us to do." This heavy burden placed on family members means they must choose between treatment options, one of which may result in losing their loved one.

Values

The emphasis on patient autonomy as a valued ethical principle is deeply embedded in the health care system of the United States. Expert medical recommendations are offered to patients and families, and they often must determine in a brief space of time whether those recommendations are aligned with their personal values. Most nurses are familiar with the scenario of families of patients in the critical care unit being told how well one body organ is functioning and trying to reconcile this "good news" with another physician communicating a poor overall prognosis. Less often, families are provided with a longer-term perspective that addresses the loss of functional status, decreased quality of life, and potential need for long-term care.

Information

Adequate, realistic information about the limits of medicine and the frailties of the body allows patients and families to make decisions that preserve a patient's dignity and respect individual autonomy. Hope is a powerful influence on decision making, and a shift from hope for recovery to hope for a peaceful death should be guided by clinicians with exemplary communication skills. Critical care nurses often interpret medical information and how it applies to personal preferences and values. The ability to respond realistically in accordance with the listener's values and culture is a learned skill. Many resources are available to develop further the necessary skills to better support patients and families through critical care unit admission to discharge. The American Association of Critical-Care Nurses (AACN) has recognized the importance of this aspect of care in the critical care unit by developing protocols for palliative and end-of-life issues in the critical care unit and by identifying palliative and end-of-life care as a major advocacy initiative.[9,10] Several other vital resources to enhance communication and elicit goals of care are discussed throughout this chapter.

Evidence

Evidence is available for the care rendered to the dying critical care patient and family through research, reports, and guidelines. One such report is from the National Consensus Project and the National Coalition for Hospice and Palliative Care,[11] in which the preferred practices of care for the imminently dying patient are discussed. Researchers have studied family and nurse perspectives to understand barriers and facilitators to quality care in various settings.[12–16] Death in the ICU has historically been a quality indicator of palliative care programs. However, White et al.[17] suggested that death in the ICU as an end-of-life quality measure bears further examination to prevent "a bias against admitting patients with acute, potentially reversible illnesses for whom there is a relatively high risk of death." Health care organizations are encouraged to identify quality indicators specific to their patient population, services, resources, and culture to improve end-of-life care.

END-OF-LIFE EXPERIENCE IN CRITICAL CARE

Attention to the end of life of hospitalized patients has increased since the publication of the Study to Understand Prognoses and Preferences for Outcomes and Risks of Treatment (SUPPORT).[18] In this major report, more than 9000 seriously ill patients in five medical centers were studied. Despite an intervention to improve communication, shortcomings were found; aggressive treatment was common, only half of the physicians knew their patients' preferences to avoid cardiopulmonary resuscitation (CPR), more than one-third of patients who died spent at least 10 days in a critical care unit, and family members of half of conscious patients reported moderate to severe pain at least half of the time.

Soon after the publication of the SUPPORT study, the Institute of Medicine (IOM) released a report, *Approaching Death: Improving Care at the End of Life*,[19] followed by an updated report in 2014.[20] Based on the growth of palliative care programs and developing research on end-of-life care, the recommendations changed to highlight new priorities. Recommendations from the IOM reports are summarized in Table 9.1, which reflects advances in the science of palliative and end-of-life care.

To describe the number of deaths in critical care units, Angus et al.[21] reviewed hospital discharge data from six states and the National Death Index. Of the more than 500,000 deaths studied, 38.3% were in hospitals, and 22% occurred after admission to

SOCIAL DETERMINANTS OF HEALTH

Health Disparities Associated With Palliative Care

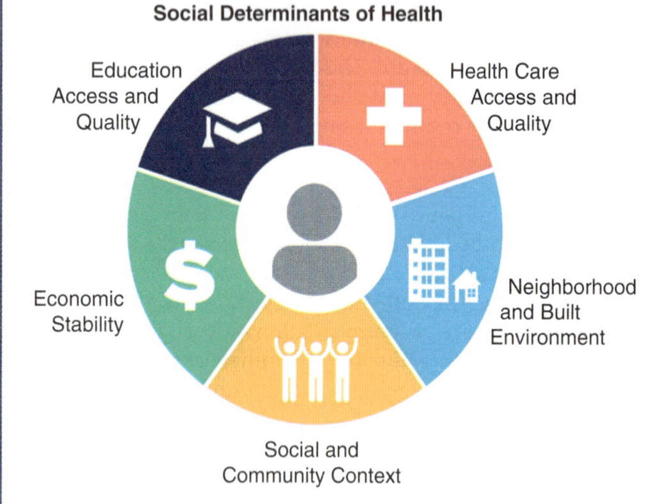

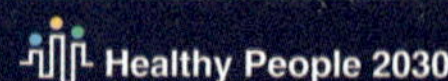

The social determinants of health can significantly affect palliative care in various ways. Socioeconomic status, insurance coverage, and geographic location can influence access to services. Individuals with lower socioeconomic status or inadequate insurance coverage may face barriers in accessing palliative care, leading to disparities in receiving appropriate symptom management and supportive care.[1,2]

Social determinants, including education level and cultural factors, can impact health literacy and communication between patients, families, and health care providers in palliative care. Limited health literacy may hinder understanding of treatment options, goals of care, and decision-making processes.

Additionally, cultural beliefs and practices can influence how individuals perceive and approach end-of-life care, impacting their engagement with palliative care services. Social support networks and resources available to caregivers play a vital role in palliative care. Caregivers may face challenges related to financial resources, availability of respite care, and emotional support. Lack of adequate support can lead to caregiver burnout, impacting the quality of care provided to the patient.

Palliative care often involves multiple health care services, including medications, medical equipment, and home care services. Financial constraints and out-of-pocket expenses can create barriers to accessing and receiving comprehensive palliative care. High costs may result in delayed or inadequate symptom management, impacting the quality of life for patients.

Palliative care should be culturally sensitive and respectful, considering diverse beliefs, values, and practices. Social determinants, including cultural factors and language barriers, can influence the provision of culturally appropriate palliative care. Understanding and respecting patients' and their families' unique cultural needs and preferences are crucial for delivering effective palliative care.

Addressing the social determinants of health in palliative care requires a holistic approach. It involves promoting equitable access to palliative care services, improving health literacy and communication, providing caregiver support, considering patients' housing and environmental needs, addressing financial concerns, and ensuring cultural sensitivity and respect. By addressing these social determinants, palliative care can be more accessible, patient-centered, and effective in enhancing the quality of life for individuals facing serious illness.

References

1. Wachterman MW, Sommers BD. Dying poor in the US-Disparities in end-of-life care. *JAMA.* 2021;325(5):423–424. https://doi.org/10.1001/jama.2020.26162.
2. Nelson KE, Wright R, Peeler A, Brockie T, Davidson PM. Sociodemographic disparities in access to hospice and palliative care: an integrative review. *Am J Hosp Palliat Care.* 2021;38(11):1378–1390. https://doi.org/10.1177/1049909120985419.

Illustration from Healthy People 2030, U.S. Department of Health and Human Services, Office of Disease Prevention and Health Promotion. Retrieved September 8, 2022, from https://health.gov/healthypeople/objectives-and-data/social-determinants-health.

TABLE 9.1 Comparison of Death in America Reports

Approaching Death Report (1997)	Dying in America Report (2014)
• Patients with fatal illnesses and their family should receive reliable, skillful, and supportive care. • Health professionals should improve care for dying patients. • Policymakers and consumers should work with health professionals to improve quality and financing of care. • Health profession education should include end-of-life content. • Palliative care should be developed, possibly as a medical specialty. • Research on end of life should be funded. • The public should communicate more about the experience of dying and options available.	• Coordinate person-centered, family-oriented end-of-life care. • Improve clinician-patient communication, including robust advance care planning processes. • Improve access to palliative care training for physicians and nurses. • Implement models of care to provide services that patients and families need that are not covered by existing insurance plans. • Implement culturally appropriate public education and public engagement strategies.

Adapted from Field MJ, Cassell CK, eds. *Approaching Death: Improving Care at the End of Life.* National Academy Press; 1997; and Dying in America and Committee on Approaching Death, Addressing Key End of Life Issues, Institute of Medicine. *Dying in America: Improving Quality and Honoring Individual Preferences Near the End of Life.* National Academies Press; 2015.

the critical care unit. Terminal admissions associated with critical care accounted for 80% of all terminal hospitalization costs. An analysis in 2014 revealed that although 90% of people would prefer to die in their own homes, more than 20% received high-tech, aggressive care before they died.[22] Improvements in completion of advance directives (ADs), hospital efforts to reduce inpatient mortality, increased availability of palliative care services, and increased hospice use have contributed to decreased deaths in hospitals and shifted place of death to community settings. Rates of critical care unit admission in the past 30 days of life increased after more Americans became insured with the Affordable Care Act but stabilized by 2015.[23]

Advance Directives

Although ADs, also known as a living will or a health care power of attorney, were intended to ensure that patients received the care they desired at the end of life, the enactment of structures and processes to support completion of ADs has been suboptimal. Traditionally, AD completion rates in adults range from 16% to 36% overall, with less than one-half of seriously or terminally ill patients having documented their wishes.[24] A 2014 study revealed that AD completion has increased to 72% with a decrease of in-hospital deaths from 45% to 35% in the older-adult study sample.[24] More recently, a study showed the COVID-19 pandemic increased the completion of ADs fivefold using a patient-facing strategy, an indication of the importance of technologies to initiate discussions with health care providers.[25] Another study demonstrated that patients with limited English proficiency (LEP) had a lower percentage of completed ADs, suggesting a disparity in care because their wishes for life-sustaining treatment were not known.[26] Most patients have expressed a desire to avoid "general life support" if dying or permanently unconscious, but few have specified preferences regarding specific life-sustaining treatments. A large study of veterans found that veterans who had living wills or who had appointed a surrogate decision maker were much less likely to experience aggressive care at the end of life.[27] Even when ADs are present, the question arises about whether they are applicable for current care decisions; in other words, is this a terminal illness? To address this problem, some states have enacted legislation that requires physicians and/or nurse practitioners and physician assistants to inform patients when a terminal illness is diagnosed and that they have a right to comprehensive information and counseling regarding end-of-life care.[28] This type of legislation supports discussion of wanted versus unwanted care during different stages of serious illness.

Physician Orders for Life-Sustaining Treatment

The Physician Orders for Life-Sustaining Treatment (POLST)[29] is different from an AD. POLST forms are medical orders that are honored across all treatment settings and are especially important to emergency responders in the community. Also, they are completed by the patient and provider in the presence of a serious chronic illness and should be incorporated into medical orders on admission to the hospital or skilled nursing facility. POLST forms are more easily read than an AD in that they are formatted as checkboxes with specific directions. States that have approved use of POLST-type forms through legislation or specific regulations have witnessed a shift in proactive discussions of patients' wishes for life-sustaining treatment.[30–32]

Preventing unwanted life-sustaining treatment through ongoing communication between patient and provider affects the critical care setting in several ways. Treatment decision making is supported when prior discussions have occurred between physicians, patients, and their loved ones regarding declining health and limits on intervention. Efficient resource utilization is maximized when inappropriate critical care unit admissions are prevented, which often begins in the emergency department. Jesus et al.[33] explored the pros and cons of admitting patients to the critical care unit who have documented DNR orders. Considering the recommendations of the Society of Critical Care Medicine regarding who should and should not be admitted to the critical care unit, the authors affirmed the importance of identifying the potential benefit of all critical care unit interventions to an individual patient and alignment of care with documented wishes.

Finally, moral distress of care providers is decreased when care is congruent with patient autonomy. Critical care nurses in states that recognize POLST forms need to be aware whether a regulatory mandate requires health care providers to honor the patient's wishes documented on the form or whether the documentation is merely a guideline. Equally important is the need to identify the POLST form when it is presented and to communicate with medical staff to ensure that stated treatment wishes are incorporated into the plan of care and physician orders.

Advance Care Planning

Although cultural influences in the United States discourage discussion of death, societal trends are shifting awareness regarding quality of life decision making and unintended consequences of aggressive medical treatment. Planning for decisions to be made at a later date if one is unable to speak for one's self is a difficult process, but this knowledge helps family members to make the treatment decisions if a patient cannot communicate. Advance care planning (ACP) for patients with chronic illness is advantageous for all involved. A systematic review of the effects of ACP on end-of-life care revealed that ACP decreases life-sustaining treatment, increases use of hospice and palliative care, and prevents hospitalization.[34] During the COVID-19 pandemic, there was an increased urgency for proactive ACP discussion and documentation with older and chronically ill adults before any hospitalization was necessary. One study demonstrated that chronically ill patients with ACP documented in the medical record had significantly fewer ICU days, lower costs, and higher hospice utilization during hospitalization.[35] When surrogates hear the patient's wishes for end-of-life care, they can be more knowledgeable and less conflicted when asked to make decisions that may result in a loved one's death during a serious illness (Box 9.1).

Communication of the patient's wishes among family members, primary care providers, and intensivists is critical. If patients have stated desires, they should be communicated when patients are entering or are transferred out of the critical care unit. If the patient has not specified his or her preferences, that information also is important and should be communicated to new health care providers; the level of care patients desire should be offered as appropriate. Families and care providers should be informed if patients decline aggressive care so that families will not be left with difficult decisions in emergency situations. Emotional support for the patient and the family is important as they discuss ACP in the critical care setting.

Ethical and Legal Issues

Ethical and legal principles guide many of our decisions in caring for dying patients and their families. The patient is respected as autonomous and able to make his or her own decisions. The Patient Self-Determination Act supports the patient's right to control future treatment in the event the individual cannot speak for himself or herself. When the patient is unable to make decisions, the same respect is usually accorded to surrogates. In many cultures, however, "...individual identity is secondary to family identity, requiring individuals to prioritize family needs over individual needs."[36] Health care providers often struggle with this altered priority, and conflict can occur as a result. When clinicians are knowledgeable and respectful about a given culture and the process of decision making, greater trust is established, and decisions may be rendered more easily.

It can be helpful to analyze conflicted situations from a basis of ethical principles (see Chapter 2). Two of the basic principles underlying the provision of health care are beneficence and nonmaleficence. Beneficence is the principle of intending to benefit the other through one's actions. Nonmaleficence means to do no harm. Sometimes in end-of-life care, these two principles are in conflict, such as when resuscitation is attempted under beneficence but causes harm to the patient, especially if resuscitation was not desired by the patient. An equally troubling situation exists when the fear of liability drives decision making from the clinician's perspective. Medical recommendations for limitation of life-sustaining treatment or comfort care often result in conflict with surrogate decision makers. Developing more effective communication with patients and families is discussed later in this chapter.

BOX 9.1 Patient-Centered Care

Principles of a Good Death

- Anticipate and be able to prepare for a good death.
- Retain some control.
- Be afforded dignity and privacy.
- Have symptom control, including pain relief.
- Choose place of death when possible.
- Have access to information and expertise when necessary.
- Have emotional and spiritual support.
- Have access to hospice care.
- Have control over who is present at death.
- Respect the wishes of the dying patient through advance directives.
- Have time to say good-bye.
- Be able to die rather than pointlessly prolonging life.

Adapted from Smith R. A good death. An important aim for health services and for us all. *BMJ.* 2000;320(7228):129–130. https://doi.org/10.1136/bmj.320.7228.129.

COMFORT CARE

The decision to withdraw life-sustaining treatments and transition to comfort care at the end of life should be made with as much involvement of the patient as possible, including physical presence of the patient in decision making or procuring paper documents if the patient is unable to participate; the patient's wishes as understood from prior discussions with the patient should guide the decision about whether to withdraw treatment. Withholding and withdrawing treatment are considered to be morally and legally equivalent.[37] However, because families experience more stress in withdrawing treatments than in withholding them,[38] treatments should not be started that the patient would not want or that would not be of benefit. Prigerson et al.[39] are currently studying surrogate decision makers of critical care unit patients in a randomized controlled trial to determine whether an intervention can reduce the stress associated with decision making and anticipatory grief and prevent the severity of post-death surrogate health outcomes and psychological stress. A standardized approach to supporting surrogate decision makers throughout the critical care unit stay is aligned with transparency in clinician-family communication and ethical principles.

Goals

The goal of withdrawal of life-sustaining treatments is to remove treatments that are not beneficial and may be uncomfortable. Any treatment in this circumstance may be withheld or withdrawn. After the goal of comfort has been chosen, each procedure and medication should be evaluated to determine whether it is necessary or causes discomfort. Treatments that cause discomfort do not need to be continued. Another defining question is whether treatments are prolonging the dying process. When disagreements arise, ethics consultations have been found to resolve conflicts regarding inappropriately prolonged, nonbeneficial, or unwanted treatments in the critical care unit, shifting the focus to more appropriate comfort care.[40]

Forgoing life-sustaining treatments is not the same as active euthanasia or assisted or self-directed suicide. Killing is an action causing another's death, whereas allowing a person to die by withholding or withdrawing life-sustaining treatment is avoiding any intervention that interferes with a natural death after illness or trauma.[41]

Cardiopulmonary Resuscitation

CPR was originally developed for patients with coronary artery disease, and those patients and those who experience cardiac arrest in the critical care unit are the most likely to survive resuscitation to discharge.[42] The benefits of resuscitation may be overestimated for survival to discharge and for the more relevant outcome of resumption of baseline functional status. Researchers have found that the rate of overall survival to discharge after in-hospital CPR ranges from approximately 15% to 20%.[43] FitzGerald et al.[44] found that functional status among almost half of the survivors of in-hospital CPR had deteriorated compared with their condition 2 months before the event. After 6 months, 30% of those patients had died, and two-thirds continued to lose function. Despite these dismal statistics, CPR is offered as an option without fully informing patients or families of the low possibility of survival, the pain and suffering involved during and after the procedure, and the potential for decline in functional status.

The AACN[45] and the Emergency Nurses Association[46] have issued position statements recommending that families be allowed to be present during CPR and invasive procedures. Family presence is a significant source of support for the patient, and there may be a benefit to the family in observing the resuscitation that can aid in the grieving process when resuscitation is unsuccessful, by knowing that all was done that could be done (Box 9.2).

Effect of Do-Not-Resuscitate Orders

As a patient clinically declines and death approaches, the decision to initiate a DNR order is influenced by many factors, including goals of care, comorbidities, pace of clinical decline, availability of surrogate decision makers, and provider practice patterns. Critical care nurses often initiate discussion of DNR status and play a key role in collaborating with physicians to identify which therapies remain useful to the patient.

Chang et al.[47] studied the effect of DNR orders in two critical care units in Taiwan and found that even though a DNR order was issued late in the clinical course, life-sustaining interventions were reduced through discussions and consent by surrogate decision makers. Nurses in Korea did not change their nursing activities substantially after receiving a DNR order, continuing to focus on maintenance, preventive, and hygiene tasks.[48] They reported becoming more passive with interventions such as central venous pressure monitoring, fluid and electrolyte balance, and reporting the patient's condition. However, the nurses were more active in communicating with the family. Results of these two studies from outside the United States highlight the challenges across the world with end-of-life care.

"DNR" and "withdrawal of life-sustaining treatment" are not synonymous. Nurses should demonstrate to families that loved ones are receiving aggressive comfort interventions and any treatments that remain part of the plan of care. Once a decision is made to withdraw life-sustaining treatment, comfort orders should be implemented before withdrawal of treatment. A best practice for minimizing pain and suffering of both the patient and family is to use standardized order sets for consistency in practice.

Prognostication and Prognostic Tools

Most patients in the critical care unit have one or more chronic illnesses that greatly affect long-term recovery from major health events such as respiratory failure, myocardial infarction, or sepsis. Because humans and their course of illness can be unpredictable, physicians' ability to prognosticate the length of time before death is limited,[49] and the time to death usually is overestimated to patients and families and in the medical record.

BOX 9.2 Evidence-Based Practice

End-of-Life Care: Fast Facts and Concepts

Cardiopulmonary resuscitation and family presence at end of life	Fast Facts 23, 24, 179, 232, 233
Recommended prognosis for specific conditions	Fast Facts 13, 141, 143, 150, 183, 184, 234
Communication	Fast Facts 6, 11, 22, 64, 76, 77, 123
Decision making	Fast Facts 55, 193, 226, 229
Family meetings	Fast Facts 16, 222, 223, 225, 227
Effective use of hospice	Fast Facts 38, 139, 140
Pain management at end of life	Fast Facts 58, 106, 107, 126, 129, 142, 161, 260
Delirium at end of life	Fast Facts 1, 60, 160

For more information on recommended best practices, visit the Palliative Care Network of Wisconsin at https://mypcnow.org/fast-facts.

Severity scoring systems belong to one of five classes: prognostic, disease-specific, single-organ failure, trauma scores, and organ dysfunction.[50] Two common tools for estimating critical care unit mortality are the Acute Physiology and Chronic Health Evaluation (APACHE) and multiple organ dysfunction score.[51,52] In addition to use of prognostic tools specific to the critical care unit, it makes sense to incorporate prognostic tools for chronic illnesses into overall decision making and the communication process with patients and families. Scoring diagnoses with a traditionally poor prognosis or a consistent trajectory of functional decline can be helpful in comparing current health status with the health status at the time of diagnosis. Recent research on frailty indexes during the COVID-19 pandemic revealed poorer survivability with ICU stays and higher 6-month post-ICU mortality in those higher-scoring patients. Investigators concluded that routine frailty assessment be incorporated into ICU care.[53] Use of prognostic scales can add meaningful information to help patients and families make informed decisions. Some more commonly used prognostic scales are listed in Table 9.2.

Despite this information and these tools, uncertainty remains a major issue in decision making for physicians, patients, and families. Because of uncertainty and because a few patients who were never thought likely to survive actually return to a critical care unit, professionals are not always confident about issues of survivability. Moreover, many families cling to small hopes of survival and recovery (see Box 9.2).

DECISION MAKING

Communication

Communication with the patient and family is critical. White et al.[54] found that shared decision making about end-of-life treatment choices in physician-family conferences was often incomplete, especially among less educated families. Families were found to go through a process in their decision making in which they considered the personal domain (rallying support and evaluating quality of life), the critical care unit environment domain (awaiting the physicians and relating to the health care team), and the decision domain (arriving at a new belief and making and communicating the decision). Higher levels of shared decision making were associated with greater

TABLE 9.2 Selected Prognostic Scales

Prognostic Scale	Disease/Clinical Condition	Prognostic Scale	Disease/Clinical Condition
Palliative Prognostic Scale (PPS)	Any hospice population; palliative care patients	Lung Cancer Prognostic Model (LCPM)	Terminal lung cancer patients
Palliative Prognostic Index (PPI)	Terminal cancer patients	Dementia Prognostic Model (DPM)	Demographic, diagnosis, laboratory, and functional data on dementia residents
Palliative Prognostic Score (PaP)	Terminal cancer patients	Prognostic Index for One-Year Mortality in Older Adults (PIMOA)	Adults older than 70 years with previous stay in hospital
Seattle Heart Failure Model; Heart Failure Risk Scoring System (HFRSS)	Acute heart failure	Cancer Prognostic Scale (CPS)	Terminal cancer patients in progressive care unit
BODE Scale	Chronic obstructive pulmonary disease	Mortality Risk Index Score (MRIS)	New admission to nursing home
Frailty Index for Elders (FIFE)[1]	All older adults with multiple medical problems	Edmonton Frailty Scale[2]	Part of a comprehensive geriatric assessment

[1]Tocchi C. Try This: Frailty Index for Elders (FIFE). HIGN. Accessed September 9, 2023. https://hign.org/consultgeri/try-this-series/try-this-frailty-index-elders-fife
[2]Frailty Index. CGA Toolkit Plus. Accessed May 8, 2024. https://www.cgakit.com/frailty-index
Adapted from Lau F, Cloutier-Fisher D, Kuziemsky C, et al. A systematic review of prognostic tools for estimating survival time in palliative care. *J Palliat Care*. 2007;23(2):93–112.

family satisfaction. More recently, Austin et al.[55] completed a systematic review of shared decision-making tools and found that several randomized controlled trials improved the clinical decision-making process and treatment received.

Simple and Realistic Terms

Regardless of the health literacy of the patient or family, explanations of life-sustaining treatments such as CPR, ventilation, and tube feedings in simple language are necessary for effective communication. Many patients and families experience a "data dump" during communication with health care providers, who focus on reporting vital statistics and odds of success. Several organizations have made available education handouts that explain life-sustaining treatments in realistic terms.[56,57] These materials are excellent visual tools during a discussion with a health care provider. Handouts are written at a low reading level and are available in several languages. Focusing on improving critical care unit communication when patients are dying increases family satisfaction, decreases family stress, and decreases days of nonbeneficial treatment.[58]

Education for Professionals

Most physicians and nurses have not been taught how to conduct this type of dialogue in their training. There are many options to gain the training and experience necessary to shift the decision making from a purely clinical perspective to a more humanistic view. Programs such as Education in Palliative and End-of-Life Care,[59] End-of-Life Nursing Education Consortium (ELNEC),[60] and Center to Advance Palliative Care Palliative Care Leadership Center[61] training are cost-effective methods to educate and support clinicians to communicate more effectively with patients and families at the end of life (see Box 9.2). In addition, VitalTalk© and Impact ICU training programs focus on incorporating palliative care into the critical care unit setting by offering advanced communication skills strategies.[62] Additional information on ethical and legal issues is provided in Chapter 2.

Patients

Patients' capacity for decision making is limited by illness severity and cognitive deficits accentuated by medications and the environment. When decision making is required, the patient is the first person to be approached if able to speak for himself or herself. When the patient is unable to safely make health care decisions because of disease progression or the therapy used for treatment, written documents such as a living will or a health care power of attorney should be obtained when possible. Additional information on power of attorney for health care can be found in the previous section on ACP. Without those documents, wishes of the patient should be ascertained from individuals closest to the patient. Some patients have neither capacity nor surrogates to assist in decision making; this was the case in 27% of deaths in one study.[63] In the absence of a surrogate decision maker, care decisions for unrepresented patients may be delayed, and discharge to another care setting can prove difficult. Only five states have empowered existing institutional committees to make decisions for unrepresented patients, illustrating the need for transparent and fair processes to be developed.[64]

Families

Family members continue to report dissatisfaction with communication and decision making.[65] Increasing the frequency of communication and sharing concerns early in the hospitalization make subsequent discussions easier for the patient, family, and health professional. Families have commonly complained about infrequent physician communication,[66] unmet communication needs in the shift from aggressive to end-of-life care, and lacking or inadequate communication.[67] Sometimes families are not ready to receive the prognosis and engage in decision making. Communication seems to be the most common source of complaints in families across studies and should be at the center of efforts to improve end-of-life care. A policy statement by the American College of Critical Care Medicine and American Thoracic Society[68] lists six recommendations for shared decision making by patients, families, and clinicians that encompasses three key elements: information exchange, deliberation, and making a treatment decision. Critical care nurses play a key role in initiating discussions, evaluating readiness, and supporting decision making.

PATIENT-CENTERED CRITICAL CARE

Family Meeting in a Critical Care Conference Room

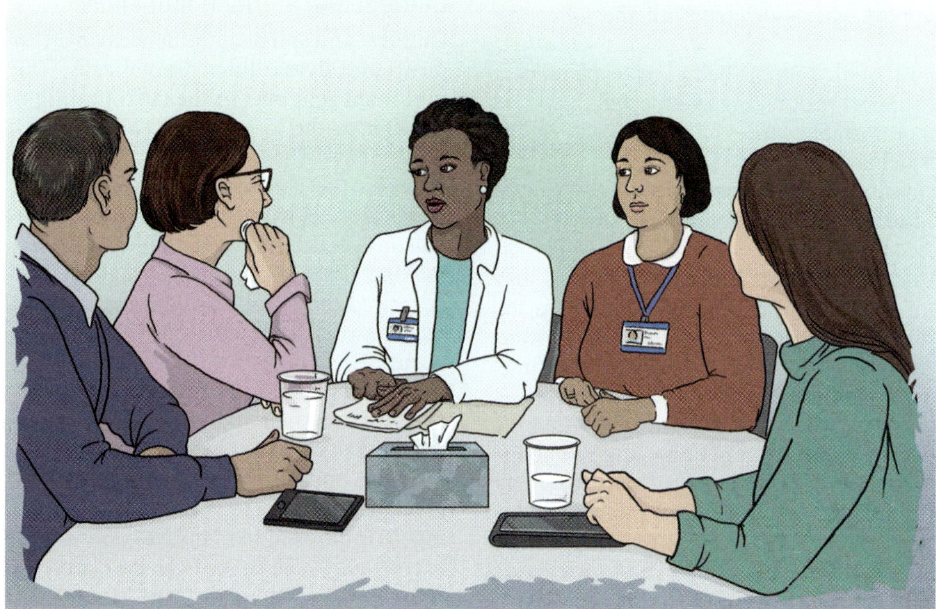

During a critical illness, a family meeting may be scheduled between the health care team and the close family when the patient is unable to express their own wishes because of the severity of the illness, cognitive impairment, intubation, or other reasons. Frequently, there are several family members in the room, and other family members may join via a conference phone or video. If there is a language barrier, a translator may be present. Sometimes there is a clergyperson or other support person for the family.

The intent of a family meeting is to facilitate open communication about the disease prognosis and to fully discuss therapeutic options. It is an opportunity for the family to share the patient's expectations and hopes for recovery. At other times family meetings focus on palliative care and the patient's preferences for end-of-life care.

The health care team can be large or small depending on the size of the hospital and the complexity of the medical care. Additional health care team members include the critical care nurse, respiratory therapist, social worker, and often members of the palliative care team.

The family meeting begins by introductions around the table, including how everyone is related to the patient, and there is a welcome to everyone involved. A physician typically describes the patient's trajectory of care up to this point and may indicate that a medical crossroads or decision point has been reached. This decision point could involve code status: cardiopulmonary resuscitation or not, need for a tracheostomy or not, or decisions about quality of life after the critical care unit. The family is asked to reflect about "What would your loved one want in this situation?"

Families vary tremendously in their responses in a family meeting. Some may say, "He is a fighter, he would want everything done"; others may say, "It is better to stop treatment as she always told us she did not want artificial life support"; others may say, "She would want the tracheostomy if there is a chance of recovery"; and others might say "I don't know, and we cannot make a decision at this point; we need more time."

Family meetings take about 30 minutes on average, although the first meeting in a series may be longer. If a patient is critically ill for several weeks, a family meeting may be held weekly. If the patient cannot express their wishes, a family member with durable power of attorney for health care (DPAHC) will act as the patient's surrogate decision maker. A weekly meeting ensures that communication between the family and the health care team remains open about the patient's progress, goals, and preferences.

Strategies to Support Shared Decision Making

Daily Rounds

Having the entire critical care unit team present for morning rounds is one method of improving communication. However, one study identified that there was low agreement among the health care team regarding patient care after daily rounds.[69] This finding indicates a need for clear goals and collaboration among care providers to decrease the chance of miscommunication to families.

Family Meetings

Family meetings in the presence of the critical care team is another method used to arrive at a common understanding of the patient's prognosis and goals for future care. A research analysis of the amount of time families were able to speak in these meetings revealed that when families had greater opportunity to talk, their satisfaction with physician communication increased, and their ratings of conflict with the physician decreased.[70,71] Abbott et al.[71] discussed families' descriptions 1 year after decisions about withdrawal of life support in relation to conflict centering on communication and the behavior of the staff. After the patient's death, greater family satisfaction with withdrawal of life support was associated with the following measures:[72]

- Process of withdrawal of life support being well explained
- Withdrawal of life support proceeding as expected
- Patient appearing comfortable
- Family and friends being prepared
- Appropriate person initiating discussion
- Adequate privacy during withdrawal of life support
- Opportunity to voice concerns

Curtis et al.[73] studied the process of family meetings and how to improve them to promote better end-of-life care for patients in the critical care unit and their families. They found that the missed opportunities that occur during these meetings were occasions to listen to family; to acknowledge and address emotions; and to pursue key tenets of palliative care such as patient preferences, surrogate decision making, and nonabandonment. How questions are asked of surrogates is extremely important. The question is not, "What do you want to do about (patient's name)?" but rather, "What would (patient's name) want if he knew he were in this situation?" These two questions have vastly different meanings and consequences for the patient and the family. The former question has a greater likelihood of engendering guilt. The latter question provides a sense of fulfilling the patient's wishes and respecting choices. This discussion is sometimes held during the family meeting, in which goals can be discussed. As families make decisions, they appreciate support for those decisions because the support can reduce the burden they experience. Sharma and Dy[65] reviewed valuable strategies for guiding clinical discussions and conducting family meetings that critical care nurses can use to focus discussions.

The health care team can reinforce the legitimacy of the family expressing feelings of disappointment, sadness, and loss. It is important that the family is made aware that the patient was more than a clinical disease and that he or she was recognized as an individual while in the critical care unit. In a German study, when relatives of critical care unit patients were provided with a brochure on bereavement and received proactive communication, they had lower negative scores on the Impact of Event Scale and on the Hospital Anxiety and Depression Scale.[74]

The Society of Critical Care Medicine (SCCM) recommends supporting the families of critical care unit patients.[75] SCCM presents 43 recommendations, including an endorsement of a shared decision-making model; family care conferencing; culturally appropriate requests for truth telling and informed refusal; spiritual support; staff education and debriefing; family presence at rounds and resuscitation; open and flexible visitation; family-friendly signs; and family support before, during, and after a death. One use of this guideline is to assess the level of family support for each critical care unit so that the most deficient recommendations could be addressed with quality-improvement actions. The categories used in this guideline are for general support of families of patients in the critical care unit. When cross-indexed with seven end-of-life domains, the needs of a family with a dying patient are decision making, spiritual and cultural support, emotional and practical support of families including visitation and family preparation for death, and continuity of care (see Box 9.2).[76,77]

Cultural and Spiritual Influences

Cultural and spiritual influences on attitudes and beliefs about death and dying differ dramatically. The cultures of the predominant religions in the surrounding community should be familiar to the local health care team. Globalization patterns have altered the cultural and religious diversity of communities in the United States, necessitating that nurses partner more closely with spiritual care resources and community liaisons to better understand family structures and decision making. These differences may affect how the health care team is viewed, how decisions are made, whether aggressive treatment is preferred, how death is met, and how grieving will occur.[78,79]

Patients who do not follow a particular religion should be assessed for their individual spiritual beliefs or lack thereof. The plan of care should also include evaluation of spiritual and religious support of the patient's family. A literature review revealed that religious or spiritual practices of families were highly important to many, yet only 4% of physicians requested a chaplain visit to critical care unit patients.[80] Identifying sources of spiritual comfort strengthens the bond between caregivers, patients, or family. Satisfaction with critical care unit care has been associated with the extent to which the family is satisfied with their spiritual care, especially when the patient is near death.[81] Staff members' own attitudes about the specific practices of a culture should be carefully monitored[82] and tempered with respect and humility. Interpreters are necessary when the patient or the family members do not speak English. A cultural and religious assessment is warranted in all situations, because cultural or religious affiliation does not imply that patients or families follow all of the tenets of that group.

Hospice Information

Although hospice care has been available for many years, patients and families often consider this method of care only in the last weeks or months of an end-stage illness, and they commonly view hospice care as "giving up," or outright abandonment. Health professionals can assist patients and families by providing information about the benefits of hospice, particularly regarding aggressive symptom management and family support. Some hospices are offering to partner with critical care units in the provision of end-of-life care and in the process of withdrawal of ventilatory support. Hospice care is an option that should be considered, especially in end-stage illness, and the benefit to surviving family members should be emphasized. In some circumstances, alert patients may express a wish to die at home. Hospice-to-home programs have demonstrated that granting this wish may be feasible with coordinated effort (see Box 9.2).

WITHDRAWAL OR WITHHOLDING OF TREATMENT

Discussions about the potential for impending death are never held early enough. The first discussion about prognosis often occurs in conjunction with the topic of the discontinuation of life support. Some family members dread such conversations but are grateful to discuss the uncertainty of their loved one's future. Physicians should give families time to adjust to this information and make preparations by providing early discussions about prognosis, goals of therapy, and the patient's wishes.

Gallagher et al.[83] described the "negotiated reorienting" that critical care nurses perform to seek consensus and emotionally support families, sometime over long periods of time. An effective approach to gaining consensus in family-clinician discussions is to take the time to identify the patient's values and preferences and incorporate them into treatment decisions. Critical care nurses greatly influence family perceptions of the quality of their loved one's dying, but measuring such a complex event can be a challenge. Several survey instruments exist to evaluate family members' attitudes toward a loved one's death and satisfaction with the critical care unit nurses during the dying process, but additional research is necessary to provide data for training and practice recommendations.[84,85]

Proactive Approach

When patients are admitted to the critical care unit with serious illnesses and are likely to die, a proactive approach to end-of-life care has been found to shorten critical care unit stays without a significant difference in mortality rates or discharge disposition.[86,87] The use of nonbeneficial resources decreases, and prolonged dying is avoided. Rapid response team daily rounds on noncritical care units have proven to be anecdotally effective in early identification of patients showing early signs of clinical deterioration. Communication with the provider at this time can avert an admission to a critical care unit, possibly even averting a Code Blue event.

Patients with assistive cardiac devices present a different challenge in discussion of withdrawal of life support. These patients often are cognitively intact and consent to removal of technology that is keeping them alive. Wiegand and Kalowes[88] outlined issues surrounding discontinuation of cardiac devices as a preventive ethics approach, with health care providers anticipating the need to shift goals of care and support patients and families through the process. To reduce confusion and distress among clinicians, protocols for discontinuation of organ-assistance devices are recommended as a standard of care.

Futility/Nonbeneficial Care Discussions

Nurses and physicians frequently disagree about the futility of interventions. Sometimes nurses consider withdrawal before physicians and patients do, and they then feel the care they are giving is unnecessary and possibly harmful. Nurses in one study were found to be more pessimistic but more often correct than physicians about the prognoses of dying patients, but the nurses also proposed treatment withdrawal for some very sick patients who survived.[89] Nurses described acknowledging futility and acting on the patient's distress, being ideally placed to advocate with specialists. At the same time, nurses describe the tension that can result in recommending palliative care or hospice to the medical staff.[90]

Steps Toward Comfort Care

Once a decision has been made to withdraw life-sustaining therapies, each intervention should be evaluated to determine whether it still provides any benefit.[91] In a patient who has received life support for a prolonged time, a staged withdrawal of interventions such as removal of ventilator support via terminal weaning allows for better symptom control. For families, seeing a loved one look peaceful as life support is withdrawn ultimately helps with grief resolution in the future. Usually, routine interventions (e.g., laboratory tests, imaging, cardiac monitoring) are removed first, followed by respiratory support devices. Withdrawal of specific treatments may have effects necessitating symptom management. Withdrawal of dialysis may cause dyspnea from volume overload, which may necessitate the use of opioids or benzodiazepines. Efforts to discontinue artificial feeding may be met with concern from the family, because offering food has great social significance. It is essential to share information with family and providers regarding the potential benefits of withholding nutrition and fluids in the days immediately before death to prevent unnecessary suffering.[92] Critical care patients who survive withdrawal of life support measures may continue to remain in critical care for a period of time before dying or being transferred to a less acute setting. During this time, various symptoms may occur that can be distressing for patients, families, and nursing staff.

PALLIATIVE CARE

An important shift in care of terminally ill patients in the critical care unit has occurred with the growth of palliative care programs in the United States. The rapid expansion of this new specialty has decreased the mortality rate in critical care units for patients followed by palliative care services through transfer to lower-acuity units and has decreased the costs associated with higher-acuity critical care beds, pharmacy, laboratory, and diagnostic costs.[93] Studies by Morrison et al.[8] reviewed hospital and Medicare data to demonstrate that hospitals with palliative care services had significant cost savings compared with hospitals providing usual care. Additionally, concurrent palliative care during a critical care unit stay has been shown to decrease critical care unit days.[94] More recent initiatives such as the IPAL-ICU have demonstrated that a focus on lifesaving interventions can be integrated with palliative care concurrently, rather than one following the failure of another.[95]

Patients who are identified as being near the end of life require aggressive care for symptom management provided by a team of health professionals. Palliative care guidelines have been released by a consortium of organizations concerned with palliative care and end-of-life care, and they may provide guidance when the usual first-line treatments do not promote comfort for critically ill patients who are near death.[96] Strategies that are based on research evidence and expert opinion for specific conditions such as delirium, opioid dose escalation, and dyspnea at the end of life are outlined on the Palliative Care Network of Wisconsin website, which provides access to evidence-based and expert-based Fast Facts that address a wide variety of clinical, ethical, and psychosocial problems that arise with the care of seriously ill and dying patients.[97] Publications such as the Quality Palliative Care guidelines and the IOM report *Improving Palliative Care for Cancer*[98] have stated that palliative care ideally begins at the time of diagnosis of a life-threatening illness and continues through cure or until death and into the family's bereavement period.

Symptom Management

It has long been in question whether critical care patients can accurately report their symptoms because of the effects of sedating medications, severe illness, and organ dysfunction. Kalowes[99] studied critical care unit patients with a diagnosis other than cancer during a daily wake-up and compared their report of symptoms with reports of their family members. Almost all patients had more than 10 symptoms, and there was 85.5% congruence between patient and family report of physiologic and psychological symptoms. Overall, patients experienced significant symptom burden near the end of life but received limited treatment to alleviate suffering.

Pain

Because many critical care patients are unconscious, assessment of pain and other symptoms becomes more difficult.[100] In sedated ventilated patients, especially patients receiving neuromuscular blocking medications, there is no systematic, reliable method to determine the presence or degree of pain.[101] Gélinas et al.[102] recommends using signs of body movements, neuromuscular signs, facial expressions, or responses to physical examination for pain assessment in patients with altered consciousness (see Chapter 7).

Because opioids provide sedation, anxiolysis, and analgesia, they are particularly beneficial in ventilated patients. Morphine is the medication of choice, and there is no upper limit in dosing. However, in higher doses, morphine metabolites can cause myoclonus, hyperalgesia, and allodynia. In a paralyzed patient, this may not be detectable, but it can be uncomfortable on some level for the patient, perhaps evident in vital signs or response to ventilator settings. Careful assessment of patients' vital signs may reveal suspected discomfort that necessitates an opioid switch to hydromorphone or fentanyl. In nonventilated patients, sedation may cause respiratory depression, and nonopioids or specific anesthetic agents may be more appropriate. Antiinflammatory medications or neuroleptic agents often provide significant comfort for inflammatory conditions or neurologic pain.

Titration of intravenous infusions to achieve maximum effect with minimum sedation is an inexact science. Critical care nurses should assume that pain is present in an immobile patient and administer routine analgesics to prevent suffering. Jacobi et al.[103] published a guideline for the sustained use of sedatives and analgesia (see Chapter 8).

Dyspnea

A systematic review and meta-analysis of cancer-related dyspnea interventions critically examined the common interventions used by many practitioners.[104] Dyspnea is best managed with close evaluation of the patient and the use of opioids, sedatives, and nonpharmacologic interventions (oxygen, positioning, and increased ambient air flow). Morphine reduces anxiety and muscle tension and increases pulmonary vasodilation but is ineffective when inhaled. Benzodiazepines, particularly midazolam, may be used in patients who are unable to take opioids or for whom the respiratory effects are minimal. Midazolam has been shown to be at least equally effective as morphine and, in some studies, superior to morphine.[105] Benzodiazepines and opioids should be titrated to effect. Oxygen did not prove to be superior in the studies reviewed, but ambient air movement of some sort often provides relief. Treatment efforts should be aimed at the patient's expression of dyspnea rather than at respiratory rates or oxygen levels.

Nausea and Vomiting

Nausea and vomiting are common and should be treated with antiemetics. The cause of nausea and vomiting may be intestinal obstruction or increased intracranial pressure. Treatment for decompression may be uncomfortable in dying patients, and its use should be weighed using a benefit-to-burden ratio. In certain circumstances, an intervention to provide percutaneous drainage for decompression may be used in a patient who is not imminently dying.

Fever and Infection

Fever and infection necessitate evaluation of the benefits of continuing antibiotics so as not to prolong the dying process. Management of fever with antipyretics may be appropriate for the patient's comfort, but other methods such as ice or hypothermia blankets should be balanced against the amount of distress the patient may experience.

Edema

Edema may cause discomfort, and diuretics may be effective if kidney function is intact. Dialysis is not warranted at the end of life. The use of fluids may contribute to the edema when kidney function is impaired and the body is slowing its functions.

Anxiety

Anxiety should be assessed verbally, if possible, or by changes in vital signs or restlessness. Benzodiazepines, especially midazolam with its rapid onset and short half-life, are commonly used. Minimizing noxious sounds and playing a patient's favorite music may help soothe anxiety.

Delirium

Delirium is commonly observed in critically ill and dying patients. Haloperidol and benzodiazepines (e.g., midazolam, lorazepam) have traditionally been used to manage delirium but have side effects that can be problematic. To ensure accurate trending of delirium, a standardized assessment tool such as the Confusion Assessment Method for the ICU is recommended to adequately assess delirium.[106] Evidence-based strategies to minimize and shorten the duration of delirium should be used.

Metabolic Derangement

Treatments for metabolic derangements, skin problems, anemia, and hemorrhage should be tempered with concerns for the patient's comfort. Only interventions promoting comfort should be performed. Patients do not necessarily feel better "when the laboratory values are right."

Near-Death Awareness

Two hospice nurses originally described the phenomenon of near-death awareness.[107] The same behaviors may be seen in conscious patients near death in the critical care unit. Having an awareness of the phenomenon enables more careful assessment of behaviors that may be interpreted as delirium, acid-base imbalance, or other metabolic derangements. These behaviors include communicating with someone who is not alive, preparing for travel, describing a place they can see, or even knowing when death will occur. Family members may find these behaviors disturbing but find comfort in understanding the phenomenon and in sharing these experiences with their loved one.

WITHDRAWAL OF MECHANICAL VENTILATION

A dramatic geographic variation exists in practices surrounding withdrawal of life-sustaining therapies. Some evidence suggests that this variation may be driven more by physicians' attitudes and biases than by factors such as patients' preferences or cultural differences. This inconsistency in care further complicates a difficult process. From clinical, ethical, and legal perspectives, standardized withdrawal from life-support order sets are recommended to direct and support nursing judgment in this complex and emotional clinical situation.

Creation of a Support Environment

At the heart of the difficulty of conversations about withdrawal of life support is the pattern and selection of language to address the decision. Selph et al.[108] taped end-of-life conversations between families and physicians and found that at least one supportive statement was provided 66% of the time during the discussion. In another study, 86% of nurses reported that they were involved in discussions of withdrawal of life-sustaining treatments and influenced the types of withdrawal interventions.[109] Recommendations for creating a supportive atmosphere during withdrawal discussions included the following:

- Taking a moment at the beginning of the conversation to inquire about the family's emotional state
- Acknowledging verbal and nonverbal expressions of emotion and using that to support families
- Acknowledging that most family members face a significant emotional burden when a loved one is critically ill or dying

Process of Withdrawing Life Support

During the family meeting in which a decision to withdraw life support is made, a time to initiate withdrawal is usually established. For example, a distant family member may need to arrive, and then the procedure will occur. When appropriate, the patient should be moved to a separate or special room. It is helpful if other staff members are alerted to the fact that a withdrawal is occurring. A neutral sign hung on the door or use of a special room may caution staff to avoid loud conversations and laughter, which is quite upsetting to grieving families. Nurses can support the family by suggesting specific measures to modify the environment and minimize symptoms that the family might perceive as suffering of their loved one.

Signs of Impending Death

After the decision to remove ventilatory support is made and the family is gathered, the family should be told what the impending death will be like. When the patient is dependent on ventilatory support or vasopressors and that support is removed, death typically follows in minutes. The patient appears as if sleeping, and the usual signs of color and skin temperature changes will not be seen before death. The opposite is true if the patient is not ventilator dependent. When the patient is to be extubated at the beginning of the withdrawal process, the family should be prepared for respiratory noises and gasping respirations. These signs are less likely when the endotracheal tube is removed near the end of the withdrawal process, as is more commonly done. When assessing how prepared family members felt for what would happen during withdrawal of life support, Kirchhoff et al.[110] found that families who did not receive preparatory information before the withdrawal of life support requested this information during interviews 2 to 4 weeks after the patient's death. Family members who received this recommended information reported they felt significantly more prepared. Providing information to families for the experience of withdrawal alerts them to what the patient may exhibit as death approaches, reducing the distress families may feel during the withdrawal process.

Pacemakers or implantable cardioverter-defibrillators should be turned off to prevent patient discomfort or distress from the shocks firing[111] and to avoid interfering with the pronouncement of death. Wiegand and Kalowes[88] provide detailed information about the conversations that should be held with the patient and how each of the specific devices are deactivated. Neuromuscular blocking agents should be discontinued before removal of ventilator support, because paralysis precludes the assessment of the patient's discomfort and the means of the patient to communicate with loved ones.[110]

The removal of monitors is usually recommended. However, physicians and nurses may use the monitor to assess the distress of the patient during the withdrawal process and to adjust the amount of medication needed for symptom management. Families may glance at the monitor to verify that electrical activity has ceased, because the appearance of death may be too subtle to detect. If not needed, monitors should be removed to make the room appear as normal as possible.

Sedation During Withdrawal of Life Support

Opioids and benzodiazepines are the most commonly administered medications, because dyspnea and anxiety are the usual symptoms related to ventilator withdrawal. Campbell[112] stated that patients who are brain dead do not require sedation and that patients with brainstem activity only may not show signs of distress or need sedation. von Gunten and Weissman[113] recommend sedating all patients, even patients who are comatose. Recommended dosing is a bolus intravenous dose of morphine (2 to 10 mg) and a continuous morphine infusion at 50% of the bolus dose per hour. An intravenous dose of midazolam (1 to 2 mg) is administered, followed by an infusion at 1 mg/h. The intent is to provide good symptom control, so doses accelerate until the patient's comfort is achieved. Additional medication should be available at the bedside for immediate administration if discomfort is observed in the patient. In one study, the use of opioids or benzodiazepines to treat discomfort after the withdrawal of life support did not hasten death in critically ill patients.[114] A standardized withdrawal order set with titration parameters minimizes variation and subjectivity among the physician's orders and the nurse's implementation of the orders.

Ventilator Settings

After the patient's comfort is achieved, ventilator settings are reduced. An experienced physician, a respiratory therapist, and a nurse should be present during this time. Ventilator alarms should be turned off. The method of withdrawal adopted is usually determined by the clinician's preference. The choice of terminal weaning as opposed to extubation is based on considerations of access for suctioning, appearance of the patient for the family, how long the patient will survive off the ventilator, and whether the patient has the ability to communicate with loved ones at the bedside.

Terminal Weaning Versus Extubation

If terminal weaning is used, positive end-expiratory pressure is reduced to normal, and then the mode is set to patient control. Next, the fraction of inspired oxygen is reduced to 0.21 (21%). All these steps are taken slowly while observing the patient for distress or anxiety. If extubation is performed immediately rather than at the end of the terminal wean, the family should be prepared for airway compromise and the appearance of the patient.

All patients do not require the same ventilator weaning or extubation protocols. For example, Campbell[112] recommended turning off the ventilator and extubating patients who are brain dead, placing patients who have brainstem-only injuries on a T-piece, and using terminal weaning for patients with altered consciousness or who are conscious. The terminal wean offers the most control over secretions, respiratory noises, and gasping.

Terminal extubation of alert patients can be difficult, because there is uncertainty about the amount and type of medications to provide. Billings outlined the issues surrounding the terminal extubation procedure.[115] Patients indicating the desire to remove life support retain the need for comfort medications to control dyspnea and secretions until death. Some health care providers may believe this is a moral "gray area" and relate the process to assisted suicide. However, patients with decisional capacity may elect to discontinue life support, which has been supported by court decisions and bioethical opinion.

PROFESSIONAL ISSUES

Health Care Settings

Professional issues surround the provision of end-of-life and palliative care within traditional acute and clinical settings. In critical care units, care may be managed by an intensivist or by a committee of specialists but seldom by the family physician who knows the patient. The use of consultants may be limited. Palliative care specialists may be available at certain times, but they are often considered "outsiders," although the trend to use this specialty service is increasing with the availability of programs in U.S. hospitals. How the consultation is arranged may vary by institution. Turf issues should not compromise patient care. Having a clear plan for withdrawal and better preparation of the family may assist the professionals involved in feeling more comfortable with the care provided.[116] Expert nurses should advocate for vulnerable patients by communicating the patient's wishes and presenting a realistic picture to family members.[117]

Some interventions have been found to be helpful for health professionals in improving patient care. Although it did not improve nurses' assessment of patients' dying experience, a standardized order form for withdrawal was found to increase the amount of medications nurses administered for sedation.[118]

Emotional Support for the Nurse

Nurses who care for dying patients need to have their work valued as highly as other high-tech functions in the critical care unit. Critical care units usually have several nurses who are looked to by other staff to provide end-of-life care or to assist with withdrawal of life support. When several deaths occur close together, those nurses may be called on frequently. Some consideration in assignment should be given when a nurse has more than one death in a shift or a week. Taking a new admission is also difficult immediately after a death, and it can occur before the family has left the unit. Nurse administrators can provide some additional resources, debriefing, or time off when the burden has been high. Hearing supportive words from colleagues has been reported by critical care nurses as helpful in coping with the death of a patient.[119]

This issue is a serious one for critical care nurses, because emotional and ethical distress can lead to burnout. Meltzer and Huckabay[120] found that the score on the emotional exhaustion subscale of the Maslach Burnout Inventory and the score on the frequency subscale on the Moral Distress Scale correlated for a group of 60 critical care nurses. Often, critical care nurses experience moral distress because of the severity of patients' illnesses and the requirement of technology to maintain vital organ function. Collaborative strategies for minimizing moral distress rely on the bedside nurse and critical care leadership to implement individual and organizational changes.[121] Nurses experience moral distress when aggressive care is offered to patients who are not expected to benefit from it. These levels of distress are high and have implications for retention of highly skilled nurses.[122]

One study showed that nurses' experience of moral distress and a negative ethical environment is more severe than that of their physician colleagues.[123] Developing a consensus about care was found to be the most helpful approach.[124] Nurses in this study had many suggestions when questioned about what could be done to improve end-of-life care, such as facilitating dying with dignity, having someone with patients who are dying, managing patients' symptoms, knowing and then following patients' wishes for end-of-life care, and promoting earlier cessation of treatment or not initiating aggressive treatment at all.

Until more recently, end-of-life content in nursing school curricula and textbooks was sparse, and continuing education was limited on this topic. ELNEC was created in 2000 to address gaps in education for nurses caring for dying patients.[60] Based on national reports, guidelines, recommendations, and research studies, ELNEC has grown into the premier source of end-of-life training for nurses all over the world. The Critical Care ELNEC course became available in 2006 and addressed topics focused on the critical care unit setting.

ORGAN DONATION

Legal Issues

The Social Security Act Section 1138 requires that hospitals have written protocols for the identification of potential organ donors.[125] The Joint Commission has a standard on organ donation, and legislation at state levels directs health care providers and organ recovery agencies.[126] Although an impending death marks a difficult time for family members, the nurse must notify the organ procurement official to approach the family with a donation request. These individuals have training to make a supportive request and are the ones to decide whether a family should not be approached based on the patient's disease. Organ donation may not be appropriate in some cases, but tissue donation remains a consideration. More information is available in Chapter 35.

Brain Death

Death may be pronounced when the patient meets a list of neurologic criteria. However, there are differences among hospital policies for certification of brain death, which may permit differences in the circumstances under which patients are pronounced dead in different U.S. hospitals.[127] Families do not always understand the meaning of brain death, and they are less likely to donate organs when they believe the patient will not be dead until the ventilator is turned off and the heart stops.[128] How these conversations are held will determine families' understanding and positively affect donation. Campbell[41] recommended not suggesting that the organs are alive while the brain is dead, but rather that the organs are functioning as a result of the machines used. Chapter 35 provides more information on the specifics of brain death.

FAMILY CARE

In this chapter, the term family means whatever the patient states is the family. An integral part of the patient-family dyad, families expect a cure for any condition the patient may have; they do not expect to receive bad news. They look for the good news in any message received from caregivers and are surprised when told that death is the only outcome possible.[129] Families need assistance in forming their expectations about outcomes. Ongoing communication about the patient's progress is preferable to waiting until the patient is near death and then communicating with the family. Most studies of families at this time are descriptive, and interventions need to be developed to help them.[130]

A number of factors affect the family experience of a loved one's decline and death in the ICU. One intervention used with families at the end of life is a grieving or comfort cart. In one critical care unit, the cart has a top drawer with English and Spanish versions of the Bible, Koran, and Book of Mormon, and pamphlets about grief and bereavement.[131] The lower portion of the cart holds paper cups, napkins, and condiments. Fresh coffee and tea are brewed on the unit and served with muffins and cookies from the cafeteria. Family responses have been positive, because they do not want to leave the bedside despite their hunger. Another strategy is to provide nursing units with supplies including religious items and music to support the emotional and spiritual needs of families at the end of life.[132,133]

Besides good communication and visitation, psychosocial and spiritual support can aid acceptance and initiation of the bereavement process. Families have also benefitted from organization-specific end-of-life programs in the ICU that provide keepsake items such as fingerprints and locks of hair to support psychologic and spiritual needs.[134] The recent COVID-19 pandemic changed a multitude of ICU processes including family presence and support for dying loved ones in the ICU. Recommendations for actions by the interdisciplinary team, coupled with virtual communication, helped staff get to know patients through family members, as well as provide compassionate care and rituals necessary for grieving.[135]

Waiting for Good News

Patients and families do not come to the critical care unit with the expectation of death. Even patients who have had previous admissions expect to be "saved." Having this in mind while talking to families may assist professionals in interpreting families' responses. Preparing families for changes in the patient as the health condition deteriorates helps them make plans. They need to know whether other family members should be called, whether someone should spend the night, or whether financial arrangements should be changed before an impending death (e.g., to enable the widow to have access to funds). Anticipated changes can be described to prepare families. Emotional support and grieving can be facilitated through discussion of the dying patient and their unique qualities and families' memories. Interactive patient education television services provide healing music and videos that help create a more comfortable environment for families as they wait for the next step in the dying process. Families often play the patient's favorite music or movies. Many services also provide access to the Internet through which family pictures or videos can be accessed. Provision of these services can be beneficial before the patient dies through visiting a shared past, making the most of the present, and hoping for an end to the patient's suffering and healing for loved ones.

Families may refuse to forgo life-supporting treatments and want "everything done" for a variety of reasons. Effective communication throughout the hospitalization and information provided throughout the stay predispose the family to better acceptance of news as the patient deteriorates. Family satisfaction is increased when they feel supported during their decision making or hear more empathic statements from physicians.[136,137]

Families in Crisis

Families may experience a sense of crisis as emergencies occur or as the patient deteriorates and dies. Responses to the news of the death vary. Family members may show anger or be quiet, exhibit emotions or stoicism. Culture or religious beliefs may affect their response to news. It is helpful to ask whether family members would like to see a chaplain or a social worker. Quiet and calm, some privacy, and support are always appreciated.

Family Presence During Cardiopulmonary Resuscitation

To be helpful, the family's presence during procedures or resuscitative attempts should be coupled with staff support.[45,46] Critical care nurses and emergency nurses have taken family members to the bedside for resuscitation or invasive procedures, but most did not have written policies for the family's presence.[138] Sometimes these experiences provide opportunities for the family to be supportive of the patient. At other times, the family may become more aware of what is involved in decisions they have made on behalf of the patient. Toronto and Larocco's[139] integrative literature review outlined studies of family member perspectives of being present during CPR on a loved one. Despite clinician concerns of psychological trauma from witnessing resuscitation activities, family members believed their presence helped them to heal, as they were aware of all that was done for their loved one.

Visiting Hours

Visiting in critical care units continues to be restricted despite national calls for increases in patient or family control over the care and evidence that family presence can decrease duration and severity of delirium.[140,141] Restricting visiting for dying patients in the critical care unit seems to be unconscionable. Providing visiting time to help family members say good-bye is important. Family members may have difficulty in seeing the person they knew among all the tubes. Coaching can be provided about how to approach the patient and about how the patient may still be able to hear despite appearing to be nonresponsive. Visitors should be permitted to the extent possible, while not interfering with other patients' privacy or rest. Children, unless they represent a significant source of infection, should be allowed to say good-bye, but they may need adult assistance in understanding the situation. Families may have religious or cultural ceremonies that are important for them to perform before the patient dies or experiences withdrawal of life support. These practices should be encouraged and facilitated as much as possible. Continuity of care by the same nurse is important, helping with families' closure and healing.

After Death

After the death, the family may wish to spend time at the bedside. Family members' time with the body should be unhurried and private. They need adequate room to sit and spend time. They can be asked if they need assistance or resources and whether they wish to be alone or have someone nearby. Frequently, the bed is needed for another patient, and juggling is required to ensure that the family has sufficient time even as another patient needs to be admitted. Supporting families after a death involves immediate bereavement support, information on what to do about the death, bereavement support for the future, contact with the family after death, and assessment of the quality of care the patient experienced.[142] Having material already prepared with the necessary after-death information is quite helpful at this time. Most hospices offer bereavement support groups that are available to any member of the community free of charge, regardless of whether a loved one was enrolled in hospice. Nurses need to be aware of their own judgment on what is an appropriate response, because individuals respond differently to the same news, even within the same family.

BOX 9.3 Evidence-Based Practice

Guidelines for End-of-Life Care in the Critical Care Unit

Key topics of the guidelines for end-of-life care in the critical care unit, based on research and expert panel review, are categorized.

Patient-Centered and Family-Centered Care and Decision Making: Comprehensive Ideal for End-of-Life Care

- Use legal standards for decision making.
- Resolve conflict.
- Communicate with families.

Ethical Principles Related to Withdrawal of Life-Sustaining Treatment

- Withholding versus withdrawing
- Killing versus allowing to die
- Intended versus merely foreseen consequences

Practical Aspects of Withdrawing Life-Sustaining Treatments in Critical Care Unit

- Procedure
- Specific issues
- Use of paralytics

Symptom Management in End-of-Life Care

- Pain and dyspnea
- Delirium
- Medications used

Considerations at Time of Death

- Notification of death
- Brain death
- Organ donation
- Bereavement and support
- Needs of interdisciplinary team

Research, Quality Improvement, and Education

- Develop interventions likely to improve quality of care.
- Develop education programs.

Data from Truog RD, Campbell ML, Curtis JR, et al. Recommendations for end-of-life care in the intensive care unit: a consensus statement by the American College [corrected] of Critical Care Medicine [published correction appears in *Crit Care Med.* 2008;36(5):1699]. *Crit Care Med.* 2008;36(3):953–963. https://doi.org/10.1097/CCM.0B013E3181659096.

COLLABORATIVE CARE

The ability to provide collaborative, compassionate end-of-life care is the responsibility of all clinicians who work with critically ill patients. Interdisciplinary collaborative efforts are associated with improvement in care.[142] In 2008, the SCCM published a revised guideline, "Recommendations for End-of-Life Care in the Intensive Care Unit," to provide guidance for end-of-life care for the team.[91] The Evidence-Based Practice feature on end-of-life care provides a summary of the topics included (Box 9.3). The Robert Wood Johnson Foundation Critical Care End-of-Life Peer Workgroup[143] identified seven end-of-life care domains for use in the critical care unit:

1. Patient-centered and family-centered decision making
2. Communication
3. Continuity of care
4. Emotional and practical support
5. Symptom management and comfort care
6. Spiritual support
7. Emotional and organizational support for critical care unit clinicians

Individuals and groups have developed online tools to improve end-of-life care.[144] Critical care unit staff can assess the quality of their care by assessing perceptions of families and staff, auditing documentation, or making observations of care. The same attention should be directed toward improving end-of-life care that is directed toward skills of electrocardiogram interpretation or hemodynamic monitoring.

ADDITIONAL RESOURCES

See Box 9.4 for Internet resources pertaining to palliative and end-of-life care.

BOX 9.4 Internet Resources

Palliative and End-of-Life Care

- American Academy of Hospice and Palliative Care Medicine (AAHPM): https://aahpm.org
- End-of-Life Nursing Education Consortium (ELNEC): https://aacnnursing.org/ELNEC
- Center to Advance Palliative Care (CAPC): https://capc.org/
- Hospice and Palliative Care Nurses Association (HPNA): https://advancing-expertcare.org
- Palliative Care Network of Wisconsin: https://mypcnow.org
- Promoting Excellence in End-of-Life Care: https://www.promotingexcellence.org/
- VitalTalk: https://vitaltalk.org

CASE STUDY 9.1 Patient at the End of Life

Brief Patient History

Mr. C is a 17-year-old African American who was involved in a motor vehicle accident. He sustained a cervical fracture at the level of C2 that transected his spinal column and both vertebral arteries. Rescue breathing was begun in the field by bystanders, and he was intubated by paramedics en route to the hospital. Mr. C's parents state that they want everything possible done and that they have faith that God will heal their son.

Clinical Assessment

Mr. C is admitted to the critical care unit from the emergency department. He is ventilator dependent. His skin is warm and dry. He is unresponsive to verbal or painful stimuli, and there is no physical movement. Mr. C's family remains at the bedside 24 hours each day throughout the week. They converse with Mr. C, speaking about all the things they are going to do when he gets home.

Diagnostic Procedures

Mr. C's vital signs are as follows: blood pressure of 120/72 mm Hg, heart rate of 120 beats/min (sinus tachycardia), no spontaneous respiration, temperature of 97.8°F, and Glasgow Coma Scale score of 3. Computed tomography scan of the head showed a global ischemic infarct involving both ventricles, and electroencephalography revealed no detectable cortical activity.

Medical Diagnosis

Mr. C is diagnosed with brain death.

Questions

1. What major outcomes do you expect to achieve for this patient?
2. What problems or risks must be managed to achieve these outcomes?
3. What interventions could be initiated to monitor, prevent, manage, or eliminate the problems and risks identified?
4. What interventions could be initiated to promote optimal functioning, safety, and well-being of the patient?
5. What technology can be used to monitor this patient and prevent complications?
6. What other interprofessional team members are needed to assist with the management of this patient?
7. What possible learning needs would you anticipate for this patient?
8. What cultural and age-related factors might have a bearing on the patient's plan of care?

KEY POINTS

- End-of-life care requires knowledge and skill, similar to any other aspect of critical care nursing.
- Realistic information about the limits of medicine and frailties of the body allows patients and families to make decisions that preserve a patient's dignity and respect individual autonomy.
- Most patients have expressed a desire to avoid "general life support" if dying or permanently unconscious, but few have specified preferences regarding specific life-sustaining treatments.
- Advanced care planning decreases life-sustaining treatment, increases use of hospice and palliative care, and prevents hospitalization. Communication of the patient's wishes between family members, primary care providers, and intensivists is critical.
- Patient-centered and family-centered decision making is key.
- Communication skills are enhanced with additional training in end-of-life conversations and early access to palliative care clinicians.
- Health professionals can assist patients and families by providing information about the benefits of hospice, particularly regarding aggressive symptom management and family support.
- Family presence during procedures or resuscitative attempts should be coupled with staff support.
- Extended visiting times are needed to help family members say good-bye.
- Proactive control of symptoms is vital for the patient's comfort.

Visit the Evolve site at http://evolve.elsevier.com/Urden/CriticalCareNursing for additional study materials.

REFERENCES

1. Rabow MW, Hardie GE, Fair JM, McPhee SJ. End-of-life care content in 50 textbooks from multiple specialties. *JAMA*. 2000;283(6):771–778. https://doi.org/10.1001/jama.283.6.771.
2. Kirchhoff KT, Beckstrand RL, Anumandla PR. Analysis of end-of-life content in critical care nursing textbook. *J Prof Nurs*. 2003;19(6):372. https://doi.org/10.1016/s8755-7223(03)00141-8.
3. Pleschberger S, Hornek A. Recognizing and defining dying: analysis of end-of-life coverage in German nursing textbooks. *Pflege*. 2011;24(4):259–269. https://doi.org/10.1024/1012-5302/a000133.
4. Peden-McAlpine C, Liachenko J, Traudt T, et al. Constructing the story: how nurses work with families regarding withdrawal of aggressive treatment in ICU – a narrative study. *Int J Nurs Stud*. 2015;57(2):1146–1156. https://doi.org/10.1016/j.ijnurstu.2015.03.015.
5. Siegel MD. End of life decision making in the ICU. *Clin Chest Med*. 2009;30(1):181–194. https://doi.org/10.1016/j.ccm.2008.11.002.
6. Prina LL. Funders' support for palliative and end of life care. *Health Aff (Millwoord)*. 2015;34(2):354. https://doi.org/10.1377/hlthaff.2014.1443.
7. Dumanovsky T, Augustin R, Rogers M, et al. The growth of palliative care in U.S. hospitals: a status report. *J Pall Med*. 2016;19(1):8–15. https://doi.org/10.1089/jpm.2015.0351.
8. Morrison RS, Penrod JD, Cassel JB, et al. Cost savings associated with U.S. hospital palliative care consultation programs. *Arch Intern Med*. 2008;168(16):1783–1790. https://doi.org/10.1001/archinte.168.16.1783.
9. Medina J, Puntillo K, eds. *AACN Protocols for Practice: Palliative Care and End of Life Issues in Critical Care*. Boston, MA: Jones & Bartlett; 2006.
10. American Association of Critical-Care Nurses. Palliative care in the acute & critical care setting. www.aacn.org/clinical-resources/palliative-end-of-life. Accessed May 8, 2024.

11. National Consensus Project for Quality Palliative Care. *Clinical Practice Guidelines for Quality Palliative Care*. 4th ed. Richmond, VA: National Coalition for Hospital and Palliative Care; 2018.
12. Teno JM, Mor V, Ward N, et al. Bereaved family member perceptions of quality of end-of-life care in U.S. regions with high and low usage of intensive care unit care. *J Am Geriatr Soc*. 2005;53(11):1905–1911. https://doi.org/10.1111/j.1532-5415.2005.53563.x.
13. Nelson JE, Angus DC, Weissfeld LA, et al. End-of-life care for the critically ill: a national intensive care unit survey. *Crit Care Med*. 2006;34(10):2547–2553. https://doi.org/10.1097/01.CCM.0000239233.63425.1D.
14. Glavan BJ, Engelberg RA, Downey L, et al. Using the medical record to evaluate the quality of end-of-life care in the intensive care unit. *Crit Care Med*. 2008;36(4):1138–1146. https://doi.org/10.1097/CCM.0b013e318168f301.
15. Beckstrand RL, Hadley KH, Luthy KE, Macintosh JLB. Providing a "good death": critical care nurses' suggestions for improving end-of-life care. Dimens. *Crit Care Nurs*. 2017;36(4):264–270. https://doi.org/10.1097/DCC.0000000000000252.
16. Mularski RA, Heine CE, Osborne ML, et al. Quality of dying in the ICU: ratings by family members. *Chest*. 2005;128(1):280–287. https://doi.org/10.1378/chest.128.1.280.
17. White DB, Ernecoff N, Billings JA, et al. Is dying in an ICU a sign of poor quality end of life care? *Am J Crit Care*. 2013;22(3):263–266. https://doi.org/10.4037/ajcc2013604.
18. Investigators SUPPORT. A controlled trial to improve care for seriously ill hospitalized patients. The Study to Understand Prognoses and Preferences for Outcomes and Risks of Treatments (SUPPORT). *JAMA*. 1995;274(20):1591–1598.
19. Field MJ, Cassell CK, eds. *Approaching Death: Improving Care at the End of Life*. Washington, DC: National Academy Press; 1997.
20. Committee on Approaching Death, Addressing Key End of Life Issues, Institute of Medicine. *Dying in America: Improving Quality and Honoring Individual Preferences Near the End of Life*. Washington DC: National Academies Press; 2015.
21. Angus DC, Barnato AE, Linde-Zwirble WT, et al. Use of intensive care at the end of life in the United States: an epidemiologic study. *Crit Care Med*. 2004;32(3):638–643. https://doi.org/10.1097/01.ccm.0000114816.62331.08.
22. Silveira M, Wiitala W, Piette J. Advance directive completion by elderly Americans: a decade of change. *J American Geri Soc*. 2014;62(4):706–710. https://doi.org/10.1111/jgs.12736.
23. Teno J, Gozalo P, Trivedi A, et al. Site of death, place of care and health care transitions among U.S. Medicare beneficiaries 2000–2015. *JAMA*. 2018;320(3):264–271. https://doi.org/10.1001/jama.2018.8981.
24. Department of Health and Human Services. Advance directives and advance care planning: report to Congress. Published August 1, 2008. https://aspe.hhs.gov/reports/advance-directives-advance-care-planning-report-congress-0. Accessed May 8, 2024.
25. Auriemma CL, Halpern SD, Asch JM, et al. Completion of advance directives and documented care preferences during the coronavirus disease 2019 (COVID-19) pandemic. *JAMA Netw Open*. 2020;3(7):e2015762. https://doi.org/10.1001/jamanetworkopen.2020.15762.
26. Barwise A, Jaramillo C, Novotny P, et al. Differences in code status and end of life decision making in patients with limited English proficiency in the intensive care unit. *Mayo Clin Proc*. 2018;93(9):1271–1281. https://doi.org/10.1016/j.mayocp.2018.04.021.
27. Silveria M, Kim S, Langa K. Advance directives and outcomes of surrogate decision making before death. *N Engl J Med*. 2015;362(13):1211–1218. https://doi.org/10.1056/NEJMsa0907901.
28. California Legislative Information. AB-2139, Eggman. End of life care: patient notification. Published September 25, 2014. http://www.leginfo.ca.gov/pub/13-14/bill/asm/ab_2101-2150/ab_2139_bill_20140925_chaptered.htm. Accessed May 8, 2024.
29. OHSU Center for Ethics & Oregon POLST Coalition. Oregon POLST. https://oregonpolst.org/. Accessed May 8, 2024.
30. Hickman SE, Nelson CA, Moss AH, et al. The consistency between treatments provided to nursing facility residents and orders on the Physician Orders for Life Sustaining Treatment form. *J Am Geriatr Soc*. 2011;59(11):2091–2099. https://doi.org/10.1111/j.1532--5415.2011.03656.x.
31. Hickman SE, Nelson CA, Perrin NA, et al. A comparison of methods to communicate treatment preferences in nursing facilities: traditional practices versus the physician orders for life-sustaining treatment program. *J Am Geriatr Soc*. 2010;58(7):1241–1248. https://doi.org/10.1111/j.1532-5415.2010.02955.x.
32. Briggs LA, Kirchoff KT, Hammes BJ, et al. Patient-centered advance care planning in special patient populations: a pilot study. *J Prof Nurs*. 2004;20(1):47–58. https://doi.org/10.1016/j.profnurs.2003.12.001.
33. Jesus J, Marshall KD, Kraus CK, et al. Should emergency department patients with end-of-life directives be admitted to the ICU? *J Emerg Med*. 2018;55(3):435–440. https://doi.org/10.1016/j.jemermed.2018.06.009.
34. Brinkman-Stoppelenburg A, Rietjens J, van der Heide A. Effects of advance care planning on end of life care: a systematic review. *Palliat Med*. 2014;228(8):1000–1025. https://doi.org/10.1177/0269216314526272.
35. Bhatia V, Geidner R, Mirchandani K, et al. Systemwide advance care planning during the Covid-19 pandemic: the impact on patient outcomes and cost. *NEJM Catal Innov Care Deliv*. 2021;2(9):1–11. https://doi.org/10.1056/CAT.21.0188.
36. Adames HY, Chavez-Duenas NY, Fuentes MA, et al. Integration of Latino/a values into palliative health care: a culture-centered model. *Palliat Support Care*. 2014;12(2):149–157. https://doi.org/10.1017/S147895151300028X.
37. Rubenfeld GD. Principles and practice of withdrawing life-sustaining treatments. *Crit Care Clin*. 2004;20(3):435–451. https://doi.org/10.1016/j.ccc.2004.03.005.
38. Tilden V, Tolle SW, Nelson CA, et al. Family decision-making to withdraw life-sustaining treatments from hospitalized patients. *Nurs Res*. 2001;50(2):105–115. https://doi.org/10.1097/00006199-200103000-00006.
39. Prigerson H, Brewin VM, et al. Enhancing and mobilizing the potential for wellness and emotional resilience (EMPOWER) among surrogate decision makers of ICU patients: study protocol for a randomized controlled trial. *Trials*. 2019;20(408):1–13. https://doi.org/10.1186/s13063-019-3515-0.
40. Voigt LP, Rajendram P, Shuman AG, et al. Characteristics and outcomes of ethics consultations in an oncologic intensive care unit. *J Intensive Care Med*. 2014;(1):436–442. https://doi.org/10.1177/0885066614538389.
41. Campbell ML. *Forgoing Life-Sustaining Therapy: How to Care for the Patient Who Is Near Death*. Aliso Viejo, CA: American Association of Critical-Care Nurses; 1998.
42. Sandroni C, Nolan J, Cavallaro F, et al. Hospital cardiac arrest: incidence, prognosis, and possible measures to improve survival. *Intensive Care Med*. 2007;33(2):237–245. https://doi.org/10.1007/s00134-006-0326-z.
43. Ramenofsky DH, Weissmen DE, Marks S: Fast fact #179: CPR survival in the hospital setting. Updated 2015. https://www.mypcnow.org/wp-content/uploads/2019/02/FF-179-CPR-Survival-inhospital.-3rd-Ed.pdf. Accessed May 8, 2024.
44. FitzGerald JD, Wenger NS, Califf RM, et al. Functional status among survivors of in-hospital cardiopulmonary resuscitation. SUPPORT investigators study to understand progress and preferences for outcomes and risks of treatment. *Arch Intern Med*. 1997;157(1):72–76.
45. American Association of Critical-Care Nurses. Family presence during CPR and invasive procedures. *Crit Care Nurse*. 2016;36(1):e11–e14. https://doi.org/10.4037/ccn2016980.
46. Vanhoy MA, Horigan A, Stapleton SJ, et al. 2017 ENA clinical practice guideline committee. Clinical practice guideline: family presence. *J Emerg Nurs*. 2019;45:76.e1–76.e29. https://doi.org/10.1016/j.jen.2018.11.012.
47. Chang Y, Huang CF, Lin CC. Do-not-resuscitate orders for critically ill patients in intensive care. *Nurs Ethics*. 2010;17(4):445–455. https://doi.org/10.1177/0969733010364893.
48. Park YR, Kim JA, Kim K. Changes in how ICU nurses perceive the DNR decision and their nursing activity after implementing it. *Nurs Ethics*. 2011;18(6):802–813. https://doi.org/10.1177/0969733011410093.
49. Christakis NA, Lamont EB. Extent and determinants of error in doctors' prognoses in terminally ill patients: prospective cohort study. *BMJ*. 2000;320(7233):469–472. https://doi.org/10.1136/bmj.320.7233.469.

50. Lau F, Cloutier-Fisher D, Kuziemsky C, et al. A systematic review of prognostic tools for estimating survival time in palliative care. *J Palliat Care*. 2007;23(2):93–112.
51. Strand K, Flaatten H. Severity scoring in the ICU: a review. *Acta Anaesthesiol Scand*. 2008;52(4):467–478. https://doi.org/10.1111/j.1399--6576.2008.01586.x.
52. Marshall JC, Cook DJ, Christou NV, et al. Multiple organ dysfunction score: a reliable descriptor of a complex clinical outcome. *Crit Care Med*. 1995;23(10):1638–1652. https://doi.org/10.1097/00003246-199510000-00007.
53. Jung C, Guidet B, Flaaten H. Frailty in intensive care medicine must be measured, interpreted and taken into account. *Intensive Care Med*. 2023;49(1):87–90. https://doi.org/10.1007/s00134-022-06887-8.
54. White DB, Braddock CH, Bereknyei S, et al. Toward shared decision making at the end of life in intensive care units: opportunities for improvement. *Arch Intern Med*. 2007;167(5):461–467. https://doi.org/10.1001/archinte.167.5.461.
55. Austin C, Mohottige D, Sudore R, et al. Tools to promote shared decision making in serious illness. *JAMA Intern Med*. 2015;175(7):1213–1221. https://doi.org/10.1001/jamainternmed.2015.1679.
56. Coalition for Compassionate Care of California. Decision Aids For Healthcare Providers. Published 2019. https://coalitionccc.org/CCCC/CCCC/Resources/Decision-Aids-for-Healthcare-Providers.aspx. Accessed May 8, 2024.
57. Family Caregiver Alliance. All Resources. Accessed May 8, 2024. https://www.caregiver.org/caregiver-resources/all-resources/.
58. Treece PD. Communication in the intensive care unit about the end of life. *AACN Adv Crit Care*. 2007;18(4):406–414. https://doi.org/10.1097/01.AACN.0000298633.38029.2d.
59. Northwestern Medicine Feinberg School of Medicine. EPEC: Education in Palliative and End-of-Life Care. www.bioethics.northwestern.edu/programs/epec/. Accessed May 8, 2024.
60. American Association of Colleges of Nursing. End-of-Life Nursing Education Consortium (ELNEC). www.aacnnursing.org/ELNEC. Accessed May 8, 2024.
61. Palliative Care Leadership Centers. Overview. https://www.capc.org/palliative-care-leadership-centers/. Accessed May 8, 2024.
62. Anderson W, Puntillo K, Cimino J, et al. Palliative care professional development for critical care nurses: a multicenter program. *Am J Crit Care*. 2017;26(5):361–372. https://doi.org/10.4037/ajcc.2017336.
63. White DB, Curtis JR, Lo B, et al. Decisions to limit life-sustaining treatment for critically ill patients who lack both decision-making capacity and surrogate decision-makers. *Crit Care Med*. 2006;4(8):2053–2059. https://doi.org/10.1097/01.CCM.0000227654.38708.C1.
64. Pope TM. Making medical decisions for patients without surrogates. *N Engl J Med*. 2013;269(21):1976–1978. https://doi.org/10.1056/NEJMp1308197.
65. Sharma RK, Dy SM. Cross-cultural communication and use of the family meeting in palliative care. *Am J Hosp Palliat Med*. 2011;28(6):437–444. https://doi.org/10.1177/1049909110394158.
66. Baker R, Wu AW, Teno JM, et al. Family satisfaction with end of-life care in seriously ill hospitalized adults. *J Am Geriatr Soc*. 2000;48(Suppl 5):S61–S69. https://doi.org/10.1111/j.1532-5415.2000.tb03143.x.
67. Curtis JR. Communicating about end-of-life care with patients and families in the intensive care unit. *Crit Care Clin*. 2004;20(3):363–380. https://doi.org/10.1016/j.ccc.2004.03.00.
68. Kon A, Davidson J, Morrison W, et al. Shared decision-making in intensive care units: an American College of Critical Care Medicine and American Thoracic Society policy statement. *Crit Care Med*. 2016;44(1):188–201. https://doi.org/10.1097/CCM.0000000000001396.
69. Have EC, Nap RE. Mutual agreement between providers in intensive care medicine on patient care after interdisciplinary care rounds. *J Intensive Care Med*. 2014;29(5):292–297. https://doi.org/10.1177/0885066613486596.
70. Curtis JR, Patrick DL, Shannon SE, et al. The family conference as a focus to improve communication about end-of-life care in the intensive care unit: opportunities for improvement. *Crit Care Med*. 2001;29(Suppl 2):N26–N33. https://doi.org/10.1097/00003246-200102001-00006.
71. Abbott KH, Sago JG, Breen CM, et al. Families looking back: one year after discussion of withdrawal or withholding of life-sustaining support. *Crit Care Med*. 2001;29(1):197–201. https://doi.org/10.1097/00003246-200101000-00040.
72. Keenan SP, Mawdsley C, Plotkin D, et al. Withdrawal of life support: how the family feels, and why. *J Palliat Care*. 2000;16(Suppl):S40–S44.
73. Curtis JR, Engelberg RA, Wenrich MD, et al. Missed opportunities during family conferences about end-of-life care in the intensive care unit. *Am J Respir Crit Care Med*. 2005;171(8):844–849. https://doi.org/10.1164/rccm.200409-1267OC.
74. Hartog CS, Schwarzkopf D, Riedemann NC, et al. End of life care in the intensive care unit: a patient-based questionnaire of intensive care unit staff perception and relatives' psychological responses. *Palliat Med*. 2015;29(4):336–345. https://doi.org/10.1177/0269216314560007.
75. Davidson JE, Powers K, Hedayat KM, et al. Clinical practice guidelines for support of the family in the patient-centered intensive care unit: American College of Critical Care Task Force 2004–2005. *Crit Care Med*. 2007;35(2):605–622. https://doi.org/10.1097/01.CCM.0000254067.14607.EB.
76. Clarke EB, Curtis JR, Luce JM, et al. Quality indicators for end-of-life care in the intensive care unit. *Crit Care Med*. 2003;31(9):2255–2262. https://doi.org/10.1097/01.CCM.0000084849.96385.85.
77. Kirchhoff KT, Faas AI. Family support at end of life. *AACN Adv Crit Care*. 2007;18(4):426–435. https://doi.org/10.1097/01.AACN.0000298635.45653.c8.
78. Degenholtz HB, Thomas SB, Miller MJ. Race and the intensive care unit: disparities and preferences for end-of-life care. *Crit Care Med*. 2003;31(Suppl 5):S373–S378. https://doi.org/10.1097/01.CCM.0000065121.62144.0D.
79. Lipson JG, Dibble SL, Minarik PA. *Culture and Nursing Care: A Pocket Guide*. San Francisco CA: University of California San Francisco Nursing Press; 1996.
80. Gordon B, Keogh M, Davidson Z, et al. Addressing spirituality during critical illness: a review of current literature. *J Crit Care*. 2018;45:76–81. https://doi.org/10.1016/j.jcrc.2018.01.015.
81. Wall RJ, Engelberg RA, Gries CJ, et al. Spiritual care of families in the intensive care unit. *Crit Care Med*. 2007;35(4):1084–1090. https://doi.org/10.1097/01.CCM.0000259382.36414.06.
82. Scheunemann L, Ernekoff N, Buddadhumaruk P, et al. Clinician-family communication about patient values and preferences in intensive care units. *JAMA*. 2019;179(5):676–684. https://doi.org/10.1001/jamainternmed.2019.0027. Available from:.
83. International Nurses' End-of-Life Decision-Making in Intensive Care Research Group, Gallagher A, Bousso R, et al. Negotiated reorienting: a grounded theory of nurses' end-of-life decision-making in the intensive care unit. *Int J Nurs Sci*. 2015;52(4):794–803. https://doi.org/10.1016/j.ijnurstu.2014.12.003.
84. Downey L, Curtis R, Lafferty W, et al. The quality of dying and death questionnaire: empirical domains and theoretical perspectives. *J Pain Symp Man*. 2010;39(1):9–22. https://doi.org/10.1016/j.jpainsymman.2009.05.012.
85. Wall R, Engelberg R, Downey L, et al. Refinement, scoring, and validation of the family satisfaction in the intensive care unit (FS-ICU) survey. *Crit Care Med*. 2010;35(1):271–279. https://doi.org/10.1097/01.CCM.0000251122.15053.50.
86. Campbell ML, Guzman JA. Impact of a proactive approach to improve end-of-life care in a medical ICU. *Chest*. 2003;123(1):266–271. https://doi.org/10.1378/chest.123.1.266.
87. Norton SA, Hogan LA, Holloway RG, et al. Proactive palliative care in the medical intensive care unit: effects on length of stay for selected high-risk patients. *Crit Care Med*. 2007;35(6):1530–1535. https://doi.org/10.1097/01.CCM.0000266533.06543.0C.
88. Wiegand DL, Kalowes PG. Withdrawal of cardiac medications and devices. *AACN Adv Crit Care*. 2007;18(4):415–425. https://doi.org/10.1097/01.AACN.0000298634.45653.81.
89. Frick S, Uehlinger DE, Zuercher Zenklusen RM. Medical futility: predicting outcome of intensive care unit patients by nurses and doctors—a prospective comparative study. *Crit Care Med*.

2003;31(2):456–461. https://doi.org/10.1097/01.CCM.0000049945.69373.7C.
90. Broom A, Kirby E, Good P, et al. Negotiating futility, managing emotions: nursing the transition to palliative care. *Qual Health Res.* 2015;25(3):299–309. https://doi.org/10.1177/1049732314553123.
91. Truog RD, Campbell ML, Curtis JR, et al. Recommendations for end of life care in the intensive care unit: a consensus statement by the American College of Critical Care Medicine. *Crit Care Med.* 2008;36(30):953–963. https://doi.org/10.1097/CCM.0B013E3181659096.
92. Hospice and Palliative Nurses Association. Artificial nutrition and hydration in end-of-life care. HPNA position paper. *Home Healthc Nurse.* 2004;22(5):341–345. https://doi.org/10.1097/00004045-200405000-00016.
93. Center to Advance Palliative Care. Palliative care programs continue rapid growth in U.S. hospitals becoming standard practice throughout the country. Published April 5, 2010. https://www.capc.org/about/press-media/press-releases/2010-4-5/palliative-care-programs-continue-rapid-growth-us-hospitals-becoming-standard-practice-throughout-country/. Accessed May 8, 2024.
94. Mercadante S, Gregoretti C, Cortegiani A. Palliative care in intensive care units: why, where, what, who, when, how. *BMC Anes.* 2018;18(106):1–6. https://doi.org/10.1186/s12871-018-0574.
95. Center to Advance Palliative Care. The IPAL-ICU. Published January 29, 2019. www.capc.org/documents/125/. Accessed May 8, 2024.
96. Abbasi J. New guidelines aim to expand palliative care beyond specialists. *JAMA.* 2019;322(3):193–195. https://doi.org/10.1001/jama.2019.5939.
97. Palliative Care Network of Wisconsin. Fast facts and concepts. https://www.mypcnow.org/fast-facts/. Accessed September 9, 2023.
98. Institute of Medicine, National Research Council. *Improving Palliative Care for Cancer: Summary and Recommendations.* Washington, DC: National Academy Press; 2001.
99. Kalowes P. *Doctoral dissertation. Symptom Burden at the End of Life in Patients With Terminal and Life Threatening Illness in Intensive Care Units.* San Diego, CA: University of San Diego; 2007.
100. Barr J, Fraser GL, Puntillo K, et al. Clinical practice guidelines for the management of pain, agitation, and delirium in adult patients in the intensive care unit. *Crit Care Med.* 2013;41(1):263–306. https://doi.org/10.1097/CCM.0b013e3182783b72.
101. Weissman C. Sedation and neuromuscular blockade in the ICU. *Chest.* 2005;128(2):477–479. https://doi.org/10.1378/chest.128.2.477.
102. Gélinas C, Fortier M, Viens C, et al. Pain assessment and management in critically ill intubated patients: a retrospective study. *Am J Crit Care.* 2004;13(2):126–135.
103. Jacobi J, Fraser GL, Coursin DB, et al. Clinical practice guidelines for the sustained use of sedatives and analgesics in the critically ill adult. *Crit Care Med.* 2002;30(1):119–141. https://doi.org/10.1097/00003246-200201000-00020.
104. Ben-Aharon I, Gafter-Gvili A, Leibovici L, et al. Interventions for alleviating cancer-related dyspnea: a systematic review and meta-analysis. *Acta Oncol.* 2012;51(8):996–1008. https://doi.org/10.3109/0284186X.2012.709638.
105. Del Fabbro E, Dalal S, Bruera E. Symptom control in palliative care, Part III: dyspnea and delirium. *J Palliat Med.* 2006;9(2):422–436. https://doi.org/10.1089/jpm.2006.9.422.
106. Vanderbilt University Medical Center. Confusion Assessment Method for the ICU (CAM-ICU): The Complete Training Manual. Published August 31, 2016. https://www.icudelirium.org/resource-downloads/cam-icu-training-manual. Accessed May 8, 2024.
107. Callanan M, Kelley P. *Final Gifts: Understanding the Special Awareness, Needs, and Communications of the Dying.* New York: Bantam Books; 1997.
108. Selph RB, Shiang J, Engelberg R, et al. Empathy and life support decisions. *J Gen Intern Med.* 2008;23(9):1311–1317. https://doi.org/10.1007/s11606-008-0643-8.
109. Kirchoff K, Kowalkowski J. Current practices for withdrawal of life support in intensive care units. *Am J Crit Care.* 2010;19(6):532–541. https://doi.org/10.4037/ajcc2009796.
110. Kirchhoff KT, Palzkill J, Kowalkowski J, et al. Preparing families of intensive care patients for withdrawal of life support: a pilot study. *Am J Crit Care.* 2008;17(2):113–122.
111. Goldstein NE, Lambert R, Bradley E, et al. Management of implantable cardioverter defibrillators in end-of-life care. *Ann Intern Med.* 2004;141(11):835–838. https://doi.org/10.7326/0003-4819-141-11-200412070-00006.
112. Campbell ML. How to withdraw mechanical ventilation: a systematic review of the literature. *AACN Adv Crit Care.* 2007;18(4):397–403. https://doi.org/10.4037/15597768-2007-4008.
113. von Gunten CF, Weissman DE. Fast facts and concepts #34. Symptom control for ventilator withdrawal in the dying patient. Updated May 2015. https://www.mypcnow.org/fast-fact/symptom-control-for-ventilator-withdrawal-in-the-dying-patient/. Accessed September 9, 2023.
114. Chan JD, Treece PD, Engelberg RA, et al. Narcotic and benzodiazepine use after withdrawal of life support: association with time to death? *Chest.* 2004;126(1):286–293. https://doi.org/10.1016/S0012-3692(15)32925-1.
115. Billings A. Terminal extubation of the alert patient. *J Palliat Care.* 2011;14(7):800–801. https://doi.org/10.1089/jpm.2011.9676.
116. Rocker GM, Cook DJ, O'Callaghan CJ. Canadian nurses' and respiratory therapists' perspectives on withdrawal of life support in the intensive care unit. *J Crit Care.* 2005;20(1):59–65. https://doi.org/10.1016/j.jcrc.2004.10.006.
117. Robichaux CM, Clark AP. Practice of expert critical care nurses in situations of prognostic conflict at the end of life. *Am J Crit Care.* 2006;15(5):480–489.
118. Treece PD, Engelberg RA, Crowley L, et al. Evaluation of a standardized order form for the withdrawal of life support in the intensive care unit. *Crit Care Med.* 2004;32(5):1141–1148. https://doi.org/10.1097/01.ccm.0000125509.34805.0c.
119. Kisorio LC, Langley GC. Intensive care nurses' experiences of end-of-life care. *Intensive Crit Care Nurs.* 2016;33:30–38. https://doi.org/10.1016/j.iccn.2015.11.002.
120. Meltzer LS, Huckabay LM. Critical care nurses' perceptions of futile care and its effect on burnout. *Am J Crit Care.* 2004;13(3):202–208.
121. American Association of Critical-Care Nurses. Resources for moral distress. https://www.aacn.org/clinical-resources/moral-distress. Accessed May 8, 2024.
122. Elpern EH, Covert B, Kleinpell R. Moral distress of staff nurses in a medical intensive care unit. *Am J Crit Care.* 2005;14(6):523–530.
123. Hamric AB, Blackhall LJ. Nurse-physician perspectives on the care of dying patients in intensive care units: collaboration, moral distress, and ethical climate. *Crit Care Med.* 2007;35(2):422–429. https://doi.org/10.1097/01.CCM.0000254722.50608.2D.
124. Badger JM. Factors that enable or complicate end-of-life transitions in critical care. *Am J Crit Care.* 2005;14(6):513–521.
125. Social Security Administration. Complication of the Social Security Laws. Hospital protocols for organ procurement and standards for organ procurement agencies. https://www.ssa.gov/OP_Home/ssact/title11/1138.htm. Accessed September 9, 2023.
126. *2023 Comprehensive Accreditation Manuals.* Oakbrook Terrace, IL: The Joint Commission; 2022.
127. Powner DJ, Hernandez M, Rives TE. Variability among hospital policies for determining brain death in adults. *Crit Care Med.* 2004;32(6):1284–1288. https://doi.org/10.1097/01.ccm.0000127265.62431.0d.
128. Siminoff LA, Mercer MB, Arnold R. Families' understanding of brain death. *Prog Transplant.* 2003;13(3):218–224. https://doi.org/10.1177/152692480301300309.
129. Wiegand D. Families and withdrawal of life-sustaining therapy: state of the science. *J Fam Nurs.* 2006;12(2):165–184. https://doi.org/10.1177/1074840706287686.
130. Whitmer M, Hurst S, Stadler K, et al. Caring in the curing environment. *J Hosp Palliat Nurs.* 2007;9(6):329–333. https://doi.org/10.1097/01.NJH.0000299318.30009.f7.
131. Davidson J. Family-centered care: meeting the needs of patients' families and helping families adapt to critical illness. *Crit Care Nurse.* 2009;29(3):28–34. https://doi.org/10.4037/ccn2009611.

132. Davidson J, Boyer ML, Casey D, et al. Gap analysis of cultural and religious needs of hospitalized patients. *Crit Care Nurs Q.* 2008;31(2):119–126. https://doi.org/10.1097/01.CNQ.0000314472.33883.d4.
133. Gries CJ, Curtis JR, Wall RJ, et al. Family member satisfaction with end-of-life decision making in the ICU. *Chest.* 2008;133(3):704–712. https://doi.org/10.1378/chest.07-1773.
134. Neville TH, Bear DK, Kao Y, et al. End-of-life care during the coronavirus disease 2019 pandemic: the 3 wishes program. *Crit Care Explor.* 2021;3(10):e549. https://doi.org/10.1097/CCE.0000000000000549.
135. Jeitziner MM, Camenisch SA, Jenni-Moser B, et al. End-of-life care during the COVID-19 pandemic-What makes the difference? *Nurs Crit Care.* 2021;26(3):212–214. https://doi.org/10.1111/nicc.12593.
136. Stapleton RD, Engelberg RA, Wenrich MD, et al. Clinician statements and family satisfaction with family conferences in the intensive care unit. *Crit Care Med.* 2006;34(6):1679–1685. https://doi.org/10.1097/01.CCM.0000218409.58256.AA.
137. MacLean SL, Guzzetta CE, White C, et al. Family presence during cardiopulmonary resuscitation and invasive procedures: practices of critical care and emergency nurses. *Am J Crit Care.* 2003;12(3):246–257.
138. Kirchhoff KT, Dahl N. American Association of Critical-Care Nurses' national survey of facilities and units providing critical care. *Am J Crit Care.* 2006;15(1):13–27.
139. Toronto CE, LaRocco SA. Family perception of and experience with family presence during cardiopulmonary resuscitation: an integrative review. *J Clin Nurs.* 2018;28(1–2):32–46. https://doi.org/10.1111/jocn.14649.
140. Berwick DM, Kotagal M. Restricted visiting hours in ICUs: time to change. *JAMA.* 2004;292(6):736–737. https://doi.org/10.1001/jama.292.6.736.
141. Shannon S. Helping families cope with death in the ICU. In: Curtis JR, Rubenfeld GD, eds. *Managing Death in the Intensive Care Unit: The Transition From Cure to Comfort.* Oxford: Oxford University Press; 2001.
142. Baggs JG, Norton SA, Schmitt MH, et al. The dying patient in the ICU: role of the interdisciplinary team. *Crit Care Clin.* 2004;20(3):525–540. https://doi.org/10.1016/j.ccc.2004.03.008.
143. Mularski RA, Curtis JR, Billings JA, et al. Proposed quality measures for palliative care in the critically ill: a consensus from the Robert Wood Johnson Foundation Critical Care Workgroup. *Crit Care Med.* 2006;34(11):S404–S411. https://doi.org/10.1097/01.CCM.0000242910.00801.53.
144. Center to Advance Palliative Care. Clinical tools for delivering high quality care. Reviewed June 22, 2020. https://www.capc.org/toolkits/clinical-tools-delivering-high-quality-care/. Accessed May 8, 2024.

10

Cardiovascular Anatomy and Physiology

Mary E. Lough

http://evolve.elsevier.com/Urden/CriticalCareNursing

ANATOMY

Discussion of the anatomy of the heart and blood vessels in this text begins on a macroscopic level with a description of the major structures and then progresses to the cellular and molecular levels for each structure.

Major Structures of the Heart

The thoracic case protects the heart, lungs, and great vessels. The heart is situated in the anterior thoracic cavity, just behind the sternum and above the diaphragm (Fig. 10.1A). Several important structures, including the esophagus, aorta, vena cava, and vertebral column, are located behind the heart. The position of the heart within the chest cavity is such that the chambers normally described as "right" and "left" are anterior and posterior. The right ventricle constitutes most of the anterior surface (closest to the chest wall) and the inferior surface (directly above the diaphragm). The left ventricle makes up the anterolateral (front and side) and posterior surfaces. The base of the heart is superior and includes the superior portion of the heart and the origin of the aorta, the vena cava, and the pulmonary arteries. The apex of the heart is inferior, situated just above the diaphragm. A lateral view of the heart is shown in Fig. 10.1B. The increasing use of digital imaging has highlighted the anatomic inaccuracy of the terms *right ventricle* and *left ventricle* because these descriptors do not relate to the position of the heart in the chest when described in the standard anatomic position (standing upright and facing the observer).[1,2]

Size, Weight, and Layers of the Heart

The size of a human heart is about the same size as that person's clenched fist. In an adult, the heart averages 12 centimeters (cm) in length and 8 to 9 cm in breadth at the broadest part. The weight of the normal heart averages 330 grams (g) in men and 245 g in women.[3,4] No significant differences exist in ventricular wall thickness between men and women. Body weight provides an approximation of heart weight, although this is not an exact relationship, because illness can lower body weight, whereas hypertension can increase the weight of the heart muscle in ventricular hypertrophy.

The four distinct layers of the heart wall are (1) the pericardium, (2) the epicardium, (3) the myocardium, and (4) the endocardium (Fig. 10.2).

Pericardium

The heart and the origins of the great vessels are surrounded and enclosed by an outer covering known as the *pericardium*. The pericardium has two layers, fibrous and serous.[5]

Fibrous pericardium. The outermost fibrous pericardium is a thick envelope of connective tissue that is tough and inelastic. Ligaments anchor the outer pericardium to the diaphragm and the great vessels such that the heart is maintained in a fixed position within the thoracic cavity. However, the heart can move freely within the pericardium.

Serous pericardium. Inside the fibrous outer layer, there is an inner, double-walled serous membrane with a potential space between the two layers, and this double-walled sac is what allows the heart to beat without friction throughout a lifetime.[5] The two serous layers are labeled *parietal* (outer layer that lines the fibrous pericardium) and *visceral* (inner layer, also known as the *epicardium*).[5] The visceral pericardium is flexible, adheres directly to the heart, and folds with the surface contours of the heart. The serosal pericardium extends over the great vessels so that the entire external surface of the heart is covered. Thus, the pericardium also provides a physical barrier against infection for the heart.

Pericardial Cavity and Fluid

The pericardial cavity is the potential space between the visceral and parietal serous layers. The space between these two layers normally contains a small amount (less than 50 mL) of serous pericardial fluid.[5,6] The fluid is secreted, is resorbed, and serves as a lubricant between the layers so that the heart can beat and move freely without friction.[5] Pericardial fluid is produced as a plasma ultrafiltrate and is drained by the lymphatic system.

In conditions where there is excess fluid, the fibrous, outer pericardial sac is noncompliant and unable to adapt to rapid increases in pericardial fluid volume and pressure. Any accumulation of excess fluid is described as a *pericardial effusion*.[7] If the fluid collection in the sac impinges on ventricular filling, ventricular ejection, or coronary artery perfusion, removal of fluid may be necessary by pericardiocentesis.[7] Inflammation of the sac is described as *pericarditis*.[7]

Phrenic nerves. The two phrenic nerves innervate the pericardium and pass between the parietal pericardium and the mediastinal pleura.[6] The pain that accompanies pericardial effusion and cardiac tamponade is sensed via phrenic nerve sensory nerve fibers.

Epicardium

The epicardium, also known as the *visceral pericardium*, is tightly adherent to the heart and to the base of the great vessels, as described earlier. The coronary arteries lie on the top of the epicardium.

Epicardial adipose tissue. The space between the epicardium (visceral pericardium) and the myocardium is where epicardial fat, also known as epicardial adipose tissue (EAT), is deposited.[8] In adults, epicardial adipose deposits are most noticeable along the surface indentations or grooves between the atrial and ventricular chambers.[5] The coronary arteries are also located in these surface grooves. Because the adipose tissue is situated so close to the major coronary arteries, the risk of coronary artery disease is increased.[8] Epicardial adipose contains smaller adipocytes compared with other fat deposits, has a different fatty acid composition, and has a higher protein content. This composition facilitates the infiltration of free fatty acids and adipokines into the coronary arteries. Autopsy data indicate that epicardial fat increases until age 20 to 40 years, but thereafter, the quantity does not depend on age. A person who is obese will usually have more epicardial adipose tissue. Because obesity is endemic in modern society, epicardial fat is receiving more attention. EAT may also increase the risk of developing atrial fibrillation.[8]

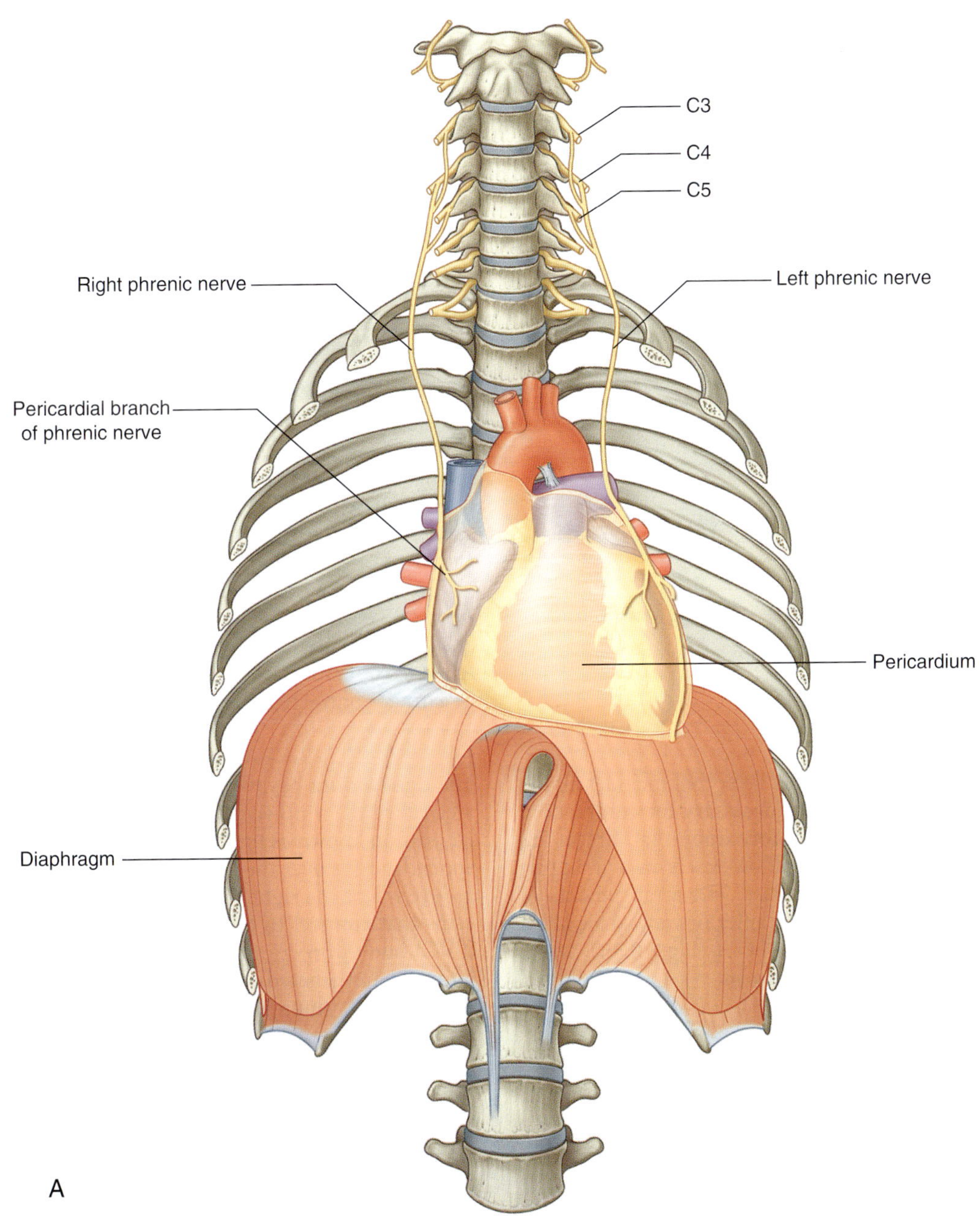

FIG. 10.1 (A) Heart situated on the diaphragm in the thoracic cavity, anterior view.

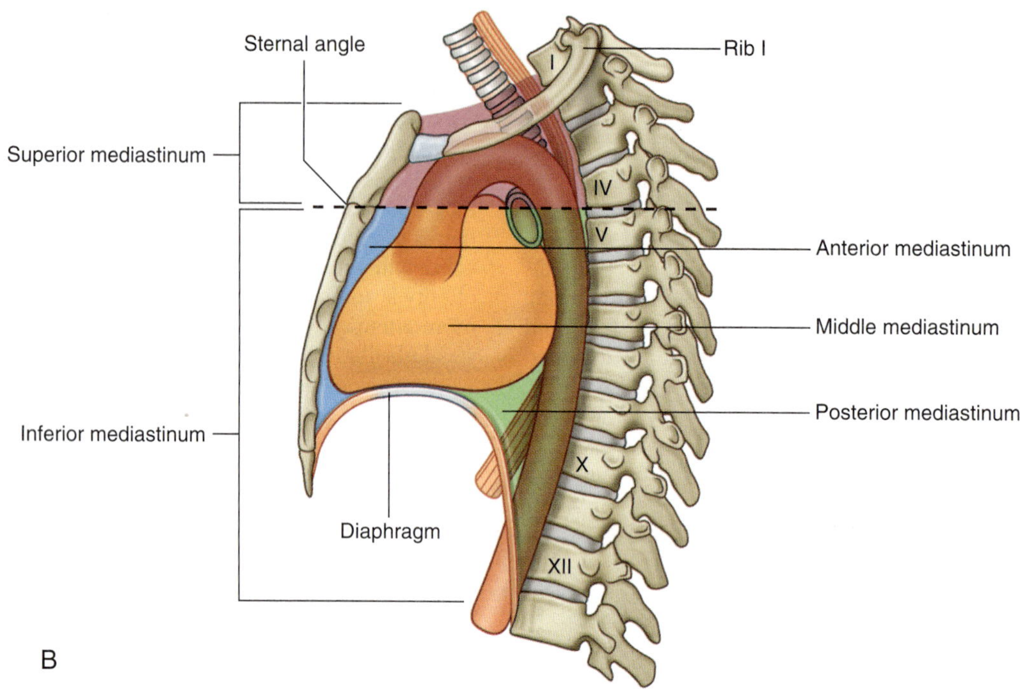

FIG. 10.1, cont'd (B) Lateral view of the heart in the thoracic cavity. (From Drake R, Vogl AW, Mitchell AWM. *Gray's Anatomy for Students*. 5th ed. Elsevier Inc; 2024.)

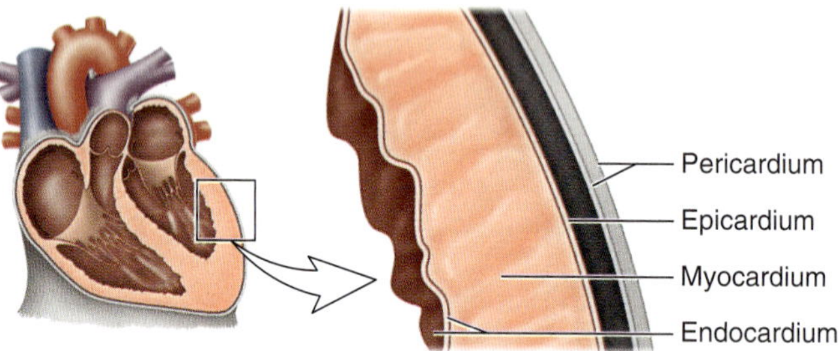

FIG. 10.2 Layers of the Heart Wall.

Myocardium

The myocardium is a thick, muscular layer that includes all the atrial and ventricular muscle fibers necessary for contraction. The fibers are organized in a spiral formation that directs the force of contraction toward the outflow tracts in a wringing motion from the apex toward the base. The arrangements of the myocardial fibers are shown in an anterior view of the heart (Fig. 10.3A), a posterior view of the heart (Fig. 10.3B), and a view from the apex of the heart (Fig. 10.3C).

Endocardium

The innermost layer of the heart is the endocardium, which is a thin layer of endothelium and connective tissue lining the inside of the heart. This layer is continuous with the endothelium of the great vessels to provide a continuous closed system. Disruption in the endothelium as a result of surgery, trauma, or congenital abnormality can predispose the endocardium to infection. Infective endocarditis is a devastating disease that, if left untreated, can lead to massive valve damage or sepsis and death.

Cardiac Chambers

The human heart has four chambers: the right atrium, the right ventricle, the left atrium, and left ventricle. The circulating blood moves through the right side of the heart (right atrium, right ventricle) and through the pulmonary circulation and returns to the left side of the heart (left atrium and left ventricle) (Fig. 10.4).

The atria are thin-walled and normally low-pressure chambers. The ventricles are muscular pumping chambers. The right and left sides are similar but not identical, and with right and left sides operating in synchrony. The physiologic mechanisms of cardiac contraction are described later in the chapter.

Right Atrium

The right atrium has two anatomical parts, a smooth posterior area called the *sinus venous,* and the anterior triangular muscular portion known as the *right atrial appendage.*[9] The right atrial appendage lies over the superior portion of the atrioventricular groove where the right coronary artery lies. There are two large veins that connect to the right atrium, the superior vena cava (SVC), and the inferior vena cava (IVC), both of which passively return deoxygenated systemic venous blood to the atrium.[9] The coronary sinus is a cardiac vein on the posterior surface of the heart that empties into the right atrium. There are two important pacemaker structures within the right atrium: the sinus node is superior-posterior, and the atrioventricular node is inferior on the floor of the right atrium. The tricuspid valve is inferior and when open allows deoxygenated blood to flow to the right ventricle.

Left Atrium

The left atrium receives oxygenated blood from the pulmonary veins and during atrial systole pumps the blood to the left

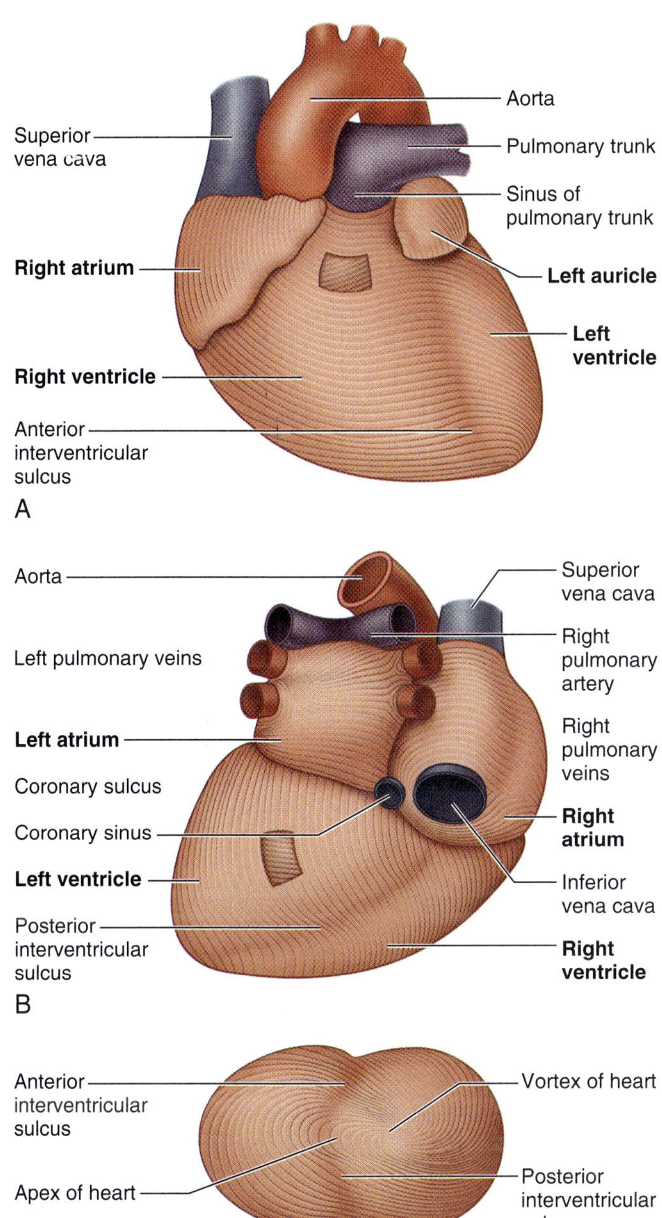

FIG. 10.3 Spiral Arrangement of Cardiac Muscles. (A) Anterior view of the heart showing spiral organization of myocardium. (B) Posterior view of the heart showing spiral organization of myocardium. (C) Spiral arrangement of the heart muscle from the apex. (From Hombach-Klonisch S, Klonisch T, Peeler J, Paulson F, Waschke J. *Sobotta Clinical Atlas of Human Anatomy*. 1st ed. Elsevier; 2019.)

ventricle via the mitral valve. The left atrium is posterior relative to the other heart chambers.[10] It is smaller than the right atrium but slightly more muscular. The back wall of the left atrium contains the openings of the four pulmonary veins. There is a *left atrial appendage* that may be described as a sac or pouch. The left atrial appendage is typically the only visible part of the left atrium, is superior, and overlies the pulmonary arterial trunk.[10] Atrial filling from the pulmonary veins is passive. The mitral valve is inferior and when open allows oxygenated blood to flow to the left ventricle, where atrial contraction, also known as *atrial kick*, adds additional volume to ventricular filling at the end of diastole.

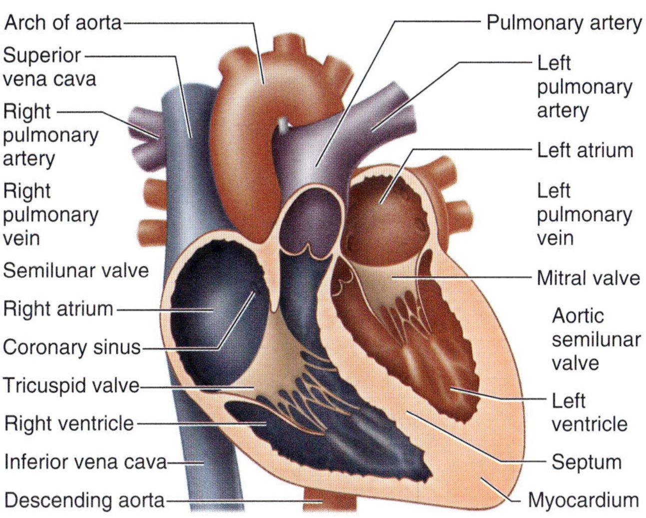

FIG. 10.4 Four Chambers of the Heart in Cross Section. Right atrium, right ventricle, left atrium, and left ventricle.

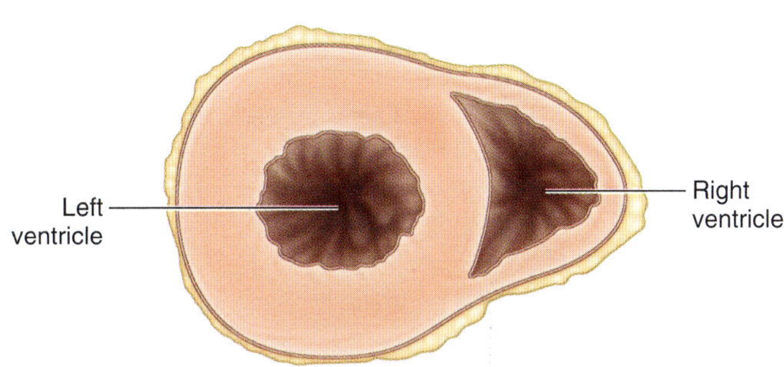

FIG. 10.5 Right and Left Ventricles in Cross Section.

Left Ventricle

The healthy left ventricle is approximately 10 to 13 mm thick, and the interior chamber appears round in cross section. The left ventricular walls are much thicker than the right ventricle (Fig. 10.5). The left ventricle must generate tremendous force to eject blood into the aorta (normal mean pressure of approximately 100 mm Hg). Because of left ventricular wall thickness and the tremendous force it generates, the left ventricle is considered the major pump of the heart.

Right Ventricle

The right ventricle is approximately 3 mm thick and appears to have a triangular shape when viewed from the side and a crescent shape when viewed in cross section (see Fig. 10.5). The right ventricle pumps deoxygenated blood into the low-pressure pulmonary circulation, which has a normal mean pressure of approximately 15 mm Hg. The RV is composed of three distinct anatomical areas:

- Inlet, which comprises the supporting structures for the tricuspid valve, chordae tendinea, and papillary muscles
- Apex, where the wall is trabeculated
- Infundibulum or outflow tract (conus), which connects to the pulmonary vascular system[11]

Cardiac Valves

Cardiac valves are composed of flexible, fibrous tissue. A normal healthy valve has the translucent appearance of a rose petal.

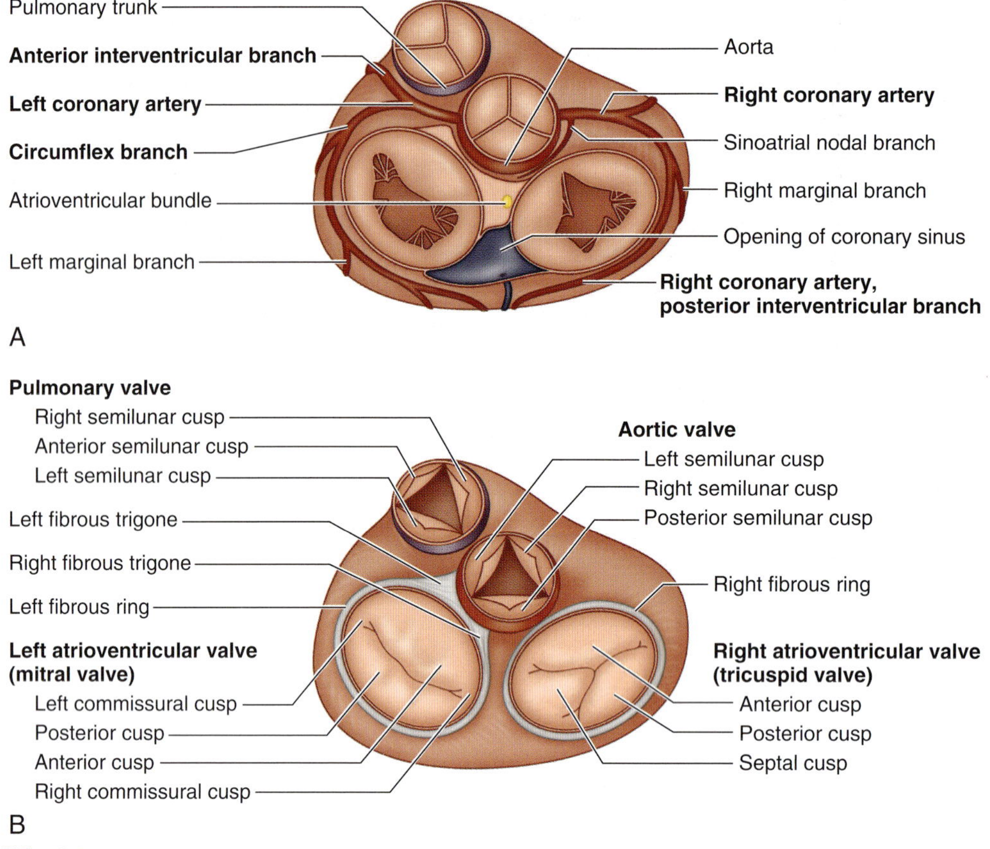

FIG. 10.6 Heart Valve Movement During Diastole and Systole. (A) Mitral and tricuspid valves are open during diastole. (B) Aortic and pulmonic valves are open during systole.

The valve structure allows blood to flow in only one direction. The opening and closing of the valves depend on the relative pressure gradients on either side of the valve. The four cardiac valves lie in an oblique plane of collagen described as the *fibrous skeleton*. Four adjacent rings of connective tissue contain and support the four cardiac valves (Fig. 10.6A).

Mitral and Tricuspid Atrioventricular Valves

The atrioventricular (AV) valves are named for their location between the atria and the ventricles. The tricuspid valve is on the left and has three leaflets (septal, anterior, posterior).[12]

The mitral valve is on the right and has two leaflets, although the "leaflets" are a continuous tissue structure.[13] The AV valves (mitral and tricuspid) are open during ventricular diastole (filling) (see Fig. 10.6A). The AV valves are attached to multiple chordae tendineae and then to papillary muscles that arise from their respective ventricle.

Papillary Muscles and Chordae Tendineae

Papillary muscles arise from the ventricular myocardium and derive their blood supply from the coronary arteries. Each papillary muscle gives rise to multiple main chordae tendineae that divide into increasingly finer chordae and attach to the valve leaflets in a variety of patterns.[13] The chordae tendineae are fibrous, avascular structures covered by a thin layer of endocardium (see Fig. 10.2). Chordae tendineae provide stability to the AV valves and prevent backflow of blood into the atria during ventricular systole (contraction) (Fig. 10.6B). Dysfunction of the chordae tendineae or of a papillary muscle may result in incomplete closure of an AV valve, resulting in backflow of blood into the atrium.

Aortic and Pulmonic Valves

The aortic and pulmonic *semilunar valves* each have three cup-like leaflets. The aortic valve (Fig. 10.7) is on the left side of the heart, and the pulmonic valve is on the right. These valves separate the ventricles from their respective outflow arteries (Table 10.1). During ventricular systole (contraction), the semilunar valves open, allowing blood to flow out of the ventricles. As systole ends and the pressure in the outflow arteries exceeds that of the ventricles, the semilunar valves close, preventing blood regurgitation back into the ventricles. The aortic and pulmonic valves do not have any additional supportive structures.

Conduction System

To analyze electrical activity within the heart, it is helpful to understand the three main areas of impulse propagation and conduction (Fig 10.8):

- Sinoatrial (SA) node
- AV node
- Bundle of His, the bundle branches, and the Purkinje fibers within the ventricles (Fig 10.8)

Sinoatrial Node

The SA node is considered the natural pacemaker of the heart because it has the highest degree of automaticity, producing the fastest intrinsic heart rate (HR) (Table 10.2). The node is described as a spindle-shaped three-dimensional structure

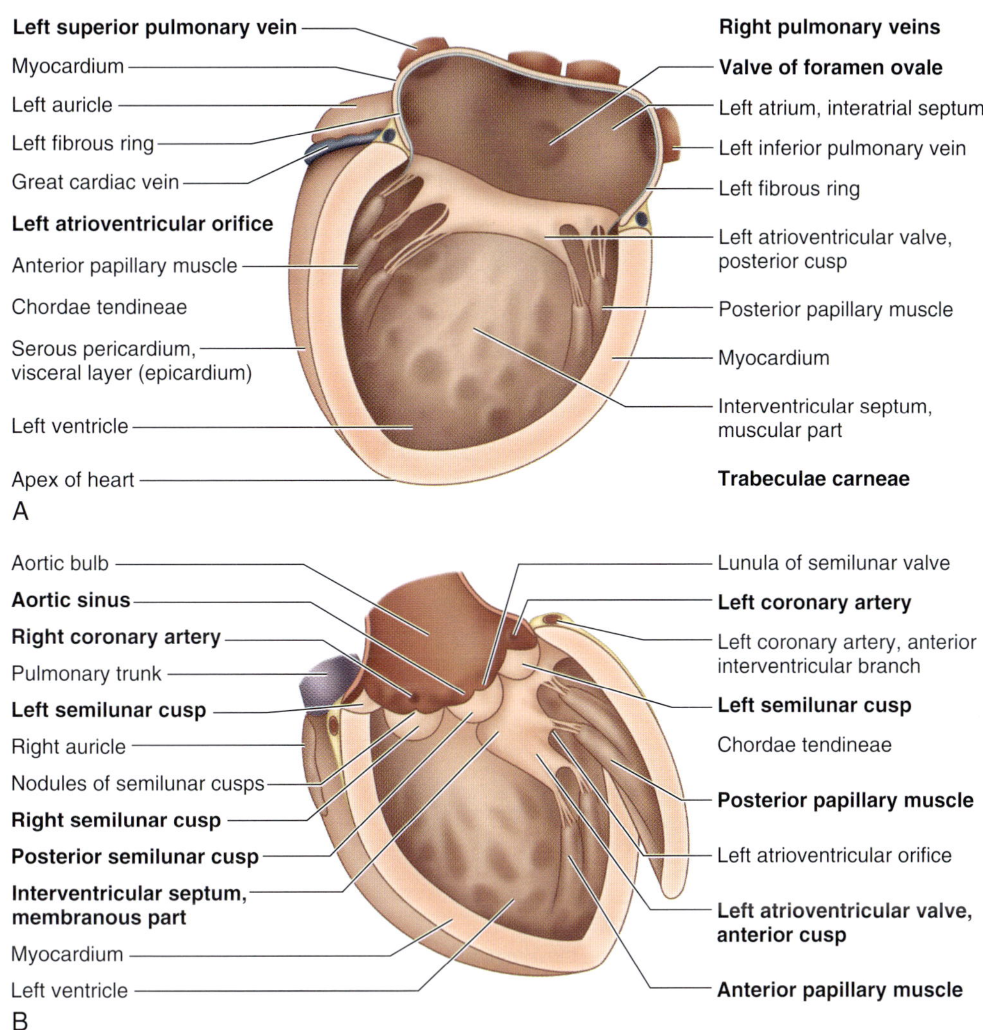

FIG. 10.7 Mitral and Aortic Valves. (A) Mitral valve separates left atrium and left ventricle. (B) Aortic valve separates left ventricle and aorta.

TABLE 10.1 Cardiac Valve Locations

Valve	Type	Situated Between
Tricuspid	Atrioventricular	Right atrium and right ventricle
Pulmonic	Semilunar	Right ventricle and pulmonary artery
Mitral	Atrioventricular	Left atrium and left ventricle
Aortic	Semilunar	Left ventricle and aorta

with multiple radiating projections.[14] It is located near the entrance of the superior vena cava, on the posterior aspect of the right atrium. Normal variability in the position and shape of the node exists. The SA node is supplied from the first branch off the right coronary system in about 50% to 60% of hearts and from the circumflex artery in approximately 40% to 50%.[14] The SA node contains two types of cells, the specialized pacemaker cells found in the node center and the border zone cells. Both cell types have inherent pacemaker properties that allow automatic depolarization 60 to 100 times per minute to produce an electrical action potential. The cells in the nodal center are the pacemakers of the heart, whereas the intrinsic depolarization capability of the fibers in the border zone are depressed by surrounding atrial tissue. Once the center nodal cells depolarize, the impulse is conducted through the border zone via transmural activation toward the AV node. An intraatrial conduction pathway known as *Bachmann's bundle* connects the superior right atrium to the superior left atrium to allow synchronous contraction of both right and left atria.[14]

Atrioventricular Node

The AV node is located on the right side of the interatrial septum on the floor of the right atrium. The AV node receives its blood supply from a branch of the right coronary artery (RCA) in almost all (90%) hearts.[14] The circumflex artery supplies the AV node in less than 10% of the population. The distal third of the AV node receives dual blood supply from the left anterior descending artery and the AV nodal artery.[14]

Because the atria and ventricles are separated by nonconductive tissue, electrical impulses initiated in the atria are conducted to the ventricles only via the AV node.[14]

The AV node performs the following four essential functions to support cardiac conduction:

- The AV node delays the conduction impulse from the atria (0.8 to 1.2 seconds) to provide time for the ventricles to fill during diastole.

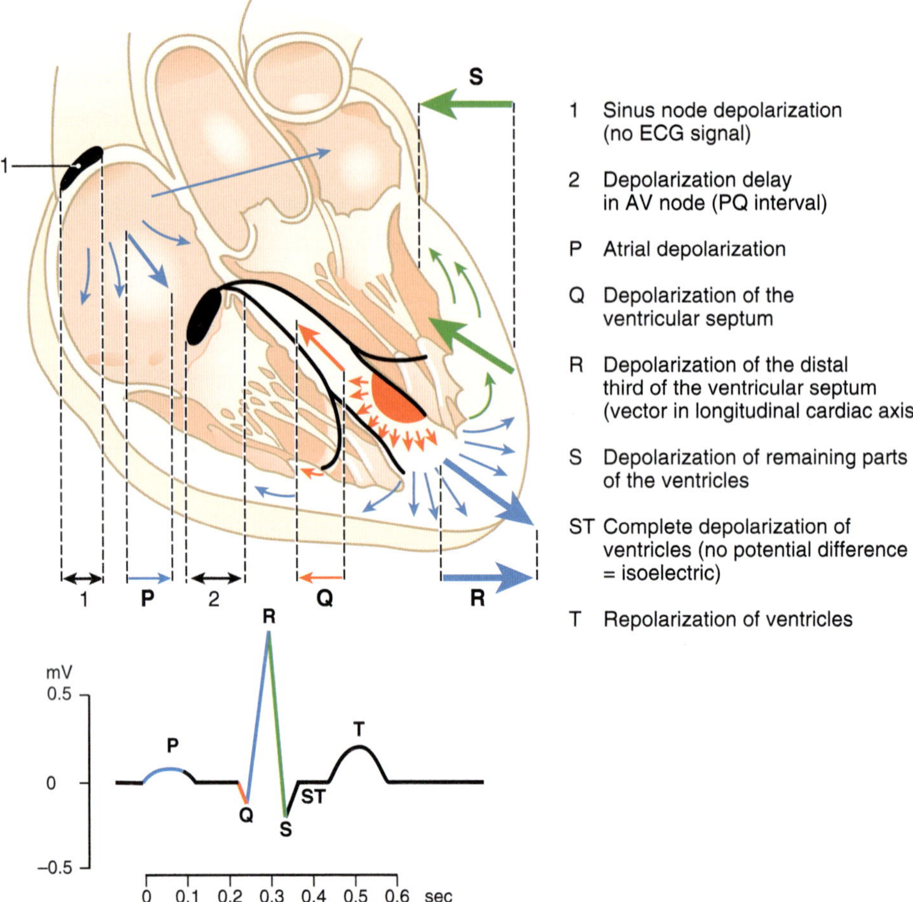

FIG. 10.8 Electrical Conduction System of the Heart Related to the Electrocardiogram *(ECG)* Waveform (PQRST). (From Hombach-Klonisch S, Klonisch T, Peeler J, Paulson F, Waschke J. *Sobotta Clinical Atlas of Human Anatomy*. 1st ed. Elsevier; 2019.)

TABLE 10.2 Intrinsic Heart Pacemaker Rates

Location	Rate (beats/min)
Sinoatrial node	60–100
Atrioventricular node	40–60
Purkinje fibers	15–40

- The AV node controls the number of impulses that are transmitted from the atria to the ventricles. This prevents rapid irregular atrial heart rhythms from destabilizing the ventricular rhythm.
- The AV node acts as a backup pacemaker if the faster SA node fails. Normally, the intrinsic AV nodal rate is slower than the SA nodal rate (see Table 10.2). When an impulse from the SA node arrives at the AV node, AV nodal tissue becomes depolarized, and the AV nodal pacemaker timing is reset. This prevents the AV node from initiating its own pacemaker impulse that would compete with the SA node.
- The AV node can conduct retrograde (backward) impulses through the node. If the SA and AV pacemaker cells fail to fire, an electrical impulse may be initiated in the ventricles and conducted backward via the AV node. Retrograde conduction time is usually longer than antegrade (forward) conduction.

Bundle of His, Bundle Branches, and Purkinje Fibers

Electrical impulses are conducted in the ventricles through the fascicles of the bundle of His, the bundle branches, and the Purkinje fibers (see Fig. 10.8). The bundle of His arises from the AV node.[14] The conduction fascicles run through the subendocardium, down the right side of the interventricular septum to the left and right bundle branches.

The left bundle branch is thicker than the right and takes off from the bundle of His and traverses the septum to the subendocardial surface of the left interventricular wall, where it divides into a thin anterior branch and a thicker posterior branch. Functionally, when one of the left branches is blocked, it is referred to as a *hemiblock*.

The right bundle branch continues down the right side of the interventricular septum toward the right apex. All the bundle branches are subject to conduction defects (bundle branch blocks) that give rise to characteristic changes in the 12-lead electrocardiogram.

The right bundle branch and the two divisions of the left bundle branch eventually divide into the Purkinje fibers, which have the fastest conduction velocity of all heart tissue. Purkinje fibers divide many times, terminating in the subendocardial surface of both ventricles. Conduction down the bundles and Purkinje fibers is followed by ventricular muscle depolarization (see Fig. 10.8).

Coronary Blood Supply

The coronary circulation consists of vessels that supply the heart structures with oxygenated blood (coronary arteries) and then return the blood to the general circulation (coronary veins). The right and left coronary arteries arise at the base of the aorta, immediately above the aortic valve (Fig. 10.9). These coronary arterial openings are called the *coronary ostia* (plural). The coronary arteries are located on the outside of the heart, above the epicardium, and lie in the natural grooves (sulci) between the chambers. To perfuse the thick heart muscle, branches from these main epicardial arteries penetrate deeply into the myocardial wall.

Right Coronary Artery

The RCA serves the right atrium and the right ventricle in most people. The sinus node artery, which supplies the SA node in approximately two-thirds of the population, arises from the RCA. The AV node is supplied via the RCA in 90% of the population. The term *dominant coronary artery* is used to describe the artery that supplies the posterior wall of the left ventricle. In most people, the RCA is dominant, supplying the posterior heart wall.

Left Coronary Artery

The left coronary artery system has several important branches. The *left main* coronary artery arises from the aortic root. It is a short but important artery that divides into two large arteries, the *left anterior descending artery* and the *circumflex artery,* that serve the left atrium and most of the left ventricle (see Fig. 10.9). The left anterior descending artery travels in the sulcus over the anterior intraventricular septum. Septal perforator branches divide off at right angles to provide blood supply to the intraventricular septal muscle.

The coronary arteries are end-arteries; that is, they supply a discrete area of the myocardium. End-arteries are susceptible to obstruction by atherosclerotic plaque or thrombus, which can result in loss of blood flow to the myocardial muscle normally supplied by that artery. Depending on the location of the obstruction, this can be fatal. Blockage of coronary arterial blood flow, especially in the left main coronary artery, usually results in death from massive infarction of the left ventricle. If the blocked artery supplies a smaller section of myocardium, the result may be infarction of a small area of myocardium, but not death.

Collateral Circulation

One of the mitigating factors when a coronary artery is partially obstructed or blocked is the extent of the coronary collateral circulation. The collateral circulation represents a rich branching vascular network and is variable among individual hearts. Collaterals are present at birth and become more prominent when a major coronary artery is blocked.

Coronary Veins

The coronary veins, carry deoxygenated blood from the myocardium, and are adjacent to the paths of the coronary arteries (Fig. 10.10). A significant difference is that the epicardial coronary veins ultimately join to form a large vein named the *coronary sinus* that travels along the posterior heart between the sulcus of the left atrium and the left ventricle.[15] The deoxygenated blood flows into the heart via the coronary sinus through the back wall of the right atrium. Coronary venous blood then mixes with the systemic venous blood in the right atrium.

Thebesian Vessels

The thebesian vessels are miniscule venous channels, without valves, that are specific to the cardiac venous circulation. The vessels facilitate drainage from the capillaries in the inner one-third of the myocardium directly into the cardiac chambers.[15] Consequently, thebesian vessels create a small physiologic shunt by contributing deoxygenated blood directly into the heart chambers.

Major Blood Vessels

Aorta

The aorta is the largest artery in the body. It carries oxygenated blood from the left ventricle to the rest of the body. The aorta is separated from the left ventricle by the aortic valve. Just above the aortic valve are two small openings that represent the origins of the right and left coronary arterial systems known as the *coronary ostia*. The aorta is labeled according to anatomical sections, the aortic root, the aortic arch, the thoracic aorta, and the abdominal aorta.[16] Major arteries branch off from the aorta at all levels. The aorta is constructed with the same three layers as all other arteries in the body (described below) with a thick muscular intima-media.[16]

Pulmonary Artery

The pulmonary artery carries deoxygenated blood from the right ventricle to the pulmonary arterioles. The pulmonary artery is separated from the right ventricle by the pulmonic valve. The main pulmonary artery divides into a right branch and a left branch, directing blood to the right and the left lung vasculature. The pulmonary artery is the only artery in the body that carries deoxygenated blood.

Pulmonary Veins

The four pulmonary veins return oxygenated blood from the lungs to the left atrium. These are the only veins in the body that carry oxygenated blood. The veins drain from the pulmonary vascular tree into the posterior wall of the left atrium. No valves inhibit the flow of blood into the left atrium. Blood flow is accomplished by simple hydrostatic pressure gradients. The pressure must be lower in the left atrium than in the pulmonary circulation for flow to occur in a forward direction.

Systemic Circulation

If the task of the heart is to generate enough pressure to pump the blood, it is the function of the vascular structures to act as conduits to carry vital oxygen and nutrients to each cell and to carry away waste products. The ability to exchange those nutrients and waste products at the cellular level is of primary importance. The vascular system acts not only as a conducting system for blood but also as a control mechanism for the pressure in the heart and vessels. The complex interplay between the heart and blood vessels maintains adequate pressure and velocity within this system for optimal functioning.

Arteries

Arteries are constructed of three layers (Fig. 10.11):

- The *tunica adventitia* is the outermost layer. It is composed largely of a connective tissue coat to provide strength and shape to the vessel.

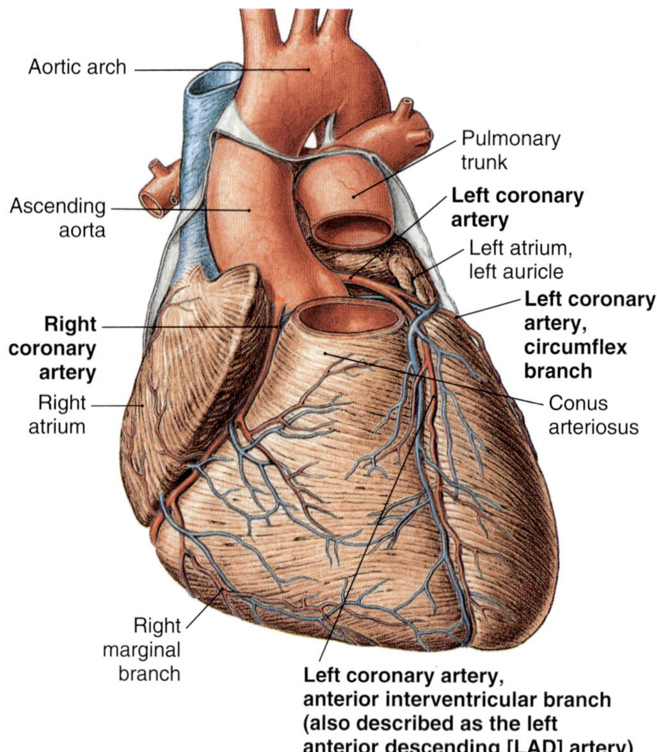

FIG. 10.9 Coronary Arteries; Anterior View of the Heart. (From Hombach-Klonisch S, Klonisch T, Peeler J, Paulson F, Waschke J. *Sobotta Clinical Atlas of Human Anatomy*. 1st ed. Elsevier; 2019.)

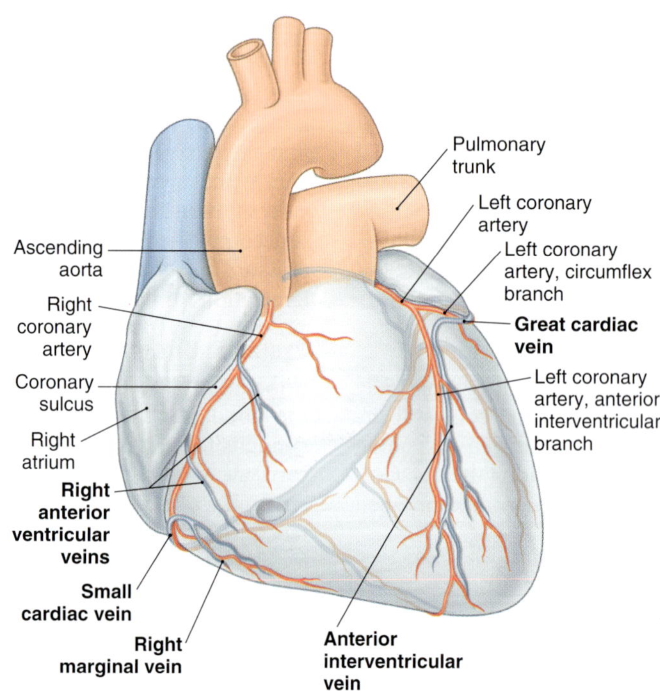

FIG. 10.10 Coronary Veins. Anterior view with posterior veins visible through the heart. (From Hombach-Klonisch S, Klonisch T, Peeler J, Paulson F, Waschke J. *Sobotta Clinical Atlas of Human Anatomy*. 1st ed. Elsevier; 2019.)

- The *tunica media*, or muscular middle layer, is made up of smooth muscle and elastic tissue. The muscular layer changes the lumen diameter as needed.
- The *tunica intima* is the innermost layer of a thin lining of endothelium and a small amount of elastic tissue. The smooth endothelial lining lowers resistance to the flowing bloodstream, minimizing the opportunity for platelet aggregation.

The intimal and the externa layers remain relatively constant in the vascular system, whereas the elastin and smooth muscle in the media vary in proportion, depending on the size and type of vessel (Fig. 10.12). The aorta contains the greatest amount of elastic tissue. This is necessary because of the sudden shifts in pressure created by the left ventricle. The arterioles, or smaller arteries, and precapillary sphincters have more smooth muscle than the larger arteries and aorta because they function to change the luminal diameter when regulating blood pressure and blood flow to tissues.

Blood Flow and Blood Pressure

The pulsatile nature of arterial flow is caused by intermittent cardiac ejection and the stretch of the ascending aorta. The pressure wave initiated by left ventricular ejection (Fig. 10.13) travels considerably faster than blood itself. When an examiner palpates a pulse, it is the propagation of the pressure wave that is perceived.

In the normal arterial system, blood flow is described as laminar, or streamlined, because the fluid moves in one direction. However, differences exist in the linear velocities within a blood vessel. The layer of blood immediately adjacent to the vessel wall moves relatively slowly because of the friction created as it encounters a motionless vessel wall. In contrast, the more central blood in the lumen travels more rapidly (Fig. 10.14). Clinical implications include conditions in which the vessel wall has an abnormality such as a small clot or plaque deposit. This disruption in the streamlined flow can set up eddy currents that may predispose the area to platelet aggregation and atherosclerosis.

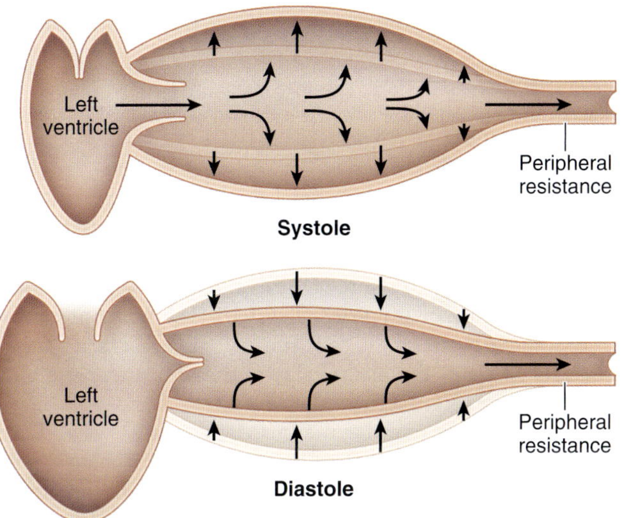

FIG. 10.13 Elastic and Recoil Properties of the Aorta.

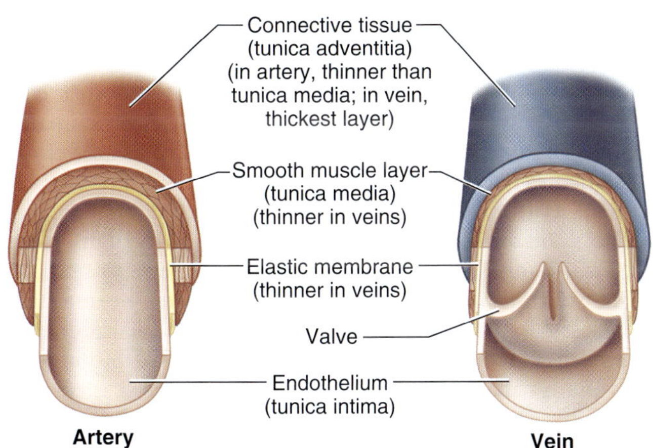

FIG. 10.11 Structure of Blood Vessels.

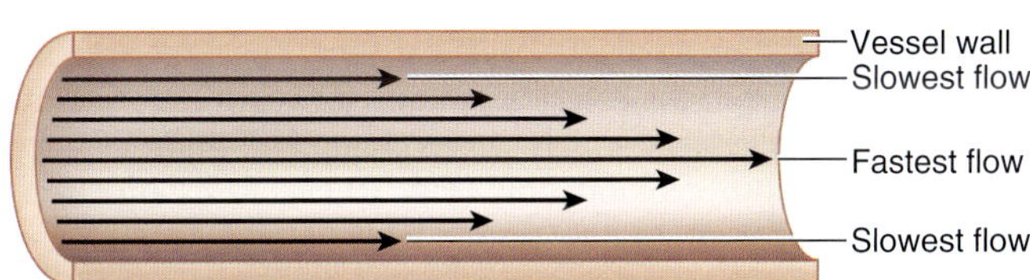

FIG. 10.14 Laminar Blood Flow in an Artery.

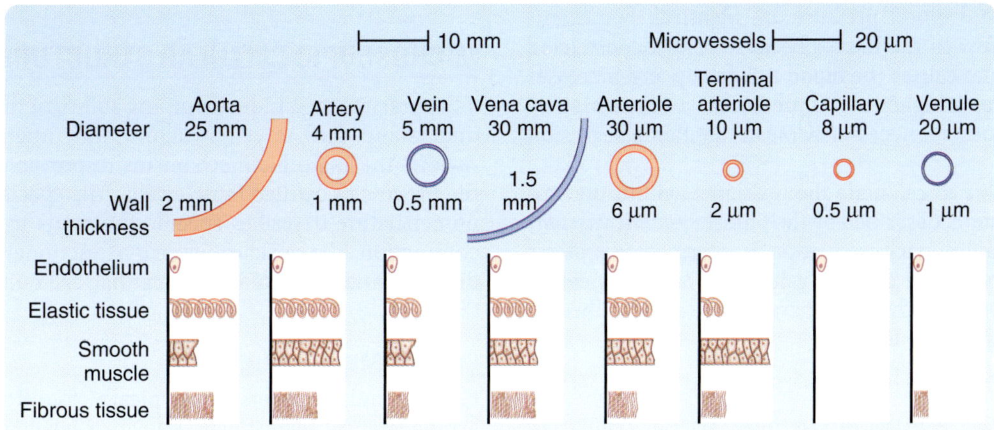

FIG. 10.12 Blood Vessel Internal Diameter and Wall Thickness: Arteries, Veins, and Capillaries. (From Koeppen BM, Stanton BA. *Berne & Levy Physiology.* 8th ed. Elsevier Inc; 2024.)

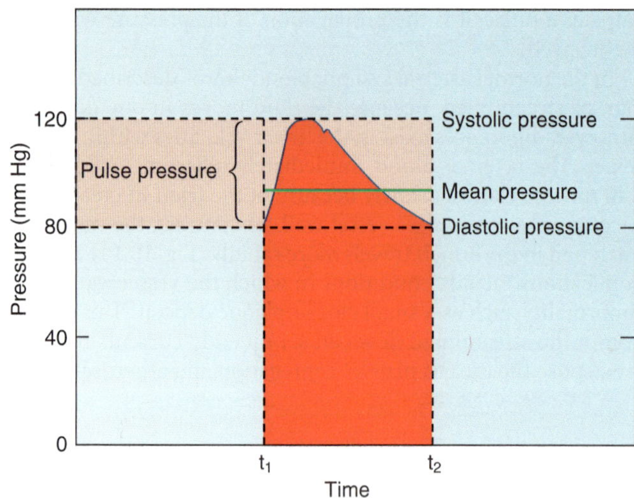

FIG. 10.15 Arterial, Systolic, Diastolic, Pulse, and Mean Arterial Pressure. (From Koeppen BM, Stanton BA. *Berne & Levy Physiology.* 8th ed. Elsevier Inc; 2024.)

Blood pressure measurement has several components. The systolic blood pressure (SBP) represents the ventricular volume ejection and the response of the arterial system to that ejection. The diastolic blood pressure (DBP) value indicates the ventricular resting state of the arterial system. The pulse pressure is the difference between the SBP and the DBP. The mean arterial pressure (MAP) is the mean value of the area under the blood pressure curve (Fig. 10.15).

Blood pressure may be measured in several ways. Direct measurement is accomplished by means of a catheter inserted into an artery. Blood pressure is measured in millimeters of mercury (mm Hg). The most common indirect method is by means of a stethoscope and sphygmomanometer (Fig. 10.16). Direct measurement is via direct cannulation of an artery as described in Chapter 12.

Vascular resistance reflects arteriolar tone. The large amount of smooth muscle in the arterioles allows for relaxation or contraction of these vessels, which causes changes in the resistance and redistribution of blood flow (Fig. 10.17). Resistance represents the opposition to flow caused by the blood vessels.

Most changes in resistance are caused by alterations in the tone of the arterial vessel walls, especially in the arterioles. The purpose of this mechanism is to maintain a constant blood pressure in the arterial system. The clinician can never assume that blood flow and blood pressure are identical. For example, poor blood flow to the tissues because of vasoconstricted peripheral arterioles causes the blood to back up and increases the blood pressure. A higher blood pressure is a compensatory mechanism but does not necessarily mean that tissue perfusion is adequate.

It is also possible to calculate the resistance within the systemic vascular system, described by the phrase *systemic vascular resistance*. In the pulmonary circulation, it is termed *pulmonary vascular resistance*. These derived values are based on calculations from other hemodynamic parameters, as described in Chapter 12 and Appendix B.

Microcirculation

The *microcirculation* consists of arterioles, arterial capillaries, venous capillaries, and venules (Fig. 10.18). Oxygen, nutrients, hormones, and waste products are exchanged between the bloodstream and adjacent cells. Lymphatic capillaries remove fluid from tissues. The microcirculation has a vital role in the regulation of oxygen supply and demand at the tissue level. The density and anatomy of the microcirculation vary depending on the metabolic needs of each tissue or organ.

Precapillary sphincters are small cuffs of smooth muscle that control blood flow at the junction of the arterioles and the capillaries. The precapillary sphincters are innervated by norepinephrine released from the sympathetic nervous system (SNS) and epinephrine released by the adrenal medulla. They selectively control blood flow into capillary beds.

As blood reaches the capillary level, the pulsatile nature of arterial flow is dampened. Although the diameter of a capillary is less than that of an arteriole, the pressure and flow velocity in the capillary bed are low because of the large cross-sectional area of the branching capillary bed. The capillary consists of a single cell layer of endothelium and is devoid of muscle or elastin. This arrangement allows solutes to diffuse in and out of the capillaries unimpeded by mechanical barriers. The capillaries normally retain larger structures, such as red blood cells, but are highly permeable to smaller solutes such as electrolytes.

Veins

As blood leaves the capillary system, it passes through the venules and into the veins. Venules and veins contain elastic tissue, smooth muscle, and fibrous tissue (see Fig. 10.17). However, the veins contain a greater percentage of smooth muscle and fibrous tissue to accommodate the large venous volume and demand for reserve capacity. Veins are referred to as *capacitance vessels* as most circulating blood is contained in the venous system (see Fig. 10.17). Approximately 70% to 75% of the total blood volume is found in the veins.[17] This enables the body to tap into a large reserve during times of need. For example, when a person changes from a supine position to a sitting position, approximately 7 to 10 mL blood per kilogram of body weight pools in the legs. Potentially, cardiac output could decrease by 20%. However, normal arterial pressure and blood flow are maintained by a combination of reflex vasoconstriction and redistribution of blood from the venous capacitance vessels. In humans, these capacitance reservoirs are greatest in the spleen, liver, and intestines. Patients with decreased blood reserves, who are dehydrated or hypovolemic, require special caution during position changes, especially from the supine position to the standing position.

MICROSCOPIC CELLULAR STRUCTURES

To appreciate the unique pumping ability of the heart, one must understand cardiac cell structure and function. This section reviews the anatomic mechanisms responsible for the contractile process in cardiac muscle cells. The specialized cardiac cell nomenclature describes specific functions to facilitate cardiac contraction. The cardiac muscle is a functional syncytium where depolarization initiated in any cardiac cell quickly spreads to all the heart.

Cardiac Muscle Fibers

Cardiac muscle fibers are typically found in a latticework arrangement. The fiber cells, known as *myofibrils*, divide, rejoin, and then separate again, but they retain distinct cellular walls and possess a single nucleus (Fig. 10.19).

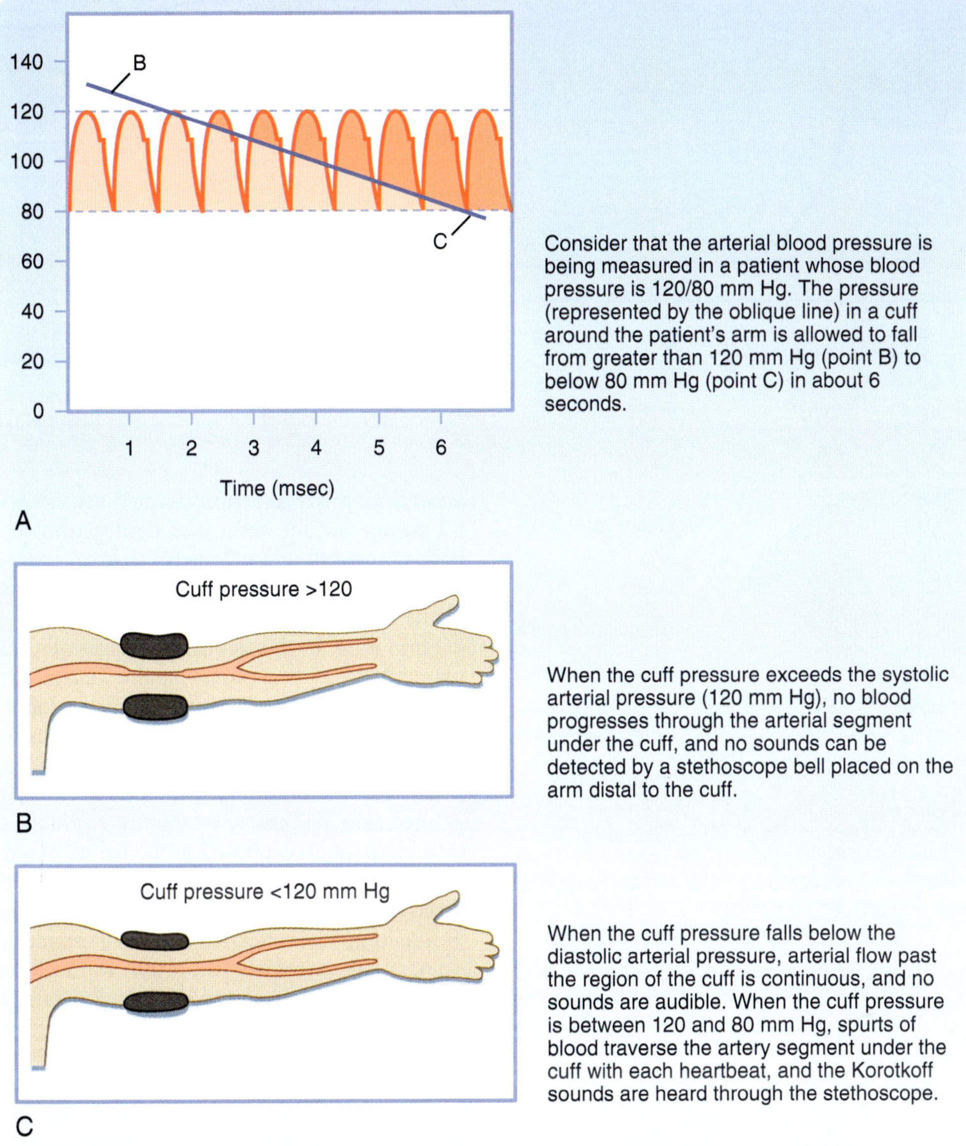

FIG. 10.16 Blood Pressure Measurement with an Arm Cuff and Sphygmomanometer. (A) An example of a blood pressure waveform with a cuff pressure of 120/80 mm Hg. (B) When the arm cuff is inflated to a pressure above the systolic value (120 mm Hg), the artery is occluded and no sounds are audible. (C) When the pressure in the arm cuff is less than the systolic arterial pressure (120 mm Hg in this example) and above the diastolic pressure (80 mm Hg), Korotkoff sounds are audible using a stethoscope or Doppler. (From Koeppen BM, Stanton BA. *Berne & Levy Physiology.* 8th ed. Elsevier Inc; 2024.)

- Myocytes: Individual cardiac muscle cells are known as *myocytes* and are interlaced into a network of cardiac muscle fibers (Fig. 10.20A).
- Sarcolemma: The cardiac cell membrane is known as the *sarcolemma.*
- Intercalated disks: Specialized junctional connector complexes called *intercalated disks* assist in propagation of depolarization. The intercalated disks are continuous with the cell membrane (sarcolemma) and separates each myocardial cell from its neighbor (Fig. 10.20B).
- Gap junction: The point at which a longitudinal branch of one cell meets the branch of another is called a *tight junction* (or *gap junction*), which is contained within the intercalated disk. The gap junctions offer much less impedance to electrical flow than the sarcolemma does, so depolarization flows easily from one cell to another.

Cardiac Cells

Each cardiac cell contains many intracellular proteins that contribute to contraction. Two important contractile proteins are actin and myosin. These proteins abound in the cell in organized longitudinal arrangements. Under electron microscopy, the myosin filaments appear thick, whereas the actin filaments, which are almost twice as prevalent, appear thin. The actin filaments are connected to a Z-line on one end, leaving the other end free to interact with the myosin cross-bridges (see Fig. 10.20). In the resting muscle cell, actin and myosin partially overlap. The ends of the myosin filament that overlap with

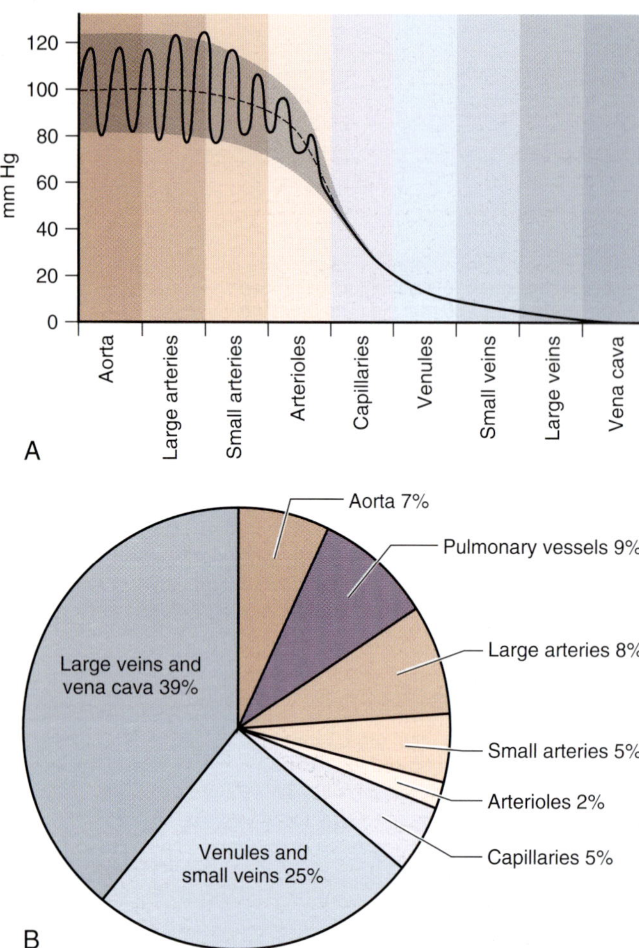

FIG. 10.17 Blood Pressure (A) and Blood Volume Percentage (B) Across the Cardiovascular System.

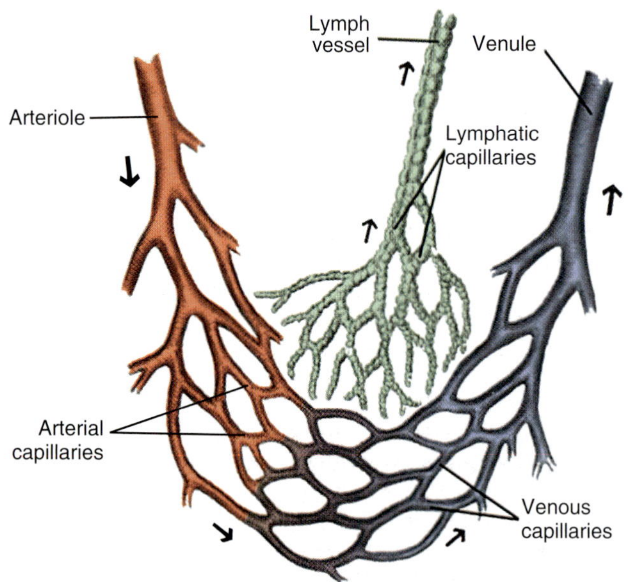

FIG. 10.18 Microcirculation With Branching Cross-Sectional Capillary Bed. (From Thompson JM, et al. *Mosby's Clinical Nursing*. 5th ed. Mosby; 2002.)

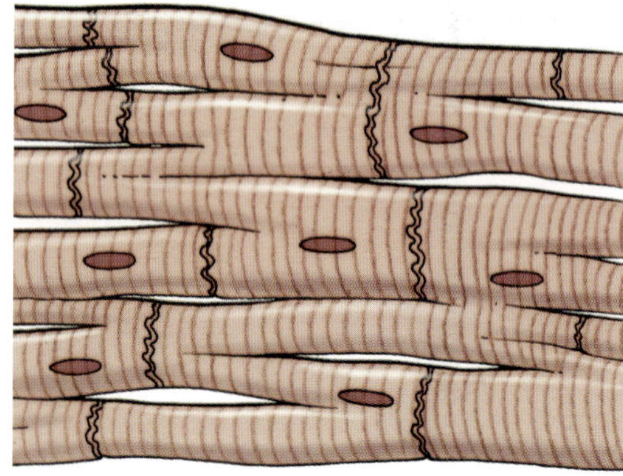

FIG. 10.19 Interconnecting Heart Muscle Fibers. (From Hall JE, Hall ME. *Guyton and Hall Textbook of Medical Physiology*. 14th ed. Elsevier Inc; 2021.)

actin have tiny projections named *myosin heads*, which contain a binding site for actin. For contraction to occur, the myosin heads must interact with actin to form cross-bridges.

The sarcomere is the functional unit of cardiac contraction. In the normal resting state, the sarcomere is approximately 2 to 2.2 mm long. Each sarcomere consists of a central *A-band* (thick filaments) and two halves of the *I-band* (thin filaments). The I-bands from two adjacent sarcomeres meet at the Z-line (also called a *Z-band* or *Z-disk*). The central portion of the A-band is the M-band, which does not contain actin. Myosin filaments are situated in the middle of the sarcomere and are attached to the Z-line of the sarcomere by the protein titan (see Fig. 10.20). The thin filament is composed of the helical chains of the actin globular proteins that coil around a long filament of tropomyosin and three troponin proteins: (1) TnT, (2) TnC, and (3) TnI. The troponin complex is attached to actin at regularly spaced intervals.

Another extremely important intracellular structure necessary for successful contraction is the sarcoplasmic reticulum. Calcium ions are stored in the sarcoplasmic reticulum and released for use after depolarization (see Fig. 10.20).

Deep invaginations into the sarcomere are called *transverse tubules*, or *T-tubules*. T-tubules are essentially an extension of the cell membrane (sarcolemma); they conduct depolarization to structures deep within the cytoplasm such as the sarcoplasmic reticulum (see Fig. 10.20). Cardiac cells abound with mitochondria, which contain respiratory enzymes necessary for oxidative phosphorylation. This enables these cells to keep up with the tremendous energy requirements of repetitive contraction. When cardiac cells are damaged by trauma, ischemia, or infarction, myocardial cells release protein biomarkers such as troponins, which, when measured by laboratory analysis, can help determine the extent of injury; for more information see Fig. 13.13 in Chapter 13.

PHYSIOLOGY

The electrical and mechanical properties of cardiac tissue include excitability, conductivity, automaticity, rhythmicity, contractility, and refractoriness. This section relates these concepts specifically to cardiac cells (Table 10.3).

Electrical Activity of the Heart

Transmembrane Potentials

Electrical potentials across cell membranes are present in essentially all the cells of the body. Cardiac cells are specialized for

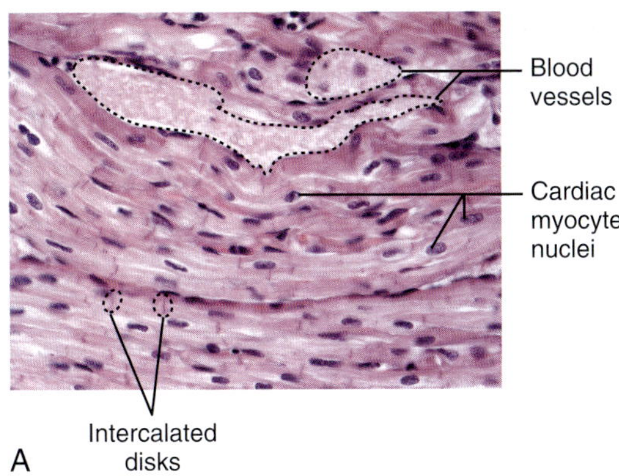

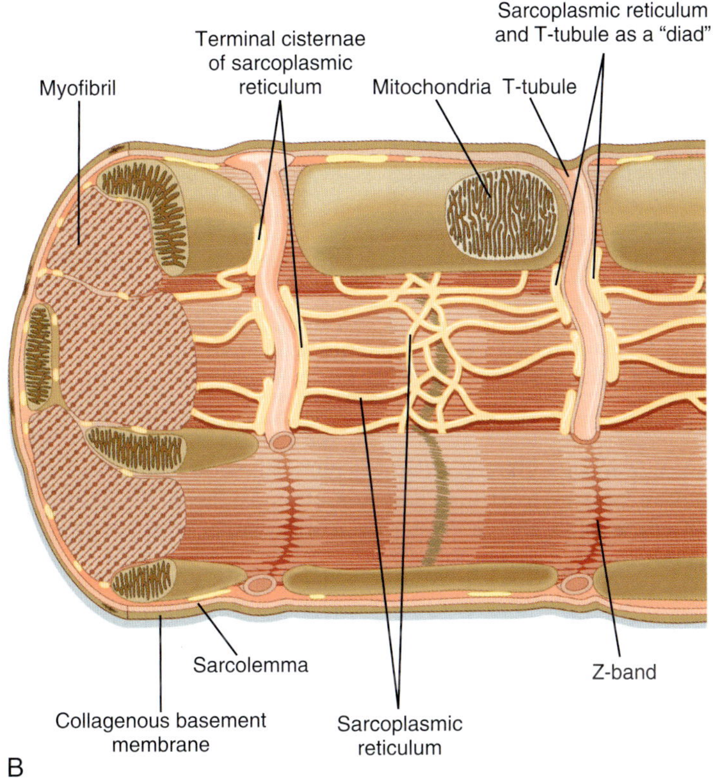

FIG. 10.20 (A) Photomicrograph of cardiac muscle cells. (B) Sarcomere within a heart muscle cell showing intercalated disks, sarcoplasmic reticulum, and T-tubules. (From Koeppen BM, Stanton BA. *Berne & Levy Physiology*. 8th ed. Elsevier Inc; 2024.)

conduction of electrical impulses. This electrical potential, or transmembrane potential, refers to the relative electrical difference between the interior of a cell and the fluid surrounding the cell. *Ionic channels* are pores in cell membranes that allow for passage of specific ions at specific times or in response to specific signals. Transmembrane potentials and ionic channels are extremely important in myocardial cells because they form the basis for electrical impulse conduction and muscular contraction. Knowledge of the normal structure and function of cardiac ion channels is increasingly important as a basis for understanding the genesis of lethal cardiac dysrhythmias and for the development of cardiac medications designed to treat these channelopathies.

Resting Membrane Potential

In a myocardial cell at rest, the normal resting membrane potential (RMP) in nonpacemaker cells is approximately −80 to −90 mV.[18] This means that the interior of the cell is relatively negative compared with the exterior medium. The relative negativity of the cell interior is created by an uneven distribution of positively and negatively charged ions. When the cell is at rest, more positively charged ions are outside the cell than are inside the cell.

When the cell is at rest, the intracellular potassium ion (K^+) concentration is high, and the intracellular sodium ion (Na^+) level is low (Table 10.4). Calcium (Ca^{2+}) has a much higher concentration outside than inside the cell when the cell is at rest. These large differences in individual ion concentrations create chemical gradients. A *chemical gradient* describes the tendency of an ion to move from an area of higher solute concentration to an area of lower concentration. However, an electrical gradient is also present, which causes the positively charged ions to move to an area of relative negativity. An important factor influencing both gradients is membrane permeability, or the

TABLE 10.3 Heart Tissue Function Definitions

Term	Definition
Excitability	Ability of cell or tissue to depolarize in response to given stimulus
Conductivity	Ability of cardiac cells to transmit a stimulus from cell to cell
Automaticity	Ability of certain cells to spontaneously depolarize ("pacemaker potential")
Rhythmicity	Automaticity generated at regular rate
Contractility	Ability of cardiac myofibrils to shorten in length in response to electrical stimulus (depolarization)
Refractoriness	State of cell or tissue during repolarization, when cell or tissue cannot depolarize regardless of intensity of the stimulus or requires a much greater stimulus than is normally required

TABLE 10.4 Electrolyte Values in a Resting Myocardial Cell

	Extracellular Electrolyte Concentration (mEq/L)	Intracellular Electrolyte Concentration (mEq/L)
Potassium (K^+)	4	135
Sodium (Na^+)	145	10
Calcium (Ca^{2+})	2	0.1

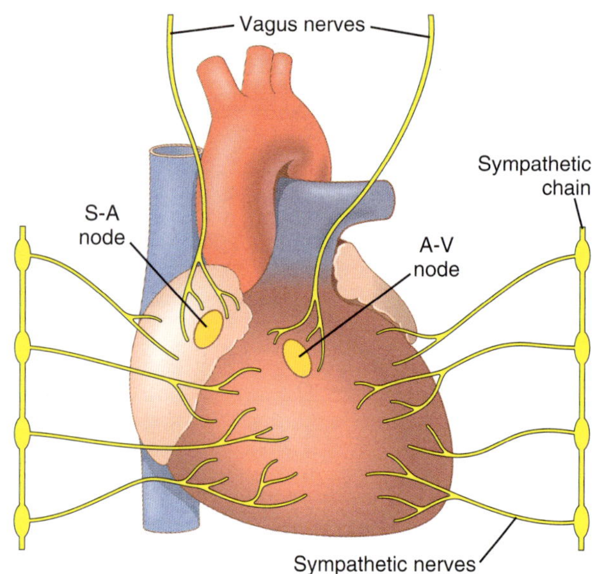

FIG. 10.21 Cardiac Muscle Depolarization and Repolarization. Role of calcium and adenosine triphosphate (ATP) in the sarcoplasmic reticulum. (From Hall JE. Hall ME. *Guyton and Hall Textbook of Medical Physiology*. 14th ed. Elsevier Inc; 2021.)

selectivity of the membrane to ionic movements. The cell membrane is approximately 50 times more permeable to K^+ than it is to Na^+. Because K^+ movement out of the cell results in greater negativity inside the cell, K^+ is the principal ion responsible for maintaining the negative RMP.

Phases of the Action Potential

In a myocardial cell, when a sudden increase in permeability of the membrane to Na^+ occurs, it is followed by a rapid sequence of events that lasts a fraction of a second. This sequence of events is termed *depolarization* (Fig. 10.21). The graphic representation of depolarization and repolarization is termed the *action potential* (AP) (Fig. 10.22). Ionic currents cause changes in electrical potentials, which are known as *AP phases 0, 1, 2, 3,* and *4.*[18] These phases give the AP a characteristic shape (Table 10.5; see Fig. 10.22).

Phase 0

The sodium crossing the cell membrane causes the cell to become depolarized and the interior of the cell to become more positive. At approximately −65 mV, the membrane reaches the threshold, the point at which the inward Na^+ current overcomes the efflux of K^+. This is accomplished by means of the fast Na^+ channels. With the fast Na^+ channels open, the inward rush of Na^+ is extremely rapid and briefly causes the inside of the cell to become slightly more positive than the outside of the cell. This series of events is graphically described as *phase 0* of the AP and is reflected in the overshoot of the AP, during which the charge is 20 to 30 mV (Fig. 10.23; see Fig. 10.22).

Phase 1

When the rapid influx of Na^+ is terminated, a brief period of partial repolarization occurs in *phase 1* as the AP slope returns toward zero as potassium leaves the cell (see Figs. 10.22 and 10.23).

Phase 2

The plateau that follows is described as *phase 2*. During this phase, the slow K^+ and Ca^{2+} channels open to allow the influx of Ca^{2+} and efflux of K^+. The Ca^{2+} entering the cell during phase 2 causes cardiac contraction (see Figs. 10.22 and 10.23).

Phase 3

The repolarization phase is described as *phase 3*, and it depends on two processes. The first is the inactivation of the slow channels, which prevents further influx of Ca^{2+}. The other is the continued efflux of K^+ out of the cell. Both processes cause the intracellular environment to become more negative, reestablishing the RMP. Phase 3 is a gradual descent during which the interior of the cell becomes more negative relative to the outside (see Figs. 10.22 and 10.23).

Phase 4

In phase 4, the AP returns to an RMP of −80 to −90 mV. The excess Na^+ that entered the cell during depolarization is removed from the cell in exchange for K^+ by means of the Na^+–K^+ pump. This mechanism returns the intracellular concentrations of Na^+ and K^+ to the levels present before depolarization in preparation for the next depolarization (see Table 10.5 and Figs. 10.22 and 10.23).

Cardiac Myocyte Conduction and Excitability

Different parts of the conduction system require different electrical currents and create individual transmembrane action potentials.[18] As a local section of the cell becomes depolarized, reaches threshold, and completely depolarizes, it affects the adjacent area of the cell and initiates depolarization in that area. The AP propagates down the cardiac fibers (nonpacemaker cells) in a wavelike fashion (Fig. 10.24). This is analogous to a trail of gunpowder. When the gunpowder is lit at one end, a

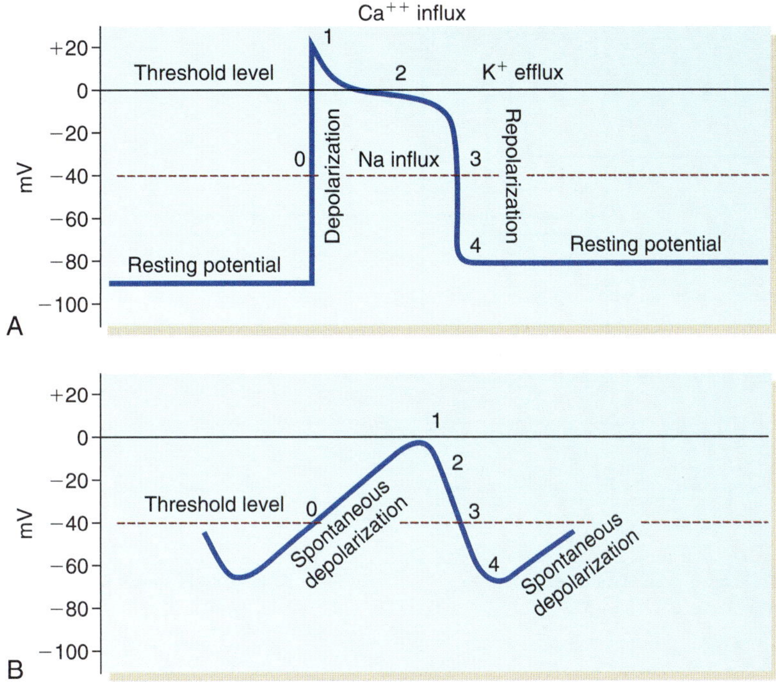

FIG. 10.22 Cardiac Action Potentials. (A) Action potential phases 0 to 4 of a cardiac nonpacemaker cell. (B) Action potential of a cardiac pacemaker cell. (From Thompson JM, et al. *Mosby's Clinical Nursing*. 5th ed. Mosby; 2002.)

TABLE 10.5 Phases 0 Through 4 of a Cardiac Cell Action Potential

Phase	Description	Ionic Movement	Mechanisms
0	Upstroke	Na^+ into cell	Fast Na^+ channels open
1	Overshoot	K^+ out of cell	Fast Na^+ channels close
2	Plateau	Ca^{2+} into cell, K^+ out of cell	Multiple channels (Ca^{2+}, Na^+, K^+) open to maintain membrane voltage
3	Repolarization	K^+ out of cell	Ca^{2+} and Na^+ channels close; K^+ channel remains open
4	Resting membrane potential	Na^+ out of cell, K^+ into cell	Na^+-K^+ pump

Ca^{2+}, Calcium; *K^+*, potassium; *Na^+*, sodium.

small area ignites, burns, and then ignites the area of gunpowder immediately adjacent to it and on down the line.

The rapid depolarization shape of the nonpacemaker action potential (Fig. 10.22A) differs in the slower depolarization profile of the SA and AV node pacemaker cells (Fig. 10.22B). The ionic transmembrane currents that produce the action potential are illustrated in Fig. 10.23.

Absolute and Relative Refractory Periods

The time from the beginning of the AP until the fiber can accept another AP is called the *absolute refractory period*. During this period, the cell cannot be depolarized regardless of the amount or intensity of the stimulus. This period lasts from the beginning of depolarization until the interior of the cell has repolarized to approximately −50 mV during phase 3. The absolute refractory period is immediately followed by the *relative refractory period*. At this time, the cell is not fully repolarized but could depolarize with a strong enough stimulus (Fig. 10.25). This period lasts from approximately −50 mV during phase 3 until the cell returns to RMP (phase 4); at that point, the cell is fully repolarized and is again ready to respond to the next stimulus. The concept of relative versus absolute refractory periods is useful for understanding the genesis of ventricular dysrhythmias. In brief, a cell cannot be stimulated to depolarize until it has at least partially recovered from the previous impulse. This is cardioprotective, as it means that an ectopic impulse cannot be propagated during the absolute refractory period.

Mechanical Myocardial Action

Excitation-Contraction Coupling

Electrical activity is the stimulus for mechanical contraction of the myocardium. As the myocardial cell is depolarized during phase 2 of the AP, extracellular Ca^{2+} ions enter the cytoplasm through the cell membrane via special Ca^{2+} channels. The entry of Ca^{2+} ions is the trigger for the release of Ca^{2+} stores from the sarcoplasmic reticulum (see Fig. 10.23). The cytoplasmic Ca^{2+} then binds with the regulatory TnC protein to induce a conformational change in TnI; this action induces a conformational change in TnT that moves the tropomyosin away from the myosin-binding site on actin. This permits actin to interact with myosin, releasing adenosine diphosphate (ADP) and an inorganic phosphate to provide the energy needed for myosin to slide along the actin molecule and initiate contraction. This mechanism is known as *cross-bridge cycling*. The result is myocardial contraction that spreads throughout the myocardium.

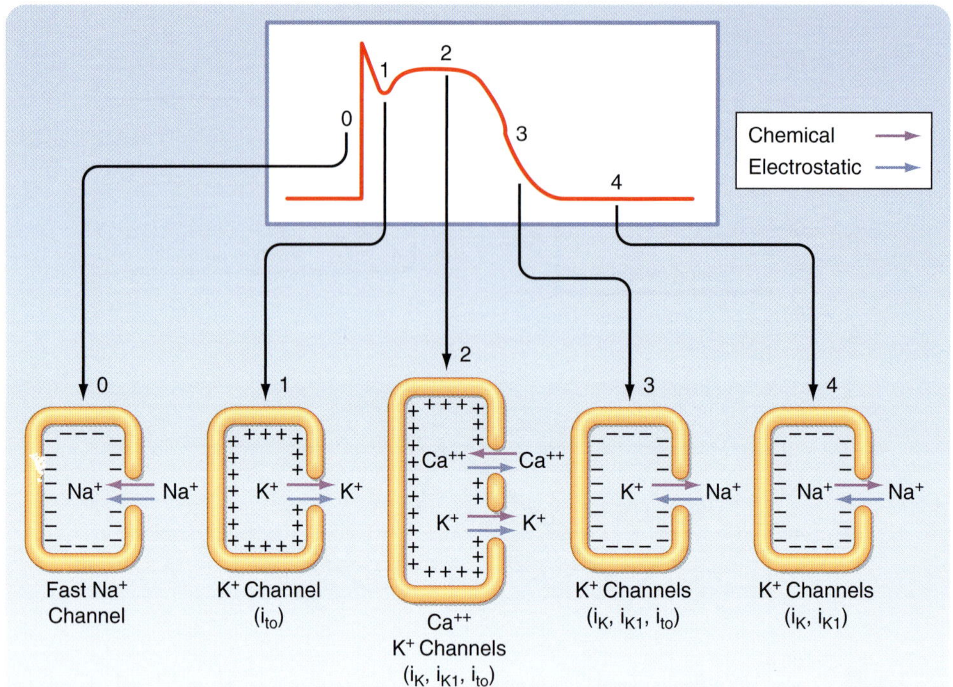

FIG. 10.23 Action Potential With Electrolyte Movement Across the Walls of the Myocardial Pacemaker Cells. (From Koeppen BM, Stanton BA. *Berne & Levy Physiology*. 8th ed. Elsevier Inc; 2024.)

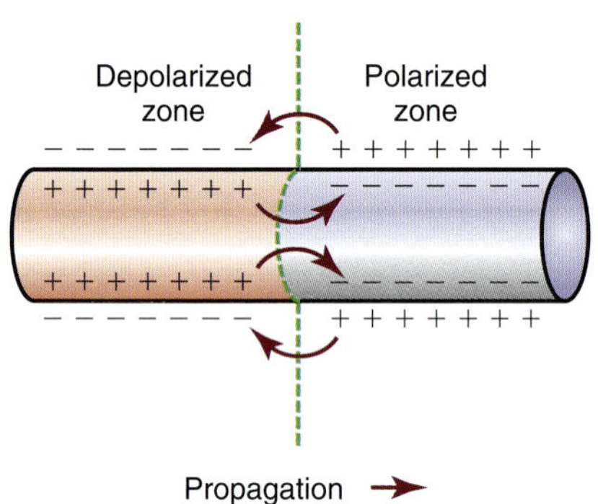

FIG. 10.24 Propagation of an Action Potential Across a Cell Wall.

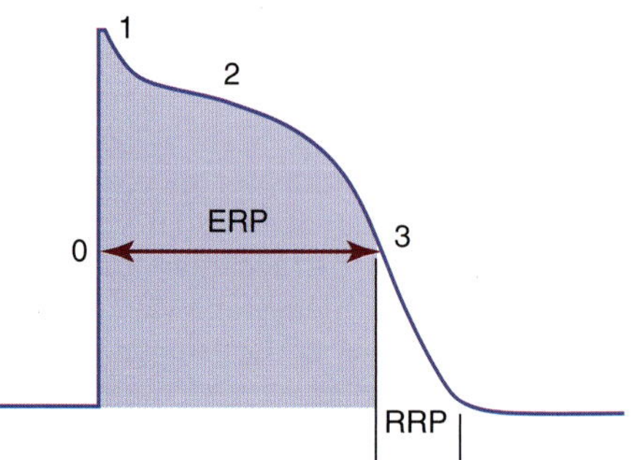

FIG. 10.25 Refractory Periods. The effective (absolute) refractory period *(ERP)* extends from phase 0 from approximately −50 mV in phase 3. The remainder of the action potential is the relative refractory period *(RRP)*. (From Conover MB. *Understanding Electrocardiography*. 8th ed. Mosby; 2002.)

Once contraction has occurred, intracellular Ca^{2+} levels are lowered by two processes. Most Ca^{2+} is taken back up into the sarcoplasmic reticulum via a Ca^{2+} and magnesium (Mg^{2+})–dependent, adenosine triphosphate (ATP)–based process. In addition, the Na^+–Ca^{2+} exchange system located in the sarcolemma moves Ca^{2+} outside the cell. This decreases the concentration of Ca^{2+} in the cytoplasm, leading to muscular relaxation.

Cardiac Cycle

The term *cardiac cycle* refers to one complete mechanical cycle of the heartbeat, beginning with ventricular contraction and ending with ventricular relaxation (Fig. 10.26).

Atrial Systole

The atria fill by passive filling from the inferior and superior vena cavae into the right atrium, and from the four pulmonary veins into the left atrium. During diastole, the mitral and tricuspid valves are open, allowing for passive filling into the ventricles (see Fig. 10.6A). After electrical depolarization of the atria (p-wave), atrial contraction (atrial systole) is initiated, causing additional blood to enter the ventricular chamber before the AV valves close. This atrial contraction at the end of atrial systole is often referred to as *atrial kick*.

Isovolumic Contraction

Ventricular depolarization from the QRS electrical stimulus depolarizes the septum and papillary muscles first. The ventricles then begin to tense, starting with the inner endocardium and traversing the myocardium toward the outer epicardium. This increases the pressure within the ventricular chambers. This is known as *isovolumic contraction*, because even though the ventricular muscle is contracting, the volume of blood within the ventricles does not change.[19] In Fig. 10.26, this is seen as a rapid increase in left ventricular pressure.

Ventricular Systole

Ventricular systole represents the ventricular ejection portion of the cardiac cycle. As ventricular tension increases,

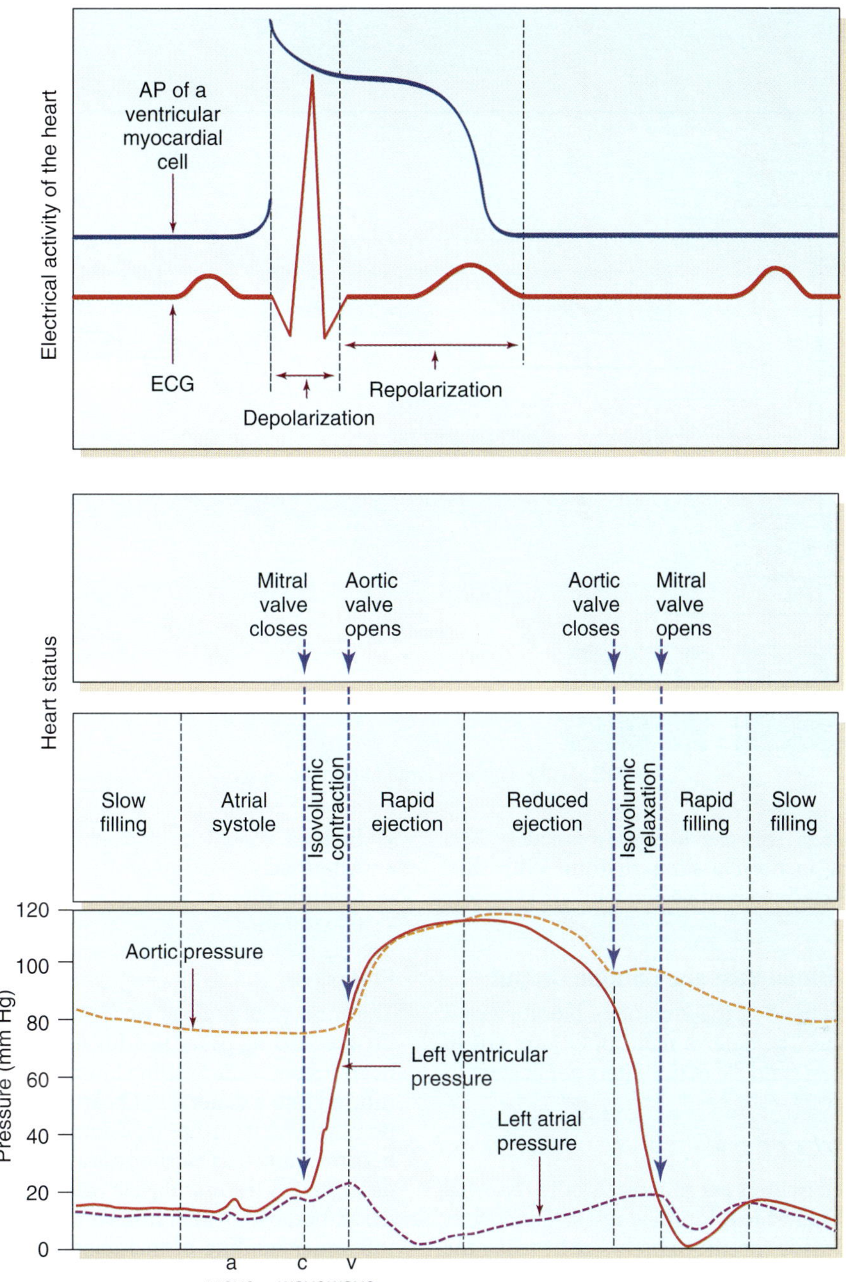

FIG. 10.26 Cardiac Cycle. *AP*, Action potential; *ECG*, electrocardiogram.

intraventricular pressures exceed the pressure in the aorta and pulmonary arteries, causing the aortic and pulmonic valves to open during systole (see Fig. 10.6B). The amount of blood ejected from the ventricles with each beat is called the *stroke volume* (SV). In a healthy heart, more than half of the total ventricular blood volume is ejected; the blood that remains in the ventricles is the residual or end-systolic volume.

The ejection fraction (EF) is the ratio of the SV ejected from the left ventricle per beat to the volume of blood remaining in the left ventricle at the end of diastole (left ventricular end-diastolic volume). EF is expressed as a percentage, and a normal value is 50% or greater. An EF of less than 35% indicates poor ventricular function (as in cardiomyopathy), poor ventricular filling, obstruction to outflow (as in some valve stenosis conditions), or a combination of these conditions.

Isovolumic Relaxation

The next phase is isovolumic relaxation, which occurs between the closure of the semilunar (aortic and pulmonic) valves and the opening of the AV (mitral and tricuspid) valves. All four valves are closed, and the pressure within the ventricular chamber falls to below atrial pressure without any change in intraventricular volume.[19] After this, the mitral and tricuspid valves open.

Ventricular Diastole

After the mitral and tricuspid valves open, most ventricular filling occurs. The next phase is a reduced ventricular filling period, during which blood flows passively from the periphery and the pulmonary vasculature into the ventricles. The last part of ventricular diastolic filling occurs during atrial contraction,

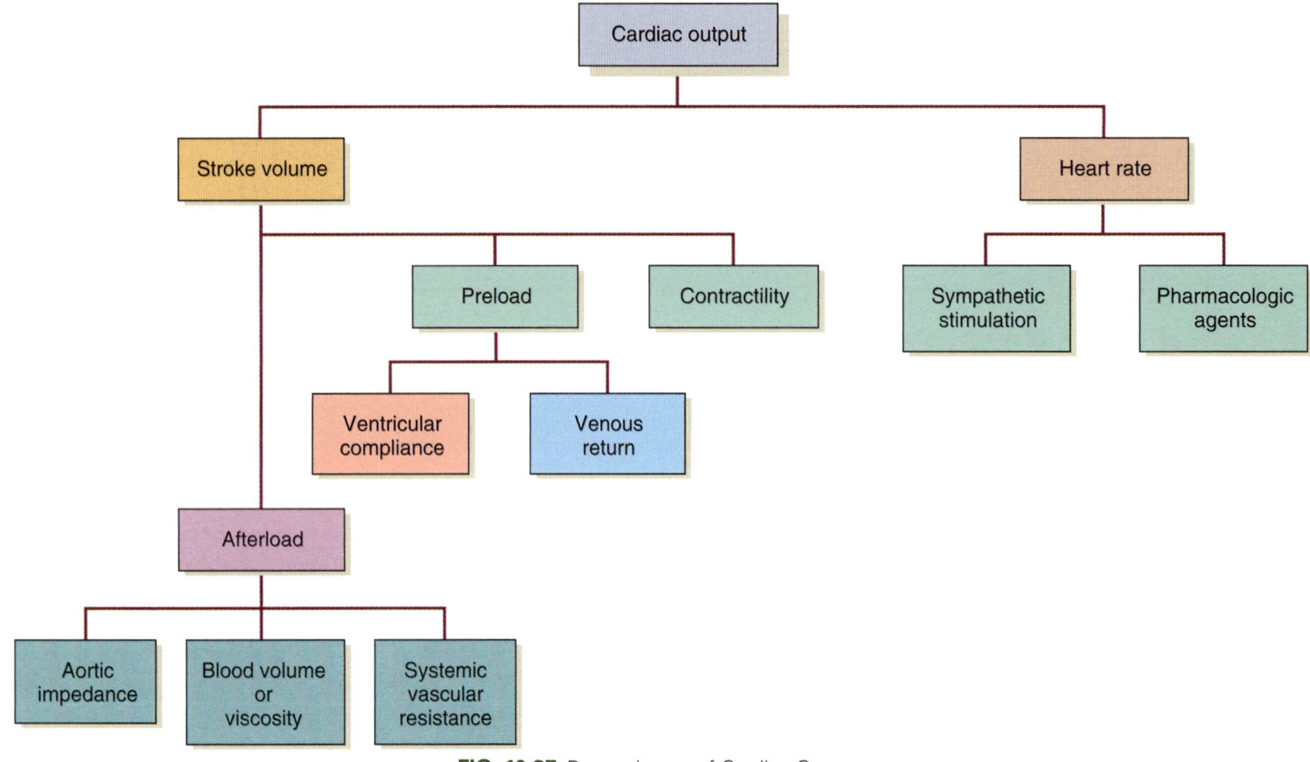

FIG. 10.27 Determinants of Cardiac Output.

also described as *atrial kick*. This provides approximately 20% of total ventricular filling in normal sinus rhythm. With this, the cycle is complete and ready to begin again with atrial systole (see Fig. 10.26).

Interplay of Heart and Blood Vessels: Cardiac Output

Cardiac output (CO) is defined as the volume of blood ejected from the heart in 1 minute. The determinants of CO are HR in beats per minute (beats/min) and SV in milliliters per beat (mL/beat). The equation is:

$$SV \times HR = CO$$

CO is usually expressed in liters per minute (L/min). Normal CO in adults is approximately 4 to 6 L/min at rest and increases with exercise. CO can be made specific to body size by using the person's height and weight to determine the cardiac index (CI). The CI is equal to CO divided by the individual's body surface area calculated from the height and weight. Body surface area is expressed in square meters (m^2); the normal range is 2.5 to 4.5 L/min per m^2. Changes in SV or HR can change CO. However, all three parameters must be individually assessed as described in the section on hemodynamics in Chapter 12.

For example, for a person with HR of 72 beats/min and SV of 70 mL/beat, the CO would be:

$$72\,\text{beats/min} \times 70\,\text{mL/beat} = 5.04\,\text{L/min}$$

If the HR were to change to 140 beats/min and the SV to 40 mL/beat in this person, the calculation would be:

$$140\,\text{beats/min} \times 40\,\text{mL/beat} = 5.6\,\text{L/min}$$

Although the CO is higher, the faster HR would not be an improvement in this situation. The decreased SV in the second instance indicates that cardiac decompensation is imminent. SV as a value is influenced by four primary factors (Fig. 10.27):

- Preload
- Afterload
- Contractility
- Heart Rate

Preload

The concept of preload was introduced in the early 1900s when Ernest Starling described his findings using an isolated canine heart preparation. Starling found that as he increased the volume infused into a denervated heart, CO increased until it reached a point at which further infusion caused CO to decrease. This has become known as *Starling's law of the heart*, and it is graphically described as the *Starling curve*, or as the *Frank-Starling function curve*, because Otto Frank, another scientist, also contributed to the understanding of this phenomenon. Frank-Starling curves are used to plot cardiac output or stroke volume relative to preload[20] (Fig. 10.28). This can be described using as a foundation the discussion of the actin and myosin cross-bridges in the myofibril.[19] As the diastolic volume increases, it stretches the actin and myosin in their resting state. As contraction occurs, contractility increases because of the increased stretch. However, if the stretch is excessive and causes actin and myosin to be stretched beyond their cross-bridging limits (>2.2 mm), contractility decreases. This is the basis for Starling's curve. With the advent of critical care units and sophisticated monitoring, this principle has acquired great significance in clinical practice. For example, after a myocardial infarction, the ability of the left ventricle to pump may be impaired. It is desirable to optimize the contractility of the remaining viable heart muscle by "stretching" it with added volume. However, if the intravascular volume exceeds the stretch limit, CO diminishes.

Preload is the volume of blood in the left ventricle at the end of diastole. The pressure created by this volume is described as the *left ventricular end-diastolic pressure*. Factors affecting left

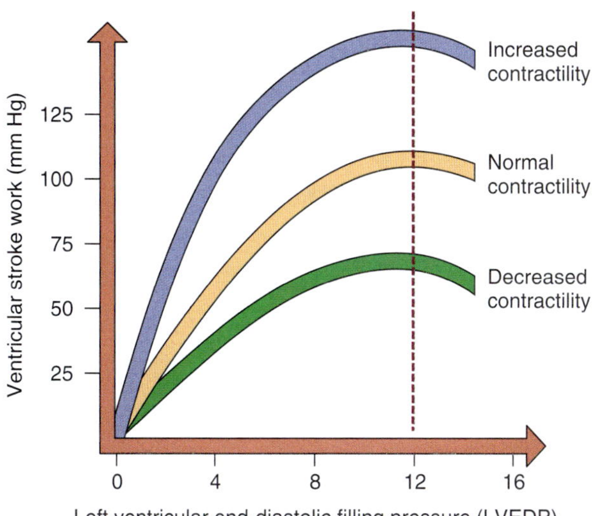

FIG. 10.28 Starling Curve. As the left ventricular end-diastolic pressure *(LVEDP)* increases, so does ventricular stroke work or contractility. When left ventricular filling pressure exceeds a maximal point, contractility and cardiac output diminish.

ventricular preload include venous return to the heart, total blood volume, and atrial kick.[17] Factors affecting the compliance (ability to stretch) of the ventricles are the stiffness and thickness of the muscular wall. One way to measure preload is by using a pulmonary artery catheter and measurement of *pulmonary artery occlusion pressure* (wedge pressure). Clinical application of pulmonary artery occlusion pressure is discussed in Chapter 12.

Afterload

Afterload can be defined as the ventricular wall tension or stress during systolic ejection. It is also described as a component of *systemic vascular resistance.* An increase in afterload usually means an increase in the work of the heart. Afterload is increased by factors that oppose ejection. Examples of increased afterload include aortic impedance (aortic stenosis), septal hypertrophy (obstruction in the outflow tract), vasoconstriction (increased systemic vascular resistance), and hypertension. Therapeutic management to decrease afterload is aimed at decreasing the work of the heart using vasodilators to decrease myocardial oxygen demand.

Contractility

Contractility refers to the heart's contractile force. It is also known as *inotropy*: "ino" for strength and "tropy" for enhancing. Contractility can be increased by Starling's mechanism to increase stretch. It also is enhanced by the SNS that innervates the heart (Fig. 10.29) and by pharmacologic agents that mimic the SNS, known as *sympathomimetics*, which are described in Chapter 14.

Heart Rate

Heart rate is controlled by several mechanisms including cerebral, metabolic and endocrine, and the autonomic nervous system as described in the following sections.

Autonomic Nervous System Control

The autonomic nervous system (ANS) is composed of two competing neurologic systems of control, the parasympathetic nervous system (PNS) and the SNS.[21] The functions of the SNS and PNS are often described by the following phrases:

- SNS "fight or flight"
- PNS "rest and digest"

These phrases are associated with the physiologic actions of the SNS and PNS[22] (see Fig. 10.29). The parasympathetic system slows HR during periods of rest, and the sympathetic system increases HR in response to physiologic stress. The effects of the divisions of the ANS on the heart are summarized in Table 10.6.

Parasympathetic fibers are concentrated near the SA and AV conduction tissue and in the atria. Specifically, this involves the right and left vagus nerves[23] (see Figs. 10.21 and 10.29). The vagus nerve is one of the pairs of cranial nerves (tenth cranial nerve) and is an important component of the PNS.[22] Vagal stimulation slows the heart rate by stimulating the SA node, which results in a decrease of sympathetic tone with resultant bradycardia.

Sympathetic nerve fibers are subepicardial and follow the path of the major coronary arteries (see Figs. 10.21 and 10.29). Stimulation of sympathetic fibers directly alters ventricular function and increases HR and contractility. Heart rate variability is a normal finding in a healthy heart.

Supplementing the ANS control of the heart are several reflexes that serve as feedback mechanisms to the brain. These reflexes maintain even blood flow, oxygenation, and perfusion in response to physiologic needs.

Baroreceptors

Baroreceptors, or strain-sensitive pressure sensors, are located in the aortic arch and the carotid sinuses[24] (Fig. 10.30). They are more sensitive to wall stretch than to the absolute blood pressure. As the receptors sense a change of shape in the arterial wall, usually from a change in pressure, the ANS is activated to raise HR (in the case of decreased pressure) or lower HR (in response to increased pressure). For example, a decrease in blood pressure alters the baroreceptor input to the vasomotor center in the medulla oblongata (brainstem), causing a reflex tachycardia. The baroreflex also initiates changes in venous tone to alter CO according to the need to increase or reduce blood return to the heart.

Chemoreceptors

Arterial chemoreceptors, known as *carotid* and *aortic bodies*, are located in the carotid arteries and at the bifurcation of the aortic arch and enjoy a rich capillary blood supply (see Fig. 10.30). Their primary function is to maintain homeostasis during hypoxemia. Chemoreceptors signal changes in oxygen tension ($PaO_2 < 80$ mm Hg) or a carbon dioxide tension ($PaCO_2$) of greater than 40 mm Hg. They do not respond to changes in acid-base balance (pH), because changes in the pH level are detected by the central chemoreceptors in the brainstem (medulla oblongata). Information about changes in these parameters is communicated to the SNS via the brainstem. Stimulation of the carotid or aortic chemoreceptors normally causes an increase in respiratory rate and depth.

Right Atrial Receptors

The Bainbridge reflex is attributed to receptors in the right and left atria. When the pressure in the right atrium increases sufficiently to stimulate the stretch receptors, it causes a reflex tachycardia. The purpose of this reflex is possibly to protect the right side of the heart from an overload state and to quickly equalize filling pressures of the right and left sides of the heart.

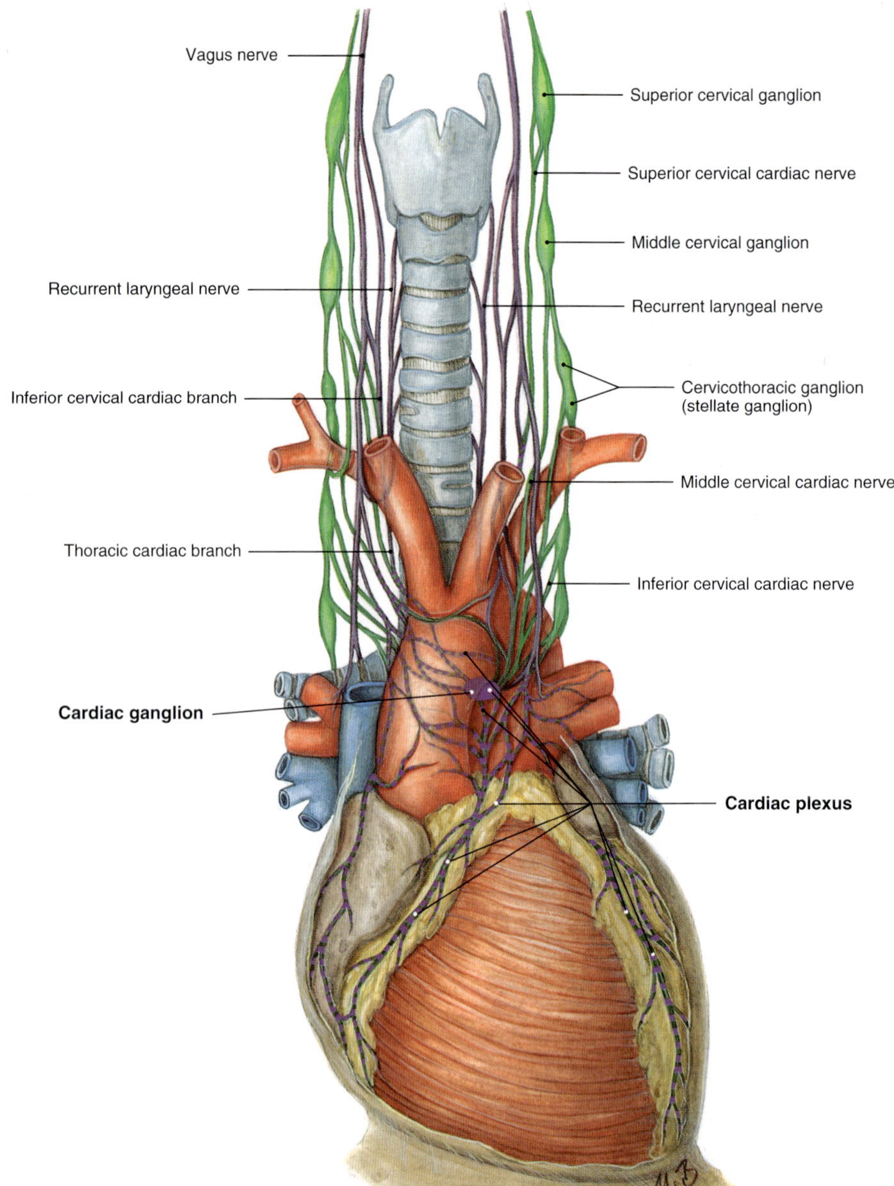

FIG. 10.29 Autonomic Nervous System: Sympathetic and Parasympathetic Innervation of the Heart. (From Hombach-Klonisch S, Klonisch T, Peeler J, Paulson F, Waschke J. *Sobotta Clinical Atlas of Human Anatomy.* 1st ed. Elsevier; 2019.)

TABLE 10.6 Autonomic Nervous System Function in Heart Tissue

Function	Parasympathetic	Sympathetic
Automaticity	Decrease	Increase
Contractility	Decrease	Increase
Conduction velocity	Decrease	Increase
Chronotropy (rate)	Decrease	Increase

Natriuretic Peptides

Another cardiac control mechanism involves the natriuretic peptide system (Fig. 10.31). The heart secretes two hormonal natriuretic peptides. The atrial myocardium secretes atrial natriuretic peptide in response to atrial stretch, and the ventricular myocardium secretes brain natriuretic peptide (also known as *b-type natriuretic peptide*) when stretch of the ventricular chamber occurs.[25] Both peptides cause vasodilation, increase natriuresis (Na^+ and water loss via the kidneys), and inhibit the SNS and the renin-angiotensin-aldosterone system (RAAS). Natriuretic peptide levels are measured to confirm a diagnosis of acute heart failure[25,26] (see Fig. 12.83 in Chapter 12).

Renin-Angiotensin-Aldosterone System

The RAAS is activated by low blood pressure or intravascular volume depletion. The juxtaglomerular cells of the kidney, located near the afferent arteriole, are activated by low renal blood flow. As shown in Table 10.7, this stimulates release of the hormone renin. Renin converts the protein angiotensinogen to angiotensin I. When angiotensin I passes through the pulmonary vascular bed, it is activated by *angiotensin-converting enzyme* (ACE) to become angiotensin II.[27]

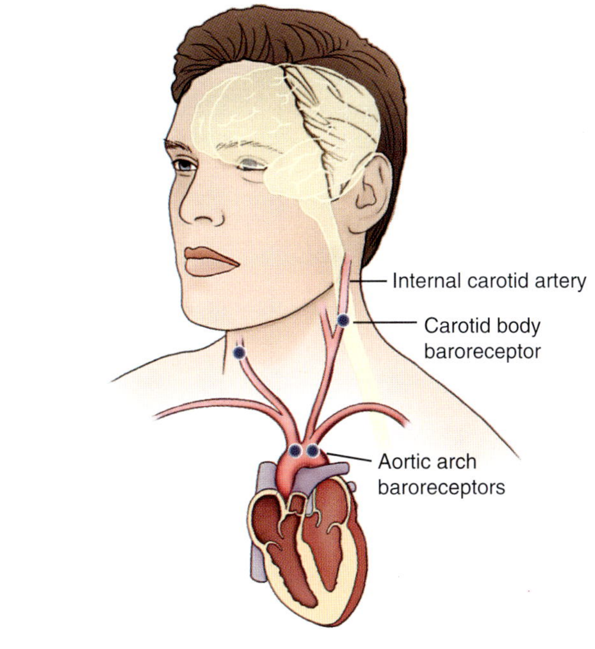

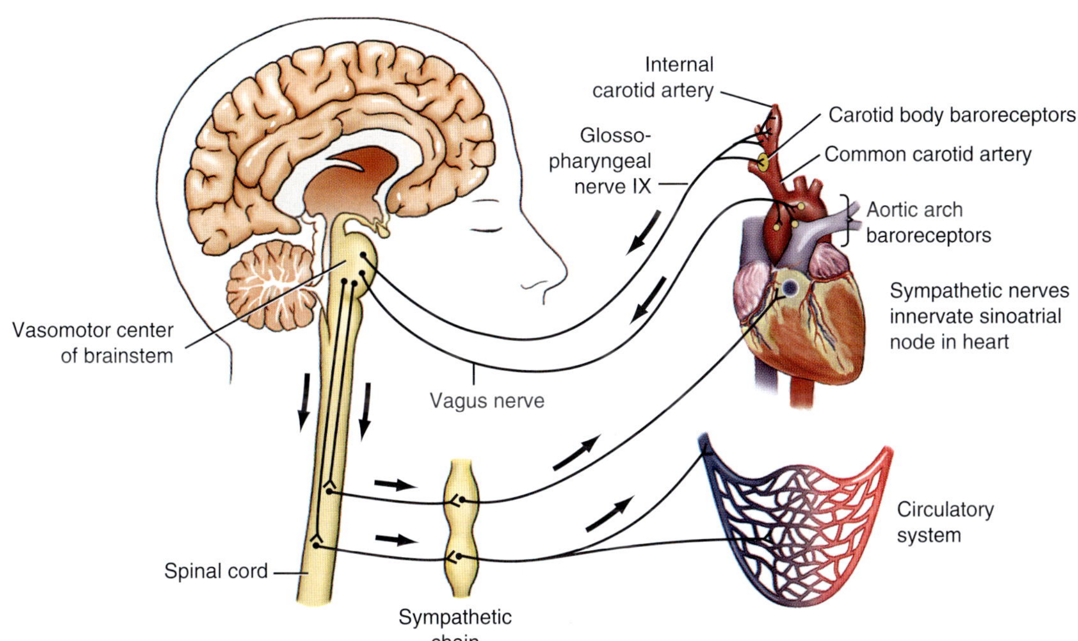

FIG. 10.30 Baroreceptors, Chemoreceptors, and the Autonomic Nervous System (ANS) Role in Regulation of Heart Rate and Contractility. (From Lough ME. *Hemodynamic Monitoring: Evolving Technologies and Clinical Practice*. Elsevier; 2016.)

Angiotensin II is a powerful agent with several actions:

- Activation of the peripheral vascular receptors to vasoconstrict the systemic arterial system
- Increases blood pressure (secondary to vasoconstriction)
- Activates the release of aldosterone from the adrenal glands.

Aldosterone works at the distal convoluted tubule in the kidney to retain sodium and, consequently, water. The role of the RAAS in heart failure is illustrated in Fig. 13.19 in Chapter 13. Many medications have been developed to manipulate the RAAS to manage symptoms of heart failure (see Table 14.24 in Chapter 14).

Respiratory Influences on Heart Rate

Normally, HR varies slightly with the respiratory cycle. The heart usually accelerates on inspiration and decelerates with exhalation (see Sinus Dysrhythmia and Fig. 12.58 in Chapter 12). Left ventricular SV decreases during normal inspiration.

Control of Peripheral Systemic Circulation

Intrinsic Control of the Systemic Circulation

Intrinsic, or local, control of the arterial peripheral circulation is most influential at the arteriolar level. Arterioles are the major resistance vessels because of the amount of smooth muscle

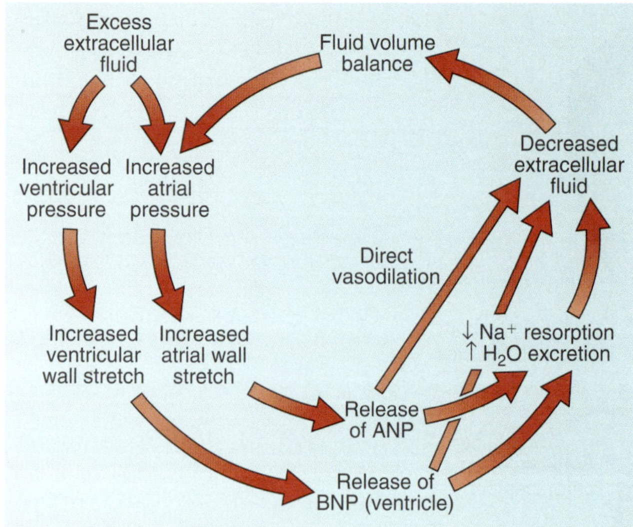

FIG. 10.31 Natriuretic Peptides. The release of atrial natriuretic peptide *(ANP)* from the atrium and brain natriuretic peptide *(BNP)* from the ventricle in response to volume overload.

TABLE 10.7 Renin-Angiotensin-Aldosterone and Antidiuretic Hormone Systems Maintain Fluid Balance

Hormone	Effect[a]
Renin ↓	Reduction in vascular volume or low arterial blood pressure stimulates renin release from juxtaglomerular cells near the kidney.
Angiotensinogen ↓	Angiotensinogen is produced in the liver.
Angiotensin I ↓	Lungs release ACE to convert angiotensin I to angiotensin II.
Angiotensin II ↓	Angiotensin II activates peripheral vascular receptors to increase SVR and raise arterial blood pressure; angiotensin II release also stimulates adrenal glands to release aldosterone.
	ADH is released from posterior pituitary when angiotensin II causes constriction of renal arterioles and when hypothalamus detects intracellular dehydration.
Aldosterone	Aldosterone acts on kidney distal tubules to retain sodium; when salt is retained, so is water.

[a]Overall effect is to increase intravascular volume and raise blood pressure.
ACE, Angiotensin-converting enzyme; *ADH*, antidiuretic hormone; *SVR*, systemic vascular resistance.

in the vessel walls. The arteriole has the potential for increasing or decreasing its lumen substantially. Several local factors influence this balance, including pharmacologic stimuli from locally released catecholamines, histamine, acetylcholine, serotonin, angiotensin, adenosine, and prostaglandins. These agents can be induced by various mechanisms such as tissue injury, hypoxemia, or hormones. For example, when red blood cells are exposed to hypoxia at the tissue level, they release the vasodilators nitric oxide and ATP to increase oxygen delivery. Other factors that influence circulation locally are temperature and carbon dioxide.

Extrinsic Control of the Systemic Circulation

Extrinsic control is mediated by two major mechanisms: (1) the ANS and (2) peripheral vascular reflexes. The ANS exerts dual control over most organ systems via sympathetic nerve fibers that cause blood vessels to constrict, and via parasympathetic fibers that allow blood vessels to dilate.[28] Stimulation of the vasomotor center in the medulla causes increases in mean arterial pressure and HR by enhancing sympathetic outflow and possibly inhibiting parasympathetic outflow. Capacitance vessels (veins) contain up to 75% of the blood volume. Increases in venous tone (venoconstriction) increase the volume of blood returning to the right side of the heart to augment SV. The most richly innervated venous beds are those in splanchnic (spleen) and cutaneous (skin) circulations. The venous and arterial vascular systems are interdependent; they dilate and constrict in unison. Table 10.8 summarizes the sympathetic receptors, including location and effects of stimulation.

TABLE 10.8 Medulla Oblongata Cardiovascular Actions

Medulla Oblongata Region	Effects
Dorsal lateral medulla (pressor region)	Vasoconstriction Cardiac acceleration Enhanced contractility
Ventromedial medulla (depressor region)	Direct spinal inhibition

KEY POINTS

- Knowledge of normal cardiovascular anatomy and physiology is vital for a complete understanding of the changes that occur in cardiac disease states.
- The major anatomic structures of the heart include the pericardium, myocardium, endocardium, coronary arteries, coronary veins, atria, ventricles, heart valves, and electrical conduction system.
- The electrical conduction system, the mechanical events of the cardiac cycle, the ANS, and the preload volume in the veins act synergistically to ensure optimal cardiac output and hemodynamic stability in a state of health.

Visit the Evolve site at http://evolve.elsevier.com/Urden/CriticalCareNursing for additional study materials.

REFERENCES

1. Mori S, Tretter JT, Spicer DE, Bolender DL, Anderson RH. What is the real cardiac anatomy? *Clin Anat*. 2019;32(3):288–309. https://doi.org/10.1002/ca.23340.
2. De Almeida MC, Spicer DE, Anderson RH. Why do we break one of the first rules of anatomy when describing the components of the heart? *Clin Anat*. 2019;32(4):585–596. https://doi.org/10.1002/ca.23356.
3. Molina DK, DiMaio VJM. Normal organ weights in men: part I-the heart. *Am J Forensic Med Pathol*. 2012;33(4):362–367. https://doi.org/10.1097/PAF.0b013e31823d298b.
4. Molina DK, DiMaio VJM. Normal organ weights in women, part I: the heart. *Am J Forensic Med Pathol*. 2015;36(3):176–181. https://doi.org/10.1097/PAF.0000000000000174.
5. Mori S, Bradfield JS, Peacock WJ, Anderson RH, Shivkumar K. Living anatomy of the pericardial space: a guide for imaging and interventions. *JACC Clin Electrophysiol*. 2021;7(12):1628–1644. https://doi.org/10.1016/j.jacep.2021.09.008.
6. Hayase J, Mori S, Shivkumar K, Bradfield JS. Anatomy of the pericardial space. *Card Electrophysiol Clin*. 2020;12(3):265–270. https://doi.org/10.1016/j.ccep.2020.04.003.

7. Kligerman S. Imaging of pericardial disease. *Radiol Clin North Am.* 2019;57(1):179–199. https://doi.org/10.1016/j.rcl.2018.09.001.
8. Iacobellis G. Epicardial adipose tissue in contemporary cardiology. *Nat Rev Cardiol.* 2022;19(9):593–606. https://doi.org/10.1038/s41569-022-00679-9.
9. Pighi M, Thériault-Lauzier P, Alosaimi H, et al. Fluoroscopic anatomy of right-sided heart structures for transcatheter interventions. *JACC Cardiovasc Interv.* 2018;11(16):1614–1625. https://doi.org/10.1016/j.jcin.2018.03.050.
10. Whiteman S, Saker E, Courant V, et al. An anatomical review of the left atrium. *Transl Res Anatomy.* 2019;17:100052. https://doi.org/10.1016/j.tria.2019.100052.
11. Sanz J, Sánchez-Quintana D, Bossone E, Bogaard HJ, Naeije R. Anatomy, function, and dysfunction of the right ventricle: JACC state-of-the-art review. *J Am Coll Cardiol.* 2019;73(12):1463–1482. https://doi.org/10.1016/j.jacc.2018.12.076.
12. Dahou A, Levin D, Reisman M, Hahn RT. Anatomy and physiology of the tricuspid valve. *JACC Cardiovasc Imaging.* 2019;12(3):458–468. https://doi.org/10.1016/j.jcmg.2018.07.032.
13. Oliveira D, Srinivasan J, Espino D, Buchan K, Dawson D, Shepherd D. Geometric description for the anatomy of the mitral valve: a review. *J Anat.* 2020;237(2):209–224. https://doi.org/10.1111/joa.13196.
14. Padala SK, Cabrera JA, Ellenbogen KA. Anatomy of the cardiac conduction system. *Pacing Clin Electrophysiol.* 2021;44(1):15–25. https://doi.org/10.1111/pace.14107.
15. Sirajuddin A, Chen MY, White CS, Arai AE. Coronary venous anatomy and anomalies. *J Cardiovasc Comput Tomogr.* 2020;14(1):80–86. https://doi.org/10.1016/j.jcct.2019.08.006.
16. Bossone E, Eagle KA. Epidemiology and management of aortic disease: aortic aneurysms and acute aortic syndromes. *Nat Rev Cardiol.* 2021;18(5):331–348. https://doi.org/10.1038/s41569-020-00472-6.
17. Persichini R, Lai C, Teboul JL, Adda I, Guérin L, Monnet X. Venous return and mean systemic filling pressure: physiology and clinical applications. *Crit Care.* 2022;26(1):150. https://doi.org/10.1186/s13054-022-04024-x.
18. Szedlak P, Steele DS, Hopkins PM. Cardiac muscle physiology. *BJA Educ.* 2023;23(9):350–357. https://doi.org/10.1016/j.bjae.2023.05.004.
19. Chung CS. How myofilament strain and strain rate lead the dance of the cardiac cycle. *Arch Biochem Biophys.* 2019;664:62–67. https://doi.org/10.1016/j.abb.2019.01.034.
20. Han J, Taberner AJ, Loiselle DS, Tran K. Cardiac efficiency and Starling's law of the heart. *J Physiol.* 2022;600(19):4265–4285. https://doi.org/10.1113/JP283632.
21. Scott-Solomon E, Boehm E, Kuruvilla R. The sympathetic nervous system in development and disease. *Nat Rev Neurosci.* 2021;22(11):685–702. https://doi.org/10.1038/s41583-021-00523-y.
22. Shanks J, Ramchandra R. Angiotensin II and the cardiac parasympathetic nervous system in hypertension. *Int J Mol Sci.* 2021;22(22):12305. https://doi.org/10.3390/ijms222212305.
23. Ruigrok TJH, Mantel SA, Orlandini L, de Knegt C, Vincent AJPE, Spoor JKH. Sympathetic components in left and right human cervical vagus nerve: implications for vagus nerve stimulation. *Front Neuroanat.* 2023;17:1205660. https://doi.org/10.3389/fnana.2023.1205660.
24. Wallbach M, Koziolek MJ. Baroreceptors in the carotid and hypertension-systematic review and meta-analysis of the effects of baroreflex activation therapy on blood pressure. *Nephrol Dial Transplant.* 2018;33(9):1485–1493. https://doi.org/10.1093/ndt/gfx279.
25. Maisel AS, Duran JM, Wettersten N. Natriuretic peptides in heart failure: atrial and B-type natriuretic peptides. *Heart Fail Clin.* 2018;14(1):13–25. https://doi.org/10.1016/j.hfc.2017.08.002.
26. Gaborit FS, Kistorp C, Kümler T, et al. Diagnostic utility of MR-proANP and NT-proBNP in elderly outpatients with a high risk of heart failure: the Copenhagen heart failure risk study. *Biomarkers.* 2020;25(3):248–259. https://doi.org/10.1080/1354750X.2020.1732466.
27. Paz OM, Riquelme JA, García L, et al. Counter-regulatory renin–angiotensin system in cardiovascular disease. *Nat Rev Cardiol.* 2020;17(2):116–129. https://doi.org/10.1038/s41569-019-0244-8.
28. Herring N, Kalla M, Paterson DJ. The autonomic nervous system and cardiac arrhythmias: current concepts and emerging therapies. *Nat Rev Cardiol.* 2019;16(12):707–726. https://doi.org/10.1038/s41569-019-0221-2.

11

Cardiovascular Clinical Assessment

Mary E. Lough

http://evolve.elsevier.com/Urden/CriticalCareNursing

Physical assessment of a patient with cardiovascular disease is an important clinical skill to master. The process is systematic and detailed as described in this chapter. Bedside assessment allows the examiner to anticipate the need for other diagnostic studies to form a complete picture of the patient's cardiovascular status.[1–3] Increasingly, the bedside physical examination is expanding in scope to include adjuncts that provide immediate physiologic information. The traditional stethoscope is the classic adjunct, followed by pulse oximetry, and more recently handheld ultrasound images.[4] These clinical tools do not replace the physical exam, rather they are actively used to enhance the physical exam findings at the bedside.

HISTORY

Data collected from a thorough, thoughtful history taking contribute to both nursing and medical decisions about therapeutic interventions.[5] For a patient in acute distress, the history taking is shortened to just a few questions about the patient's chief complaint, precipitating events, and current medications (Box 11.1). For a patient who is not in obvious distress, the history focuses on the following four areas:

- Review of present illness
- Overview of general cardiovascular status, including previous cardiac diagnostic studies, interventional procedures, cardiac surgeries, and current medications, including cardiac, noncardiac, and over-the-counter medications
- Review of general health status, including family history of coronary artery disease (CAD), hypertension, diabetes, peripheral arterial disease, or stroke
- Survey of relevant lifestyle factors, including risk factors for CAD

Evaluating Chest Pain

One unique challenge in cardiovascular assessment is identifying when "chest pain" is of cardiac origin and when it is not.[6,7] Each year 6.5 million visits to hospital emergency departments are for chest pain.[6] However, only 5% of these patients are experiencing an acute coronary event.[6] In most cases, the chest pain is from another cause such as gastroesophageal reflux disease. For this reason, accurately identifying the patients who are experiencing an acute coronary syndrome is crucial.[6]

The following safety information should always be considered:

- If any evidence of CAD or risk of heart disease exists, assume that the chest pain is caused by myocardial ischemia until proven otherwise.[8]
- Questions to elicit the nature of the chest pain cover five areas:
  - Quality of the pain
  - Location of the pain
  - Duration of the pain
  - Factors that provoke the pain
  - Factors that relieve the pain
- Questions that may help elicit additional information are listed in Table 11.1.
- Little correlation may exist between the severity of chest discomfort and the gravity of its cause. This is a result of the subjective nature of pain and the unique presentation of ischemic disease in women, older patients, and patients with diabetes.
- Subjective descriptors vary greatly among individuals. Not all patients use the word "pain"; some may describe their problem as "pressure," "heaviness," "discomfort," or "indigestion."[6]
- Other nonpainful symptoms that may signal cardiac dysfunction are dyspnea, palpitations, cough, fatigue, edema, ischemic leg pain, nocturia, cyanosis, and a history of syncope.[6]
- In the evaluation of acute chest pain, a 12-lead electrocardiogram to diagnose ST segment changes must be obtained within 10 minutes of arrival at the emergency department.[6,9]

PHYSICAL EXAMINATION

A comprehensive physical assessment is fundamental to arriving at an accurate diagnosis. A nurse who has developed the skills of *inspection, palpation*, and *auscultation* can be confident when assessing patients with cardiovascular disease. *Percussion*, another physical assessment skill, is not used when assessing the cardiovascular system.

Inspection

Face

The face is observed for skin color (i.e., cyanotic, pale, or jaundiced) and for an apprehensive or painful expression as part of the initial visual inspection of the patient.[10] The skin, lips, tongue, and mucous membranes are inspected for pallor or cyanosis. *Central cyanosis* is a bluish discoloration of the tongue and sublingual area. Central cyanosis is a medical emergency indicating hypoxemia. Pulse oximetry, arterial blood gas analysis, and treatment with oxygen must be instituted immediately.

New information about pulse oximeter values obtained from attaching a finger probe is relevant to the clinical

BOX 11.1 DATA COLLECTION

Cardiovascular History

Common Cardiovascular Symptoms
- Chest pains
- Palpitations
- Dyspnea
- Cough, hemoptysis
- Nausea
- Nocturia
- Edema
- Dizziness, syncope, visual changes
- Leg claudication (pain) or paresthesia
- Fatigue

Patient Lifestyle
- Baseline cognitive functioning
- Health habits
- Use of tea and coffee, over-the-counter medication use, smoking, exercise, sleep, dietary habits
- Use of illegal drugs (e.g., cocaine)
- Use of alcohol (daily quantity)
- Lifestyle pattern and responsibilities
- Working, relaxing, coping, cultural habits
- Social support systems
- Recent life changes within past 12 months
- Emotional state
- Evidence of psychological stress, anger, anxiety, depression
- Perception of illness and its meaning for the future

Cardiovascular Risk Factors
- Sex
- Age
- Cultural identity
- Family history of premature CAD (age 65 years or younger)
- Smoking history
- Hypertension
- Hyperlipidemia
- Sedentary lifestyle
- Diabetes mellitus
- Obesity
- Kidney failure

Medical History

Child
- Murmurs, cyanosis, streptococcal infections, rheumatic fever

Adult
- Diseases and abnormalities
- Heart failure (right- or left-sided), CAD, heart valve disease, mitral valve prolapse, myocardial infarction, peripheral vascular disease (arterial or venous), diabetes mellitus, hypertension, hyperlipidemia, dysrhythmias, murmurs, endocarditis, visual defects, recent weight changes, psychiatric illnesses, thrombophlebitis, deep vein thrombosis, systemic or pulmonary emboli
- Surgical history
- *Cardiovascular:* Coronary artery bypass grafting, valvular placement, peripheral vascular bypasses or repairs, pacemaker, defibrillator implant (ICD)
- *Other body systems:* Neurologic, gastrointestinal, musculoskeletal, pulmonary, renal, immunologic, hematologic
- Allergies, especially to emergency medications (lidocaine, morphine), radiographic contrast agents, or iodine (shellfish)
- Recent dental work or infection

Family History
- CAD at age 65 years or younger
- Myocardial infarction
- Early death of unknown origin
- Hypertension
- Stroke
- Diabetes mellitus
- Lipid disorders
- Collagen vascular disease

Current Medication Use
- Angiotensin-converting enzyme (ACE) inhibitors
- Anticoagulants
- Antidysrhythmics
- Antihypertensives
- Antiplatelet agents
- Angiotensin-receptor blockers
- Beta-blockers
- Calcium channel blockers
- Cholesterol-lowering agents
- Digitalis
- Diuretics
- Nitrates
- Hormone replacement therapy
- Oral contraceptives
- Potassium, calcium
- Nonprescription medications or herbal remedies

Cardiac Studies or Interventions Completed in the Past
- Cardiac catheterization
- Electrophysiology study
- Cardiac ultrasound (echocardiogram)
- 12-lead electroencephalogram
- Exercise ECG (stress test)
- Myocardial imaging with radiographic isotopes (e.g., thallium, dipyridamole, dobutamine)
- Fibrinolytic therapy
- Percutaneous transluminal coronary angioplasty
- Atherectomy
- Stent placement
- Valvuloplasty

ACE, Angiotensin-converting enzyme; *CAD*, coronary artery disease; *ECG*, electrocardiogram; *ICD*, implantable cardioverter defibrillator.

examination. The pulse oximeter provides adjunctive information about oxygen saturation; however, in the setting of cyanosis visible in the nail beds, the finger reading is not recommended, and the earlobe may provide a more accurate value. Additionally, if a patient has pigmented skin that is black or brown, the finger probe pulse oximeter has been shown to underestimate hypoxemia in patients who self-report as black or Hispanic compared to white patients.[11] This is significant because the underestimation of hypoxemia in patients with darker skin tones has been associated with less supplemental oxygen in critical care units[12] and longer delays in treatment related to COVID-19.[13] Adjuncts to clinical assessment, such as pulse oximetry, are helpful in the physical examination but must always be evaluated in the context of the patient's clinical presentation and any evidence of cyanosis or cardiopulmonary distress.

TABLE 11.1 Clarifying Chest Pain Symptoms by Asking Specific Questions

Determine	Typical Question
Location, radiation	Where is it? Does it move or stay in one place?
Quality	What is it like?
Quantity	How severe is it? How frequent is it? How long does it last?
Chronology	When did it begin? How has it progressed? What are you doing when it occurs? What do you do to get rid of it?
Associated findings	Do you feel any other symptoms at the same time?
Treatment sought and effect	Have you seen a physician in the past for this same problem? What was the treatment?
Personal Perception	What do you think this is from? Why do you think it happened now?

Nail Beds and Cyanosis

The nail beds are inspected for signs of discoloration or cyanosis.

Clubbing in the nail bed is a sign associated with long-standing central cyanotic heart disease or pulmonary disease with hypoxemia. Clubbing of the nail refers to a nail that has lost the normal angle between the finger and the nail root; the nail becomes wide and convex. The terminal phalanx of the finger also becomes bulbous and swollen. Clubbing is rare and is a sign of severe central cyanosis (Fig. 11.1).

Peripheral cyanosis, or a bluish discoloration of the nail bed, is a more common sign. Peripheral cyanosis results from a reduction in the quantity of oxygen in the peripheral extremities from arterial disease or decreased cardiac output. Clubbing never occurs because of peripheral cyanosis.

A finding of cyanosis visible in the nail beds indicates the digits should not be used for pulse oximetry and the earlobe should be used instead.

Clubbing of Nail Beds

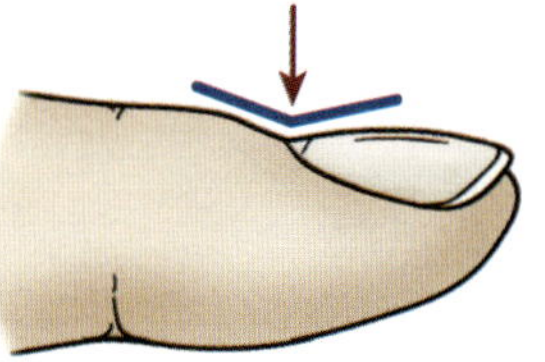

Normal Finger and Nail Bed

Normal nail shows a slight angle between root of nail bed and finger.

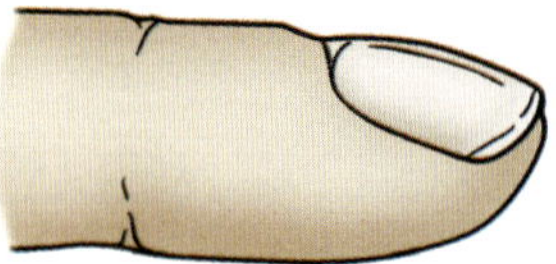

Early Clubbing

Early clubbing shows loss of angle at root of nail bed. Fingertip is of normal size.

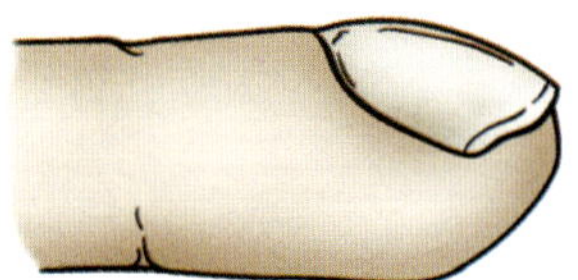

Moderate Clubbing

Moderate clubbing shows bulging of angle at root of nail bed. Distal finger/toe is enlarged.

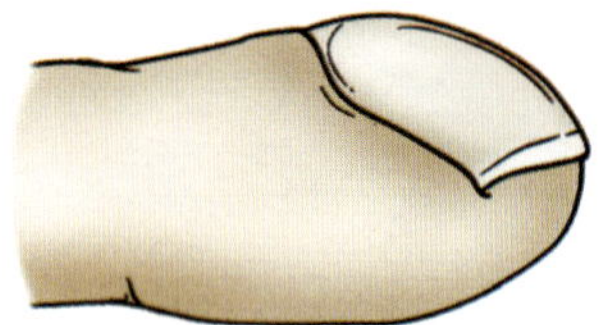

Advanced Clubbing

Advanced clubbing shows bulging and widening of nail bed. Distal finger/toe is bulbous.

FIG. 11.1 Clubbing of Nail Beds.

Thorax

The anterior thorax and posterior thorax are inspected for skeletal deformities that may displace the heart and cause cardiac compromise. The skin on the chest wall and abdomen is inspected for scars, bruises, wounds, and bulges associated with pacemaker or defibrillator implants. Respiratory rate, pattern, and effort are also observed and recorded.

Abdomen

The abdomen is assessed for signs of distention or ascites, which may be associated with right-sided heart failure. Abdominal adiposity is a known risk factor for CAD.

Lower Extremities

Legs are inspected for both signs of peripheral arterial disease and venous disease. Peripheral arterial disease (PAD) is the third most prevalent cardiovascular disease and is encountered in both high-income and low-income countries.[14] PAD affects more than 23 million people worldwide.[14] The visible signs of peripheral arterial vascular disease include pale, shiny legs with sparse hair growth.[15] Research suggests that women can have peripheral atherosclerosis with less obvious signs of peripheral arterial disease.[16] There is also a strong association between diabetes and PAD.[14] If untreated, peripheral arterial disease can lead to critical limb ischemia, decreased quality of life, and premature death.[17]

Venous disease is caused by failure of the valves in the veins leading to bleeding into the surrounding tissues, although symptoms and timeline of venous changes are highly variable.[18] Increasing venous pressure in the tissues causes edema, brown skin discoloration from red blood cell destruction, dependent rubor, and frequently nonhealing leg ulcers.

A comparison of typical assessment findings in arterial and venous diseases is presented in Table 11.2.

Posture

Body posture can provide information about the amount of effort it takes to breathe. For example, sitting upright to breathe may be necessary for a patient with acute heart failure. Leaning forward may be the least painful position for a patient with pericarditis.

TABLE 11.2 **Comparison of Arterial and Venous Disease in Legs**

Signs and Symptoms	Peripheral Arterial Disease	Venous Insufficiency
Skin	Shiny dry appearance Pallor with elevation	Brown patches on skin at ankles and lower leg Mottled rubor (brown/red) appearance, especially when dependent Skin texture may be hard and fibrotic Flaking skin, dermatitis
Hair on leg	Decreased hair growth	Decreased hair growth
Ulcers on leg or foot	Foot or toe wounds (ulcers) that do not heal Gangrene on toes	Venous ulcers at ankle or lower leg Moist with copious drainage
Nails	Slow nail growth Thick, opaque nails	Normal
Varicose veins	No	Present
Temperature	Cold compared with rest of the body	Warm
Capillary refill	Slow (≥3 sec)	Normal (<3 sec)
Edema	None	Legs and feet are swollen and edematous
Pulses	Weak or absent	Normal
Pain	Burning sensation in feet Leg cramps when walking: intermittent claudication Leg cramps at rest: ischemic claudication Numbness	Legs can feel heavy, aching, tired, with burning or itching from swelling
Associated conditions	Diabetes Atherosclerotic disease	Diabetes Varicose veins

Weight

Body weight in proportion to height is assessed to determine whether the patient is obese, a risk factor for cardiovascular disease,[19] or severely underweight (cachectic).[20]

Mentation

The patient is observed for signs of confusion or lethargy that may indicate hypotension, low cardiac output, or hypoxemia.

Jugular Veins

The jugular veins of the neck are inspected to noninvasively estimate intravascular volume.[10,21]

- ***JVP visualization.*** Elevated jugular venous pressure (JVP) is best observed in the *right internal jugular vein.*[21] If the vein is visible and distended, it is described as *jugular venous distention* (JVD), and this suggests volume overload is present (Fig. 11.2). The right IJV is preferred because of its anatomical proximity to the superior vena cava and right atrium. The procedure to visualize JVD is described in Box 11.2.
- ***JVP measurement.*** The right internal jugular vein can be palpated to permit noninvasive estimation of elevated right atrial pressure (RAP), central venous pressure (CVP) in centimeters (cm) as described in Fig. 11.3 and Box 11.3. With normal fluid volume status, the internal jugular veins are not visible.[10] Thus, a distended right IJV is a cause for concern and any elevation greater than 8 cm is considered high.[21]
- ***JVP assessment by ultrasound.*** Bedside handheld ultrasound, also known as Point of Care Ultrasound (POCUS), is increasingly used to assess and measure jugular vein distention in critical care units and in the emergency department.[22,23] A combination of peripheral edema and JVD identifies a high-risk profile for poor clinical outcomes.[10,24]

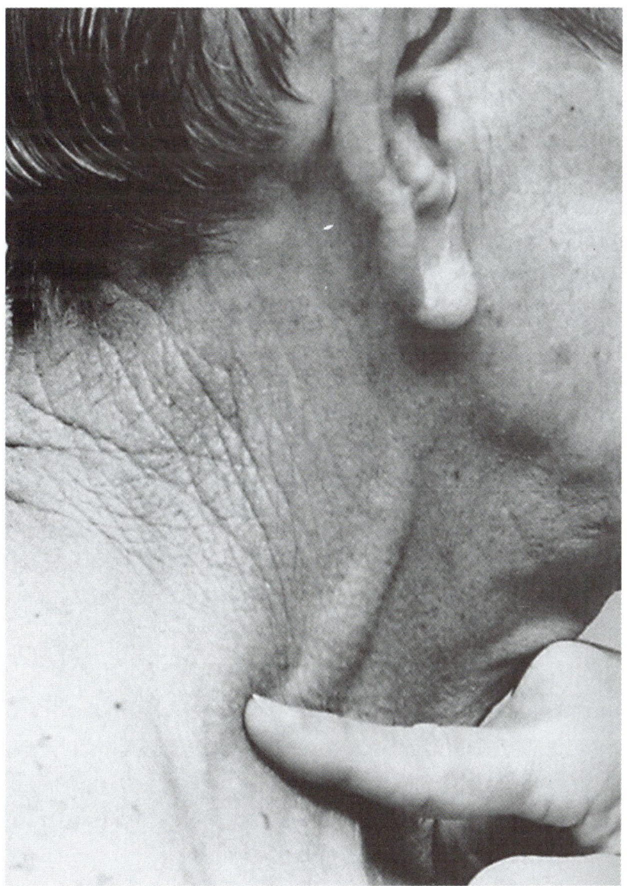

FIG. 11.2 Assessment of Jugular Vein Distention. Applying light finger pressure over the sternocleidomastoid muscle, parallel to the clavicle, helps identify the external jugular vein by occluding flow and distending it. The finger pressure is released, and the patient is observed for true distention. If the patient's trunk is elevated to 30 degrees or more, jugular vein distention should not be present.

Abdominojugular Reflux

The abdominojugular reflux sign can assist with the diagnosis of right ventricular failure. This noninvasive test is used in conjunction with measurement of JVP. The procedure for assessing abdominojugular reflux is described in Box 11.4. A positive abdominojugular reflux sign is an increase in the JVP (CVP equivalent) of 4 cm or more sustained for at least 10 seconds.[3,21] Additionally, point of care handheld ultrasound can be used to assess volume in the inferior vena cava and right heart function.[4,22,24]

Thoracic Reference Points

The thoracic cage is divided with imaginary vertical lines (sternal, midclavicular, axillary, vertebral, and scapular), and the intercostal spaces are divided by imaginary horizontal lines to serve as reference points in locating or describing cardiac findings (Fig. 11.4). The ribs are numbered from 1 (the first rib below the clavicle) to 12. The intercostal space below each rib is given the same number as the rib that lies above it. The second rib is the easiest to locate because it is attached to the sternum at the angle of Louis. This angle (also called the *sternal angle*) is the bony ridge on the sternum that lies approximately 2 inches below the sternal notch (see Fig. 11.4A). After the second rib has been located, it can be used as a reference point to count off the other ribs and intercostal spaces.

BOX 11.2 Procedure for Assessing Jugular Vein Distention

1. The patient reclines at 30- to 45-degree angle.
2. The examiner stands on the patient's right side and turns the patient's head slightly toward the left.
3. If the jugular vein is not visible, light finger pressure is applied across the sternocleidomastoid muscle just above and parallel to the clavicle. This pressure fills the external jugular vein by obstructing flow (see Fig. 11.2).
4. After the location of the vein has been identified, the pressure is released, and the presence of JVD is assessed.
5. Because inhalation decreases venous pressure, JVD should be assessed at end-exhalation.
6. Any fullness in the vein extending more than 3 cm above the sternal angle is evidence of increased venous pressure. Generally, the higher the sitting angle of the patient when JVD is visualized, the higher is the central venous pressure.
7. *Documentation:* JVD is reported by including the angle of the head of the bed at the time JVD was evaluated (e.g., "Presence of JVD with head of bed elevated to 45 degrees").

JVD, Jugular vein distention.

Apical Impulse

The anterior thorax is inspected for the apical impulse, sometimes referred to as the *point of maximal impulse.* The apical impulse occurs as the left ventricle contracts during systole and rotates forward, causing the left ventricular apex of the heart to hit the chest wall. The apical impulse is a quick, localized, outward movement normally located just lateral to the left midclavicular line at the fifth intercostal space in an adult patient (Fig. 11.5).[21] The apical impulse is the only normal pulsation visualized on the chest wall. In a patient without cardiac disease, point of maximal impulse may not be noticeable (see Fig. 11.5).

Palpation

Palpation is a technique that uses the sense of touch in the tips of the fingers and the palm of the hand.

Arterial Pulses

Seven pairs of bilateral arterial pulses are normally palpated. The examination incorporates bilateral assessment of the carotid, brachial, radial, ulnar, popliteal, posterior tibial, and dorsalis pedis arterial pulses. The pulses are palpated separately and compared bilaterally to check for consistency. Pulse volume is graded on a scale of 0 to 3+ (Box 11.5). The abdominal aortic pulse can also be palpated.

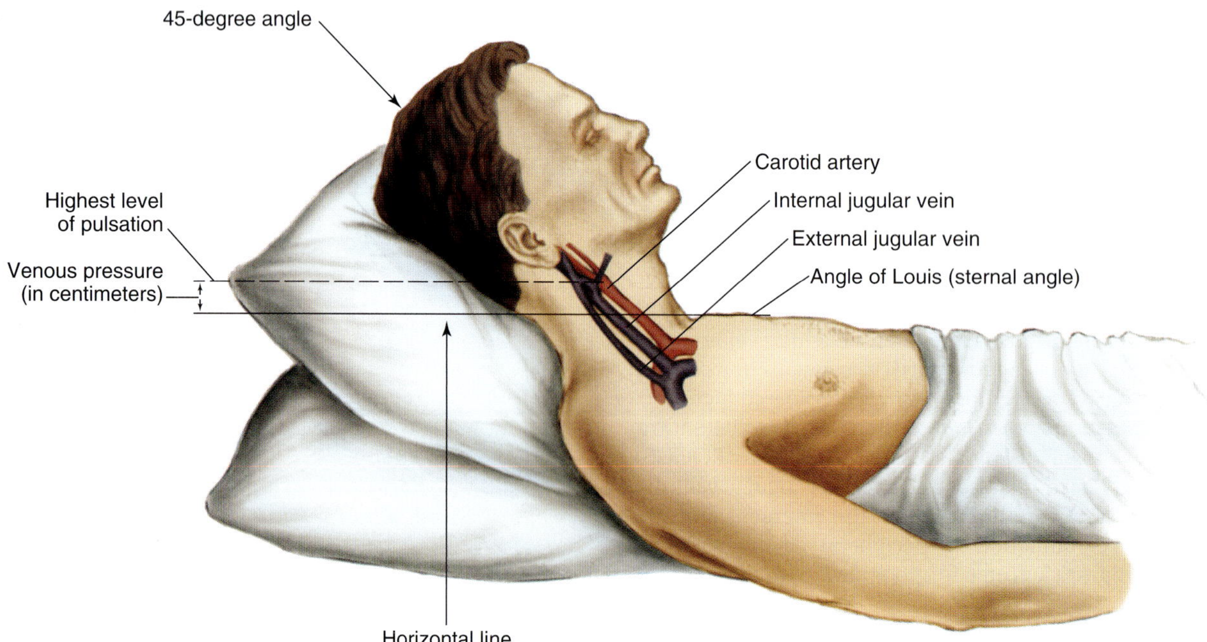

FIG. 11.3 Position of Internal and External Jugular Veins. Pulsation in the internal jugular vein can be used to estimate central venous pressure. (Modified from Thompson JM, McFarland GK. *Mosby's Clinical Nursing.* 5th ed. Mosby; 2002.)

BOX 11.3 Procedure for Assessing Central Venous Pressure

1. The patient reclines in the bed. The highest point of pulsation in the internal jugular vein is observed during exhalation.
2. The vertical distance between this pulsation (top of the fluid level) and the sternal angle is estimated or measured in centimeters.
3. This number is added to 5 cm for an estimation of CVP; 5 cm is the approximate distance of the sternal angle above the level of the right atrium (see Fig. 11.3).
4. *Documentation:* The degree of elevation of the patient is included in the report (e.g., "CVP estimated at 13 cm, using internal jugular vein pulsation, with head of bed elevated 45 degrees").

CVP, Central venous pressure.

BOX 11.4 Procedure for Assessing Abdominojugular Reflux

1. Ask the patient to relax and breathe normally through an open mouth.
2. Measure JVD in the patient's right internal jugular vein, following the procedure described in Box 11.2.
3. Apply firm pressure of approximately 20 to 35 mm Hg to the patient's midabdomen for 15 to 30 seconds and remeasure JVD during the compression.
4. Measure the right JVD a third time after compression is released.
5. Ask the patient not to tense or hold the breath during the test. (Doing so increases venous return to the heart and may produce a false-positive result.)
6. A positive abdominojugular reflux is identified when abdominal compression causes a sustained JVD increase of 4 cm or more. This sign is indicative of right-sided heart failure.
7. A normal abdominojugular reflux is reported if there is no increase in JVD, a transient (<10 s) increase in JVD, or an increase in JVD less than or equal to 3 cm sustained throughout compression.

JVD, Jugular vein distention.

Carotid Pulses

The carotid arteries are assessed at the medial midneck region. If blood flow through the carotid arteries is compromised by atherosclerotic plaque, firm palpation could cause total occlusion. The touch is light, and the carotid arteries are palpated gently and only one at a time. This pulse is also checked during cardiac arrest and cardiopulmonary resuscitation (CPR).[25] As in other areas of the physical examination, the use of ultrasound technology is being studied, especially in the assessment of cardiac arrest.[26]

Brachial, Ulnar, and Radial Pulses

The brachial pulse is assessed by gently palpating the inner aspect of the slightly bent elbow with the fingers. The radial pulse is palpated in the medial area of the wrist (thumb side). The ulnar artery is palpated at the opposite side of the wrist (little finger side). The radial and ulnar arterial pulses must be assessed before an arterial line is inserted; this test, known as the modified *Allen test,* is described in Box 11.6.

Femoral Pulses

The femoral arteries are palpated by pressing deeply into the groin beneath the inguinal ligament, approximately midway between the anterior superior iliac spine and the symphysis pubis. Recent studies have compared the effectiveness of manual femoral pulse palpation with Doppler ultrasound during cardiac arrest and CPR.[27] As with other areas of the physical examination, technology is increasingly being used to conform the results or to provide a digital record of the findings in clinical situations.

Popliteal Pulses

The popliteal pulse is lightly palpated using the fingertips. The patient's leg is very slightly bent, and the clinician's two hands gently cup the patient's knee with the thumbs on top of the kneecap and the fingertips behind the knee.

Dorsalis Pedis and Posterior Tibial Pulses

The pulses of the lower leg and foot are assessed to determine blood flow to the limb and to assess adequacy of cardiac output to the extremities. The dorsalis pedis pulse is located on the upper aspect of the foot. The posterior tibial pulse is located behind the medial malleolus (inner ankle bone) of the lower leg.

Descending Aorta Pulse

When the patient is in the supine position, the abdominal aortic pulsation is located in the epigastric area and can be felt as a forward movement when firm fingertip pressure is applied above the umbilicus. If prominent or diffuse, the pulsation may indicate an abdominal aneurysm.

A diminished or absent pulse may indicate low cardiac output, arterial stenosis, or occlusion proximal to the site of the examination. An abnormally strong or bounding pulse may suggest the presence of an aneurysm or an occlusion distal to the examination site. If a distal pulse cannot be palpated by using light finger pressure, a Doppler ultrasound stethoscope may enhance diagnostic accuracy. It is important to mark the location of the audible signal with an indelible ink marker pen for future evaluation of pulse quality.

Capillary Refill

Capillary refill assessment is an important assessment technique that uses the patient's nail beds to evaluate arterial circulation to the extremity and determine overall perfusion. The nail bed is compressed to produce blanching, after which release of the pressure should result in the return of blood flow and baseline nail color in less than 2 seconds. Capillary refill time of greater than 3 seconds has been associated with poor outcomes in cardiogenic shock.[28] Capillary refill time is a standard component of the cardiovascular physical examination, and as with other aspects of bedside assessment, point of care technologies are being developed to measure capillary refill.[29]

Edema

Edema is fluid accumulation in the extravascular spaces of the body. The dependent tissues within the legs and sacrum are particularly susceptible. Edema may be dependent, unilateral, or bilateral, and pitting or nonpitting. The amount of edema is quantified by measuring the circumference of the limb or by pressing the skin of the feet, ankles, and shins against underlying bone. Edema is a symptom associated with several diseases, and further diagnostic evaluation is required to determine the cause. Although no universal scale for pitting edema exists, typical scales use a system ranging from 0 to 4+ (Table 11.3).

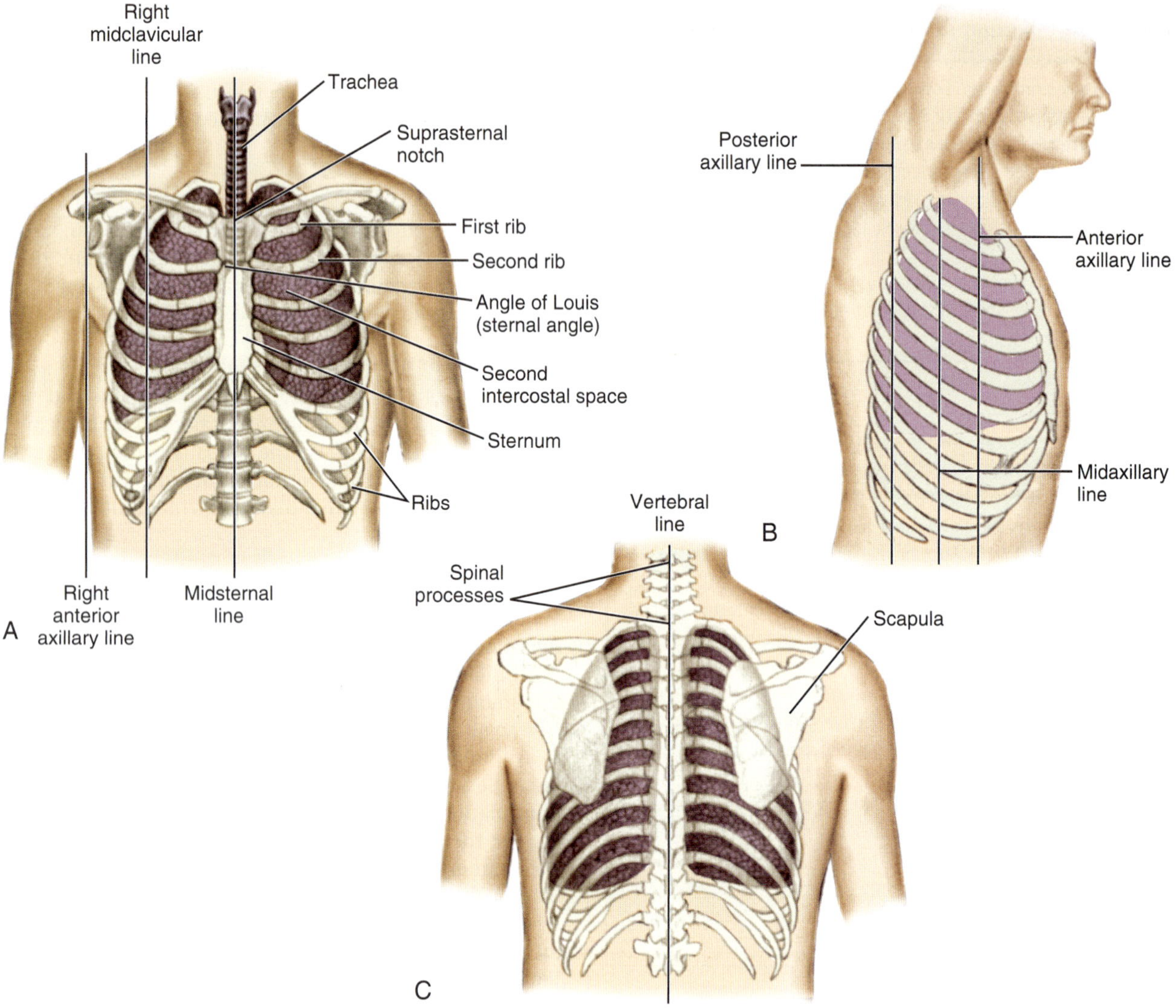

FIG. 11.4 Thoracic Landmarks. (A) Anterior thorax. (B) Right lateral thorax. (C) Posterior thorax.

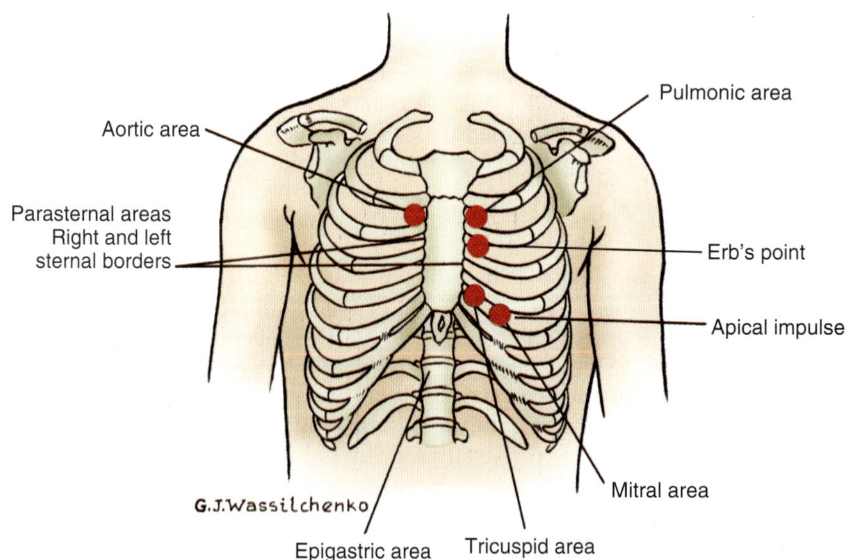

FIG. 11.5 Thoracic Palpation and Auscultation Points.

Auscultation

Auscultation is a vital skill to master in the physical examination. Generally, auscultation involves use of a stethoscope.[30] While most health care professionals use a traditional biaural stethoscope, electronic and digital technologies are increasingly available, and are used in some assessments.[31]

Handheld ultrasound devices are the latest adjunct to the physical examination and are used in critical care and the emergency department for rapid triage and serial assessment in emergency situations.[32] International guidelines recommend that pocket-sized ultrasound images be reported as part of the physical examination, that images be stored in the patient's electronic health care record, and that handheld ultrasound not replace a formal echocardiogram as the images are of lesser quality.[32–34]

BOX 11.5 Pulse Palpation Scale

0	Not palpable
1+	Faintly palpable (weak and thready)
2+	Palpable (normal pulse)
3+	Bounding (hyperdynamic pulse)

BOX 11.6 Procedure for Assessment of Arterial Blood Supply to the Hand: Allen Test

Before a radial artery is punctured or cannulated, the Allen test is performed to assess blood flow to the hand and to ensure that it is adequate.

Allen Test by Visual Inspection

1. If the patient is alert and cooperative, he or she is asked to repeatedly make a tight fist to squeeze the blood out of the hand.
2. The radial artery is compressed with firm thumb pressure by the examiner.
3. The patient is requested to open the hand palm side up while the radial artery is still occluded.
4. Pressure is released, and the time it takes for color to return to the hand is noted.

If the ulnar artery is patent, color will return within 3 seconds. The patient may describe a tingling in the palm as blood flow returns. Delayed color return (a "failed" Allen test) implies that the ulnar artery is inadequate. This means the radial artery is the only reliable source of arterial blood flow to the hand, and therefore it must not be punctured or cannulated.

Allen Test with Pulse Oximetry

1. If the patient is unable to cooperate to make a fist, an alternative approach is to use a pulse oximeter that displays a pulse waveform.
2. Place the pulse oximeter on the patient's middle finger, and establish an adequate pulse amplitude display on the monitor.
3. Simultaneously compress the radial and ulnar arteries until the waveform clearly decreases or vanishes.
4. Release pressure off the ulnar artery only. If the ulnar artery is patent, the pulse amplitude recovers its normal appearance.
5. Repeat the procedure with the radial artery.
6. Arterial catheterization of the radial artery can be accomplished safely only if blood supply to the hand is adequate.

Blood Pressure Measurement

Auscultation of blood pressure (BP) is a noninvasive measurement and is an essential component of every complete physical examination. BP is an important modifiable risk factor for prevention of cardiovascular disease–related premature mortality.[35]

Current BP management guidelines stratify antihypertensive medication treatment goals by age ranges and specific diseases.[35]

- Age 60 years and older, a BP less than 150/90 mm Hg[35]
- Age 30 to 59 years, a BP less than 140/90 mm Hg[35]
- Chronic kidney disease, a BP less than 140/90 mm Hg[35]
- Diabetes, a BP less than 140/90 mm Hg[35]

The JNC8 guideline BP targets were challenged after the results of a breakthrough clinical trial, known as the SPRINT study, that randomized 9361 patients to a systolic BP target of either 140 mm Hg or 120 mm Hg.[36] Patients in this study were older than 50 years, did not have type 2 diabetes, and were representative of the general population of the United States. After 3.3 years follow-up the patients randomized to the lower BP target had fewer major cardiovascular events and lower mortality.[36]

Hypertension requiring treatment is defined by the American Heart Association (AHA) and other cardiac societies as:

- BP higher than 130/80 (Stage 1 hypertension)[37]
- BP higher than 140/90 (Stage 2 hypertension)[37]

Pharmacological treatment for hypertension should be started when the BP is +20 mm Hg (systolic) or +10 mm Hg (diastolic) above goal.[38]

In the critical care setting, systemic BP can be measured directly or indirectly. Direct BP measurement is via an invasive arterial catheter and is discussed in detail in Chapter 12. Indirect BP measurement is with a stethoscope and sphygmomanometer or electronic measuring devices. Ideally, indirect BP values closely reflect direct measurements (within 1 to 3 mm Hg). The following discussion reviews the essential elements of noninvasive BP monitoring.

Noninvasive Blood Pressure Monitoring

The most common peripheral locations for BP monitoring are the bilateral brachial arteries. The pressure is measured in both arms to rule out subclavian arterial stenosis. Normally, the difference in pressure between the arms is expected to be less than 10 mm Hg.[39,40] A higher difference between the bilateral arm pressures suggests arterial obstruction on the side with the lower pressure. Furthermore, data from the Framingham study

TABLE 11.3 Pitting Edema Scale

		Indentation Depth		
Scale	Edema	English Units	Metric Units	Time to Baseline
0	None	0	0	
1+	Trace	0–0.25 inch	<6.5 mm	Rapid
2+	Mild	0.25–0.5 inch	6.5–12.5 mm	10–15 s
3+	Moderate	0.5–1 inch	12.5 mm–2.5 cm	1–2 min
4+	Severe	>1 inch	>2.5 cm	2–5 min

BOX 11.7 Measurement of Postural (Orthostatic) Vital Signs

Guidelines

1. Record BP and HR in each position.
2. Do not remove cuff between measurements.
3. Record all associated signs and symptoms.
4. Document patient position.

Lying

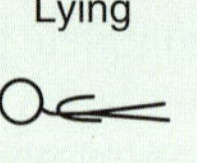

Standing

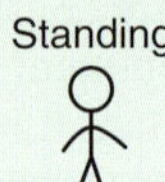

Technique

1. Patient supine and resting: Obtain initial BP and HR measurements.
2. Patient standing: Measure BP and HR after 1 minute and 3 minutes standing.

Results

Positive Orthostasis

- Decrease in systolic BP by more than 20 mm Hg.
- Decrease in diastolic BP by more than 10 mm Hg within 3 minutes standing.

BP, Blood pressure; *HR*, heart rate.

suggest that a difference in BP between the two arms is a predictor for the development of cardiovascular disease.[41]

Correct positioning of the extremity being measured is essential. BP can be measured in any position as long as the arm or the leg is at the level of the heart. Falsely elevated readings are obtained if the arm is at a level lower than the heart, and falsely low pressures are obtained when the arm is at a level higher than the heart.

Orthostatic Hypotension

Postural (orthostatic) hypotension occurs when the systolic BP falls more than 20 mm Hg or the diastolic BP falls more than 10 mm Hg with a change in position from supine to a standing position (Box 11.7).[42–44] After standing, measure BP and HR at 1-minute and at 3-minute intervals.[44] Orthostatic hypotension is typically accompanied by dizziness, lightheadedness, or syncope. It is also an independent predictor of mortality[45] and may be caused by an underlying problem with the autonomic nervous system.[42] In critical care, orthostatic vital sign changes (i.e., decrease in BP and increase in heart rate) may be precipitated by changes in intravascular volume or vascular tone.

- Intravascular volume depletion or fluid loss caused by bleeding, diuresis, or fever.
- Inadequate vascular vasoconstrictor mechanisms to constrict the arterial bed, which can occur after prolonged immobility or as a result of spinal cord injury.
- Autonomic insufficiency caused by administration of pharmacologic agents such as beta-blockers, angiotensin-converting enzyme inhibitors, and calcium channel blockers.

Blood Pressure Cuff Size

Correct size and placement of the BP cuff are essential to obtain accurate BP values. Most BP measurements are now obtained using automated oscillometric devices. Research shows that if the cuff is too large or too small inaccurate BP values are recorded.[46] The cuff should be long enough to encircle at least 80% of the width of the upper arm (or leg). Cuffs that are too small produce falsely high readings, and cuffs that are too large give falsely low readings.[46] Box 11.8 lists the key points to observe when obtaining BP readings.

When the automatic cuff is set to cycle frequently, such as every 15 minutes, cuff placement should be rotated frequently to avoid local skin irritation.

BOX 11.8 Obtaining Accurate Blood Pressure Readings

- Compare right and left measurements.
- Position the extremity at the level of the heart.
- Document the position of the patient.
- Ensure proper cuff size.
- Measure readings at eye level at the top of the meniscus.

Korotkoff Sounds

Obtaining systemic BP readings involves auscultation of *Korotkoff sounds*, the sounds created by turbulence of blood flow within a vessel caused by constriction of the BP cuff. The pressure in the cuff is inflated above the normal systolic pressure. As the pressure in the cuff is reduced, Korotkoff sounds change in quality and intensity. These sounds are divided into five stages. The systolic BP is the highest point at which initial tapping occurs. Diastolic BP is equated with the complete disappearance of Korotkoff sounds. Often, a muffling of diastolic sounds occurs before these sounds completely disappear. This has caused debate about which diastolic value to record. Because complete disappearance of Korotkoff sounds corresponds more closely to intraarterial catheter measurement, it is the value that should be recorded.

Auscultatory Gap

In older patients with systolic hypertension, the presence of an *auscultatory gap* is common. It is important to inflate the cuff to greater than the patient's normal systolic pressure to avoid this gap and underestimation of systolic BP. Use of an initial palpation estimate of the systolic BP taken before auscultation with a stethoscope is one recommended method to accurately determine the upper systolic BP.

Pulse Pressure

Pulse pressure describes the difference between systolic and diastolic values. The normal pulse pressure is 40 mm Hg (i.e., the difference between a systolic BP of 120 mm Hg and a diastolic BP of 80 mm Hg). In a critically ill patient, a low BP is frequently associated with a narrow pulse pressure.

For example, a patient with a BP of 90/72 mm Hg has a pulse pressure of 18 mm Hg. The narrowed pulse pressure is a temporary compensatory mechanism caused by arterial vasoconstriction resulting from volume depletion or heart failure. The narrow pulse pressure ensures that the mean arterial pressure (78 mm Hg in this example) remains in a therapeutic range to provide adequate organ perfusion.

In contrast, a hypotensive patient with sepsis who exhibits vasodilation has a wide pulse pressure and inadequate organ perfusion. If the BP is 90/36 mm Hg, the pulse pressure is 54 mm Hg, and the mean arterial pressure is an inadequate 54 mm Hg. In both of these examples, the systolic BP is the same (90 mm Hg); the difference in pulse pressure is a function of intravascular volume and vascular tone.

Pulsus Paradoxus

In normal physiology, the strength of the pulse fluctuates throughout the respiratory cycle. When the "pulse" is measured using the SBP, the pressure is observed to decrease slightly during inspiration and to increase slightly during respiratory exhalation. The normal difference is 2 to 4 mm Hg. In some clinical conditions such as cardiac tamponade, the BP decline is abnormally large during inspiration. In general, an inspiratory decline of systolic BP greater than 10 mm Hg is considered diagnostic of pulsus paradoxus. The techniques for measuring pulsus paradoxus using a sphygmomanometer, BP cuff, and pulse oximetry waveform are described in Box 11.9. If the patient is hypotensive, pulsus paradoxus is more accurately assessed in the critical care unit by monitoring a pulse oximetry waveform or an indwelling arterial catheter waveform.

Pulsus Alternans

Pulsus alternans describes a regular pattern of pulse amplitude changes that alternate between stronger and weaker beats. This finding is suggestive of end-stage left ventricular heart failure.

Vascular Bruits

The carotid and femoral arteries are auscultated for bruits. A bruit, a high-pitched "sh-sh" sound, is an extracardiac vascular sound that vacillates in volume with systole and diastole. An abnormal bruit is produced as blood flows through a partially occluded vessel. Auscultation of a bruit can expedite the diagnosis of suspected arterial obstruction.

Normal Heart Sounds

Auscultation of the heart with a stethoscope is considered the most challenging part of the cardiac physical examination. Electronic, digital, and ultrasound devices are increasingly used at the bedside as adjuncts to improve cardiac auscultation technique.[47,48] While technology will continue to enhance the physical examination, especially when digital findings can be preserved in the electronic health record, an understanding of the underlying principles of cardiac anatomy, physiology, and auscultation will always be required to accurately interpret heart sounds and murmurs.

A summary of the advice given by most experts to effectively acquire the skills of cardiac auscultation using the traditional stethoscope include:

- Auscultate systematically across the precordium.
- Visualize the cardiac anatomy under each point of auscultation, expecting to hear the physiologically associated sounds.
- Memorize the cardiac cycle to enhance the ability to hear abnormal sounds.
- Practice, practice, practice.

First and Second Heart Sounds

Normal heart sounds are referred to as the *first heart sound* (S_1) and the *second heart sound* (S_2). S_1 is the sound associated with mitral and tricuspid valve closure and is heard most clearly in the mitral and tricuspid areas. S_2 (aortic and pulmonic closure) can be heard best at the second intercostal space to the right and left of the sternum (see Fig. 11.5). Both sounds are high pitched and heard best with the diaphragm of the stethoscope (Box 11.10). Each sound is loudest in an auscultation area located downstream from the actual valvular component of the sound, as shown in Fig. 11.6.

Physiologic Splitting of S_1 and S_2

Each normal heart sound has two components: right and left. Mitral valve closure and tricuspid valve closure are responsible for S_1, and aortic valve closure and pulmonic valve closure are responsible for S_2. All the components of the split sounds are high pitched and best heard with the diaphragm of the stethoscope (Fig. 11.7). Normally, sounds emitted from the left side are louder than sounds from the right because left ventricular contraction occurs milliseconds before right ventricular contraction. Physiologic splitting is accentuated by inspiration and usually disappears on expiration. This splitting is most easily detected on inspiration, because there is an increased amount of blood return to the right side of the heart and a decreased amount of blood return to the left side of the heart. As a result, pulmonic valve closure is delayed because of the extra time needed for the increased blood volume to pass through the pulmonic valve, and aortic valve closure is early because of the relatively smaller amount of blood ejected from the left ventricle.

BOX 11.9 Procedure for Measuring Pulsus Paradoxus

Measurement With Sphygmomanometer

1. The patient should be lying supine in a comfortable position.
2. The breathing pattern should be of normal depth and rate to avoid excessive respiratory interference.
3. BP is measured following standard procedures (see Boxes 11.7 and 11.8). The sphygmomanometer cuff is inflated to a pressure greater than systolic BP, and Korotkoff sounds are auscultated over the brachial artery while the cuff is deflated at a rate of approximately 2 to 3 mm Hg per heartbeat.
4. The peak systolic BP during expiration (i.e., pressure at which Korotkoff sounds are heard only during expiration) should be identified and then reconfirmed.
5. The cuff is deflated slowly to establish systolic BP at which Korotkoff sounds become audible during both inspiration and expiration.
6. If the auscultated difference between these two systolic BP values exceeds 10 mm Hg during quiet respiration, a paradoxical pulse is present.

Measurement by Waveform Analysis

1. A pulse oximetry sensor with a visible pulse waveform can be used as an additional measurement device.
2. In the critical care unit, an arterial waveform from an indwelling arterial catheter (if present) can be used to measure the difference in systolic BP between expiration and inspiration.

BP, Blood pressure.

BOX 11.10 Characteristics of First and Second Heart Sounds

First Heart Sound (S_1)	Second Heart Sound (S_2)
High pitched	High pitched
Loudest in mitral area (apex)	Loudest in aortic area (base)
Split S_1	Split S_2
Normal split less than 20 ms	Normal split less than 30 ms
Split heard best in tricuspid area	Split heard best in pulmonic area
Important to differentiate between split S_1 and S_4	↑ Split with inhalation
Occurs immediately before carotid upstroke	↓ Split with exhalation

↑, Increased; ↓, decreased, *ms*, milliseconds.

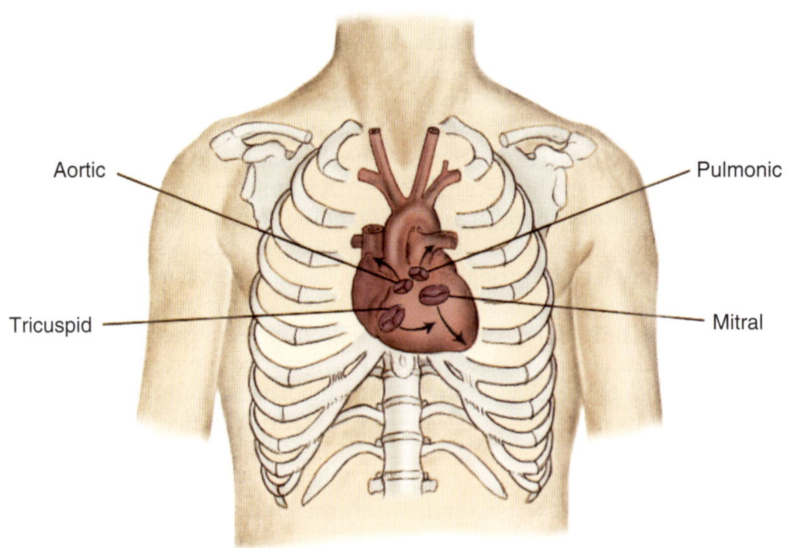

FIG. 11.6 Transmission of Heart Sounds to Thorax and Their Relationship to Anatomic Position of Heart Valves.

	HEART SOUNDS		AREA BEST HEARD
A	S_1 S_2	Intense first sound	Mitral
B	S_1 M T S_2	Split first sound	Tricuspid
C	S_1 S_2	Intense second sound	Aortic
D	S_1 S_2	Physiologic splitting—S_2 Expiration	Pulmonic
	S_1 S_2 A P	Inspiration	
E	S_1 S_2 S_3	Third sound (ventricular gallop)	Mitral
F	S_4 S_1 S_2	Fourth sound (atrial gallop)	Mitral
G	S_1 S_2 $S_{3\text{-}4}$	Summation gallop	Mitral

FIG. 11.7 Characteristics of Normal and Abnormal Heart Sounds and Auscultatory Areas: Where Each Is Best Heard With a Stethoscope.

The resulting heart sound is a split S_2 (the closure of each valve is audible because there is more time between left and right contractions) (see Fig. 11.7).

Pathologic Splitting of S_1 and S_2

A variety of abnormalities can alter the intensity and timing of split heart sounds. For example, during auscultation in the pulmonic area, a pathologic split is audible with a stethoscope if the pulmonic valve closure occurs after the aortic valve closure. Pathologic splitting of S_1 and S_2 is associated with specific cardiovascular conditions such as pulmonary hypertension, pulmonic stenosis, and right ventricular failure and with electrical conduction disturbances such as right bundle branch block and premature ventricular contractions.

Abnormal Heart Sounds

Recognition of abnormal heart sounds is a skill that requires practice, patience, and a quiet environment as these are low-pitched sounds and only audible in the setting of heart failure of volume overload.

Third and Fourth Heart Sounds

Abnormal heart sounds are known as the *third heart sound* (S_3) and the *fourth heart sound* (S_4). These are referred to as *gallops* when auscultated during an episode of tachycardia. These low-pitched sounds occur during diastole and are best heard with the bell of the stethoscope positioned lightly over the apical impulse.[49] The characteristics of S_3 and S_4 are described in detail in Box 11.11. The presence of S_3 may be normal in children, young adults, and pregnant women because of rapid filling of the ventricle in a young, healthy heart. However, auscultation of an S_3 in the presence of cardiac symptoms suggests advanced heart failure, a noncompliant ventricle, and fluid overload.

Auscultation of S_4 leads the examiner to suspect heart failure and decreased ventricular compliance. Also referred to as an *atrial gallop*, S_4 occurs at the end of diastole (just before S_1), when the ventricle is full.[49] It is associated with atrial contraction, also called *atrial kick*.

BOX 11.11 Characteristics of Third and Fourth Heart Sounds

Third Heart Sound (S_3)	Fourth Heart Sound (S_4)
Physiologic Causes	
Related to diastolic motion and rapid filling of ventricles in early diastole	Related to diastolic motion and ventricular dilation with atrial contraction in late diastole
Can be normal in children and young adults (<40 years old)	May occur with or without cardiac decompensation
	Ventricular hypertrophy with decrease in ventricular compliance (CAD, systemic hypertension, cardiomyopathy, aortic or pulmonary stenosis, increase in intensity with acute MI or angina)
Pathologic Causes	
Ventricular dysfunction with increase in end-systolic volume (MI, heart failure, valvular disease, systemic or pulmonary hypertension)	Hyperkinetic states (anemia, thyrotoxicosis, arteriovenous fistula)
Hyperdynamic states (anemia, thyrotoxicosis, mitral or tricuspid regurgitation)	Acute valvular regurgitation
Rhythmic Word Association	
"Kentucky": S_1, S_2, S_3	"Tennessee": S_4, S_1, S_2
Synonyms	
Ventricular gallop	Atrial gallop
Protodiastolic gallop	Presystolic gallop

CAD, Coronary artery disease; *MI*, myocardial infarction.

Heart Murmurs

Heart valve murmurs are prolonged extra sounds that occur during systole or diastole and are typically a sign of either ventricular dysfunction or valvular heart disease.[50–52] Mortality is increased with multivalve disease.[53]

Murmurs are produced by turbulent blood flow through the chambers of the heart, from forward flow through narrowed or irregular valve openings, or backward regurgitant flow through an incompetent valve. Murmurs occur in both systole and diastole. Most murmurs are caused by structural cardiac changes. The steps to auscultate effectively and accurately for cardiac murmurs are listed in Box 11.12. Murmurs are characterized by specific criteria:

- *Timing:* Place in the cardiac cycle (systole/diastole)
- *Location:* Where the sound is auscultated on the chest wall (mitral or aortic area)
- *Radiation:* How far the sound spreads across the chest wall
- *Quality:* Whether the murmur is blowing, grating, or harsh
- *Pitch:* Whether the tone is high or low
- *Intensity:* Loudness is graded on a scale of 1 to 6; the higher the number, the louder the murmur (Box 11.13)

The four most common valvular murmurs auscultated in adults are briefly discussed in the following sections. For more information on valvular anatomy, refer to Chapter 10; for information on valvular heart disease diagnostic procedures, see Chapter 12; for valve-related therapeutic interventions, see Chapters 13 and 14.

Mitral Stenosis Murmur

The term *mitral stenosis* refers to narrowing of the mitral valve orifice. This narrowing produces a low-pitched murmur, which varies in intensity and harshness depending on the degree of valvular stenosis. It occurs during diastole, is auscultated at the mitral area (fifth intercostal space, midclavicular line), and does not radiate. A prolonged duration of the murmur during diastole suggests that the mitral stenosis is severe.[21] As mitral stenosis progresses, left atrial enlargement occurs, often leading to atrial fibrillation and development of left atrial thrombi. The increased left atrial pressure increases pressure in the pulmonary vasculature. This causes a moist cough, decreased exercise tolerance, and breathlessness (dyspnea), especially with exercise.

Mitral Regurgitation Murmur

Mitral regurgitation is described as acute or chronic. Causes of *acute mitral regurgitation* include rupture of a papillary muscle after an acute myocardial infarction (MI) and rupture of one or more chordae tendineae. As a result, when the ventricle contracts during systole, a jet of blood is sent in a retrograde manner to the left atrium, causing a sudden increase in left atrial pressure, acute pulmonary edema, and low cardiac output leading to cardiogenic shock.

BOX 11.12 Technique of Auscultation of Heart Sounds and Murmurs

1. Stethoscope
   - Diaphragm
   - Larger surface area
   - Brings out higher frequency and filters out lower frequency
   - Use for listening to S_1/S_2 (split S_1/S_2), loud murmurs, pericardial friction rubs
   - Bell
   - Smaller surface area
   - Filters out high-frequency sounds and accentuates low-frequency sounds
   - Rest lightly on area (or else it becomes a diaphragm)
2. Location: Heart sounds auscultated at *APTM*
   A: Aortic area (second right ICS along sternal border)
   P: Pulmonic area (second left ICS along sternal border)
   T: Tricuspid area (fourth left ICS along sternal border)
   M: Mitral area (fifth ICS at MCL)
3. "Know your bases"
   - Base of the heart refers to the right and left second ICS beside the sternum S_2 where the aortic or pulmonic sounds are auscultated
   - Apex or left ventricular area refers to the fifth ICS along the MCL
   - Most commonly referred to as PMI
   - Also referred to as mitral area
   - S_1 and mitral sounds are loudest here
   - Erb's point: Second aortic area (third left ICS along sternal border); pericardial friction rubs are heard best here
4. Palpation
   - Location
   - Palpate carotid pulse (or watch ECG to identify S_1 and S_2)
5. Be quiet and patient
   - Listen for S_1 and S_2 first, ignoring all other sounds
   - Inching technique
   - After you are sure which is S_1 or S_2, try to determine when the other sound comes in
   - Is it systolic or diastolic?
   - S_3 and S_4 are best heard with patient in left lateral decubitus position; note the location (suggests origin of sound)
   - Note the timing (S_4 comes just before S_1, and S_3 comes just after S_2)
6. Interpret the sounds based on the clinical condition

ECG, Electrocardiogram; *ICS*, intercostal space; *MCL*, midclavicular line; *PMI*, point of maximal impulse.

BOX 11.13 Grading of Cardiac Murmurs

Grade	Description
1	Very faint; may be heard only in quiet environment
2	Quiet but clearly audible
3	Moderately loud
4	Loud; may be associated with palpable thrill
5	Very loud; thrill easily palpable
6	Very loud; may be heard with stethoscope off the chest Thrill palpable and visible

Causes of *chronic mitral regurgitation* may be caused by deterioration of the valve structures (leaflets, chordae tendineae). It occurs in older adults from loss of valvular connective tissue and in younger adults from degenerative valve changes associated with mitral prolapse. The murmur of mitral regurgitation is auscultated in the mitral area and occurs during systole. It is high pitched and blowing, although the pitch and intensity vary depending on the degree of regurgitation. As mitral regurgitation progresses, the murmur radiates more widely. The murmur of mitral regurgitation can also occur when a dilated ventricle impedes the mitral valve from closing completely during systole. One can detect the murmur with auscultation but not identify the cause of mitral regurgitation.[54]

Aortic Stenosis Murmur

The term *aortic stenosis* describes narrowing of the aortic valve orifice. As a result, the left ventricle faces increasing difficulty in ejecting blood to the aorta. The ventricle responds by increasing intraventricular pressure and adding muscle mass (left ventricular hypertrophy).[55] Over time, because of the pressure load and the increasingly restricted aortic valve outflow, the left ventricle fails and loses contractile force. The decreased blood volume entering the aorta during systole means that the coronary arteries do not fill efficiently, and chest pain is a common symptom of aortic stenosis. This chest pain can be difficult to differentiate from angina caused by CAD. Other symptoms include dizziness, syncope, and breathlessness secondary to left ventricular heart failure. After symptoms occur, the clinical course is poor unless the aortic valve is replaced. The murmur of aortic stenosis occurs during systole. It is auscultated at the aortic area (second intercostal space, right sternal border). Aortic stenosis produces a low-pitched murmur that does not radiate, although the tone of the murmur varies, depending on the degree of valvular obstruction. Because a strong correlation does not exist between the loudness of the murmur, clinical symptoms, and the severity of the stenosis, especially if critical illness and hypotension are present, it is important to use ultrasound color Doppler and transthoracic echocardiography to visualize the valve after an aortic stenosis murmur is detected.[55]

Aortic Insufficiency Murmur

The term *aortic regurgitation* describes an incompetent aortic valve. Also commonly known as *aortic insufficiency*, it is often described in layperson's terms as a "leaking valve." After the left ventricle has ejected blood into the aorta, the valve normally closes, maintains a tight seal, and prevents blood from moving back into the left ventricle. If the valve cusps do not maintain this seal, the sound of blood flowing back into the left ventricle during diastole is heard as a decrescendo, high-pitched, blowing murmur. This early diastolic murmur is initially audible at the aortic area (second intercostal space, right sternal border), but as the aortic regurgitation progresses, it can be auscultated along the length of the left sternal border. As with all valvular murmurs, the pitch and intensity vary with the degree of regurgitation. A prolonged murmur indicates more severe regurgitation is present.[56] Physical assessment findings are initially investigated noninvasively by echocardiography.[50–52] Box 11.14 lists expected abnormal findings at each of the key auscultation areas; Table 11.4 compares the features of the most common valvular murmurs.

Innocent Murmurs

In children, adolescents, and healthy young adults, systolic "high-flow" murmurs are common and are a result of vigorous ventricular contraction. These nonpathologic murmurs are termed *innocent murmurs*. They are always systolic, have a low

BOX 11.14 Auscultation of the Cardiac Valves

Aortic Area
- S_2 loud
- Aortic systolic murmur

Tricuspid Area
- S_1 split
- Right ventricular S_3 and S_4
- Tricuspid valve murmurs
- Murmur of ventricular septal defect

Pulmonic Area
- S_2 loud and split with inhalation
- Pulmonic valve murmurs

Mitral Area
- S_1 loud
- Left ventricular S_3 and S_4
- Mitral valve murmurs

Erb's Point
- S_2 split with inhalation
- Aortic diastolic murmur
- Pericardial friction rub

to medium pitch (heard best with the bell of the stethoscope), and are of grade 1 to 2 intensity with a blowing quality. They are often heard best in the tricuspid area and do not radiate (Box 11.15).

Murmurs Associated With Myocardial Infarction

At the bedside, the nurse may be the first person to auscultate a new murmur. Holosystolic or pansystolic murmurs that can occur acutely as a complication of MI are good examples.

Papillary Muscle Rupture Murmur

The auscultation of a new, high-pitched, holosystolic, blowing murmur at the cardiac apex heralds mitral valve regurgitation resulting from papillary muscle dysfunction. This murmur may be soft (grade 1 or 2) and may occur only during ischemic episodes when papillary muscle contractility is impaired, but its presence is associated with persistent

TABLE 11.4 Characteristics of Some Murmurs

Defects	Timing in Cardiac Cycle	Pitch; Intensity; Quality	Location; Radiation
Systolic Murmurs			
Mitral regurgitation	S_1 S_2	High; harsh; blowing	Mitral area; may radiate to axilla
Tricuspid regurgitation	S_1 S_2	High; often faint, but varies; blowing	Tricuspid RLSB, apex, LLSB, epigastric areas; little radiation
Ventricular septal defect	S_1 S_2	High; loud; blowing	Left sternal border
Aortic stenosis	S_1 S_2	"Chhhh hh;" medium; rough, harsh	Aortic area to suprasternal notch, right side of neck, apex
Pulmonary stenosis	S_1 S_2	Low to medium; loud; harsh, grinding	Pulmonic area; no radiation
Diastolic Murmurs			
Mitral stenosis	Atrial kick S_2 S_1	Low; quiet to loud with thrill; rough rumble	Mitral area; usually no radiation
Tricuspid stenosis	Atrial kick S_2 S_1	Medium; quiet; louder with inspiration; rumble	Tricuspid area or epigastrium; little radiation
Aortic regurgitation	S_2 S_1	High; faint to medium; blowing	Aortic area to LLSB and aorta; Erb's point
Pulmonic regurgitation	S_2 S_1	Medium; faint; blowing	Pulmonic area; no radiation

LLSB, Left lower sternal border; *RLSB*, right lower sternal border.

BOX 11.15 Description of Innocent Murmurs

- Always systolic
- Soft, short (grade 1 or 2, low pitched)
- Modified by change in position
- Normal S_2
- Most common at left sternal border

pain, ventricular failure, and higher mortality. If the murmur is loud (grade 5 or 6), harsh, and radiating in all directions from the apex, the papillary muscle or the chordae tendineae may have ruptured. The clinical auscultation of a new murmur is always confirmed by transthoracic or transesophageal echocardiography.[55] Papillary muscle rupture is an emergency situation requiring immediate medical and surgical intervention.

Ventricular Septal Rupture Murmur

Ventricular septal rupture is a rare emergency situation that can occur after an acute MI. Ventricular septal rupture describes a new opening in the septum between the two ventricles. It creates a harsh, holosystolic murmur that is loudest (by auscultation) along the lower left sternal border.[57] The murmur does not vary with respiration.[21] The clinical picture associated with acute ventricular septal rupture is that of acute ventricular failure and cardiogenic shock. Immediate diagnosis and treatment are necessary to prevent death.[57]

Pericardial Friction Rub

A pericardial friction rub is a sound that can occur 2 to 7 days after an MI. The friction rub results from pericardial inflammation (pericarditis).[4,57] A pericardial friction rub can be auscultated in many cases. Classically, a pericardial friction rub is a grating or scratching sound that is both systolic and diastolic, corresponding with cardiac motion within the pericardial sac. It is often associated with chest pain, which can be aggravated by deep inspiration, coughing, swallowing, and changing position.[58] It is important to differentiate pericarditis from acute myocardial ischemia, and the detection of a pericardial friction rub through auscultation, or handheld ultrasound imaging at the bedside, can assist in this differentiation, leading to effective diagnosis and treatment.[4,57]

KEY POINTS

- An accurate history from the patient or from a family member or significant other who knows the individual's current state of health is essential. Signs and symptoms experienced by the patient offer clues as to the underlying causes of the cardiac condition. If the patient exhibits obvious signs of acute distress (shortness of breath, pink-frothy sputum, hypotension, tachycardia, pallor, sweating) or complains of chest pain or pressure, the questions are brief and focused to quickly identify the immediate problem.
- Inspection is used to determine whether the patient is anxious or relaxed. Inspection is also used to identify serious conditions such as cyanosis, clubbing of fingernails, or significant peripheral edema.
- Palpation of the major pulses is a routine part of the cardiovascular physical examination. Normally, pulses are equal bilaterally. The loss of a pulse on one side may indicate the presence of atherosclerotic arterial vascular disease.
- Auscultation of heart sounds and murmurs is a skill that takes time and practice to master. When performed skillfully, auscultation can reveal much about cardiac function and blood flow.
- Physical examination findings are being augmented by point of care technology, specifically handheld ultrasound and electronic/digital stethoscopes.

Visit the Evolve site at http://evolve.elsevier.com/Urden/CriticalCareNursing for additional study materials.

REFERENCES

1. Lekic M, Lekic V, Riaz IB, Mackstaller L, Marcus FI. The cardiovascular physical examination – is it still relevant? *Am J Cardiol*. 2021;149:140–144. https://doi.org/10.1016/j.amjcard.2021.02.042.
2. Drazner MH. Insights from the history and physical examination in HFpEF or HFrEF: similarities and differences. *JACC Heart Fail*. 2021;9(5):398–400. https://doi.org/10.1016/j.jchf.2021.02.009.
3. Thibodeau JT, Drazner MH. The role of the clinical examination in patients with heart failure. *JACC Heart Fail*. 2018;6(7):543–551. https://doi.org/10.1016/j.jchf.2018.04.005.
4. Henning RJ. Handheld ultrasound as an adjunct to physical examination in the diagnosis of cardiopulmonary disease. *Future Cardiology*. 2022;18(7):585–600. https://doi.org/10.2217/fca-2021-0142.
5. Weinstock C, Wagner H, Snuckel M, Katz M. Evidence-based approach to palpitations. *Med Clin North Am*. 2021;105(1):93–106. https://doi.org/10.1016/j.mcna.2020.09.004.
6. Gulati M, Levy PD, Mukherjee D, et al. 2021 AHA/ACC/ASE/CHEST/SAEM/SCCT/SCMR guideline for the evaluation and diagnosis of chest pain: a report of the American College of Cardiology/American Heart Association Joint Committee on Clinical Practice Guidelines. *Circulation*. 2021;144(22):e368–e454. https://doi.org/10.1161/CIR.0000000000001029.
7. Wertli MM, Dangma TD, Müller SE, et al. Non-cardiac chest pain patients in the emergency department: do physicians have a plan how to diagnose and treat them? A retrospective study. *PLoS One*. 2019;14(2):e0211615. https://doi.org/10.1371/journal.pone.0211615.
8. Kontos MC, de Lemos JA, Deitelzweig SB, et al. 2022 ACC expert consensus decision pathway on the evaluation and disposition of acute chest pain in the emergency department: a report of the American College of Cardiology Solution Set Oversight Committee. *J Am Coll Cardiol*. 2022;80(20):1925–1960. https://doi.org/10.1016/j.jacc.2022.08.750.
9. Bhatt DL, Lopes RD, Harrington RA. Diagnosis and treatment of acute coronary syndromes: a review. *JAMA*. 2022;327(7):662–675. https://doi.org/10.1001/jama.2022.0358.
10. Seitz MP, Minhas S, Khouzam A, Khouzam N, Harper Y. The face is the mirror of the soul. The cardiovascular physical exam is not yet dead. *Curr Probl Cardiol*. 2021;46(3):100644. https://doi.org/10.1016/j.cpcardiol.2020.100644.
11. Wong AKI, Charpignon M, Kim H, et al. Analysis of discrepancies between pulse oximetry and arterial oxygen saturation measurements by race and ethnicity and association with organ dysfunction and mortality. *JAMA Netw Open*. 2021;4(11):e2131674. https://doi.org/10.1001/jamanetworkopen.2021.31674.
12. Gottlieb ER, Ziegler J, Morley K, Rush B, Celi LA. Assessment of racial and ethnic differences in oxygen supplementation among patients in the intensive care unit. *JAMA Intern Med*. 2022;182(8):849–858. https://doi.org/10.1001/jamainternmed.2022.2587.
13. Fawzy A, Wu TD, Wang K, et al. Racial and ethnic discrepancy in pulse oximetry and delayed identification of treatment eligibility among patients with COVID-19. *JAMA Intern Med*. 2022;182(7):730. https://doi.org/10.1001/jamainternmed.2022.1906.

14. Criqui MH, Matsushita K, Aboyans V, et al. Lower extremity peripheral artery disease: contemporary epidemiology, management gaps, and future directions: a scientific statement from the American Heart Association. *Circulation*. 2021;144(9):e171–e191. https://doi.org/10.1161/CIR.0000000000001005.
15. Gogalniceanu P, Lancaster RT, Patel VI. Clinical assessment of peripheral arterial disease of the lower limbs. *N Engl J Med*. 2018;378(18):e24. https://doi.org/10.1056/NEJMvcm1406358.
16. Coke LA, Dennison-Himmelfarb C. Peripheral arterial disease prevention in women: awareness and action. *J Cardiovasc Nurs*. 2019;34(6):427–429. https://doi.org/10.1097/JCN.0000000000000617.
17. Aboyans V, Ricco JB, Bartelink MLEL, et al. 2017 ESC guidelines on the diagnosis and treatment of peripheral arterial diseases, in collaboration with the European Society for Vascular Surgery (ESVS): document covering atherosclerotic disease of extracranial carotid and vertebral, mesenteric, renal, upper and lower extremity arteries. Endorsed by: the European Stroke Organization (ESO). The Task Force for the Diagnosis and Treatment of Peripheral Arterial Diseases of the European Society of Cardiology (ESC) and of the European Society for Vascular Surgery (ESVS). *Eur Heart J*. 2018;39(9):763–816. https://doi.org/10.1093/eurheartj/ehx095.
18. De Maeseneer MG, Kakkos SK, Aherne T, et al. European Society for Vascular Surgery (ESVS) 2022 clinical practice guidelines on the management of chronic venous disease of the lower limbs. *Eur J Vasc Endovasc Surg*. 2022;63(2):184–267. https://doi.org/10.1016/j.ejvs.2021.12.024.
19. Powell-Wiley TM, Poirier P, Burke LE, et al. Obesity and cardiovascular disease: a scientific statement from the American Heart Association. *Circulation*. 2021;143(21):e984–e1010. https://doi.org/10.1161/CIR.0000000000000973.
20. Bielecka-Dabrowa A, Ebner N, Dos Santos MR, Ishida J, Hasenfuss G, von Haehling S. Cachexia, muscle wasting, and frailty in cardiovascular disease. *Eur J Heart Fail*. 2020;22(12):2314–2326. https://doi.org/10.1002/ejhf.2011.
21. Higgins JP. Physical examination of the cardiovascular system. *Int J Clin Cardiol*. 2015;2(1). https://clinmedjournals.org/articles/ijcc/ijcc-2-019.pdf.
22. Jassim HM, Naushad VA, Khatib MY, et al. IJV collapsibility index vs IVC collapsibility index by point of care ultrasound for estimation of CVP: a comparative study with direct estimation of CVP. *Open Access Emerg Med*. 2019;11:65–75. https://doi.org/10.2147/OAEM.S176175.
23. Vaidya GN, Kolodziej A, Stoner B, et al. Bedside ultrasound of the internal jugular vein to assess fluid status and right ventricular function: the POCUS-JVD study. *Am J Emerg Med*. 2023;70:151–156. https://doi.org/10.1016/j.ajem.2023.05.042.
24. Pellicori P, Platz E, Dauw J, et al. Ultrasound imaging of congestion in heart failure: examinations beyond the heart. *Eur J Heart Fail*. 2021;23(5):703–712. https://doi.org/10.1002/ejhf.2032.
25. Badra K, Coutin A, Simard R, Pinto R, Lee JS, Chenkin J. The POCUS pulse check: a randomized controlled crossover study comparing pulse detection by palpation versus by point-of-care ultrasound. *Resuscitation*. 2019;139:17–23. https://doi.org/10.1016/j.resuscitation.2019.03.009.
26. Rolston DM. Time is running out for manual pulse checks as ultrasound races past. *Resuscitation*. 2022;179:59–60. https://doi.org/10.1016/j.resuscitation.2022.07.031.
27. Cohen AL, Li T, Becker LB, et al. Femoral artery Doppler ultrasound is more accurate than manual palpation for pulse detection in cardiac arrest. *Resuscitation*. 2022;173:156–165. https://doi.org/10.1016/j.resuscitation.2022.01.030.
28. Merdji H, Curtiaud A, Aheto A, et al. Performance of early capillary refill time measurement on outcomes in cardiogenic shock: an observational, prospective multicentric study. *Am J Respir Crit Care Med*. 2022;206(10):1230–1238. https://doi.org/10.1164/rccm.202204-0687OC.
29. Sheridan DC, Cloutier RL, Samatham R, Hansen ML. Point-of-care capillary refill technology improves accuracy of peripheral perfusion assessment. *Front Med*. 2021;8:694241. https://doi.org/10.3389/fmed.2021.694241.
30. Choudry M, Stead TS, Mangal RK, Ganti L. The history and evolution of the stethoscope. *Cureus*. 2022;14(8):e28171. https://doi.org/10.7759/cureus.28171.
31. Luo H, Lamata P, Bazin S, et al. Smartphone as an electronic stethoscope: factors influencing heart sound quality. *EHJDH*. 2022;3(3):473–480. https://doi.org/10.1093/ehjdh/ztac044.
32. Atkinson P, Bowra J, Milne J, et al. International Federation for Emergency Medicine consensus statement: sonography in hypotension and cardiac arrest (SHoC): an international consensus on the use of point of care ultrasound for undifferentiated hypotension and during cardiac arrest. *CJEM*. 2017;19(06):459–470. https://doi.org/10.1017/cem.2016.394.
33. Sicari R, Galderisi M, Voigt JU, et al. The use of pocket-size imaging devices: a position statement of the European Association of Echocardiography. *Eur J Echocardiogr*. 2011;12(2):85–87. https://doi.org/10.1093/ejechocard/jeq184.
34. European Society of Radiology (ESR). ESR statement on portable ultrasound devices. *Insights Imaging*. 2019;10(1):89. https://doi.org/10.1186/s13244-019-0775-x.
35. James PA, Oparil S, Carter BL, et al. 2014 evidence-based guideline for the management of high blood pressure in adults: report from the panel members appointed to the Eighth Joint National Committee (JNC 8). *JAMA*. 2014;311(5):507–520. https://doi.org/10.1001/jama.2013.284427.
36. SPRINT Research Group, Lewis CE, Fine LJ, et al. Final report of a trial of intensive versus standard blood-pressure control. *N Engl J Med*. 2021;384(20):1921–1930. https://doi.org/10.1056/NEJMoa1901281.
37. Whelton PK, Carey RM, Aronow WS, et al. 2017 ACC/AHA/AAPA/ABC/ACPM/AGS/APhA/ASH/ASPC/NMA/PCNA guideline for the prevention, detection, evaluation, and management of high blood pressure in adults: a report of the American College of Cardiology/American Heart Association Task Force on Clinical Practice Guidelines. *Hypertension*. 2018;71(6). https://doi.org/10.1161/HYP.0000000000000065.
38. Flack JM, Adekola B. Blood pressure and the new ACC/AHA hypertension guidelines. *Trends Cardiovasc Med*. 2020;30(3):160–164. https://doi.org/10.1016/j.tcm.2019.05.003.
39. Clark CE, Warren FC, Boddy K, et al. Associations between systolic interarm differences in blood pressure and cardiovascular disease outcomes and mortality: individual participant data meta-analysis, development and validation of a prognostic algorithm: the INTERPRESS-IPD collaboration. *Hypertension*. 2021;77(2):650–661. https://doi.org/10.1161/HYPERTENSIONAHA.120.15997.
40. Clark CE, Warren FC, Boddy K, et al. Higher arm versus lower arm systolic blood pressure and cardiovascular outcomes: a meta-analysis of individual participant data from the INTERPRESS-IPD collaboration. *Hypertension*. 2022;79(10):2328–2335. https://doi.org/10.1161/HYPERTENSIONAHA.121.18921.
41. Weinberg I, Gona P, O'Donnell CJ, Jaff MR, Murabito JM. The systolic blood pressure difference between arms and cardiovascular disease in the Framingham Heart Study. *Am J Med*. 2014;127(3):209–215. https://doi.org/10.1016/j.amjmed.2013.10.027.
42. Freeman R, Abuzinadah AR, Gibbons C, Jones P, Miglis MG, Sinn DI. Orthostatic hypotension: JACC state-of-the-art review. *J Am Coll Cardiol*. 2018;72(11):1294–1309. https://doi.org/10.1016/j.jacc.2018.05.079.
43. Fedorowski A, Ricci F, Hamrefors V, et al. Orthostatic hypotension: management of a complex, but common, medical problem. *Circ Arrhythm Electrophysiol*. 2022;15(3):e010573. https://doi.org/10.1161/CIRCEP.121.010573.
44. Centers for Disease Control and Prevention (CDC). *Measuring Orthostatic Hypotension*. 2017. www.Cdc.Gov/Steadi/Pdf/STEADI-Assessment-MeasuringBP-508.Pdf.
45. Wahba A, Shibao CA, Muldowney JAS, Peltier A, Habermann R, Biaggioni I. Management of orthostatic hypotension in the hospitalized patient: a narrative review. *Am J Med*. 2022;135(1):24–31. https://doi.org/10.1016/j.amjmed.2021.07.030.
46. Ishigami J, Charleston J, Miller ER, Matsushita K, Appel LJ, Brady TM. Effects of cuff size on the accuracy of blood pressure readings: the cuff(SZ) randomized crossover trial. *JAMA Intern Med*. 2023:e233264. https://doi.org/10.1001/jamainternmed.2023.3264. Published online August 7.

47. Price S, Platz E, Cullen L, et al. Echocardiography and lung ultrasonography for the assessment and management of acute heart failure. *Nat Rev Cardiol.* 2017;14(7):427–440. https://doi.org/10.1038/nrcardio.2017.56.
48. Chowdhury MEH, Khandakar A, Alzoubi K, et al. Real-time smart-digital stethoscope system for heart diseases monitoring. *Sensors (Basel).* 2019;19(12):2781. https://doi.org/10.3390/s19122781.
49. Reimer-Kent J. Heart sounds: are you listening? Part 1. *Can J Cardiovasc Nurs.* 2013;23(2):3–6.
50. Nishimura RA, Otto CM, Bonow RO, et al. 2014 AHA/ACC guideline for the management of patients with valvular heart disease: a report of the American College of Cardiology/American Heart Association Task Force on Practice Guidelines. *J Am Coll Cardiol.* 2014;63(22):e57–185. https://doi.org/10.1016/j.jacc.2014.02.536.
51. Nishimura RA, Otto CM, Bonow RO, et al. 2017 AHA/ACC focused update of the 2014 AHA/ACC guideline for the management of patients with valvular heart disease: a report of the American College of Cardiology/American Heart Association Task Force on Clinical Practice Guidelines. *Circulation.* 2017;135(25):e1159–e1195. https://doi.org/10.1161/CIR.0000000000000503.
52. Otto CM, Nishimura RA, Bonow RO, et al. 2020 ACC/AHA guideline for the management of patients with valvular heart disease: executive summary: a report of the American College of Cardiology/American Heart Association Joint Committee on Clinical Practice Guidelines. *Circulation.* 2021;143(5):e35–e71. https://doi.org/10.1161/CIR.0000000000000932.
53. Unger P, Clavel MA, Lindman BR, Mathieu P, Pibarot P. Pathophysiology and management of multivalvular disease. *Nat Rev Cardiol.* 2016;13(7):429–440. https://doi.org/10.1038/nrcardio.2016.57.
54. Del FB, De Bonis M, Agricola E, et al. Mitral valve regurgitation: a disease with a wide spectrum of therapeutic options. *Nat Rev Cardiol.* 2020;17(12):807–827. https://doi.org/10.1038/s41569-020-0395-7.
55. Jentzer JC, Ternus B, Eleid M, Rihal C. Structural heart disease emergencies. *J Intensive Care Med.* 2021;36(9):975–988. https://doi.org/10.1177/0885066620918776.
56. Reimer-Kent J. Heart sounds: are you listening? Part 2. *Can J Cardiovasc Nurs.* 2013;23(3):3–9.
57. Montrief T, Davis WT, Koyfman A, Long B. Mechanical, inflammatory, and embolic complications of myocardial infarction: an emergency medicine review. *Am J Emerg Med.* 2019;37(6):1175–1183. https://doi.org/10.1016/j.ajem.2019.04.003.
58. McNamara N, Ibrahim A, Satti Z, Ibrahim M, Kiernan TJ. Acute pericarditis: a review of current diagnostic and management guidelines. *Future Cardiol.* 2019;15(2):119–126. https://doi.org/10.2217/fca-2017-0102.

12

Cardiovascular Diagnostic Procedures

Mary E. Lough, Sarah J. Berger, Amy Larsen, and Cass Piper Sandoval

http://evolve.elsevier.com/Urden/CriticalCareNursing

Numerous cardiovascular diagnostic procedures are used in the diagnosis and management of critically ill patients. This chapter explores hemodynamic monitoring, electrocardiography, laboratory tests, and diagnostic procedures in critical care.

HEMODYNAMIC MONITORING

Hemodynamic monitoring follows a spectrum of very invasive, moderately invasive, minimally invasive, and noninvasive methods (Fig. 12.1).[1] Every method has advantages and disadvantages, and all require an understanding of the physiologic principles that guide diagnostic assessment and management. In clinical practice, there is tremendous variation in the technologies used depending on the setting and patient acuity. In general, cardiovascular surgical units use more invasive hemodynamic monitoring, whereas nonsurgical critical care areas begin with less-invasive monitoring, adding invasive technologies based on the patient's physiologic requirements. Hemodynamic technologies are discussed in this chapter following a more-invasive to less-invasive trajectory.

Hemodynamic Monitoring Equipment

A traditional invasive hemodynamic monitoring system has four component parts (Fig. 12.2):

- An invasive catheter and high-pressure tubing connect the patient to the transducer.
- The transducer receives the physiologic signal from the catheter and tubing and converts it into electrical energy.
- The flush system maintains patency of the fluid-filled system and catheter.
- The bedside monitor contains the amplifier with recorder, which increases the volume of the electrical signal and displays it on an oscilloscope and on a digital scale in millimeters of mercury (mm Hg).

Although many different types of invasive catheters can be inserted to monitor hemodynamic pressures, all such catheters are connected to similar equipment (see Fig. 12.2). However, there is variation in the way different hospitals configure their hemodynamic systems. The basic setup consists of the following:

- A bag of 0.9% sodium chloride (also sometimes known as *normal saline*) is used as a flush solution. In some hospitals, heparin is added as an anticoagulant. A pressure infusion cuff covers the bag of flush solution and is inflated to 300 mm Hg.
- The system contains intravenous (IV) tubing, three-way stopcocks, and an in-line flow device attached for continuous fluid infusion and manual flush. High-pressure tubing must be used to connect the invasive catheter to the transducer to prevent damping (flattening) of the waveform.
- A pressure transducer is used. Transducers are disposable and use a silicon chip.

Heparin

The use of the anticoagulant heparin added to the normal saline flush setup to maintain catheter patency is controversial.[2,3] Although some critical care units do add heparin to flush solutions, many avoid heparin because of concern about development of heparin-induced antibodies that can trigger an autoimmune condition known as heparin-induced thrombocytopenia (HIT). HIT is associated with a decrease in platelet count of more than 50% accompanied by thrombus formation.[4] If heparin is used in the flush infusion, ongoing monitoring of the platelet count is recommended.

Flush solutions, lines, stopcocks, and disposable transducers are changed every 96 hours per current U.S. Centers for Disease Control and Prevention guidelines.[5,6] It is essential to be familiar with the specific written procedures that concern hemodynamic monitoring equipment in each critical care unit. Dextrose solutions are not recommended as flush solutions in monitoring catheters.[5,6]

Calibration of Hemodynamic Monitoring Equipment

To ensure accuracy of hemodynamic pressure readings, two baseline measurements are necessary:

1. Calibration of the system to atmospheric pressure, known as *zeroing the transducer.*
2. Identify anatomic location to be level with transducer height, known as *levelling the transducer.*

Zeroing the Transducer

To calibrate the equipment to atmospheric pressure, referred to as *zeroing the transducer*, the three-way stopcock nearest to the transducer is turned simultaneously to open the transducer to air (atmospheric pressure) and to close it to the patient and the flush system. The monitor is adjusted so that "0" (zero) is displayed, which equals local atmospheric pressure. Atmospheric pressure is not zero; it is 760 mm Hg at sea level. Using zero to represent current atmospheric pressure provides a convenient baseline for hemodynamic measurement purposes.[2]

Some monitors also require calibration of the upper scale limit while the system remains open to air. At the end of the calibration procedure, the stopcock is returned to the closed position, and a closed cap is placed over the open port. At this point, the patient's waveform and hemodynamic pressures are displayed.

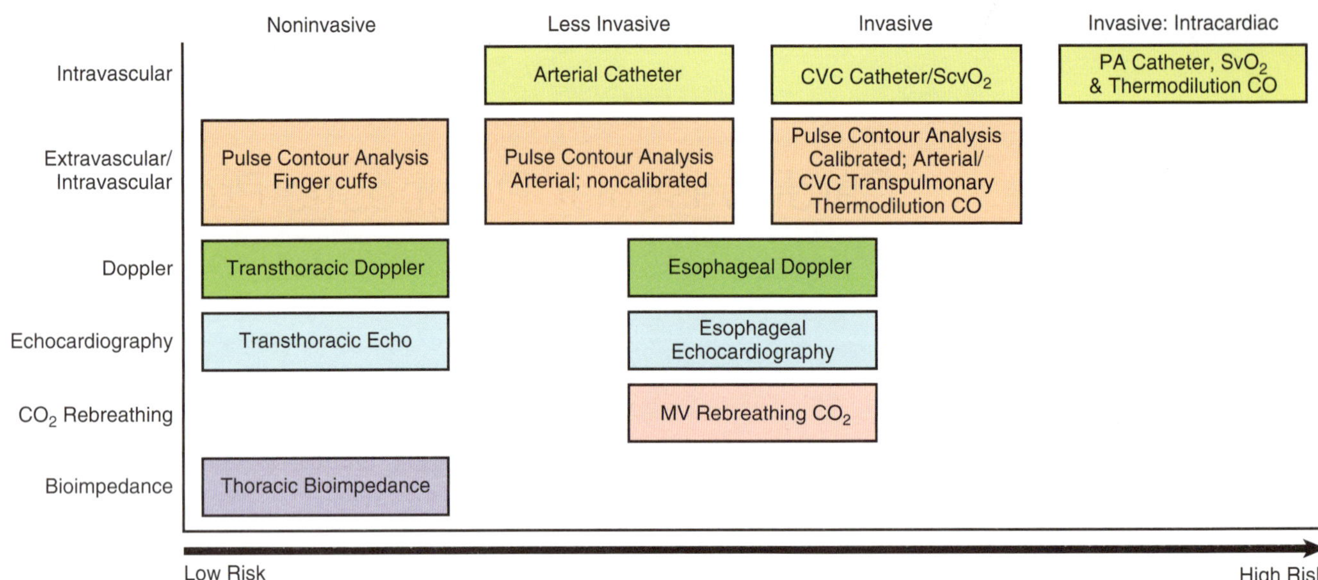

FIG. 12.1 Overview of options for hemodynamic monitoring in critical care from noninvasive to highly invasive, from low risk to high risk, and listing the different monitoring options that are available. *CO*, Cardiac output; *CO_2*, carbon dioxide; *CVC*, central venous catheter; *MV*, mechanical ventilation; *$ScvO_2$* central venous oxygen saturation; *SvO_2* mixed venous oxygen saturation.

Disposable transducers are very accurate, and after they are calibrated to atmospheric pressure, drift from the zero baseline is minimal. Although in theory this means that repeated calibration is unnecessary, clinical protocols in most units require the nurse to calibrate the transducer at the beginning of each shift for quality assurance.

Midaxillary Line

The midaxillary line, also called the *phlebostatic axis*, is a reference line on the side of the chest that is used as a baseline for consistent transducer height placement. To locate the axis, a theoretical line is drawn from the fourth sternal intercostal space, where it joins the sternum, to a theoretical line on the side of the chest that is one-half of the depth of the lateral chest wall. This theoretical line approximates the level of the atria, as shown in Fig. 12.2. It is used as the reference mark for central venous pressure (CVP) and pulmonary artery (PA) catheter transducers. The level of the transducer "air reference stopcock" approximates the position of the tip of an invasive hemodynamic monitoring catheter within the chest.

Levelling the Transducer

Leveling the transducer is different from zeroing. This process aligns the transducer air-reference stopcock with the level of the left atrium, especially for PA or CVP monitoring (described later). The purpose is to line up the air-fluid interface with the left atrium to correct for changes in hydrostatic pressure in blood vessels above and below the level of the heart.[7]

A carpenter's level or laser-light level can be used to ensure that the transducer is parallel with the midaxillary line (phlebostatic axis). Research suggests that placement of the "air reference stopcock" relative to the midaxillary line varies among clinicians, and this can lead to inaccurate placement and inaccurate hemodynamic values.[7–9]

Errors in measurement can occur if the transducer is placed below the midaxillary line, because the fluid in the system weighs on the transducer, creating additional hydrostatic pressure, and produces a falsely high reading. For every inch the transducer is below the tip of the catheter, the fluid pressure in the system increases the measurement by 1.87 mm Hg. For example, if the transducer is positioned 6 inches below the tip of the catheter, this falsely elevates the displayed pressure by 11 mm Hg.

If the transducer is placed above this atrial level, gravity and lack of fluid pressure give an erroneously low reading. For every inch the transducer is positioned above the catheter tip, the measurement is 1.87 mm Hg less than the true value. If several clinicians are taking measurements, the reference point can be marked on the side of the patient's chest to ensure accurate measurements. When there is a change in the patient's position, the transducer must be leveled again to ensure that accurate hemodynamic pressure measurements are recorded.[7]

Patient Position During Hemodynamic Monitoring

The position of the patient during hemodynamic monitoring would not be an issue if critical care patients remained supine. The emphasis on raising the head of the bed above 30 degrees to prevent aspiration, and position changes to prevent sacral skin pressure injury, require a reevaluation of transducer level immediately following each change in the patient's position.

Head of Bed Backrest Position

Nurse researchers have determined that the CVP, pulmonary artery pressure (PAP), and pulmonary artery occlusion pressure (PAOP), also known as *pulmonary artery wedge pressure*, can be reliably measured at head of bed backrest positions from 0 (flat) to 60 degrees if the patient is lying on their back (supine).[7] If the patient is normovolemic and hemodynamically stable, raising the head of the bed usually does not affect hemodynamic pressure measurements. If the patient is so hemodynamically unstable or hypovolemic that raising the head of the bed negatively affects intravascular volume distribution, the priority is to correct the hemodynamic instability and leave the patient in a lower backrest position. Most patients do not need the head of the bed to be lowered to 0 degrees to obtain accurate CVP, PAP,

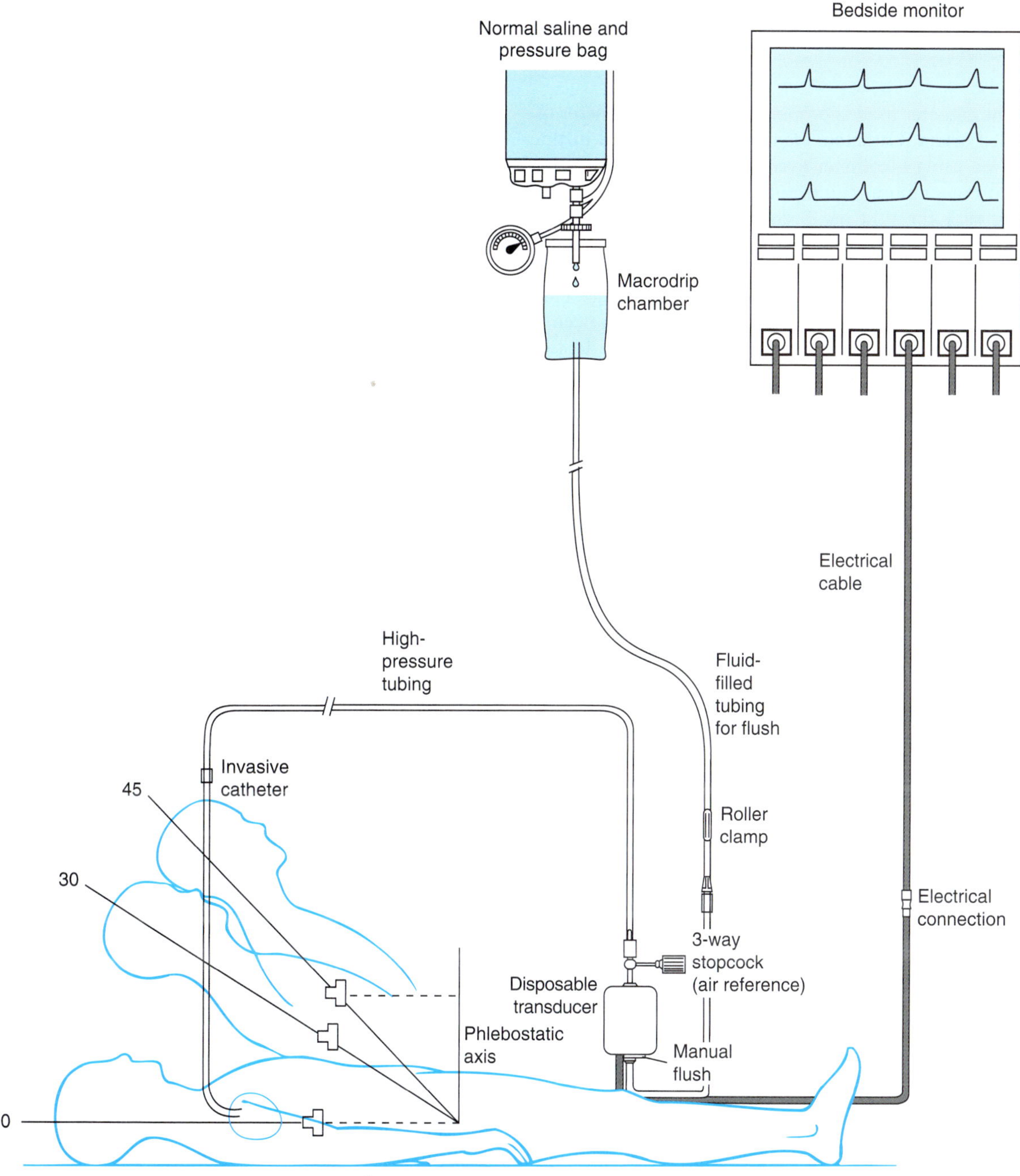

FIG. 12.2 The four parts of a hemodynamic monitoring system include an invasive catheter attached to high-pressure tubing to connect to the transducer; a transducer; a flush system, including a manual flush; and a bedside monitor.

or PAOP readings, as long as the midaxillary line is used as the reference point.[7]

Lateral Position

Researchers have evaluated hemodynamic pressure measurement readings from a 20-degree to a 90-degree lateral position and found the measurements to be reliable as long as the air-reference stopcock is in the correct position. It is important to know that measurements can be recorded in nonsupine positions, because critically ill patients must be turned to prevent skin pressure injury and other complications of immobility.

Intraarterial Blood Pressure Monitoring

Indications

Intraarterial blood pressure monitoring is considered minimally invasive compared with catheters placed into a central artery or central vein. Arterial blood pressure monitoring is indicated for any major medical or surgical condition that has the potential to alter blood pressure or cardiac output (CO), tissue perfusion, or fluid volume status. The system is designed for continuous measurement of three blood pressure parameters: systole, diastole, and mean arterial pressure (MAP). Additionally, direct arterial access is helpful in the management of patients with acute lung failure who require frequent arterial blood gas measurements.

Catheters

The size of the catheter used is proportionate to the diameter of the cannulated artery. Catheters are most often inserted in the smaller arteries, using a "catheter-over-needle" unit in which the needle is used as a temporary guide for catheter placement. With this method, after the unit has been inserted into the artery, the needle is withdrawn, leaving the supple plastic catheter in place.[10] To insert a catheter into a larger artery, the Seldinger technique is typically used,[10] which involves the following steps:

1. Entry into the artery at a 30 to 45 degree angle, using a needle
2. Passage of a supple guidewire through the needle into the artery
3. Removal of the needle
4. Passage of the catheter over the guidewire
5. Removal of the guidewire, leaving the catheter in the artery

Insertion and Allen Test

Several peripheral arteries are suitable for receiving a catheter and for long-term hemodynamic monitoring. The most frequently used site is the radial artery. The femoral artery is a larger vessel that is also frequently cannulated. Other smaller arteries such as the dorsalis pedis, axillary, or brachial arteries are used only when other arterial access is unavailable.

The major advantage of the radial artery is the supply of collateral circulation to the hand provided by the ulnar artery through the palmar arch in most people.

Before radial artery cannulation, collateral circulation is assessed by using Doppler flow or by the modified Allen test according to institutional protocol. In the modified Allen test, the radial and ulnar arteries are compressed simultaneously. The patient is asked to clench and unclench the hand until it blanches. One of the arteries is then released, and the hand should immediately flush from that side. The same procedure is repeated for the remaining artery. Studies indicate that complications with arterial cannulation are low even when the modified Allen test is inconclusive.

Nursing Management

Intraarterial blood pressure monitoring is designed for continuous assessment of arterial perfusion to the major organ systems of the body. MAP is the clinical parameter most often used to assess perfusion, because MAP represents perfusion pressure throughout the cardiac cycle. Because one-third of the cardiac cycle is spent in systole and two-thirds is spent in diastole, the MAP calculation must reflect the greater amount of time spent in diastole. This MAP formula can be calculated by hand or with a calculator, where diastole times 2 plus systole is divided by 3, as shown in the following formula:

$$\frac{(\text{Diastole} \times 2) + (\text{Systole} \times 1)}{3} = \text{MAP}$$

A blood pressure of 120/60 mm Hg produces a MAP of 80 mm Hg. However, the bedside hemodynamic monitor may show a slightly different digital number, because bedside monitoring computers calculate the area under the curve of the arterial line tracing (Table 12.1).

Infection

Infection was once believed to be rare in arterial catheters because of the rapid arterial blood flow. Evidence suggests that arterial catheters are associated with the same risk of bloodstream infections as central venous catheters.[11] Therefore, infection prevention measures must be just as meticulous for arterial catheters as for central catheters.[11]

Perfusion Pressure

A MAP greater than 60 mm Hg is necessary to perfuse the coronary arteries. A higher MAP may be required to perfuse the brain and the kidneys. A MAP between 70 and 90 mm Hg is preferable for a patient with heart disease to decrease left ventricular (LV) workload. After carotid endarterectomy or neurosurgery, a higher MAP of 90 to 110 mm Hg may be more appropriate to increase cerebral perfusion pressure. Systolic and diastolic pressures are monitored in conjunction with the MAP as a further guide to the accuracy of perfusion. If CO decreases, the body compensates by constricting peripheral vessels to maintain the blood pressure. In this situation, the MAP may remain constant, but the pulse pressure (difference between systolic and diastolic pressures) narrows. The following examples explain this point:

- Mr. A: Blood pressure 90/70 mm Hg; MAP 76 mm Hg
- Mr. B: Blood pressure 150/40 mm Hg; MAP 76 mm Hg

Both patients have a perfusion pressure of 76 mm Hg, but they are clinically very different. Mr. A is peripherally vasoconstricted, as is demonstrated by the narrow pulse pressure (90/70 mm Hg). His skin is cool to touch, and he has weak peripheral pulses. Mr. B has a wide pulse pressure (150/40 mm Hg), warm skin, and normally palpable peripheral pulses. Nursing assessment of a patient with an arterial line includes comparison of clinical findings with arterial line readings including perfusion pressure and MAP.

Pulse Pressure

Clinical Exemplar: A clinical example of hemodynamic nursing assessment is helpful for understanding pulse pressure. The patient is JW, 1 day after coronary artery bypass graft (CABG) surgery. JW recently has been weaned from dopamine and sodium nitroprusside and received an IV diuretic, 20 mg of furosemide (Lasix). He has voided 800 mL of urine via the urinary catheter during the past 2 hours. JW's MAP remains at 80 mm Hg, but his pulse pressure has narrowed by 30 mm Hg from 120/60 to 100/70 mm Hg. His heart rate (HR) has increased from 90 to 110 beats/min. This clinical situation is expected after furosemide administration, but the narrowed pulse pressure and increased HR may indicate hypovolemia. The nurse caring for JW will monitor the trend of the MAP. If the MAP begins to decrease and JW shows signs of a low CO, the physician will be notified. In most nonemergency situations, following the trend of the arterial pressure is more valuable than an isolated measurement.

Noninvasive Cuff Blood Pressure

If the arterial line becomes unreliable or dislodged, a cuff pressure can be used as a reserve system. However, research studies indicate that often, a noninvasive cuff blood pressure, whether intermittent or continuous, does not produce the same values as an intraarterial catheter.[12] Other challenges to obtaining accurate measurements with a cuff include obesity and cuff location on the arm. Any difference between cuff and arterial line pressures becomes significant when a patient has a low CO or is in shock. The concern is that the cuff pressure may be unreliable because of peripheral vasoconstriction. It is usual practice to compare a cuff pressure after the arterial line is inserted to identify and document any difference in pressure readings.

TABLE 12.1 Hemodynamic Pressures and Calculated Hemodynamic Values

Hemodynamic Pressure	Definition and Explanation	Normal Range
MAP	Average perfusion pressure created by arterial blood pressure during the cardiac cycle. The normal cardiac cycle is one-third systole and two-thirds diastole. These three components are divided by 3 to obtain the average perfusion pressure for the whole cardiac cycle.	70–100 mm Hg
CVP	Pressure created by volume in the right side of the heart. When the tricuspid valve is open, the CVP reflects filling pressures in the right ventricle. Clinically, the CVP is often used as a guide to overall fluid balance.	2–5 mm Hg 3–8 cm H_2O
LAP	Pressure created by the volume in the left side of the heart. When the mitral valve is open, the LAP reflects filling pressures in the left ventricle. Clinically, the LAP is used after cardiac surgery to determine how well the left ventricle is ejecting its volume. In general, the higher the LAP, the lower the ejection fraction from the left ventricle.	5–12 mm Hg
PAP	Pulsatile pressure in the pulmonary artery measured by an indwelling catheter.	
PAS		20–30 mm Hg
PAD		5–10 mm Hg
PAP_M		10–15 mm Hg
PAOP[a]	Pressure created by the volume in the left side of the heart. When the mitral valve is open, the PAOP reflects filling pressures in the pulmonary vasculature, and pressures in the left side of the heart are transmitted back to the catheter "wedged" into a small pulmonary arteriole.	5–12 mm Hg
CO	Amount of blood pumped out by a ventricle over 1 min. Clinically, it can be measured using the thermodilution CO method, which calculates CO in L/min.	4–6 L/min (at rest)
CI	CO divided by BSA, with tailoring of CO to individual body size. A BSA conversion chart is necessary to calculate CI, which is considered more accurate than CO because it is individualized to height and weight. CI is measured in L • min • m^2 of BSA.	2.2–4.0 L • min • m^2
SV	Amount of blood ejected by the ventricle with each heartbeat, expressed in mL. Hemodynamic monitoring systems calculate SV by dividing CO (in L/min) by HR and then multiplying the answer by 1000 to change L to mL.	60–70 mL
SI	SV indexed to the BSA.	40–50 mL/m^2
SVR	Mean pressure difference across the systemic vascular bed divided by blood flow. Clinically, SVR represents the resistance against which the left ventricle must pump to eject its volume. This resistance is created by the systemic arteries and arterioles. As SVR increases, CO falls. SVR is measured in Wood units or dyn • s • cm^{-5}. If the number of Wood units is multiplied by 80, the value is converted to dyn • s • cm^{-5}.	10–18 Wood units or 800–1400 dyn • s • cm^{-5}
SVRI	SVR indexed to BSA.	2000–2400 dyn • s • cm^{-5}
PVR	Mean pressure difference across pulmonary vascular bed divided by blood flow. Clinically, PVR represents the resistance against which the right ventricle must pump to eject its volume. This resistance is created by the pulmonary arteries and arterioles. As PVR increases, the output from the right ventricle decreases. PVR is measured in Wood units or dyn • s • cm^{-5}. PVR is normally one-sixth of SVR.	1.2–3.0 Wood units or 100–250 dyn • s • cm^{-5}
PVRI	PVR indexed to BSA.	225–315 dyn • s • cm^{-5}
LCWI	Amount of work the left ventricle does *each minute* when ejecting blood. The hemodynamic formula represents pressure generated (MAP) multiplied by volume pumped (CO). A conversion factor is used to change mm Hg to kg-m. LCWI is always represented as an indexed volume (BSA chart). LCWI increases or decreases because of changes in pressure (MAP) or volume pumped (CO).	3.4–4.2 kg-m/m^2
LVSWI	Amount of work the left ventricle performs with *each heartbeat*. The hemodynamic formula represents pressure generated (MAP) multiplied by volume pumped (SV). A conversion factor is used to change mL/mm Hg to g-m. LVSWI is always represented as an indexed volume. LVSWI increases or decreases because of changes in the pressure (MAP) or volume pumped (SV).	50–62 g-m/m^2
RCWI	Amount of work the right ventricle performs *each minute* when ejecting blood. The hemodynamic formula represents pressure generated (PAP_M) multiplied by volume pumped (CO). A conversion factor is used to change mm Hg to kg-m. RCWI is always represented as an indexed value (BSA chart). Similar to LCWI, RCWI increases or decreases because of changes in the pressure (PAP_M) or volume pumped (CO).	0.54–0.66 kg-m/m^2
RVSWI	Amount of work the right ventricle does *each heartbeat*. The hemodynamic formula represents pressure generated (PAP_M) multiplied by volume pumped (SV). A conversion factor is used to change mm Hg to g-m. RVSWI is always represented as an indexed value (BSA chart). Similar to LVSWI, RVSWI increases or decreases because of changes in the pressure (PAP_M) or volume pumped (SV).	7.9–9.7 g-m/m^2

[a]Pulmonary artery occlusion pressure (PAOP) was formerly called *pulmonary capillary wedge pressure* (PCW or PCWP) or *pulmonary arterial wedge pressure* (PAWP).

BSA, Body surface area; *CI*, cardiac index; *CO*, cardiac output; *CVP*, central venous pressure; *HR*, heart rate; *LAP*, left atrial pressure; *LCWI*, left cardiac work index; *LVSWI*, left ventricular stroke work index; *MAP*, mean arterial pressure; *PAD*, pulmonary artery diastolic; *PAOP*, pulmonary artery occlusion pressure; *PAP*, pulmonary artery pressure; PAP_M, mean pulmonary artery pressure; *PAS*, pulmonary artery systolic; *PVR*, pulmonary vascular resistance; *PVRI*, pulmonary vascular resistance index; *RCWI*, right cardiac work index; *RVSWI*, right ventricular stroke work index; *SI*, stroke volume index; *SV*, stroke volume; *SVR*, systemic vascular resistance; *SVRI*, systemic vascular resistance index.

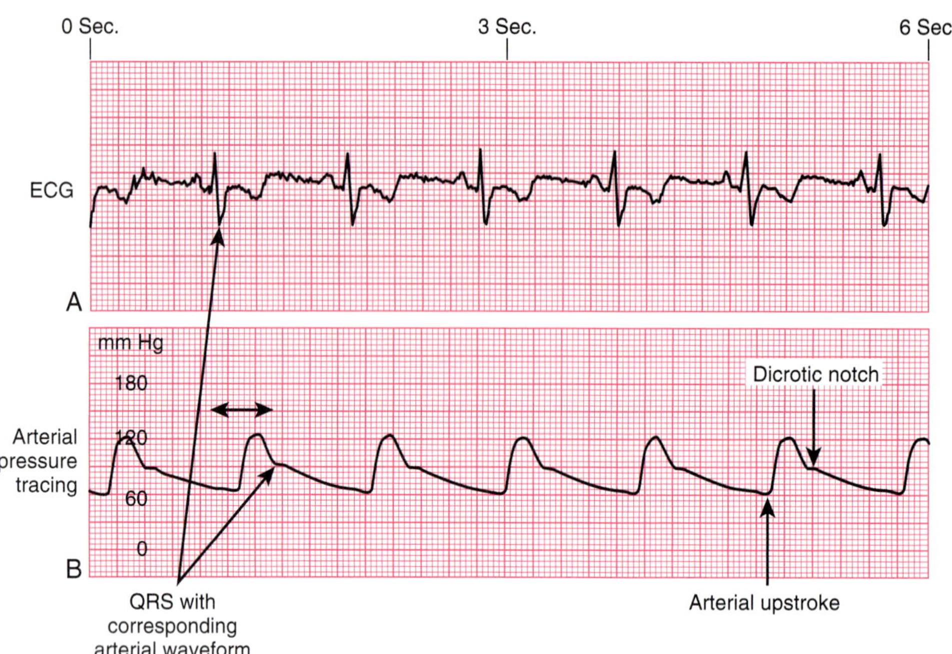

FIG. 12.3 Simultaneous electrocardiogram *(ECG)* (A) and normal arterial pressure (B) tracings.

Arterial Pressure Waveform Interpretation

As the aortic valve opens, blood is ejected from the left ventricle and is recorded as an increase of pressure in the arterial system on the arterial waveform. The highest point recorded is called *systole.* After peak ejection (systole), the force decreases, and the pressure falls. A notch (dicrotic notch) may be visible on the downstroke of this arterial waveform, representing closure of the aortic valve. The *dicrotic notch* signifies the start of blood flow into the arterial vasculature. The lowest point recorded is called *diastole.* A normal arterial pressure tracing is shown in Fig. 12.3. Electrical stimulation (QRS) is always first, and the arterial pressure tracing follows the initiating QRS complex.

Decreased Arterial Perfusion

Specific problems with heart rhythm can translate into poor arterial perfusion if CO decreases. Poor perfusion may be seen as a single, nonperfused beat after a premature ventricular contraction (PVC) (Fig. 12.4) or as multiple, nonperfused beats (Fig. 12.5). In ventricular bigeminy, every second beat is poorly perfused (Fig. 12.6). A disorganized atrial baseline resulting from atrial fibrillation creates a variable arterial pulse because of the differences in stroke volume (SV) between each beat (Fig. 12.7). All these examples illustrate that when two beats are close together, the left ventricle does not have time to fill adequately, and the second beat is inadequately perfused or is not perfused at all.

Pulse Deficit

A pulse deficit occurs when the apical HR and the peripheral pulse are not equal. In the critical care unit, this can be seen on the bedside monitor. Normally, there is one arterial upstroke for each QRS complex, and if there are more QRS complexes than arterial upstrokes, a pulse deficit is present, as shown in Figs. 12.4 and 12.7. To identify a pulse deficit in an unmonitored patient, a stethoscope is placed over the apex of the heart. The heartbeat can be heard, but it cannot be felt as a radial pulse. To determine whether a pulse deficit is significant, it is necessary to evaluate the clinical effect on the patient and whether any change in MAP or pulse pressure has occurred. Generally, the more nonperfused beats, the more serious the problem.

Pulsus Paradoxus

Pulsus paradoxus is a decrease of more than 10 mm Hg in the arterial waveform that occurs during inhalation (inspiration). This is caused by a physiologic decrease in CO as a result of negative intrathoracic pressure during spontaneous inspiration (inhalation). As pressure within the thorax decreases, blood pools in the large veins of the lungs and thorax, and this reduces the volume returned to the right heart and consequently lowers SV. The procedure for identification of pulsus paradoxus is described in Chapter 11 (see Box 11.9).

In certain clinical conditions, the pulsus paradoxus is obvious and can be clearly seen on an arterial waveform. It can be used as a clinical diagnostic test for a patient with cardiac tamponade, pericardial effusion, or constrictive pericarditis.[13]

Respiratory physiology is altered when the patient is receiving positive pressure ventilation. Because the ventilator uses positive pressure to deliver a breath, this increases intrathoracic pressure during the inspiratory phase. Pulsus paradoxus may be observed in patients who are mechanically ventilated with larger tidal volumes, as seen in the arterial waveform in Fig. 12.4.

Pulsus Alternans

In pulsus alternans, every other arterial pulsation is weak. This sometimes occurs in advanced LV heart failure.

Overdamped Waveform

If the arterial monitor shows a low blood pressure, it is important to determine whether the problem is related to the patient (hypotension) or to the monitoring equipment, as described in Table 12.2.

An overdamped arterial waveform is rounded, without a dicrotic notch, compared with a normal waveform. A low arterial blood pressure waveform is shown in Fig. 12.8. By

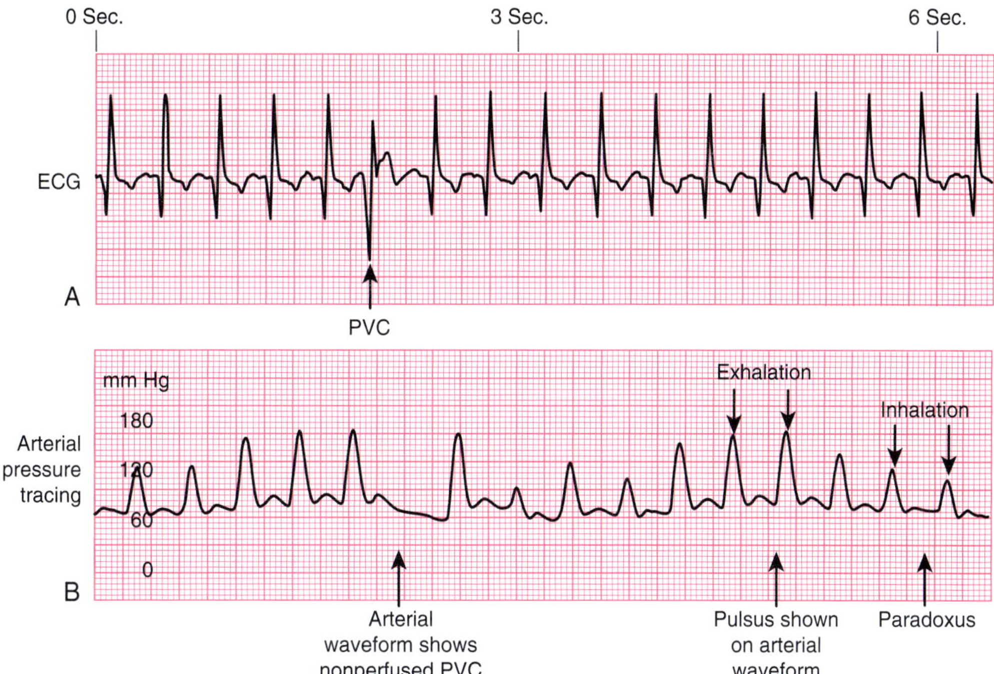

FIG. 12.4 Simultaneous electrocardiogram *(ECG)* (A) and arterial pressure (B) tracings show normal arterial waveform with nonperfused premature ventricular contraction *(PVC)*. The arterial waveform also shows evidence of pulsus paradoxus in a patient who is mechanically ventilated.

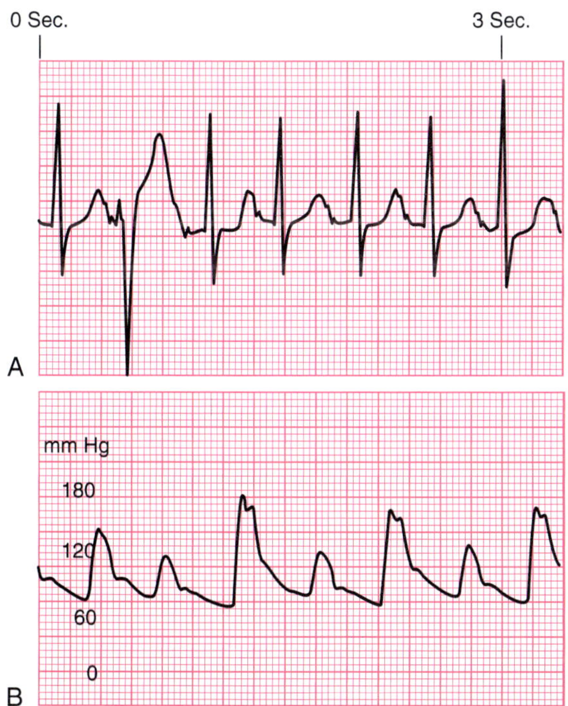

FIG. 12.5 Simultaneous electrocardiogram (A) and arterial pressure (B) tracings show pulsus alternans. A nonperfused premature ventricular contraction is also present.

comparison, an overdamped (flattened) arterial waveform is shown in Fig. 12.9.

An overdamped waveform occurs when communication from the artery to the transducer is interrupted and produces falsely lower values on the monitor and oscilloscope.[10] Damping can be caused by a biofilm-fibrin "tail" that partially occludes the tip of the catheter, by kinks in the catheter or tubing, or by air bubbles in the system. Troubleshooting techniques are used to find the origin of the problem and to remove the cause of overdamping (see Table 12.2).

Underdamped Waveform

Another cause of arterial waveform distortion is underdamping.[10] This is recognized by a narrow upward systolic peak that produces a falsely high systolic reading compared with the patient's cuff blood pressure, as shown in Fig. 12.10. The overshoot is caused by an increase in dynamic response or increased oscillations within the system.

Fast-Flush Square Waveform Test

The dynamic response of the monitoring system can be verified for accuracy at the bedside by the fast-flush square waveform test, also called the *dynamic frequency response test*.[7] The nurse performs this test to ensure that the patient pressures and waveform shown on the bedside monitor are accurate.[7] The test makes use of the manual flush system on the transducer. Normally, the flush device allows only 3 mL of fluid per hour. With the normal waveform displayed, the manual fast-flush procedure is used to generate a rapid increase in pressure, which is displayed on the monitor oscilloscope (Fig. 12.11).

- *Square wave is normal in appearance*: The normal dynamic response waveform has a square pattern with one or two oscillations before the return of the arterial waveform.
- *Square wave overdamped*: If the system is overdamped, a sloped (rather than square) pattern is seen.
- *Square wave underdamped*: If the system is underdamped, additional oscillations, or vibrations, are seen on the fast-flush square wave test.

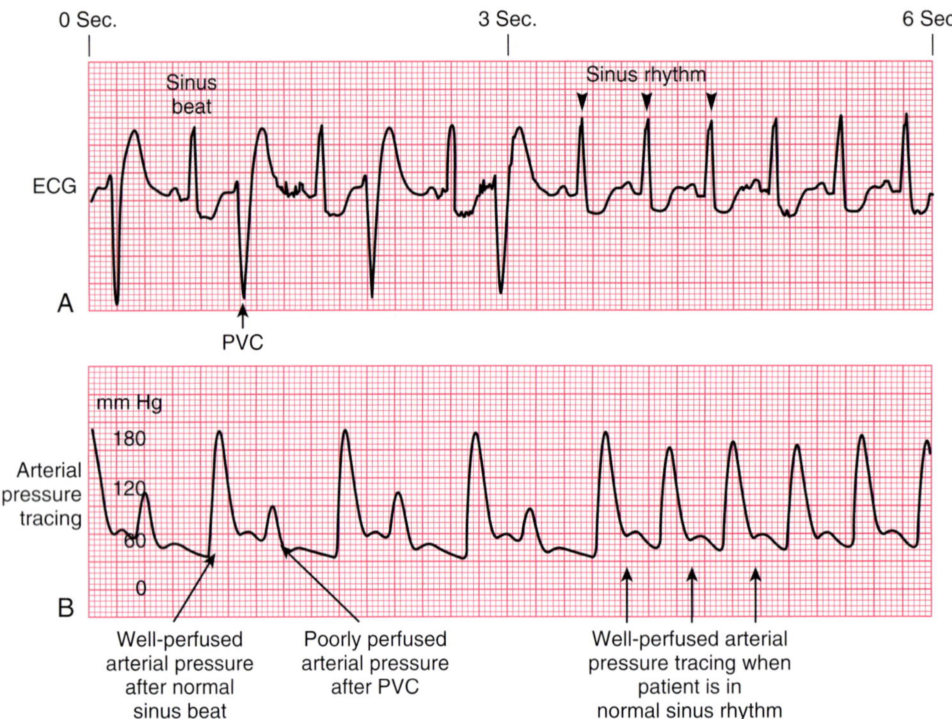

FIG. 12.6 Simultaneous electrocardiogram *(ECG)* (A) and arterial pressure (B) tracings show ventricular bigeminy. Every other ventricular beat is poorly perfused on the arterial pressure waveform. A well-perfused arterial pressure tracing is depicted (B) as the patient converts to normal sinus rhythm. *PVC,* Premature ventricular contraction.

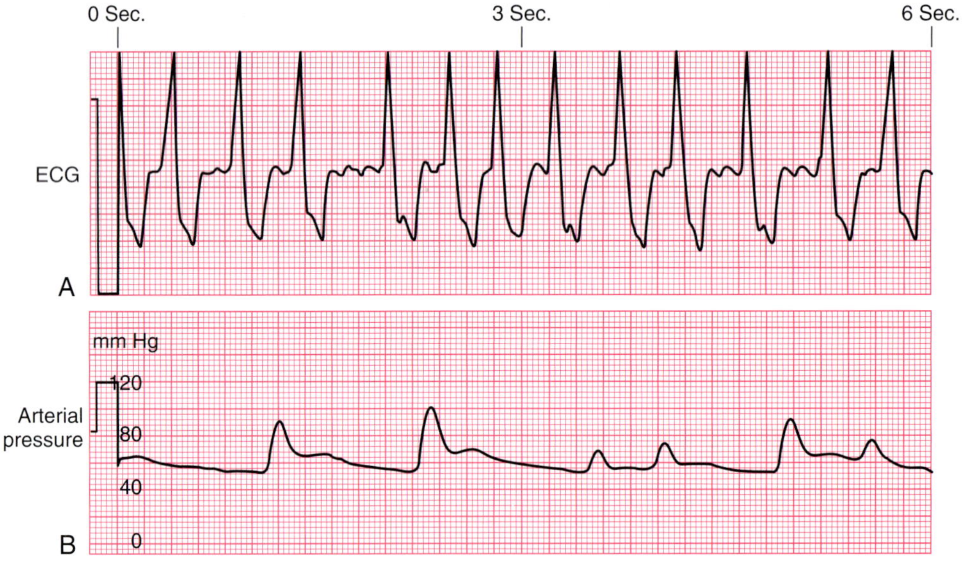

FIG. 12.7 Simultaneous electrocardiogram *(ECG)* (A) and arterial pressure (B) tracings show atrial fibrillation, which results in irregular atrial pulsations. The irregular pulsations create differences in beat-to-beat ventricular upstroke volume, resulting in diminished or absent ventricular output, as seen on the arterial waveform.

This test can be performed with any hemodynamic monitoring system. If air bubbles, clots, or kinks are in the system, the waveform becomes damped, or flattened, and this is reflected in the square waveform result.

This is an easy test to perform and is incorporated into nursing care procedures at the bedside when the hemodynamic system is first set up, at least once per shift, after opening the system for any reason, and when there is concern about the accuracy of the waveform. If the pressure waveform is distorted or the digital display is inaccurate, the troubleshooting methods described in Table 12.2 can be implemented. The nurse caring for a patient with an arterial line must be able to assess whether a low MAP or narrowed perfusion pressure represents decreased arterial perfusion or equipment malfunction. Assessment of the arterial

TABLE 12.2 **Nursing Measures to Ensure Patient Safety and to Troubleshoot Problems With Hemodynamic Monitoring Equipment**

Problem	Prevention	Rationale	Troubleshooting
Overdamping of waveform	Provide continuous infusion of pressurized 0.9% sodium chloride solution at 1–3 mL/hour.	Ensure that recorded pressures and waveform are accurate, because a damped waveform gives inaccurate readings.	Before insertion, completely flush the line and/or catheter. In a line attached to a patient, back flush through the system to clear bubbles from tubing or transducer.
Underdamping ("overshoot" or "fling")	Use short lengths of noncompliant tubing. Use fast-flush square wave test to demonstrate optimal system damping. Verify arterial waveform accuracy with the cuff blood pressure.	If the monitoring system is underdamped, the systolic and diastolic values will be overestimated by the waveform and the digital values. False high systolic values may lead to clinical decisions based on erroneous data.	Perform the fast-flush square wave test to verify optimal damping of the monitoring system.
Clot formation at end of the catheter	Provide continuous infusion of pressurized 0.9% sodium chloride solution 1–3 mL/hour using an in-line flush device.	Any foreign object placed in the body can cause local activation of the patient's coagulation system as a normal defense mechanism. The clots that are formed may be dangerous if they break off and travel to other parts of the body.	If a clot in the catheter is suspected because of a damped waveform or resistance to forward flush of the system, gently aspirate the line using a small syringe inserted into the proximal stopcock. Flush the line again after the clot is removed, and inspect the waveform. It should return to a normal pattern.
Hemorrhage	Use Luer-Lock (screw) connections in line setup. Close and cap stopcocks when not in use.	A loose connection or open stopcock creates a low-pressure sump effect, causing blood to back into the line and into the open air. If a catheter is accidentally removed, the vessel can bleed profusely, especially with an arterial line or if the patient has abnormal coagulation factors or has hypertension.	After a blood leak is recognized, tighten all connections, flush the line, and estimate blood loss.
	Ensure that the catheter is sutured or securely taped in position.		If the catheter has been inadvertently removed, put pressure on the cannulation site. When bleeding has stopped, apply a sterile dressing, estimate blood loss, and inform the physician. If the patient is restless, an armboard may protect lines inserted in the arm.
Air emboli	Ensure that all air bubbles are purged from a new line setup before attachment to an indwelling catheter.	Air can be introduced at several times, including when CVP tubing comes apart, when a new line setup is attached, or when a new CVP or PA line is inserted. During insertion of a CVP or PA line, the patient may be asked to hold their breath at specific times to prevent drawing air into the chest during inhalation.	Because it is impossible to get the air back after it has been introduced into the bloodstream, prevention is the best cure.
	Ensure that the drip chamber from the bag of flush solution is more than one-half full before using the in-line, fast-flush system.	In-line, fast-flush devices are designed to permit clearing of blood from the line after withdrawal of blood samples.	If air bubbles occur, they must be vented through the in-line stopcocks, and the drip chamber must be filled.
	Some sources recommend removing all air from the bag of flush solution before assembling the system.	If the chamber of the intravenous tubing is too low or empty, the rapid flow of fluid will create turbulence and cause flushing of air bubbles into the system and into the bloodstream.	The LAP line setup is the only system that includes an air filter specifically to prevent air emboli.
Normal waveform with *low* digital pressure	Ensure that the system is calibrated to atmospheric pressure.	This will provide a zero-baseline relative to atmospheric pressure.	Recalibrate the equipment if transducer drift has occurred.
	Ensure that the transducer is placed at the level of the midaxillary line (phlebostatic axis).	If the transducer has been placed *higher* than the midaxillary line (phlebostatic level), gravity and the lack of hydrostatic pressure will produce a false *low* reading.	Reposition the transducer at the level of the midaxillary line phlebostatic axis). Misplacement can occur if the patient moves from the bed to the chair or if the bed is placed in a Trendelenburg position.

Continued

TABLE 12.2 Nursing Measures to Ensure Patient Safety and to Troubleshoot Problems With Hemodynamic Monitoring Equipment—cont'd

Problem	Prevention	Rationale	Troubleshooting
Normal waveform with *high* digital pressure	Ensure that the system is calibrated to atmospheric pressure.	This will provide a zero-baseline relative to atmospheric pressure.	Recalibrate the equipment if transducer drift has occurred.
	Ensure that the transducer is placed at the level of the midaxillary line.	If the transducer has been placed *lower* than the midaxillary line., the weight of hydrostatic pressure on the transducer will produce a false *high* reading.	Reposition the transducer at the level of the midaxillary line.
			This situation can occur if the head of the bed was raised and the transducer was not repositioned. Some centers require attachment of the transducer to the patient's chest to avoid this problem.
Loss of waveform	Always have the hemodynamic waveform monitored so that changes or loss can be quickly noted.	The catheter may be kinked, or a stopcock may be turned off.	Check the line setup to ensure that all stopcocks are turned in the correct position and that the tubing is not kinked. Sometimes the catheter migrates against a vessel wall, and having the patient change position restores the waveform.

CVP, Central venous pressure; *LAP*, left atrial pressure; *PA*, pulmonary artery.

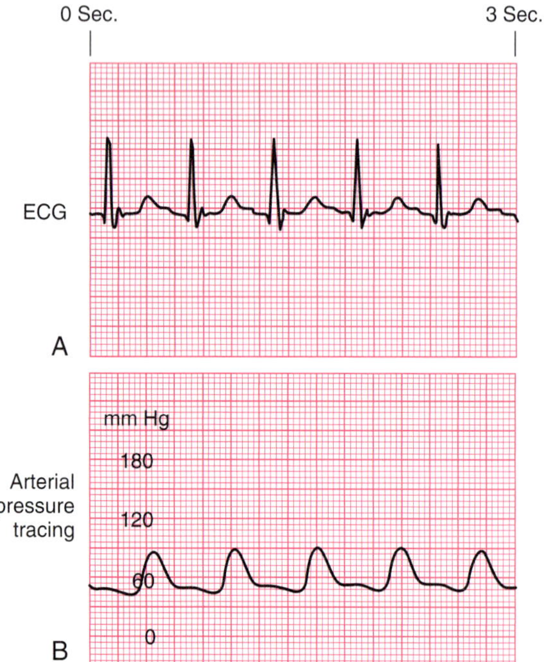

FIG. 12.8 Simultaneous electrocardiogram *(ECG)* (A) and arterial pressure (B) tracings show low arterial pressure waveform.

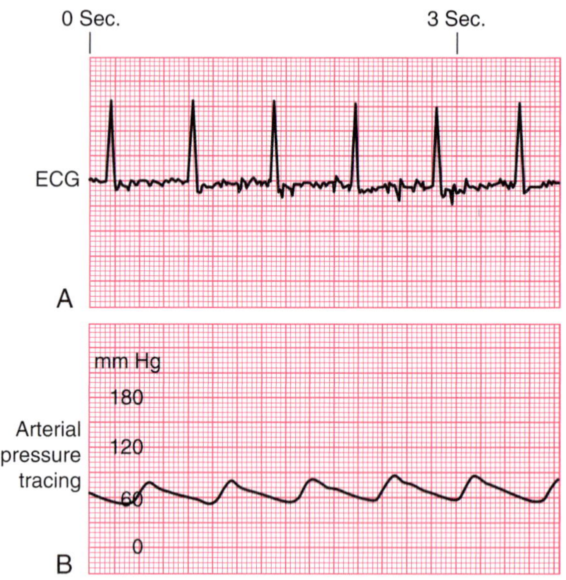

FIG. 12.9 Simultaneous electrocardiogram *(ECG)* (A) and arterial pressure (B) tracings show damped arterial pressure waveform.

waveform on the oscilloscope, in combination with clinical assessment, and use of the square waveform test will yield the answer.

Hemodynamic Monitoring Alarms

All critically ill patients must have the hemodynamic monitoring alarms on and adjusted to produce an audible alarm if the patient should experience a change in blood pressure, HR, respiratory rate, and any other significant monitored variable. Managing alarms and reducing alarm fatigue is an important National Patient Safety Goal.[14] Alarm limits must be customized to the patient's physiologic baseline to reduce false-positive alarms. The key issues concerning clinical monitor alarms are presented in Box 12.1.

Invasive Hemodynamic Monitoring

Invasive hemodynamic monitoring refers to monitoring situations where catheters are placed into central veins or pass

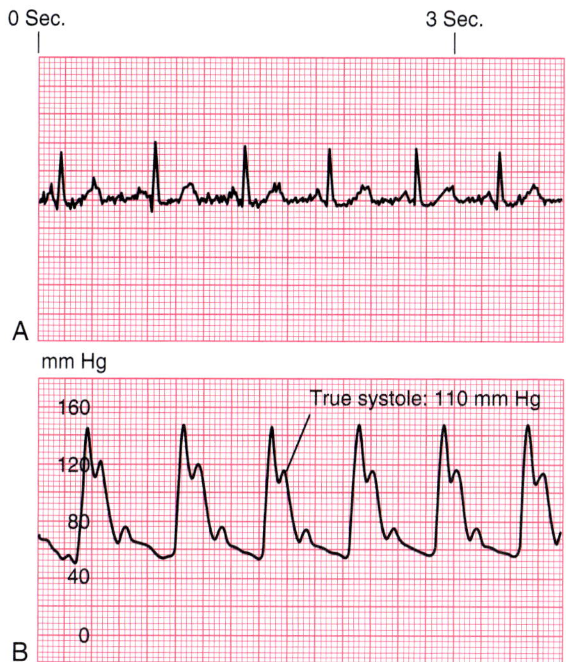

FIG. 12.10 Simultaneous electrocardiogram (A) and arterial pressure (B) tracings show the overshoot, or fling, caused by a heightened dynamic response in the monitoring system. The monitor recorded an arterial line blood pressure of 141/51 mm Hg. The patient's true blood pressure with a cuff was 110/54 mm Hg. The 110 mm Hg cuff systolic pressure is consistent with the arterial line tracing without overshoot.

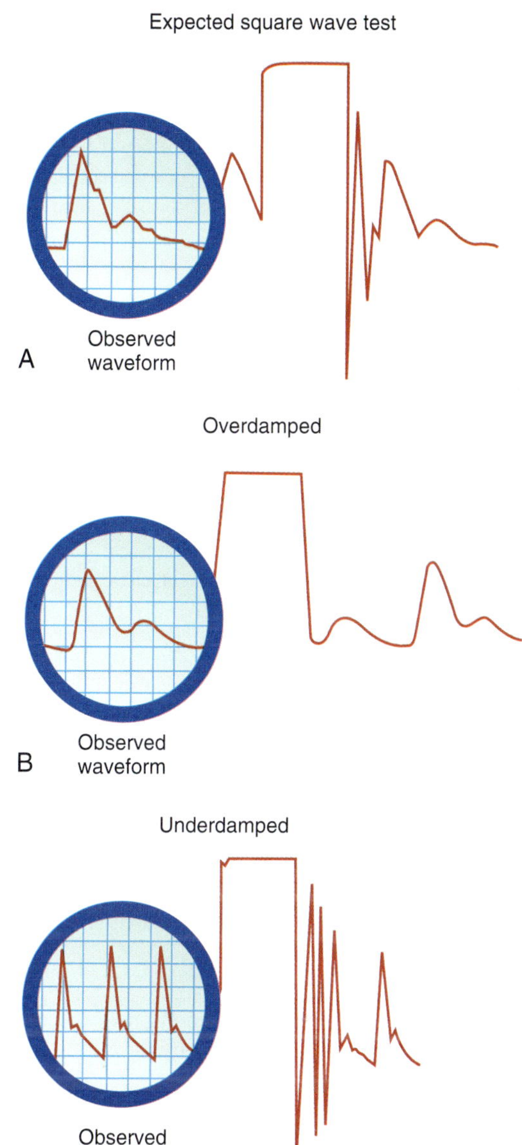

FIG. 12.11 Square Wave Test. (A) Expected square wave test result. (B) Overdamped. (C) Underdamped. (From Darovic GO. *Hemodynamic Monitoring: Invasive and Noninvasive Clinical Application.* 3rd ed. Saunders; 2002.)

through the right heart chambers (see Fig. 12.1). This predominantly describes central venous catheters, pulmonary artery catheters, thermodilution CO, and continuous mixed-venous oxygen saturation monitoring.[1] Some of the newer monitoring methods that combine arterial and central venous monitoring systems also are considered invasive (see Fig. 12.1).

CENTRAL VENOUS PRESSURE MONITORING

Monitoring of CVP may be indicated whenever a patient has a significant alteration in fluid volume (see Table 12.1). The CVP is often used as a guide for fluid volume replacement in hypovolemia. In addition to clinical signs and symptoms, CVP is also monitored in hypervolemia to assess the effect of diuresis after diuretic administration. When a major IV line is required for volume replacement, a central venous catheter (CVC) is used, because large volumes of fluid can be delivered easily. Because of the risks associated with central lines during insertion and maintenance, this is considered an invasive form of hemodynamic monitoring.

Central Venous Catheter Lumen Options

The range of available CVC options includes single-lumen, double-lumen, triple-lumen, and quad-lumen infusion catheters, depending on the specific needs of the patient. CVCs are made from a variety of materials ranging from polyurethane to silicone; most are soft and flexible. Antimicrobial coated catheters, in conjunction with CVC-infection-prevention bundles, are associated with a lower rate of bloodstream infections.[15]

Specialized Central Venous Catheters

A CVC that incorporates a fiberoptic sensor to continuously measure central venous oxygen saturation ($ScvO_2$) can be used as a traditional CVC and additionally used to follow the trend of venous oxygen saturation.[16] The physiology underlying use of this fiberoptic technology is discussed later in sections on monitoring mixed venous oxygen saturation (SvO_2) and $ScvO_2$.

Site Selection

The large veins of the upper thorax, the subclavian (SC) and internal jugular (IJ), are most used for percutaneous CVC line insertion. The femoral vein in the groin area is used when the thoracic veins are not accessible. All three major sites have different advantages and disadvantages.

Internal Jugular Vein

The IJ vein is a frequently used access site for CVC insertion. Disadvantages to the IJ vein include patient discomfort when moving the head or neck and risk of contamination of the IJ

BOX 12.1 Safety

Clinical Alarm Systems

Clinical Alarm System Effectiveness

1. Implement regular preventive maintenance and testing of alarm systems.
2. Ensure that alarms are activated with appropriate settings and are sufficiently audible with respect to distances and competing noise within the unit.

Clinical Alarm Safety Alarm Identification

1. Audible and visual indication should be present for any condition that poses a risk to the patient. Indicators should be visible from at least 10 ft (3 m).
2. Cause of the alarm must be easily identifiable by the health care practitioner.
3. Life-threatening conditions should be clearly differentiated from noncritical alarm situations.
4. High-priority alarms should override low-priority alarms.
5. Alarm must be sufficiently loud or distinctive to be heard over the environmental noise of a busy critical care unit.
6. It should never be possible to turn the volume control to "off."

Disabling and Silencing Alarms

1. Alarm silence must have visual indicator to clearly show it is disabled.
2. Critical alarms should not be permanently overridden (turned "off").
3. New, life-threatening alarm conditions should override a silenced alarm.

Power

Battery units should initiate an alarm before a unit stops working effectively.

Alarm Limits

1. Alarm limits can be adjusted to meet the clinical needs of a patient. The system should default to standard settings between patients.
2. Alarm limits should preferably be displayed on the monitor.

insertion site from oral or tracheal secretions, especially if the patient is intubated or has a tracheostomy.

Subclavian Vein

The SC position has the lowest infection rate compared to other sites.[5,6] The SC site has the least patient discomfort from the catheter. The disadvantages are that the SC vein is more difficult to access and carries a higher risk of iatrogenic pneumothorax or hemothorax. However, this risk varies greatly depending on the experience and skill of the physician or the advanced practice provider that is inserting the catheter.

Femoral Vein

The femoral vein is considered the easiest cannulation site because there are no curves in the insertion route. The large diameter of the femoral vein is advantageous for specialized procedures such as continuous renal replacement therapy or plasmapheresis. Because there is a higher rate of nosocomial infection with femoral catheters, this site is not recommended for routine access.[5,6] If a femoral venous access has been used, the CVC should be changed to either the SC or IJ location as soon as the patient is hemodynamically stable.

Insertion of a Central Venous Catheter

During insertion of a catheter in the SC or IJ vein, the patient may be placed in a Trendelenburg position if clinically tolerable. Placing the head in a dependent position causes the IJ veins in the neck to become more prominent, facilitating line placement. To minimize the risk of air embolus during the procedure, the patient may be asked to "take a deep breath and hold it" any time the needle or catheter is open to air. The tip of the catheter is designed to remain in the vena cava and should not migrate into the right atrium. Because many patients are awake and alert when a CVC is inserted, a brief explanation about the procedure can minimize patient anxiety and result in cooperation during the insertion. This cooperation is important, because CVC insertion is a sterile procedure and because the supine or Trendelenburg position may be uncomfortable for many patients. The electrocardiogram (ECG) should be monitored during CVC insertion because of the associated risk of dysrhythmias.

All CVCs are designed for placement by percutaneous injection after skin preparation and administration of a local anesthetic. Visualization of the vessel using bedside ultrasound before insertion is recommended to reduce CVC placement attempts. A prepackaged CVC kit typically is used for the procedure. The standard CVC kit contains sterile towels, chlorhexidine and alcohol for skin preparation, a needle introducer, a syringe, a guidewire, and a catheter. The Seldinger technique, in which the vein is located by using a "seeking" needle and syringe, is the preferred method of placement. A guidewire is passed through the needle, the needle is removed, and the catheter is passed over the guidewire. After the tip of the catheter is correctly placed in the vena cava, the guidewire is removed. Sterile intravenous tubing with solution is attached, and the catheter is sutured in place. A chest radiograph is obtained after upper thoracic CVC placement to verify placement and the absence of an iatrogenic hemothorax or pneumothorax, especially if the SC vein was accessed.

Complications

The CVC is an essential tool in care of a critically ill patient, but it is associated with some risks, and it is the responsibility of all clinicians to be informed about these hazards and to follow hospital procedures to avoid iatrogenic complications. CVC complications include air embolus, catheter-associated thrombus formation, and infection.

Air Embolus

The risk of air embolus, although rare, is always present for a patient with a central venous line in place.[17] Air can enter during insertion through a disconnected or broken catheter, or by means of an open stopcock, or air can enter along the path of a removed CVC. This is more likely when a patient is spontaneously breathing and is in an upright position, as air can be pulled into the venous system during inspiration (inhalation) as a result of the negative intrathoracic pressure during the inspiratory phase. If a large volume of air is inadvertently infused rapidly, it can become trapped in the right ventricular outflow tract, stopping blood flow from the right side of the heart to the lungs.[17] If the air embolus is large, the patient experiences respiratory distress and cardiovascular collapse. An auscultatory clinical sign specifically associated with a large venous air embolism is called a *mill wheel murmur*. A mill wheel murmur is a loud, churning sound heard over the middle chest, caused by a large obstruction to right ventricular outflow. Treatment involves immediately occluding the external site where air is entering, administering 100% oxygen, and placing the patient on the left side with the head downward *(left lateral Trendelenburg position)*. This position displaces the air from the right ventricular outflow tract to the apex of the heart, where the air may be aspirated by catheter intervention or gradually absorbed by the bloodstream as the patient remains in the left lateral Trendelenburg position. Precautions to prevent an air embolism in a central line include using only screw (Luer-Lock) connections and using only closed-top screw caps on all three-way stopcocks.

Thrombus Formation

Clot formation (thrombus) at the CVC site is common. Thrombus formation is not uniform; a thrombus can form at the catheter tip or be attached directly to the vessel wall. Risk factors include injury to the vessel wall during insertion and interruption of laminar blood flow. The use of ultrasound guided insertion reduces repeated insertion attempts and may decrease risk of vessel injury. Gradual thrombus formation may lead to "sudden" CVC occlusion as it becomes more difficult to withdraw blood from the CVC, or the waveform becomes intermittently damped over a period of hours or days. Patient risk factors include older age and carcinoma. CVC complications can be additive; for example, the risk of catheter-related infection is increased in the presence of thrombi, where the thrombus likely serves as a culture medium for bacterial growth.

Infection

Bloodstream infection related to the use of CVCs is a major risk. Described as a *central line bloodstream infection (CLABSI)*, the infection incidence strongly correlates with the length of time the CVC has been inserted, with longer insertion times associated with higher infection rates.[5,6] CVC-related infection is identified at the catheter insertion site or as a bloodstream infection (septicemia). Systemic manifestations of infection can be present without inflammation at the catheter site. No decrease in bloodstream infections was found when catheters were routinely changed, and this practice is no longer recommended.[5,6] When a CVC has redness at the site or signs of infection, it must be removed, and a new catheter must be inserted in a different site. If a catheter infection is suspected, the CVC should not be changed over a guidewire because of the risk of transferring the infection.[5,6]

Most infections are transmitted from the skin, and infection prevention begins before insertion of the CVC. Insertion guidelines state that the physician must use effective handwashing procedures, clean the insertion site with 2% chlorhexidine gluconate in 70% isopropyl, use sterile technique during catheter insertion, and maintain maximal sterile barrier precautions.[16,17] In most hospitals, the nurse is authorized to stop the insertion procedure if these insertion infection control guidelines are not followed. A daily review to determine whether the central line is still required is recommended to ensure that CVCs are removed promptly when no longer needed (Box 12.2).[5,6] All clinicians must use good handwashing technique and follow aseptic procedures during site care and any time the CVC system is entered to withdraw blood, give medications, or change tubing. Site dressings impregnated with chlorhexidine are recommended to reduce CVC infection rates.[17] To decrease the infection risk, most hospitals routinely audit use of CVCs to reduce the CVC duration to the absolute minimum, as fewer insertion days means fewer CLABSIs.

Nursing Management

In a critically ill patient, the CVC is used to monitor the venous pressure and waveform. The CVC access is used to measure the filling pressures of the right side of the heart. During diastole, when the tricuspid valve is open and blood is flowing from the right atrium to the right ventricle, the CVP accurately reflects right ventricular end-diastolic pressure. Normal CVP is 2 to 5 mm Hg.

Central Venous Pressure—Volume Assessment

Use of the CVP value alone to assess volume status is considered inaccurate.[18] A landmark systematic review of the literature revealed a weak relationship between the CVP measurement and patient blood volume.[18] Furthermore, a low CVP value is not always reliable in predicting which patients will respond to a fluid challenge. Overall, only approximately half of critically ill patients respond as expected to a fluid challenge. In this situation, it is essential to consider other indices of poor tissue perfusion, such as an elevated lactate level, low base deficit, or decreased urine output.

Passive Leg Raise

Another method to assess fluid responsiveness is to passively raise and support the patient's legs to allow the venous blood from the lower extremities to flow rapidly into the vena cava and return to the right heart. This method has the advantage of not infusing any IV fluid. If this maneuver significantly increases the CVP, this may suggest that the patient would have a positive response to an IV fluid bolus. However, change in the CVP value after a passive leg maneuver has not been consistently associated with a reduction in mortality or difference in other treatment outcomes.[19]

Removal of a CVC

Removal of the CVC usually is a nursing responsibility. Complications are uncommon, and the ones to anticipate are bleeding and air embolus. Recommended techniques to avoid air embolus during CVC removal include removing the catheter when the patient is supine in bed and placing the patient flat if the patient's clinical condition permits this maneuver. Patients with heart failure, pulmonary disease, and neurologic conditions with raised intracranial pressure should not be placed flat supine. Some hospitals recommend the Trendelenburg position (head downward) for CVC removal to reduce the risk of air embolus. If the patient is alert and able to cooperate, they are asked to take a deep breath to raise intrathoracic pressure during removal. After removal, to decrease the risk of air entering by a residual track, an occlusive dressing is applied to the site. If bleeding at the site occurs after removal, firm pressure is applied. If a patient has prolonged coagulation times, fresh frozen plasma or platelets may be prescribed before CVC removal.

Patient Position

To achieve accurate CVP measurements, the midaxillary line (phlebostatic axis) is used as a reference point on the body, and the transducer must be level with this point. If the midaxillary line is used and the transducer is correctly aligned, any head of bed position may be used for accurate CVP readings for most patients. Elevating the head of the bed is especially helpful for a patient with cardiopulmonary problems who cannot tolerate a flat supine position.

Central Venous Pressure Waveform

The normal right atrial (CVP) waveform has three positive deflections—a, c, and v waves—that correspond to specific atrial events in the cardiac cycle (Fig. 12.12).

BOX 12.2 Safety

1. Education, Training, and Staffing
   a. Nurses and other health care providers should receive education about indications for central venous catheter (CVC) use, maintenance, and infection prevention.
   b. Only trained personnel should insert and maintain CVCs.
   c. Adequate staffing levels in critical care units are associated with fewer catheter-related bloodstream infections (CRBSIs).
2. Selection of Catheters and Sites
   a. Use subclavian site rather than jugular or femoral insertion sites to minimize infection risk.
   b. Use ultrasound guidance to place CVCs.
   c. Remove any catheter that is no longer essential.
   d. If a CVC was placed in a medical emergency when aseptic technique was not assured, replace CVC within 48 h.
3. Hand Hygiene and Aseptic Technique
   a. Perform hand hygiene procedures by washing hands with soap and water or alcohol-based hand rub (ABHR) before and after palpating the CVC site, dressing the site, or any other intervention.
   b. New sterile gloves must be worn by the professional inserting the CVC.
   c. New sterile gloves must be donned before touching a new catheter for CVC exchange over a guidewire.
   d. Wear clean or sterile gloves when changing the catheter dressing.
4. Maximal Sterile Barrier Precautions
   a. For insertion, use maximal sterile barrier precautions including cap, mask, sterile gown, sterile gloves, and full-body drape.
5. Skin Preparation
   a. Prepare clean skin with greater than 0.5% chlorhexidine preparation with alcohol before CVC insertion.
   b. Antiseptics should be allowed to dry according to the manufacturer's recommendation before CVC insertion.
6. Catheter Site Dressing Regimens
   a. Transparent, semipermeable polyurethane dressings permit continuous visualization of the CVC insertion site.
   b. Replace transparent dressings on CVC sites at least every 7 days.
   c. Monitor the site when changing the dressing or by palpation through an intact dressing.
   d. Replace catheter site dressing whenever the dressing becomes damp, loose, or soiled.
   e. Do not use topical antibiotic ointment or creams on insertion sites (except for dialysis catheters) because of increased fungal infection risk.
   f. Use a chlorhexidine-impregnated sponge dressing at CVC site if CRBSI rate is not decreasing by other means (no recommendation for other types of chlorhexidine dressings).
7. Patient Cleansing
   a. Use 2% chlorhexidine wash for daily skin cleaning to reduce CRBSIs.
8. Catheter Securement Device
   a. Use a sutureless catheter securement device to reduce catheter movement, which may reduce infection risk.
9. Antimicrobial Strategies
   a. Use an antimicrobial-impregnated CVC when catheters are expected to remain in place for longer than 5 days.
   b. Do not administer systemic antimicrobial prophylaxis to prevent CRBSIs.
   c. Do not routinely use anticoagulant therapy to prevent CRBSIs.
10. No Routine CVC Replacement
    a. Do not routinely replace CVCs.
    b. Do not replace CVCs on the basis of fever alone.

From O'Grady P, Alexander M, Burns LA, et al. Guidelines for the prevention of intravascular catheter-related infections. *Am J Infect Control.* 2011;39(4):S1–S34.

- The *a wave* reflects atrial contraction and follows the P wave seen on the ECG. The downslope of this wave is called the *x descent* and represents atrial relaxation.
- The *c wave* reflects the bulging of the closed tricuspid valve into the right atrium during ventricular contraction; this wave is small and not always visible but corresponds to the QRS–T interval on the ECG.
- The *x descent* represents atrial relaxation. When the *c wave* is present, it interrupts the downward slope of the *x descent* and may be labeled x^1 (before the c wave) and x^2 (after the c wave, as shown in Fig. 12.12).
- The *v wave* represents atrial filling and increased pressure against the closed tricuspid valve in early diastole. The downslope of the v wave is named the *y descent.*
- The *y descent* represents the fall in pressure as the tricuspid valve opens and blood flows from the right atrium to the right ventricle.

This pattern may also be described as the right atrial waveform. When the tip of the CVC is positioned correctly within the superior vena cava (SVC), there are no obstructions or valves between the right atrium and the tip of the catheter. Therefore, the CVC waveform is an accurate reflection of the right atrial a, c, v, pressure waves described above.

Cannon Waves

Dysrhythmias can change the pattern of the CVP waveform. In a junctional rhythm or following a PVC, the atria are depolarized after the ventricles when retrograde conduction to the atria occurs. This may be seen as a retrograde P wave on the ECG and as a large, combined *ac* or *cannon wave* on the CVP waveform (Fig. 12.13). These cannon waves are observed as large pulses in the jugular veins. Other pathologic conditions, such as advanced right ventricular failure or tricuspid valve insufficiency, allow regurgitant backflow of blood from the right ventricle to the right atrium during ventricular contraction, producing large v waves on the right atrial waveform. In atrial fibrillation, the CVP waveform has no recognizable pattern because of the disorganization of the atrial contractions.

PULMONARY ARTERY PRESSURE MONITORING

The PA catheter is the most invasive of the critical care monitoring catheters (see Fig. 12.1). It is historically known as a *right heart catheter* or *Swan-Ganz catheter* (named after the catheter's inventors).[20] PA catheters are less frequently inserted now, except during open-heart surgery, [21,22] or in management of cardiogenic shock to monitor circulatory support.[23] The PA catheter is invasive. It previously seemed intuitive that the diagnostic information provided would confer a survival advantage over less-invasive methods, but research has shown this is not the case. Consequently, routine use of the PA catheter has decreased dramatically. One of the criticisms of the PA catheter is that the data it provides may result in overtreatment.

In noncardiac critical care units, the PA catheter has been replaced by less-invasive technologies, discussed later in this chapter.

The thermodilution PA catheter is reserved for the most hemodynamically unstable patients for the diagnosis and evaluation of cardiogenic shock, pulmonary hypertension,

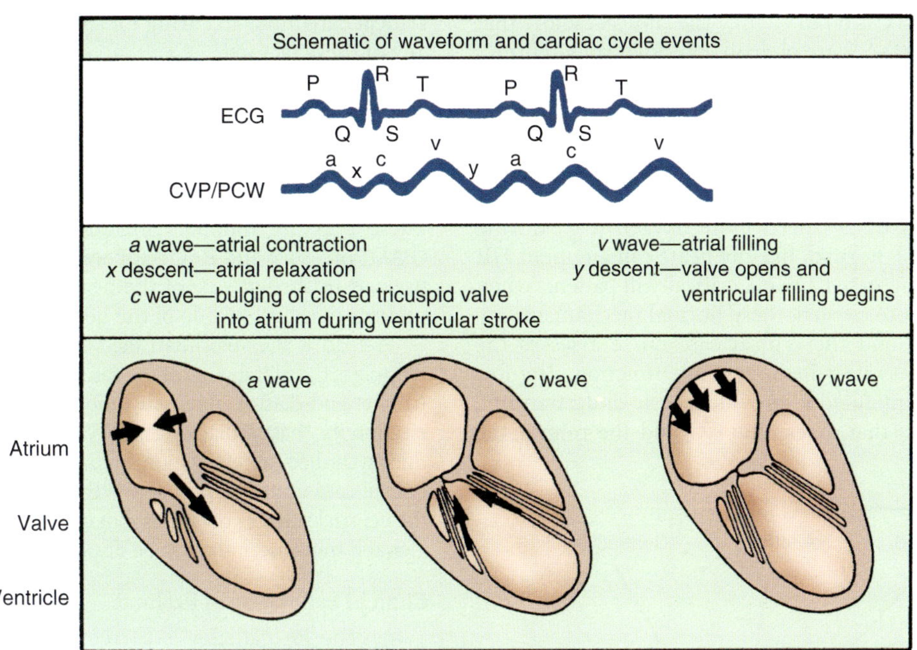

FIG. 12.12 Cardiac Events That Produce Central Venous Pressure Waveform With a, c, and v Waves. The a wave represents atrial contraction. The x descent represents atrial relaxation (it may be interrupted by the c wave). The c wave represents the bulging of the closed tricuspid valve into the right atrium during ventricular systole. The v wave represents atrial filling. The y descent represents opening of the tricuspid valve and filling of the ventricle. *CVP*, Central venous pressure; *ECG*, electrocardiogram; *PCW*, pulmonary capillary wedge pressure.

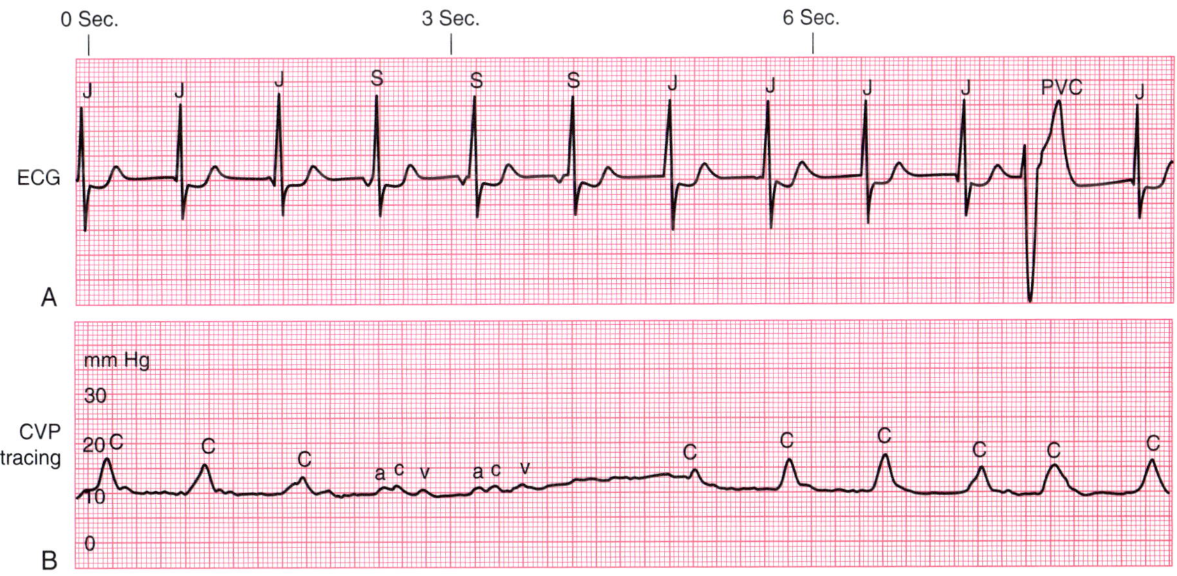

FIG. 12.13 Simultaneous electrocardiogram *(ECG)* (A) and central venous pressure *(CVP)* (B) tracings. The CVP waveform shows large cannon waves corresponding to the junctional beats or premature ventricular contractions *(bottom strip)*. As the patient converts to sinus rhythm, the CVP waveform has a normal configuration. *ac*, Normal right atrial pressure tracing; *C*, cannon waves on CVP tracing; *J*, junctional rhythm followed by cannon waves on CVP waveform; *PVC*, premature ventricular contraction followed by cannon wave on CVP; *S*, sinus rhythm followed by normal CVP tracing with a, c, and v waves.

and management during and after heart surgery.[21,23] The PA catheter can provide information about PA pressures (systolic, diastolic, mean), PAOP (wedge pressure), and CO. The location of the tip of the PA catheter in the pulmonary artery can provide access for measurement of mixed venous oxygen saturation.

Cardiac Output Determinants

CO is the product of HR multiplied by SV.

SV is the volume of blood ejected by the heart during each beat (reported in milliliters).

$$HR \times SV = CO$$

The normal adult SV is 60 to 70 mL. The clinical factors that contribute to the heart's SV are preload, afterload, and contractility and may be monitored using the PA catheter (Fig. 12.14). Another contributor to CO is HR, which is usually recorded from the ECG leads.

Oxygen Supply and Demand

When the peripheral tissues need more oxygen (e.g., during exercise or sepsis), the normal, healthy heart can augment HR and SV and greatly increase CO. In a critically ill patient, when the tissues require more oxygen, these normal mechanisms are often nonfunctional, and the critical care nurse assesses the need for and then optimizes hemodynamic function. The following discussion is intended to provide a basic understanding of the clinical factors that determine CO and the role of the critical care nurse in caring for the patient with an alteration in any of these factors.

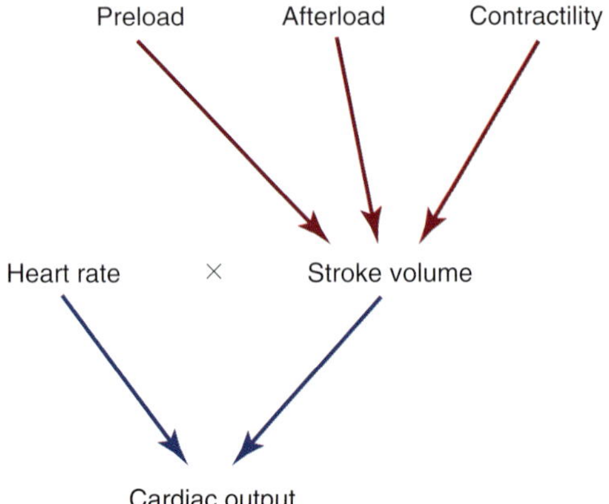

FIG. 12.14 Preload, afterload, and contractility contribute to stroke volume. Stroke volume × Heart rate = Cardiac output.

Preload

Clinicians commonly describe the hemodynamic numbers related to preload as *filling pressures*. These values refer to the pressures resulting from the volumes in the atria and ventricles. These pressure numbers include pulmonary artery diastolic (PAD) pressure and PAOP (or wedge pressure), which measure preload in the left side of the heart, and CVP, which measures preload in the right side of the heart.

Preload is the volume in the ventricle at end-diastole. Because diastole is the filling stage of the cardiac cycle, the volume in the ventricle at end-diastole represents the presystolic volume available for ejection for that cardiac cycle. LV volume can be measured directly during cardiac catheterization, but it is not generally measured in the critical care unit. The principle is that the presence of blood within the ventricle creates pressures that can be measured by the PA catheter and transducer and can be displayed on the bedside monitor.

Clinical Estimation of Preload

When the PA catheter is correctly positioned with the tip in one of the large branches of the PA, the only valve between the PA catheter tip and the left ventricle is the mitral valve. During diastole, when the mitral valve is open, no vascular obstruction exists between the tip of the PA catheter and the left ventricle (Fig. 12.15). The LV preload volume creates left ventricular end-diastolic pressure (LVEDP). Using a PA catheter, preload is estimated by measuring the PAOP or wedge pressure. Normal left atrial pressure or PAOP is 5 to 12 mm Hg.

Frank-Starling Law of the Heart

The PAOP has clinical significance, because a change in LV volume (preload) is reflected by a change in the measured PAOP

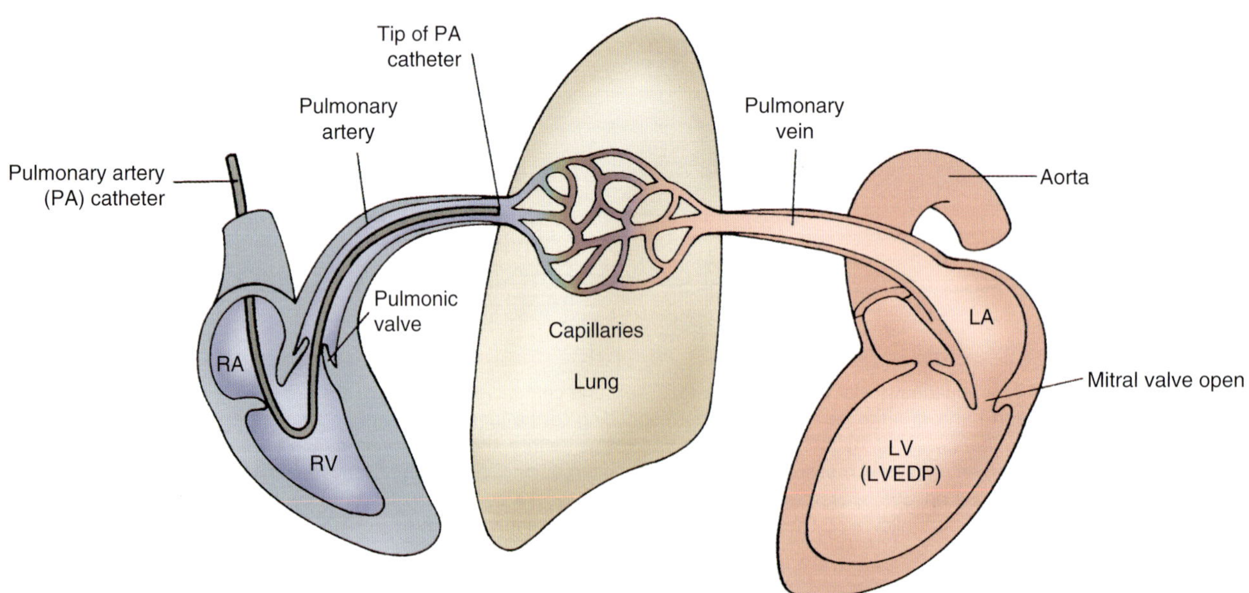

FIG. 12.15 Relationship of Pulmonary Artery Occlusion Pressure (PAOP) to Left Ventricular End-Diastolic Pressure *(LVEDP)*. In most clinical situations, PAOP (i.e., wedge pressure) accurately reflects LVEDP (i.e., preload). During diastole, when the mitral valve is open, there are no other valves or other obstructions between the tip of the catheter and the left ventricle *(LV)*. The pressure exerted by the volume in the LV is reflected through the left atrium *(LA)*, through the pulmonary veins, and to the pulmonary capillaries. *PA*, Pulmonary artery; *RA*, right atrium; *RV*, right ventricle.

(wedge pressure). Change in preload relies on the Frank-Starling law of the heart.[24] This law states that the force of ventricular ejection is directly related to the following two elements:

- Volume in the ventricle at end-diastole (preload)
- Amount of myocardial stretch placed on the ventricle muscle

If the volume in the left ventricle is low, CO is also suboptimal. If IV fluids (volume) are infused, CO increases as LV volume and myocardial fiber stretch increase. This is true up to a point. Past this point, more fluid volume overdistends the ventricle and stretches the myocardial fibers so much that CO decreases. This scenario is seen clinically in the setting of acute heart failure with pulmonary edema. The increased volume in the overdistended left ventricle raises pressure in the left ventricle, left atrium, and pulmonary veins (that drain into the left atrium), and this ultimately raises pulmonary capillary pressures, measured as increased wedge pressure (PAOP). The effect of preload on CO is represented in Figs. 12.16 and 12.17 using the Frank-Starling curve as a model.[24]

Ejection Fraction

The relationship of preload to the CO is complex, because not all of the preload volume is ejected with every heartbeat. The percentage of preload volume ejected from the left ventricle per beat is measured during cardiac catheterization and is described as the ejection fraction (EF). A normal EF in a vigorous healthy heart is approximately 70%. In clinical practice, most cardiologists accept an EF of greater than 50% as normal. The volume ejected from the left ventricle with each beat is known as the stroke volume (SV), which can be calculated at the bedside by dividing the CO by the HR per minute (SV = CO ÷ HR).

Preload and Ventricular Dysfunction

A significant relationship exists between LVEDP and cardiac muscle dysfunction. As a rule, the higher the pressure inside the left ventricle, the greater the degree of cardiac dysfunction. The pressure rises at end-diastole (end of filling) because the compromised ventricle cannot eject all the preload blood volume. For example, in a patient with heart failure, the preload volume may be 100 mL. However, the SV ejected may be only 30 mL. The EF in this patient is 30% (normal EF is greater than 50%). The remaining preload volume (70 mL in this example) significantly elevates LV pressures. When the mitral valve opens at the beginning of diastole, the pressure in the left atrium needs to be slightly higher than pressures in the left ventricle to allow filling. The 70 mL remaining in the ventricle produces high LV diastolic pressures. This elevates the left atrial filling pressure and consequently elevates the PAOP (wedge pressure). In this example, the left ventricle is overstretched by excessive preload, and CO is below normal. The myocardial dysfunction eventually leads to heart failure symptoms, which are discussed further in Chapter 13.[25]

Pulmonary Artery Diastolic Pressure and Pulmonary Artery Occlusion Pressure Relationship

LVEDP can be estimated by indirect measures using the PA catheter by two methods.

- **PAOP**: *pulmonary artery occlusion pressure*, which is informally known as the *wedge pressure* when the catheter balloon is inflated and wedged into a small pulmonary artery. This is the most accurate method to measure LVEDP.
- **PAD pressure**: *pulmonary artery diastolic pressure*, is used when the balloon is not in an optimal position to wedge when inflated. In this situation the PAD pressure can be used to estimate LVEDP. The underlying physiology is that during diastole the normal PAD pressure is only 1 to 3 mm Hg higher than the mean PAOP (wedge). Thus, in many patients the PAD pressure may be used to estimate LVEDP (Table 12.3, illustration A).

Even in the setting of heart failure, the PAD pressure may be used to estimate LVEDP when the PA catheter balloon is not optimally positioned to wedge. In left-sided heart failure with a low SV and low CO, intracardiac filling pressures are elevated in the left ventricle, the left atrium, and in the pulmonary vasculature. Consequently, both the PAOP (wedge) and the PAD pressure are elevated. This is illustrated in (Table 12.3, illustration B) which shows elevated PAOP and PAD pressures and illustrates their close relationship. This pathophysiology is further explained in the preceding section titled "Preload and Ventricular Dysfunction." It is physiologically impossible for the PAOP (wedge pressure) be higher than the PAD pressure. The system

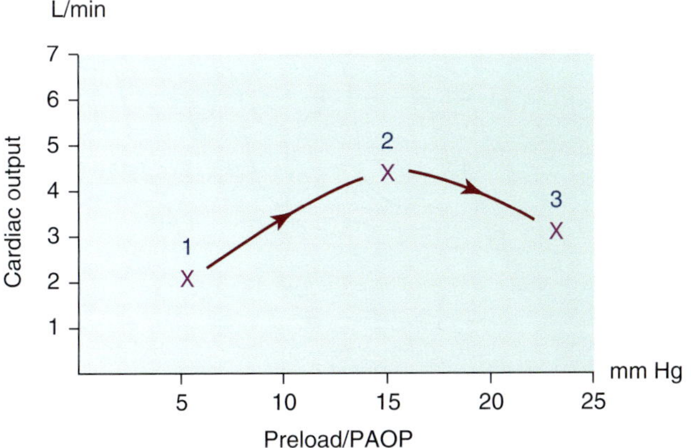

FIG. 12.16 Effect of Preload on Cardiac Output (CO). *1,* Poor cardiac output with low preload as a result of hypovolemia. *2,* Hypovolemia is corrected after administration of 2 L of intravenous fluid. The preload volume in the ventricle is increased, and pulmonary artery occlusion pressure *(PAOP)* has risen. Because of the increased fiber stretch from the increase in preload, CO also has risen. *3,* After infusion of an additional 2 L of intravenous solution, the myocardial fibers are overdistended, preload (PAOP) has increased, and CO has fallen as the volume in the left ventricle rises.

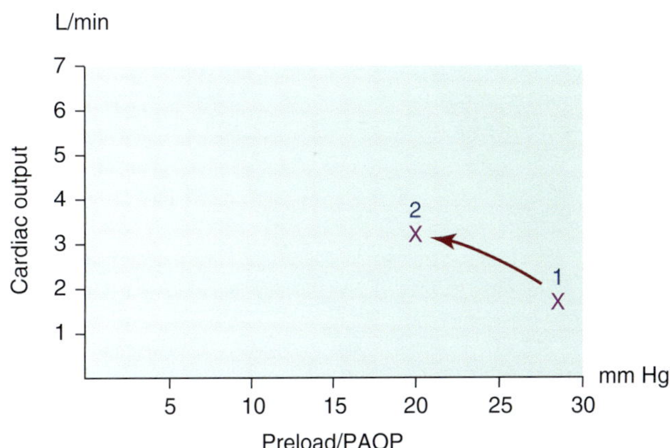

FIG. 12.17 Effect of Preload and Venodilation on Cardiac Output (CO). *1,* After an acute anterior wall myocardial infarction that has created significant left ventricular dysfunction, this patient has left ventricle pump failure with low CO and elevated filling pressures identified by an elevated pulmonary artery occlusion pressure *(PAOP)*. One of the clinical problems faced by this patient is too much preload. *2,* After administration of diuretics to reduce volume and nitroglycerin to dilate the venous system, preload is reduced, and CO rises.

must be recalibrated to troubleshoot the monitoring system if this appears to occur (see Table 12.2).

Pulmonary Hypertension and PAD-PAOP

Specific clinical conditions can alter the normal PAD-PAOP relationship, most notably pulmonary hypertension and acute right heart failure. In pulmonary hypertension, the pulmonary arterial systolic and diastolic pressures are independently raised above the LV pressures.[26] In this clinical situation, the PAD pressure does not accurately reflect function of the left side of the heart as illustrated in Table 12.3, illustration C. Additional information about pulmonary hypertension is provided in Chapter 13.

Valvular Heart Disease and PAD-PAOP

In failure of the left side of the heart, the PAD and PAOP (wedge) are both elevated and approximately equal (see Table 12.3, illustration B). If the mitral valve is stenotic, pressures in the left atrium and the pulmonary vasculature will increase, while the left ventricle will have lower pressures due to reduced blood flow through the narrowed valve.

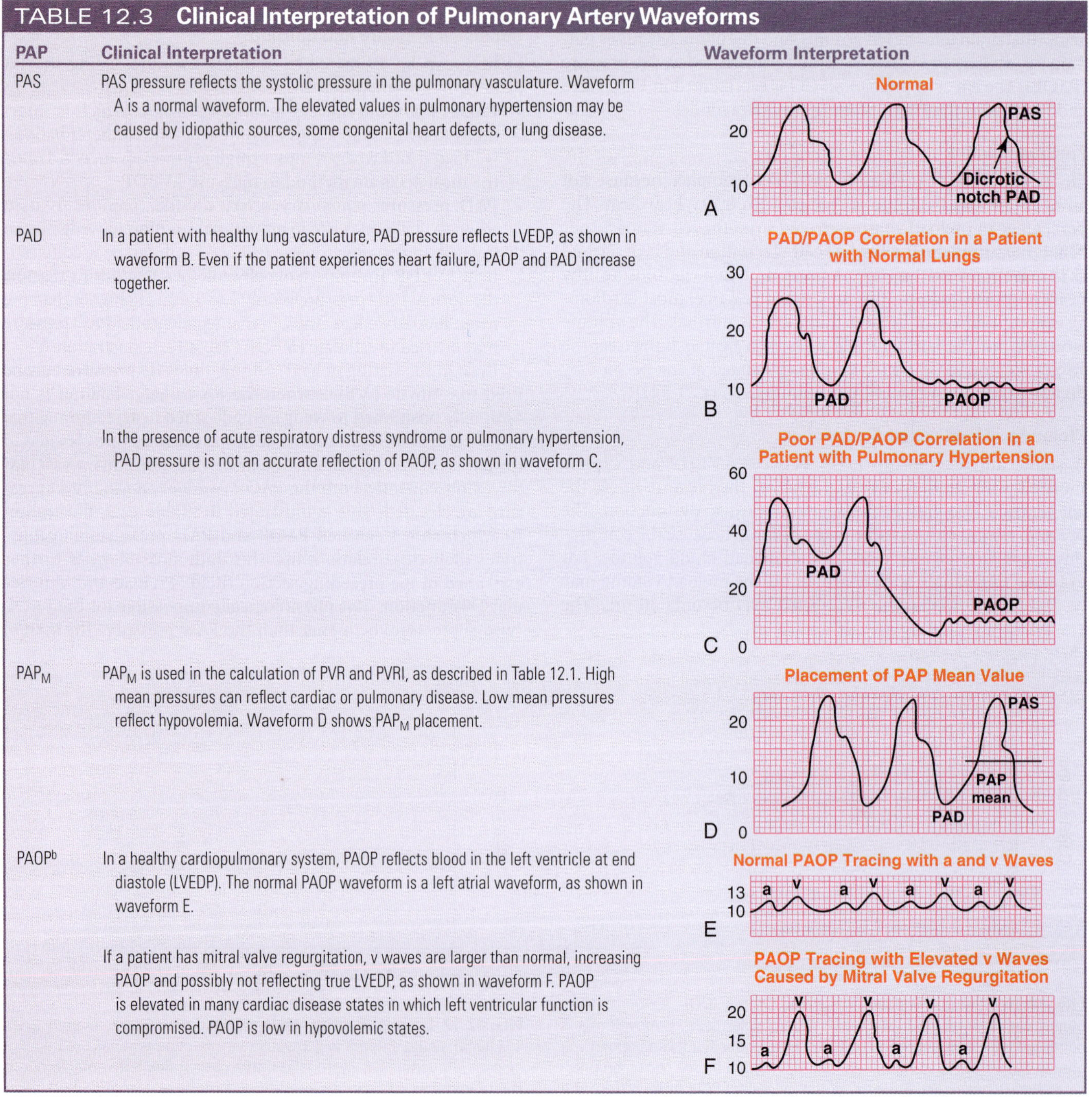

TABLE 12.3 Clinical Interpretation of Pulmonary Artery Waveforms

PAP	Clinical Interpretation	Waveform Interpretation
PAS	PAS pressure reflects the systolic pressure in the pulmonary vasculature. Waveform A is a normal waveform. The elevated values in pulmonary hypertension may be caused by idiopathic sources, some congenital heart defects, or lung disease.	A: Normal (20, 10; PAS; Dicrotic notch PAD)
PAD	In a patient with healthy lung vasculature, PAD pressure reflects LVEDP, as shown in waveform B. Even if the patient experiences heart failure, PAOP and PAD increase together.	B: PAD/PAOP Correlation in a Patient with Normal Lungs (30, 20, 10; PAD; PAOP)
	In the presence of acute respiratory distress syndrome or pulmonary hypertension, PAD pressure is not an accurate reflection of PAOP, as shown in waveform C.	C: Poor PAD/PAOP Correlation in a Patient with Pulmonary Hypertension (60, 40, 20, 0; PAD; PAOP)
PAP_M	PAP_M is used in the calculation of PVR and PVRI, as described in Table 12.1. High mean pressures can reflect cardiac or pulmonary disease. Low mean pressures reflect hypovolemia. Waveform D shows PAP_M placement.	D: Placement of PAP Mean Value (20, 10, 0; PAS; PAP mean; PAD)
PAOP[b]	In a healthy cardiopulmonary system, PAOP reflects blood in the left ventricle at end diastole (LVEDP). The normal PAOP waveform is a left atrial waveform, as shown in waveform E.	E: Normal PAOP Tracing with a and v Waves (13, 10; a, v, a, v, a, v, a, v)
	If a patient has mitral valve regurgitation, v waves are larger than normal, increasing PAOP and possibly not reflecting true LVEDP, as shown in waveform F. PAOP is elevated in many cardiac disease states in which left ventricular function is compromised. PAOP is low in hypovolemic states.	F: PAOP Tracing with Elevated v Waves Caused by Mitral Valve Regurgitation (20, 15, 10; v, a, v, a, v, a, v, a)

[a]Pressures on the y axis are given in mm Hg.
[b]Or pulmonary artery occlusion pressure (PAOP).

LVEDP, Left ventricular end-diastolic pressure; *PAD*, pulmonary artery diastolic; *PAOP*, pulmonary artery occlusion pressure; *PAP*, pulmonary artery pressure; *PAP_M*, mean pulmonary artery pressure; *PAS*, pulmonary artery systolic; *PVR*, pulmonary vascular resistance; *PVRI*, pulmonary vascular resistance index

Mitral Regurgitation and PAD-PAOP

In patients with a mitral valve regurgitation (MR), the mean PAOP (wedge) reading is artificially elevated because of abnormal backflow of blood from the left ventricle to the left atrium during systole. The causes of MR are diverse because of the complex architecture of the mitral valve.[27] Degenerative valve disease damages the valve leaflets, and myocardial infarction (MI) can cause rupture of the papillary muscles or chordae tendineae.

Acute MR is notable for very large v waves on the PAOP (wedge) tracing (see Table 12.3, illustration F). The size of the v wave is related to the amount of regurgitation during systole and the compliance of the left atrium, although individual cardiac anatomy results in considerable variation between patients.[28] Reading the PAOP tracing in the presence of MR can be very challenging without the context of a cardiac history and symptoms.

If MR is chronic and the left atrium is compliant and enlarged, the v waves may be small.

In the setting of acute MR after infarction of a papillary muscle, a smaller noncompliant or stiff atrium may result in larger v waves on the wedge tracing. If the v waves are large (acute MR), they cannot be used to accurately estimate LV preload. If the v wave is small (chronic MR), the mean PAOP may be used to estimate LV preload (LVEDP), which would be elevated. Echocardiography is increasingly used to confirm the presence of MR. [28]

Afterload

Afterload is defined as the pressure the ventricle generates to overcome the resistance to ejection created by the arteries and arterioles. It is a calculated measurement derived from information obtained from the PA catheter. As a response to increased afterload, ventricular wall tension rises. After a decrease in afterload, wall tension is lowered. The technical name for afterload is *systemic vascular resistance (SVR).*

Systemic Vascular Resistance

Resistance to ejection from the left side of the heart is estimated by calculating the SVR. The calculation represents the pressure difference between the average arterial pressure (MAP) and venous pressure (CVP) divided by flow (CO). The formula, normally calculated by the bedside computer, is as follows:

$$SVR = \frac{MAP - CVP}{CO} = 80$$

The normal value is 800 to 1200 dyn • sec • cm^{-5}. To index this value to the patient's body surface area, the cardiac index (CI) is placed in the formula in the same position as the CO. The critical care nurse frequently manipulates prescribed vasoactive medications to therapeutically alter SVR. In general, the lower the SVR value (arteries more dilated), the higher the CO.

Systemic Vascular Resistance and Afterload Reduction

Pharmacologic manipulation of SVR to improve cardiac performance is commonly used in critically ill patients.

Low SVR. If the SVR is extremely low (e.g., less than 500 dyn • sec • cm^{-5}), as may occur in sepsis, the CO will be elevated, and MAP will be low. In this situation, volume and vasopressors are infused to increase MAP and SVR. After adequate volume resuscitation, the Surviving Sepsis Campaign guidelines recommend norepinephrine (Levophed) administered via a CVC, which increases MAP by vasoconstriction of the peripheral vasculature to increase SVR.[29] Frequent assessment of the peripheral circulation is required when medications that increase SVR are used, because excessive vasoconstriction will decrease tissue perfusion.

For a person with a normal heart without cardiac dysfunction, an elevated SVR may have only a small effect on CO. The importance of SVR on CO is related to the functional quality of the myocardium. However, when the heart muscle is globally damaged (cardiomyopathy) or regionally damaged (MI), small changes in SVR can produce significant changes in CO.

High SVR. When the SVR is elevated, continuous infusions of vasodilators such as sodium nitroprusside or high-dose nitroglycerin may be used to reduce SVR.

Clinical Exemplar: Mr. T had a large anterior wall MI 2 days ago. As a result, he has symptoms of acute heart failure, an elevated SVR of 1840 dyn • sec • cm^{-5}, and a low CO of 2.8 L/min. In a heart with decreased contractility after an acute MI, an SVR measurement above the normal range lowers CO. To optimize Mr. T's cardiac function, systemic vasodilators (afterload-reducing medications) are infused to lower the SVR into the normal range. After the administration of sodium nitroprusside (1 to 4 mcg/kg per minute), Mr. T's SVR decreased to 970 dyn • sec • cm^{-5}, and his CO increased to 4.1 L/min. In this situation, decreasing the SVR greatly increased the amount of blood ejected from the left ventricle.

Pulmonary Vascular Resistance

Resistance to ejection from the right side of the heart is estimated by calculating the pulmonary vascular resistance (PVR). The PVR value is normally one-sixth of the SVR. Normal PVR is 100 to 250 dyn • sec • cm^{-5}. The formula to calculate PVR is listed in Appendix B. Acute pulmonary hypertension, identified as an elevated mean PA pressure can occur as a sequela of severe acute respiratory distress syndrome (ARDS).[30] The acute rise in PVR may cause the right ventricle to fail, although LV pressures may remain within the normal range. Traditionally, a PA catheter was used to monitor vasodilator therapy and fluid management, although this is no longer recommended. Current guidelines on ARDS management do not even mention the PA catheter.[31]

Contractility

Many factors impact contractility, including preload volume as measured by PAOP, SVR, myocardial oxygenation, electrolyte balance, positive and negative inotropic medications, and amount of functional myocardium available to contribute to contraction. These factors can have a positive inotropic effect, enhancing contractility, or a negative inotropic effect, decreasing contractility. Significant factors related to contractility that can be measured by the PA catheter include preload filling pressures, SVR, and CO. Additional contractility numbers can be calculated and are displayed in the hemodynamic profile on the bedside monitor. These include left and right ventricular stroke work index values. These values estimate the force of cardiac contraction (see Table 12.1).

Preload contributes to contractility using the Starling mechanism.[24] As volume in the ventricle rises, contractility increases up to a point. If the ventricle is overdistended with volume, contractility falls (see Figs. 12.16 and 12.17). SVR alters contractility by changes in resistance to ventricular ejection.

- When SVR is high, ventricular contractility is reduced.
- When SVR is low, ventricular contractility is augmented.

Hypoxemia acts as a negative inotrope, because the myocardium must have oxygen for the cells to contract efficiently.

Optimizing Contractility

IV medications such as dopamine, dobutamine, and milrinone are prescribed for their positive inotropic effect. The nurse considers the effect of these pharmacologic agents on contractility when following the trend of the patient's hemodynamic profile. No single hemodynamic number reflects contractility. However, if LV contractility is increased in response to treatment, this effect is frequently reflected by changes in PAOP (wedge pressure) and by an increase in CO.

Pulmonary Artery Catheters

The traditional PA catheter, invented by Swan and Ganz, has four lumens for measurement of right atrial pressure, PA pressures, PAOP, and CO (Fig. 12.18A). Multifunction catheters may have additional lumens, which can be used for IV infusion (Fig. 12.18B) and to measure continuous SvO_2, right ventricular volume, and continuous CO (Fig. 12.18C). Other PA

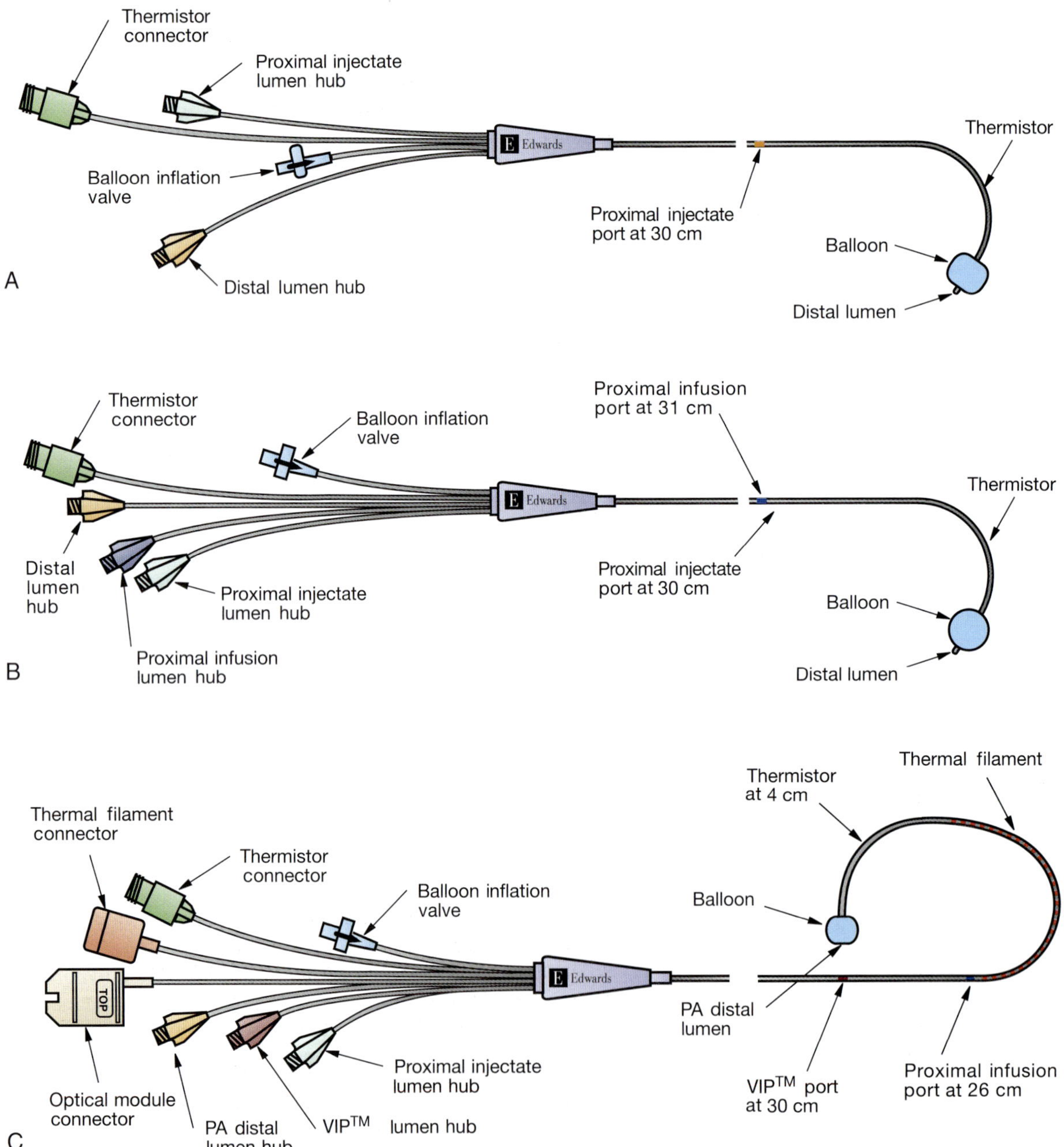

FIG. 12.18 Types of Pulmonary Artery Catheters. (A) Four-lumen catheter. (B) Five-lumen catheter that includes additional venous infusion port *(VIP)* into the right atrium. (C) Seven-lumen catheter that includes a VIP port and two additional lumens, as well as a thermal filament for continuous cardiac output (CCO) and internal fiberoptic strands for continuous mixed venous oxygen saturation (SvO_2) monitoring (i.e., optical module connector). An additional option is to combine the use of the CCO filament and the thermistor response time to calculate continuous right ventricular end-diastolic volume and right ventricular ejection fraction. *PA*, Pulmonary artery. (Copyright 2001 Edwards Lifesciences LLC. All rights reserved. Reprinted with permission of Edwards Lifesciences, Swan-Ganz is a trademark of Edwards Lifesciences Corporation, registered in the US Patent and Trademark Office.)

catheters include transvenous pacing electrodes to pace the heart if needed.

The PA flow-directed catheter is 110 cm long. The most used sizes are 7.5 or 8.0 Fr, although 5.0 and 7.0 Fr sizes are available. Each of the four lumens exits into the heart or pulmonary artery at a different point, graduated along the catheter length (see Fig. 12.18A).

Right Atrial Lumen

The proximal lumen is situated in the right atrium and is used for IV infusion, right atrial pressure measurement, withdrawal of venous blood samples, and injection of fluid for CO determinations. This port is often described as the *right atrial port.*

Pulmonary Artery Lumen

The distal PA lumen is located at the tip of the PA catheter and is situated in the pulmonary artery. It is used to record pressures within the artery and can be used for withdrawal of blood samples to measure mixed venous blood gases.

Balloon Lumen

The third lumen opens into a balloon at the end of the catheter that can be inflated with 0.8 mL (7 Fr) to 1.5 mL (7.5 Fr) of air. The balloon is inflated during catheter insertion after the catheter reaches the right atrium to assist in forward flow of the catheter and to minimize right ventricular ectopy from the catheter tip. The balloon is also inflated to obtain the PAOP (wedge) measurements when the PA catheter is correctly positioned in the pulmonary artery.

Thermistor Lumen

The fourth lumen is a thermistor (temperature sensor) used to measure changes in blood temperature. It is located 4 cm from the catheter tip and is the calculation of thermodilution CO.

Additional PA Catheter Features

If continuous SvO_2 is measured, the catheter has an additional fiberoptic lumen that exits at the tip of the catheter (see Fig. 12.18C).

If cardiac pacing is used, two PA catheter methods are available:

- PA catheter with three atrial (A) and two ventricular (V) pacing electrodes that can be connected to a pacemaker for atrioventricular (AV) pacing.
- Transvenous pacing wire is passed through an additional catheter lumen to exit into the right ventricle if ventricular pacing is required.

A right ventricular volumetric PA catheter measures SV in the right ventricle.

Insertion of the Pulmonary Artery Catheter

If a PA catheter is to be inserted into a patient who is awake, some brief explanations about the procedure are helpful to ensure that the patient understands what is going to happen. The initial insertion techniques used for placement of a PA catheter are similar to those described for CVC insertion. Because the PA catheter passes within the right heart chambers and pulmonary artery, the catheter insertion is monitored using fluoroscopy or waveform analysis on the bedside monitor (Fig. 12.19). In most insertions, the PA catheter floats into the right pulmonary artery.

Before inserting the catheter into the vein, the physician—using sterile technique—tests the balloon for inflation and flushes the catheter with physiologic saline to remove any air. The PA catheter is then attached to the bedside hemodynamic line setup and monitor so that the waveforms can be visualized while the catheter is advanced through the right side of the heart (see Fig. 12.19). A larger introducer sheath (8.5 Fr), which has the tip positioned in the vena cava and has an additional IV side-port lumen, is often used to cannulate the vein first. This introducer sheath is known by several different names in clinical practice, including

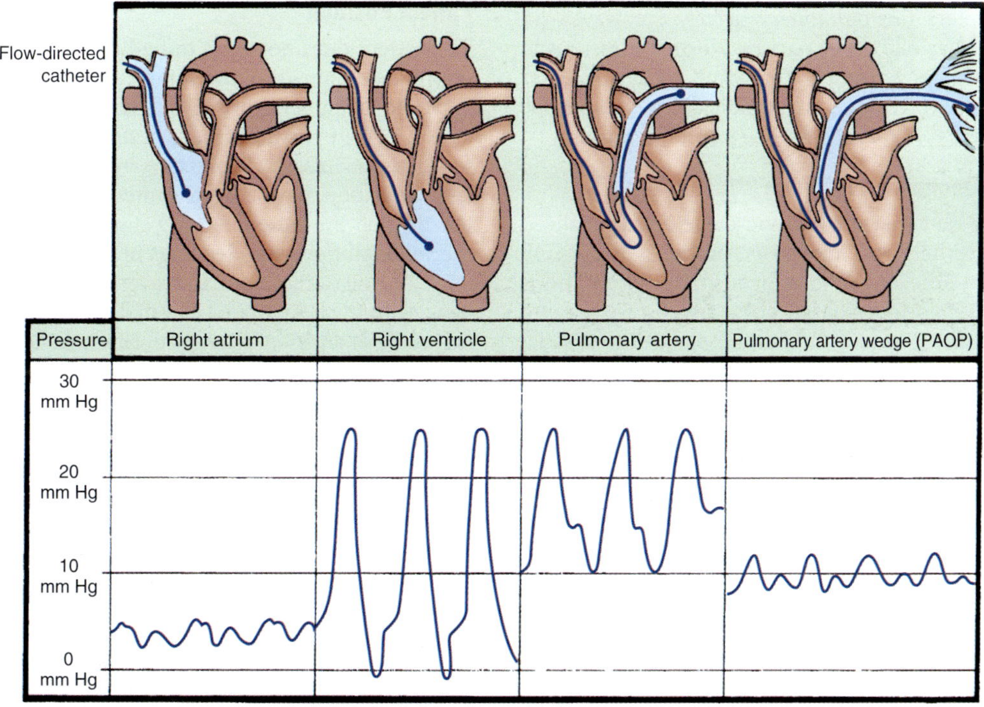

FIG. 12.19 Pulmonary Artery Catheter Insertion With Corresponding Waveforms.

sheath, cordis, introducer, or *side port.* This introducer sheath remains in place, and the supple PA catheter is threaded through it into the vena cava and into the right side of the heart.

Pulmonary Artery Waveform Interpretation

Each chamber of the heart has a distinctive waveform with recognizable characteristics. It is the responsibility of the critical care nurse to recognize each waveform displayed on the bedside monitor when the catheter enters the corresponding chamber during insertion and during routine monitoring.

Right Atrial Waveform

As the PA catheter is advanced into the right atrium during insertion, a right atrial waveform should be visible on the monitor, with recognizable a, c, and v waves (see Fig. 12.19). Normal mean pressure in the right atrium is 2 to 5 mm Hg. Before passage through the tricuspid valve, the balloon at the tip of the catheter is inflated for two reasons.

- The balloon cushions the pointed tip of the PA catheter during its passage through the ventricle. This minimizes myocardial irritability and lowers the risk of ventricular dysrhythmias.
- Balloon inflation allows the catheter to float with the flow of blood from the right ventricle into the pulmonary artery.

Because of these features and the balloon, PA catheters are described as *flow-directional catheters.*

Right Ventricular Waveform

The right ventricular waveform is distinctly pulsatile, with distinct systolic and diastolic pressures. Normal right ventricular pressures are 20 to 30 mm Hg systolic and 0 to 5 mm Hg diastolic. Even with the balloon inflated, it is common for ventricular ectopy to occur during passage through the right ventricle. All patients who have a PA catheter inserted must have simultaneous ECG monitoring, with defibrillator and emergency resuscitation equipment nearby.

Pulmonary Artery Waveform

As the catheter enters the pulmonary artery, the waveform again changes. The diastolic pressure rises. Normal pressures in the pulmonary artery range from 20 to 30 mm Hg systolic over 10 mm Hg diastolic. A dicrotic notch, visible on the downslope of the waveform, represents closure of the pulmonic valve.

Pulmonary Artery Occlusion Waveform (Wedge)

While the balloon remains inflated, the catheter is advanced into the wedge position. This maneuver produces the PAOP left atrial waveform. The PAOP waveform small in size and is nonpulsatile, reflecting a normal left atrial tracing with a and v wave deflections (the c wave is difficult to see in the left atrial tracing). This is known as a *wedge tracing* because the balloon is "wedged" into a small pulmonary vessel, but it is technically described as the PAOP (see Fig. 12.19) or sometimes a PAWP (PA wedge pressure). The balloon occludes the pulmonary vessel so that the PA catheter tip and lumen are exposed only to left atrial pressure and are protected from the pulsatile influence of the right ventricle and PA. When the balloon is deflated, the catheter should spontaneously float back into the PA. When the balloon is reinflated, the catheter should move forward into a small artery and the wedge tracing should be visible on the monitor. Normal PAOP ranges from 5 to 12 mm Hg.

After insertion, the introducer is sutured to the skin, and the catheter, which lies within the introducer, is secured with a catheter securement device. A chest radiograph is taken to verify placement. If the catheter is advanced too far into the pulmonary bed, the patient is at risk for pulmonary infarction. If the PA catheter is not advanced sufficiently into the pulmonary artery, it will not be useful for PAOP readings. However, in many critical care units, if the patient's PAD pressure and PAOP values approximate (within 1 to 3 mm Hg), the PAD pressure is reliably used to follow the trend of LV filling pressure (preload). This practice prevents possible trauma from frequent balloon inflation; in such a situation, the PA catheter is consciously pulled back into a safe position within the pulmonary artery so that wedging cannot occur.

After insertion of the catheter, a chest radiograph or fluoroscopy is used to verify the PA catheter position to ensure that it is not looped or knotted in the right ventricle and to rule out pneumothorax or hemorrhagic complications. A thin plastic sleeve is placed on the outside of the catheter when it is inserted to maintain sterility of the part of the PA catheter that exits from the patient.[32] If the PA catheter is not in the desired position or if it migrates out of position, it can be repositioned within the plastic sleeve.

Medical Management

Controversy exists in the medical community over the use of PA catheters, and rates of use have declined in response to lack of benefit demonstrated in clinical trials.[1] Medical goals of hemodynamic monitoring include assessment of adequacy of perfusion in stable patients, early detection of decreased perfusion, titration of therapy to meet specific therapeutic outcomes, and differentiation of different organ system dysfunctions.

Nursing Management

The more knowledgeable the critical care nurse can become about use of the PA catheter, the more accurate and effective the nursing management interventions will be.[7] Factors that affect PA measurement are the head-of-bed backrest position and lateral body position relative to transducer height placement, respiratory variation, and use of positive end-expiratory pressure (PEEP).

Patient Position

The patient does not need to be flat for accurate pressure readings to be obtained. In the supine position, when the transducer is placed at the level of the midaxillary line (phlebostatic axis), a head-of-bed position from flat up to 60 degrees is appropriate for most patients.[7] PAD pressure and PAOP measurements in the lateral position may be significantly different from measurements taken when the patient is lying supine. If there is concern about the validity of pressure readings in a particular patient turned to one side, measurements can be verified with the patient on their back, with the head of bed elevated from flat to 60 degrees as tolerated. After a patient changes position, a stabilization period of 5 to 15 minutes is recommended before taking pressure readings.[7]

Respiratory Variation

All PAD pressure and PAOP (wedge) tracings are subject to respiratory interference, especially when the patient is on a positive-pressure, volume-cycled ventilator.[33] During the positive-pressure inhalation phase, the increase in intrathoracic pressure may "push up" the PA tracing, producing an artificially high reading, especially if larger tidal volumes are used (Fig. 12.20A). During inhalation with spontaneous breaths, negative intrathoracic pressure "pulls down" the waveform, producing an erroneously low measurement (Fig. 12.20B). To minimize the effect of respiratory variation, the PAD pressure is read at end-expiration, which is the most stable point in the respiratory cycle because intrapleural pressures are close to zero.[32] If the digital number fluctuates with respiration, a printed readout on paper can be obtained to verify true PAD pressure. In some clinical settings, ECG signals or airway pressure and flow are recorded simultaneously with the PAD-PAOP tracing to identify end-expiration.[7]

Positive End-Expiratory Pressure and PAOP (Wedge)

Some clinical diagnoses, such as ARDS, require the use of high levels of PEEP set with the ventilator to treat refractory hypoxemia.[31] If a PEEP of greater than 10 cm H_2O is used, PAOP (wedge) and PA pressures will be artificially elevated, and CO may be negatively affected. However, it is important *not* to disconnect a patient from the ventilator just to record PA pressures measurements, because this will close alveoli, will decrease the patient's oxygenation level, and may result in persistent hypoxemia.

Because patients remain on PEEP for treatment, they remain on it during measurement of PA pressures. In this situation, the trend of PA readings is more important than one individual

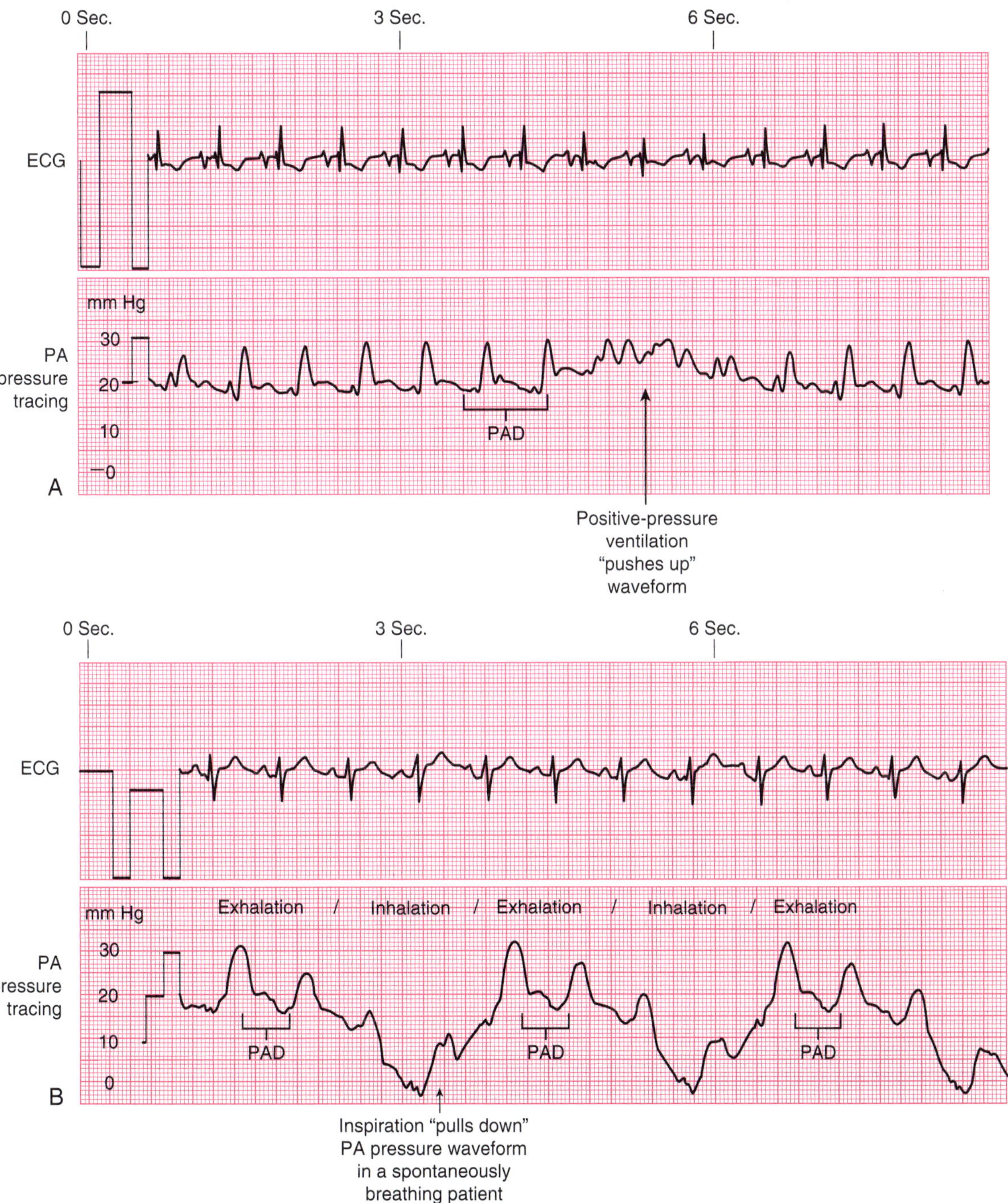

FIG. 12.20 Pulmonary Artery *(PA)* Waveforms That Demonstrate the Effect of Mechanical Ventilation on PA Pressures. For accuracy, PA pressures are read at the end of exhalation. (A) In positive-pressure ventilation, the increase in intrathoracic pressure during inhalation "pushes up" the PA waveform, creating a falsely high reading. (B) In spontaneous breathing, the decrease in intrathoracic pressure during normal inhalation "pulls down" the PA waveform, creating a falsely low reading. *ECG*, Electrocardiogram; *PAD*, pulmonary artery diastolic pressure.

measurement. The trend of the measurements is used as a basis for clinical interventions to support and improve cardiopulmonary function in the critically ill patient.

Avoiding Complications With PA Catheters

Potential cardiac complications include ventricular dysrhythmias, endocarditis, valvular damage, myocardial rupture, and cardiac tamponade. Potential pulmonary complications include rupture of a PA, PA thrombosis, embolism or hemorrhage, and infarction of a segment of lung. The PA catheter tracing is continuously monitored to ensure that the catheter does not migrate forward into a spontaneous PAOP (wedged) position. A segment of lung can infarct if the wedged catheter occludes a segment of the lung vasculature for a prolonged period. If the catheter is spontaneously wedged, the catheter must be gently pulled back out of the wedge position to prevent pulmonary infarction.

Infection is always a risk with a PA catheter. The risks are similar to those discussed in the section on CVCs (see Box 12.2).

Pulmonary Artery Catheter Removal

PA catheters can be safely removed from the patient by critical care nurses competent in this procedure.[7] Removal is not usually associated with major complications. Rarely, PVCs occur as the catheter is pulled through the right ventricle.[7]

Cardiac Output Measurement With a Pulmonary Artery Catheter

The PA catheter measures CO using an intermittent (bolus) or a continuous CO method.

Thermodilution Cardiac Output Bolus Measurement

The bolus thermodilution method is performed at the bedside and results in CO calculated in liters per minute. Three CO values that are within a 10% mean range are obtained at one time and are averaged to calculate CO. The thermodilution CO is very accurate when several injectate values are averaged. A known amount, usually 10 mL, of room temperature physiologic saline solution is injected into the proximal lumen of the PA catheter. The injectate exits into the right atrium and travels with the flow of blood past the thermistor (temperature sensor) located at the distal end of the catheter in the PA. The injectate can be delivered by hand injection using individual syringes of saline. Frequently, a closed in-line system attached to a 500-mL bag of 0.9% saline is used as a reservoir to deliver the individual injections.

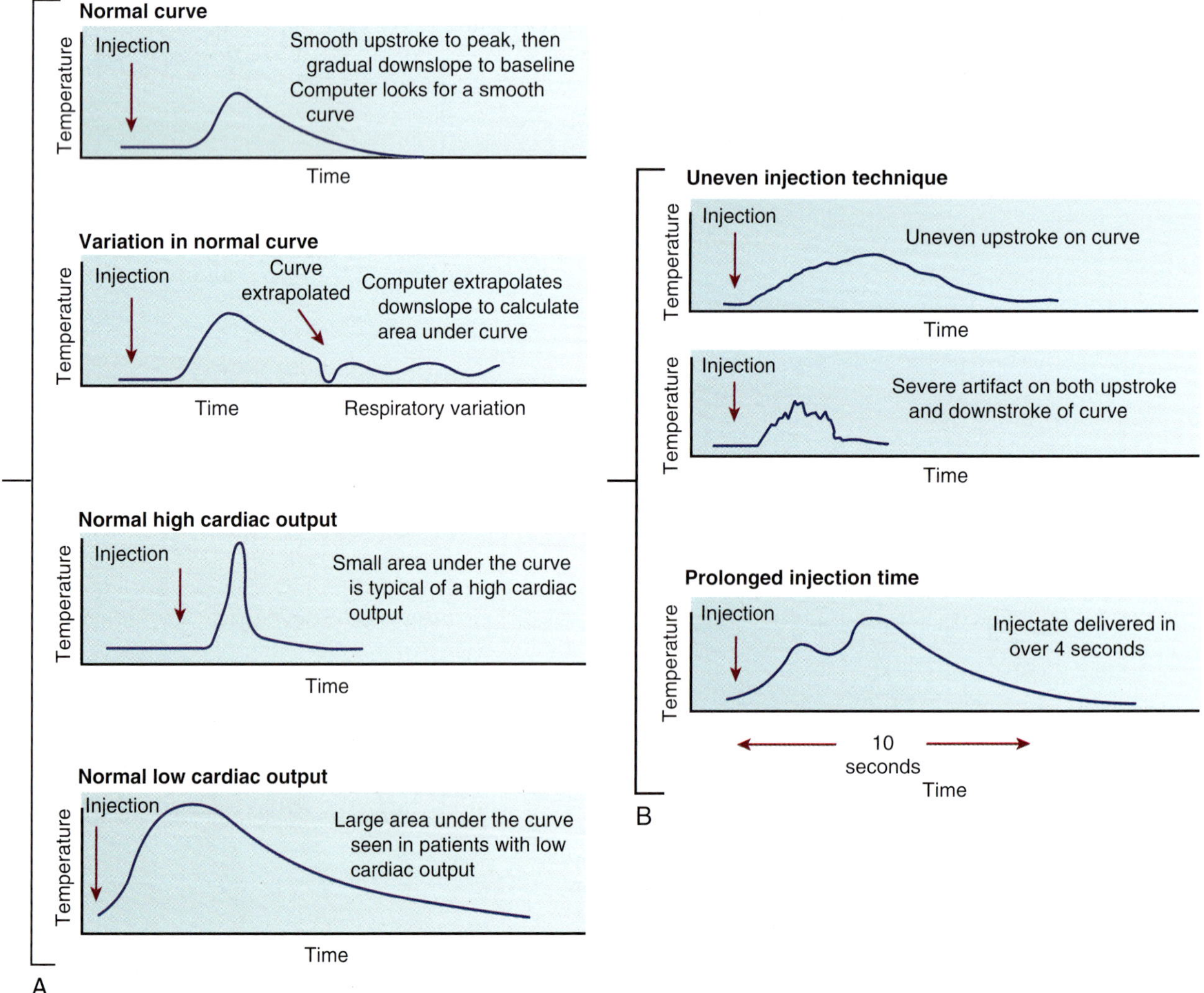

FIG. 12.21 (A) Variations in normal cardiac thermodilution bolus output curve. (B) Abnormal cardiac output (CO) curves produce erroneous CO values.

Cardiac Output Curve

The thermodilution CO method uses the indicator-dilution method, in which a known temperature is the indicator. It is based on the principle that the change in temperature over time is inversely proportional to blood flow. Blood flow can be diagrammatically represented as a CO curve on which temperature is plotted against time (Fig. 12.21A). Most hemodynamic monitors display this CO curve, which must then be interpreted to determine whether the CO injection is valid. The normal curve has a smooth upstroke, with a rounded peak and a gradually tapering downslope. If the curve has an uneven pattern, it may indicate faulty injection technique, and the CO measurement must be repeated. Patient movement or coughing also alters the CO measurement (Fig. 12.21B).

Injectate Temperature

If the CO is within the normal range, it is equally accurate whether iced or room temperature injectate is used. However, if the CO values are extremely high or very low, iced injectate may be more precise. To ensure accurate readings, the difference between injectate temperature and body temperature must be at least 10° C, and the injectate must be delivered within 4 seconds, with minimal handling of the syringe to prevent warming of the solution. This is particularly important if iced injectate is used. With all delivery systems, the injectate is delivered at the same point in the respiratory cycle, usually end-exhalation.

Patient Position and Cardiac Output

In a normovolemic, stable patient, reliable CO measurements can be obtained in a supine position (patient lying on his or her back) with the head of the bed elevated up to 60 degrees. If the patient is hypovolemic or unstable, leaving the head of the bed only slightly elevated, in a flat position is the most clinically appropriate choice. CO measurements performed when the patient is turned to the side are not considered as accurate as measurements performed with the patient in the supine position.

Clinical Conditions That Alter Cardiac Output

Two clinical conditions produce errors in the thermodilution CO measurement: tricuspid valve regurgitation and ventricular septal rupture.

- Tricuspid valve regurgitation: With tricuspid valve regurgitation, the expected flow of blood from the right atrium to the pulmonary artery is disrupted by backflow from the right ventricle to the right atrium. The bolus indicator (normal saline) injected into the RA may take longer to flow to the PA thermistor producing a lower CO measurement.
- Ventricular septal rupture: With an intracardiac left-to-right shunt, as occurs after ventricular septal rupture the new opening in the septum allows blood from the high pressure LV to flow to the low pressure RV during systole. The thermodilution CO measures this increase in RV volume and records a higher CO than the patients true systemic output.[34]

Continuous Thermodilution Cardiac Output Measurement

Continuous CO monitoring using a PA catheter is also frequently used in clinical practice. One method uses a thermal filament incorporated into the PA catheter. The thermal filament emits small thermal-energy signals (the indicator) into the bloodstream. These signals are then detected by the thermistor near the tip of the PA catheter. An indicator curve is created, and a CO value is calculated from these data.

Calculated Hemodynamic Profiles Using a Pulmonary Artery Catheter

For a patient with a thermodilution PA catheter in place, additional hemodynamic information can be calculated using routine vital signs, CO, and body surface area. These measurements are calculated using specific formulas that are indexed to a patient's body size.

The calculated values used in the hemodynamic profiles are described in Table 12.1. Clinical use of these profiles is described in two case studies. In Hemodynamic Profile 1 (Box 12.3), the example is a step-by-step interpretation of the hemodynamic profile to familiarize the reader with use of calculated values. In Hemodynamic Profile 2 (Box 12.4), the example uses only values indexed to body weight and illustrates the effect of treatment on these values over time.

Continuous Monitoring of Mixed Venous Oxygen Saturation and Central Venous Oxygen Saturation

Continuous monitoring of venous oxygen saturation is indicated for a critically ill patient who has the potential to develop an imbalance between oxygen supply and metabolic tissue demand.[35,36] Continuous venous oxygen monitoring permits a calculation of the balance achieved between arterial oxygen supply (SaO_2) and oxygen demand at the tissue level by sampling desaturated venous blood from the PA catheter distal tip. This sample is called *mixed venous oxygen saturation* (SvO_2) because it is a mixture of all of the venous blood drained from many body tissues. The same fiberoptic technology has been used in combination with a fiberoptic triple-lumen CVC. In this situation, the venous blood is sampled from the superior vena cava, just above the right atrium, and the $ScvO_2$ is measured.

Under normal conditions, the cardiopulmonary system achieves a balance between oxygen supply and demand. The following four factors contribute to this balance:

1. CO
2. Hemoglobin
3. Arterial oxygen saturation (SaO_2)
4. Tissue oxygen metabolism (VO_2)

Three of these factors (CO, hemoglobin, and SaO_2) contribute to the supply of oxygen to the tissues. Tissue metabolism (VO_2) determines oxygen consumption, or the quantity of oxygen extracted at tissue level that creates the demand for oxygen (Fig. 12.22). The relationships of these factors to tissue oxygen utilization are illustrated in Fig. 12.23.

In addition to measurement of venous oxygen saturation, it is possible to calculate the quantity of oxygen (in mL/min) that is provided to the tissues by the cardiopulmonary system and to assess the amount of oxygen consumed by the body tissues.[36] These calculations rely on principles of oxygen transport physiology and are the basis for calculation of SvO_2. These formulas are explained in greater detail in Table 12.4 and are listed in Appendix B.

The type of catheter used to measure venous oxygen saturation is defined by where the fiberoptic tip is located, either at the tip of a CVC or on the distal tip of a PA catheter.

SvO_2 Catheter

The pulmonary arterial SvO_2 catheter has the traditional four lumens plus a lumen containing two or three optical fibers. The fiberoptics are attached to an optical module that is connected to a small bedside computer. The optical module transmits a narrow band of light down one optical fiber. This light is reflected off the hemoglobin in the blood and returns to the

BOX 12.3 Hemodynamic Profile 1

Admission

Mr. SR has a medical history of cardiomyopathy and chronic obstructive pulmonary disease (COPD). He is admitted to a coronary care unit because of an exacerbation of biventricular heart failure. He has been complaining about anginal pain and shortness of breath. His nursing diagnoses are Decreased Cardiac Output and Impaired Gas Exchange.

Height	163 cm	PAD	27 mm Hg	PVR	322 dyn • s • cm^{-5}
Weight	79 kg	PAP_m	36 mm Hg	PVRI	612 dyn • s • cm^{-5}/m^2
BSA	1.9 m^2	PAOP	26 mm Hg	LCW	2.1 kg-m
		CVP	24 mm Hg	LCWI	1.1 kg-m/m^2
HR	104 beats/min	CO	2.48 L/min	LVSW	2.4 g-m
ABP		CI	1.31 L/min/m^2	LVSWI	10.7 g-m/m^2
Systolic	88 mm Hg	SV	23.8 mL	RCW	1.21 kg-m
Diastolic	51 mm Hg	SI	12.5 mL/m^2	RCWI	0.64 kg-m/m^2
MAP	63 mm Hg	SVR	1257 dyn • s • cm^{-5}	RVSW	11.7 g-m
PAS	55 mm Hg	SVRI	2388 dyn • s • cm^{-5}/m^2	RVSWI	6.2 g-m/m^2

Analysis of Hemodynamic Profile[a]

Profile	Analysis
HR	HR of 104 beats/min is above normal limits (normal, 60–100 beats/min).
ABP	Narrow pulse pressure of 88/51 mm Hg with low mean arterial pressure (MAP) of 63 mm Hg (normal MAP, 65–90 mm Hg).
PAP	Pulmonary artery pressures are elevated (55/27 mm Hg), consistent with diagnosis of cardiomyopathy, failure of left side of heart, and COPD (normal PAP, 25/10 mm Hg).
PAOP	Elevated PAOP (26 mm Hg), consistent with diagnosis of cardiomyopathy and failure of left side of heart (normal PAOP, 5–12 mm Hg).
CVP	Elevated CVP (24 mm Hg), consistent with diagnosis of cardiomyopathy, failure of right side of heart, and COPD (normal CVP, 4–6 mm Hg).
CO and CI	Poor CO and CI (CO, 2.48 L/min; CI, 1.31 L/min/m^2). Both values are below normal (normal CO, 4–6 L/min; normal CI, 2.2–4 L/min/m^2).
SV and SI	SV and SI are low (SV, 23.8 mL; SI, 12.5 mL/m^2). These results would be anticipated from the low CO (normal SV, 60–70 mL; normal SI, 40–50 mL/min/m^2).
SVR and SVRI	SVR and SVRI are at the upper normal range (SVR, 1257 dyn • s • cm^{-5}; SVRI, 2388 dyn • s • cm^{-5}/m^2). These values are not contributing to the low CO at this time (normal SVR, 800–1400 dyn • s • cm^{-5}; normal SVRI, 2000–2400 dyn • s • cm^{-5}/m^2).
PVR and PVRI	PVR and PVRI are elevated (PVR, 322 dyn • s • cm^{-5}; PVRI 612 dyn • s • cm^{-5}/m^2). High PVR may be contributing to the low CO (normal PVR, 100–250 dyn • s • cm^{-5}; normal PVRI, 225–315 dyn • s • cm^{-5}/m^2).
LCWI and LVSWI	Both LCWI and LVSWI are below normal (LCWI, 1.1 kg-m/m^2; LVSWI, 10.7 g-m/m^2), indicating that left ventricular myocardial damage may be present. This is consistent with Mr. SR's diagnosis of cardiomyopathy (normal LCWI, 3.4–4.2 kg-m/m^2; normal LVSWI, 50–62 g-m/m^2).
RCWI and RVSWI	RCWI is normal, but RVSWI is below normal (RCWI, 0.64 kg-m/m^2; RVSWI, 6.2 g-m/m^2), indicating that right ventricular myocardial damage may be present. This is consistent with Mr. SR's diagnosis of cardiomyopathy and history of COPD (normal RCWI, 0.54–0.66 kg-m/m^2; normal RVSWI, 7.9–9.7 g-m/m^2).
Nursing impression	The hemodynamic data confirm the nursing clinical diagnosis of poor CO. The goal is to improve CO within the limits of Mr. SR's myocardial dysfunction and COPD. As CO improves and PA pressures decrease, the patient will have less pulmonary congestion, which will improve alveolar gas exchange.

[a] Formulas and normal values. The hemodynamic values are given in Table 12.1 and in Appendix B.

ABP, Arterial blood pressure; *BSA*, body surface area; *CI*, cardiac index; *CO*, cardiac output; *CVP*, central venous pressure; *HR*, heart rate; *LCWI*, left cardiac work index; *LVSW*, left ventricular stroke work; *LVSWI*, left ventricular stroke work index; *MAP*, mean arterial pressure; *PAD*, pulmonary artery diastolic pressure; *PAOP*, pulmonary artery occlusion pressure; *PAPM*, pulmonary artery mean pressure; *RCW*, right cardiac work; *RCWI*, right cardiac work index; *RVSW*, right ventricular stroke work; *RVSWI*, right ventricular stroke work index; *SI*, stroke volume index; *SV*, stroke volume; *SVR*, systemic vascular resistance; *SVRI*, systemic vascular resistance index.

optical module through the receiving fiberoptic. The SvO_2 signal is recorded on a continuous display.

$ScvO_2$ Catheter

The central venous $ScvO_2$ technology is incorporated into a multilumen CVC. The fiberoptic catheter tip is positioned in a central vein, such as the superior vena cava. The technology used to measure the venous saturation is identical in both types of catheters, and the same continuous display module is used for both catheters.

The values obtained from the traditional PA (SvO_2) catheter and the central venous ($ScvO_2$) catheter are very similar, although the $ScvO_2$ values are slightly higher. The trend of parallel measurements (up or down as patient condition changes) is in the same direction in most cases.

SvO_2 or $ScvO_2$ Calibration

The catheter is calibrated before insertion into the patient through a standardized color reference system, which is part of the catheter package. Insertion technique and sites are identical

BOX 12.4 Hemodynamic Profile 2

Admission

Mrs. JL has been admitted to the critical care unit with pulmonary edema. She has a history of anterior wall myocardial infarction and severe chronic obstructive pulmonary disease (COPD).

Height	159 cm	MAP	106 mm Hg	SI	9.9 mL/m^2
Weight	45.8 kg	PAS	53 mm Hg	SVRI	5351 dyn • s • cm^{-5}/m^2
BSA	1.40 m^2	PAD	27 mm Hg	PVRI	1046 dyn • s • cm^{-5}/m^2
		PAP_M	44 mm Hg	LCWI	1.9 kg-m/m^2
HR	131 beats/min	PAOP	27 mm Hg	LVSWI	14.3 g-m/m^2
ABP		CVP	19 mm Hg	RCW	0.78 kg-m/m^2
Systolic	160 mm Hg	CO	1.82 L/min	RCWI	5.9 g-m/m^2
Diastolic	80 mm Hg	CI	1.3 L/min/m^2		

Analysis of the Hemodynamic Profile on Admission[a]

In the hemodynamic profile, notice the fast HR; high MAP; high PA and CVP filling pressures; low CI, SI, LVSWI, and RVSWI; and high SVRI and PVRI. These values are consistent with a diagnosis of failure of the left side of the heart causing pulmonary edema, which may lead to cardiogenic shock. Treatment is focused on increasing the CI by lowering SVRI and PVRI and using intravenous (IV) sodium nitroprusside and IV nitroglycerin in continuous infusion.

Three Hours Later

Height	159 cm	MAP	83 mm Hg	SI	16.5 mL/m^2
Weight	45.8 kg	PAS	41 mm Hg	SVRI	3088 dyn • s • cm^{-5}/m^2
BSA	1.40 m^2	PAD	26 mm Hg	PVRI	300 dyn • s • cm^{-5}/m^2
		PAP_M	33 mm Hg	LCWI	2.1 kg-m/m^2
HR	113 beats/min	PAOP	26 mm Hg	LVSWI	18.6 g-m/m^2
ABP		CVP	11 mm Hg	RCWI	0.84 kg-m/m^2
Systolic	104 mm Hg	CO	2.61 L/min	RVSWI	7.4 g-m/m^2
Diastolic	69 mm Hg	CI	1.86 L/min/m^2		

Analysis of Hemodynamic Profile After 3 Hours

Results 3 hours after sodium nitroprusside administration showed improving hemodynamic values demonstrated as normal MAP and lower intracardiac filling pressures (PA and CVP). However, CI and SI remain low, and SVRI is above normal. Mrs. JL remains in severe left ventricular failure because of her low CI.

The Next Day

Height	159 cm	MAP	77 mm Hg	SI	22.5 mL/m^2
Weight	45.8 kg	PAS	31 mm Hg	SVRI	2423 dyn • s • cm^{-5}/m^2
BSA	1.40 m^2	PAD	15 mm Hg	PVRI	273 dyn • s • cm^{-5}/m^2
		PAP_M	23 mm Hg	LCWI	2.4 kg-m/m^2
HR	104 beats/min	PAOP	15 mm Hg	LVSWI	22.9 g-m/m^2
ABP		CVP	4 mm Hg	RCWI	0.74 kg-m/m^2
Systolic	111 mm Hg	CO	3.28 L/min	RVSWI	7.1 g-m/m^2
Diastolic	60 mm Hg	CI	2.34 L/min/m^2		

Analysis of Hemodynamic Profile the Next Day

The next day, Mrs. JL's hemodynamic values have improved with continued use of sodium nitroprusside and nitroglycerin. The CI value is in the low-normal range, and SVRI and PVRI values are in the high-normal range. LVSWI remains low, reflecting the patient's compromised left ventricle from a prior anterior wall myocardial infarction.

[a] Formulas and normal values for the hemodynamic values are given in Table 12.1 and in Appendix B.

ABP, Arterial blood pressure; *BSA*, body surface area; *CI*, cardiac index; *CO*, cardiac output; *CVP*, central venous pressure; *HR*, heart rate; *LCWI*, left cardiac work index; *LVSWI*, left ventricular stroke work index; *MAP*, mean arterial pressure; *PAD*, pulmonary artery diastolic pressure; *PAOP*, pulmonary artery occlusion pressure; *PAPM*, pulmonary artery mean pressure; *PAS*, pulmonary artery systolic pressure; *RCW*, right cardiac work; *RCWI*, right cardiac work index; *SI*, stroke volume index; *SV*, stroke volume; *SVRI*, systemic vascular resistance index.

to those used for placement of conventional PA or CVC catheters. Waveform analysis or venous saturation measurement, or both, can be used for accurate placement. After the catheter is inserted, recalibration is unnecessary unless the catheter becomes disconnected from the optical module.

To recalibrate the fiberoptic module to verify accuracy when the catheter is already inserted in a patient, a mixed venous blood sample (SvO_2) or central venous sample ($ScvO_2$) must be withdrawn from the appropriate catheter tip and sent to the laboratory for oxygen saturation analysis. In many critical care units, this is a standard daily procedure to ensure that readings used to guide patient care remain accurate.

Nursing Management

$ScvO_2$ monitoring provides a continuous assessment of the balance of oxygen supply and demand for an individual patient. Nursing assessment includes evaluation of the SvO_2 or $ScvO_2$ value and evaluation of the four factors (SaO_2, CO, hemoglobin, and VO_2) that maintain the oxygen supply-demand balance.

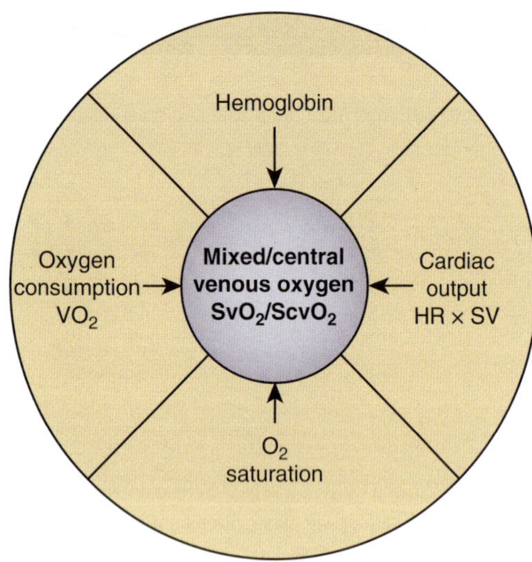

FIG. 12.22 Determinants of Venous Oxygen Saturation: Cardiac Output, Hemoglobin, Arterial Oxygen Saturation, and Tissue Oxygen Metabolism *(VO_2)*. *HR*, Heart rate; *SV*, stroke volume; *$ScvO_2$*, central venous oxygen saturation; *SvO_2*, mixed venous oxygen saturation. (From Lough ME. *Hemodynamic Monitoring: Evolving Technologies and Clinical Practice*. Elsevier; 2016.)

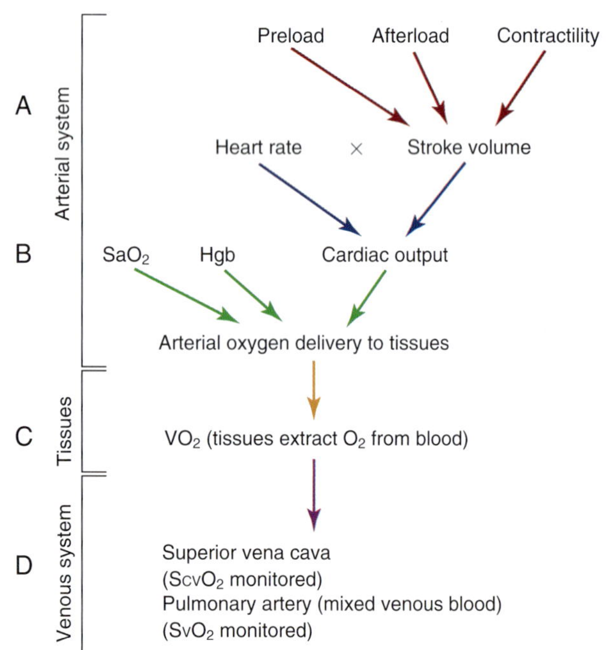

FIG. 12.23 Factors That Contribute to Mixed Venous Oxygen Saturation *(SvO_2)* Value. (A) Cardiac output (CO) is determined by heart rate × stroke volume. (B) Oxygen saturation *(SaO_2)*, hemoglobin (Hgb) level, and CO contribute to arterial oxygen delivery at the tissue level. (C) Tissues extract and use the oxygen carried in the blood. This process of cellular oxygen consumption is tissue oxygen metabolism *(VO_2)*. (D) Blood returns to the superior vena cava (recorded as central venous oxygen saturation [$ScvO_2$]) and then to the pulmonary artery, where the mixed venous blood is recorded as SvO_2.

Normal SvO_2 Values

Normal SvO_2 is approximately 75% in a healthy individual (range, 60% to 80%). In critically ill patients, an SvO_2 value between 60% and 80% is evidence of adequate balance between oxygen supply and demand.

Normal $ScvO_2$ Values

Normal values for the $ScvO_2$ catheter are slightly higher than $ScvO_2$ values. This is because the reading is taken before the blood enters the right heart chambers, where the cardiac sinus vein delivers venous blood drained from the myocardium into the right atrium. The heavily desaturated myocardial blood decreases the oxygen saturation by about 5%. For this reason, SvO_2 values are always slightly lower than $ScvO_2$ readings in the same patient.[36]

SvO_2 or $ScvO_2$ and Arterial Oxygen Saturation

A change in SvO_2 or $ScvO_2$ may be caused by a change in SaO_2.

- If the SaO_2 is increased because supplemental oxygen is being administered, the SvO_2 also will increase.
- If the oxygen supply is decreased and SaO_2 is decreased, SvO_2 will decrease.

The SvO_2 can be decreased by any action or disease that reduces oxygen supply, including ARDS, endotracheal suctioning, removing a patient from the ventilator, or removing supplementary oxygen. Fig. 12.24 demonstrates a decrease in SvO_2 that occurred during suctioning in a patient with ARDS. Transient decreases in SvO_2 or $ScvO_2$ related to a nursing action such as endotracheal suctioning are not usually a cause for concern. Some patients may be slow to resaturate up to the presuction level of SvO_2 or $ScvO_2$. In this case an appropriate nursing intervention is to wait until the venous oxygen saturation has again returned to baseline before initiating other nursing activities.

One clinical tip is to subtract 30 from the SaO_2, and the resulting value should represent the SvO_2 percentage value. For example,

$$SaO_2 \text{ is } 100\% - 30\% = 70\% \, SvO_2$$

$$SaO_2 \text{ is } 95\% - 30\% = 65\% \, SvO_2$$

If the SvO_2 or $ScvO_2$ value changes by more than 10% and this change is maintained for more than 10 minutes, it is important to determine which of the four factors is affecting SvO_2.

SvO_2 or $ScvO_2$ and Cardiac Output

A change in SvO_2 or $ScvO_2$ may be caused by an alteration in CO. Changes in one or more of the following four individual hemodynamic factors affect CO: preload, SVR, contractility, and HR (see Fig. 12.22).

- Volume
- Administration and Changes in Heart Rate: Fig. 12.25 shows an improvement in a patient's SvO_2 concentration from 70% to 80% after volume administration that increased preload (point A). This patient's CO later fell abruptly during a short run of ventricular tachycardia (VT) (point B). Any major loss of HR causes a decrease in CO. Alterations in contractility, preload, and afterload (SVR) also have the potential to alter CO.

Because CO is an important component of the continuous SvO_2 value, researchers investigated whether SvO_2 could be substituted for thermodilution CO as a monitoring tool. Studies of adult patients after cardiac surgery and acute MI indicate that a sustained change in the SvO_2 value does not automatically mean there has been a change in CO. No consistent or reliable correlation was found between SvO_2 and CO. Instead, a change in SvO_2 indicates a need to check CO at the bedside to determine the cause of the change in venous oxygen saturation. The SvO_2 measurement is very sensitive and serves as an early warning for changes in patient condition, regardless of whether the change is the result of an alteration in CO. Monitoring SvO_2

TABLE 12.4 Calculations of Oxygen Transport Physiology

Name	Formula	Normal Value	Explanation
Arterial oxygen saturation (SaO_2)		>96%	SaO_2 is determined by the amount of oxygen (O_2) bound to hemoglobin (Hgb), termed *oxyhemoglobin* ($HgbO_2$). $HgbO_2$ is divided by the total hemoglobin (Hgb + $HgbO_2$). Normally, 96% of O_2 is bound to hemoglobin.
Blood oxygen content	(O_2 dissolved) + (O_2 saturation)	19–20 mL/dL	Blood O_2 content is the amount of O_2 dissolved in 100 mL (1 dL) of blood. It can be calculated for arterial blood (CaO_2) and for venous blood (CvO_2). Measured in units of mL/dL, it is the combination of dissolved O_2 (PaO_2) and O_2 saturation (SaO_2).
CaO_2 (arterial) CvO_2 (venous)	$(PO_2 \times 0.003) + (1.34 \times Hgb \times SaO_2)$	12–15 mL/dL	
Blood oxygen transport (i.e., oxygen delivery)	$CO \times CaO_2 \times 10$ (arterial)	1000 mL/min	O_2 transport represents the amount (mL) of O_2 transported to or from the tissues each minute (mL/min). Arterial O_2 transport is a measure of the O_2 delivered to the tissues. Venous O_2 transport reflects the venous return to the right side of the heart.
	$CO \times CvO_2 \times 10$ (venous)	750 mL/min	O_2 transport is calculated by multiplying the cardiac output (CO) by the O_2 content (CaO_2 or CvO_2) and by the number 10. The difference between normal arterial and normal venous O_2 return represents O_2 consumption by the tissues.
Tissue oxygen consumption (VO_2)	Arterial O_2 transport minus venous O_2 transport $(CO \times CaO_2 \times 10) - (CO \times CvO_2 \times 10)$	250 mL/min	O_2 consumption is the amount of O_2 consumed by the tissues in 1 minute. To calculate VO_2, the arterial O_2 transport and venous O_2 transport values (calculated in mL/min) must be known. The difference is VO_2.
Arterial-venous oxygen difference (a-v O_2 difference)	Arterial O_2 content minus venous O_2 content $CaO_2 - CvO_2$	3.0–5.5 mL/dL	The a-v O_2 difference is the difference between the arterial O_2 content (CaO_2) and the venous O_2 content (CvO_2). Because CaO_2 and CvO_2 are measured in mL/dL, the a-v O_2 difference is also measured in mL/dL.
Mixed venous oxygen saturation (SvO_2)	Arterial O_2 transport minus tissue O_2 consumption equals venous O_2 return $(CO \times CaO_2 \times 10) - VO_2$	60%–80%	SvO_2 is the venous O_2 return that is bound (saturated) to hemoglobin. Saturation is measured as a percentage (%). The SvO_2 value is a function of the amount of O_2 delivered to the tissues minus the amount of O_2 consumed by the tissues (VO_2) and is measured in mL/min. The higher the amount (mL) of O_2 in the venous return, the greater the hemoglobin saturation.

CO, Cardiac output.

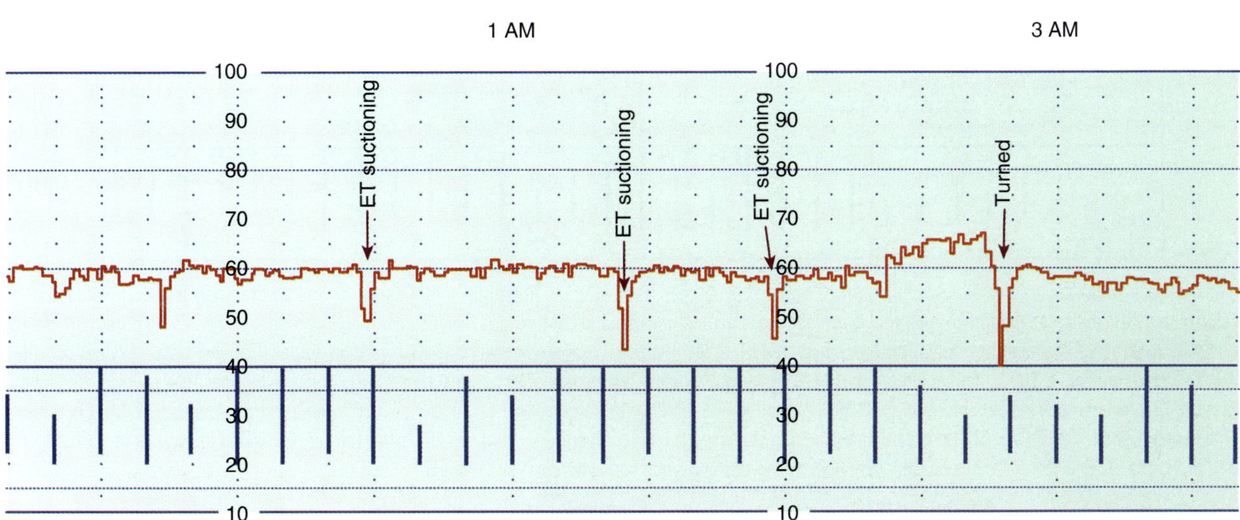

FIG. 12.24 The mixed venous oxygen saturation (SvO_2) value decreases during endotracheal (ET) suctioning. The ET suction decreases the oxygen saturation level. The baseline SvO_2 value is low (60%) because the patient has acute respiratory distress syndrome and is hypoxemic.

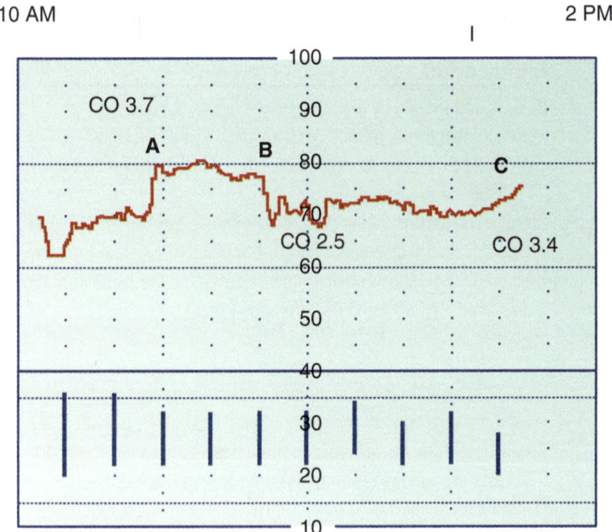

FIG. 12.25 Effect of Changes in Cardiac Output *(CO)* on Mixed Venous Oxygen Saturation (SvO_2) Values. *Point A:* Just before point A, SvO_2 readings are low, because CO and pulmonary artery pressures were low as a result of excessive diuresis. Infusion of 500 mL of colloid solution and 1000 mL of lactated Ringer solution crystalloid increased SvO_2 level and improved CO, which rose to 3.7 L/min. *Point B:* A short run of ventricular tachycardia caused CO to fall abruptly to 2.5 L/min and decreased SvO_2 value. *Point C:* The beginning of an upward trend in SvO_2 is related to administration of fluids and to improvement in CO and in filling pressures. CO is now 3.4 L/min. The graph represents a 4-h printout; the space between each dotted line represents 20 min.

is an additional level of hemodynamic monitoring but does not replace thermodilution CO.

- This principle that a change in SvO_2 is not always related to alterations in CO is clearly illustrated in the SvO_2 Hemodynamic Profile 3 (Box 12.5), in which an increase in SvO_2 is not associated with a significant rise in CO. The rationale and explanation for this finding is also discussed in the section on assessment of oxygen consumption.

SvO_2 or $ScvO_2$ and Hemoglobin

Hemoglobin is the transport mechanism for oxygen in the blood. If the hemoglobin level falls as a result of bleeding or red blood cell (RBC) destruction, the body maintains oxygen transport by increasing CO and using oxygen reserves in the venous blood return. The body can compensate efficiently for anemia in the absence of illness. In a healthy person, the hemoglobin concentration must be extremely low before SvO_2 decreases. However, in an anemic patient with a compromised cardiovascular system who cannot adequately increase CO, SvO_2 or $ScvO_2$ declines as venous oxygen reserves are depleted.

SvO_2 or $ScvO_2$ and Oxygen Consumption

VO_2 describes the amount of oxygen the body tissues normally consume in 1 minute. If the body's metabolic demands increase because of exercise or increased metabolic rate, the body increases CO to augment oxygen supply and uses reserve oxygen in the venous system.

Normal oxygen delivery to the tissues is 1000 mL (1 liter) of oxygen per minute. At rest, a person may consume one-fourth of the available oxygen, or 250 mL of oxygen per minute. This

BOX 12.5 Hemodynamic Profile 3

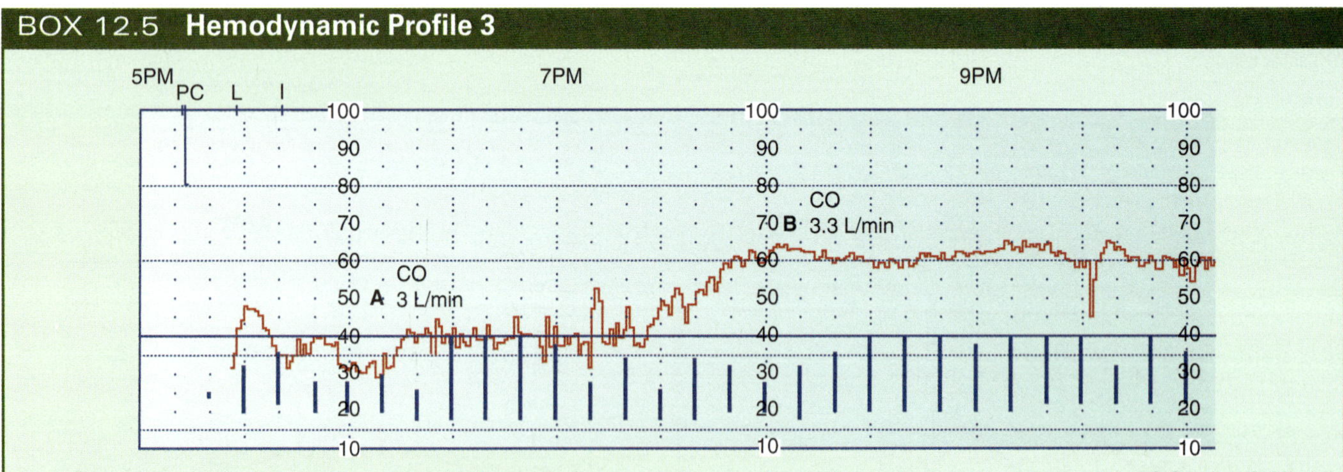

Mr. EH has just been admitted to the cardiovascular critical care unit after open heart surgery. At point A in the figure, he has an extremely low SvO_2 value of 40%. An SvO_2 value below 40% indicates that the oxygen supply is inadequate to meet the demands of the body tissues, resulting in metabolic acidosis. To determine the reason for the low SvO_2 level, values must be known for the hemoglobin (Hgb) level, arterial oxygen saturation (SaO_2), cardiac output (CO), and tissue oxygen consumption (VO_2). Mr. EH's Hgb value is 11.6 g/dL (normal male Hgb, 13.5 – 18.0 g/dL), which is acceptable after major surgery; SaO_2 is 99.6% (normal, 97%), which is high because Mr. EH started receiving mechanical ventilation with 70% oxygen immediately after surgery; and CO is low at 3.15 L/min (normal, 4–6 L/min). Mr. EH is receiving dopamine (5 mcg/kg/min) for his low CO. He is cold and shivering because his body temperature is only 35.2° C after the surgery. Using the values of Hgb of 11.6 g/dL, SaO_2 of 99.6%, and CO of 3.15 L/min, it is possible to calculate the tissue oxygen consumption (VOO_2) for EH.

Arterial Supply **Venous Return**

$$CO\,(PaO_2 \times 0.003) + (1.34 \times Hgb \times SaO_2)\,10 - CO\,(PvO_2 \times 0.0031) + (1.34 \times Hgb \times S\bar{v}O_2)\,10 = \dot{V}O_2$$

To calculate arterial oxygen supply, the oxygen in the venous return, VO_2, and the difference between the arterial (a) and venous (v) oxygen content (a-v O_2 difference), insert Mr. EH's values (shown in boldface below) into the previous formula.

BOX 12.5 Hemodynamic Profile 3—cont'd

Arterial Supply	Venous Return	$\dot{V}O_2$	a-v O_2 Difference
3.15 (**354** × 0.003) + (1.34 × **11.6** × **0.99**) 10 −	**3.15** (**20** × 0.003) + (1.34 × **11.6** × **0.38**) 10		
3.15 (1.0 + 15.3) 10	**3.15** (0.06 + 5.90) 10		
3.15 (16.3) 10	**3.15** (5.90) 10		
505 mL/min (see preceding illustration)	183 mL/min	= 322 mL/min	10.4 mL/dL

At point A in the figure, the arterial oxygen supply to the tissues is 505 mL/min (normal, 1000 mL/min), whereas the oxygen returned in the venous blood is only 183 mL/min (normal, 750 mL/min). Mr. EH's VO_2 is elevated at 322 mL/min (normal, 250 mL/min). The clinical goals for this patient would be to (1) increase the CO and (2) use sedation or muscle relaxants to decrease oxygen consumption by controlling the patient's shivering. The difference between the oxygen content in the arterial (a) and the venous (v) blood (a-v O_2 difference) is very large at 10.4 mL/dL (normal, 3.5–5.0 mL/dL). These calculated values confirm there is ineffective tissue perfusion with a decreased CO.

Two hours later, at point B in the figure, Mr. EH's SvO_2 has improved to a low-normal value of 60%. Additional inotropic medications have been administered. At this time, Hgb is 10.8 g/dL, SaO_2 is 99.6%, and CO remains low at 3.3 L/min. The improvement in SvO_2 has not been caused by a dramatic increase in CO. When Mr. EH's oxygen consumption is calculated at point B, it becomes evident that the decrease in physical activity after sedation with morphine to reduce shivering has improved the SvO_2. Mr. EH's values are in boldface in the formula below.

Arterial Supply	Venous Return

$$CO\,(PaO_2 \times 0.003) + (1.34 \times Hgb \times SaO_2)\,10 - CO\,(PvO_2 \times 0.003) + (1.34 \times Hgb \times S\overline{v}O_2)\,10 = \dot{V}O_2$$

Arterial Supply	Venous Return	$\dot{V}O_2$	a-v O_2 Difference
3.3 (**266** × 0.003) + (1.34 × **10.8** × **0.99**) 10 −	**3.3** (**28** × 0.003) + (1.34 × **10.8** × **0.60**) 10		
3.3 (0.82 + 14.32) 10	**3.3** (0.86 + 8.6) 10		
3.3 (15.1) 1	**3.3** (9.4) 10		
498 mL/min	300 mL/min	= 198 mL/min	5.7 mL/dL

At point B in the figure, Mr. EH's arterial oxygen supply is still low at 498 mL/min, and the oxygen in his mixed venous blood return remains low at 300 mL/min. VO_2 is now lower than normal (typical after sedation) at 198 mL/min. At this time, the a-v O_2 difference is almost within normal limits at 5.7 mL/dL. These findings are confirmed by the low-normal SvO_2 value of 60% at point B. This patient profile illustrates the point that tissue oxygen consumption (oxygen demand) can be as important as CO and oxygenation (oxygen supply) in determining SvO_2 in a patient with a compromised cardiovascular system.

See Table 12.1, Box 12.3, and Appendix B for explanations of abbreviations and of hemodynamic values.

leaves a venous oxygen reserve of 750 mL of oxygen per minute (see Table 12.4). For a normal individual, the combination of increased CO and use of considerable venous oxygen reserve provides adequate compensation for increased metabolic needs. However, for a critically ill patient with cardiac or respiratory dysfunction, an increase in activity leading to increased oxygen consumption may overwhelm the cardiopulmonary system and oxygen reserves.

In a critically ill patient, nursing procedures can increase VO_2 by 10% to 36% (Table 12.5). The critical care nurse can observe the effect of increased VO_2 during routine nursing care and under conditions that increase metabolic rate. Activities such as turning, giving a backrub, or getting a patient out of bed are often accompanied by a sudden, temporary decrease in the patient's continuous SvO_2 or $ScvO_2$ reading (Table 12.5). After the physical activity is finished, most patients resaturate up to their prior venous oxygen saturation level within a few minutes. In critical illness, it may take 5 minutes for resaturation (increase in SvO_2 or $ScvO_2$) to occur. In this situation, the appropriate nursing action is to observe the patient clinically in conjunction with monitoring SvO_2 or $ScvO_2$ and to postpone additional maneuvers until the venous saturation has returned to baseline.

Many clinical conditions that dramatically increase VO_2 consumption are common in critical care units. Conditions such as sepsis, multiple-organ dysfunction syndrome, burns, head injury, seizures, and shivering can more than double the normal oxygen tissue requirements (see Table 12.5). Such dramatic increases in VO_2 translate into a low SvO_2 or $ScvO_2$ value, even if the CO is normal.

- Increased VO_2: A dramatic increase in VO_2 situation is demonstrated in Hemodynamic Profile 3, in which intense shivering resulted in increased tissue oxygen consumption causing a low initial SvO_2 value (point A); after sedation, and when the shivering stopped, the SvO_2 value increased secondary to the normalization of tissue oxygen requirements (point B).

Normal SvO_2 or $ScvO_2$

If SvO_2 or $ScvO_2$ is within the normal range of 60% to 80% and the patient is not clinically compromised, it is reasonable to assume that oxygen supply and demand are balanced. The situation becomes out of balance when a decrease in oxygen delivery (SaO_2) occurs because of changes in CO or hemoglobin concentration, or an increase in oxygen demand (increased VO_2) occurs.

Low SvO_2 or $ScvO_2$

If SvO_2 or $ScvO_2$ falls below 60% and is sustained, the clinician must assume that oxygen supply is not equal to demand (Table 12.6). It is helpful to assess the cause of decreased SvO_2 or $ScvO_2$ in a logical sequence that reflects knowledge of the meaning of the venous saturation value. The following is one such assessment sequence:

- Clinically assess the patient.
  - Assess whether the decreased SvO_2 or $ScvO_2$ is caused by low oxygen supply. Verify the effectiveness of the ventilator or oxygen mask or check SaO_2 from arterial blood gas values.
  - Assess cardiac function by performing a CO measurement.

TABLE 12.5 Alterations in Oxygen Consumption

Condition or Activity	% Increase Over Resting VO_2	% Decrease Under Resting VO_2
Clinical Conditions That Increase VO_2		
Fever	10% (for each 1° C above normal)	
Skeletal injuries	10%–30%	
Work of breathing	40%	
Severe infection	60%	
Shivering	50%–100%	
Burns	100%	
Routine postoperative procedures	7%	
Nasal intubation	25%–40%	
Endotracheal tube suctioning	27%	
Chest trauma	60%	
Multiple-organ dysfunction syndrome	20%–80%	
Sepsis	50%–100%	
Head injury, with patient sedated	89%	
Head injury, with patient not sedated	138%	
Critical illness in emergency department	60%	
Nursing Activities That Increase VO_2		
Dressing change	10%	
Electrocardiogram	16%	
Agitation	18%	
Physical examination	20%	
Visitor	22%	
Bath	23%	
Chest radiograph examination	25%	
Position change	31%	
Chest physiotherapy	35%	
Weighing on sling scale	36%	
Conditions That Decrease VO_2		
Anesthesia		25%
Anesthesia in burn patients		50%

VO_2, Oxygen consumption.
Modified from White KM, Winslow EH, Clark AP, Tyler DO. The physiologic basis for continuous mixed venous oxygen saturation monitoring. *Heart Lung.* 1990;19(5 Pt 2): 548–551.

- Assess hemoglobin value by checking recent laboratory results or by withdrawing a blood sample for laboratory analysis.
- Assess whether the decreased SvO_2 or $ScvO_2$ is the result of a recent patient movement or nursing action that may have temporarily increased VO_2.

The concept of target values has been helpful when designing protocols for hemodynamic monitoring. Target values for venous oximetry are SvO_2 of 70% or greater and $ScvO_2$ of 65% or greater. Patients with values below these targets are at greater risk for organ hypoperfusion and increased mortality. This was seen in a study of intraoperative and postoperative surgical patients, in whom $ScvO_2$ below 65% was associated with increased mortality.[36]

If SvO_2 or $ScvO_2$ falls below 40% and is maintained at this low value, the imbalance of oxygen supply and demand will be inadequate to meet tissue needs at the cellular level. At some point, the cells change from an aerobic to anaerobic mode of metabolism, which results in the production of lactic acid and is representative of a shock state in which cellular injury or cell death may result. At this point, every attempt must be made to determine the cause of the low SvO_2 or $ScvO_2$ and to correct the oxygen supply-demand imbalance.

High SvO_2

In certain clinical conditions, SvO_2 or $ScvO_2$ may increase to an above-normal level (greater than 80%). This occurs during times of low oxygen demand (decreased VO_2), such as during anesthesia or hypothermia. In some cases of septic shock, the tissue cells cannot use the oxygen supplied to them, and the oxygen is not extracted from the blood at the tissue level. In this situation, the venous oxygen reserve remains elevated, and the SvO_2 or $ScvO_2$ value is higher than normal (see Table 12.6).

If the SvO_2 PA catheter drifts into a wedged position (into a pulmonary artery), the SvO_2 increases because the fiberoptic tip of the catheter is in contact with freshly oxygenated blood.[36] The associated waveform will display a wedged left atrial pattern as described previously. The intervention is to ensure that the balloon is not inflated and to gently pull back the PA into a nonwedge position. The catheter position can also be verified by a chest radiograph.

Less-Invasive Hemodynamic Monitoring

Tremendous progress has been made in the development of less-invasive methods of hemodynamic monitoring. The newer monitoring methods range from completely noninvasive to methods that, although less invasive than a PA catheter, involve insertion of intravascular catheters or esophageal probes to gather monitoring information (Table 12.7). All newer monitoring methods that estimate CO have been compared with the PA catheter thermodilution CO method.

The latest innovation is to provide a suite of hemodynamic monitoring options using similar technologies with different ranges of invasiveness, as diagramed in Fig. 12.1. This range of hemodynamic options allows the critical care team to tailor the invasiveness and diagnostic capabilities of the monitoring system to the clinical needs of the patient.

ARTERIAL WAVEFORM–BASED HEMODYNAMIC MONITORING SYSTEMS

Arterial pressure–based systems are revolutionizing hemodynamic monitoring as proprietary technologies from different companies showcase new technologies with options ranging from noninvasive, minimally invasive, or invasive (see Fig. 12.1 and Table 12.7).

Noninvasive—Finger Cuff Hemodynamic Monitoring Systems

Finger cuff systems are noninvasive and trend continuous blood pressure, SV, stroke volume variation (SVV), and CO. Finger-cuff systems are designed for short-term use to assess hemodynamics without inserting invasive catheters. They are the first step in a suite of devices that use arterial waveform analysis (Fig. 12.26).[37] Finger-cuff systems are noncalibrated and noninvasive and are not recommended for monitoring of critically ill patients.[38,39] However, finger cuff devices are helpful during initial hemodynamic assessment or when invasive

TABLE 12.6 Measurements of Mixed Venous Oxygen Saturation

SvO_2 Measurement	Physiologic Basis for Changes in $SvO_2/ScvO_2$	Clinical Diagnosis and Rationale
High SvO_2 (80%–95%)	Increased oxygen supply Decreased oxygen demand	Patient receiving more oxygen than required by clinical condition Anesthesia, which causes sedation and decreased muscle movement Hypothermia, which lowers metabolic demand (e.g., during cardiopulmonary bypass) Sepsis caused by decreased ability of tissues to use oxygen at a cellular level False high-positive result because pulmonary artery catheter is wedged in a pulmonary arteriole (SvO_2 only)
Normal $ScvO_2/SvO_2$ (60%–80%)	Normal oxygen supply and metabolic demand	Balanced oxygen supply and demand
Low $SvO_2/ScvO_2$ (<60%)	Decreased oxygen supply caused by Low Hgb Low SaO_2 Low CO Increased VO_2	Anemia or bleeding with compromised cardiopulmonary system Hypoxemia resulting from decreased oxygen supply or lung disease Cardiogenic shock caused by LV pump failure Metabolic demand exceeding oxygen supply in conditions that increase muscle movement and increase metabolic rate, including physiologic states such as shivering, seizures, and hyperthermia and nursing interventions such as being weighed on a bed scale and turning

CO, Cardiac output; *Hgb*, hemoglobin; *LV*, left ventricular; *SaO_2*, arterial saturation; *$ScvO_2$*, Central venous oxygen saturation; *SvO_2*, mixed venous oxygen saturation; *VO_2*, oxygen consumption.

TABLE 12.7 Cardiac Output Measurement

Device Name	Probe Placement	Method	Cardiac Output Calculation	Clinical Issues
Noninvasive Methods				
Bioimpedance	External electrodes placed on the neck and chest	Thoracic electrical bioimpedance	A small alternating current is applied across the chest by skin electrodes.	Noninvasive
Pressure and Pulse Contour (ClearSight, Edwards Lifesciences, CA)	Fingers	External Finger Cuffs	Pulsatile changes in thoracic blood volume result in changes in electrical impedance. The rate of change of impedance during systole is measured and used to calculate CO. Pulsatile changes on finger arteries are used to calculate BP, CO, SVV.	Less accurate with low body temperature. One cuff used up to 8 hours on a finger. With two cuffs, change fingers each hour.
Minimally Invasive Methods				
Pulse Contour Waveform Methods				
LiDCO (LiDCO Ltd., Cambridge, United Kingdom)	Requires a venous access catheter (central or peripheral) and an arterial catheter with a lithium-monitoring sensor attached (calibrated)	Pulse contour waveform analysis method (calibrated)	Independent calibration with a lithium dilution technique is initially required. A small, subtherapeutic dose of isotonic lithium chloride is injected through the venous catheter. The lithium is detected at the arterial sensor (femoral artery), where a fixed flow pump ensures constant flow. A concentration-time curve is produced for lithium before recirculation. CO is calculated based on lithium dose given and the measurement of the area under the curve. A noncalibrated system is also available.	Easy to set up; uses conventional venous and arterial catheters Can measure extravascular lung water for patients with pulmonary edema CO measurement affected by artifact on arterial waveform and by irregular and damped arterial waveforms Can be used in conscious and in unresponsive patients Requires calibration at least every 8 h to maintain accuracy; cannot be used in patients on lithium therapy because this interferes with calibration

Continued

TABLE 12.7 Cardiac Output Measurement—cont'd

Device Name	Probe Placement	Method	Cardiac Output Calculation	Clinical Issues
PiCCO (Pulsion Medical Systems, Munich, Germany)	Requires a central venous access catheter and uses a specialized arterial thermistor-tipped catheter in the femoral artery	Pulse contour waveform analysis method that uses transpulmonary thermodilution	A set volume of cold saline is injected through the central venous catheter. The arterial thermistor-tipped catheter detects the blood temperature change. Continuous CO measurements are achieved by analyzing the systolic component of the arterial waveform. A noncalibrated system is also available.	CO measurement affected by artifact on arterial waveform and irregular arterial waveforms Three calibrations required initially; frequent recalibration required to maintain accuracy
FloTrac, Vigileo (Edward Lifesciences, Irvine, CA)	Requires a functional arterial catheter	Pulse contour waveform analysis method (does not require calibration)	Calculates CO by use of arterial pressure waveform analysis in conjunction with patient data (age, sex, height, weight). Uses an internal proprietary algorithm based on the principle that pulse pressure (difference between systolic and diastolic pressure) is proportional to SV and inversely proportional to aortic compliance. Aortic pressure is sampled at 100 Hz and is updated every 20 s.	Does not require external calibration, but requires zeroing of the transducer Lack of calibration procedures controversial
Esophageal Probe Methods				
Esophageal Doppler	Ultrasound probe placed in the lower esophagus	SV calculated by measurement of the aortic blood velocity in the descending thoracic aorta (by continuous wave Doppler) plus calculation of the cross-sectional area of the aorta; CO calculated based on these values	The aorta cross-sectional area, measured using M-mode ultrasound, is multiplied by blood velocity to calculate flow or CO. The value of total CO is derived from a nomogram using aortic blood velocity, height, weight, and age.	Useful in the operating room or with deeply sedated patients Stiff probe; placement not well tolerated by conscious patients
TEE	Ultrasound probe placed in esophagus	Probe placement allows imaging of LV outflow tract; SV measured by Doppler	The LV outflow tract area is measured; this value is squared and multiplied by the velocity time interval of blood flow and HR. LV SV can be measured, as can HR to use the SV × HR = CO formula.	Useful in the operating room or with deeply sedated patients Stiff probe; placement not well tolerated by conscious patients Requires skill to accurately position probe to visualize LV outflow tract
Partial CO_2 Rebreathing Method				
$NICO_2$ (Philips, Respironics) Amsterdam, Netherlands	Addition of partial CO_2 rebreathing circuit to ventilator	Partial CO_2 rebreathing method	CO measurement is based on changes in respiratory CO_2 concentration obtained from a short period of rebreathing. CO_2 elimination is calculated by sensors that measure flow, airway pressure, and CO_2 concentration. These variables are used in the Fick partial rebreathing formula to calculate CO.	Can be used only in intubated and ventilated patients Specialized additional tubing setup on ventilator Cannot be used in patients who cannot tolerate hypercapnia (elevated CO_2) CO measurement altered by intrapulmonary shunt

BP, Blood pressure; *CO*, cardiac output; *CO_2*, carbon dioxide; *HR*, heart rate; *LV*, left ventricular; *SV*, stroke volume; *SVV*, stroke volume variation; *TEE*, transesophageal echocardiography.

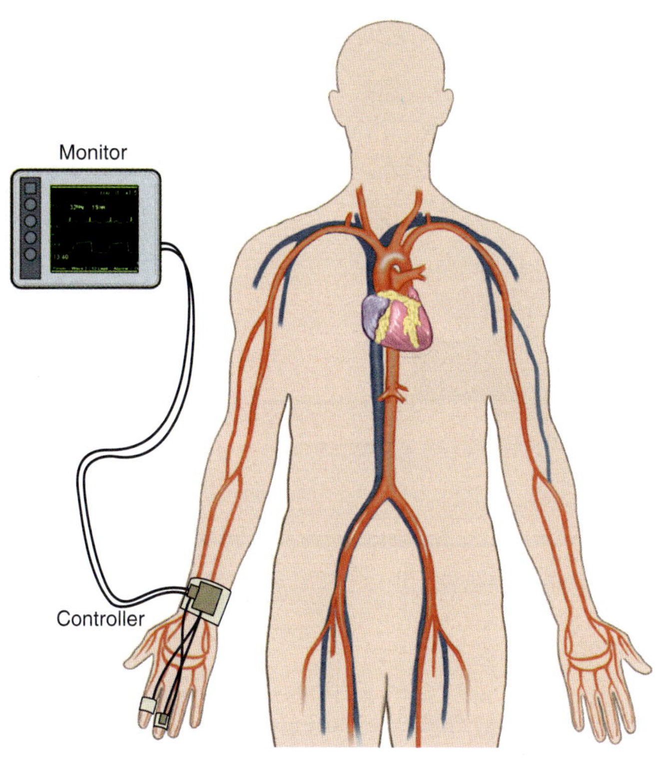

FIG. 12.26 Finger Cuff Arterial Pressure-Based Monitoring. Noninvasive systems can measure blood pressure and heart rate and calculate stroke volume variation and cardiac output using finger cuff technology. (From Lough ME. *Hemodynamic Monitoring: Evolving Technologies and Clinical Practice*. Elsevier; 2016.)

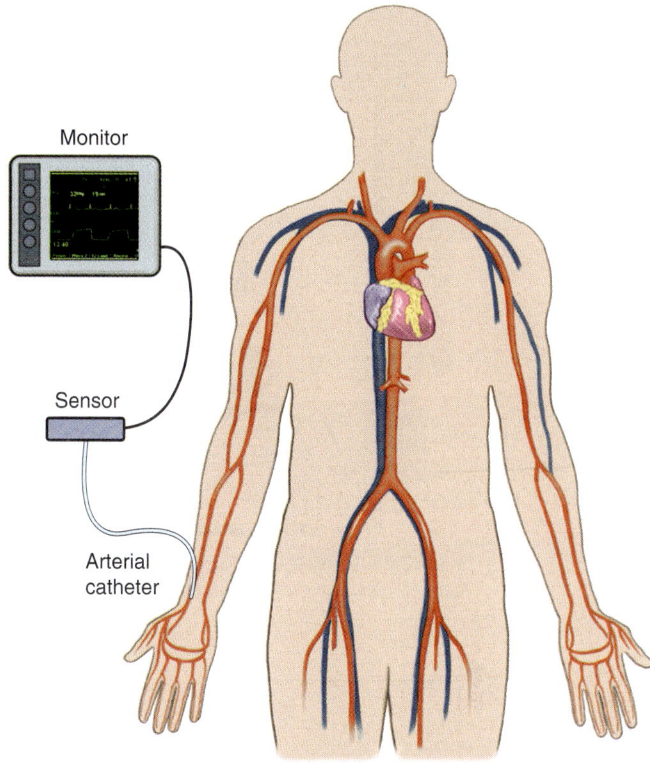

FIG. 12.27 Arterial Waveform and Pressure-Based Monitoring. Less-invasive systems that use a specialized transducer and arterial catheter sensor to calculate stroke volume, stroke volume variation, cardiac output, and cardiac index. Both calibrated and noncalibrated hemodynamic systems are available. (From Lough ME. *Hemodynamic Monitoring: Evolving Technologies and Clinical Practice*. Elsevier; 2016.)

monitoring is not readily available. To protect the skin, the finger cuffs must be moved to different fingers, at least every 8 hours.[40]

Minimally Invasive—Pulse Wave Analysis Hemodynamic Monitoring Systems

Arterial waveform–based systems require insertion of an arterial catheter fitted with specialized sensors that use arterial pressure and the arterial waveform contour to provide real-time data. The systems use proprietary thermistors, software, and bedside computer systems (Fig. 12.27) and are internally calibrated.[41] The different technologies and the systems may be described as *pulse contour analysis*, *pulse wave analysis*, or *pulse power analysis*. Because an arterial catheter is inserted these are considered minimally invasive.[41] Arterial pressure–based systems trend continuous blood pressure, SV, SVV, pulse pressure variation, and CO. A significant advantage is that the patient does not have to be intubated or sedated to tolerate the monitoring system. Another advantage is that the CO values are recorded in real time and change with breathing pattern and fluid volume interventions.[41] The continuous SVV and CO values are sometimes referred to as *functional hemodynamics*. These values can be used in the assessment of *fluid volume responsiveness* using the *passive leg raise* maneuver (Fig. 12.28).[19] Real-time hemodynamic monitoring systems are especially well suited to this bedside examination. The increase in central blood volume as the legs are raised should increase SV and decrease SVV if a patient is fluid responsive (Fig. 12.29).

The nursing management of an arterial catheter described in the earlier section on arterial pressure monitoring also applies here. If the arterial waveform is not pristine, the hemodynamic data will be compromised. A fast-flush square wave test should be performed to verify the accuracy of the arterial waveform.[40] Frequent dysrhythmias will change the shape of the pulse waveform and decrease accuracy. The position of the transducer is also important. If the transducer level is misaligned by more than 4 inches (10 cm), inaccurate measurements can result.[42]

Invasive—Transpulmonary Thermodilution Monitoring Systems

Transpulmonary thermodilution monitoring systems are calibrated and more invasive, as they require both arterial and central venous access (see Fig. 12.1). As explained earlier, the system may be described as pulse wave, or pulse contour, depending on the manufacturer. Transpulmonary thermodilution systems are used when more exact (calibrated) information is required. The calibration methods vary from cold saline to lithium depending on the system used and manufacturer guidelines.[41]

To obtain a CO using the transpulmonary thermodilution technique, a bolus of cold saline is injected into the CVC and measured at a femoral arterial thermistor-tipped catheter. Injectate temperature and transit time are used to generate a thermodilution temperature curve to calculate CO (Fig. 12.30).

The transpulmonary thermodilution method uses a CVC and an arterial catheter but avoids placing a catheter into the

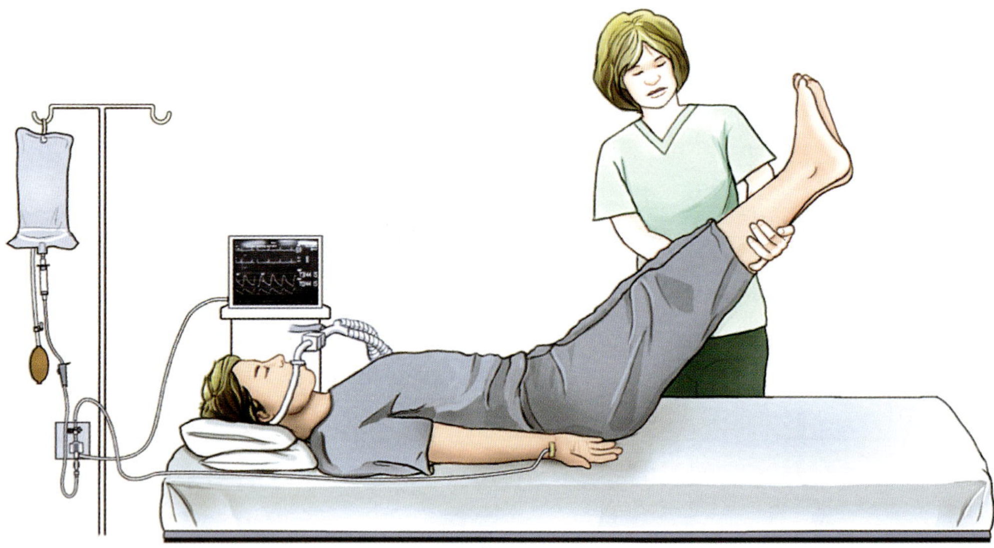

FIG. 12.28 Passive Leg Raise in Intubated Patient. (From Lough ME. *Hemodynamic Monitoring: Evolving Technologies and Clinical Practice.* Elsevier; 2016.)

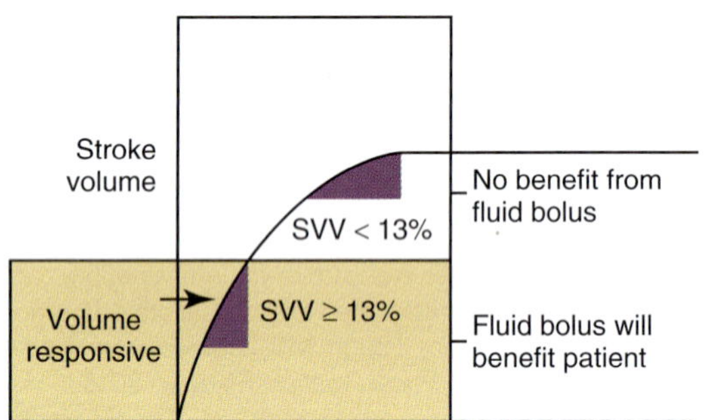

FIG. 12.29 Stroke Volume Variation *(SVV)* in Response to a Volume Challenge. (From Lough ME. *Hemodynamic Monitoring: Evolving Technologies and Clinical Practice.* Elsevier; 2016.)

right heart chambers, which is considered a benefit because it is less invasive. Transpulmonary thermodilution systems also provide different data from the traditional PA catheter. The *extravascular lung water index* measures the volume and percentage of water in lung tissue; a higher index value is a marker of pulmonary edema.[43] Lung water content increases in conditions such as heart failure and ARDS. Higher lung water content is associated with higher mortality. Knowledge of extravascular lung water may influence whether to administer diuretics or administer volume.

Pulse contour analysis enables the use of SVV to assess volume status. SVV measures the difference between the highest and lowest SV over the previous 30 seconds. The caveat is that for this to be considered truly accurate, the patient must be mechanically ventilated and not over-breathing the ventilator. This requirement restricts accurate SVV monitoring to patients during anesthesia, deep sedation, or pharmacologic paralysis.

VISUAL HEMODYNAMIC MONITORING SYSTENS

Transesophageal Echocardiography

Traditionally, echocardiography would not have been described as a primary hemodynamic monitoring modality, although this has changed in many settings.[44] This is because transesophageal echocardiography (TEE) monitoring during cardiac surgery has increased, with more patients returning to the cardiac critical care unit with an esophageal probe in place.[45] Generally, surgical patients monitored with TEE are mechanically ventilated and anesthetized after surgery. Because of the close anatomic relationship between the heart and the esophagus, TEE produces images of very high quality of the heart chambers, heart valves, and thoracic aorta without the interference of the chest wall, bone, or air-filled lung (Fig. 12.31). TEE has the advantage of displaying a real-time image of the heart in motion. This allows real-time assessment of LV cardiac contractility. Additional information specific to noninvasive transthoracic echocardiography (TTE) is provided later in this chapter.

Ultrasound-Based Hemodynamic Monitoring

Handheld ultrasound has become an essential noninvasive component of beside hemodynamic assessment in many critical care units. Critical care societies now recommend that all medical trainees learn the basic skills of ultrasonography. One of the most useful ultrasound skills is the assessment of fluid volume status by examination of the inferior vena cava (IVC) during the respiratory cycle.[46]

- **IVC with mechanical ventilation.** In a mechanically ventilated patient, intrathoracic pressure is highest during inspiration and lowest at end-expiration. At the point of lowest pressure, preload volume is rapidly drawn into the right atrium, causing the IVC to "collapse." This collapse is more obvious in a patient with hypovolemia. In a patient with normal volume status or hypervolemia, the IVC walls have less movement with breathing (Fig. 12.32).
- **IVC with spontaneous breathing.** In a spontaneously breathing patient, the respiratory mechanics are different. The lowest pressure occurs during inspiration; with hypovolemia, the IVC walls may be seen to collapse. This measure is considered less reliable in a spontaneously breathing patient.

Many ultrasound protocols have been developed to guide clinical management. These validated protocols are often a first-line level of hemodynamic assessment in an unstable patient.

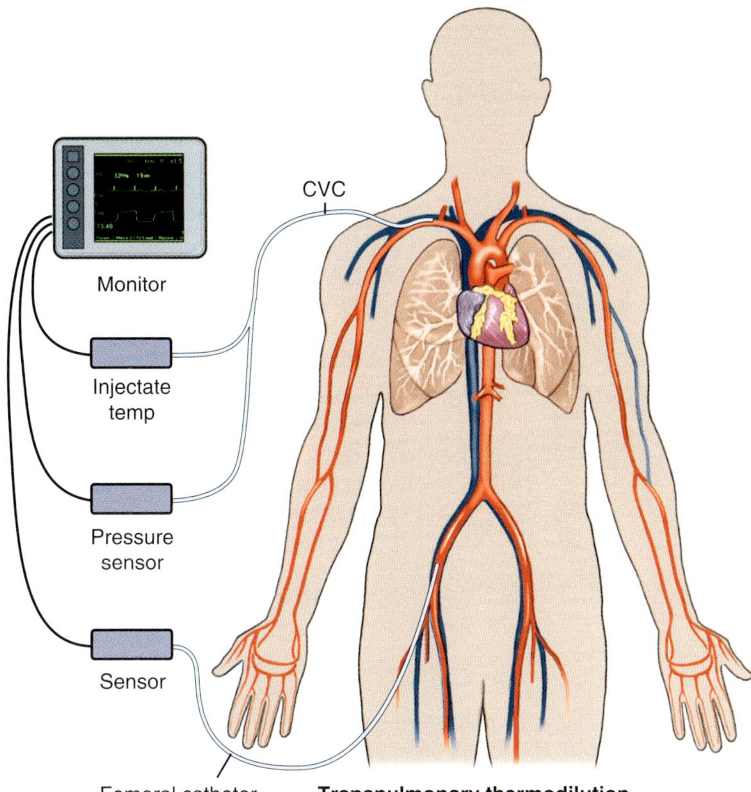

FIG. 12.30 Transpulmonary Thermodilution Arterial Waveform Pressure-Based Monitoring. More invasive calibrated systems that use an arterial catheter and central venous catheter *(CVC)* to obtain a transpulmonary thermodilution cardiac output (CVC through pulmonary vascular system to arterial catheter with sensor). (From Lough ME. *Hemodynamic Monitoring: Evolving Technologies and Clinical Practice.* Elsevier; 2016.)

Ultrasound is a frequency greater than 20,000 Hz, which is above the range of human hearing. Ultrasound is reflected visibly at interfaces between tissues that have different densities. Protocols are used to ensure that all practitioners use ultrasound-guided diagnosis in a consistent manner.

- **Focused assessment by sonography for trauma.** One of the earliest uses was in trauma, where focused assessment by sonography for trauma (FAST) is used to evaluate intraabdominal blood. Chapter 33 has additional information about use of FAST for trauma assessment (see Fig. 32.17).

Doppler-Based Hemodynamic Monitoring Methods

Doppler offers another method to trend CO. This modality can be noninvasive or invasive. The esophagus is used as the invasive monitoring site for patients who are deeply sedated or are under general anesthesia in the operating room. The esophageal Doppler probe is less invasive than a PA catheter (Fig. 12.33). Insertion of the esophageal Doppler probe is similar to insertion of a gastric tube, although the probe is relatively inflexible and stiff. The probe is inserted 35 to 40 cm from the teeth. The tip of the probe rests near T5-T6 on the vertebral column, where the esophagus typically is parallel with the descending aorta. When the probe is correctly placed, this method has a high degree of accuracy for CO measurement. Because of advances in Doppler technology, noninvasive Doppler is more frequently used in conjunction with echocardiography.

ELECTROCARDIOGRAPHY

Electrocardiography is a complex and vitally useful skill to master. Detailed evaluation of an ECG can provide a wealth of cardiac diagnostic information and often provides the basis on which other, definitive diagnostic tests are selected. The following sections discuss the many clinical factors that the critical care nurse considers when using ECG monitoring, specific dysrhythmias commonly encountered in clinical practice, and the skills needed for 12-lead ECG analysis. The intent is to provide a sound basis for understanding the value of the many clinical applications of electrocardiography.

Basic Principles of Electrocardiography

The ECG records electrical changes in heart muscle caused by an action potential. It does not record the mechanical contraction, which usually follows electrical depolarization immediately. A brief discussion of the cardiac action potential is provided to explain the concept that electrical changes occurring during electrical stimulation of the myocardial cell produce the deflections seen on the ECG tracing (Fig. 12.34).

Phase 0

During phase 0 (depolarization), the electrical potential changes rapidly from a baseline of −90 mV to +20 mV and stabilizes at approximately 0 mV. Because this is a significant electrical change, it appears as a wave on the ECG as the QRS complex.

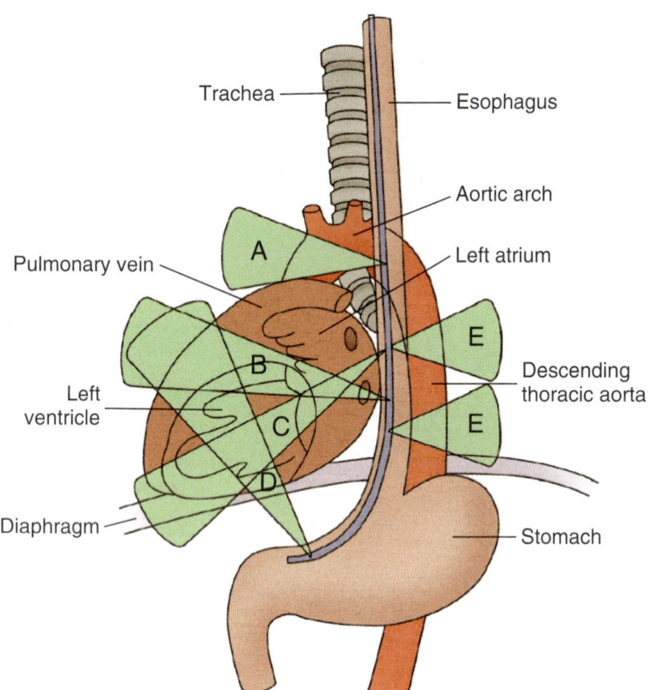

FIG. 12.31 Diagram of Common Scan Planes During a Transesophageal Echocardiogram With a Two-Dimensional View. (A) Horizontal scan plane of the aortic arch and distal portion of aorta. (B) Basal short-axis (transverse), long-axis (sagittal), and short-axis views of both atria. (C) Four-chamber and left atrioventricular long-axis views. A sagittal scan plane can image a cross section of the left ventricle. (D) Transgastric, short-axis view of the left and right ventricles. (E) Transverse and sagittal scan sections of the descending aorta.

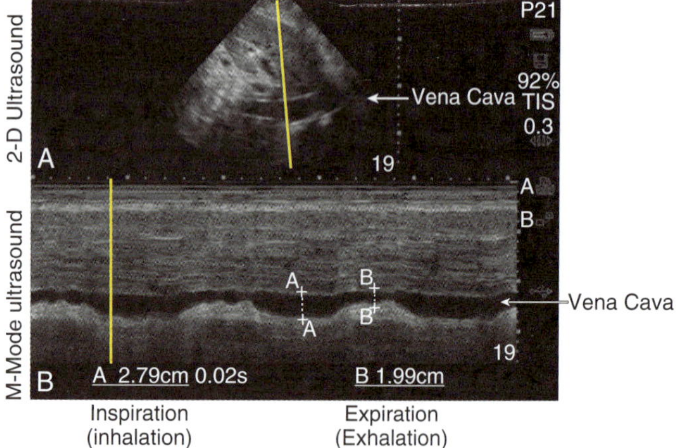

FIG. 12.32 Respiratory Changes in Intrathoracic Pressure on Inferior Vena Cava (IVC) Diameter Viewed by Handheld Ultrasound. (A) The upper image shows a two-dimensional ultrasound of the IVC from the subxiphoid view in a spontaneously breathing patient. The open appearance of the vena cava indicates it is filled with blood, suggesting the patient has taken a deep breath. A yellow line passes through the vena cava to take a measurement. (B) The lower image shows M-mode ultrasound showing changes in the IVC diameter with breathing over time. The yellow line passing through the vena cava is in the same position as in the upper image.

- Position measurement A-A is obtained during inspiration (inhalation) when the IVC measures 2.79 cm apart (wider).
- Position measurement B-B is taken during expiration (exhalation) when the IVC measures 1.99 cm apart (narrower).

(From Lough ME. *Hemodynamic Monitoring: Evolving Technologies and Clinical Practice*. Elsevier; 2016.)

Phases 1 and 2

During phases 1 and 2, an electrical plateau is created, and mechanical contraction occurs during this plateau. Because there is no significant electrical change, no waveform appears on the ECG (the recorded tracing is isoelectric with baseline).

Phase 3

During phase 3 (repolarization), the electrical potential again changes, this time a little more slowly, from 0 mV back to −90 mV. This is another major electrical event and is reflected on the ECG as a T wave.

Phase 4

During phase 4 (resting period), the chemical balance is restored by the sodium pump, but because positively charged ions are exchanged on a one-for-one basis, no electrical activity is generated, and no visible change occurs on the ECG tracing. For more information on the cardiac action potential, see Phases of the Action Potential in Chapter 10.

Electrocardiogram Leads

All electrocardiographs use a system of one or more leads. The basic three-lead system consists of three bipolar electrodes that are applied to the chest wall and labeled *right arm (RA)*, *left arm (LA)*, and *left leg (LL)*. The term *bipolar* means that each created ECG lead has a positive and a negative pole. A third electrode acts as a ground. The function of the ground electrode is to prevent the display of background electrical interference on the ECG tracing. Electrodes do not transmit any electricity to the patient; rather, they sense and record intrinsic cardiac electrical activity from the body's surface. Lead wires can be disposable or reusable.[47] There is no difference in infection rates as long as the nondisposable ECG lead wires and connectors are thoroughly cleaned between each patient use.[48] The ECG skin electrode patch that touches the patient's skin is always disposable. Disposable leads or electrodes should be changed or replaced per manufacturer's guidelines. It is important to properly prepare the patient's skin before placing the electrodes because this will improve signal quality, thereby decreasing erroneous alarms. Proper preparation includes washing the electrode area with soap and water and wiping with a washcloth or gauze.[49–51] Do not use alcohol for skin preparation because it dries out the skin. Excessive hair at the electrode site should be clipped.[49] Alarm fatigue is a serious patient safety issue that has direct effects on nursing practice and care. See Box 12.6 for more information on alarm management.

The positive electrode on the skin is similar to an "eye" that provides the "point of view" of the positive electrode as a component of the ECG tracing. If the wave of depolarization travels toward the positive electrode, an upward stroke, or positive deflection, is written on the ECG paper (Fig. 12.35A). If the wave of depolarization travels away from the positive electrode, a downward line, or negative deflection, is recorded on the ECG paper or monitor (Fig. 12.35B). When depolarization moves both toward and away from the positive electrode, a biphasic complex occurs. Sometimes the complex may even appear almost flat, or isoelectric, if the electrical forces traveling in opposite directions are equal and have the effect of canceling each other out (Fig. 12.35C). The size of the muscle mass being depolarized also has an effect, with larger muscle mass (usually the left ventricle) producing a higher amplitude tracing.

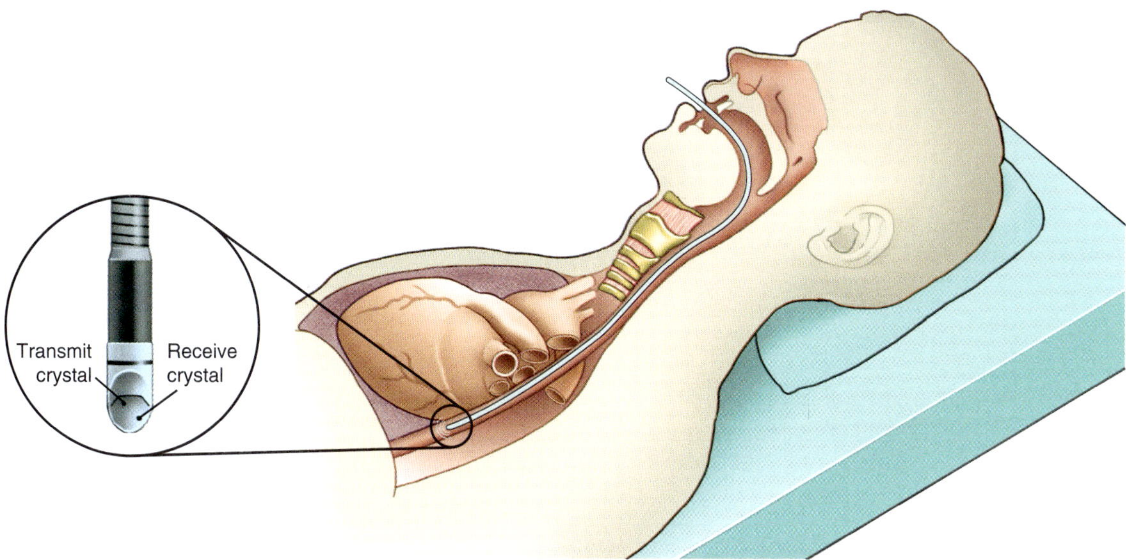

FIG. 12.33 Esophageal Doppler probe with tip positioned in the esophagus, parallel to the descending aorta. (From Lough ME. *Hemodynamic Monitoring: Evolving Technologies and Clinical Practice*. Elsevier; 2016.)

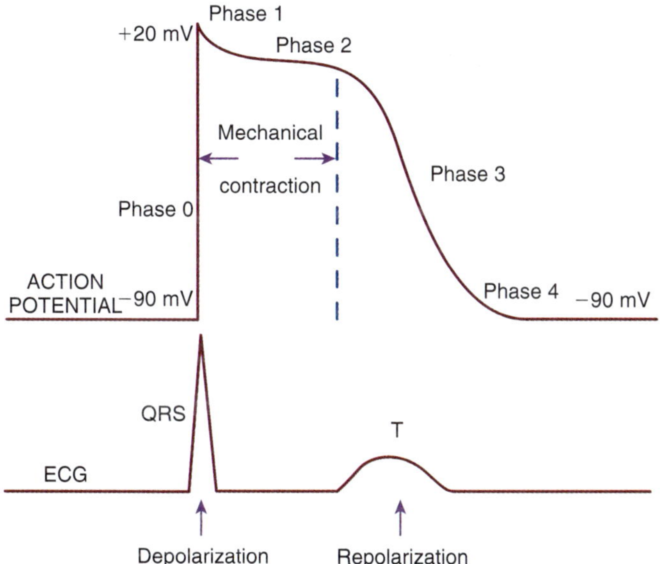

FIG. 12.34 Correlation of Action Potential of a Ventricular Myocardial Cell With Electrical Events Recorded on Surface Electrocardiogram *(ECG)*. The ECG pattern is "silent" during phase 2 of the action potential. Mechanical contraction is occurring, but no significant electrical activity is present.

The wave of ventricular depolarization in the healthy heart travels from superior to inferior and slightly leftward. The appearance of the ECG waveforms, positive or negative, is different in various ECG leads depending on the location of the positive electrode.

12-Lead Electrocardiogram Leads

The standard 12-lead ECG provides a picture of the electrical activity in the heart using 10 different electrode positions to create 12 unique views of electrical activity occurring within the heart.[51,52] A standard 12-lead ECG contains six limb lead images and six chest (precordial) lead images, and the correct placement of these leads is vitally important to avoid misdiagnosis. For a 12-lead ECG, the limb electrodes are typically placed on the muscle of the limb, avoiding bone, and the patient is asked to remain still during recording. In the critical care unit, the electrodes are typically placed on the torso (Mason-Likar configuration), near the origin of the limb, avoiding the clavicular bone (LA and RA) and the pelvic bone (LL and RL), as shown in Fig. 12.36A. This arrangement is used because patients wear the electrodes continuously (hours or days), and limb movement would distort the electrical baseline and cause artifact. Practically, this means that ECG waveforms on the bedside monitor will not be identical to the waveforms obtained by a standard 12-lead ECG unless limb leads are moved to the standard 12-lead placement location on the wrist and ankles.[52]

BOX 12.6 Safety

Alarm Fatigue

Alarm fatigue is a significant patient safety risk. Adverse patient events, including death, have occurred as the result of improper alarm management in the acute care setting. Recent studies have demonstrated that over 85% (and possibly even up to 99%) of alarms are clinically nonactionable, resulting in desensitization to alarms. The concern over alarm fatigue needs to be balanced with the need to continuously monitor patients that are critically ill. Evidence-based strategies to reduce alarm fatigue include:

- Following proper skin preparation steps when applying ECG monitoring leads. Replace leads on a routine basis as outlined by institutional guidelines.
- Personalizing alarm parameters for individual patients based on patient condition and institutional guidelines.
- Diligent use of continuous monitoring. Once no longer clinically indicated, continuous monitoring should be discontinued.

American Association of Critical Care Nurses (AACN). Managing Alarms in Acute Care Across the Lifespan: Electrocardiography and Pulse Oximetry: AACN Practice Alert. *Crit Care Nurse*. 2018;38(2):e16–e20.

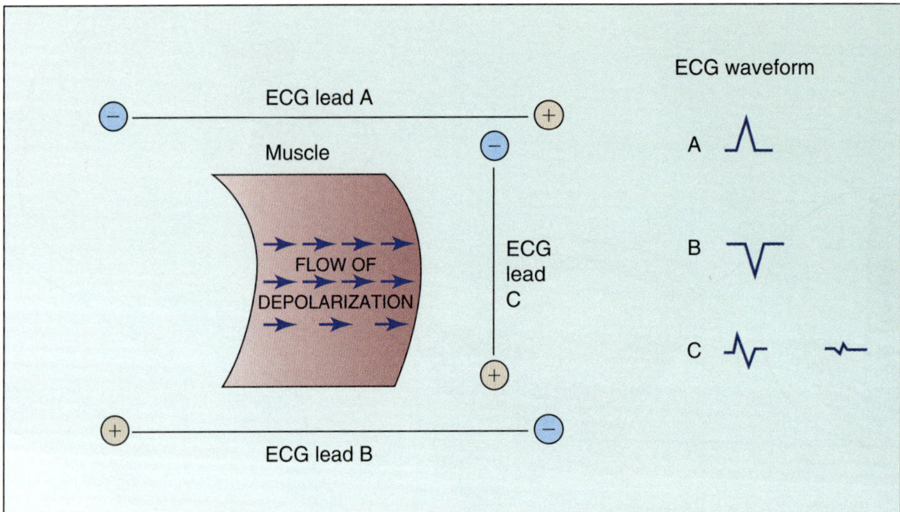

FIG. 12.35 Effect of Lead Position on an Electrocardiogram *(ECG)* Tracing. (A) Flow of depolarization toward the positive electrode results in a positive deflection on the ECG. (B) Flow of depolarization away from the positive electrode results in a negative deflection on the ECG. (C) Flow of depolarization perpendicular to the positive electrode results in a biphasic or nearly isoelectric deflection on the ECG. This basic principle applies to the P wave and the QRS complex.

Standard Limb Leads

The limb lead tracings are obtained by placing electrodes on all four extremities: LA, RA, LL, and RL. Leads I, II, and III are bipolar limb leads that use limb lead electrodes paired as the positive and negative poles (see Fig. 12.36A). The electrodes are placed in a static position on the body, and the polarity is switched within the cardiograph machine to achieve the desired view. This can be done manually on the critical care bedside monitor or transport monitor or, most commonly, automatically by the electrocardiography machine:

- Lead I: Positive electrode at LA and negative electrode at RA
- Lead II: Positive electrode at LL and negative electrode at RA
- Lead III: Positive electrode at LL and negative electrode at LA

This configuration means that the three limb leads are linked in a circuit. The information obtained from the three limb leads is used to create a central reference potential that reflects the average potential of the RA, LA, and LL electrodes.[52] The central reference potential shown at the center of the electrode triangle in Fig. 12.36A is used to calculate the augmented vector leads.

Augmented Vector Leads

The augmented vector leads, labeled aVR (right arm), aVL (left arm), and aVF (left foot), are derived using the bipolar electrode pairs previously described (Leads I, II, III). These augmented leads have only one positive electrode (see Fig. 12.36A), with the calculated central reference potential (center of triangle) acting as a negative electrode. Under these circumstances, the ECG tracing obtained is ordinarily very small, so the machine enhances, or augments (hence the "a" designation) it by adding enough voltage to render the waveform amplitudes roughly equivalent to the other lead views. The term *vector* refers to directional force. The augmented vector leads are used in the interpretation of myocardial injury and infarction. Combined, the limb leads and the augmented vector leads are derived from the four limb electrodes. They constitute the frontal plane axis of the 12-lead ECG. The frontal plane QRS axis is used to determine the overall direction of ventricular depolarization.[53]

Precordial Leads

The six precordial, or left chest, leads are labeled as V leads and are distributed in an arc around the left side of the chest. They are positioned to detect electrical forces traveling from right to left or from front to back. Each of the V leads is independent of the other precordial electrodes and provides a unique view of the cardiac electrical system (Fig. 12.36B). The six electrodes are placed on the chest in the following locations[52]:

V_1: Fourth intercostal space at the right sternal border
V_2: Fourth intercostal space at the left sternal border
V_3: Midway between V_2 and V_4
V_4: Fifth intercostal space in the midclavicular line
V_5: In the horizontal plane of V_4 at the anterior axillary line or, if the anterior axillary line is ambiguous, midway between V_4 and V_6
V_6: In the horizontal plane of V_4 at the midaxillary line

Right Ventricular Precordial Leads

Additional leads sometimes are helpful in evaluating the extent of myocardium involved in an acute MI. The right ventricle and the posterior wall of the heart are areas that are not clearly seen on a standard 12-lead ECG. The right ventricle can be visualized more fully by adding right-sided chest leads (Fig. 12.36C). Labeled V_1R, V_2R, V_3R, V_4R, V_5R, and V_6R, they are added to the standard 12-lead ECG when right ventricular infarction is suspected. Right ventricular infarction is commonly accompanied by inferior and posterior wall infarction. The use of the six right ventricular leads expands the diagnostic accuracy of the 12-lead ECG and is sometimes called an *18-lead ECG*.[52]

Posterior Wall Leads

The posterior wall of the heart can be assessed using posterior chest leads (Fig. 12.36D). These leads are labeled

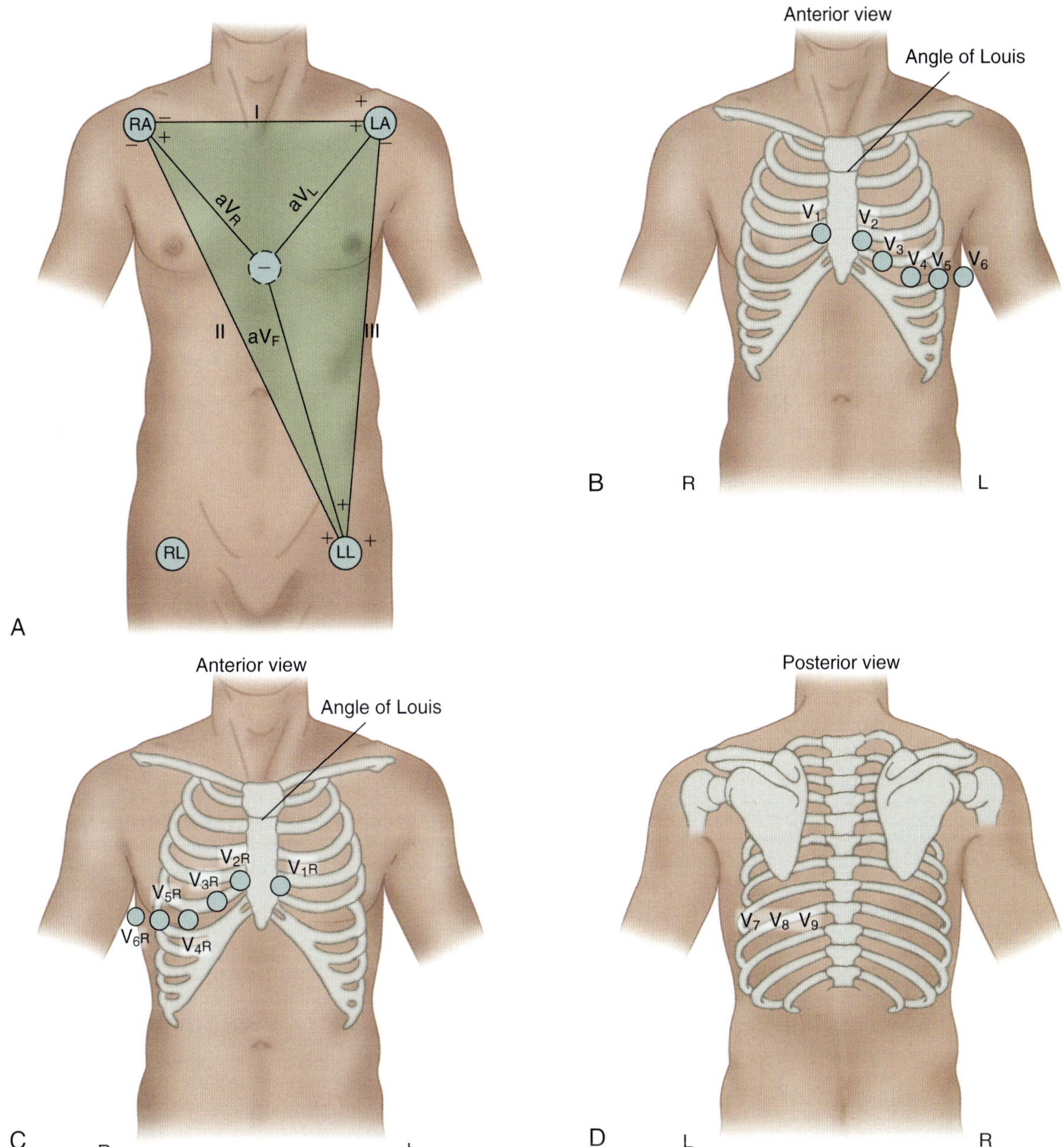

FIG. 12.36 (A) Standard limb leads. Leads are located on the extremities: right arm (*RA*), left arm (*LA*), and left leg (*LL*). The right leg electrode serves as a ground. Leads I, II, and III are bipolar, with each using a positive electrode and a negative electrode. Leads aVR, aVL, and aVF are augmented unipolar leads that use the calculated center of the heart as their negative electrode. (B) Precordial leads. V_1 to V_6 are the six standard precordial leads and are placed as follows: V_1, fourth intercostal space, right sternal border; V_2, fourth intercostal space, left sternal border; V_3, equidistant between V_2 and V_4; V_4, fifth intercostal space, left midclavicular line; V_5, anterior axillary line, same horizontal level as V_4; V_6, midaxillary line, same horizontal level as V_4. (C) The right precordial leads V_1R to V_6R are shown. They are not part of a standard 12-lead ECG but are used when a right ventricular infarction is suspected. Their placement is identical to V_3 to V_6 except that they are placed on the right side of the chest rather than on the left. (D) Posterior precordial leads V_7, V_8, and V_9 are placed on the patient's left posterior chest at the same horizontal level as V_4 (fifth intercostal space). V_7 is on the posterior axillary line, V_8 is on the scapular line, and V_9 is on the spinal border. These leads may be added to the standard 12-lead electrocardiogram when a posterior wall infarction is suspected.

V_7, V_8, and V_9. Although posterior lead placement can be technically challenging, the information obtained may influence decisions regarding clinical management. The use of the posterior leads expands the diagnostic accuracy of the 12-lead ECG and can be described as a *15-lead ECG*.[52]

Baseline Distortion

The ECG tracing must have a flat baseline, which is the portion of the tracing between the various waveforms. Two forms of artifact can distort the baseline: 60-cycle interference and muscular movement. The 60-cycle (Hertz) interference artifact (Fig. 12.37A) results from leakage of ambient electrical current

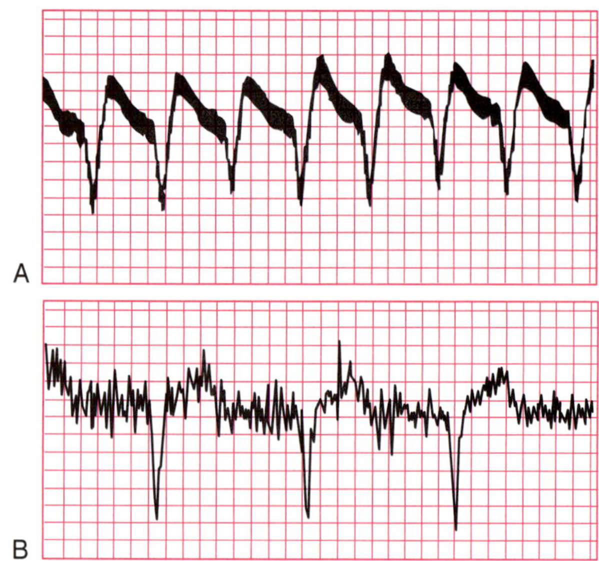

FIG. 12.37 (A) Artifact from 60-cycle interference. (B) Artifact caused by muscular movement.

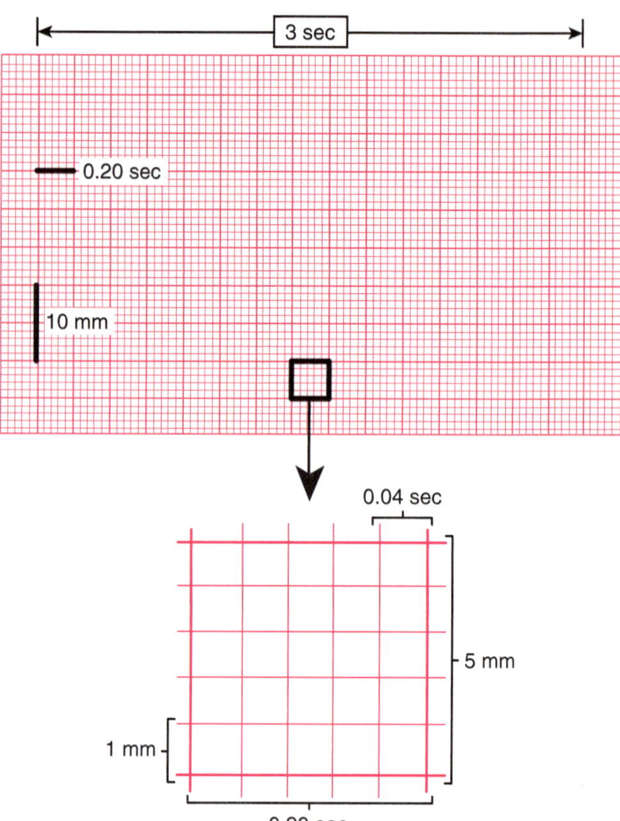

FIG. 12.38 Electrocardiogram Graph Paper. The horizontal axis represents time, and the vertical axis represents the magnitude of voltage. Horizontally, each small box is 0.04 second, and each large box is 0.20 second. Vertically, each large box is 5 mm. Markings are present every 3 seconds at the top of the paper for ease in calculating heart rate.

in the immediate environment, or devices in contact with the patient's body (e.g., warming/cooling blanket left ventricular assist device) and appears as a generalized thickening of the baseline. Ambient electrical current can usually be resolved by ensuring that all electrical equipment at the bedside is electrically grounded. Moving the offending device away from the patient may help, or occasionally it may be necessary to unplug one piece of equipment at a time until the offending device is found. Muscular movement (Fig. 12.37B) is displayed as a coarse, erratic disturbance of the baseline. In most cases, asking the patient to lie quietly while the ECG is obtained is sufficient. If movement is caused by shivering or seizure activity, it is best to wait until the activity subsides before obtaining the 12-lead ECG, if possible. When baseline tremor is present, resolution of artifact may be impossible. Electrical artifact disrupts accurate interpretation of the tracing and may mimic lethal ventricular dysrhythmias.

Electrocardiogram Analysis

Specialized Electrocardiogram Paper

ECG paper records the speed and magnitude of electrical impulses on a grid composed of small and large boxes (Fig. 12.38). Every large square box contains 25 small boxes within it. Each small box is 1 millimeter (mm) wide and 1 mm high. At a standard paper speed of 25 mm/s, looking at the ECG paper from left to right, one small box (1 mm wide) is equivalent to 0.04 second, and one large box (5 mm wide) is equivalent to 0.20 second in time. These ECG boxes represent the time it takes for the electrical impulse to travel through a particular part of the heart and are described in seconds rather than in millimeters or number of boxes. The vertical scale represents the magnitude, or amplitude, of the electrical signal. The vertical scale is standardized to a specific calibration.

Calibration

At standard calibration, one small square equals 0.1 millivolt (mV), or 1 mm in height. One large square equals 0.5 mV, or 5 mm in height. It is important to look for the standardization mark, which is usually located at the beginning of the tracing (Fig. 12.39A). The mark indicates that in response to a standard electrical signal of 1 mV, the calibration signal rises vertically the equivalent of two large square boxes to make a calibration mark. ECGs are sometimes run at different calibrations. If some complexes are so tall that they run off the paper at standard calibration, the ECG recording is repeated at one-half standard (Fig. 12.39B), and the calibration mark rises only one large box. If all the complexes on a standard tracing are very small, it may be repeated at double standard, with the calibration mark going up four large boxes (Fig. 12.39C). In any case, the calibration must be clearly marked on the tracing, because some diagnostic conclusions (e.g., QRS amplitude, ST segments) are based on the magnitude of specific portions of the ECG complex.

ECG Waveforms

The analysis of waveforms and intervals provides the basis for ECG interpretation (Fig. 12.40).

P Wave

The P wave represents atrial depolarization.

QRS Complex

The QRS complex represents ventricular depolarization, corresponding to phase 0 of the ventricular action potential. It is referred to as a *complex* because it consists of several different waves.

- ***Q*** is used to describe an initial negative deflection; the first deflection from the baseline is labeled a Q wave only if it is negative.
- ***R*** applies to any positive deflection from baseline. If there are two positive deflections in one QRS complex, the second is

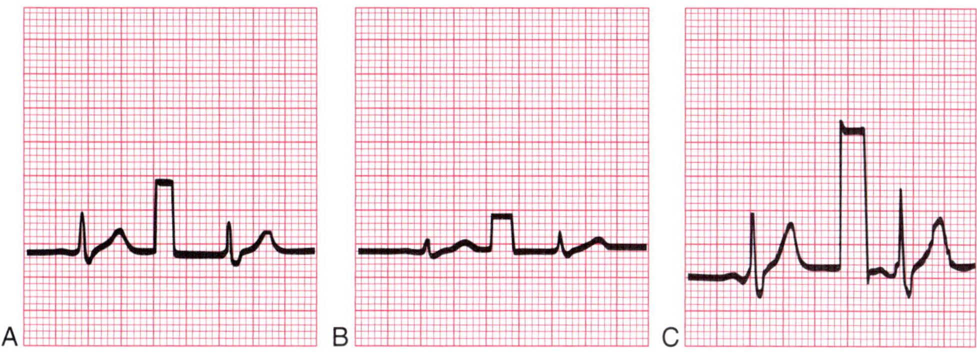

FIG. 12.39 (A) The machine is calibrated so that the normal standardization mark is 10 mm tall. (B) Half standardization is used when QRS complexes are too tall to fit on the paper. (C) Twice normal standardization is used when QRS complexes are too small to be adequately analyzed.

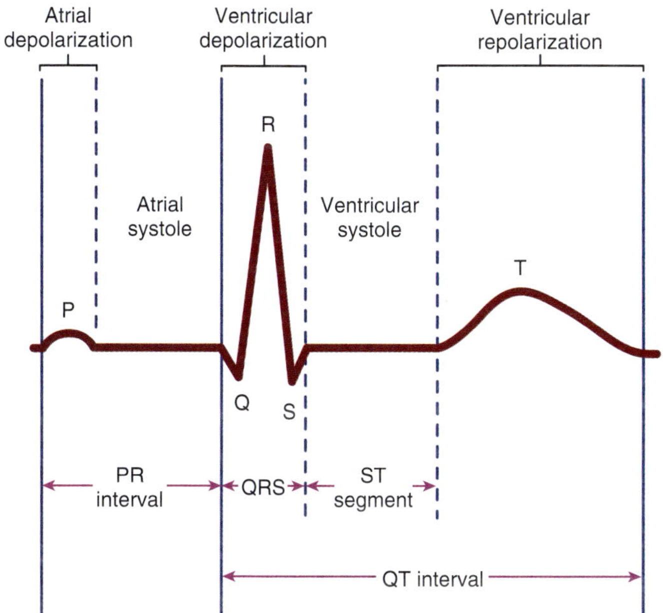

FIG. 12.40 Normal Electrocardiogram (ECG) Waveforms, Intervals, and Correlation with Events of the Cardiac Cycle. The *P wave* represents atrial depolarization, followed immediately by atrial systole. The *QRS complex* represents ventricular depolarization, followed immediately by ventricular systole. The *ST segment* corresponds to phase 2 of the action potential, during which time the heart muscle is completely depolarized and contraction normally occurs. The *T wave* represents ventricular repolarization. The *PR interval*, measured from the beginning of the P wave to the beginning of the QRS complex, corresponds to atrial depolarization and impulse delay in the atrioventricular node. The *QT interval*, measured from the beginning of the QRS complex to the end of the T wave, represents the time from initial depolarization of the ventricles to the end of ventricular repolarization.

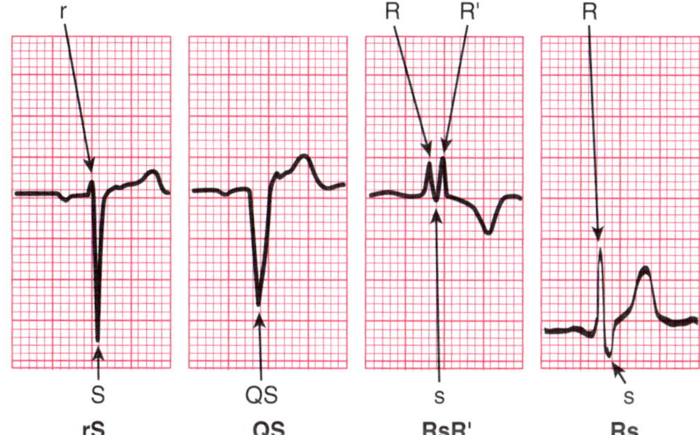

FIG. 12.41 Examples of QRS Complexes. Small deflections are labeled with lowercase letters, and uppercase letters are used for larger deflections. A second upward deflection is labeled R′.

labeled *R′* ("R prime") and is commonly seen in lead V_1 in patients with right bundle branch block (RBBB).

- ***S*** refers to any subsequent negative deflections. Any combination of these deflections can occur and is collectively called the *QRS complex* (Fig. 12.41). The QRS complex duration is normally less than 0.11 second (2.5 small boxes).

T Wave

The T wave represents ventricular repolarization, corresponding to phase 3 of the ventricular action potential. The onset of the QRS complex to approximately the midpoint or peak of the T wave represents an absolute refractory period, during which the heart muscle cannot respond to another stimulus no matter how strong that stimulus may be (Fig. 12.42). From the midpoint to the end of the T wave, the heart muscle is in the relative refractory period. The heart muscle has not yet fully recovered, but it can be depolarized again if a strong enough stimulus is received. This can be a particularly dangerous time for ventricular ectopy to occur, especially if any portion of the myocardium is ischemic, because the ischemic muscle takes even longer to fully repolarize. An impulse arriving during this period is known as *R on T* and may cause disorganized, self-perpetuating depolarizations of various sections of the myocardium and lead to VT or ventricular fibrillation (VF).

Intervals Between Waveforms

The intervals between waveforms are evaluated to determine the time it takes for cardiac activation (see Fig. 12.40).

PR Interval

The PR interval is measured from the beginning of the P wave to the beginning of the QRS complex. The PR interval is normally 0.12 to 0.20 seconds long and represents the time it takes for the electrical impulse to travel from the SA node to the AV node. Because this period includes any delay of the impulse within the AV node to initiate ventricular depolarization, the PR interval is an indicator of AV node function.

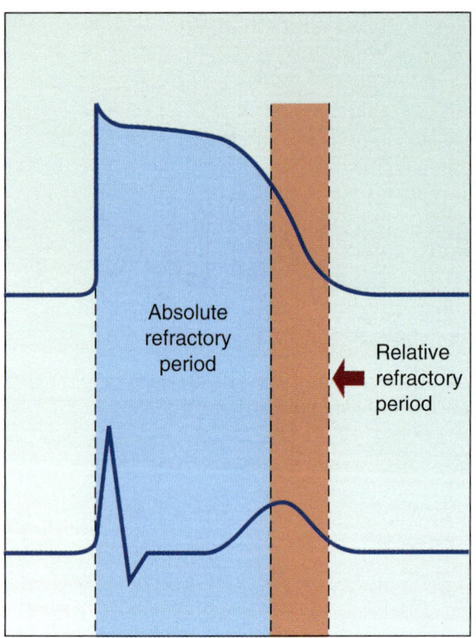

FIG. 12.42 Absolute and relative refractory periods are correlated with the cardiac muscle action potential and with an electrocardiogram tracing.

QRS Duration

As mentioned previously, the QRS complex duration is normally less than 0.11 second (2.5 small boxes). The QRS duration is widened in bundle branch block (BBB; right or left) or ventricular preexcitation, as would be present in Wolff-Parkinson-White syndrome. Ventricular paced rhythms also cause a wide QRS complex.

ST Segment

The ST segment is the portion of the ECG waveform that extends from the end of the QRS complex to the beginning of the T wave. Its duration is not measured. Instead, its shape and amplitude are evaluated. The ST segment is normally flat and at the same level as the isoelectric baseline measured at the PR segment or the TP segment. Any change (i.e., elevation or depression) from baseline is expressed in millimeters and may indicate myocardial ischemia (one small box equals 1 mm). ST segment elevation of 1 to 2 mm is associated with acute myocardial injury, preinfarction, and pericarditis. ST segment depression (decrease from baseline more than 1 to 2 mm) is associated with myocardial ischemia.[54] The ST segment must be monitored carefully in high-risk patients (described later).

QT Interval

The QT interval is measured from the beginning of the QRS complex to the end of the T wave and indicates the total time from the onset of ventricular depolarization to the completion of ventricular repolarization. While there is no established bedside monitoring lead recommended for measuring the QT interval, the lead with the longest T wave should be selected, typically lead V2 or V3. It is also suggested to avoid leads with U waves, because it can be difficult to determine the end of the QT interval.[51,55] The important point is that each clinician measures the QT interval using the same ECG lead.[51] At a normal HR, the QT interval is less than one-half of the R-R interval when measured from one QRS complex to the next. However, the length of a QT interval depends on the HR and must be adjusted according to the HR to be evaluated in a clinically meaningful way.

Because the QT interval shortens at faster HRs and lengthens with slower HRs, it is often written as a "corrected" value (QTc), meaning the QT value was mathematically corrected to a HR of 60 beats/min. This allows comparison of the QTc interval across a range of HRs. The QTc interval is usually calculated by Bazett's formula, which divides the measured QT interval (in seconds) by the square root of the R-R cycle length.[51] It should be noted that Bazett's formula has been shown to overestimate QTc in patients with faster HRs. Alternative calculations include the Hodges, Framingham, and Fridericia, although there is no consensus on which is most accurate.[51] A QTc interval of greater than 0.47 second (470 ms) in women and greater than 0.45 seconds (450 ms) in men is considered prolonged.[51] A prolonged QTc interval is significant because it can predispose the patient to the development of polymorphic VT, known also as *torsades de pointes*.

A long QT interval can be congenital, as a result of genetic inheritance, or it can be acquired from an electrolyte imbalance or medications.[56,57] Many antidysrhythmic medications can prolong the QT interval, notably class Ia antidysrhythmics (quinidine, procainamide, disopyramide) and class III antidysrhythmics (amiodarone, dronedarone, ibutilide, dofetilide, sotalol). Not all QT-prolonging medications are antidysrhythmics. Other classes of medications known to cause QT prolongation include anesthetics, antibiotics, antidepressants, antiemetics, antipsychotics, opioids, and sedatives.

When medications associated with a high risk of QT prolongation are started, it is important to record the premedication baseline QTc interval and to regularly monitor and record the QTc interval during treatment. The risk of torsades de pointes is increased with prolongation of the QTc interval beyond 0.5 second (500 ms) or an increase of 60 ms compared with the baseline QTc interval.[58]

The risk of torsades de pointes is intensified with electrolyte abnormalities, including hypokalemia, hypomagnesemia, and hypocalcemia.[56] Risk increases in the presence of bradycardia, heart block with pauses, and premature ventricular beats with short-long-short cycles (Box 12.7).[56] Another risk factor may be genetics; 10% to 15% of patients with acquired long QT syndrome (medication induced) carry a genetic predisposition for the syndrome.[56]

Acute therapy is directed at increasing the HR, which shortens the QT interval, stopping culprit medications, and correcting electrolyte abnormalities. It may also include placement of a temporary pacemaker and administering IV magnesium, especially if serum levels of magnesium are low.

QRS Axis

Electrical impulses spread through cardiac muscle tissue in many directions at once when the ventricular muscle is depolarized. Using the 12-lead ECG, all these individual forces can be averaged to describe the overall direction that current is traveling, which is called the *mean vector*. This mean vector represents the general direction of the wave of depolarization within the heart. The mean vector can be plotted on a circular graph known as the *hexaxial reference system* (Fig. 12.43), and a degree value can be assigned to it. This degree represents the overall QRS axis.[53] The QRS axis helps determine whether the electrical current is moving in the expected direction. It can also verify correct lead placement and aides in differentiation of

BOX 12.7 Risk Factors for Torsades de Pointes

Prolonged QTc Interval
QTc interval ≥ 500 ms
Medications
Use of QT interval–prolonging medications
Rapid intravenous infusion of QT interval–prolonging medications
Diuretics
Structural Heart Conditions
Heart failure
Myocardial infarction
Metabolic Conditions
Hypokalemia
Hypomagnesemia
Hypocalcemia
Liver failure with decreased medication metabolism
Bradycardia
Sinus bradycardia
Complete heart block
Incomplete heart block with pauses
Premature complexes leading to short-long-short cycles
Genetic Predisposition
Occult (latent) congenital long-QT syndrome
Genetic polymorphisms (reduced repolarization reserve)
Age and Sex
Advanced age
Female sex

Torsades de pointes risk increases with a higher number of risk factors, some of which may be clinically silent and difficult to detect.

From Drew BJ, Ackerman MJ, Funk M, et al. Prevention of torsade de pointes in hospital settings: a scientific statement from the American Heart Association and the American College of Cardiology Foundation. *Circulation.* 2010;121(8):1047–1060. https://doi.org/10.1161/CIRCULATIONAHA.109.192704.

sources of arrhythmias, for example, VT versus wide complex tachycardia with aberrancy.

Parameters for normal QRS axis in degrees are −30 to +90 degrees.[53] Right-axis deviation is present if the heart's electrical axis falls between +90 and +180 degrees. Right-axis deviation can be further delineated as moderate right-axis deviation when it is between +90 and +120 degrees and marked right-axis deviation when it is between +120 and +180 degrees.[53]

Left-axis deviation is present if the axis falls between −30 and −90 degrees. Moderate left-axis deviation describes an axis between −30 and −45 degrees. Marked left-axis deviation describes an axis between −45 and −90 degrees.[53]

Fig. 12.43 shows how these points are located on the hexaxial reference system. If the axis plots in the upper left portion of the circle, also known as the *extreme quadrant* or *northwest quadrant*, it is called an *indeterminate axis*. This axis occurs rarely but can be seen when the wave of depolarization starts at the bottom of the ventricle, near the point of maximal impulse or apex of the ventricle, and spreads upward toward the atria. Clinically, this can be seen in beats of ventricular origin, such as PVCs and some pacemaker-initiated beats.

Calculating the QRS Axis

The QRS axis is calculated using the six limb leads (leads I, II, III, aVR, aVL, aVF) in the following three steps:

- Step 1. Find the limb lead with the smallest QRS complex, which is the one that is the most equiphasic (equal portions above and below the baseline). In Fig. 12.44, lead aVF is the equiphasic.
- Step 2. Using the hexaxial reference system (see Fig. 12.43), locate the lead that is perpendicular to the one that had the smallest complex. For example, perpendicular to lead aVF is lead I, so the mean vector lies parallel with lead I.
- Step 3. The third step is to determine whether the QRS complex is positive or negative in the lead parallel to the mean vector (in this case, lead I). If the QRS complex is positive, the mean vector is directed *toward* the positive electrode. If the QRS complex is negative, the mean vector is directed *away*

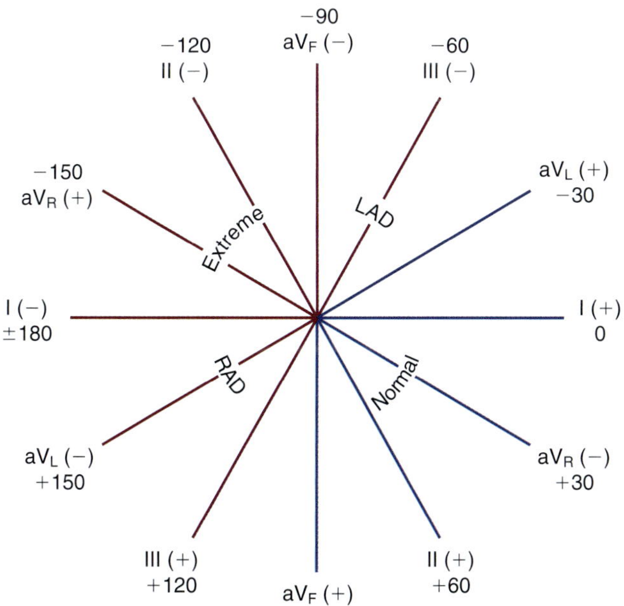

FIG. 12.43 Hexaxial Reference System. *LAD*, Left-axis deviation; *RAD*, right-axis deviation.

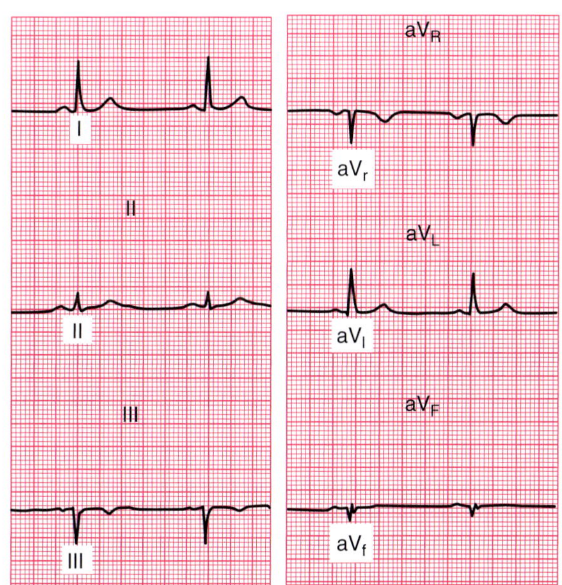

FIG. 12.44 Leads of Normal Electrocardiogram Illustrating Normal Axis of 0 Degrees.

BOX 12.8 Steps in Determining the Axis

1. Find the most isoelectric limb lead.
2. Using the hexaxial reference system, find the lead that is perpendicular to the lead identified in step 1.
3. Determine whether the QRS complex is positive or negative in the perpendicular lead.
4. Look at the corresponding positive or negative pole of the perpendicular lead on the hexaxial reference system.
5. The degree listed on the hexaxial reference system is the axis.

from the positive electrode. In Fig. 12.44, the QRS complex deflection in lead I is upright or positive. The positive pole of lead I is at the right midpoint of the hexaxial reference system and corresponds to a numeric degree of zero, which is within the normal range (Box 12.8; see Fig. 12.44).

Cardiac Monitor Lead Analysis

During continuous cardiac monitoring, adhesive, pre-gelled electrodes are used to obtain an ECG tracing that is similar to one or more leads of a 12-lead ECG. At minimum, this requires three electrodes. One of the electrodes acts as a positive pole, one acts as a negative pole, and one acts as a ground. In most critical care units, five electrodes are used. Five electrode systems allow the clinician to monitor six leads simultaneously and permit selection of typically two leads to display on the physiologic monitor. Typical placement of the five electrodes in a multilead system is RA, LA, LL, and RL, with one chest lead that usually is placed in the V_1 position, as illustrated in Fig. 12.45.

The choice of monitoring lead should take into consideration the patient's clinical condition and recent clinical history, as well as organizational standards and procedures.[51] If the patient has experienced ST segment elevation associated with acute coronary syndrome (ACS), percutaneous coronary intervention (PCI), or recent cardiac surgery, the leads that exhibited ST segment elevation should be used to guide selection of the optimal ECG monitoring leads.[51] The nurse verifies correct electrode placement and appropriate lead selection at the beginning of each shift. Daily replacement of electrodes is recommended to reduce artifact and erroneous alarms.[54] Skin prep should be conducted in the same manner as for standard 12-lead ECGs.

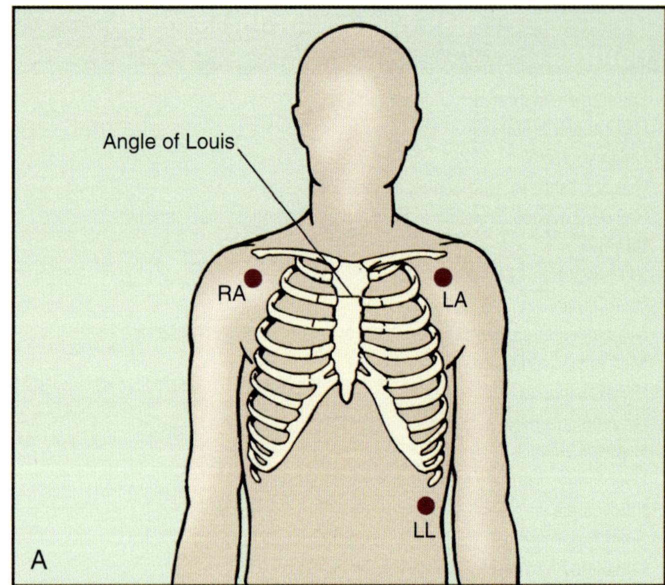

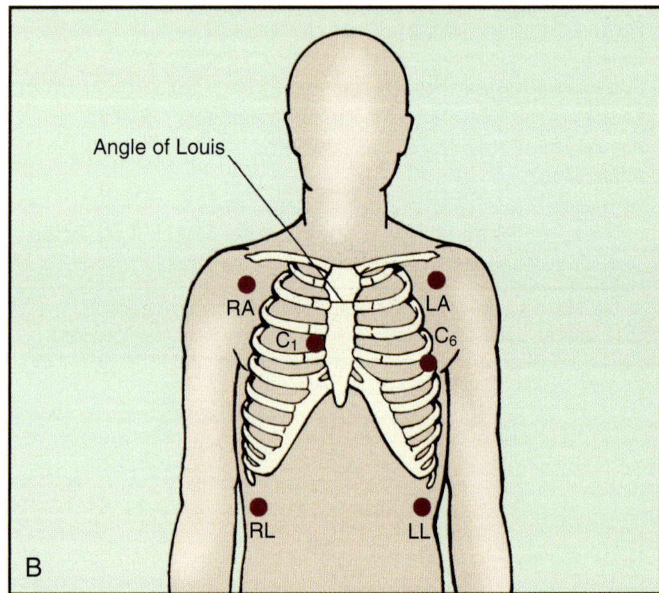

FIG. 12.45 (A) Three electrodes and lead-wire cables allow monitoring of three of the limb leads (I, II, and III). (B) In the multilead monitoring system, five electrodes and lead-wire cables allow monitoring of any of the six standard limb leads (I, II, III, aVR, aVL, or aVF) and any one precordial lead (V_1 or V_6). C_1 indicates the proper position of the chest electrode for monitoring lead V_1, and C_6 indicates the proper position of the chest electrode for monitoring V_6. Color-coded cable attachments allow quick identification and accurate electrode placement.

Lead II

On a standard 12-lead ECG, lead II is formed by a positive electrode attached to the left leg, a negative electrode attached to the right arm, and a ground electrode attached to the right leg. It is not practical to connect electrodes to the arms and legs during continuous monitoring, so the electrodes are placed on the torso near the origin of the limbs (see Fig. 12.45). If the monitored heart has a normal electrical axis, lead II displays a waveform that is predominantly upright, with a positive P wave and positive QRS complex waveform (Fig. 12.46). P waves are usually easy to identify in lead II, and this lead is recommended for monitoring of atrial dysrhythmias. However, it is difficult to identify RBBB and left bundle branch block (LBBB) in lead II because this is a vertical lead that does not clearly display horizontal interventricular conduction changes. Lead II is also nondiagnostic in differentiating VT from supraventricular tachycardia (SVT) with aberrant conduction. More information on differentiating VT from wide complex SVT is provided later in this chapter.

Lead V_1

The V_1 electrode is placed at the fourth intercostal space to the right of the sternal border. Most of the electrical activity of the heart is directed toward the left ventricle and away from the V_1 electrode. For this reason, the normal QRS complex in lead V_1 is mostly negative. Any abnormal electrical activity directed toward the right ventricle, such as in RBBB, results in an upright QRS complex, often in an RSR′ pattern.

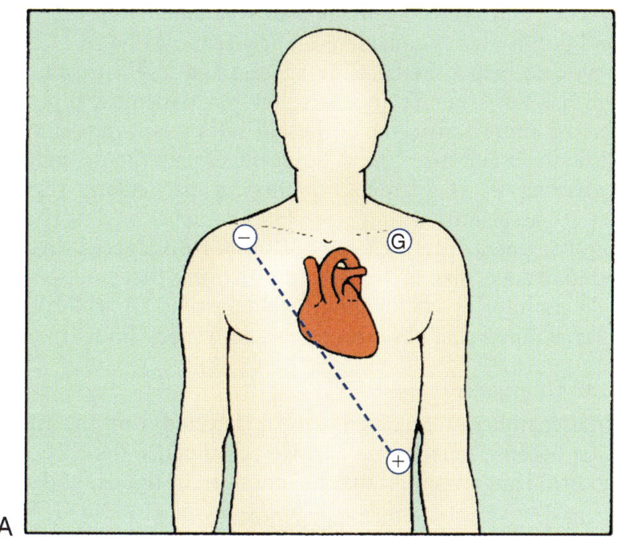

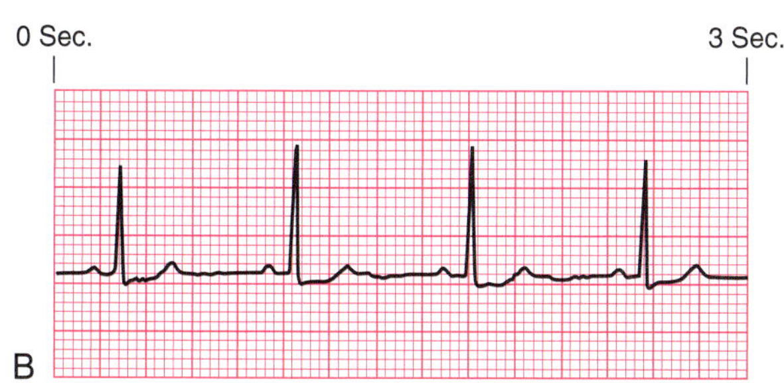

FIG. 12.46 Monitoring Lead II. (A) Electrode placement. The negative electrode is placed below the right shoulder; the positive electrode is placed on the lower left torso, preferably below the rib cage; and the ground electrode *(G)* is placed on the left shoulder. (B) Typical electrocardiogram tracing in lead II.

V_1 is the optimal lead to select if the critical care nurse needs to analyze ventricular ectopy. V_1 provides information to facilitate differentiation between a RBBB versus LBBB pattern, to distinguish between VT and SVT with aberrant conduction, to determine whether PVCs originate in the right or left ventricle, and to clarify when ST segment changes are caused by the RBBB and when they are the result of ischemia. More information on the criteria used to identify these rhythms using the V_1 lead is provided later.

Electrocardiogram Lead Selection for Optimal Bedside Monitoring

In the early years of critical care nursing, the primary goals of cardiac monitoring were HR surveillance, detection of "warning" ventricular dysrhythmias (mostly PVCs), and early detection of lethal dysrhythmias. Although these are still goals of ECG monitoring, advances in monitoring technology allow for surveillance of more complex conditions. For example, not all wide QRS complex tachycardias are ventricular in origin; they may be supraventricular with aberrant ventricular conduction. ST segment monitoring can recognize ischemia even in the absence of clinical symptoms. This is especially valuable for patients undergoing reperfusion therapy involving PCI, stent, or fibrinolysis. Diagnostic accuracy is diminished if limb electrodes are moved too close to the heart.

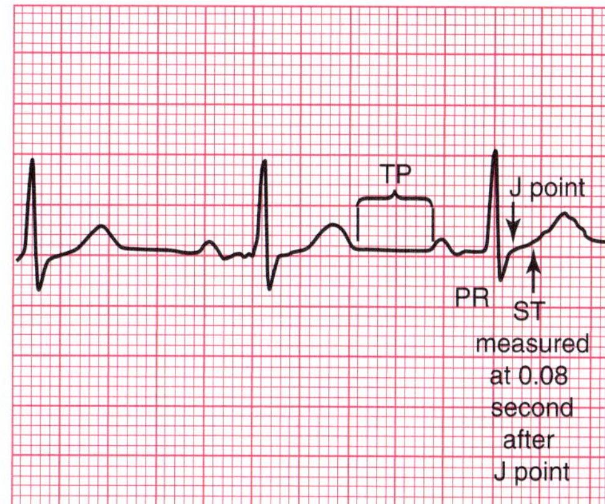

FIG. 12.47 The TP segment is used as the reference point for the isoelectric line if the heart rate is slow enough for the TP segment to be clearly seen. If not, the PR interval can be used.

Continuous Dysrhythmia Monitoring

Patients with serious cardiac diseases such as acute MI, heart failure, and cardiomyopathy are at risk for the development of BBBs, complex ectopy, and wide complex tachycardias. These patients need to be monitored with lead V_1 because it documents interventricular conduction changes. The six frontal plane (limb and augmented lead) tracings also offer several monitoring choices that can be individualized to the clinical needs of the patient. Leads I and aVF are selected to detect a sudden change in ventricular axis. If ST segment monitoring is required, the lead is selected according to the area of ischemia. If the ischemic area is known, leads V_3 and III are recommended to detect ST segment ischemia.[54] In inferior wall injury, leads II, III, and aVF are chosen; if lateral ischemia is present, lead I or aVL should be selected.

Continuous ST Segment Monitoring

A key responsibility of the critical care nurse is monitoring for myocardial ischemia via ECG ST segment changes.[54] Continuous ST segment monitoring is increasingly available via bedside physiologic monitors. Bedside monitoring systems incorporate ST segment analysis software to detect myocardial ischemia or injury. ST segment changes may be accompanied by classic symptoms such as chest pain, or they may be "silent," without any clinical symptoms except ST segment depression or elevation seen on the ECG monitor.[59] Risk of progression from silent ischemia to overt cardiac events has been documented in patients with diabetes mellitus.[60]

The best way to choose a lead for monitoring the ST segment to detect ischemia is to look at the patient's 12-lead ECG during an episode of ischemia, if available. Under normal (nonischemic) conditions, the ST segment is at the same level as the TP segment (segment of the isoelectric line that begins at the end of the T wave to the start of the next P wave),[55] also known as the *isoelectric line* (Fig. 12.47). The standard 12-lead ECG obtained during an episode of chest pain or during a PCI will demonstrate the leads with greatest ST segment deviation from the isoelectric line.[51]

Patients at risk for *silent ischemia* include patients experiencing an ACS even if treated with fibrinolytics, nitrates, or anticoagulation therapy.[59] Patients undergoing a PCI are at risk for coronary artery repeat occlusion or spasm, reflected by ST segment changes similar to those seen during PCI balloon inflation.

Any patient with a history of prior MI, angina, diabetes, or kidney failure is a candidate for ST segment monitoring.[51]

ST segment deviation can have nonischemic causes and can create a false-positive alarm. Common culprits include hyperkalemia, pericarditis, hypokalemia, hypomagnesemia, hypothermia, ventricular aneurysm, hypothyroidism, pulmonary infarction, BBB (right or left), and medications such as quinidine and digitalis. Patients with subarachnoid hemorrhage often demonstrate ST segment changes believed to be caused by excess release of norepinephrine from the myocardial sympathetic nerves. The degree of myocardial necrosis and ST segment elevation depends on the severity of neurologic injury.[61]

ST segment deviation is measured as the number of millimeters of ST segment vertical displacement from the isoelectric line or from the patient's baseline. Because ST segments may slope or arc, the best measurement position is 60 milliseconds (ms) to the right of the J point (Fig. 12.48).[54] The J point is chosen to avoid monitoring the upstroke of the T wave. On the bedside monitor, ST segment elevation is displayed as a positive number, whereas ST segment depression is indicated as a negative number (see Fig. 12.48). To be clinically significant, the J point of the ST segment must be displaced up or down from the isoelectric baseline by at least 1 or 2 mm (one or two small boxes on ECG paper) on the ECG lead being monitored.[62]

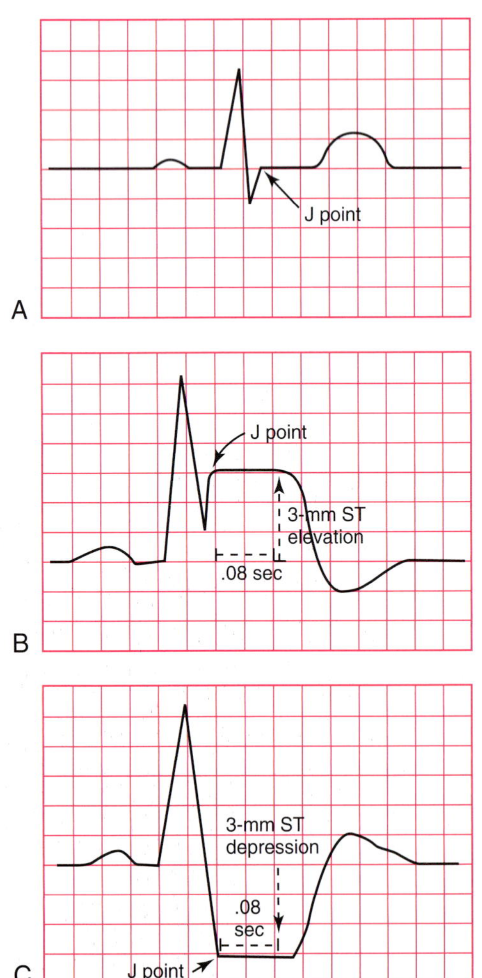

FIG. 12.48 (A) Normal position of J point. (B) A 3-mm ST segment elevation. (C) A 3-mm ST segment depression. ST segment changes are measured 60 to 80 ms (0.06 to 0.08 s) after the J point.

When setting ST segment alarm parameters, the patient's condition is always considered. The alarm may be set at 1 mm above and below the baseline ST segment level in patients at high risk for ischemia. In stable, low-risk patients and patients who are more active, the suggested setting is 2 mm above or below the isoelectric line.[51] Some ECG patterns do not lend themselves to ST segment monitoring, particularly rhythms that are associated with a wide QRS complex or distortion of the ST segment. This includes LBBB and RBBB, paced rhythms, and idioventricular rhythms. Other rhythms that make ST segment monitoring challenging include erratic atrial fibrillation or atrial flutter that obscures the isoelectric baseline.[51]

Atrial Enlargement

Atrial chamber enlargement can be detected from the 12-lead ECG, because muscle size and shape influence the ECG tracing. Atrial abnormalities may be identified by the size and shape of the P waves and are usually most obvious in lead II. Wide, m-shaped P waves are classically seen in left atrial enlargement (Fig. 12.49A). Tall, peaked P waves are seen with right atrial enlargement (Fig. 12.49B). However, current ECG guidelines emphasize that P wave abnormalities can be caused by many conditions and can occur without atrial enlargement. For this reason, the ECG is not considered definitive in the identification of atrial hypertrophy.[63] The less specific term *atrial abnormality* is suggested for P wave abnormalities when the underlying pathology is unknown.[63]

Ventricular Hypertrophy

Ventricular hypertrophy describes an increase in the size and muscle mass of one or both ventricles. Because a larger muscle is being depolarized, a greater amount of electrical activity is recorded on the ECG during depolarization. In ventricular hypertrophy, the increased muscle mass results in increased QRS complex voltages, particularly in the precordial leads. Upright QRS complexes become taller, and negative QRS complexes become even more negative. The QRS complex often

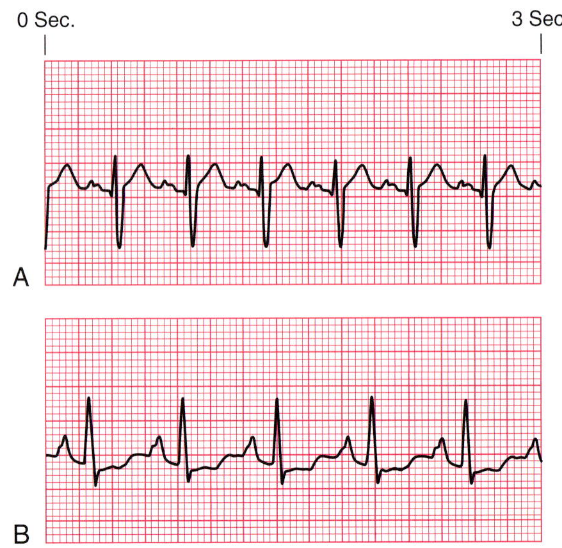

FIG. 12.49 Atrial Hypertrophy. (A) In left atrial hypertrophy, the P wave is broad and notched and is sometimes called *P mitrale*, because it is often associated with mitral valve disease. (B) In right atrial hypertrophy, the P wave is tall and peaked and is sometimes called *P pulmonale*, because it is often associated with pulmonary disease.

becomes slightly wider because it takes longer to depolarize a larger muscle. The QRS complex axis often shifts toward the enlarged ventricle because a greater portion of the total electrical activity of the heart occurs there. Although the 12-lead ECG can suggest hypertrophy, the echocardiogram is the most reliable diagnostic device, because it can visualize ventricular wall thickness and motion.[63]

Myocardial Ischemia and Infarction

Ischemia occurs when the delivery of oxygen to the tissues is insufficient to meet metabolic demand. Cardiac ischemia, or angina, can be considered stable or unstable. Cardiac ischemia in an unstable form occurs because of a sudden decrease in supply, such as when the artery is blocked by a thrombus or when coronary artery spasm occurs.[64,65] Stable angina can occur when a stenotic coronary artery is unable to adapt to a sudden increase in demand created by exercise. Ischemia is by nature a transient process; when the balance of supply versus demand is restored, the cardiac muscle tissue recovers. Conversely, when the imbalance in myocardial oxygen demand and delivery becomes so great that the tissues can no longer survive, myocardial cells infarct and become necrotic.

Infarction refers to the death and disintegration of muscle cells and their eventual replacement by fibrotic scar tissue. After infarction has occurred, the process cannot be reversed. Thus, careful ECG monitoring and swift intervention to restore myocardial perfusion before infarction can take place is critically important.

Electrocardiogram Changes Indicating Ischemia and Infarction

Ischemia and infarction cause changes in the way cardiac muscle cells respond to electrical stimuli. These changes are best seen in a 12-lead ECG tracing since multiple myocardial areas are examined.

ST segment elevation is seen when the positive electrode lies directly over an area of transmural (full-wall thickness) injury (Fig. 12.50A). The ST segment changes on the surface ECG are caused by differences in voltage gradients between ischemic and healthy myocardium, referred to as *injury currents*.[62] This represents a preinfarction state, and interventions to unblock the occluded coronary artery must be initiated to prevent death of myocardium. ST segment elevation is a precursor to an ST elevation myocardial infarction (STEMI).[65] STEMI is discussed in further detail in Chapter 13.

Not every myocardial infarction is heralded by ST segment elevation. When the patient has an MI without ST segment elevation, it is described as a non–ST elevation myocardial infarction (NSTEMI). The diagnosis can be considerably more challenging without the signature ST segment changes seen on the ECG.[64] For further information on NSTEMI, refer to Chapter 13.

ST segment depression occurs when the reduction of blood flow is limited to the endocardium and some normal muscle tissue remains between the ischemic area and the positive electrode (Fig. 12.50B). ST segment depression is seen because the positive electrode on the body surface is separated from the ischemic area (endocardium) by normal tissue. T waves most commonly flatten or become inverted.

Infarction involves necrosis (death) of muscle cells with eventual formation of scar tissue. These cells can no longer be depolarized when an impulse reaches them. If the infarction involves the epicardial (outer) layer of the heart muscle or the entire thickness of the heart wall (transmural lesion), the QRS complex changes. Abnormal Q waves often develop in the leads overlying the infarcted area; however, not all patients will develop Q waves. Occasionally, the entire QRS complex becomes smaller without development of Q waves. Non–Q wave infarctions may be diagnosed based on symptomatic clinical presentation and/or biomarkers and cardiac catheterization. STEMI is typically associated with a Q wave infarction. Conversely, NSTEMI is more likely to result in a non–Q wave infarction (see Fig. 13.12 in Chapter 13).

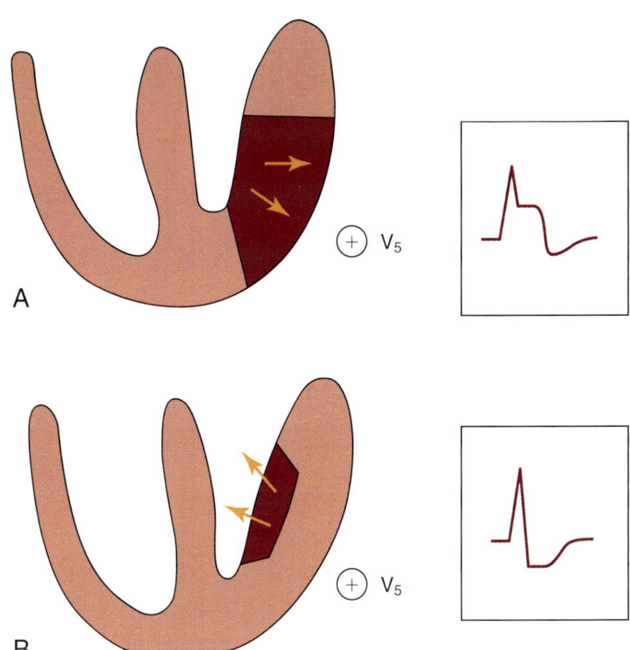

FIG. 12.50 (A) Acute transmural ischemia. The electrical forces *(arrows)* responsible for the ST segment are directed outward through the entire thickness of the heart muscle wall, causing ST segment elevation in leads directly over the ischemic area. (B) Acute subendocardial ischemia. The electrical forces responsible for the ST segment are deviated toward the inner layer of the heart, resulting in ST segment depression in leads directly over that area of the heart muscle wall.

Infarct Location by 12-Lead Electrocardiogram

The location of the infarction can be roughly determined by noting the specific leads in which the ST segment and T wave changes are seen on the 12-lead ECG. Table 12.8 summarizes the anticipated 12-lead ECG changes. Chapter 13 provides a more in-depth discussion of ECG changes with myocardial infarction.

Right ventricular infarction and posterior wall infarction are particularly difficult to identify on a standard 12-lead ECG, because none of the standard leads directly view these areas. A right ventricular infarction may be suspected and investigated in the setting of an acute inferior wall MI.[66] To avoid missing this diagnosis, right-sided precordial leads (see Fig. 12.36C) can be placed, and a 12-lead ECG can be obtained for any patient with a suspected inferior right ventricular wall MI. Early identification of right ventricular infarction is important, because it requires special management and carries a greater in-hospital mortality risk.[66] Nitrates and other vasodilatory agents, commonly administered in acute infarction of the left ventricle, can cause profound hypotension with negative effect on preload and CO when the infarcted area is in the right ventricle.[67]

TABLE 12.8 Electrocardiogram Changes During Myocardial Infarction

Location of Infarction	Artery Involved	Leads Involved	ECG Changes
Anterior wall	LAD	V_3–V_4	Q waves, ST↑,T↓
Inferior wall	RCA or LCx	II, III, aVF	Q waves, ST↑,T↓
Ventricular septum	LAD	V_1–V_2	Q waves, ST↑,T↓
Lateral wall	LCx	V_5–V_6, I, aVL	Q waves, ST↑,T↓
Posterior wall	RCA or LCx	V_1–V_3 (anterior[a]); V_7–V_9 (posterior[b])	Tall, upright R; ST↓; upright T with ST↑ V_7–V_9
Right ventricle	Proximal RCA	V_4R (right[c])	ST ↑

[a]See Fig. 12.36B for ECG lead placement.
[b]See Fig. 12.36D for ECG lead placement.
[c]See Fig. 12.36C for ECG lead placement.
LAD, Left anterior descending; *LCx*, left circumflex; *RCA*, right coronary artery.

A posterior wall infarction may be suspected in a patient with an occluded right coronary artery (posterior descending branch) or the left circumflex coronary artery when there is ST segment depression in leads V_1, V_2, and V_3 on the standard 12-lead ECG. Tall, upright R waves may also be present. Posterior wall involvement can be verified by adding posterior precordial leads V_7, V_8, and V_9 (see Fig. 12.36D), although this is uncommon, mainly because the posterior leads have low voltage, making changes difficult to see ST segment changes.

Infarction Progression on Electrocardiogram

When blood flow in a coronary artery is suddenly occluded, the entire area of heart muscle normally perfused by that artery becomes ischemic. Collateral arterioles usually exist that overlap and supply the perimeter of this area and may prevent necrosis of some of the affected tissue. At the center of the ischemic area, collateral blood flow is minimal or does not exist at all. Within a few hours, this tissue begins to die. On the ECG tracing, this process is illustrated as follows: Within minutes of the onset of infarction, ST segment elevation occurs in the leads directly overlying the affected heart wall. This ST segment elevation persists for a period of hours to 1 day, gradually becoming less severe. Within the first few hours, T waves may become tall and symmetric. They are known as *hyperacute T waves*, and they indicate acute ischemia. Meanwhile, usually within 4 to 24 hours from the onset of the infarction, abnormal Q waves begin to develop in the affected leads, and T waves begin to invert. Sometimes, instead of Q waves developing, the R waves become smaller. This still indicates necrosis of muscle tissue. The ST segments become isoelectric again in a few days, and the T wave becomes symmetric and deeply inverted in the affected leads. The T waves usually return to normal within several days. The Q waves may persist for the remainder of the patient's life, or they may get smaller over time and disappear altogether in some individuals. Table 12.9 summarizes the timing of these changes.

Intraventricular Conduction Defects

Intraventricular conduction defects are the result of an abnormal pathway of conduction through the ventricles. Normally, conduction to the ventricles spreads rapidly from the AV node to the bundle of His and down the right and left bundle branches. The right bundle branch is long and thin and terminates in a mass of Purkinje fibers, which spread the wave of depolarization into surrounding right ventricular muscle. After only a short distance, the left bundle branch divides into the left anterior fascicle, the left posterior fascicle, and many people have an additional left septal fascicle near the septum (Fig. 12.51). The terms *fascicle* and *bundle* are often used interchangeably when describing the anatomy of the conduction system. Each of these fascicles causes depolarization of separate areas of the left ventricle. If any part of the conduction system fails, the muscle cells in that area still depolarize, but not as quickly. Depolarization must then spread from cell to cell, a slower process than activation through specialized conduction pathways.

On the ECG, intraventricular conduction defects cause a widening of the QRS complex because of the slower spread of depolarization. The affected muscle tissue begins the slower cell-to-cell depolarization just as the other areas in the ventricle are almost finished. This later depolarization is then tacked onto the end of the normal QRS complex, making it prolonged and altering its shape.

Any part of the conduction system can be affected. The term *bundle branch block* refers to complete interruption of conduction through the right bundle or the entire left bundle branch.

TABLE 12.9 Timing of Electrocardiogram Changes With Ischemia/Infarction

Time Frame	Electrocardiogram Change
Immediate	ST segment elevation in leads over area of infarction
Within a few hours	Giant, upright T waves
Several hours	ST segment normalizes; T waves invert symmetrically
Several hours to days	Q waves or reduced R waves; voltage may remain low permanently

Right and Left Bundle Branch Blocks

The chest leads are the most useful in identifying complete RBBB and LBBB. V_1 and V_6 are the best leads from which to identify forces traveling in a horizontal direction, because they are located on the right and left sides of the heart, respectively. Fig. 12.52A shows the normal sequence of ventricular activation and the usual shape of the QRS complex in V_1 and V_6.

Recognition of BBBs can be done at the bedside if the patient is being monitored with leads V_1 and V_6. However, definitive diagnosis of BBB should be made via a 12-lead ECG. In sinus rhythm, a BBB exists when the P wave is followed by a QRS complex that is wider than 0.12 second (120 ms) with other features of the block.[53] The presence of the P wave indicates that the QRS complex did not originate from the ventricles. Patients with atrial fibrillation can also have a BBB but a discernable P wave will not be present. Examining a prior 12-lead ECG can be helpful to determine if atrial fibrillation is the underlying rhythm or evaluation of the medical record for documentation of a prior history. One quick method to determine which bundle branch is blocked is to look at the last part of the QRS complex just before it returns to the baseline in leads V_1 and V_6. If upright in V_1 and negative in V_6, a RBBB exists. If negative in V_1 and upright in V_6, a LBBB is present.

Right Bundle Branch Block

In complete RBBB, the QRS complex is wider than 0.12 second (120 ms) (Fig. 12.52B). This is because the right ventricle is not activated through the normal rapid conduction system. Instead, it must be activated slowly, from one cell to the next. Electrical

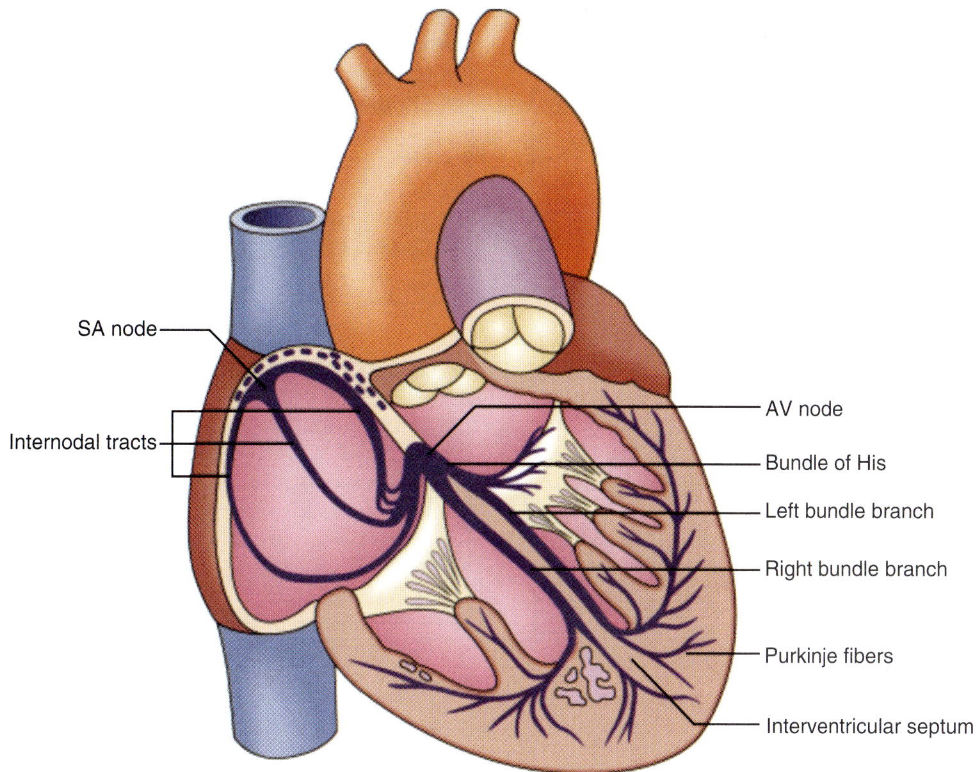

FIG. 12.51 Cardiac Conduction System. *AV*, Atrioventricular; *SA*, sinoatrial. (From Nash J, Court DS, eds. *Medical Sciences*. 3rd ed. Elsevier; 2019.)

forces that are not counterbalanced by opposing forces from the left side of the heart travel toward the right at the end of the ventricular activation. The septum is depolarized first in a normal manner from left to right. Next, the wave of depolarization spreads through the left ventricle and is recorded in lead V_1 as a tiny negative deflection. The final portion of the QRS complex is wide and upright, indicating final electrical forces traveling toward the right. This represents right ventricular depolarization that occurs after LV depolarization is almost complete. In V_1, this QRS complex represents a classic pattern that is labeled rsR′ in V_1.[53] The ST segment, representing repolarization, is also abnormal and makes recognition of ST segment changes related to ischemia difficult to detect by ECG monitoring. The presence of a RBBB is associated with a higher risk of cardiac events.[68]

In lead V_6 the positive electrode is on the left side of the chest, and the waveforms are reversed. The final forces of the QRS complex are negative because they are traveling toward the right and away from the positive electrode of V_6. The final negative deflection in V_6 is smaller than the final upright deflection in lead V_1, because the positive electrode in V_6 is at a greater distance from the right ventricle.

Left Bundle Branch Block

In complete LBBB (Fig. 12.52C), the conduction through the left ventricle must spread from cell to cell, which results in a prolonged QRS complex duration, longer than 0.12 second (120 ms).[53] Because a portion of the common left bundle normally initiates depolarization of the septum, the septum is depolarized in an abnormal direction, from right to left. In lead V_1, this is recorded as an initial negative deflection. Next, the right ventricle is depolarized, which is identified as a small upright notch in the QRS complex as the forces travel briefly toward the positive electrode of V_1. Sometimes this notch is absent in patients with a prior septal wall MI. The final forces travel toward the left as the left ventricle is being depolarized. The left ventricle is a very large muscle mass, and these final electrical forces are large and wide. In lead V_1, the final deflection is a deep, negative deflection (S wave), whereas in lead V_6 these final forces inscribe a tall, upright deflection (R wave).

The presence of an LBBB makes diagnosis of an acute anterior wall MI extremely difficult, because the change in repolarization masks ST segment elevation. Perhaps related to this difficulty in interpreting injury, patients with ACS in the presence of LBBB have double the in-hospital mortality risk compared with patients with ACS without LBBB.[69]

Hemiblocks

Hemiblocks involve conduction failure of only part of the left bundle branch. In left anterior fascicular block, also called *left anterior hemiblock*, LV depolarization begins in the left posterior fascicle and spreads anteriorly through Purkinje fibers distal to the block. The QRS complex is of normal duration, meaning it is less than 0.12 second. However, the frontal plane axis changes dramatically and becomes more negative than −30 degrees, indicating left-axis deviation (axis between −45 degrees and −90 degrees) (Boxes 12.9 and 12.10).[53,70]

Left posterior fascicular block is also a hemiblock and is also known by the term *left posterior hemiblock*. The QRS complex duration is within normal limits (less than 0.12 second).[53] The block in the posterior fascicle changes the normal conduction pathway so that the anterior portion of the left ventricle is depolarized first. Conduction spreads slowly to the right, inferiorly and posteriorly. The axis then swings entirely in the other direction and becomes greater than +90 degrees, indicating right-axis deviation (axis between 90 degrees and 180 degrees).[53] Isolated posterior hemiblock is rare, and it is

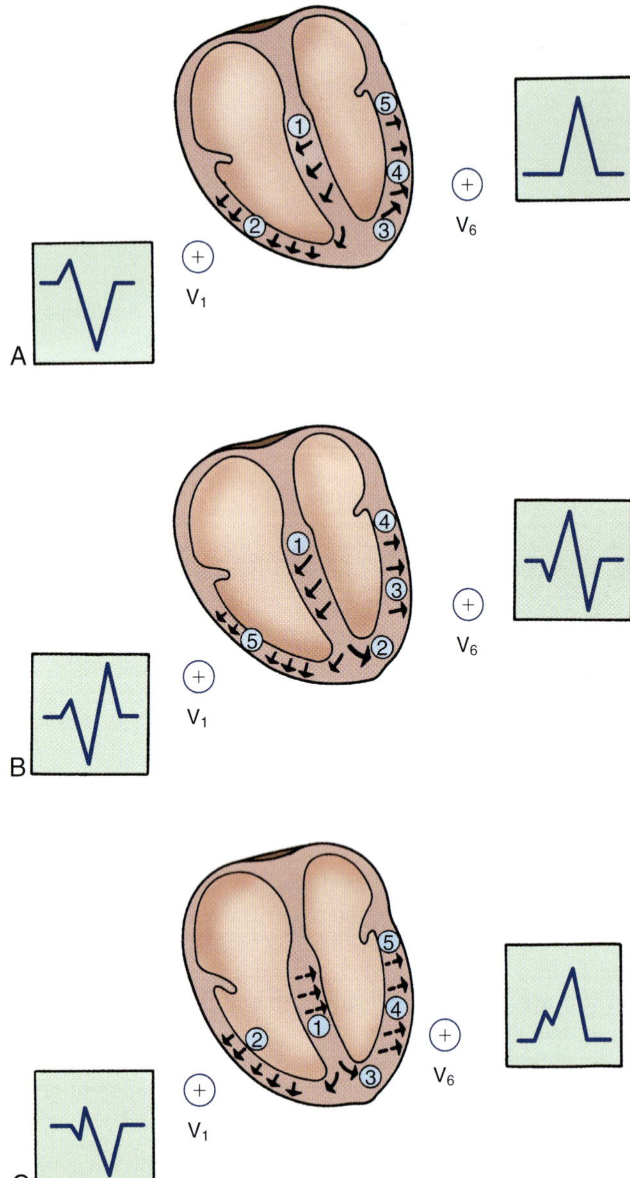

FIG. 12.52 (A) Sequence of ventricular depolarization and resulting QRS complex, as seen in leads V_1 and V_6. (B) Sequence of ventricular depolarization for a right bundle branch block and resulting QRS complex, as seen in leads V_1 and V_6. (C) Sequence of ventricular depolarization for a left bundle branch block and resulting QRS complex, as seen in leads V_1 and V_6.

almost always associated with concomitant RBBB[70] (see Box 12.10).

Bifascicular Block

Blockage of either of the two branches of the LV conduction system plus RBBB constitutes a bifascicular block. Any combination of these conduction disturbances can occur and can evolve into complete heart block. Normally, bifascicular block (hemiblock plus RBBB) is well tolerated, and no intervention is necessary. The exception is bifascicular block that develops during an acute MI. An evolving infarct with bifascicular block may warrant placement of a temporary pacemaker because conduction tissue ischemia may progress to complete heart block.

BOX 12.9 Causes of Left-Axis Deviation

- Normal variation
- Mechanical shifts: exhalation; high diaphragm caused by pregnancy, ascites, or abdominal tumor
- Left anterior hemiblock
- Left ventricular hypertrophy
- Wolff-Parkinson-White syndrome
- Hyperkalemia
- Cardiomyopathy

BOX 12.10 Causes of Right-Axis Deviation

- Normal variation
- Mechanical shifts: inhalation, emphysema
- Left posterior hemiblock
- Right ventricular hypertrophy
- Lateral wall myocardial infarction
- Right bundle branch block
- Dextrocardia

Dysrhythmia Interpretation

In clinical practice, the terms *dysrhythmia* and *arrhythmia* often are used interchangeably. Which is more accurate is a common debate. Both terms are correct, and either may be used in practice. In this textbook, dysrhythmia is the more commonly used term. A dysrhythmia is any disturbance in the normal cardiac conduction pathway. Dysrhythmias can be detected on a 12-lead ECG, but they often occur only sporadically. For this reason, patients in a critical care unit are monitored continuously using a five-lead ECG system, and rhythm strips are routinely recorded per organization standards. Dysrhythmias occur frequently in cardiac and noncardiac critically ill patients. A systematic approach to assess a rhythm disturbance is an indispensable skill. Steps to accurately interpret a rhythm strip are introduced first, followed by specific criteria to evaluate common dysrhythmias encountered in clinical practice.

Heart Rate Determination

The first thing to assess when evaluating a rhythm strip is the ventricular rate. Regardless of the dysrhythmia involved, the ventricular rate and blood pressure are key to whether a patient can tolerate the dysrhythmia (i.e., maintain CO and mentation). Once the patient can no longer tolerate the dysrhythmia, often a ventricular rate greater than 200 or less than 30, emergency measures must be started to correct the condition. A detailed analysis of the underlying rhythm disturbance can proceed later once the patient's clinical condition has stabilized.

ECG paper is usually marked at the top in 3-second increments, making it easy to manually calculate a heart rate (Fig. 12.53A) as follows:

- Number of R-R intervals in 6 seconds times 10 (between two 3-second markers)
- Number of large boxes between QRS complexes divided into 300
- Number of small boxes between QRS complexes divided into 1500

In a healthy heart, the atrial rate and the ventricular rate are the same. However, in many dysrhythmias, the atrial and ventricular rates are different, and both must be calculated. To find

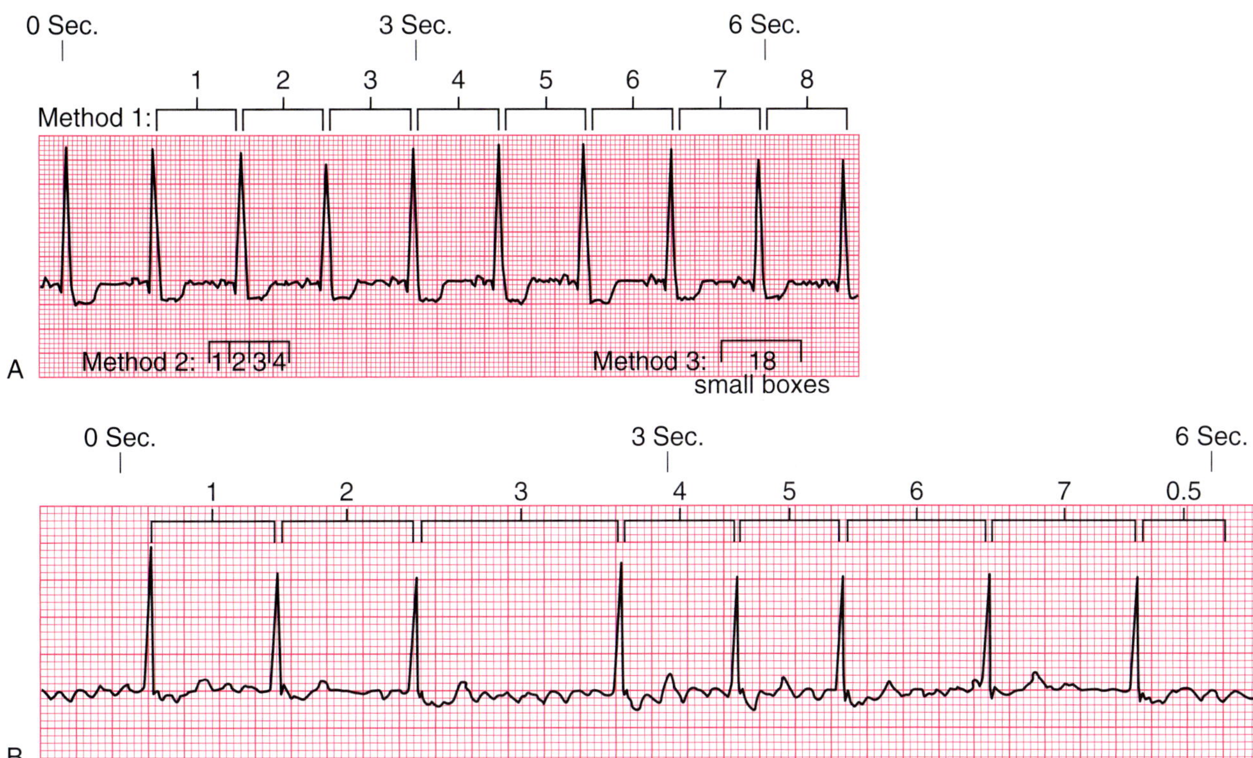

FIG. 12.53 (A) Calculation of heart rate if the rhythm is regular. Method 1: Number of R-R intervals in 6 s multiplied by 10 (e.g., 8 × 10 = 80/min). Method 2: Number of large boxes between QRS complexes divided into 300 (e.g., 300 ÷ 4 = 75/min). Method 3: Number of small boxes between QRS complexes divided into 1500 (e.g., 1500 ÷ 18 = 84/min). (B) Rate calculation if the rhythm is irregular. Only method 1 can be used (e.g., 7.5 intervals × 10 = 75/min).

the atrial rate, the P-P interval, instead of the R-R interval, is used in one of the three methods listed for determining rate.

The choice of method for calculating the HR depends on the regularity of the rhythm. If the rhythm is irregular, the first method (R-R intervals in 6 seconds times 10) is the only method that can be used (Fig. 12.53B). If the rhythm is regular, any method can be used.

Rhythm Determination

The term *rhythm* refers to the regularity with which the P waves or R waves occur. Calipers assist in determining rhythm. One point of the calipers is placed on the beginning of one R wave, and the other point is placed on the next R wave. Leaving the calipers “set” at this interval, each succeeding R-R interval is checked to be sure it is the same width as the first one measured.

In describing the rhythm, three terms are used. If the rhythm is *regular*, the R-R intervals are the same, within 10%. If the rhythm is *regularly irregular*, the R-R intervals are not the same, but some sort of pattern is involved, which could be grouping, rhythmic speeding up and slowing down, or any other consistent pattern (Fig. 12.54). If the rhythm is *irregularly irregular*, the R-R intervals are not the same, and no pattern can be found.

P Wave Evaluation

The P wave is analyzed by considering whether the P wave is present or absent. If present, is each P wave associated with a QRS complex? It is expected that one P wave will be in front of every QRS. Sometimes, two, three, or four P waves may be in front of every QRS complex. If this pattern is consistent, the P waves and QRS are still associated, although not on a 1:1 basis.

PR Interval Evaluation

The duration of the PR interval, which normally is 0.12 to 0.20 seconds (120 to 200 ms), is measured first. This is measured from the start of a visible P wave to the beginning of the next QRS complex (Fig. 12.55). All PR intervals on the strip are verified to be sure they have the same duration as the original interval.

QRS Complex Evaluation

The entire ECG strip must be evaluated to ascertain that the QRS complexes are consistently the same shape and width. The normal QRS complex duration is 0.06 to 0.10 second (60 to 110 ms). Any QRS longer than 0.10 second is considered abnormal. If more than one QRS shape is visible on the strip, each QRS complex must be measured. The QRS complex is measured from where it leaves the baseline to where it returns to the baseline (see Fig. 12.55).

QT Interval Evaluation

The length of the QT interval varies with the HR. The QT interval is shorter when the HR is faster. A QT interval corrected for HR (QTc interval) that is longer than 0.50 second (500 ms) is of concern, as discussed earlier in the section on QT interval.

Sinus Rhythms

The cardiac cycle begins when an impulse originates in the sinus node. The wave of depolarization spreading through the atria results in a P wave on the ECG. The impulse is delayed briefly in the AV node, which corresponds to the PR interval on the ECG. After leaving the AV node, the wave of depolarization spreads

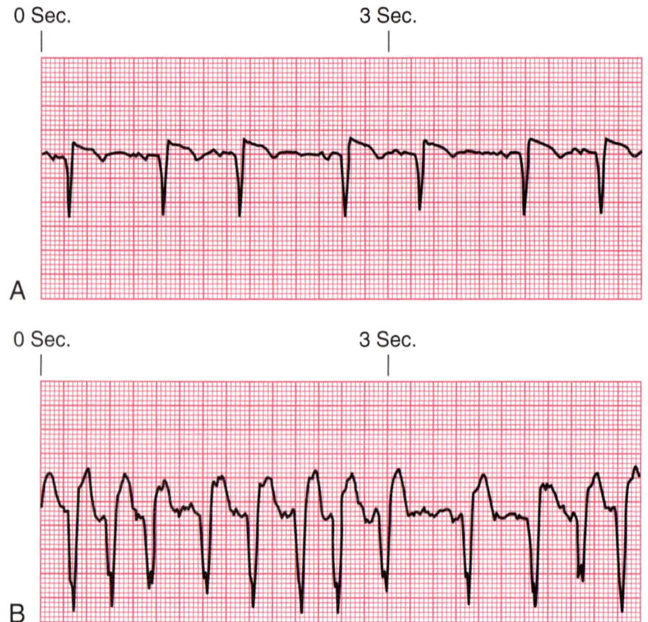

FIG. 12.54 (A) This regularly irregular rhythm is irregular but has a consistent pattern in that every other beat is premature. (B) This irregularly irregular rhythm is irregular with no consistent pattern.

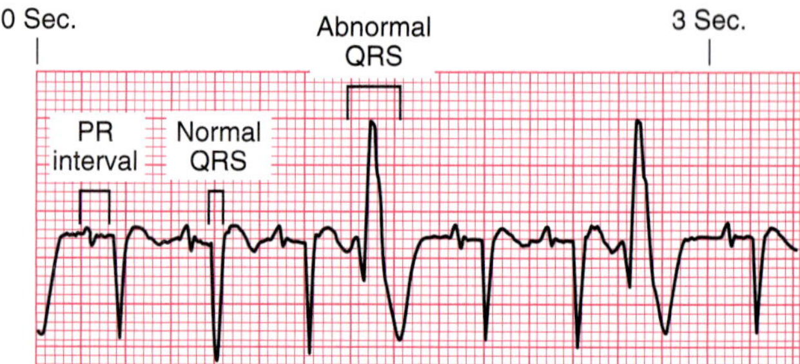

FIG. 12.55 PR Interval Measurement, From the Beginning of the P Wave to the Beginning of the QRS Complex. The PR interval on this tracing is 0.20 s; the QRS complex duration illustrates normal and abnormal intervals. The narrow QRS complexes measure 0.08 s, which is normal. The wide QRS complexes measure 0.20 s and are caused by ventricular ectopy.

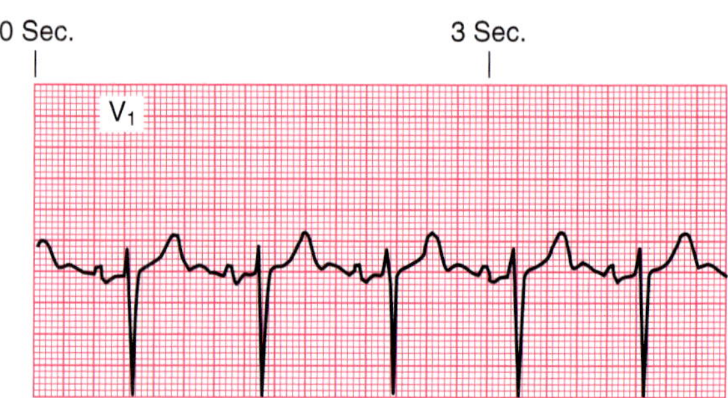

FIG. 12.56 Normal Sinus Rhythm. The rate is 70, and the rhythm is regular. One P wave is present before each QRS complex. The PR interval is 0.18 s and does not vary throughout the strip. The QRS complex duration is 0.08 s. All evaluation criteria are within normal limits.

rapidly through the bundle of His and the bundle branches and causes ventricular depolarization, which is recorded as a QRS complex by the ECG. Contraction immediately follows depolarization. Contraction is terminated by repolarization, which is demonstrated as a T wave on the ECG.

Normal Sinus Rhythm

If all the events described for sinus rhythms occur in their normal sequence with normal rates and intervals, the patient is in normal sinus rhythm. The criteria for normal sinus rhythm are as follows:

Rate: The intrinsic rate of the sinus node is 60 to 100 beats/min. External factors such as medications, fever, or exercise can affect the intrinsic rate.

Rhythm: The rhythm must be regular, within 10%.

P wave: P waves must be present, and only one must precede every QRS complex.

PR interval: The PR interval represents the expected delay in the AV node. In normal sinus rhythm, the PR interval is 0.12 to 0.20 second.

QRS complex: All QRS complexes must look alike. However, QRS complex size and shape may vary in sinus rhythms and often depend on lead placement and gain adjustments on the monitor. If conduction through the ventricles is normal, the QRS complex duration is 0.06 to 0.10 second. Fig. 12.56 is an example of normal sinus rhythm in V_1.

Sinus Bradycardia

Sinus bradycardia meets all the criteria for normal sinus rhythm except that the rate is less than 60 beats/min (Table 12.10). It is normally seen in well-trained athletes at rest or in other individuals during sleep. Other conditions in which sinus bradycardia occurs include vagal stimulation, increased intracranial pressure, medication therapy with digoxin or beta-blockers, and ischemia of the sinus node caused by an acute MI. Sinus bradycardia usually is not treated unless the patient displays symptoms of hypoperfusion, such as hypotension, dizziness, chest pain, or changes in level of consciousness.

Sinus Tachycardia

Sinus tachycardia meets all the criteria for normal sinus rhythm except that the rate is greater than 100 beats/min (see Table 12.10). Rates may be 180 to 200 beats/min in healthy young adults during strenuous exercise. However, in the absence of exercise, any sinus tachycardia with a rate greater than 150 beats/min should lead to a search for a triggering focus other than the sinus node. For example, atrial flutter waves may be difficult to see at first glance because of baseline distortion caused by the high ventricular rate (Fig. 12.57).

Sinus tachycardia can be caused by a wide variety of factors, such as medications with a beta-agonist effect, exercise, emotion, pain, fever, hemorrhage, shock, heart failure, and thyrotoxicosis.[71] Illegal stimulant drugs such as cocaine, MDMA (Ecstasy/molly), and amphetamines can raise the resting HR significantly. Tachycardia is detrimental to anyone with ischemic heart disease because it decreases the time for ventricular filling, decreases SV, and compromises CO. Tachycardia increases heart work and myocardial oxygen demand, while decreasing oxygen supply by decreasing coronary artery filling time.

If the cause of the tachycardia can be determined, such as fever or pain, the cause is treated rather than trying to lower the HR directly. Several medications are available to decrease the HR if needed. Calcium-channel blockers and beta-blockers are widely used for this purpose. However, a word of caution is warranted. Both HR and SV contribute to the CO (see Fig.12.14). If

TABLE 12.10 **Sinus Rhythms**

Parameter	Normal Sinus Rhythm	Sinus Bradycardia	Sinus Tachycardia	Sinus Dysrhythmia
Rate	60–100 beats/min	<60 beats/min	>100 beats/min	Variable
Rhythm	Regular	Regular	Regular	Irregular; respiratory variation
P wave	Present, with 1 per QRS complex	Present, with 1 per QRS complex	Present, with 1 per QRS complex	Present, with 1 per QRS complex
PR interval	0.12–0.20 s and constant	0.12–0.20 s and constant	0.12–0.20 s and constant	0.12–0.20 s and constant
QRS complex	0.06–0.10 s	0.06–0.10 s	0.06–0.10 s	0.06–0.10 s

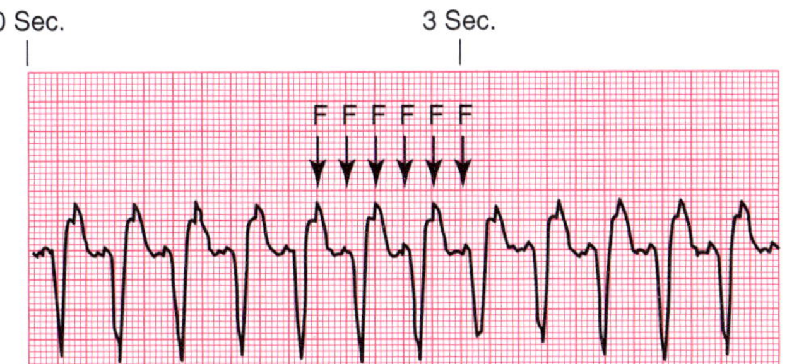

FIG. 12.57 Although the tracing may be confused with sinus tachycardia, it is atrial flutter with 2:1 conduction. It is difficult to see the extra flutter waves *(F)* that are hidden in the QRS complexes.

an injured heart can no longer maintain an adequate SV, HR can be increased to maintain CO and supply an adequate blood flow to vital body tissues. If a medication is administered to force the sinus node to slow, severe and relatively immediate heart failure can result. The sinus node is controlled by many neural and humoral influences in the body, and the rate is set to try to meet the perceived demands; a close examination of the reason for the tachycardia is mandatory before treatment decisions are made.

Sinus Dysrhythmia

Sinus dysrhythmia, commonly called *sinus arrhythmia* in clinical practice, meets all the criteria for normal sinus rhythm except that the rhythm is irregular (see Table 12.10). This irregularity coincides with the respiratory pattern; HR increases with inhalation and decreases with exhalation (Fig. 12.58). Sinus dysrhythmia often occurs in children and young adults, and the incidence decreases with age. No treatment is required. To avoid being misled by other rhythm disturbances, the examiner must look at all P waves closely to verify that they are the same shape and that the PR intervals are consistent.

Atrial Dysrhythmias

Atrial dysrhythmias originate from an ectopic focus in the atria somewhere other than the sinus node. The ectopic impulse occurs prematurely, before the normal sinus impulse occurs. The premature atrial depolarization may initiate a normal QRS complex, an abnormal or aberrant pattern, or an SVT. Huge advances have been made in the understanding of the pathogenesis and management of atrial dysrhythmias.

Premature Atrial Contractions

Premature atrial contractions (PACs) are isolated early beats from an ectopic focus in the atria. The underlying rhythm is usually sinus. The regular sinus rhythm is interrupted by an early, abnormally shaped atrial P wave. The early atrial wave usually looks different from the sinus P wave and may be inverted. The PR interval may be longer, shorter, or the same as the PR interval of a sinus impulse. The QRS complex that follows the ectopic atrial P wave can vary in shape depending on the degree of refractoriness of the AV node.

- *Normal narrow QRS complex:* If the atrial impulse arrives in the AV node after the AV node is fully repolarized, the impulse is conducted to the ventricles as a normal QRS complex. If the ventricles are also fully repolarized, conduction through the bundle branches is expected, and a normal QRS complex is recorded on the ECG (Fig. 12.59A).
- *Wide QRS complex:* Occasionally, the early ectopic P wave can be conducted through the AV node, but part of the conduction pathway through the ventricular bundle branches is blocked. Because the right bundle branch normally has the longest refractory period, it is usually the right bundle branch that is still blocked when the early impulse arrives. This produces a QRS that is wider than 0.12 second (120 ms), with a shape consistent with RBBB (Fig. 12.59B). Conduction through the ventricles that is different from normal is referred to as *aberrant.* Consequently, these early, abnormally conducted PACs are described as *aberrantly conducted PACs.*
- *Pause with no QRS complex:* The ectopic P wave sometimes arrives so early that the AV node is still in its absolute refractory period. In this case the wave of depolarization does not move past the AV node, and no QRS complex follows. All that is seen on the ECG is an early, abnormal P wave followed by a pause until the next sinus P wave occurs (Fig. 12.59C). This is called a *nonconducted PAC.* Usually, these P waves are so early that they are superimposed on the T wave of the previous beat, making them difficult to find. The pause that follows is still clearly seen. Whenever an unexpected pause occurs in a rhythm, the T wave preceding the pause must be examined very carefully and compared with other T waves on the same strip to locate distortions that may reveal a hidden early P wave.

PACs can occur in individuals with normal hearts. PACs may be exacerbated by emotional upheaval, nicotine, caffeine, and digitalis. Mitral valve prolapse is associated with an increased frequency of atrial dysrhythmias. Heart failure can cause PACs because of increased pressure within the atria. As atrial pressure begins to rise, the atrial walls are stretched, causing irritability of atrial cells and the occurrence of PACs.

Supraventricular Tachycardia

Supraventricular tachycardia or SVT describes a varied group of dysrhythmias that originate above the AV node. SVT is not a specific term; it includes sinus tachycardia, atrial tachycardia, multifocal atrial tachycardia, atrial flutter, atrial fibrillation, and junctional tachycardia. Each of these entities has a distinct

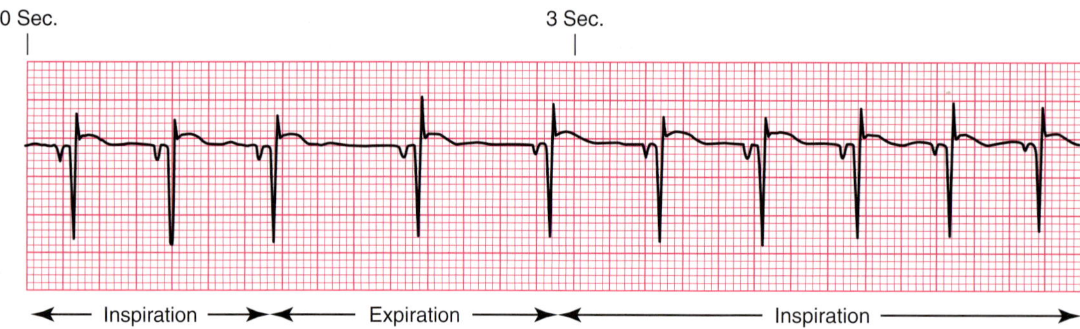

FIG. 12.58 Sinus Dysrhythmia. The heart rate is increased during inspiration and decreased during expiration.

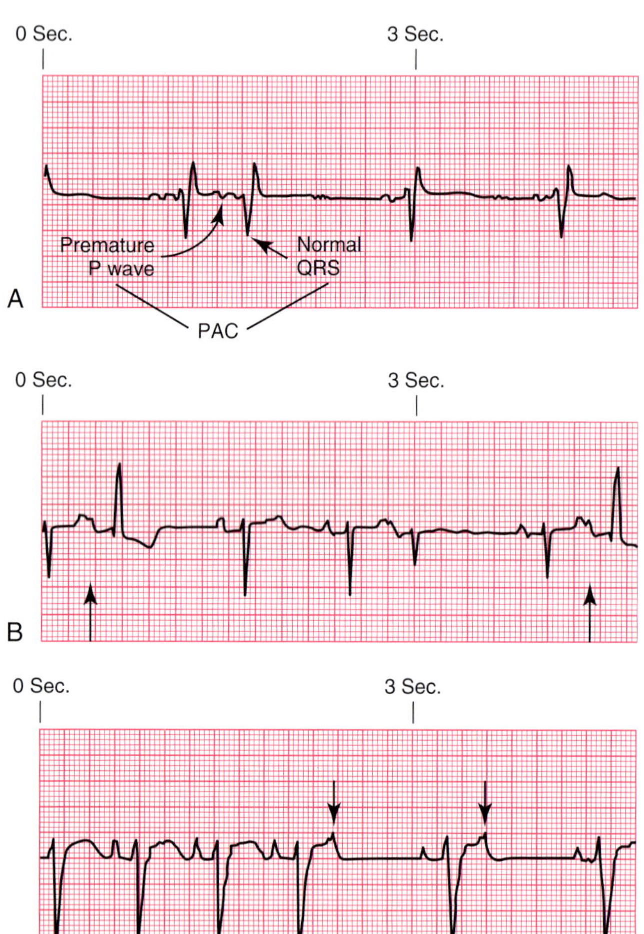

FIG. 12.59 Premature Atrial Contractions *(PACs)*. (A) Normally conducted PAC. The early P wave is indicated by the *arrow*, and the QRS complex that follows has a normal shape and duration. (B) Aberrantly conducted PAC. Early PACs that are abnormally conducted, identified by arrows, are described as *aberrantly conducted PACs*. (C) Nonconducted PACs. The early P waves arrive at the AV node too early to be conducted and distort the T waves, making them appear peaked compared with the normal T waves. These are known as *nonconducted* or *blocked PACs* and are indicated by *arrows*.

pathophysiology, specific therapy, and expected outcome. SVT may also be described as a *narrow complex tachycardia*, defined as a QRS complex that is less than 0.12 second (120 ms).[71] After the specific dysrhythmia is identified, it usually is referred to by a specific name, such as atrial fibrillation with a rapid ventricular response. SVT describes a rapid, sustained atrial or junctional tachycardia when the exact mechanism is unknown. Women are affected by episodic SVT at approximately twice the rate of men.[71]

In an acute situation, a rapid dysrhythmia may be difficult to identify precisely. SVT can cause hemodynamic instability. It is important to differentiate VT from SVT; the focus then can be directed toward rate control until the acute situation is resolved and hemodynamic stability is restored. At that point, a more careful analysis is needed to determine the specific dysrhythmia responsible for the SVT. The differentiation of wide complex SVT from VT requires specific knowledge of the relevant ECG criteria (discussed later).

SVT is not always benign. Approximately 14% of people with SVT report that they have experienced syncope (lost consciousness) while driving, and 50% have experienced symptoms of near-syncope.[71] Medications are used to limit the SVT rate and prevent "blackouts" or syncope. SVT that is persistent for weeks or months may lead to a tachycardia-mediated cardiomyopathy. A baseline 12-lead ECG is helpful, and a 12-lead ECG should be obtained during the palpitations when possible.[71]

Supraventricular Tachycardia With Aberrant Conduction

If the QRS complex in SVT is wider than 0.12 second, it is important to differentiate between SVT with aberrant conduction and VT (discussed later). SVT with aberrant conduction includes SVT with a BBB and SVT that uses an anomalous congenital additional fiber (accessory pathway), such as Wolff-Parkinson-White syndrome. Patients with SVT with aberrant conduction are frequently misdiagnosed, and evaluation by a specialist is highly recommended.[71]

Paroxysmal Supraventricular Tachycardia

Paroxysmal means starting and stopping abruptly. *Paroxysmal supraventricular tachycardia (PSVT)* refers to the sudden interruption of sinus rhythm by an atrial ectopic focus that fires repetitively at a rate of 150 to 250 beats/min and eventually stops as suddenly as it began (Fig. 12.60).

The rhythm of PSVT is perfectly regular because the reentry loop has a specific length; each circuit through the loop requires exactly the same amount of time to complete. Reentry within the atria itself or involving the AV node is the mechanism responsible for most SVTs, including PSVT. Other common underlying mechanisms include abnormal automaticity and triggered activity. P waves are present and abnormally shaped, although they may be difficult to identify, because they often blend in with the previous T wave as a result of the rapid rate. It is most helpful if the beginning of the PSVT run is captured and recorded on ECG paper, because the early, abnormal P wave is often easiest to identify in front of the first beat of the run. The

PR interval should be the same for each cycle in the run, but it will probably be different from the PR interval of the patient's own normal sinus rhythm. As with PACs, the QRS complex is usually normal, because after the impulse passes through the AV node, conduction through the ventricles follows the usual pathway (Table 12.11). However, in PSVT (as discussed for SVT), aberrant conduction, often in the form of LBBB or RBBB, can occur with a wide QRS complex (greater than 0.12 second); this creates difficulty in differentiating relatively benign PSVT from its more serious counterpart, VT.

Because of refractoriness in the AV node, sometimes not all of the ectopic P waves are conducted to the ventricles. Usually, at least every other P wave conducts a QRS complex, described as a 2:1 ratio, but occasionally the conduction may drop to three P waves for every QRS complex (3:1 ratio).

PSVT has essentially the same causal factors as PACs. PSVT has greater clinical significance because it may be sustained for long periods and because it occurs at such a rapid rate. As stressed in the discussion of sinus tachycardia, rapid rates decrease ventricular filling time, increase myocardial oxygen consumption, and decrease oxygen supply. Heart failure, angina, or MI can result. PSVT usually responds rapidly to medical management, which initially includes the use of vagal maneuvers.[71]

Vagal maneuvers used in critical care include the following:

- *Valsalva maneuver:* The patient is asked to "bear down," as if going to the bathroom.
- *Carotid sinus massage:* This maneuver is performed on only one side of the neck over the carotid artery by a physician on a patient with a monitored ECG. It is not used on older patients who may have atherosclerotic disease of the carotid arteries.
- *Modified Valsalva maneuver:* A newer method of Valsalva maneuver has shown increased efficacy for converting PSVT to normal sinus rhythm. This method involves performing the standard Valsalva by asking the patient to bear down; then, immediately after, the patient is positioned flat and a passive leg raise of 45° for 15 seconds is performed.[72]

If vagal maneuvers are unsuccessful in terminating the PSVT, the next step usually is the use of IV medications if the patient is hemodynamically stable. The IV medication of choice to briefly block conduction through the AV node is adenosine.[71] In PSVT, adenosine alone is often sufficient to restore normal sinus rhythm, but if not, it will unmask the ectopic P waves and confirm or provide strong clues to diagnose the SVT. The usual dose is 6 mg given intravenously by rapid push, followed by a normal saline flush. If the 6 mg adenosine does not create a temporary AV block or restore sinus rhythm, a 12-mg IV dose is administered. Continuous cardiac monitoring is essential when administering adenosine. Potential dysrhythmic side effects of adenosine include a 1% to 15% chance of initiating atrial fibrillation. Adenosine should be used with caution for patients with severe asthma or chronic obstructive pulmonary disease (COPD).

Other IV medications that may be used to slow the rate in PSVT include amiodarone, a class III antidysrhythmic with a rapid onset and a short half-life. Beta-blockers, such as metoprolol, are also commonly used to slow conduction. Alternatively, diltiazem, a class IV calcium-channel blocker in the nondihydropyridine group, can be administered. However, extreme caution should be taken when administering calcium-channel blockers if any beta-blockade has already been administered, and vice versa. The action of these medications is to slow conduction

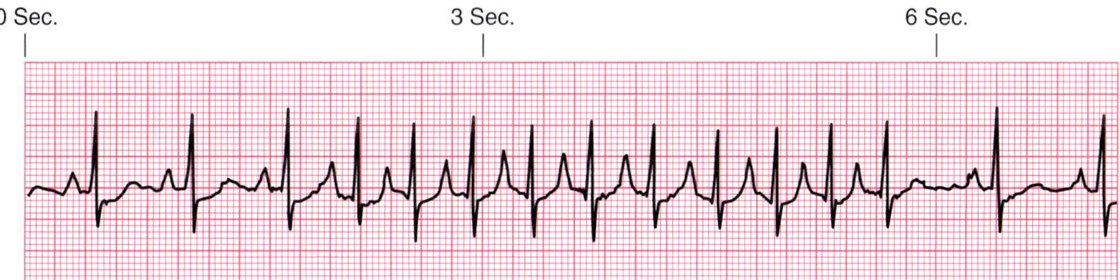

FIG. 12.60 Paroxysmal Supraventricular Tachycardia. The atrial rate during tachycardia is 158 beats/min. The run starts and stops abruptly.

TABLE 12.11 Atrial Dysrhythmias

Parameter	Paroxysmal Supraventricular Tachycardia	Multifocal Atrial Tachycardia	Atrial Flutter	Atrial Fibrillation
Rate				
Atrial	150–250 beats/min	100–160 beats/min	250–350 beats/min	>350 beats/min (unable to count it)
Ventricular	Same or less	Same	250–350 beats/min, one half or less	100–180 beats/min (uncontrolled); <100 beats/min (controlled)
Rhythm	Regular	Irregular	Atrial, regular; ventricular, may or may not be regular	Irregularly irregular
P wave	Present; abnormally shaped	Present; 3 or more different shapes	F waves	Fibrillatory baseline
PR interval	May be normal or prolonged	Variable	Conduction ratio: flutter waves per QRS complex	Absent
QRS complex	0.06–0.10 s	0.06–0.10 s	0.06–0.10 s	0.06–0.10 s

through the AV node. If IV medications do not convert the PSVT or sustained SVT, or if the patient becomes hemodynamically unstable, the next step is electrical cardioversion.[71]

Focal Atrial Tachycardia

Focal atrial tachycardia occurs when there is a nonsinus focus that is firing rapidly. This dysrhythmia can be managed with the same medications used for other atrial dysrhythmias (amiodarone, diltiazem, verapamil, beta-blockers); flecainide or propafenone is used in patients without structural heart disease. Focal atrial tachycardia can be permanently eliminated using catheter ablation.[71]

Multifocal Atrial Tachycardia

Multifocal atrial tachycardia (MAT) refers to numerous irritable atrial foci that intermittently fire and generate an impulse (Fig. 12.61). The atrial rate is greater than 100 beats/min but usually does not exceed 160 beats/min. The atrial feature that distinguishes MAT on the ECG is that there are at least three different P wave shapes, indicating at least three different irritable foci within the atria. MAT is always irregular and is frequently misdiagnosed and confused with atrial fibrillation. MAT is associated with pulmonary disease, pulmonary hypertension, coronary disease, and valvular heart disease.[71] All of these conditions may cause chronically elevated right ventricular and right atrial pressures. The abnormally high right atrial pressure causes stretching of the right atrial muscle cells and chronic irritability. Pharmacologic management of recurrent symptomatic MAT includes beta-blockers or verapamil.[71] Treatment is focused on management of the underlying disorder. When the underlying cause cannot be resolved, MAT is described as *refractory to treatment.* There is no role for electrical cardioversion or catheter ablation.[71]

Atrial Flutter

Atrial flutter is recognized on the ECG by the *sawtooth* atrial pattern. These sawtooth-shaped atrial wavelets are not P waves; they are more appropriately called F waves (atrial flutter waves), as shown in Fig. 12.62. The AV node does not allow conduction of all these impulses to the ventricles.

Pathogenesis of Atrial Flutter

Atrial flutter can be started by any isolated atrial impulse, but to be maintained, the atrial flutter requires a reentry circular pathway around macroscopic structures in the atria. Typically, these structures are in the right atrium and in 75% of cases involve the vena cava and the tricuspid valve in an area known as the *cavotricuspid isthmus.*[71]

The *reentry loop* can circle counterclockwise around the tricuspid valve, circle the inferior vena caval opening, or encircle the IVC and the tricuspid valve. To maintain a viable, self-perpetuating reentry pathway, the loop must avoid the sinoatrial node and be large enough to always meet tissue that is ready to be depolarized (accept a new electrical stimulus). The atrial reentry rate in atrial flutter is typically between 250 beats/min and 330 beats/min, producing the classic sawtooth or flutter wave pattern.[71] The atrial flutter wavelet always appears regular, because the circuit is always the same length and requires exactly the same amount of time to complete the reentry loop.

Atrial and Ventricular Rates in Atrial Flutter

When evaluating the rate of atrial flutter, it is important to calculate both atrial and ventricular rates. The ventricular rhythm is regular when the same number of flutter waves occurs between each QRS complex, indicating that the degree of block at the AV node remains constant. Sometimes, the refractoriness in the AV node changes from beat to beat, resulting in an irregular ventricular response. When describing atrial flutter, the term *PR interval* no longer applies; instead, a conduction ratio, such as 3:1 or 4:1 (ratio of atrial waves to QRS complexes), is used. In normal sinus rhythm, measuring the PR interval allows evaluation of the speed of conduction through the AV node; in atrial flutter, the number of flutter waves that arrive at the AV node before one is allowed to pass through to the ventricles is a measure of AV nodal conduction. After the impulse has passed the AV node, conduction through the ventricles is unaltered. The QRS complex duration remains normal or at least the same as it was in normal sinus rhythm (see Table 12.11). Atrial flutter and atrial fibrillation often coexist in the same patient.[71]

The major factor underlying atrial flutter symptoms is the ventricular response rate. If the atrial rate is 300 beats/min and the AV conduction ratio is 4:1, the ventricular response rate is 75 beats/min and should be well tolerated. However, if the atrial rate is 300 beats/min but the AV conduction ratio is 2:1, the corresponding ventricular rate of 150 beats/min may cause angina, acute heart failure, or other signs of cardiac decompensation. An atrial rate of 250 beats/min with a 1:1 AV conduction ratio yields a ventricular response rate of 250 beats/min; the patient is extremely symptomatic, and emergency measures are needed to decrease the ventricular rate.

Sometimes it is difficult to identify the flutter waves, especially if the conduction ratio is 2:1 (see Fig. 12.62A). Vagal maneuvers or adenosine can be useful diagnostic tools to allow better visualization of the flutter waves. Vagal maneuvers or IV adenosine cannot terminate atrial flutter but do create a temporary AV

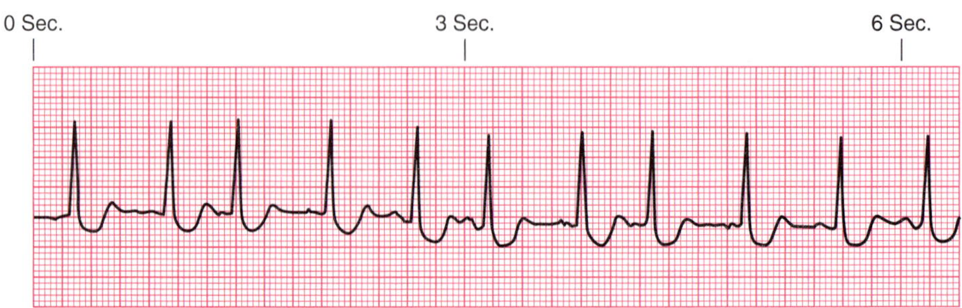

FIG. 12.61 Multifocal Atrial Tachycardia. There are several differently shaped P waves, and the PR intervals vary.

block to permit visualization of the atrial waveform and thereby facilitate accurate diagnosis, as seen in Fig. 12.62B.

Atrial Flutter Management

Antidysrhythmic medications are prescribed in two ways to treat atrial flutter: to convert the rhythm to sinus rhythm (rhythm control) and to slow conduction through the AV node (rate control). The most effective medications for rhythm control are amiodarone, dofetilide, and sotalol; flecainide or propafenone can be used in the absence of structural heart disease. Medications that slow conduction through the AV node are used to control the ventricular rate, including calcium-channel blockers and beta-blockers.[71] Amiodarone shares both properties. It can slow conduction through the AV node and convert the atrial dysrhythmia. Amiodarone is preferred when the atrial flutter creates hemodynamic instability.[71] If at any time a patient with atrial flutter becomes hemodynamically unstable, electrical cardioversion is the recommended emergency intervention.[71]

Nonpharmacologic interventions to convert atrial flutter to sinus rhythm are the most effective; they include catheter ablation and electrical synchronized cardioversion. If atrial flutter has been present for more than 48 hours, one-third of patients will have thrombi in the atria, and anticoagulation is mandated before pharmacologic or electrical cardioversion.[71]

For patients with atrial flutter unrelated to an acute disease process, permanent termination of the atrial flutter circuit can be achieved by radiofrequency catheter ablation. Catheter ablation is used to create a line of conduction block across one or more sections of the reentry pathway. The most frequent location in atrial flutter is a narrow band of tissue between the IVC and the tricuspid anulus known as the *cavotricuspid isthmus*.[71] Table 14.17 in Chapter 14 contains additional information about antidysrhythmic medications.

Atrial Fibrillation

Atrial fibrillation is the most common dysrhythmia in the developed world (Fig. 12.63).[73,74] This dysrhythmia affects 2.7 million to 6.1 million adults in the United States; this number is expected to double in the next 25 years.[73] Treatment of atrial fibrillation adds approximately $8700 per patient per year in health care costs.[73] When first detected, atrial fibrillation may be described as *paroxysmal* (duration less than 7 days from onset), *persistent* (duration more than 7 days), or *long-standing persistent* (duration more than 12 months). When all attempts at conversion to sinus rhythm have failed and there is an acceptance by the patient that atrial fibrillation is not reversible, it is described as *permanent atrial fibrillation*.[73] The etiology of atrial fibrillation is either associated with structural heart disease such as a mitral valve stenosis or described as *nonvalvular atrial fibrillation*.[73]

Atrial fibrillation may be classified under the broad category of SVT, because the HR is rapid and many patients have symptoms of hypotension and breathlessness during paroxysmal atrial fibrillation when uncontrolled by medication. Uncoordinated atrial electrical activity leads to a rapid deterioration in atrial mechanical function. The ECG tracing in atrial fibrillation is notable for an uneven atrial baseline that lacks clearly defined P waves and instead shows rapid oscillations or fibrillation wavelets that vary in size, shape, and frequency. The atrial fibrillation waves are particularly visible in the inferior ECG leads II, III, and AVF.

The ventricular response to atrial fibrillation is influenced by several factors, including the efficiency of the AV node and autonomic nervous system activity. Autonomic activity is directly influenced by the level of sympathetic nervous system (SNS) input, which will increase HR (see Fig. 10.21 in Chapter 10) or from parasympathetic nervous system (PNS) input via the vagus nerve, which will slow the HR (see Figs. 10.29 and 10.30 in Chapter 10). AV node efficiency is also affected by medications that increase or slow conduction through the AV node and bundle branch conduction system. In addition, various structural heart conditions such as cardiomyopathy and heart failure can affect the ventricular response.[73] Atrial fibrillation displays irregular R-R intervals (different timing intervals between the QRS complexes) that do not show any logical pattern. The ability of the AV node and bundle branches to conduct or block the fibrillating atrial impulses is key to the appearance of the QRS complex on the ECG. In atrial fibrillation, the QRS complex shape is usually narrow and normal in appearance as long as the pathway through the ventricles is intact after the impulse leaves the AV node. The AV node acts as a filter to protect the ventricles from the hundreds of atrial impulses that occur each minute, although the AV node does not receive all these atrial impulses. When the atrial muscle tissue immediately surrounding the AV node is in a refractory state, impulses generated in

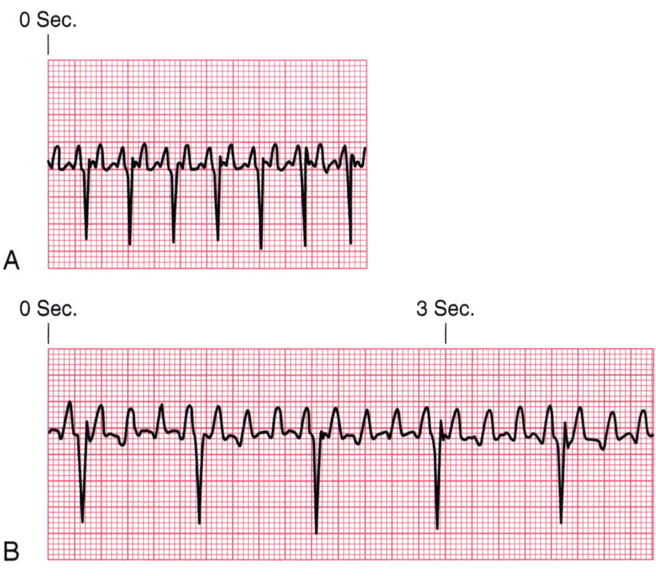

FIG. 12.62 (A) The initial strip shows atrial flutter with 2:1 conduction through the atrioventricular (AV) node. (B) During carotid sinus massage, the AV conduction rate is decreased, revealing the flutter waves more clearly.

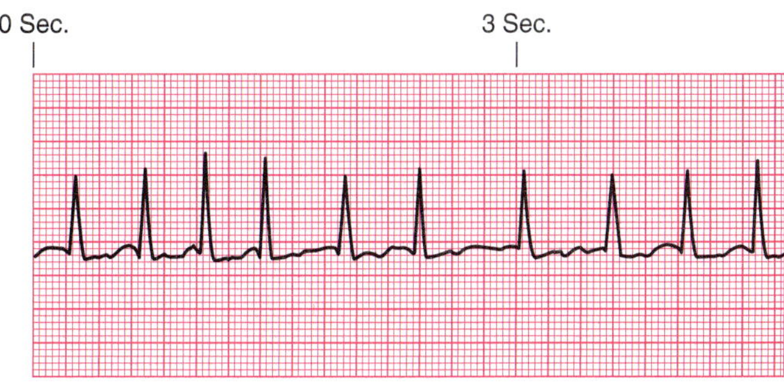

FIG. 12.63 Atrial Fibrillation. The ventricular rhythm is irregularly irregular.

other areas of the atria cannot reach the AV node, which helps explain the wide variation in R-R intervals during atrial fibrillation (see Table 12.11).

Pathogenesis of Atrial Fibrillation

The pathogenesis of atrial fibrillation has traditionally been ascribed to random electrical foci firing in the atria. Research using high-density atrial mapping, high-speed video recordings, and ECG analysis has uncovered distinct spatial organization within the atria.[73] Atrial fibrillation involves several reentry circuits within the atria, and in some cases, they originate at specific anatomic sites. The four pulmonary veins that drain into the left atrium are a trigger site for early atrial foci to initiate and propagate reentry circuits to maintain atrial fibrillation.[73] The earliest atrial ectopic foci have been electrically mapped 2 to 4 cm within the pulmonary veins. The affected pulmonary veins contain thin myocardial sleeves that project into the pulmonary veins from the left atrium. This ectopic tissue resembles discontinuous fingerlike projections approximately 5 mm thick that extend 4.5 cm into one or more pulmonary veins. The tissue ultimately becomes part of the venous wall. The spread of atrial fibrillation to the rest of the atria is thought to occur through multiple reentry wavelets that are maintained in perpetual motion by a dominant reentry circuit, which functions at a higher frequency and perpetuates the atrial fibrillation.

When a single focus can be identified, it is possible to encircle that area and isolate that site using radiofrequency catheter ablation. Several different catheter ablation designs are used to isolate foci that originate in the four pulmonary veins, encircling all four veins together or isolating individual or pairs of pulmonary veins.[73,74]

The atria demonstrate other pathologic changes in atrial fibrillation, typically atrial fibrosis and loss of atrial muscle mass.[73] Any change in atrial architecture increases the risk of atrial fibrillation.[73] An enlarged atrium is an independent risk factor for atrial fibrillation. Conversely, ongoing atrial fibrillation can contribute to pathologic atrial enlargement.

It is probable that there are several different types of atrial fibrillation involving different mechanisms. As electrophysiologic mapping techniques become more advanced, the mystery surrounding the origins of atrial fibrillation will become clearer. Although atrial fibrillation may look disorganized on the ECG baseline tracing, an electrical pattern exists within the atria. Knowledge of this pattern will ultimately lead to treatments that can help cure or control atrial fibrillation.

Atrial Fibrillation Risk Factors

Atrial fibrillation is most common in older adults. Less than 1% of adults younger than 60 years have atrial fibrillation. In contrast, almost one-third of adults older than 80 years have atrial fibrillation.[73] Atrial fibrillation is the most common cardiac dysrhythmia in the United States and is responsible for most dysrhythmia-related hospital admissions. There are known risk factors that increase the risk of developing atrial fibrillation, notably structural heart disease, including hypertension, ischemic heart disease, hyperlipidemia, and heart failure. Other disease states associated with higher risk include diabetes mellitus, chronic kidney disease, anemia, arthritis, and COPD.[73]

Atrial Fibrillation Management

Debate continues about the most effective treatment approach for atrial fibrillation. In the past, the gold standard goal has been to convert the patient out of atrial fibrillation back to sinus rhythm. However, for many older adults, remaining out of atrial fibrillation is an unattainable goal. The major therapeutic decision is whether it is possible to achieve *rhythm* control or ventricular *rate* control.[75] The risk of stroke increases fivefold with atrial fibrillation.[73] Therefore all patients with atrial fibrillation require anticoagulation to prevent development of atrial thrombi, thrombotic embolism, and stroke.[73]

Atrial Fibrillation Rhythm Control

For a hospitalized patient with new-onset atrial fibrillation with unstable hemodynamic values, the primary focus is generally on rhythm control (conversion to sinus rhythm) using antidysrhythmic medications or electrical cardioversion. Emergency medications used to convert atrial fibrillation to sinus rhythm, also known as a *chemical cardioversion*, include amiodarone and ibutilide. Antidysrhythmic medications used long-term to maintain sinus rhythm include amiodarone, dronedarone, disopyramide, flecainide, propafenone, quinidine, sotalol, and dofetilide. Selection of the optimal medication depends on whether the patient has underlying structural heart disease.[73-76] Even with medication therapy, recurrence of atrial fibrillation is likely. Electrical cardioversion may be successful in converting the atria to sinus rhythm if attempted within a few days or weeks of the onset of atrial fibrillation. Success is less likely if atrial fibrillation has existed for a long time.[73]

Surgical Procedures to Manage Atrial Fibrillation

The Cox-Maze III procedure (typically called the *maze procedure*) is an open-heart surgical operation. The surgery is suitable for only a tiny fraction of the patients who have atrial fibrillation, usually those who have lone atrial fibrillation, meaning without other structural heart disease. This surgery is designed to permanently cure atrial fibrillation by "cut and sew" insertion of strategic scar lines into the atria. The success rate, measured as freedom from atrial fibrillation, is 75% to 95% up to 15 years after surgery.[77,78] The surgical maze procedure is now rarely performed, as it has been replaced by catheter-based techniques.

Catheter Procedures to Manage Atrial Fibrillation

Many factors must be considered before choosing radiofrequency catheter ablation. Type of atrial fibrillation, degree of symptoms, presence of structural heart disease, candidacy for alternative options, candidacy for anticoagulation, and patient preference must all be assessed. The goal of radiofrequency catheter ablation is to reduce clinical symptoms associated with atrial fibrillation. Based on the results of published studies, 57% of patients have reduced symptoms after ablation even without antidysrhythmic medications.[79] When multiple ablation procedures are performed, the success rate increases to 71% without antidysrhythmic medications and to 77% with antidysrhythmics.[79]

Atrial Fibrillation Rate Control

The most prescribed medications used to control the ventricular rate in atrial fibrillation include calcium-channel blockers, beta-blockers, and digoxin. These medications work to slow conduction through the AV node. They have no effect on the fibrillating atria. In the past, it was assumed that rate control was an inferior strategy, because the patient stayed in atrial fibrillation, lost "atrial kick," and was presumed to have an increased risk of embolic stroke. Two multicenter trials have altered that perception: the *A*trial *F*ibrillation *F*ollow-up: *I*nvestigation of

*R*hythm *M*anagement (AFFIRM) and the *RA*te Control vs. *E*lectrical Cardioversion for Persistent Atrial Fibrillation (RACE). These two trials found similar morbidity, mortality, and quality of life in patients treated with rhythm conversion or rate control. For long-term management of permanent atrial fibrillation, rate control is the recommended approach, and therapeutic anticoagulation to prevent embolic stroke is mandatory.[80] Antidysrhythmic and antithrombotic medications used to manage atrial fibrillation are listed in Table 14.17 in Chapter 14.

Stroke Risk Assessment and Antithrombotic Therapy in Atrial Fibrillation

Atrial fibrillation, because of the development of thrombi in the atria, greatly increases the risk of embolic stroke. Electrical and chemical (medication-induced) forms of cardioversion entail the threat of precipitating emboli into the systemic circulation. During atrial fibrillation, the atria do not contract effectively, and blood may pool and promote clots that attach to the atrial walls (mural thrombi). If cardioversion is successful and normal sinus rhythm is restored, the atria again contract forcibly and, if thrombus formation has occurred, may send clots traveling through the pulmonary or systemic circulation.

To prevent embolic stroke, it is important to pay attention to the 48-hour rule. Patients who have been in atrial fibrillation for greater than 48 hours, or unknown, must be adequately anticoagulated with an oral vitamin K antagonist (warfarin) to a goal INR of 2.0 to 3.0, a factor Xa inhibitor, or a direct thrombin inhibitor for at least 3 weeks before elective cardioversion.[81] After successful cardioversion, patients should be anticoagulated for an additional 4 weeks. [80]

TEE is helpful in identifying the presence or absence of thrombi in fibrillating atria and is recommended as a screening tool before elective cardioversion.[80] It is especially helpful for patients in atrial fibrillation for less than 48 hours who, in the absence of atrial thrombi, may undergo cardioversion without anticoagulation.[80] TEE is described in more detail later in this chapter.

Patients who experience episodes of rapid atrial fibrillation for only a few hours or days at a time and then convert back to sinus rhythm spontaneously (paroxysmal atrial fibrillation) are also at risk for embolic stroke. Several scoring mechanisms have been developed to help predict which patients with atrial fibrillation require prophylactic anticoagulation; the most used are the CHADS2 and CHA2DS2-VASc, discussed in the following sections. The atrial fibrillation antithrombotic recommendations apply equally to patients with atrial flutter.[78,80]

CHADS2

The acronym *CHADS2* is an easy-to-remember risk assessment tool used to predict stroke risk in atrial fibrillation and to guide antithrombotic therapy (Box 12.11). The letters stand for *cardiac failure, hypertension, age, diabetes, stroke* (double points).[80] The score ranges from 0 to 6.

CHA2DS2-VASc

Other scoring systems such as the CHA2DS2-VASc have expanded the risk factor profile to include acute heart failure, hypertension, age 75 years or older (double points), diabetes, stroke (double points), vascular disease, age 65 to 74 years, and sex (female) (see Box 12.11).[77,78] Anticoagulant therapy is based on risk stratification score and patient-specific comorbidities. The CHA2DS2-VASc scoring system has demonstrated increased specificity and is more widely used.

Junctional Dysrhythmias

Only certain areas of the AV node have the property of automaticity. The entire area around the AV node is collectively called the *junction*; impulses generated there are called *junctional impulses*. After an ectopic impulse arises in the junction, it spreads in two directions at once. One wave of depolarization spreads upward into the atria and depolarizes them, causing the recording of a P wave on the ECG. This is called *retrograde (backward) conduction*, and the P wave is inverted when viewed in lead II. At the same time, another wave of depolarization spreads downward into the ventricles through the normal conduction pathway, producing a normal QRS complex. This is called *antegrade (forward) conduction*. Depending on timing, the P wave (1) may be seen in front of the QRS complex, with a short PR interval of less than 0.12 second; (2) may be obscured entirely by the QRS complex; or (3) may immediately follow the QRS complex.

Premature Junctional Contraction

If only a single ectopic impulse originates in the junction, it is simply called a *premature junctional contraction*. On the ECG, the rhythm is regular from the sinus node except for one early QRS complex of normal shape and duration. The P wave can be entirely absent. If a P wave can be found, it very closely precedes or follows the QRS complex. In lead II, the P wave appears inverted (having a negative deflection) because the atria are being depolarized from the AV node upward, which is the opposite direction from the wave of depolarization that occurs when triggered by the sinus node. If the P wave appears before the QRS complex, the PR interval is less than 0.12 second. Premature junctional contractions have virtually the same clinical significance as PACs. However, if the patient is receiving digoxin, digitalis toxicity may be suspected. Although digoxin slows conduction through the AV node, it also increases automaticity in the junctional area.

BOX 12.11 CHADS2 and CHA2DS2-VASc Score

CHADS2

Letter	Risk Factor	Score
C	Chronic heart failure	1
H	Hypertension	1
A	Age >75 years	1
D	Diabetes mellitus	1
S	Stroke or TIA	2

CHA2DS2-VASc

Letter	Risk Factor	Score
C	Chronic heart failure	1
H	Hypertension	1
A	Age >75 years	2
D	Diabetes mellitus	1
S	Stroke or TIA	2
V	Vascular disease	1
A	Age 65–74	1
Sc	Sex category (female)	1

TIA, Transient ischemic attack.

Junctional Escape Rhythm

Sometimes the junction becomes the dominant pacemaker of the heart (Table 12.12). The intrinsic rate of the junction normally is 40 to 60 beats/min. The intrinsic rate of the sinus node is 60 to 100 beats/min. Under normal conditions, the junction never has a chance to escape and depolarize the heart, because it is overridden by the sinus node. However, if the sinus node fails, the junctional impulses can depolarize completely and pace the heart. This is called a *junctional escape rhythm*, and it is a protective mechanism to prevent asystole in the event of sinus node failure. Generally, a junctional escape rhythm (Fig. 12.64) is well tolerated hemodynamically, although efforts must be directed toward restoring sinus rhythm. A pacemaker sometimes is inserted as a protective measure because of concern that the AV junction may also fail.

Junctional Tachycardia and Accelerated Junctional Rhythm

A junctional rhythm can also occur at a faster rate (see Table 12.12). As with sinus rhythm, the term *tachycardia* is reserved for rates greater than 100 beats/min. *Junctional tachycardia* is a narrow complex rhythm that arises from the AV junction nearer to the bundle of His area. The rate is rapid (120 to 220 beats/min).[71] Junctional tachycardia may cause hemodynamic compromise, depending on the rate and the patient's underlying cardiac reserve.

When the junctional rate is greater than 60 beats/min and less than 100 beats/min, it is described as an *accelerated junctional rhythm*. Blood pressure is usually maintained in an accelerated junctional rhythm, because the HR is within the normal range to provide adequate diastolic filling time.

Junctional tachycardia and accelerated junctional rhythms are uncommon in adults, apart from those caused by digoxin toxicity.[71] Digoxin toxicity is always a concern in patients taking this medication, because digoxin enhances automaticity of the AV node. The optimal strategy in these cases is to measure the digoxin serum level and withhold digoxin until the dysrhythmia resolves. When digoxin toxicity is life-threatening, the fastest-acting antidote is digoxin immune Fab.[82]

Ventricular Dysrhythmias

Ventricular dysrhythmias result from an ectopic focus in any portion of the ventricular myocardium. The usual conduction pathway through the ventricles is not used, and the wave of depolarization must spread from cell to cell. As a result, the QRS complex is prolonged and is always greater than 0.12 second. The width of the QRS complex, not the height, is important in the diagnosis of ventricular ectopy. In general, ventricular dysrhythmias have more serious implications than atrial or junctional dysrhythmias and occur only rarely in healthy individuals.

Premature Ventricular Contraction

A PVC is a single ectopic impulse originating in the ventricles. Some PVCs are very small in height but remain wider than 0.12 second. If there is doubt, a different lead is evaluated. The shape of the QRS complex depends on the location of the ectopic focus. If the ectopic focus arises from the right ventricle, the impulse spreads from right to left, and the QRS complex resembles a LBBB pattern, because the left ventricle is the last to be depolarized. In V_1, this is a wide negative QRS complex (Fig. 12.65A). If the ectopic focus is in the LV free wall, the wave of depolarization spreads from left to right (Fig. 12.65B).

Because the ectopic focus may be any cell in the ventricle, the QRS complex can manifest in an unlimited number of shapes or patterns.

Unifocal: When all the ventricular ectopic beats look the same in a particular lead, they are called *unifocal*, and all probably arise from the same irritable focus (Fig. 12.66A).

Multifocal: Conversely, if the ventricular ectopic beats are of various shapes in the same lead, they are called *multifocal* (Fig. 12.66B). Multifocal ventricular ectopic beats are more serious than unifocal ventricular ectopic beats, because they indicate a greater area of irritable myocardial tissue and are more likely to deteriorate into VT or VF.

A PVC originates in a ventricular cell that has become abnormally permeable to sodium, usually as a result of damage. Because of this new permeability to sodium, the cell reaches depolarization

TABLE 12.12 Junctional Rhythms

Parameter	Junctional Escape Rhythm	Accelerated Junctional Rhythm	Junctional Tachycardia
Rate	40–60 beats/min	60–100 beats/min	>100 beats/min
Rhythm	Regular	Regular	Regular
P waves	May be present or absent; inverted in lead II	May be present or absent; inverted in lead II	May be present or absent; inverted in lead II
P-R interval	<0.12 s	<0.12 s	<0.12 s
QRS complex	0.06–0.10 s	0.06–0.10 s	0.06–0.10 s

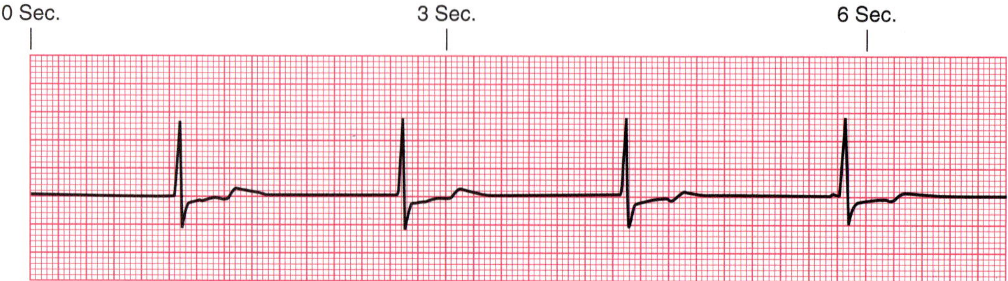

FIG. 12.64 Junctional Escape Rhythm. The ventricular rate is 38 beats/min. P waves are absent, and the QRS complex has a normal width.

threshold before an impulse is received from the sinus node. After the depolarization threshold is reached, the cell automatically depolarizes, initiating total ventricular depolarization. Ordinarily, the ventricular impulse does not conduct back through the AV node; the sinus node is not disturbed and continues to depolarize the atria, resulting in a normal P wave, which will likely be hidden within the PVC. Conduction from the sinus node does not proceed into the ventricles if they are in a refractory state. Assuming there is no further ventricular ectopy, the next sinus beat conducts normally through the AV node and into the ventricles.

Compensatory Pause

When the impulse from the sinus node is interrupted by a PVC, a compensatory pause occurs. A full compensatory pause is shown and described in Fig. 12.67A. The conduction of the SA node is not disturbed; therefore, the R-R intervals before and after the PVC will be the same. Because this does not usually occur in PACs or premature junctional contractions, when present, it is diagnostic of ventricular ectopy. If the normal sinus P wave that occurs immediately after the PVC finds the ventricles sufficiently recovered to accept another impulse, a normal QRS complex results, and the PVC is sandwiched between two normal beats (Fig. 12.67B). This PVC is referred to as *interpolated* (meaning "between"). Interpolated PVCs usually occur when the PVC is very early, or the normal sinus rate is relatively slow.

The ventricular impulse occasionally spreads backward across the AV node to depolarize the atria. When this occurs, the sinus node is reset, and no full compensatory pause occurs.

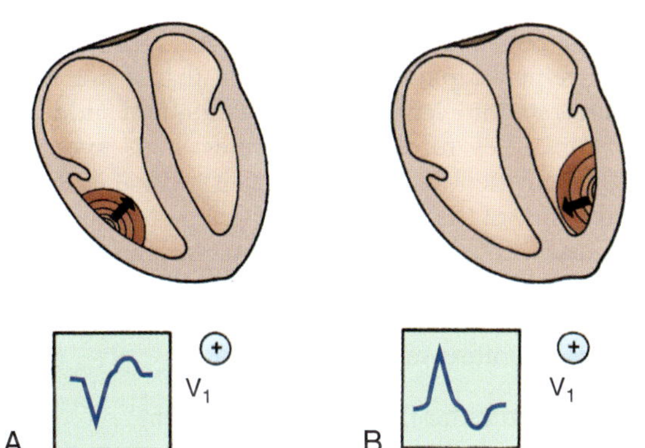

FIG. 12.65 (A) Right ventricular premature ventricular contraction (PVC). The spread of depolarization is from right to left, away from the positive electrode in lead V_1, resulting in a wide, negative QRS complex. (B) Left ventricular PVC. The spread of depolarization is from left to right, toward the positive electrode in lead V_1. The QRS complex is wide and upright.

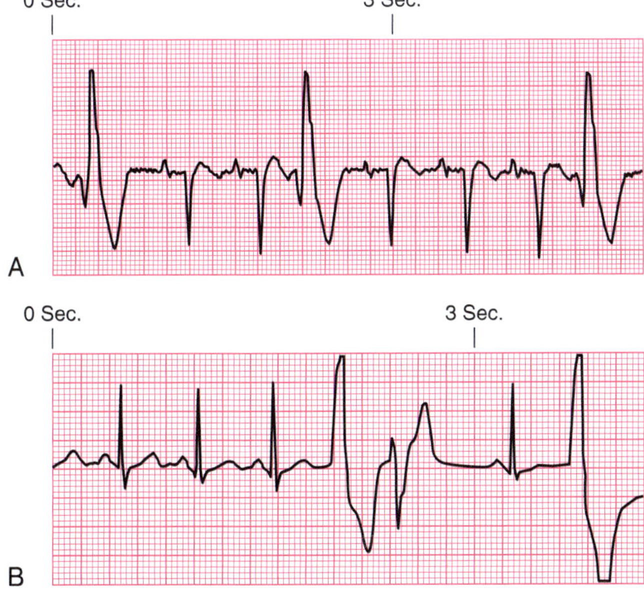

FIG. 12.66 (A) Unifocal premature ventricular contractions (PVCs). (B) Multifocal PVCs.

Describing Ventricular Ectopy

PVCs can develop concurrently with any supraventricular dysrhythmia. It is not sufficient to describe a patient's rhythm as "frequent PVCs" or even "frequent unifocal PVCs." The underlying rhythm must always be described first, such as "sinus bradycardia with frequent unifocal PVCs" or "atrial fibrillation with occasional multifocal PVCs." Timing of PVCs can also be described. When a PVC follows each normally conducted beat, *ventricular bigeminy* is present (Fig. 12.68). If a PVC follows every two normal beats, it is called *ventricular trigeminy*. Two consecutive PVCs are described as a *couplet*, and three consecutive PVCs are called a *triplet* or a *three-beat run of VT*.

In individuals with underlying heart disease, PVCs or episodes of self-terminating VT are potentially malignant. Nonsustained VT is defined as three or more consecutive premature ventricular beats at a rate faster than 110 beats/min lasting less than 30 seconds.

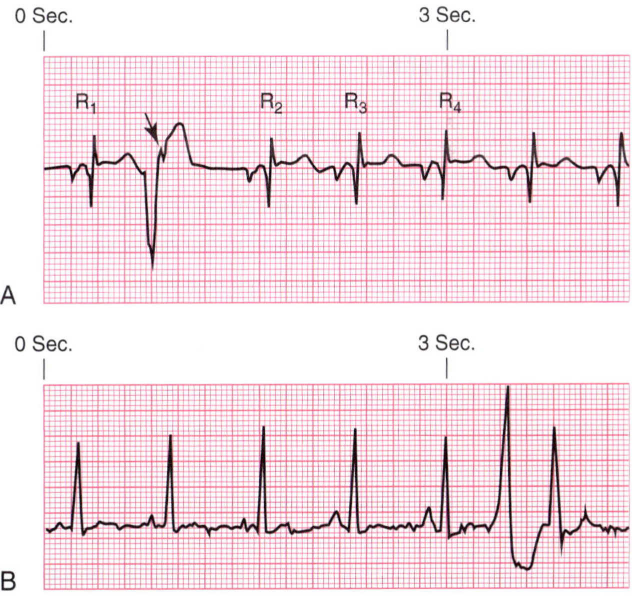

FIG. 12.67 (A) Premature ventricular contraction (PVC) with fully compensatory pause. The interval between the two sinus beats that surround the PVC (R_1 and R_2) is exactly two times the normal interval between sinus beats (R_3 and R_4). The fully compensatory pause occurs because the sinus node continues to pace despite the PVC. The sinus P wave *(arrow)* is hidden in the ST segment of the PVC. This P wave did not conduct through to the ventricles because they had just been depolarized and were still in the absolute refractory period. (B) Interpolated PVC. The PVC falls between two normal QRS complexes without disturbing the rhythm. The RR interval between sinus beats remains the same.

Premature Ventricular Complex Timing

The timing of PVCs can be important. The relative refractory period, represented on the ECG by the last half of the T wave, is a particularly vulnerable time for ectopy to occur, because repolarization is incomplete. If a PVC occurs at this critical point when only a part of the muscle is repolarized, individual segments of muscle can depolarize separately from each other, resulting in ventricular dysrhythmias. This is called the *R-on-T phenomenon* (Fig. 12.69). This phenomenon can be particularly problematic for patients with ischemic tissue. Repolarization is even more delayed in ischemic tissue, so various portions of the ventricular muscle are not repolarized simultaneously.

Causes of Premature Ventricular Contractions

PVCs can result from many causes. They can occur in healthy individuals with no evidence of heart disease. The critical care nurse has an important role in identifying factors that may be causing or contributing to PVCs. Acute ischemia is the most dangerous cause of ventricular ectopy. Ischemia causes cell membrane permeability to change, giving rise to early depolarization and the initiation of ectopic impulses. Ventricular ectopy that occurs during an acute ischemic event may require treatment with IV amiodarone or other antidysrhythmic medications.

Metabolic abnormalities are common causes of PVCs. Hypokalemia, hypoxemia, and acidosis predispose the cell membrane to instability and may cause ventricular ectopy. Treatment is directed toward identifying the metabolic disturbance and correcting it. The ability of oxygen and potassium values to change very rapidly in a critically ill patient must not be underestimated. For example, if PVCs develop during suctioning of an intubated patient, a few additional breaths of 100% oxygen usually are sufficient to restore adequate oxygenation and may eliminate the ventricular ectopy.

Any form of structural heart disease can lead to ventricular ectopy. Patients with cardiomyopathy or ventricular aneurysms can have chronic, severe ventricular ectopy, which may prove to be refractory to antidysrhythmic agents. Invasive procedures, such as insertion of a PA catheter or cardiac catheterization, can cause PVCs by mechanically irritating the ventricular muscle. In these situations, the ectopy usually resolves with removal or advancement of the catheter.

Certain medications can cause ventricular ectopy. Digitalis toxicity may precipitate PVCs, which are resistant to conventional antidysrhythmic therapy. Some class I antidysrhythmic medications can cause more serious dysrhythmias than the dysrhythmias they were intended to treat. This is called a *prodysrhythmic effect* (also described as a *proarrhythmic effect*), and it can sometimes be fatal. Class 1a medications prolong the QT interval by lengthening the ventricular refractory period. This is a therapeutic effect, but when the QT interval prolongation becomes excessive, a characteristic form of polymorphic VT called *torsades de pointes* can develop (Fig. 12.70). In this dysrhythmia, the ventricular rate is very rapid, and QRS complexes appear to twist in a spiral pattern around the baseline, so called "twisting of the points" or the French term torsades de pointes. Torsades de pointes results in hemodynamic instability because of the extremely rapid ventricular rate that if not terminated can deteriorate into ventricular fibrillation and sudden cardiac death. Sometimes torsades de pointes stops spontaneously, although the patient may experience a syncopal episode or seizure at the time of the dysrhythmia. Because torsades de pointes is associated with a lengthened QT interval, careful and consistent measurement of the QT interval in critically ill patients can identify patient at increased risk. Risk factors for development of torsades de pointes are listed in Box 12.7.

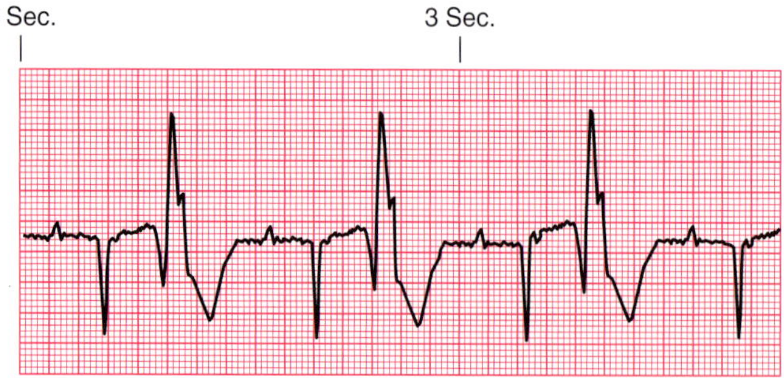

FIG. 12.68 Ventricular Bigeminy.

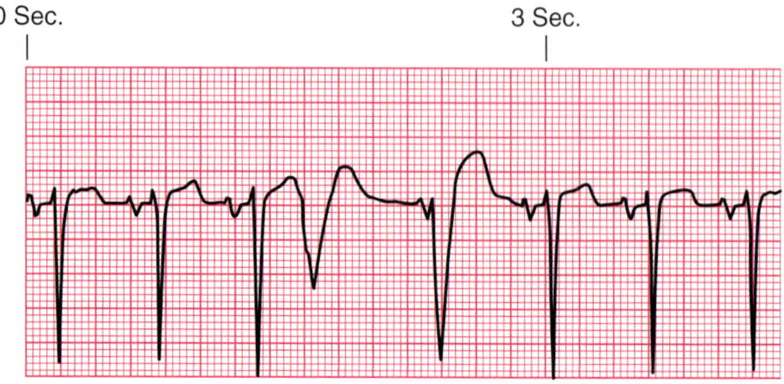

FIG. 12.69 R-on-T Phenomenon.

Premature Ventricular Complex Management

Not all ventricular ectopy requires treatment. In individuals without significant underlying heart disease, isolated PVCs do not represent an increased risk for sudden death and are considered benign. If the patient complains of palpitations or becomes symptomatic, therapy includes reassurance and correction of any potentially contributing factor(s). During an acute MI, antidysrhythmic medications such as amiodarone or beta-blockers may be used to decrease the risk of isolated PVCs progressing to VT. In contrast, if a patient with PVCs has a healthy heart, antidysrhythmic medications, specifically medications that increase the incidence of VT, are used as a last resort because of the risk of prodysrhythmia. Chapter 14 provides further information about antidysrhythmic medications (see Table 14.17).

Idioventricular Rhythms

Sometimes an ectopic focus in the ventricle can become the dominant pacemaker of the heart (Table 12.13). If the sinus node and the AV junction fail, the ventricles depolarize at their own intrinsic rate of 20 to 40 times per minute. This is called an *idioventricular rhythm* and is a naturally protective mechanism. Rather than trying to abolish the ventricular beats, the aim of treatment is to increase the effective HR and reestablish dominance of a higher pacing site such as the sinus node or the AV junction. Usually, a temporary pacemaker is used to increase the HR until the underlying problems that caused failure of the other pacing sites can be resolved.

An accelerated idioventricular rhythm (AIVR) occurs when a ventricular focus assumes control of the heart at a rate greater than its intrinsic rate of 40 beats/min but less than 100 beats/min (Fig. 12.71). Although relatively benign[83] in and of itself,

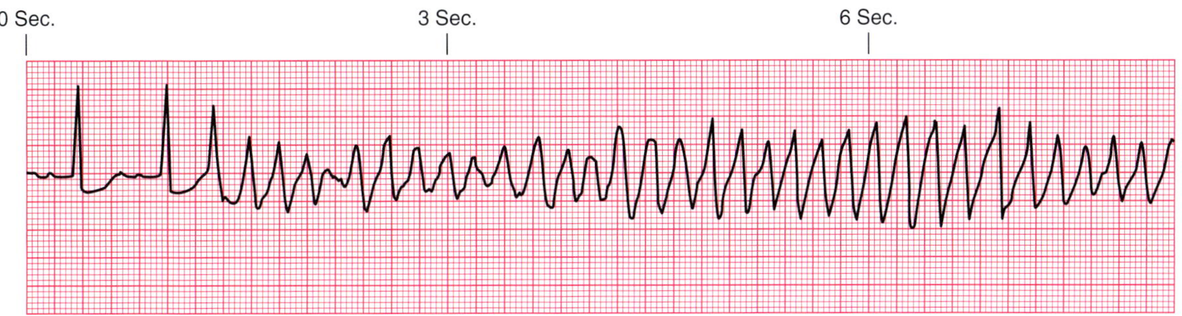

FIG. 12.70 Torsades de Pointes.

TABLE 12.13 Ventricular Rhythms

Parameter	Idioventricular Rhythm	Accelerated Idioventricular Rhythm	Ventricular Tachycardia	Ventricular Fibrillation
Rate	20–40 beats/min	40–100 beats/min	>100 beats/min	None
Rhythm	Usually regular	Usually regular	Usually regular	Irregular
P waves	Absent or retrograde	Absent or retrograde	Absent or retrograde	None
PR interval	None	None	None	None
QRS complex	>0.12 s	>0.12 s	>0.12 s	Fibrillatory waves

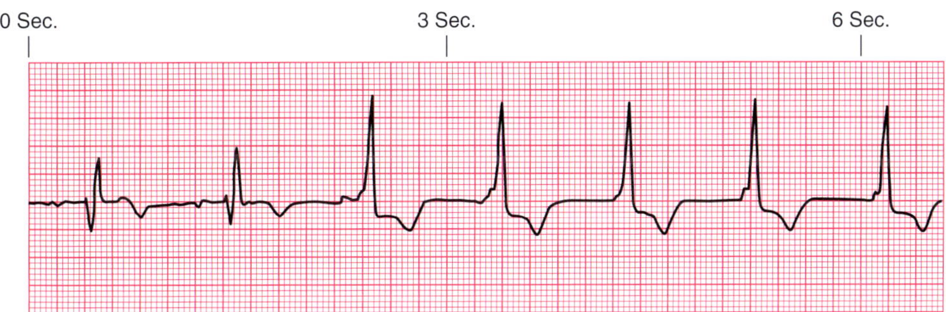

FIG. 12.71 Accelerated Idioventricular Rhythm. The QRS complex duration is 0.14 s, and the ventricular rate is 65 beats/min.

this rhythm must be closely observed for any increase in rate, and the patient must be observed for hemodynamic deterioration. Usually, AIVR is not typically treated pharmacologically if well tolerated with a stable blood pressure, though temporary ventricular pacing should be available as a precaution should sudden hemodynamic deterioration occur. IV lidocaine must never be administered to a patient with an idioventricular rhythm, because it suppresses the ventricular pacemaker and can convert the rhythm to asystole.

Ventricular Tachycardia

VT is caused by a ventricular pacing site firing at a rate of 100 beats or more per minute, usually maintained by a reentry mechanism within the ventricular tissue (Fig. 12.72). The complexes are wide, and the rhythm may be slightly irregular, often accelerating as the tachycardia continues (see Table 12.13). In most cases, the sinus node is not affected, and it continues to depolarize the atria on schedule. Therefore, P waves can sometimes be seen on the ECG tracing. However, they are not related (disassociated) from the QRS complex and may even appear to conduct a normal impulse to the ventricles if their timing is just right. A brief episode with a duration less than 30 seconds is termed *nonsustained VT*.

If the sinus impulse and the ventricular ectopic impulse meet in the middle of the ventricles, a fusion beat results. Fusion beats are narrower than ventricular beats and look like a cross between the patient's sinus QRS complex and the ventricular ectopic QRS complex (Fig. 12.73). When present, P waves and fusion beats are helpful in verifying the diagnosis of VT as opposed to SVT. Differentiation between VT and SVT is discussed earlier in this chapter.

Most VT occurs in the presence of structural cardiac disease, such as myocardial ischemia, congenital heart disease, valvular dysfunction, and/or cardiomyopathy. Other triggers include medication toxicities, electrolyte disturbances, and certain antidysrhythmic medications (prodysrhythmia). Sustained VT is a life-threatening dysrhythmia and must be treated quickly. The rapid ventricular rate decreases blood pressure, and the patient may lose consciousness. The loss of the synchronized timing of atrial contraction, which normally adds volume to the ventricles just before contraction and enhances the force of contraction, is lost, greatly reducing CO. If not terminated quickly, VT can degenerate into VF and death.

Clinical management of VT depends on whether the patient is stable or unstable and whether a pulse and/or adequate blood pressure are present. Pulseless VT is a life-threatening

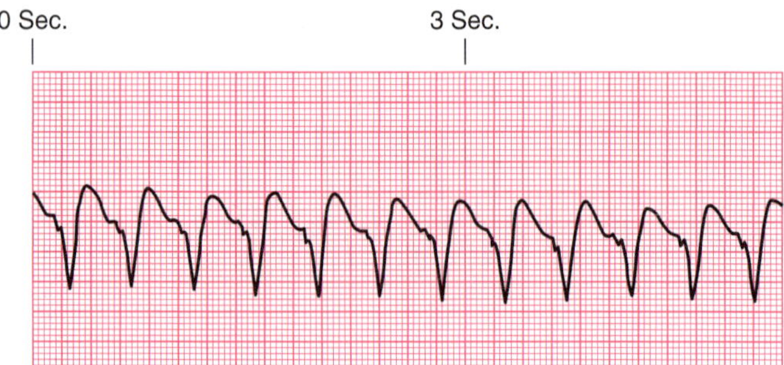

FIG. 12.72 Ventricular Tachycardia.

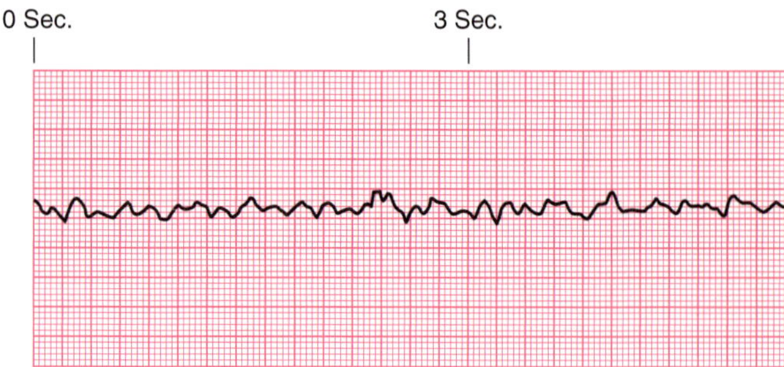

FIG. 12.74 Ventricular Fibrillation.

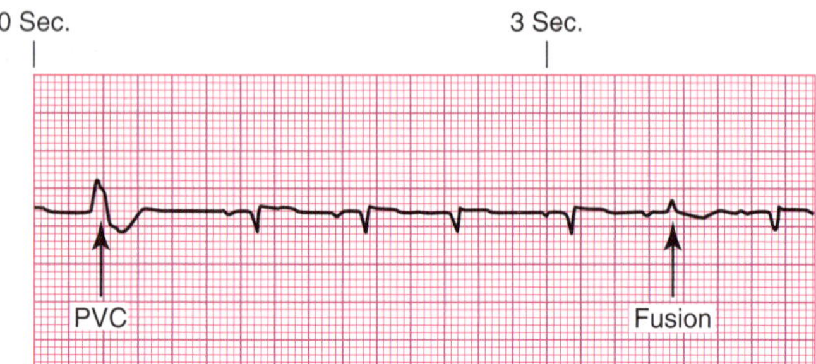

FIG. 12.73 Ventricular Fusion Beat *(arrows)*. The QRS complex duration is only 0.08 s, and the shape represents the normal QRS complex and the previous premature ventricular contraction *(PVC)*.

condition. In this case, the patient loses consciousness and needs immediate cardiopulmonary resuscitation and defibrillation as described in the American Heart Association protocols for advanced cardiac life support. Patients with stable or wide complex "slow VT" who have a HR below 150 beats/min, palpable pulse, and stable blood pressure may be treated pharmacologically and/or with synchronized cardioversion as described in the advanced cardiac life support protocols.

After the acute episode is over, patients who have already experienced sustained VT or cardiac arrest continue to be at risk for sudden cardiac death. An extensive clinical evaluation of these patients is warranted, including cardiac catheterization and electrophysiologic testing with programmed ventricular stimulation. Therapy is aimed at preventing a recurrence of sustained VT or VF. It may include treating the underlying cause, administering antidysrhythmic medications, performing ablation of the reentrant pathway within the ventricle, or inserting an implantable cardioverter defibrillator (ICD). Chapter 14 provides more information on ICDs (see Fig. 14.9).

Ventricular Fibrillation

VF is the result of chaotic electrical activity in the ventricles from repetitive, small areas of reentry or a series of rapid discharges from various foci within the ventricular myocardium. This electrical activity causes the ventricles to be unable to contract completely and effectively. The ventricles merely quiver, and no forward flow of blood occurs. Without forward flow, no palpable pulse or audible apical heart tones are present. Clinically, VF can be indistinguishable from asystole (absence of electrical activity). On the ECG, VF appears as a continuous, undulating pattern without clear P waves, QRS complexes, or T waves (Fig. 12.74). When VF occurs in the setting of an acute ischemic event and is accompanied by a significant amount of myocardial damage, the survival rate is poor. Resuscitation is often unsuccessful; recurrence rates are high for patients who are resuscitated. VF is seen on the ECG as large, erratic undulations of the baseline (coarse VF) or as a mild tremor (fine VF). In VF, the patient does not have a pulse, no blood is being pumped forward, and defibrillation is the only definitive therapy. Defibrillation is more likely to be successful with coarse VF. The American Heart Association ACLS protocol should be followed. As with any cardiac arrest situation, supportive measures such as cardiopulmonary resuscitation, intubation, and correction of metabolic abnormalities are performed concurrently with definitive therapy.

Differential Diagnosis of Wide QRS Complex Tachycardia

Wide complex tachycardias may be caused by a variety of mechanisms (Table 12.14). VT is the most common reason for a sudden-onset wide complex tachycardia; however, an atypical SVT with an ectopic atrial or junctional focus arising from an irritable site above the ventricles may also be the cause. Typical SVT has a narrow QRS complex (less than 0.12 second duration) because the electrical impulse enters the ventricle through the AV node and continues down the normal conduction pathway by means of the bundle branches through the ventricles. VT always has a wide QRS complex (longer than 0.12 second) because the impulse begins somewhere within the ventricles and depolarization is slower, moving from cell to cell, without the benefit of the usual conduction pathways. Typical SVT versus VT can be determined by QRS complex width alone since SVT results in a narrow QRS whereas VT results in a wide QRS. However, not all SVTs result in a narrow QRS complex. SVT manifests with a wide QRS complex in three situations:

- The patient may have an existing RBBB or LBBB, resulting in a wide QRS rhythm even during sinus rhythm. If the patient develops an atrial or junctional tachycardia, the shape of the BBB is unchanged, and the QRS complex is still wide.
- A supraventricular impulse may arrive in the ventricles so early that only part of the conduction system is repolarized. In this case, one of the bundle branches is still refractory (unable to conduct), causing the wave of depolarization to spread abnormally (aberrantly) through the ventricles and resulting in a wide QRS complex.
- Occasionally, an anatomic variant occurs in which the patient has a small strip of muscle tissue connecting the atria with the ventricles and bypassing the AV node. This is called an *accessory pathway* or *bypass tract*, the most common of which occurs in Wolff-Parkinson-White syndrome.[71]

This does not pose a hemodynamic problem in normal sinus rhythm, although it sometimes causes subtle ECG

TABLE 12.14 Differential Diagnosis of Wide–QRS Complex Tachycardia

Mechanism
• Ventricular tachycardia
• SVT with preexisting bundle branch block or intraventricular conduction defect
• SVT with aberrant conduction because of tachycardia (normal QRS when in sinus rhythm)
• SVT with wide QRS related to electrolyte or metabolic disorder
• SVT with conduction over an accessory pathway (preexcitation)
• Paced rhythm
• Artifact

SVT, Supraventricular tachycardia.

From Page RL, Joglar JA, Caldwell MA, et al. 2015 ACC/AHA/HRS guideline for the management of adult patients with supraventricular tachycardia: a report of the American College of Cardiology/American Heart Association Task Force on Clinical Practice Guidelines and the Heart Rhythm Society. *J Am Coll Cardiol*. 2016;67(13):e27–e115.

changes that make it easier to be detected. However, when rapid atrial dysrhythmias occur, they can be conducted directly to a portion of the ventricular myocardium without the normal AV delay. Depolarization through the ventricles then proceeds from cell to cell rather than through the normal and efficient pathway of the conduction system, resulting in a wide QRS complex tachycardia that closely resembles VT.

Significance of Wide QRS Complex Tachycardia

SVT is treated with a variety of medications that work by blocking the AV node conduction pathway: diltiazem, verapamil, amiodarone, or digoxin.[71] However, a problem occurs if the SVT has occurred as a result of the presence of an accessory pathway and the narrow complex tachycardia is treated with verapamil or other medications that block the AV node but do not block the Wolff-Parkinson-White accessory pathway.[71] This can result in an extremely fast wide complex tachycardia through the accessory pathway with acute, severe hypotension or loss of consciousness requiring immediate cardioversion. For this reason, it is important to be sure of the cause of the wide complex tachycardia in individuals who are relatively hemodynamically stable before treatment is initiated.

Regardless of the site of origin, a rapid wide QRS complex tachycardia may not be well tolerated, largely because of the fast HR and decreased CO. Hemodynamic deterioration is evidenced by syncope, severe hypotension, or ischemic symptoms. In this case, emergency external cardioversion must be performed regardless of whether the tachycardia is of ventricular or supraventricular origin. Correct differentiation of a wide QRS complex tachycardia is important for long-term management. Depending on the clinical situation, the patient may require long-term antidysrhythmic therapy. If there is a history of VT or sudden cardiac death and the patient is already on antidysrhythmic therapy, a recurrent episode of VT indicates that the current treatment regimen is not effective, and the therapy needs to be changed.

Clinical Differentiation of VT from SVT

Contrary to popular belief, hemodynamic stability or instability does not help differentiate between VT and SVT with a wide QRS complex. In theory, SVT is better tolerated, especially if atrial contraction is still occurring before each ventricular contraction (AV synchrony). However, clinically this is often variable. VT may be well tolerated, especially if the rate is less than 150 beats/min. Some patients can be in sustained VT for long periods of time without significant hemodynamic compromise. Conversely, because AV synchrony is lost in atrial fibrillation or atrial flutter and the ventricular response rate may be very rapid, ventricular filling and CO can be severely compromised.[71]

The most reliable bedside method of diagnosing a wide QRS complex tachycardia is through careful analysis of the ECG. HR and heart rhythm are evaluated first, although they are not the only diagnostic indicators. The tracing is examined closely for the presence of P waves. If P waves can be identified and they do not correlate on a 1:1 basis with the QRS complexes, AV dissociation exists and strongly suggests VT. Although P waves may be found in any lead, they are generally most readily visible in leads V_1 or II. The shape of the QRS complex in the right precordial lead V_1 and the left precordial lead V_6 can be diagnostic of VT or SVT with aberrant conduction. Table 12.15 summarizes these ECG criteria. If the QRS complex is entirely positive from V_1 through V_6 or entirely negative, this strongly suggests VT. This phenomenon is known as *precordial concordance*.[71]

When the sinus node remains in control of the atria and a ventricular ectopic focus is in control of the ventricles, it is likely that at some point the timing will be coordinated, and, by chance, the sinus impulse will conduct through the AV node and begin to depolarize the ventricles just as the ventricular ectopic focus fires. The resulting QRS complex is a fusion beat (see Fig. 12.73), which resembles a blend of the patient's normal QRS complex and the wide QRS complex of the ventricular dysrhythmia. The presence of fusion beats also strongly suggests VT.

Atrioventricular Blocks

On the ECG, the ability of the AV node to conduct is evaluated by measuring the PR interval and the relationship of P waves to QRS complexes (Table 12.16). The normal PR interval, measured from the beginning of the P wave to the beginning of the QRS complex, ranges from 0.12 to 0.20 second. When the normal conduction of the AV node is impaired, the PR interval will be greater than 0.2 second, resulting in a heart block.

First-Degree Atrioventricular Block

When all atrial impulses are conducted to the ventricles and the PR interval is greater than 0.20 second, a condition known as *first-degree AV block* exists (Fig. 12.75). First-degree AV block can be chronic or acute, and it may be caused by a multitude of conditions. Chronic first-degree block may occur related to fibrosis and sclerosis of the conduction system, lack of blood supply to the conduction system secondary to coronary artery disease (CAD), valvular heart disease, myocarditis, and various cardiomyopathies. First-degree heart block that develops acutely is of much greater concern. Causes include medication toxicity related to digoxin, beta-blockers, or amiodarone administration; acute myocardial ischemia or MI; hyperkalemia; edema after valvular heart surgery; and increased vagal tone. If the associated QRS complex is narrow, it is likely that the only conduction abnormality is in the AV node. However, if the associated QRS complex is widened, it is likely that there is also damage to the bundle branches as a result of sclerosis, ischemia, or infarction.

Second-Degree Atrioventricular Block

Second-degree AV block can be broadly defined as a condition in which some atrial impulses are conducted to the ventricles, but others are "blocked" at the AV node. This description of intermittent AV conduction covers two patterns with markedly different clinical significance: Second-degree AV block is divided into Mobitz type I (also known as *Wenckebach block*) and Mobitz type II.

TABLE 12.15 Electrocardiographic Criteria to Differentiate Ventricular Tachycardia From Supraventricular Tachycardia in Wide-Complex Tachycardia

Findings or Leads on Electrocardiogram Assessed	Interpretation
QRS complex in leads V1-V6 (Brugada criteria)	Lack of any R-S complexes implies VT. R-S interval (onset of R wave to nadir of S wave) >100 ms in any precordial lead implies VT.
QRS complex in aVR (Vereckei algorithm)	Presence of initial R wave implies VT. Initial R or Q wave >40 ms implies VT. Presence of a notch on the descending limb at the onset of a predominantly negative QRS implies VT.
AV dissociation[a]	Presence of AV dissociation (with ventricular rate faster than atrial rate) or fusion complexes implies VT
QRS complexes in precordial leads all positive or all negative (concordant)	Implies VT
QRS in tachycardia that is identical to sinus rhythm	Suggests SVT
R-wave peak time in lead II	R-wave peak time ≥50 ms suggests VT

[a]AV dissociation is also a component of the Brugada criteria.
AV, Atrioventricular; *SVT*, supraventricular tachycardia; *VT*, ventricular tachycardia.
From Page RL, Joglar JA, Caldwell MA, et al. 2015. ACC/AHA/HRS guideline for the management of adult patients with supraventricular tachycardia: a report of the American College of Cardiology/American Heart Association Task Force on Clinical Practice Guidelines and the Heart Rhythm Society. *J Am Coll Cardiol.* 2016;67(13):e27–e115.

Mobitz Type I

In Mobitz type I block, the AV conduction times progressively lengthen until a P wave is not conducted. This typically occurs in a pattern of *grouped beats* and is observed on the ECG by a gradual lengthening of the PR interval, until ultimately the final P wave in the group fails to conduct. In Mobitz type I, the QRS complex is generally of normal width and appearance. Several criteria must be present for Mobitz I (Wenckebach) to be diagnosed, as follows:

1. The sinus node is functional and generates impulses that conduct to the AV node at a constant rate. On the ECG, the measured P-P interval is regular.
2. As each successive atrial impulse arrives earlier into the *relative refractory period* of the impaired AV node, more time is needed to conduct the impulse. On the ECG, this is seen as an incremental increase in the length of each PR interval. The R-R interval usually becomes shorter with each beat.
3. The PR interval is shortest in the first beat.
   a. The initial PR interval is often, but not always, of normal length. If first-degree block coexists, the initial PR interval will be prolonged, but this initial P-R interval will still have the shortest measured interval of the group.
   b. The initial PR interval is shorter, because the AV node has had enough time to fully repolarize secondary to the final nonconducted P wave in the group, as subsequently described.
4. The final P wave of the group is not conducted. The atrial impulse arrives during the absolute refractory period of the AV node and is not conducted. This is seen on the ECG by a P wave that is *not* followed by a QRS complex (Fig. 12.76).

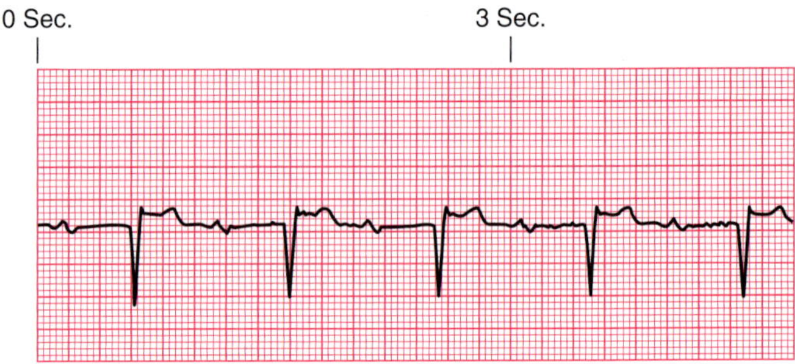

FIG. 12.75 First-Degree Atrioventricular Block. The PR interval is prolonged to 0.44 s.

TABLE 12.16 Atrioventricular Block

Parameter	First-Degree	Second-Degree Mobitz I (Wenckebach)	Second-Degree Mobitz II	Third-Degree (Complete)
PR interval	>0.20 s and constant	Increases with each consecutively conducted P wave	Constant	Varies randomly
P waves	1 P wave for each QRS complex	Intermittently not conducted, yielding more P waves than QRS complexes	Intermittently not conducted, yielding more P waves than QRS complexes	P waves independent and not related to QRS complexes
QRS complex	0.06–0.10 s	0.06–0.10 s	May be normal, but usually coexists with BBB (>0.12 s)	0.06–0.10 s if junctional escape pacemaker activates ventricles >0.12 s if ventricular escape pacemaker activates ventricles

BBB, Bundle branch block.

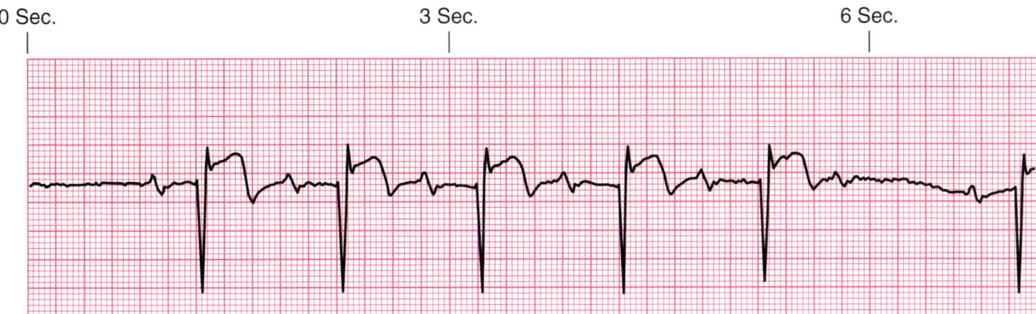

FIG. 12.76 Mobitz type I (Wenckebach) Second-Degree Atrioventricular Block. The PR intervals gradually increase from 0.36 to 0.46 s until a P wave is not conducted to the ventricles.

Mobitz I block has a specific, repeating pattern that catches the eye. The expected groups are 3:2, 4:3, or 5:4. For example, if four P waves are conducted to the ventricles and the fifth one is not, a 5:4 conduction ratio is present (five P waves to four QRS complexes). The nonconducted P wave ends a group. After the pause, the cycle repeats itself.

Mobitz type I does not generally cause significant hemodynamic compromise as long as the ventricular HR is maintained. However, in the presence of ischemia and infarction, it may progress to a more severe level of block. When Mobitz type I occurs in the setting of an acute inferior wall infarction, the patient must be closely monitored and precautionary measures such as placement of a temporary pacemaker may be warranted.

Mobitz Type II

Mobitz type II block is always anatomically located below the AV node in the bundle of His, in the bundle branches, or in the Purkinje fibers. This results in an all-or-nothing situation with respect to AV conduction. When conduction does occur, all PR intervals are the same. Because of the anatomic location of the block, the PR interval is constant and the QRS complexes are wide on the ECG (Fig. 12.77).

Mobitz II block is more ominous clinically than Mobitz I and may progress to complete AV block. If the block involves the Purkinje fibers, an escape rhythm may not develop. For this reason, it is important to prepare for transcutaneous cardiac pacing (TCP), external pacing from outside the chest wall. Consider the possibility that the patient will need a temporary transvenous pacemaker inserted and possibly require a permanent pacemaker before hospital discharge.

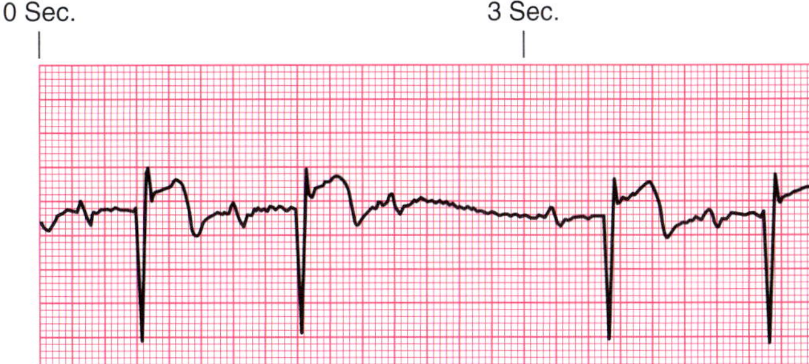

FIG. 12.77 Mobitz Type II Second-Degree Atrioventricular Block. The PR intervals remain constant.

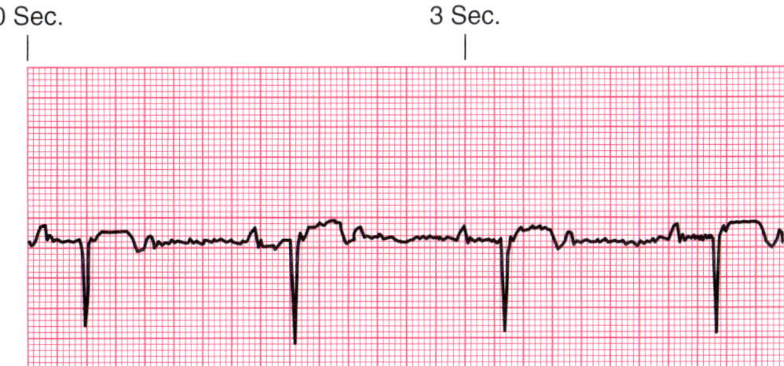

FIG. 12.78 A 2:1 Atrioventricular (AV) Block. Because no two consecutive P waves are conducted, it is impossible to determine with certainty whether this is a Mobitz I or Mobitz II second-degree AV block.

2:1 Conduction

Occasionally, only every other P wave is conducted through the AV node (Fig. 12.78). This pattern may indicate Mobitz type I or Mobitz type II, because consecutive conduction of P waves, which reveal a lengthening or constant PR interval, does not occur. In Mobitz I, the conduction ratios may have decreased from 4:3 to 3:2 to 2:1, but the site and type of block have not changed. The change in conduction ratio may be caused by an increase in atrial rate, or it may change spontaneously.

In 2:1 conduction, it is impossible to be certain whether the block is Mobitz type I or type II from the ECG. If it occurs along with other Mobitz I ratios, it is probably still Mobitz I. If it is an isolated occurrence with no other strips for comparison, the QRS complex width and the PR interval offer valuable clues to the site of the block. In Mobitz I, the QRS complex is usually normal, and the PR interval is usually prolonged. In Mobitz II, the QRS complex is usually wide, and the PR interval is usually normal. During an acute inferior MI, Mobitz type I AV block with 2:1 conduction is much more common than type II.

Third-Degree Atrioventricular Block

Third-degree, or complete, AV block is a condition in which no atrial impulses can conduct from the atria to the ventricles. This condition is also described by the terms *complete heart block* or *AV dissociation* to indicate that different cardiac pacemakers control the atrial rate and the ventricular rate. The block can be located at the level of the AV node or below the node within the bundle of His or the bundle branches. It can be caused by infarction, digitalis toxicity, or age-related degeneration of the conduction system in older patients. It is hoped that a junctional focus or ventricular focus depolarizes spontaneously at its intrinsic rate of 20 to 40 beats/min and that ventricular contraction continues. Pacemaker support is often necessary to maintain an adequate CO.

On the ECG, P waves are present and usually occur at regular intervals. If a junctional focus is pacing the heart, normal QRS complexes are present but occur at a rate and timing interval totally independent of the P waves. The PR intervals vary widely, because the P wave and QRS complex are not related to each other. If a ventricular focus is pacing the heart, the QRS complex is wide and unrelated to the P waves (Fig. 12.79).

Management of Atrioventricular Block

Clinically, the consequences of AV block range from benign to life threatening. First-degree AV block is seldom of immediate concern but requires close observation for progression of the conduction disturbance. Second-degree Mobitz I (Wenckebach) is usually benign as long as the patient is not bradycardic. If hemodynamic compromise is present or deemed likely, a temporary pacemaker can be inserted prophylactically. Second-degree Mobitz II is more serious and often precedes complete AV block. Use of a temporary pacemaker is recommended, but its insertion can be elective if the patient remains hemodynamically stable. Complete heart block causes AV dissociation and is associated with a low CO that requires use of a pacemaker.

LABORATORY TESTS

Laboratory assessment of cardiovascular status is obtained through studies of blood serum. Accurate interpretation of these laboratory studies, along with the clinical picture, enables the critical care team to diagnose, treat, and assess the response to therapeutic interventions.

Laboratory studies of blood serum are performed to assess the following:

1. Electrolyte levels that can alter cardiac muscle contraction
2. Cardiac biomarkers that reflect myocardial cellular integrity or infarction
3. Hematologic status to evaluate risk of anemia and infection
4. Coagulation times
5. Serum lipid levels
6. Status of other organ systems that can secondarily affect cardiac function

Electrolytes

Potassium

During depolarization and repolarization of nerve and muscle fiber, potassium and sodium exchange occurs intracellularly and extracellularly. The potassium gradient across the cell membrane determines conduction velocity and helps confine pacing activity to the sinus node. Excess or deficiency of potassium can alter myocardial muscle function. If alterations in potassium level are suspected, serum potassium levels must be drawn. Normal serum potassium (K^+) levels are generally 3.5 to 4.5 mEq/L, although definitions may vary slightly between institutions. Table 12.17 lists electrolyte values that affect cardiac contractility.

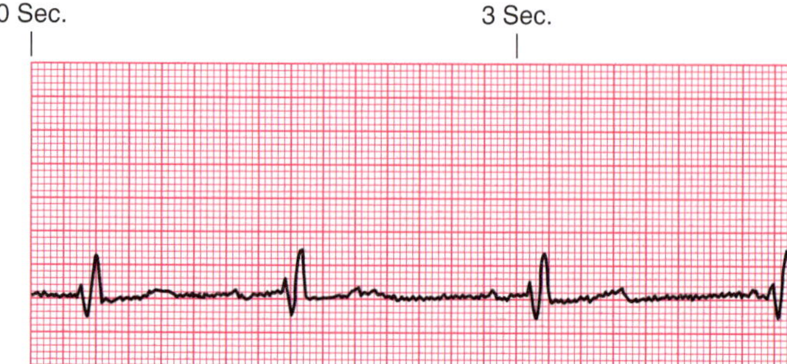

FIG. 12.79 Third-Degree (Complete) Heart Block.

Hyperkalemia

Elevated serum potassium (higher than 4.5 mEq/L), called *hyperkalemia*, can be caused by various conditions, including excess potassium administration, extensive skeletal muscle destruction (rhabdomyolysis), tumor lysis syndrome, and kidney failure. Some medications may induce hyperkalemia, including potassium-sparing diuretics, angiotensin-converting enzyme inhibitors, and angiotensin-receptor blockers.[84]

Hyperkalemia can elicit significant changes in the ECG because it decreases AV conduction velocity, slows ventricular depolarization, and accelerates repolarization. As the serum levels of potassium rise, tall, narrow peaked T waves may be seen and are followed by prolongation of the PR interval, loss of the P wave, widening of the QRS complex, heart block, and eventually asystole (Fig. 12.80A). Severely elevated serum potassium (greater than 8 mEq/L) causes a wide QRS complex tachycardia, as shown in the 12-lead ECG in Fig. 12.80B. If not corrected, severe hyperkalemia can lead to VF or cardiac standstill. Evidence of hyperkalemia is not always visible on the ECG, and research has shown that ECG waveform changes are not a sensitive indicator of elevated potassium levels.

Extreme hyperkalemia can be acutely managed with IV insulin to drive the potassium inside the cell and temporarily out of the plasma. Glucose must be administered at the same time to avoid hypoglycemia as a secondary complication. Potassium is permanently removed from the bloodstream by cation-exchange resin products, such as sodium polystyrene sulfonate (Kayexalate), placed into the gastrointestinal tract or is removed directly from the blood by hemodialysis.[85] Coexisting low serum sodium, calcium, or pH levels potentiate the cardiac effects of hyperkalemia.

Hypokalemia

A low serum potassium level, called *hypokalemia* (less than 3.5 mEq/L), is commonly caused by diuretic therapy with

TABLE 12.17 Electrolyte Values That Affect Cardiac Contractility and Conduction

	NORMAL RANGES[a]		
Electrolyte	mEq/L	mg/dL	mmol/L
Potassium (K^+)	3.5–4.5		3.50–4.50
Ionized calcium (Ca)		4.0–5.0	1.00–1.30
Total calcium (Ca^{2+})		8.5–10.5	2.00–2.60
Magnesium (Mg^{2+})	1.5–2.0	1.8–2.4	0.70–1.10

[a]Laboratory values may be reported as mEq/L, mg/dL, or mmol/L. Each measurement parameter used produces a different value. Some electrolytes are reported with more than one reference value. Different clinical laboratories use different reference values, and the cited reference values may vary slightly between hospital laboratories.

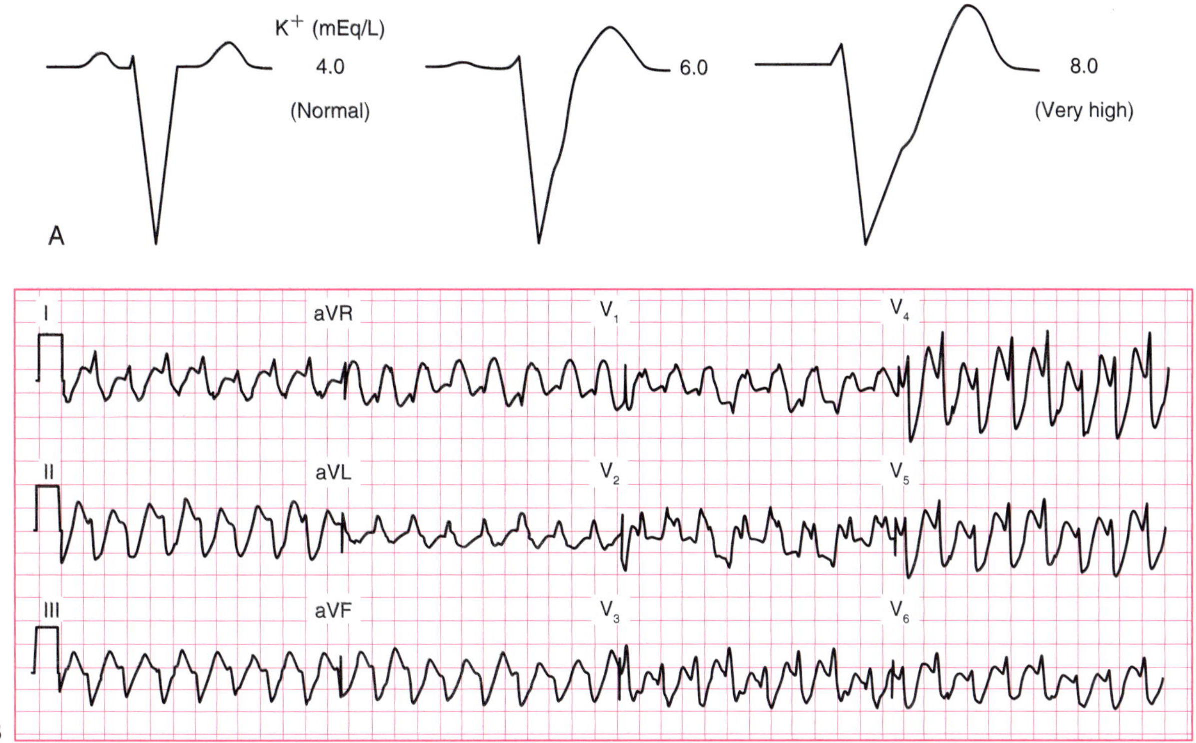

FIG. 12.80 Effects of Hyperkalemia on an Electrocardiogram (ECG). (A) Stages in hyperkalemia from normal potassium levels to plasma levels of 8 mEq/L. At approximately 6 mEq/L, the P wave flattens, the QRS complex broadens, and the ST segment disappears, with the S wave flowing into the tall, tented T wave. (B) A 12-lead ECG of a patient with a serum potassium level of 9.1 mEq/L.

insufficient replacement, gastrointestinal losses, and some medications.[85] Hypokalemia is also reflected by changes on the ECG (Fig. 12.81). The earliest ECG change is often PVCs, which can deteriorate into VT or VF without appropriate potassium replacement.

Hypokalemia impairs myocardial conduction and prolongs ventricular repolarization; this can be seen by a prominent U wave (a positive deflection after the T wave on the ECG). The U wave is not totally unique to hypokalemia, but its presence is a signal for the clinician to check the serum potassium level. Serum potassium levels must be closely monitored and replacement administered as needed. Great care must be taken with administration of concentrated electrolytes to prevent complications. Potassium is a high-alert medication, and additional safety procedures are recommended for replacement of this electrolyte (Box 12.12).

Calcium

Calcium (Ca^{2+}) is an important cation in the body. Calcium metabolism is controlled by many factors, including normal parathyroid hormone function, calcitonin, and vitamin D acting on target organs such as the kidney, bone, and gastrointestinal tract. Calcium is an important mediator of many cardiovascular functions because of its effect on vascular tone, myocardial contractility, and cardiac excitability.

Serum calcium values can be recorded in three ways, depending on the hospital laboratory: milliequivalents per liter (mEq/L), milligrams per deciliter (mg/dL), or millimoles per liter (mmol/L). In the bloodstream, approximately 50% of calcium is biologically active, known as *ionized calcium*.[86] The remaining calcium is bound to protein (primarily albumin) and inorganic ions such as sulfate and phosphate. Calcium is not biologically active in its bound state.[86] The normal values for total and ionized serum calcium levels are listed in Table 12.17. The normal serum concentration of ionized calcium is maintained within very narrow limits; changes in ionized calcium level are responsible for the clinical effects of hypercalcemia and hypocalcemia. The only accurate way to determine the level of ionized calcium, described as *physiologically active, unbound,* or *free,* is to measure the ionized serum value with a laboratory assay.[86] The mathematically calculated values that extrapolate ionized calcium from total calcium and serum albumin levels have been shown to be inaccurate and should not be used with critically ill patients.[86]

Hypercalcemia

Hypercalcemia is defined as increased amounts of ionized calcium (greater than 4.8 mg/dL or 1.30 mmol/L) or increased amounts of total serum calcium (greater than 10.5 mg/dL or 2.60 mmol/L). Serum calcium levels are increased by bone tumors; primary hyperparathyroidism caused by elevated parathyroid hormone levels; excessive intake of supplemental calcium and vitamin D, usually in oral antacids; hypomagnesemia; and as a complication of kidney failure from decreased excretion of calcium. Hypercalcemia affects many organs; causes smooth muscle relaxation; and can lead to neurologic changes such as lethargy, confusion, and even coma. Cardiovascular effects of elevated serum calcium include

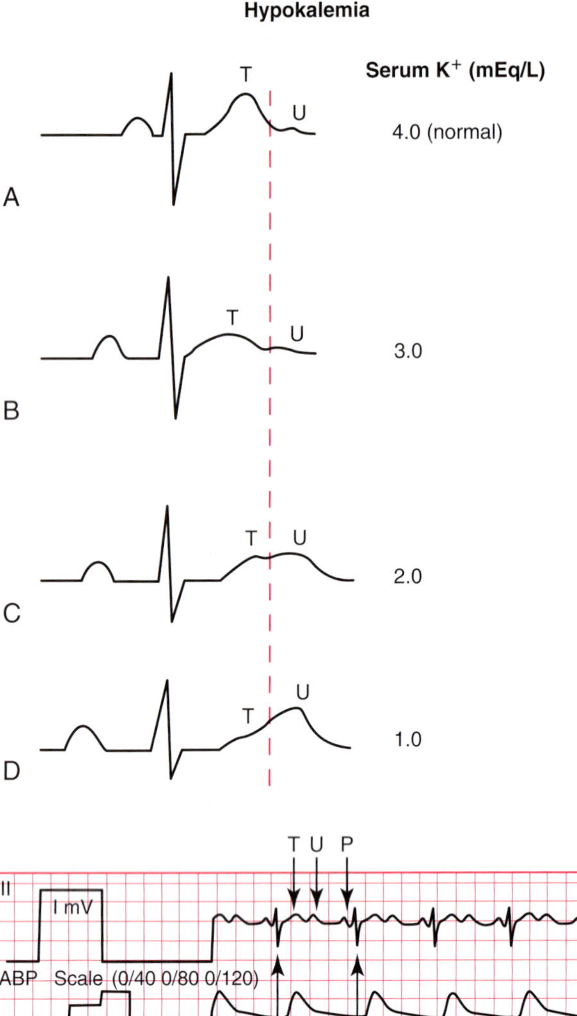

FIG. 12.81 Effects of Hypokalemia on an Electrocardiogram (ECG). (A) At a normal serum concentration of 3.5 to 4.5 mEq/L, the amplitude of the T wave is appreciably greater than that of the U wave. (B) By the time the serum potassium level has decreased to 3 mEq/L, the amplitudes of the T and U waves are approaching each other. (C and D) With a further decrease in the level of potassium, the U wave begins to tower over and fuse with the T wave. (E) ECG tracing from a patient with a serum potassium of 2.6 mEq/L shows a prominent U wave.

strengthening contractility and shortening ventricular repolarization, demonstrated on the ECG by a shortened Q-Tc interval. Rhythm disturbances may include bradycardia; first-degree, second-degree, and third-degree heart block; and BBB. Hypercalcemia can potentiate the effects of digitalis and cause hypertension.[86]

Management of symptomatic hypercalcemia involves promotion of calcium excretion by diuretics and infusion of a large volume of normal saline if tolerated by the heart, lungs, and kidneys. Patients who cannot tolerate this clinical regimen may receive hemodialysis using a low-calcium dialysate.

Hypocalcemia

Hypocalcemia is defined as an ionized calcium level below normal (less than 1.05 mmol/L) or a low total serum calcium level. Hypocalcemia (measured by ionized calcium) is a common finding and was found in 55% of critically ill patients on admission to the critical care unit in one study.[86] The more severe the patient's illness, the greater the risk of developing hypocalcemia.[86] Transfusions of blood from the blood bank lower serum calcium levels, because the citrate used as an anticoagulant in banked blood binds to the calcium.[86] This is called *citrate chelation*. If citrate is used during hemodialysis or plasmapheresis, it has the same calcium-binding (chelating) effect. Phosphate also binds to calcium and can lower the serum calcium level. Metabolic alkalosis often coexists with hypocalcemia. The cardiovascular effects of hypocalcemia include decreased myocardial contractility, decreased CO, and hypotension. Rhythm disturbances with severe hypocalcemia are variable, ranging from bradycardia to VT and asystole. When ionized calcium is low, the ECG may show a prolonged QTc interval (Fig. 12.82). A prolonged QTc predisposes a patient to torsades de pointes.

Management of hypocalcemia, especially when ionized calcium is low, involves infusion of IV calcium chloride or IV calcium gluconate.[86]

- Calcium chloride provides 27 mg of elemental calcium/mL (272 mg in 10 mL).
- Calcium gluconate provides 9 mg of elemental calcium/mL (90 mg in 10 mL).

Magnesium

Magnesium (Mg^{2+}) is essential for many enzyme, protein, lipid, and carbohydrate functions in the body and is critical for the production and use of energy.[87] The body stores most magnesium in bone (50% to 60%), muscle, and soft tissues, with less than 1% present in blood.[87] As with other electrolytes, the ionized portion of serum magnesium is the biologically active component that is available for biochemical processes. Due to limited availability, only 2% of clinical laboratories in the United States measure ionized magnesium; routine blood tests measure total serum magnesium.[87] Serum magnesium can be reported in units of mEq/L, mg/dL, or mmol/L, depending on the laboratory running the analysis. The normal serum range is 1.5 to 2 mEq/L, 1.8 to 2.4 mg/dL, or 0.7 to 1.1 mmol/L. Normal reference values vary between hospital laboratories.

Hypermagnesemia

Hypermagnesemia is generally considered a serum magnesium level above 1.1 mmol/L. While generally considered to be rare in critical care patients, it results from kidney failure, tumor lysis syndrome, or iatrogenic overtreatment. Hypermagnesemia can cause nausea, vomiting, lethargy, headache, or flushing.[87]

Hypomagnesemia

Hypomagnesemia is generally considered as a total serum magnesium concentration less than 0.75 mmol/L. It is commonly associated with other electrolyte imbalances, most notably alterations in potassium, calcium, and phosphorus. Low serum magnesium levels can result from many causes. Aggressive diuresis with loop diuretics can lower serum levels.[87] Diarrhea can be a significant cause of magnesium loss, because lower gastrointestinal fluids contain up to 15 mEq/L of magnesium; vomiting or gastric suction causes less depletion,

BOX 12.12 Safety

Medication Administration

1. Accurate Patient Identification
   - Use at least two patient identifiers (not the patient's room number) when taking blood samples or administering medications or blood products. Examples include the patient's name or date of birth.
2. Effective Communication Among Caregivers
   - An organizational method to decrease the number of medication errors is the use of *computerized physician order entry.*
   - Hospitals should have a process for taking verbal or telephone orders that requires a verification "read back" of the complete order by the person receiving the order.
   - The Institute of Safe Medication Practices (ISMP) maintains a list of medications with similar-sounding names, as name confusion can lead to medication errors. The list is available on the ISMP website at www.ismp.org/tools/confuseddrugnames.pdf. Medication errors can be reported to the **Medication Errors Reporting Program.**
   - Standardize the abbreviations, acronyms, and symbols used throughout the organization, including a list of abbreviations, acronyms, and symbols not to use.
   - Examples of problematic abbreviations include "U" for units and "μg" for micrograms. When handwritten, a capital U can be mistaken for a zero (0); in numerous case reports, an insulin dosage written in U was interpreted as 0. Using the abbreviation "μg" instead of "mcg" for micrograms is also problematic; when handwritten, the Greek letter μ can look like an "m." The error-prone abbreviations list is available on the ISMP website at www.ismp.org/tools/errorproneabbreviations.pdf
   - Use of trailing zeros (e.g., 2.0 versus 2) and use of a leading decimal point without a leading zero (e.g., .2 instead of 0.2) are dangerous prescription-writing practices. Misinterpretation has caused 10-fold dosing errors.

High-Alert Medication Safety

- In the first 2 years after enacting a *sentinel event reporting mechanism,* the most common category was medication errors, and the most frequently implicated medication was KCl.
- The Joint Commission reviewed 10 incidents of patient death resulting from misadministration of KCl. Eight deaths were the result of direct infusion of concentrated KCl. In six of the eight cases, KCl was mistaken for another medication, primarily because of similarities in packaging and labeling. Most often, KCl was mistaken for sodium chloride, heparin, or furosemide (Lasix).
- The Joint Commission suggests that health care organizations *not* make concentrated KCl available outside the pharmacy unless appropriate, specific safeguards are in place.
- Remove concentrated electrolytes (including, but not limited to, potassium chloride [KCl], potassium phosphate, and hypertonic sodium chloride) from patient care units.
- Standardize and limit the number of medication concentrations available in the organization.
- A list of high-alert medications is available on the ISMP website www.ismp.org.

Infusion Pump Safety

- Ensure free-flow protection on all general-use and patient-controlled analgesia intravenous (IV) infusion pumps in the organization.
  - *Free flow* occurs when IV solution flows freely under the force of gravity without being controlled by the infusion pump. Free flow typically occurs after the administration set is temporarily removed from the pump to transfer a patient to another area, change a patient's gown, or place a patient on a radiography table. Clinicians can greatly reduce this risk by using administration sets with set-based anti–free-flow mechanisms that prevent gravity free flow by closing off the IV tubing to prohibit flow when the administration set is removed from the pump.

Hospital Safety

- The Joint Commission develops Hospital National Patient Safety Goals each year that incorporate medication safety requirements.

because upper gastrointestinal fluids contain approximately 1 mEq/L. Another cause of magnesium depletion is rapid administration of citrated blood products, which results in citrate chelation. Insufficient dietary magnesium intake and chronic alcohol abuse are also risk factors. Hypomagnesemia can also occur in patients who take proton-pump inhibitor medications to reduce production of gastric acid. This condition improves when the proton-pump inhibitors are stopped. In chronic hypomagnesemia, serum levels are replenished from the bone stores.[87]

In hypomagnesemia, the ECG changes are similar to changes seen with hypokalemia and hypocalcemia: prolonged PR and QTc intervals, presence of U waves, T wave flattening, and widened QRS complex. Cardiac dysrhythmias may be supraventricular or ventricular and include the polymorphic ventricular rhythm torsades de pointes. In cardiac arrest with pulseless VT with torsade de pointes, protocol is to administer IV magnesium, 1 to 2 g diluted in 10 mL solution (5% dextrose or normal saline), over 15 minutes.[88] It is important to evaluate kidney function when administering magnesium to avoid precipitating hypermagnesium states.

Cardiac Biomarker Studies

Cardiac Biomarkers in Acute Coronary Syndrome

Cardiac biomarkers are the factors, hormones, and proteins released from damaged myocardial cells.[89] When myocardial cells are damaged, they release detectable proteins into the bloodstream, so an increase in biomarkers can be correlated with heart muscle injury. The biomarkers that are routinely measured include cardiac troponin I and cardiac troponin T. Table 12.18 summarizes the cardiac biomarkers related to myocardial injury and MI.

Troponin T and Troponin I

Cardiac troponins are the most specific and sensitive biomarkers of myocardial ischemia or necrosis. There are three isoforms of cardiac troponins: I, C, and T. The elevation of troponin I and troponin T occurs 3 to 6 hours after acute myocardial damage.[89] Troponin levels are measured at symptom onset in the hospital or upon arrival to the emergency department. Serial troponin values are measured at time intervals per institutional protocol until values peak.

Because troponin I is found only in cardiac muscle, it is a highly specific biomarker for myocardial damage. The advantage to using a more sensitive biomarker test is that more patients with ACS will be identified, although this will not eliminate the requirement for astute clinical assessment because of the many other conditions associated with elevated troponin levels.[64] A negative high-sensitivity troponin result eliminates acute MI as a diagnosis in 99% of cases.[64]

Natriuretic Peptide Biomarkers in Heart Failure

Natriuretic peptides are biomarkers that provide additional information for accurate evaluation of a patient with acute shortness of breath.[89] It can be difficult to identify whether a patient with shortness of breath has a primary pulmonary problem or has symptoms of acute heart failure with pulmonary edema. In decompensated heart failure, ventricular distention from volume overload, or pressure overload, causes myocytes in the ventricle to release B-type natriuretic peptide (BNP). Several laboratory assays are commercially available to measure BNP, including a point-of-care test, a central laboratory test for BNP, and a laboratory test to measure the N-terminal fragment of proBNP (NT-proBNP).[89] BNP has a half-life of approximately

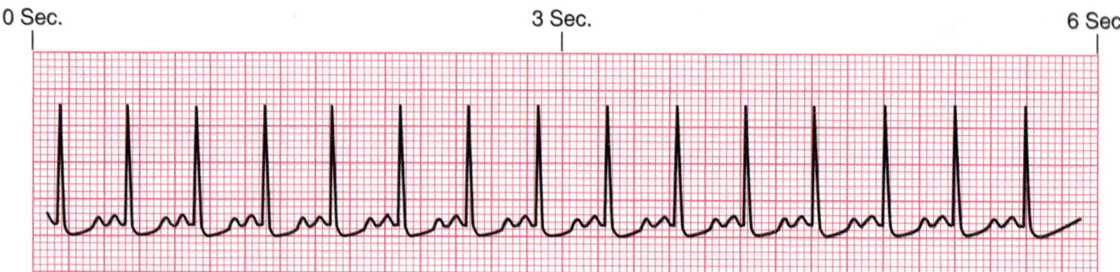

FIG. 12.82 Abnormal QT Prolongation in a Hypocalcemic Patient. A 50-year-old woman was admitted to the critical care unit with a diagnosis of alcoholic liver disease and malnourishment. Total calcium concentration is 5.1 mg/dL, and the albumin level is 1.3 mg/dL. The QT interval (0.55 s) is markedly prolonged for the heart rate (HR) (100 beats/min). The QT interval varies with the HR and can be corrected ($Q–T_c$) as if the HR were 60 beats/min using the formula $\sqrt{QT / RR} = Q - T_c$. The $Q–T_c$ should be 0.44 s or less. The $Q–T_c$ in the ECG tracing shown is 0.55 s. Hypocalcemia lengthens ventricular repolarization. A quick method for assessing the QT interval is to remember that it is usually less than half of the R-R interval. If it is more than one-half of the R-R interval, it is prolonged. (From Yucha CB, Toto KH. Calcium and phosphorus derangements. *Crit Care Nurs Clin North Am*. 1994;6[4]:747.)

TABLE 12.18 Serum Biomarkers After Acute Myocardial Infarction

Serum Biomarker	Time to Initial Elevation (hours[a])	Peak Elevation[b] (ha)	Return to Baseline (days[a])
Cardiac troponin I	3–12	24	5–10
Cardiac troponin T	3–12	12–48	5–14
CK-MB[c]	3–12	24	2–3

[a]Time periods represent average reported values.
[b]Does not include patients who have had reperfusion therapy.
[c]The creatine kinase *(CK)* enzyme consists of two subunits, the brain type *(B)* and the muscle type *(M)*.

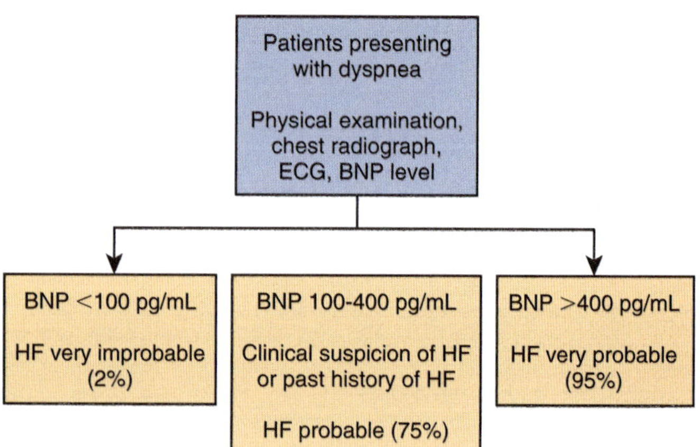

FIG. 12.83 Brain Natriuretic Peptide *(BNP)* Algorithm in the Diagnosis of Heart Failure *(HF)*.

20 minutes, whereas NT-proBNP has a longer half-life of 1 to 2 hours.

With greater ventricular wall stress, more natriuretic peptide is released from the myocardium, reflected as an elevated BNP/NT-proBNP blood level. This value is combined with the physical examination, 12-lead ECG, and chest radiograph to increase the accuracy of heart failure diagnosis (Fig. 12.83). The choice of test generally depends on what is available in the hospital clinical laboratory.

B-Type Natriuretic Peptide

A symptomatic patient with a BNP level less than 100 pg/mL is unlikely to be in heart failure. Conversely, a patient with a BNP level greater than 400 pg/dL is almost definitely in heart failure. BNP is an excellent test to rule out acute heart failure. The challenge lies in interpreting the results of patients with a BNP level of 100 to 400 pg/mL, sometimes described as the *gray zone* (see Fig. 12.83). This gray zone highlights the importance of using a spectrum of clinical and diagnostic tests. As the symptoms of heart failure are successfully treated, the BNP level usually decreases toward the normal range.

N-Terminal Fragment of Pro-B-Type Natriuretic Peptide

A symptomatic patient with a NT-proBNP below 300 pg/mL is unlikely to be in heart failure. Notably, NT-proBNP is often stratified by age, and threshold values may vary by clinical laboratory. For example, in a patient younger than 50 years, a NT-proBNP level of 450 pg/mL suggests heart failure. In a patient older than 50 years, the threshold for heart failure rises to 900 pg/mL. In a patient older than 75 years, the NT-proBNP threshold as an indicator of heart failure rises to 1800 pg/mL.

There are some caveats to the use of natriuretic peptides as biomarkers principally because they are not unique to the heart. Natriuretic peptides are also released from the endothelium and from the kidney, and this can alter the measured BNP levels. Filtration by the kidney is one of the mechanisms by which BNP is cleared from the bloodstream. BNP levels are higher in patients with kidney failure, especially if the glomerular filtration rate is less than 60 mL/min/1.7 m^2.

Hematologic Studies

Hematologic laboratory studies that are routinely ordered for the management of patients with altered cardiovascular status are RBC or erythrocyte level, hemoglobin level, hematocrit level, and white blood cell (WBC) or leukocyte level.

Red Blood Cells

The normal amount of RBCs in a person varies between males and females, and is also influenced by age, exposure to high altitudes, and exercise. Men produce 4.5 to 6 million RBCs/mm^3, whereas the normal level for women is 4 to 5.5 million RBCs/mm^3. Anemia is the clinical condition that occurs when insufficient RBCs are available to carry oxygen to the tissues. Polycythemia is the condition that occurs when excess RBCs are produced.

Hemoglobin. Hemoglobin is a measure of the oxygen carrying capacity of the red blood cells. Hemoglobin levels normally range from 14 to 18 g/dL in men and from 12 to 16 g/dL in women.

Hematocrit. The hematocrit is the volume percentage of RBCs in whole blood. The value is 40% to 54% for men and 38% to 48% for women.

White Blood Cells

Most inflammatory processes that produce necrotic tissue within the heart muscle, such as rheumatic fever, endocarditis, and MI, increase the WBC, or leukocyte, level. The WBC level also increases in response to infection. The normal WBC level for men and women is 5000 to 10,000 cells/mm^3.

Platelets

The normal platelet count is 150,000 to 400,000 cells/mm^3. Less commonly, the normal platelet count range is written as 150 to 400×10^9/L. There is no routine test available that can evaluate platelet functionality. The reported lab value is simply a total count of platelets. Platelets are important because they are the first cells to be activated when the coagulation system is stimulated. Many medications inhibit platelet function and make the platelets "slippery" so that they do not clump together to activate the clotting process. The antiplatelet action of a medication sometimes is its intended role, such as with aspirin used to prevent ACS, or it can be an unintended side effect. A low platelet count is called *thrombocytopenia.*

Blood Coagulation Studies

Coagulation studies are ordered to evaluate the function of the clotting cascade in the body. Depending on the clinical scenario, clinicians may need to support anticoagulating the blood, or supporting coagulation; therefore, anticoagulants and clotting factors are often administered in critical care units. It is essential to understand the laboratory tests that are used to monitor the effectiveness of therapeutic anticoagulation.

Prothrombin Time

Prothrombin time (PT) evaluates the function of the extrinsic coagulation pathway and is the time necessary for the sample to form a clot. Normal PT varies between laboratories but is generally considered to be between 11 to 13 seconds. Because of the lack of standardization of PT between laboratories, the result of this test is reported with the standardized international normalized ratio (INR).[90] For patients on warfarin (Coumadin) therapy, it is the INR, not direct PT, that is used to determine the dosages of warfarin (Coumadin) necessary to achieve therapeutic anticoagulation.

International Normalized Ratio

The INR was developed by the World Health Organization (WHO) in 1982 to standardize PT results among clinical laboratories worldwide. Target INR range for therapeutic anticoagulation with warfarin is 2 to 3 (also in Table 12.19).[91]

Activated Partial Thromboplastin Time

The activated partial thromboplastin time (aPTT) evaluates the function of the intrinsic coagulation pathway and is used to measure the effectiveness of IV or subcutaneous unfractionated heparin therapy or direct oral anticoagulants.[91] Therapy using subcutaneous low-molecular-weight heparin does not require monitoring with aPTT because lower levels of plasma protein binding mean the aPTT is not prolonged, regardless of therapeutic status. Normal aPTT varies between laboratories but is generally considered to be between 25 and 35 seconds.

Activated Clotting Time

The activated clotting time (ACT) is a point-of-care test that is performed outside of the laboratory setting in areas such as the cardiac catheterization laboratory, operating room, or critical care unit. Normal and therapeutic values for ACT coagulation studies are shown in Table 12.19.

Anti-Factor Xa Assay

For patients in whom aPTT may not be accurate due to physiologic factors (clotting factor deficiencies, liver disease, kidney impairment, obesity, and lupus, among others), anti-Factor Xa monitoring may provide more accurate assessment of anticoagulation status. Anti-Factor Xa measures plasma heparin levels and may be used to monitor unfractionated heparin. Therapeutic ranges for anti-Factor Xa for unfractionated heparin are 0.3 to 0.7 IU/mL.[92]

Serum Lipid Studies

Four primary blood lipid levels are important in evaluating an individual's risk of developing or having progression of CAD: total cholesterol, low-density lipoprotein cholesterol (LDL-C), triglycerides, and high-density lipoprotein cholesterol (HDL-C). When levels of cholesterol low-density lipoproteins (LDLs) and triglycerides are elevated or the level of high-density lipoproteins (HDLs) is low, the patient is considered at risk for developing or having progression of CAD and is offered intensive interventions involving diet therapy, exercise prescription, and medication therapy.[93] More information on cholesterol management with CAD is provided in Chapter 13. The following lipid biomarkers are commonly ordered together as a "lipid panel."

Total Cholesterol

Cholesterol is a type of lipid (sterol) that is present in cell membranes, is produced by the liver, and is a precursor of bile

TABLE 12.19 Normal and Therapeutic Coagulation Values

Test	Normal Value	Therapeutic Anticoagulant Target Value
INR	<1.0	2.0–3.0
aPTT	28–38 s	1.5–2.5 × normal
PTT	60–90 s	1.5–2.0 × normal
ACT[a]	0–120 s	150–300 s
Anti-Xa	0	0.35–0.7 IU/mL for unfractionated heparin 0.5–1.0 IU/mL for low-molecular-weight heparin

[a]ACT is normal, but therapeutic values may vary with type of activator used.
ACT, Activated coagulation time; *aPPT,* activated partial thromboplastin time; *INR,* international normalized ratio; *PTT,* partial thromboplastin time.

acids and steroid hormones. The cholesterol level in the blood is determined partly by genetics and partly by acquired factors such as diet, calorie balance, and level of physical activity. Cholesterol in excess amounts (greater than 200 mg/dL) in the serum accelerates the progression of atherosclerosis (atherogenesis).

Low-Density Lipoproteins

Approximately 60% to 70% of the total serum cholesterol is carried in the bloodstream, complexed as LDL-C. The LDL-C and total serum cholesterol levels are directly correlated with risk for CAD, and high levels of each are significant predictors of future acute MI in individuals with established coronary artery atherosclerosis. LDL-C is the major atherogenic lipoprotein and is the primary target for cholesterol-lowering efforts.[93] Guidelines recommend maintaining an LDL-C level below 130 mg/dL for a patient with no history of atherosclerotic disease. A patient with known CAD but who is not high risk should aim for an LDL-C level below 100 mg/dL. The recommended target LDL-C level for high-risk patients with CAD or diabetes is 70 mg/dL.[93]

Very-Low-Density Lipoproteins and Triglycerides

Very-low-density lipoproteins contain 10% to 15% of the total serum cholesterol along with most of the triglycerides in fasting serum.

High-Density Lipoproteins

HDLs are particles that carry 20% to 30% of the total serum cholesterol. Although higher levels of HDL seem to carry a relation to reduced atherosclerotic risk, the evidence is not currently conclusive.[94]

Triglycerides

Triglycerides are another form of lipid in the bloodstream that is normally included in the lipid assessment panel. Current guidelines recommend beginning medical management for triglyceride levels greater than 150 mg/dL.[93] Elevated triglyceride levels are associated with diabetes mellitus and an increased risk of atherosclerotic disease.

CARDIAC DIAGNOSTIC PROCEDURES

Cardiac Catheterization and Coronary Arteriography

Cardiac catheterization and coronary arteriography are routine diagnostic procedures for patients with known or suspected heart disease. Clinical indications for cardiac catheterization include ACS, positive findings on noninvasive cardiac stress testing or imaging, after cardiac arrest with unclear etiology, pulmonary hypertension, pericardial disease, heart failure with a history suggestive of CAD, cardiomyopathy or valvular heart disease, and congenital heart disease. Cardiac catheterization is also common as part of the perioperative evaluation before cardiac and noncardiac surgery. Cardiac catheterization is used to describe anatomic and hemodynamic findings and to provide a baseline for medical or surgical therapy.[95–97]

Left-Heart Catheterization

During catheterization of the left side of the heart, hemodynamic pressure measurements are taken in the aortic root, the left ventricle, and the left atrium. Access is obtained via the radial, brachial, or femoral artery.[98] Radiopaque contrast dye is used to visualize the left ventricle (ventriculogram). This information is also used to calculate the LV ejection fraction. The coronary arteries are visualized, and contrast dye is injected directly into each arterial system. The general term for vessel imaging is *angiogram* (veins and arteries), but the more specific term used to describe visualization of the coronary arteries is *arteriogram.*

Right-Heart Catheterization

Catheterization of the right side of the heart is performed using a thermodilution PA catheter. Access is obtained via the brachial, IJ, or femoral vein. Information obtained includes hemodynamic pressure measurements in the right atrium, the right ventricle, the PA, and the PA occlusion wedge position, as well as the measurement of CO, calculated hemodynamic values, and oxygen saturations. An angiogram of the right-heart chambers using radiopaque contrast dye may also be performed.

Cardiac Catheterization Procedure

Before catheterization, the patient meets with the cardiologist to discuss the purpose, benefits, and risks of the study. For many patients, cardiac catheterization is the first major invasive procedure after a diagnosis of possible heart disease. The patient is often very anxious and has many questions. It is important that nursing and medical staff fully address patients' questions about the catheterization experience.

The morning of the procedure the patient fasts, except for ingesting prescribed cardiac medications.[98] Anticoagulants are usually held before the procedure per institutional protocols that are based on the type of anticoagulant, the patient's renal function, the catheter insertion site, and whether venous and/or arterial access is required.[98] If there is a history of allergy to contrast dye, an antihistamine and corticosteroid may be administered to prevent any adverse reactions. Procedural sedation is often given to keep patients comfortable and able to lie still during the procedure.[98] Throughout the cardiac catheterization, the patient remains awake and able to respond. He or she is positioned on a hard table with a C-shaped camera arm overhead or to the side. This arm can be positioned to view the heart from several different angles.

Cardiac catheterization catheters, which are available in a variety of designs and sizes, are placed in the vein or artery after the patient receives a local anesthetic. The choice of catheter and location is based on the cardiologist's experience and the diagnostic study required. The femoral, radial, or brachial artery is used to catheterize the left side of the heart, including the coronary arteries. The brachial, femoral, or IJ vein can be used as the access vessel to pass catheters to the right side of the heart. During the study, the patient receives heparin systemically to reduce the risk of emboli. Many patients also receive nitroglycerin to control chest pain, particularly when the coronary arteries are full of contrast material during the coronary arteriographic procedure. The patient may also experience bradycardia or hypotension at this time. To move the contrast dye more quickly and minimize the vagal effect on HR and blood pressure, the patient may be asked to cough. If bradycardia persists, atropine or occasionally a transvenous pacemaker may be used. If hypotension continues, IV fluids are administered as a bolus. These reactions are rare and occur less frequently when low-osmolar contrast agents are used. At the end of the study, the catheters are removed from the vessels. After catheterization, when the patient is stable, the cardiologist meets with the patient and family to discuss the findings and plan of care.

Nursing Management

Access Site Care

After the diagnostic catheters (and the sheaths through which they are inserted) are removed from the artery or vein, pressure is applied to the vessel until bleeding has stopped. Most bleeding occurs within the first 2 to 3 hours after the procedure. During this time, the site is checked frequently for evidence of bleeding or hematoma. Three methods may be used to control bleeding at the puncture site after catheter or sheath removal. The most basic method is manual pressure, in which a clinician holds pressure directly on the vessel until bleeding stops. The second method uses an external mechanical compression device over the site. The third method is for the cardiologist to use a vascular closure device (VCD) at the end of the catheterization procedure. VCD types include percutaneous suture-type devices that are designed to suture the artery closed as the sheath is removed; collagen-based biosealants that involve placement of a collagen plug into the track of the sheath insertion site; and staple and clip devices that pull together the edges of the arteriotomy. All these methods are effective. After routine diagnostic cardiac catheterization procedures, there is no difference in the rate of femoral arterial site complications for the different closure methods. After femoral artery catheterization specifically, the patient remains flat for up to 6 hours to allow the puncture site to form a stable clot (time varies by institutional protocol and catheter size). The patient is asked to lie still and not to bend at the hip. It usually takes approximately 40 minutes for a stable clot to form, but it can take longer in some patients, including patients with a large body surface area. Radial access sites have fewer vascular and bleeding complications; however, femoral access is still often required for patients with small or tortuous radial vessels or for interventional procedures that are high risk and may require large-bore catheters.[99]

Peripheral Pulses

The peripheral pulses located distal to the arterial access site are monitored closely by the critical care nurse. If the femoral artery has been used, dorsal pedal and posterior tibial pulses are assessed. If the radial artery is used, the radial pulse is assessed. Pulses are assessed every 15 minutes for the first hour after the catheterization and every 30 minutes to 1 hour thereafter. The limb corresponding to the catheterization site is assessed for changes in color, temperature, pain, or paresthesia to detect early evidence of acute arterial occlusion.

Rehydration

The patient is encouraged to drink large amounts of clear liquids, and the IV fluid rate is increased to promote rehydration because the radiopaque contrast material acts as an osmotic diuretic. Rehydration is also used to prevent contrast-induced nephropathy (CIN) or damage to the kidney from the contrast dye used to visualize the heart structures. Though the risk of CIN has been decreasing over the last decade, certain categories of patients remain at increased risk for injury. These include patients diagnosed with STEMI or cardiogenic shock and those with chronic kidney disease, especially when combined with diabetes. Strategies to reduce the risk of CIN include discontinuing metformin and other nephrotoxic medications in the periprocedural window, the use of preprocedure and postprocedure IV volume expansion with isotonic crystalloids, and the use of as low as reasonably achievable (ALARA) low-osmolar contrast. There is some early evidence that the use of preprocedure statin medications and the discontinuation of angiotensin-converting enzyme inhibitors and angiotensin-receptor blockers may protect against CIN.[100]

Angina

The patient is assessed for chest pain after the procedure. Sublingual nitroglycerin usually is sufficient to relieve the pain, discomfort, or pressure. Not all patients describe their angina as "pain," and many other descriptors, such as "pressure," may be used. Patients are encouraged to use the 0-to-10 pain scale to quantify the angina. A 12-lead ECG must be obtained immediately to identify the coronary arteries involved, and the cardiologist is notified. If the chest pain persists, this may indicate that a clot has formed in a coronary artery, and the patient may need to return to the cardiac catheterization laboratory for an interventional cardiology procedure. Chapter 14 provides more information about PCI in the section on catheter interventions for coronary artery disease (see Figs. 14.11, 14.12, and 14.13).

Dysrhythmias

Dysrhythmias are always a concern after an invasive cardiovascular diagnostic procedure. They result from the underlying cardiac disease and the low potassium levels that can occur after excessive diuresis. Baseline potassium levels, along with other chemistries, blood counts, and clotting times, are always checked before the procedure to determine whether it is safe to proceed.

Patient and Family Education

Because of the invasive nature of cardiac catheterization, many patients express considerable anxiety. Relevant information to provide patients concerns the sensory details of the procedure, such as potential discomfort from lying flat and immobile on a hard table for up to several hours and sometimes experiencing a feeling of warmth when the dye is injected. Pain is uncommon, because opiate analgesics and sedative medications are usually provided. Information about possible outcomes—positive and negative—and possible complications must be provided to the patient. Postcatheterization requirements such as lying still and drinking large quantities of fluids are explained. The basic information can be provided using written and audiovisual material, but it is vital to individualize the content and answer any specific concerns or questions. Patients are also asked to report any other unusual symptoms, such as chest pain or nausea.

Electrophysiology Study

An electrophysiology study (EPS) is an invasive diagnostic procedure used to record intracardiac electrical activity. A person may have an EPS because of a history of a syncopal episode (loss of consciousness); rapid wide complex tachycardia; or other cardiac electrical problems not diagnosed by noninvasive diagnostic studies such as the 12-lead ECG, treadmill stress test, signal-averaged ECG, or Holter monitoring. Information from the study helps rule out a dysrhythmia or determine how best to treat one if present—usually with medication, catheter ablation, or placement of a pacemaker or internal cardioverter device.

EPS Procedure

An EPS is performed in a specially equipped cardiac catheterization or electrophysiology laboratory.[101] Before an EPS, written and verbal education is provided to the patient and family to increase their sense of security and to decrease stress and anxiety. All antidysrhythmic medications are discontinued several days before the study so that any ventricular dysrhythmias may be readily induced during the EPS. Anticoagulants, especially warfarin, are also stopped before an EPS. The patient should fast for at least 6 hours before the study, because procedural sedation will be administered to induce a relaxed state. The patient is conscious during the procedure and receives sedative agents (e.g., midazolam or propofol) at regular intervals. The patient lies supine on a hard table with a C-shaped or U-shaped camera arm to the side or directly overhead to verify the position of the EPS catheters in the heart.

Electrophysiology equipment for stimulation of dysrhythmias and monitoring is usually positioned nearby. A peripheral IV access line and surface ECG leads are placed, and electrophysiology catheters are inserted into the femoral or IJ vein and advanced to the right side of the heart under fluoroscopy. These catheters, similar to pacing catheters, are placed at specific anatomic sites within the heart to record the earliest electrical activity. The catheter placements are demonstrated in Fig. 12.84, with catheter tip positions shown at the following locations:

1. High right atrium near the sinoatrial node
2. Coronary sinus behind the left atrial/ventricular border
3. Bundle of His near the tricuspid valve
4. Right ventricle near the apex

During an EPS, programmed electrical stimulation is used to trigger the dysrhythmia. This technique delivers pulses of early paced beats via a specific catheter to the selected area of myocardium. The electrophysiologist simultaneously looks for a site of early electrical activation that stimulates the myocardium before the sinoatrial node. The goal of an EPS is to discover the origin of dysrhythmias that cannot be evaluated from the surface ECG alone.

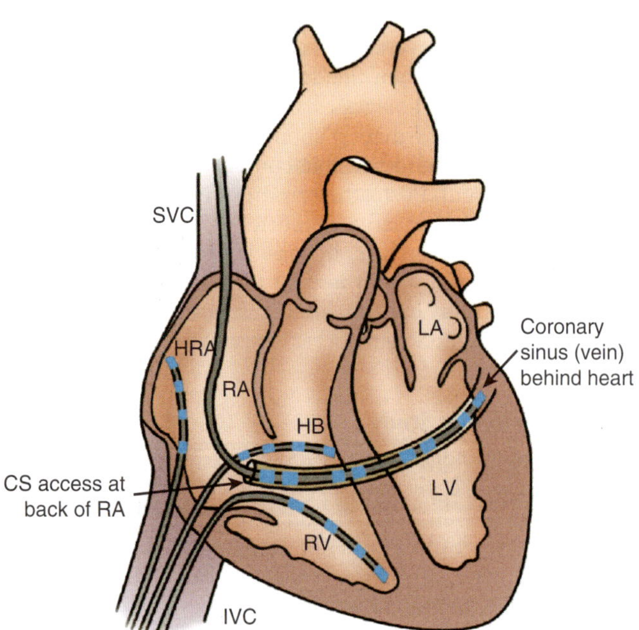

FIG. 12.84 Catheter Placement Within the Heart During an Electrophysiology Study. *CS*, Coronary sinus; *HB*, His bundle; *HRA*, high right atrium; *IVC*, inferior vena cava; *LA*, left atrium; *LV*, left ventricle; *RA*, right atrium; *SVC*, superior vena cava.

Atrial Measurements

Typical measurements during EPS include sinus node recovery time and sinoatrial conduction time plus atrial pacing to measure the atrial and AV node refractory periods. Coronary sinus pacing is used to induce left atrial tachydysrhythmias. Atrial pacing usually is performed after the ventricular study to reduce the risk of putting the patient into atrial fibrillation or flutter because of retrograde conduction up the bundle of His and AV node.

Ventricular Measurements

Programmed electrical stimulation is used to induce the ventricular dysrhythmia, especially in patients who have experienced sustained or nonsustained VT or survived a sudden cardiac death episode. To measure the retrograde V-to-A interval and stimulate the myocardium, a right ventricular catheter is used to rapidly pace the right ventricle; the catheter then is moved to the right ventricular outflow tract (near the pulmonary valve), and the pacing stimulation is repeated. This protocol produces VT in most patients with a known history of VT or VF.

After the dysrhythmia is induced and diagnosed, it can be converted to normal sinus rhythm by 10 to 15 paced beats delivered at a rate faster than the VT or by cardioversion and defibrillation plus IV antidysrhythmic medications. At the end of the study, all the electrophysiology catheters are removed before the patient returns to the nursing unit.

Implantable Cardioverter Defibrillator

When a follow-up EPS is required for a patient with an ICD, the device can substitute for the electrophysiology catheters. The ICD has sensing leads, pace termination, backup bradycardia pacing, and cardioversion and defibrillation capabilities. The EPS can also be performed via the external ICD programmer in the electrophysiology laboratory. Chapter 14 provides more information on the therapeutic uses of ICDs.

Chest Radiography for the Cardiovascular System

Chest radiography, often referred to as a chest x-ray, is the oldest noninvasive method for visualizing images of the heart, and it remains a frequently used and valuable diagnostic tool. Information about cardiac anatomy and physiology can be obtained with ease and safety at a relatively low cost. In the critical care unit, the nurse may be the first person to view the chest radiograph of an acutely ill patient. Critical care nurses also have an important role in ensuring the quality of the film through proper positioning and instruction of the patient. For these reasons, it is crucial to understand the basics of chest radiography techniques and interpretation as they apply to the cardiovascular and pulmonary systems.

Tissue Densities on Radiography

As x-rays travel through the chest from the emitting tube to the film plate, they are absorbed to various degrees by the tissues

TABLE 12.20 **Intrathoracic Radiographic Densities**

Metal or Bone (White)	Fluid (Gray)	Air (Black)
Bone	Blood visualized in	Air visualized in
Calcium deposits in arteries	• Heart	• Lung
	• Veins	• Other tissues
Implants	• Arteries	
• Surgical wires or clips	Effusion	
	• Pericardium	
• Prosthetic valves	• Pleura	
• Pacemaker wires	Edema	
• ICD/Pacemaker	• Lung	

ICD, Implantable cardioverter defibrillator.

through which they pass (Table 12.20). Very dense tissue, such as bone, absorbs almost all the x-rays, leaving the film unexposed, or white. The heart, aorta, and pulmonary vessels and the blood they contain are moderately dense structures, appearing as gray areas on the radiographic film. These vascular structures are surrounded by air-filled lung that allows the greatest penetration of x-rays, resulting in fully exposed (black) areas on the film. Thoracic structures can be studied best by examining their borders. Two structures with the same density, when located next to each other, have no visible border. If a structure is located next to a contrasting density (e.g., vascular structures next to an air-filled lung), even subtle changes in size and shape can be seen.

Standard Views

In most institutions, a standard radiographic examination of the heart and lungs consists of posteroanterior and left lateral films. The standard film is taken in the radiology department with the patient in an upright position. The film is exposed during a deep, sustained inhalation, and the x-ray tube is aimed horizontally 6 feet from the film. This is referred to as a *posteroanterior film* because the beam traverses the patient from posterior to anterior.

Portable Chest Radiography

Because most patients in critical care units are too ill to go to the radiology department, chest radiographs are routinely obtained by using portable radiographic machines with the patient sitting upright or lying supine, depending on the patient's clinical condition and the judgment of the nurse. The film plate is placed behind the patient's back, and an anteroposterior projection is used, in which the x-ray beam enters from the front of the chest. For the supine film, with the patient lying flat on the bed, the x-ray tube can be only approximately 36 inches from the patient's chest because of ceiling height and radiographic equipment construction. This results in a lower quality film from a diagnostic standpoint because the images of the heart and great vessels are magnified and not as sharply defined. Whenever possible, the upright (anteroposterior) film is preferred to the supine (flat) one, because it provides a more accurate image, it shows more of the lung because the diaphragm is lower, and the thoracic structures appear sharper and less magnified. Information about the chest radiograph from a pulmonary perspective is presented in Chapter 17.

Nursing Interventions to Produce an Optimal Chest Radiograph

The critical care nurse can have a big effect on the quality of the radiographic film. Several key elements must be considered, as follows:

- The radiograph is taken when the patient has taken a deep breath (inspiration). During exhalation, the lungs are less full of air, which can make the lung tissue appear cloudy as if there is additional lung water. The heart also appears larger during exhalation. This could lead to an erroneous diagnosis of heart failure. Alert patients are encouraged to take in a deep breath and hold it while the exposure is obtained. For patients receiving mechanical ventilatory support, the exposure must be timed to coincide with maximal inhalation.
- It is important to remove extrinsic tubing and other movable objects from the patient's thorax to permit optimal visualization of the chest. Hands or arms should not be across the chest while the radiograph is obtained.
- The patient should sit upright in bed if the clinical condition permits this position. Upright radiograph views have a sharper focus, because the distance from the patient to the x-ray tube is closer to the standard 72 inches (6 feet).
- The nurse should ensure that the patient is straight in the bed rather than turned or twisted; this permits clearer visualization of the major thoracic structures.

Chest Radiograph Indications

The prior emphasis on daily chest radiographs in critical care is slowly changing to the use of on demand radiographs only.[102] The American College of Radiology (ACR), the Society for Pediatric Radiology (SPR), and the Society of Thoracic Radiology (STR) recently collaboratively revised their recommendations for the use of portable chest radiography when PA and lateral examinations cannot be performed. The indications in critical illness include:

- Cardiac or thoracic surgery or major trauma
- Life-support devices
- Unable to be transported for standard chest radiography
- Pneumothorax following an interventional procedure in the chest or abdomen
- Intraoperative assessment of a newly placed catheter, device or retained foreign bodies[103]

Chest Radiograph Analysis: Cardiac Factors

A wealth of physiologic data can be gleaned from a chest radiograph. To be valid, this information must be interpreted in the context of a thorough physical examination and clinical knowledge of the patient's condition.

Heart Size

Comparison of the cardiothoracic ratio (Fig. 12.85) can be used to assess heart size. The normal heart size is less than one-half of the diameter of the chest viewed on the radiograph. Patients with chronic heart failure often have cardiomegaly (enlarged heart), which can dramatically occupy much of the thoracic diameter on the film.

Pulmonary Edema

Pulmonary edema is a common finding in heart failure and in critical illness. The lungs look "wet" on the chest radiograph and appear as white, dense, cloudy areas and may accentuate pulmonary vascular markings. Pulmonary edema shows up

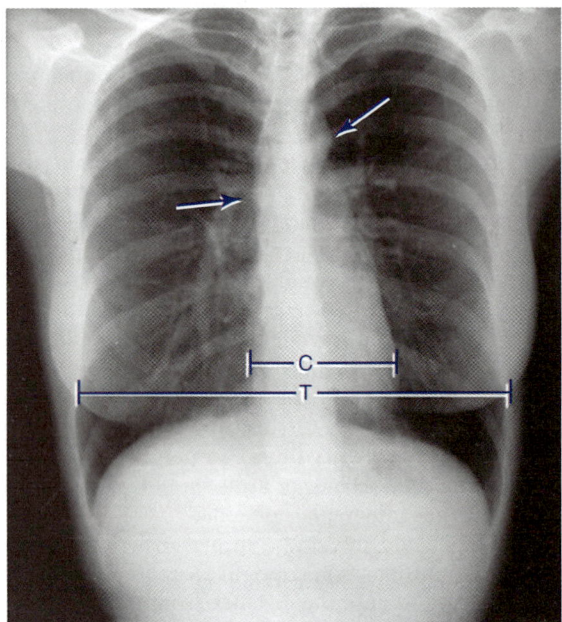

FIG. 12.85 Determining the cardiothoracic ratio is a technique for estimating heart size on a posteroanterior chest radiograph. Normally, the cardiac diameter is 50% or less of the thoracic diameter when measured during full inhalation. The width of the vascular pedicle *(arrows)* is a more accurate indicator of systemic blood volume. *C*, Maximal cardiac diameter; *T*, maximal thoracic diameter measured to the inside of the ribs.

very clearly on the chest radiograph, although in the absence of a clinical history the radiograph is insufficient to determine whether the pulmonary edema is from a cardiac or a pulmonary cause. If the pulmonary edema is caused by heart failure, sometimes described as *hydrostatic pulmonary edema*, the fluid may be in a "bat-wing" distribution, with the white areas concentrated in the hilar region (origin of the major pulmonary vessels). However, as heart failure progresses, the quantity of fluid in the alveolar spaces increases, and the white, fluffy appearance is visible throughout the lung.

If the pulmonary edema is caused by ARDS, also known as noncardiogenic pulmonary edema, the fluid is randomly distributed and may be described as diffuse bilateral infiltrates[104] (see Chapter 18 for information on ARDS).

Chest Radiograph Analysis: Cardiac Lines and Tubes

Evaluation of a chest film is a systematic process. All thoracic invasive tubes and lines must be located and identified. Major thoracic structures including the lungs, pleural space, mediastinum, diaphragm, and vascular structures are assessed and compared with previous films, if available. Variations from previous films can alert the clinician to possible complications and provide information about the patient's hemodynamic status.

Central venous catheter. CVCs are seen on the chest film as moderately radiopaque tubes extending centrally from a SC or IJ vein insertion site. The ideal location of the catheter tip is within the superior vena cava above the right atrium. CVC misplacement during insertion may result in inadvertent arterial cannulation and extravascular placement with pneumothorax or hemothorax.[104]

Pulmonary artery catheter. A chest radiograph is required after insertion of a PA catheter, also known as a *Swan-Ganz catheter*. The primary clinical reason for the chest radiograph is to determine the position of the tip of the PA catheter. To wedge correctly, the catheter tip (balloon deflated) must rest in the right or left pulmonary artery and not extend beyond the hilum of the lung.[104]

Endotracheal tube. A chest radiograph is always requested after endotracheal intubation, because physical examination is not sufficiently sensitive to determine endotracheal tube position. The tip of the endotracheal tube should be 2 to 4 cm above the carina: the anatomic location where the trachea divides into the right main bronchus and left main bronchus. Inadvertent intubation of the right bronchus is the most common malposition.[104]

Enteric tube. Because the consequences of delivering enteral nutrition into a nongastric space are so severe, a chest radiograph is required after placement of a feeding tube, and before beginning enteral nutrition.

Chest tube. Chest tubes contain a radiopaque line that makes them clearly visible on the chest radiograph. Chest tubes are located within the pleural or mediastinal space. Mediastinal chest tubes are placed during cardiac surgery. Pulmonary chest tubes are placed to treat pneumothorax or hemothorax. Most pneumothoraces in the critical care unit are iatrogenic, caused by ventilator barotrauma, from a complication of CVC placement, or after cardiothoracic surgery. Approximately 10% of chest tubes are malpositioned.[104]

Intra-aortic balloon catheter. An intra-aortic balloon pump (IABP) provides mechanical support for the failing heart. The catheter that is evaluated on the chest radiograph is a 26- to 28-mm long inflatable balloon that surrounds a catheter inserted into the descending aorta, usually percutaneously through the femoral or axillary artery. A chest radiograph must be obtained immediately after insertion to evaluate the position of the IABP catheter. The distal tip of the IABP catheter contains a small radiopaque marker that is helpful in determining its position on the chest film. The balloon must lie below the origin of the left SC artery in the descending thoracic aorta (just below the aortic arch). Even when inserted properly, there is a risk of aortic dissection. Aortic dissection is a life-threatening complication. It can be seen on the chest radiograph as a loss of sharpness of the borders of the descending thoracic aorta. Other types of mechanical circulatory support, such as ventricular assist devices or extracorporeal life support, have drivelines or cannulas that can be seen on chest radiograph but are beyond the scope of this discussion.

Pacemaker or implantable defibrillator. Pacemakers and ICDs are cardiovascular devices that can be visualized on a chest film. There is considerable variety in the range of pacing electrodes that are encountered in critical care patients. If the pacemaker is permanently implanted, the entire system is seen on the chest film. With temporary pacemakers, the pulse generator is external to the body and is not seen on the chest radiograph. The pacing electrodes are radiopaque and, on a radiograph, they appear as white wires extending transvenously into the right side of the heart. Pacing wires sutured on the epicardium during cardiac surgery are visible on the right atrium or right ventricle or both. Patients with a history of heart failure may have an additional pacing wire inserted into the coronary sinus (vein) to pace the left ventricle in addition to a right ventricular wire (biventricular pacing). Table 12.21 summarizes the most common cardiovascular devices and their correct position as seen on the chest radiograph.

TABLE 12.21 **Cardiovascular Devices**

Device	Function	Position
Pulmonary artery catheter	Measures pulmonary artery occlusion pressure and right-heart pressures	Tip in right or left pulmonary artery
Central venous catheter	Measures central venous pressure	Tip in the superior vena cava
Mediastinal chest tubes	Mediastinal fluid evacuation	Anterior mediastinum, posterior pericardium
Pacemaker leads	Cardiac pacing	Over right heart
Intra-aortic balloon catheter	Assists left ventricular function	Tip just below top of aortic arch

Digital Radiography

Digital radiography systems are standard in hospitals. In a digital radiograph, the image is divided into discrete elements (pixels) that are assigned a specific value and are available for display on a computer screen. Digital systems have many advantages. No film development is necessary, and the image can be expanded to show greater detail. Digital systems can be used for computer-assisted diagnosis or artificial intelligence (AI) analysis, where the image is analyzed to detect and quantify pathologic findings. If a baseline film has been digitally recorded, it can be "subtracted" from the current film, highlighting any areas of change, such as increased heart size or new pulmonary infiltrates.

Ambulatory Electrocardiography

Before coming to the critical care unit, a patient might have had other ECG tests to determine the degree of cardiovascular disease. Ambulatory electrocardiography is a technique that records the ECG of patients while they perform their usual activities. It is designed to document abnormal cardiac rhythms that occur randomly or that are induced by specific circumstances such as emotional stress or physical activity. Clinical indications include palpitations, dizziness, syncope, and pacemaker evaluation. Two types of recording systems are available: continuous and intermittent. Many intermittent systems have a short memory loop that permits capture of recent antecedent ECG rhythms that may have precipitated the symptoms of concern. They can be worn externally or placed subcutaneously, and some can automatically transmit recordings for immediate evaluation.

Continuous Electrocardiogram Recording Systems

Holter monitors are the most widely used continuous recording systems for patients with daily symptoms. The patient wears skin electrodes and carries a small box that contains a digital recorder. The monitor is carried by a shoulder strap or clipped to a belt or pocket for 24 hours or longer and then is returned to the hospital or clinic for reading. This is a totally noninvasive procedure with no adverse effects. All Holter monitors record between 3 and 12 leads to minimize inaccurate interpretation caused by artifact. Most systems have an event marker, which the patient can press to indicate the onset of symptoms. The patient is asked to keep a diary of activities, symptoms, and any medications that are taken. Patch monitors are a newer generation that continuously records the ECG for up to 14 days. These are small adhesive devices that are more convenient than Holter monitors but can only record in one or two leads.

Continuous recording systems are the most thorough form of ambulatory electrocardiography, because they record every heartbeat. They do not require active participation of the patient (although a detailed patient log is helpful) and do not miss asymptomatic ECG changes or dysrhythmias that may be accompanied by a loss of consciousness. When dysrhythmias occur that correlate with symptoms or symptoms occur in the absence of dysrhythmias, one of the primary goals of continuous monitoring has been achieved. Most patients do not have typical symptoms daily. If no significant dysrhythmias or symptoms occur during the continuous monitoring period, the test is unhelpful. The only activities that are restricted while wearing a continuous monitor are activities that would get the chest electrodes or monitor wet, including swimming and taking a shower or tub bath.

Intermittent Electrocardiogram Recording Systems

A portable monitor that does not record the ECG continuously can also be used to diagnose dysrhythmias. These are also be described as *event recorders*. The patient wears external electrodes, but the device is not constantly recording. The patient is instructed to press a button when experiencing symptoms to initiate the recording manually in real time, or the monitor may start recording when it senses an automatic trigger such as a dysrhythmia. The big advantages of the intermittent recording system are the ability to wear the recorder for weeks and the ability to trigger recording when symptoms such as heart palpitations occur.[105]

Remote Temporary ECG Monitoring Patches

Many companies have developed ECG monitoring systems, where, instead of leads, a patch is worn on the chest for up to 30 days to detect dysrhythmias. At the end of the diagnosis period the patch is mailed back to the company for analysis.

Implantable Loop Recorder

For patients who require longer periods of follow-up to diagnose syncope or intermittent dysrhythmias, a small, continuous implantable loop recorder may be inserted under the skin of the upper chest. The recorder is approximately 2 inches × 1 inch × 1 inch. Insertion takes approximately 20 minutes under local anesthetic. It is especially useful if prior short-term ambulatory ECG recordings have failed to reveal an underlying problem. The inserted loop recorder continuously monitors the ECG rhythm for up to 3 years with automatic downloads scheduled every 3 months. Data can be collected through a proprietary application on a smartphone. During a dysrhythmia or after a syncopal episode (loss of consciousness), the patient or a family member can add a note about the pre-event activity or symptoms.

Smart Watch Heart Rate and Rhythm Monitors

Software algorithms built into electronic wristbands or smartwatches can detect rapid HRs or irregular rhythms.

Some devices record single-lead ECGs. Studies evaluating their effectiveness are currently in progress.[106] While smartwatch and other wearable devices are extremely helpful in health-monitoring, concerns have been raised about economic disparity, as not everyone can affort wearable technologies.

SOCIAL DETERMINANTS OF HEALTH

Health Disparities Associated With Using Wearables

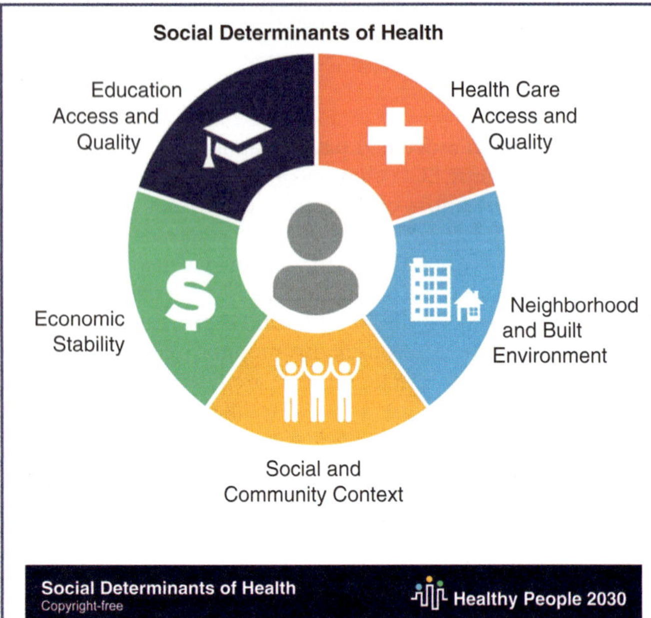

Wearables, such as fitness trackers and smartwatches, can provide valuable data for managing and improving health, but their effectiveness can be affected by various social factors.

- **Income and Socioeconomic Status**: Affordability is crucial in adopting wearable devices. Individuals with higher incomes are more likely to afford these devices, which can provide them with valuable health data. Individuals with lower-incomes may struggle to purchase wearables, limiting access to these health-monitoring tools.
- **Access to Technology**: Owning and using wearable devices requires access to technology, including smartphones or tablets. People in underserved or rural areas with limited access to technology may not be able to leverage these monitoring tools fully.
- **Education and Health Literacy**: Understanding how to use wearable devices effectively and interpret the data they provide can be influenced by a person's level of education and health literacy. Individuals with lower health literacy may struggle to use wearables fully.
- **Geographic Location**: Geographic disparities can impact wearables' availability and internet connectivity quality necessary for syncing and sharing data. People in remote or underserved areas may have limited access to these devices and may not benefit from real-time monitoring.
- **Cultural and Language Factors**: Cultural beliefs and language barriers can affect the acceptance and understanding of wearable technology. Culturally sensitive and language-appropriate education and support materials may be needed to ensure effective use.
- **Social Support**: Support from family and peers can encourage the use of wearables and adherence to health monitoring routines. Conversely, a lack of social support may result in decreased motivation and engagement with these devices.
- **Privacy and Data Security Concerns**: People with concerns about data privacy may be hesitant to use wearables or may limit the sharing of their health data.
- **Access to Health Care**: Wearables can complement health care by providing continuous health data. However, access to health care providers and services remains critical for interpreting and acting on this data effectively.

To ensure equitable access to the benefits of wearable health monitoring, health care systems, policymakers, and technology companies need to implement strategies such as subsidies for low-income individuals, targeted education and outreach efforts, community-based support programs, and data privacy protections. Additionally, considering social factors in designing and marketing wearable devices can help make these technologies more inclusive and effective for diverse populations.

References:

Smith B, Magnani JW. New technologies, new disparities: The intersection of electronic health and digital health literacy. *Int J Cardiol.* 2019;292:280–282. https://doi.org/10.1016/j.ijcard.2019.05.066.

Illustration from Healthy People 2030, U.S. Department of Health and Human Services, Office of Disease Prevention and Health Promotion. Retrieved August 23, 2023, from https://health.gov/healthypeople/objectives-and-data/social-determinants-health.

Stress Tests: Exercise With Electrocardiogram Monitoring

Exercise stress testing is a noninvasive procedure. It consists of recording an ECG tracing during a period of physiologic stress on the heart muscle and its blood supply to uncover and diagnose ischemia that is not apparent at rest. Physiologic stress is created by asking the patient to walk on a treadmill or to ride a stationary bicycle.[107]

Physiology of Exercise on the Cardiovascular System

Exercise places unique demands on the cardiovascular system. Systemic oxygen consumption increases markedly, requiring the heart to increase CO to meet these demands. Myocardial contractility increases, resulting in greater SV and systolic blood pressure. HR is increased because of circulating catecholamines. Normally, as HR and SV rise, CO is increased dramatically, and the tissue needs for oxygen are met. This enhanced myocardial performance is not without a penalty. Even at rest, the heart muscle extracts 70% of the oxygen available in the circulating blood. When the myocardial demand for oxygen increases during exercise, coronary blood flow must increase to maintain an adequate oxygen supply. In patients with CAD, coronary blood flow cannot increase sufficiently to meet the high metabolic needs of the myocardium during exercise, and ischemia results.

Stress Test Protocols

Exercise is performed by using a treadmill on which the speed and slope can be varied or by using a stationary bicycle. Numerous protocols have been developed using a treadmill. Two popular ones are the Bruce protocol, in which the grade and speed are varied every 3 minutes, and the Balke protocol, in which speed remains constant and grade is gradually increased every minute. Regardless of the protocol used, the ECG is monitored continuously. Blood pressure is also measured and recorded every minute.[107]

Heart Rate Criteria in Treadmill Stress Test

The treadmill test is stopped when a target level, based on the patient's maximal stress test HR, is reached. The maximal predicted HR is estimated using the formula 220 − Patient age.[107]

Increasing the HR to 85% to 90% of the predicted maximum is preferred, and this level of exercise is sufficient in most patients to unmask any significant CAD. The diagnostic value of the test is based on the maximal HR achieved, *not* on the length of time that the patient remains on the treadmill. A well-trained athlete may be able to stay on the treadmill for 15 minutes, whereas an older or sedentary person may tolerate it for only 3 to 5 minutes; however, if 85% of the predicted maximal HR is achieved, both tests are equally diagnostic. A person who is taking beta-blockers may be unable to reach his or her age-adjusted targeted HR because of the bradycardic effect of this class of medications.

Clinical Reasons to Stop a Treadmill Test

A treadmill test may be aborted before maximal HR is reached if symptoms occur. Reasons to halt the test include the development of moderate to severe angina (chest pain), signs of pallor or poor perfusion, and the patient asking to stop the test. Other signs that can alert the nurse to stop the test include ST segment elevation equal to or greater than 1.0 mm (one small box), ST depression equal to or greater than 2.0 mm (2 small boxes), cardiac dysrhythmias or a marked shift in ventricular axis, and increased symptoms such as breathlessness or fatigue or a fall in blood pressure of 10 mm Hg or more from baseline. Blood pressure is expected to rise during exercise, but a systolic blood pressure greater than 250 mm Hg or a diastolic blood pressure greater than 115 mm Hg is an indication to stop the test.[107]

Signal-Averaged Electrocardiogram

The signal-averaged electrocardiogram (SAECG) is used to identify late potentials within the QRS complex. These low-amplitude waveforms cannot be detected on a standard surface ECG but can be recorded as an SAECG. Late potentials indicate slow conduction within the ventricular myocardium that can be a substrate for ventricular dysrhythmias and put the individual at risk for sudden cardiac death. The SAECG is used to assess risk of SCD.

SAECG is a noninvasive test. The patient lies in a supine position and is asked to keep muscle movement to a minimum. Cardiac electrode leads are applied to the anterior and posterior chest walls, and the leads are connected to an SAECG computer. This computer produces a high-resolution, high-magnification ECG signal. This "noise-free" ECG is analyzed for QRS complex duration and for the presence, duration, and measurement of late myopotentials. After computer analysis, the SAECG is described as negative (normal) or positive (abnormal). A positive SAECG in combination with other specific indicators is a predictor of increased risk for sudden cardiac death.

Many patients with a positive SAECG (abnormal) produce a normal SAECG when placed on antidysrhythmic medications. The SAECG is not analyzed in isolation. It is used in conjunction with other cardiac diagnostic tests, including the EPS. It is a helpful adjunct to the EPS but does not replace it.

ECHOCARDIOGRAPHY

Echocardiography uses waves of ultrasound to obtain and display images of cardiac structures. Normal human hearing occurs at a sound frequency of 20 to 20,000 cycles per second (Hz). Ultrasound uses sound frequencies above 20,000 Hz. Ultrasound is reflected best at interfaces between tissues that have different densities. In the heart, these are the blood, cardiac valves, myocardium, and pericardium. Because all these structures differ in density, their borders can be seen on the echocardiogram. Echocardiography is used to detect structural heart abnormalities such as mitral valve stenosis and regurgitation, prolapse of mitral valve leaflets, aortic stenosis and insufficiency, hypertrophic cardiomyopathy, atrial septal defect, thoracic aortic dissection, cardiac tamponade, and pericardial effusion. There are several methods for obtaining images of cardiac structures with echocardiography, including:

- Transthoracic (TTE)
- Transesophageal (TEE)
- Intravascular ultrasound (IVUS)
- Intracardiac echocardiography (ICE)

There are also several basic modes of echocardiography used to image the heart: two dimensional, three dimensional, motion mode (M-mode), and Doppler. Echocardiography can also be performed during stress testing to noninvasively evaluate patients for ischemic heart disease.

Transthoracic Echocardiography

The TTE is a noninvasive test used to examine heart function, contractility, and valve motion. When TTE is performed, the patient is in a supine, left lateral, or semirecumbent position. The position used depends on the patient's clinical condition and on which structures are to be examined. A transducer is placed on the skin, with lubricant between the transducer and the skin to improve contact and reduce artifact. The active element in the transducer is a piezoelectric crystal. *Piezoelectric* refers to the ability to transform electrical energy into mechanical energy (in this case, sound energy). The transducer emits ultrasound waves and receives a signal from the reflected sound waves. Periods of sound transmission alternate with periods of sound reception.

Ultrasonic waves do not travel through air very well, and they cannot penetrate very dense structures such as bone. In adults, the transducer is usually placed in the third or fourth intercostal space to the left of the sternum, because at that point the pericardium is in direct contact with the chest wall, and the ultrasonic waves are not obstructed by air or bone. Other positions are sometimes used if the standard location does not provide adequate visualization of the cardiac structures. In the critical care unit, the echocardiograph machine is usually brought to the bedside. The lighting in the room can be dimmed to improve the visual clarity of the images displayed on the screen.

Nursing care consists of monitoring the patient during the procedure, which is usually performed by an echocardiography technician. TTE is completely noninvasive; the nurse explains this and the purpose of the test to the patient and family. The procedure is not uncomfortable, but it may be tiring for certain patients because of the length of the procedure, which is usually 30 to 60 minutes.

Transesophageal Echocardiography

The TEE is an invasive test used to examine heart function, contractility and valve motion as it provides extremely clear images. TEE is a technique in which the transducer (single-plane, biplane, or multiplane device) is mounted on a flexible shaft similar to an endoscope and advanced into the esophagus, from where cardiac structures can be more clearly visualized. The multiplane transducer has a single array of crystals that can be rotated in a 180-degree arc, requiring less manipulation of the probe within the esophagus. Because of the close anatomic relationship between the heart and the esophagus, TEE produces high-quality images of intracardiac structures and the thoracic aorta without the interference of the chest wall, bone, or air-filled lung.

The insertion procedure is similar to upper gastrointestinal endoscopy. The patient is asked to fast for a minimum of 6 hours before TEE to prevent nausea and vomiting. For an elective TEE, medication is usually given to inhibit salivary secretions, reducing the risk of aspiration. Analgesic and sedative agents are administered to reduce fear and anxiety and to provide retrograde amnesia. Routine antibiotic prophylaxis against bacteremia and endocarditis is unnecessary, although it is considered for high-risk patients, such as patients with prosthetic valves, previous endocarditis, or very poor dentition. The oropharyngeal region is anesthetized with topical lidocaine to lessen the gag reflex and prevent retching and laryngospasm. The patient is usually placed in the left lateral decubitus position, although the supine position can be used in the critical care setting if necessary. A soft bite block is inserted between the teeth to prevent damage to the echoscope. As the echoscope is inserted, the patient is asked to swallow. The echoscope is advanced to 25 cm from the mouth, and imaging is begun (see Fig. 12.31). TEE is also used intraoperatively during cardiac surgery for monitoring valve repair and replacement. The images obtained by TEE are superior to transthoracic views in a variety of ways. The entire thoracic aorta can be visualized clearly. Both atrial chambers are clearly seen with TEE, and the left atrial appendage is particularly well visualized, making TEE the procedure of choice for detection of left atrial thrombus. Diagnosis and quantification of atrial septal defects is possible with this method, and the addition of Doppler capabilities allows assessment of atrial shunting. TEE is useful in evaluating patients with valvular disorders, including visualizing vegetations on the valve leaflets in a patient with infective endocarditis.

Manipulation of the TEE probe within the esophagus can cause a vasovagal response, producing bradycardia and hypotension. The most serious risk of the procedure is esophageal bleeding. Individuals with liver cirrhosis or esophageal varices and patients on anticoagulants are also at risk for esophageal bleeding. During TEE, the patient's vital signs are closely monitored with ECG, blood pressure, and clinical observation. If esophageal entry is difficult, it should not be forced. Emergency resuscitation equipment must be present in case of a severe vasovagal episode, typically bradycardia and hypotension. Suction equipment must be at the bedside in the event that the patient vomits or has difficulty handling oral secretions.

Intravascular Ultrasound

Intravascular ultrasound (IVUS) is used as an adjunct diagnostic technique during coronary angiography or during a percutaneous coronary procedure. A miniature, flexible ultrasound catheter that incorporates a high-frequency transducer (20 to 40 MHz) provides high-resolution images of the coronary arterial wall. This technology is not an alternative to angiography but is used as a complementary diagnostic technique. IVUS permits an anatomic view of the interior of the coronary artery. The cardiologist can visualize the exact location of atherosclerotic plaque or see whether a coronary stent has deployed (expanded) correctly against the vessel wall.

Intracardiac Ultrasound

The use of intracardiac ultrasound, also known as intracardiac echo (ICE), is increasing. Flexible ultrasound catheters can be directed into the atria and ventricles. Diagnostic uses include direct visualization of intracardiac structures, replacement for TEE during interventional or selected surgical procedures, and views of the atrial or ventricular septum during a repair procedure.

Two-Dimensional and Three-Dimensional Echocardiograms

The two-dimensional echocardiogram uses crystals in the transducer to create a cross-sectional imaging plane. Sections of the heart are then viewed from numerous different angles. The picture is displayed on an oscilloscope, and digital photographs are taken to serve as a permanent record. The two-dimensional echocardiogram images a whole "slice" of the heart at once and is used for direct measurement of LV volumes and wall mass. The two-dimensional slice also permits visualization of the cardiac structures in relation to each other and readily identifies valvular dysfunction and wall-motion abnormalities after MI. A more recent innovation is a real-time three-dimensional echocardiogram. It produces more realistic images, especially when imaging cardiac valves or congenital anomalies.

Two-Dimensional Motion-Mode Echocardiography

M-mode two-dimensional echocardiography is noninvasive and allows visualization of specific cardiac structures over time. A hand-held crystal transducer is placed against the chest wall to direct a thin beam of ultrasound through the heart. As the ultrasound beam encounters different interfaces, it is reflected back (echo) as a dot and recorded as the heart beats. Fig.12.86A shows the labeled structures and Fig.12.86B shows the ultrasound visualization via the line of the transducer. In M-mode, each echo-dot becomes a line on an oscilloscope recording motion and measurement of the mitral valve, the intraventricular septum, and other structures the ultrasound beam encounters over time (Fig. 12.86C). M-mode echocardiograms are particularly useful in detecting small pericardial effusions and cardiac tamponade.

Phonocardiogram

Phonocardiography is combined with echocardiography to evaluate valvular dysfunction. A phonocardiogram (*phono* [sound], *cardio* [heart], and *gram* [recording]) provides a graphic display of the sounds that occur in the heart and great vessels. The transducer is placed on the chest wall to record heart sounds that correspond to auscultation with a traditional stethoscope. Chapter 11 provides more information on heart sounds (see Fig. 11.6) and heart murmurs (see Table 11.4).

Color-Flow Doppler Echocardiography

Doppler echocardiography provides a special kind of echocardiogram that assesses blood flow. It uses a pulsed or continuous wave of ultrasound that records frequency shifts of

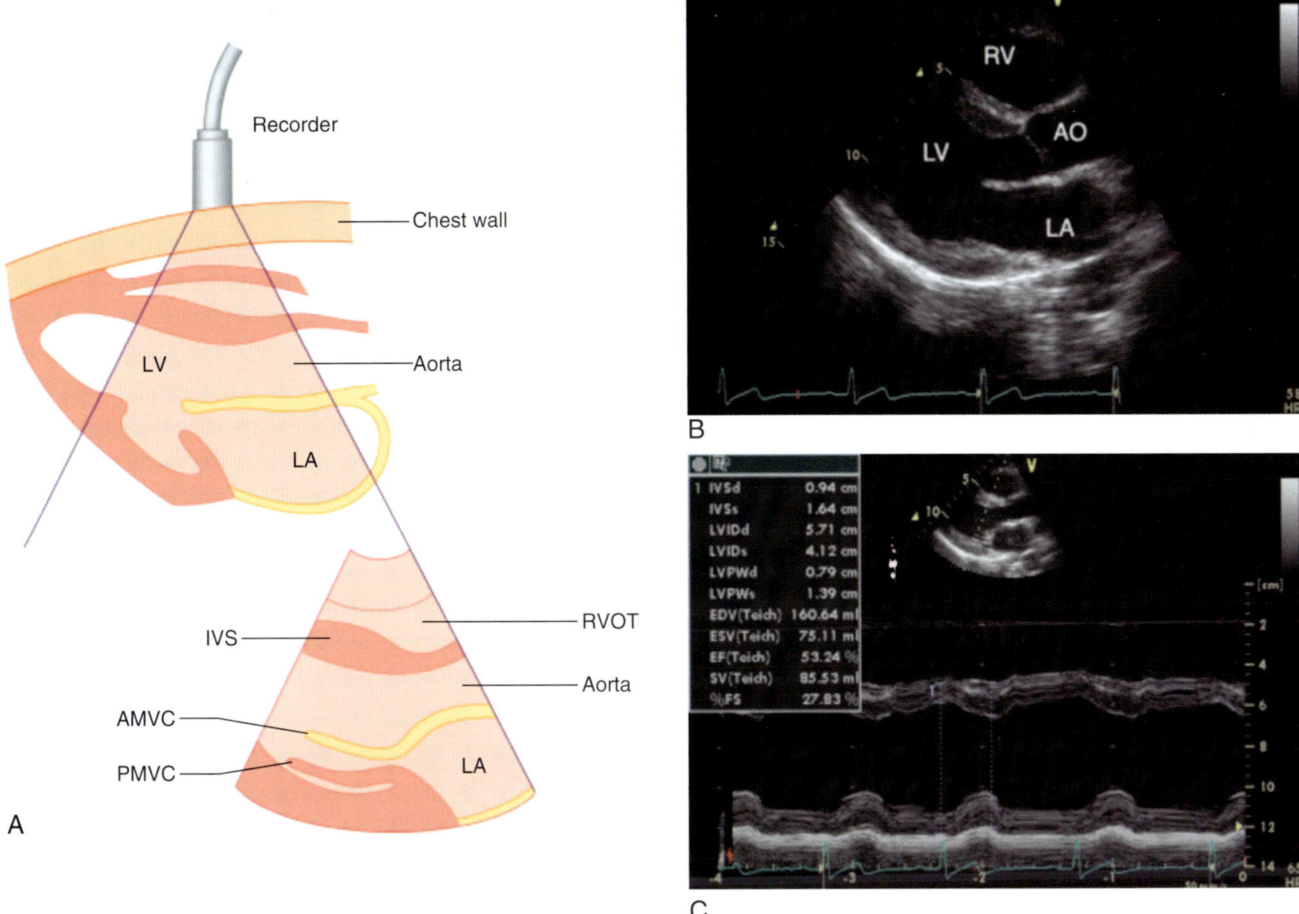

FIG. 12.86 Two-Dimensional Echocardiography and M-Mode Echocardiography (A) Schematic of long-axis view of normal cardiac structures traversed by a two-dimensional ultrasound beam, as the heart beats. The transducer is repositioned on the chest to allow visualization of different structures. (B) Two-dimensional echocardiography recording of a normal heart. (C) M-mode echocardiograph recording of a normal heart. The transducer ultrasound beam traverses the left ventricle slightly below the mitral valve. *AMVC,* Anterior mitral valve cusp; *AO,* aorta; *IVS,* interventricular septum; *LA,* left atrium; *LV,* left ventricle; *LV(d),* left ventricular end-diastolic dimensions; *LV(s),* left ventricular end-systolic dimensions; *MV,* mitral valve; *PM,* papillary muscle; *PMVC,* posterior mitral valve cusp; *PVW,* posterior ventricular wall; *RA,* right atrium; *RV,* right ventricle; *RVOT,* right ventricular outflow tract. (From Kumar P, Clark M, eds. *Kumar and Clarke's Clinical Medicine.* 9th ed. Elsevier; 2017.)

reflected sound waves, showing velocity and direction of blood flow relative to the transducer. Doppler signals are usually displayed in color. Known as *color-flow mapping* or *imaging,* this technique analyzes Doppler signals from multiple intracardiac sites simultaneously. The Doppler tracing for each site is displayed in a color-coded format superimposed on a real-time two-dimensional echocardiographic image. Flow toward the transducer is displayed in one color, whereas flow away from the transducer is displayed in a contrasting color. The brightness of the color varies to signify different flow velocities.

Doppler echocardiography is especially useful in individuals with valvular heart disease. The blood flow associated with regurgitation and stenosis can be detected, and estimates can be made of the severity of the disease. Doppler can accurately estimate right ventricular systolic pressure. When several valves are involved, the Doppler technique can clarify the extent of damage to the individual valves. Other uses for Doppler echocardiography include evaluation of congenital shunts, measurement of volume flow and CO, and assessment of new structural abnormalities after acute MI. By measuring flow velocity in the right ventricular outflow tract, mean PAP can also be estimated.

Stress Echocardiography

Stress echocardiography is a noninvasive test used to examine heart function, contractility, and valve motion under stress, either physical (treadmill) or pharmacologic (inotropic medications). Stress echocardiography is often used in the outpatient setting to evaluate stable angina.[97] It provides a very accurate picture of the ischemic effect of CAD on the myocardium. Stress echocardiography can diagnose regional (ischemia) and global (cardiomyopathy) abnormalities. It may also be used after MI to evaluate the effect of necrosis on viable heart muscle tissue. Physiologic stress from increased exercise can create an imbalance between myocardial oxygen supply and demand. This causes ischemia and eventually results in wall-motion abnormalities, which are detectable with an echocardiogram. During the test, physiologic stress can be triggered either by exercise or via pharmacologic agents given to stimulate the heart. For exercise stress, either the treadmill or stationary bicycle is used for physical exertion. The protocols used for echocardiographic exercise stress testing are very similar to the protocols used in the ECG stress test setting previously described (Table 12.22).

Pharmacologic Stress Test

When patients are unable to exercise to raise the HR sufficiently to evaluate myocardial response, pharmacologic agents may be used. Dobutamine, a beta-1 agonist, is the most common and is discussed here. However, alternative agents may be selected to provoke an accelerated HR for the study, including the vasodilators adenosine and dipyridamole, as well as regadenoson (an adenosine A2A receptor agonist). Choice of agent is based on the patient's concomitant disease states and clinical status.

Pharmacologic stress is most frequently incited with a dobutamine infusion beginning at 5 mcg/kg/min. The infusion is increased every 3 minutes until a maximum dose has been achieved (typically 40 mcg/kg/min) or a primary endpoint has been reached, usually 85% of the patient's maximal HR.[107] Dobutamine may cause myocardial ischemia through a dramatic increase in myocardial oxygen demand due to an increase in HR, contractility, and systemic blood pressure. Potential side effects include hypotension, hypertension, dysrhythmias, nausea, headache, anxiety, and tremor. Atropine is also administered if the dobutamine infusion alone does not cause an adequate increase in HR.

Magnetic Resonance Imaging

Magnetic resonance imaging (MRI) is a noninvasive imaging technique that can obtain specific biochemical information from body tissue without the use of ionizing radiation. The procedure does not present any known hazard to living cells. In many respects, the image created is superior to radiography and ultrasonography because bone does not interfere with MRI.

Magnetic Resonance Imaging Physics

The physics behind MRI scanning is complex, but the basic concept is simple. Certain atoms within molecules act as tiny bar magnets with north and south poles. The nuclei spin around this axis like a spinning top. Under normal conditions, these small atomic magnets are arranged at random. If a patient is placed within a strong magnetic field, many of the nuclei line up in the same direction as the magnetic force. When a radiofrequency wave is sent, some of the nuclei absorb this energy, causing them to fall out of alignment and wobble like a gyroscope that is winding down. This wobbling out of alignment is called

TABLE 12.22 Stress Testing Methods

Test Parameters	Stress Electrocardiography	Stress Echocardiography	Stress Radionuclide Imaging
Exercise stress test	3-, 5-, or 12-lead ECG leads are attached to the chest and limbs to monitor the ECG *during* exercise protocol.	Patient exercises according to protocol. Echocardiogram is recorded immediately *after* exercise.	Radiopharmaceutical (thallium-201 or technetium-99m) is injected before exercise. Patient exercises according to the protocol. Heart is scanned *after* exercise to view uptake of radiotracer.
Pharmacologic stress test	Patient is at rest. IV medications stimulate HR and contractility: Dosage starts with dobutamine at 5 mcg/kg/min and is increased as needed to increase HR. ECG pattern is monitored during the medication infusions. Other medications include adenosine, regadenoson, and dipyridamole.	Patient is at rest. IV medications stimulate HR and contractility: Dosage starts with dobutamine at 5 mcg/kg/min and is increased as needed to increase HR. Echocardiogram is recorded during and after the medication infusions. Other medications include adenosine, regadenoson, and dipyridamole.	Patient is at rest. IV medications simulate exercise: Dosage starts with dobutamine 5 mcg/kg/min and is increased as needed to increase HR. Radionuclide image is scanned during and after pharmacologic stress. Other medications include adenosine, regadenoson, and dipyridamole.
Clinical indications	Used to rule out CAD. Not as helpful if patient has a distorted ECG pattern at baseline owing to LBBB, RBBB, or internal ventricular pacemaker because ST segment changes are obscured.	Useful for patients with LBBB, RBBB, and implanted pacemaker because the wall motion is visualized directly.	Helpful for patients with LBBB, RBBB, and implanted pacemaker. It is useful before CABG to determine whether bypass graft will supply blood to an ischemic area. There is no benefit in grafting an artery to an infarcted area.
Clinical outcome of a positive test result	Chest pain develops. ST segment ECG pattern changes.	Chest pain develops. Wall-motion abnormalities are visualized.	Areas of the heart that do not take up radiotracer are called *cold spots*. A cold spot is ischemic or infarcted tissue. A follow-up scan later the same day (or the next day with some radiotracers) shows whether the cold spot has filled in; if yes, the area is ischemic; if it remains cold, the area is infarcted.

CABG, Coronary artery bypass graft; *CAD*, coronary artery disease; *ECG*, electrocardiogram; *HR*, heart rate; *IV*, intravenous; *LBBB*, left bundle branch block; *RBBB*, right bundle branch block.

resonance. The process of returning to alignment with the magnetic field after the radiofrequency signal is turned off is called *relaxation*. These energy changes can be detected and recorded by the scanner.

Each type of atom has its own unique resonance and relaxation pattern. The easiest one to record is the hydrogen ion, although other atoms such as phosphorus, sodium, and carbon are being studied. Because there are two hydrogen ions per molecule of water, MRI is especially sensitive to changes in tissue water content. Myocardial ischemic injury results in predictable increases in regional myocardial water content, allowing differentiation between normal and ischemic tissue. Infarction leads to myocardial scarring, and because the scar tissue has lower water content, it can be identified on an MRI scan as an area of decreased intensity.

Metal Objects

MRI is a safe procedure. The main hazard is related to the presence of metal substances in the environment. Because the magnetism used is approximately 40,000 times stronger than the magnetic field of the earth, metal objects such as IV-line poles, infusion pumps, or oxygen tanks can become projectiles if they come close enough to the magnet's pull. No metal objects are permitted in the area of the MRI scanner. The patient must be asked about the presence of any metallic implants or other metal (residual bullet or shrapnel) that may be moved by the magnetic force during the scan. Aneurysm clips are composed of ferromagnetic materials and can experience significant torque when exposed to the magnetic field. Most contemporary cardiac electronic devices that are implanted are MRI safe, but older pacemakers or ICDs may malfunction during exposure to the strong magnetic field.

MRI Limitations

MRI has significant limitations that affect patients in the critical care setting. One of the challenges is that patients must leave the unit and be transported to the MRI scanner. Standard ventilators, monitoring equipment, and infusion pumps cannot be used because these machines contain metal parts. Special ventilators with nonmagnetic accessories are available, as are nonmetal ECG, pulse oximetry sensors, and infusion pumps.

The narrow size of the magnet bore (tube or tunnel) requires the patient to lie flat and motionless for long periods. The close quarters inside the magnet bore tend to provoke claustrophobia in anyone already predisposed to it, and sedation may be required. A claustrophobic patient needs considerable reassurance and education before lying supine and motionless inside the MRI tube. A more recent innovation is the use of open MRI scanners. The MRI tube is open at both ends so that the patient's head is not enclosed while the body is scanned; however, imaging quality may be reduced.

Cardiac MRI

Cardiac MRI, also known as *cardiovascular magnetic resonance (CMR)*, can provide information about tissue integrity, anatomic structure, cardiac wall-motion abnormalities, aneurysms, EF, CO, patency of proximal coronary arteries, and flow rates through CABG sites. CMR is useful in diagnosing complications of MI such as pericarditis or pericardial effusion, valvular dysfunction, ventricular septal rupture, aneurysm, and intracardiac thrombus. Blood that is actively flowing does not emit a magnetic resonance signal; it provides a natural dark contrast material in the lumen of proximal coronary arteries. As a result, abnormalities of lumen size such as narrowing, which may provide evidence of obstruction, can be visualized. Pharmacologic stress imaging can also be done during CMR using an inotrope such as dobutamine or alternate vasodilating agents.

MRI works best for structures that have little or no motion, such as the brain. Cardiac applications have been limited because of the constant motion of the heart. In an attempt to overcome this limitation, various gating or slicing techniques have been used to time the images at exact phases of the cardiac cycle. The gating can be timed from the R wave of the ECG or from the arterial pulse tracing. Either method is satisfactory as long as the patient is in normal sinus rhythm. With any irregularity of the rhythm, the gating technique becomes much less helpful and image quality is reduced.

Cardiac Computed Tomography Angiogram

Cardiac CT is a widely available noninvasive examination that is usually used to evaluate patients for coronary artery disease but can also be used to assess LV function, morphology, and myocardial perfusion.

When used to assess the coronary arteries, it is known as *coronary CT angiography (CCTA)*. Before CCTA, sublingual nitroglycerin is used to dilate the coronary arteries, and beta-blockers may be administered to reduce the HR to allow for better visualization. During the study, IV contrast dye is injected to help outline the presence of plaques or stenosis within the coronary arteries. Patients must be able lie still and hold their breath periodically. Contraindications include kidney injury due to the use of contrast.

Coronary Artery Calcium Score

Cardiac CT is also used to calculate the coronary artery calcium score (CACS).[108] The quantity of calcium in atherosclerotic plaque is measured using multidetector computed tomography, and then the CACS is calculated. A score less than 100 is considered low risk, whereas a score greater than 300 indicates high risk of a future coronary event. Clinically, the CACS is considered along with other risk factor information to evaluate individual risk from atherosclerotic coronary disease.

Cardiac Radionuclide Imaging Studies

Several types of radionuclide imaging tests are available. As with diagnostic ECG and echocardiography, many of the radionuclide tests can be performed both at rest and during exercise.[107]

Purpose of Radionuclide Scans

- The purpose of a radionuclide scan, also known as *nuclear myocardial perfusion imaging*, is to determine whether there is a perfusion defect in cardiac muscle (Fig. 12.87). A scan is indicated for a symptomatic patient with known or suspected CAD. The radionuclide scan is especially helpful for a patient who has a coexisting LBBB or a permanent pacemaker where the QRS complex shape is distorted. Both situations make interpretation of acute angina or equivalent symptoms challenging to interpret accurately on the 12-lead ECG or during ECG stress testing. This has opened a window of opportunity for radionuclide imaging, in which the myocardial ability to receive blood flow is visualized directly.

Blockage of an artery can lead to a discrete myocardial perfusion defect, meaning that the blood supply to this area is decreased (ischemic) or absent (infarcted). Although coronary

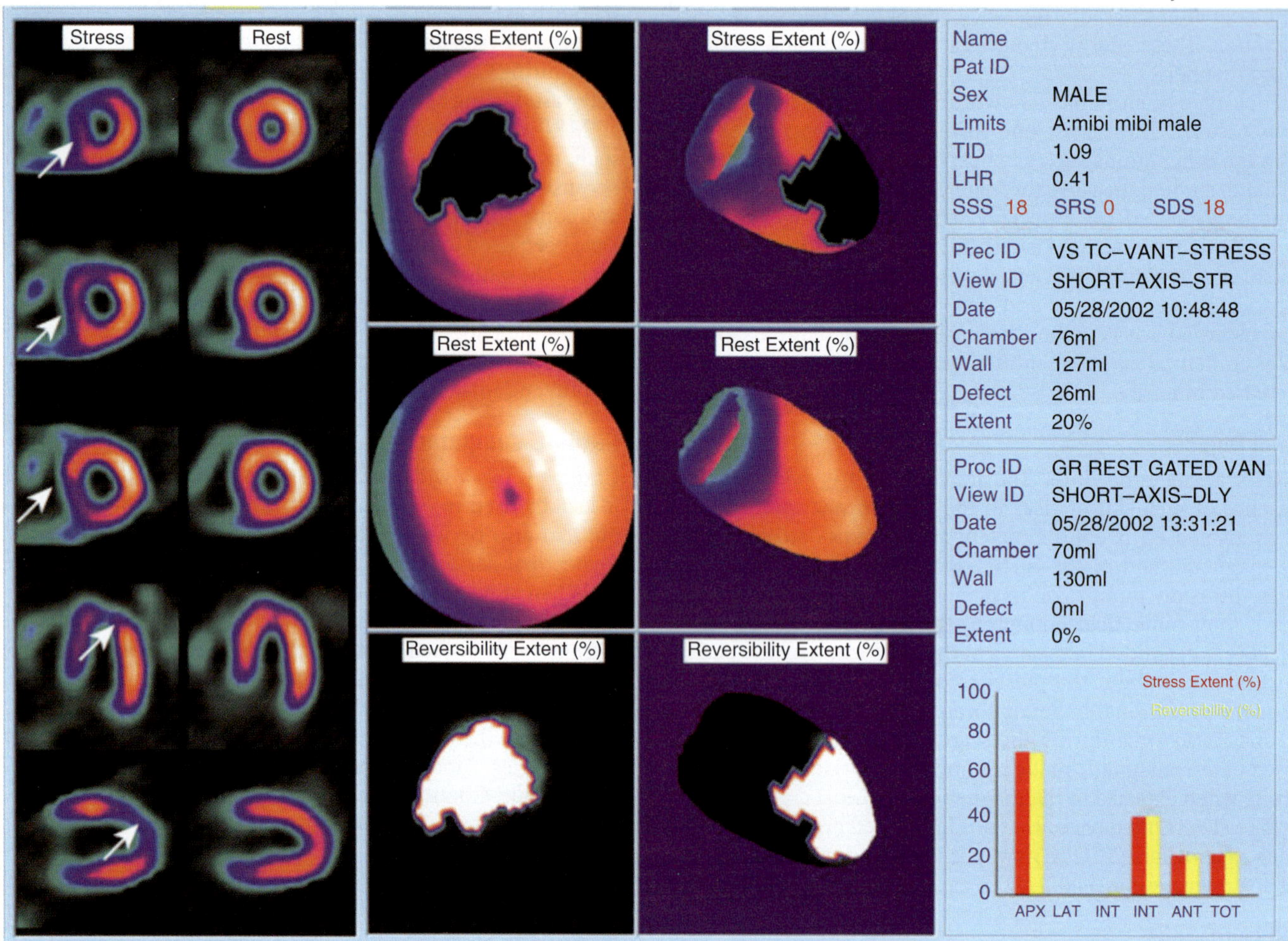

FIG. 12.87 Radionuclide Isotope and Myocardial Perfusion Viability. Left panel: From top to bottom, three short-axis views and two vertical-axis views of the heart after stress. The *white arrow* shows areas of poor myocardial perfusion. The matching scans are taken after rest and reinjection of the tracer. The images at rest show normal perfusion and tracer uptake. Bright orange indicates normal myocardial uptake, while blue-purple indicates ischemic tissue with poor tracer uptake. Middle panel: From top to bottom, polar maps of the entire myocardium localize the ischemic area normally supplied by the left anterior descending artery. Right panel: Quantitative analysis of myocardial viability. (From Kumar P, Clark M, eds. *Kumar and Clarke's Clinical Medicine*. 9th ed. Elsevier; 2017.)

arteriography defines the anatomy of the coronary arteries, it does not show how effectively the arteries perfuse the portion of cardiac muscle they supply. Radionuclide imaging can help determine whether there are ischemic areas of the heart that are still viable and amenable to revascularization.

Radionuclide Isotopes

The radioisotopes used in cardiac diagnostic imaging are very different from the radioisotopes used in oncology for tumor ablation. Diagnostic isotopes have a short half-life (minutes to hours) and are used in very small amounts to minimize radioactivity risk. Patients do not need to be isolated, and no specific precautions are required for blood, urine, stool, or other body fluids.

Thallium-201. Thallium-201 (^{201}Tl) is a low-energy radioactive isotope. It is an analog of potassium and acts like potassium when injected into the bloodstream. Thallium is similar to potassium, in that it is absorbed from the bloodstream by cardiac muscle cells as part of the sodium-potassium adenosine triphosphatase (ATPase) pump. Thallium uptake depends on two factors: the patency of the coronary arteries and the amount of healthy myocardium with a functional sodium-potassium ATPase pump. Areas of infarcted myocardium (dead tissue) do not take up thallium. After thallium has been injected, a specialized scintillation camera and associated computer system are used to scan the myocardium.

Technetium-99m. Technetium-99m (^{99m}Tc) is also used frequently. It is often attached to other trace substances for diagnostic imaging (^{99m}Tc-sestamibi or ^{99m}Tc-tetrofosmin). These substances may be described as *radiopharmaceuticals*. ^{99m}Tc tracers are highly suited to imaging myocardium during ACS because the tracers do not redistribute over time (they remain in myocardium), allowing a second scan to be performed many hours later if needed (see Fig. 12.87).

Stress Myocardial Perfusion Imaging

A stress myocardial perfusion imaging (MPI) scan is conducted in a specialized nuclear medicine department. It can be performed using single-photon emission computed tomography (SPECT) (see Fig. 12.87) or positron emission tomography (PET) and using exercise or pharmacologic stress. The walls of the testing space are normally lined with lead to prevent any radioactivity dispersal to other areas. A patent IV line is required. A radioisotope flow agent (^{201}Tl or ^{99m}Tc) is injected into the bloodstream before exercise to permit identification of perfused versus nonperfused (cold) areas. A specialized perfusion-scanning camera is used to scan the heart. As with the other cardiac stress tests, the options to increase the HR and myocardial blood flow are physical exercise by the patient or infusion of a medication to achieve the same effect (see Table 12.22).

Exercise Stress Myocardial Perfusion Imaging Procedure

Before an exercise stress MPI, the procedure is fully explained to the patient, including a description of the equipment (ECG monitoring equipment, cardiovascular exercise treadmill or stationary bicycle, and an Anger gamma scintillation camera). The patient is usually fasting, because the scan involves vigorous exercise. Vasodilating medications that may alter the uptake of the radioisotope (nitrates, theophylline, and related medications) are held before any baseline study. A patent IV line is inserted before the test. In the laboratory, the patient is asked to exercise vigorously for 1 minute or more or until angina or fatigue develops. At this point, the isotope is injected into the bloodstream. After the injection, the patient is asked to exercise vigorously for another minute to stress the heart and circulate the radioisotope. As soon as possible after exercise (within 10 minutes), the patient is asked to lie on the examination table for the first perfusion scan by the scintillation camera. The camera examines the heart from three angles, anterior, left anterior oblique, and left lateral oblique, to increase accuracy. On the camera screen, the heart image looks like a circle with a hole (doughnut shape). The myocardium appears, but the fluid-filled center does not.

Pharmacologic Stress Myocardial Perfusion Imaging Procedure

A patient who cannot tolerate an exercise MPI stress test can undergo a pharmacologic MPI stress test at rest. The test can be performed with ^{201}Tl or ^{99m}Tc. Similar to the protocol for an ECG stress test, a dobutamine infusion is used to increase coronary artery and myocardial blood flow. The goal is to drive the HR to the 85% maximal HR predicted for that individual; if needed, atropine is added to achieve the desired HR. After the first scan, the patient is removed from the scanner, and the HR is allowed to return to baseline. After approximately 5 to 10 minutes, the patient is asked to return to the scanner to ensure the LV wall motion has also returned to baseline.

Radionuclide Test Results

If no perfusion defect is seen, the test is complete for that patient. If a perfusion defect (dark area) is observed in the myocardium, the patient is asked to return for a repeat scan 2 to 4 hours later or the next day, depending on the radioisotope tracer that was used. If a perfusion defect is present 4 hours later, the area is infarcted. This is sometimes described as a *cold spot* or as a *fixed lesion*. If the perfusion defect has taken up the radioisotope since the first test (redistribution), the area is ischemic. An ischemic defect is amenable to reperfusion therapy such as a CABG or a catheter-based procedure to open a coronary artery.

BOX 12.13 Internet Resources

Cardiovascular Diagnostic Procedures

- American Association of Critical Care Nurses (AACN): https://www.aacn.org
- American Heart Association (AHA): https://www.heart.org/en/professional

ADDITIONAL RESOURCES

See Box 12.13 for Internet resources related to cardiovascular diagnostic procedures.

KEY POINTS

Hemodynamic Monitoring

- Hemodynamic monitoring is a major reason for admission to a critical care unit.
- Hemodynamic monitoring and CO measurement now incorporates not only invasive catheter-based and thermodilution methods but also less invasive and noninvasive (ultrasound/Doppler) systems.
- Continuous monitoring of venous oxygen saturation (SvO_2 and $ScvO_2$) is indicated for a critically ill patient who has the potential to develop an imbalance between oxygen supply and metabolic tissue demand, although use of this technology is now less common.

Electrocardiography

- Accurate ECG lead placement and interpretation of ECG rhythms in the context of a clinical diagnosis yields relevant information that contributes to optimal patient outcomes. This includes recognition of ischemia and infarction on a 12-lead ECG and knowledge of atrial dysrhythmias, ventricular dysrhythmias, and heart blocks.

Laboratory Tests

- Laboratory studies required in cardiac care include electrolyte levels (potassium, sodium, calcium), cardiac biomarkers (troponin and creatine kinase-MB), hematologic status (hemoglobin, hematocrit, WBC, platelets), coagulation times (INR, activated partial thromboplastin time), serum lipid levels (LDL-C, HDL-C, triglycerides), and laboratory values associated with the status of other organ systems that can secondarily affect cardiac function.

Diagnostic Procedures

- Specialized diagnostic studies include cardiac catheterization to assess the heart chambers and intracardiac pressures, angiography to assess the coronary arteries, and electrophysiology to assess the heart's electrical system.
- Interpretation of the chest radiograph is used to noninvasively locate catheters, tubes, and implantable devices and to detect heart-related complications such as pulmonary edema.
- Echocardiography is commonly used in the critical care unit for rapid assessment of change in cardiac function. Point-of-care ultrasound use has increased as this technology has become smaller and more portable.
- Ambulatory diagnostic tests include remote ECG monitoring, treadmill or pharmacologic stress tests, signal-averaged ECG, MRI, and CT.

Visit the Evolve site at http://evolve.elsevier.com/Urden/CriticalCareNursing for additional study materials.

REFERENCES

1. Pinsky MR, Cecconi M, Chew MS, et al. Effective hemodynamic monitoring. *Crit Care.* 2022;26(1):294. https://doi.org/10.1186/s13054-022-04173-z.
2. Lough ME. *Arterial pressure monitoring. Hemodynamic Monitoring: Evolving Technologies and Clinical Practice.* 1st ed. Elsevier; 2016:55–88. chap 3.
3. Robertson-Malt S, Malt GN, Farquhar V, Greer W. Heparin versus normal saline for patency of arterial lines. *Cochrane Database Syst Rev.* 2014;(5):CD007364. https://doi.org/10.1002/14651858.CD007364.pub2.
4. Cuker A, Arepally GM, Chong BH, et al. American Society of Hematology 2018 guidelines for management of venous thromboembolism: heparin-induced thrombocytopenia. *Blood Adv.* 2018;2(22):3360–3392. https://doi.org/10.1182/bloodadvances.2018024489.
5. O'Grady NP, Alexander M, Burns LA, et al. Guidelines for the prevention of intravascular catheter-related infections. *Am J Infect Control.* 2011;39(4 suppl 1):S1–34. https://doi.org/10.1016/j.ajic.2011.01.003.
6. Centers for Disease Control and Prevention. Guidelines for the Prevention of Intravascular Catheter-Related Infections. Updated 2017. Accessed September, 2023. https://www.cdc.gov/infectioncontrol/guidelines/bsi/updates.html#print.
7. Barros L, Bridges E., Cockerham M, Greco S, Herrera F, N. S. Pulmonary Artery / Central Venous Pressure Monitoring in Adults. American Association of Caritical Care Nurses (AACN). Accessed September, 2023. https://www.aacn.org/~/media/aacn-website/clincial-resources/practice-alerts/pap2017practicealert.pdf.
8. Crowther M, Ricker J, Frank L, et al. Arterial monitoring system leveling method, transducer location, and accuracy of blood pressure measurements. *Am J Crit Care.* 2022;31(3):250–254. https://doi.org/10.4037/ajcc2022890.
9. Oh C, Lee S, Jeon S, et al. Errors in pressure measurements due to changes in pressure transducer levels during adult cardiac surgery: a prospective observational study. *BMC Anesthesiol.* 2023;23(1):8. https://doi.org/10.1186/s12871-023-01968-7.
10. Saugel B, Kouz K, Meidert AS, Schulte-Uentrop L, Romagnoli S. How to measure blood pressure using an arterial catheter: a systematic 5-step approach. *Crit Care.* 2020;24(1):172. https://doi.org/10.1186/s13054-020-02859-w.
11. O'Horo JC, Maki DG, Krupp AE, Safdar N. Arterial catheters as a source of bloodstream infection: a systematic review and meta-analysis. *Crit Care Med.* 2014;42(6):1334–1339. https://doi.org/10.1097/CCM.0000000000000166.
12. Kamboj N, Chang K, Metcalfe K, Chu CH, Conway A. Accuracy and precision of continuous non-invasive arterial pressure monitoring in critical care: a systematic review and meta-analysis. *Intensive Crit Care Nurs.* 2021;67:103091. https://doi.org/10.1016/j.iccn.2021.103091.
13. Hamzaoui O, Monnet X, Teboul JL. Pulsus paradoxus. *Eur Respir J.* 2013;42(6):1696–1705. https://doi.org/10.1183/09031936.00138912.
14. Dee SA, Tucciarone J, Plotkin G, Mallilo C. Determining the impact of an alarm management program on alarm fatigue among ICU and telemetry RNs: an evidence based research project. *SAGE Open Nurs.* 2022;8:23779608221098713. https://doi.org/10.1177/23779608221098713.
15. Wang H, Tong H, Liu H, et al. Effectiveness of antimicrobial-coated central venous catheters for preventing catheter-related blood-stream infections with the implementation of bundles: a systematic review and network meta-analysis. *Ann Intensive Care.* 2018;8(1):71. https://doi.org/10.1186/s13613-018-0416-4.
16. Oliveira B, Prasanna M, Lemyze M, Tronchon L, Thevenin D, Mallat J. A comparison between measured and calculated central venous oxygen saturation in critically ill patients. *PLoS One.* 2018;13(11):e0206868. https://doi.org/10.1371/journal.pone.0206868.
17. Chaaban N, Mallick AK, Shaheen W, Kshatriya S. Isolated right ventricular air embolism. *Radiol Case Rep.* 2022;17(9):3043–3045. https://doi.org/10.1016/j.radcr.2022.05.026.
18. Marik PE. Obituary: pulmonary artery catheter 1970 to 2013. *Ann Intensive Care.* 2013;3(1):38. https://doi.org/10.1186/2110-5820-3-38.
19. Azadian M, Win S, Abdipour A, Kim CK, Nguyen HB. Mortality benefit from the passive leg raise maneuver in guiding resuscitation of septic shock patients: a systematic review and meta-analysis of randomized trials. *J Intensive Care Med.* 2022;37(5):611–617. https://doi.org/10.1177/08850666211019713.
20. Kubiak GM, Ciarka A, Biniecka M, Ceranowicz P. Right heart catheterization-background, physiological basics, and clinical implications. *J Clin Med.* 2019;8(9). https://doi.org/10.3390/jcm8091331.
21. Beydoun HA, Beydoun MA, Eid SM, Zonderman AB. Association of pulmonary artery catheter with in-hospital outcomes after cardiac surgery in the United States: National Inpatient Sample 1999-2019. *Sci Rep.* 2023;13(1):13541. https://doi.org/10.1038/s41598-023-40615-6.
22. Brown JA, Aranda-Michel E, Kilic A, et al. The impact of pulmonary artery catheter use in cardiac surgery. *J Thorac Cardiovasc Surg.* 2022;164(6):1965–1973.e6. https://doi.org/10.1016/j.jtcvs.2021.01.086.
23. Saxena A, Garan AR, Kapur NK, et al. Value of hemodynamic monitoring in patients with cardiogenic shock undergoing mechanical circulatory support. *Circulation.* 2020;141(14):1184–1197. https://doi.org/10.1161/circulationaha.119.043080.
24. Han JC, Taberner AJ, Loiselle DS, Tran K. Cardiac efficiency and starling's law of the heart. *J Physiol.* 2022;600(19):4265–4285. https://doi.org/10.1113/jp283632.
25. Heidenreich PA, Bozkurt B, Aguilar D, et al. 2022 ACC/AHA/HFSA guideline for the management of heart failure. *J Card Fail.* 2022;28(5):e1–e167. https://doi.org/10.1016/j.cardfail.2022.02.010.
26. Barnett CF, O'Brien C, De Marco T. Critical care management of the patient with pulmonary hypertension. *Eur Heart J Acute Cardiovasc Care.* 2022;11(1):77–83. https://doi.org/10.1093/ehjacc/zuab113.
27. Coffey S, Roberts-Thomson R, Brown A, et al. Global epidemiology of valvular heart disease. *Nat Rev Cardiol.* 2021;18(12):853–864. https://doi.org/10.1038/s41569-021-00570-z.
28. Hayashi H, Abe Y, Morita Y, et al. The accuracy of a large V wave in the pulmonary capillary wedge pressure waveform for diagnosing current mitral regurgitation. *Cardiology.* 2018;141(1):46–51. https://doi.org/10.1159/000493007.
29. Evans L, Rhodes A, Alhazzani W, et al. Executive summary: surviving sepsis campaign: international guidelines for the management of sepsis and septic shock 2021. *Crit Care Med.* 2021;49(11):1974–1982. https://doi.org/10.1097/ccm.0000000000005357.
30. Calcaianu G, Calcaianu M, Gschwend A, Canuet M, Meziani F, Kessler R. Hemodynamic profile of pulmonary hypertension (PH) in ARDS. *Pulm Circ.* 2018;8(1):2045893217753415. https://doi.org/10.1177/2045893217753415.
31. Grasselli G, Calfee CS, Camporota L, et al. ESICM guidelines on acute respiratory distress syndrome: definition, phenotyping and respiratory support strategies. *Intensive Care Med.* 2023;49(7):727–759. https://doi.org/10.1007/s00134-023-07050-7.
32. Bootsma IT, Boerma EC, de Lange F, Scheeren TWL. The contemporary pulmonary artery catheter. Part 1: placement and waveform analysis. *J Clin Monit Comput.* 2022;36(1):5–15. https://doi.org/10.1007/s10877-021-00662-8.
33. Corp A, Thomas C, Adlam M. The cardiovascular effects of positive pressure ventilation. *BJA Educ.* 2021;21(6):202–209. https://doi.org/10.1016/j.bjae.2021.01.002.
34. Pahuja M, Schrage B, Westermann D, Basir MB, Garan AR, Burkhoff D. Hemodynamic effects of mechanical circulatory support devices in ventricular septal defect. *Circ Heart Fail.* 2019;12(7):e005981. https://doi.org/10.1161/circheartfailure.119.005981.
35. Christensen M. Mixed venous oxygen saturation monitoring revisited: thoughts for critical care nursing practice. *Aust Crit Care.* 2012;25(2):78–90. https://doi.org/10.1016/j.aucc.2011.10.001.

36. Leeper B. Venous oxygen saturation monitoring. In: Lough ME, ed. *Hemodynamic Monitoring: Evolving Technologies and Clinical Practice*. 1st ed. Elsevier; 2016:205–229.
37. Saugel B, Hoppe P, Nicklas JY, et al. Continuous noninvasive pulse wave analysis using finger cuff technologies for arterial blood pressure and cardiac output monitoring in perioperative and intensive care medicine: a systematic review and meta-analysis. *Br J Anaesth*. 2020;125(1):25–37. https://doi.org/10.1016/j.bja.2020.03.013.
38. Jedrzejewski D, McFarlane E, Lacy PS, Williams B. Pulse wave calibration and implications for blood pressure measurement: systematic review and meta-analysis. *Hypertension*. 2021;78(2):360–371. https://doi.org/10.1161/hypertensionaha.120.16817.
39. Saugel B, Kouz K, Scheeren TWL, et al. Cardiac output estimation using pulse wave analysis-physiology, algorithms, and technologies: a narrative review. *Br J Anaesth*. 2021;126(1):67–76. https://doi.org/10.1016/j.bja.2020.09.049.
40. Berndsen M. Noninvasive and minimally invasive cardiac output monitoring: a nursing perspective. *Dimens Crit Care Nurs*. 2022;41(3):121–123. https://doi.org/10.1097/dcc.0000000000000524.
41. Thomsen KK, Kouz K, Saugel B. Pulse wave analysis: basic concepts and clinical application in intensive care medicine. *Curr Opin Crit Care*. 2023;29(3):215–222. https://doi.org/10.1097/mcc.0000000000001039.
42. He HW, Liu DW, Long Y, Wang XT, Zhao ML, Lai XL. The effect of variable arterial transducer level on the accuracy of pulse contour waveform-derived measurements in critically ill patients. *J Clin Monit Comput*. 2016;30(5):569–575. https://doi.org/10.1007/s10877-015-9756-x.
43. Rasch S, Schmidle P, Sancak S, et al. Increased extravascular lung water index (EVLWI) reflects rapid non-cardiogenic oedema and mortality in COVID-19 associated ARDS. *Sci Rep*. 2021;11(1):11524. https://doi.org/10.1038/s41598-021-91043-3.
44. Boissier F, Bagate F, Mekontso Dessap A. Hemodynamic monitoring using trans esophageal echocardiography in patients with shock. *Ann Transl Med*. 2020;8(12):791. https://doi.org/10.21037/atm-2020-hdm-23.
45. Metkus TS, Thibault D, Grant MC, et al. Transesophageal echocardiography in patients undergoing coronary artery bypass graft surgery. *J Am Coll Cardiol*. 2021;78(2):112–122. https://doi.org/10.1016/j.jacc.2021.04.064.
46. Pastore MC, Ilardi F, Stefanini A, et al. Bedside ultrasound for hemodynamic monitoring in cardiac intensive care unit. *J Clin Med*. 2022;11(24). https://doi.org/10.3390/jcm11247538.
47. Albert NM, Murray T, Bena JF, et al. Differences in alarm events between disposable and reusable electrocardiography lead wires. *Am J Crit Care*. 2015;24(1):67–73. https://doi.org/10.4037/ajcc2015663.
48. Albert NM, Slifcak E, Roach JD, et al. Infection rates in intensive care units by electrocardiographic lead wire type: disposable vs reusable. *Am J Crit Care*. 2014;23(6):460–467. https://doi.org/10.4037/ajcc2014362.
49. Block 3rd FE, Block Jr FE. Decreasing false alarms by obtaining the best signal and minimizing artifact from physiological sensors. *Biomed Instrum Technol*. 2015;49(6):423–431. https://doi.org/10.2345/0899-8205-49.6.423.
50. Shue McGuffin K, Ortiz S. Daily Electrocardiogram electrode change and the effect on frequency of nuisance alarms. *Dimens Crit Care Nurs*. 2019 Jul/Aug;38(4):187–191. https://doi.org/10.1097/DCC.0000000000000362.
51. Sandau KE, Funk M, Auerbach A, et al. Update to practice standards for electrocardiographic monitoring in hospital settings: a scientific statement from the American heart association. *Circulation*. 2017;136(19):e273–e344. https://doi.org/10.1161/CIR.0000000000000527.
52. Kligfield P, Gettes LS, Bailey JJ, et al. Recommendations for the standardization and interpretation of the electrocardiogram: part I: the electrocardiogram and its technology: a scientific statement from the American Heart Association Electrocardiography and Arrhythmias Committee, Council on Clinical Cardiology; the American College of Cardiology Foundation; and the Heart Rhythm Society Endorsed by the International Society for Computerized Electrocardiology. *Circulation*. 2007;115(10):1306–1324. https://doi.org/10.1161/CIRCULATIONAHA.106.180200.
53. Surawicz B, Childers R, Deal BJ, et al. AHA/ACCF/HRS recommendations for the standardization and interpretation of the electrocardiogram: part III: intraventricular conduction disturbances: a scientific statement from the American Heart Association Electrocardiography and Arrhythmias Committee, Council on Clinical Cardiology; the American College of Cardiology Foundation; and the Heart Rhythm Society: endorsed by the International Society for Computerized Electrocardiology. *Circulation*. 2009;119(10):e235–e240. https://doi.org/10.1161/CIRCULATIONAHA.108.191095.
54. American Association of Critical Care Nurses (ACCN). ST segment monitoring: AACN Practice Alert. Accessed 9/21/2023. http://www.aacn.org/wd/practice/docs/practicealerts/st-segment-monitoring.pdf?menu=aboutus
55. Rautaharju PM, Surawicz B, Gettes LS, et al. AHA/ACCF/HRS recommendations for the standardization and interpretation of the electrocardiogram: part IV: the ST segment, T and U waves, and the QT interval: a scientific statement from American Heart Association Electrocardiography and Arrhythmias Committee, Council on Clinical Cardiology; the American College of Cardiology Foundation; and the Heart Rhythm Society Endorsed by the International Society for Computerized Electrocardiology. *Circulation*. 2009;119(10):e241–e250. https://doi.org/10.1161/CIRCULATIONAHA.108.191096.
56. Drew BJ, Ackerman MJ, Funk M, et al. Prevention of torsade de pointes in hospital settings: a scientific statement from the American Heart Association and the American College of Cardiology Foundation. *Circulation*. 2010;121(8):1047–1060. https://doi.org/10.1161/CIRCULATIONAHA.109.192704.
57. Pickham D, Helfenbein E, Shinn JA, et al. High prevalence of corrected QT interval prolongation in acutely ill patients is associated with mortality: results of the QT in Practice (QTIP) Study. *Crit Care Med*. 2012;40(2):394–399. https://doi.org/10.1097/CCM.0b013e318232db4a.
58. Sommargren CE, Drew BJ. Preventing torsades de pointes by careful cardiac monitoring in hospital settings. *AACN Adv Crit Care*. 2007;18(3):285–293.
59. Pelter MM, Loranger DL, Kozik TM, et al. Among unstable angina and non-ST-elevation myocardial infarction patients, transient myocardial ischemia and early invasive treatment are predictors of major in-hospital complications. *J Cardiovasc Nurs*. 2016;31(4):E10–E19. https://doi.org/10.1097/JCN.0000000000000310.
60. Zellweger MJ, Maraun M, Osterhues HH, et al. Progression to overt or silent CAD in asymptomatic patients with diabetes mellitus at high coronary risk: main findings of the prospective multicenter BARDOT trial with a pilot randomized treatment substudy. *JACC Cardiovasc Imaging*. 2014;7(10):1001–1010. https://doi.org/10.1016/j.jcmg.2014.07.010.
61. Behrouz R, Sullebarger JT, Malek AR. Cardiac manifestations of subarachnoid hemorrhage. *Expert Rev Cardiovasc Ther*. 2011;9(3):303–307. https://doi.org/10.1586/erc.10.189.
62. Wagner GS, Macfarlane P, Wellens H, et al. AHA/ACCF/HRS recommendations for the standardization and interpretation of the electrocardiogram: part VI: acute ischemia/infarction: a scientific statement from the American Heart Association Electrocardiography and Arrhythmias Committee, Council on Clinical Cardiology; the American College of Cardiology Foundation; and the Heart Rhythm Society Endorsed by the International Society for Computerized Electrocardiology. *Circulation*. 2009;119(10):e262–e270. https://doi.org/10.1161/CIRCULATIONAHA.108.191098.
63. Hancock EW, Deal BJ, Mirvis DM, et al. AHA/ACCF/HRS recommendations for the standardization and interpretation of the electrocardiogram: part V: electrocardiogram changes associated with cardiac chamber hypertrophy: a scientific statement from the American Heart Association Electrocardiography and Arrhythmias Committee, Council on Clinical Cardiology; the American College of Cardiology Foundation; and the Heart Rhythm Society Endorsed by the International Society for Computerized Electrocardiology. *Circulation*. 2009;119(10):e251–e261. https://doi.org/10.1161/CIRCULATIONAHA.108.191097.
64. Amsterdam EA, Wenger NK, Brindis RG, et al. 2014 AHA/ACC guideline for the management of patients with non-ST-elevation acute coronary

syndromes: a report of the American College of Cardiology/American Heart Association Task Force on Practice Guidelines. *Circulation.* 2014;130(25):e344–426. https://doi.org/10.1161/CIR.0000000000000134.
65. O'Gara PT, Kushner FG, Ascheim DD, et al. 2013 ACCF/AHA guideline for the management of ST-elevation myocardial infarction: a report of the American College of Cardiology Foundation/American Heart Association Task Force on Practice Guidelines. *Circulation.* 2013;127(4):e362–425. https://doi.org/10.1161/CIR.0b013e3182742cf6.
66. Goldstein JA. Acute right ventricular infarction. *Cardiol Clin.* 2012;30(2):219–232. https://doi.org/10.1016/j.ccl.2012.03.002.
67. Peters A, Lakhter V, Bashir R. Under-pressure: right ventricular infarction. *Am J Med.* 2015;128(9):966–969. https://doi.org/10.1016/j.amjmed.2015.05.007.
68. Xiong Y, Wang L, Liu W, Hankey GJ, Xu B, Wang S. The prognostic significance of right bundle branch block: a meta-analysis of prospective cohort studies. *Clin Cardiol.* 2015;38(10):604–613. https://doi.org/10.1002/clc.22454.
69. Erne P, Iglesias JF, Urban P, et al. Left bundle-branch block in patients with acute myocardial infarction: presentation, treatment, and trends in outcome from 1997 to 2016 in routine clinical practice. *Am Heart J.* 2017;184:106–113. https://doi.org/10.1016/j.ahj.2016.11.003.
70. Elizari MV, Chiale PA. The electrocardiographic features of complete and partial left anterior and left posterior hemiblock. *J Electrocardiol.* 2012;45(5):528–535. https://doi.org/10.1016/j.jelectrocard.2012.06.012.
71. Page RL, Joglar JA, Caldwell MA, et al. 2015 ACC/AHA/HRS guideline for the management of adult patients with supraventricular tachycardia: a report of the American College of Cardiology/American Heart Association Task Force on Clinical Practice Guidelines and the Heart Rhythm Society. *Circulation.* 2016;133(14):e506–e574. https://doi.org/10.1161/CIR.0000000000000311.
72. Appelboam A, Reuben A, Mann C, et al. Postural modification to the standard Valsalva manoeuvre for emergency treatment of supraventricular tachycardias (REVERT): a randomised controlled trial. *Lancet.* 2015;386(10005):1747–1753. https://doi.org/10.1016/S0140-6736(15)61485-4.
73. January CT, Wann LS, Alpert JS, et al. 2014 AHA/ACC/HRS guideline for the management of patients with atrial fibrillation: a report of the American College of Cardiology/American Heart Association Task Force on practice guidelines and the Heart Rhythm Society. *Circulation.* 2014;130(23):e199–267. https://doi.org/10.1161/CIR.0000000000000041.
74. Joglar JA, Chung MK, Armbruster AL, et al. 2023 ACC/AHA/ACCP/HRS Guideline for the Diagnosis and Management of Atrial Fibrillation: A Report of the American College of Cardiology/American Heart Association Joint Committee on Clinical Practice Guidelines [published correction appears in Circulation. 2024 Jan 2;149(1):e167] [published correction appears in Circulation. 2024 Feb 27;149(9):e936]. *Circulation.* 2024;149(1):e1–e156. https://doi.org/10.1161/CIR.0000000000001193.
75. Sardar MR, Saeed W, Kowey PR. Antiarrhythmic drug therapy for atrial fibrillation. *Cardiol Clin.* 2014;32(4):533–549. https://doi.org/10.1016/j.ccl.2014.07.012.
76. Zimetbaum P. Antiarrhythmic drug therapy for atrial fibrillation. *Circulation.* 2012;125(2):381–389. https://doi.org/10.1161/CIRCULATIONAHA.111.019927.
77. Camm AJ, Kirchhof P, Lip GY, et al. Guidelines for the management of atrial fibrillation: the task force for the management of atrial fibrillation of the European society of Cardiology (ESC). *Europace.* 2010;12(10):1360–1420. https://doi.org/10.1093/europace/euq350.
78. Camm AJ, Lip GY, De Caterina R, et al. 2012 focused update of the ESC Guidelines for the management of atrial fibrillation: an update of the 2010 ESC Guidelines for the management of atrial fibrillation. Developed with the special contribution of the European Heart Rhythm Association. *Eur Heart J.* 2012;33(21):2719–2747. https://doi.org/10.1093/eurheartj/ehs253.
79. Calkins H. Catheter ablation to maintain sinus rhythm. *Circulation.* 2012;125(11):1439–1445. https://doi.org/10.1161/CIRCULATIONAHA.111.019943.
80. You JJ, Singer DE, Howard PA, et al. Antithrombotic therapy for atrial fibrillation: Antithrombotic Therapy and Prevention of Thrombosis, 9th ed: American College of Chest Physicians Evidence-Based Clinical Practice Guidelines. *Chest.* 2012;141(2 Suppl):e531S–e575S. https://doi.org/10.1378/chest.11-2304.
81. January CT, Wann LS, Calkins H, et al. 2019 AHA/ACC/HRS focused update of the 2014 AHA/ACC/HRS guideline for the management of patients with atrial fibrillation: a report of the American College of Cardiology/American Heart Association Task Force on Clinical Practice Guidelines and the Heart Rhythm Society. *J Am Coll Cardiol.* 2019;74(1):104–132. https://doi.org/10.1016/j.jacc.2019.01.011.
82. Roberts DM, Gallapatthy G, Dunuwille A, Chan BS. Pharmacological treatment of cardiac glycoside poisoning. *Br J Clin Pharmacol.* 2016;81(3):488–495. https://doi.org/10.1111/bcp.12814.
83. Suba S, Sandoval CP, Zegre-Hemsey JK, Hu X, Pelter MM. Contribution of electrocardiographic accelerated ventricular rhythm alarms to alarm fatigue. *Am J Crit Care.* 2019;28(3):222–229. https://doi.org/10.4037/ajcc2019314.
84. Raebel MA. Hyperkalemia associated with use of angiotensin-converting enzyme inhibitors and angiotensin receptor blockers. *Cardiovasc Ther.* 2012;30(3):e156–e166. https://doi.org/10.1111/j.1755-5922.2010.00258.x.
85. Kovesdy CP. Management of hyperkalemia: an update for the internist. *Am J Med.* 2015;128(12):1281–1287. https://doi.org/10.1016/j.amjmed.2015.05.040.
86. Melchers M, van Zanten ARH. Management of hypocalcaemia in the critically ill. *Curr Opin Crit Care.* 2023;29(4):330–338. https://doi.org/10.1097/mcc.0000000000001059.
87. Reddy ST, Soman SS, Yee J. Magnesium balance and measurement. *Adv Chronic Kidney Dis.* 2018;25(3):224–229. https://doi.org/10.1053/j.ackd.2018.03.002.
88. Neumar RW, Otto CW, Link MS, et al. Part 8: adult advanced cardiovascular life support: 2010 American Heart Association Guidelines for Cardiopulmonary Resuscitation and Emergency Cardiovascular Care. *Circulation.* 2010;122(18 suppl 3):S729–S767. https://doi.org/10.1161/CIRCULATIONAHA.110.970988.
89. Wang XY, Zhang F, Zhang C, Zheng LR, Yang J. The biomarkers for acute myocardial infarction and heart failure. *BioMed Res Int.* 2020;2020:2018035. https://doi.org/10.1155/2020/2018035.
90. Hirsh J, Poller L. The international normalized ratio. A guide to understanding and correcting its problems. *Arch Intern Med.* 1994;154(3):282–288. https://doi.org/10.1001/archinte.154.3.282.
91. Dager WE, Gulseth MP, Nutescu EA. *Anticoagulation Therapy: A Clinical Practice Guide*; 2018. https://doi.org/10.37573/9781585284900.
92. Witt DM, Nieuwlaat R, Clark NP, et al. American Society of Hematology 2018 guidelines for management of venous thromboembolism: optimal management of anticoagulation therapy. *Blood Adv.* 2018;2(22):3257–3291. https://doi.org/10.1182/bloodadvances.2018024893.
93. Grundy SM, Stone NJ, Bailey AL, et al. 2018 AHA/ACC/AACVPR/AAPA/ABC/ACPM/ADA/AGS/APhA/ASPC/NLA/PCNA guideline on the management of blood cholesterol: a report of the American College of Cardiology/American Heart Association Task Force on Clinical Practice Guidelines. *J Am Coll Cardiol.* 2019;73(24):e285–e350. https://doi.org/10.1016/j.jacc.2018.11.003.
94. Rosenson RS. The high-density lipoprotein puzzle: why classic epidemiology, genetic epidemiology, and clinical trials conflict? *Arterioscler Thromb Vasc Biol.* 2016;36(5):777–782. https://doi.org/10.1161/ATVBAHA.116.307024.
95. Patel MR, Bailey SR, Bonow RO, et al. ACCF/SCAI/AATS/AHA/ASE/ASNC/HFSA/HRS/SCCM/SCCT/SCMR/STS 2012 appropriate use criteria for diagnostic catheterization: a report of the American College of Cardiology Foundation Appropriate Use Criteria Task Force, Society for Cardiovascular Angiography and Interventions, American Association for Thoracic Surgery, American Heart Association, American Society of Echocardiography, American Society of Nuclear Cardiology, Heart Failure Society of America, Heart Rhythm Society, Society of Critical Care Medicine, Society of Cardiovascular Computed Tomography, Society for Cardiovascular Magnetic Resonance, and Society of Thoracic Surgeons. *J Am Coll Cardiol.* 2012;59(22):1995–2027. https://doi.org/10.1016/j.jacc.2012.03.003.

96. Sanborn TA, Tcheng JE, Anderson HV, et al. ACC/AHA/SCAI 2014 health policy statement on structured reporting for the cardiac catheterization laboratory: a report of the American College of Cardiology Clinical Quality Committee. *Circulation*. 2014;129(24):2578–2609. https://doi.org/10.1161/CIR.0000000000000043.
97. Virani SS, Newby LK, Arnold SV, et al. 2023 AHA/ACC/ACCP/ASPC/NLA/PCNA guideline for the management of patients with chronic coronary disease: a report of the American Heart Association/American College of Cardiology Joint Committee on Clinical Practice Guidelines. *Circulation*. 2023;148(9):e9–e119. https://doi.org/10.1161/cir.0000000000001168.
98. Bangalore S, Barsness GW, Dangas GD, et al. Evidence-Based Practices in the Cardiac Catheterization Laboratory: A Scientific Statement From the American Heart Association. *Circulation*. 2021;144(5):e107–e119. https://doi.org/10.1161/CIR.0000000000000996.
99. Sandoval Y, Burke MN, Lobo AS, et al. Contemporary arterial access in the cardiac catheterization laboratory. *JACC Cardiovasc Interv*. 2017;10(22):2233–2241. https://doi.org/10.1016/j.jcin.2017.08.058.
100. Ronco F, Tarantini G, McCullough PA. Contrast induced acute kidney injury in interventional cardiology: an update and key guidance for clinicians. *Rev Cardiovasc Med*. 2020;21(1):9–23. https://doi.org/10.31083/j.rcm.2020.01.44.
101. Haines DE, Beheiry S, Akar JG, et al. Heart Rythm Society expert consensus statement on electrophysiology laboratory standards: process, protocols, equipment, personnel, and safety. *Heart Rhythm*. 2014;11(8):e9–51. https://doi.org/10.1016/j.hrthm.2014.03.042.
102. Laroia AT, Donnelly EF, Henry TS, et al. ACR appropriateness Criteria® intensive care unit patients. *J Am Coll Radiol*. 2021;18(5s):S62–s72. https://doi.org/10.1016/j.jacr.2021.01.017.
103. American, College, of, Radiology. ACR–SPR–STR practice parameter for the performance of portable (Mobile Unit). *Chest Radiography*. 2022. Accessed 9/20, 2023 https://www.acr.org/-/media/ACR/Files/Practice-Parameters/Port-Chest-Rad.
104. Bentz MR, Primack SL. Intensive care unit imaging. *Clin Chest Med*. 2015;36(2):219–234. https://doi.org/10.1016/j.ccm.2015.02.006. viii.
105. Steinberg JS, Varma N, Cygankiewicz I, et al. 2017 ISHNE-HRS expert consensus statement on ambulatory ECG and external cardiac monitoring/telemetry. *Heart Rhythm*. 2017;14(7):e55–e96. https://doi.org/10.1016/j.hrthm.2017.03.038.
106. Varma N, Cygankiewicz I, Turakhia M, et al. 2021 ISHNE/HRS/EHRA/APHRS collaborative statement on mHealth in Arrhythmia Management: Digital Medical Tools for Heart Rhythm Professionals: From the International Society for Holter and Noninvasive Electrocardiology/Heart Rhythm Society/European Heart Rhythm Association/Asia Pacific Heart Rhythm Society. *J Arrhythm*. 2021;37(2):271–319. https://doi.org/10.1002/joa3.12461.
107. Fletcher GF, Ades PA, Kligfield P, et al. Exercise standards for testing and training: a scientific statement from the American Heart Association. *Circulation*. 2013;128(8):873–934. https://doi.org/10.1161/CIR.0b013e31829b5b44.
108. Cheong BYC, Wilson JM, Spann SJ, Pettigrew RI, Preventza OA, Muthupillai R. Coronary artery calcium scoring: an evidence-based guide for primary care physicians. *J Intern Med*. 2021;289(3):309–324. https://doi.org/10.1111/joim.13176.

13

Cardiovascular Disorders

Corey Fry, Juliana Liu, and Mary E. Lough

http://evolve.elsevier.com/Urden/CriticalCareNursing

Cardiovascular disease (CVD) remains the leading cause of death in the United States.[1,2] The impact is significant for both health economics and individuals, as the average cost of CVD in the United States was over $407 billion for 1 year (2018 to 2019).[1] CVD is a global disease that causes more than 19 million deaths each year.[1]

POPULATION LEVEL HEART-HEALTH PROMOTION

Because CVD is a global disease, population-level health promotion is of major importance. The *American Heart Association* (AHA) and *National Institutes of Health* (NIH) collect statistics and generate guidelines that have expanded beyond disease prevention to promoting a healthy lifestyle for everyone.

A healthy lifestyle is made up of core health behaviors and health factors, defined as the AHA's *Life's Essential 8*.[1]

- Core health behaviors include not smoking, physical activity, sleep, healthy diet, and healthy weight.
- Core health factors are cholesterol, blood pressure (BP), and glucose control.

Population-level health promotion aims to improve the cardiovascular health of the public. The prevalence of CVD, which includes coronary heart disease (CHD), heart failure (HF), stroke, and hypertension in adults (>20 years old) was 48.6% (127.9 million people) in 2020. Hypertension has the greatest association with CVD, with 24.3 million people affected.[2]

The *World Health Organization* (WHO) global action plan targets preventable risk factors (tobacco and alcohol use, salt intake, obesity, elevated BP and glucose) to reduce premature mortality by 25% by 2025, also known as the *25 by 25 campaign*.[3]

The critical care nurse is uniquely positioned in the inpatient setting to manage CVD outcomes and educate the public on modifiable risk factors that promote a healthy lifestyle. Current guidelines for primary prevention of CVD include estimation of the *10-year Atherosclerotic Cardiovascular Disease risk* (ASCVD).[4] This measure allows team focus on promoting healthy behaviors and working within the individual's *social determinants of health* (SDOH). These determinants include housing instability, food insecurity, transportation, access to exercise activities, and personal safety, all of which are essential for CVD prevention.[3] Care delivery of clinical guidelines is evolving to a *person-centered approach* that considers the patient's environment, resources, culture, and personality in symptom management and health behavior change.[4,5]

An understanding of the pathology of CVD processes and clinical management allows the critical care nurse to anticipate and plan interventions. This chapter focuses on cardiac disorders commonly seen in the critical care environment.

CORONARY ARTERY DISEASE

Description and Etiology

The biggest contributor to cardiovascular system–related morbidity and mortality is *coronary artery disease* (CAD). *Atherosclerosis* is a progressive disease that affects arteries throughout the body. In the heart, atherosclerotic changes are clinically known as *CAD*. This disease process is also known as CHD because other heart structures ultimately become involved in the disease process.

Risk Factors

Research and epidemiologic data collected during the past 50 years have identified preventable (*modifiable*) risk factors, and nonpreventable (*nonmodifiable*) risk factors, that contribute to the development of CAD[2,6] (Box 13.1).

The nonmodifiable risk factors are:

- Age[7]
- Sex (males affected at younger ages than females)[7]
- Family history[8]
- Race[9]

The salient modifiable risk factors for CAD include:

- Diabetes (Table 13.1)[10–12]
- Hyperlipidemia (Table 13.2)[13–15]
- Hypertension (Table 13.3)[16–18]
- Tobacco/Cigarette smoking, including e-cigarettes, second-hand smoke[1,19]
- Obesity[20]
- Physical inactivity (Box 13.2)[1,4,21]

Controlling BP, with a systolic BP < 130 mm Hg, and lowering low-density lipoprotein (LDL) are primary targets to reduce CAD risk.[4] Other risk factors include elevated C-reactive protein[22] (Table 13.4), which is a marker of inflammation. There are also two CAD disease risk-equivalent conditions: chronic kidney disease and diabetes. See Box 13.3 for a summary of all the currently recommended target levels to prevent and manage CAD risk.

Women and Heart Disease Risk

Substantial progress has been made in the awareness, treatment, and prevention of CVD in women.[23] CVD still causes approximately more than one-third of female deaths in the United States.[24] After age 65 years, a higher percentage of women than men have hypertension. Average body weight continues to

BOX 13.1 Modifiable and Nonmodifiable Coronary Artery Disease Risk Factors

Nonmodifiable Risk Factors

- Age
- Sex
- Family history
- Race

Modifiable Risk Factors

- Elevated serum lipids
- Hypertension
- Cigarette smoking
- Prediabetes or diabetes mellitus
- Diet high in saturated fat, cholesterol, and calories
- Elevated homocysteine level
- Metabolic syndrome
- Obesity
- Physical inactivity

TABLE 13.1 Fasting Blood Glucose and Risk for Coronary Artery Disease

Blood Glucose Level	Fasting Plasma Glucose Level[a] (mg/dL)
Normal	70–100
Prediabetes	101–125
Diabetes	126 or greater

[a]Values greater than normal increase the risk for coronary artery disease and kidney failure.

increase. Nearly two out of every three women in the United States older than age 20 years are overweight or obese.[23] The average age for first acute myocardial infarction (MI) in men is 65 years; in women, it is 71.8 years.[24]

Heart Disease and Pregnancy

Pregnancy-related hypertensive disorders and gestational diabetes during pregnancy may raise a women's risk of heart disease later in life.[1]

Heart Disease and Menopause

The *Nurses' Health Study* identified that early menarche (monthly period onset) younger than 10 years old increased CVD risk, but more recent studies consider that genetic and other health factors are also important in age of menarche.[25] Women who experience early-onset menopause (below age 40) have a 40% higher risk of developing CHD compared with women who do not experience early-onset menopause.[26] The incidence of CVD is higher among postmenopausal women. In the past, it seemed logical to prescribe *hormone replacement therapy* (HRT) to treat the symptoms of menopause.[26] Current guidelines do not recommend the use of HRT for primary or secondary prevention of CVD.[26] Diabetes, smoking, and hyperlipidemia all increase the cardiovascular risk for women.[26] Data from the *Framingham Heart Study* indicate the lifetime risk for CVD is more than one in two for women.[27,28] Optimum prevention strategies for women following the AHA's *Life's Essential 8* are often delayed or inadequate.[27] Overall, women are 10 years older than men when they experience major CVD events, and 20 years older for MI and sudden cardiac death (SCD).

TABLE 13.2 Treatment of Blood Cholesterol to Decrease Atherosclerotic Cardiovascular Risk Disease

Patient Characteristics	Intensity of Statins Needed
Age 75 y or less and no safety concerns	High-intensity statin
Age more than 75 y or safety concerns	Moderate-intensity statin
Primary Prevention for LDL-C >190 mg/dL	
Age >21 y	High-intensity statins to achieve 50% decrease in LDL-C; consider nonstatin therapy
Diabetes; age 40–75 y; LDL-C 70–189 mg/dL	Moderate-intensity statins; high-intensity statins when 10-y ASCVD risk is greater than 7.5%
No diabetes; age 40–75 y; LDL-C 70–189 mg/dL	Moderate-intensity statins; if 10-y ASCVD risk is more than 7.5%, moderate- to high-intensity statins; if 10-y ASCVD risk is 0.5%–7.5%, moderate-intensity steroids
Other Factors to Consider	
LDL-C ≥160 mg/dL	Family history; premature ASCVD; hs-CRP 2 or greater; CAC Agatston score >300; ABI <0.9; or lifetime ASCVD risk
LDL-C <190 mg/dL	Age less than 40 y or greater than 75 y; or <5% 10-y ASCVD risk
Clinical ASCVD Risk Factors	
ACS	
History of MI	
Stable or unstable angina	
Coronary or other arterial revascularization	
Stroke	
TIA	
PAD	

ABI, Ankle-brachial index; *ACS*, acute coronary syndrome; *ASCVD*, atherosclerotic cardiovascular disease; *CAC*, coronary artery calcium; *hs-CRP*, high-sensitivity C-reactive protein; *LDL-C*, low-density lipoprotein cholesterol; *MI*, myocardial infarction; *PAD*, peripheral artery disease; *TIA*, transient ischemic attack.
Data from Grundy SM, Stone NJ, Bailey AL, et al. Guidelines on Management of blood cholesterol: Executive Summary. *Circulation.* 2018;2018(139):e1046–e1081.

TABLE 13.3 Hypertension Management Guidelines

General Population (No Diabetes or CKD)		Diabetes or CKD Present	
Age ≥60 y	Age <60 y	All ages; diabetes present; no CVD	All ages; CKD present with or without diabetes
BP goal[a]: SBP <150 DBP <90	BP goal: SBP <140 DBP <90	BP goal: SBP <140 DBP <90	BP goal: SBP <140 DBP <90

BP, Blood pressure; *CKD*, chronic kidney disease; *CVD*, cardiovascular disease; *DBP*, diastolic blood pressure; *SBP*, systolic blood pressure. A BP value greater than normal increases the risk for coronary artery disease and heart failure. All BP values are reported in mm Hg.
Data from James PA. Evidence-based guidelines for the management of high blood pressure in adults. Report from the panel members appointed to the Eighth Joint National Committee (JNC8). *JAMA.* 2014;311(5):507–520.

BOX 13.2 Detailed Coronary Artery Disease Risk Factors

Age
- Coronary artery disease (CAD) disease generally first manifests after age 45 years.
- Men tend to develop CAD symptoms 10 years earlier than women.
- Rate of cardiovascular disease (CVD) in women increases after age 75 years.
- CAD rate is two to three times greater postmenopause than before menopause.

Family History
- Positive family history is defined as a close blood relative who has a myocardial infarction (MI) or stroke before age 60 years.
- Family history suggests genetic or lifestyle predisposition for development of CAD.
- Patients with CAD family history have a 50% greater risk of having an MI.

Diabetes Mellitus
- Elevated blood glucose is a known risk factor for development of vascular inflammation associated with atherosclerosis.
- The American Diabetes Association recommends use of the hemoglobin A_{1c} test with a threshold of 6.5% or greater, fasting blood glucose 126 mg/dL or greater, or 2-hour plasma glucose 200 mg/dL during an oral glucose tolerance test to diagnose diabetes.
- Diabetics have increased risk of developing CAD and worse clinical outcomes after acute coronary syndrome (ACS) events.
- See Table 13.1 for fasting blood glucose levels and risk for CAD.

Physical Activity/Sedentary Lifestyle
- A sedentary lifestyle has negative effects regardless of age, sex, body mass index (BMI), and smoking status.
- Regular physical activity using large muscle groups promotes adaptation to aerobic exercise, which can prevent or delay development of CAD and reduce symptoms in patients with established CVD.
- Exercise decreases low-density lipoprotein (LDL) and triglyceride levels, and increased high-density lipoprotein (HDL) cholesterol reduces insulin resistance at the cellular level, lowering the risk for developing type 2 diabetes.
- Lifelong physical activity is necessary to prevent atherosclerotic CAD and stroke.

Obesity
- Two-thirds of U.S. adults are overweight.
- BMI greater than 30 kg/m^2 is considered obese.
- Obesity is associated with a sedentary lifestyle, calories consumed, and portion size.
- Normal BMI is 18.5–25 kg/m^2 (Weight/Height^2)

Fat Pattern Distribution
- Higher weight carried in the abdominal area has greater risk of CAD.
- Large waist (apple body shape)—excess abdominal adiposity—indicates added fat around the abdominal organs.
- Smaller waist and larger hips (pear body shape) is associated with lower risk of CAD.
- Goal waist measurements are less than 40 inches for men, and less than 35 inches for women.

High-Fat Diet
- A diet rich in saturated fats leads to elevated cholesterol levels.
- A low-fat, high-fiber diet and increased physical activity are the first line of treatment.
- If lifestyle changes are ineffective, lipid-lowering medications are indicated.
- Many patients do not reach their LDL target value.

Hyperlipidemia
- Hyperlipidemia causes severe atherosclerosis and development of CAD.
- Total cholesterol is the sum of HDL, LDL, and VLDL cholesterol (goal <200 mg/dL).

HDL (Goal >40 mg/dL for Men; >50 mg/dL for Women)
- HDL is known as *good cholesterol*; a higher serum level protects against atherosclerotic events.
- HDL promotes efflux of cholesterol from cells.
- HDL has anti-inflammatory and antioxidant effects on the arterial wall.[6]

LDL (Goal <100 mg/dL)
- LDL is known as *bad cholesterol* because high serum levels are associated with increased risk of ACS, stroke, and peripheral artery disease.
- LDL initiates atherosclerosis by infiltrating the vessel wall and inflammatory vessel effects.
- Initial efforts to decrease LDL are based on weight loss, smoking cessation, low-fat diet, physical exercise, and maintaining normal body size.
- If lifestyle changes are not effective in decreasing LDL, the medication category of choice is statins.
- See Table 13.2 for lipid guidelines and risk for CAD.

Triglycerides (Ideal Goal <100 mg/dL)
- Triglyceride level greater than 150 mg/dL increases risk for heart disease and stroke.

Lipoprotein(a) (Goal <30 mg/dL)
- Lp(a) is one of the lipid particles that makes up total LDL value.
- Lp(a) is described verbally as "LP little a."
- It is manufactured in the liver and circulates bound to a large glycoprotein called *apolipoprotein A*.
- Lp(a) is elevated in the presence of inflammation.
- Lp(a) stimulates atheroma and clot formation in inflamed arteries.
- Elevated Lp(a) is the most frequently encountered genetic lipid disorder in families with premature CAD. There are no approved medications effective at lowering Lp(a) and clinical trials are ongoing.

Metabolic Syndrome
- *Metabolic syndrome* refers to clustering of risk factors associated with CVD and type 2 diabetes.
- Approximately one-third of people in the United States have metabolic syndrome.
- Risk factors include:
  - Fasting plasma glucose ≥100 mg/dL
  - HDL cholesterol ≤40 mg/dL in men and ≤50 mg/dL in women
  - Triglycerides ≥150 mg/dL
  - Waist circumference ≥40 inches (102 cm) in men or ≥35 inches (88 cm) in women
  - Blood pressure (BP) ≥130/80 mm Hg

Tobacco/Cigarette Smoking
- Smoking unfavorably alters lipid profile by decreasing HDL and increasing LDL and triglyceride levels.
- The greater number of cigarettes smoked per day, the greater risk of developing CAD, acute MI, and stroke.
- Smoking fewer than five cigarettes per day increases risk.
- Smokers are two to four times more likely to develop CAD compared with nonsmokers.

BOX 13.2 Detailed Coronary Artery Disease Risk Factors—cont'd

- Passive secondhand smoke exposure also increases CVD risk for nonsmoking adults.
- Within 1 year of giving up cigarettes, an ex-smoker's risk of developing CAD decreases significantly.
- Nicotine is addictive, and giving up smoking is difficult.
- People need tremendous support to be able to "kick the habit."

Hypertension

- Hypertension is defined as BP greater than 130/80 mm Hg.
- Increased systolic pressure damages endothelium, leading to vascular inflammation and plaque development.
- Hypertension is known as the silent killer many people with and without CAD are unaware of having hypertension.
- Initial treatments aim at lifestyle changes including physical activity, low sodium diet, limiting alcohol intake, and achieving normal body weight.
- Most patients are started on a diuretic; if this is insufficient, an angiotensin-converting enzyme inhibitor, angiotensin receptor blocker, beta-blocker, or calcium channel blocker may be added.
- Most patients require at least two medications from different classifications to normalize their BP.
- See Table 13.3 for BP guidelines and CAD risk.

Risk Equivalents for CAD

- Medical conditions in which patients have as much risk of experiencing a coronary event as if they already had CAD include:
  - Chronic kidney disease—risk for death from acute MI rises as serum creatinine level increases
  - Diabetes mellitus
  - Peripheral artery disease
  - Cerebrovascular disease

Prevention of Heart Disease in Women

The 2011 AHA *Effectiveness-Based Guidelines for the Prevention of CVD in Women*[23] stratified CVD risk for women into the following three categories:

- *Women at high risk:* Documented CHD, CVD, peripheral artery disease, abdominal aortic aneurysm, diabetes mellitus, end-stage or chronic kidney disease, or 10-year predicted CVD risk greater than 10%.
- *Women at risk:* Cigarette smoking; systolic BP 120 mm Hg or greater, diastolic BP 80 mm Hg or greater, or treated hypertension; total cholesterol 200 mg/dL or greater, high-density lipoprotein C (HDL-C) less than 50 mg/dL, or treated for dyslipidemia; obesity, particularly central adiposity; poor diet; physical inactivity; family history of premature CVD occurring in first-degree relatives in men younger than 55 years old or women younger than 65 years old; metabolic syndrome; evidence of advanced subclinical atherosclerosis (e.g., coronary calcification, carotid plaque, or thickened intimal mean thickness); systemic autoimmune collagen vascular disease (e.g., lupus or rheumatoid arthritis); history of preeclampsia, gestational diabetes, or pregnancy-induced hypertension; or poor exercise tolerance with treadmill testing
- *Women's ideal cardiovascular health (presence of all of these):* total cholesterol <200 mg/dL (untreated), BP <120/<80 mm Hg

TABLE 13.4 C-Reactive Protein and Risk for Coronary Artery Disease

Category	hs-CRP Level[a] (mg/L)
Low risk (normal)	<1
Moderate risk	1–3
High risk	>3

[a]Values ≥1 mg/dL increase the risk for coronary artery disease, but test results are not valid in the presence of infection or other inflammatory condition. Normal values may vary slightly between clinical laboratories; however, values <1 mg/dL are usually considered normal. A test result >10 mg/L suggests a noncoronary source of inflammation or infection.

hs-CRP, High-sensitivity C-reactive protein.

Data from Ramasamy I. Biochemical markers in acute coronary syndrome. *Clin Chim Acta.* 2011;412:1279.

BOX 13.3 Characteristics of Angina Pectoris

Location

- Beneath sternum, radiating to neck and jaw
- Upper chest
- Beneath sternum, radiating down left arm
- Epigastric
- Epigastric, radiating to neck, jaw, and arms
- Neck and jaw
- Left shoulder, inner aspect of both arms
- Intrascapular

Duration

- Less than 5 minutes (stable)
- Longer than 5 minutes or worsening symptoms without relief from rest or sublingual nitroglycerin indicates preinfarction symptoms (unstable)

Quality

- Sensation of pressure or heavy weight on the chest
- Feeling of tightness like a vise
- Visceral quality (deep, heavy, squeezing, aching)
- Burning sensation
- Shortness of breath, with feeling of suffocation
- Most severe pain ever experienced

Radiation

- Medial aspect of left arm
- Jaw
- Left shoulder
- Right arm

Precipitating Factors

- Exertion or exercise
- Cold weather
- Exercising after large, heavy meal
- Emotional upset
- Fear, anger
- Coitus

Medication Relief

- Usually within 1 to 5 minutes after sublingual nitroglycerin administration

(untreated), fasting blood glucose <100 mg/dL (untreated), body mass index (BMI) <25 kg/m², abstinence from smoking, physical activity at goal for adults >20 years of age: ≥150 minutes/week moderate intensity or ≥75 minutes/week vigorous intensity, and healthy DASH-like diet.

Mortality From Heart Disease for Women

Almost 400,000 women die of CVD annually in the United States. Mortality rates for women after an acute MI are higher than for men: 26% compared with 15%.[29] The risk factors hypertension, diabetes mellitus, alcohol intake, and physical inactivity are more strongly associated with acute MI in women than in men.[23,27] Many reasons contribute to the higher mortality from acute MI in women, including waiting longer to seek medical care, having smaller coronary arteries, being older when symptoms occur, and experiencing very different symptoms from those of men of similar age.[27,28]

Increased focus on sex differences with CVD has led to more female enrollment in studies and female-focused studies. Female-specific predictors of increased risk include pregnancy-related outcomes such as: preeclampsia, gestational diabetes, gestational hypertension, preterm delivery, and low birth weight for estimated age. Collaboration between the *American College of Obstetrics and Gynecology* (ACOG) and AHA led to guidelines to address female CV risk across the lifespan.[29] These guidelines include recognition of the female-specific risk profile and identify the need for early and continued healthy heart behaviors as primary prevention. Many women use their obstetrician/gynecologist as a primary care provider. This collaborative emphasis on healthy heart behaviors for women across the lifespan is essential for all health care providers. The future of successful prevention and CVD treatment for women depends on collaborative work across physician specialties with ongoing studies and preventive treatment plans.[29]

Major Adverse Cardiac Event—Multifactorial Risk

The goal of guideline management for patients with CCD is to reduce the risk of a *major adverse cardiac event* (MACE) through risk stratification that is patient-centered, addresses comorbid conditions, and incorporates cardiac testing results.[19] The following indicate increased risk of MACE in patients with CCD:

- *Demographics and socioeconomic status*: age, male sex, poor social support, and poverty or lack of health care access (SDOH)
- *Past or concurrent medical, mental health conditions*: elevated BMI, previous MI, percutaneous coronary intervention (PCI), or coronary artery bypass graft (CABG) surgery, heart failure, atrial fibrillation or flutter, diabetes, dyslipidemia, chronic kidney disease, current or former smoker, peripheral artery disease, depression, and poor adherence with guideline-directed pharmacotherapy.
- *Ancillary cardiac testing or imaging*: inability to exercise, angina with stress, 12-lead ECG with left bundle branch block (LBBB), left ventricular hypertrophy (LVH), high resting heart rate. Echocardiography: reduced left ventricular ejection fraction (LVEF), LVH; *exercise stress testing* (EST): high resting heart rate, achieved heart rate < 85% predicted, stress echocardiography; positron emission testing (PET), coronary computed tomography angiography (CCTA), high calcium score, and cardiovascular magnetic resonance (CMR) imaging.
- *Biomarkers*: elevated high-sensitivity troponins, elevated B-type natriuretic peptides.

Chronic Coronary Disease

In 2023, the AHA, the *American College of Cardiology* (ACC), and the Joint Commission updated guidelines for the management of stable ischemic heart disease with *Guidelines for the Management of Patients With* **Chronic Coronary Disease** (CCD).[19] CCD is an organizing term to describe obstructive and nonobstructive CAD with or without MI or revascularization, ischemic heart disease diagnosed by noninvasive testing, and chronic angina syndromes with heterogenous etiologies.

The new guidelines reflect the increasing complexity of comorbid disease management, advances in diagnostic evaluation, development of new medications, and *Goal-Directed Medical Therapy* (GDMT).[19] Risk stratification for patients with CCD should include all available patient information, invasive and noninvasive diagnostic testing results, and validated risk scores.

Primary Versus Secondary Prevention of Coronary Artery Disease

If a person has symptoms of CAD or has previously had a prior cardiovascular event, the goal of any lifestyle change or medication is called *secondary prevention*, or preventing another acute MI.[14,30] If a person matches the risk profile described previously but does *not* have symptoms of CAD or has *not* had an acute MI, the treatment plan is described as *primary prevention*.[4] The constellation of cardiac risk factors is well established and can predict development of CAD for most populations in the developed world.[7]

PATHOPHYSIOLOGY OF CORONARY ARTERY DISEASE

Vascular Inflammation

The link between vascular inflammation and atherosclerotic disease is well established.[22]

CAD is a progressive atherosclerotic disorder of the coronary arteries that results in narrowing or complete occlusion. *Atherosclerosis* affects the medium-sized arteries that perfuse the heart and other major organs. Normal arterial walls are composed of three layers:

- Intima (inner lining)
- Media (middle muscular layer)
- Adventitia (outer coat)

Development of Atherosclerosis

Atherosclerosis is a chronic inflammatory disorder that is characterized by an accumulation of macrophages and T lymphocytes in the arterial intimal wall. One of the triggers of vascular inflammation is a high LDL cholesterol concentration. The inflammation injures the wall, allowing the LDL cholesterol to infiltrate into the vessel wall below the endothelial surface.[31] Blood monocytes adhere to endothelial cells and migrate into the vessel wall. Within the artery wall, some monocytes differentiate into macrophages that unite with and then internalize LDL cholesterol. The *foam cells* that result are marker cells of atherosclerosis.[31]

Elevated LDL cholesterol levels promote low-level endothelial inflammation, which allows lipoproteins to infiltrate the intimal vessel wall.[31] After it has infiltrated under the endothelium, LDL cholesterol tends to stay within the vessel wall rather than return to the circulation. This contrasts with the actions of HDL cholesterol, which enters the vessel wall, helps efflux cholesterol from cells, and then returns to the circulation.[32] The actions of HDL cholesterol may help minimize the number of foam cells in the artery wall.[32]

Atherosclerotic Plaque Rupture

When a mature atherosclerotic plaque develops, it is not uniform in composition. It has a lipid liquid center filled with procoagulant factors. A connective tissue *fibrous cap* covers the top of the fluid lipid center. The abrupt rupture of this cap allows procoagulant lipids to flood into the vessel lumen and rapidly form a coronary thrombosis, as shown in Table 13.5. As the enlarging clot blocks blood flow through the coronary artery, an MI will occur unless adequate collateral circulation from other coronary vessels occurs. Symptoms and suggested cardiac interventions at appropriate stages in development of CAD are listed in Table 13.5.

Plaques that are likely to rupture are saturated with macrophages and other inflammatory cells. These *vulnerable plaques* are usually not obstructive and are situated at bends or branch points in the arterial tree.[33] It is unknown what factors increase erosion or rupture of the fibrous cap. As deep fissures in the cap expose the procoagulant factors to the blood plasma, an unstoppable cycle is put into motion. When platelets in the bloodstream are exposed to the combination of collagen, necrotic debris, von Willebrand factor, and thromboxane, a clot is formed and can occlude the coronary artery. Highly fibrotic plaques do not rupture. The type of atherosclerotic plaque that is prone to rupture has a weak fibrous cap and a large amount of liquid cholesterol within the core (see Table 13.5).

Plaque Regression

A reduction in blood cholesterol can decrease atherosclerotic plaque size by decreasing the amount of liquid cholesterol within the plaque core.[14] Lowering cholesterol levels does not change the dimensions of the fibrous or calcified portions of the plaque. However, lower cholesterol levels reduce vascular inflammation and make vulnerable plaque less likely to rupture.

C-Reactive Protein

The inflammatory biomarker most frequently cited is *C-reactive protein* (CRP). It is measured as high-sensitivity CRP (hs-CRP).[22] CRP is associated with an increased risk for development of other cardiovascular risk factors, including diabetes, hypertension, and weight gain. The higher the hs-CRP value, the greater the risk of a coronary event, especially if all other potential causes of systemic inflammation, such as infection, can be ruled out. Value ranges for hs-CRP are shown in Table 13.4. If other systemic inflammatory conditions such as bronchitis or urinary tract infection are present, the hs-CRP test loses all predictive value. CRP and other inflammatory markers are used to estimate the probability of future acute coronary events.[22,34,35] During acute coronary syndrome (ACS) events, there is widespread activation of neutrophils in the cardiac circulation (measured from the coronary sinus), which suggests that inflammation is not limited to one unstable plaque.[22]

ACUTE CORONARY SYNDROME

Description and Etiology

Acute coronary syndrome (ACS) is used to describe the array of clinical presentations of CAD that range from unstable angina to acute MI (Fig. 13.1).[19] An acute MI is generally described by patients as a "heart attack." This section discusses the range of manifestations of CAD and is outlined in a visual concept map (Fig. 13.1). A patient who presents with angina is evaluated to identify the severity of their underlying coronary disease. This can range from partial occlusion to complete blockage of a coronary artery.

Angina

Angina pectoris, or chest pain, caused by myocardial ischemia is not a separate disease but rather a symptom of CAD.[19] It is caused by a blockage or spasm of a coronary artery, leading to diminished myocardial blood supply. The lack of oxygen causes myocardial ischemia, which is felt as chest discomfort, pressure, or pain. Angina may occur anywhere in the chest, neck, arms, or back, and is commonly described as pain or pressure behind the sternum. The pain often radiates to the left arm but can also radiate down both arms and to the back, shoulder, jaw, or neck (Fig. 13.2). Angina symptoms are not the same for all individuals. Many patients may describe pressure or discomfort rather than pain, and presenting symptoms can be highly individualized, as described in Box 13.3. Patients and their families must be taught that angina does not always present in the dramatic heart attack scenario as often portrayed on television and in movies, in which the person clutches the throat or chest and exhibits extreme distress.[19,36]

Angina Symptom Equivalents

Men and women should be informed of angina symptom equivalents, such as unexpected shortness of breath; breaking out in a cold sweat; or sudden fatigue, nausea, or lightheadedness.[19,36] These symptom equivalants may occur in the absence of pain.

Women and Angina

Many women experience a variety of symptoms before an acute MI and during the acute event, as shown in Box 13.4.[27] The recognition and publicity about the fact that many women have atypical symptoms but do not experience "crushing chest pain" is important to understand to avoid a woman's symptoms being trivialized by health care clinicians.[27] It is vital that women are made aware of the *angina symptom equivalents* of unexplained shortness of breath; breaking out in a cold sweat; or sudden fatigue, nausea, or lightheadedness. More women die every year in the United States of ACS compared with men, a fact that is largely unknown by health care providers.[27]

Stable Angina

Stable angina is predictable and caused by similar precipitating factors each time; typically, it is exercise induced. Stable angina falls into the category of chronic coronary disease.[19] Patients become used to the pattern of this type of angina and may describe it as "my usual chest pain." Pain control should be achieved within 5 minutes of rest and by taking sublingual

TABLE 13.5 Coronary Artery Disease: Pathogenesis, Symptoms, Diagnosis and Management Timeline

Pathology of CAD	Symptoms of CAD	Diagnosis of CAD	Management of CAD
Normal coronary artery seen in young healthy children	No symptoms	None	• Healthy lifestyle • Obesity prevention
Fatty streaks on intima of aorta and coronary arteries in many young adults	No symptoms	None	Preventive measures with a focus on a healthy lifestyle
Atherosclerotic plaque increases in size but does not occlude blood flow	• No symptoms • Most adults are unaware they have CAD	None	Cardiac risk factor management
Atherosclerotic plaque occludes more than 70% of coronary artery lumen. Stable cap on lipid plaque interior.	Stable Angina • Chest pain or pressure with exertion or exercise	ECG stress test Elective coronary arteriogram	• Aggressive risk factor management • Sublingual nitroglycerin for angina • Elective PCI with stent
Atherosclerotic plaque becomes fibrous and calcified. Plaque has a large procoagulant lipid core. Cap has thinned with cracks, allowing platelets and fibrin to aggregate.	Unstable angina/ACS • Change in chest pain/pressure symptoms • Chest pain/pressure at rest • Symptoms not relieved by NTG	• 12-lead ECG • Coronary arteriogram • Biomarkers	• Emergency PCI with stent • Aggressive risk factor management • Aggressive risk factor management
Atherosclerotic cap ruptures and the procoagulant lipid core is released, forming a thrombosis that blocks blood flow.	STEMI or NSTEMI • Abrupt onset of chest pain or pressure or symptoms at rest • Angina not relieved by NTG • Sudden shortness of breath, cold sweat	• Emergency 12-lead ECG • Emergency coronary arteriogram • Biomarkers	• Emergency PCI with stent • Aggressive risk factor management

ACS, Acute coronary syndrome; *ECG*, electrocardiogram; CAD, coronary artery disease; *NSTEMI*, non–ST segment elevation myocardial infarction; *NTG*, nitroglycerin; *PCI*, percutaneous coronary intervention; *STEMI*, ST segment elevation myocardial infarction.

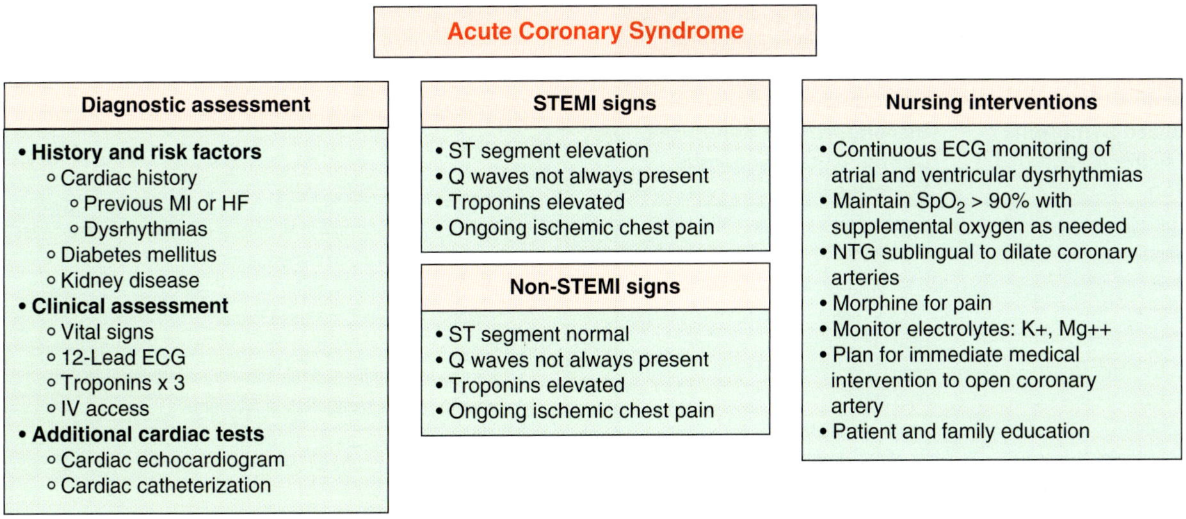

Acute Coronary Syndrome

Diagnostic assessment

- **History and risk factors**
  - Cardiac history
    - Previous MI or HF
    - Dysrhythmias
  - Diabetes mellitus
  - Kidney disease
- **Clinical assessment**
  - Vital signs
  - 12-Lead ECG
  - Troponins x 3
  - IV access
- **Additional cardiac tests**
  - Cardiac echocardiogram
  - Cardiac catheterization

STEMI signs

- ST segment elevation
- Q waves not always present
- Troponins elevated
- Ongoing ischemic chest pain

Non-STEMI signs

- ST segment normal
- Q waves not always present
- Troponins elevated
- Ongoing ischemic chest pain

Nursing interventions

- Continuous ECG monitoring of atrial and ventricular dysrhythmias
- Maintain SpO_2 > 90% with supplemental oxygen as needed
- NTG sublingual to dilate coronary arteries
- Morphine for pain
- Monitor electrolytes: K+, Mg++
- Plan for immediate medical intervention to open coronary artery
- Patient and family education

FIG. 13.1 Summary of Key Concepts Related to Acute Coronary Syndrome. *BNP*, brain natriuretic peptide; *ECG*, electrocardiogram; HF, heart failure; *HTN*, hypertension; *IV*, intravenous; *K^+*, potassium; *Mg^{++}*, magnesium; *MI*, myocardial infarction; *NTG*, nitroglycerin; *NSTEMI*, non-ST segment elevation myocardial infarction; *SpO_2*, pulse oximetry oxygen saturation; *STEMI*, ST segment elevation myocardial infarction.

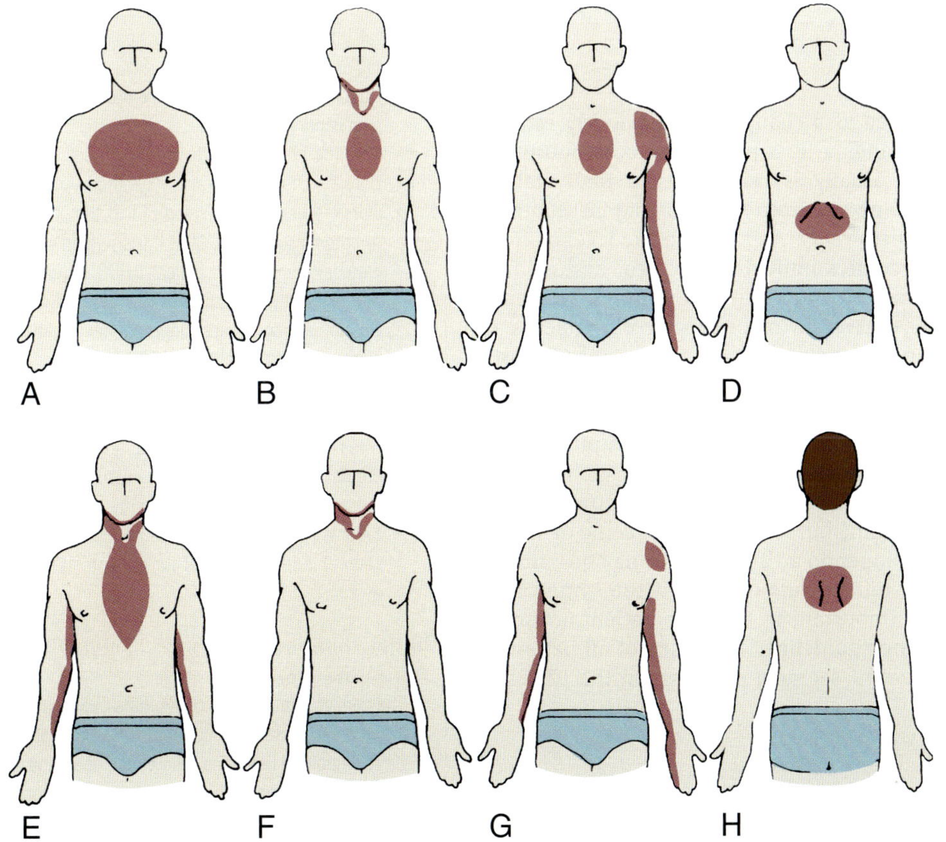

FIG. 13.2 Common Sites for Anginal Pain. (A) Upper part of chest. (B) Beneath sternum, radiating to neck and jaw. (C) Beneath sternum, radiating down left arm. (D) Epigastric. I Epigastric, radiating to neck, jaw, and arms. (F) Neck and jaw. (G) Left shoulder. (H) Intrascapular.

BOX 13.4 Cardiovascular Symptoms Experienced by Women Before Acute Myocardial Infarction

Generalized Symptoms Before Acute Myocardial Infarction	Discomfort/Pain Symptoms During Acute Myocardial Infarction
Unusual fatigue	Centered high in chest
Dizzy or faint	Left breast
Hot, flushed	Back/between shoulder blades
Indigestion	Neck/throat
Heart racing	Generalized chest
Numbness in hands/fingers	Leg(s)
Vomiting	Both arms
Loss of appetite	Top of shoulders
New vision problems	Right arm or shoulder
Headache	Jaw/teeth
Coughing	
Choking sensation	

Data from McSweeney JC. Preventing and experiencing ischemic heart disease as a woman: state of the science. A scientific statement from the American Heart Association. *Circulation.* 2016;133:1302.

nitroglycerin. Ischemia and chest pain occur when myocardial demand from exertion exceeds the fixed blood oxygen supply. Additional information on CAD and stable angina is provided in Box 13.5.

Unstable Angina

Unstable angina is defined as a change in a previously established stable pattern of angina. It is part of the continuum of ACS. Unstable angina usually is more intense than stable angina, may awaken the person from sleep, or may necessitate more than nitrates for pain relief. A change in the level or frequency of symptoms requires immediate medical evaluation. Severe angina that persists for more than 5 minutes, worsens in intensity, and is not relieved by one nitroglycerin tablet is a medical emergency, and the patient or a family member must call 911 immediately.[37]

Unstable angina is an indication of atherosclerotic plaque instability. It can signal atherosclerotic plaque rupture and thrombus formation that can lead to MI.

A patient who comes to the emergency department with recent-onset unstable angina but who has nonspecific or nonelevated ST segment changes on a 12-lead ECG may be admitted to the critical care unit to rule out MI. If the symptoms are typical of MI, it is important to treat the patient according to the latest published guidelines, because not all patients who experience MI have ST segment elevation on the 12-lead ECG.[37]

Call 911

The 911 *emergency medical services* (EMS) system is available to 98% of the population of the United States.[36] Family and friends are discouraged from driving a person experiencing unstable angina to the hospital and instead are urged to call 911. Patients should be instructed never to drive themselves but to contact the EMS by calling 911. Delay in reperfusion, cardiac arrest in a personal car, and mortality are all increased when EMS is not called.[36]

BOX 13.5 Evidence-Based Practice

Coronary Artery Disease and Stable Angina

Strong evidence exists that lifestyle interventions can help prevent coronary artery disease (CAD).

- Diet:
  - Diet low in salt and high in fiber, fruit, vegetables, and grains
  - All dietary fat less than 30% of total calories; saturated fat less than 7%
  - Limit glucose in diet (simple sugars)
  - Limit calories if overweight
  - Omega-3 fatty acids included in diet
- Exercise:
  - Start by walking more often and increase physical exercise from there.
  - Refer to cardiac rehabilitation program.
- Obesity:
  - Achieve healthy body weight.
- Addiction:
  - Stop cigarette smoking.
  - Avoid exposure to environmental (secondhand) tobacco smoke at home and at work.
  - Limit alcohol intake.
- Strong evidence exists that the following diagnostic procedures are helpful for the diagnosis.
- When a patient presents with chest pain, quickly obtaining a detailed history of symptoms, focused physical examination, and risk factor assessment to determine whether the probability of CAD is low, intermediate, or high.
- Initial laboratory tests include hemoglobin, fasting blood glucose, lipid panel, and cardiac biomarkers.
  - Obtain a baseline 12-lead electrocardiogram (ECG) at rest, even if chest pain is not present.
  - Obtain a 12-lead ECG during an episode of chest pain.
  - Obtain a chest radiograph if symptoms of heart failure are present.
  - Obtain an exercise 12-lead ECG if the patient's condition is stable and symptoms suggest CAD or if the patient's condition is stable with complete left bundle branch block (LBBB) or right bundle branch block (RBBB) that makes the ECG difficult to interpret for ischemia.
  - Obtain cardiac echocardiography for a patient with a systolic murmur suggestive of aortic stenosis.
  - Use cardiac echocardiography to determine the extent of left ventricular (LV) hypertrophy or dysfunction.
  - Stress cardiac echocardiography is recommended for patients with greater than 1 mm of ST segment depression at rest (stress may be induced by physical exercise or by pharmacologic stimulation).
  - Coronary angiography (typically as part of a cardiac catheterization procedure) is recommended for patients at high risk for adverse coronary events.

Initial Pharmacologic and Lifestyle Treatment Recommendations

- The goal of treatment is to eliminate chest pain.
- The most important elements of CAD and stable angina management can be remembered using the following A-to-E mnemonic:

  A—Aspirin and antianginal medications: Prescribe daily low-dose (75–325 mg) aspirin, oral nitrates, and sublingual nitroglycerin for episodes of angina.

  B—Beta-blockers and blood pressure: Use angiotensin-converting enzyme inhibitors and beta-blockers to decrease blood pressure to less than 140/90 mm Hg if no other CAD risk factors are present and to less than 130/80 mm Hg if diabetes or kidney disease is present.

BOX 13.5 Evidence-Based Practice—cont'd

Coronary Artery Disease and Stable Angina

C—Cholesterol and cigarettes: Obtain a fasting lipid profile. Recommend diet or lipid reduction medication therapy (statin) to lower low-density lipoprotein cholesterol (LDL-C) to less than 100 mg/dL (<70 mg/dL if achievable), increase high-density lipoprotein cholesterol to more than 40 mg/dL for men or more than 50 mg/dL for women, and reduce triglycerides to less than 150 mg/dL. Always ask about tobacco use, and strongly recommend smoking cessation; encourage nicotine replacement therapy (nicotine patches or gum) as needed.

D—Diet and diabetes: Prescribe a low-fat, calorie-appropriate diet and provide nutritional consultation as needed to achieve a fasting blood glucose level of 70 to 100 mg/dL and hemoglobin A_{1c} of less than 6.5%.

E—Education and exercise: Provide education about risk factor modification and the CAD disease process; recommend daily exercise for 30 to 60 min (ideal) or at least seven times each week (minimum of 5 days per week). A body mass index between 18.5 kg/m^2 and 24.9 kg/m^2 and waist circumference less than 40 inches for men or less than 35 inches for women should be recommended. Treat depression, if present. Hormone replacement therapy is not recommended as a treatment for symptoms of coronary heart disease. Influenza vaccination is recommended.

Interventional and Surgical Recommendations for Stable High-Risk Patients

Patients are risk are stratified according to their symptoms and the results of cardiac diagnostic tests.

- Percutaneous catheter intervention (PCI):
- PCI is more frequently performed than open heart surgery for relief of anginal symptoms.
- Coronary artery bypass graft surgery:
  - For patients with left main occlusion or multivessel disease
  - For patients with two-vessel disease who have significant proximal left anterior descending coronary artery stenosis and an LV ejection fraction less than 50%

References

O'Gara PT, Kushner FG, Ascheim DD, et al. 2013 ACCF/AHA Guideline for the Management of ST-Elevation Myocardial Infarction: A Report of the American College of Cardiology Foundation/American Heart Association Task Force on Practice Guidelines. *Circulation*. 2013;127(4):e362–e425. https://doi.org/10.1161/CIR.0b013e3182742cf6.

Amsterdam EA, Wenger NK, Brindis RG, et al. 2014 AHA/ACC Guideline for the Management of Patients With Non–ST-Elevation Acute Coronary Syndromes: Executive Summary: A Report of the American College of Cardiology/American Heart Association Task Force on Practice Guidelines. *Circulation*. 2014;130(25):2354–2394. https://doi.org/10.1161/CIR.0000000000000133.

Virani SS, Newby LK, Arnold SV, et al. 2023 AHA/ACC/ACCP/ASPC/NLA/PCNA Guideline for the Management of Patients With Chronic Coronary Disease: A Report of the American Heart Association/American College of Cardiology Joint Committee on Clinical Practice Guidelines. *Circulation*. 2023;148(9):e9–e119. https://doi.org/10.1161/CIR.0000000000001168.

Arnett DK, Blumenthal RS, Albert MA, et al. 2019 ACC/AHA Guideline on the Primary Prevention of Cardiovascular Disease: A Report of the American College of Cardiology/American Heart Association Task Force on Clinical Practice Guidelines. *Circulation*. 2019;140(11):e596–e646. https://doi.org/10.1161/CIR.0000000000000678.

BOX 13.6 Clinical Characteristics of Silent Ischemia

- Objective electrocardiogram (ECG) evidence of myocardial ischemia without any chest pain or symptoms.
- No anginal symptoms after previous myocardial infarction (MI), but objective ECG evidence of myocardial ischemia continues.
- Symptoms of angina with some episodes of ischemia and no symptoms with other ischemic events; patient may or may not have had previous MI.

BOX 13.7 Factors to Consider When Assessing Chest Pain

- **Onset:** Was onset of pain sudden or gradual?
- **Duration:** Did pain last seconds or minutes? How soon after onset did the patient call for help?
- **Precipitating factors:** Was the patient up and moving around?
- **Location:** Was pain substernal? Was it located in the same area as previous pain?
- **Radiation:** Did pain radiate to the jaw, neck, arm, or shoulder?
- **Quality:** Was pain similar to previous anginal pain? Was pain more intense or less intense?
- **Intensity:** On a scale of 0 to 10, where would the patient rate the pain?
- **Relieving factors:** What made the pain better—changing position, nitroglycerin, oxygen, the presence of the nurse?
- **Aggravating factors:** Did things such as the environment, telephone calls, or waiting for help worsen the pain?
- **Associated symptoms:** Was the pain accompanied by nausea, vomiting, diaphoresis, or dyspnea?
- **Emotional response:** Was there an emotional response that intensified the pain—anxiety, fear, anger?

Variant Angina

Variant angina, also known as *Prinzmetal angina*, is caused by a dynamic obstruction from intense vasoconstriction of a coronary artery.[38] Spasm can occur with or without atherosclerotic lesions. Vasospasm is suspected when angina is a symptom, and the coronary arteries are visualized as "open" and are not obstructed by plaque on a coronary angiogram.[39,40]

Variant angina commonly occurs when the individual is at rest, and it is often cyclic, occurring at the same time every day. Smoking, alcohol use, and illegal stimulant drug (cocaine, methamphetamine) use may precipitate spasm. A definitive diagnosis of variant angina is made during a cardiac catheterization study. Signs of spasm include ST segment elevation and chest pain. Coronary artery vasospasm is treated with nitroglycerin or calcium channel blockers to vasodilate the coronary arteries.

Silent Ischemia

Silent ischemia describes a situation in which objective evidence of ischemia is observed on an ECG monitor, but the person does not complain of anginal symptoms. Silent ischemia can occur in many clinical situations, as described in Box 13.6. One-third of patients who are having an MI do not report chest pain as a symptom.[19] Patients with diabetes are at particular risk for silent ischemia. Many patients who had type 2 diabetes for more than 10 years have developed *autonomic neuropathy*, which decreases their ability to experience chest pain. Patients with diabetes may misinterpret angina symptom equivalents such as nausea, vomiting, and diaphoresis as signaling a disruption in glucose control rather than a sign of myocardial ischemia.

Medical Management

Accurate assessment of chest pain symptoms is essential if unstable angina is to be recognized and treated effectively. Factors to consider when assessing chest pain are listed in Box 13.7. An important reason to ask questions about the chest

BOX 13.8 DIAGNOSIS AND PATIENT CARE MANAGEMENT

Coronary Artery Disease and Angina

- Acute pain due to transmission and perception of cutaneous, visceral, muscular, or ischemic impulses
- Ineffective tissue perfusion due to decreased myocardial blood flow
- Activity intolerance due to cardiopulmonary dysfunction
- Powerlessness due to lack of control over current situation or disease progression
- Anxiety due to threat to biologic, psychologic, or social integrity
- Lack of knowledge of treatment regime due to lack of previous exposure to information (see Box 13.9, Patient and Family Education Plan: Coronary Artery Disease and Angina)

Patient Care Management plans are located in Appendix A.

pain is to differentiate between stable and unstable angina. The change from stable to unstable angina is potentially life threatening for the patient. If the ST segments are elevated or a newly documented LBBB is seen on the 12-lead ECG, the patient should be treated for acute MI.[36] However, if these classic ECG signs are missing and the chest pain continues, the current pharmacologic treatment of choice is aspirin. If the patient cannot tolerate aspirin, a thienopyridine such as clopidogrel can be given.

Patients with definite unstable angina or non–ST segment elevation myocardial infarction (NSTEMI) should receive loading doses of antiplatelet and anticoagulation medications irrespective of initial treatment strategy.[37] Antiplatelet therapy includes the gold standard aspirin, P2Y12 inhibitors (clopidogrel, prasugrel, and ticagrelor), and glycoprotein (GP) IIb/IIIa inhibitors (eptifibatide, tirofiban). Therapeutic anticoagulation incudes low-molecular-weight heparin (LMWH), direct thrombin inhibitor bivalirudin, and factor X inhibitor fondaparinux. Aspirin is the gold standard for antiplatelet therapy and is the only agent proven to reduce recurrent MI risk and improve patient mortality.[37] Patients undergoing noninvasive treatment should receive aspirin and a P2Y12 inhibitor (clopidogrel, prasugrel, or ticagrelor) for 1 month and ideally up to 1 year. If symptoms persist, diagnostic angiography is performed. Noninvasive cardiac stress testing is recommended to evaluate unstable angina in patients who do not receive coronary angiography and are free from ischemia for 48 hours.

Nursing Management

Nursing care management for a patient with CAD and angina incorporates a variety of patient care diagnoses (Box 13.8). Nursing interventions focus on early identification of myocardial ischemia, control of chest pain, recognition of complications, maintenance of a calm environment, and patient and family education. See Appendix A for patient care management plans specific to patients with CAD.

Recognizing Myocardial Ischemia

Complaints of chest discomfort (angina) must be evaluated quickly because angina is an indicator of myocardial ischemia (see Box 13.7). The patient is asked to rate the intensity of the chest discomfort on a scale of 0 to 10. Pain levels must be assessed with sensitivity to differences in cultural manifestations of pain. The term *chest pain* is not to be used exclusively, because some patients describe their angina as "pressure" or "heaviness."

It is important to document the characteristics of the pain and the patient's heart rate and rhythm, BP, respirations, temperature, skin color, peripheral pulses, urine output, mentation, and overall tissue perfusion. A 12-lead ECG is used to identify the area of ischemic myocardium. The major concern is that the chest pain may represent pre-infarction angina, and early identification is essential so that the patient can be immediately treated. Treatment may include transfer to the cardiac catheterization laboratory for a coronary arteriogram and opening of a blocked artery. If the hospital does not have a cardiac catheterization laboratory, therapeutic anticoagulation with LMWH, or GP IIb/IIIa receptor blockers, may be initiated to prevent the evolution of the acute MI before transfer.[19,36,37]

Relieving Chest Pain

In the critical care unit, control of angina is achieved by a combination of supplemental oxygen, nitrates, analgesia, and surveillance of angina and of the effects of pharmacologic therapy.

- *Oxygen:* All patients with acute ischemic pain are administered supplemental oxygen to increase myocardial oxygenation. Pulse oximetry is used to guide therapy and maintain oxygen saturation above 90% unless the patient has a history of chronic obstructive pulmonary disease and is a carbon dioxide retainer.
- *Nitrates:* Administer 3 sublingual nitroglycerin tablets (0.4 mg) 1 at a time, spaced 5 minutes apart, or 1 aerosol spracy under tongue every 5 minutes for 3 doses to treat persistent chest pain.

  An intravenous infusion of nitroglycerin can be titrated to chest pain relief if the patient does not have hypotension or recent use of phosphodiesterase inhibitors (e.g., medications for erectile dysfunction).

  A combination of intravenous and sublingual nitroglycerin is used to vasodilate the coronary arteries and decrease pain. After nitrate administration, the critical care nurse closely observes the patient for relief of chest pain, for return of the ST segment to baseline, and for the potential development of unwanted side effects such as hypotension and headache. Administration of a nitrate is avoided if the systolic BP is less than 90 mm Hg.
- *Analgesia:* Morphine (2 to 4 mg given intravenously) is the analgesic opiate of choice for preinfarction angina that is not relieved by nitrate therapy. It relieves pain and decreases fear and anxiety. After administration, the critical care nurse assesses the patient for pain relief and the development of unwanted side effects such as hypotension and respiratory depression.[37]
- *Aspirin:* Chewing an oral non–enteric-coated aspirin (162 to 325 mg) at the beginning of chest pain has been shown to reduce mortality. The nonenteric formulation is preferred because it increases absorption in the mouth when chewed, not swallowed.[19,37]

Maintaining a Calm Environment

Patients admitted to a critical care unit with unstable angina experience extreme anxiety and fear of death. The critical care

PATIENT-CENTERED CRITICAL CARE

Multidisciplinary Team Rounds in the Cardiac Intensive Care Unit

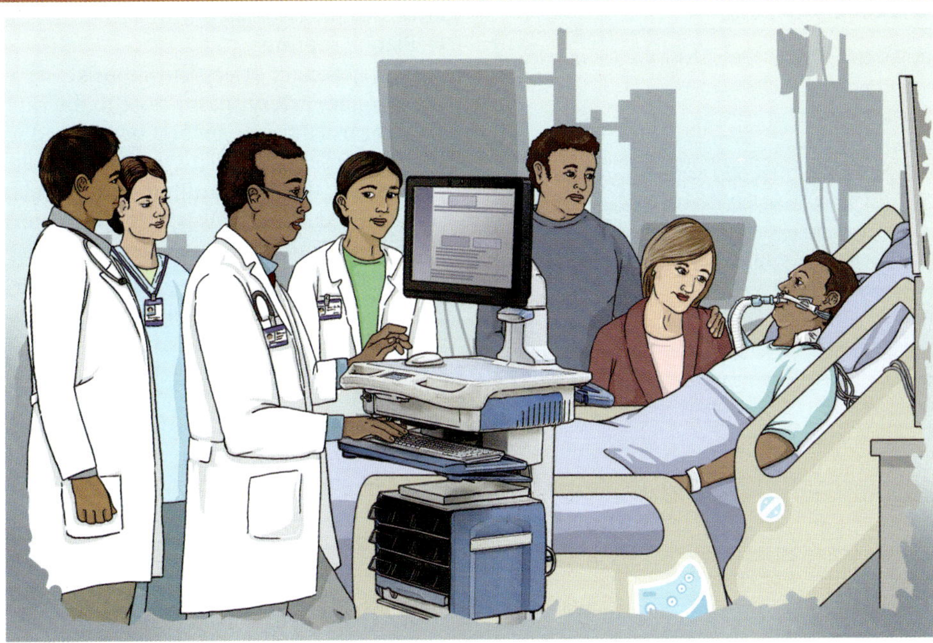

Patient-centered care, shared decision making, and informed consent in the management of coronary artery disease are recommended by the American Heart Association/American College of Cardiology (AHA/ACC) and Joint Commission.[33] Daily multidisciplinary bedside rounds are a best practice recommended by the AHA/ACC and other critical care organizations to enhance communication, improve safety, and support patient-centered care for critically ill patients in the critical care unit.[41] Rounds can involve large or small numbers of health care professionals depending on the size of the hospital and whether it is an academic/teaching hospital or a community hospital.

In larger teaching hospitals, the team at morning rounds will include professionals from multiple disciplines. These may include medical staff (attending physician, fellows, residents, medical students) and the primary nurse. The team may also include advanced practice providers (nurse practitioners, physician assistants, clinical nurse specialists), respiratory therapists, pharmacists, dietitians, rehabilitation therapists, and medical social workers. Consulting teams for specialty care may also participate in morning rounds when care needs are complex. Consequently, for some patients, the rounding teams will have 10 to 20 people at the bedside. In an academic/teaching hospital, the morning rounds often include education about disease processes and interventions so that rounds are also a learning opportunity.

In a smaller hospital, the team has fewer members and may include the attending physician (medicine or surgical specialty), advanced practice providers, and the bedside nurse. A respiratory therapist and other professionals may also be present.

With the national movement toward patient-centered care and greater family involvement in critical care, it is natural to include family participation in bedside rounds, especially when the patient is unable to communicate because of intubation, sedation, critical illness, or cognitive impairment. When family members are present, it is helpful to begin with introductions in which everyone present at rounds states their name and role. Although the discussion is often rapid and includes technical-medical terms, there is generally time at the end of rounds to answer family questions and explain the plan for the day in everyday language.

Team rounds may be a few minutes longer with the family present. However, when patients and family members understand the plan for the day and agree with the plan, this is beneficial for communication and patient outcomes.

nurse is faced with the challenge of ensuring that the elements of a calm environment to alleviate the patient's fear and anxiety are maintained, while always being ready to respond to an acute emergency such as a cardiac arrest or to assist with emergency intubation or insertion of hemodynamic monitoring catheters.

Educating the Patient and Family

In the critical care unit, the patient's ability to retain educational information is severely affected by stress and pain. Education topics that should be discussed when the clinical condition has stabilized are listed in Box 13.9. It is essential to teach avoidance of the Valsalva maneuver, which is defined as forced expiration against a closed glottis. This can be explained to the patient as "bearing down" during defecation or breath holding when repositioning in bed. The Valsalva maneuver causes an increase in intrathoracic pressure, which decreases venous return to the right side of the heart and can be associated with low BP and symptomatic bradycardia.

BOX 13.9 PATIENT AND FAMILY EDUCATION

Coronary Artery Disease and Angina

Before discharge, the patient should be able to teach back the following topics:

- Angina: Describe signs and symptoms such as pain, pressure, and heaviness in chest, arms, or jaw.
- Preinfarction or unstable angina: Any chest pain that is not relieved by a sublingual nitroglycerin (NTG) tablet taken 5 min apart times three doses provides a reason to call 911 (emergency services).
- Use of the 0-to-10 pain scale: Notify critical care nurse or emergency personnel of any changes in pain intensity.
- Use of sublingual NTG for angina: Pain intensity should decrease on pain scale after NTG administration. At home, NTG must be kept in a dark, airtight container, or it loses its potency. To ensure potency, the NTG supply must be replaced approximately every 6 months. Active NTG has a slight burning sensation when placed under the tongue.
- Avoid Valsalva maneuver.
- Risk factor modification tailored to the patient's individual risk factor profile:
  - Decrease fat intake to 30% of total calories a day.
  - Stop smoking.
  - Reduce salt intake.
  - Control hypertension.
  - Treat diabetes and control blood glucose levels (if patient has diabetes).
  - Increase physical activity; achieve ideal body weight.
- Intention to attend a cardiac rehabilitation program
- Medication teaching about indications and side effects
- Follow-up care after discharge
- Symptoms to report to a health care professional
- Discussion of how to handle emotional stress and anger

After the anginal pain is controlled, longer-term education of the patient and the family can begin. Education points to cover include (1) risk factor modification, (2) signs and symptoms of angina, (3) when to call the physician, (4) medications, and (5) dealing with emotions and stress. However, because the acute hospital length of stay for uncomplicated angina is usually less than 3 days, referral to a cardiac rehabilitation program for a controlled exercise program and risk factor modification after discharge may be the most helpful teaching intervention a critical care nurse can provide. Clinical practice guidelines for the management of CAD and stable angina are listed in Box 13.6.

MYOCARDIAL INFARCTION

Description and Etiology

Myocardial infarction is the term used to describe irreversible myocardial necrosis (cell death) that results from an abrupt decrease or total cessation of coronary blood flow to a specific area of the myocardium. In the hospital, this is often referred to as an *acute MI*, indicating the sudden onset and the life-threatening nature of the event. An acute MI is described in relation to whether ST segment elevation is seen on a diagnostic 12-lead ECG.

- *acute NSTEMI* (non-ST segment elevation myocardial infarction)[37]
- *acute STEMI* (ST segment elevation myocardial infarction)[41,42]

Pathophysiology of Acute Myocardial Infarction

Three mechanisms can block the coronary artery and are responsible for the acute reduction in oxygen delivery to the myocardium associated with a STEMI:

- Plaque rupture
- New coronary artery thrombosis
- Coronary artery spasm close to the ruptured plaque

Myocardial tissue can best be salvaged within the first 2 hours after the onset of anginal symptoms, as illustrated in Fig. 13.3.[33] The earlier the myocardium is revascularized, the better the chances of survival. This is why it is important that patients with chest pain be urgently evaluated. However, many people do not seek treatment until the acute phase has passed because they do not realize that their symptoms are due to thrombosis of a coronary artery.

Ischemia

The outer region of the infarcted myocardial area is the *zone of ischemia*, or penumbra, as illustrated in Fig. 13.4. It is composed of viable cells. Priority interventions are targeted to save this viable muscle. Repolarization in this zone is temporarily impaired but eventually is restored to normal. Repolarization of the cells in this area manifests as T-wave inversion on the ECG (Fig. 13.5).

Injury

The infarcted zone is surrounded by injured but still potentially viable tissue in an area known as the *zone of injury* (see Fig. 13.4). Cells in this area do not fully repolarize because of the deficient blood supply. This is recorded on the ECG as elevation of the ST segment (Fig. 13.5C). The visual clue of ST segment elevation on the 12-lead ECG is often key to early recognition of a STEMI.

Infarction

The area of dead muscle (necrosis) in the myocardium is known as the *zone of infarction* (see Fig. 13.4). On the ECG, evidence of this zone is seen as new pathologic Q waves, which reflect a lack of depolarization from the cardiac surface involved in the MI (Fig. 13.5D). As healing takes place, the cells in this area are replaced by scar tissue.

Q Wave Myocardial Infarction

Myocardial infarctions are classified according to the location on the myocardial surface and the muscle layers affected. Not all infarctions cause necrosis in all layers, as shown in Fig. 13.6. A transmural MI involves all three cardiac layers: *endocardium*, *myocardium*, and *epicardium*. A transmural (full-thickness) MI usually provokes significant ECG changes (see Fig. 13.5). This is also described as a *Q wave MI*. Not every acute MI produces a recognizable series of Q waves on the 12-lead ECG. Some patients who had a demonstrated Q wave on a 12-lead ECG from an acute MI lose the Q wave months or years later. The reasons for this are unknown, but it may represent the development of collateral circulation.

Twelve-Lead Electrocardiogram Changes

The ECG changes produced by an MI demonstrate alteration in myocardial depolarization (QRS complex) and repolarization (ST segment). The changes in repolarization are seen by the presence of new Q waves. These new, pathologic Q waves

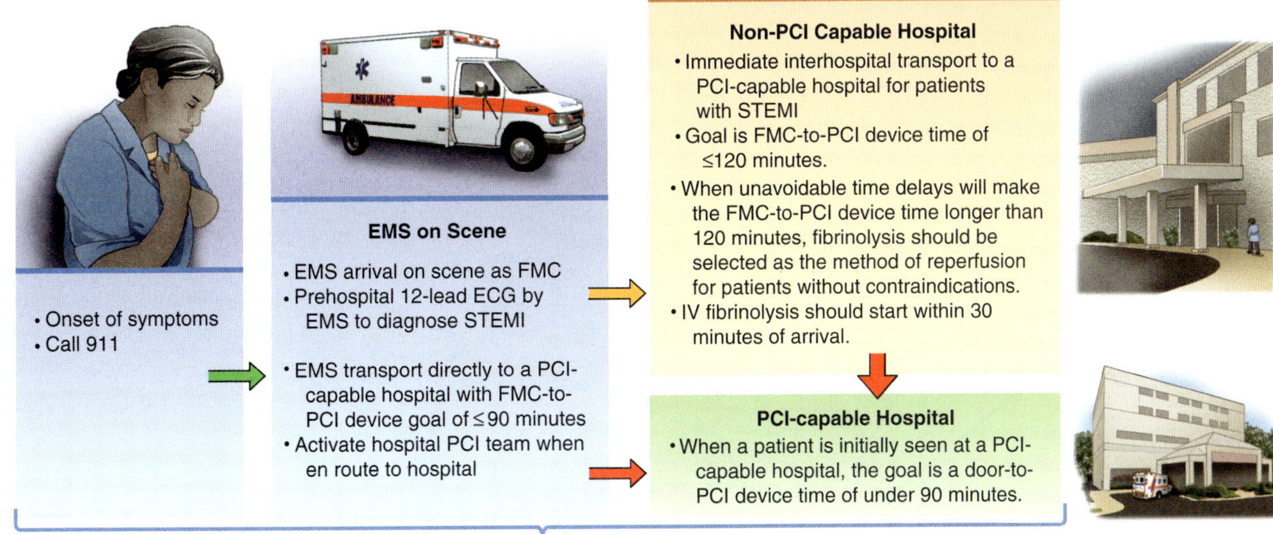

FIG. 13.3 Evaluation of Prehospital Chest Pain and Acute Coronary Syndrome and Treatment Options. The first step is to call 911 *(green arrow)*. Transport to a PCI-capable hospital is always the optimal first choice when available *(red arrows)*. Transport to a non-PCI-capable hospital is considered when other options are unavailable *(yellow arrow* and *yellow box)*. *ECG*, Electrocardiogram; *EMS*, emergency medical services; *FMC*, first medical contact; *PCI*, percutaneous coronary intervention; *STEMI*, ST segment elevation myocardial infarction.

are deeper and wider than the tiny Q waves found on a normal 12-lead ECG.

Myocardial Infarction Location

The location of infarction is determined by correlating the ECG leads with Q waves and the ST segment and T wave abnormalities (Table 13.6). The ECG manifestations that are used to diagnose MI and pinpoint the area of damaged ventricle include inverted T waves, ST segment elevation, and pathologic Q waves in specific lead groupings, as described subsequently.

Anterior Wall Infarction

Anterior wall infarction results from occlusion of the proximal left anterior descending artery (Table 13.7). ST segment elevation is expected in leads V_1 through V_4 on the 12-lead ECG, as shown in Fig. 13.7. If the left main coronary artery is occluded, the ECG manifestations will involve almost all precordial leads V_1 through V_6 and leads I and aVL (see Table 13.7). These specific groups of ECG changes that help locate the part of the heart that is experiencing infarction are called *indicative changes*. A large anterior wall MI may be associated with LV pump failure, cardiogenic shock, or death.

Left Lateral Wall Infarction

Left lateral wall infarction occurs from occlusion of the circumflex coronary artery. On a 12-lead ECG, new Q waves and ST segment T wave changes are seen in leads I, aVL, V_5, and V_6 (Fig. 13.8). In clinical practice, very few patients present with only lateral wall ECG changes, and often anterior wall leads (V_3 and V_4) also show evidence of injury or infarction.

Inferior Wall Infarction

Inferior wall infarction occurs with occlusion of the right coronary artery (RCA). This infarction manifests by ECG changes in leads II, III, and aV_F (Fig. 13.9). Conduction disturbances are expected with an inferior wall MI and are related to the anatomy of the coronary arterial supply. Because the RCA perfuses the sinoatrial node in slightly more than half of the population and supplies the proximal bundle of His and the atrioventricular (AV) node in more than 90% of individuals, heart block and other conduction disturbances should be anticipated.

Right Ventricular Infarction

Infarction of the right ventricle occurs when a blockage occurs in a proximal section of the RCA. This places the entire right ventricle and inferior wall at risk. Right ventricular ischemia can be demonstrated in one-half of inferior wall STEMIs, although only 10% to 15% show the hemodynamic abnormalities associated with classic infarction of the right ventricle. If massive infarction occurs, the patient can experience cardiogenic shock, which carries a mortality rate of more than 50% in this population.[43]

The ECG leads on the 12-lead ECG also correlate with the coronary arteries. Leads can also be placed on the right side of the chest to assist in the diagnosis of right ventricular infarction and posteriorly to show a posterior infarction. To detect a right ventricular infarction, specific ECG lead placement is used. Electrodes are placed over the right precordium (chest) in a mirror image of the conventional left-sided leads. It is important to write R on the 12-lead ECG (e.g., V_1R through V_6R) in front of the recorded right ventricular chest leads to ensure that the lead location is clear. The limb leads are not affected. Fig. 12.36C in Chapter 12 shows the correct position of the right-sided precordial leads used to diagnose an acute right ventricular MI. The ECG voltage is much lower in the V_1R through V_6R leads; when detected, ST segment elevation is usually seen in V_4R (Fig. 13.10).[36] The right ventricle has a very thin wall, which means that ST segment elevation is detected only in the right ventricular leads during the acute phase of the infarction.

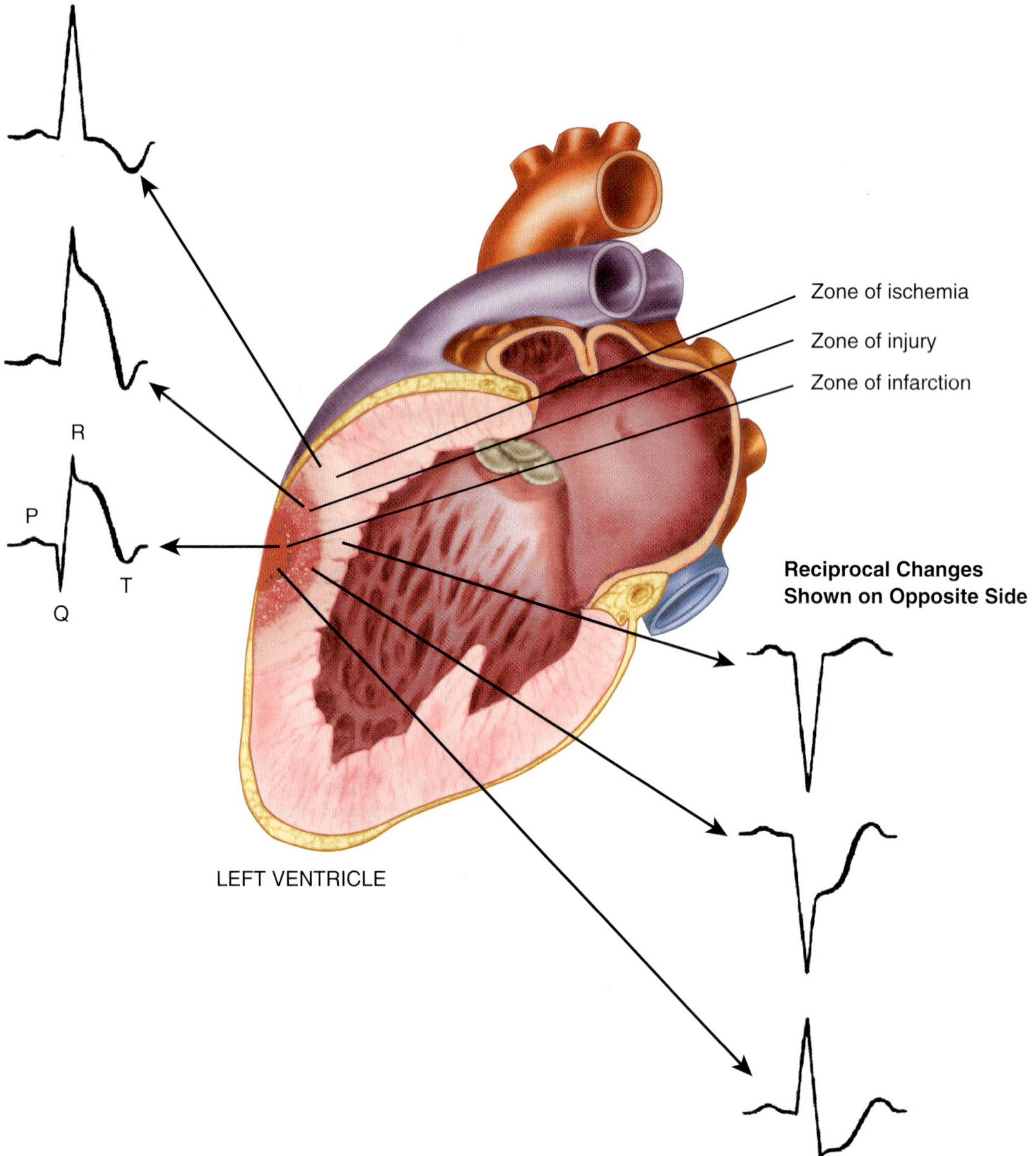

FIG. 13.4 Zone of ischemia, zone of injury, and zone of infarction are shown through electrocardiogram waveforms and reciprocal waveforms corresponding to each zone.

Posterior Wall Infarction

Infarction in the posterior wall can occur because of a blockage in the RCA or in the circumflex artery. This occurs because both arteries supply this section of the heart, although the RCA is generally the dominant vessel. A posterior wall MI is difficult to detect but may be identified either by specific leads placed in the left scapular area or by very tall R waves in leads V_1 and V_2 (Fig. 13.11). Fig. 12.36D in Chapter 12 shows the correct placement of the left posterior leads used to diagnose an acute posterior MI.

Non–ST Segment Elevation Myocardial Infarction

The 12-lead ECG is a highly useful diagnostic tool. For many years, it was considered the gold standard when diagnosing acute MI. However, the ST segment is not elevated in every acute MI. One reason for the lack of ST segment elevation may be that the infarction and subsequent necrosis are not full-thickness lesions. When ST segment elevation is not present on the 12-lead ECG, this is diagnostically known as an *NSTEMI*.[37] This type of MI is also less likely to develop Q waves on a subsequent 12-lead ECG after the acute phase has passed.

NSTEMI condition has previously been described by several names including nontransmural MI, non–Q wave MI, and subendocardial MI. Because patients who sustain an NSTEMI do have CAD, it is important that they be treated aggressively to minimize the size of the infarcted area. Without the visual clue of ST segment elevation on the 12-lead ECG, the patients cannot receive immediate intravenous fibrinolytic agents, but they can be appropriately managed in an interventional catheterization laboratory and receive GP IIb/IIIa inhibitor therapy, as illustrated in the timeline in Fig. 13.3.

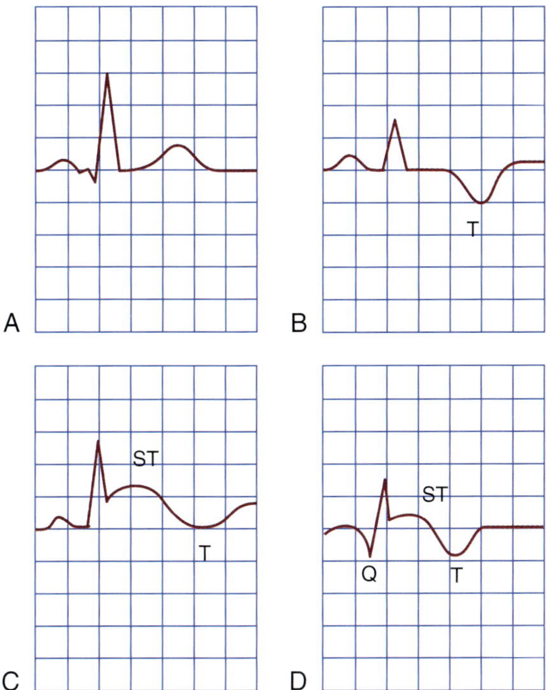

FIG. 13.5 Electrocardiogram (ECG) Changes Indicative of Ischemia, Injury, and Infarction (necrosis) of the Myocardium. (A) Normal ECG. (B) Ischemia indicated by inversion of the T wave. (C) Ischemia and current of injury indicated by T-wave inversion and ST segment elevation. The ST segment may be elevated above or depressed below the baseline, depending on whether the tracing is from a lead facing toward or away from the infarcted area and depending on whether epicardial or endocardial injury occurs. Epicardial injury causes ST segment elevation in leads facing the epicardium. (D) Ischemia, injury, and myocardial necrosis. The Q wave indicates necrosis of the myocardium.

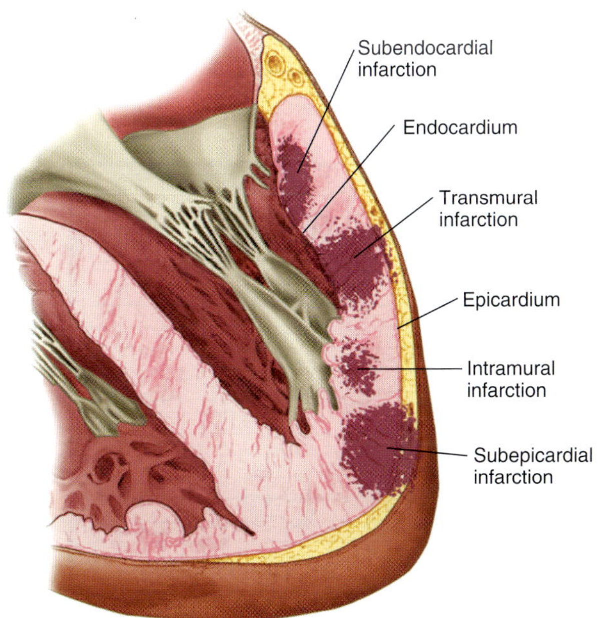

FIG. 13.6 Location of Infarctions in Myocardium.

The 12-lead ECG plays a vital role in identifying the treatment plan for a patient with ACS. Visualizing ST segment elevation when present is helpful. Patients without ST segment elevation may still be at risk for becoming unstable and should be monitored (Fig. 13.12). In this case, the definitive diagnosis may be made in the cardiac catheterization laboratory or by elevation of specific cardiac biomarkers.

TABLE 13.6 New York Heart Association Functional Classification of Heart Failure

Class	Definition
I	Normal daily activity does not initiate symptoms
II	Normal daily activities initiate onset of symptoms, but symptoms subside with rest
III	Minimal activity initiates symptoms, patients are usually symptom free at rest
IV	Any type of activity initiates symptoms, and symptoms are present at rest

TABLE 13.7 Correlations Among Ventricular Surfaces, Electrocardiogram Leads, and Coronary Arteries

Surface of Left Ventricle	ECG Leads	Usually Involved
Inferior	II, III, aVF	Right coronary artery
Lateral	V_5 and V_6, I, aVL	Left circumflex artery
Anterior	V_2, V_3, V_4	Left anterior descending artery
Anterior lateral	V_1 through V_6, I, aVL	Left main coronary artery
Septal	V_1 and V_2	Left anterior descending artery
Posterior	V_1 and V_2 V_7, V_8, V_9 (direct)	Left circumflex or right coronary artery (reciprocal changes)

I lateral	aVR	V_1 septal	V_4 anterior
II inferior	aVL lateral	V_2 septal	V_5 lateral
III inferior	aVF inferior	V_3 anterior	V_6 lateral

ECG, Electrocardiogram.

Cardiac Biomarkers During Myocardial Infarction

Cardiac biomarkers are released in the presence of damage and necrosis of the myocardium. The most recent AHA guidelines recommend testing with *high-sensitivity cardiac troponins* (hs-cTn).[44] These tests are highly accurate and offer a rapid turnaround time.[42]

To confirm the diagnosis of acute MI, the serum biomarkers troponin I or troponin T are measured by a blood test. Troponins begin to rise within 2 to 4 hours of STEMI and are detectable for 7 to 14 days.[44] If the coronary artery is opened by fibrinolytic therapy or by a percutaneous catheter intervention (PCI), the biomarkers exhibit a more rapid increase and dramatic decrease (Fig. 13.13). Information on biomarkers is also presented in Table 12.18 in Chapter 12.

Complications of Acute Myocardial Infarction

Many patients experience complications occurring early or late in the post-STEMI.[45] These complications may result from electrical dysfunction or from a cardiac contractility problem.

- Electrical dysfunctions include bradycardia, bundle branch blocks, and various degrees of heart block.
- Pumping complications can cause heart failure, pulmonary edema, and cardiogenic shock.
- Structural complications involving the septum, heart valves, myocardium, or pericardium.

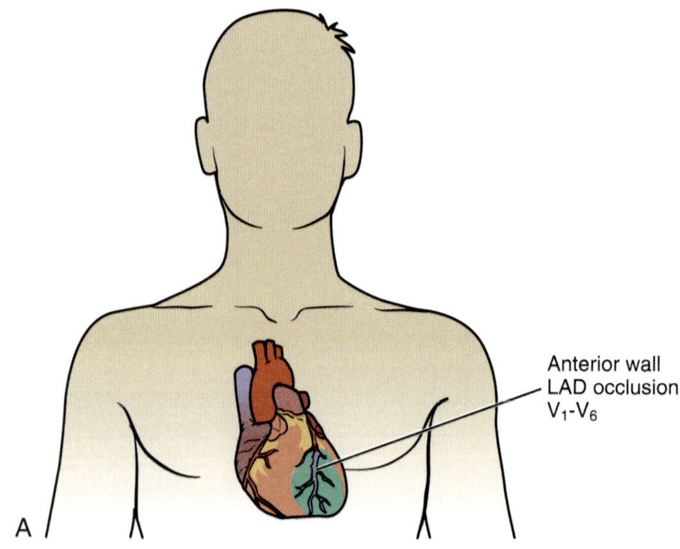

LIMB LEADS		PRECORDIAL LEADS	
Lead I	AVR	V1	V4
Lead II	AVL	V2	V5
Lead III	AVF	V3	V6

B

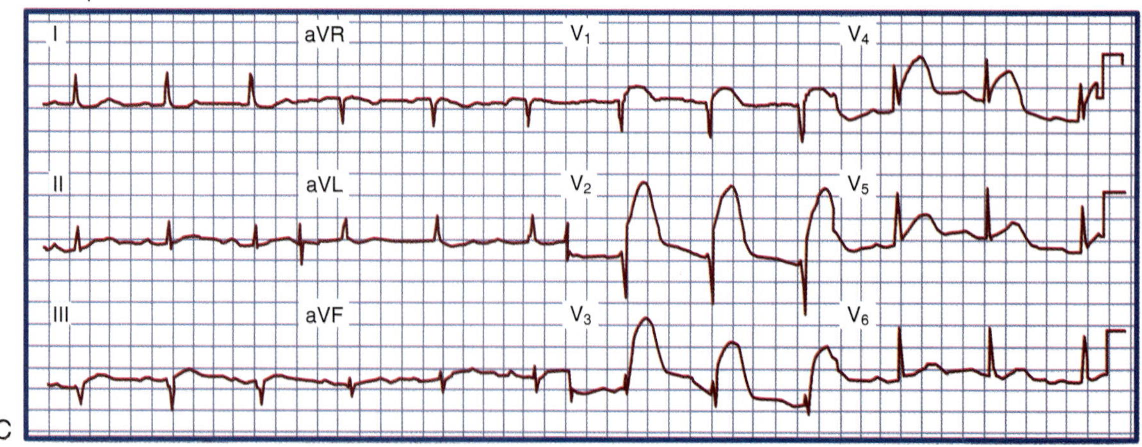

FIG. 13.7 Changes Seen on 12-Lead Electrocardiogram (ECG) With Anterior Wall Myocardial Infarction (MI). (A) Infarction location on the cardiac wall. (B) ECG leads with expected ST segment elevation. (C) A 12-lead ECG from a patient experiencing left anterior wall MI. *LAD*, left anterior descending artery.

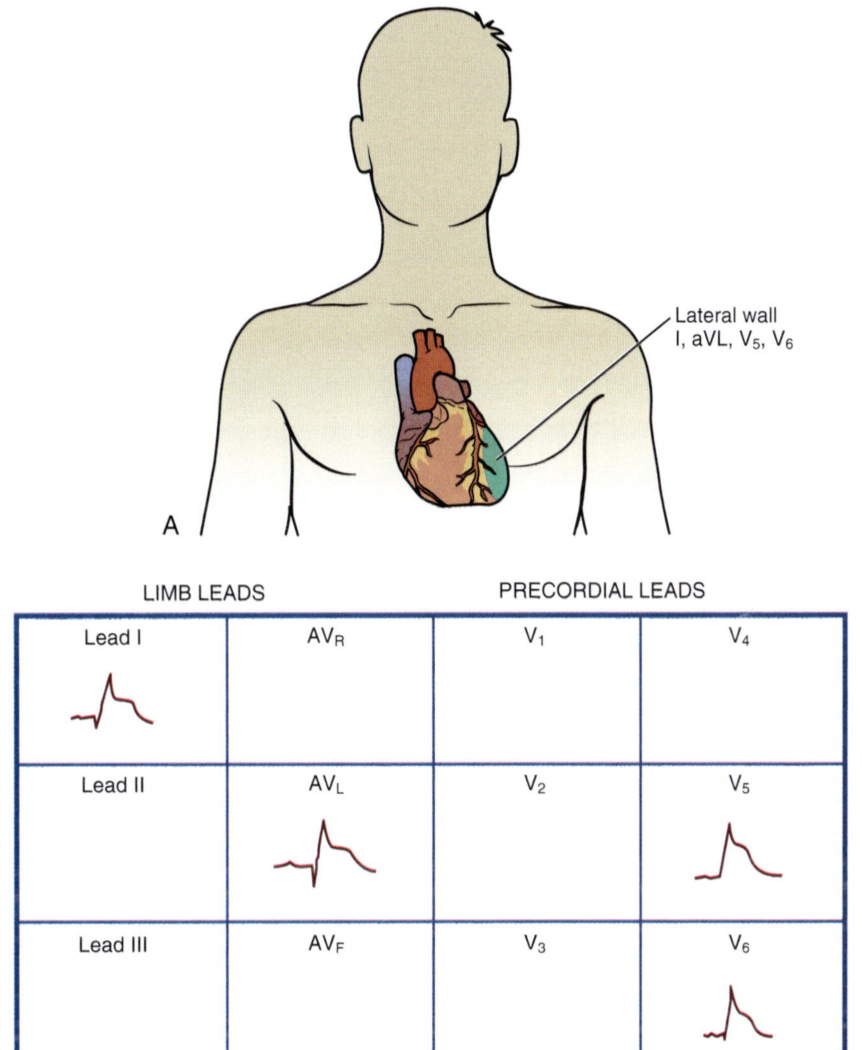

FIG. 13.8 Changes Seen on 12-Lead Electrocardiogram (ECG) With Lateral Wall ST Segment Elevation Myocardial Infarction. (A) Infarction location on the cardiac wall. (B) ECG leads with expected ST segment elevation.

The presence of a new murmur in a patient with a STEMI warrants special attention, as it may indicate a structural complication such as rupture of the papillary muscle or of the intraventricular septum. A new murmur can be indicative of severe damage and impending complications such as heart failure, or pulmonary edema.

Sinus Bradycardia

Sinus bradycardia (heart rate less than 60 beats/min) occurs frequently in patients who sustain an acute MI. It is more prevalent with an inferior wall infarction in the first hour after STEMI. Symptomatic bradycardia with hypotension and low cardiac output is treated with atropine (0.5 to 1.0 mg by intravenous push), repeated every 3 to 5 minutes to a maximum dose of 0.03 mg/kg (e.g., 2 mg for a person who weighs 70 kg) per advanced cardiac life support guidelines.

Sinus Tachycardia

Sinus tachycardia (heart rate greater than 100 beats/min) most often occurs with an anterior wall MI. Anterior infarction impairs LV pumping ability, reducing the ejection fraction and the stroke volume. To maintain cardiac output, the heart rate increases. Sinus tachycardia is corrected by treating the underlying cause, as it greatly increases myocardial oxygen consumption, leading to further ischemia.

Atrial Dysrhythmias

Premature atrial contractions occur frequently in patients who sustain an acute MI. Atrial fibrillation is also common and may occur spontaneously or may be preceded by premature atrial contractions. With the onset of atrial fibrillation, the loss of organized atrial contraction decreases cardiac output by up to 20%. Patients with new-onset or preexisting atrial fibrillation have higher morbidity rates than patients in sinus rhythm during an ACS event. Patients with ACS and new-onset atrial fibrillation experience a greater number of in-hospital adverse events, such as reinfarction, shock, pulmonary edema, bleeding, and stroke. Management of atrial fibrillation includes both rate control and rhythm control.[46]

Ventricular Dysrhythmias

Premature ventricular contractions are seen in almost all patients within the first few hours after MI. They are initially controlled through administration of oxygen to reduce myocardial hypoxia and by correcting acid-base or electrolyte

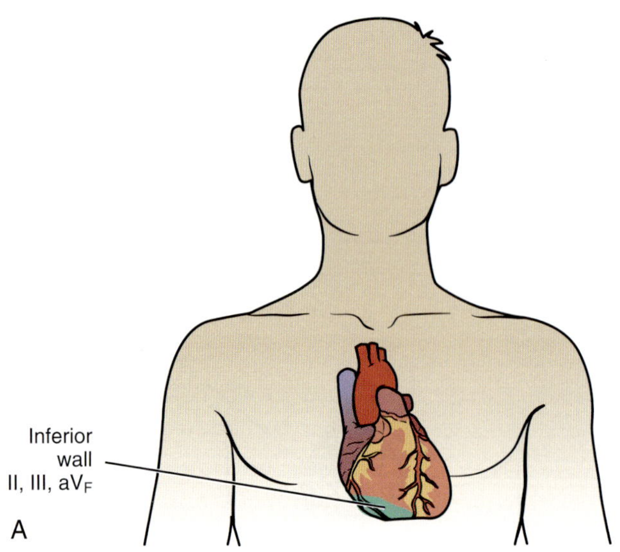

LIMB LEADS		PRECORDIAL LEADS	
Lead I	aV$_R$	V$_1$	V$_4$
Lead II	aV$_L$	V$_2$	V$_5$
Lead III	aV$_F$	V$_3$	V$_6$

B

Example of an Acute Inferior Wall MI

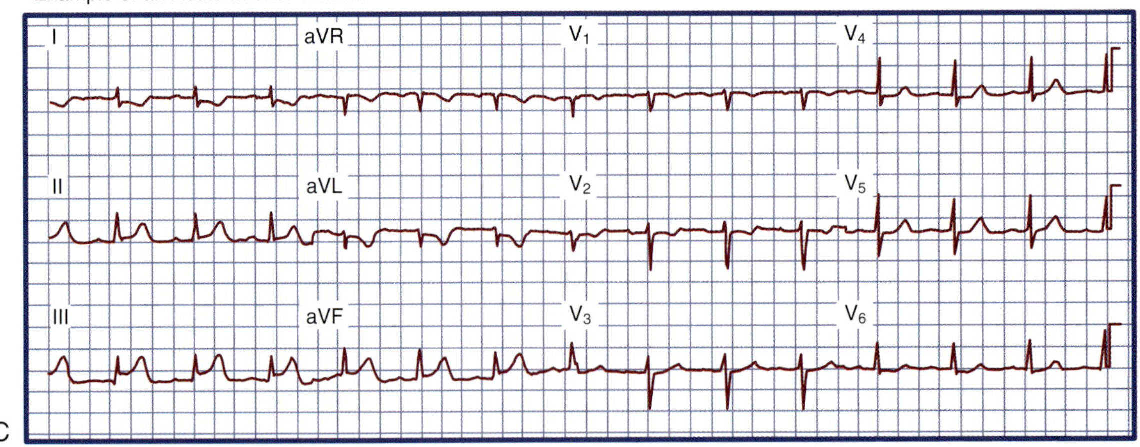

FIG. 13.9 Changes Seen on 12-Lead Electrocardiogram (ECG) With Inferior Wall Myocardial Infarction (MI). (A) Infarction location on the cardiac wall. (B) ECG leads with expected ST segment elevation. (C) A 12-lead ECG from a patient experiencing inferior wall MI.

imbalances. In the setting of an acute MI, premature ventricular contractions are pharmacologically treated if they have the following characteristics: frequent (more than six per minute), closely coupled (R-on-T phenomenon), multiform shapes, and occurrence in bursts of three or more, increasing the risk of sustained ventricular tachycardia (VT). Ventricular fibrillation (VF) is a life-threatening dysrhythmia associated with high mortality in acute MI. Beta-blockers are prescribed after acute MI to decrease mortality from ventricular dysrhythmias.

Atrioventricular Heart Block During Myocardial Infarction

Complete heart block occured in 2% of patients with STEMI in one series and was associated with increased in-hospital mortality.[47] In STEMI, AV block most often occurs after an inferior wall MI. Because the RCA supplies the AV node in 90% of the population, RCA occlusion leads to ischemia and infarction of the AV node cells.

The development of complete heart block has become less common because most patients receive fibrinolysis or undergo PCI to open the occluded vessel. Complete heart block is an emergency, and transcutaneous pacing is the primary intervention; transvenous pacemakers are used less frequently.

Ventricular Aneurysm After Myocardial Infarction

A ventricular aneurysm (Fig. 13.14) is a noncontractile, thinned LV wall that results from an acute transmural infarction. It most often occurs in the setting of an acute left anterior descending artery occlusion with a wide area of infarcted myocardium. The most effective prevention is early reperfusion of the myocardium, accomplished by opening the thrombosed coronary artery. The most common complications of a ventricular aneurysm are acute heart failure, systemic emboli, angina, and VT. Treatment is directed toward management of these complications and surgical repair of LV aneurysm. The affected area may be described as:

- Hypokinetic—contracts poorly
- Akinetic—noncontractile scar tissue
- Dyskinetic—scar tissue that moves in the opposite direction to normal contractile myocardium

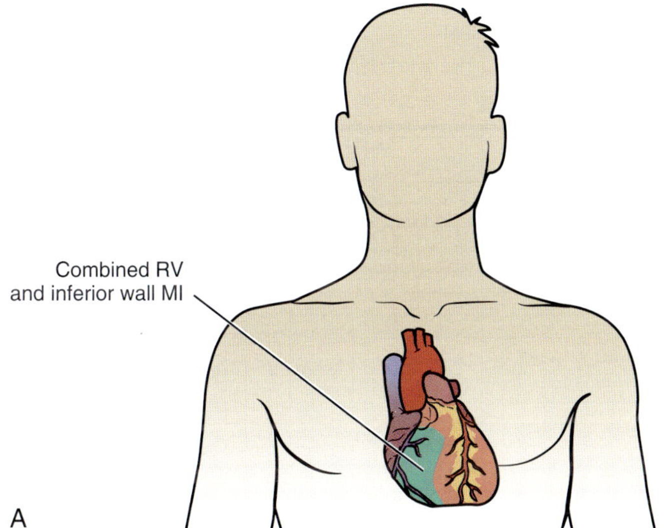

FIG. 13.10 Changes Seen on 12-Lead Electrocardiogram (ECG) With Inferior Right Ventricular (RV) ST Segment Elevation Myocardial Infarction (MI). (A) Image of an RV wall MI. (B) Acute inferior wall MI with the right coronary artery (RCA) occluded. (C) Example of an acute inferior RV wall MI with conventional 12-lead ECG. (D) Example of an acute RV wall MI with a right-sided 12-lead ECG. Both 12-lead ECGs are taken from the same patient.

Example of an Acute Inferior Wall and RV Wall MI. Shows ST elevation in leads II, III, AV_F, and reciprocal changes (ST depression) in anterior and lateral leads.

#1

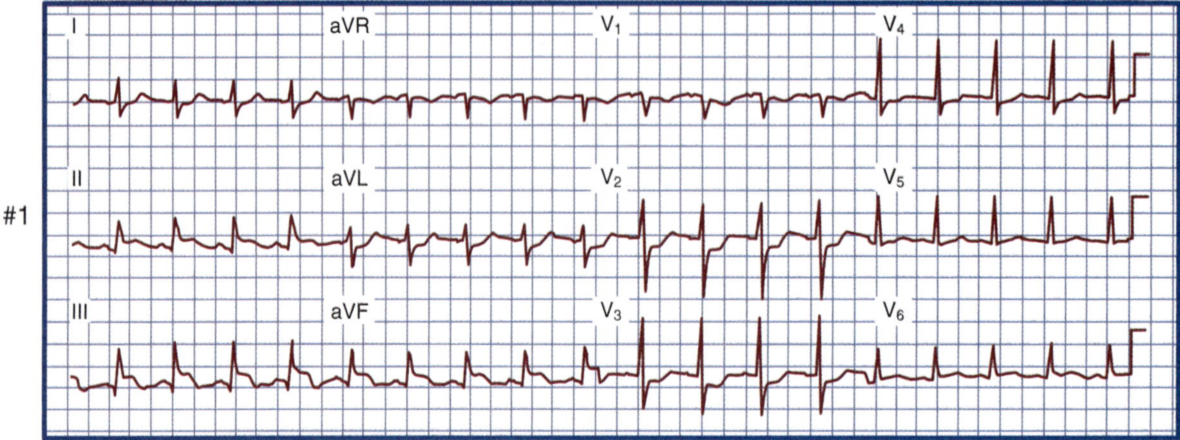

Reciprocal changes seen in V_1, V_2, V_3, V_4, I, and aVL, which provides a clue as to the extent of the MI.
Angiographic changes associated with an occlusion of the RCA.
These findings can range from:

- Proximal occlusion (near origin of RCA) that will produce inferior MI, posterior MI, and RV MI
- Middle RCA occlusion that will produce posterior and inferior MI
- Distal RCA occlusion that will produce inferior wall MI

C

Example of an Acute RV MI in right precordial leads.

#2

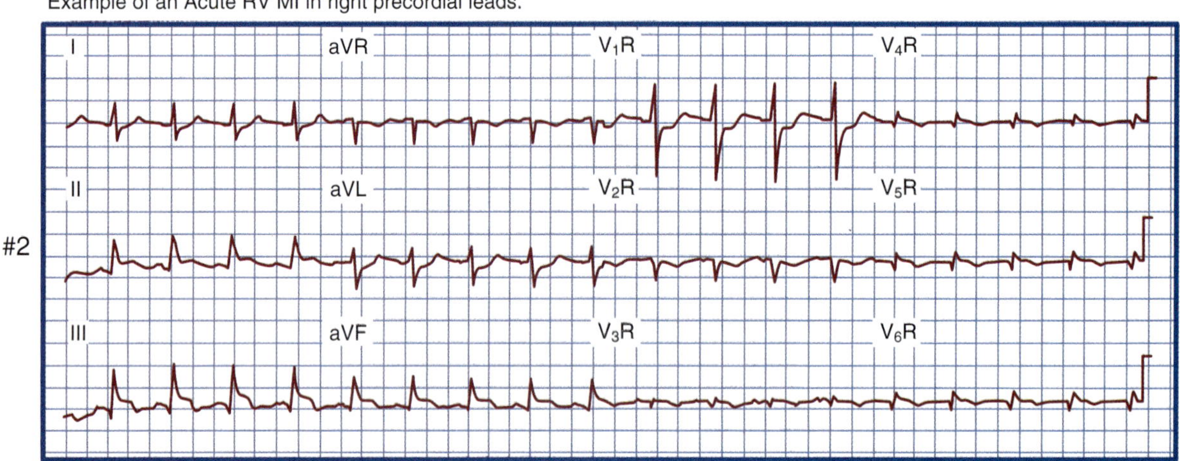

ECG shows ST elevation in right precordial leads (V_3R to V_6R), indicating RV wall injury/infarct.
Note limb leads are identical in both ECGs.

D

These two 12-lead ECGs are from the same patient with RV MI.

FIG. 13.10, cont'd

The prognosis depends on the size of the aneurysm, the level of overall LV dysfunction, and the severity of coexisting CAD.[45]

Ventricular Septal Rupture After Myocardial Infarction

Rupture of the ventricular septal wall after MI is a rare but potentially lethal complication of an acute anterior wall MI (Fig. 13.15). *Ventricular septal rupture* creates a pathological opening between the right and left ventricle. Studies report this complication occurs in 0.3% of all STEMI.[45] The incidence has declined because most patients with STEMI have the blocked coronary artery opened through PCI or fibrinolysis within a short time frame after diagnosis.[33] Nevertheless, rupture of the ventricular septum carries an extremely high mortality rate. Mortality rates are very high, almost 80% at 30 days.[45] Most patients with septal rupture also have signs and symptoms of cardiogenic shock.[45] Ventricular septal rupture manifests as severe chest pain, syncope, hypotension, and sudden hemodynamic deterioration caused by shunting of blood from the high-pressure left ventricle into the low-pressure right ventricle through the new septal opening. A holosystolic murmur can be auscultated along the left sternal border and is often accompanied by a thrill palpable on the chest. Rupture of the septum is a medical and surgical emergency.

The patient's condition is stabilized with vasodilators and an intra-aortic balloon pump (IABP) to decrease afterload. The goal of afterload reduction in this patient population is to decrease the amount of blood being shunted to the right side of the heart and consequently to increase the flow of blood to the systemic circulation. Survival improves if the septal rupture is very small

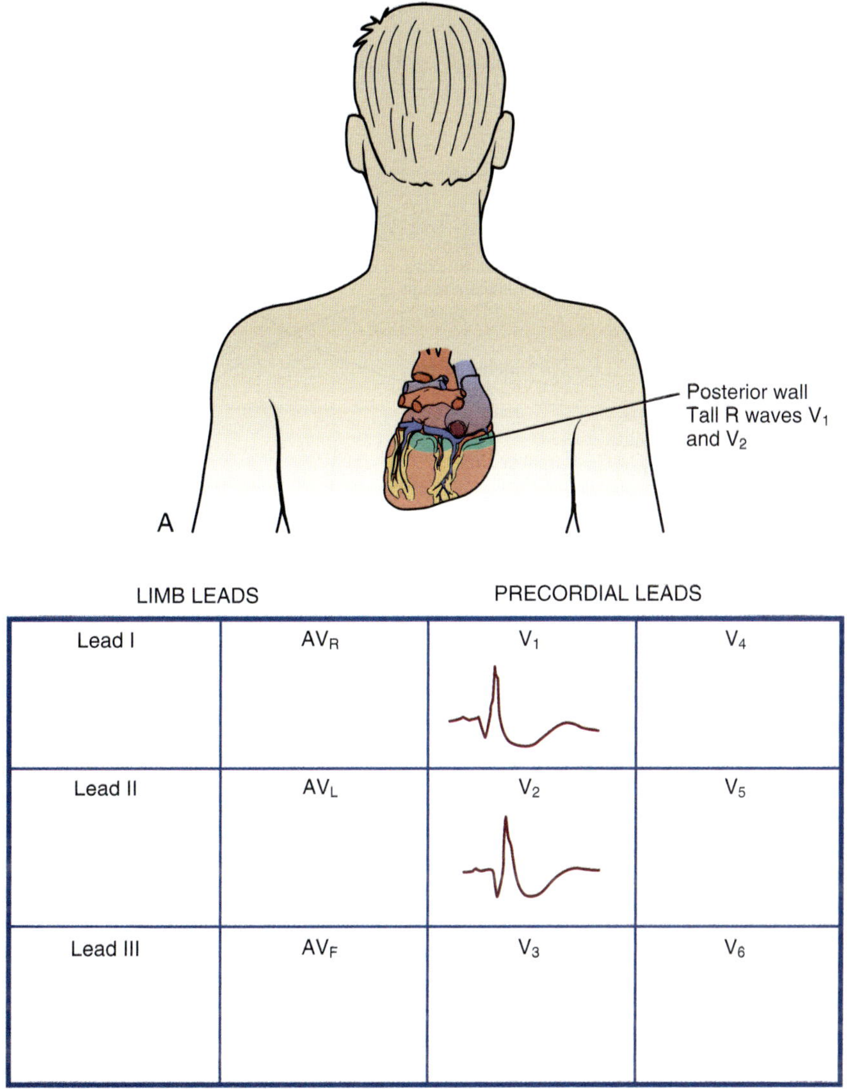

FIG. 13.11 Changes Seen on 12-Lead Electrocardiogram (ECG) With ST Segment Elevation Myocardial Infarction (STEMI). Infarction location on the cardiac wall. (B) ECG leads with expected ST segment elevation in posterior wall STEMI.

and the patient's condition is sufficiently stable to wait for scar tissue to form before surgical repair. When the septal opening is large, the massive left-to-right shunt across the septum makes the chances of survival dismal with or without surgery.[45]

Papillary Muscle Rupture After Myocardial Infarction

Papillary muscle rupture can occur when the infarct involves the area around one of the papillary muscles that support the mitral valve. Infarction of the papillary muscles results in ineffective mitral valve closure, and blood is forced back into the low-pressure left atrium during ventricular systole. The rupture may be partial or complete. Complete rupture is catastrophic and precipitates severe acute mitral regurgitation, cardiogenic shock, and high risk of death. This complication is encountered less frequently as early reperfusion of the coronary arteries has prevented STEMI sequelae.[45]

Partial rupture (Fig. 13.16) also results in mitral regurgitation, but the condition can be stabilized with aggressive medical management using an IABP and vasodilators. Urgent surgical intervention is required to replace the mitral valve.[45]

Cardiac Wall Rupture After Myocardial Infarction

The incidence of cardiac wall rupture has two peak times. The first occurs within the first 24 hours, and the second occurs between 3 and 5 days after infarction, when leukocyte scavenger cells are removing necrotic debris, thinning the myocardial wall. The onset is sudden and usually catastrophic. Bleeding into the pericardial sac results in cardiac tamponade, cardiogenic shock, pulseless electrical activity, and death. Survival is rare. If rupture occurs in the hospital, emergency pericardiocentesis is required to relieve the tamponade until a surgical repair can be attempted. The best prevention is early reperfusion of the myocardium.[45]

Pericarditis After Myocardial Infarction

Pericarditis is inflammation of the pericardial sac. It can occur after an acute MI, but also from viral or bacterial causes.[48] From all causes of pericarditis, 20% are classified as postcardiac injury.[48] After an STEMI if the damaged epicardium becomes rough and inflamed it may irritate the pericardium lying adjacent to it, precipitating pericarditis. Pain is the most common symptom of pericarditis, and a pericardial friction rub is the

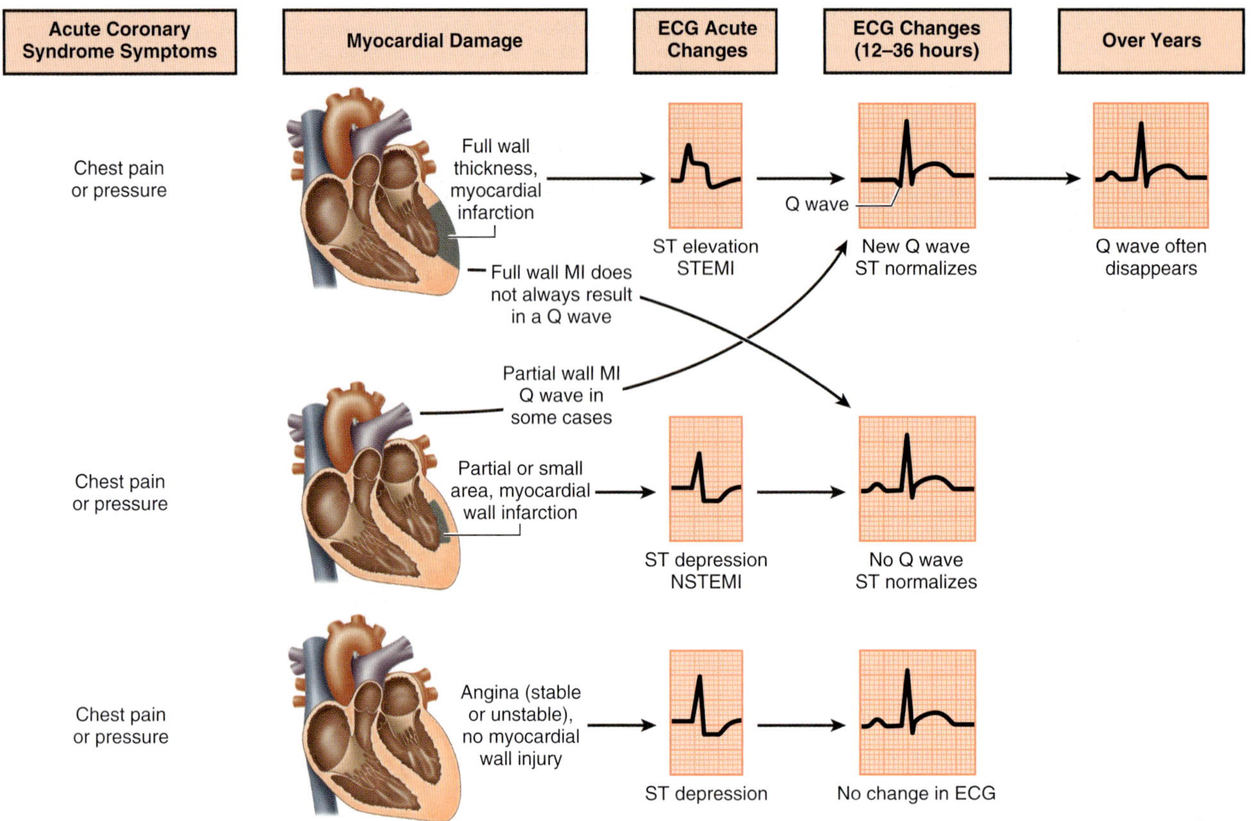

FIG. 13.12 Acute Coronary Syndrome: STEMI, NSTEMI, Unstable Angina, Electrocardiography Changes Over Time.

most common initial sign. The friction rub is best auscultated with a stethoscope at the sternal border and is described as a grating, scraping, or leathery scratching. Pericarditis frequently produces a pericardial effusion.[48] After the effusion occurs, the friction rub may disappear. On a 12-lead ECG, pericarditis may manifest as elevation of the ST segment in all the typically upright leads.[48] Pericarditis is treated with antiinflammatory medications, acetylsalicylic acid (aspirin), and rest.[48]

Pericarditis that occurs as a late complication of acute MI is also known as *Dressler syndrome* and is suspected when blood cultures are sterile and there is recent myocardial injury or infarction.[49]

Heart Failure and Acute Myocardial Infarction

Many patients with acute STEMI also have acute heart failure on admission to the hospital. These patients have often waited longer to come to the hospital and are older and more likely to be female. Compared with patients with acute MI but not heart failure, these patients have a higher risk of adverse in-hospital events and have longer lengths of stay and higher in-hospital mortality rates. More detailed information about heart failure is presented later in this chapter.

Medical Management

Adherence to the guidelines developed by the ACC and the AHA decreases in-hospital mortality after STEMI.[33] The guidelines are research based and are designed to improve the outcome of patients admitted to the hospital with acute MI. Clinical guidelines address the issues of interventions to open the coronary artery, anticoagulation, prevention of dysrhythmias, intensive glucose control, and prevention of ventricular remodeling after STEMI.

To facilitate rapid coronary artery revascularization in STEMI, hospitals are encouraged to develop a coordinated patient transfer strategy between *PCI-capable* and *non–PCI-capable* hospitals, as illustrated in Fig. 13.3.[33]

Recanalization of Coronary Arteries

The essential immediate interventions for a patient with an acute STEMI are fibrinolytic therapy or PCI to open the occluded artery.[33] All clinical guidelines emphasize the need for patients with symptoms of ACS to be rapidly triaged and treated.[33] See Chapter 14 for more information on mechanisms to reopen an occluded coronary artery.

Anticoagulation

In the acute phase after STEMI, heparin is administered in combination with fibrinolytic therapy to recanalize (open) the coronary artery.[33] For patients who will receive fibrinolytic therapy, an initial heparin bolus of 50–70 units/kg (maximum 5000 units) is given intravenously, followed by a continuous heparin drip at 12 units/kg per hour (maximum 1000 units/h) to maintain an activated partial thromboplastin time (aPTT) between 50 and 70 seconds (1.5 to 2.0 times control) for 48 hours or until revascularization.[33]

It Is also prudent to administer intravenous unfractionated heparin (UFH), or subcutaneous LMWH, if the patient is at risk for thrombus development. For patients with known heparin-induced thrombocytopenia, or as an alternative to LMWH or UFH, a third class of antithrombotic medications is available: direct antithrombotic agents (e.g., bivalirudin, argatroban). Risk for thrombotic emboli comes from anterior wall infarction, atrial fibrillation, cardiomyopathy, cardiogenic shock, and patients with a history of prior embolic events.

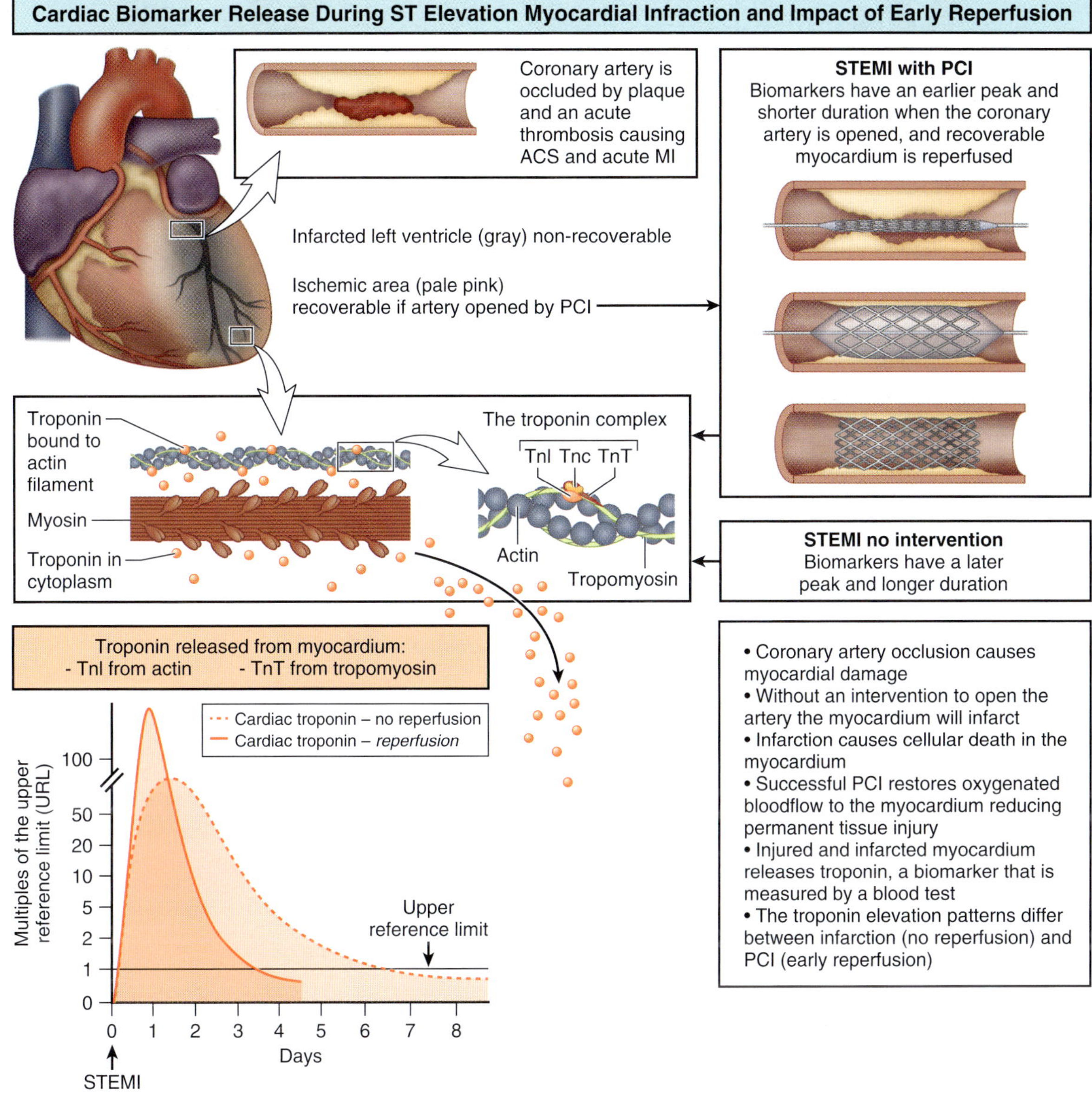

FIG. 13.13 Cardiac Biomarkers During ST Elevation Myocardial Infarction and the Effect of Early Reperfusion. *ACS*, Acute coronary syndrome; *MI*, myocardial infarction; *PCI*, percutaneous coronary intervention; *STEMI*, ST segment elevation myocardial infarction; *TnC*, troponin C; *TnI*, troponin I; *TnT*, troponin T.

Antiplatelet Therapy

Antiplatelet therapy with aspirin and P2Y12 inhibitors is administered in conjunction with anticoagulation therapy. Dual antiplatelet therapy (DAPT) prevents platelet adhesion and aggregation implicated in the formation of occlusive coronary disease. Selection of P2Y12 inhibitor therapy depends on the reperfusion strategy, patient characteristics, and local practice.

Dysrhythmia Prevention

The antidysrhythmic with the best safety record after STEMI is amiodarone. Beta-blockers are another class of antidysrhythmics that are recommended for all patients after STEMI. Beta-blockers prevent ventricular dysrhythmias, lower BP, and prevent reinfarction, especially in patients with LV dysfunction.[33]

Prevention of Ventricular Remodeling

Many patients are at risk for development of heart failure after STEMI. Vasodilating medications, including an angiotensin-converting enzyme inhibitor (ACEi), or angiotensin II receptor blocker (ARBs), can stop or limit the ventricular remodeling that leads to heart failure. *Ventricular remodeling* refers to progressive changes in the size, architecture, and shape of the myocardium and occurs because of an injury such as STEMI. Ventricular remodeling is modulated by catecholamines and activation of neurohormonal compensatory mechanisms. The heart chamber walls ultimately become dilated, thinned, and poorly contractile. An ACEi or, if this is not tolerated, an ARB is indicated for all patients after STEMI.[33] Information about the clinical effects of heart failure is provided later in this chapter.

Nursing Management

Nursing care management for a patient with an acute MI incorporates a variety of patient diagnoses (Box 13.10). Nursing interventions focus on achieving a balance between myocardial oxygen supply and demand, preventing complications, and providing

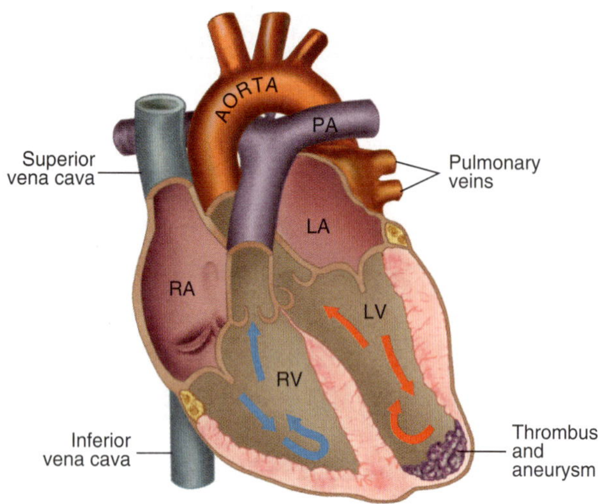

FIG. 13.14 Ventricular Aneurysm After Acute Myocardial Infarction. *LA,* Left atrium; *LV,* left ventricle; *PA,* pulmonary artery; *RA,* right atrium; *RV,* right ventricle.

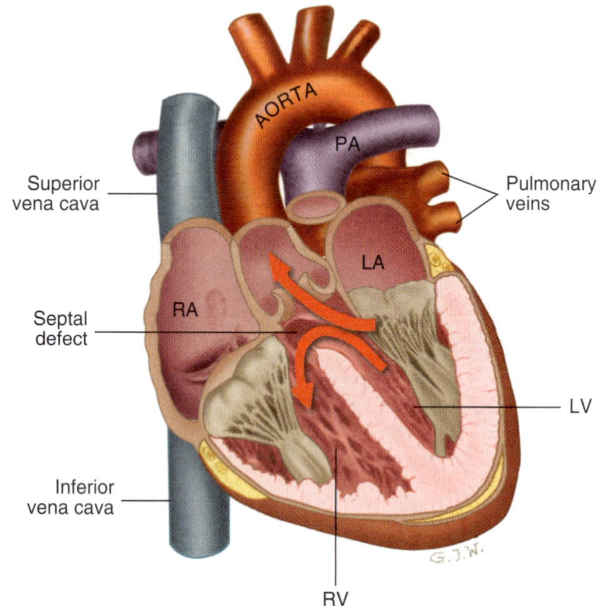

FIG. 13.15 Ventricular Septal Rupture After Acute Myocardial Infarction. *LA,* Left atrium; *LV,* left ventricle; *PA,* pulmonary artery; *RA,* right atrium; *RV,* right ventricle.

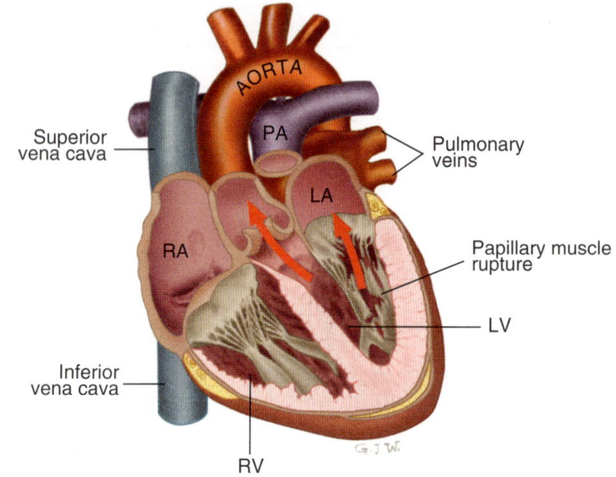

FIG. 13.16 Papillary Muscle Rupture After Acute Myocardial Infarction. *LA,* Left atrium; *LV,* left ventricle; *PA,* pulmonary artery; *RA,* right atrium; *RV,* right ventricle.

BOX 13.10 DIAGNOSIS AND PATIENT CARE MANAGEMENT

Myocardial Infarction

- Acute pain due to transmission and perception of cutaneous, visceral, muscular, or ischemic impulses
- Impaired cardiac output due to alterations in preload
- Impaired cardiac output due to alterations in afterload
- Impaired cardiac output due to alterations in contractility
- Impaired cardiac output due to alterations in heart rate or rhythm
- Impaired cardiac output due to sympathetic blockade
- Ineffective tissue perfusion due to decreased myocardial blood flow
- Activity intolerance due to cardiopulmonary dysfunction
- Impaired sleep due to fragmented sleep
- Anxiety due to threat from biologic, psychologic, or social integrity
- Lack of knowledge of treatment regime due to lack of previous exposure to information (see Box 13.12, Patient and Family Education Plan: Myocardial Infarction)

Patient Care Management plans are located in Appendix A.

patient and family education. See Appendix A for patient care management plans specific to patients with acute MI.

Balance of Myocardial Oxygen Supply and Demand

In the acute period, if severe heart muscle damage has occurred, myocardial oxygen supply is increased by the administration of supplemental oxygen to prevent tissue hypoxia. This imbalance manifests as many clinical signs (Box 13.11). Cardiac medications play an increasingly important role in balancing supply and demand, and the critical care nurse administers and monitors the effectiveness of these agents. For a patient with a low cardiac output, positive inotropic medications such as dobutamine, dopamine, or both may be administered.

Milrinone, a phosphodiesterase inhibitor that increases contractility by improving sarcolemma calcium uptake and causes positive inotropic effects in the myocardium, may also be used. In contrast to dobutamine and dopamine, milrinone does not compete for receptor sites in patients taking beta-blockers. These inotropic agents are used to increase cardiac contractility in the healthy areas of the heart (increasing oxygen supply) while avoiding damage to the recently infarcted areas.

Myocardial oxygen supply can be further enhanced using coronary artery vasodilators. Nitroglycerin is often administered for the first 48 hours to increase vasodilation and prevent myocardial ischemia. Research evidence supports the administration of early beta-blockade therapy to decrease myocardial workload and to prevent dysrhythmias. However, if the patient is in cardiogenic shock, beta-blockers are withheld until the cardiac output has improved.[33] Other interventions to decrease cardiac workload and myocardial oxygen consumption include bed rest, only beginning mobilization when the patient is clinically stable.

Prevention of Complications

A thorough grasp of the range of potential complications that can occur after STEMI is essential. Cardiac monitoring for early

BOX 13.11 Clinical Manifestations of Acute Myocardial Infarction

- Tachycardia with or without ectopy
- Bradycardia
- Normotension or hypotension
- Tachypnea
- Diminished heart sounds, especially S_1
- If left ventricular dysfunction present, may have S_3, S_4, or both
- Systolic murmur
- Pulmonary crackles
- Pulmonary edema
- Air hunger
- Orthopnea
- Frothy sputum
- Decreased cardiac output
- Decreased urine output
- Decreased peripheral pulses
- Slow capillary refill
- Restlessness
- Delirium
- Anxiety
- Agitation
- Denial
- Anger

detection of ventricular dysrhythmias is ongoing. Assessment for signs of continued ischemic pain is important because angina is a warning sign of the myocardium being at risk. In response to angina, a 12-lead ECG is obtained to determine whether an extension of the infarct exists, nitroglycerin is administered, and the physician is notified immediately so that interventions may be initiated to limit the size of the MI.

Heart failure is a serious complication after STEMI. When the patient's BP is stable, an ACEi is initiated. These vasodilators are used to prevent LV remodeling and dilation that occurs in many patients after STEMI. Hypotension is a potential complication of ACEi, especially with the first dose. It is an important nursing responsibility to monitor BP and patient symptoms after taking an ACEi. Surveillance to detect obvious and subtle signs of bleeding is also a priority, because so many patients with acute MI receive antiplatelet, anticoagulant, and fibrinolytic medications.

Prevention of hospital-acquired complications such as pneumonia, deep vein thrombosis (DVT), and hospital acquired infections (HAIs) is essential.[41] Early mobilization is also encouraged.[41]

Raising the head of the bed upright to 30 degrees or more facilitates decrease in venous return, lowering of preload, and decrease in the workload of the myocardium. Stool softeners may be given to lessen the risk of constipation from analgesics and bed rest and to decrease the risk of straining and increasing intraabdominal pressure. Providing a calm and quiet environment that is patient centered assists in recovery.[5]

Depression After Myocardial Infarction

Depression is a condition that occurs across a wide spectrum of human experiences. When depression is appropriately treated, there is no difference in outcomes.[50] However, untreated depression is associated with an increased mortality after STEMI.[50] Key symptoms of depression mentioned frequently by patients are fatigue, change in appetite, and sleep disturbance.

BOX 13.12 PATIENT AND FAMILY EDUCATION PLAN

Myocardial Infarction

Before discharge, the patient should be able to teach back the following topics:

- Pathophysiology of coronary artery disease, angina, and acute myocardial infarction
- Angina: Describe signs and symptoms such as pain, pressure, or heaviness in chest, arms, or jaw.
- Use of 0-to-10 pain scale: Notify critical care nurse or emergency personnel of any changes in chest pain intensity.
- Avoid Valsalva maneuver.
- Risk factor modification tailored to the patient's individual risk factor profile:
  - Decrease daily fat intake to less than 30% of total calories.
  - Reduce total serum cholesterol to less than 200 mg/dL.
  - Reduce low-density lipoprotein cholesterol to less than 70 mg/dL.
  - Stop smoking.
  - Reduce salt intake.
  - Control hypertension.
  - Control diabetes (if patient has diabetes).
  - Increase physical activity.
  - Achieve ideal body weight, if overweight.
- Referral to cardiac rehabilitation program
- Medication teaching about indications and side effects
- Follow-up care after discharge
- Symptoms to report to a health care professional
- Discussion of how to handle emotional stress and anger

Educating the Patient and Family

After the acute phase of an MI, patient and family education becomes a priority. Education focuses on the following key elements: (1) risk factor reduction, (2) manifestations of angina, (3) when to call a physician or emergency services, (4) medications, and (5) resumption of physical and sexual activities (Box 13.12). It is recommended that a referral be made to a cardiac rehabilitation program to reinforce education that was initiated during hospitalization.[51,52] Clinical practice guidelines for multidisciplinary care of a patient with an acute MI are listed in Box 13.13.

SUDDEN CARDIAC DEATH

Description

Sudden cardiac arrest and associated SCD annually account for 50% of all cardiovascular deaths, and for 25% this is their first symptom of heart disease.[53] SCD incidence is higher in men than women, although this disparity decreases with advancing age.[53]

When the onset of symptoms is rapid, the most likely mechanism of SCD is VT, which degenerates into VF. Despite aggressive cardiopulmonary resuscitation (CPR) initiated outside the hospital, few individuals who sustain an out-of-hospital cardiac arrest survive to hospital discharge. Strategies that have been shown to improve resuscitation survival involve huge community-wide programs to teach laypersons CPR and how to use an automated external defibrillator. These programs assist with survival to hospital discharge.[53]

BOX 13.13 Evidence-Based Practice

Acute Coronary Syndrome and Acute Myocardial Infarction (Non-STEMI and STEMI)

Prevention of Acute Coronary Syndrome

The term *acute coronary syndrome* (ACS) is used to define the life-threatening consequences of coronary artery disease (CAD), notably unstable angina, non–ST segment elevation myocardial infarction (non-STEMI), and ST segment elevation myocardial infarction (STEMI):

- *Unstable angina* is a term that denotes chest pain that is not relieved by sublingual nitroglycerin or rest within 5 min.
- Non-STEMI is an acute myocardial infarction (MI) *without* ST segment elevation on the 12-lead electrocardiogram (ECG).
- STEMI is an acute MI *with* ST segment elevation on the 12-lead ECG.

All recommendations are class I, meaning that there is strong research evidence to support these recommendations.

Recommendations That Decrease Risk of Developing Non-STEMI and STEMI

- Primary care providers should evaluate CAD risk factors for all patients every 3 to 5 years using a validated risk assessment scoring tool.
- The 10-year risk of ACS and acute MI should be assessed for all patients who have more than two major risk factors through the use of evidence-based risk assessment tools.
- An intensive risk factor modification program is recommended for patients with established CAD or high-risk equivalents such as diabetes or chronic kidney disease.

Recommendations About Emergency ACS Symptoms

- A patient who has previously diagnosed CAD should take one sublingual nitroglycerin dose, and the patient (if alone) or a friend or relative should call 911 if chest pain or discomfort is unrelieved or worsening in 5 min.
- The same recommendation applies to a patient without known CAD. If pain is unrelieved with rest or worsening at 5 min, the patient (if alone) or a friend or relative should call 911.
- Patients with chest discomfort should be transported to the hospital by ambulance rather than be driven by a friend or relative.
- Family members should be advised to take a cardiopulmonary resuscitation (CPR) course before an ACS emergency occurs. This course teaches CPR skills, demonstrates use of an automated external defibrillator (AED), and educates participants about the "chain of survival" concept.

Recommendations for Prehospital EMS Paramedic First Responders

- First responders such as emergency medical services (EMS) paramedics can provide early defibrillation and advanced cardiac life support (ACLS) for patients in cardiac arrest.
- EMS personnel should administer 162 to 325 mg of nonenteric aspirin (chewed, not swallowed) to patients with chest pain and suspected STEMI.
- A prehospital fibrinolysis protocol is reasonable for patients with STEMI if there are physicians in the ambulance or if there is a well-organized EMS service with full-time paramedics plus 12-lead ECG transmission capability and online medical direction.
- Patients older than 75 years and patients with cardiogenic shock should be transported to a hospital with the capability to provide fibrinolytics, emergency percutaneous coronary intervention (PCI), or emergency coronary artery bypass graft (CABG) surgery.
- Patients with STEMI who have a contraindication to fibrinolytic therapy should be brought to a hospital with the capability to provide emergency PCI or CABG surgery. At the scene, the door-to-departure time should be *less than 30 min.* PCI should be initiated *within 90 min* after initial medical contact.

Recommendations for Initial Emergency Clinical Management

- Hospitals should establish multidisciplinary teams to facilitate rapid triage of patients who present to the emergency department (ED) with chest pain.
- Use of written protocols is recommended to standardize care. An immediate cardiology consultation is advised if the patient's symptoms fall outside the written protocol.

STEMI

- *Fibrinolytics for STEMI:* Time from coming into contact with the health care system (paramedics or ED) to receiving fibrinolytics should be *less than 30 min.* A brief, focused neurologic examination to determine prior stroke or presence of cognitive defects is necessary before administration of fibrinolytics.
- *PCI for STEMI:* Time from coming into contact with the health care system (paramedics or ED) to balloon inflation PCI should be *less than 90 min.*

Non-STEMI

- If the level of risk for a patient with non-STEMI is not immediately apparent, a "chest pain unit" within the ED permits close surveillance by competent clinicians without immediate hospital admission.
- Glycoprotein lib/IIIa inhibitors for non-STEMI, in addition to aspirin and heparin, are indicated if cardiac catheterization or PCI is planned.
- PCI may be indicated for non-STEMI.

Recommendations for Initial Emergency Physical Assessment

Vital Signs

- Heart rate, blood pressure, respiratory rate, temperature, oxygen saturation with pulse oximetry (SpO_2), and ECG monitoring to detect presence of dysrhythmias are obtained.

Physical Assessment

- Assess for warm or cool skin, color, capillary refill, and peripheral pulses.
- Auscultate heart for cardiac murmur or new S_3 or S_4.
- Auscultate lungs for air entry plus crackles and wheezes.
- Observe for breathlessness and frothy pink sputum (pulmonary edema).
- Ask patient, family, or significant others for relevant history.

Recommendations for Emergency Diagnostics

12-Lead ECG

- For all patients with chest discomfort or angina-equivalent symptoms, a 12-lead ECG should be obtained and shown to the ED physician within 10 min after the patient's arrival in the ED.
- If the first ECG is normal, but the patient continues to have symptoms of chest pain or discomfort, the 12-lead ECG should be repeated at 5- to 10-min intervals, *or* continuous 12-lead ECG monitoring can be used.
- In patients with inferior wall infarction, right ventricular infarction must be suspected and right-sided ECG leads recorded. V_4R is the diagnostic lead of choice to diagnose ST segment elevation in the right ventricle.

Laboratory Studies

- Laboratory tests should be performed as part of the general management of STEMI but should not delay the administration of reperfusion therapy.

Cardiac Biomarkers

- Measurement of cardiac-specific troponins is recommended for patients with coexistent skeletal muscle injury. Clinicians are advised not to wait for results of the biomarker assay before initiating reperfusion therapy. Point-of-care (handheld) biomarker assay results can be used for rapid

 BOX 13.13 **Evidence-Based Practice—cont'd**

Acute Coronary Syndrome and Acute Myocardial Infarction (Non-STEMI and STEMI)

determination of treatment, but subsequent biomarker assays should be done by quantitative laboratory analysis.

Imaging Studies

- *Portable chest radiograph:* Obtaining a chest radiograph must not delay reperfusion therapy unless a major complication such as aortic dissection is suspected.
- Portable echocardiography (transthoracic echocardiogram or transesophageal echocardiogram) or magnetic resonance imaging: A scan should be obtained to distinguish aortic dissection from STEMI for patients in whom the symptoms are unclear.

Recommendations for Care

Prevent Hypoxia

- Supplemental oxygen is administered to maintain oxygen saturation greater than 90%.

Coronary Vasodilation

- Sublingual nitroglycerin (0.4 mg every 5 min × 3 doses) is administered. If chest pain or discomfort is ongoing, start a peripheral intravenous (IV) line. Administer IV nitroglycerin for relief of chest pain, control of hypertension, or relief of pulmonary congestion.

Pain Control

- Intravenous morphine sulfate (2–4 mg) is administered; dosage can be increased by 2- to 8-mg IV increments at 5- to 15-min intervals for STEMI pain control.

Anti-Platelet Therapy

- Discontinue nonsteroidal nti-inflammatory drugs (NSAIDs; except for aspirin), both nonselective and cyclooxygenase 2 selective agents, at time of presentation with STEMI because of increased risk of mortality, reinfarction, hypertension, heart failure, and myocardial rupture associated with NSAID use.
- Aspirin 162–325 mg non-enteric coated should be chewed for rapid buccal absorption.
- Additional antiplatelet therapy includes the P2Y12 inhibitors:
  - Ticagrelor loading dose of 180 mg.
  - Prasugrel loading dose of 60 mg (if no contraindications: prior stroke or TIA, or relative contraindications for prasugrel such as those age 75 years or older, weight less than 60 kg).
  - Clopidogrel 600 mg is given to patients at high risk of bleeding or when prasugrel or ticagrelor cannot be used.

Beta-Blockers

- Oral beta-blocker therapy is administered to patients with STEMI who do not have contraindications to beta blockade, regardless of fibrinolytic or primary PCI reperfusion.
- Contraindications for beta blockade with STEMI include signs of heart failure, low cardiac output, cardiogenic shock risk, heart block or prolonged P–R interval (>0.24 s), and active asthma or reactive airways disease.
- While considering the options for reperfusion, beta-blockers are given if the patient has tachycardia or hypertension; otherwise, they are started as soon as possible after STEMI.

Angiotensin-Converting Enzyme Inhibitors

- Oral angiotensin-converting enzyme inhibitors (ACEi) are indicated within the first 24 hours after STEMI unless contraindicated.

Recommendations for Emergency Interventions for STEMI

Fibrinolytic Medications

- Fibrinolytic medications are administered to patients with STEMI (if PCI is unavailable) with ST segment elevation greater than 0.1 mV (1 mm or one small box) in two contiguous precordial (chest) leads *or* two adjacent limb leads, new left bundle branch block (LBBB) or presumed new LBBB, and onset of symptoms less than 12 h earlier.
- Before administration of fibrinolytic therapy, rule out neurologic contraindications.
- Rule out facial trauma, uncontrolled hypertension, or ischemic stroke within the past 3 months.
- If contraindications to fibrinolysis are present, PCI is the preferred method of reperfusion.

PCI

- Emergency diagnostic coronary angiography should be performed to identify blocked coronary artery before PCI.
- Emergency PCI is recommended over fibrinolytic therapy if symptom onset was longer than 3 h ago.
- Emergency PCI can be performed within 12 h after symptom onset for patients with new LBBB or presumed new LBBB.
- Emergency PCI balloon inflation should be done within 90 min after arrival at the hospital.

Cardiac Surgery

Emergency CABG Surgery is Undertaken for Specific Indications in STEMI:

- Failed PCI with persistent pain or hemodynamic instability
- Recurrent ischemia refractory to medical therapy in patients with suitable anatomy who are not candidates for PCI
- Post-MI ventricular septal rupture or papillary muscle rupture, both of which frequently lead to cardiogenic shock
- Cardiogenic shock less than 36 h after MI, in patients younger than 75 years with ST segment elevation, or in patients with new LBBB who have multivessel or left main disease
- Recurrent ventricular dysrhythmias in patients with 50% or greater left main coronary artery lesion or triple-vessel disease or both

Recommendations for Secondary Prevention of Complications

Medications

- ACEi to prevent ventricular remodeling
- Beta-blocker to prevent ventricular dysrhythmias
- Diuretic if heart failure has developed
- Antihyperlipidemic if total cholesterol, low-density lipoprotein cholesterol, or triglycerides are elevated

Recommendations for Management of Complications After STEMI

Cardiogenic Shock

- Intra-aortic balloon pump for patients with hypotension (blood pressure of 90 mm Hg or systolic blood pressure of 30 mm Hg below baseline).

Ventricular Arrhythmias

- Ventricular fibrillation (VF) or pulseless ventricular tachycardia (VT) is managed by standard ACLS criteria.
- Patients with hemodynamically significant VT more than 2 days after STEMI who have ongoing ventricular dysrhythmias are considered for implantation of an implantable cardioverter defibrillator (ICD).
- Patients with an ejection fraction (EF) between 30% and 40% at 1 month after STEMI should undergo an electrophysiology study; if they are inducible to VT/VF, an ICD is recommended to reduce risk of sudden cardiac death (SCD).

Continued

BOX 13.13 Evidence-Based Practice—cont'd

Acute Coronary Syndrome and Acute Myocardial Infarction (Non-STEMI and STEMI)

- Patients with an EF of less than 30% at 1 month after STEMI are at high risk for SCD.

AV Block

- Transvenous pacemaker (emergency) or permanent pacemaker (later elective) is inserted for symptomatic second-degree or third-degree atrioventricular block.
- All patients who require permanent pacing after STEMI should also be evaluated for ICD indications.

Provide Relevant Education

Medications

- Provide written and verbal instructions about medication dosages, administration, and side effects.

Emergency Information

- Give the patient and family information about calling 911 if pain/angina-equivalent symptoms persist or worsen after 5 min.
- Family members of high-risk patients are advised to take a CPR class and learn about AEDs.

Risk Factors

- Provide education to reduce risk factors including education on smoking cessation, hypertension control, weight control, normal blood glucose, low-fat diet, and normal lipid panel.
- Patients are advised to increase physical activity.
- Women are advised to avoid new hormone replacement therapy.

Cardiac Rehabilitation

- Participation in a cardiac rehabilitation program will help the patient continue the process of risk factor and lifestyle modification.

Systems of Care

- Updating systems of care to reach more people in the community and to decrease delays to receiving treatment for STEMI.

References

Amsterdam EA, Wenger NK, Brindis RG, et al. 2014 AHA/ACC Guideline for the management of patients with non-ST elevation acute coronary syndromes. A report of the American College of Cardiology/American Heart Association Task Force on practice guidelines. *Circulation.* 2014;130:e344–e426. https://doi.org/10.1161/CIR.0000000000000134.

Jacobs AK, Ali MJ, Best PJ, et al. Systems of care for ST-segment-elevation myocardial infarction: a policy statement from the American Heart Association. *Circulation.* 2021;144(20):e310–e327. https://doi.org/10.1161/CIR.0000000000001025.

O'Gara PT, Kushner FG, Ascheim DD, et al. 2013 ACCF/AHA guideline for the management of ST-elevation myocardial infarction: a report of the American College of Cardiology Foundation/American Heart Association Task Force on Practice Guidelines. *Circulation.* 2013;127(4):e362–e425. https://doi.org/10.1161/CIR.0b013e3182742cf6.

BOX 13.14 Causes of Sudden Cardiac Death

Most patients with sudden cardiac death (SCD) are older adults and have a history of coronary artery disease (CAD), myocardial infarction (MI), and subsequent heart failure.

- Heart failure:
- Ejection fraction less than 30%
- Heart structure is abnormal (systolic or diastolic ventricular dysfunction).
- CAD and a history of MI that has produced scar tissue is the most common cause of ventricular tachycardia (VT)/ventricular fibrillation (VF) leading to SCD.
- Cardiomyopathy (dilated or ischemic):
- Patients who are inducible for VT/VF in electrophysiology study[43] are at highest risk.
- Risk is decreased by implantation of an implantable cardioverter defibrillator (ICD) and antidysrhythmic medication therapy.

Genetic SCD Risk

Genetic cardiovascular disease accounts for 40% of SCD in young adults.

- Brugada syndrome:
- Electrocardiogram (ECG) signs: Coved-type ST segment elevation (>2 mm) in right precordial leads, although ECG variations occur.
- Heart structure appears normal.
- High risk of VT or VF in otherwise young healthy adults.
- VT/VF also occurs at night or at rest.
- Represents up to 20% of genetic SCD patients.
- Hereditary: Autosomal-dominant genetic transmission.
- Five times more common in men.
- Patients who are inducible in EPS are at increased risk.
- Risk reduced by implantation of an ICD.
- Wolff-Parkinson-White (WPW) syndrome:
- Congenital accessory conduction pathway connects atria and ventricles.
- Accessory pathway is *in addition* to the normal conduction system.
- Accessory pathway allows very rapid transmission of impulses leading to "preexcitation" of the ventricle that can degenerate into VT/VF, especially if atrial dysrhythmias are present.
- WPW syndrome is usually identified when the patient is a teenager or young adult.
- WPW syndrome is often recognized during exercise by palpitations or breathlessness.
- Cure is possible in many cases by radiofrequency ablation of the accessory pathway.
- Hypertrophic cardiomyopathy (HCM):
- Risk of VT/VF with exercise exists.
- The obstructive form of HCM can be cured in many cases by myectomy or alcohol ablation of the enlarged ventricular septum.
- For other patients with HCM, the risk is reduced by implantation of an ICD.
- Long QT syndrome:
- Risk of VT/VF with exercise exists.
- Risk is reduced by implantation of an ICD.

Etiology

Most SCD incidents occur in patients with preexisting ventricular dysfunction resulting from cardiac disease. The most common SCD risk factor is extensive coronary atherosclerosis with or without a history of acute MI, but other structural conditions also may be causative. These include dilated or hypertrophic cardiomyopathy, valvular heart disease, autonomic nervous system abnormalities, electrical system abnormalities such as AV block, Wolff-Parkinson-White syndrome, long QT syndrome, and Brugada syndrome.[53] In addition, taking medications that prolong the Q–T interval increases SCD risk.[53] An ejection fraction less than 30% and a history of ventricular dysrhythmias are powerful predictors of SCD. Other risk factors are listed in Box 13.14. Many people are unaware of their risk of cardiac arrest and how to identify them before a SCD event remains an ongoing concern.[53]

Medical Management

Depending on the length of time the patient was unconscious because of cardiac arrest, cognitive defects may be present because of the lack of cerebral blood flow and resultant

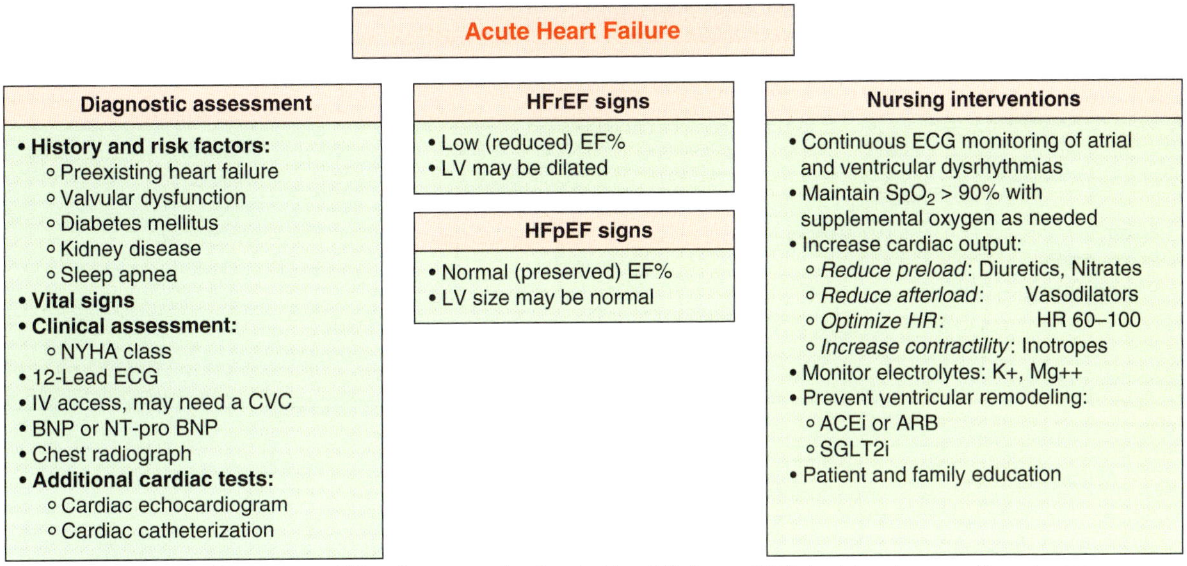

Acute Heart Failure

Diagnostic assessment

- **History and risk factors:**
  - Preexisting heart failure
  - Valvular dysfunction
  - Diabetes mellitus
  - Kidney disease
  - Sleep apnea
- **Vital signs**
- **Clinical assessment:**
  - NYHA class
- 12-Lead ECG
- IV access, may need a CVC
- BNP or NT-pro BNP
- Chest radiograph
- **Additional cardiac tests:**
  - Cardiac echocardiogram
  - Cardiac catheterization

HFrEF signs

- Low (reduced) EF%
- LV may be dilated

HFpEF signs

- Normal (preserved) EF%
- LV size may be normal

Nursing interventions

- Continuous ECG monitoring of atrial and ventricular dysrhythmias
- Maintain SpO_2 > 90% with supplemental oxygen as needed
- Increase cardiac output:
  - *Reduce preload*: Diuretics, Nitrates
  - *Reduce afterload*: Vasodilators
  - *Optimize HR*: HR 60–100
  - *Increase contractility*: Inotropes
- Monitor electrolytes: K+, Mg++
- Prevent ventricular remodeling:
  - ACEi or ARB
  - SGLT2i
- Patient and family education

FIG. 13.17 Summary of Key Concepts for Acute Heart Failure. *ACEi*, Angiotensin converting enzyme inhibitor; *ARB*, angiotensin receptor blocker, *ARNi*, angiotensin receptor neprilysin inhibitors; *BNP*, brain natriuretic peptide; *EF*, ejection fraction; *ECG*, electrocardiogram; *HFrEF*, heart failure with reduced ejection fraction; *HFpEF*, heart failure with preserved ejection fraction; *HR*, heart rate; *IV*, intravenous; K^+, potassium; Mg^{++}, magnesium; *GL2i*, sodium glucose cotransporter-2 inhibitor; SpO_2, pulse oximetry, oxygen saturation.

hypoxia.[54] For comatose patients at high risk for hypoxic brain injury after cardiac arrest, therapeutic hypothermia (targeted temperature management) is initiated to preserve brain function. Prevention of SCD focuses on identification and treatment of high-risk cardiac patients (see the sections on Implantable Cardioverter Defibrillator and Antidysrhythmic Medications in Chapter 14).

HEART FAILURE

Description and Etiology

The number of patients with heart failure is increasing.[1] There are now 6.7 million adults (older than age 20 years) in the United States with heart failure.[1] It is estimated that by 2030, an additional 3 million more people will be diagnosed with heart failure. Fig. 13.17 is a summary of key concepts of heart failure.

Pathophysiology

Heart failure is a response to cardiac dysfunction, a condition in which the heart cannot pump blood at a volume required to meet the body's needs. Any condition that impairs the ability of the ventricles to fill or eject blood can cause heart failure. STEMI with resultant necrotic damage to the left ventricle is the underlying cause of heart failure in many patients. Other major conditions that lead to heart failure include valvular dysfunction, infection (myocarditis or endocarditis), cardiomyopathy, and uncontrolled hypertension.[55]

Assessment and Diagnosis

Heart failure signs and symptoms are classified in several ways.

- New York Heart Association I–IV, functional categories with degree of physical activity that elicits symptoms (see Table 13.6).
- Stages of heart failure A–D, organized by increasing severity of symptoms and intensity of clinical interventions (Fig. 13.8). Stage C is further classified by degree of LV dysfunction and ejection fraction.[55]
- LVEF percentage is classified by degree of dysfunction and potential clinical interventions for those with Stage C heart failure[55]
  - LVEF ≤ 40%
  - LVEF 41%–49%
  - LVEF ≥ 50%

Heart failure is progressive, and symptoms manifest how far ventricular remodeling and dysfunction have advanced. The first step in the diagnosis is to identify the underlying structural abnormality creating the LV dysfunction. Heart failure may be discovered because of a known clinical syndrome such STEMI or be discovered during admission for an unrelated condition.

Various imaging tests are available to visualize cardiac anatomy, and laboratory tests are used to evaluate the effect of hormonal or electrolyte imbalance. The results of these tests permit the cardiology team to design a treatment plan to control symptoms and possibly correct the underlying cause.

Left Ventricular Failure—Signs and Symptoms

When the heart failure affects the left side of the heart this leads to vasoconstriction of the arterial bed that increases *systemic vascular resistance* (SVR), a condition also described hemodynamically as "high afterload" and this leads to backpressure into the pulmonary circulation and alveoli causing pulmonary edema and breathlessness. Other clinical manifestations of LV failure and low cardiac output include decreased peripheral perfusion with weak or diminished pulses, cool and pale extremities, and in later stages peripheral cyanosis (Table 13.8).

TABLE 13.8 Clinical Manifestations of Right-Sided and Left-Sided Heart Failure

LEFT VENTRICULAR FAILURE		RIGHT VENTRICULAR FAILURE	
Signs	**Symptoms**	**Signs**	**Symptoms**
Tachypnea	Fatigue	Peripheral edema	Weakness
Tachycardia	Dyspnea	Hepatomegaly	Anorexia
Cough	Orthopnea	Splenomegaly	Indigestion
Bibasilar crackles	Paroxysmal nocturnal dyspnea	Hepatojugular reflux	Weight gain
Gallop rhythms (S_3 and S_4)	Nocturia	Ascites	Mental changes
Increased pulmonary artery pressures		Jugular venous distention	
Hemoptysis		Increased central venous pressure	
Cyanosis		Pulmonary hypertension	
Pulmonary edema			

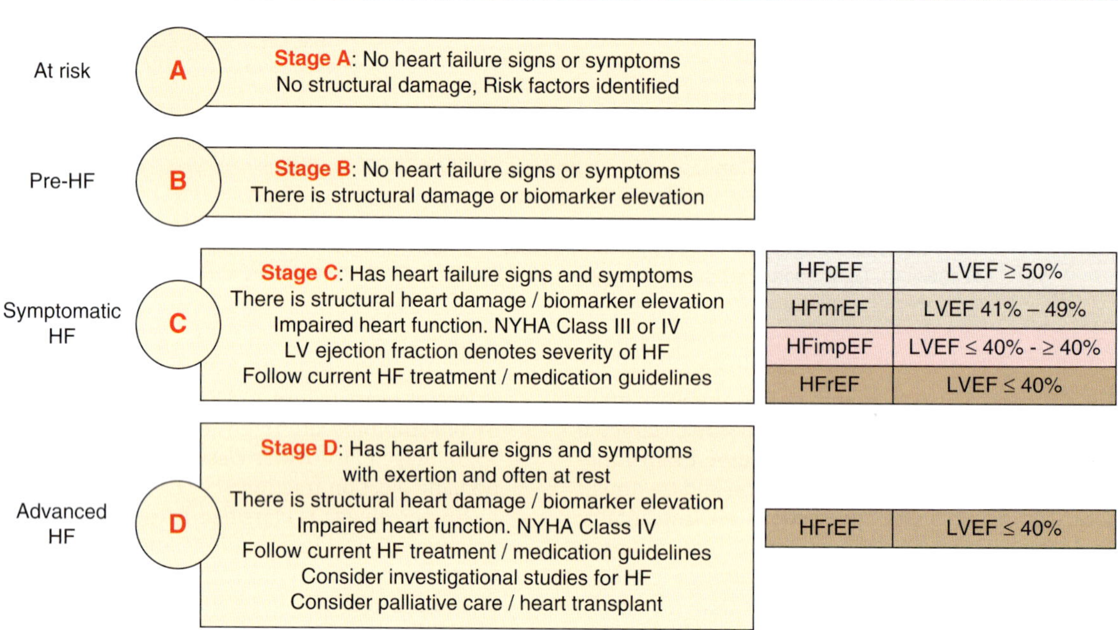

FIG. 13.18 Heart Failure Stages. *HF*, Heart failure; *HFimpEF*, heart failure with improved ejection fraction; *HFmrEF*, heart failure with mildly reduced ejection fraction; *HFpEF*, heart failure with preserved ejection fraction; *HFrEF*, heart failure with reduced ejection fraction; *LVEF*, left ventricular ejection fraction; *NYHA*, New York Heart Association.

Right Ventricular Failure—Signs and Symptoms

Failure of the right side describes ineffective right ventricular contractile function. This is most often secondary to failure of the left side of the heart that developed after elevated pulmonary vascular pressures made right ventricular contraction ineffective. The classic manifestations of right ventricular failure are jugular venous distention, elevated central venous pressure, weakness, peripheral or sacral edema, hepatomegaly (enlarged liver), jaundice, and liver tenderness. Gastrointestinal symptoms include poor appetite, anorexia, nausea, and an uncomfortable feeling of fullness (see Table 13.8). Isolated failure of the right ventricle is not common, but can be caused by a pulmonary embolus, right ventricular infarction, or from pulmonary hypertension (described later in this chapter).

Heart Failure Stages

The AHA guidelines for heart failure are classified into four stages (Fig 13.18).[55]

- **Stage A—At risk for heart failure** without any signs or symptoms. Stage A includes individuals with diabetes, obesity, or a strong family history.
- **Stage B—Pre-heart failure** without any signs or symptoms. Stage B includes individuals with structural heart disease, elevated LV filling pressures, or elevated biomarkers.
- **Stage C—Symptomatic heart failure** with signs and symptoms. Stage C is further subclassified by degree of LV dysfunction.
- **Stage D—Advanced heart failure** with obvious signs and symptoms. Stage D is often associated with multiple repeat hospital admissions.

Left Ventricular Dysfunction—Stage C Heart Failure

For patients diagnosed with Stage C heart failure, there is a further subdivision to classify the trajectory of heart failure signs and symptoms.[55]

- New onset heart failure
- Resolution of heart failure
- Persistent heart failure
- Worsening heart failure

Furthermore, heart failure is defined by the degree of LVEF percentage, with a lower percentage denoting more severe LV dysfunction.[55] There is a simplified diagram in Fig. 13.18 although for greater detail it is recommended to consult the AHA 2022 Heart Failure guidelines.[55] The LVEF categories are listed below.

- LVEF ≤ 40% *Heart failure with reduced ejection fraction* (HFrEF)[55]
- LVEF ≤ 40% and on repeat test ≥40% *Heart failure with improved ejection fraction* (HFimpEF) with treatment[55]

- LVEF 41%–49% *Heart failure with mildly reduced ejection fraction* (HFmrEF)[55]
- LVEF ≥ 50% *Heart failure with preserved ejection fraction* (HFpEF)[55]

Heart Failure With a Reduced Ejection Fraction

Patients with a diagnosis of *heart failure with HFrEF* have signs and symptoms of heart failure combined with a below-normal ejection fraction (LVEF ≤ 40%).[55] Symptoms of HFrEF include dyspnea, exercise intolerance, and fluid volume overload.

In HFrEF, the ventricular chambers will hypertrophy or dilate and ultimately become less efficient. This detrimental trajectory is termed *ventricular remodeling* and is different from the dysfunction caused by myocardial ischemia and infarction. Interventions and medications used to treat heart failure are discussed in Chapter 14.

Heart Failure With a Mildly Reduced Ejection Fraction

Patients with a diagnosis of *heart failure with HFmrEF* have some signs and symptoms of heart failure combined with a reduced ejection fraction (LVEF 41%–49%).[55] Diagnosis of HFmrEF requires evidence that LV filling pressures are elevated at rest, [55] that symptoms are precipitated during an exercise stress test, or that biomarkers such as B-type natriuretic peptide (BNP) or NT-proBNP are elevated.[55]

Heart Failure With Improved Ejection Fraction

The diagnosis of *heart failure with HFimpEF* indicates improvement with treatment.[55] This includes patient who initially have a low LVEF ≤40% and with treatment following current clinical guidelines the repeat LVEF is ≥40%.

Heart Failure With a Preserved Ejection Fraction

The diagnosis of *heart failure with HfpEF* may be difficult to establish.[55] Shortness of breath, in the context of diabetes, obesity, and advanced age, without another cardiac structural cause, often indicate the need for further diagnostic tests.[55]

Left Ventricular Dysfunction—Stage D Heart Failure

For patients with advanced heart failure and a reduced ejection fraction (Stage C and Stage D HFrEF with LV ≤ 40%), and there are additional steps and treatment options.[55]

- Step 1—Start medications.
- Step 2—Triage to appropriate medication dose.
- Step 3—Individualize to each patient.
- Step 4—For dysrhythmias, consider an implantable device.
- Step 5—Reassess symptoms and treatment.
- Step 6—Assess for heart transplant, palliative care, investigational studies.

Neurohormonal Compensatory Mechanisms in Heart Failure

When the heart begins to fail and the cardiac output is no longer sufficient to meet the metabolic needs of tissues, the body activates several major compensatory mechanisms: the sympathetic nervous system, the *renin-angiotensin-aldosterone system* (RAAS), and, if hypertension is present, the development of ventricular hypertrophy. This process ultimately reshapes the ventricle in a process described as *ventricular remodeling*.[56] These pathophysiologic processes are described in this section.

Heart Failure and Sympathetic Nervous System Activation

The sympathetic nervous system compensates for low cardiac output by increasing heart rate and BP. As a result, levels of circulating catecholamines are increased, leading to peripheral vasoconstriction. In addition to increasing BP and heart rate, catecholamines cause shunting of blood from nonvital organs such as the skin to vital organs such as the heart and brain. This mechanism, although initially helpful, may become a negative factor if elevation of heart rate increases myocardial oxygen demand while shortening the amount of time for diastolic filling and coronary artery perfusion.

Heart Failure and Renin Angiotensin Aldosterone System Activation

Activation of the RAAS in heart failure promotes fluid retention.[56] The RAAS is activated by low cardiac output that causes the hormone *renin* to be secreted by the kidneys (Fig.13.19). A physiologic chain of events is then set in motion that leads to volume overload. The renin acts on *angiotensinogen* in the bloodstream and converts it to angiotensin I; when angiotensin passes through the lung tissues, it is activated by *angiotensin-converting enzyme*, an enzyme that converts angiotensin I to *angiotensin II*, a powerful vasoconstrictor that increases SVR, BP, and the workload of the left ventricle; the increased SVR further decreases cardiac output.

The mineralocorticoid hormone *aldosterone* is released from the adrenal glands and stimulates sodium retention via the distal tubules of the kidney. In response to the low cardiac output, the renal arterioles constrict, decrease glomerular filtration, and increase reabsorption of sodium from the proximal and distal tubules. To break the RAAS cycle of fluid retention in heart failure, multiple medications are prescribed with different synergistic actions. See later in this section and in Table 14.23 in Chapter 14).

Heart Failure and Ventricular Hypertrophy

Ventricular hypertrophy is a compensatory mechanism. It is also strongly associated with preexisting hypertension. Because myocardial hypertrophy increases the force of contraction, hypertrophy helps the ventricle overcome an increase in afterload. When this mechanism is no longer efficient for the ventricle, it will remodel by dilation.

Heart Failure and Prevention of Ventricular Remodeling

Ventricular remodeling occurs because of the previously described pathologic mechanisms. The shape of the ventricle changes, or remodels, to resemble a round bowl. A dilated ventricle has poor contractility and is enlarged without hypertrophy. Synergistic use of medications from different categories—ACEi (or ARB, ARNi), mineralocorticoid receptor antagonists (MRA), beta-blockade, and SGLT2i—are designed to slow the progression of heart failure remodeling.[55,56]

Heart Failure and Atrial Dysrhythmias

Atrial fibrillation is common in heart failure. Atrial fibrillation does not cause heart failure, but heart failure increases the likelihood of atrial fibrillation developing.[55] Because of the association of atrial thrombus and risk of stroke, patients with atrial fibrillation must receive anticoagulation.

- Warfarin was the traditional anticoagulant used to decrease interatrial thrombus formation although it is less frequently used today because warfarin requires frequent blood tests to

monitor anticoagulant effectiveness and has many drug-food interactions that make management challenging.
- *Direct acting oral anticoagulant* (DOAC) medications that inhibit factor Xa, or directly inhibit thrombin, are now often prescribed instead of traditional warfarin. These classes of medications have the advantage of no requirement for routine anticoagulation blood tests, which patients perceive as a major benefit.[55]

Digoxin is an older medication that is now used less frequently. It may be prescribed for atrial fibrillation to control ventricular heart rate. Digoxin does not prolong life, but if symptoms are not effectively managed with other medications, it may be considered with caution as some patients feel less symptomatic.[46,55]

Heart Failure and Ventricular Dysrhythmias

A ventricular ejection fraction less than 40% and a heart failure diagnosis of Stage C/D or New York Heart Association (NYHA) class III–IV is strongly associated with ventricular dysrhythmias and higher mortality.[55] Because sustained VT or VF initiates SCD, high-risk patients with severe heart failure are prescribed anti-dysrhythmic medications and have an implantable cardioverter defibrillator (ICD) inserted.[55]

Heart Failure and Natriuretic Peptide Biomarkers

Diagnostic blood tests are available to assist clinicians in differentiating whether a patient's shortness of breath is caused by heart failure or by pulmonary complications. BNP, a cardiac neurohormone released by the ventricles in response to volume expansion and pressure overload, is elevated in heart failure.[55]

Heart failure increases LV wall tension because of the excess preload in the ventricles. When the BNP blood level is greater than 100 pg/mL, the dyspnea is most likely related to heart failure rather than pulmonary failure.[57] A BNP greater than 200 pg/mL is required to diagnose heart failure. It is important to know that other systemic conditions alter the interpretation of BNP results. If there is concomitant kidney disease, the BNP will be elevated because of the kidney failure.[57] In general, the more severe the heart failure, the higher the BNP value.[56]

An associated blood test is NT-proBNP which is a similar natriuretic peptide test with higher cut-off values. Either BNP or NT-proBNP can be used for diagnosis, as elevation in either test result indicates an increased likelihood of heart failure.[55–57]

Heart Failure and Pulmonary Complications

The clinical manifestations of acute heart failure result from tissue hypoperfusion and organ congestion and are progressive. The severity of clinical symptoms increases as heart failure worsens. Initially, breathlessness occurs only with exertion, but eventually, shortness of breath also occurs at rest.

Heart Failure and Breathlessness

In heart failure, the feeling of being short of breath first comes with exertion, but as heart failure worsens, symptoms are present at rest.

Breathlessness in heart failure is described by these terms:
- *Dyspnea:* sensation of shortness of breath from pulmonary vascular congestion and decreased lung compliance
- *Orthopnea:* difficulty breathing when lying flat because of an increase in venous return that occurs in the supine position
- *Paroxysmal nocturnal dyspnea:* severe form of orthopnea in which the patient awakens from sleep gasping for air
- *Cardiac asthma:* dyspnea with wheezing, a nonproductive cough, and pulmonary crackles that progress to the gurgling sounds of pulmonary edema

Heart Failure and Pulmonary Edema

Pulmonary edema, or protein-laden fluid in the alveoli, inhibits gas exchange by impairing the diffusion pathway between the alveolus and the capillary (Fig. 13.20A). It is caused by increased left atrial and ventricular pressures and results in an excessive accumulation of serous or serosanguineous fluid in the interstitial spaces and alveoli of the lungs. The formation of pulmonary edema has two stages.

The first stage is not as severe and is characterized by interstitial edema, engorgement of the perivascular and peribronchial spaces, and increased lymphatic flow (Fig. 13.20B). The later stage is characterized by alveolar edema resulting from fluid moving into the alveoli from the interstitium (Fig. 13.20C). Eventually, blood plasma moves into the alveoli faster than the lymphatic system can clear it, interfering with diffusion of oxygen, depressing the arterial partial pressure of oxygen (PaO_2), and leading to tissue hypoxia (Fig. 13.20D).

Patients experiencing heart failure and pulmonary edema are extremely breathless and anxious with a sensation of suffocation. They expectorate pink, frothy sputum and feel as if they are drowning. A patient may sit bolt upright, gasp for breath, or thrash about. The respiratory rate is rapid, and accessory muscles of ventilation are used, with nasal flaring and bulging neck muscles. Respirations are characterized by loud inspiratory and expiratory gurgling sounds. Diaphoresis is profuse, and the skin is cold, ashen, and sometimes cyanotic. This reflects low cardiac output, increased sympathetic stimulation, peripheral vasoconstriction, and desaturation of arterial blood and is life-threatening.

Arterial blood gases in pulmonary edema. Arterial blood gas values are variable. In the early stage of pulmonary edema, respiratory alkalosis may be present because of hyperventilation, which eliminates carbon dioxide. As the pulmonary edema progresses and gas exchange becomes impaired, acidosis (pH less than 7.35) and hypoxemia ensue. A chest radiograph usually confirms an enlarged cardiac silhouette, pulmonary venous congestion, and interstitial edema.

Cardiogenic pulmonary edema versus noncardiogenic pulmonary edema. In the critical care unit, sometimes when a patient develops pulmonary edema, it is often a challenge to determine whether the cause is cardiac, known as *cardiogenic pulmonary edema*, or pulmonary or systemic in origin. The latter is referred to as *noncardiogenic pulmonary edema* or, more commonly, *acute respiratory distress syndrome* (ARDS). Options to determine the cause of the pulmonary edema include use of the serum BNP level or insertion of a pulmonary artery catheter. The pulmonary artery catheter is used to determine the patient's pulmonary artery occlusion pressure. It is essential to understand the different causes of pulmonary edema because the treatments are disease specific. Chapter 18 provides more information on the management of ARDS.

Pharmacologic Management in Heart Failure

RAAS Inhibitor Medications

- *ACEi* block the conversion of angiotensin I to angiotensin II and thus inhibit arterial vasoconstriction, lower BP and SVR, and decrease the amount of ventricular remodeling that occurs with heart failure.
- *ARBs* inhibit angiotensin II directly and also counteract RAAS activation.[55,56,58]

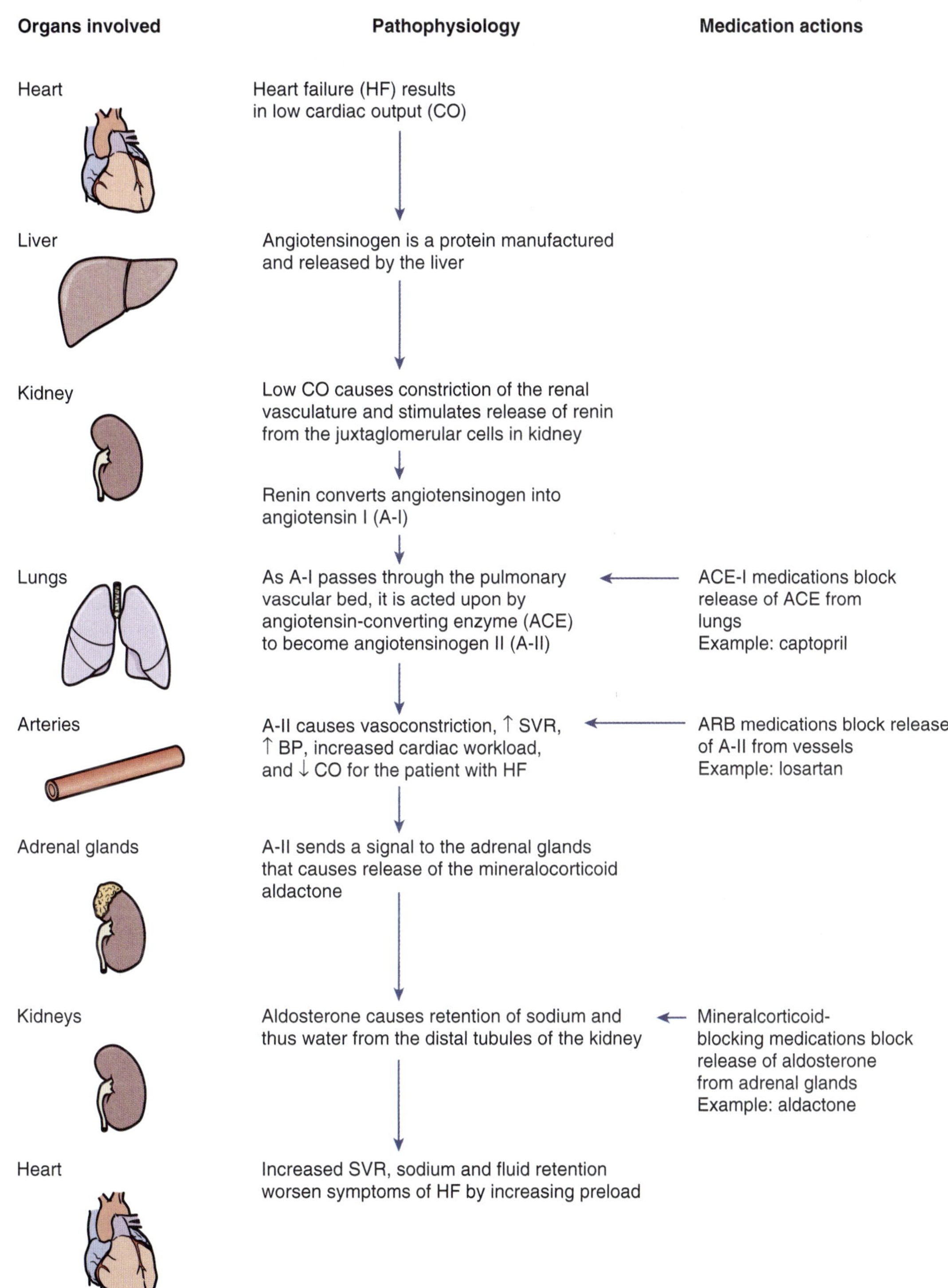

FIG. 13.19 Renin-Angiotensin-Aldosterone System, Role in Heart Failure, and Medication Actions. *ARB*, Angiotensin receptor blocker; *BP*, blood pressure; *CO*, cardiac output; *SVR*, systemic vascular resistance.

- *Angiotensin receptor neprilysin inhibitors* (ARNi) are a newer class of RAAS-blocking medication that reduce vasoconstriction and lower BP in patients with HFrEF.[55,58]

Mineralocorticoid Receptor Antagonists

MRA, such as spirolactone, inhibit sodium retention from the distal tubules of the kidney[55,58] (Fig. 13.19).

Beta-Blockers

Beta-blockers are used to decrease myocardial oxygen demand and block activation of the sympathetic nervous system. Beta-blockers also reduce heart rate and dysrhythmias.[55,58] Low-dose beta-blockers such as carvedilol may be added although strict surveillance is required to anticipate and avoid untoward negative inotropic effects.

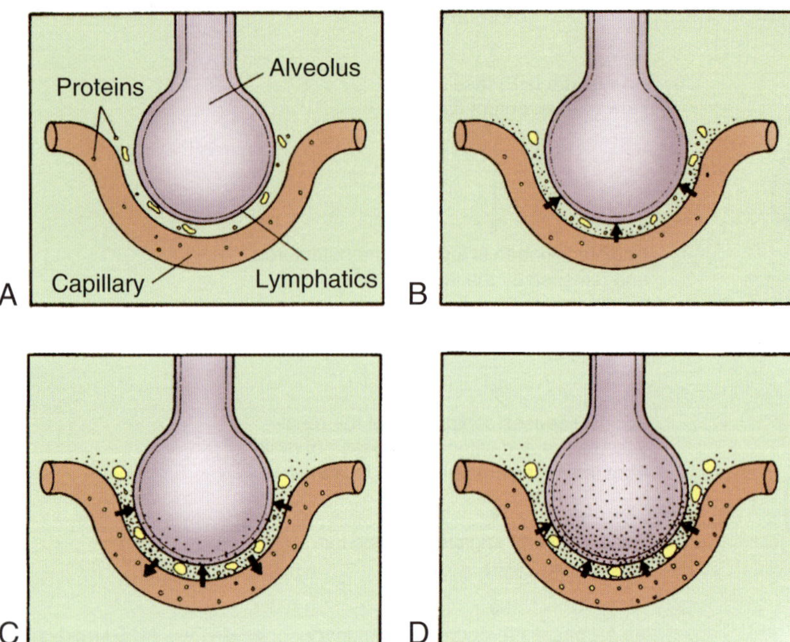

FIG. 13.20 Development of Pulmonary Edema. As pulmonary progresses, it inhibits oxygen and carbon dioxide exchange at the alveolar capillary interface. (A) Normal relationship. (B) Increased pulmonary capillary hydrostatic pressure causes fluid to move from the vascular space into the pulmonary interstitial space. (C) Lymphatic fow increases in an attempt to pull fluid back into the vascular or lymphatic space. (D) Failure of lymphatic flow and worsening of left-sided heart failure results in further movement of fluid into the interstitial space and the alveoli.

Sodium Glucose Cotransporter-2 Inhibitors

Sodium glucose cotransporter-2 inhibitors (SGLT2i) have been shown to reduce acute cardiovascular events, hospitalizations, and mortality across the spectrum of heart failure symptoms and stages.[59] Many patients with heart failure also have type 2 diabetes, and the SGLT2i medications facilitate glycemic control.[55,58,59] However, even without diabetes, patients with heart failure have better outcomes when an SGLT2i is added to the regimen.[59] This suggests that SGLT2i have additional beneficial mechanisms, not yet understood, that help to reduce adverse cardiovascular outcomes.[55] Addition of an SGLT2i is recommended for heart failure management even when the patient does not have diabetes.[55]

Diuretics

Diuretics are a cornerstone of heart failure management.[60] Loop diuretics, oral or IV, are typically first-line therapies, and dosages are increased as heart failure symptoms and fluid retention increases. Over time diuretic resistance may develop caused by changes in kidney function and then additional classes of diuretics are added.[60] When there is poor diuretic efficacy the clinical outcomes are worse.[60] There is more information about diuretics in Table 25.8 and Fig. 25.3 in Chapter 25.

Medical Management

The goals of the medical management of heart failure are to relieve symptoms, enhance cardiac performance, and correct known precipitating causes.

Symptom Relief

Control of symptoms involves management of fluid overload and improvement of cardiac output by decreasing SVR and increasing contractility.

- Diuretics are administered to decrease preload and to eliminate excess fluid from the body.[60] If pulmonary edema develops, additional diuretics are used.
- Afterload is decreased by vasodilators such as sodium nitroprusside (SNP). SNP is a balanced vasodilator medication that relaxes arterial resistance and venous capacitance vessels. By reducing both preload and afterload, cardiac output may improve, particularly in patients with increased SVR. It is useful in favorably redistributing total LV stroke volume in patients with either mitral or aortic insufficiency such that regurgitant flow is reduced while forward flow is increased.
- Nitrates are used to decrease preload and vasodilate the coronary arteries if CAD is an underlying cause of the acute heart failure. Subinguinal nitroglycerin is used to provide immediate relief for anginal pain.
- Morphine is given to decrease anxiety and facilitate vasodilation.

Enhancement of Cardiac Output

In the critical care unit, contractility is initially increased by continuous infusion of positive inotropic medications (dopamine) or by combination inodilators such as dobutamine or milrinone, which have both inotropic and vasodilatory effects.

After the acute exacerbation is resolved, the patient is transitioned to oral agents and weaned off the intravenous medications.

Heart Failure and Nonpharmacologic Interventions

Nonpharmacologic interventions that are increasingly used include *cardiac resynchronization therapy* (CRT).[61] CRT is biventricular pacing, where the right and left ventricles each

BOX 13.15 **DIAGNOSIS AND PATIENT CARE MANAGEMENT**

Acute Heart Failure

- Impaired gas exchange due to ventilation/perfusion mismatching or intrapulmonary shunting
- Impaired cardiac output due to alterations in preload
- Impaired cardiac output due to alterations in contractility
- Impaired cardiac output due to alterations in afterload (pulmonary circulation)
- Impaired cardiac output due to alterations in heart rate or rhythm
- Activity intolerance due to cardiopulmonary dysfunction
- Anxiety due to threat from biologic, psychologic, or social integrity
- Ineffective tissue perfusion due to decreased myocardial blood flow
- Lack of knowledge of treatment regime due to lack of previous exposure to information (see Box 13.16, Patient and Family Education Plan: Acute Heart Failure)

Patient Care Management plans are located in Appendix A.

have a pacing lead in contact with the myocardium. In patients with heart failure, CRT has a beneficial effect on clinical symptoms, exercise capacity, and systolic LV performance for patients with Stage C heart failure on optimal pharmacological support.[61]

An ICD is beneficial for patients with nonischemic heart failure and ventricular dysrhythmias[62] (see Fig. 14.9 in Chapter 14). The ICD does not improve the symptoms or progression of heart failure but contributes to longer survival by reducing the incidence of SCD.[62]

Ablation of ectopic foci in the pulmonary arteries may be considered for patients with atrial fibrillation as described in Chapter 14.

Heart Failure and Palliative Care

Heart failure is a progressive disease, and patients do not recover.[55,63] At a point in their trajectory of heart failure, many patients with NYHA class IV or Stage D heart failure become candidates for palliative care, especially when repeat hospitalizations occur.[55,63] The primary aim of palliative care is symptom management, relief of suffering, and ongoing discussion about how to achieve an optimal health-related quality of life. Transparency and shared decision making with the patient and their significant others is essential.[55] If the patient has a cardiac implantable device (ICD, pacemaker) or is dependent on inotropes this should be discussed as these are not incompatible with end-of-life treatments. Other cardiac medications are optimized to manage symptoms according to current guidelines.[55] Advanced heart failure carries a high symptom burden including dyspnea, pain, and fatigue, related to low cardiac output and fluid overload.[63] See Chapter 9 for in-depth information on palliative care.

Nursing Management

Nursing care management for a patient with heart failure incorporates a variety of patient diagnoses (Box 13.15). Nursing interventions are designed to achieve optimal cardiopulmonary function, promote comfort and emotional support, monitor the effectiveness of pharmacologic therapy, ensure nutrition intake is sufficient, and provide patient and family education. See Appendix A for patient care management plans specific to patients with heart failure.

Optimizing Cardiopulmonary Function

The patient's ECG is evaluated for dysrhythmias that may be present as a result of medication toxicity or electrolyte imbalance. Patients with heart failure are prone to additional complications because of decreased renal perfusion and electrolyte imbalances. Breath sounds are auscultated frequently to determine the adequacy of respiratory effort and to assess for onset or worsening of pulmonary congestion. Oxygen is administered through a nasal cannula to relieve dyspnea. Diuretics or vasodilators are used to decrease excessive preload and afterload. If the patient is not hypotensive, morphine may be administered to decrease hyperventilation and anxiety. If the patient's ventilatory status worsens, the nurse must be prepared for endotracheal intubation and mechanical ventilation. Obtaining daily weights is important until the weight stabilizes at a "dry" weight. Generally, the daily weight is used in fluid management, and a weekly weight is optimally used for tracking body weight (e.g., muscle, fat).

Promoting Comfort and Emotional Support

Activity must be restricted during periods of breathlessness. Bed rest usually is prescribed for the patient, who is positioned with the head of the bed elevated to allow for maximal lung expansion. The arms can be supported on pillows so that no undue stress is placed on the shoulder muscles. The legs may be placed in a dependent position to encourage venous pooling, decreasing venous return. Rest periods must be carefully planned and adhered to, and independence within the patient's activity prescription must be fostered. Vital signs are recorded before an activity is begun and after it is completed. Signs of activity intolerance such as dyspnea, fatigue, sustained increase in pulse, and onset of dysrhythmias are documented and reported to the physician. Activity is gradually increased according to the patient's tolerance. Skin breakdown is a risk because of the combination of bed rest, inadequate nutrition, peripheral edema, and decreased perfusion to the skin and subcutaneous tissue. Frequent position changes and mobilization can help provide comfort and prevent this complication.

Monitoring Effects of Pharmacologic Therapy

Patients experiencing acute heart failure require aggressive pharmacologic therapy.[55] The critical care nurse must know the action, side effects, and therapeutic levels of diuretics and venodilation used to decrease preload; positive inotropic agents used to increase ventricular contractility; vasodilators used to decrease afterload; and any antidysrhythmics used to control heart rate and prevent dysrhythmias. The patient's hemodynamic response to these agents is closely monitored. Fluid intake and output balances are tabulated daily or hourly in the critical care unit.

Nutritional Intake

Patients experiencing heart failure often have decreased appetite and nausea.[57] Small, frequent meals may be more appropriate than the standard three large meals. Food must be as tasty as possible. Favorite foods and foods from home may be incorporated into the diet as long as the foods are compatible with nutritional restrictions such as low sodium to decrease

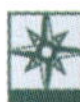

BOX 13.16 PATIENT AND FAMILY EDUCATION PLAN

Acute Heart Failure

The patient should be able to teach back the following topics:

- Heart failure: pathophysiology of heart failure
- Fluid balance: low-salt diet to reduce fluid retention; intake and output measurement; signs of fluid overload such as peripheral edema
- Daily weight: Increase or loss of 1 to 2 lb in a few days is a sign of fluid gain or loss, not true weight gain or loss.
- Breathlessness: Increasing shortness of breath, wheezing, and sleeping upright on pillows or in a recliner are symptoms that must be monitored and reported to a health care professional.
- Activity: activity conservation with rest periods as heart failure progresses
- Medications: As medications are complex, information must be given in writing and orally.
    - Preload: purpose of diuretics, increased urine output, and control of fluid volume
    - Afterload: purpose of vasodilators or angiotensin-converting enzyme inhibitors in decreasing workload of the heart
    - Heart rate: The purpose of digoxin is to control atrial fibrillation, a frequent dysrhythmia in heart failure.
    - Contractility: With the exception of digoxin, no oral contractility medications are approved by the U.S. Food and Drug Administration.
    - Anticoagulation: Patients with distended atria and enlarged ventricles or with atrial fibrillation may be prescribed an anticoagulant such as warfarin (Coumadin); risks of bleeding, importance of correct dosages, prothrombin times, international normalized ratio, and nutritional-pharmacologic interactions are emphasized.
- Follow-up care
- Symptoms to report to a health care professional

fluid retention. Each patient must be assessed for nutritional imbalance individually. Not all patients with heart failure have the same nutritional needs. See Chapter 7 for an in-depth discussion of nutrition in heart disease.

Educate the Patient and Family

The nurse assesses the patient's and family's understanding of the pathophysiology and individual risk factor profile for heart failure. Primary topics of education include (1) the importance of a daily weight, (2) fluid restrictions, (3) written information about the multiple medications used to control the symptoms of heart failure, (4) physical activity, and (5) when to call a health care provider (Box 13.16). Many patients with a diagnosis of heart failure also require education about lifestyle changes such as smoking cessation, weight loss, energy conservation, and how to incorporate exercise and sodium restriction into their daily lives.[64] Achieving the optimal outcomes for a patient with heart failure requires contributions from a team of educated health care clinicians (Box 13.17).

BOX 13.17 Evidence-Based Practice

Heart Failure

A collaborative heart failure management team provides an integrated approach to care to achieve clinical stability for the patient.

- Ensure systematic assessment and management:
- To optimize a patient's condition at the best "stage" possible when in the hospital
- To maintain same stability once discharged home and to avoid hospital readmission
- Counsel and educate patient and family after discharge from hospital. Patients and families should understand:
- Heart failure disease process
- Heart failure medications, dosages, medication schedule, medication side effects
- Fluid balance related to salt-restriction diet (2 g/day of sodium), daily weight, diuretic regimen
- When to call health care provider
- Risk of additional complications: sudden cardiac death; progressive heart failure; need for other cardiac procedures (pacemaker, implantable cardioverter-defibrillator, percutaneous coronary intervention) or cardiac surgery (coronary artery bypass graft, valve replacement); mechanical assist device or heart transplantation, as needed by some patients
- Purpose of advance directive for health care decisions
- Promote patient compliance with treatment regimen:
- Patient needs support from concerned companions and health care professionals.
- Patient should remain physically active and involved with life.
- Facilitate hospital discharge; implement outpatient models of health care delivery:
- Close communication between inpatient and outpatient health care providers is essential.

References

Heidenreich PA, Bozkurt B, Aguilar D, et al. 2022 AHA/ACC/HFSA Guideline for the Management of Heart Failure: A Report of the American College of Cardiology/American Heart Association Joint Committee on Clinical Practice Guidelines. *Circulation.* 2022;145(18). https://doi.org/10.1161/CIR.0000000000001063.

Bozkurt B, Coats AJS, Tsutsui H, et al. Universal definition and classification of heart failure: a report of the Heart Failure Society of America, Heart Failure Association of the European Society of Cardiology, Japanese Heart Failure Society and Writing Committee of the Universal Definition of Heart Failure: Endorsed by the Canadian Heart Failure Society, Heart Failure Association of India, Cardiac Society of Australia and New Zealand, and Chinese Heart Failure Association. *Eur J Heart Fail.* 2021;23(3):352–380. https://doi.org/10.1002/ejhf.2115.

CARDIOMYOPATHY

Description and Etiology

Cardiomyopathy is a disease of the heart muscle (*cardio-* [heart], *-myo-* [muscle], and *-pathy* [pathology]). Cardiomyopathies are primarily classified by their structural heart disease features and the genotype/phenotype, if known. All types of cardiomyopathies are associated with development of heart failure as symptoms advance.[55,57]

Cardiomyopathy structural categories are illustrated in Fig. 13.21.

- Hypertrophic cardiomyopathy
- Dilated cardiopathy
- Restrictive cardiomyopathy

Hypertrophic Cardiomyopathy

Hypertrophic cardiomyopathy (HCM) describes a hypertrophied, stiff, noncompliant left ventricle, that is sometimes hypertrophied asymmetrically in the upper septum. In about a third of cases, HCM is caused by a known genetic mutation that affects the myocardial sarcomere; 14 genes with multiple variants have been identified so far.[65–67]

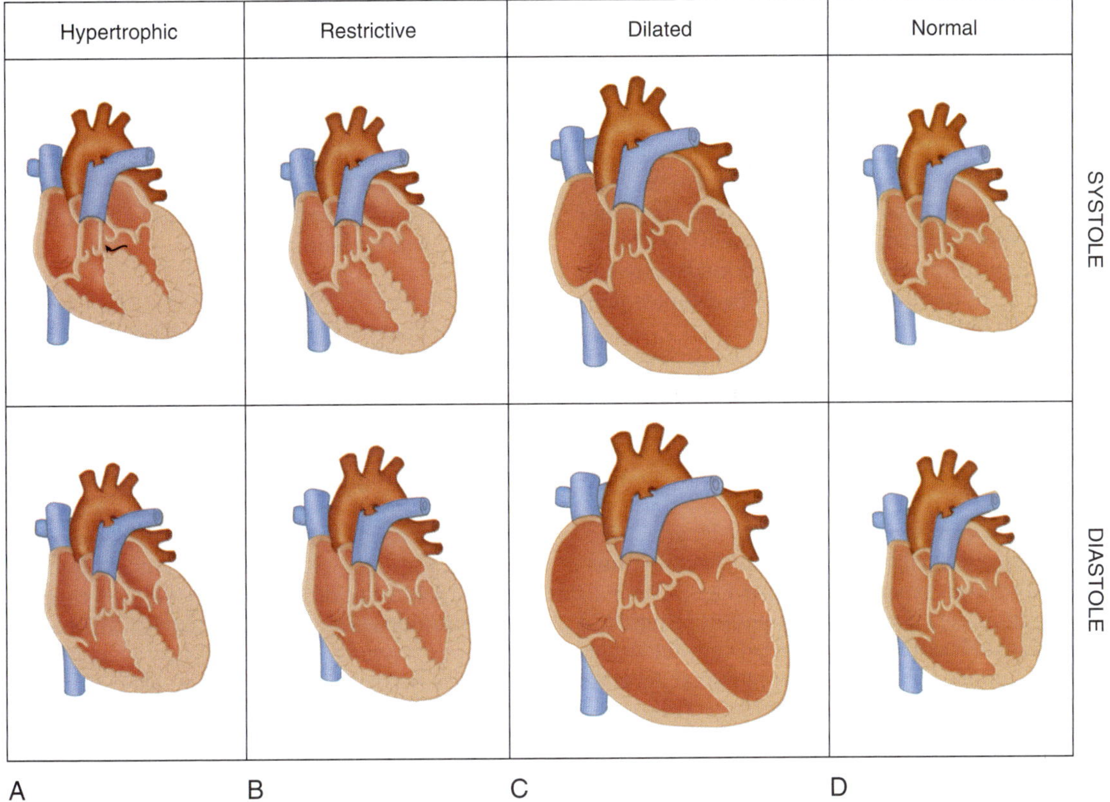

FIG. 13.21 Types of Cardiomyopathies and Differences in Ventricular Diameter During Systole and Diastole Compared with a Normal Heart. (A) Hypertrophic. (B) Restrictive. (C) Dilated. (D) Normal.

HCM occurs in two forms:

- Generalized LV hypertrophy (nonobstructive)
- Septal LV hypertrophy (obstructive)

The degree of hypertrophy of the LV wall can range from mild, ≤15 mm, to ≥30 mm, which is considered massive.[65] In generalized HCM the LV is hypertrophied, but the septum is not more enlarged than other areas of myocardium. This is the nonobstructive form. HCM causes significant diastolic dysfunction because the muscle-bound, stiff, noncompliant heart muscle does not relax to allow adequate filling during diastole.

HCM with hypertrophy of the upper ventricular septum obstructs LV outflow through the aortic valve during systole, especially during exercise (see Fig. 13.21A). It also pulls the papillary muscle out of alignment, causing mitral regurgitation. This is the obstructive form of HCM.

HCM Imaging

Technological advances have increased diagnostic accuracy for HCM. This includes 12-lead ECG, echocardiography, and CMR imaging.[65,66] Echocardiography (at rest or as an exercise stress test) is noninvasive and can provide initial images and measurements of ventricular wall thickness, septal anatomy, ventricular wall motion, and septal movement. CMR imaging provides additional detail.[65]

HCM Genotype and Phenotype

The second major advance comes from genetic testing with the ability to identify which patients with LV hypertrophy have a genetic mutation, versus not. Fourteen genotypes are now identified with HCM, and almost one-third of patients have a known pathologic sarcomere gene-variant.[65,67] The most frequently identified genes are *MYBPC3* and *MYH7*.[65,67]

Familial HCM can be inherited as an autosomal dominant trait. Therefore, when a pathologic variant is detected, genetic testing of other family members is recommended with construction of a family pedigree for HCM.[65] One challenge is that the clinical manifestations of HCM are highly variable. The clinical expression of a genetic condition is known as the *phenotype*, and this is described in more detail in Chapter 3. Thus, a positive genotype does not automatically mean all affected persons will have the same phenotype or develop symptoms at the same time. For this reason, and because of the risk of SCD, ongoing follow-up for gene-positive individuals is recommended at 2- to 3-year intervals.[65,66]

Equally important, if a family member does not have the genotype, they will not develop the phenotype and do not require follow-up.[65] Genetic counseling is important to help families understand the implications of their specific genotype-phenotype pattern and risks of genetic transmission.[66] For more information about genetics see Chapter 3. HCM is also associated with several other syndromic conditions.

HCM Symptoms

Progression of LV hypertrophy leads to heart failure. The symptoms are similar to those seen with heart failure, with the addition of myocardial ischemia, supraventricular tachycardia, VT, syncope, and stroke. Symptoms usually are more intense with physical exercise, especially in the obstructive form of HCM, in which the aortic outflow tract is obstructed by the enlarged LV septum. Because a known association exists between HCM and SCD, limitation of physical activity may be recommended. SCD risk is thought to stem from ventricular dysrhythmias and atrial fibrillation.

HCM Management

Pharmacologic management includes beta-blockers to decrease LV workload, medications to control and prevent atrial and ventricular dysrhythmias, anticoagulation if atrial fibrillation or LV thrombi are present to prevent stroke, and medications to manage heart failure. An ejection fraction ≤50% denotes poor systolic function and a higher risk of SCD.[66]

Interventional procedures include:

- ICD to decrease risk of SCD[67,68]
- Percutaneous alcohol ablation of the intraventricular septum[67,68]
- Surgical myectomy of the septal wall[67,68]

Dilated Cardiomyopathy

Dilated cardiomyopathy (DCM) is characterized by gross dilation of both ventricles and depressed contractility, without muscle hypertrophy and without hypertension[69] (see Fig. 13.20C). In DCM, the myocardial muscle fibers contract poorly, resulting in global LV dysfunction, low cardiac output, atrial and ventricular dysrhythmias, blood pooling that leads to ventricular thrombi and embolic episodes, progression to refractory heart failure, and premature death. As an indicator of disease severity, DCM is the most common reason for heart transplant.[70]

Multiple conditions can contribute to DCM. Traditionally, DCM was categorized as ischemic versus nonischemic. However, as more information has become available about genetic causes and other linked diseases, there is recognition that DCM can result from numerous causes. The origin may vary, but the final outcome is the same, whether the DCM results from valvular dysfunction, illegal drugs, dysrhythmias, infiltrates, infection, genetic or systemic causes.[69,70]

Ischemic Dilated Cardiomyopathy

Ischemic DCM results from repeated myocardial injury or infarction resulting in a reduced ejection fraction. This is the most common cause of DCM in the United States. The patient has signs and symptoms of advanced heart failure and a low ejection fraction. Treatment follows the advanced heart failure guidelines for HFrEF (Stage C/D and NYHA class III and IV).[55]

Familial Genetic Dilated Cardiomyopathy

Over 50 genes have been reported to have a role in the genetic transmission of DCM.[70] In some cases multiple genes may overlap to contribute to DCM and the genes do not have the same inheritance patterns in different family groups.[70] Thus, much research remains to be done. In general, if two closely related family members both meet the criteria for DCM (where no other cause is identified) genetic testing can be conducted using DCM-gene panels that test for multiple causative gene variants.[71] Research indicates that the genetic picture is highly individualized for different family groups, even if the clinical picture appears similar.

Acquired or Nonischemic Dilated Cardiomyopathy

Many nonischemic, nongenetic, noncardiac causes of DCM exist, these are acquired through exposure to toxins, systemic diseases, or infections, with origins that are highly varied, as listed below.

- Alcohol abuse[69–71]
- Illegal drugs: Cocaine, methamphetamines[69–71]
- Chemotherapeutic agent toxicity[69–71]
- Peripartum[69–71]
- Autoimmune: Systemic lupus erythematosus (SLE)[69–71]
- Infections—bacterial, fungal, viral: Human immunodeficiency virus (HIV), COVID-19[69–71]
- Inflammation: Myocarditis[69–71]

The variety of identified cases of DCM now implies that there will be further categorization of DCM, with perhaps varied treatment options in the future.

Idiopathic Dilated Cardiomyopathy

When the cause of the DCM cannot be identified, it is described as *idiopathic DCM*.

Restrictive Cardiomyopathy

Restrictive cardiomyopathy (RCM) is the least commonly encountered cardiomyopathy in developed countries (see Fig. 13.21B). As with the other cardiomyopathies, RCM can be idiopathic or can have a known cause. RCMs involve abnormalities of diastolic function with preserved systolic (contractile) function. Low cardiac output, dyspnea, orthopnea, and liver engorgement are the most common clinical manifestations of RCM. An elevated jugular venous pressure, S_4, and late S_3 may be present. Both ventricles are typically small with decreased volumes and large atria. The atrial septum and cardiac valves may be thickened, and pericardial effusion may be present.

Medical Management of Cardiomyopathy

The goals of medical management of all cardiomyopathies resemble the goals for symptomatic and advanced heart failure: improvement of myocardial contractility, removal of excess fluid, control of heart failure symptoms, anticipation and management of complications, and prevention of SCD.[55]

Nursing Management

Nursing care management for a patient with cardiomyopathy incorporates a variety of patient diagnoses related to symptoms of heart failure (Box 13.18). Nursing interventions are individualized according to the type of cardiomyopathy and are focused on achievement of a stable fluid balance, monitoring the effects of pharmacologic therapy, safely increasing mobility, and providing patient and family education.[64] As with heart failure, a collaborative team of compassionate, knowledgeable professionals is required to provide effective

BOX 13.18 DIAGNOSIS AND PATIENT CARE MANAGEMENT

Cardiomyopathy

- Impaired cardiac output due to alterations in preload
- Impaired cardiac output due to alterations in afterload
- Impaired cardiac output due to alterations in contractility
- Impaired cardiac output due to alterations in heart rate or rhythm
- Ineffective tissue perfusion due to decreased myocardial blood flow
- Impaired gas exchange due to intrapulmonary shunting
- Activity intolerance due to cardiopulmonary dysfunction
- Anxiety due to threat from biologic, psychologic, or social integrity
- Lack of knowledge of treatment regime due to lack of previous exposure to information (see Box 13.19, Patient and Family Education Plan: Cardiomyopathy)

Patient Care Management plans are located in Appendix A.

BOX 13.19 **PATIENT AND FAMILY EDUCATION PLAN**

Cardiomyopathy

Before discharge, the patient should be able to teach back the following topics:

Cardiomyopathy produces symptoms of heart failure; patient education covers many of the same issues discussed for heart failure.

- Cardiomyopathy: Explain pathophysiology of cardiomyopathy and heart failure.
- Fluid balance: low-salt diet to reduce fluid retention; intake and output measurement; signs of fluid overload such as peripheral edema
- Daily weight: Increase or loss of 1 to 2 lb in a few days is a sign of fluid gain or loss, not true weight gain or loss.
- Breathlessness: Increasing shortness of breath, wheezing, and sleeping upright on pillows are symptoms that must be monitored and reported to a health care professional.
- Activity: activity conservation with rest periods as heart failure progresses
- Medications: As medications are complex, information must be given in writing and orally.
  - Preload: purpose of diuretics, increased urine output, and control of fluid volume
  - Afterload: purpose of vasodilators or angiotensin-converting enzyme inhibitors in decreasing the workload of the heart
  - Heart rate: Purpose of digoxin is to control atrial fibrillation, a frequent dysrhythmia in heart failure; purpose of amiodarone is to control ventricular and atrial dysrhythmias, which are common in heart failure.
  - Contractility: With the exception of digoxin, no oral contractility medications are approved by U.S. Food and Drug Administration.
  - Decrease sympathetic response: Purpose of carvedilol (beta-blocker) is to lower cardiac response to adrenergic stimulation.
  - Anticoagulation: Patients with distended atria, enlarged ventricles, or atrial fibrillation may be prescribed anticoagulants such as warfarin (Coumadin) or aspirin or both; risk of bleeding, importance of correct dosages, prothrombin times, international normalized ratio, and nutritional-pharmacologic interactions are emphasized.
- Follow-up care
- Symptoms to report to a health care professional

care and education for these patients facing challenging health issues. See Appendix A for patient care management plans specific to patients with cardiomyopathy.

Educate the Patient and Family

Education is tailored to the type of cardiomyopathy and to any associated conditions (Box 13.19). The education is focused on the specific form of cardiomyopathy (HCM, DCM, RCM) and management is similar to care of the patient with heart failure.

PULMONARY HYPERTENSION

Pulmonary hypertension (PH) can lead to a progressive and ultimately fatal disease. Several contributing factors cause elevations in pulmonary pressures and can result in refractory right heart failure and ultimately death.

Pulmonary Arterial Hypertension

Within all causes of PH, a specific subset of patients is considered to have pulmonary arterial hypertension, or PAH. In PAH, vascular proliferation, inflammation, and remodeling of the small pulmonary arterial vessels culminate in an increased and fixed elevation in pulmonary vascular resistance. Also referred to "precapillary" pulmonary hypertension, the etiology of PAH is predominantly in the pulmonary arterial system.

PAH Definition

PAH is defined by the following hemodynamic criteria[72]:

- Mean pulmonary artery pressure ≥20 mm Hg
- Pulmonary artery occlusion (wedge) pressure ≤15 mm Hg
- Pulmonary vascular resistance ≥3 Woods units

PAH and PH may arise as isolated conditions or be associated with other diseases. PH is discussed with CVD because it not only affects cardiac function but can also be affected by other cardiac conditions. It is a true cardiopulmonary disease.

World Health Organization Classification of Pulmonary Hypertension

The WHO classification of PH was updated most recently in 2018 at the Sixth World Symposium of Pulmonary Hypertension (WSPH). The next update is anticipated following the *Seventh World Symposium of Pulmonary Hypertension* in 2024. This updated model groups disorders according to similarities in pathophysiology and treatment (Table 13.9).[72] Whatever the cause, the presence of PH significantly increases morbidity and mortality of any underlying cardiac or pulmonary disease. PH is a serious and frequently life-threatening condition that requires aggressive treatment.

WHO Functional Classification of Pulmonary Hypertension

A functional classification describes a grouping of physical symptoms that limit a patient's activity as a result of their disease condition. The AHA has used a functional classification for heart failure symptoms for many years (see Table 13.6). The NYHA heart failure classification was used for PAH symptoms until 2003, when a new PAH disease-specific functional classification was developed (Table 13.10). The premise is the same, where a higher number means the patient is more symptomatic, has greater limitation of activity, and risks higher mortality. The functional classification level strongly predicts mortality and is used to guide PH therapy.

WHO Group I—Idiopathic Pulmonary Arterial Hypertension

If the cause of PH is unknown, it is called *idiopathic PAH* (IPAH) and is classified as WHO group I (see Table 13.9).

IPAH is characterized by these features (Fig. 13.22):

- Intimal endothelial cell proliferation and medial thickening as a result of vascular smooth muscle cell proliferation, resulting in vasoconstriction and luminal narrowing
- Muscularization of precapillary arterioles
- Angioproliferative plexiform lesions of the endothelial cells develop from proliferation and fibrosis of the endothelium and increase obstruction.

IPAH is rare, with a prevalence estimated at 5 to 15 cases per million people, with a greater than 4:1 female to male ratio. Yet, in almost 50% of PH cases, the cause is unknown and classified as IPAH.[73] The onset of PH is insidious, and diagnosis is often difficult because of the nonspecific nature of symptoms (e.g., dyspnea, fatigue). Frequently, by the time a firm diagnosis is made, the patient is highly symptomatic with anginal chest pain, near-syncope or syncope, and right ventricular heart failure.

WHO Group I—Heritable Pulmonary Arterial Hypertension—Genetics

Heritable PAH, previously known as familial pulmonary artery hypertension, is a condition with genetic mutations classified in WHO group I (see Table 13.9).

TABLE 13.9 World Health Organization Classification of Pulmonary Hypertension

Group 1	**PAH**	
	1.1	Idiopathic PAH
	1.2	Heritable *PAH*
	1.3	Drug- and toxin-induced PAH
	1.4	PAH associated with:
	1.4.1	Connective tissue diseases
	1.4.2	HIV infection
	1.4.3	Portal hypertension
	1.4.4	Congenital heart disease
	1.4.5	Schistosomiasis
	1.5	PAHlong-termresponderstocalciumchannelblockers
	1.6	PAHwithovertfeaturesofvenous/capillaries(PVOD/PCH) involvement
	1.7	Persistent PH of the newborn syndrome
Group 2	**PH due to left heart disease**	
	2.1	PH due to heart failure with preserved LVEF
	2.2	PH due to heart failure with reduced LVEF
	2.3	Valvular heart disease
	2.4	Congenital/acquiredcardiovascularconditionsleadingto postcapillary PH
Group 3	**PH due to lung diseases and/or hypoxia**	
	3.1	Obstructive pulmonary disease
	3.2	Restrictive lung disease
	3.3	Other lung disease with mixed restrictive/obstructive pattern
	3.4	Hypoxia without lung disease
	3.5	Developmental lung disorders
Group 4	**PH due to pulmonary artery obstructions**	
	4.1	Chronic thromboembolic PH
	4.2	Other pulmonary artery obstructions
Group 5	**PH with unclear mechanisms and/or multifactorial mechanisms**	
	5.1	Hematological disorders
	5.2	Systemic disorders and metabolic disorders
	5.3	Others
	5.4	Complex congenital heart disease

HIV, Human immunodeficiency virus; *PAH*, pulmonary arterial hypertension; *PH*, pulmonary hypertension, *PVOD*, pulmonary venoocclusive disease; *PCH*: pulmonary capillary hemangiomatosis; *LVEF*, left ventricular ejection fraction.
Information from Gérald Simonneau, David Montani, David S. Celermajer, Christopher P. Denton, Michael A. Gatzoulis, Michael Krowka, Paul G. Williams, Rogerio Souza,Haemodynamic definitions and updated clinical classification of pulmonary hypertension.Reproduced with permission of the © ERS 2024:European Respiratory Journal 53 (1) 1801913; DOI: 10.1183/13993003.01913-2018 Published 24 January 2019.

Several genes associated with heritable PAH have been implicated including: *BMPR2, ALK1, ACVRL1, CAV1, KCNK3, 5HTT, ENG, TBX4, SMAD.* [74]

Most significantly, *BMPR2* is the associated genetic abnormality in 80% of these cases. Transmission of the *BMPR2* mutation leads to alteration of apoptosis (programmed cell death) that favors cellular proliferation.[75] In families with this gene, the children of patients have a 50% risk of inheriting the gene. However, not everyone who inherits the gene will exhibit the signs and symptoms of the disease, the reasons for which are not understood. More information about patterns of genetic inheritance is available in Chapter 3.

In heritable PAH, the pathogenesis of PAH is thought to be caused by multiple genetic and environmental stimuli. This has led to the development of a "multiple-hit hypothesis." This hypothesis suggests that modifier genes and environmental stimuli influence primary gene abnormalities such as the *BMPR2* variant to develop into clinically evident PAH.

TABLE 13.10 World Health Organization Functional Classification of Pulmonary Hypertension

Class	Symptoms
I	Patients with PH but without resulting limitation of physical activity; ordinary physical activity does not cause undue dyspnea of fatigue, chest pain, or near syncope
II	Patients with PH resulting in slight limitation of physical activity; they are comfortable at rest; ordinary physical activity causes undue dyspnea or fatigue, chest pain, or near syncope
III	Patients with PH resulting in marked limitation of physical activity; they are comfortable at rest; less than ordinary activity causes undue dyspnea or fatigue, chest pain, or near syncope
IV	Patients with PH with inability to carry out any physical activity without symptoms; these patients manifest signs of right heart failure; dyspnea and/or fatigue may be present at rest; discomfort is increased by any physical activity

PH, Pulmonary hypertension.
Information from Zamanian RT, Kudelko KT, Sung YK, de Jesus Perez V, Liu J, Spiekerkoetter E. Current clinical management of pulmonary arterial hypertension. *Circ Res.* 2014;115:131.

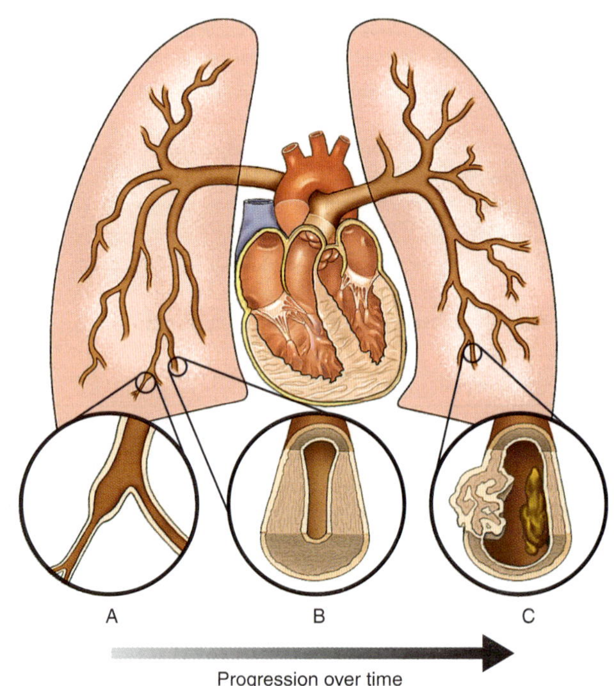

FIG. 13.22 Pulmonary Hypertension Progression Over Time. Pulmonary hypertension is a progressive disease. (A) Vasoconstriction. (B) Hypertrophy and hyperplasia of all three layers of the small pulmonary arteries. (C) Development of plexiform vascular lesions and localized thrombosis contribute to progressive narrowing of the peripheral pulmonary vessels. (From Lough ME. *Hemodynamic Monitoring: Evolving Technologies and Clinical Practice.* Elsevier; 2016.)

WHO Group I—Pulmonary Arterial Hypertension

Associated conditions that lead to PAH are classified as WHO group I disease (see Table 13.9). They all share the common pathology where the precapillary pulmonary vascular bed is the primary site of the disease.

TABLE 13.11 Drugs and Toxins Associated With PAH

Definite PAH Association	Possible PAH Association
Aminorex	Cocaine
Fenfluramine	Phenylpropanolamine
Dexfenfluramine	L-tryptophan
Benfluorex	St John's wort
Methamphetamines	Amphetamines
Dasatinib	Interferon-α and -β
Toxic rapeseed oil	Alkylating agents
	Bosutinib
	Direct-acting antiviral agents against hepatitis C virus
	Leflunomide
	Indirubin (Chinese herb Qing-Dai)

Some associated conditions include connective tissue disease (such as scleroderma or systemic lupus erythematosus), congenital heart disease, HIV infection, portal hypertension, and schistosomiasis.[72]

Drugs and toxin-induced PAH. Drugs and toxin-induced PAH comprise a significant portion of patients with WHO group I PAH. The first identified group included aminorex and fenfluramine derivatives used for weight loss. An epidemic of PH cases in the 1960s in Europe identified the link between developing PH and specific weight loss medications. In the United States, the first cases of fenfluramine or dexfenfluramine (commonly referred to as Fen-Phen) associated PAH appeared in 1997. Ultimately those agents were removed from the U.S. market in 1997 after the discovery that they caused valvular heart disease. Since the last WHO World Symposium, other agents have been moved from the possible to the definite association category (Table 13.11).

Most notably, methamphetamines are now considered to have a definite association with PAH.[72] These patients typically have worse hemodynamics at diagnosis, worse outcomes, and were less likely to be female.[76] The care of methamphetamine-associated PAH patients can be challenging due to the complex psychosocial factors that may inhibit adherence to therapy. Other agents with a possible association with the development of PAH are listed in Table 13.11.

Long-term responders to calcium channel blockers and PAH. Another group added to WHO Group I PAH is *Long-Term Responders to Calcium Channel Blockers.* These are patients who responded favorably to their initial vasoreactivity testing, treated on calcium channel blockers, and maintained their favorable response for at least 1 year. A description of vasoreactivity testing is found in the assessment and diagnosis section. These responders shared a specific blood signature and different gene variants than IPAH patients, thus leading to a hypothesis that they are a separate phenotype that possess better prognosis than those with IPAH.[77]

WHO Group I—Pulmonary Venoocclusive Disease and Pulmonary Capillary Hemangiomatosis

Pulmonary venoocclusive disease (PVOD) and *pulmonary capillary hemangiomatosis* (PCH) demonstrate the same hemodynamics and symptoms as IPAH, but the pathology in the vessels is found predominantly in the pulmonary veins. Therefore, typical treatments used for IPAH may in fact worsen the condition at high doses, and these patients may need to be referred for lung transplantation earlier than other PAH patients.

PVOD genetics. One significant discovery is that mutations in the eukaryotic translation initiation factor 2-alpha kinase 4 (*EIF2AK4*) gene leads to the development of PVOD. Although sporadic cases can occur, those with the *EIF2AK4* mutation carry a definitive diagnosis of PVOD.[78] Thus, the clinical team can make an earlier recommendation for transplantation should this gene mutation be identified.

WHO Group II—Pulmonary Hypertension Caused by Left Heart Disease

PH that results from left heart disease is classified as a WHO group II (see Table 13.9). This is the most common form of PH, with heart failure with preserved LVEF (HFpEF), heart failure with reduced LVEF (HFrEF), valvular disease, and congenital/acquired cardiovascular conditions (such as left heart inflow/outflow tract obstruction and congenital cardiomyopathies) composing distinct etiologies.[72]

PH caused by left heart disease can be thought of as pulmonary venous hypertension or postcapillary PH. That is, PH occurs because of elevated pressures in the left side of the heart that passively raises the left-sided filling pressure in the pulmonary circulation. Patients with pulmonary venous hypertension have a history of CAD, acute MI, valvular disease, heart failure, or DCM. Prolonged pressure elevation leads to an increase in pulmonary arteriolar resistance and persistent vascular changes. This is particularly difficult to treat since many of the medications used to treat PAH worsen pulmonary venous hypertension. Strategies to treat this group beyond addressing the underlying left heart disease have not been well established.

WHO Group III—Pulmonary Hypertension Due to Lung Disease and/or Hypoxia

In this group, which is classified as WHO group III (see Table 13.9), PH is caused by alveolar hypoxia secondary to lung disease, sleep apnea, impaired control of breathing, or chronic exposure to high altitude.[72] When exposed to hypoxia, the body's natural response is to vasoconstrict in order to decrease the area of perfusion in the lung to compensate for the low levels of oxygen. This results in a temporary rise in pulmonary pressures. However, when exposed to chronic hypoxia, this temporary compensatory mechanism leads to fixed elevations in pulmonary pressures or PH. Typically, patients with chronic lung disease or PH related to sleep apnea have mild levels of PH. The latter can be improved with positive airway pressure treatment. However, all patients with chronic obstructive pulmonary disease (COPD) and PH have worse survival rates than with the lung disease alone.[79] For this reason it is imperative to screen patients with lung disease to see if there might be underlying PH. Pulmonary function tests and sleep studies are performed as part of the diagnostic work-up for patients with PH and lung disease.

WHO Group IV—Pulmonary Hypertension Due to Pulmonary Artery Obstructions

PH that results from pulmonary artery obstructions such as from chronic thromboembolism is classified as WHO group IV (see Table 13.9). PH can occur acutely in response to a large pulmonary embolus that blocks flow to the pulmonary vascular bed. PH can also occur after multiple microemboli, or thrombi that obstruct the smaller pulmonary arteries. Chronic thromboembolic pulmonary hypertension (CTPH) has an incidence of up to 4% after acute pulmonary emboli.[80] If the risk of pulmonary emboli is recognized in a patient with hypercoagulability, this condition is potentially preventable. When PH is diagnosed, a ventilation-perfusion scan be performed to determine the presence or absence of pulmonary emboli. Treatment in a center of excellence with experience in *pulmonary thromboendarterectomy* (PTE) is recommended for this condition because skill in the procedure and required support systems are essential.[80] Increasingly, pulmonary balloon angioplasty is being offered as an alternative to PTE for those with medical comorbidities that may preclude surgical excision.[80]

WHO Group V—Pulmonary Hypertension With Unclear and/or Multifactorial Mechanisms

Group V in the WHO classification (see Table 13.9) comprises miscellaneous conditions, including hematologic disorders (chronic hemolytic anemia, or sickle cell disease, myeloproliferative disorders, splenectomy), systemic disorders (sarcoidosis, neurofibromatosis, lymphangioleiomyomatosis, pulmonary Langerhans cell histiocytosis), and metabolic disorders (glycogen storage disease, Gaucher disease, thyroid disorders).

Pathophysiology of Pulmonary Hypertension

The pulmonary vascular bed is normally a high-flow, low-pressure, low-resistance system that easily adjusts to changes in cardiac output, oxygen demand, and exercise. When these characteristics are deranged, pulmonary hypertension results. Progressive and sustained elevation of pulmonary pressures with increased pulmonary vascular resistance leads to increased pressure on the right ventricle, increased right ventricular workload, right ventricular hypertrophy, heart failure, and death.

The major components in the pathogenesis of chronic PH are:

- Endothelial dysfunction and vasoconstriction
- Vascular remodeling
- Thrombosis
- Plexiform lesions that irreversibly obliterate the pulmonary arterioles (see Fig. 13.22)

Impaired endothelial cell function results in vasoconstriction caused by a decrease in endothelial cell–derived *nitric oxide* (NO), a decrease in prostacyclin, and an increase in the vasoconstrictor endothelin. This results in thrombi within the pulmonary arterioles from increased thrombosis and diminished thrombolysis. Overproduction of substances that cause vasoconstriction, such as thromboxane and endothelin; a decrease in endothelial factors that cause vasodilation, specifically endothelial prostacyclin, and NO; or a combination of these factors may be the catalyst.

Assessment and Diagnosis

The diagnosis of PH is difficult. PH is often a diagnosis of exclusion when all other diagnostic theories are exhausted. The clinical symptoms of PH are nonspecific in the early stages. Symptoms of advanced disease reflect the inability of the pulmonary vascular bed to accommodate increased cardiac output with exercise. These factors support findings that symptoms are often present more than 2 years before diagnosis. Furthermore, unlike the left ventricle, the cardiac output of the right ventricle is exquisitely sensitive to even small increments of change in pulmonary pressure. Hence the care of the critically ill patient with PH must focus on preventing any deterioration as even a small incremental rise in pulmonary pressures can precipitate acute right heart failure.

Physical Assessment

The severity of PH clinical symptoms is classified using WHO pulmonary hypertension functional classes I to IV (see Table 13.9). Physical examination clues that reveal right ventricular failure include elevated jugular venous pressure, a palpable right ventricular heave, hepatomegaly, ascites, and peripheral edema. Auscultation of heart sounds reveals a prominent pulmonic component to S_2 and a holosystolic blowing murmur from tricuspid regurgitation. Pulmonary edema suggests LV dysfunction.

Signs and symptoms early in PAH include fatigue and shortness of breath caused by impaired oxygen transport and reduced cardiac output. Later symptoms include syncope from systemic hypotension because of low cardiac output and angina from the underfilled right and left ventricles. Patients may have intestinal edema, which can cause constipation, abdominal pain, malabsorption, and anorexia.

Diagnostic Tests for PAH

Diagnostic tests that can assist with PAH diagnosis include a 12-lead ECG, echocardiogram, and right heart catheterization. The most helpful noninvasive test is the echocardiogram. Echocardiography can estimate right atrial pressure and pulmonary arterial pressure (PAP), and it can determine the degree of right ventricular dysfunction. Signs of significant disease include right ventricular dilation and hypertrophy; septal bowing into the left ventricle, creating a D-shaped left ventricle; right ventricular hypokinesis; tricuspid regurgitation; right atrial enlargement; and a dilated inferior vena cava.

The 12-lead ECG is a noninvasive test that may show right-axis deviation and right ventricular hypertrophy resulting from PAH. The 12-lead ECG is an adjunct test that can indicate strain on the right ventricle, but a diagnosis of PH cannot be made from the ECG alone.

The diagnostic standard is the right heart catheterization because it can not only provide actual pressure measurements in the pulmonary arteries but also assess the pulmonary artery occlusion pressure (PAOP or wedge pressure) which can delineate the type of PH. To diagnose PAH, the mean PAP must be ≥20 mm Hg; PAOP (wedge) ≤15 mm Hg; with a pulmonary vascular resistance greater ≥3 Wood units.[72]

Precise analysis of mixed venous oxygen saturation (SvO_2) during insertion and passage of the pulmonary artery catheter through the cardiac chamber can allow diagnosis of intracardiac shunts. A pulmonary artery wedge pressure ≤15 mm Hg rules out LV heart disease. Information on diagnostic use of the pulmonary artery catheter and SvO_2 is included in the section Hemodynamics in Chapter 13.

Vasoreactivity Test

The ability of the pulmonary vessels to vasodilate in response to administration of a pulmonary artery vasodilator, called a *positive vasoreactivity test*, is an important component of the cardiac catheterization study. Vasoactive medications used in the test include inhaled NO (iNO), the preferred agent, intravenous adenosine, or intravenous epoprostenol (prostacyclin). A positive response is a reduction in mean PAP of at least 10 mm Hg to achieve a mean PAP less than 40 mm Hg with an increased or unchanged cardiac output. Only approximately 10% to 20% of patients with PH have a positive response to vasodilators. Patients with vasoreactive pulmonary vasculature may be able to be treated with calcium channel blockers alone and have an excellent prognosis. Vasoreactive responders share a specific gene variant unlike other IPAH patients, leading to a hypothesis that they are a separate phenotype and possesses better prognosis than those with IPAH.[77]

If diagnostic tests are performed when PH is advanced, the PAP may almost equal the systemic aortic pressure and the pulmonary arterioles may not vasodilate in response to vasodilator medications. In this scenario, the enlarged right ventricle puts pressure on the intraventricular septum and compresses the left ventricle. The smaller, compressed left ventricle has a greatly reduced LV stroke volume and cardiac output.

Exercise Tolerance Assessment

Formal assessment of exercise tolerance is important for evaluation and ongoing treatment of PH. The *6-minute walk distance* (6MWD) is used for this evaluation. In the 6MWD, the patient walks as far as possible for 6 minutes. The distance walked in 6 minutes has a strong association with mortality among patients with IPAH. Evaluation of serial 6MWD tests can monitor the severity, response to treatment, or progression of the disease.

Medical Management

Medical management focuses on the use of appropriate pharmacologic therapies and prevention of complications. Goals of therapy include alleviation of symptoms, improvements in quality of life, and survival. Improvements are measured by changes in functional class and exercise tolerance. Clinical practice guidelines recommend referral to a medical center specializing in the management of PH.

Pharmacologic Management of Pulmonary Hypertension

Table 13.12 lists PH medications. Most patients are maintained on multiple medications that include oral endothelin receptor antagonists, phosphodiesterase-5 inhibitors, pulmonary vasodilators such as prostacyclin derivatives, and in the early stages,

TABLE 13.12 PHARMACOLOGIC MANAGEMENT

Pulmonary Hypertension Medications

Medication	Dosage	Action	Special Considerations
Endothelin Receptor Antagonist			
Bosentan (Tracleer)	62.5–125 mg PO BID	Blocks vasoconstriction and smooth muscle proliferation	Monitor LFTs Teratogenic
Ambrisentan (Letairis)	5–10 mg PO daily	NO pathway leads to vasodilation	Teratogenic
Macitentan (Opsumit)	10 mg PO daily		Teratogenic
Riociguat (Adempas)	0.5–2.5 mg PO TID		
Phosphodiesterase-5 Inhibitors			
Sildenafil (Revatio)	20 mg PO TID IV bolus 10 mg TID	Pulmonary vasodilation and decreases smooth muscle proliferation	Concomitant use with nitrates can result in hypotension
Tadalafil (Adcirca)	40 mg PO daily		Concomitant use with nitrates can result in hypotension
Soluble Guanylate Cyclase Stimulators			
Riociguat (Adempas)	0.5 mg PO TID–2.5 mg PO TID	Sensitizes sGC to endogenous NO, directly stimulates sGC receptors which result in vasorelaxation and antiproliferative effects	Teratogenic May cause hypotension. Needs BP monitoring when starting dose
Pulmonary Vasodilator			
Inhaled NO (iNO)			
Prostacyclin Analogue/Receptor Agonist			
Epoprostenol (Flolan) (Veletri)	Start at 2 ng/kg/min continuous IV infusion. Chronic dose varies but usually in 20–40 ng/kg/min range	Dilates pulmonary and peripheral vessels; antiplatelet	Rebound pulmonary hypertension if abruptly discontinued or dose decreased. 6 minute half-life
Treprostinil (Remodulin)	Start at 1.25 ng/kg/min subcutaneous or IV infusion Chronic dose varies but usually in 40–80 ng/kg/min range	Prostacyclin analogue. Dilates pulmonary and peripheral vessels	3–4 hour half life
Treprostinil Oral (Orenitram)	0.125 mg TID or 0.25 mg BID Titrate by 0.125 mg TID or by 0.25 mg or 0.5 mg BID every 3–4 days as tolerated		Avoid abrupt cessation
Treprostinil Inhaled (Tyvaso)	3 breaths QID. Increase by 3 breaths per treatment every week as tolerated up to 9–12 breaths QID		Nebulized drug only administered via Tyvaso Inhalation System.
Tyvaso DPI	1 cartridge QID		
Activin Signaling Inhibitors			
Sotatercept (Winrevair)	Start at 0.3 mg/kg by subcutaneous injection. Then 0.7 mg/kg every 3 weeks	Fusion protein that traps activins and growth differentiation factors to improve the balance between pro- and antiproliferative signaling.	Monitor hemoglobin and platelets prior to every treatment for the first five doses. Monitor for signs and symptoms of hyperviscosity or thromboembolic events. Monitor for signs of bleeding.

BID, Two times a day; *BP*, blood pressure; *LFT*, liver function test; *NO*, nitric oxide; *PO*, by mouth; *QID*, four times a day; *sGC*, soluble guanylate cyclase stimulator; *TID*, three times a day.

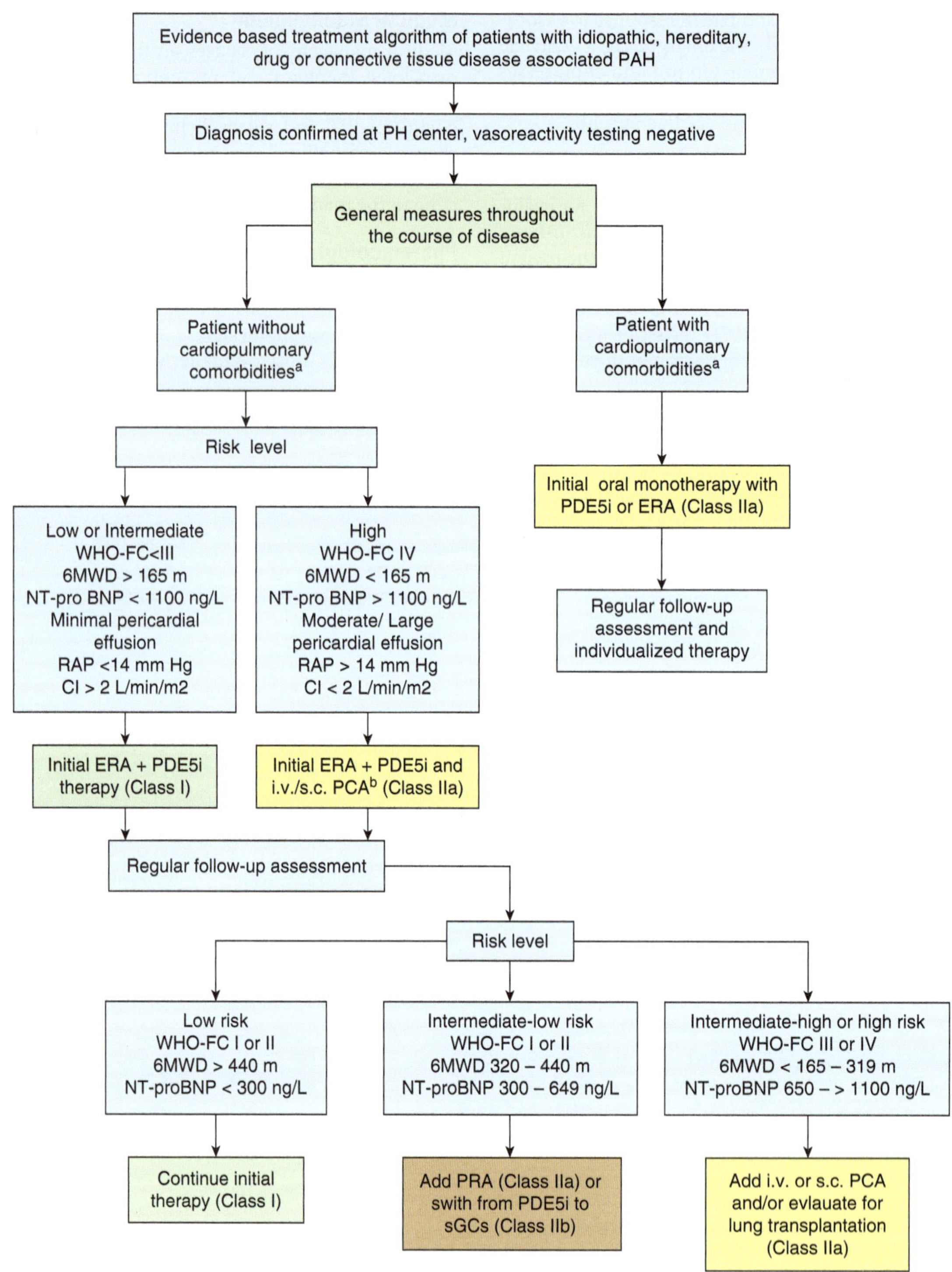

FIG. 13.23 Combination Medication Therapy Used to Treat Pulmonary Hypertension. Treatment recommendations adapted from ERS 2022. *6MWD,* 6-Minute walk distance; *CI,* cardiac index; *ERA,* endothelin receptor antagonist; *i.v.,* intravenous; *NT-pro BNP,* N-terminal pro-brain natriuretic peptide; *PAH,* pulmonary arterial hypertension; *PCA,* prostacyclin analogue; *PDE5i,* phosphodiesterase type 5 inhibitor; *PH,* pulmonary hypertension; *PRA,* prostacyclin receptor agonist; *RAP,* right atrial pressure; *WHO-FC,* World Health Organization functional class; *s.c.,* subcutaneous; *sGC,* soluble guanylate cyclase stimulator; *WHO-FC,* World Health Organization functional class. (Data from Humbert M, Kovacs G, Hoeper MM, et al. 2022 ESC/ERS Guidelines for the diagnosis and treatment of pulmonary hypertension. *Eur Respir J.* 2023;61(1):2200879. https://doi.org/10.1183/13993003.00879-2022.)

calcium channel blockers. Fig. 13.23 provides an example of how these medications can be combined as part of the treatment regimen.

Calcium Channel Blockers

Calcium channel blockers improve survival of patients with PH who demonstrate positive vasoreactivity test result during right heart catheterization. Long-acting calcium channel blockers include nifedipine, diltiazem, and amlodipine. Most patients with PH are nonresponders and are more effectively managed with agents specifically designed to treat PAH (Table 13.12).

Endothelin Receptor Antagonists

Endothelin receptor antagonists (ERA) are oral agents used for treating PH. Endothelin 1 is a potent vasoconstrictor and smooth muscle mitogen capable of inducing smooth muscle cell hypertrophy. Two types of endothelin receptors are *endothelin A*, which causes vasoconstriction and smooth muscle proliferation, and *endothelin B*, which causes vasodilation and is involved in clearance of endothelin.

There are three types of ERAs currently approved by the U.S. Food and Drug Administration (FDA) (Table 13.12). In order of approval dates, these are:

- Bosentan (Tracleer)
- Ambrisentan (Letairis)
- Macitentan (Opsumit)

Bosentan is approved for WHO functional classes III and IV patients. Studies have shown that it improves symptoms, functional class, hemodynamics, and exercise capacity measured by 6MWD. Notably, patients on bosentan can develop hepatotoxicity. Therefore, careful monthly monitoring of liver transaminases is required.

Ambrisentan (Letairis) also improves symptoms, time to clinical worsening, exercise capacity, and functional class. It appears to not have significant hepatotoxity. Thus, monthly liver function testing is not mandatory.

Macitentan (Opsumit) improved both morbidity and mortality and had significant improved time to clinical worsening compared to placebo in clinical trials.

All ERAs are teratogenic, and thus strict birth control methods need to be deployed for any females of childbearing potential taking this class of medication.

Phosphodiesterase Inhibitors and Soluble Guanylate Cyclase Stimulators

Phosphodiesterase inhibitors are designed to inhibit the degradation of cGMP. These medications promote pulmonary vasodilation and decrease vascular smooth muscle cell proliferation. Sildenafil and tadalafil (Adcirca) are potent inhibitors of phosphodiesterase-5; both agents are used to treat erectile dysfunction and are effective treatment options for PAH.

Soluble guanylate cyclase (sGC) *stimulators* (riociguat) work by stimulating sGC to induce *cyclic guanosine monophosphate* (cGMP) release. This affects the NO pathway, increasing vasodilation and resulting in improved exercise tolerance and pulmonary hemodynamics. This medication was the first to test its effects not only on WHO group I PAH patients but also WHO Group IV chronic thromboembolic PH patients (Table 13.12).

Nitric Oxide

NO is a potent *vasodilator* that dilates the pulmonary vasculature in ventilated lung units. It improves oxygenation and reduces PAP. In critically ill mechanically ventilated patients, iNO is useful especially in combination with dobutamine or milrinone. Abrupt withdrawal of iNO can lead to methemoglobinemia, nitrogen dioxide production, and rebound PH with hemodynamic collapse, which limits iNO use (Table 13.12).

Prostacyclin Analogs and Prostacyclin Receptor Agonists

Prostacyclins are potent vasodilators that affect the pulmonary and systemic circulations, and they have antiproliferative and antiplatelet aggregatory effects. Prostacyclin analog medications are known as *prostanoids*. There are six prostanoid analog or *prostacyclin receptor agonist* medications approved by the FDA[81]:

1. Epoprostenol (Flolan)
2. Treprostinil (Remodulin)
3. Inhaled treprostinil (Tyvaso)
4. Oral treprostinil (Orenitram)
5. Oral selexipag (Uptravi)
   - *Epoprostenol* (Flolan) is used in patients with advanced PH and right ventricular failure; long-term therapy with intravenous epoprostenol can be lifesaving. Epoprostenol therapy is started in the hospital and continued long term at home. Epoprostenol has a short elimination half-life of less than 6 minutes. Patients who are critically ill and have functional class IV symptoms should be started on epoprostenol, because it is the most rapidly effective therapy. Epoprostenol provides a sustained survival benefit of about 70%.
   - *Treprostinil:* Treprostinil sodium is administered by a subcutaneous or intravenous infusion catheter and pump and has a half-life of 3 to 4 hours. Subcutaneous administration is safe and effective and avoids the risks associated with the indwelling catheter. However, it is associated with injection site pain, which may not be tolerated. These prostacyclin analogs do not cure PH, but all vasodilate the pulmonary vascular bed, control symptoms, and prolong life in responsive patients.
   - *Tyvaso (inhaled treprostinil):* Tyvaso is an inhaled prostanoid administered with a handheld nebulizer four times daily. Tyvaso improved 6MWD when used in combination therapy with bosentan or sildenafil therapy. The Dry Powder Inhaler (DPI) formulation was recently approved. The BREEZE trial showed that patients on stable doses of nebulized Tyvaso were able to safely transition to the DPI formulation.[82] Inhaled treprostinil is the first PH-specific therapy that had been FDA approved for WHO group I PAH and WHO group III PH, associated with interstitial lung disease (Table 13.12).

Activin Signaling Inhibitors

Sotatercept was approved by the FDA in March of 2024, and represents the newest class of medication to be approved for the treatment of WHO group I PAH. It is a subcutaneous injection administered once every 3 weeks. Sotatercept is an *activin signaling inhibitor*, a fusion protein that traps activins and growth differentiation factors thought to improve the balance between pro- and antiproliferative signaling that regulates vascular cell proliferation in PAH (Table 13.12).

In the Phase 3 STELLAR clinical trial, sotatercept was given to adult patients with PAH who were already on background PAH therapy.[83] Compared to placebo, those on sotatercept increased the 6MWD by 41 meters and reduced risk of death from any cause, or experienced less PAH clinical worsening events.[83]

Sotatercept has side effects. It can cause an increase in hemoglobin and can lead to erythrocytosis, which can be severe. This can be linked to thromboembolic events or hyperviscosity syndrome. It can also decrease platelets that can lead to severe thrombocytopenia, thus increasing the risk of bleeding. This was observed more frequently in patients on concomitant prostacyclin infusions. Therefore the manufacturer recommends monitoring hemoglobin and platelets before initiation of therapy and subsequently for the first five doses.

Because this therapy is so new, current treatment guidelines have not yet commented on when to use this therapy. The 7th World Symposium of Pulmonary Hypertension in June 2024 will likely comment on where sotatercept falls within current treatment protocols.

Diuretics

Diuretics are used to prevent right ventricular volume overload, edema, ascites, and malabsorption associated with bowel edema. Serum electrolytes and kidney function are closely monitored (Table 13.12).

Supplemental Oxygen

Supplemental oxygen use is a key component of therapy for chronic PH. Chronic hypoxemia from impaired cardiac output results in mixed venous desaturation. Hypoxemia can also be related to right-to-left shunting through *patent foramen ovale* (PFO) or other cardiopulmonary shunts. Oxygen inhalation decreases PAP and improves cardiac output. Hypoxia is a potent pulmonary vasoconstrictor. Oxygen saturation is preferably maintained above 90%.

Acute Decompensated Right Ventricular Failure

Patients who are refractory to pharmacologic management may be admitted to the critical care unit with *acute decompensated right ventricular failure* (ADRVF). Developing treatments for end-stage PH include continuous inhaled vasodilators, mechanical assist devices, and transplant. Inhaled nitric oxide, a potent vasodilator, was often used in these patients to decrease mean PAP (mPAP) with high risk and cost incurred. Studies comparing use of iNO and inhaled epoprostenol (iEPO) demonstrated implementing iEPO significantly decreased cost with same decrease in mPAP.

The use of venoarterial *extracorporeal membrane oxygenator* (ECMO) in awake end-stage PH patients has successfully bridged patients to lung transplant. Either bilateral lung or heart-lung transplant is the surgical option for end-stage PH treatment. Detailed information on heart-lung transplantation is provided in Chapter 35.

Nursing Management

Care management for a patient with PH incorporates a variety of patient diagnoses related to the symptoms of breathlessness and right-sided heart failure as listed in Box 13.20. Nursing actions are individualized according to how advanced the symptoms of PH are. Interventions focus on lowering PAP, administering pharmacologic therapy, monitoring the effects and safety of all medications, treating pain that can occur at the site of injection (subcutaneous treprostinil), and providing patient and family education. See Appendix A for patient care management plans specific to patients with PH.

Educate the Patient and Family

If the cause for PH is known, the patient can receive tailored education to their diagnosis before discharge. All patients should be provided with a written medication list with the name and purpose of all their medications. Specific education topics include: (1) use and care of a handheld nebulizer, tunneled intravenous catheter, or subcutaneous pump for medication administration; (2) infection prevention; (3) sterile preparation of the prostacyclin analog medication; (4) name of the health care professional to contact for questions related to PH (Box 13.21). A collaborative team of empathetic, educated professionals is essential to provide effective care for patients with pulmonary hypertension (Box 13.22).

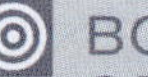

BOX 13.20 DIAGNOSIS AND PATIENT CARE MANAGEMENT

Pulmonary Artery Hypertension

- Impaired gas exchange due to ventilation-perfusion mismatching or intrapulmonary shunting
- Activity intolerance due to cardiopulmonary dysfunction
- Impaired cardiac output due to alterations in preload
- Impaired cardiac output due to alterations in contractility
- Impaired cardiac output due to alterations in heart rate or rhythm
- Risk for infection
- Anxiety due to threat from biologic, psychologic, or social integrity
- Impaired adaptation due to situational crisis and personal vulnerability
- Lack of knowledge of treatment regime due to lack of previous exposure to information (see Box 13.21, Patient and Family Education Plan: Pulmonary Artery Hypertension)

Patient Care Management plans are located in Appendix A.

BOX 13.21 PATIENT AND FAMILY EDUCATION PLAN

Pulmonary Artery Hypertension

The patient should be able to teach back the following topics:

- Pathophysiology of pulmonary artery hypertension and disease process
- Symptoms: dyspnea at rest or, more commonly, with exertion
- Activity conservation with scheduled rest periods
  - Medications: purpose, side effects, special considerations
  - Epoprostenol (Flolan): intravenous (IV) by pump, half-life of 2 to 3 min
  - Treprostinil (Remodulin): IV or subcutaneous (SC) by pump, half-life of 3 h
  - Bosentan (Tracleer): oral
  - Sildenafil (Viagra): oral concomitant use with nitrates contraindicated, as may result in profound hypotension
- Pain management at insertion site of IV or SC catheter
- Anticoagulation: purpose of international normalized ratio; monitoring of skin, gums, urine, and stool for signs of bleeding; precautions to prevent bleeding when on anticoagulation (e.g., use soft toothbrush, use electric razor when shaving, avoid contact sports)
- Follow-up care after discharge
- Symptoms to report to a health care professional

ENDOCARDITIS

Description and Etiology

Endocarditis is an inflammation on the endothelial surface of the heart, with thrombotic fibrin vegetations on the heart valves. Endocarditis is most often related to an infectious organism. The older term *bacterial endocarditis* has been replaced by the term *infectious endocarditis* (IE) because nonbacterial organisms can also be the infective source. IE is fatal if not treated and carries a 1-year mortality rate of 30%.[84] Among intravenous drug abusers, the incidence of IE is even higher.[84]

BOX 13.22 **Evidence-Based Practice**

Pulmonary Artery Hypertension

Recommendations for Early Detection and Screening for Pulmonary Artery Hypertension

- Relatives of patients with heritable pulmonary artery hypertension (PAH) are recommended to undergo prenatal genetic testing before any pregnancy.
- Pregnancy is not recommended for female patients with PAH.
- If PAH is suspected, a 12-lead electrocardiogram (ECG) is required as an early screening test to rule out other possible cardiac anomalies; the ECG is not diagnostic for PAH.
- If PAH is suspected, a chest radiograph can reveal features supportive of a PAH diagnosis.
- If PAH is suspected, Doppler echocardiography is recommended to noninvasively evaluate right ventricular systolic pressures and to assess for anatomic abnormalities such as right atrial or right ventricular enlargement, left ventricular involvement, and intracardiac shunting.

Recommendations for Diagnostic Tests to Further Evaluate Pulmonary Artery Hypertension

- In patients with unexplained PAH, testing for connective tissue disease and human immunodeficiency virus infection is recommended.
- In patients with probable connective tissue PAH, a ventilation-perfusion scan is recommended to identify perfusion blocks and severity of disease progression.
- Pulmonary function tests are recommended to rule out other causes of lung disease.
- Lung biopsy is not recommended; it carries a high risk and low diagnostic yield.
- Right-sided heart catheterization is recommended, as is acute vasoreactivity testing using a short-acting agent such as intravenous (IV) epoprostenol, IV adenosine, or inhaled nitrous oxide.
- Serial assessments of functional class and endurance on a 6-min walk are recommended.

Recommendations for General Management of Pulmonary Artery Hypertension

- Anticoagulation with warfarin (Coumadin) should be considered.
- Diuretics should be administered, as indicated.
- Supplemental oxygen should be used as necessary to maintain oxygen saturation values higher than 90% at all times.
- Referral to a center that specializes in treatment of PAH is strongly recommended.

Recommendations for Medications to Treat Pulmonary Artery Hypertension

- A calcium channel blocker is recommended for patients with positive vasoreactivity testing.
- All patients should be considered for long-term therapy with a combination of the following medications (see Fig. 13.23):
  - Endothelin receptor antagonists:
    - Bosentan (oral)
    - Ambrisentan (oral)
    - Macitentan (oral)
  - Soluble guanylate cyclase sensitizer:
    - Riociguat
  - Phosphodiesterase inhibitors:
    - Sildenafil
    - Tadalafil
  - Prostanoids:
    - Epoprostenol (IV)
    - Treprostinil (subcutaneous, IV, inhaled)
- Patients with PAH in functional class IV are candidates for long-term treatment with IV epoprostenol.

References

Humbert M, Kovacs G, Hoeper MM, et al. 2022 ESC/ERS Guidelines for the diagnosis and treatment of pulmonary hypertension. *Eur Respir J.* 2023;61(1):2200879. https://doi.org/10.1183/13993003.00879-2022.

Simonneau G, Montani D, Celermajer DS, et al. Haemodynamic definitions and updated clinical classification of pulmonary hypertension. *Eur Respir J.* 2019;53(1):1801913. https://doi.org/10.1183/13993003.01913-2018.

IE is the fourth most common cause of life-threatening infectious syndromes (after urosepsis, pneumonia, and intraabdominal sepsis).[85] The risk of acquiring IE is higher among patients with congenital heart disease, valvular heart disease, and prosthetic heart valves.[86] Approximately 75% of patients have a preexisting structural abnormality of the involved heart valve. The increasing incidence of invasive health care interventions such as implantable pacemakers and ICDs, body piercings, intravenous drug abuse (IVDA), and an increase in the number of older patients with degenerative valve disease increase the numbers at risk for IE. Additional risk factors include being male and poor dentition.[84] Involvement of right heart valves is highly suspicious for IVDA.[85]

Development of IE depends on these events:

- Presence of a nonbacterial thrombotic lesion on a cardiac valve or endothelium
- Bacteremia (bacteria in bloodstream)
- Bacteria attach to a nonbacterial thrombotic lesion.
- Proliferation of bacteria on and within the lesion that may develop into a vegetation.

Research suggests the source of the organism is less likely to be related to a specific invasive procedure such as a urogenital procedure or dental work. Rather, IE can result from the confluence of multiple daily bacteremic events in the presence of a susceptible cardiac lesion.[85]

Pathophysiology

IE results from a bacterial or fungal organism in the bloodstream that successfully colonizes the cardiac endothelium. Bacterial organisms, typically streptococci, staphylococci, and enterococci, are the most common pathogens. *Staphylococcus viridans* used to be the most common organism, but this has now been replaced by *Staphylococcus aureus.*[84,86]

An increase in multidrug-resistant organisms has led to increased numbers of patients, more serious complications, and higher mortality rates.[8]

Sites where endocarditis vegetations occur often correlate with aberrant intracardiac flow caused by valvular damage or septal defects. After the vegetations have colonized, organisms multiply at a rapid rate inside a protective platelet-fibrin casing that sequesters the infection.[80]

Assessment and Diagnosis

Diagnosis must be made as soon as possible to initiate treatment and identify patients at high risk for complications. Diagnosis is guided by classic manifestations of bacteremia or fungemia, evidence of active valvulitis, peripheral emboli, and immunologic vascular phenomena.

Modified Duke Criteria

The 2015 AHA scientific statement on IE[85] supports use of the modified Duke criteria for diagnosis, early identification, and treatment of IE (Table 13.13). This system stratifies patients with suspected IE into three categories: (1) definite cases, (2) possible cases, and (3) rejected cases. A definite diagnosis of IE involves:

- Microbiologic criteria: microorganisms in a vegetation or positive blood cultures
- Imaging criteria: imaging shows endocardial involvement

Blood Cultures

Initial symptoms include fever sometimes accompanied by rigor (shivering), fatigue, and malaise; up to 50% of patients report myalgias and joint pain. Blood cultures are drawn during periods of elevated temperature to detect the infective organism. At least 10 mL of venous blood should be placed in each of the blood culture containers to ensure that the organism will be detected.[85] Culture-negative endocarditis occurs in up to one-third of cases and usually is related to prior antibiotic use, or infection by a "fastidious" organism, which does not proliferate under conventional laboratory culture conditions.[85] White blood cell counts are typically elevated, and the symptoms are identified in the Duke criteria (see Table 13.13).

Chest Radiograph

Cough and pleuritic chest pain are often present. The first noninvasive test is often a chest radiograph to detect nodular infiltrates, cardiomegaly, and enlarged pulmonary vessels.

Echocardiogram

The other essential noninvasive test is an echocardiogram of the heart valves to visualize vegetations. Transthoracic echocardiography (TTE) may be performed initially, but transesophageal echocardiography is more valuable because of the clarity of the heart valve images. Transesophageal echocardiography is more sensitive in detection of vegetations and abscesses.[85] Color-flow mapping is especially useful to visualize the severity of valvular regurgitation.

Complications

Heart failure is the most frequent complication of IE and the most frequent cause of death. Embolic complications are the second most common complication, occurring in up to half of IE cases; 65% of the emboli occur in the central nervous system (CNS) and can cause a stroke. Pulmonary embolism (PE) occurs in 66% to 75% of IVDA cases that involve vegetations on the tricuspid valve. Other organs affected by emboli include liver, spleen, kidney, abdominal mesenteric artery, and peripheral vessels. Septic emboli may be visible on the fingers and toes. Rate of emboli formation rapidly declines with appropriate IV antimicrobial administration.[85] Risk of death increases with the development of emboli and decreased arterial perfusion to vital organs. Even with appropriate treatment, mortality is almost 30% at 1 year.[84] Clinical manifestations of IE that may be discovered on physical examination are often nonspecific and are listed in Box 13.23.

Medical Management

Treatment requires prolonged intravenous therapy with adequate doses of antimicrobial agents tailored to the specific IE microbe. The antibiotic management of native valve endocarditis is frequently different from treatment of prosthetic valve endocarditis, or IVDA endocarditis. Antibiotic treatment, administered in high doses intravenously, is prolonged and may involve combination therapy.[85] Best outcomes are achieved if antimicrobial therapy is initiated before hemodynamic compromise.

TABLE 13.13 Modified Duke Criteria

Major Criteria

Blood Culture Positive for IE

- Microorganism consistent with IE from two separate blood cultures:
  - Viridans streptococci
  - *Streptococcus bovis*
- HACEK group (***H****aemophilus* species, ***A****ggregatibacter* species, ***C****ardiobacterium hominis*, ***E****ikenella corrodens*, and ***K****ingella* species)
- Staphylococcus aureus
- Community-acquired enterococci without a known primary focus

OR

- Microorganisms consistent with IE from persistently positive blood cultures:
- At least two positive cultures from blood samples drawn at least 12 hours apart
- Four separate blood cultures (with first and last sample drawn at least 1 hour apart)
- 1 positive blood culture for *Coxiella nti-infl* or antiphase-I immunoglobulin G (IgG) antibody titer >1:800

Echocardiogram Positive for IE

- TEE/TTE to visualize heart valves
- TEE recommended for prosthetic valves
- Oscillating intracardiac mass on valve
- Intracardiac abscess
- New partial dehiscence of prosthetic valve
- New valvular regurgitation

Minor Criteria

Predisposition: Heart condition or an injectable drug user
Fever: Temperature >38°C
Vascular phenomena: Major arterial emboli, septic pulmonary infarcts, mycotic aneurysm, intracranial hemorrhage, conjunctival hemorrhages, and Janeway lesions
Immunologic phenomena: Glomerulonephritis, Osler nodes, Roth spots, rheumatoid factor
Microbial evidence: Positive blood culture that does not meet any major criterion (as described) or serologic evidence of active infection with an organism consistent with IE

Possible Rejection Criteria for IE

- Firm alternative diagnosis for IE
- Resolution of IE symptoms with antibiotics ≤4 days
- No pathologic evidence of IE at surgery or autopsy with antibiotics for ≤4 days.

IE, Infective endocarditis; *TEE*, transesophageal echocardiography; *TTE*, transthoracic echocardiography.

BOX 13.23 Clinical Manifestations of Endocarditis

- Fever
- Splenomegaly
- Hematuria
- Petechiae
- Cardiac murmurs
- Easy fatigability
- Osler nodes are small, raised, tender areas most commonly found in pads of fingers and toes.
- Splinter hemorrhages in nail beds
- Roth spots are round or oval spots consisting of coagulated fibrin; seen in the retina and can lead to hemorrhage.

In many cases, antimicrobial medications are insufficient to cure the IE. Cardiac surgery to excise the damaged native or prosthetic valve is required for persistent vegetation, valve dysfunction, perivalvular extension, and aggressive fungal or antibiotic-resistant bacteria. Valve surgery usually is delayed until the patient is stable. Early surgery is indicated for patients with signs of heart failure, large mobile vegetations, or persistent symptomatic infection lasting longer than 5 to 7 days with ongoing positive blood cultures despite appropriate antibiotics.[87,88] For patients who cannot undergo surgery, the use of *percutaneous vegetectomy* to remove or debulk large vegetations has been described.[89]

Patients with uncomplicated IE are being discharged earlier than in the past and are continuing IV antimicrobial therapy at home with a surgically or peripherally implanted long-term central venous catheter.

Nursing Management

Nursing care management of a patient with IE incorporates a variety of patient diagnoses (Box 13.24). Nursing interventions focus on timely antimicrobial administration to resolve the infection, prevent complications, provide pain medication, and individualize patient education. See Appendix A for patient care management plans specific to patients with IE.

Resolving the Infection

IE requires a long course (usually 4 to 6 weeks) of intravenous antibiotics. Treatment is begun in the hospital and continued at home with an indwelling central catheter after the patient is in stable condition. Nursing assessment includes monitoring for complications and possible signs of worsening infection, such as persistent temperature elevation, malaise, weakness, easy fatigability, night sweats, or new emboli on hands or feet (see Box 13.24).

Preventing Complications

Complications occur in 20% to 50% of patients with IE.[87] The nursing assessment is attuned to the early detection of changes, such as shortness of breath or chest pain with hemoptysis. As valvular dysfunction accelerates, acute heart failure develops. Cardiac assessment includes auscultation of heart sounds to detect the presence of or change in a cardiac murmur. Murmurs can be caused by worsening heart failure or by pulmonary emboli. Changes in level of consciousness, visual changes, or complaints of headache should always be reported immediately because of the risk of emboli.

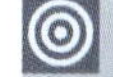

BOX 13.24 DIAGNOSIS AND PATIENT CARE MANAGEMENT

Endocarditis

- Impaired cardiac output due to alterations in preload
- Impaired cardiac output due to alterations in afterload
- Impaired cardiac output due to alterations in contractility
- Impaired cardiac output due to alterations in heart rate or rhythm
- Activity intolerance due to cardiopulmonary dysfunction
- Acute pain due to transmission and perception of cutaneous, visceral, muscular, or ischemic impulses
- Risk for infection
- Anxiety due to threat from biologic, psychologic, or social integrity
- Lack of knowledge of treatment regime due to lack of previous exposure to information (see Box 13.25, Patient and Family Education Plan: Endocarditis)

Patient Care Management plans are located in Appendix A.

BOX 13.25 PATIENT AND FAMILY EDUCATION PLAN

Endocarditis

Before discharge, the patient should be able to teach back the following topics:

- Pathophysiology of endocarditis
- Medications: importance of long-term intravenous antibiotics for eradication
- Temperature: daily temperature monitoring
- Infection control: prophylactic antibiotics related to dental work or other invasive procedures after current medical crisis is controlled
- Activity tolerance: increased activity as tolerated and rest periods as needed
- Heart failure: If symptoms of heart failure are present, education is provided on fluid and sodium restriction, fluid balance, diuretic management, daily weight, and controlling breathlessness.
- Follow-up care after discharge
- Symptoms to report to a health care professional

Evaluation of liver and kidney function is essential to monitor the health of those organs because of the risk of emboli. Because of the complex and prolonged antibiotic therapy required for treating IE, adverse medication reactions are another important consideration.

Educate the Patient and Family

A patient with IE needs to know the manifestations of infection, how to take an oral temperature, and what medical procedures increase risk for recurrence of IE. A written list of all medications must be supplied (Box 13.25). It is essential to reinforce to patients the need to provide a comprehensive endocarditis history to their other health care providers such as their dentist or podiatrist.[85,86] Multidisciplinary support for the patient to meet the challenges of opiate withdrawal and psychologic dependence is essential to prevent a relapse. Many clinicians participate in the care of a patient with IE (Box 13.26).

VALVULAR HEART DISEASE

Description and Etiology

The term *valvular heart disease* describes structural and functional abnormalities of single or multiple cardiac valves. The result is an alteration in blood flow across the valve. The two types of valvular lesions are *stenotic* and *regurgitant*. These are described in this section with reference to the specific cardiac valves involved.

Admission with valvular disease to the critical care unit is generally related to surgical valve replacement, transcatheter valve replacement, or an exacerbation of heart failure.

Pathophysiology

Mitral Valve Stenosis

The term mitral valve stenosis describes a progressive narrowing of the mitral valve orifice. The primary cause is rheumatic endocarditis, with rare occurrences related to congenital malformations. Mitral stenosis occurs in twice as many women as men. Symptoms occur when the normal valve size is reduced to 1.5 cm^2 or less.[90] Narrowing is caused by aging valve tissue or by acute rheumatic valvulitis (Table 13.14). The diffuse valve leaflets fibrose and fuse, reducing mobility and thickening the chordae tendineae. As a result, the mitral valve can no longer open or close passively in response to left atrial and ventricular pressure changes. Blood flow across the valve is impeded. Mitral stenosis increases the risk of developing atrial fibrillation because of the high pressures in the left atrium that stimulate left atrial remodeling and enlargement. Development of atrial fibrillation significantly increases symptoms and may increase the need for surgical replacement of the valve.

Mitral Valve Regurgitation

Mitral valve regurgitation may result from rheumatic disease, aging of the valve, endocarditis, collagen vascular disease, or papillary muscle dysfunction (see Table 13.14). In mitral regurgitation, the valve anulus, leaflets, chordae tendineae, and papillary muscles all may be dysfunctional, or the dysfunction may be isolated to just one component of the valve. Mitral valve regurgitation results in a retrograde flow of blood into the left atrium with each ventricular contraction. It is always described as chronic or acute because of the very different effect on the left-sided chambers.

In chronic mitral valve regurgitation, the left atrium has dilated to accommodate the additional regurgitant volume, whereas the left ventricle has hypertrophied (increased muscle) to maintain an adequate stroke volume and cardiac output.

In contrast, acute mitral valve regurgitation is precipitated by chordae tendineae or papillary muscle rupture resulting from STEMI or IE. This is a medical emergency. The left atrium cannot accommodate the sudden increase in volume and pressure, and use of an IABP and inotropic and afterload-reducing pharmacologic support are often required to increase forward output and to reduce pulmonary congestion.

After the acute condition has stabilized, surgical replacement or repair of the incompetent valve is performed. A transcatheter mitral valve repair may be considered for a patient with chronic severe MR and NYHA class III or IV symptoms. Percutaneous mitral valve repair using the MitraClip (Abbot Vascular) device provides a minimally invasive transcatheter means of mitral valve repair. This procedure has reduced severity of MR, improved symptoms, and led to reverse LV remodeling. Clinical studies are in progress to evaluate other new transcatheter mitral valve replacement systems.

BOX 13.26 Evidence-Based Practice

Infective Endocarditis

Diagnosis of IE

The Modified Duke Criteria are recommended to guide diagnosis of infective endocarditis (IE) (see Table 13.13).

Endocarditis Prophylaxis is Recommended for:

- Patients with high and intermediate risk of IE
  - High risk
    - Previous history of IE
    - Prosthetic heart valves and cardiac valve repair
    - Congenital heart disease
    - Destination therapy ventricular assist devices
  - Intermediate risk
    - Rheumatic heart disease
    - Non-rheumatic degenerative valve disease
    - Bicuspid aortic valve disease
    - Cardiovascular implanted electronic devices
    - Hypertrophic cardiomyopathy

Antimicrobial Therapy

- Antimicrobial therapy administered for IE is characterized by six features:
  1. It is prolonged
  2. It is bactericidal
  3. It is parenteral for critically ill patients
  4. It can be parenteral or oral for stable patients
  5. It is high dosage
  6. It is guided by blood cultures and serum antibiotic levels

Complications From IE

- Embolic events
- Acute heart failure
- Intra-cardiac complications (leaflet perforation and chordal rupture)
- Cerebrovascular complications
- Uncontrolled infection and septic shock

Complications From Antibiotics

- Toxicity from the high doses of antibiotics may impair kidney function or vestibular function (balance).
- Diarrhea and colitis can be caused by a reaction to the antibiotic therapy or by overgrowth by *Clostridioides difficile*.
- Rash, fever, neutropenia, and liver function abnormalities can be caused by prolonged antibiotic use.

Indications for Surgery

- Emergent (within 24 hours)
  - NYHA class IV heart failure with cardiogenic shock and pulmonary edema
- Urgent (within 3–5 days)
  - Uncontrolled infection with local complications (abscess, fistula, enlarging vegetation)
  - High risk of embolism or established embolism
  - Vegetation size greater than 10 mm and emboli despite appropriate antibiotic therapy

References

Baddour LM, Wilson WR, Bayer AS, et al. Infective endocarditis in adults: diagnosis, antimicrobial therapy, and management of complications: a scientific statement for healthcare professionals from the American Heart Association. *Circulation*. 2015;132(15):1435–1486.

Delgado V, et al. ESC Scientific Document Group. 2023 ESC Guidelines for the management of endocarditis. *Eur Heart J*. 2023;44(39):3948–4042.

Pettersson GB, Hussain ST, Current AATS guidelines on surgical treatment of infective endocarditis. *Ann Cardiothorac Surg*. 2019;8(6):630–644.

Wilson WR, Gewitz M, Lockhart PB, et al. Prevention of viridans group streptococcal infective endocarditis: a scientific statement from the American Heart Association. *Circulation*. 2021;143(20):e963–e978.

Aortic Valve Stenosis

The term *aortic valve stenosis* describes a narrowing of the aortic valve area. It can result from aging, rheumatic valvulitis, or deterioration of a congenital bicuspid valve (see Table 13.14).[90–93] The pathologic hallmarks are inflammation, fibrous valvular thickening, and tissue calcification.[90–92] Aortic stenosis is the most common valvular heart disease in North America and Europe, due to aging populations.[94]

Cardiac catheterization or Doppler echocardiography are used to measure the valve area and the gradient across the valve. The *gradient* represents the difference in systolic pressure between the left ventricle and the aorta. A significant pressure difference inhibits forward flow and is a diagnostic of aortic stenosis. The impedance of LV ejection into the aorta results in increased LV systolic pressure, LVH, and eventually LV dilation.

- *Mild aortic stenosis.* When the aortic valvular opening is reduced to less than 1.5 cm^2, the condition is classified as mild with a gradient of less than 25 mm Hg across the valve.

TABLE 13.14 Heart Valve Dysfunction

	Pathophysiology	Clinical Manifestations	Physical Signs
Mitral Valve Stenosis A: Mitral valve stenosis; dashed arrow indicates stenosis	Left atrium must generate more pressure to propel blood beyond lesion; rise in left atrial pressure and volume reflected retrograde into pulmonary vessels; right ventricular hypertrophy; right ventricular failure	Dyspnea on exertion; fatigue and weakness; pronounced respiratory symptoms (e.g., orthopnea, paroxysmal nocturnal dyspnea); mild hemoptysis with bronchial capillary rupture; susceptibility to pulmonary infections	• Chest radiograph: pulmonary congestion, redistribution of blood flow to upper lobes • ECG: atrial fibrillation and other atrial dysrhythmias • Auscultation: diastolic murmur, accentuated S_1, opening snap • Catheterization: elevated pressure gradient across valve; increased left atrial pressure, pulmonary artery occlusion pressure, and pulmonary artery pressure; low cardiac output
Mitral Valve Regurgitation B: Mitral valve regurgitation; cloud indicates backward flow from a valve that is leaking or regurgitant	LV dilation and hypertrophy; left atrial dilation and hypertrophy	Weakness and fatigue; exertional dyspnea; palpitations; severe symptoms precipitated by LV failure, with consequent low output and pulmonary congestion	• Chest radiograph: left atrial and LV enlargement, variable pulmonary congestion • ECG: P mitrale, LV hypertrophy, atrial fibrillation • Auscultation: murmur throughout systole • Catheterization: opacification of left atrium during LV injection, v waves, increased left atrial and LV pressures • Variable elevations of pulmonary pressures
Aortic Valve Stenosis C: Aortic valve stenosis; dashed arrow indicates stenosis	LV hypertrophy; progressive failure of ventricular emptying; pulmonary congestion; failure of right side of heart, with systemic venous congestion; sudden cardiac death	Exertional dyspnea; exercise intolerance; syncope; angina; heart failure (LV failure)	• Chest radiograph: poststenotic aortic dilation, calcification • ECG: LV hypertrophy • Auscultation: systolic ejection murmur • Catheterization: significant pressure gradient, increased LV end-diastolic pressure

Continued

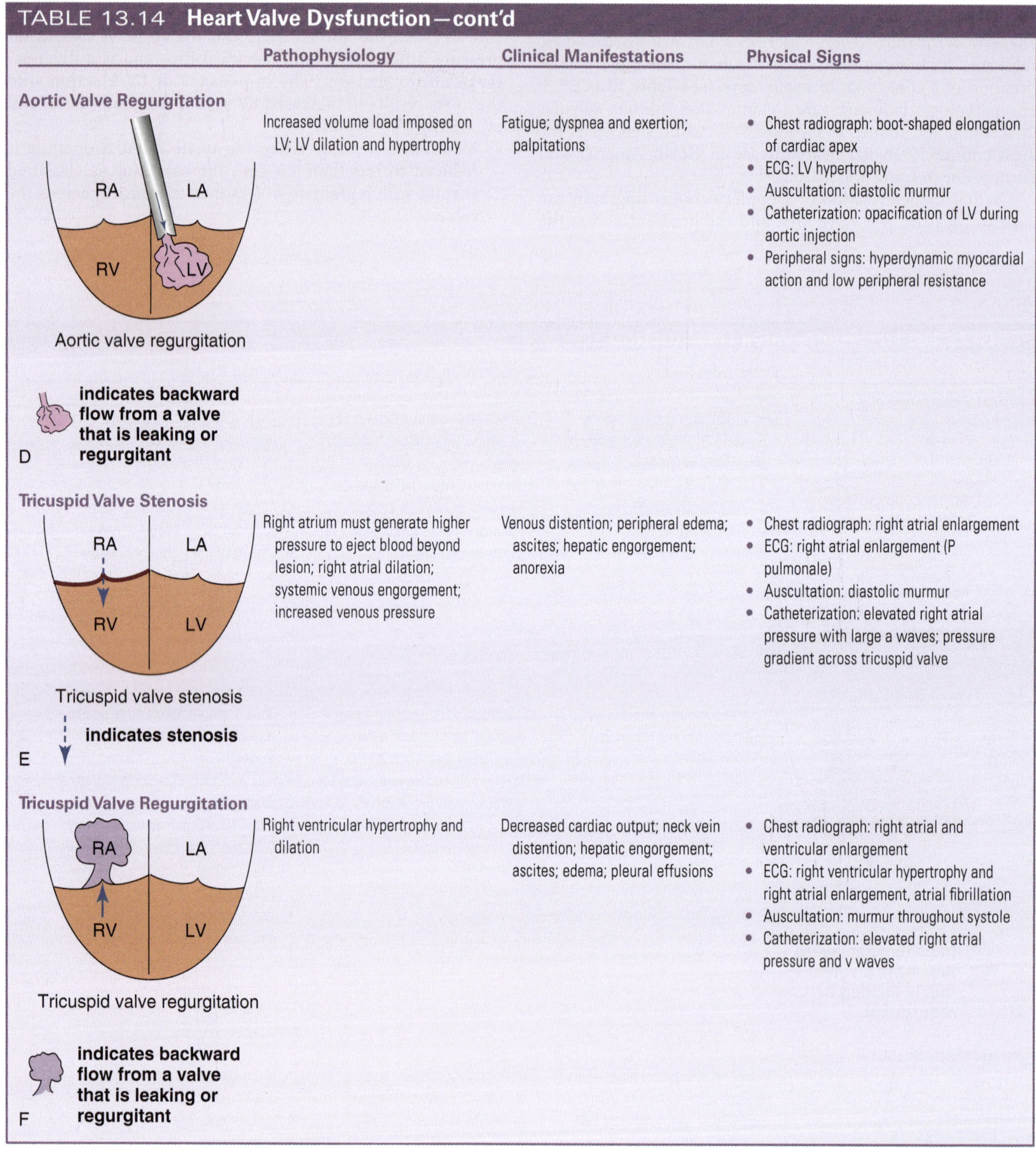

TABLE 13.14 Heart Valve Dysfunction—cont'd

	Pathophysiology	Clinical Manifestations	Physical Signs
Aortic Valve Regurgitation	Increased volume load imposed on LV; LV dilation and hypertrophy	Fatigue; dyspnea and exertion; palpitations	• Chest radiograph: boot-shaped elongation of cardiac apex • ECG: LV hypertrophy • Auscultation: diastolic murmur • Catheterization: opacification of LV during aortic injection • Peripheral signs: hyperdynamic myocardial action and low peripheral resistance
Tricuspid Valve Stenosis	Right atrium must generate higher pressure to eject blood beyond lesion; right atrial dilation; systemic venous engorgement; increased venous pressure	Venous distention; peripheral edema; ascites; hepatic engorgement; anorexia	• Chest radiograph: right atrial enlargement • ECG: right atrial enlargement (P pulmonale) • Auscultation: diastolic murmur • Catheterization: elevated right atrial pressure with large a waves; pressure gradient across tricuspid valve
Tricuspid Valve Regurgitation	Right ventricular hypertrophy and dilation	Decreased cardiac output; neck vein distention; hepatic engorgement; ascites; edema; pleural effusions	• Chest radiograph: right atrial and ventricular enlargement • ECG: right ventricular hypertrophy and right atrial enlargement, atrial fibrillation • Auscultation: murmur throughout systole • Catheterization: elevated right atrial pressure and v waves

ECG, Electrocardiogram; *LV*, left ventricular; *P mitrale*, m-shaped P waves that occur in left atrial hypertrophy and are often caused by mitral stenosis; *P pulmonale*, tall, peaked P waves that occur in right atrial hypertrophy and are often caused by chronic pulmonary disease.

- *Severe aortic stenosis.* When the valve orifice has narrowed to less than 1 cm^2, the gradient will typically be greater than 40 mm Hg, and the diagnosis will be upgraded to severe aortic valve stenosis.[95]

When symptoms such as angina, dyspnea, syncope, and other indicators of heart failure develop, it is critical to intervene to prevent further damage to the left ventricle. Aortic valve replacement is indicated. Congenitally abnormal valves may require replacement by the fourth to sixth decades, whereas the degenerative changes are often tolerated until the seventh decade of life.[90–92]

For patients with severe aortic stenosis and high to intermediate surgical risk, percutaneous transcatheter aortic valve replacement (TAVR) procedures have proven safe and effective. Studies of these percutaneous procedures have demonstrated decreased mortality, improved quality of life, and cost effectiveness.[94]

Aortic Valve Regurgitation

Aortic regurgitation, also known as *aortic insufficiency*, may occur from numerous causes not limited to rheumatic fever, systemic hypertension, Marfan syndrome, syphilis, rheumatoid arthritis, aging valve tissue, discrete subaortic stenosis, or as a complication of a transcatheter procedure (Table 13.14). Aortic valve incompetence results in a reflux of blood back into the left ventricle during ventricular diastole. To accommodate this extra volume, the left ventricle initially dilates and then enlarges to meet the needs of the peripheral circulation. Aortic valve replacement is recommended for symptomatic patients with well-preserved or moderate LV dysfunction.[90–92]

Tricuspid Valve Stenosis

Tricuspid valve stenosis is rarely an isolated lesion (Table 13.14). It often occurs in conjunction with mitral or aortic disease or congenital disease. The origin most often is rheumatic fever or a complication of IVDA and resultant IE.[96] Tricuspid valve stenosis increases the pressure and work of the usually low-pressure right atrium, resulting in right atrial hypertrophy. The right atrium dilates to accommodate the residual right atrial volume and the incoming venous return. As a result, systemic venous congestion occurs, the consequences of which include jugular venous congestion, liver failure, hepatomegaly, ascites, and peripheral edema.

Tricuspid Valve Regurgitation

Tricuspid valve regurgitation usually results from advanced failure of the left side of the heart that eventually affects the right side of the heart, severe PH, or as a complication of IE. Other causes include carcinoid, rheumatoid arthritis, radiation therapy, trauma, and Marfan syndrome (see Table 13.14).

Pulmonary Valve Disease

Pulmonary valve disease is an uncommon disorder in adults. It is most often related to congenital anomalies and produces failure of the right side of the heart. Acquired cases are most often related to carcinoid or rheumatic fever pathologies. Initial symptoms include dyspnea, and symptoms of severe heart failure occur with disease progression. Balloon valvuloplasty has proven successful for treatment of these patients, although there is a high recurrence rate. More recent studies have proved percutaneous pulmonary valve and valve conduits as successful replacements for the pulmonary valve apparatus.

Mixed Valvular Lesions

Many persons have *mixed valvular lesions* as an element of stenosis and regurgitation. Mixed lesions can accentuate the severity of a condition. For example, when combined, aortic stenosis and aortic regurgitation increase LV volume and pressure and multiply the LV workload.

Medical Management

Management of valvular disorders includes pharmacologic therapy to control symptoms of heart failure and cardiac surgical repair or replacement of the affected valve. When surgery is not feasible, balloon dilation is a rare option selected for patients too ill to undergo a major cardiac surgical procedure. Percutaneous valve devices including stent valves and mitral clips are being used as a less invasive alternative.[90–92,94]

Nursing Management

Nursing care management for a patient with valvular heart disease incorporates a variety of patient diagnoses (Box 13.27). Nursing interventions focus on achievement of adequate cardiac output, maintenance of fluid balance, and patient and family education. See Appendix A for patient care management plans specific to patients with valvular heart disease.

Cardiac Output

Low cardiac output is a common finding in patients with valvular heart disease. It can occur because of decreased forward flow through a stenotic valve, bidirectional flow across an incompetent valve, or associated heart failure. Vital signs and the effect of positive inotropic and afterload-reducing agents are assessed and documented. If the patient has hemodynamic catheters inserted, cardiac output and hemodynamic parameters are measured and evaluated. Patient care activities are carefully planned to provide adequate rest periods to prevent fatigue.

Fluid Balance

Fluid status is evaluated by auscultation of breath sounds for crackles, heart sounds for presence of S_3, daily weights to trend a "sudden weight gain," and presence of peripheral edema. The appearance of pulmonary crackles or an S_3 heart sound confirms volume overload. The jugular vein is assessed for signs of increased distention. Diuretics and vasodilators are administered to counteract excess fluid retention. A weight is obtained daily and assessed against the recorded fluid intake and output.

Educate the Patient and Family

Education for a patient with acute or chronic heart failure caused by valvular dysfunction includes (1) information related to diet, (2) fluid restrictions, (3) the actions and side effects of heart failure medications, (4) the need for prophylactic antibiotics before undergoing any invasive procedures, and (5) when

BOX 13.27 DIAGNOSIS AND PATIENT CARE MANAGEMENT

Valvular Heart Disease

- Impaired cardiac output due to alterations in preload
- Impaired cardiac output due to alterations in afterload
- Impaired cardiac output due to alterations in contractility
- Impaired cardiac output due to alterations in heart rate or rhythm
- Activity intolerance due to cardiopulmonary dysfunction
- Lack of knowledge of treatment regime due to lack of previous exposure to information (see Box 13.28, Patient and Family Education Plan: Valvular Heart Disease)

Patient Care Management plans are located in Appendix A.

to call the health care provider to report a negative change in cardiac symptoms (Box 13.28).

Many patients also require information about valvular heart surgery or percutaneous replacement procedures. Achieving optimal outcomes for a patient with valve disease requires contributions from a team of educated health care clinicians. Collaborative multidisciplinary priorities are listed in Box 13.29. In Chapter 14, the section on valvular surgery provides more information on surgical management.

ACUTE AORTIC SYNDROMES

Description and Etiology

Two acute aortic conditions are described: aortic aneurysm and aortic dissection. In most cases, aortic conditions are the result of progressive atherosclerotic disease. However, thoracic aortic aneurysms may have a heritable cause in up to 20% of cases.[97] *Acute aortic syndrome* is a more recent term that encompasses the growing understanding that there are multiple ways injury to the aorta can occur.[97–99]

Most patients with an acute aortic syndrome have a history of systemic hypertension. Causative factors include atherosclerotic changes in the thoracic and abdominal aorta encompassing the same risk factors as other atherosclerotic diseases. Other nonatherosclerotic risks for aortic injury include blunt trauma, Marfan syndrome, and pregnancy.[99]

BOX 13.28 PATIENT AND FAMILY EDUCATION PLAN

Valvular Heart Disease

Before discharge, the patient should be able to teach back the following topics:

- Pathophysiology of valvular disease
- Infection control: prophylactic antibiotics related to dental work or other invasive procedures
- Heart failure: If symptoms of heart failure are present, education is provided on fluid and sodium restriction, fluid balance, diuretic management, daily weight, and controlling breathlessness.
- Surgery: If open-heart surgery was performed, information about postsurgical recovery is provided.
- Medications: Medications may be complex, and information must be given in writing and orally:
  - Preload: purpose of diuretics, increased urine output, and control of fluid volume
  - Afterload: purpose of vasodilators or angiotensin-converting enzyme inhibitors in decreasing the workload of the heart
  - Heart rate: purpose of digoxin is to control the rate in atrial fibrillation, a frequent dysrhythmia in heart failure
  - Contractility: With the exception of digoxin, no oral contractility medications are approved by U.S. Food and Drug Administration.
  - Anticoagulation: Patients with distended atria, enlarged ventricles, atrial fibrillation, or mechanical valves may be prescribed anticoagulants, which increase risk of bleeding. Monitoring depends on the specific anticoagulant prescribed.
- Follow-up care after discharge
- Symptoms to report to a health care professional

BOX 13.29 Evidence-Based Practice

Valvular Heart Disease

Class I recommendations with strong evidence are provided.

Recommendations for Detection and Surveillance of Valvular Disease by Echocardiography

- Echocardiography is noninvasive and is used for all initial diagnostic and serial follow-up evaluations.

Recommendations for Aortic Stenosis

- Echocardiography is the primary diagnostic tool.
- Coronary arteriography is used before aortic valve replacement (AVR) if coronary artery disease (CAD) is suspected.
- AVR is recommended for symptomatic patients with severe aortic stenosis; AVR can be combined with coronary artery bypass graft (CABG) surgery when CAD is present.

Recommendations for Aortic Regurgitation

- Echocardiography is the primary diagnostic tool.
- Cardiac catheterization is used if noninvasive tests are inconclusive.
- AVR is indicated for symptomatic patients with severe AR regardless of left ventricular (LV) systolic function.
- AVR is indicated for nonsymptomatic patients with severe AR with LV systolic dysfunction (ejection fraction <0.5 [50%]); AVR can be combined with CABG surgery if CAD is present.

Recommendations for Mitral Stenosis

- Echocardiography is the primary diagnostic tool.
- Anticoagulation is indicated in patients with mitral stenosis (MS) and atrial fibrillation (paroxysmal, persistent, or permanent) and in patients with MS in sinus rhythm with a prior embolic event or left atrial thrombus.
- Cardiac catheterization if noninvasive tests are inconclusive.
- Mitral valve repair (preferable) or mitral valve replacement is indicated for symptomatic (New York Heart Association functional class III or IV) moderate or severe MS if percutaneous mitral balloon valvuloplasty is contraindicated.

Recommendations for Mitral Regurgitation

- Echocardiography is the primary diagnostic tool.
- Cardiac catheterization if noninvasive tests are inconclusive or if additional hemodynamic measurements are required.
- Mitral valve repair is the operation of choice over valve replacement in most patients with chronic mitral regurgitation.

See Box 13.26 for recommendations related to management of patients with valve disease and prosthetic valves.

References

Otto CM, Nishimura RA, Bonow RO, et al. 2020 ACC/AHA Guideline for the management of patients with valvular heart disease: Executive Summary: A Report of the American College of Cardiology/American Heart Association Joint Committee on Clinical Practice Guidelines. *Circulation.* 2021;143(5):e35–e71. https://doi.org/10.1161/CIR.0000000000000932.

Vahanian A, Beyersdorf F, Praz F, et al. 2021 ESC/EACTS Guidelines for the management of valvular heart disease. *Eur Heart J.* 2022;43(7):561–632. https://doi.org/10.1093/eurheartj/ehab395.

Nishimura RA, Otto CM, Bonow RO, et al. 2017 AHA/ACC Focused Update of the 2014 AHA/ACC Guideline for the Management of Patients With Valvular Heart Disease: A Report of the American College of Cardiology/American Heart Association Task Force on Clinical Practice Guidelines. *Circulation.* 2017;135(25):e1159–e1195. https://doi.org/10.1161/CIR.0000000000000503.

Nishimura RA, Otto CM, Bonow RO, et al. 2014 AHA/ACC guideline for the management of patients with valvular heart disease: a report of the American College of Cardiology/American Heart Association Task Force on Practice Guidelines. *J Am Coll Cardiol.* 2014;63(22):e57–185. https://doi.org/10.1016/j.jacc.2014.02.536.

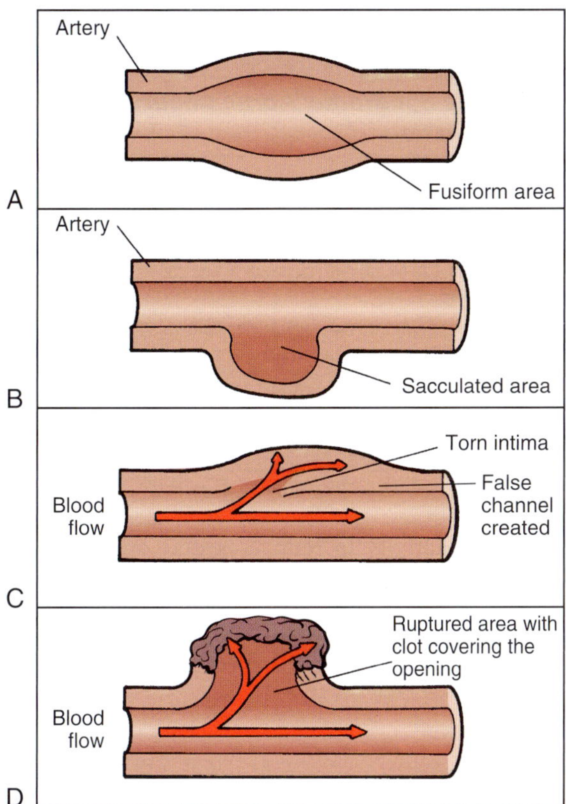

FIG. 13.24 Types of Vascular Injury. In a fusiform aneurysm, an entire segment of an artery is dilated, taking on a spindle or bulbous shape. Fusiform aneurysms occur most often in the abdominal aorta and result from atherosclerosis. (B) A sacculated aneurysm involves only one side of an artery and usually is located in the ascending aorta. (C) Dissection occurs because of a tear in the Intima, resulting in the shunting of blood between the intima and media of a vessel. (D) A pseudoaneurysm can result from arterial trauma from an arterial introducer sheath or intra-aortic balloon catheter, when the arterial opening does not heal normally and is covered by a clot that may rupture at any time.

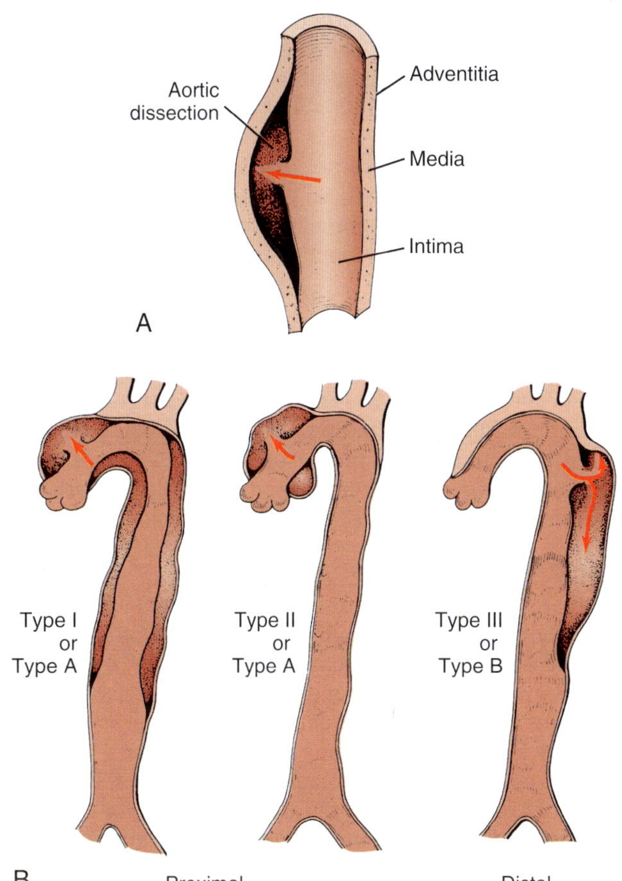

FIG. 13.25 Aortic Dissection. (A) Separation of vascular layers. (B) Classification of aortic dissection. (Modified from Price SA, Wilson LM. *Pathophysiology: clinical concepts of disease processes*. 5th ed. Mosby; 1997.)

Aortic Aneurysm

An *aortic aneurysm* is a localized dilation of the arterial wall that results in an alteration in vessel shape and blood flow. There are two types of vascular aneurysms, fusiform and sacculated (Fig. 13.24A and B). Aortic aneurysm is diagnosed mostly in older adults.

An aortic aneurysm does not always produce symptoms. It may be detected during routine abdominal examination as a palpable, pulsatile mass located in the umbilical region of the abdomen to the left of the midline.

Aortic Aneurysm Size

A thoracic aneurysm may be identified on a routine chest radiograph. An aneurysm less than 4 cm in diameter can be managed on an outpatient basis with frequent BP monitoring and ultrasound testing to document any changes in the size of the aneurysm.

An aneurysm sized between 4 cm and 4.5 cm should stimulate discussion and shared decision making to plan treatment options.[97] An aortic aneurysm between 5 cm and 5.5 cm in diameter requires evaluation for surgical repair or placement of an aortic stent to eliminate the risk of rupture[97] (see Chapter 14).

Aortic Dissection

An *aortic dissection* occurs when a column of blood separates the vascular layers. This creates a *false lumen*, which communicates with the true lumen through a tear in the intima (Fig. 13.24C).

Aortic dissections are classified according to the origin of the site of the tear.[97] Two classification systems are commonly used in clinical practice with either the letters A and B or the numerals I, II, or III, as shown in Fig. 13.25.

- Type A (proximal) also called Type I or II
- Type B (distal) also called Type III

The classic clinical presentation is the sudden onset of intense, severe, tearing pain, which may be localized initially in the chest, abdomen, or back. As the aortic tear (dissection) extends, pain radiates to the back or distally toward the lower extremities. However, many patients with a thoracic aortic dissection do not present with pain.[99]

Cardiovascular warning signs may include severe hypertension, fleeting peripheral pulses, limb ischemia, or a new murmur indicative of aortic regurgitation.

- An ascending aortic dissection typically creates pain in the central chest or midscapular region of the back.

- A descending aortic dissection typically creates pain that radiates down the back, abdomen, or legs.

The location of the dissection may be estimated according to the site of pain, although this does not eliminate the need for diagnostic procedures.

Many patients with dissections have hypertension on initial presentation, and the focus is on control of BP and postponing operation. Higher surgical mortality is found among patients who present with shock, hypotension, and signs of poor organ perfusion.

Assessment and Diagnosis

Several diagnostic tests are available including TTE, computed tomography (CT), intravascular ultrasound, and magnetic resonance Imaging (MRI).[97] All permit detailed visualization of aortic structures. Diagnostic findings that identify high-risk patients include a widened mediastinum or an excessively dilated aorta.[99] The definitive invasive diagnostic procedure is an aortogram (aortic angiogram with radiopaque contrast agent).[99]

Medical Management

Medical management of an aortic aneurysm and aortic dissection depends on what symptoms are seen, and if the condition is emergent. Management is focused on controlling hypertension and educating the patient about the need for corrective surgery before the aneurysm is ≥5.5 cm wide.[97] In other words, plan surgery before a life-threatening emergency occurs. If there is an acute aortic dissection, management involves immediate control of hypertension with intravenous medications and control of pain with opiates. In an emergency, progression of the dissection is evaluated by the patient's report of worsening or new pain, and changes in hemodynamics.

If the patient presents with hypotension or in cardiogenic shock, BP support measures to maintain tissue perfusion are initiated. In such cases, emergency surgery may be performed. Surgery is usually required for dissections that involve the ascending aorta to prevent death from cardiac tamponade (type A or type I and type II, see Fig. 13.25). The surgical procedure includes resection of the affected area, followed by graft placement and restoration of blood flow to major branches of the aorta. The aortic valve is replaced if the dissection involves the valve.[97]

Dissections that involve the descending aorta (type B or type III) do not always require surgery. Another option for this population is percutaneous endovascular repair, which provides a less invasive option instead of traditional surgery.[97]

Nursing Management

Nursing care management for a patient with an aortic aneurysm or aortic dissection incorporates a variety of patient diagnoses (Box 13.30). Nursing interventions are directed toward control of hypertension, pain control, prevention of complications, and education of the patient and family. See Appendix A for patient care management plans specific to patients with an aortic aneurysm or aortic dissection.

Hypertension Management

The cardiovascular status is assessed hourly, including monitoring BP in both arms, checking peripheral pulses bilaterally, auscultating for an aortic murmur, and monitoring the ECG for ischemic changes or dysrhythmias. Patients usually require an arterial line and receive potent antihypertensive medications such as labetalol, which combines beta-blocking activity to reduce cardiac output and lower BP and peripheral alpha-blocking activity to vasodilate the arteries and decrease BP. Another medication that has been shown to provide rapid control of BP in patient with aortic aneurysms is clevidipine, a dihydropyridine calcium channel blocker.

> **BOX 13.30 DIAGNOSIS AND PATIENT CARE MANAGEMENT**
>
> ***Acute Aortic Syndrome: Aortic Aneurysm and Aortic Dissection***
>
> - Impaired cardiac output due to alterations in preload
> - Acute pain due to transmission and perception of cutaneous, visceral, muscular, or ischemic impulses
> - Impaired peripheral tissue perfusion due to decreased blood flow
> - Risk for infection
> - Anxiety due to threat from biologic, psychologic, or social integrity
> - Lack of knowledge of treatment regime due to lack of previous exposure to information (see Box 13.31, Patient and Family Education Plan: Aortic Aneurysm and Aortic Dissection)
>
> Patient Care Management plans are located in Appendix A.

Pain Control

Acute pain is a classic sign of aortic dissection. Opiates and sedatives are administered to control pain, decrease anxiety, and increase comfort. Because these medications can mask the pain of further dissection, they are administered judiciously. The patient's neurovascular status is assessed hourly. Documentation includes the presence and distribution of pain, pallor, paresthesia, paralysis, and movement of the limb. Due to the risk for paralysis and paresthesia, a lumbar drain may be used to allow management of cord edema. See Chapter 7 for more in-depth information on pain management.

Educate the Patient and Family

In the acute period, education is limited to an explanation of the critical care environment and the importance of BP control (Box 13.31). Recommendations for prevention and treatment of atherosclerotic aortic aneurysm and dissection are listed in Box 13.32.

PERIPHERAL ARTERY DISEASE

Description and Etiology

Lower extremity arterial disease (LEAD), also known as *peripheral arterial disease* (PAD), is a common atherosclerotic cause of arterial occlusion in older adults. PAD may require critical care admission for an *acute thrombotic occlusion* or for a vascular surgical procedure. PAD can occur in any peripheral artery and is especially painful in the arteries that supply the lower extremities. The following descriptions relate to PAD.

Pathophysiology

Atherosclerosis is the most common cause of arterial disease. Most patients with PAD have at least one risk factor that predisposes them to development of CAD.[100,101] Diabetes, smoking, hypertension, hyperlipidemia, and male sex

BOX 13.31 PATIENT AND FAMILY EDUCATION PLAN

Acute Aortic Syndrome: Aortic Aneurysm and Aortic Dissection

Before discharge, the patient should be able to teach back the following topics:

- Pathophysiology of atherosclerotic aortic disease: aortic aneurysm or aortic dissection
- Hypertension control: Hypertension increases the risk of aneurysm rupture or aortic dissection.
- Pain control: use of 0-to-10 pain scale; information about availability of pain medications for acute pain
- Preprocedure teaching for aortic angiogram, computed tomography scan, or transesophageal echocardiogram
- Preoperative teaching for aortic surgical repair
- Risk factor modification: After the acute episode, if the cause of the aortic aneurysm or aortic dissection is atherosclerosis, an individual risk factor profile is developed for each patient. Strategies to discuss include decrease daily fat intake to less than 30% of total calories, achieve total blood cholesterol level of less than 200 mg/dL, stop smoking, reduce salt intake, control hypertension, treat diabetes if patient has diabetes, increase physical activity, achieve and maintain ideal body weight.
- Symptoms to report to a health care professional: pain, signs, and symptoms of infection
- Follow-up care after discharge

BOX 13.32 Evidence-Based Practice

Acute Aortic Syndrome: Aortic Aneurysm and Aortic Dissection

Recommendations for Prevention of Atherosclerotic Aortic Aneurysm and Dissection

- Hypertension is a major risk factor. There are no specific recommendations related to blood pressure (BP) control and aortic disease. Reduction of BP to less than 130/80 mm Hg is consistent with recommendations for other atherosclerotic diseases (coronary and cerebrovascular).
- Cigarette smoking is a major risk factor for aortic disease; smoking cessation is essential.
- Routine use of statins has been found to decrease the aneurysm rupture rate and may be effective in decreasing abdominal aortic aneurysm (AAA) growth rate.
- Aortic dissection also occurs as a complication of blunt chest trauma from high-speed motor vehicular trauma.

Recommendations for Treatment of Aortic Dissection

- Admission to the critical care unit for monitoring of heart rate and BP
- Reduction of systolic BP using intravenous (IV) beta-blockers (esmolol) or beta-blocker plus alpha-blocker combination (labetalol); beta-blockers are recommended because they reduce the force of blood ejected from the ventricle against the weakened aortic wall.
- If further systolic BP reduction is necessary, IV vasodilators (sodium nitroprusside) are added in addition to beta-blockers.
- Intubation and mechanical ventilation are recommended if profound hemodynamic instability exists.
- Pain relief (morphine sulfate) and sedation are recommended.
- Diagnosis of aortic dissection is made by clinical signs and location of the site of the tear and false lumen. Computed tomography is the most common diagnostic test in an emergency. Magnetic resonance imaging is often used for chronic stable dissections. Transthoracic echocardiography followed by transesophageal echocardiography may also be used.
- Treatment recommendations depend on the classification of the dissection:
- Type A (type I, type II) dissections that involve the aortic arch are repaired surgically to prevent aortic rupture or cardiac tamponade.
- Type B (type III) dissections are recommended for medical treatment. Surgery or endovascular repair is recommended only in cases of persistent chest pain, aortic expansion, periaortic hematoma, or mediastinal hematoma.
- Type A aortic dissection is a high-risk diagnosis with an overall hospital mortality rate of 25%. Patients with type A dissections who are admitted to the hospital with hypotension have a higher risk of adverse events.

Recommendations for Treatment of Elective Abdominal Aortic Aneurysm

- Formation of AAA or dissection before the sixth decade of life is uncommon.
- Based on current evidence, a 5.5-cm aneurysm diameter is the best threshold for repair in the "average" male patient. Vascular surgery experts recommend that women have elective repair of an aneurysm 4.5 to 5 cm. Individual anatomy, patient age, and physical size must also be considered.
- Until the results of long-term randomized trials are available, the choice between endoluminal repair (stent) and open abdominal surgery depends on patient and physician preferences.

References

Isselbacher EM, Preventza O, Hamilton Black J, et al. 2022 ACC/AHA Guideline for the Diagnosis and Management of Aortic Disease: A Report of the American Heart Association/American College of Cardiology Joint Committee on Clinical Practice Guidelines. *Circulation.* 2022;146(24):e334–e482. https://doi.org/10.1161/CIR.0000000000001106.

Kaji S. Acute medical management of aortic dissection. *Gen Thorac Cardiovasc Surg.* 2019;67(2):203.

Bossone E, Eagle KA. Epidemiology and management of aortic disease: aortic aneurysms and acute aortic syndromes. *Nat Rev Cardiol.* 2021;18(5):331–348. https://doi.org/10.1038/s41569-020-00472-6.

increase the risk of peripheral artery occlusion.[100,101] As with CAD, the presence of kidney disease and diabetes increase the likelihood of concomitant PAD.[100,101] The most affected vessels in the lower extremities are the superficial femoral artery and the popliteal artery in the legs, followed by the distal aorta and iliac arteries.

Assessment and Diagnosis

Ankle-Brachial Index

The *ankle-brachial index* is a noninvasive test used to estimate the severity of arterial disease in the leg by comparing the arterial pressure in the leg with the measured arterial pressure in the arm.[100,101] The systolic BP is measured with a cuff on the arm and twice on the leg just above where the pulse is measured.[102]

- Directly above the ankle for the *dorsalis pedis pulse*
- Directly above the knee for the *popliteal pulse*
- Directly above the elbow for the *brachial pulse*

$$\text{Ankle Brachial Index(ABI)} = \frac{\text{Lower extremity systolic pressure}}{\text{Brachial artery systolic pressure}}$$

The systolic BP can be palpated with the fingers or generally is auscultated using a handheld 5- to 7-MHz Doppler device.[102] To calculate the ABI, the arm systolic BP is divided into the ankle systolic BP. The formula and values are shown below.[100,101]

- ABI value ≥ 1.4 high and abnormal—Stiff, noncompressible arteries
- ABI value between 1.0 and 1.4—Peripheral arteries normal
- ABI value between 0.9 and 1.0—Borderline
- ABI value ≤0.9 is abnormal—PAD is present
  - ABI between 0.71 and 0.9—mild PAD
  - ABI between 0.41 and 0.7—moderate PAD
  - ABI ≤ 0.4—severe PAD, limb-threatening ischemia.

As the ABI value decreases, symptoms of peripheral ischemia increase.[100–102]

Intermittent Claudication

Arterial occlusion obstructs blood flow to the distal extremity. The lack of blood flow produces ischemic muscle pain known as *intermittent claudication*. This cramping, aching pain while walking is often the first symptom of PAD. The pain is relieved by rest and may remain stable in occurrence and intensity for many years. As with other atherosclerotic conditions, symptoms do not occur until more than 75% of the vessel lumen is occluded. PAD is typically asymptomatic until the disease process is well advanced.

Rest Pain

As PAD progresses, patients may develop pain at rest. Pain at rest threatens the viability of the limb and requires immediate catheter or surgical intervention to relieve the blockage and restore circulation to the extremity.

Acute Occlusion

The symptoms of acute occlusion from thrombosis are sudden onset of severe pain, loss of pulses, collapse of superficial veins, coldness, pallor, and impaired motor and sensory function. As with rest pain, acute occlusion requires immediate intervention to open the artery.

Atrophic Tissue Changes

Skin changes associated with PAD include thickening of the nails and drying of the skin. Hair loss is common on the lower leg, feet, and toes. Pallor and a temperature gradient may be present as a line of demarcation between areas that have adequate arterial perfusion and areas that have poor perfusion. Wasting of muscle or soft tissue may be seen. As atherosclerotic arterial disease progresses, skin ulcerations and gangrene can occur.

Medical Management

Medical therapy is geared toward controlling or eliminating risk factors and suggesting alterations in lifestyle to promote rest and pain relief. Pharmacologic management may include the use of anticoagulants, vasodilators, antiplatelet agents, anti-lipid agents, and similar medications used to treat other atherosclerotic conditions.[100–102] If pharmacological therapies do not produce positive results, the patient may be a candidate for interventional, or surgical procedures. Percutaneous transluminal angioplasty or stent placement is effective when the lesion (blockage) is discrete and localized. However, if the arterial disease is diffuse, bypass surgery is usually performed. If gangrene (cell death) is present, limb or partial limb amputation is required.

BOX 13.33 DIAGNOSIS AND PATIENT CARE MANAGEMENT

Peripheral Artery Disease

- Acute pain due to transmission and perception of cutaneous, visceral, muscular, or ischemic impulses
- Impaired peripheral tissue perfusion due to decreased blood flow
- Activity intolerance due to prolonged immobility or deconditioning
- Anxiety due to threat from biologic, psychologic, or social integrity
- Lack of knowledge of treatment regime due to lack of previous exposure to information (see Box 13.34, Patient and Family Education Plan: Peripheral Artery Disease)

Patient Care Management plans are located in Appendix A.

Nursing Management

Nursing care management for a patient with PAD incorporates a variety of patient diagnoses (Box 13.33). Nurses assess the quality of the peripheral artery pulses, intervene to maintain skin integrity, to control pain, and to educate the patient and family about peripheral arterial disease. See Appendix A for patient care management plans specific to patients with PAD.

Arterial Pulses

Assessments of peripheral pulses, limb color, and temperature are critical for the evaluation of an ischemic limb. Arterial pulses are typically diminished, or absent distal to the site of occlusion. Patients with diabetes have a much higher incidence of peripheral vascular disease (arterial and venous) compared with the general population. Most hospitals use a standard scale to improve documentation of pulses. If the pulse cannot be palpated, Doppler ultrasonography may be used to assess blood flow.

Skin Integrity

Care is taken to protect the limb from injury and development of pressure injuries. Healing is often impaired because of poor arterial blood flow or diabetes. Feet may be protected from injury by cotton or lamb's wool placed between the toes or by a bed cradle. However, for an acute ischemic limb, emergent removal of the thrombus is the only treatment that can salvage ischemic tissue.

Pain Control

The term *intermittent claudication* refers to pain during exercise in the presence of PAD. Leg pain that occurs after exercise, caused by increased muscle oxygen demand, can be effectively managed by stopping the exertion. However, pain at rest (without exercise) is a warning sign of an anoxic limb. The pain of an acute ischemic limb is extreme, and morphine is used for pain control. Ultimately, removal of the arterial obstruction is the only method to eliminate the pain. See Chapter 7 for more in-depth information on pain management.

Educate the Patient and Family

Education topics include risk factor modification that emphasizes similar lifestyle changes to those recommended for patients with CAD, including smoking cessation, promoting exercise, maintenance of ideal body weight, inspection of the feet and legs, foot care, avoidance of foot trauma, and medications. Many patients with PAD underestimate their risk of stroke or STEMI and do not understand that the risk factors for PAD are

BOX 13.34 PATIENT AND FAMILY EDUCATION PLAN

Peripheral Artery Disease

Before discharge, the patient should be able to teach back the following topics:

- Pathophysiology of peripheral artery disease
- Daily inspection and care of feet and legs
- Avoidance of trauma to feet or legs
- Increase walking distance gradually
- Risk factor modification: After the acute episode, if the cause of peripheral artery disease is atherosclerosis, an individual risk factor profile is developed for each patient. Strategies to discuss include decrease daily fat intake to less than 30% of total calories, achieve total blood cholesterol level of less than 200 mg/dL, stop smoking, reduce salt intake, control hypertension, control diabetes if patient has diabetes, increase physical activity, achieve and maintain ideal body weight.
- Preprocedure teaching about angiogram, percutaneous angioplasty, or stent placement in the lower extremities
- Risks and benefits of fibrinolytic therapy for acute peripheral artery occlusion
- Preoperative teaching for revascularization surgery
- Rehabilitation education, if amputation is indicated
- Medications:
  - Antithrombotic therapy: usually aspirin to decrease platelet adhesiveness
  - Low-density lipoprotein cholesterol lipid-lowering agents: Statins
  - Antihypertensive agents: antihypertensive medications and how to self-monitor blood pressure
- Symptoms to report to a health care professional: pain (chest or legs), leg or foot trauma
- Follow-up care after discharge

the same risk factors for all of the cardiovascular atherosclerotic diseases.[100–102] Walking is good exercise for increasing blood flow to the lower extremities and is highly recommended for patients with PAD.[100–102]

If a surgically implanted prosthetic bypass graft is in place, teaching must include information about IE precautions. If the patient has diabetes, education about diabetes management is included in the education plan. Box 13.34 lists the salient points to include when teaching patients and families about PAD. Symptoms of PAD are listed in Box 13.35.

CAROTID ARTERY DISEASE

Description and Etiology

The bifurcation of the carotid arteries is a common site of atherosclerotic plaque development (Fig. 13.26). Because these arterioles carry the blood supply to the brain, when they are obstructed, the presenting symptoms are neurologic. Treating carotid artery disease, a readily treatable obstruction, can prevent a stroke. Blood supply to the brain is provided by two separate arterial systems: (1) the vertebral arteries and (2) the internal carotid arteries, whose branches anastomose to form the circle of Willis. Any abrupt interruption in circulation for 4 to 6 minutes can produce permanent brain damage. When circulation to an area is impaired gradually, collateral circulation is often able to develop and maintain an adequate supply of blood to that area of the brain. Abrupt interruption in blood supply leads to an area of brain tissue becoming ischemic and often permanently damaged.

BOX 13.35 Evidence-Based Practice

Peripheral Artery Disease

Peripheral artery disease (PAD) affects millions of older adults in the United States. An international multidisciplinary group of clinicians summarized evidence from clinical trials develop clinical guidelines.

Recommendations to Increase Awareness of PAD and Its Consequences

- Patients who are at highest risk of developing PAD are patients who smoke cigarettes, have diabetes, and are older. In screening asymptomatic patients in high-risk groups, 30% to 50% of patients have PAD and do not know it.
- Other PAD risk factors include hypertension, hyperlipidemia, male sex, elevated C-reactive protein levels, elevated plasma fibrinogen levels, elevated blood glucose, prior myocardial infarction (MI), heart failure, and history of transient ischemic attack or stroke.
- Patients with symptomatic PAD had a four to five times increased risk of stroke and a 20% to 60% increased risk of MI with a twofold to sixfold increased risk of death from coronary heart disease compared with patients without PAD.
- Many patients are unaware of the link between PAD and cardiac and cerebrovascular atherosclerotic disease.

Recommendations to Improve Identification of Patients With Symptomatic PAD

- Because PAD is asymptomatic in the early stages of the disease, the ankle-brachial index is recommended as a screening tool in high-risk patients. (See text for information on how to measure the ABI.)
- If the diagnosis is not made until the patient complains of intermittent claudication (pain with walking), the disease is already at an advanced stage.

Recommendations to Treat Risk Factors Associated With PAD

- Smokers should stop smoking. This is not easy to do. Physician advice with frequent follow-up and pharmacologic therapy (nicotine replacement and bupropion) demonstrate 1-year success rates of 5%, 16%, and 30%.
- If the patient is hyperlipidemic, a normal lipid panel needs to be achieved: Reduce total serum cholesterol to less than 200 mg/dL and low-density lipoprotein cholesterol to less than 70 mg/dL.
- Studies have not specifically examined the effect of controlling hypertension and diabetes on rates of PAD. However, extrapolating from the cardiac literature, researchers recommend reducing blood pressure to less than 130/80 mg Hg and maintaining blood glucose within the normal range (70–110 mg/dL; hemoglobin A_{1c} ≤7%).
- Low-dose aspirin or another platelet inhibitor medication is recommended.
- Exercise rehabilitation is recommended with promotion of daily walking. The goal is to increase the ability of the patient to walk longer distances without leg pain.

References

Aboyans V, Ricco JB, Bartelink MLEL, et al. 2017 ESC Guidelines on the Diagnosis and Treatment of Peripheral Arterial Diseases, in collaboration with the European Society for Vascular Surgery (ESVS): Document covering atherosclerotic disease of extracranial carotid and vertebral, mesenteric, renal, upper and lower extremity arteries. Endorsed by: the European Stroke Organization (ESO)The Task Force for the Diagnosis and Treatment of Peripheral Arterial Diseases of the European Society of Cardiology (ESC) and of the European Society for Vascular Surgery (ESVS). *Eur Heart J.* 2018;39(9):763–816. https://doi.org/10.1093/eurheartj/ehx095.

Abramson BL, Al-Omran M, Anand SS, et al. Canadian Cardiovascular Society 2022 Guidelines for Peripheral Arterial Disease. *Can J Cardiol.* 2022;38(5):560–587. https://doi.org/10.1016/j.cjca.2022.02.029.

Kearon C, Akl EA, Comerota AJ, et al. Antithrombotic therapy for VTE diseases, antithrombotic therapy and prevention of thrombosis, 9th ed. American College of Chest Physicians evidence-based clinical practice guidelines. *Chest.* 2012;141(Suppl 2):e419S.

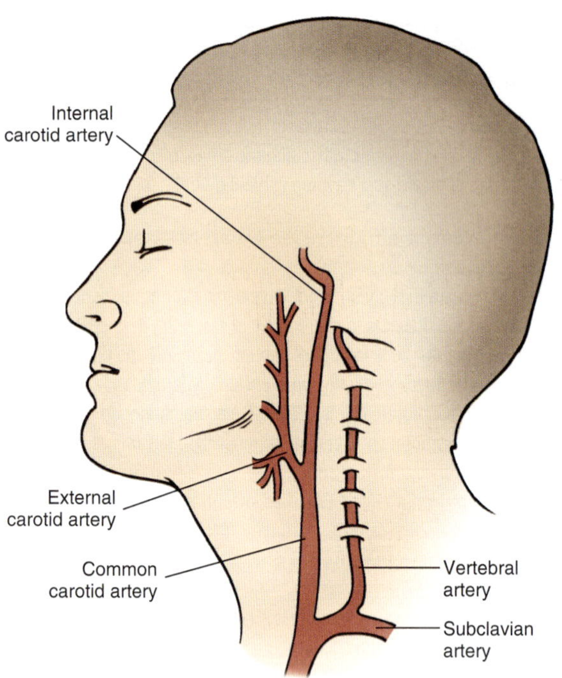

FIG. 13.26 Common, Internal, and External Carotid Arteries. Atherosclerotic Plaque develops in the Common Carotid Artery at the Bifurcation into the Internal and External Carotid Arteries. Plaque can develop in the common, Internal, and External Carotid Arteries.

Pathophysiology

The most common cause of carotid artery disease is atherosclerosis.[103] Uncommon causes include fibromuscular dysplasia, irradiation, and arteritis. The risk factors for development of atherosclerotic carotid artery disease and stroke are similar to those for CAD and PAD. Patients with any of these conditions must be educated about the other disease processes as well.

Modifiable risk factors include uncontrolled hypertension (systolic BP greater than 160 mm Hg), atrial fibrillation, smoking, diabetes, and hyperlipidemia.[103] The incidence of carotid stenosis increases with age and coexisting CAD increases the incidence of stroke for both men and women.[103] Women taking estrogen supplements after menopause also increased their risk of stroke.[103]

Atherosclerotic changes in the carotid arteries create ischemic symptoms are embolization and thrombosis. Ulcerated carotid lesions with accumulated platelet and fibrin produce thrombi that travel along with cholesterol deposits to become emboli to the brain. Stenotic areas in the carotid arteries are prone to thrombosis because of sluggish flow across the lesions. Doppler studies can examine the carotid arteries noninvasively. If a stroke is suspected, an emergency CT scan of the head is the appropriate diagnostic test.[103]

Carotid artery disease can remain asymptomatic for many years. After emboli are dislodged, the manifestations of carotid artery disease are neurologic and include hemiparesis, dysphasia, dysarthria, global aphasia, diplopia, vertigo, syncope, confusion, and monocular blindness. Neurologic symptoms that resolve completely within a short time are classified as *transient ischemic attacks* (TIAs). Symptoms that do not resolve are described as ischemic strokes.[103] Additional information on the neurologic management of the patient experiencing a stroke is provided in Chapter 22. Screening for asymptomatic carotid artery stenosis is not recommended.[104]

BOX 13.36 DIAGNOSIS AND PATIENT CARE MANAGEMENT

Carotid Artery Disease

- Acute pain due to transmission and perception of cutaneous, visceral, muscular, or ischemic impulses
- Ineffective tissue perfusion due to decreased cerebral blood flow
- Anxiety due to threat from biologic, psychologic, or social integrity
- Lack of knowledge of treatment regime due to lack of previous exposure to information (see Box 13.37, Patient and Family Education Plan: Carotid Artery Disease)

Patient Care Management plans are located in Appendix A.

Medical Management

Medical management is focused on reducing the atherosclerotic risk factors that can be controlled by the patient. This includes regulation of hypertension, smoking cessation, seeking medical attention for treatable cardiac abnormalities such as atrial fibrillation, reducing weight, and reducing the cholesterol level to less than 200 mg/dL. Antithrombotic therapy is prescribed for atrial fibrillation because of the risk of embolic stroke.[46,103]

Both coronary stent placement and coronary artery endarterectomy (CEA) can successfully restore carotid artery patency,[105] and both reduce the risk of future stroke.[106] Patients with carotid artery stenosis need to be informed about the risks involved with any procedure and their risk for future cerebrovascular events such as stroke.

Nursing Management

Nursing care management for a patient with carotid artery disease incorporates a variety of patient diagnoses (Box 13.36). Nursing management is focused on assessment of adequate cerebral perfusion, represented by vital signs, respiratory pattern, level of consciousness, pupil reaction, pupil size, and possible cranial nerve deficits manifested by difficulty in swallowing, loss of gag reflex, changes in speech, and loss of facial symmetry. The *National Institutes of Health Stroke Scale* (NIHSS) is used to predict patient outcome on initial and ongoing assessment of TIA and stroke-related symptoms in the critical care unit. The nurse educates the patient and family about the causes of the current event and provides information on preventing further cerebrovascular events. See Appendix A for patient care management plans specific to patients with carotid artery disease.

Neurologic Assessment

Neurologic assessment of a patient with carotid artery disease is divided into two parts: (1) level of consciousness, mental alertness, and cerebral perfusion and (2) cranial nerve function. A neurologic assessment is performed to ensure that the patient has not experienced a TIA or stroke. Questions to ascertain level of consciousness relate to time and place and reason for hospital admission. Mental alertness is assessed by the patient's ability to respond to these and other questions. The person is asked to move all four limbs on command. To assess specific cranial nerves, the patient is asked to make a grimace, which should

BOX 13.37 PATIENT AND FAMILY EDUCATION PLAN

Carotid Artery Disease

Before discharge, the patient should be able to teach back the following topics:

- Pathophysiology of atherosclerotic carotid artery disease
- Pathophysiology of embolic stroke (emboli from carotid artery)
- Warning signs of impending stroke
- Risk factor modification: After the acute episode, if the cause of carotid artery disease is atherosclerosis, an individual risk factor profile is developed for each patient; strategies to discuss include decrease daily fat intake to less than 30% of total calories, achieve total blood cholesterol level of less than 200 mg/dL, stop smoking, reduce salt intake, control hypertension, control diabetes if patient has diabetes, increase physical activity, achieve and maintain ideal body weight.
- Signs and symptoms to report to a health care professional
- Follow-up care after discharge

demonstrate bilateral facial symmetry; to stick out the tongue to ensure it is midline; and to swallow and speak, which should be done without difficulty (see Cranial Nerves in Chapter 20 and Rapid Neurologic Examination in Chapter 21).

Educate the Patient and Family

If a patient who has known carotid artery disease and has not had a cerebrovascular event is admitted to a critical care unit, preventive education is essential. It is important to discuss the mechanism of stroke in carotid artery disease. A stroke is most often caused by an embolic thrombus that has traveled in the bloodstream to a specific area of the brain. The thrombus may have originated in the atria during an episode of atrial fibrillation or in the carotid arteries. In the carotid arteries, a thrombus can develop across the narrowed carotid artery lumen, reducing flow and causing widespread cerebral hypoperfusion. Many patients who have atherosclerotic carotid artery disease also have CAD or PAD and diabetes or hypertension.[103] The major areas of patient education are listed in Box 13.37. Recommendations for prevention of carotid artery disease are listed in Box 13.38.

BOX 13.38 Evidence-Based Practice

Carotid Artery Disease

Recommendations for Prevention of Carotid Artery Disease

- Smokers should stop smoking and avoid exposure to environmental tobacco smoke (secondhand tobacco smoke); smoking doubles the risk of stroke.
- Achieve a normal blood pressure (BP), preferably less than 120/80 mm Hg, for individuals at high risk of stroke. Oral antihypertensive medications are prescribed if the target BP is not met with diet and exercise alone. Reduction of BP greatly reduces stroke incidence.
- Achieve and maintain normal weight. The target weight-to-height ratio is a body mass index (BMI) between 18.5 kg/m^2 and 24.9 kg/m^2. Obesity is defined as a BMI above 25 kg/m^2. Obese patients are also identified as having a large waist circumference—more than 40 inches for men or more than 35 inches for women.
- Have serum lipids checked and attain a normal lipid profile. Many patients are prescribed lipid-lowering medications to achieve these goals:
- Total cholesterol goal below 200 mg/dL
- Low-density lipoprotein cholesterol goal below 70 mg/dL if patient has cardiovascular disease risk factors (all patients with carotid artery disease are likely to fall in this category), diabetes, or kidney disease
- Triglycerides goal below 150 mg/dL
- Normal fasting blood glucose level goal should be between 70 mg/dL and 110 mg/dL. If the patient has diabetes, hemoglobin A_{1c} should be near normal or less than 7%.
- A healthy diet should be instituted. Reduce saturated fat and add fruits and vegetables. Add omega-3 fatty acids as part of the treatment regimen to lower elevated triglycerides.
- Regular exercise is essential. The goal is at least three times weekly.

Recommended Medications for Carotid Artery Disease

- Aspirin (50–325 orally each day) or other platelet-inhibitor medications are recommended. The combination of aspirin plus extended-release dipyridamole and clopidogrel monotherapy are acceptable options for initial antiplatelet therapy.
- The statin class of medications is recommended to aggressively lower lipid levels.
- Antihypertensive medications are used to lower BP into normal range.

Recommended Interventions for Carotid Artery Disease

Asymptomatic Patients

- Medical therapy without revascularization is recommended for low-grade carotid stenosis, which is defined as a carotid artery narrowed to less than 60% in asymptomatic patients.
- Carotid endarterectomy and optimal medical therapy are recommended for carotid stenosis greater than 60% in asymptomatic patients with low operative risk.

Symptomatic Patients

- Medical therapy without revascularization is recommended for low-grade carotid stenosis, defined as a carotid artery narrowed to less than 50% in patients with symptoms.
- Carotid endarterectomy and optimal medical therapy are recommended for carotid stenosis greater than 50% in patients with symptoms.

References

Brott TG, Howard G, Roubin GS, et al. Long-term results of stenting versus endarterectomy for carotid-artery stenosis. *N Engl J Med.* 2016;374:1021–1031.

Meschia JF, Bushnell C, Boden-Albala B, et al. Guidelines for the primary prevention of stroke: a guideline for healthcare professionals from the American Heart Association/American Stroke Association. *Stroke.* 2014;45(12):3754–3832.

VENOUS THROMBOEMBOLISM

Description and Etiology

Venous thromboembolism (VTE) comprises two related conditions, DVT and PE. DVT is a clot (thrombus) that forms in a large vein in the leg, pelvis, and, less commonly, the arm. It is often accompanied by inflammation, pain, tenderness, and redness at the site of the thrombus. The concern is that the thrombus may migrate as a VTE through the venous circulation to the pulmonary vascular bed, causing a PE, development of pulmonary hypertension, or death.[107–109]

Etiology

VTE is the third most frequent acute cardiovascular event on a global scale, after acute MI and stroke.[108] Patients in the critical care are at high risk from invasive procedures, immobility, and vascular inflammation, including from sepsis.[110] Other risk factors for thrombus formation include advanced age, obesity, immobility, trauma, spinal cord injury, active cancer, major surgery, pregnancy, family history, heart failure, and sepsis. The incidence is similar for men and women, unless a person is taking a contraceptive pill or estrogen supplements with higher doses carrying increased thrombotic risk.[110]

Inherited coagulation disorders and hypercoagulability, also called *genetic thrombophilia*, confer a propensity for thrombus formation and increase the DVT risk in patients with this genetic inheritance.[110] More detailed information on heritable thrombophilias is found in Chapter 3.

Three major predisposing factors are traditionally described as *Virchow triad*:

- Stasis of blood
- Endothelial injury
- Hypercoagulability

Two of these three conditions usually must be present for thrombosis to occur. Patients in critical care units generally have several risk factors that predispose them to the development of a venous thrombus. The incidence of DVT increases with age and consequently increases the risk for acute PE[108] (see Pulmonary Embolism in Chapter 18).

Assessment and Diagnosis

Development of DVT is often the first risk factor for VTE. The DVT may be insidious and asymptomatic. Pain, if present, is described as an aching or throbbing sensation, which worsens with ambulation. A positive *Homans sign*, which is pain in the calf on dorsiflexion of the foot, heightens the suspicion of a DVT but is not considered a reliable marker. If DVT is present in the upper extremity, the entire arm swells. Other clinical manifestations include redness with swelling, increased skin temperature, dilation of superficial veins, and mottling and cyanosis caused by stagnant blood flow. In patients in the critical care unit, symptoms are often masked by intubation, sedation, and altered levels of consciousness.

Venous Ultrasound and d-Dimer

When DVT is suspected, noninvasive venous ultrasonography typically is performed to evaluate vein patency. If the thrombus is large and the vein is easy to visualize, the presence of a DVT can be confirmed by ultrasound alone. However, when the results are inconclusive, the addition of the d-dimer blood test increases diagnostic accuracy.

The d-dimer test measures the presence of cross-linked fibrin derivatives in the serum. If the normal d-dimer serum value is elevated, it signifies the presence of clots, but the thrombi could be located anywhere in the body. Ultrasonography can help localize the DVT. Together, these two tests represent a useful and powerful diagnostic strategy. When the d-dimer value is normal (not elevated), a DVT (or other thrombosis) can safely be ruled out.[108,110]

Diagnosis of Pulmonary Embolism

If PE is suspected, a CT scan of the thorax may be obtained. *Computed tomography pulmonary arteriography* (CTPA) with contrast has the greatest sensitivity and specificity for detecting emboli in the pulmonary arteries.[108] CTPA has now replaced traditional pulmonary angiography to diagnose PE.[108]

Ventilation-perfusion scintography (V/Q scan) can be helpful in the diagnosis if the lung fields are clear, but it is less helpful in critically ill patients with ARDS or pulmonary congestion. A normal perfusion scan result effectively rules out acute PE.[108]

Current guidelines recommend evaluating the risk factors for each patient on an individual basis. Maintaining a high index of suspicion and using thromboprophylaxis prevention for at-risk patients is essential. If VTE is suspected, clinical assessment, venous ultrasound, and d-dimer assay results can rapidly confirm or negate the presence of VTE.

Medical Management

Prevention of Venous Thromboembolism

Major therapeutic emphasis is placed on prophylaxis for critically ill patients at high risk for VTE.[104] Pharmacologic preventive measures include prophylactic anticoagulation with *subcutaneous LMWH* or IV UFH. Prevention also includes early mobility versus bed rest and use of sequential compression devices placed on the lower extremities.

Normally, the simple action of walking helps return blood to the right side of the heart and prevents venous stasis that may lead to development of venous thrombi. For critically ill patients, immobility is often imposed because of severity of the illness. Once over the critical period, most patients are assisted out of bed and helped to walk to restore the circulatory pump.

Management of Diagnosed Venous Thromboembolism

Initially, bed rest with elevation of the limb and anticoagulation therapy are recommended. Analgesics are prescribed to reduce discomfort.

Anticoagulation

Anticoagulants are prescribed to reduce further clotting. The risks and benefits of therapeutic anticoagulation are discussed with the patient and family before therapy begins. In the acute phase, VTE can be treated with IV heparin or subcutaneous LMWH. Recent guidelines recommend the direct-acting anticoagulant agents (DAOC) apixaban, dabigatran, edoxaban, or rivaroxaban instead of the traditional vitamin K antagonist (VKA) warfarin.[109] Antiplatelet therapy with aspirin or other medications may be added to prevent VTE recurrence; however, antiplatelet therapy alone does not provide protection against development of VTE. None of the antithrombotics described above will dissolve an existing clot; the intent is to prevent new thrombi from forming.

In an emergency, with a large acute PE and hemodynamic deterioration, thrombolytic therapy is an option.[108,109]

Catheter-directed fibrinolytic therapy has been used to lyse a thrombus in the ileofemoral artery when there is limited risk of bleeding.[110]

For patients who cannot be anticoagulated insertion of an *inferior vena cava filter* is an option. Clinical guidelines do not recommend combining anticoagulation and a filter.[109]

Nursing Management

Management for a patient with VTE incorporates a variety of patient diagnoses (Box 13.39). The focus of nursing interventions is to prevent the development of DVT. For patients with DVT, interventions include rest of the affected extremity, prevention of complications that may result from VTE, and monitoring of anticoagulant therapy. See Appendix A for patient care management plans specific to patients with VTE.

Activity With Deep Vein Thrombosis

Previously, it was thought that physical activity should be limited in a patient who has developed a DVT to prevent

BOX 13.39 DIAGNOSIS AND PATIENT CARE MANAGEMENT

Venous Thromboembolism

- Acute pain due to transmission and perception of cutaneous, visceral, muscular, or ischemic impulses
- Activity intolerance due to prolonged immobility or deconditioning
- Anxiety due to threat from biologic, psychologic, or social integrity
- Lack of knowledge of treatment regime due to lack of previous exposure to information (see Box 13.40, Patient and Family Education Plan: Venous Thromboembolism)

Patient Care Management plans are located in Appendix A.

BOX 13.40 PATIENT AND FAMILY EDUCATION PLAN

Venous Thromboembolism

Before discharge, the patient should be able to teach back the following topics:

- Pathophysiology of deep vein thrombosis
- Discuss risk of pulmonary embolus and need for antiembolism stockings or pneumatic compression devices on legs; avoid trauma to legs; report any chest pain, breathlessness, or increased respiratory rate
- Medications: anticoagulants to prevent formation of new thrombus at the site; aspirin to decrease platelet aggregation

dislodgment of emboli. Findings from more recent studies with support from updated treatment guidelines indicate that during the acute phase, self-care activities need not be limited once anticoagulation is initiated, and graduated ambulation is encouraged. Range-of-motion exercises can be performed with any unaffected limb. The patient is instructed to avoid bending at the knees or hips because this impedes venous return. Antiembolism stockings that have been custom fitted can be used. It is unclear when it is safe to resume normal activity such as walking after DVT. It is usually resumed after a Doppler study shows no evidence of DVT in the extremity and after symptoms have abated. Prevention strategies become important because the patient remains at risk for a recurrence. In general, early ambulation after surgery or other procedures and avoidance of bed rest are the most effective prevention strategies.

Risk of Pulmonary Embolism

The patient with a VTE is closely monitored for signs of PE and instructed to report immediately any chest pain, dyspnea, hemoptysis, or tachypnea. Risk factors for VTE are almost identical to risk factors for PE. For patients who must remain immobile because of their clinical condition, external pneumatic compression devices and low-dose heparin are commonly used. Complaints or observation of dyspnea or chest pain must be quickly evaluated to assess the risk of PE.

Anticoagulation

Anticoagulant therapy is monitored by obtaining daily coagulation values based on the specific anticoagulant.[103] Signs of bleeding are monitored, and symptoms treated promptly. For a critically ill patient, hemoglobin levels and hematocrit are monitored daily. Avoidable mechanical trauma is minimized. The alert patient should be instructed to use a soft toothbrush and, if needed, an electric razor.

Patients receiving anticoagulation therapy require careful assessment for bleeding, including testing stool and urine for the presence of occult blood; inspecting gums for bleeding; and when endotracheal suctioning is required, being gentle and assessing for the presence of blood in the aspirate.

Educate the Patient and Family

Patient education emphasizes VTE prevention for all patients who are immobile in the critical care unit for any length of time. This includes explanations about activity prophylaxis such as early ambulation after major surgery, external pneumatic compression boots, and low-dose heparin.

For patients who have a diagnosed DVT, education is focused on identifying symptoms to report, avoidance of trauma to the limb, and elevation of the limb to decrease venous pooling and increase blood flow. If the patient is on anticoagulation medications, the risks and benefits of this therapy are discussed along with the risk of VTE and pulmonary embolus. The patient is instructed to report any chest pain, shortness of breath, or respiratory distress (Box 13.40). A collaborative team of clinicians who are aware of current clinical recommendations is essential to provide effective care for all critical care patients at risk for VTE (Box 13.41).

HYPERTENSIVE EMERGENCIES

Description

Hypertensive emergency is defined as an acute severe increase in BP, higher than 180/120 mm Hg that results in acute end-organ damage.[104] Hypertensive emergency is life threatening and there is often a recognizable underlying cause. Additionally, with the advent of so many categories of antihypertensive medications, hypertensive emergencies can be effectively managed in the critical care setting.

These two forms of acute hypertension are recognized:

- *Hypertensive emergencies* pose a risk of end-organ damage and are life-threatening conditions. The target organs most often affected are the brain, heart, or the kidney.
- *Hypertensive urgencies* are characterized by a serious elevation in BP but without end-organ damage.

Etiology

The organs and conditions associated with hypertensive emergency are listed below[111]:

- Neurologic events (ischemic stroke; subarachnoid or intracerebral hemorrhage)
- Cardiovascular: Heart failure and pulmonary edema; Aortic dissection
- Pregnancy-induced eclampsia[112]
- Acute kidney failure[113]
- Drug-induced hypertension: Illegal drugs (cocaine or amphetamines)

Pathophysiology

The exact trigger of a hypertensive crisis may be unknown. However, most patients have been diagnosed with hypertension before the event, and the sudden rise in BP is often related to the underlying disease process. Clinical manifestations of hypertensive emergency are listed in Table 13.15.

BOX 13.41 Evidence-Based Practice

Venous Thromboembolism

Summary of Evidence-Based Recommendations for VTE Prevention

Strong evidence exists for the following:

- For highest risk patients, combine pharmacologic and mechanical prevention methods.
- All patients admitted to the critical care unit must be assessed for risk of venous thromboembolism (VTE).
- Most critically ill patients require thromboprophylaxis.
- Aspirin *alone* should not be used for VTE prophylaxis for any patient group.
- Pharmacologic thromboprophylaxis with low-dose unfractionated heparin *or* low-molecular-weight heparin (subcutaneous administration), fondaparinux *or* rivaroxaban
- Oral vitamin K agonists (warfarin) used to achieve a target international normalized ratio of 2.5 (INR range, 2–3). Warfarin may be replaced by an anticoagulant that does not require such intensive follow-up.
- Mechanical prophylaxis: graduated compression stockings or intermittent pneumatic compression devices
- Patients at highest risk for VTE include patients undergoing open urologic surgery, gynecologic surgery, or total hip or knee procedures; all trauma patients with at least one risk factor; and medical patients with acute heart failure or acute respiratory failure. Others included in this group are immobile patients confined to bed who have at least one risk factor.

References

Stevens SM, Woller SC, Kreuziger LB, et al. Antithrombotic therapy for VTE disease: second update of the CHEST guideline and expert panel report. *Chest.* 2021;160(6):e545–e608. https://doi.org/10.1016/j.chest.2021.07.055.

Konstantinides SV, Meyer G, Becattini C, et al. 2019 ESC Guidelines for the diagnosis and management of acute pulmonary embolism developed in collaboration with the European Respiratory Society (ERS): The Task Force for the diagnosis and management of acute pulmonary embolism of the European Society of Cardiology (ESC). *Eur Respir J.* 2019;54(3):1901647. https://doi.org/10.1183/13993003.01647-2019.

Kearon C, Akl EA, Comerota AJ, et al. Antithrombotic therapy for VTE disease: antithrombotic therapy and prevention of thrombosis, 9th ed: American College of Chest Physicians Evidence-Based Clinical Practice Guidelines. *Chest.* 2012;141(Suppl 2):e419s.

TABLE 13.15 Hypertensive Emergencies

Signa and Symptoms	Possible Causes
Cardiovascular	
Chest pain	Acute coronary syndrome (ACS), aortic dissection
Acute heart failure	Myocardial infarction, pulmonary edema
Neurologic	
Headache, papilledema, agitation, lethargy, delirium, seizures, coma	Hypertensive encephalopathy—ischemic stroke; subarachnoid hemorrhage (SAH); intracerebral hemorrhage (ICH); increased intracranial pressure (ICP)
Other Conditions	
Pregnancy	Eclampsia
Kidney failure	Dialysis missed—fluid overload. Malignant hypertension.
Catecholamine excess	Pheochromocytomas—adrenal tumor that secretes epinephrine/ norepinephrine
Medication related	Abrupt withdrawal of antihypertensive medications such as clonidine, guanabenz, or beta-blockers

Assessment and Diagnosis

Hypertensive emergency symptoms depend on the target organ involved, most frequently:

- Neurologic: Headache, blurred vision, change in level of consciousness, coma
- Cardiovascular: Chest pain, heart failure, pulmonary edema, aortic dissection
- Kidney: No urine output

Emergent diagnostic studies include taking BP measurement in both arms, as in aortic dissection there may be a marked difference between the two arms, and placement of an intraarterial line for close arterial pressure monitoring. A 12-lead ECG is taken to evaluate for STEMI or LVH.

Medical Management

Hypertensive Emergencies

Hypertensive emergencies are defined as an acute BP elevation greater than 180/120 mm Hg complicated by impending or progressive target organ dysfunction. Hypertensive emergencies necessitate admission to the critical care unit, where IV antihypertensive therapy can be administered, and BP monitored continuously with an arterial line.[114]

Initial goals of therapy in hypertensive emergencies are to reduce BP without compromising organ function.[115] Depending on the cause, this may involve lowering mean arterial BP by no more than 20% to 25% over a period of several minutes to several hours. This variability depends on the affected target organ and disease-specific guidelines for treatment. Guidelines for treating stroke do not recommend a rapid reduction of BP.

For a patient with CAD experiencing a hypertensive emergency, the need to maintain adequate diastolic BP to allow for coronary artery filling is paramount. If vasodilator therapy decreases the diastolic pressure too much, when coronary artery filling occurs, myocardial ischemia may result.

The question of how much to decrease the BP in a hypertensive emergency is not simply a matter of reading the number on the monitor from the patient's arterial line; it involves an assessment of the underlying pathology and an appreciation of the physiologic requirements of the affected target organ. If potent antihypertensive medications such as sodium nitroprusside or labetalol are being used, an arterial line must be inserted, and the medications must be infused through an infusion pump.[114]

Hypertensive Urgencies

Hypertensive urgencies may not necessitate admission to a critical care unit because organ damage is not evident, and the patient may be treated with rapid-acting oral antihypertensive agents. Many medication categories are available, including ACEi, ARBs, calcium channel blockers, and beta-blockers. A loop diuretic (e.g., furosemide) often is prescribed in addition to the antihypertensive agents when the patient has fluid retention.

Nursing Management

Nursing care management for a patient with hypertensive crisis is to return the BP to the desired range without introducing other complications because of therapy.[115] After hypertension is controlled, the underlying factors that resulted in this life-threatening condition must be controlled. Several patient diagnoses are associated with hypertensive crisis (Box 13.42). See Appendix A for patient care management plans specific to patients with hypertensive crises.

BOX 13.42 DIAGNOSIS AND PATIENT CARE MANAGEMENT

Hypertensive Emergency

- Ineffective tissue perfusion due to decreased cerebral blood flow
- Ineffective tissue perfusion due to decreased kidney blood flow
- Anxiety due to threat from biologic, psychologic, or social integrity
- Lack of knowledge of treatment regime due to lack of previous exposure to information (see Box 13.43, Patient and Family Education Plan: Hypertensive Emergency)

Patient Care Management plans are located in Appendix A.

BOX 13.43 PATIENT AND FAMILY EDUCATION PLAN

Hypertensive Emergency

Before discharge, the patient should be able to teach back the following topics:

- Pathophysiology of hypertensive crisis
- Normal and abnormal blood pressure values
- Self-monitoring of blood pressure at home
- Connection between hypertension and other atherosclerotic diseases such as coronary artery disease, peripheral artery disease (PAD), and cerebrovascular disease
- Warning signs of a "heart attack" or myocardial infarction
- Warning signs of a "stroke"
- Warning signs of intermittent claudication or PAD
- Risk factors modification: After the acute episode, if the cause of carotid artery disease is atherosclerosis, an individual risk factor profile is developed for each patient. Strategies to discuss include decrease daily fat intake to less than 30% of total calories, achieve total blood cholesterol level of less than 200 mg/dL, stop smoking, reduce salt intake, control hypertension, control diabetes if patient has diabetes, increase physical activity, achieve and maintain ideal body weight
- Medications: Antihypertensive medications, rationale, and side effects
- Signs and symptoms to report to a health care professional
- Follow-up care after discharge

Educate the Patient and Family

Patient education during the acute phase of a hypertensive emergency is limited to an explanation of the need to control BP and the purpose of the equipment used in the critical care unit. After the hypertensive crisis is resolved, the focus of education is on lifestyle changes to modify risk factors.[4] Hypertension is emphasized as a risk factor for atherosclerotic disease of the heart, brain, and peripheral artery system. The major points to discuss with the patient are listed in Box 13.43. Management of hypertensive emergencies and urgencies are presented in Box 13.44.

BOX 13.44 Evidence-Based Practice

Hypertensive Emergencies

Definition

Hypertensive emergency is defined as an acute blood pressure (BP) elevation greater than 180/120 mm Hg complicated by impending or progressive target organ dysfunction.

Recommendations

- Early identification of hypertensive emergency in the emergency department and admission to a critical care unit is recommended.
- Patients with hypertensive emergency should have continuous BP monitoring.
- Intravenous (IV) medications are used to reduce BP (not necessarily to normal) to prevent or limit target organ damage.
- Decreasing BP gradually is recommended to avoid cerebral, coronary, or kidney ischemia.
- Medications that cause rapid falls in BP are not recommended in the management of acute hypertensive emergency.
- Further gradual reductions in BP can be achieved by following target-organ guidelines.

Special Situations: Hypertension and Acute Ischemic Stroke

- For patients admitted with an ischemic stroke, no clinical evidence exists to support rapid reduction in BP.
- For patients with systolic blood pressure (SBP) greater than 220 mm Hg or DBP between 120 mm Hg and 140 mm Hg, BP should be lowered cautiously by 10% to 15% only.
- If DBP is greater than 140 mm Hg, sodium nitroprusside is recommended to cautiously lower SBP by approximately 10%.
- If SBP is greater than 185 mm Hg or DBP is greater than 110 mm Hg, the use of fibrinolytic therapy (tissue plasminogen activator [tPA]) is contraindicated within the first 3 h after an acute ischemic stroke. BP must be lowered before administration of tPA.
- Careful monitoring of the patient for signs of neurologic deterioration related to the lower BP is mandatory in all situations.

Ultimate Blood Pressure Target Goal

- Target BP is 130/80 mm Hg or lower for patients with known hypertension, kidney failure, diabetes, or cardiovascular disease. Almost all patients with these conditions require oral medications to achieve their target BP. Many patients require two or more oral medications.

References

Siddiqi TJ, Usman MS, Rashid AM, et al. Clinical outcomes in hypertensive emergency: a systematic review and meta-analysis. *J Am Heart Assoc.* 2023;12(14):e029355. https://doi.org/10.1161/JAHA.122.029355.

Garovic VD, Dechend R, Easterling T, et al. Hypertension in pregnancy: Diagnosis, blood pressure goals, and pharmacotherapy: a scientific statement from the American Heart Association. *Hypertension.* 2022;79(2):e21–e41. https://doi.org/10.1161/HYP.0000000000000208.

BOX 13.45 Internet Resources

Cardiovascular Disorders

- American Heart Association (AHA). Patient Education Resources: www.heart.org/en/professional/quality-improvement/ascvd/resources-for-healthcare-professionals
- American Thoracic Society. Pulmonary Hypertension Patient Education Resources: https://www.thoracic.org/patients/patient-resources/resources/pulmonary-hypertension.pdf
- Centers for Disease Control (CDC) and Prevention. Hypertension Patient Education Resources: https://www.cdc.gov/bloodpressure/materials_for_patients.htm

ADDITIONAL RESOURCES

Internet resources related to cardiovascular disorders are found in Box 13.45.

KEY POINTS

- The number of patients with CVD in the United States continues to grow.
- Research and clinical progress have clarified the diagnosis and management of many cardiac conditions.
- Atherosclerosis provides a common link among CAD, atherosclerotic aortic disease, PAD, and carotid artery disease. The risk factors and general management strategies for all these diseases are the same.
- STEMI, NSTEMI, aortic aneurysm, aortic dissection, and embolic stroke are acute manifestations of chronic disease progression.
- Heart failure is a consequence of damaged heart muscle that results from MI, cardiomyopathy, valve disease, or hypertension.

Coronary Artery Disease

- Progressive atherosclerotic buildup in coronary arteries results in narrowing of lumens and decreasing flow.
- Medical management focuses on lifestyle changes and symptom management, including anticoagulants and vasodilators to increase flow.
- Nursing management focuses on treating symptoms and providing patient education.

Acute Coronary Syndrome

- ACS is an umbrella term for the clinical presentation of ischemic coronary artery events.
- Medical management includes vasodilators and anticoagulation.
- Nursing management focuses on managing pain and symptoms, maintaining a calm environment, and providing patient and family education.

Myocardial Infarction

- MI is irreversible myocardial necrosis secondary to an abrupt decrease of total blood flow through coronary arteries.
- Medical management focuses on reestablishing flow through the arteries and preventing ventricular remodeling.
- Nursing management focuses on improving myocardial oxygen supply or decreasing myocardial demand, preventing complications, and providing patient and family education.

Cardiomyopathy

- Cardiomyopathy is a disease caused by structural abnormalities of the heart that affect cardiac function.
- Medical management focuses on relieving symptoms and preventing arrhythmias.
- Nursing management focuses on maintaining fluid balance, monitoring medication effects, improving mobility, and providing patient and family education.

Sudden Cardiac Death

- SCD refers to sudden death without previous symptoms of disease. The mechanism is most likely VT that evolves to VF.
- Medical management focuses on using hypothermia after a cardiac arrest procedure to protect the brain and rhythm management with probable insertion of an ICD device.
- Nursing management focuses on monitoring treatment effects, preventing complications, and providing patient and family education.

Heart Failure

- Heart failure is a response to cardiac dysfunction that results in impaired ability to eject blood from the ventricle.
- Medical management focuses on relieving symptoms, enhancing cardiac performance, and correcting the precipitating cause.
- Nursing management focuses on supporting optimal cardiopulmonary function, promoting comfort, providing emotional support, and providing patient and family education.

Pulmonary Hypertension

- PH is a progressive sustained increase in pulmonary pressures with resultant right heart failure and ultimately death.
- Medical management focuses on pharmacologic therapies and prevention of complications.
- Nursing management focuses on managing symptoms and providing education on medications and treatments, including intravenous site care.

Endocarditis

- IE is an infection on the endocardial surface of the heart, heart valves, or both.
- Medical management requires prolonged treatment with intravenous antibiotics. Some patients require excision of the involved valve for eradication of infection.
- Nursing management includes monitoring for worsening symptoms and providing patient and family education on the need for prolonged medication for treatment including intravenous site care.

Valvular Heart Disease

- Valvular heart disease comprises structural and functional abnormalities of cardiac valves.
- Medical management includes medications to control symptoms and surgical interventions to repair or replace involved valves.

- Nursing management focuses on titrating medications to improve flow through involved valves, monitoring patient symptoms and responses to treatment, and organizing patient care activities to prevent fatigue.

Atherosclerosis of the Aorta

- Aortic disease results from progressive atherosclerosis and hypertension and includes aneurysmal and local dilation of the wall and aortic dissection where blood separates the vascular layers.
- Medical management depends on symptoms and hemodynamics. Corrective surgery is indicated for aneurysms more than 5 cm wide. Acute dissection requires immediate control of hypertension and pain, and surgical correction is required for dissection of the ascending aorta.
- Nursing management focuses on monitoring for changes in cardiovascular status and administering medications for significant BP reduction and pain control.

Peripheral Artery Disease

- PAD includes chronic venous disease and acute arterial changes.
- Medical management focuses on controlling or eliminating risk factors; pharmacologic management including anticoagulants, vasodilators, and antiplatelets; and surgical interventions including percutaneous transluminal coronary angioplasty, stent placement, or vascular bypass.
- Nursing care includes assessment of pulses, maintenance of skin integrity, and pain control.

Carotid Artery Disease

- Carotid artery disease results in obstruction of the major extracranial arterial supply to the brain.
- Medical management focuses on limiting risks and performing surgical endarterectomy when obstruction is greater than 60%.
- Nursing management focuses on monitoring neurologic assessment and educating patients and family about stroke symptoms.

Venous Thromboembolism

- VTE includes DVT and PE with clot formation and obstruction of large vessels.
- Medical management focuses on prevention and treatment with anticoagulation.
- Nursing management focuses on prevention, encouraging early mobility as soon as possible, and monitoring the effects of anticoagulation.

Hypertensive Emergency

- Hypertensive emergency is defined as acute BP elevation greater than 180/120 mm Hg and is associated with end-organ damage causing stroke, subarachnoid or intracerebral hemorrhage, pulmonary edema and heart failure, or acute kidney failure.
- Medical management is aimed at use of appropriate medications to initially decrease BP by no more than 20% to 25% over several hours.
- Nursing management is focused on close monitoring of symptoms with judicious use of BP-lowering medications.

Visit the Evolve site at .elsevier.com/UrdenCCN for additional study materials.

REFERENCES

1. Tsao CW, Aday AW, Almarzooq ZI, et al. Heart disease and stroke statistics—2023 update: a report from the American Heart Association. *Circulation*. 2023;147(8). https://doi.org/10.1161/CIR.0000000000001123.
2. Benjamin EJ, Muntner P, Alonso A, et al. Heart disease and stroke statistics-2019 update: a report from the American Heart Association. *Circulation*. 2019;139(10):e56–e528. https://doi.org/10.1161/CIR.0000000000000659.
3. Vikulova DN, Grubisic M, Zhao Y, et al. Premature atherosclerotic cardiovascular disease: trends in incidence, risk factors, and sex–related differences, 2000 to 2016. *JAHA*. 2019;8(14):e012178. https://doi.org/10.1161/JAHA.119.012178.
4. Arnett DK, Blumenthal RS, Albert MA, et al. 2019 ACC/AHA guideline on the primary prevention of cardiovascular disease: a report of the American College of Cardiology/American Heart Association Task Force on Clinical Practice Guidelines. *Circulation*. 2019;140(11). https://doi.org/10.1161/CIR.0000000000000678.
5. Rossi LP, Granger BB, Bruckel JT, et al. Person-centered models for cardiovascular care: a review of the evidence: a scientific statement from the American Heart Association. *Circulation*. 2023;148(6):512–542. https://doi.org/10.1161/CIR.0000000000001141.
6. Pencina MJ, Navar AM, Wojdyla D, et al. Quantifying importance of major risk factors for coronary heart disease. *Circulation*. 2019;139(13):1603–1611. https://doi.org/10.1161/CIRCULATIONAHA.117.031855.
7. Timmis A, Kazakiewicz D, Townsend N, Huculeci R, Aboyans V, Vardas P. Global epidemiology of acute coronary syndromes. *Nat Rev Cardiol*. 2023;20(11):778–788. https://doi.org/10.1038/s41569-023-00884-0.
8. Wahrenberg A, Magnusson PK, Discacciati A, et al. Family history of coronary artery disease is associated with acute coronary syndrome in 28,188 chest pain patients. *Eur Heart J Acute*. 2020;9(7):741–747. https://doi.org/10.1177/2048872619853521.
9. Graham G. Racial and ethnic differences in acute coronary syndrome and myocardial infarction within the United States: from demographics to outcomes. *Clin Cardiol*. 2016;39(5):299–306. https://doi.org/10.1002/clc.22524.
10. Arnold SV, Bhatt DL, Barsness GW, et al. Clinical management of stable coronary artery disease in patients with type 2 diabetes mellitus: a scientific statement from the American Heart Association. *Circulation*. 2020;141(19). https://doi.org/10.1161/CIR.0000000000000766.
11. Fox CS, Golden SH, Anderson C, et al. Update on prevention of cardiovascular disease in adults with type 2 diabetes mellitus in light of recent evidence: a scientific statement from the American Heart Association and the American Diabetes Association. *Diabetes Care*. 2015;38(9):1777–1803. https://doi.org/10.2337/dci15-0012.
12. Joseph JJ, Deedwania P, Acharya T, et al. Comprehensive management of cardiovascular risk factors for adults with type 2 diabetes: a scientific statement from the American Heart Association. *Circulation*. 2022;145(9):e722–e759. https://doi.org/10.1161/CIR.0000000000001040.
13. Budoff M. Triglycerides and triglyceride-rich lipoproteins in the causal pathway of cardiovascular disease. *Am J Cardiol*. 2016;118(1):138–145. https://doi.org/10.1016/j.amjcard.2016.04.004.
14. Grundy SM, Stone NJ, Bailey AL, et al. 2018 AHA/ACC/AACVPR/AAPA/ABC/ACPM/ADA/AGS/APhA/ASPC/NLA/PCNA guideline on the management of blood cholesterol: a report of the American College of Cardiology/American Heart Association Task Force on Clinical Practice Guidelines. *Circulation*. 2019;139(25). https://doi.org/10.1161/CIR.0000000000000625.
15. Miller M, Stone NJ, Ballantyne C, et al. Triglycerides and cardiovascular disease: a scientific statement from the American Heart Association. *Circulation*. 2011;123(20):2292–2333. https://doi.org/10.1161/CIR.0b013e3182160726.
16. James PA, Oparil S, Carter BL, et al. 2014 evidence-based guideline for the management of high blood pressure in adults: report from the panel members appointed to the Eighth Joint National Committee (JNC 8). *JAMA*. 2014;311(5):507–520. https://doi.org/10.1001/jama.2013.284427.
17. Rosendorff C, Lackland DT, Allison M, et al. Treatment of hypertension in patients with coronary artery disease: a scientific statement from the American Heart Association, American College of Cardiology, and American Society of Hypertension. *Hypertension*. 2015;65(6):1372–1407. https://doi.org/10.1161/HYP.0000000000000018.

18. Mancia G, Kreutz R, Brunström M, et al. 2023 ESH guidelines for the management of arterial hypertension the Task force for the management of arterial hypertension of the European Society of Hypertension: Endorsed by the International Society of Hypertension (ISH) and the European Renal Association (ERA). *J Hypertens*. Published online June 21, 2023. https://doi:10.1097/HJH.0000000000003480
19. Virani SS, Newby LK, Arnold SV, et al. 2023 AHA/ACC/ACCP/ASPC/NLA/PCNA guideline for the management of patients with chronic coronary disease: a report of the American Heart Association/American College of Cardiology Joint Committee on Clinical Practice Guidelines. *Circulation*. 2023;148(9). https://doi.org/10.1161/CIR.0000000000001168.
20. Powell-Wiley TM, Poirier P, Burke LE, et al. Obesity and cardiovascular disease: a scientific statement from the American Heart Association. *Circulation*. 2021;143(21):e984–e1010. https://doi.org/10.1161/CIR.0000000000000973.
21. Piercy KL, Troiano RP, Ballard RM, et al. The physical activity guidelines for Americans. *JAMA*. 2018;320(19):2020–2028. https://doi.org/10.1001/jama.2018.14854.
22. Soeki T, Sata M. Inflammatory biomarkers and atherosclerosis. *Int Heart J*. 2016;57(2):134–139. https://doi.org/10.1536/ihj.15-346.
23. Mosca L, Benjamin EJ, Berra K, et al. Effectiveness-based guidelines for the prevention of cardiovascular disease in women—2011 update: a guideline from the American Heart Association. *Circulation*. 2011;123(11):1243–1262. https://doi.org/10.1161/CIR.0b013e31820faaf8.
24. Benjamin EJ, Muntner P, Alonso A, et al. Heart disease and stroke statistics—2019 update: a report from the American Heart Association. *Circulation*. 2019;139(10). https://doi.org/10.1161/CIR.0000000000000659.
25. Luijken J, van der Schouw YT, Mensink D, Onland-Moret NC. Association between age at menarche and cardiovascular disease: a systematic review on risk and potential mechanisms. *Maturitas*. 2017;104:96–116. https://doi.org/10.1016/j.maturitas.2017.07.009.
26. El Khoudary SR, Aggarwal B, Beckie TM, et al. Menopause transition and cardiovascular disease risk: implications for timing of early prevention: a scientific statement from the American Heart Association. *Circulation*. 2020;142(25). https://doi.org/10.1161/CIR.0000000000000912.
27. McSweeney JC, Rosenfeld AG, Abel WM, et al. Preventing and experiencing ischemic heart disease as a woman: state of the science: a scientific statement from the American Heart Association. *Circulation*. 2016;133(13):1302–1331. https://doi.org/10.1161/CIR.0000000000000381.
28. Mehta LS, Beckie TM, DeVon HA, et al. Acute myocardial infarction in women: a scientific statement from the American Heart Association. *Circulation*. 2016;133(9):916–947. https://doi.org/10.1161/CIR.0000000000000351.
29. Brown HL, Warner JJ, Gianos E, et al. Promoting risk identification and reduction of cardiovascular disease in women through collaboration with obstetricians and gynecologists: a presidential advisory from the American Heart Association and the American College of Obstetricians and Gynecologists. *Circulation*. 2018;137(24). https://doi.org/10.1161/CIR.0000000000000582.
30. Goff DC, Lloyd-Jones DM, Bennett G, et al. 2013 ACC/AHA guideline on the assessment of cardiovascular risk. *J Am Coll Cardiol*. 2014;63(25):2935–2959. https://doi.org/10.1016/j.jacc.2013.11.005.
31. Jebari-Benslaiman S, Galicia-García U, Larrea-Sebal A, et al. Pathophysiology of atherosclerosis. *Int J Mol Sci*. 2022;23(6):3346. https://doi.org/10.3390/ijms23063346.
32. Arora S, Patra SK, Saini R. HDL—a molecule with a multi-faceted role in coronary artery disease. *Clin Chim Acta*. 2016;452:66–81. https://doi.org/10.1016/j.cca.2015.10.021.
33. Lawton JS, Tamis-Holland JE, Bangalore S, et al. 2021 ACC/AHA/SCAI guideline for coronary artery revascularization: a report of the American College of Cardiology/American Heart Association Joint Committee on Clinical Practice Guidelines. *Circulation*. 2022;145(3). https://doi.org/10.1161/CIR.0000000000001038.
34. Aydin S, Ugur K, Aydin S, Sahin İ, Yardim M. Biomarkers in acute myocardial infarction: current perspectives. *VHRM*. 2019;15:1–10. https://doi.org/10.2147/VHRM.S166157.
35. Lupton JR, Quispe R, Kulkarni K, Martin SS, Jones SR. Serum homocysteine is not independently associated with an atherogenic lipid profile: the Very Large Database of Lipids (VLDL-21) study. *Atherosclerosis*. 2016;249:59–64. https://doi.org/10.1016/j.atherosclerosis.2016.03.031.
36. O'Gara PT, Kushner FG, Ascheim DD, et al. 2013 ACCF/AHA guideline for the management of ST-elevation myocardial infarction: a report of the American College of Cardiology Foundation/American Heart Association Task Force on Practice Guidelines. *Circulation*. 2013;127(4). https://doi.org/10.1161/CIR.0b013e3182742cf6.
37. Amsterdam EA, Wenger NK, Brindis RG, et al. 2014 AHA/ACC guideline for the management of patients with non–ST-elevation acute coronary syndromes: executive summary: a report of the American College of Cardiology/American Heart Association Task Force on Practice Guidelines. *Circulation*. 2014;130(25):2354–2394. https://doi.org/10.1161/CIR.0000000000000133.
38. De Luna AB, Cygankiewicz I, Baranchuk A, et al. Prinzmetal angina: ECG changes and clinical considerations: a consensus paper. *Noninvasive Electrocardiol*. 2014;19(5):442–453. https://doi.org/10.1111/anec.12194.
39. Pepine CJ. ANOCA/INOCA/MINOCA: open artery ischemia. *Am Heart J*. 2023;26:100260. https://doi.org/10.1016/j.ahjo.2023.100260.
40. Woudstra J, Vink CEM, Schipaanboord DJM, et al. Meta-analysis and systematic review of coronary vasospasm in ANOCA patients: prevalence, clinical features and prognosis. *Front Cardiovasc Med*. 2023;10:1129159. https://doi.org/10.3389/fcvm.2023.1129159.
41. Fordyce CB, Katz JN, Alviar CL, et al. Prevention of complications in the cardiac intensive care unit: a scientific statement from the American Heart Association. *Circulation*. 2020;142(22). https://doi.org/10.1161/CIR.0000000000000909.
42. Gulati M, Levy PD, Mukherjee D, et al. 2021 AHA/ACC/ASE/CHEST/SAEM/SCCT/SCMR guideline for the evaluation and diagnosis of chest pain: a report of the American College of Cardiology/American Heart Association Joint Committee on Clinical Practice Guidelines. *Circulation*. 2021;144(22):e368–e454. https://doi.org/10.1161/CIR.0000000000001029.
43. Namana V, Gupta SS, Abbasi AA, Raheja H, Shani J, Hollander G. Right ventricular infarction. *Cardiovasc Revasc Med*. 2018;19(1):43–50. https://doi.org/10.1016/j.carrev.2017.07.009.
44. Sandoval Y, Apple FS, Mahler SA, et al. High-sensitivity cardiac troponin and the 2021 AHA/ACC/ASE/CHEST/SAEM/SCCT/SCMR guidelines for the evaluation and diagnosis of acute chest pain. *Circulation*. 2022;146(7):569–581. https://doi.org/10.1161/CIRCULATIONAHA.122.059678.
45. Damluji AA, Van Diepen S, Katz JN, et al. Mechanical complications of acute myocardial infarction: a scientific statement from the American Heart Association. *Circulation*. 2021;144(2). https://doi.org/10.1161/CIR.0000000000000985.
46. January CT, Wann LS, Calkins H, et al. 2019 AHA/ACC/HRS focused update of the 2014 AHA/ACC/HRS guideline for the management of patients with atrial fibrillation: a report of the American College of Cardiology/American Heart Association Task Force on Clinical Practice Guidelines and the Heart Rhythm Society in collaboration with the society of thoracic surgeons. *Circulation*. 2019;140(2). https://doi.org/10.1161/CIR.0000000000000665.
47. Harikrishnan P, Gupta T, Palaniswamy C, et al. Complete heart block complicating ST-segment elevation myocardial infarction: temporal trends and association with in-hospital outcomes. *JACC Clin Electrophysiol*. 2015;1(6):529–538. https://doi.org/10.1016/j.jacep.2015.08.007.
48. Chiabrando JG, Bonaventura A, Vecchié A, et al. Management of acute and recurrent pericarditis: JACC state-of-the-art review. *J Am Coll Cardiol*. 2020;75(1):76–92. https://doi.org/10.1016/j.jacc.2019.11.021.
49. Campos ID, Salgado A, Azevedo P, Vieira C. Dressler's syndrome: are we underdiagnosing what we think to be rare? *BMJ Case Rep*. 2019;12(5):e227772. https://doi.org/10.1136/bcr-2018-227772.
50. Smolderen KG, Buchanan DM, Gosch K, et al. Depression treatment and 1-year mortality after acute myocardial infarction: insights from the TRIUMPH registry (translational research investigating

underlying disparities in acute myocardial infarction patients' health status). *Circulation*. 2017;135(18):1681–1689. https://doi.org/10.1161/CIRCULATIONAHA.116.025140.

51. Beatty AL, Beckie TM, Dodson J, et al. A new era in cardiac rehabilitation delivery: research gaps, questions, strategies, and priorities. *Circulation*. 2023;147(3):254–266. https://doi.org/10.1161/CIRCULATIONAHA.122.061046.
52. Dibben G, Faulkner J, Oldridge N, et al. Exercise-based cardiac rehabilitation for coronary heart disease. *Cochrane Database Syst Rev*. 2021;11(11):CD001800. https://doi.org/10.1002/14651858.CD001800.pub4.
53. Al-Khatib SM, Stevenson WG, Ackerman MJ, et al. 2017 AHA/ACC/HRS guideline for management of patients with ventricular arrhythmias and the prevention of sudden cardiac death: a report of the American College of Cardiology/American Heart Association Task Force on Clinical Practice Guidelines and the Heart Rhythm Society. *Circulation*. 2018;138(13). https://doi.org/10.1161/CIR.0000000000000549.
54. Sawyer KN, Camp-Rogers TR, Kotini-Shah P, et al. Sudden cardiac arrest survivorship: a scientific statement from the American Heart Association. *Circulation*. 2020;141(12). https://doi.org/10.1161/CIR.0000000000000747.
55. Heidenreich PA, Bozkurt B, Aguilar D, et al. 2022 AHA/ACC/HFSA guideline for the management of heart failure: a report of the American College of Cardiology/American Heart Association Joint Committee on Clinical Practice Guidelines. *Circulation*. 2022;145(18). https://doi.org/10.1161/CIR.0000000000001063.
56. Schwinger RHG. Pathophysiology of heart failure. *Cardiovasc Diagn Ther*. 2021;11(1):263–276. https://doi.org/10.21037/cdt-20-302.
57. Bozkurt B, Coats AJS, Tsutsui H, et al. Universal definition and classification of heart failure: a report of the Heart Failure Society of America, Heart Failure Association of the European Society of Cardiology, Japanese Heart Failure Society and Writing Committee of the Universal Definition of Heart Failure: Endorsed by the Canadian Heart Failure Society, Heart Failure Association of India, Cardiac Society of Australia and New Zealand, and Chinese Heart Failure Association. *Eur J Heart Fail*. 2021;23(3):352–380. https://doi.org/10.1002/ejhf.2115.
58. Baker C, Perkins SL, Schoenborn E, Biondi NL, Bowers RD. Pharmacotherapy considerations in heart failure with mildly-reduced ejection fraction. *J Pharm Pract*. 2023;36(1):155–163. https://doi.org/10.1177/08971900211027315.
59. Monzo L, Ferrari I, Cicogna F, et al. Sodium-glucose co-transporter 2 inhibitors in heart failure: an updated evidence-based practical guidance for clinicians. *Eur Heart J Suppl*. 2023;25(Suppl C):C309–C315. https://doi.org/10.1093/eurheartjsupp/suad055.
60. Felker GM, Ellison DH, Mullens W, Cox ZL, Testani JM. Diuretic therapy for patients with heart failure: JACC state-of-the-art review. *J Am Coll Cardiol*. 2020;75(10):1178–1195. https://doi.org/10.1016/j.jacc.2019.12.059.
61. Ojo A, Tariq S, Harikrishnan P, Iwai S, Jacobson JT. Cardiac resynchronization therapy for heart failure. *Interv Cardiol Clin*. 2017;6(3):417–426. https://doi.org/10.1016/j.iccl.2017.03.010.
62. Wasiak M, Tajstra M, Kosior D, Gąsior M. An implantable cardioverter-defibrillator for primary prevention in non-ischemic cardiomyopathy: a systematic review and meta-analysis. *Cardiol J*. 2023;30(1):117–124. https://doi.org/10.5603/CJ.a2021.0041.
63. Von Schwarz ER, He M, Bharadwaj P. Palliative care issues for patients with heart failure. *JAMA Netw Open*. 2020;3(2):e200011. https://doi.org/10.1001/jamanetworkopen.2020.0011.
64. Fabbri M, Murad MH, Wennberg AM, et al. Health literacy and outcomes among patients with heart failure: a systematic review and meta-analysis. *JACC Heart Fail*. 2020;8(6):451–460. https://doi.org/10.1016/j.jchf.2019.11.007.
65. Maron BJ, Desai MY, Nishimura RA, et al. Diagnosis and evaluation of hypertrophic cardiomyopathy: JACC state-of-the-art review. *J Am Coll Cardiol*. 2022;79(4):372–389. https://doi.org/10.1016/j.jacc.2021.12.002.
66. Ommen SR, Mital S, Burke MA, et al. 2020 AHA/ACC guideline for the diagnosis and treatment of patients with hypertrophic cardiomyopathy: executive summary: a report of the American College of Cardiology/American Heart Association Joint Committee on Clinical Practice Guidelines. *J Am Coll Cardiol*. 2020;76(25):3022–3055. https://doi.org/10.1016/j.jacc.2020.08.044.
67. Ottaviani A, Mansour D, Molinari LV, et al. Revisiting diagnosis and treatment of hypertrophic cardiomyopathy: current practice and novel perspectives. *J Clin Med*. 2023;12(17):5710. https://doi.org/10.3390/jcm12175710.
68. Ommen SR, Mital S, Burke MA, et al. 2020 AHA/ACC guideline for the diagnosis and treatment of patients with hypertrophic cardiomyopathy: executive summary: a report of the American College of Cardiology/American Heart Association Joint Committee on Clinical Practice Guidelines. *Circulation*. 2020;142(25):e533–e557. https://doi.org/10.1161/CIR.0000000000000938.
69. Bozkurt B, Colvin M, Cook J, et al. Current diagnostic and treatment strategies for specific dilated cardiomyopathies: a scientific statement from the American Heart Association. *Circulation*. 2016;134(23):e579–e646. https://doi.org/10.1161/CIR.0000000000000455.
70. Orphanou N, Papatheodorou E, Anastasakis A. Dilated cardiomyopathy in the era of precision medicine: latest concepts and developments. *Heart Fail Rev*. 2022;27(4):1173–1191. https://doi.org/10.1007/s10741-021-10139-0.
71. Schultheiss HP, Fairweather D, Caforio ALP, et al. Dilated cardiomyopathy. *Nat Rev Dis Primers*. 2019;5(1):32. https://doi.org/10.1038/s41572-019-0084-1.
72. Simonneau G, Montani D, Celermajer DS, et al. Haemodynamic definitions and updated clinical classification of pulmonary hypertension. *Eur Respir J*. 2019;53(1):1801913. https://doi.org/10.1183/13993003.01913-2018.
73. Ling Y, Johnson MK, Kiely DG, et al. Changing Demographics, epidemiology, and survival of incident pulmonary arterial hypertension: results from the pulmonary hypertension registry of the United Kingdom and Ireland. *Am J Respir Crit Care Med*. 2012;186(8):790–796. https://doi.org/10.1164/rccm.201203-0383OC.
74. Morrell NW, Aldred MA, Chung WK, et al. Genetics and genomics of pulmonary arterial hypertension. *Eur Respir J*. 2019;53(1):1801899. https://doi.org/10.1183/13993003.01899-2018.
75. Fessel JP, Loyd JE, Austin ED. The genetics of pulmonary arterial hypertension in the *post–BMPR2* era. *Pulm Circ*. 2011;1(3):305–319. https://doi.org/10.4103/2045-8932.87293.
76. Zamanian RT, Hedlin H, Greuenwald P, et al. Features and outcomes of methamphetamine-associated pulmonary arterial hypertension. *Am J Respir Crit Care Med*. 2018;197(6):788–800. https://doi.org/10.1164/rccm.201705-0943OC.
77. Hemnes AR, Trammell AW, Archer SL, et al. Peripheral blood signature of vasodilator-responsive pulmonary arterial hypertension. *Circulation*. 2015;131(4):401–409. https://doi.org/10.1161/CIRCULATIONAHA.114.013317.
78. Hadinnapola C, Bleda M, Haimel M, et al. Phenotypic characterization of *EIF2AK4* mutation carriers in a large cohort of patients diagnosed clinically with pulmonary arterial hypertension. *Circulation*. 2017;136(21):2022–2033. https://doi.org/10.1161/CIRCULATIONAHA.117.028351.
79. Vizza CD, Hoeper MM, Huscher D, et al. Pulmonary hypertension in patients with COPD. *Chest*. 2021;160(2):678–689. https://doi.org/10.1016/j.chest.2021.02.012.
80. Wiedenroth CB, Pruefer D, Adameit MSD, Mayer E, Guth S. Chronic thromboembolic pulmonary hypertension-medical, interventional, and surgical therapy. *Herz*. 2023;48(4):280–284. https://doi.org/10.1007/s00059-023-05172-8.
81. Humbert M, Kovacs G, Hoeper MM, et al. 2022 ESC/ERS Guidelines for the diagnosis and treatment of pulmonary hypertension. *Eur Respir J*. 2023;61(1):2200879. https://doi.org/10.1183/13993003.00879-2022.
82. Spikes LA, Bajwa AA, Burger CD, et al. BREEZE: open–label clinical study to evaluate the safety and tolerability of treprostinil inhalation powder as Tyvaso DPI™ in patients with pulmonary arterial hypertension. *Pulm Circ*. 2022;12(2):e12063. https://doi.org/10.1002/pul2.12063.
83. Hoeper MM, Badesch F, Ghofrani HA, et al. Phase 3 trial of sotatercept for treatment of pulmonary arterial hypertension. *N Engl J Med*. 2023;388(16):1478–1490. https://doi.org/10.1056/NEJMoa2213558.

84. Harky A, Zaim S, Mallya A, George JJ. Optimizing outcomes in infective endocarditis: a comprehensive literature review. *J Card Surg.* 2020;35(7):1600–1608. https://doi.org/10.1111/jocs.14656.
85. Baddour LM, Wilson WR, Bayer AS, et al. Infective endocarditis in adults: diagnosis, antimicrobial therapy, and management of complications: a scientific statement for healthcare professionals from the American Heart Association. *Circulation.* 2015;132(15):1435–1486. https://doi.org/10.1161/CIR.0000000000000296.
86. Wilson WR, Gewitz M, Lockhart PB, et al. Prevention of viridans group streptococcal infective endocarditis: a scientific statement from the American Heart Association. *Circulation.* 2021;143(20):e963–e978. https://doi.org/10.1161/CIR.0000000000000969.
87. Pettersson GB, Hussain ST. Current AATS guidelines on surgical treatment of infective endocarditis. *Ann Cardiothorac Surg.* 2019;8(6):630–644. https://doi.org/10.21037/acs.2019.10.05.
88. Alexis SL, Malik AH, George I, et al. Infective endocarditis after surgical and transcatheter aortic valve replacement: a state of the art review. *J Am Heart Assoc.* 2020;9(16):e017347. https://doi.org/10.1161/JAHA.120.017347.
89. Riasat M, Hanumanthu BKJ, Khan A, et al. Outcomes and survival of patients undergoing percutaneous vegetectomy for right heart endocarditis. *Int J Cardiol Heart Vasc.* 2023;47:101231. https://doi.org/10.1016/j.ijcha.2023.101231.
90. Otto CM, Nishimura RA, Bonow RO, et al. 2020 ACC/AHA guideline for the management of patients with valvular heart disease: executive summary: a report of the American College of Cardiology/American Heart Association Joint Committee on Clinical Practice Guidelines. *Circulation.* 2021;143(5):e35–e71. https://doi.org/10.1161/CIR.0000000000000932.
91. Nishimura RA, Otto CM, Bonow RO, et al. 2014 AHA/ACC guideline for the management of patients with valvular heart disease: a report of the American College of cardiology/American heart association Task force on practice guidelines. *J Am Coll Cardiol.* 2014;63(22):e57–e185. https://doi.org/10.1016/j.jacc.2014.02.536.
92. Nishimura RA, Otto CM, Bonow RO, et al. 2017 AHA/ACC focused update of the 2014 AHA/ACC guideline for the management of patients with valvular heart disease: a report of the American College of Cardiology/American Heart Association Task Force on Clinical Practice Guidelines. *Circulation.* 2017;135(25):e1159–e1195. https://doi.org/10.1161/CIR.0000000000000503.
93. Michelena HI, Della Corte A, Evangelista A, et al. Summary: international consensus statement on nomenclature and classification of the congenital bicuspid aortic valve and its aortopathy, for clinical, surgical, interventional, and research purposes. *J Thorac Cardiovasc Surg.* 2021;162(3):781–797. https://doi.org/10.1016/j.jtcvs.2021.05.008.
94. Vahanian A, Beyersdorf F, Praz F, et al. 2021 ESC/EACTS Guidelines for the management of valvular heart disease. *Eur Heart J.* 2022;43(7):561–632. https://doi.org/10.1093/eurheartj/ehab395.
95. Eleid MF, Nkomo VT, Pislaru SV, Gersh BJ. Valvular heart disease: new concepts in pathophysiology and therapeutic approaches. *Annu Rev Med.* 2023;74(1):155–170. https://doi.org/10.1146/annurev-med-042921-122533.
96. Shmueli H, Thomas F, Flint N, Setia G, Janjic A, Siegel RJ. Right-sided infective endocarditis 2020: challenges and updates in diagnosis and treatment. *J Am Heart Assoc.* 2020;9(15):e017293. https://doi.org/10.1161/JAHA.120.017293.
97. Isselbacher EM, Preventza O, Hamilton Black J, et al. 2022 ACC/AHA guideline for the diagnosis and management of aortic disease: a report of the American Heart Association/American College of Cardiology Joint Committee on Clinical Practice Guidelines. *Circulation.* 2022;146(24):e334–e482. https://doi.org/10.1161/CIR.0000000000001106.
98. Vilacosta I, San Román JA, di Bartolomeo R, et al. Acute aortic syndrome revisited: JACC state-of-the-art review. *J Am Coll Cardiol.* 2021;78(21):2106–2125. https://doi.org/10.1016/j.jacc.2021.09.022.
99. Bossone E, Eagle KA. Epidemiology and management of aortic disease: aortic aneurysms and acute aortic syndromes. *Nat Rev Cardiol.* 2021;18(5):331–348. https://doi.org/10.1038/s41569-020-00472-6.
100. Aboyans V, Ricco JB, Bartelink MLEL, et al. 2017 ESC Guidelines on the Diagnosis and Treatment of Peripheral Arterial Diseases, in collaboration with the European Society for Vascular Surgery (ESVS): document covering atherosclerotic disease of extracranial carotid and vertebral, mesenteric, renal, upper and lower extremity arteriesEndorsed by: the European Stroke Organization (ESO)The Task Force for the Diagnosis and Treatment of Peripheral Arterial Diseases of the European Society of Cardiology (ESC) and of the European Society for Vascular Surgery (ESVS). *Eur Heart J.* 2018;39(9):763–816. https://doi.org/10.1093/eurheartj/ehx095.
101. Abramson BL, Al-Omran M, Anand SS, et al. Canadian cardiovascular society 2022 guidelines for peripheral arterial disease. *Can J Cardiol.* 2022;38(5):560–587. https://doi.org/10.1016/j.cjca.2022.02.029.
102. Street TK. Ankle-brachial index for the assessment of peripheral arterial disease in the emergency department. *Adv Emerg Nurs J.* 2022;44(1):34–40. https://doi.org/10.1097/TME.0000000000000385.
103. Meschia JF, Bushnell C, Boden-Albala B, et al. Guidelines for the primary prevention of stroke: a statement for healthcare professionals from the American Heart Association/American Stroke Association. *Stroke.* 2014;45(12):3754–3832. https://doi.org/10.1161/STR.0000000000000046.
104. US Preventive Services Task Force, Krist AH, Davidson KW, et al. Screening for asymptomatic carotid artery stenosis: US Preventive Services Task Force Recommendation Statement. *JAMA.* 2021;325(5):476–481. https://doi.org/10.1001/jama.2020.26988.
105. Halliday A, Bulbulia R, Bonati LH, et al. Second asymptomatic carotid surgery trial (ACST-2): a randomised comparison of carotid artery stenting versus carotid endarterectomy. *Lancet.* 2021;398(10305):1065–1073. https://doi.org/10.1016/S0140-6736(21)01910-3.
106. Mueller C, McDonald K, de Boer RA, et al. Heart Failure Association of the European Society of Cardiology practical guidance on the use of natriuretic peptide concentrations. *Eur J Heart Fail.* 2019;21(6):715–731. https://doi.org/10.1002/ejhf.1494.
107. Kearon C, Akl EA, Comerota AJ, et al. Antithrombotic therapy for VTE disease: Antithrombotic Therapy and Prevention of Thrombosis, 9th ed: American College of Chest Physicians Evidence-Based Clinical Practice Guidelines. *Chest.* 2012;141(2 Suppl):e419S–e496S. https://doi.org/10.1378/chest.11-2301.
108. Konstantinides SV, Meyer G, Becattini C, et al. 2019 ESC Guidelines for the diagnosis and management of acute pulmonary embolism developed in collaboration with the European Respiratory Society (ERS): the Task Force for the diagnosis and management of acute pulmonary embolism of the European Society of Cardiology (ESC). *Eur Respir J.* 2019;54(3):1901647. https://doi.org/10.1183/13993003.01647-2019.
109. Stevens SM, Woller SC, Kreuziger LB, et al. Antithrombotic therapy for VTE disease: second update of the CHEST guideline and expert panel report. *Chest.* 2021;160(6):e545–e608. https://doi.org/10.1016/j.chest.2021.07.055.
110. Chopard R, Albertsen IE, Piazza G. Diagnosis and treatment of lower extremity venous thromboembolism: a review. *JAMA.* 2020;324(17):1765. https://doi.org/10.1001/jama.2020.17272.
111. Siddiqi TJ, Usman MS, Rashid AM, et al. Clinical outcomes in hypertensive emergency: a systematic review and meta-analysis. *J Am Heart Assoc.* 2023;12(14):e029355. https://doi.org/10.1161/JAHA.122.029355.
112. Garovic VD, Dechend R, Easterling T, et al. Hypertension in pregnancy: diagnosis, blood pressure goals, and pharmacotherapy: a scientific statement from the American heart association. *Hypertension.* 2022;79(2):e21–e41. https://doi.org/10.1161/HYP.0000000000000208.
113. Pothuru S, Chan WC, Mehta H, et al. Burden of hypertensive crisis in patients with end-stage kidney disease on maintenance dialysis: insights from United States renal data system database. *Hypertension.* 2023;80(4):e59–e67. https://doi.org/10.1161/HYPERTENSIONAHA.122.20546.
114. El Hussein MT, Dolynny A. Hypertensive emergencies: common presentations and pharmacological interventions. *Crit Care Nurs Q.* 2023;46(2):145–156. https://doi.org/10.1097/CNQ.0000000000000447.
115. Mathews EP, Newton F, Sharma K. CE: hypertensive emergencies: a review. *Am J Nurs.* 2021;121(10):24–35. https://doi.org/10.1097/01.NAJ.0000794104.21262.86.

14

Cardiovascular Therapeutic Management

Mary E. Lough, Nikki Taylor, Brandi Holcomb, and Daniel L. Arellano

http://evolve.elsevier.com/Urden/CriticalCareNursing

This chapter spans a wide arc of cardiac therapeutic devices and treatments. The content complements the previous cardiac disorders chapter, with an emphasis on nursing care management for each cardiac treatment, citing the latest evidence. The interventions encompass implanted devices for dysrhythmias and heart failure; percutaneous interventions to treat coronary, valvular, aortic, and peripheral arterial disease; surgical considerations; and medications for cardiovascular disease management. Because of the diversity of the content and the huge number of abbreviations used in cardiac care, a summary list of abbreviations and specialized acronyms is provided at the end of this chapter. This is in alignment with current cardiac guidelines published by professional societies that also now include an abbreviation summary list with all new guidelines.

PACEMAKERS

A pacemaker can initiate a heartbeat when the intrinsic electrical system of the heart cannot effectively generate a rate adequate to support cardiac output.[1] Pacemakers may be used temporarily, either supportively or prophylactically, until the condition responsible for the rate or conduction disturbance resolves. They also may be used on a permanent basis if the patient's condition persists despite adequate interventions. The use of permanent pacemakers as a form of device-based therapy has expanded significantly.[2]

This section emphasizes temporary pacemakers because the critical care nurse is responsible for preventing, assessing, and managing pacemaker malfunctions when these devices are used in the clinical setting. A brief discussion of permanent pacemakers is provided, and similarities between implanted and temporary pacemakers are presented where appropriate.

Therapeutic Indications for Temporary Pacing

The purpose of temporary cardiac pacing is to ensure or restore an adequate heart rate and rhythm. The clinical indications for instituting temporary pacemaker therapy are similar regardless of the cause of the rhythm disturbance that necessitates the placement of a pacemaker (Box 14.1).

The causes range from treatment of symptomatic bradycardia, electrolyte imbalances, bridge for permanent cardiac pacing, or for other indications such as myocardial infarction (MI) and injury to the conduction system following structural heart procedure such as transcatheter aortic valve implantation or cardiac surgery.[3–5] Dysrhythmias that are unresponsive to medications and result in compromised hemodynamic status are a definite indication for pacemaker therapy. Pacemakers function by electrically stimulating the myocardium to increase the heart rate for the treatment of bradyarrhythmias or to prevent or treat tachyarrhythmia.[6]

Prevent Conduction Disturbances

The goal of therapy in bradyarrhythmias is to increase the ventricular rate and enhance cardiac output. Temporary pacing may be used in the treatment of symptomatic bradycardia or progressive heart block that occurs as a result of acute myocardial ischemia, medication overdose, toxic agents, or intragenic causes.[7] After cardiac surgery, temporary pacing is used to improve a transiently depressed, rate-dependent cardiac output. Conduction disturbances that occur after valvular surgery can be managed effectively with temporary pacing.[3]

Overdrive Pacing

Overdrive pacing can be used to decrease the rate of a rapid supraventricular or ventricular tachyarrhythmia. This rapid pacing of the heart (i.e., overdrive pacing) functions to prevent the breakthrough ectopy that can result from a slow rate or to interrupt an ectopic focus and allow the natural pacemaker to regain control.[3]

Diagnostic Indications for Temporary Pacing

Temporary pacing is used during diagnostic studies to provoke and assess dysthymias. An electrophysiology study (EPS) is performed in a specialized cardiac catheterization laboratory that is equipped with pacing equipment. During the EPS, catheters with pacing electrodes are inserted to diagnose a patient's potential for dysrhythmias.[2] The electrodes are used to induce a dysrhythmia in patients with recurrent symptomatic tachycardias; this allows the physician to closely evaluate the dysrhythmia and determine appropriate therapy.

For patients who have ventricular tachycardias (VAs) that are refractory to conventional antiarrhythmic therapy, radiofrequency (RF) current catheter ablation of the responsible tissue can be done safely and effectively in the electrophysiology laboratory. After a mapping procedure has localized the site of arrhythmia formation, short bursts of RF current are delivered through the catheter, destroying the offending tissue with heat.

Ablation has also been shown to be an effective treatment for patients with symptomatic supraventricular tachycardia (SVT) that results from atrioventricular (AV) node reentry or accessory pathways. Catheter ablation is recommended for selected eligible patients with atrial fibrillation.[8,9]

BOX 14.1 Indications for Temporary Pacing

- Bradydysrhythmias
  - Sinus bradycardia and arrest
  - Sick sinus syndrome
  - Heart blocks
- Tachydysrhythmias
  - Supraventricular
  - Ventricular
- Permanent pacemaker failure
- Support of cardiac output after cardiac surgery
- Diagnostic studies
- Electrophysiology studies
- Atrial electrograms

Atrial Electrograms

Intracardiac electrograms are recordings of cardiac electrical activity obtained from pacing electrodes. These can provide useful diagnostic information. The *atrial electrogram* is an amplified recording of atrial activity that can be obtained using an atrial pacing electrode or an esophageal pill electrode and a standard electrocardiogram (ECG) machine. It may be used after cardiac surgery to facilitate the diagnosis of supraventricular dysrhythmias in patients with temporary atrial epicardial wires already in place.[10]

Pacemaker System

A pacemaker system is a simple electrical circuit consisting of a pulse generator and a pacing lead (an insulated electrical wire) with one, two, or three electrodes.

Pacing Pulse Generator

The pulse generator is designed to generate an electrical current that travels through the pacing lead and exits through an electrode (exposed portion of the wire) that is in direct contact with the myocardium. The electrical current initiates a myocardial depolarization. The current then seeks to return by one of several pathways to the pulse generator to complete the circuit.

The power source for a temporary external pulse generator is a standard alkaline battery inserted into the generator. Implanted permanent pacemaker batteries are usually long-lived lithium cells.

Pacing Lead Systems

The pacing lead used for temporary pacing may be bipolar or unipolar. In a bipolar system, two electrodes (positive and negative) are located within the heart, whereas in a unipolar system, only one electrode (negative) is in direct contact with the myocardium. In both systems, the current flows from the negative terminal of the pulse generator, down the pacing lead to the negative electrode, and into the heart. The current is then picked up by the positive electrode (ground) and flows back up the lead to the positive terminal of the pulse generator.

Bipolar lead systems. The bipolar lead used in transvenous pacing has two electrodes on one catheter (Fig. 14.1). The distal, or negative, electrode is at the tip of the pacing lead and is in direct contact with the heart, usually inside the right atrium (RA) or right ventricle (RV). Approximately 1 centimeter (cm) from the negative electrode is a positive electrode. The negative electrode is attached to the negative terminal, and the positive electrode is attached to the positive terminal of the pulse generator, either directly or by means of a bridging cable (see Fig. 14.1B).

An epicardial lead system is often used for temporary pacing after cardiac surgery. The bipolar epicardial lead system has two separate insulated wires (one negative and one positive electrode) that are loosely secured with sutures to the cardiac chamber to be paced. Both leads are in contact with the myocardial tissue, so either wire may be used as the negative, or pacing, electrode. The remaining wire is then used as the positive, or ground, electrode.

Unipolar lead systems. A unipolar pacing system (epicardial or transvenous) has only one electrode (the negative electrode) that makes contact with the heart. For a permanent pacemaker, the positive electrode can be created by the metallic casing of the subcutaneously implanted pulse generator (Fig. 14.2), or as is the case with a unipolar epicardial lead system, the positive electrode can be formed by a piece of surgical steel wire sewn into the subcutaneous tissue of the chest or the metal portion of a surface ECG electrode.

Because the unipolar pacing system has a wide sensing area because of the relatively long distance between the negative and positive electrodes, it has better sensing capabilities than a bipolar system. However, this feature makes the unipolar system more susceptible to sensing extraneous signals, such as the electrical artifacts created by normal muscle movements (i.e., myopotentials) or by external electromagnetic interference (EMI), which may result in inappropriate inhibition of the pacing stimulus.[11,12] This problem is of more concern in permanent pacing systems, in which the outer casing of the pacemaker generator may be used as a part of the pacing circuit. Because the pacemaker is located near a large muscle mass, upper body movement can result in the inappropriate sensing of myopotentials.

Pacing Routes

Several routes are available for temporary cardiac pacing (Box 14.2). Permanent pacing usually is accomplished transvenously, although when a thoracotomy is otherwise indicated, as in cardiac surgery, the physician may elect to insert permanent epicardial pacing wires.

Transcutaneous Cardiac Pacing

Transcutaneous cardiac pacing describes temporary external pacing using two large skin electrodes, one placed anteriorly and the other posteriorly on the chest; these are connected to an external temporary pulse generator.[13] This is a rapid, noninvasive procedure that nurses can perform in the emergency setting and is recommended in the Advanced Cardiac Life Support (ACLS) algorithm for the treatment of symptomatic bradycardia that does not respond to atropine. Improved technologies related to stimulus delivery and the development of large electrode pads that help disperse the energy have helped reduce the pain associated with cutaneous nerve and muscle stimulation. Discomfort may still be an issue for some patients, particularly when higher energy levels are required to achieve capture. This route is typically used as a short-term therapy until the situation resolves or another route of pacing can be established.[13]

Epicardial Pacing

The insertion of temporary epicardial pacing wires is a routine procedure during many cardiac surgical cases.[3,4] Ventricular and, in many cases, atrial pacing wires are loosely sewn to the epicardium. The terminal pins of these wires are pulled through

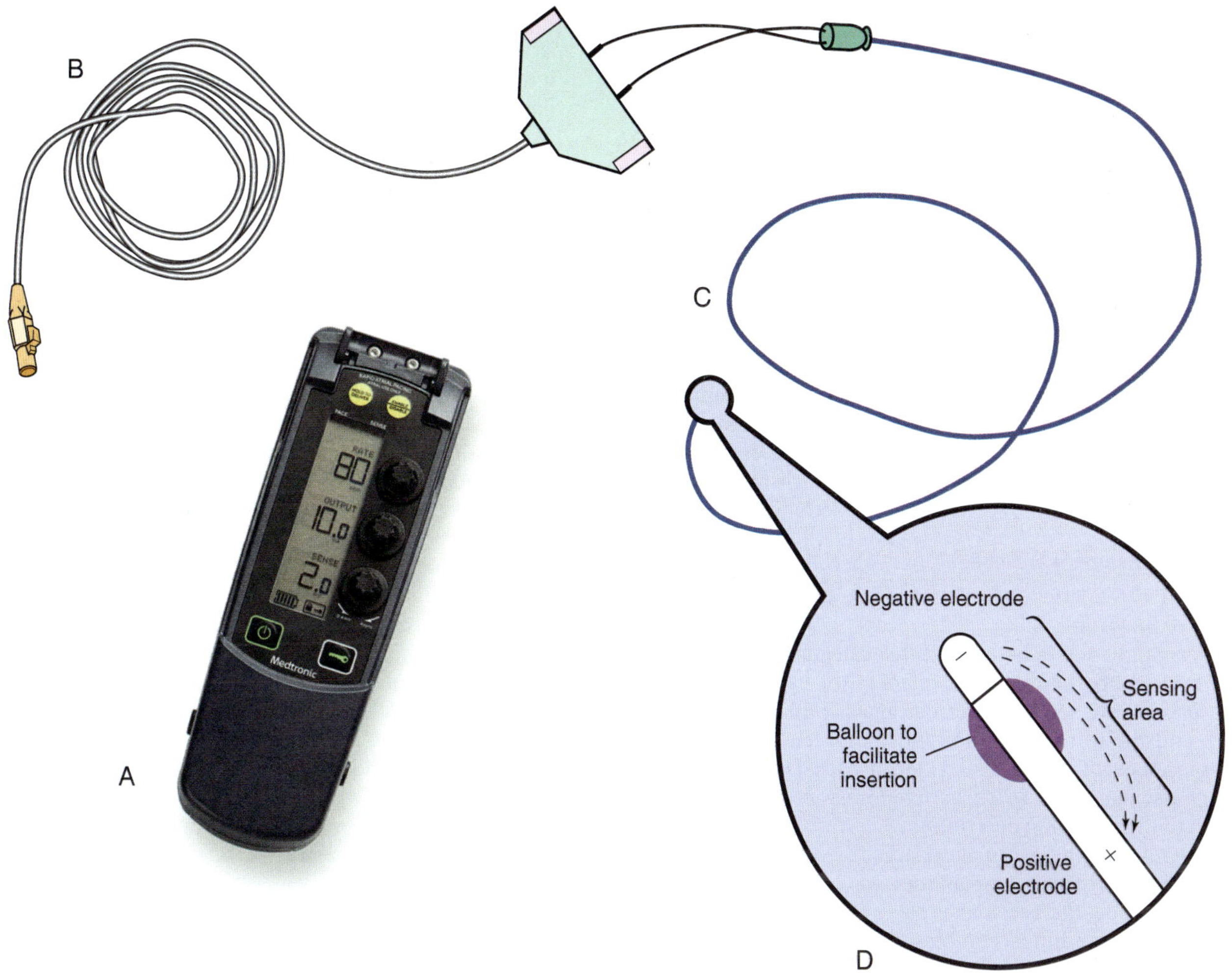

FIG. 14.1 (A) Single-chamber temporary (external) pulse generator (Medtronic model #53401). (B) Bridging cable. (C) Pacing lead. (D) Enlarged view of pacing lead tip. (©2024 Medtronic. All rights reserved. Used with the permission of Medtronic.)

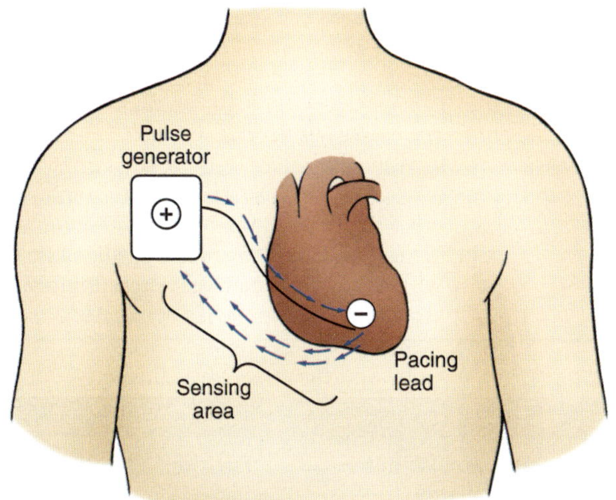

FIG. 14.2 Components of a Permanent Unipolar Transvenous Pacing System.

the skin before the chest is closed. If both chambers have pacing wires attached, the atrial wires exit subcostally to the right of the sternum, and the ventricular wires exit in the same region but to the left of the sternum. These wires can be removed several days after surgery by gentle traction at the skin surface.[4] Generally there is minimal risk of bleeding but complications can occur, the most serious being cardiac tamponade.[3]

BOX 14.2 Routes for Temporary Pacing

Transcutaneous
Emergency pacing is achieved by depolarizing the heart through the chest by means of two large skin electrodes.

Epicardial
Pacing electrodes are sewn to the epicardium during cardiac surgery.

Transvenous (Endocardial)
The pacing electrode is advanced through a vein into the right atrium and/or right ventricle.

Transvenous Endocardial Pacing

Temporary transvenous endocardial pacing is accomplished by advancing a pacing electrode wire via an introducer through a vein, often the subclavian or internal jugular vein, and into the RA or RV. Insertion can be facilitated through direct visualization with ultrasound, fluoroscopy, or using a standard ECG. In some cases, the pacing wire is inserted through a special pulmonary artery (PA) catheter by means of a port that exits in the RA or RV.[14]

Five-Letter Pacemaker Codes

In the 1960s, pacemaker terminology was limited to *fixed-rate* and *demand* pacing; *AV sequential* pacing was introduced in the early 1970s. Although these terms are still useful for understanding pacemaker function (Box 14.3), the continued expansion of functional capabilities of pulse generators has made it necessary to develop a more precise classification system. In 1974, the Inter-Society Commission for Heart Disease adopted a three-letter code for describing the various pacing modalities available. The code has since undergone several revisions, including the addition of two more letters representing programming characteristics and multisite pacing functions, to accommodate the development of newer devices that are rate responsive or that pace from more than one site within the atria and the ventricles. Table 14.1 describes the current five-letter code.[15]

Three-Letter Pacemaker Code

The original three-letter code is adequate to describe temporary pacemaker function.

The original code is based on three categories, each represented by a letter. The first letter refers to the cardiac chamber that is paced. The second letter designates which chamber is sensed, and the third letter indicates the pacemaker response to the sensed event. These three letters are used to describe the mode of pacing. Table 14.2 lists temporary pacing modes in addition to the following descriptions.

- In VOO mode, the pacemaker paces the ventricle at a fixed rate and has no sensing capabilities.
- In DOO mode, the pacemaker paces the atrium and ventricle at a fixed rate and has no sensing capabilities (emergency mode in cardiac arrest).
- In VVI mode, the pacemaker paces the ventricle when the pacemaker fails to sense an intrinsic ventricular depolarization and can sense a spontaneous ventricular depolarization that will inhibit ventricular pacing.
- In DDD mode, there are both atrial and ventricular leads used for both pacing and sensing.

In DDD mode, the pacemaker functions in both the atrium and the ventricle.

- **DDD Mode in the Atrium:** In response to sensed atrial activity (a sensed P wave), the atrial pacing circuit is inhibited from firing. A sensed P wave may also be used to trigger a ventricular pacing stimulus if normal conduction through the AV node is impaired. With no atrial activity, the pacemaker will fire.
- **DDD Mode in the Ventricle:** In response to sensed ventricular activity (a sensed R wave) inhibits the ventricular pacing circuit is inhibited from firing. With no ventricular activity, the pacemaker will fire.

Physiologic Pacing Modes

Cardiac physiologic pacing has traditionally been used to describe modes in which the normal physiologic, or sequential, relationship between atrial and ventricular stimulation and contraction is maintained. AV synchrony increases the volume in the ventricle before contraction and helps improve cardiac output. This may be achieved with atrial pacing in patients who have an intact conduction system or by dual-chamber pacing when atrial-to-ventricular conduction is impaired (i.e., during heart block).

BOX 14.3 Pacemaker Terminology

Fixed-Rate (Asynchronous)
Delivers a pacing stimulus at a set (fixed) rate regardless of the occurrence of spontaneous myocardial depolarization; occurs in nonsensing modes

Demand (Synchronous)
Delivers a pacing stimulus only when the heart's intrinsic pacemaker fails to function at a predetermined rate; the pacing stimulus is either inhibited or triggered by the sensing of intrinsic activity

Atrioventricular Sequential (Dual-Chamber)
Delivers a pacing stimulus to atrium and ventricle in physiologic sequence with sufficient atrioventricular delay to permit adequate ventricular filling

TABLE 14.2 Examples of Temporary Pacing Modes

Pacing Mode	Description
Asynchronous	
AOO	Atrial pacing, no sensing
VOO	Ventricular pacing, no sensing
DOO	Atrial and ventricular pacing, no sensing
Synchronous	
AAI	Atrial pacing, atrial sensing, inhibited response to sensed P waves
VVI	Ventricular pacing, ventricular sensing, inhibited response to sensed QRS complexes
DVI	Atrial and ventricular pacing, ventricular sensing; both atrial and ventricular pacing are inhibited if spontaneous ventricular depolarization is sensed
DDD	Both chambers are paced and sensed; inhibited response of pacing stimuli to sensed events in their respective chambers; triggered response to sensed atrial activity to allow for rate-responsive ventricular pacing

TABLE 14.1 NASPE/BPEG Generic Code

Position I: Chambers Paced	Position II: Chambers Sensed	Position III: Response to Sensing	Position IV: Rate Modulation	Position V: Multisite Pacing
0 = None	0 = None	0 = None	0 = None	0 = None
A = Atrium	A = Atrium	T = Triggered	R = Rate modulation	A = Atrium
V = Ventricle	V = Ventricle	I = Inhibited		V = Ventricle
D = Dual (A + V)	D = Dual (A + V)	D = Dual (T + I)		D = Dual (A + V)

BPEG, British Pacing and Electrophysiology Group; *NASPE*, North American Society of Pacing and Electrophysiology.
Modified from Bernstein AD, et al. The revised NASPE/BPEG generic pacemaker code for antibradycardia, adaptive-rate and multisite pacing. *Pacing Clin Electrophysiol.* 2002;25:260.

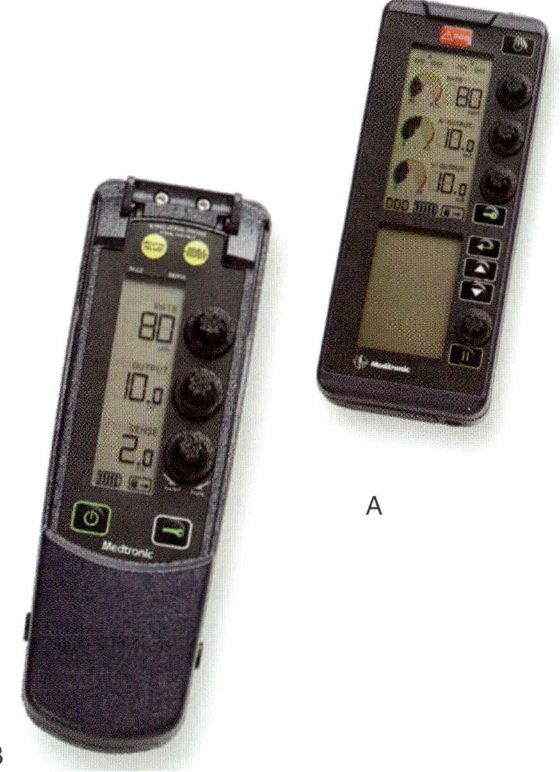

FIG. 14.3 Temporary Pulse Generators (External). (A) Dual-chamber pulse generator (Medtronic model #5392). (B) Single-chamber pulse generator (Medtronic model #53401). (©2024 Medtronic. All rights reserved. Used with the permission of Medtronic.)

BOX 14.4 Determining Temporary Pacemaker Pacing Threshold

1. Adjust pacemaker rate setting so that patient is 100% paced. It may be necessary to increase the pacing rate to achieve this setting.
2. Gradually decrease the output (milliampere) setting until 1:1 capture is lost. The pacing threshold is the point at which capture is lost.
3. Slowly increase the output setting until 1:1 capture is reestablished. With a properly positioned pacing electrode, the pacing threshold should be less than 1 mA.
4. Set the output setting two to three times higher than measured threshold because thresholds tend to fluctuate over time.
5. If a dual-chamber pulse generator is being used, evaluate pacing thresholds for the atrial and ventricular leads separately.

BOX 14.5 Determining Temporary Pacemaker Sensitivity Threshold

1. Set sensitivity control to its most sensitive setting.
2. Adjust the pulse generator rate to 10 beats/min less than patient's intrinsic rate (flash indicator should flash regularly).
3. Reduce the generator output to the minimal value to eliminate the risk of competing with the intrinsic rhythm.
4. Gradually increase the sensitivity value until the sense indicator stops flashing and the pace indicator starts flashing.
5. Decrease sensitivity until the sense indicator begins to flash again; this is the sensitivity threshold.
6. Adjust the sensitivity setting on the generator to half of threshold value; restore the generator output and rate to their original values.

More recently, physiologic pacing has evolved to include the maintenance of ventricular synchrony.[2] Strategies to achieve this include minimizing the use of ventricular pacing (VVI), and instead synchronizing pacing of both the RV and left ventricle (LV), and direct conduction system pacing of the bundle of His.[2]

Pacemaker Settings

The controls on all external temporary pulse generators are similar. Their functions must be thoroughly understood so that pacing can be initiated quickly in an emergency and troubleshooting can be facilitated quickly if pacemaker problems arise.

Pacemaker Rate Control

The *rate control* (Fig. 14.3) regulates the number of impulses that can be delivered to the heart per minute. The rate setting depends on the physiologic needs of the patient, but it usually is maintained between 60 and 80 beats/min. Pacing rates for overdrive suppression of tachyarrhythmias may greatly exceed these values. Some generators have special controls for overdrive pacing that allow for rates of 800 stimuli per minute. If the pacemaker is operating in a dual-chamber mode, the ventricular rate control also regulates the atrial rate.

Pacemaker Output Control

The *output dial* regulates the amount of electrical current, measured in milliamperes (mA), that is delivered to the heart to initiate depolarization. The point at which depolarization occurs, called *threshold*, is indicated by a myocardial response to the pacing stimulus (i.e., capture). Threshold can be determined by gradually decreasing the output setting until 1:1 capture is lost. The output setting is then slowly increased until 1:1 capture is reestablished; this threshold to pace is less than 1 mA with a properly positioned pacing electrode. The output is set two to three times higher than threshold because thresholds tend to fluctuate over time. Box 14.4 details the procedure for measuring pacing thresholds. Separate output controls for atrium and ventricle are used with a dual-chamber pulse generator.

Pacemaker Sensitivity Control

The *sensitivity control* regulates the ability of the pacemaker to detect the heart's intrinsic electrical activity. Sensitivity is measured in millivolts (mV) and determines the size of the intracardiac signal that the generator will recognize. If the sensitivity is adjusted to its most sensitive setting, a setting of 0.5 to 1 mV, the pacemaker can respond even to low-amplitude electrical signals coming from the heart. Turning the sensitivity to its least sensitive setting (i.e., adjusting the dial to a setting of 20 mV or to the area labeled *async*) results in inability of the pacemaker to sense any intrinsic electrical activity and causes the pacemaker to function at a fixed rate. A sense indicator (often a light) on the pulse generator signals each time intrinsic cardiac electrical activity is sensed. A pulse generator may be designed to sense atrial activity or ventricular activity or both. Box 14.5 describes the procedure for measuring sensitivity. The sensitivity is set at half of the value of the sensitivity threshold to ensure that all appropriate intrinsic cardiac signals are sensed. For example, if the measured sensitivity threshold is 3.0 mV, the generator is set at 1.5 mV. The sensing ability of the pacemaker can be quickly evaluated by observing for a change in pacing rhythm in response to spontaneous depolarizations.

Pacemaker AV Interval Control

The *AV interval control* (available only on dual-chamber generators) regulates the time interval between the atrial and ventricular pacing stimuli. This interval is analogous to the P–R interval that occurs in the intrinsic ECG. Accurate adjustment of this interval to between 150 and 250 milliseconds (ms) preserves AV synchrony and permits maximal ventricular stroke volume and enhanced cardiac output. Because the AV interval is limited by the length of the cardiac cycle, modern temporary generators automatically adjust the AV delay based on the programmed heart rate.

Pacemaker Upper and Lower Rate Controls

Temporary dual-chamber pacemakers have other settings that are required in the DDD mode (see Fig. 14.3B). The *lower rate*, or *base rate*, determines the rate at which the generator will pace when intrinsic activity falls below the set rate of the pacemaker. The *upper rate* determines the fastest ventricular rate the pacemaker will deliver in response to sensed atrial activity. This setting is needed to protect the patient's heart from being paced in response to rapid atrial dysrhythmias.

There also is an *atrial refractory period*, programmable from 150 to 500 ms, which regulates the length of time, after a sensed or paced ventricular event, during which the pacemaker cannot respond to another atrial stimulus.

Pacemaker Emergency Pacing

An emergency button is available on most models to allow for rapid initiation of asynchronous (DOO) high-output pacing during an emergency.

Pacemaker Safety Features

On all temporary pacemakers, an on/off switch is provided with a safety feature that prevents the accidental termination of pacing. There is also generally a locking feature to prevent unintended changes to the prescribed settings.

Pacing Artifacts

All patients with temporary pacemakers require continuous ECG monitoring. The pacing artifact is the spike that is seen on the ECG tracing as the pacing stimulus is delivered to the heart. A *P wave* is visible after the pacing artifact if the atrium is being paced (Fig. 14.4A). Similarly, a *QRS complex* follows a ventricular pacing artifact (Fig. 14.4B). With dual-chamber pacing, a pacing artifact precedes both the P wave and the QRS complex (Fig. 14.4C).

Not all paced beats look alike. For example, the artifact (spike) produced by a unipolar pacing electrode is larger than the artifact produced by a bipolar lead (Fig. 14.5). The QRS complex of paced beats appears different depending on the location of the pacing electrode. If the pacing electrode is positioned in the RV, a left bundle branch block pattern is displayed on the ECG. A right bundle branch block pattern is visible if the pacing stimulus originates from the LV.

Pacemaker Malfunction

Most pacemaker malfunctions can be categorized as abnormalities of pacing or of sensing. Problems with pacing can involve failure of the pacemaker to deliver the pacing stimulus, a pacing stimulus that fails to depolarize the heart, or an incorrect number of pacing stimuli per minute.

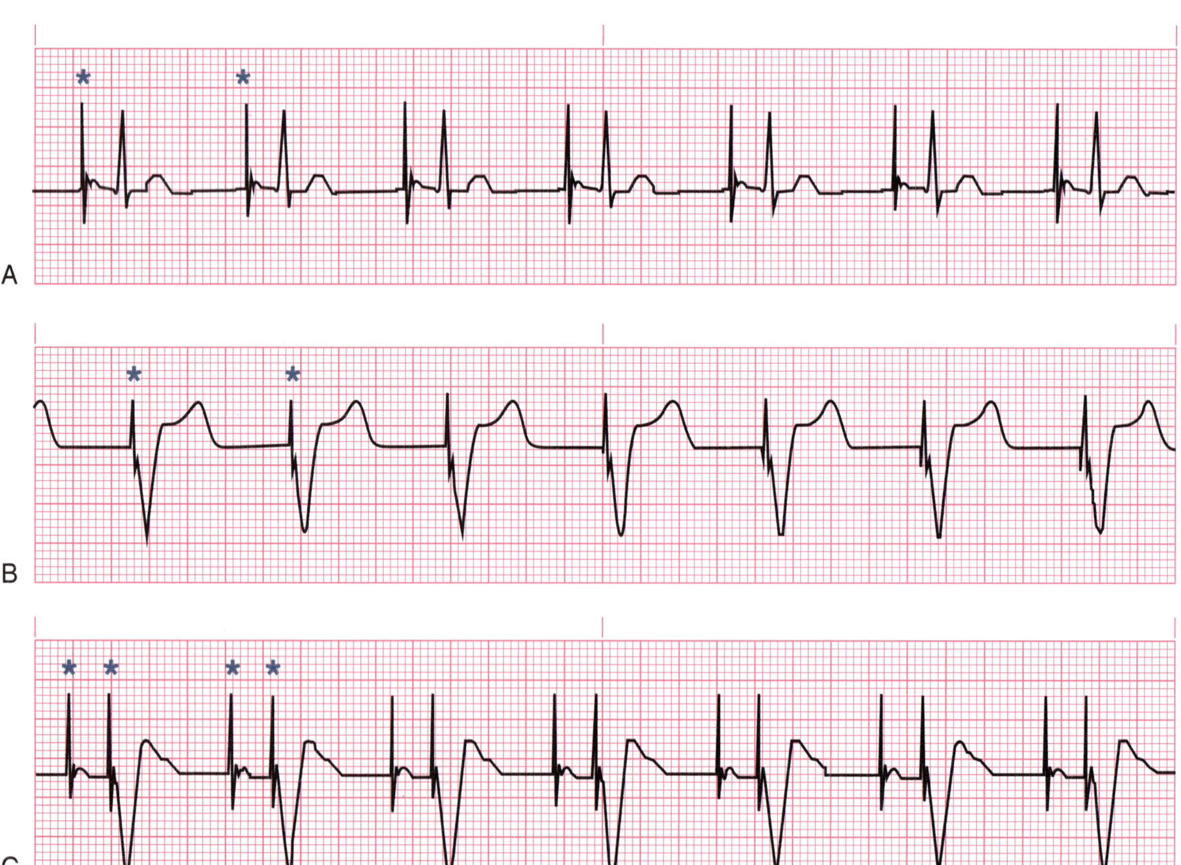

FIG. 14.4 **Pacing Examples.** (A) Atrial pacing. (B) Ventricular pacing. (C) Dual-chamber pacing. Each asterisk represents a pacemaker impulse.

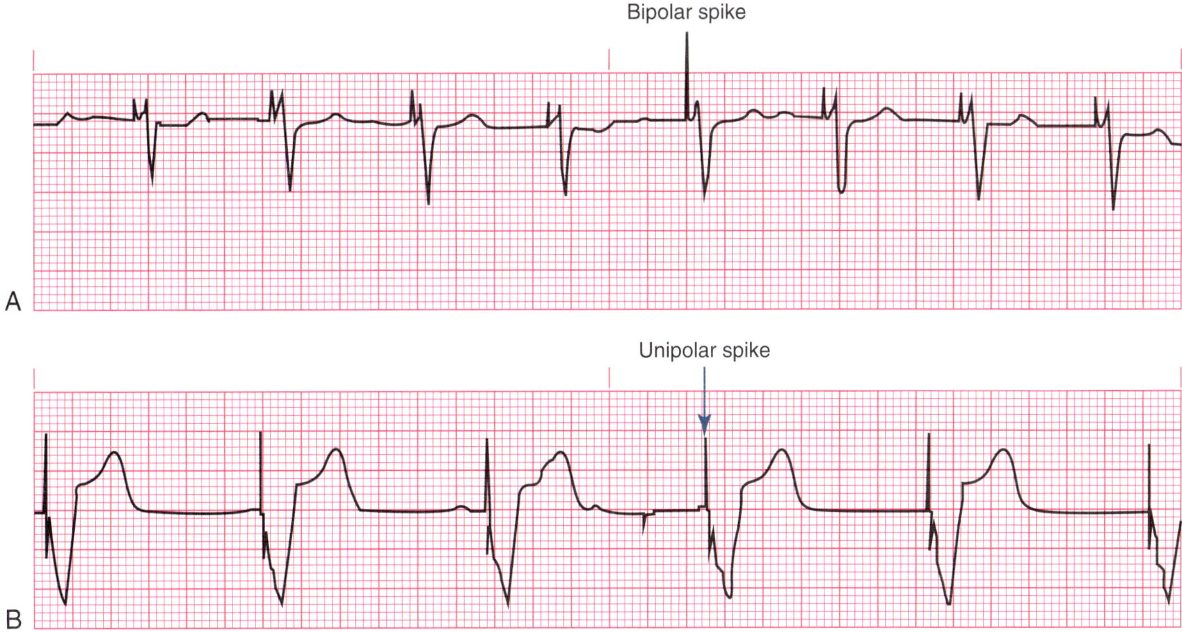

FIG. 14.5 Bipolar and Unipolar Pacing. (A) Bipolar pacing artifact. (B) Unipolar pacing artifact. (Modified from Conover MB. *Understanding Electrocardiography*. 8th ed. Mosby; 2003.)

Pacing Malfunction—Failure to Pace

Failure of the pacemaker to deliver the pacing stimulus results in disappearance of the pacing artifact even if the patient's intrinsic rate is less than the set rate on the pacer. This can occur intermittently or continuously and can be attributed to failure of the pulse generator or its battery, a loose connection between the various components of the pacemaker system, broken lead wires, or stimulus inhibition because of EMI.[4] Tightening connections, replacing the batteries or the pulse generator itself, or removing the source of EMI may restore pacemaker function.

Pacing Malfunction—Loss of Capture

If the pacing stimulus fires but fails to initiate a myocardial depolarization, a pacing artifact will be present but will not be followed by the expected P wave or QRS complex, depending on the chamber being paced (Fig. 14.6). This *loss of capture* can be attributed most often to displacement of the pacing electrode or to an increase in threshold (the electrical stimulus necessary to elicit a myocardial depolarization) because of medications, metabolic disorders, electrolyte imbalances, fibrosis, or myocardial ischemia at the site of electrode placement.[4,16] The pacing output is measured in milliamperes (mA). In many cases, increasing the mA output elicits capture.

For loss of capture with transvenous lead pacing, repositioning the patient onto their left side may improve lead contact and restore capture.[5]

Pacing can occur at inappropriate rates. For example, impending battery failure in a permanent pacemaker can result in a gradual decrease in the paced rate, also referred to as *rate drift*. Inappropriate stimuli from a pacemaker may result in pacemaker-mediated tachycardia; this usually is caused by sensing of inappropriate signals in a dual-chamber pacemaker that is in a trigger mode, such as DDD.[16] In a permanent pacemaker, the tachycardia can be terminated by placing a magnet over the generator to transiently suspend sensing.[12]

Sensing Malfunction—Undersensing

Sensing abnormalities include undersensing and oversensing.

Undersensing is the inability of the pacemaker to sense spontaneous myocardial depolarizations. Often the pacemaker sensitivity setting is set too high.[4] Undersensing results in competition between paced complexes and the heart's intrinsic rhythm. This malfunction is manifested on the ECG by pacing artifacts that occur after or are unrelated to spontaneous complexes (Fig. 14.7). Undersensing can result in the delivery of pacing stimuli into a relative refractory period of the cardiac depolarization cycle (see Fig. 10.25 in Chapter 10). A ventricular pacing stimulus delivered into the downslope of the T wave (R-on-T phenomenon) is a real danger with this type of pacer aberration because it may precipitate a lethal dysrhythmia. Identification of the cause to initiate appropriate interventions must happen quickly. The cause often can be attributed to inadequate wave amplitude (height of the P or R wave). If this is the case, the situation can be promptly remedied by increasing the sensitivity by moving the sensitivity toward a lower setting (lower numbers are more sensitive). Other possible causes include inappropriate (asynchronous) mode selection, lead displacement or fracture, loose cable connections, and pulse generator failure.

Sensing Malfunction—Oversensing

Oversensing occurs because of inappropriate sensing of extraneous electrical signals that leads to unnecessary triggering or inhibition of stimulus output, depending on the pacer mode. The source of these electrical signals can range from tall-peaked T waves to EMI in the critical care environment.[4] Because most temporary pulse generators are programmed in demand modes, oversensing results in unexplained pauses in the ECG tracing as the extraneous signals are sensed and inhibit pacing. Moving the sensitivity dial toward 20 mV (higher numbers are less sensitive) often stops the pauses.

With permanent pacemakers, a magnet may be placed over the generator to restore pacing to an asynchronous mode

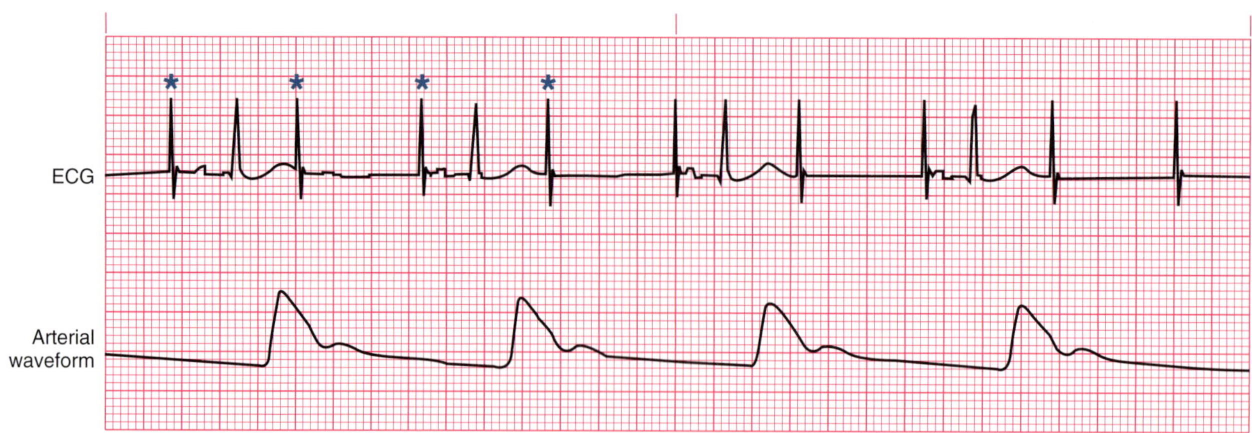

FIG. 14.6 Pacemaker Malfunction: Failure to Capture. Atrial pacing and capture occur after pacer spikes 1, 3, 5, and 7. The remaining pacer spikes fail to capture the tissue, resulting in loss of the P wave, no conduction to the ventricles, and no arterial waveform. Each asterisk represents a pacemaker impulse.

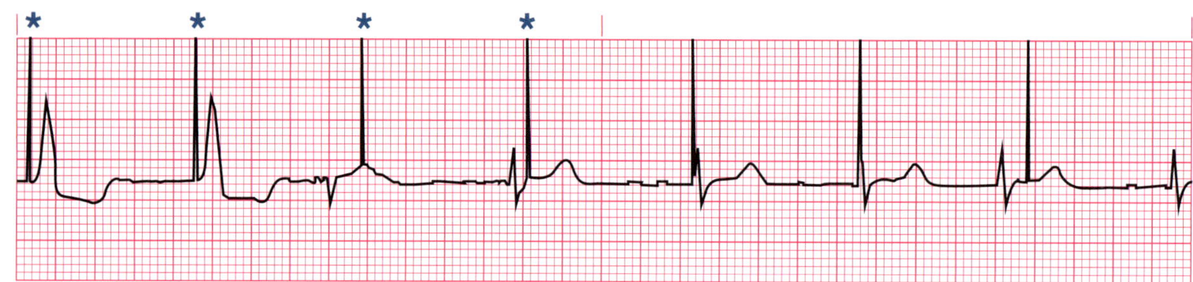

FIG. 14.7 Pacemaker Malfunction: Undersensing. After the first two paced beats, a series of intrinsic beats occurs; the pacemaker unit fails to sense these intrinsic QRS complexes. These spikes do not capture the ventricle because they occur during the refractory period of the cardiac cycle. Each asterisk represents a pacemaker impulse.

until appropriate changes in the generator settings can be programmed.[12]

Medical Management

If the patient is undergoing heart surgery, epicardial leads are often electively placed at the end of the operation to facilitate temporary pacing. The surgeon places the epicardial pacing lead or leads, repositioning them as needed, to obtain adequate pacing and sensing thresholds.[3] Decisions regarding lead placement may later limit the pacing modes available to the clinician. For example, to perform dual-chamber pacing, both atrial and ventricular leads must be placed. After lead placement, the initial settings for output and sensitivity in atria and ventricles are determined, the pacing rate and mode are selected, and the response to the pacing stimulus is evaluated. Pacemaker settings are typically listed as part of the hospital postoperative and postprocedure protocols.

Nursing Management

Nursing responsibilities in the care of a patient with a temporary pacemaker are associated with several patient problems and can be combined into four primary areas: assessment and prevention of pacemaker malfunction, protection against microshock, surveillance for complications such as infection, and patient education.

Prevention of Pacemaker Malfunction

Continuous ECG monitoring is essential to facilitate prompt recognition of and appropriate intervention for pacemaker malfunction. Proper care of the pacing system can prevent pacing abnormalities.

The temporary pacing lead and bridging cable must be properly secured to the body with tape or securement device to prevent accidental displacement of the electrode, which can result in failure to pace or sense. The external pulse generator can be secured to the patient's waist with a strap or placed in a pouch for a mobile patient. If the patient is on a regimen of bed rest, the pulse generator can be suspended by using the pouch or with twill tape from an intravenous pole mounted that is attached to the bed or overhead ceiling. This positioning prevents tension on the lead while the patient is moved (given adequate length of bridging cable) and alleviates the possibility of accidentally dropping the pulse generator.

The nurse inspects for loose connections between the leads and pulse generator on a regular basis. Replacement batteries and pulse generators must always be available on the unit. Although the battery has an anticipated life span of 1 month, it probably is sound practice to change the battery if the pacemaker has been operating continually for several days. Newer generators provide a low-battery signal 24 hours before complete loss of battery function occurs to prevent inadvertent interruptions in pacing. Change the batteries according to the institution's policy and procedure.

The pulse generator may be labeled with the date on which the battery was replaced.

It is important to be aware of all sources of EMI within the critical care environment that may interfere with the function of the temporary pacemaker. Sources of EMI in the clinical area include electrocautery, defibrillation current, radiation therapy, magnetic resonance imaging (MRI) scanners, and transcutaneous electrical nerve stimulation (TENS) units. In most cases, if EMI is suspected of precipitating pacemaker malfunction, conversion to the asynchronous mode (fixed rate) can maintain pacing until the cause of the EMI is removed.[11]

Microshock Protection

Because the pacing electrode provides a direct, low-resistance path to the heart, the nurse takes special care while handling the external components of the pacing system to avoid conducting stray electrical current from other equipment. Even a small amount of stray current transmitted through the pacing lead could precipitate a lethal dysrhythmia. The possibility of microshock can be minimized by wearing gloves when handling the pacing wires and by proper insulation of terminal pins of pacing wires when they are not in use (Box 14.6). The latter precaution can be accomplished using caps provided by the manufacturer or by improvising with a plastic syringe or section of disposable rubber glove. The wires are taped securely to the patient's chest to prevent accidental electrode displacement.

Infection Risk

Infection at the lead insertion site is a rare but serious complication associated with temporary pacemakers. The site is carefully inspected for purulent drainage, erythema, and edema, and the patient is observed for signs of systemic infection. Site care is performed according to the institution's policies and procedures. Although most infections remain localized, endocarditis can occur in patients with endocardial pacing leads. A less common complication associated with transvenous pacing is myocardial perforation, which can result in rhythmic hiccoughs or cardiac tamponade.

Educate the Patient and Family

Teaching for a patient with a temporary pacemaker emphasizes the prevention of complications (Box 14.7). The patient is instructed not to handle any exposed portion of the lead wire and to notify the nurse if the dressing over the insertion site becomes soiled, wet, or dislodged. The patient also is advised not to use any electrical devices brought in from home that could interfere with pacemaker functioning. Patients with temporary transvenous pacemakers need to be taught to restrict movement of the affected extremity to prevent lead displacement.

BOX 14.6 Safety

Prevention of Microshock

- Wear gloves when handling pacing wires.
- Secure all connections between pulse generator, pacing cable, and leads.
- Insulate lead tips with nonconducting materials when not attached to generator (manufacturer's cap, finger cot, plastic syringe).
- Keep dressings and pacing equipment dry.
- Ensure all electrical equipment is properly grounded.
- Use battery-operated shavers.

BOX 14.7 PATIENT AND FAMILY EDUCATION PLAN

Temporary Pacemaker

Before discharge, the patient should be able to teach back the following topics:

- Description of pacemaker therapy
- Care of pacemaker system
- Minimize handling of leads or cables
- Notify nurse if dressing becomes wet or loose
- Activity restrictions (minimize upper extremity movement with transvenous leads)
- Electrical safety precautions (no electric razors)
- Symptoms to report (dizziness)

PERMANENT PACEMAKERS

Many patients with cardiac disease have an implanted permanent pacemaker and nurses will frequently encounter these devices in their clinical practice. Permanent pacemakers were originally designed to provide an adequate ventricular rate in patients with symptomatic bradycardia. Today, the goal of pacemaker therapy is to simulate, as much as possible, normal physiologic cardiac depolarization and conduction. Thus, the most common indications for implantation of a permanent pacemaker are for the management of sinus node dysfunction and second-degree and third-degree AV blocks.[1]

Sophisticated generators permit rate-responsive pacing, effecting responses to sensed atrial activity (DDD) or to various physiologic sensors (body motion or minute ventilation). For patients who do not have a functional sinus node that can increase their heart rate, rate-responsive pacemakers may improve exercise capacity and quality of life.[2] Table 14.3 describes the types of rate-responsive pacing generators in clinical use. The concept of physiologic pacing continues to evolve because studies have indicated that pacing initiated from the RV apex alone, even in a dual-chamber mode, may promote heart failure in patients with permanent pacemakers.[17,18] Further research has been conducted to identify alternative sites for pacing and modes that can maximize intrinsic AV conduction and minimize ventricular pacing.[2]

A patient who undergoes implantation of a permanent pacemaker is usually in the hospital for less than 24 hours. Longer lengths of stay are expected for patients with serious comorbidities or complications such as MI or cardiogenic shock.

Technologic advances in the computer industry have had a major impact on permanent pacemakers. Microprocessors have allowed for the development of increasingly smaller generators despite the incorporation of more complex features. Current generators are smaller, more energy efficient, and more reliable than previous models. A transvenous pacemaker is shown in Fig. 14.8A.

Cardiac Implantable Electronic Devices

A permanent pacemaker is classified as a *cardiac implantable electronic device* (CIED). These are devices that can regular heart rate and rhythm. One of the major concerns with cardiac implantable devices is the risk for infection arising from the transvenous leads, or from the generator pocket where the device is inserted.[19–21] Based on a variety of sources, the CIED infection risk is approximately 1% to 3%.[19] Signs and symptoms associated with CIED infection may be localized to the pocket site, with erythema (redness), warmth, swelling, pain erosion, ulceration, or drainage; or signs may be systemic with elevated temperature, chills, and positive blood cultures. If infection is present, the entire pacemaker system is explanted (removed) and appropriate antibiotics are administered.

Leadless Pacemakers

Newer innovations include *leadless pacemakers*. The first leadless device (Micra™; Medtronic) was a single-chamber unit placed in the RV via the femoral vein programmed for VVI mode capability.[22–24] A newer leadless pacemaker from the same device company allows for AV synchrony with leadless units placed into both right atrial and right ventricular chambers. Leadless pacemakers have a small cylindrical shape that contains the electrodes and the generator in a single unit. They are about 2.5 cm (approximately 1 inch) in length, are placed percutaneously via the femoral vein, and have a long battery life estimated at 16 years. Examples of leadless pacemakers are shown in Fig. 14.8B.

These devices eliminate the need for a subcutaneous pocket and transvenous leads that account for the majority of complications associated with transvenous permanent pacemakers.[23] Several new pacemaker generators are also compatible with MRI.[25,26] A rapidly expanding role for permanent pacemakers is for adjunctive treatment of heart failure, used in conjunction with heart failure pharmacotherapy[2,11] (see Chapter 13 section on heart failure management).

TABLE 14.3 Permanent Pacemaker Rate-Response Pacing Modes

Pulse Generator	Description
AAIR	AAI features plus rate-responsive pacing; used for patients with symptomatic bradycardia who have a paceable atrium and intact atrioventricular conduction
VVIR	VVI features plus rate-responsive pacing; used for patients with atrium that is unpaceable as a result of chronic atrial fibrillation
DDDR	DDD features plus rate-responsive pacing; used for patients with symptomatic bradycardia in which the atrium is paceable but atrioventricular conduction is, or may become, unreliable

Cardiac Resynchronization Therapy

Approximately one-third of patients with severe heart failure have ventricular conduction delays (prolonged QRS duration or bundle branch block).[27] These conduction delays have been shown to create a lack of synchrony between the contractions of the LV and RV. The hemodynamic consequences of this dyssynchrony include impaired ventricular filling with decreased ejection fraction (EF) and lower cardiac output. Cardiac resynchronization therapy (CRT), also known as biventricular pacing, uses atrial pacing plus synchronous pacing stimulation in both the LV and RV to optimize atrial and ventricular mechanical activity.[2,11] The CRT device uses three pacing leads:

- A lead in the RA
- A lead in the RV
- A transvenous lead inserted through the *coronary sinus* to pace the LV.

Because many patients with heart failure are also at risk for sudden cardiac death, defibrillation and CRT may be combined. To distinguish between the types of CRT, the letter P (pacing) or D (defibrillation) is added to the name.

- CRT-P: Cardiac resynchronization therapy with pacing
- CRT-D: Cardiac resynchronization therapy with defibrillation

Numerous clinical trials have shown that CRT improves symptoms and functional status, reduces mortality in patients with moderate to advanced heart failure, and slows progression of heart failure.[2,11]

The use of CRT has been associated with improved EF, decreased heart failure events, improvement in the class of heart failure, and reduction in mortality. The greatest benefit appears to be in patients with a confirmed left bundle branch block and a QRS duration greater than 150 ms.[11,28]

Medical Management

Permanent pacemakers may be implanted with the patient under local anesthesia in the cardiac catheterization laboratory. Transvenous leads usually are inserted through the cephalic or subclavian vein and positioned in the RA or RV or both, with

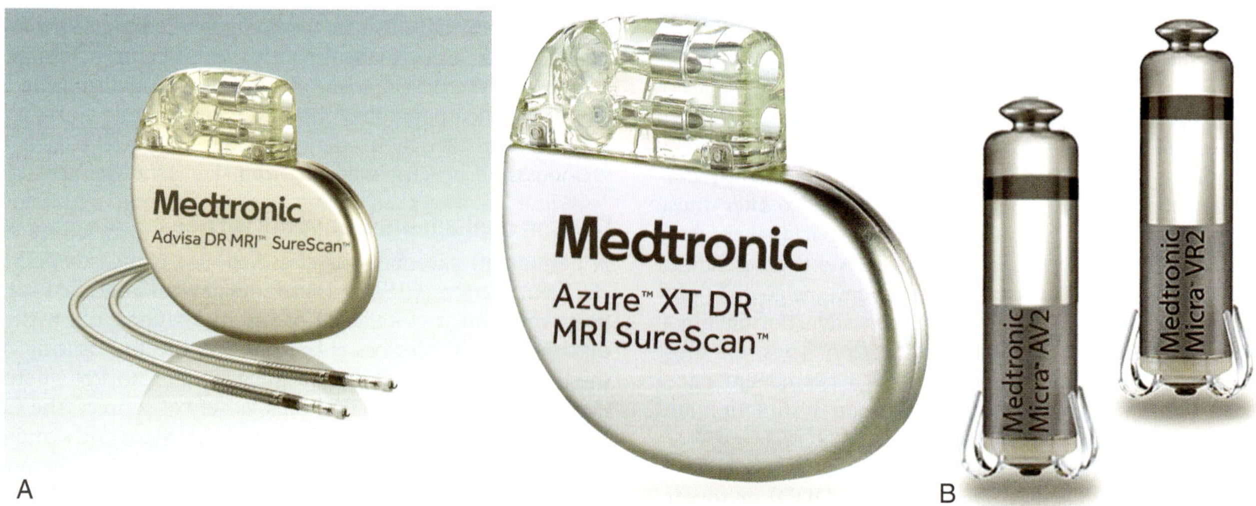

FIG. 14.8 (A) Permanent pacemakers with transvenous leads (Medtronic Advisa™ DR MRI SureScan™ and Medtronic Azure™ XT DR MRI SureScan™). (B) Permanent leadless pacemakers, Medtronic Micra™ AV2 (AV synchrony) and Medtronic Micra™ V2 (ventricular single chamber). Leadless pacemakers are much smaller than a conventional pacemaker and approximate 2.5 cm or 1 inch in length. (©2024 Medtronic. All rights reserved. Used with the permission of Medtronic.)

fluoroscopic guidance. Satisfactory lead placement is determined by testing the stimulation and sensitivity thresholds with a pacing system analyzer. The leads are then attached to the generator, which is inserted into a surgically created pocket in the subcutaneous tissue below the clavicle. The generator is placed between the subcutaneous tissue and pectoral fascia of the left upper chest. The leads are inserted transvenous through the subclavian, axillary, or cephalic veins.

Ongoing assessment of pacemaker function after discharge can be performed remotely, using wireless technology via the Internet or a cellular network. Remote monitoring reduces the number of clinic visits and provides early detection of patient or pacemaker problems.[29,30]

Nursing Management

Nursing management for patients after permanent pacemaker implantation includes monitoring for complications related to insertion and for pacemaker malfunction.[31] Postoperative complications are rare but include cardiac perforation and tamponade, pneumothorax, lead displacement, hematoma, and infection.[20,21] A hematoma in the pacemaker pocket greatly increases the risk of infection.[20]

The process for identification of permanent pacemaker malfunction is the same as the process described previously for temporary pacemakers. Information about the type of pacemaker that has been implanted will include the manufacturer, the programmed pacing mode, and the lower rate setting, all of which should be documented in the electronic health record (EHR) or readily available at the bedside.

With permanent pacemakers, settings are adjusted noninvasively through a specialized programmer that uses pulsed magnetic fields or a RF signal. If a pacemaker problem is suspected, ECG strips are obtained and the physician or nurse practitioner is notified so that the pacemaker settings can be reprogrammed as needed. If a patient experiences symptoms of decreased cardiac output, support with temporary transcutaneous pacing may be required until the problem is corrected.

The foregoing discussion is an introduction to the basic concepts of pacemaker therapy. Nurses who care for patients with permanent or temporary pacemakers must be familiar with modes of pacemaker function, infection risk, and other potential complications in order to care for patients safely and effectively.

IMPLANTABLE CARDIOVERTER DEFIBRILLATORS

An implantable cardioverter defibrillator (ICD) is an electronic device that is used in the treatment of tachydysrhythmias. ICDs are programmed to monitor, identify, and terminate life-threatening ventricular arrhythmias. The ICD is placed in the subcutaneous tissue of the pectoral region in the upper chest (Fig. 14.9). As with permanent pacemakers, ICDs are implantable cardiac devices classified as CIEDs.

Indications for ICD

Initially, an ICD was recommended only for patients who had survived an episode of cardiac arrest caused by ventricular fibrillation (VF) or VT or in whom lethal arrhythmias could be induced during EPS. In current practice, the ICD is an integral component of management for patients with not only ventricular dysrhythmias but also advanced heart failure to reduce the risk of death from cardiac arrest.[32,33]

Prevention of Sudden Cardiac Death

The ICD is implanted for primary prevention of sudden cardiac death (SCD) in patients at high risk of a fatal dysrhythmia and who have a life expectancy of longer than 1 year. This includes patients with ischemic heart disease and a low LVEF (less than 35%) despite optimal medical management for heart failure.[32,33] Patients with genetic or familial conditions that predispose them to life-threatening tachydysrhythmias, such as long QT syndrome or hypertrophic cardiomyopathy, are also candidates for an ICD.[32]

Implantable Cardioverter Defibrillator System

The basic ICD system consists of leads and a generator, and while it shares similarities with pacemakers, there are some key differences in the leads, generator, and functions.

- The leads contain not only electrodes for sensing and pacing but also integrated defibrillator coils capable of delivering a shock.
- The generator is larger, to accommodate a more powerful battery, a high-voltage capacitor, and the microprocessor.
- The generators have pacemaker capabilities.
- Programmable ICD options include:
  - Antitachycardia pacing
  - Bradycardia backup pacing
  - Low-energy cardioversion
  - High-energy defibrillation

The ICD response to a dysrhythmia depends on the type of device and how it is programmed. Options include:

- **Antitachycardia pacing** is often the first line of treatment for VT using programmed bursts of fast pacer discharges. If the VT is successfully "pace terminated," the patient will not receive a shock from the generator and may not even realize that the ICD terminated the dysrhythmia.
- **Cardioversion** is used for VT within programmed rate limits. The patient will experience a shock as the ICD discharges.
- **Defibrillation** is used if the dysrhythmia deteriorates into VF. The patient will experience a shock.
- **No discharge** (no shock) if the dysrhythmia terminates spontaneously.
- **Bradycardia backup pacing** if the electrical rhythm deteriorates to asystole or a slow idioventricular rhythm.

Implantable Cardioverter Defibrillator Leads

ICDs are dual-chamber devices with multiple leads and functions.

- Dual leads in both atria and ventricles can deliver dual-chamber pacing.
- Atrial leads for atrial sensing to discriminate more accurately between SVT and VT to decrease the incidence of inappropriate shocks.
- Triple-lead ICDs have leads in one atrium and both ventricles to allow for CRT pacing and defibrillation in one device.

Some studies suggest the addition of CRT may improve heart failure over time and thus reduce the number of shocks required from the ICD.[34] Other developments in ICD technology include improved diagnostic and telemetry functions, to provide real-time electrograms obtained from the ICD electrodes or the ability to perform remote device interrogation using cellular or wireless technology.[11]

Transvenous Implantable Cardioverter Defibrillator Implant

The majority of ICDs use transvenous leads that are positioned in the heart under fluoroscopy and then attached to a generator implanted in the tissue of the upper chest. Procedural complications are infrequent but may include hematoma, pneumothorax,

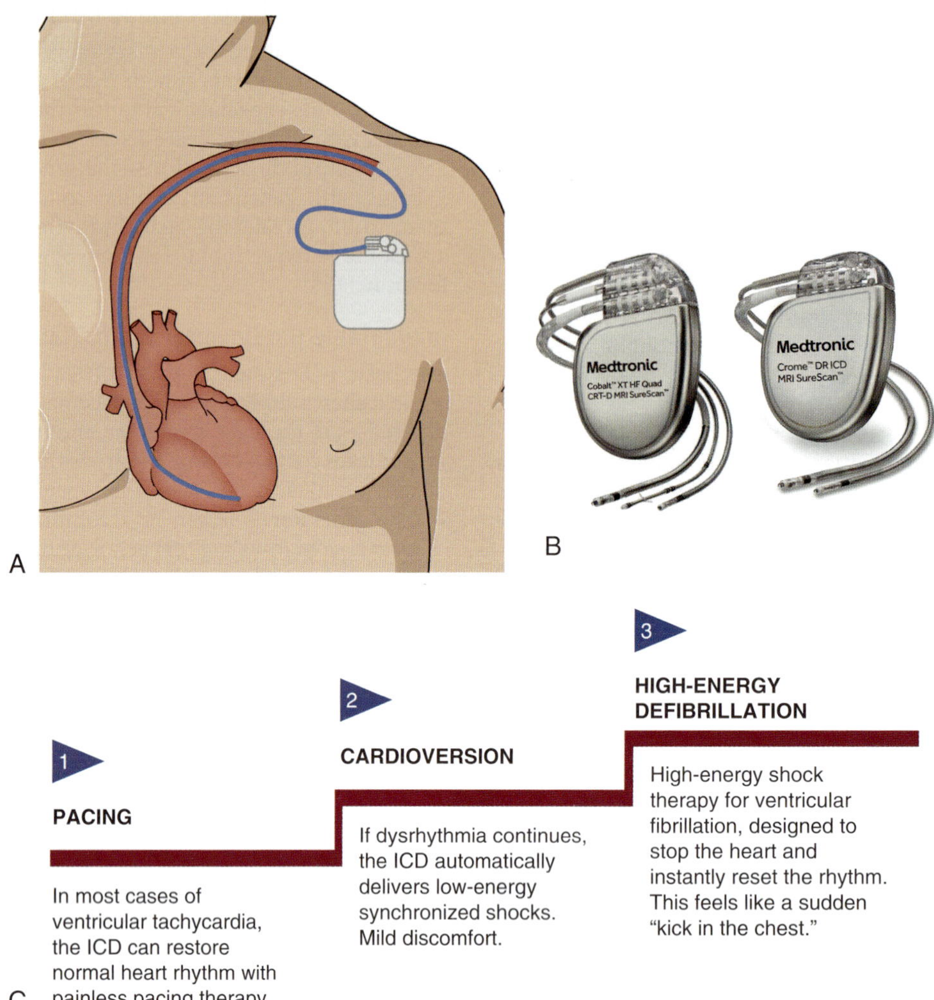

FIG. 14.9 Placement of Implantable Cardioverter Defibrillator (ICD) and/or a Cardiac Resynchronization Therapy (CRT) With ICD and a Transvenous Lead System. (A) The generator is placed in a subcutaneous "pocket" in the pectoral region. The pacing, cardioversion, and defibrillation functions all are contained in a lead (or leads) inserted into the right atrium and ventricle. (B) Example of ICD types that may be implanted: Dual chamber ICD (Medtronic Cobalt™ HF quad CRT-D MRI SureScan™) with tiered therapy and pacing capabilities; or a CRT-Defibrillator Crome™ DR ICD MRI SureScan™). (C) Tiered therapy is designed to use increasing levels of intensity to terminate ventricular dysrhythmias. (B: ©2024 Medtronic. All rights reserved. Used with the permission of Medtronic.)

cardiac tamponade, or lead dislodgment. This configuration may be referred to as a transvenous-ICD (TV-ICD).[35]

Subcutaneous Implantable Cardioverter Defibrillator Implant

The subcutaneous ICD (S-ICD) is a more recent innovation. The S-ICD consists of a generator implanted in the left axillary area and a single lead that is only subcutaneous (not transvenous) that connects with the heart.[35] The subcutaneous lead can detect ventricular dysrhythmias and deliver defibrillation shock therapy but is unable to provide pacing therapies.

The S-ICD offers an alternative for patients who need defibrillation but not pacing. The subcutaneous design avoids complications associated with transvenous leads.[35]

Medical Management

Medical management in a patient with an ICD begins before implantation with a thorough evaluation of the patient's risk for life-threatening ventricular dysrhythmias and underlying cardiac function. Patients will undergo EPS to determine the origin of the arrhythmia and the effect of antiarrhythmic agents in suppressing or altering the rate of the dysrhythmia.

Comprehensive Diagnostic Evaluation

Further assessment of cardiac status is made to determine whether additional interventions, such as revascularization or CRT, are indicated to improve cardiac function. This part of the work-up may include cardiac catheterization, stress testing, and echocardiography. Based on the evaluation, decisions are made regarding the optimal implantation approach, either transvenous or subcutaneous, along with the types of therapy included, such as antitachycardia pacing, cardioversion, defibrillation, and resynchronization therapy.

Current guidelines recommend that ICD implantation not be performed within 40 days of an MI[36] or within 90 days of revascularization, to allow time for ventricular recovery. In some of these patients an external wearable cardioverter defibrillator may be used to address the risk of sudden cardiac death during the waiting period.[36,37]

Programming the ICD

A cardiology electrophysiologist performs the initial programming of the device at the time of implantation. Defibrillation efficacy of the ICD may be assessed by inducing the dysrhythmia and then evaluating the ability of the device to terminate it.

Although defibrillation testing was routinely performed at the time of implant with early devices, clinical trials have failed to demonstrate an improvement in shock efficacy or clinical outcomes related to this practice, and it is not required today.[38–40] Modern ICDs are more reliable and offer higher energy levels than in the past, and generally the high-output setting for defibrillation is used. See the previous description of ICD lead functions for other programable functions.

There is one exception for implantation testing, which concerns S-ICD implants where the lead is subcutaneous. Defibrillation testing is still the standard of care for S-ICD implants.[41]

Avoiding Inappropriate Shocks

Other adjustments in programming may be performed to decrease unnecessary shocks, including aggressive use of antitachycardia pacing and withholding shocks for SVT or nonsustained ventricular dysrhythmias.[42] ICD follow-up is typically conducted on an outpatient basis, with remote monitoring options to monitor the number of discharges and the battery life of the device.[29]

Nursing Management

If the ICD system was implanted during open-heart surgery, postoperative nursing management resembles care for any patient who has undergone cardiac surgery.

If an endocardial lead system is implanted, nursing management is less intense and the hospital stay is shorter. The nursing management of a patient with an ICD includes assessing for dysrhythmias and monitoring for complications related to insertion. In the case of a ventricular dysrhythmia, it is important to know the type of ICD implanted, how the device functions, and whether it is activated (turned "on"). If the patient experiences a shockable rhythm, the nurse should be prepared to defibrillate in the rare event that the device fails. During external defibrillation, the paddles or patches should never be placed directly over the ICD generator. For recurring shocks, patients should be assessed for underlying causes such as electrolyte imbalance, ischemia, or worsening heart failure.

Most patients continue to take antidysrhythmic medications to decrease the number of shocks required and to slow the rate of the tachycardia. Some patients will undergo percutaneous catheter ablation in the ventricle to eliminate ectopic foci.[43]

Complications associated with an ICD include broken leads, sensing of supraventricular tachydysrhythmias resulting in unneeded discharges, and infection risk from the implanted system.[20]

Educate the Patient and Family

To facilitate a positive psychologic adjustment to the ICD, education of the patient and family about the device is vital (Box 14.8). Preoperative teaching for a patient with an ICD includes information about how the device works and what to expect during the implantation procedure. After implantation, education is focused on aspects of living with an ICD. Patients need information pertaining to device follow-up, technology used for remote monitoring, and instructions about what to do if they experience a shock. Many institutions have successfully used family support groups for this patient population. Finally, because the ICD is an adjunctive treatment rather than a cure for heart failure, patients need to understand the importance of continued risk factor modification and adherence taking prescribed medications.[33]

BOX 14.8 PATIENT AND FAMILY EDUCATION PLAN

Implantable Cardioverter Defibrillator

Before discharge, the patient should be able to teach back the following topics:

- Pathophysiology of the underlying disease process, including sudden cardiac death, ventricular dysrhythmias, and heart disease
- Information regarding how the implantable cardioverter defibrillator is programmed to function
- Actions to take if a shock occurs
- Importance of continuing antidysrhythmic and heart failure medications
- Activity limitations related to driving and avoiding strong magnetic fields
- Signs and symptoms of device failure
- Follow-up schedule for remote monitoring and office visits
- Cardiopulmonary resuscitation training for family members

FIBRINOLYTIC THERAPY

Fibrinolytic therapy is an important clinical intervention for patients experiencing acute ST segment elevation myocardial infarction (STEMI) when cardiac catheterization and percutaneous coronary intervention (PCI) therapies are not available. Timely reperfusion can limit the size of the infarction in jeopardized myocardium by restoring blood flow through the thrombosed vessel. Two options are available for opening the artery: fibrinolytics and mechanical percutaneous interventions. Numerous studies have demonstrated that catheter-based interventions are preferred because of better outcomes when performed in a timely fashion,[44] but not all hospitals have this capability.[45] If cardiac catheterization and catheter-based therapies to open the occluded artery within 120 minutes are not available, intravenous (IV) fibrinolytic therapy is administered.[46] In the United States, hospitals are grouped by regional STEMI systems of care to facilitate transfer from non-PCI to PCI-capable hospitals.[45] This is also described in Chapter 13 in Fig. 13.3.

Fibrinolytic Actions

The administration of a fibrinolytic agent results in lysis of the acute thrombus, resulting in recanalization, or opening, of the obstructed coronary artery and restoration of blood flow to the affected tissue. In addition to restoring perfusion, adjunctive measures (anticoagulants and antiplatelet therapy) are taken to prevent further clot formation and repeat occlusion. Within 24 hours after fibrinolysis is complete, transfer to a PCI-capable hospital for early angiography and possible PCI is recommended.[46]

Following the rupture of an atherosclerotic plaque a thrombus forms, which is composed of aggregated platelets bound together with fibrin strands; this occludes the coronary artery and deprives the myocardium of oxygen previously supplied by that artery causing an acute coronary syndrome (ACS) as described in Chapter 13 (Fig. 13.13). Fibrinolytic therapy lyses the fibrin strands within the thrombus to open the artery. Fibrinolysis is followed by administration of anticoagulant and antiplatelet medications to maintain patency.

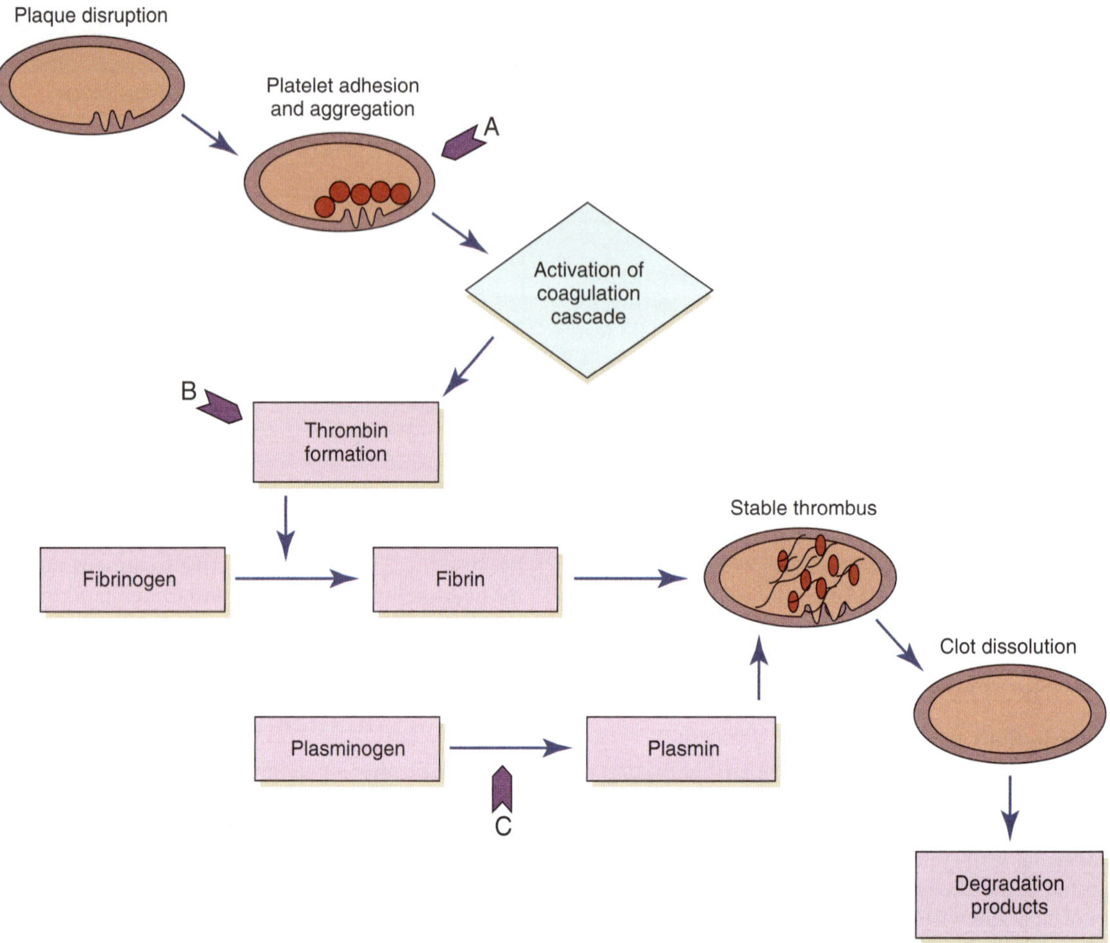

FIG. 14.10 Thrombus Formation and Site of Action of Medications Used in the Treatment of Acute Myocardial Infarction. (A) Site of action of antiplatelet agents such as aspirin, thienopyridines, and glycoprotein IIb/IIIa inhibitors. (B) Heparin bonds with antithrombin III and thrombin to create an inactive complex. (C) Fibrinolytic agents convert plasminogen to plasmin, an enzyme responsible for degradation of fibrin clots.

Eligibility Criteria

For patients who present with a STEMI at a non-PCI capable hospital, the multidisciplinary heart team must determine whether the "first medical contact-to-device" time will exceed 120 minutes for any reason (e.g., time to transfer to a PCI-capable facility) and if so, then fibrinolytics are recommended.[46] Patients with recent onset of chest pain (less than 12 hours' duration) and persistent ST segment elevation (greater than 0.1 mV in two or more contiguous leads) are considered candidates for fibrinolytic therapy.[47] Patients who present with bundle branch blocks on the ECG pose a challenge because this may obscure ST segment elevation. It is essential to elicit any history suggestive of an acute MI to accurately identify candidates for therapy. The goal of therapy is to administer fibrinolytic therapy within 30 minutes after presentation ("door-to-needle") because early reperfusion yields the greatest benefit.[47] See Myocardial Infarction in Chapter 13, specifically Fig. 13.3. Other criteria for the use of fibrinolytic therapy are presented in Box 14.9.

Exclusion Criteria for Fibrinolytic Therapy

Exclusion criteria are usually based on the increased risk of bleeding incurred from the use of fibrinolytics. Patients who have stable clots that might be disrupted by fibrinolytic therapy (recent surgery, facial or head trauma), uncontrolled hypertension, or ischemic stroke in the past 3 months are usually are not considered candidates for fibrinolytic therapy.[48] The major concern with fibrinolytic therapy is intracerebral hemorrhage.[45]

Fibrinolytic therapy is not indicated for patients with unstable angina or a NSTEMI.[49] Instead, these patients are treated with IV antiplatelet (GPIIb/IIIa inhibitors) and antithrombotic agents (heparin) followed by oral antiplatelet agents:

- GPIIb/IIIa inhibitors: abciximab, eptifibatide, and tirofiban (IV)
- Cyclooxygenase inhibitors: aspirin (oral)
- P2Y12 receptor antagonists: clopidogrel, prasugrel, ticagrelor (oral)

> **BOX 14.9 Fibrinolytic Therapy Selection Criteria**
>
> - No more than 12 hours from onset of chest pain and preferably within 30 minutes of diagnosis of ST segment elevation myocardial infarction
> - ST segment elevation on electrocardiogram or new-onset left bundle branch block
> - Ischemic chest pain unresponsive to sublingual nitroglycerin
> - No conditions that might cause a predisposition to hemorrhage

TABLE 14.4 PHARMACOLOGIC MANAGEMENT

Fibrinolytic Agents for Use in Acute Myocardial Infarction

Medication	Dosage	Actions	Special Considerations
Clot-Specific			
tPA (alteplase)	IV: 100 mg total 15 mg given as a bolus over 2 min followed by 50 mg IV infusion over 30 min then 35 mg IV infusion over 60 min (dose is adjusted based on weight for patients ≤67 kg)	Binds to fibrin at clot and promotes activation of plasminogen to plasmin	Anticoagulants are given concurrently. DAPT is begun with administration and continued daily.
rPA (reteplase)	IV: 10 units given as a bolus over 2 min, repeated in 30 min	Binds to fibrin at clot and promotes activation of plasminogen to plasmin	Anticoagulants are given concurrently. DAPT is begun with administration and continued daily.
Tenecteplase (TNKase)	IV: 30–50 mg based on body weight, given as a single bolus	Binds to fibrin at clot and promotes activation of plasminogen to plasmin	Anticoagulants are given concurrently. DAPT is begun with administration and continued daily.

DAPT, Dual antiplatelet therapy; *IV*, intravenous; *rPA*, recombinant plasminogen activator; *tPA*, tissue plasminogen activator.

Fibrinolytic Agents

Several fibrinolytic agents are available for intravenous treatment of acute STEMI. All these agents stimulate lysis of the clot by converting inactive plasminogen to plasmin, an enzyme responsible for degradation of fibrin (see Fig. 14.10). The first-generation fibrinolytic agents (e.g., streptokinase, urokinase) had their primary effect on circulating plasminogen. Newer fibrinolytic agents (e.g., alteplase, reteplase, tenecteplase) have a greater effect on clot plasminogen than on circulating plasminogen and are considered clot selective. Currently approved fibrinolytic agents are compared in Table 14.4. Because patients with an area of plaque disruption are still at risk for clot formation and reocclusion, fibrinolytic therapy is used in conjunction with anticoagulants and antiplatelet agents. Current guidelines recommend that anticoagulant therapy be administered for a minimum of 48 hours after reperfusion.[47] Unfractionated heparin traditionally has been used, but low-molecular-weight heparin and fondaparinux are also acceptable options and are preferred when anticoagulation is planned for more than 48 hours after fibrinolytic therapy.[47] Antiplatelet therapy with clopidogrel is recommended for at least 14 days up to 1 year, and aspirin should be continued indefinitely.[47]

Streptokinase

Streptokinase is a fibrinolytic agent derived from beta-hemolytic streptococci, which, when combined with plasminogen, catalyzes the conversion of plasminogen to plasmin, the enzyme responsible for clot dissolution in the body. Because streptokinase is a bacterial protein, it can produce various allergic reactions, including anaphylaxis. In addition, the fibrinolytic action of streptokinase is systemic (non–clot specific) and prolonged (half-life of 20 to 25 minutes), increasing the risk for bleeding complications. Because of these issues, streptokinase is no longer commercially available in the United States, although it is available in some other countries.

Tissue Plasminogen Activator

Tissue plasminogen activator (tPA), or alteplase (Activase), is a naturally occurring enzyme (i.e., nonantigenic) that is clot specific and has a very short half-life (3 to 4 minutes). It converts plasminogen to plasmin after binding to the fibrin-containing clot. This clot-specific action results in an increased concentration and activity of plasmin at the site of the clot, where it is needed. Several different intravenous dosing regimens have been proposed and tested in the clinical setting, but accelerated dose tPA is considered the most effective means of establishing early patency of the occluded vessel.

Recombinant Plasminogen Activator

Recombinant plasminogen activator, or reteplase, is a variant of the natural human enzyme tPA. Reteplase is less fibrin selective and has a longer half-life than tPA, making it suitable for bolus administration rather than as a continuous infusion. This new-generation plasminogen activator is given as a double bolus and then followed with adjunctive therapies. In contrast to tPA, reteplase does not require weight-based dosing. Studies have shown that reteplase is as effective as tPA in the treatment of acute STEMI and is easier to administer.

Tenecteplase

Tenecteplase (TNKase) is a genetically engineered variant of alteplase with slower plasma clearance and better fibrin specificity. Studies have shown that tenecteplase is as effective as alteplase, and the two agents have similar rates of bleeding complications. Tenecteplase requires only a single bolus injection, which may help facilitate more rapid treatment both inside and outside the hospital. Although the need for weight-based dosing is a potential disadvantage of this medication, tenecteplase is a widely used fibrinolytic agent in the United States at the present time.

Outcomes of Fibrinolytic Therapy

The benefit of fibrinolytic therapy correlates with the degree of restoration of normal blood flow in the infarct-related artery. Coronary artery patency is defined by angiographic perfusion grades developed by the *Thrombolysis in Myocardial Infarction (TIMI)* study group in 1985 (Table 14.5).[50] Achievement of TIMI grade 3 flow is associated with the best long-term survival. Studies also indicate that rapid restoration of normal blood flow, within 90 minutes after treatment, results in improved LV function and reduced mortality. The three fibrin-specific fibrinolytics achieve TIMI grade 2 or grade 3 flow in 73% to 84% of patients at 90 minutes.[50] Fibrinolytic therapy continues to evolve, and medication dose ranges and regimens are subject to change when research findings are updated.

TABLE 14.5 Flow in Infarct-Related Artery as Described in Thrombolysis in Myocardial Infarction Trial

Perfusion Grades	Flow in the Infarct-Related Artery
TIMI 3	Normal or brisk flow through coronary artery
TIMI 2	Partial flow, slower than in normal vessels
TIMI 1	Sluggish flow with incomplete distal filling
TIMI 0	No flow beyond point of occlusion

TIMI, Thrombolysis in Myocardial Infarction Trial.
Data from the TIMI Study Group. The Thrombolysis in Myocardial Infarction (TIMI) trial: phase I findings. *N Engl J Med.* 1985;312:932.

Evidence of Reperfusion

Several phenomena may be observed after reperfusion of an artery that has been completely occluded by a thrombus (Box 14.10). Although recognition of these noninvasive markers of recanalization is important for assessing the patient's response to fibrinolytic therapy, they are less reliable than angiography in determining whether reperfusion has been successful.

BOX 14.10 Noninvasive Evidence of Reperfusion

- Cessation of chest pain
- Reperfusion dysrhythmias, primarily ventricular
- Return of elevated ST segments to baseline
- Early and marked peaking of cardiac troponins

Pain and Reperfusion Dysrhythmias

One possible sign of reperfusion is the abrupt cessation of chest pain as blood flow is restored to the ischemic myocardium. Another potential indicator of reperfusion is the appearance of various reperfusion dysrhythmias. A variety of dysrhythmias can occur—premature ventricular contractions, bradycardias, heart block, VT—but accelerated idioventricular rhythms have shown the best correlation with reperfusion. Reperfusion dysrhythmias are usually self-limiting or nonsustained, and aggressive antidysrhythmic therapy is not required. However, vigilant monitoring of the patient's ECG is essential because dysrhythmias associated with ongoing ischemia could deteriorate rapidly and may necessitate emergency treatment.

ST Segment Monitoring Leads

Another noninvasive marker of recanalization is rapid return to baseline of the elevated ST segments, which indicates restoration of blood flow to previously ischemic myocardial tissue. A monitoring lead should be chosen that clearly demonstrates ST segment elevation before initiation of therapy (see Continuous ST Segment Monitoring in Chapter 12). The inability to achieve 50% to 70% resolution of ST segment elevation within 60 to 90 minutes of administering the medication is considered an indication of failure of fibrinolytic therapy.[47,50]

Cardiac Biomarkers After Fibrinolytic Therapy

Serial measurement of serum biomarkers may serve as further evidence of successful reperfusion after fibrinolytic therapy. Cardiac-specific creatine kinase and troponin increase rapidly and then decrease markedly after reperfusion of the ischemic myocardium. This phenomenon is called *washout* because it is thought to result from the rapid readmission of substances released by damaged myocardial cells into the circulation after restoration of blood flow (see Cardiac Biomarker Studies in Chapter 12; and Fig. 13.13 in Chapter 13).

Residual Coronary Artery Stenosis

Fibrinolytic therapy has been determined to be a successful strategy for reopening occluded coronary arteries in the setting of a STEMI. It limits infarct size, salvages myocardium, and significantly reduces morbidity and mortality associated with cardiogenic shock and VF. However, once the thrombus is lysed, residual coronary artery stenosis resulting from the atherosclerotic process will remain, even after successful fibrinolysis.

Subsequent prevention of reocclusion is critical to preserving myocardial function and preventing the risk of late complications. Therefore, fibrinolytic therapy is recognized as an emergency procedure to restore patency until more definitive therapy can be initiated to effectively reduce the degree of stenosis. Current guidelines recommend that patients who receive fibrinolytic therapy be transferred to a facility capable of performing PCI procedures and angiography within the first 3 to 6 hours to allow for additional interventions as warranted.[47]

BOX 14.11 Signs of Inadequate Hemostasis Related to Fibrinolytic Therapy

- Bleeding or hematoma at puncture sites
- Hematuria, hematemesis, hemoptysis, melena, epistaxis
- Bruising or petechiae (pinpoint hemorrhages)
- Flank ecchymoses with complaints of low back pain (suggestive of retroperitoneal bleeding)
- Gingival bleeding
- Change in neurologic status (intracranial bleeding)
- Deterioration in vital signs, decreased hematocrit values (internal bleeding)

Nursing Management

Nursing management of patients undergoing fibrinolytic therapy begins with identifying potential candidates. In many institutions, checklists are used to facilitate the rapid identification of patients who are candidates for fibrinolytics. The nurse prepares the patient for fibrinolytic therapy by starting IV lines and obtaining baseline laboratory values and vital signs. Throughout the administration of the fibrinolytic agent, assessment of the patient continues for clinical indicators of reperfusion and complications related to therapy.

Monitoring for Bleeding

The most common complication related to thrombolysis is bleeding, which is related to the fibrinolytic therapy itself and anticoagulation therapy that patients routinely receive to minimize the possibility of rethrombosis. The nurse must continually monitor for clinical manifestations of bleeding (Box 14.11). Mild gingival bleeding and oozing around venipuncture sites is common and not a cause of concern. Should serious bleeding occur, such as intracranial or internal bleeding, all fibrinolytic and antithrombotic therapies are discontinued, and volume expanders, coagulation factors, or both are administered.

Prevention of Bleeding

In addition to accurate assessment of the patient for evidence of bleeding, nursing management includes preventive measures to minimize the potential for bleeding. For example, handling of the patient is limited, injections are avoided if possible, and additional pressure is provided to ensure hemostasis at venipuncture and arterial puncture sites. Intravenous lines are placed before lytic therapy is administered, and a saline lock may be used for obtaining laboratory specimens during treatment.

Educate the Patient and Family

Education for the patient receiving fibrinolytic therapy includes information regarding the actions of fibrinolytic agents, with emphasis on precautions to minimize bleeding (Box 14.12). For example, the patient is cautioned against vigorous toothbrushing and told to refrain from using straight-edge razors. Information is provided regarding ongoing risk factor management in the prevention of atherosclerotic coronary artery disease (CAD) (see Chapter 13, Box 13.9).

PERCUTANEOUS CORONARY INTERVENTIONS

Percutaneous coronary intervention, abbreviated as PCI, has become the gold standard in the treatment of acute coronary disease used to reverse ongoing ischemia and infarction. Advances in device technology, along with more effective anticoagulant and antiplatelet regimens, have reduced complication rates and improved procedural outcomes. As a result, elective PCI is often performed as a short-stay or outpatient procedure.

In the setting of emergency PCI associated with acute myocardial ischemia, patients are hospitalized depending on the cardiovascular work-up that is required.

Coronary angiography is an essential component of PCI to provide anatomical information about critical coronary stenoses for PCI.[44]

Percutaneous transluminal coronary angioplasty (PTCA), frequently abbreviated to *balloon angioplasty*, was introduced in 1977 as an alternative to coronary surgical revascularization. PTCA avoided many of the risks associated with cardiac surgery (general anesthesia, sternotomy, extracorporeal circulation, and mechanical ventilation [MV]), but its success was hampered by complications related to the procedure (e.g., acute closure, dissection) and restenosis or renewed narrowing of the artery after the procedure.

Continued research led to the development of several interventional devices to overcome the limitations of conventional angioplasty and further expanded the use of catheter-based interventions. Current PCI procedures include PTCA, atherectomy, thrombectomy, and stent implantation and many adjunctive devices used to facilitate successful revascularization in coronary vessels.

Indications for Percutaneous Coronary Interventions

Indications for catheter-based interventions have been considerably broadened since the initial application of PTCA. Current guidelines recommend that when a patient presents with a STEMI, the "first medical contact-to-device" time should be less than 90 minutes for patients presenting to a PCI-capable site and less than 120 minutes for patients presenting to an outside facility who need to be transferred to a PCI-capable hospital.[47] See Fig. 13.3 in Chapter 13.

In non–ST elevation myocardial infarction (NSTEMI), PCI is used where there is nonocclusive but anatomically significant disease, generally greater than 70% occlusion, to revascularize the vessel, treat intractable angina, and to prevent further vessel occlusion.

BOX 14.12 PATIENT AND FAMILY EDUCATION PLAN

Fibrinolytic Therapy

Before discharge, the patient should be able to teach back the following topics:
- Pathophysiology of atherosclerosis
- Risk factor management
- Description of fibrinolytic agent and how it works
- Measures to minimize bleeding and bruising associated with fibrinolytic therapy
- Recognition and actions to take for recurrent ischemic symptoms
- Information regarding prescribed medications (antiplatelet agents, anticoagulants)

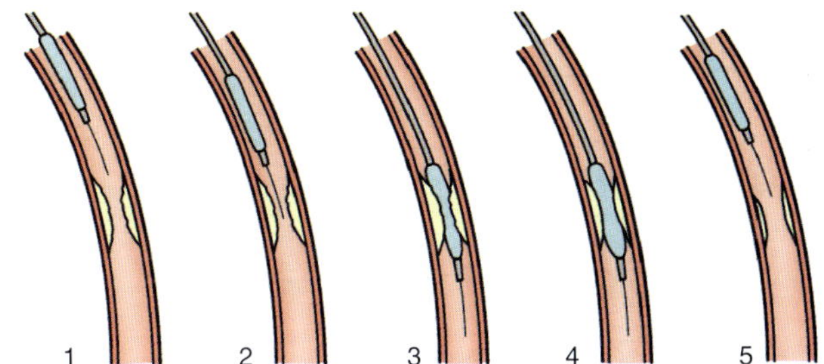

FIG. 14.11 Percutaneous Transluminal Coronary Angioplasty (PTCA). (1–2) Catheter is advanced over a guidewire; (3) catheter crosses the atherosclerotic plaque; (4) balloon is expanded; and (5) catheter is withdrawn. PTCA is used to open a stenotic vessel occluded by atherosclerosis.

Percutaneous Transluminal Coronary Angioplasty

PTCA involves the use of a balloon-tipped catheter that, when advanced through an atherosclerotic lesion (atheroma), can be inflated intermittently for the purpose of dilating the stenotic area and improving blood flow through it (Fig. 14.11). The high inflation pressure of the balloon stretches the vessel wall, fractures the plaque, and enlarges the vessel lumen. After balloon deflation, the vessel wall exhibits some elastic recoil.

Although PTCA has relatively high success rates in initially opening occluded vessels, the technique by itself has major limitations, including the risk of acute vessel closure and a high frequency of restenosis. For these reasons, coronary balloon angioplasty is usually combined with stent implants.

Balloon catheters now incorporate modifications of the balloon surface. Cutting balloons and scoring balloons are two types of available devices and are useful in facilitating lesion dilation. Currently, there are no trials showing any difference in recurrent restenosis between patients treated with cutting-balloon or standard-balloon angioplasty.[51]

Drug-coated balloon (DCB) angioplasty adds an antiproliferative medication coating to the balloon along with an excipient to avoid drug transfer, which may help prevent restenosis. Studies are still investigating whether use of DCB angioplasty alone is a feasible strategy to avoid the potential disadvantages of stent implantation.[51]

Intravascular Ultrasound

Intravascular ultrasound (IVUS) is helpful to assess the characteristics of the lesion from inside the vessel.[44] Intracoronary imaging allows for greater definition of the lesion morphology before a procedure, especially in higher-risk cases.[52]

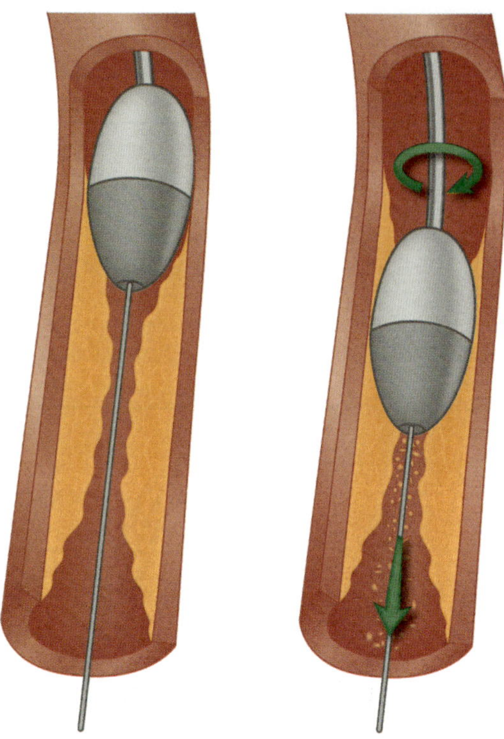

FIG. 14.12 Rotational Atherectomy Catheter.

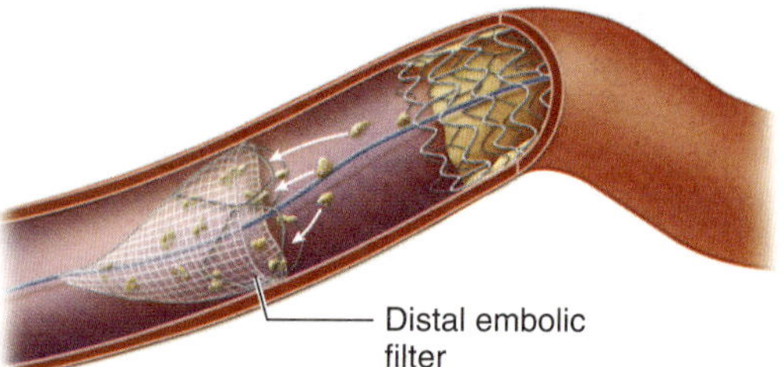

FIG. 14.13 Embolic Protection Device.

Atherectomy

Calcified lesions do not respond well to primary PTCA or to stent placement because a calcified coronary artery, or a densely fibrotic artery, is difficult to dilate.[44,53] Hence the importance of atherectomy, which is the excision and removal of atherosclerotic plaque by cutting, shaving, or grinding.[44] Atherectomy alone does not open the artery enough to treat severe CAD.[44] Instead, the role of atherectomy is to prepare the artery for stent deployment. The removal of calcification by rotational and orbital atherectomy is essential to facilitate stent delivery and optimal expansion.[44]

Rotational Atherectomy

Rotational atherectomy systems (Boston Scientific) have a high-speed, rotating, diamond-coated burr that drills through the plaque, creating tiny particles (Fig. 14.12). The particulate matter is carried through the bloodstream and disposed of by the reticuloendothelial system. Rotational atherectomy is designed to cut through calcified plaque.[44]

Orbital Atherectomy

Orbital atherectomy (Diamondback 360) has an eccentrically mounted crown, coated with diamonds, that rotates along the axis of the drive shaft and orbits along the vessel walls. Complications are rare, with the most serious being coronary perforation.[54]

Thrombectomy

Thrombectomy catheters are used to decrease the risk of thrombotic emboli by removing large thrombi from the vessel before the intervention. These devices are recommended primarily for use in PCI patients with a large thrombus burden.

Embolic Protection Devices

Initial devices for performing PCI were designed to optimize flow at the point of the lesion or blockage within the coronary artery. However, despite evidence of procedural success on angiography, some patients still exhibited signs of compromised distal perfusion. This is termed "no reflow" and is believed to be caused by distal embolization of atherosclerotic plaque or thrombus at the time of the procedure. Several adjunctive tools have been developed to help protect the microvasculature during PCI procedures. Embolic protection devices consist of balloons or filters that are positioned beyond the lesion to trap and remove debris that might be released during the intervention. One type of distal filter is shown in Fig. 14.13.

Coronary Stents

A major development in the field of interventional cardiology has been the coronary stent.[55] A stent is a metal structure that is introduced into the coronary artery over a guidewire and expanded into the vessel wall at the site of the lesion. Bare metal stents (BMS) were first used to treat acute or threatened vessel closure after failed PTCA. The stent acted as a scaffold to tack dissection flaps against the vessel wall and provided mechanical support to minimize elastic recoil. Subsequent studies confirmed the clinical benefits of stents, which led to elective coronary stent placement as a primary procedure. Stent implantation was initially limited to large vessels (greater than 3 mm) with proximal, discrete lesions. Improvements in stent design and operator technique allow for deployment in smaller vessels with diffuse disease, vessels with lesions at bifurcations, and vessels with thrombus.

Multiple stents may be implanted sequentially within a vessel to fully cover the area of the lesion. Numerous types of stents are available. They are composed of various types of metal (stainless steel, cobalt, or platinum chromium alloys) and come in a variety of configurations (mesh, coil).[55] Although initially composed of metal alone, contemporary stents incorporate various polymer coatings and medications to improve long-term patency of the vessel. Most stents are balloon expandable[55] (Fig. 14.14).

Drug-Eluting Stents

The drug-eluting stents (DESs) were developed to minimize in-stent restenosis and hyperplasia.[55] These stents have polymer coatings impregnated with medications that are released slowly into the endothelium at the site of stent placement to inhibit cellular proliferation. Current DESs (second-generation everolimus-eluting stents and zotarolimus-eluting stents) have proven superior outcomes compared with first-generation stents.[44] Even with the development of biodegradable polymer

DES, and stents with bioresorbable vascular scaffolding, second-generation metallic DESs are the most used in PCI today. BMS have declined in use due to the superior performance of DES[55] (Table 14.6).

Bioresorbable Stents

Bioresorbable stents or nonmetallic "scaffolds" were developed to avoid a metal stent remaining permanently in the artery. The scaffold was designed to create a temporary mechanical support for the arterial wall and then to biodegrade over time.[55] However, in early trials the scaffolds were assocated with higher stent thrombosis compared to DES.[56] Despite early challenges, research and development to find bioresorbable solutions continues.[55,56]

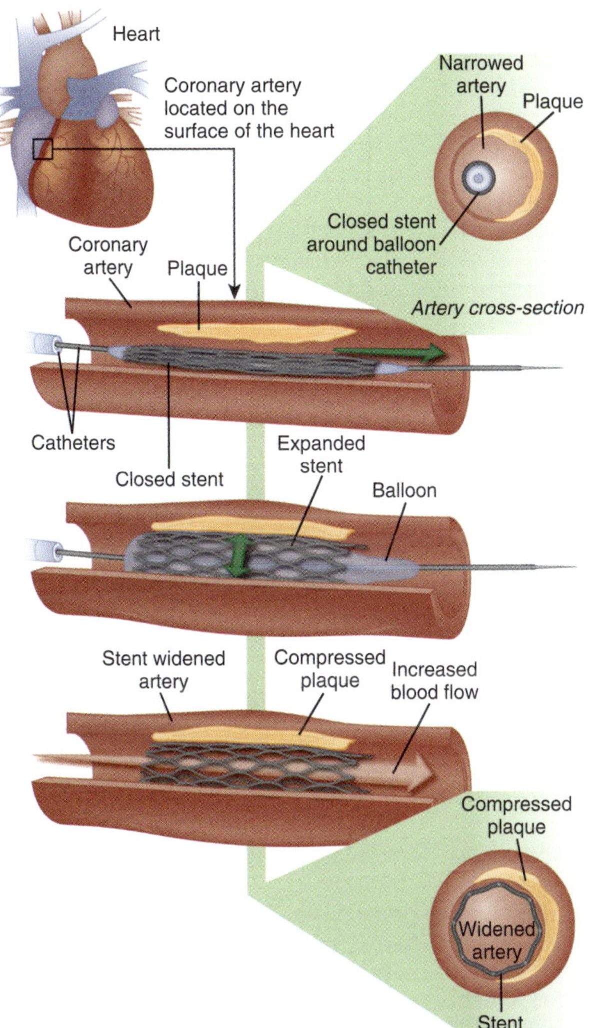

FIG. 14.14 The Intracoronary Stent Is a Balloon-Expandable Stent.

Stent Thrombosis

Early use of stents was hampered by a high incidence of subacute stent thrombosis: abrupt occlusion of a previously patent vessel secondary to clot formation. Later it was found that stent thrombosis was caused in part by inadequate stent expansion within the vessel, which could be remedied by applying high-pressure balloon inflations within the stent during deployment.

Antiplatelet Therapy After Stent Deployment

Antithrombotic therapy, including dual antiplatelet therapy (DAPT) and anticoagulation, is important to prevent stent thrombosis.[44,48] Because platelet activation is a complex process involving multiple pathways, combination therapy with two or more agents has proven most effective.[44] The current standard of care for PCI typically includes dual antiplatelet therapy with aspirin and a P2Y12 inhibitor.[44,57] These oral agents are administered before the procedure and continued at discharge.[44] Oral antiplatelet agents are described in Table 14.7.

Cangrelor is an intravenous P2Y12 inhibitor option for patients unable to take oral antiplatelet agents or for patients scheduled for immediate surgery. Platelet inhibition takes place within 20 minutes and returns when the intravenous infusion is stopped. Although it is a seemingly ideal antiplatelet agent, both availability and cost have limited its use in the United States.[57]

GPIIb/IIIa inhibitors, which are more potent intravenous antiplatelet agents, could be considered in patients who have inadequate P2Y12 receptor inhibitor loading or a large thrombus burden.[48] These medications act on the GPIIb/IIIa receptors on the platelet membrane to inhibit the final phase of platelet aggregation and prevent platelets from binding with fibrinogen. Intravenous antiplatelet agents are described in Table 14.8.

In-Stent Restenosis

Stents have been shown to decrease the incidence of restenosis compared with balloon angioplasty, most likely from achieving the largest possible lumen diameter at the time of the intervention. Successful stent implantation should result in less than 10% residual stenosis and optimally as close to zero as possible. However, stents have not proved to be the cure for restenosis, as was once hoped. Restenosis within the stent is caused by intimal hyperplasia and can occur in a diffuse pattern throughout the stent, as discrete lesions within the body of the stent, or at the stent margins. In contrast to thrombosis, restenosis is a gradual process that generally occurs within the first 6 to 12 months and manifests clinically as recurrent angina. Factors that increase the risk of in-stent restenosis are listed in Box 14.13.

TABLE 14.6 Comparison of Bare Metal and Drug-Eluting Stents

Characteristics	Bare Metal Stent	Drug-Eluting Stent
Restenosis rate (at 6 months)	15%–20%	5%–10%
Cost	$	$$$
Duration of dual antiplatelet therapy	Minimum of 1 month for non-ACS patients, at least 12 months for stents implanted for ACS	Minimum of 6 months for either non-ACS or ACS patients and longer if tolerated
Recommended lesion features	Short lesions <20 mm Large vessel diameter >3 mm	Longer lesions >20 mm Small vessel diameter <3.5 mm

ACS, Acute coronary syndrome; *mm* millimeters.

TABLE 14.7 PHARMACOLOGIC MANAGEMENT

Oral Antiplatelet Agents

Medication	Dosage	Action	Special Considerations
COX Inhibitor			
Aspirin	81–325 mg initial dose 81 mg maintenance dose	Inhibits synthesis of thromboxane A_2 resulting in irreversible inhibition of platelet activation	Lower doses are recommended when given with other antithrombotics
P2Y12 Inhibitors			
Clopidogrel (Plavix)	600 mg loading dose 75 mg maintenance	Irreversibly inhibits ADP P2Y12 platelet receptor to block platelet activation	Onset of action 2–4 hours Should be held 5–7 days before elective surgery to decrease risk of bleeding Some patients may have a genetic resistance to clopidogrel, resulting in inadequate platelet inhibition
Prasugrel (Effient)	60 mg loading dose 10 mg daily maintenance	Irreversibly inhibits ADP P2Y12 platelet receptor to block platelet activation	Onset of action 15–30 min Should be held 5–7 days before elective surgery to decrease risk of bleeding Contraindicated in patients with prior TIA or stroke; not recommended in patients age >75 years
Ticagrelor (Brilinta)	180 mg loading dose 90 mg twice daily maintenance	Reversibly inhibits ADP P2Y12 platelet receptor to block platelet activation	Onset of action 30 min Should be held 5 days before elective surgery to decrease risk of bleeding Contraindicated in patients with history of ICH or severe hepatic impairment Maintenance aspirin dose >100 mg reduces effectiveness

ADP, Adenosine diphosphate; *ICH*, intracranial hemorrhage; *TIA*, transient ischemic attack.

TABLE 14.8 PHARMACOLOGIC MANAGEMENT

Intravenous Antiplatelet Agents

Medication	Dosage	Action	Special Considerations
P2Y12 Inhibitor			
Cangrelor	30 mcg/kg IV bolus over 1 minute then 4 mcg/kg/min IV infusion for at least 2 hours or duration of PCI	Reversibly inhibits ADP P2Y12 platelet receptor to block platelet activation	Platelet inhibition in 20 minutes with return of platelet function with the cessation of IV infusion
GP 11b/111a Inhibitor			
Abciximab (ReoPro)	ACS: 0.25 mg/kg IV over 5 minutes followed by 0.125 mcg/kg/min (max 10 mcg/min) IV infusion for 12 hours. PCI: 0.25 mg/kg IV over 5 min followed by IV infusion of 10 mcg/min for 18–24 hours concluding 1 hour after PCI	Inhibits GPIIb/IIIa receptors responsible for platelet aggregation	Used concomitantly with aspirin and anticoagulants May affect platelet function for 48 hours after infusion
Eptifibatide (Integrilin)	ACS: 180 mcg/kg IV bolus, followed by continuous infusion of 2 mcg/kg/min up to 72 hours PCI: 180 mcg/kg IV bolus immediately before PCI (repeat after 10 min) followed by continuous infusion of 2 mcg/kg/min for 12–24 h	Reversibly binds to GPIIb/IIIa platelet receptor and inhibits platelet aggregation	Concomitant aspirin and anticoagulants may be administered Platelet function returns to baseline within 6–8 hours Contraindicated in patients with significant kidney dysfunction
Tirofiban (Aggrastat)	ACS: 25 mcg/kg within 5 min, then continued at 0.15 mcg/kg/min for up to 18 hours	Reversibly binds to GPIIb/IIIa platelet receptor and inhibits platelet aggregation	Platelet function returns to baseline within 4–8 hours Dosage should be reduced in patients with kidney dysfunction

ACS, Acute coronary syndrome; *GP*, glycoprotein; *IV*, intravenous; *PCI*, percutaneous coronary intervention.

PCI Procedure

PCI is performed in the cardiac catheterization laboratory under fluoroscopy. Patients typically receive antiplatelet therapy (a P2Y12 inhibitor and aspirin) before beginning the procedure. An introducer catheter, or sheath, is inserted percutaneously into an artery to provide access to the coronary arteries. Access via the radial artery (transradial access) has become the preferred method because studies show that it results in lower rates of bleeding complications, is associated with earlier ambulation, and demonstrates improved outcomes.[58] The femoral artery is still used when larger catheters are needed or because of anatomic limitations when the catheter cannot be advanced from the radial artery. In some cases, a venous sheath is inserted and used to perform a right heart catheterization. A catheter with pacing capabilities may be indicated if dilation of the right coronary artery or circumflex artery is anticipated because the blood supply to the conduction system of the heart may be interrupted, requiring emergency pacing.

The patient is systemically anticoagulated to prevent clots from forming on or in any of the catheters. Unfractionated heparin has been used traditionally, initiated with a weight-based bolus, and then titrated to achieve a target activated clotting time. Other anticoagulants may be selected if the patient cannot tolerate heparin. Options for anticoagulant agents are described in Table 14.9.

BOX 14.13 Risk Factors for In-Stent Restenosis

Patient Factors

- Age
- Diabetes mellitus
- Chronic kidney failure

Anatomic Factors

- Longer lesions (>20 mm)
- Small vessel diameter (<3 mm)
- Complex, branched lesions

Procedural Factors

- Inadequate stent expansion
- Stent design (bare metal stent vs. drug-eluting stent)
- Gaps in sequential stent placement in the artery

A special guiding catheter, designed to engage the coronary ostia, is inserted through the arterial sheath and advanced in a retrograde manner through the aorta. Nitroglycerin, calcium channel blockers, or adenosine may be given at this time to prevent coronary artery spasm and to maximize coronary vasodilation during the procedure. A guidewire is then advanced down the coronary artery and negotiated across the occluding atheroma. The balloon catheter is advanced over this guidewire and positioned across the lesion. The balloon is inflated and deflated repetitively until evidence of dilation is demonstrated on an angiogram (Fig. 14.15). For lesions that do not respond well to angioplasty, additional plaque or thrombus removal may be done with an adjunctive device.

In most procedures, vessel dilation is followed by deployment of an intracoronary stent. A stent is positioned at the target site, the stent is expanded, and the catheter is removed, leaving the stent in place. IVUS is used by many clinicians to evaluate the vessel lumen diameter after stent deployment to ensure optimal expansion. Information obtained by ultrasound provides a better estimate of residual plaque than information provided by angiography because contrast material may surround the latticework of the stent, giving the appearance of a large lumen even when the stent is not fully open.

To facilitate early sheath removal, heparin or other anticoagulants are usually discontinued immediately after the procedure.

TABLE 14.9 PHARMACOLOGIC MANAGEMENT

Anticoagulants

Medication	Dosage	Action	Special Considerations
Unfractionated Heparin			
Heparin sodium	Initial bolus 60 units/kg (maximum dose 4000 units), followed by 12 units/kg/h infusion	Enhances activity of antithrombin III, a natural anticoagulant, to prevent clot formation	Effectiveness of treatment may be monitored by aPTT or ACT Response is variable because of binding with plasma proteins Effects may be reversed with protamine sulfate Risk of developing HIT Should not be given to patients already receiving therapeutic SC enoxaparin
Low-Molecular-Weight Heparin			
Enoxaparin (Lovenox)	30 mg IV bolus, followed by 1 mg/kg SC every 12 h For patients already on SC dosing, an additional bolus of 0.3 mg/kg is given if last dose was >8 h before PCI	Enhances activity of antithrombin III	More predictable response than heparin because enoxaparin is not largely bound to protein No need for aPTT or ACT monitoring Lower risk of HIT than with UFH Significant reduction in dosage needed when CrCl <30 mL/min Administer within 30 min of initiation of fibrinolytic therapy
Direct Thrombin Inhibitors			
Bivalirudin (Angiomax)	0.75 mg/kg IV bolus, followed by infusion at 1.75 mg/kg/h during PCI	Directly inhibits thrombin	May be administered alone or in combination with GPIIb/IIIa inhibitors Produces dose-dependent increase in aPTT and ACT Coagulation times return to baseline within 1 h after stopping infusion Dose should be reduced for patients with kidney dysfunction No reversal agent is available May be used instead of UFH for patients with HIT
Argatroban	Loading dose of 100 mcg/kg IV bolus over 1 min, followed by infusion of 1–3 mcg/kg/min for 6–72 hours	Directly inhibits thrombin	May be used instead of UFH for patients with HIT ACT is monitored during PCI; aPTT is used during prolonged infusion Abrupt discontinuation may lead to rebound hypercoagulable state
Factor Xa Inhibitor			
Fondaparinux (Arixtra)	2.5 mg IV, followed by 2.5 mg SC once daily	Selective inhibitor of factor Xa	May be used in conjunction with fibrinolytics For PCI, must be administered with another anticoagulant (i.e., UFH) to prevent catheter thrombosis Long half-life (>17 h) Contraindicated in patients with kidney failure

ACT, Activated clotting time; *aPTT*, activated partial thromboplastin time; *CrCl*, creatinine clearance; *GP*, glycoprotein; *HIT*, heparin-induced thrombocytopenia; *IV*, intravenous/intravenously; *MI*, myocardial infarction; *PCI*, percutaneous coronary intervention; *SC*, subcutaneous/subcutaneously; *UFH*, unfractionated heparin.

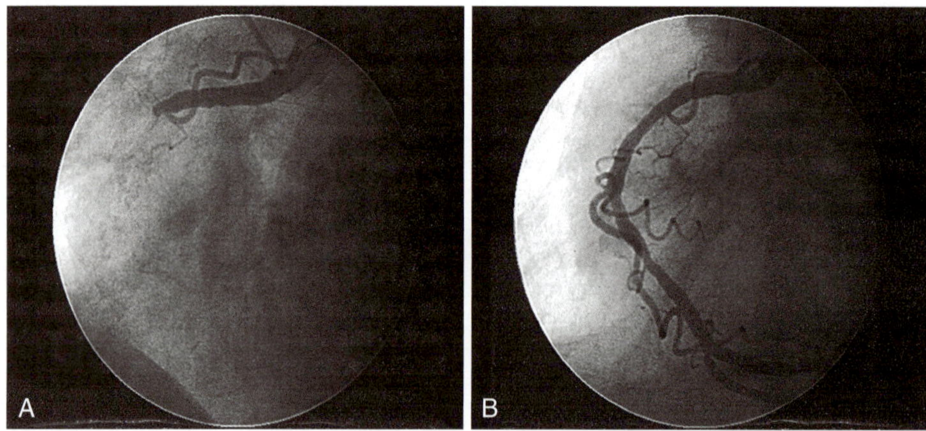

FIG. 14.15 (A) Coronary arteriogram of an acute proximal total occlusion of the right coronary artery. The patient had sudden onset of chest pain at home and was emergently admitted to the cardiac catheterization laboratory. (B) The same vessel as in (A) after successful coronary atherectomy and intracoronary fibrinolytic therapy to open the occluded artery. Symptoms of chest pain resolved after the procedure.

Sheaths are removed when the activated clotting time returns to normal in heparinized patients or sooner if other anticoagulants or a vascular closure device (VCD) is used. If GPIIb/IIIa inhibitors were initiated during the procedure, they may be continued for 12 to 24 hours, depending on the agent used. Dual antiplatelet therapy (DAPT) with aspirin and a P2Y12 inhibitor (clopidogrel, prasugrel, or ticagrelor) is routinely prescribed at discharge. Recommendations for P2Y12 inhibitor administration vary based on the type of stent used (see Table 14.6), whereas aspirin is continued indefinitely.

Acute Complications After PCI

The incidence of serious cardiac complications after PCI, including coronary spasm, coronary artery dissection, and acute coronary thrombosis, has decreased significantly with improvements in technology. Stents have proved efficacious in the repair of coronary dissections, decreasing the need for emergency bypass surgery. Acute thrombosis has decreased with the established use of dual antiplatelet agents known as DAPT. Bleeding and complications at the site of vascular cannulation (hematoma, compromised blood flow to the involved extremity, and retroperitoneal bleeding with femoral access) occur infrequently but are associated with increased morbidity and lengthened hospitalization. Other complications that can occur in the period immediately after PCI include contrast-induced acute kidney injury (CI-AKI), dysrhythmias, and vasovagal response (hypotension, bradycardia, and diaphoresis) during manipulation or removal of introducer sheaths.

Nursing Management

Nursing management after PCI focuses on accurate assessment of the patient's condition and prompt intervention. The nurse at the bedside is in a unique position to continuously monitor for clinical manifestations of potential problems and to take quick and appropriate action to minimize the deleterious effects of complications related to the interventional catheter procedure.

Monitoring for Angina

It is essential that the nurse observes the patient for recurrent angina or ST segment elevation, which are clinical indicators of myocardial ischemia. Monitoring leads should be selected that will reflect ischemia in the vessels that were treated during the intervention. Angina after a coronary interventional procedure may be caused by transient coronary vasospasm, or it may signal a more serious complication: acute thrombosis. In any case, the nurse must act quickly to assess for manifestations of myocardial ischemia and initiate clinical interventions as indicated. Nitroglycerin (IV) can be titrated to alleviate chest pain. Continued angina despite maximal vasodilator therapy usually rules out transient coronary vasospasm as the source of ischemic pain, and a return to the cardiac catheterization laboratory must be considered.

Prevention of Contrast-Induced Acute Kidney Injury

Patients undergoing PCI are exposed to significant amounts of contrast dye (radiopaque dye), with its associated risk of nephrotoxicity. *Contrast-induced acute kidney injury* (CI-AKI) is recognized by a decline in kidney function within days following contrast administration. Because there is no specific treatment for CI-AKI, protective strategies should be implemented before the procedure, especially for patients with evidence of baseline kidney impairment.[59] First, the avoidance of unnecessary contrast administration is important to prevent CI-AKI. This means limiting the quantity of contrast and using low-osmolality or iso-osmolality contrast.[59] Whenever possible, avoid concomitant use of other nephrotoxic drugs such as nonsteroidal antiinflammatory drugs (NSAIDs) and metformin. Absolutely avoid dehydration and ensure adequate hydration before and after the procedure. Controversy remains as to the optimal IV solution for hydration and whether there are medications that can prevent CI-AKI and research is ongoing in this area.[59]

Vascular Site Care—Radial Artery

Radial arterial access for PCI is associated with a lower rate of complications than the traditional femoral arterial approach.[60] Ultrasound is used to guide access.[61] After obtaining radial access, peripheral circulation may be assessed by monitoring the plethysmography waveform from a pulse oximeter probe placed on the thumb of the affected extremity. A splint may be used to prevent flexion of the wrist.

Vascular Site Care—Femoral Artery

If a femoral approach was used, while the sheath is in place or after its removal, bleeding or hematoma at the insertion site may occur secondary to the effects of anticoagulation. Frequent assessments of the puncture site for signs of bleeding or swelling or for changes in vital signs such as hypotension or tachycardia are required. Additionally, patient symptoms of back pain could indicate retroperitoneal bleeding from the internal arterial puncture site.

After sheath removal, direct pressure is applied to the puncture site for 15 to 30 minutes until hemostasis is achieved. If direct pressure is inadequate or the patient is at higher risk for bleeding, an external hemostatic device may be used to apply continuous pressure for 1 to 2 hours to ensure adequate hemostasis. Patients usually are allowed to resume ambulation 4 to 8 hours after the procedure or sooner if a VCD is employed.[62]

Vascular Closure Devices—Femoral Artery

Many products have been introduced to facilitate adequate hemostasis at the femoral access site after sheath removal. These products are known as vascular closure devices, and different devices are used depending on cardiologist preference, vessel size, catheter size (French size), and procedure (Fig. 14.16).[62–64] The types of closure devices are broadly grouped as:

- Suture-based closure
- Plug-based closure—collagen/sealant/gel
- Clip/staple closure
- Manual compression devices

Advantages of VCDs include a reduced time to hemostasis, earlier ambulation, and patient comfort.[62] Table 14.10 describes various vascular closure systems.[62] Disadvantages associated with VCDs include risk of device failure or malfunction, infection, potential limb ischemia, bleeding/hematoma, embolization, and device cost.[62] Generally, a larger sheath/catheter size is associated with a higher risk of complications. A recent nursing meta-analysis assessed VCD failure rates as a percentage per 100 cases compared to manual compression.[63]

- Suture based: 6.84%
- Plug sealant/gel based: 7.22%
- Plug collagen based: 3.15%
- Clip/staple closure: 3.28%

Peripheral Ischemia

Peripheral ischemia can occur secondary to cannulation of an artery, so nursing care includes frequent assessment of the adequacy of circulation to the involved extremity (Box 14.14). The patient is instructed to keep the limb straight and minimize movement. For femoral access, the head of the bed is not elevated more than 30 degrees while the sheath is in place (to prevent dislodgment) and for a period after its removal (to prevent bleeding). Additional activity restrictions vary depending on the size and location of the sheath, type of anticoagulation, the method used to achieve hemostasis, and institutional protocols.

Educate the Patient and Family

In most cases, patients undergoing elective angioplasty, atherectomy, or stent procedures are hospitalized for less than

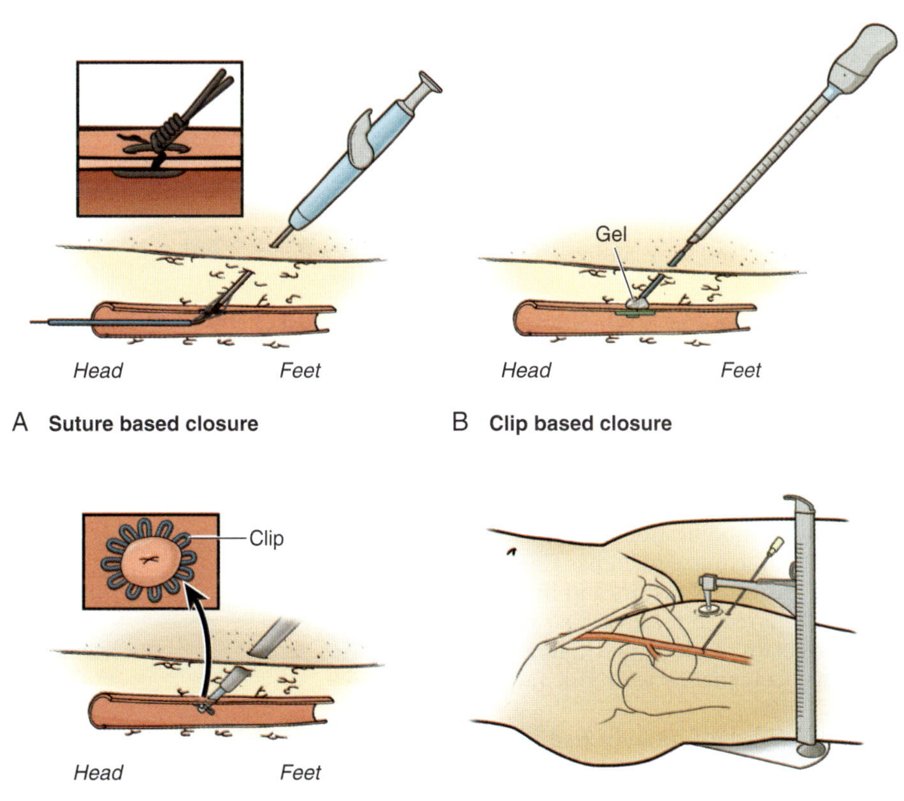

FIG. 14.16 Vascular Closure Devices for the Femoral Artery. (A) Suture-based closure. (B) Clip-/staple-based closure. (C) Plug sealant-/gel-/collagen-based closure. (D) External compression device closure. (Courtesy Perclose, Inc., Redwood City, CA.).

TABLE 14.10 **Vascular Closure Devices**

Device Category	Device Name	Puncture Size, F	Comments
Suture Based			
Clip or staple	StarClose SE	5,6	Extravascular nitinol clip over arteriotomy site
Suture	Prostar XL	8.5–10	Percutaneous braided polyester suture delivered, for procedures requiring larger sheaths
Suture	ProGlide ProStyle	5–21	A suture loop is formed to close the arteriotomy. Two devices and a preclose technique are required for sheath sizes >8F
Plug Based			
Collagen based	Angio-Seal	5/6, 7/8	An absorbable collagen plug deployed over the arteriotomy site expands in subcutaneous tissue, it is connected to an endoluminal bioresorbable toggle.
Collagen based	MANTA	14, 18	Suitable for large bore femoral access, available in 14F and 18F sizes. Delivers a collage hemostatic plug outside the arterial puncture site.
Collagen based	Vascade Vascular Closure System	5–7	A low-profile disc is deployed intraluminally to abut the wall as a collagen plug is deployed extraluminally over the arteriotomy site
Sealant or gel based	MYNXGRIP	5–7	Small, semicompliant balloon is inflated intraluminally to serve as an anchor as the sealant is deployed over the arteriotomy
Sealant or gel based	Exoseal	5–7	A bioabsorbable polyglycolic acid plug is deployed extraluminally over the arteriotomy
Sealant or gel based	Closer Vascular Sealing System	5–7	Absorbable intraluminal patch and extraluminal spheres that are cinched together with absorbable stitch
Sealed or gel based	FISH CombiClose (Femoral Introducer Sheath and Hemostasis)	5–8	The introducer sheath is used to position the patch. A bioabsorbable matrix patch is deployed through the arteriotomy that straddles the arterial wall.
External Hemostasis Devices – Compression Based			
External compression	FemoStop	Any size	Transparent inflatable bubble placed over the puncture site and belt wrapped around patient for stabilization
	CompressAR	Any size	Hands-free stand with transparent disc that is placed over puncture site and adjusted to height.
	QuicKlamp	Any size	Hands-free stand with compression discs with or without calcium alginate pad, adjusted to height and amount of pressure provided.

Data obtained from: Noori VJ, Eldrup-Jørgensen J. A systematic review of vascular closure devices for femoral artery puncture sites. *J Vasc Surg.* 2018;68(3):887–899; Noble S, Mauler-Wittwer S. Vascular closure for large-bore access: Plug-based or sutured-based vascular closure devices? *Can J Cardiol.* 2023;39(11):1535–1538.

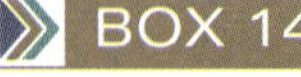

BOX 14.14 **Safety**

Peripheral Ischemia

- Maintain head of bed 30 degrees or lower for femoral access
- Keep cannulated extremity straight (use immobilizer or splint as needed)
- Monitor distal perfusion (pulse strength, capillary refill) frequently
- Assess color, sensation, and temperature in involved extremity

24 hours. All patients require education about their medication regimen and about risk factor modification (Box 14.15). Because of the short hospital stay, the nurse often has time to do little more than identify the major risk factors and initiate basic instruction. Patients are referred to local cardiac rehabilitation centers for more extensive teaching and follow-up to facilitate understanding and compliance with risk factor modification.

Another point of instruction that must be addressed is the patient's knowledge deficit related to discharge medications. Patients are sent home on a regimen of antiplatelet medications and medications for secondary prevention, such as lipid-lowering agents and blood pressure medications. A nitrate such as isosorbide may be prescribed to promote vasodilation, or, if the patient has demonstrated evidence of a vasospastic component to the disease, calcium channel blockers may be used. It is essential that the patient clearly understands the rationale for therapy and the potential side effects of each medication. Patients also need to understand the importance of adherence to their antiplatelet therapy because premature discontinuation of these agents is associated with increased risk of death from stent thrombosis.

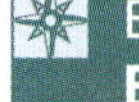

BOX 14.15 **PATIENT AND FAMILY EDUCATION PLAN**

Percutaneous Transluminal Coronary Angioplasty, Coronary Atherectomy, and Stent Placement

Before discharge, the patient should be able to teach back the following topics:

- Pathophysiology of atherosclerosis
- Risk factor modification (diet, exercise, smoking cessation, weight loss)
- Information about prescribed medications (e.g., antiplatelet agents, antihypertensives, nitrates, calcium channel blockers, lipid-lowering medications)
- Symptoms to report to the health care professional (chest pain, shortness of breath, bleeding or drainage from the access site)
- Follow-up appointments

PERCUTANEOUS VALVE REPAIR

Percutaneous catheter technology has been adapted for management of valvular heart disease. There are catheter interventions for mitral regurgitation and for aortic stenosis. There are approximately 10,000 transcatheter mitral valve repairs and 78,000 transcatheter aortic implantations each year in the United States.[65] Annual procedural minimal volume per site is recommended at 50 procedures per year to maintain competence with the procedure.[66]

Mitral Regurgitation—Transcatheter Repair

The mitral valve has a complex anatomical structure (leaflets, chordae tendinea, and papillary muscles) and mitral regurgitation can occur from primary valve dysfunction or secondary to LV dysfunction or enlargement. Because of the variation in presentations, the options for transcatheter repair interventions are also varied, depending on the valve pathophysiology.[67] These include the edge-to-edge repair, annuloplasty, chordal implant, and transcatheter mitral valve replacement.[67]

Transcatheter edge-to-edge repair (TEER) is recommended for patients with severe degenerative mitral regurgitation who have advanced heart failure, are very symptomatic, have extreme surgical risk, and have a life expectancy of at least 1 year.[68] A preprocedure transoesophageal echocardiogram (TEE) is used to assess the mitral valve leaflets and the position of the regurgitant jet. The *MitraClip*™ edge-to edge repair has been widely studied. The clip approximates (brings together) the anterior and posterior mitral leaflets, creating two openings for blood to flow through from atria to ventricle. Postprocedure nursing management is very similar to other transcatheter cardiac procedures.

Mitral Stenosis—Balloon Valvuloplasty

Balloon valvuloplasty, also known as a *percutaneous mitral balloon commissurotomy* (PMBC), is performed in the cardiac catheterization laboratory.[69] A preprocedure TEE is done to ensure the left atrium is free of thrombus and to calculate the mitral valve area, which is often $\leq 1.5\ cm^2$ in mitral stenosis.[68]

A balloon is placed across the stenotic valve and inflated to separate the commissures (valve leaflets) and increase the opening size. Regurgitant flow can result after mitral valvuloplasty and may require emergent valve replacement if severe.

The risks of balloon valvuloplasty resemble the risks inherent in most cardiac catheterization procedures and include perforations, thromboembolic events, dysrhythmias, and vascular complications caused by the sheath. Nursing management after the procedure is very similar to nursing care for other percutaneous heart catheter procedures.

Aortic Stenosis—Transcatheter Aortic Valve Implantation

Transcatheter aortic valve implantation (TAVI) also known as *transcatheter aortic valve replacement* (TAVR) is a transformational therapy for patients who have severe aortic valve stenosis. Patient inclusion criteria has been expanded from high-risk surgical candidates to now include patients with lower surgical risk.[65,68,70] TAVI can be done with spinal or general anesthesia in a hybrid-equipped cardiac surgery operating room. Access is generally via the femoral artery using a large bore sheath (14F-18F).[65]

The TAVI procedure consists of positioning a bioprosthetic valve that has been loaded on a stent within the native aortic valve and then expanding the stent to anchor the valve within the aortic annulus. Different approaches are used to deploy the device. Correct location is checked by echocardiography, hemodynamic assessment, and/or aortography.

Postprocedural monitoring includes mental status assessment, telemetry, vital signs, volume status, and possible clinical laboratory tests.[70] Vascular access complications can be significant after TAVI, requiring close monitoring of the insertion site to detect possible bleeding, hematoma formation, or limb ischemia. Recommendations are for patients to continue on dual antiplatelet therapy for 3 to 6 months to prevent thromboembolism and ensure that the valve is endothelialized.[70]

CARDIAC SURGERY

Nursing management of a patient undergoing cardiac surgery is demanding but exciting work that requires the talents of an experienced team of critical care nurses. This section introduces basic cardiac surgical techniques along with principles of cardiopulmonary bypass (CPB) and highlights the key points about postoperative care of adult patients who require valve replacement, coronary artery revascularization, or other cardiac surgical procedures.

Coronary Artery Bypass Graft Surgery

Since its introduction over 60 years ago, coronary artery bypass graft (CABG) surgery has proved to be safe and effective in relieving angina symptoms and improving survival in most patients. Although there has been a great deal of evolution involving less invasive techniques, improved pharmacologic therapy, and expanded education regarding lifestyle modifications, CABG surgery continues to have an important role in the treatment of CAD. Information on CAD is presented in Chapter 13, and catheter-based interventions for CAD are discussed earlier in this chapter.

Surgical revascularization has been shown to be more efficacious than PCI in patients with multivessel or left main coronary disease.[44] It has been shown that coronary artery bypass surgery is very effective in relieving angina, in many cases is able to delay infarction, and in most cases can improve patient survival. Bypass surgery may allow for more complete revascularization because it can be used on vessels that are not amenable to treatment with a percutaneous approach, such as vessels with total occlusions or excessive tortuosity. However, as medical therapy and surgical procedures continue to evolve, updated studies and evaluations are required to guide optimal treatment.

Myocardial revascularization involves the use of a conduit, or channel, designed to bypass an occluded coronary artery. Surgeons must evaluate which conduits would provide the best graft patency and long-term outcomes for their patients. The long saphenous vein graft (SVG) is the most frequently used conduit for CABG surgery. Saphenous vein grafting involves the anastomosis of an excised portion of the saphenous vein proximal to the aorta and distal to the coronary artery below the obstruction. Vein-graft harvesting can be done via either an open or endoscopic approach (Fig. 14.17).

Use of arterial conduits has dramatically improved long-term graft patency. The internal thoracic artery (ITA), which usually remains attached to its origin at the subclavian artery, is swung down and anastomosed distal to the coronary

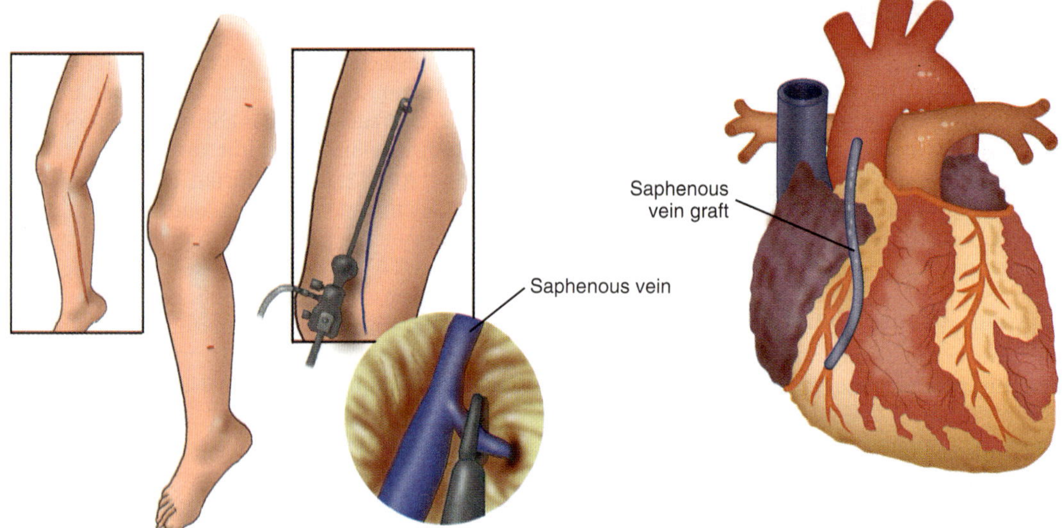

FIG. 14.17 (A) Saphenous vein graft removal from the leg either surgically (longer incisions) or endoscopic (small incisions), also showing closure of smaller side-branching veins. (B) Saphenous vein graft in situ from the aorta distal to bypass the atherosclerotic occlusion. (Leg illustration from Moser D, Riegel B. *Cardiac Nursing: A Companion to Braunwald's Heart Disease*. Philadelphia: Saunders; 2007.)

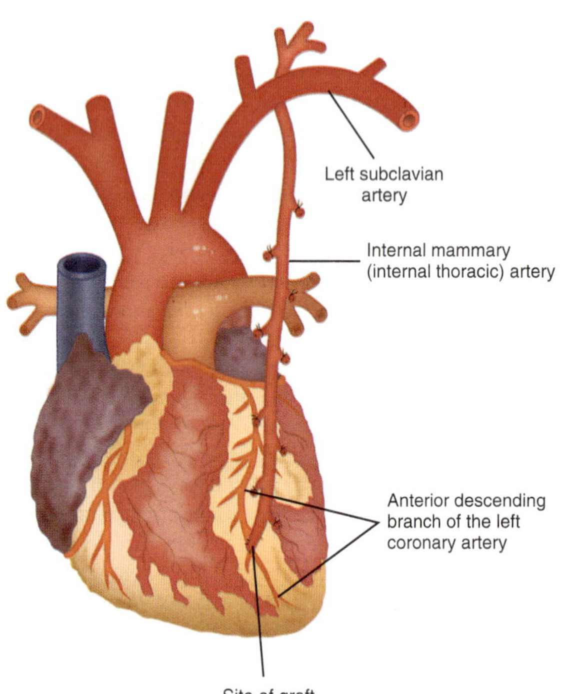

FIG. 14.18 Internal Thoracic Artery Graft.

artery (Fig. 14.18). The left ITA is considered the gold standard conduit in CABG and has been shown to increase graft patency, survival, and freedom from cardiac events compared with SVG conduits.[71] Radial artery conduits in CABG are typically used as adjuncts to the left ITA. Graft patency has increased with improved harvesting techniques, adjunctive medication strategies (statins and antiplatelet agents), and aggressive risk factor modification such as smoking cessation. Conduits used for myocardial revascularization are compared in Table 14.11.

Valvular Heart Surgery

Valvular disease results in various hemodynamic dysfunctions that can usually be managed medically as long as the patient remains symptom free. There is reluctance to intervene surgically early in the course of this disease because of the surgical risks and long-term complications associated with prosthetic valve replacement. However, these consequences must be weighed against the possibility of irreversible deterioration in LV function that may develop during the compensated asymptomatic phase (see Valvular Heart Disease and Table 13.14 in Chapter 13).

- Aortic valve. Surgical options for aortic valve disease are limited to aortic valve replacement
- Mitral valve. Surgical options for mitral valve disease include both valve repair and mitral valve replacement

Mitral valve repair is preferred over valve replacement to avoid the complications inherent with a prosthetic valve, including the risk of thromboembolic events and sometimes the need for long-term anticoagulation. If reconstruction of the mitral valve is impossible, it is replaced.

There are two categories of prosthetic valves:

- Mechanical heart valve (MHV)
- Bioprosthetic heart valve (BHV)

MHVs are made from combinations of metal alloys, pyrolytic carbon, Dacron, and Teflon and have rigid occluding devices (Fig. 14.19). Their construction renders them highly durable, but all patients with mechanical valves require anticoagulation to reduce the incidence of thromboembolism.

BHVs are constructed from animal or human cardiac tissue and have flexible occluding mechanisms. Because of their low thrombogenicity, tissue valves offer the patient freedom from therapeutic anticoagulation. However, their durability is limited by their tendency toward early calcification. Various valvular prostheses are described in Box 14.16.

A discussion regarding the risks and benefits of different prosthetic valves should be had between the patient and the physician.[68] Because MHVs are more durable, they may be

TABLE 14.11 Conduits Used for Coronary Artery Bypass Grafts

Type of Graft	Advantages	Disadvantages
Saphenous vein	Easily harvested Length allows for multiple grafts No anatomic limitations to graft sites	Long-term patency less than arterial grafts Requires at least two anastomosis sites
Internal thoracic artery (ITA)	Proven patency rates Requires only one anastomosis	Requires extensive dissection and may not be accessible for emergency bypass Potential increased risk of sternal wound infections with bilateral ITAs Anatomic limitations to bypassing some areas of the heart
Radial artery	Improved patency rates Easily harvested No anatomic limitations to graft sites	Requires adequate collateral flow to hand through the ulnar artery Higher rates of vasospasm require pharmacologic prophylaxis Requires two anastomosis sites

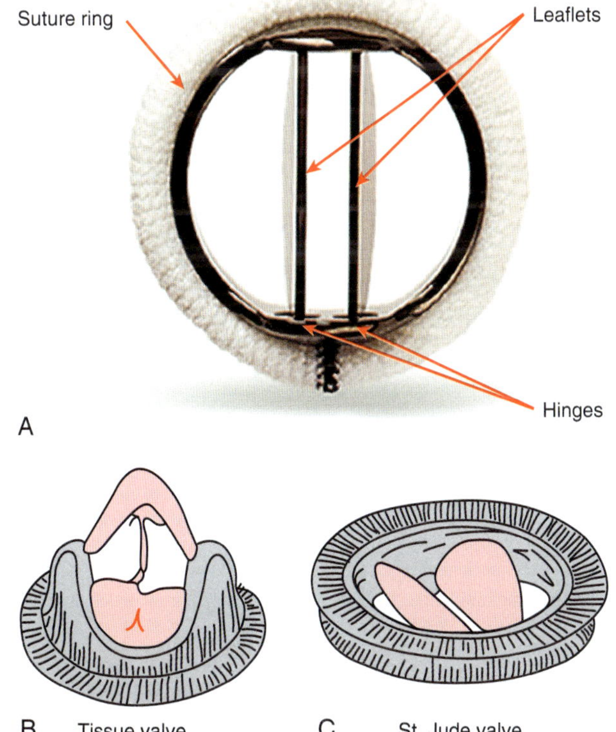

FIG. 14.19 (A) Mechanical bileaflet valve. (B) Prosthetic tissue valve. (C) Mechanical bileaflet valve (St. Jude). (A courtesy St. Jude Medical.)

preferred for a young person who is anticipated to have a relatively long life span ahead. A BHV may be chosen for an older adult patient; the valve has a reduced longevity, but this disadvantage is offset by the older patient's shorter life expectancy. The optimal valve selection is discussed between the patient

BOX 14.16 Classification of Prosthetic Cardiac Valves

Mechanical Valves

- *Tilting-disk:* A free-floating, lens-shaped disk mounted on a circular sewing ring (Medtronic Hall)
- *Bileaflet:* Two semicircular leaflets mounted on a circular sewing ring that opens centrally (St. Jude)

Biologic or Tissue Valves (Bioprostheses)

- *Stented* (porcine xenograft or pericardial xenograft)
- *Stentless* (porcine xenograft or pericardial xenograft)
- *Homograft:* A human heart valve (aortic or pulmonic) harvested from a donated heart and cryopreserved; may or may not be mounted on a support ring

Percutaneous

- Expanded over a balloon (Edwards SAPIEN)
- Self-expandable (CoreValve)

and the surgeon.[68] For patients with medical contraindications to anticoagulation and for patients whose past compliance with medications has been questionable, a BHV may be selected. Technical considerations, such as the size of the annulus (or the anatomic ring in which the valve sits), can also influence the choice of valve; for example, a bioprosthesis may be too big for a small aortic root.

Infective endocarditis continues to be a significant clinical problem associated with high mortality rates. Destruction of valve leaflets, invasion of surrounding myocardial tissue, systemic embolization of valvular vegetations, persistent sepsis, or acute heart failure can be the result of infective endocarditis.[72] Considerations for the timing of surgery, if required, are made with the surgeon along with aggressive antibiotic therapy and the removal of devices.[68]

Cardiopulmonary Bypass

CPB is a mechanical means of circulating and oxygenating a patient's blood while diverting most of the circulation from the heart and lungs during cardiac surgical procedures. The extracorporeal circuit consists of cannulas that drain off venous blood; an oxygenator that oxygenates the blood; and a pump head that propels the arterialized blood back to the ascending aorta, which has been cross clamped to prevent the back flow of blood into the heart. CPB is accompanied by normovolemic hemodilution and nonpulsatile flow.

Several adjunctive strategies are used to facilitate circulation and oxygenation while the patient is on bypass (on-pump). The patient is systemically heparinized (activated clotting time >400) before initiation of bypass to prevent clotting within the bypass circuit.[73] After the patient is taken off the CPB machine, protamine sulfate is given to reverse the anticoagulant effects of the heparin.

Rapidly stopping the heart in diastole by perfusing the coronary arteries with a potassium cardioplegic (heart-paralyzing) agent assists with intraoperative myocardial protection. The cardioplegia solution must be reinfused at regular intervals during CPB to keep the heart in an arrested state so that the surgeon can operate while the heart is stopped and to minimize myocardial oxygen requirements.

Systemic hypothermia during bypass can reduce tissue oxygen requirements to 50% of normal, which affords the major organs additional protection from ischemic injury. Lowering the body temperature to approximately 28°C (82.4°F) is accomplished through a heat exchanger incorporated into the pump. The blood is warmed back to normal body temperature before bypass is discontinued.

The technique of hemodilution is also used to enhance tissue oxygenation by improving blood flow through the systemic and pulmonary microcirculation during bypass. *Hemodilution* refers to the dilution of the patient's own (autologous) blood with the isotonic crystalloid solution used to prime the circuit. This hemodilution enhances capillary perfusion by reducing blood viscosity (stickiness) and decreasing the risk of microthrombi formation. At the completion of CPB, the large quantities of "pump blood" that remain in the bypass circuit can be collected and used for initial postoperative volume replacement.

Numerous clinical sequelae can result from CPB (Table 14.12). Knowledge of these physiologic effects allows the nurse to anticipate problems and to intervene effectively in the postoperative period.

Off-Pump Coronary Artery Bypass Graft Surgery

The principal reason to perform off-pump CABG (OP-CABG) surgery is to avoid the potential complications associated with CPB and to avoid cross-clamping of a calcified aorta.[44] OP-CABG surgeries account for less than 15% of all CABG procedures in the United States.[74] Several techniques are used to stabilize the operative area during an OP-CABG procedure. Immobilization devices that use compression or suction to create an immobile area have been developed to stabilize cardiac wall motion at the site of the anastomosis. Medications that temporarily decrease the heart rate (e.g., esmolol, diltiazem) or cause transient cardiac asystole (e.g., adenosine) may also be used to further limit cardiac motion. Although the OP-CABG procedure was developed to decrease complications associated with CPB, there are no convincing data that OP-CABG surgery is superior to on-pump CABG surgery.[75] Long-term graft patency, complete revascularization, and overall survival may be better with conventional CABG surgery.[76]

TABLE 14.12 Physiologic Effects of Cardiopulmonary Bypass

Effects	Causes
Intravascular fluid deficit (hypotension)	Third spacing Postoperative diuresis Sudden vasodilation (medications, rewarming)
Third spacing (weight gain, edema)	Decreased plasma protein concentration Increased capillary permeability
Myocardial depression (decreased cardiac output)	Hypothermia Increased systemic vascular resistance Prolonged cardiopulmonary bypass pump run Preexisting heart disease Inadequate myocardial protection
Coagulopathy (bleeding)	Systemic heparinization Mechanical trauma to platelets Decreased release of clotting factors from liver as a result of hypothermia
Pulmonary dysfunction (decreased lung mechanics and impaired gas exchange)	Decreased surfactant production Pulmonary microemboli Interstitial fluid accumulation in lungs
Hemolysis (hemoglobinuria)	Red blood cells damaged in pump circuit
Hyperglycemia (rise in serum glucose concentration)	Decreased insulin release Stimulation of glycogenolysis
Hypokalemia (low serum potassium concentration)	Intracellular shifts during bypass and postoperative diuresis
Hypomagnesemia (low serum magnesium concentration)	Postoperative diuresis resulting from hemodilution
Neurologic dysfunction (decreased level of consciousness, motor/sensory deficits)	Inadequate cerebral perfusion Microemboli to brain (air, plaque fragments, fat globules)
Hypertension (transient increase in blood pressure)	Catecholamine release and systemic hypothermia causing vasoconstriction

Nursing Postoperative Management After Coronary Artery Bypass Graft Surgery

Medical and nursing management of postoperative cardiac surgery patients is collaborative. Patient transfer from the operating room suite to the intensive care unit bed presents potential for airway and ventilation problems, sudden hypotension or hypertension, dysthymias, inadvertent medication changes, and unidentified problems with invasive catheters, monitoring, and bleeding. Immediate attention should be given to getting the patient connected to bedside monitors and the ventilator, ensuring patient safety.

The physician prescribes therapeutic interventions and identifies specific hemodynamic endpoints to maintain adequate organ perfusion and oxygen delivery. The nurse is responsible for applying these therapies to maintain the patient's hemodynamic parameters within the desired range. In most institutions, standard protocols are used to facilitate the postoperative nursing diagnoses and management of cardiac surgical patients (Box 14.17).

BOX 14.17 DIAGNOSIS AND PATIENT CARE MANAGEMENT

Open Heart Surgery

- Impaired cardiac output due to alterations in preload
- Impaired cardiac output due to alterations in afterload
- Impaired cardiac output due to alterations in contractility
- Impaired cardiac output due to alterations in heart rate or rhythm
- Impaired cardiac output due to sympathetic blockade
- Impaired gas exchange due to alveolar hypoventilation
- Impaired gas exchange due to ventilation–perfusion mismatching or intrapulmonary shunting
- Impaired airway clearance due to excessive secretions or abnormal viscosity of mucus
- Activity intolerance due to cardiopulmonary dysfunction
- Activity intolerance due to prolonged immobility or deconditioning
- Risk for infection
- Acute pain due to transmission and perception of cutaneous, visceral, muscular, or ischemic impulses
- Anxiety due to threat to biologic, psychologic, or social integrity
- Impaired sleep due to fragmented sleep
- Lack of knowledge of treatment regime due to lack of previous exposure to information (see Box 14.19, Patient and Family Education Plan: Open Heart Surgery).

Patient Care Management Plans are located in Appendix A.)

Cardiovascular Support

Postoperative cardiovascular support often is indicated because of a low-output state. The most common causes of cardiac dysfunction after cardiac surgery are mechanical complications, physiologic complications, MI, and dysrhythmias. Cardiac output can be maximized by adjustments in heart rate, preload, afterload, and contractility with utilization of vasopressor and inotropic agents as well as colloidal and crystalloid solutions.

Heart Rate Optimization

In the presence of low cardiac output, the heart rate can be appropriately regulated via temporary pacing or medication therapy. Temporary atrial or ventricular epicardial pacing is usually instituted when the heart rate decreases to less than 60 beats/min and the patient is hypotensive, requiring a supportive rate of 80 to 100 beats/min. In the case of tachycardia, intravenous beta-blockers (esmolol) or calcium channel blockers (diltiazem) may be used in the acute postoperative period to slow supraventricular rhythms. Obtaining a 12-lead ECG to assess dysrhythmias further may also be indicated. Electrolyte disturbances such as hypokalemia, hypomagnesemia, hypocalcemia, and hypercalcemia must be closely monitored and corrected to prevent postoperative dysrhythmias.

Atrial fibrillation is the most common adverse event after cardiac surgery. It occurs in 30% to 50% of patients after cardiac surgery.[77,78] The peak occurance is within the first few postoperative days after surgery, and patients with atrial fibrillation have a longer postoperative course with a longer stay in the critical care unit.[78] This rhythm may also induce hemodynamic compromise and increase the patient's risk of stroke.[78] Prophylactic administration of beta-blockers is recommended to decrease the incidence of atrial fibrillation after cardiac surgery.[9,44,78] Amiodarone is an alternative for patients who have contraindications to beta-blockers.[9,44,78,79] Initial management of atrial fibrillation involves slowing of the ventricular rate and stabilization of hemodynamics. Pharmacological restoration of sinus rhythm using antidysrhythmic drugs or cardioversion is recommended, with imaging to ensure the left atrial appendage (LAA) does not contain thrombi.[9,79] Persistent ventricular arrhythmias are uncommon and a reason to suspect and investigate for ongoing myocardial ischemia.[80]

Preload Optimization

In most patients, reduced preload is the cause of low postoperative cardiac output. The most common causes of decreased preload are hypovolemia from bleeding, fluid shifts caused by the systemic inflammatory response, increased vascular capacitance with rewarming, and elevated cardiac preload requirements. Appropriate volume resuscitation immediately postoperatively is one of the most important interventions and should be a first-line therapy for hemodynamic instability. To enhance preload, volume may be administered in the form of crystalloid, colloid, or packed red cells. Crystalloids are preferred for fluid resuscitation; the type of crystalloid depends on institutional preference. Preload is often evaluated by intermittent pressure readings obtained from catheters placed in the RA or PA. A growing body of research suggests that static indices such as central venous pressure (CVP) and pulmonary artery occlusion pressure (PAOP) have a very weak relationship with the patient's intravascular volume and are not helpful in predicting if a patient will respond to fluid resuscitation. Volume resuscitation should be done in the context of the full patient picture because excessive fluid administration can lead to adverse events. Approximately 2 to 3 L of crystalloid will suffice for most patients.

Afterload Optimization

Patients who have had cardiac surgery may demonstrate postoperative hypertension. Although it is transient, postoperative hypertension can precipitate or exacerbate bleeding from the mediastinal chest tubes.

Elevated systemic vascular resistance. The high systemic vascular resistance (SVR) (afterload) resulting from the intense vasoconstriction can increase LV workload. Vasodilator therapy with intravenous sodium nitroprusside or nitroglycerin often is used to reduce afterload, control hypertension, and improve cardiac output. Increased afterload may be partially caused by the peripheral vasoconstrictive effects of hypothermia, which can be managed with careful rewarming.

Vasodilation.

Low systemic vascular resistance. A significant percentage of patients experience hypotension after CPB secondary to peripheral vasodilation. This condition is believed to occur in part because of the systemic inflammatory response to CPB, surgical trauma, ischemia, or reperfusion. Therapy for hypotension after cardiac surgery usually includes volume loading and vasopressors. Typical vasopressor agents include norepinephrine and vasopressin in patients with excessive vasodilation. Phenylephrine should be used cautiously because it increases afterload and decreases graft flow. These medications are administered via a central line and smart pumps for patient safety.

Contractility Optimization

The patient's EF should be used to inform the treatment plan. If the adjustments in heart rate, preload, and afterload fail to produce significant improvement in cardiac output, contractility can be enhanced with positive inotropic support. There is a great deal of variability in the choice of vasoactive agents used with few data guiding decision making. Epinephrine, norepinephrine, dopamine, and dobutamine are commonly used inotropic catecholamines. Mechanical circulatory support (MCS) may also need to be added to help augment circulation (discussed later).

Mechanical Complications

Different mechanical complications after cardiac surgery include cardiac tamponade, hematomas, vasospasm of a coronary artery graft, prosthetic valve paravalvular regurgitation, and systolic anterior motion of the mitral valve. Some mechanical complications are noncardiac, such as pneumothorax, hemothorax, and endotracheal tube malposition. Identifying and intervening are important to quickly prevent any further dysfunction.

Temperature Regulation

Hypothermia can contribute to depressed myocardial contractility, vasoconstriction, and ventricular dysrhythmias in a patient who has undergone cardiac surgery. Hypothermia may also contribute to postoperative bleeding because the functioning of clotting factors is depressed. After surgery, patients may be rewarmed with the use of warm blankets or forced-air warming devices. Excessive temperature elevations must be avoided, with the goal of maintaining a target body temperature of 36°C to 37°C (96.8°F to 98.6°F).

Control of Bleeding

Postoperative bleeding from the mediastinal chest tubes can be caused by inadequate hemostasis, disruption of suture lines, coagulopathy associated with CPB, residual heparin effect, clotting factor depletion, thrombocytopenia, or hypothermia, along with other less frequent factors. Blood conservation strategies should be used to limit the number of transfusions because the administration of packed red blood cells has been independently associated with increased complications and increased mortality. At the present time, blood transfusions are not recommended for a hemoglobin greater than 10 grams per deciliter (g/dL), but transfusions are reasonable in most postoperative patients whose hemoglobin is less than 7 g/d.[81]

Clotting factors (fresh frozen plasma, fibrinogen, and platelets), protamine, or desmopressin may be administered. Medications used in the treatment of postoperative bleeding are described in Table 14.13. To help guide the selection of appropriate factors or medications, laboratory values such as prothrombin time/international normalized ratio, partial thromboplastin time, platelets, fibrinogen, and thrombin time are obtained.

Rewarming the patient reverses the depressed manufacture and release of clotting factors that results from hypothermia. There is little evidence to support other interventions, such as targeted low systolic pressures or use of higher positive end-expiratory pressures to limit postoperative blood loss.[82]

Although no exact definition exists for excessive bleeding, amounts greater than 200 mL/h often require further interventions. Persistent mediastinal bleeding, usually greater than 500 mL in 1 hour, or 300 mL/h for 2 consecutive hours despite normalization of clotting studies, is an indication for reexploration of the surgical site.

Chest Tube Patency

Chest tube stripping to maintain patency of the tubes is controversial because of the high negative pressure generated by vigorous methods of stripping as this can result in tissue damage that can contribute to bleeding. This risk must be carefully weighed against the real danger of cardiac tamponade if blood is not effectively drained from around the heart. There is variation in practice and often more gentle techniques such as fan-folding of the mediastinal chest tube is recommended for routine postoperative care. Research is ongoing into the development of automated chest tube clearance systems to safely manage mediastinal chest tube drainage after cardiac surgery.[83]

TABLE 14.13 Medications Used to Treat Postoperative Bleeding

Medication	Dose	Action and Side Effects
Aminocaproic acid (Amicar)	Loading dose: 4–5 g over 1 h, followed by continuous infusion of 1 g/h for 8 h or until bleeding is controlled	Inhibits conversion of plasminogen to plasmin to prevent fibrinolysis, helping to stabilize clots
Desmopressin acetate (DDAVP)	0.3 mcg/kg IV over 20–30 min	Improves platelet function by increasing levels of factor VIII Side effects include facial flushing, tachycardia, headache, and hypotension
Protamine sulfate	25–50 mg IV slowly over 10 min	Neutralizes anticoagulant effect of heparin Can cause hypotension, bradycardia, and allergic reactions

IV, Intravenously.

Cardiac Tamponade

Cardiac tamponade is a potentially lethal complication that may occur after surgery if blood accumulates in the mediastinal space, impairing the heart's ability to pump. Signs of tamponade include elevated and equalized filling pressures (e.g., CVP, PA diastolic pressure, PAOP), decreased cardiac output, decreased blood pressure, jugular venous distention, pulsus paradoxus, muffled heart sounds, sudden cessation of chest tube drainage, and a widened cardiac silhouette on radiographs. A bedside echocardiogram is helpful to confirm tamponade. Interventions for tamponade may include emergency sternotomy in the critical care unit or a return to the operating room for surgical evacuation of the clot.

Pulmonary Care

MV is used initially to provide adequate alveolar oxygenation and ventilation in the postoperative period. Protocol-based multidisciplinary initiatives that facilitate early extubation (less than 6 hours after surgery) have been implemented in most institutions and have been shown to decrease pulmonary complications after cardiac surgery.[84] Early extubation requires a multidisciplinary approach that incorporates anesthesiologists, surgeons, advance practice providers, nurses, and respiratory therapists. Potential candidates must be identified before surgery so that the anesthetic regimen supports early extubation.[85]

In a global study of MV in 4809 patients after cardiac surgery, 86% were extubated in under 6 hours with a mortality rate of less than 1%.[85] Conversely, 14% required prolonged mechanical ventilatory support, experienced multiple postoperative complications, and had a mortality rate of 14% at 30 days postsurgery.[85] MV is often associated with a higher level of critical illness and more serious complications.

After surgery, patients are evaluated for hemodynamic stability, adequate control of bleeding, normothermia, and the ability to follow commands. Once these criteria have been met, most institutions have a weaning protocol to follow that often involves a spontaneous breathing trial to evaluate the patient's readiness for extubation. Patients who exhibit hemodynamic instability or intraoperative complications or who have underlying pulmonary disease may require longer periods of MV. After extubation, supplemental oxygen is administered and patients are medicated for incisional pain to facilitate aggressive pulmonary hygiene and early mobility, which is essential to help prevent postoperative complications.

Neurologic Complications

The neurologic dysfunction often seen in patients who have undergone cardiac surgery has been attributed to decreased cerebral perfusion, cerebral microemboli, hypoxia, and the systemic inflammatory response. Neurological dysfunction can range from subtle cognitive changes to signs of acute stroke.

Early recognition of neurologic changes is important so that prompt initiation of therapy may prevent worsening of complications. Delirium is a frequent complication following cardiac surgery and is associated with older age, advanced heart disease, prolonged MV, and longer length of stay in a critical care unit.[86,87] Delirium is associated with long-term negative outcomes such as higher mortality, decreased cognitive function, and reduced quality of life (see Delirium in Chapter 8 for more information).

Infection

Postoperative fever is common after CPB. However, persistent temperature elevation to greater than 101°F (38.3°C) must be investigated. Sternal wound infections and infective endocarditis are the most devastating infectious complications, but leg wound infections, pneumonia, and urinary tract infections also can occur. Infection rates are greater in patients with diabetes, malnutrition, chronic diseases, obesity, and in patients requiring emergent or prolonged surgery.

Blood Glucose Control

Using a continuous insulin infusion to maintain blood glucose concentrations below 180 mg/dL while avoiding hypoglycemia can reduce the incidence of adverse events, including deep sternal wound infections.[44]

Acute Kidney Injury

AKI is recognized as a significant problem after cardiac surgery because of a very complex pathogenesis. Prevention of *cardiac surgery–associated acute kidney injury* (CSA-AKI) is a major goal of postoperative management, and for patients at risk a *nephroprotective care bundle* should be implemented.[88,89] The nephroprotective actions include ensuring that hemodynamics are optimal with adequate blood pressure, cardiac output, and intravascular volume. It is also important to avoid known insults such as hyperglycemia, hypotension, nephrotoxic medications, and radiopaque contrast whenever possible.[88]

Because of postoperative fluid retention, diuresis is used to help mobilize fluids from the interstitial to the intravascular space and may be done with the administration of medications or may be allowed to occur naturally. Frequent monitoring of urine output and serum creatinine levels is required. The patient's potassium levels may be depleted with the diuresis, requiring that levels be closely monitored and replaced. Research studies to identify biomarkers for early detection and prevention of CSA-AKI are ongoing. This is important because reducing CSA-AKI will also reduce mortality and morbidity.[88,89] See Acute Kidney Injury in Chapter 25 for more information on AKI.

Resuscitation of Patients Who Arrest After Cardiac Surgery

The incidence of cardiac arrest after cardiac surgery is relatively low. After cardiac surgery, patients have comparatively good outcomes given the high incidence of reversible causes of cardiac arrest. Special guidelines have been developed by the Society of Thoracic Surgeons on the resuscitation of patients who arrest after cardiac surgery, focusing on the differences in this patient population. These guidelines differ from the Advanced Cardiac Life Support (ACLS) guidelines in several ways. Specific recommendations include:[90,91]

- Patients who arrest with VF or pulseless VT should receive three sequential attempts at defibrillation before external cardiac massage.
- Patients with asystole or extreme bradycardia should undergo an attempt to pace if wires are available before external cardiac massage, using maximum pacemaker settings.
- Patients with pulseless electrical activity should have quickly reversible causes excluded (such as tamponade or bleeding) followed by emergency resternotomy.
- Patients with three unsuccessful defibrillation attempts for VF or pulseless VT should receive an IV bolus of amiodarone 300 mg.

Finally, because of the danger of extreme hypertension if a reversible cause is rapidly identified, full-dose epinephrine is not recommended unless directed by a senior physician.[90,91] Although there are several special caveats with this patient population, the importance of early emergency resternotomy (within 5 minutes) is a major recommendations.[90,91]

Guidelines for Coronary Artery Bypass Graft Surgery

The American College of Cardiology and the American Heart Association have developed a set of clinical practice guidelines for the care of patients undergoing CABG surgery.[44] These guidelines are designed to support clinical decision making with research evidence (Box 14.18).

Educate the Patient and Family

Patient and family education includes information related to the surgical procedure, risk factor management, and prevention of atherosclerosis. Patients who have undergone valve surgery may also require information regarding the need for antibiotic prophylaxis before invasive procedures and specific instructions pertaining to their anticoagulation regimen (Box 14.19).

Minimally Invasive Cardiac Surgery

Continuously evolving techniques have expanded the options for patients undergoing cardiac surgery. To avoid common complications associated with traditional CABG surgery, *minimally invasive direct CABG* (MIDCAB) was developed. MIDCAB is performed via a left anterior mini thoracotomy as a sternal-sparing approach. However, there are many limitations with this approach concerning the extent of revascularization. Improvements in technology have led to endoscopic techniques coming to the forefront.

Totally Endoscopic Coronary Artery Bypass—Robotic Assisted

Totally endoscopic coronary artery bypass (TECAB) or robotic-assisted surgery is the least invasive version. The main advantage of this procedure is the avoidance of a thoracotomy or sternotomy. Robotically controlled surgical instruments are inserted through five dime-size incisions and are controlled by the surgeon from the surgical console, allowing more degrees of freedom than conventional surgical instruments.

Postoperative care of patients following TECAB is very similar to that of the standard CABG patient.[44] A few differences include the fact that early extubation may occur in the operating room. Acute pain from the telemanipulation port sites may require early initiation of patient-controlled analgesia (PCA) to assist with pain management. Because the sternum has been preserved, there are no requirements for sternal precautions, which allows for physical activity to be quickly advanced.

A hybrid operating room allows for the combination of PCI and surgical coronary artery revascularization. The goal is to combine the best of both worlds: excellent long-term patency

BOX 14.18 Evidence-Based Practice

Coronary Artery Bypass Graft Surgery

Levine GN, Bates ER, Bittl JA, Brindis RG, Fihn SD, Fleisher LA, Granger CB, Lange RA, Mack MJ, Mauri L, Mehran R, Mukherjee D, Newby LK, O'Gara PT, Sabatine MS, Smith PK, Smith SC Jr. 2016 ACC/AHA guideline focused update on duration of dual antiplatelet therapy in patients with coronary artery disease: a report of the American College of Cardiology/American Heart Association Task Force on Clinical Practice Guidelines: an update of the 2011 ACCF/AHA/SCAI guideline for percutaneous coronary intervention, 2011 ACCF/AHA guideline for coronary artery bypass graft surgery, 2012 ACC/AHA/ ACP/AATS/PCNA/ SCAI/STS guideline for the diagnosis and management of patients with stable ischemic heart disease, 2013 ACCF/AHA guideline for the management of ST-elevation myocardial infarction, 2014 ACC/AHA guideline for the management of patients with non–ST-elevation acute coronary syndromes, and 2014 ACC/ AHA guideline on perioperative cardiovascular evaluation and management of patients undergoing noncardiac surgery. Circulation. 2016;134:e123–e155.

A summary is provided of evidence and evidence-based review recommendations for management of patients undergoing coronary artery bypass graft (CABG) surgery.

Lawton JS, Tamis-Holland JE, Bangalore S, Bates ER, Beckie TM, Bischoff JM, Bittl JA, Cohen MG, DiMaio JM, Don CW, Fremes SE, Gaudino MF, Goldberger ZD, Grant MC, Jaswal JB, Kurlansky PA, Mehran R, Metkus TS Jr, Nnacheta LC, Rao SV, Sabik JF, Sellke FW, Sharma G, Yong CM, Zwischenberger BA. 2021 ACC/AHA/SCAI guideline for coronary artery revascularization: a report of the American College of Cardiology/American Heart Association Joint Committee on Clinical Practice Guidelines. Circulation. 2022;145:e18–e114. https://doi.org/10.1161/CIR.0000000000001038

Strong Evidence to Support the Following

Coronary Artery Bypass Graft Surgery for Patients

- Emergency CABG surgery has a limited role during/after acute ST elevation myocardial infarction (STEMI) and its use continues to decrease in this situation.
- Emergency CABG surgery is indicated for patients undergoing surgical repair of postinfarction mechanical complications, patients with cardiogenic shock, or patients with life-threatening ventricular dysrhythmias in the presence of left main stenosis or three-vessel coronary artery disease (CAD).
- CABG surgery is indicated for patients undergoing noncoronary cardiac surgery if 50% or greater stenosis of left main or 70% or greater stenosis of other major coronary arteries.
- CABG surgery is indicated for patients with significant (50% or greater) stenosis of left main coronary artery.
- CABG surgery is indicated for patients with significant (70% or greater) stenosis in three major coronary arteries or in the proximal left anterior descending (LAD) artery plus one other major coronary artery.
- CABG surgery or percutaneous coronary intervention (PCI) is indicated in patients with one or more significant (70% or greater) coronary artery stenoses with unacceptable angina despite guideline-directed medical therapy.
- Patients undergoing CABG surgery who have at least moderate aortic stenosis should undergo aortic valve replacement.
- Patients undergoing CABG surgery who have severe ischemic mitral valve regurgitation not likely to resolve with revascularization should undergo mitral valve repair or replacement.

Anesthetic Considerations

- Anesthetic management should be directed toward early postoperative extubation and accelerated recovery of low-risk to medium-risk patients.

Bypass Graft Conduits

- Internal thoracic arteries (ITAs) should be used to bypass the LAD artery when bypass of the LAD is indicated.

Antiplatelet Therapy

- Discontinuation of P2Y12 inhibitors for a few days before cardiovascular operations is recommended to reduce bleeding, especially in high-risk patients.
- For stable nonbleeding patients, aspirin should be given within 6 to 24 hours to optimize graft patency.

Management of Hyperlipidemia

- All patients should receive statin therapy unless contraindicated.

Blood Glucose Management

- Continuous intravenous insulin is administered to maintain early postoperative blood glucose concentration 180 mg/dL or less while avoiding hypoglycemia to reduce adverse events.

Dysrhythmia Management

- Beta-blockers should be administered for at least 24 hours before CABG surgery, reinstituted as soon as possible after surgery, and prescribed at discharge unless contraindicated to reduce the incidence and clinical sequelae of atrial fibrillation.

Angiotensin-Converting Enzyme Inhibitors and Angiotensin-Receptor Blockers

- Angiotensin-converting enzyme inhibitors and angiotensin-receptor blockers should be instituted or restarted postoperatively and continued indefinitely for patients with left ventricular ejection fraction (LVEF) 40% or less, hypertension, diabetes, or chronic kidney disease.

Smoking Cessation

- All patients who smoke should receive educational counseling and be offered smoking cessation therapy during hospitalization for CABG surgery.

Cardiac Rehabilitation

- Cardiac rehabilitation should be offered to all eligible patients after CABG surgery.

Reduction in Risk of Infection

- Antibiotics should be administered preoperatively in all patients to reduce the risk of postoperative infection.

Bleeding and Transfusions

- Aggressive attempts at blood conservation are indicated to reduce the need for red blood cell transfusions.

Moderate Evidence to Support the Following

Coronary Artery Bypass Graft Surgery for Patients

- CABG surgery or PCI is indicated for selected patients age 75 y or older with ST segment elevation or left bundle branch block who are suitable for revascularization regardless of the time interval from STEMI to the onset of cardiogenic shock.
- Emergency CABG surgery is indicated after failed PCI to retrieve a foreign body in a crucial anatomic location or for hemodynamic compromise in patients with impairment of the coagulation system and without previous sternotomy.
- CABG surgery is indicated in patients with significant (70% or greater) stenosis in two major coronary arteries with extensive myocardial ischemia or target vessels supplying a large area of viable myocardium.
- CABG surgery is indicated in patients with mild to moderate left ventricular systolic dysfunction (LVEF 35% to 50%) and significant (70% or greater stenosis) multivessel CAD or proximal LAD stenosis with viable myocardium present.
- CABG surgery is indicated in patients with complex three-vessel CAD (SYNTAX score greater than 22) with or without involvement of the proximal LAD artery who are good candidates for CABG surgery.

BOX 14.18 Evidence-Based Practice—cont'd

Coronary Artery Bypass Graft Surgery

- CABG surgery is preferred over PCI to improve survival in patients with multivessel CAD and diabetes mellitus, particularly if a left internal thoracic artery graft can be anastomosed to the LAD artery.
- Patients undergoing CABG surgery who have moderate ischemic mitral valve regurgitation not likely to resolve with revascularization should undergo mitral valve repair or replacement.

Hybrid Coronary Revascularization

- The planned combination of the left internal thoracic artery (ITA)-to-LAD artery grafting and PCI of one or more non-LAD coronary arteries is reasonable for (1) limitations to CABG surgery such as heavily calcified proximal aorta or poor target vessels for CABG surgery, (2) lack of suitable graft conduits, and (3) unfavorable LAD artery for PCI.

Antiplatelet Therapy

- For patients on DAPT (dual antiplatelet therapy) a daily aspirin 81 mg is recommended.
- In patients who cannot take aspirin, clopidogrel 75 mg daily is a reasonable alternative.

Beta-Blockers

- Preoperative beta-blockers, particularly in patients with an ejection fraction greater than 30%, can reduce the risk of in-hospital mortality.
- Preoperative beta-blockers can reduce the incidence of perioperative myocardial ischemia.

Emotional Dysfunction and Psychosocial Considerations

- Cognitive-behavioral therapy or collaborative care for patients with clinical depression after CABG surgery can be beneficial to reduce objective measures of depression.

Carotid Artery Disease

- For patients with a previous transient ischemic attack or stroke and significant (50% to 99%) carotid artery stenosis, carotid revascularization should be considered in conjunction with CABG surgery. Sequence and timing (staged or simultaneous) should be determined by the relative magnitude of cerebral and myocardial dysfunction.

Infection Prevention

- Leukocyte-filtered blood can be useful to reduce the rate of overall perioperative infection and in-hospital death.

Adjuncts to Myocardial Protection

- Insertion of an intra-aortic balloon pump is reasonable to reduce the mortality rate in patients undergoing CABG surgery who are considered to be at high risk (e.g., LVEF less than 30% or left main CAD).
- Assessment of cardiac biomarkers in the first 24 h after CABG surgery may be considered.

Dysrhythmia Management

- For patients who cannot take beta-blockers, amiodarone is an alternative to reduce the incidence of postoperative atrial fibrillation.
- Beta-blockers, nondihydropyridine calcium channel blockers, and amiodarone can be used to control the ventricular rate in the setting of atrial fibrillation.

Data from Hillis LD, Smith PK, Anderson JL, et al. 2011 ACCF/AHA guideline for coronary artery bypass graft surgery: Executive summary: a report of the American College of Cardiology Foundation/American Heart Association Task Force on Practice Guidelines. *Circulation*. 2011;124(23):2610;

BOX 14.19 PATIENT AND FAMILY EDUCATION PLAN

Open Heart Surgery

Before discharge, the patient should be able to teach back the following topics:

- Pathophysiology of disease (coronary artery or valvular disease)
- Risk factor modification to prevent coronary artery disease (smoking cessation, regular exercise, weight loss)
- Postoperative incisional care
- Activity limitations (no lifting, pushing, or pulling anything heavier than 10 lb for 6 to 8 weeks; no driving for 6 to 8 weeks)
- Recommended exercise progression after surgery
- Recommended diet after surgery
- Information regarding prescribed medications (including prescribed pain medication)
- Anticipated mood changes after surgery
- Follow-up appointment for clinic or primary physician
- Additional information for patients with valve procedures
- Symptoms of endocarditis
- Antibiotic prophylaxis before invasive procedures
- Information regarding anticoagulant therapy and follow-up

and improved survival of the ITA grafting and minimally invasive nature of PCI.[44]

Surgical Treatment of Atrial Fibrillation

Surgical techniques have assumed a more prominent role in the treatment of atrial fibrillation as surgical ablation has demonstrated effectiveness, not only in reducing atrial fibrillation but also in improving quality of life for patients. Surgical ablation of atrial fibrillation can be done with either an open or closed surgical cardiac procedure and as a stand-alone surgical atrial fibrillation ablation.[92] The most frequent choice of surgical ablation is in combination with a surgical mitral valve replacement.[9] Hybrid percutaneous and surgical procedures are also an option.[9]

The surgical Cox-Maze procedure has evolved over the years but still involves a series of scars that are made in the atrial tissue to create an electrical maze that disrupts the reentrant pathways and directs the sinus impulse through the AV node. The procedure also includes surgical isolation of the pulmonary veins, which are frequently the source for the initiation of atrial fibrillation, and removal of the left and right atrial appendages. The goal of treatment is not only to prevent the recurrence of atrial tachydysrhythmias but also to restore sinus rhythm and AV synchrony, if possible. Patients require continued monitoring for arrhythmias, as atrial fibrillation is common for months afterward while the scar tissue fully matures. Medications such as amiodarone are often continued for 2 to 3 months after surgical ablation to prevent dysrythmias.[93] Full anticoagulation is continued until sustained sinus rhythm is established.[93]

Left Atrial Appendage Surgical Occlusion

The LAA is a cylindrical structure that opens into the left atrium and has been shown to be one potential source for blood clots that can cause strokes. For those patients who

PATIENT-CENTERED CRITICAL CARE

Debriefing After a Code in the Critical Care Unit

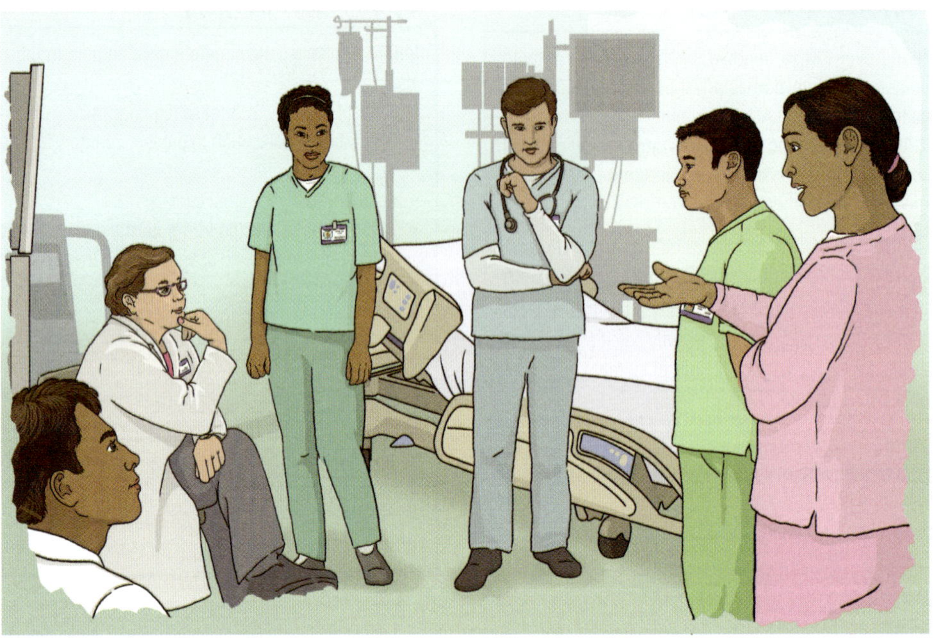

Cardiac arrest, when cardiopulmonary resuscitation (CPR) and advanced cardiac life support (ACLS) are provided, is a high-stress situation. The adrenaline is surging during the resuscitation as everyone works as a team to save the patient's life. Afterward there may be a feeling of deflation mixed with concern that everything was done correctly. There may be feelings of sadness if the patient did not survive the code.

A short debriefing session for health care team members, immediately or soon after the code, has multiple goals. It is a safe place for staff members to express feelings about the patient outcome after the code. In addition, the team leader may describe the correct actions that were taken and evaluate what was not done correctly. Sometimes the team discusses how the resuscitation could be improved at a system level.

A separate responsibility is helping family members debrief after a code. Often family members are present in the room and witness the arrest and resuscitation. Guidelines from professional organizations recommend that an empathetic staff member stand with the family to explain what is happening during the code. This could be a nurse, a social worker, or a hospital chaplain of any faith. It is important that family members are not left alone during the code. Afterward, many families need to ask questions and debrief about what they have witnessed.

may be at higher risk for long-term anticoagulation use, surgical occlusion of the left atrial appendage is an option.[8,94] There are a number of specialized LAA devices that may applied during any cardiac surgery.[95] Surgical closure of the appendage is associated with a lower risk of embolic stroke in combination with postoperative anticoagulation.[94]

Percutaneous Treatment of Atrial Fibrillation

Atrial fibrillation originates in the pulmonary veins from tissue that produces sustained rapid discharges that causes disorganized fibrillatory waves in the atria.[96] A percutaneous catheter-based option to manage atrial fibrillation is called *pulmonary vein isolation* (PVI), where the pulmonary veins are walled off using catheter ablative techniques to isolate the pulmonary veins from the rest of the atria.[97] In multiyear follow-up studies PVI has been shown to be long lasting with 25% of patients remaining in sinus rhythm.[97] This implies that PVI can also reverse the structural abnormalities that accompany atrial fibrillation if the ablation can be performed at an early stage.[96] If PVI is not an option, in some situations an AV nodal ablation is performed and a pacemaker is inserted to provide dual-chamber synchronized pacing.[98]

MECHANICAL CIRCULATORY SUPPORT

MCS devices are an integral part of the cardiovascular therapeutic management of patients. The primary goals of MCS devices are to decrease myocardial workload, maintain adequate perfusion to vital organs, reduce pulmonary congestion, augment coronary perfusion, provide circulatory support during procedures, and limit infarction size.[80]

If the acute heart failure is reversible, a short duration of ventricular assistance is used to allow the myocardium time to recover. If the condition is irreversible, MCS may be used as a bridge to heart transplantation for qualified candidates or as destination therapy for patients who have no other surgical options.[99]

Intra-Aortic Balloon Pump

The intra-aortic balloon pump (IABP) is the most frequently used temporary percutaneous circulatory assist device used in hemodynamically unstable patients (Box 14.20). Because the IABP is relatively easy to insert and has few complications,[100] IABPs represent 70% of all MCS placed.[99] However, the number is decreasing because of the availability of alternative MCS devices that provide more cardiac support.[99]

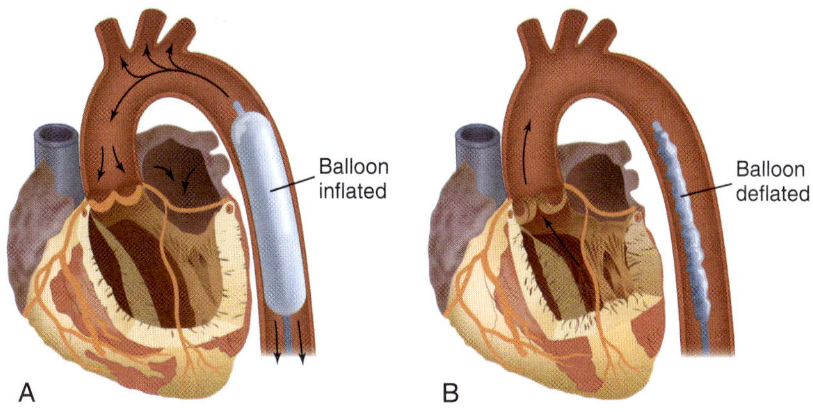

FIG. 14.20 Mechanisms of Action of Intra-aortic Balloon Pump. (A) Diastolic balloon inflation augments coronary blood flow. (B) Systolic balloon deflation decreases afterload.

The intra-aortic balloon (IAB) catheter consists of a single sausage-shaped polyurethane balloon that is wrapped around the distal end of a vascular catheter and positioned in the descending thoracic aorta just distal to the takeoff of the left subclavian artery.

Counterpulsation Physiology in IABP

Counterpulsation is the key mechanism for the IABP. The therapeutic effects are based on the hemodynamic principles of diastolic augmentation and afterload reduction (Box 14.21).

Initially, as the balloon is inflated in diastole concurrent with aortic valve closure, the blood in the aortic arch above the level of the balloon is displaced retrograde (backward) toward the aortic root, augmenting diastolic coronary arterial blood flow and increasing myocardial oxygen supply (Fig. 14.20A). The blood volume in the aorta below the level of the balloon is propelled forward toward the peripheral vascular system, which enhances systemic perfusion. Subsequently, the deflation of the balloon just before the opening of the aortic valve creates a potential space or vacuum in the aorta, toward which blood flows unimpeded during ventricular ejection (Fig. 14.20B).

This decreased resistance to LV ejection, or decreased afterload, facilitates ventricular emptying and reduces myocardial oxygen demands. The overall physiologic effect of IABP therapy is an improvement in the balance between myocardial oxygen supply and demand. Contraindications to IABP include aortic aneurysm, significant aortic valve insufficiency, and severe peripheral vascular disease.[101]

Intra-Aortic Balloon Insertion

The IAB may be inserted in the operating room, the cardiac catheterization laboratory, or the critical care unit. The IAB catheter is usually inserted percutaneously through the femoral artery and advanced to the correct position in the descending thoracic aorta. After insertion, the balloon is attached to the console and filled with the prescribed volume of helium and pumping is initiated.

Nursing Management

The management of the pumping console and its timing functions may be performed by the nurse caring for the patient or delegated to specially trained personnel. Multiple factors may affect the efficacy of the IABP, including position of the balloon within the aorta; balloon displacement volume; inflation and deflation timing; signal quality; the patient's cardiac function; and hemodynamic variables, which include circulating blood volume, blood pressure, and vascular resistance.[102] Clinicians need to be aware of these factors to adequately assess for and ensure optimal IABP performance.

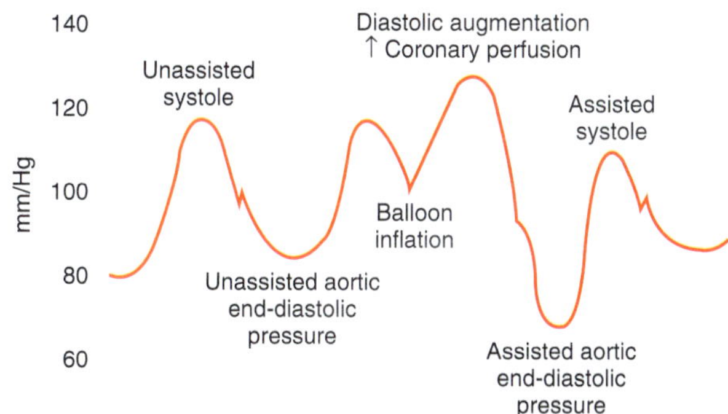

FIG. 14.21 Timing and Effect of Balloon Counterpulsation. Timing is adjusted by synchronizing balloon inflation with the dicrotic notch on the arterial waveform, resulting in an elevated diastolic pressure. Inflation is maintained throughout diastole to augment coronary perfusion. Deflation occurs just before the next systole, resulting in a reduced systolic pressure and decreased afterload.

Timing the IABP

The IABP depends on proper timing to ensure optimal hemodynamic benefits. Although systems now adjust the timing automatically, clinicians must still be aware of how to set the timing, understand the method used, and evaluate its effects. The ECG and arterial pressure tracings are constantly monitored to verify the timing and effect of balloon counterpulsation (Fig. 14.21). For counterpulsation to occur, the pump must receive a trigger signal to identify the beginning and end of the cardiac cycle. The trigger can be the R wave of the ECG, the upstroke of the arterial pressure waveform, or a pacemaker spike.

Complications With IABP

Vascular complications include lower extremity ischemia resulting from occlusion of the femoral artery by the catheter itself or by emboli caused by thrombus formation on the balloon. Evaluation of peripheral circulation remains an important nursing assessment. Signs of diminished perfusion must be reported immediately. Anticoagulation (e.g., heparin infusion) may be prescribed to decrease the incidence of thrombosis. Other vascular complications associated with IABP include acute aortic dissection and the development of pseudoaneurysms at the catheter insertion site.

BOX 14.20 Suggested Indications for Percutaneous Mechanical Circulatory Support

- Severe heart failure in the setting of nonischemic cardiomyopathy
- Failure to wean from cardiopulmonary bypass
- Acute cardiac allograft failure
- Post-transplant right ventricular failure
- Prophylactic use for high-risk percutaneous coronary intervention
- Complications of acute myocardial infarction
- Cardiogenic shock
- Papillary muscle dysfunction or rupture with mitral regurgitation
- Refractory arrhythmias
- Bridge to definitive therapy: cardiac transplantation or ventricular assist device

BOX 14.21 Physiologic Effects of Intra-aortic Balloon Pump

Increased
- Coronary blood flow
- Cardiac output
- Urine output
- Improved mentation

Decreased
- Signs of myocardial ischemia: angina, ST segment changes, ventricular dysrhythmias
- Afterload
- Preload
- Myocardial oxygen demand
- Pulmonary congestion
- Heart rate

Balloon complications can include balloon perforation and malpositioning. A balloon leak is evidenced by a gas leak alarm from the pump console or the presence of blood in the IAB tubing. If a balloon leak is detected, pumping is stopped, and the physician is immediately notified so that the balloon can be removed. If the balloon is not promptly removed or pumping is attempted after the perforation, the IAB may become entrapped as the blood hardens within the catheter, creating a mass. If this occurs, the balloon must be surgically removed. The balloon catheter must be maintained in proper position to optimize its effectiveness and minimize complications. The balloon may migrate proximally and occlude the left subclavian artery or the carotids, or it may move distally, compromising renal and mesenteric circulation. Careful assessment of the left radial pulse, level of consciousness, urinary output, and gastrointestinal symptoms is essential along with a daily chest radiograph to evaluate IAB position. Measures to prevent accidental displacement of the balloon catheter include ensuring that the IAB is secured to the patient's skin, bed rest with the head of the bed elevated no more than 30 degrees, and no flexion of the involved hip.

Further complications include thrombocytopenia, which may occur because of mechanical destruction of the platelets by the pumping action of the balloon. Platelet counts are closely monitored, and the patient is observed for evidence of bleeding. Patients must also be monitored for signs of stroke and infections.

Weaning From the Intra-Aortic Balloon Pump

Weaning from the IABP is considered after hemodynamic stability has been achieved with no, or only minimal, pharmacologic support. Weaning is accomplished by reducing the ratio of augmented to nonaugmented beats from 1:1 to 1:2 or 1:3, as tolerated. A less common weaning method involves a gradual decrease in balloon volume. To prevent thrombus formation on the balloon surface, the IABP must remain at a minimal pumping ratio (or volume) until its removal.

BOX 14.22 PATIENT AND FAMILY EDUCATION PLAN

Intra-aortic Balloon Pump

Before discharge, the patient should be able to teach back the following topics:
- Description of why an intra-aortic balloon pump was necessary
- Activity restrictions (minimize leg movement)
- Symptoms to report to the health care professional (pain in the back, leg, or chest)

Educate the Patient and Family

Patient education for a patient with an IAB is presented in Box 14.22. Many IABP manufacturers provide educational booklets designed for patients and families.

Short-Term Mechanical Circulatory Support Devices

Short-term MCS devices provide hemodynamic support for the management of cardiogenic shock, decompensated heart failure, cardiopulmonary arrest, or even prophylactic insertion for high-risk invasive coronary artery procedures[99,100] (Box 14.20). Several temporary MCS devices are available with different mechanical properties (Table 14.14).

- Axial flow pumps
- Centrifugal pumps

Not all MCS devices are available in all settings; therefore, which device to use is primarily a choice of the surgeon and institutional resources. Many ventricular assist devices (VADs) cannot be inserted in the critical care unit, which limits how quickly therapy can be initiated. Another consideration is that many VADs provide only single ventricular support, which would necessitate a second device in the setting of biventricular failure.

TandemHeart—Left Atria to Aorta Assist Device

The TandemHeart (Cardiac Assist, Inc.; Pittsburgh, PA, USA) uses a continuous-flow *centrifugal pump* with an inflow and outflow cannula that can be configured in different ways to achieve percutaneous or minimally invasive surgical approaches. The device pumps blood from the left atrium to the lower aorta/ileofemoral arterial system and requires a transseptal atrial catheter for drainage.[100] The increase in cardiac output and arterial blood pressure provides support for systemic perfusion up to 5 L/minute. Frequently, LV contraction will virtually cease, resulting in a flat mean arterial pressure (MAP) curve. Adequate RV function is required to maintain left atrial filling volumes. Complications are related to the need for anticoagulation, transseptal puncture, thromboembolism or air embolism, and hemolysis. Care must be taken to prevent catheter dislodgement, which could lead to systemic desaturation or device malfunction.

Impella—Left Ventricle to Aorta Mechanical Assist Device

Impella (Abiomed, Danvers, MA, USA) has a suite of MCS devices. Impella is a nonpulsatile axial flow pump that draws blood from the LV and ejects it proximally into the ascending aorta (Fig. 14.22). Different versions are available in different sizes.

TABLE 14.14 Mechanical Circulatory Support Devices

Type	Indications	Description
Temporary		
CentriMag	Short-term univentricular or biventricular support For central or peripheral VA-ECMO and VV-ECMO	Continuous-flow pump that produces blood flow from 0–10 L/min Blood flow is produced by rotation of a magnetically suspended impeller, eliminating contact between components Placed either through an open chest or by percutaneous methods
Impella CP and Impella 5.0	Short-term left ventricular support	Continuous-flow pump that has a percutaneously inserted catheter, allowing flows of ≥3.5 L/min or 5 L/min for the version that requires a surgical cut-down for implantation The catheter is placed retrograde across the aortic valve to pull blood from the left ventricle, which is returned to the ascending aorta
TandemHeart	Short-term left or right ventricular support	Percutaneously inserted device that provides continuous flow up to 5 L/min LVAD: Inflow is obtained from a catheter positioned in the left atrium (by a transseptal approach), and outflow is through the femoral artery RVAD: Inflow is obtained from a catheter positioned in the right atrium, and outflow is through the pulmonary artery Device allows for transport to a center for long-term therapy
Long-Term		
HeartWare	Long-term left ventricular support FDA approved for BTT and DT	A continuous flow rotary pump with centrifugal design that produces nonpulsatile flow Its small size allows for placement above the diaphragm in the pericardial space The pump has no points of mechanical contact, which reduces damage to red blood cells
HeartMate II	Long-term left ventricular support FDA approved for BTT and DT	An electrically driven axial continuous-flow pump that produces nonpulsatile flow Anticoagulation and antiplatelet therapy are required
HeartMate 3	Long-term left ventricular support FDA approved for BTT and DT	Magnetically levitated centrifugal-flow pump that produces nonpulsatile flow Anticoagulation and antiplatelet therapy are required Improved outcomes over HeartMate II in regard to pump replacement and survival free of disabling stroke

BTT, Bridge to transplant; *DT*, destination therapy; *FDA*, U.S. Food and Drug Administration; *LVAD*, left ventricular assist device; *RVAD*, right ventricular assist device; *VA-ECMO*, venoarterial extracorporeal membrane oxygenation; *VV-ECMO*, venovenous extracorporeal membrane oxygenation.

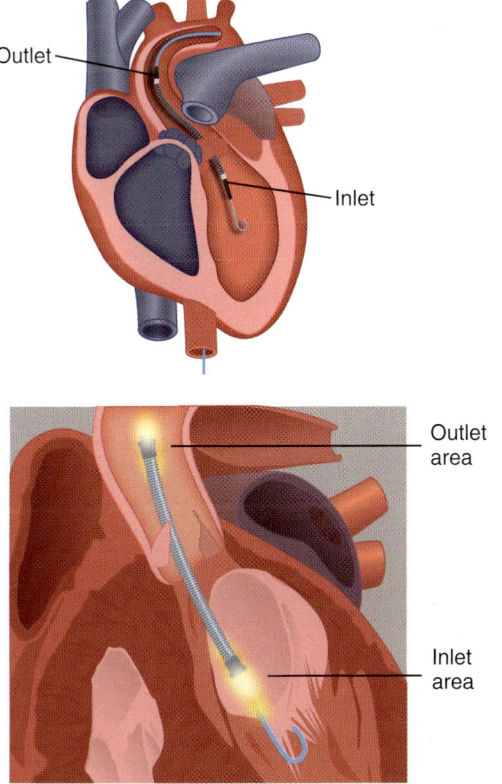

FIG. 14.22 Impella Ventricular Assist Device. Blood is pulled into the catheter from the left ventricle and returned to the ascending aorta.

The smaller device (Impella CP) can be quickly placed percutaneously, providing 3.0 to 4.0 L/min of support, whereas the larger device (Impella 5.0) requires a surgical cut-down to provide flow rates of 5.0 L/min. The Impella is contraindicated in patients with mechanical aortic valves. Monitoring for catheter migration is an import aspect of care to prevent hemolysis and ensure proper pump functioning.

Right Ventricular Assist Devices

RV failure carries a high mortality, especially in cardiogenic shock. MCS devices are now being developed specifically to support the failing RV.[99,100] The percutaneously inserted *Impella RP* catheter takes blood from the inferior vena cava and delivers it into the outlet opening in the pulmonary artery (PA) with flow of up to 4 L/min.[100] However, complications and mortality rates have caused the FDA to issue an advisory concerning patient selection and timing.[100,103]

A different option is the dual limen *Protek Duo* catheter that is inserted percutaneously into the internal jugular vein and advanced via the RA and RV to the main PA visualized by TEE or fluoroscopy.[104] When optimally positioned, the proximal holes (openings) are positioned within the RA, and the distal holes are in the PA. When connected to an extracorporeal circulatory pump such as the TandemHeart, the venous blood is drained from the RA, via the extracorporeal pump, and returned to the main PA, thus unloading the RV.[100,105] The blood flow is 4.5 L/minute depending on the cannula size.[100,105] A separate oxygenator can be added to the system if needed.[100,104,105]

Extracorporeal Membrane Oxygenation System

Extracorporeal membrane oxygenation (ECMO) is being used with increasing frequency in critical care units. The primary indication for ECMO is acute severe heart or lung failure with high mortality risk despite conventional treatment.[99] There are two types of ECMO:

- ECMO venoarterial (VA)
- ECMO venovenous (VV)

ECMO Hemodynamic Support

Both types provide pulmonary support, but only VA-ECMO provides hemodynamic support.

VA-ECMO can be initiated quickly at the bedside by either a direct right atrial cannulation (via a preexisting sternotomy) or peripherally using a percutaneous technique (Fig. 14.23). Once the patient is connected to the ECMO circuit and hemodynamic parameters are satisfactory, vasoactive drugs can be weaned to minimal levels to allow the myocardium to rest. Anticoagulation is

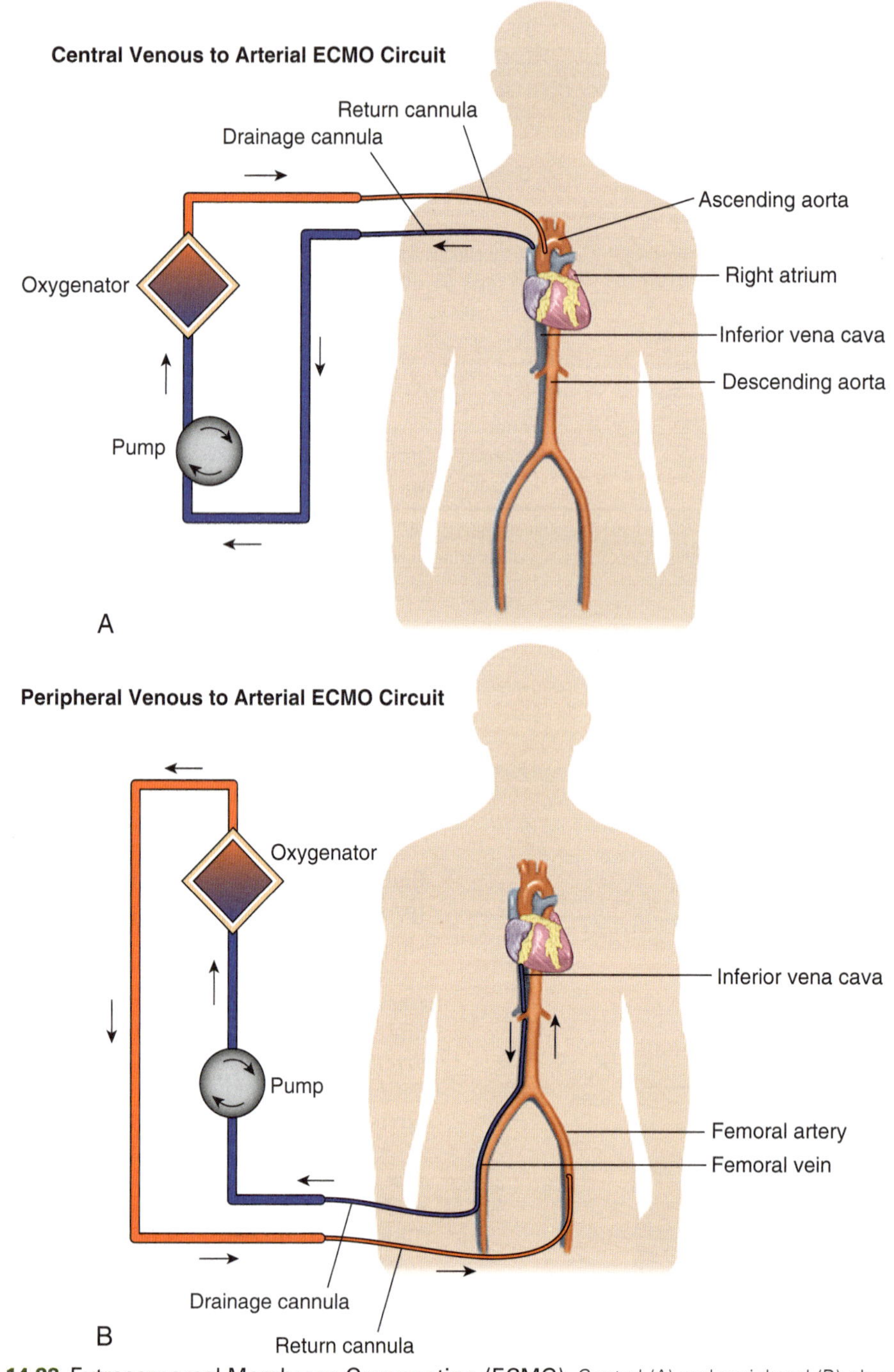

FIG. 14.23 Extracorporeal Membrane Oxygenation (ECMO). Central (A) and peripheral (B) placement of an ECMO circuit. (Modified from Hung M, Vuylsteke A, Valchanov K. Extracorporeal membrane oxygenation coming to an ICU near you. *J Intensive Care Soc.* 2012;13(1):31–38.)

required for most venoarterial ECMO support because of the risk of venous and arterial thromboembolization. However, consideration must also be given to the fact that bleeding is the most common complication, often requiring transfusions after placement.

ECMO Pulmonary Support

ECMO is also used to support gas exchange for patients with acute respiratory distress syndrome (ARDS) where support with mechanical ventilation is insufficient.[106] A recent randomized controlled trial (RCT) of prone positioning while on ECMO found the addition of proning did not improve survival.[107] VV-ECMO has also been used to remove high levels of carbon dioxide (CO_2) that can occur as a consequence of low tidal volumes and lung protective ventilation strategies.[108]

ECMO Safety

To safely manage ECMO requires a highly trained interdisciplinary team to maintain the ECMO circuit and to monitor for other complications, such as cardiac tamponade, multiorgan failure, sepsis, limb ischemia, and pulmonary complications. Once evidence of cardiopulmonary function has returned, weaning trials can be conducted to assess if the patient can be maintained with conventional support.

The major limitations of ECMO are its limited availability, short duration of usage, need for highly trained personnel, and risk of complications related to vascular access, thromboembolism, hemorrhage, or infection.

LONG-TERM VENTRICULAR ASSIST DEVICES

The VAD is designed to support or replace a failing natural heart with flow assistance. Clinical use of the continuous flow left ventricular assist device (LVAD) continues to increase due to limited heart transplantation options and improvements in survival rates and quality of life for LVAD patients with heart failure.[109,110]

Long-term MCS devices are currently placed for two types of clinical indications.

- Bridge to transplantation
- Destination therapy

The first category, called *bridge to transplantation* (BTT), includes patients with decompensated chronic heart failure who need circulatory support until heart transplantation can be performed. The second category, called *destination therapy* (DT), includes patients with severe heart failure who are not candidates for heart transplantation and for whom all other medical options have been exhausted. There is no single ideal system, so device selection is often based on individual VAD capabilities and institutional preference (see Table 14.14).

All devices consist of a blood pump, cannula, controller, and some type of power source. They differ in the mechanism by which they move blood, either through centrifugal flow or axial flow.[110] Inlet cannulas that divert blood from the heart to the LVAD for LV support are placed in the left atrium or the LV apex, with the outlet cannula attached to the ascending aorta or femoral artery (Fig. 14.24). The LVAD is used most because LV failure occurs more often than RV failure. However, RV failure can happen in the immediate postoperative phase or even months after LVAD implantation, which can lead to additional clinical challenges. Another option for biventricular failure is the total artificial heart, which can be used as a bridge to transplant.

Nursing Management of a Patient With a Left Ventricular Assist Device

Nursing management for a patient with a VAD includes monitoring for hemodynamic changes and for complications related to the device. The same interventions that are used for cardiac surgery patients to optimize cardiac output by manipulation of heart rate, preload, afterload, and contractility apply to patients with a VAD.

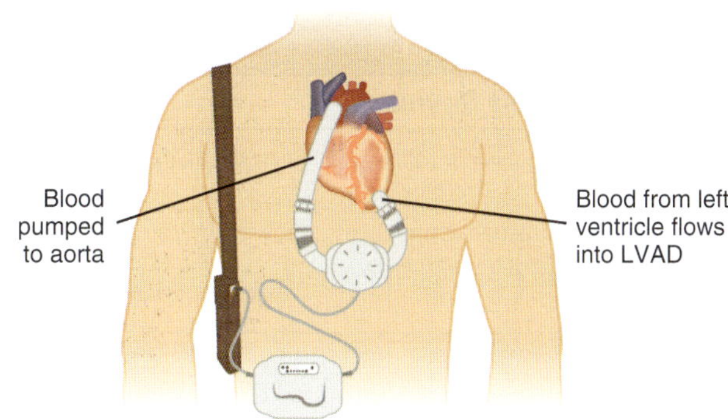

FIG. 14.24 Left Ventricular Assist Device (LVAD) System.

Adequate filling volumes are essential to maintain pump flow. Afterload reduction may be needed to improve output from the unassisted ventricle when univentricular support is used. Although complication rates vary among the different models, complications common to all types of VADs include bleeding, infection, stroke, thromboembolism, respiratory failure, arrhythmias, and device failure.[99] On physical examination, patients with continuous-flow VADs may not have palpable pulses; this can make measurement of blood pressure difficult and will require an invasive arterial catheter for the initial postoperative period. An occlusive pressure obtained with a manual blood pressure cuff and Doppler at the brachial artery is the best reflection of MAP.[111]

Arterial blood gas analysis may be required because pulse oximetry may be unreliable with little or no pulse. While in VT or VF, not all patients with an LVAD will be unconscious. Cardioversion and defibrillation should be performed for the same indications as other patients.[111] Nurses must often rely on basic assessments such as circulation, mentation, and urine output to determine whether the patient is receiving adequate support.

Assist Device Failure

Although the incidence of device failure continues to decrease, it is a life-threatening event because of the nature of this therapy. The two most common causes of pump failure involve failure of the driveline and power disconnection. VAD designs vary considerably, and troubleshooting methods for device failure are unique to each device. The nurse must be aware of signs of device malfunction and patient factors (volume status, dysrhythmias, RV failure) that may affect VAD function.

Anticoagulation

Anticoagulation protocols vary with the device, individual patient, and institution. Both antiplatelet agents and warfarin are commonly used. Although bleeding is the most frequent complication, thrombotic events can also be a problem leading to stroke and device failure. Coagulation studies must be frequently monitored during support.

Infection

Patients with a VAD are at considerable risk for localized and septicemic infections. Infectious risks are posed by the presence of invasive catheters and the surgically implanted VAD. Infection is prevented using strict aseptic techniques with all invasive tubing and dressing changes. Site care varies depending on institutional protocols and the type of VAD that is used. Nurses monitor patients

BOX 14.23 PATIENT AND FAMILY EDUCATION PLAN

Ventricular Assist Device

Before discharge, the patient should be able to teach back the following topics:

- Description of the specific ventricular assist device (VAD) and how it works
- Activity restrictions during VAD therapy
- Symptoms to report to a health care professional

for infection by measuring temperatures, inspecting insertion sites and incisions, and obtaining daily leukocyte counts. If an infection is suspected, cultures of blood, urine, and sputum are taken, using the results to guide appropriate antibiotic therapy.

Educate the Patient and Family

The rapid and acute nature of cardiogenic shock limits the nurse's ability to prepare patients and families for VAD insertion. Despite the critical nature of the illness, nurses explain the reason for the use of the VAD and provide information about the critical care environment and equipment (Box 14.23). The number of patients with VADs discharged to home continues to increase.[112] These patients and their families require education related to care of the device and reinforcement on the components of heart failure management.

VASCULAR SURGERY

Vascular surgery may be used as a treatment for arterial occlusive disease or to correct structural abnormalities such as aneurysms. With the evolution in endovascular technology, many patients with vascular disease can now be effectively treated with percutaneous procedures. The choice between an open surgical procedure and an endovascular intervention depends on many factors, including the type and location of the vascular lesion, life expectancy, comorbid conditions, and patient preference. Because atherosclerosis is a diffuse disease that affects both the peripheral vessels and the coronary arteries, patients undergoing arterial vascular surgery are at high risk for perioperative cardiac events. The nursing care of patients after vascular surgery focuses not only on observations for surgical complications such as hematoma or reocclusion but also on prompt recognition and appropriate treatment of complications that may arise from the impact of the procedure on preexisting cardiac, pulmonary, or kidney disease.

Carotid Endarterectomy

Carotid stenosis is a narrowing of the carotid artery, often around the bifurcation of the internal and external carotid arteries.[113] The stenotic narrowing results from atherosclerosis and is *extracranial*, meaning it is external to the brain and skull. Stenosis at the bifurcation accounts for 8% to 15% of ischemic strokes.[114] Treatment options include medical management, endovascular stent placement, and surgery depending on the degree of stenosis and symptoms.[115]

Symptomatic Carotid Stenosis

Symptomatic patients with a carotic stenosis greater than 50% are at high risk of experiencing an embolic stroke and are recommended to have surgery to reduce the stenosis.[115]

Asymptomatic Carotid Stenosis

Not all patients are symptomatic, but stenosis in the carotid artery increases with time and consequently increases the risk of embolic stroke. In general, asymptomatic patients have a more favorable outcome than patients with symptoms.[116]

Carotid Endarterectomy Indications

In current guidelines a carotid endarterectomy (CEA) is recommended over maximal medical therapy in the following situations:[115]

- Symptomatic patients with carotid artery stenosis of 50% to 99%
- Asymptomatic patients with carotid artery stenosis of 70% to 99%

If a patient also has symptomatic CAD, it is recommended that the CEA be performed before the CABG surgery.[115]

Carotid Endarterectomy Procedure

The carotid endarterectomy procedure is performed through a neck incision that allows for visualization of the vessel. The plaque is removed and the vessel is closed directly or with a patch composed of saphenous vein or a prosthetic material. A small percutaneous drain may be placed at the end of the procedure to minimize hematoma formation. Complications after carotid endarterectomy include perioperative MI, cerebral ischemia or infarction, bleeding, and cranial nerve damage.

Postoperative Management After Carotid Endarterectomy

Patients require 12 to 24 hours of intensive nursing assessment in the period immediately after carotid endarterectomy. Complications are rare but some may be life threatening and require rapid intervention. Serial assessments are performed to assess neurologic status, blood pressure, bleeding, or hematoma. The surgeon is promptly notified of significant changes in the patient's status.

Neurologic Assessment

Frequent neurologic assessments are performed as the patient awakens from anesthesia and then hourly for the first 12 hours. These assessments should include level of consciousness, orientation, pupil response, motor function, and evaluation of cranial nerve function by asking the patient to swallow, stick out his or her tongue, and smile or grimace while the nurse looks for evidence of a facial droop.[113] Other signs of cranial nerve injury include an impaired gag reflex or a hoarse voice.[113] Compression, traction, or inadvertent severing can damage nerves that lie in or near the surgical field. The most common injuries are damage to the vagus and hypoglossal nerves.[117] Most cranial nerve dysfunction resolves within a short time.[117] The major procedural risks of disabling stroke or death are rare, with 1% equivalent occurance after either CEA or carotid artery stent.[118]

Bleeding

Bleeding is assessed by observation of the dressing for drainage or swelling and measurement of output from the neck drain if present. If hematoma formation occurs internally, it may impinge on the trachea, so the patient is also monitored for signs of a compromised airway. In addition to monitoring respiratory rate and oxygen saturation, the nurse assesses the patient for tracheal deviation and for symptoms of upper airway obstruction such as stridor or wheezing. A small venous hematoma may respond to manual pressure, but larger arterial hematomas that expand rapidly require emergent return to the operating room for reexploration and evacuation.

Cardiovascular Monitoring

Continuous ECG with ST segment monitoring is used to detect myocardial ischemia after carotid endarterectomy. Bradycardia is not uncommon because of baroreceptor stimulation during the operative procedure, but this is usually hemodynamically tolerated provided the patient's blood pressure is stable.

Arterial Pressure Monitoring

Manipulation of the carotid bulb during surgery often results in hemodynamic instability in the immediate postoperative period. An arterial line may be placed to allow for prompt detection and treatment of hypotension or hypertension. Adequate blood pressure control in the postoperative period is of paramount importance. Hypertension increases the risk of bleeding at the suture line and is typically treated with short-acting vasodilators such as sodium nitroprusside. Relative hypotension compared with the patient's baseline value results in inadequate cerebral perfusion and potential neurologic deficits, and vasopressors such as phenylephrine may be used to maintain an adequate blood pressure.

Carotid Stents

Although carotid endarterectomy has been the gold standard for treatment of patients with significant carotid stenosis, carotid artery stent (CAS) is a less invasive alternative for patients with appropriate anatomy.[119] The procedure is performed with the use of local anesthesia and percutaneous cannulation similar to that used in coronary stent placement.

The most serious complication associated with carotid artery stenting is stroke, especially within the first 30 days after the procedure.[119] Risk factors include lesion morphology and age older than 70 years.[119] Embolic protection devices are used to trap and remove embolic particles generated during the procedure, but there is always a risk of minor stroke from catheter manipulation and hypoperfusion. Compared with CEA, carotid stent placement has a lower periprocedural risk of cranial nerve injury and bleeding at the carotid site.[116] Over the long term, RCT studies show no significant difference in stroke incidence between CEA and CAS.[116,118,119]

Neurological nursing assessment of patients after carotid stent placement is similar to care provided after carotid endarterectomy. Patients require intensive nursing for a brief time to allow for frequent neurologic assessments and treatment of hemodynamic instability. Patients are also monitored for potential complications related to femoral vascular access sheaths.

AORTIC ANEURYSM AND DISSECTION REPAIR

Aortic aneurysm and aortic dissection are two of the conditions that fall under the umbrella term *acute aortic syndromes*[120] as described in Chapter 13.

Aortic Aneurysm Assessment

Asymptomatic patients with an aortic abdominal aneurysm (AAA) are monitored medically over time to evaluate risks and benefits of elective repair versus ongoing medical management and surveillance.[121] As the aneurysm enlarges, the likelihood of complications and rupture increase. Significantly, a ruptured AAA carries a mortality of 80% to 90%. as many patients will not arrive at the hospital before demise and others experience complications leading to higher mortality after the procedure.[122]

To prevent AAA rupture, annual monitoring is recommended for an aortic aneurysm of 4.0 cm to 4.9 cm diameter.[123] For an aneurysm between 5.0 cm and 5.4 cm an elective repair is discussed with the patient, because there is an increase in aneurysmal complications with an aortic diameter above 6.0 cm.[121] Monitoring may involve ultrasound or contrast-enhanced computed tomography (CT).

Aortic disease progression varies according to the underlying disease process and the interplay of genetics and environment.[121] Risk factors for development of an AAA include older age, smoking, male sex, positive family history (first degree relative affected), and aneurysmal disease in other large vessels.[122] For thoracic aortic disease, there are additional genetic risk factors such as Marfan disease.[121]

Aortic Dissection Assessment

Medical management of aortic dissection depends on the site of the dissection and whether it is classified as chronic or acute.[120] See Fig. 13.24 in Chapter 13 for a description of the different types of aortic dissection.

- Type A dissection involves the aortic arch and requires generally an open cardiac surgery operation.
- Type B dissection involves the descending aorta and may be treated with an open surgical approach or an endovascular stent. Type B dissections may be acute or chronic.

Endovascular Stents for Abdominal Aneurysm or Dissection

Endovascular aneurysm repair (EVAR) is placement of a stent graft within the aortic aneurysmal sac. This is a less invasive approach that avoids the abdominal incision associated with open surgical aneurysm repair.[122] EVAR is increasingly employed for elective repair and has replaced open abdominal surgery in many settings.[124,125] In the EVAR procedure, a sutureless vascular graft is implanted into the abdominal aorta using fluoroscopy or ultrasound guidance. The insertion site is generally percutaneous via the femoral artery.[122,126] The stent isolates the aneurysmal wall from intraluminal blood pressure to prevent further expansion or rupture of the aneurysm. The EVAR procedure can be performed with the patient under epidural anesthesia with minimal blood loss and a shorter length of stay.

Studies have shown that short-term (30-day) operative mortality is lower with endovascular stents, but for longer term outcomes (6 years), the mortality, morbidity, and reintervention are higher compared to open surgical aneurysm repair.[127] Thus, surveillance over time is essential after EVAR because late complications such as endoleak and device migration can occur, necessitating reintervention.[127] After, the EVAR patients need to commit to annual check-ups to ensure stent and aortic wall integrity.

Endovascular stent is the recommended approach to treat a ruptured aneurysm, with a door to procedure time of under 90 minutes.[123]

Surgical Procedure for Abdominal Aneurysm or Dissection

Surgery is performed with the patient under general anesthesia and involves a midline abdominal incision or a flank incision (retroperitoneal approach). Clamping of the aorta proximal and distal to the dilated area isolates the aneurysm. The aneurysmal portion of the aorta is replaced with a prosthetic graft, which is then enclosed within the aneurysmal sac.

Postoperative complications can include myocardial ischemia or infarction, bleeding, AKI, and distal embolization.

Rarely, colon or spinal cord ischemia may occur because of interruption of blood flow during aortic cross-clamping or embolization. Urinary catheters are removed as soon as possible. After the surgical procedure, patients are monitored in the critical care unit for 24 to 48 hours, with a total hospital length of stay of approximately 5 days. The open abdominal surgical option is much less frequently used today because of the advances in endovascular stent procedures.[124,125]

Postoperative Nursing Management After Aortic Repair

Nursing assessment of vital signs and peripheral perfusion is performed frequently after the procedure, which may be open surgical or endovascular. Continuous ECG monitoring with ST segment analysis is used to detect myocardial ischemia. An arterial line may be in place to allow for prompt detection and treatment of hypotension or hypertension.

- Hypertension increases the risk of bleeding at the suture lines and is often treated with short-acting vasodilators such as sodium nitroprusside.
- Hypotension may result in compromised perfusion to organs or the extremities and is treated with volume replacement and vasopressors as needed.

Hourly assessment of urine output is performed to evaluate kidney function. If urine output is less than 30 mL/h, diuretics may be used after correction of hypovolemia. The urinary drainage catheter is removed as soon as possible to avoid infection. The abdominal dressing is assessed for bleeding and signs of internal hemorrhage from the graft site. Hypotension or complaints of back pain are further evaluated with serial hematocrit measurements. Management of serum glucose to avoid hypo- or hyperglycemia is considered best practice.[128]

PERIPHERAL VASCULAR PROCEDURES

Atherosclerosis of the lower extremities can result in progressive obstruction of large to medium arteries. These occlusive lesions commonly occur at bifurcations of the abdominal aorta and the iliac, femoral, popliteal, tibial, and peroneal arteries.

Peripheral Arterial Disease Symptoms

Peripheral arterial disease (PAD) may go undetected for long periods until symptoms appear. PAD is often associated with *intermittent claudication* (leg pain with exercise), but this only affects 5% to 10% of patiens with PAD.[129] Often the presentation is less obvious with atypical back or lower limb pain. Intermittent claudication is a warning sign, but it differs from *critical limb ischemia* manifested by rest pain, ulceration, or gangrene, which are limb threatening and may result in amputation if revascularization is not performed.[129]

Patients with PAD are likely to have significant cardiovascular atherosclerotic symptoms such as CAD and may have undergone other cardiac procedures.[122,129] There is also a strong association with diabetes and kidney failure.[129] One inexpensive method to evaluate PAD is the ankle-brachial index (ABI), which is described in Chapter 13.

Lifestyle and Pharmacologic Management

Initial treatment focuses on lifestyle modification, such as smoking cessation, exercise therapy, blood glucose control, treatment of hypertension, and pharmacologic management of dyslipidemia, heart failure, and other comorbidities.[130] Because there are many endovascular and surgical options a shared decision between provider and patient is recommended.

The risks of a surgical procedure need to be weighed against the anticipated benefits, including long-term patency and options for further treatment if needed. Consensus guidelines have been issued that include treatment recommendations based on lesion morphology, but practice continues to evolve with improvements in technology and operator expertise.[129,131]

Revascularization for Peripheral Arterial Disease

Elective revascularization can be either percutaneous or surgical and is based on the patient's symptoms, the ABI, and vascular imaging studies as explained in Chapter 13. The goals of treatment are to relieve symptoms of *intermittent claudication*, improve walking, and improve quality of life.[132]

Acute arterial occlusion occurs when an artery is blocked due to thrombosis, emboli, trauma, or compression, and this requires an emergency intervention. Left untreated, acute ischemia may lead to amputation of the affected limb.

Percutaneous Interventions for Peripheral Arterial Disease

Percutaneous interventions used in the coronary arteries—angioplasty, atherectomy, and stent placement—can be performed to treat occlusion or narrowing in the peripheral vasculature. Advances in catheter design and the development of intravascular stents have resulted in a dramatic increase in the number of endovascular procedures performed for peripheral artery disease.[133] Endovascular therapy is best suited to the treatment of short, focal stenoses and is routinely used as first-line therapy in the iliac and femoral arteries.[133]

Percutaneous transluminal balloon angioplasty (PTA) is an option to widen a stenosed vessel. Because large peripheral vessels are often calcified rotational atherectomy is effective to widen the lumen.[132] Intravascular stents may be used in combination with PTA, depending on lesion morphology and location. The larger arteries are well suited to stent placement.[133] Complications of interventional vascular procedures include hematoma formation at the site of the arteriotomy, formation of a pseudoaneurysm at the vascular access site, distal embolization, and thrombotic occlusion.

Percutaneous fibrinolytic medications and thrombectomy catheter interventions may be used to remove a clot and recanalize an acutely occluded artery. In the setting of limb-threatening ischemia, both surgical and endovascular interventions have acceptable rates of limb salvage and survival.

Surgical Revascularization for Peripheral Arterial Disease

Surgical revascularization uses graft material to bypass the diseased portion of the vessel, improving distal blood flow. Surgeries are usually performed under general anesthesia, although regional anesthesia may be used in some cases. Conduits available for peripheral vascular bypass include vein grafts (reversed saphenous vein, arm vein, or human umbilical vein) and synthetic grafts made of polytetrafluoroethylene.

As in CABG surgery, the type of conduit used has an impact on the patency rate of the graft. Although synthetic grafts perform well in larger vessels (higher flow), veins are preferred for smaller vessels because of better patency rates.[131] Types of peripheral vascular procedures are shown in Fig. 14.25.

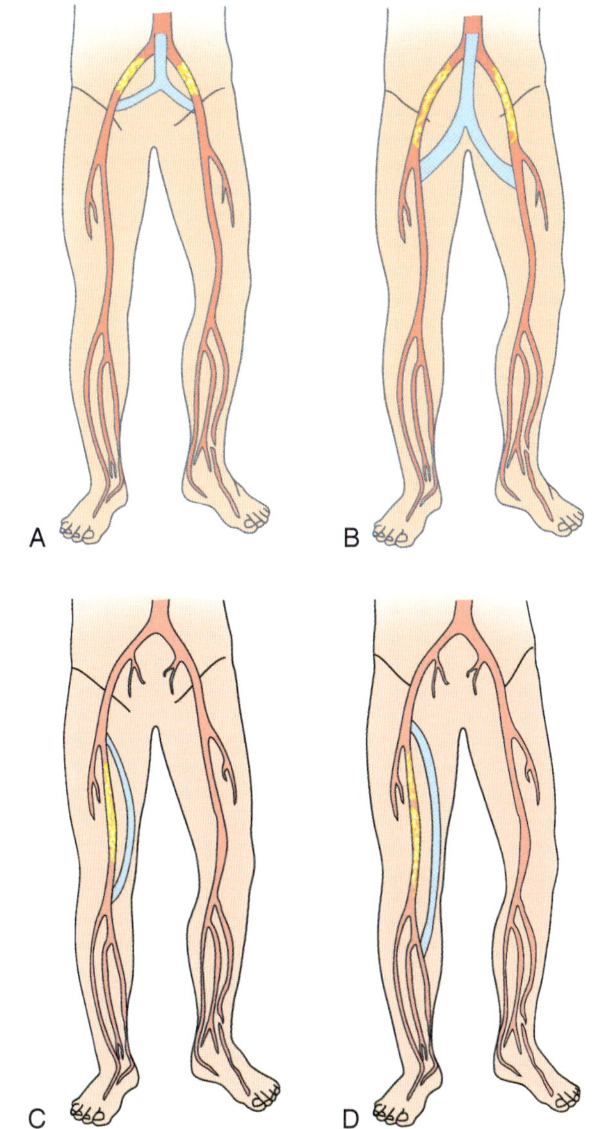

FIG. 14.25 Peripheral Arterial Bypass Procedures. (A) Aortoiliac bypass, (B) aortobifemoral bypass, (C) femoropopliteal bypass, (D) femorotibial bypass.

Nursing Management Following Peripheral Vascular Procedures

The primary focus of nursing care in the immediate postprocedural period is assessment of the adequacy of perfusion to the affected limb and early identification of complications. Pulse checks are performed frequently, and the physician is notified of any decrease in the strength of the Doppler signal. Adequate blood pressure is essential to maintain perfusion through the repaired vessel or graft. Because distal perfusion is compromised in PAD, nursing measures to prevent skin breakdown (e.g., sheepskin, frequent repositioning, foot cradles) are implemented. Urinary catheters are rarely required after peripheral vascular procedures, and if present, are removed promptly. To prevent thrombotic complications early mobility and use of antithrombotic and antiplatelet regimes are recommended.[130] Patients with atherosclerotic PAD are at high risk for cardiac events, and continuous cardiac ST segment monitoring on the ECG is performed to detect episodes of myocardial ischemia throughout the perioperative period.[130]

CARDIOVASCULAR MEDICATIONS

Multiple medications are used in the treatment of critically ill cardiovascular patients. The critical care nurse is responsible for administration of these pharmacologic therapies and often is required to titrate the dose based on the patient hemodynamic response. The Joint Commission recently clarified criteria to enable nurses trained for critical care and procedural areas to use their clinical judgment in titration of vasoactive medications.[134]

Specific parameters must be delineated in a medication order that include the name, route, and initial/maximum rate or dose of the infusion, as well as the incremental units and time interval for increasing or decreasing the drug in response to a defined clinical measure (e.g., blood pressure, heart rate). The new regulation also provides for documentation over a specified block of time to address periods in which rapid titration of infusions is needed to manage urgent changes in the patient's condition.[134] Smart Infusion Pumps as described in Box 14.24 are used to increase medication safety.

New functionality in IV Smart Infusion Pumps allows medication rate and dose changes to be transmitted to the EHR without the nurse manually documenting the rate/dose change, which makes documentation of medication escalation and titration in real-time highly accurate.[135]

The medications used to treat cardiovascular disease are rapidly changing and expanding as more is learned about the pathophysiology of cardiac disease and as improved formulas are developed by pharmaceutical companies. The critical care nurse with an understanding of the mechanisms of action of the various pharmacologic classifications can readily apply this knowledge to new medications within the same classification.

This section provides a concise review of medications commonly administered to support cardiovascular function in the critical care setting. The emphasis is on intravenously administered medications that are used for acute cardiovascular conditions, with discussion of oral medications started as the IV infusions are discontinued.

Antidysrhythmic Medications

Antidysrhythmic medications comprise a diverse category of pharmacologic agents used to terminate or prevent an array of abnormal cardiac rhythms. These agents are commonly classified according to their primary effect on the action potential of cardiac cells (Fig. 14.26). The classification scheme shown in Table 14.15 is the most frequently used system. Classification of newer agents is more difficult because some of these agents have characteristics of more than one class, and others have no characteristics of the current system.

Class I—Sodium Channel Blockers

Class I agents are sodium channel blockers that decrease the influx of sodium ions through "fast" channels during phase 0 depolarization. This prolongs the absolute (effective) refractory period, decreasing the risk of premature impulses from ectopic foci. These medications also depress automaticity by slowing the rate of spontaneous depolarization of pacemaker cells during the resting phase (phase 4).

BOX 14.24 Informatics

Smart Infusion Pumps

Smart infusion pumps are medical devices used to deliver fluids and medications to patients in a controlled and precise manner. These pumps have evolved over the years to incorporate various intelligent features that enhance patient safety and improve the accuracy of medication delivery.[1]

- **Smart Medication Dosing.** One of the primary advantages of smart pumps is their ability to provide accurate medication dosing. They can calculate and deliver the exact amount of medication, reducing the risk of human error.
- **Medication Library.** Many smart infusion pumps come with a library containing a database of medications and their dosing guidelines. Health care professionals can select the medication from the library, and the pump will automatically set the appropriate parameters, such as infusion rate and concentration.
- **Wireless Connectivity.** Some advanced smart pumps are equipped with wireless connectivity, allowing them to communicate with electronic health records (EHR) systems. Integration with barcode scanning technology ensures that the right medication is administered to the right patient, reducing the risk of medication errors. This process enables real-time monitoring of infusions and automatic documentation of medication administration.
- **Reduce Adverse Events.** Smart pumps can monitor the infusion rate and detect variations or deviations from the prescribed rate. If a deviation occurs, the pump can automatically adjust to maintain the correct rate. They can enforce dose limitations to prevent administering medications at rates that exceed safe limits, reducing the risk of
- **Quality Control.** Smart infusion pumps often require user authentication through PINs or biometric verification to ensure that only authorized personnel can operate them. These pumps typically store a log of infusion data, including start and stop times, flow rates, and any alarms or alerts triggered during the infusion. These data can be valuable for auditing and quality control. Smart pumps have significantly improved the safety and precision of medication delivery in healthcare settings.

Smart infusion pumps are crucial in reducing medication errors and improving patient outcomes. Health care professionals must stay updated on the latest technology and best practices in using smart pumps to ensure optimal performance and patient safety.

Data from Alamer F, Alanazi AT. The impact of smart pump technology in the healthcare system: A scope review. *Cureus*. 2023;15(3):e36007. https://doi.org/10.7759/cureus.36007.

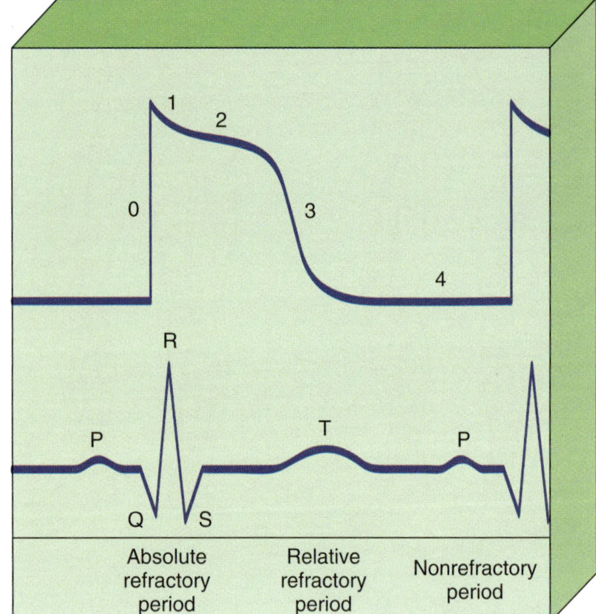

FIG. 14.26 Phases of the Cardiac Action Potential and Their Relationship to Refractory Periods of the Heart. *Phase 0*, depolarization with rapid influx of sodium. *Phase 1*, rapid repolarization with rapid efflux of potassium ions and decreased sodium conductance. *Phase 2*, plateau with slow influx of sodium and calcium ions. *Phase 3*, repolarization with continued efflux of potassium ions. *Phase 4*, resting phase with restoration of ionic balance by sodium and potassium pumps.

TABLE 14.15 Classification and Actions of Antidysrhythmic Agents

Class	Action on Receptors	Medications
I	Blocks sodium channels (stabilizes cell membrane)	
IA	Blocks sodium channels and delays repolarization, lengthening duration of the action potential	Quinidine Procainamide Disopyramide
IB	Blocks sodium channels and accelerates repolarization, shortening duration of the action potential	Lidocaine Mexiletine
IC	Blocks sodium channels and slows conduction through His-Purkinje system, prolonging QRS duration	Flecainide Propafenone
II	Blocks beta-receptors	Esmolol Metoprolol Propranolol
III	Slows repolarization and prolongs duration of the action potential	Amiodarone Dronedarone Dofetilide Ibutilide Sotalol
IV	Blocks calcium channels	Diltiazem Verapamil

Class I antidysrhythmic medications can be subdivided further into three groups according to their potency as sodium channel inhibitors and their effect on phase 3 repolarization.

- Class IA agents may depress myocardial contractility, with disopyramide having the most potent negative inotropic effect.
- Class IA agents—quinidine, procainamide, and disopyramide—block both the fast sodium channels and phase 3 repolarization, prolonging the action potential duration. Clinically, this may result in measurable increases in the QRS duration and lengthening of the Q–T interval.[136]
- Class IA agents—flecainide and propafenone—are proarrhythmic and have negative inotropic effects, which limits their use in patients with heart failure.[136]
- Class IB agents have only a moderate effect on sodium channels and accelerate phase 3 repolarization to shorten the action potential duration; lidocaine and mexiletine belong in this group.
- Class IC agents are the most potent sodium channel blockers and have little effect on repolarization. Class IC agents increase the P–R and QRS intervals.

Class II—Beta-Blockers

Class II agents are beta-adrenergic blockers (beta-blockers).[136] They inhibit dysrhythmias mediated by the sympathetic nervous system by competing with endogenous catecholamines for available receptor sites. As a result, spontaneous depolarization during the resting phase (phase 4) is depressed and AV conduction is slowed. Antidysrhythmic medications in this class can be further subdivided into groups:

- Cardioselective agents that block only beta-1-receptors
- Noncardioselective agents that block both beta-1-receptors, and beta-2-receptors

Knowledge of the effects of adrenergic-receptor stimulation allows for anticipation of both the therapeutic responses brought about by beta-blockade and the potential adverse effects of these agents (Table 14.16). For example, bronchospasm can be precipitated by noncardioselective beta-blockers in a patient with chronic obstructive pulmonary disease caused by blockade of the effects of beta-2-receptors in the lungs. Beta-blockers also are negative inotropes and must be used cautiously in patients with LV dysfunction. However, in patients after MI who did not have heart failure, beta-blockers reduced mortality for those under 75 years of age.[137]

Although numerous beta-blockers are available, only esmolol, metoprolol, and propranolol are approved as IV agents for the treatment of acute dysrhythmias. Of these, esmolol (Brevibloc) offers significant advantages for critically ill patients because of its short half-life (approximately 9 minutes). Esmolol is used in the treatment of SVTs, such as atrial fibrillation and atrial flutter.[9,138]

Class III—Potassium Channel Blockers

Class III agents block potassium channels to slow the rate of phase 3 repolarization, increasing the effective refractory period and the action potential duration.[136]

Class III agents include amiodarone, dronedarone, dofetilide, ibutilide, and sotalol.[136] Although the effects on the action potential are similar, these medications differ greatly in their mechanism of action and their side effects.

- Amiodarone as an intravenous medication is effective for management of SVT and serious ventricular dysrhythmias refractory to other medications.[138] It is administered as an IV bolus followed by a continuous infusion.[138]
- Dronedarone resembles amiodarone but has fewer extracardiac side effects.
- Dofetilide (Tikosyn) is a newer class III antidysrhythmic agent used for the conversion to and maintenance of normal sinus rhythm in patients with highly symptomatic atrial fibrillation or atrial flutter. Because dofetilide prolongs the refractoriness of both atrial and ventricular tissue, prolongation of the Q–T interval can occur and is associated with an increased risk of torsades de pointes. As a result, therapy with dofetilide is initiated in a hospital setting with mandatory ECG monitoring.[136]
- Ibutilide (Covert) is a short-term antidysrhythmic agent used for the rapid conversion of acute atrial fibrillation or atrial flutter to sinus rhythm. Ibutilide is administered as a 10-minute infusion in a carefully monitored clinical setting.[136] The most serious side effect of ibutilide is its potential for inducing life-threatening dysrhythmias, especially torsades de pointes[136] (Table 14.17).
- Sotalol not only blocks potassium channels but also has properties of a noncardioselective beta-blocker and should be used cautiously in patients with heart failure.[136]

TABLE 14.16 Effects of Adrenergic Receptors

Receptor	Location	Response to Stimulation
Alpha	Vessels of skin, muscles, kidneys, and intestines	Vasoconstriction of peripheral arterioles
Beta-1	Cardiac tissue	Increased heart rate Increased conduction Increased contractility
Beta-2	Vascular and bronchial smooth muscle	Vasodilation of peripheral arterioles Bronchodilation

Class IV—Calcium Channel Blockers

Class IV agents are calcium channel blockers that inhibit the influx of calcium through slow calcium channels during the plateau phase (phase 2). In the heart, this effect occurs primarily in tissue in which slow calcium channels predominate, primarily the sinus node, AV node, and in atrial tissue (Table 14.18).

There are two categories of calcium channel blockers. One group targets the heart (nondihydropyridines) described here, and the other group causes vasodilation of blood vessels (dihydropyridines) that are described later.

- Verapamil was the first medication in the nondihydropyridine category available as an intravenous antidysrhythmic. It depresses sinus and AV node conduction and is effective in terminating SVTs caused by AV nodal reentry.[138]
- Diltiazem (Cardizem) is available as an IV infusion form and is effective in treating supraventricular dysrhythmias.[138]

Because accessory pathways are not affected by many of the medications that slow AV node conduction (verapamil, diltiazem, amiodarone, digoxin, adenosine, beta-blockers), these medications must be avoided when treating atrial tachycardias in patients with accessory conduction pathways.[9]

Unclassified Antidysrhythmics

Adenosine (Adenocard) is an antidysrhythmic agent that remains unclassified under the current system. Adenosine occurs endogenously in the body as a building block of adenosine triphosphate. Given in intravenous boluses, adenosine slows conduction through the AV node, causing transient AV block. It is used clinically to convert SVTs and to facilitate differential diagnosis of rapid dysrhythmias. Because of its short half-life, adenosine is administered intravenously as a rapid bolus followed by a saline flush. The bolus is delivered as centrally as possible so that the medication reaches the heart before it is metabolized. Side effects are transient because adenosine is rapidly taken up by the cells and is cleared from the body within 10 seconds.[138]

Magnesium is also unclassified under the present system. Although its action as an antidysrhythmic agent is not entirely understood, observational studies suggest that it may reduce the incidence of both ventricular and supraventricular dysrhythmias in selected patient populations. It is considered the treatment of choice in patients with *torsades de pointes*.[139] For acute treatment, 1 to 2 g of magnesium is administered over 1 to 2 minutes. In patients with confirmed hypomagnesemia, this bolus may be followed with repeated infusions.

TABLE 14.17 **PHARMACOLOGIC MANAGEMENT**

Antidysrhythmic Agents

Medication	Dosage	Actions	Special Considerations
Adenosine	6 mg IV rapid push; if unsuccessful, repeat with 12 mg over 1–2 s; follow with IV fluid 10 mL flush (NS or D_5W)	Blocks AV node to terminate SVT, PSVT	Transient; flushing, dyspnea, hypotension
Digoxin	0.5–1 mg loading dose in divided doses; maintenance dose of 0.125–0.25 mg daily	Conversion and/or rate control in SVT, AFib, AF	Bradycardia, heart block Toxicity: CNS and GI symptoms
Diltiazem	Bolus dose of 0.25 mg/kg IV over 2 min, followed by infusion of 5–15 mg/h	Conversion and/or rate control in SVT, AFib, AF	Bradycardia, hypotension, AV block
Esmolol	Loading dose of 500 mcg/kg over 1 min, followed by infusion of 50 mcg/kg/min for 4 min; repeat procedure every 5 min, increasing infusion by 25–50 mcg/kg/min to maximum of 200 mcg/kg/min	Conversion and/or rate control in SVT, AFib, AF Also used to decrease rate of sinus tachycardia	Hypotension, bradycardia, heart failure
Ibutilide	0.010–0.025 mg/kg infused over 10 min (may repeat once) or 1 mg diluted in 50 mL infused over 10 min (may repeat once)	Conversion of AFib, AF	Minimal side effects except for rare polymorphic VT (torsades de pointes)
Verapamil	5–10 mg IV over at least 2 min, may repeat in 15–30 min	Conversion and/or rate control in SVT	Hypotension, bradycardia, heart failure
Lidocaine	1–1.5 mg/kg bolus, followed by continuous infusion of 1–4 mg/min	Treatment of ventricular dysrhythmias (PVCs, VT, VF)	CNS toxicity, nausea, vomiting with repeated doses
Amiodarone	*VT/VF arrest:* 300 mg IV push; may repeat with 150 mg in 3–5 min (maximum dose, 2.2 g/24 h) *Pulsatile VT, AFib, AF:* 150 mg IV over 10 min, followed by 360 mg over 6 h (1 mg/min); maintenance infusion of 0.5 mg/min	Treatment of atrial (AFib, AF, SVT) and ventricular (PVCs, VT, VF) dysrhythmias	Hypotension, abnormal liver function tests
Procainamide	Loading dose of 12–17 mg/kg at a rate of 20 mg/min, followed by infusion of 1–4 mg/min	Treatment of atrial (AFib, AF, SVT) and ventricular (PVCs, VT) dysrhythmias	Hypotension, GI effects widening of QRS and Q–T lengthening

AF, Atrial flutter; *AFib,* atrial fibrillation; *AV,* atrioventricular; *CNS,* central nervous system; *D_5W,* 5% dextrose in water; *GI,* gastrointestinal; *IV,* intravenous/intravenously; *NS,* normal saline; *PSVT,* paroxysmal supraventricular tachycardia; *PVCs,* premature ventricular contractions; *ST,* sinus tachycardia; *SVT,* supraventricular tachycardia; *VF,* ventricular fibrillation; *VT,* ventricular tachycardia.

Antidysrhythmic Medication Side Effects

Antidysrhythmic medications carry the risk of serious side effects, some of which can be life threatening. The major side effects and special considerations of intravenous antidysrhythmic agents are listed in Table 14.17. The most severe complication is the potential for a prodysrhythmic effect.[140] This may result in worsening of the underlying dysrhythmia, the occurrence of a new dysrhythmia, or the development of a bradydysrhythmia. For example, torsades de pointes is caused by many medications that prolong the Q–T interval on the ECG.[140]

Because the development of a dysrhythmia is unpredictable, the nurse plays an important role in evaluating ECG changes, monitoring serum medication levels, and assessing patient symptoms. Antidysrhythmic agents may also alter the amount of energy required for defibrillation and pacing. For example, increases in the dose of an antidysrhythmic medication may increase the amount of output (mA) required to depolarize the myocardium.

Antidysrhythmic Medications and Atrial Fibrillation

The three goals of pharmacologic therapy to reduce symptoms caused by atrial fibrillation are[9]:

- Rhythm control and reestablishing and maintaining sinus rhythm
- Rate control by decreasing the rapid ventricular response during episodes of rapid atrial fibrillation
- Prevention of thromboembolism using antithrombotic therapy

Table 14.18 reviews current medications used in the treatment of atrial fibrillation. If rate and rhythm control are not attainable with medications, interventional therapies are considered.[8,9,98,141]

Selection of a treatment strategy should consider the patient's age, severity of symptoms, duration of the arrhythmia, other comorbidities.

Antithrombotic Medications for Atrial Fibrillation

Although warfarin has been the traditional choice for antithrombotic therapy, direct-acting oral anticoagulant (DOAC) agents are now preferred for embolism prophylaxis for patients with nonvalvular atrial fibrillation in the United States and Europe.[8,9,98,141] See Table 14.7 and Table 14.18.

- Dabigatran inhibits thrombin directly.
- Rivaroxaban inhibits factor Xa.
- Apixaban inhibits factor Xa.
- Edoxaban inhibits factor Xa.

The DOAC agents have a rapid onset of therapeutic effect, fewer medication and food interactions than warfarin, and do not require routine laboratory monitoring.[8,98,141] DOAC agents are considerably more expensive than warfarin, and when cost is a barrier to a patient receiving treatment, warfarin is recommended for stroke prevention in atrial fibrillation.[9]

DOAC anticoagulant effects can be reversed with medication-specific reversal agents.[9,142]

- Idarucizumab is a reversal agent for dabigatran
- Andexanet alfa is a reversal agent for factor Xa inhibitor agents

TABLE 14.18 Atrial Fibrillation—Medication Classifications

Treatment Goal	Classification and Medications	Special Considerations
Conversion or maintenance of sinus rhythm	**Class IA** Quinidine Procainamide (Pronestyl) Disopyramide (Norpace)	Class IA agents prolong Q–T intervals and may cause torsades de pointes. Rate control should be achieved before initiation of therapy.
	Class IC Flecainide (Tambocor) Propafenone (Rythmol)	Class IC agents are prodysrhythmic in patients with CAD or previous MI and should be avoided in these patients.
	Class III—Potassium Channel Blockers Amiodarone (Cordarone) Dofetilide (Tikosyn) Dronedarone (Multaq) Ibutilide (Corvert) Sotalol (Betapace)	Amiodarone and sotalol also have beta-blocking properties and may help with rate control. Treatment with dofetilide requires careful monitoring for prodysrhythmic effects. Ibutilide is an IV agent and is used for conversion only.
Control of ventricular rate	**Class II—Beta-blockers** Esmolol (Brevibloc) Metoprolol (Lopressor) Propranolol (Inderal)	IV esmolol used in acute settings to control ventricular rate. Oral agents are used for maintenance therapy and provide good rate control.
	Class IV—Calcium channel blockers Diltiazem (Cardizem) Verapamil (Isoptin)	Intravenous calcium channel blockers may be used in emergency situations, followed by oral agents for maintenance therapy.
	Digitalis compounds Digoxin (Lanoxin)	Digoxin is not first-line treatment, only used when other antidysrhythmics are ineffective. Toxicity and higher mortality associated with higher serum levels.
Atrial Fibrillation—Anticoagulants and Antithrombotics		
Prevention of thromboembolism	Heparin	Heparin may be used in emergency situations before cardioversion.
	Vitamin K Agonist Warfarin (Coumadin)	Warfarin requires monitoring to achieve an INR of 2–3. It is less frequently used because DOACs have fewer side effects.
	DOACs Dabigatran (Pradaxa) Rivaroxaban (Xarelto) Apixaban (Eliquis) Edoxaban (Savaysa)	Dabigatran is an oral direct thrombin inhibitor approved to reduce risk of thromboembolism in patients with nonvalvular AFib. Dabigatran does not require routine anticoagulant monitoring. Rivaroxaban, apixaban, and edoxaban are factor Xa inhibitors that reduce risk of thromboembolism in patients with nonvalvular AFib. Factor Xa inhibitors do not require routine anticoagulant monitoring.

AFib, Atrial fibrillation; *CAD*, coronary artery disease; *DOAC*, direct-acting oral anticoagulants; *INR*, international normalized ratio; *IV*, intravenous; *MI*, myocardial infarction.

If needed, nonspecific DOAC reversal agents are available.[9,142]

- Four-factor prothrombin complex concentrates
- Activated prothrombin complex concentrate
- Recombinant activated factor VII

Warfarin can be reversed with four-factor prothrombin complex concentrates plus IV Vitamin K.[9,143]

Inotropic Medications

Critically ill patients with compromised cardiac function often require medications to enhance myocardial contractility (positive inotropy). Clinically available inotropes classes include:

- Sympathomimetics
- Phosphodiesterase inhibitors

These agents increase myocardial contractility, resulting in improved cardiac output, more complete emptying of the ventricles, and decreased filling pressures.

Sympathomimetic Agents

Sympathomimetic agents stimulate adrenergic receptors, simulating the effects of sympathetic nerve stimulation.

Included in this category are naturally occurring catecholamines (epinephrine, dopamine, and norepinephrine) and synthetic catecholamines (dobutamine and isoproterenol). The cardiovascular effects of these medications vary according to their selectivity for specific receptor sites, and effects are often dose dependent. Because these drugs target beta-1 adrenergic receptors, they do not work well for patients taking beta-blocker medications.[144] Sympathomimetic infusions are typically administered using an IV smart pump and the dose is calculated according to body weight in micrograms per kilogram per minute (mcg/kg/min). Table 14.19 describes the cardiovascular effects of sympathomimetic agents at various dosages.

Dopamine

Dopamine (Intropin) was one of the most widely used medications in the critical care setting. It is an endogenous precursor of norepinephrine.[144] The actions of dopamine are dose related through stimulation of beta-1 adrenergic (β1) receptors at low dose and alpha-1 adrenergic (α1) receptors at higher dosages. However, there is overlap in effects between the range margins.

- Low-dose dopamine 1 to 2 mcg/kg/min stimulates selective dopaminergic receptors, causing vasodilation in the renal and mesenteric vasculature.[144] The resultant increase in renal perfusion increases urinary output. However, this increase in urine output does not confer protection against the development of AKI.

TABLE 14.19 Physiologic Effects of Sympathomimetic Agents

		RECEPTOR ACTIVATED[a]				CARDIOVASCULAR EFFECTS		
Medications	**Dose Ranges**	**Alpha**	**Beta-1**	**Beta-2**	**Dopa**	**CO**	**HR**	**SVR**
Dobutamine	Low	0	↑↑↑	↑	0	↑↑	↑	↓↓
	Medium-High	0	↑↑↑	↑↑	0	↑↑↑	↑↑↑	↓↓
Dopamine	Low	0	↑	↑	↑↑↑	0/↑	0/↑	0
	Medium	↑↑	↑↑↑	↑	↑↑↑	↑↑↑	↑	↑
	High	↑↑↑	↑↑↑	↑	↑↑	↑↑	↑↑	↑↑↑
Epinephrine	Low	0	↑	↑↑	0	0/↑	0/↑	↓
	Medium	↑↑	↑↑↑	↑↑	0	↑↑↑	↑↑	↑
	High	↑↑↑	↑↑↑	↑↑	0	↑↑	↑↑	↑↑↑
Isoproterenol	Low-High	0	↑↑↑	↑↑↑	0	↑↑↑	↑↑↑	↓↓↓
Norepinephrine	Low	↑↑↑	↑↑	0	0	↑	0/↑	↑↑↑
	Medium High	↑↑↑↑	↑↑	0	0	↓	↑	↑↑↑↑
Phenylephrine	Low-High	↑↑↑↑	0	0	0	0	↓	↑↑↑

[a]See Table 14.15 and Table 14.16 for actions of receptors. See Table 14.23 for specific medication dosages.
0, No effect; ↑, increased (number of arrows indicates degree of effect); ↓, decreased (number of arrows indicates degree of effect); *CO*, cardiac output; *Dopa*, dopamine receptor; *HR*, heart rate; *SVR*, systemic vascular resistance.

- Moderate dose dopamine 3 to 5 mcg/kg/min stimulates beta-1 receptors that increase contractility. The alpha-1 adrenergic effects cause vasocontraction and may raise afterload.[144]
- High-dose dopamine 5 mcg/kg/min or greater predominantly stimulates alpha-receptors, resulting in vasoconstriction that often negates both the beta-adrenergic and the dopaminergic effects.[144]

Dobutamine

Dobutamine (Dobutrex) is a synthetic catecholamine with predominantly beta-1 adrenergic effects.[144] This results in inotropy (increased contractility), chronotropy (increased heart rate), and lower LV filling pressures.[144] It also produces some beta-2 stimulation, resulting in mild vasodilation.

Dobutamine is as effective as dopamine in increasing myocardial contractility and is useful in the treatment of heart failure, especially in hypotensive patients who cannot tolerate vasodilator therapy.[144] The usual dosage range is 2 to 20 mcg/kg/min, titrated on the basis of hemodynamic parameters.[144]

Epinephrine

Epinephrine (adrenaline) is endogenously produced by the adrenal gland as part of the body's response to stress. When infused as a medication, epinephrine can stimulate both alpha-1 receptors, beta-1 receptors, and beta-2 receptors, depending on the dose administered (see Table 14.19).

- Low-dose epinephrine at 0.05 to 0.5 mcg/kg/min binds with beta-1 receptors to increase heart rate, cardiac conduction, inotropy/contractility. It binds with beta-2 receptors to produce vasodilation. This combination will increase cardiac output.[144]
- Higher dose epinephrine binds to alpha-receptors, resulting in increased vascular resistance and increased blood pressure.[144] At higher doses, the impact of epinephrine on cardiac output depends on the ability of the heart to pump against the increased afterload.

Epinephrine has side effects related to beta-1 and alpha-1 adrenergic activation including accelerating the sinus rate, angina, ventricular dysrhythmias, restlessness, and headache.

Epinephrine is also administered as part of the ACLS cardiac arrest guidelines 1 mg IV every 3 to 5 minutes.[145]

Norepinephrine

Norepinephrine (Levophed) is an endogenous catecholamine that is similar to epinephrine in that it stimulates beta-1 receptors and alpha-1 receptors.[144] However, norepinephrine lacks the beta-2 (vasodilation) effects.

- Low-dose norepinephrine 0.02 to 1.0 mcg/kg/min has a strong inotropic effect, stimulating beta-1 receptors to increase inotropy/contractility, increasing cardiac output.[144]
- High-dose norepinephrine 0.25 to 0.5 mcg/kg/min stimulates alpha-1 receptors to produce marked vasoconstriction.[146] Clinically, norepinephrine is first-line therapy as a vasopressor to elevate blood pressure in sepsis and shock states.[146]

Isoproterenol

Isoproterenol (Isuprel) is a pure beta-receptor stimulant with no alpha-adrenergic effects. It produces dramatic increases in heart rate, conduction, and contractility through beta-1 stimulation and vasodilation through beta-2 stimulation. Isoproterenol also produces vasodilation of the PAs and bronchodilation. It greatly increases the automaticity of cardiac cells and frequently precipitates dysrhythmias such as premature ventricular contractions and VT. These effects limit its usefulness in most patients, and it is rarely used.

Phosphodiesterase Inhibitors

Medications in this classification inhibit the enzyme phosphodiesterase, resulting in increased levels of cyclic adenosine monophosphate and intracellular calcium.[144] Phosphodiesterase inhibitors are both inotropic agents and potent vasodilators (inodilators). Improvement in cardiac output occurs because of increased contractility and decreased afterload.

Milrinone (Primacor), a second-generation drug in this category, is used in the treatment of patients with acute decompensated heart failure. Milrinone side effects include hypotension and dysrhythmias.[144]

TABLE 14.20 **Hormone Vasoactive Infusion Cardiovascular System Actions**

Medication	Dosage	Receptor Activated	CARDIOVASCULAR EFFECTS		
			CO	HR	SVR
Vasopressin	0.01–0.04 units/min	V1 receptors	0	0	↑↑
Angiotensin II	10 ng/kg/min-80 ng/kg/min	Angiotensin II receptor type 1	0	0	↑↑↑

CO, Cardiac output; *HR*, heart rate; *SVR*, systemic vascular resistance.

Vasopressor Medications

Vasopressors include both sympathomimetic agents that mediate peripheral vasoconstriction and hormones that increase SVR (afterload). Some of these medications (epinephrine and norepinephrine) also stimulate beta-1 receptors, as previously described (see Table 14.16). Vasopressors are not used for primary treatment of cardiac illnesses because the dramatic increase in afterload is taxing to a damaged heart. However, vasopressors are used to maintain organ perfusion in shock states in all critical care units.[147]

Other vasopressors infusions are also available, including vasopressin and angiotensin II.

Hormone Vasoactive Agents—Vasopressin and Angiotensin II

Exogenous administration of naturally occurring vasoactive hormones offers another vasopressor strategy (see Table 14.20). Vasopressin and angiotensin II are the most common drugs administered in the hormone vasoactive category. Unlike the sympathomimetic agents, these drugs do not have significant arrhythmogenic effects on the heart. The receptor sites and cardiovascular effects of these hormone vasoactive medications are described in Table 14.20.

Vasopressin

Vasopressin acts primarily upon vasopressin-1 receptors located in the vascular smooth muscle. Stimulation triggers vasoconstriction and higher blood pressure due to an increase in intracellular calcium. Vasopressin-2 receptors are also stimulated and act on the kidneys to retain more water, thereby increasing blood pressure.

Vasopressin, also known as antidiuretic hormone, has become popular in the critical care setting for its vasoconstrictive effects. A one-time IV dose of 40 units was previously administered for treatment of cardiac arrest but several RCTs described in the ACLS guidelines found vasopressin offered no advantage over administration of epinephrine alone.[145]

In early septic shock, vasopressin levels have been reported to be lower than anticipated for a shock state.[146] Vasopressin is a recommended as a secondary infusion that can be added to the norepinephrine infusion in adult patients with refractory septic shock with an inadequate MAP. Vasopressin is added to avoid increasing the norepinephrine above the 0.25 to 0.5 mcg/kg/min range.[146] Patients must be assessed for side effects such as heart failure caused by the antidiuretic effects and monitored for increased risk of ischemia in the myocardium, spleen, and periphery. Vasopressin should be infused through a central line to avoid the risk of peripheral extravasation and resultant tissue necrosis. Placement of an arterial line is recommended in shock states to monitor blood pressure and SVR.

Angiotensin II

Angiotensin II is a component of the renin–angiotensin-aldosterone system and acts as a potent vasoconstrictor to increase blood pressure. This hormone triggers the release of aldosterone, which encourages sodium retention by the kidneys. This medication was approved by the FDA in December 2017 and is used to treat *distributive shock* in sepsis and vasoplegia after cardiovascular surgery.[148,149] Vasoplegia is a form of distributive shock where the arterial system has massively vasodilated producing a low SVR, low MAP, and a high or preserved cardiac output. Vasoplegia is most often encountered in sepsis and following cardiac surgery with CPB.[150]

Angiotensin II offers an alternative pathway to pharmacologic vasoconstriction without triggering adrenergic receptors (Table 14.20). This helps to ensure a multimodal pathway to increase afterload in the patient with hypotension.[148,149]

Vasodilator Medications

Vasodilators are pharmacologic agents that improve cardiac performance by various degrees of arterial or venous dilation or both (Table 14.21). The goal of vasodilator therapy may be reduction of preload, afterload, or both. Afterload reduction is accomplished by vasodilation of arterial vessels. This results in decreased resistance to LV ejection and may improve cardiac output without increasing myocardial oxygen demands. Reduction of preload is accomplished by dilation of venous vessels to increase capacitance. This results in decreased filling pressures for a failing heart. These vasodilatory medications may be classified by their mechanism of action (Table 14.21).

Direct Smooth Muscle Relaxants

Direct-acting vasodilators include sodium nitroprusside, nitroglycerin, and hydralazine. These medications produce relaxation of vascular smooth muscle through the activation of nitric oxide, which results in decreased peripheral vascular resistance. Hypotension may occur as a result of peripheral vasodilation, and headaches may be caused by cerebral vasodilation. Compensatory mechanisms can occur in response to the decrease in blood pressure. These mechanisms include baroreceptor activation that causes reflex tachycardia and activation of the renin-angiotensin-aldosterone system (see Fig. 13.18 in Chapter 13), with resultant sodium and water retention.

Sodium Nitroprusside

Sodium nitroprusside (Nipride) is a potent, rapidly acting venous and arterial vasodilator that is particularly suitable for rapid reduction of blood pressure in hypertensive emergencies

TABLE 14.21 PHARMACOLOGIC MANAGEMENT

Vasodilator Agents

Medication	Dosage	Action	Special Considerations
Smooth Muscle Relaxants			
Sodium nitroprusside (Nipride, Nitropress)	0.3–10 mcg/kg/min IV infusion	Potent arterial and moderate venous dilation	May cause hypotension and reflex tachycardia, thiocyanate toxicity with prolonged infusions, or kidney dysfunction
Nitroglycerin (Tridil)	5–200 mcg/min IV infusion	Potent venodilator, with arterial effects at higher doses	May cause headache, reflex tachycardia, hypotension
Calcium Channel Blockers			
Clevidipine (Cleviprex)	1–2 mg/h IV infusion, titrated to 32 mg/h (max 1000 mg/24 h)	Potent arterial dilator, with no effect on venous capacitance (preload)	Hypotension, reflex tachycardia, nausea, vomiting, rebound hypertension
Nicardipine (Cardene)	5 mg/h IV, titrated to 15 mg/h	Potent arterial dilator, no effect on preload	Hypotension, headache, reflex tachycardia
ACEi			
Enalaprilat (Vasotec)	0.625–1.25 mg IV over 5 min, then every 6 h	Moderate dilation of arteries and veins	Hypotension, elevation of liver enzymes
Alpha-Adrenergic Blockers			
Labetalol (Normodyne)	20–80 mg IV bolus every 10 min, then 1–8 mg/min infusion	Moderate dilation of arteries and veins	Orthostatic hypotension, bronchospasm, AV block
Phentolamine (Regitine)	5 mg IV slowly every 6 h	Moderate dilation of arteries and veins	Hypotension, tachycardia

ACEi, Angiotensin-converting enzyme inhibitors; *AV*, atrioventricular; *IV*, intravenous/intravenously; *PO*, by mouth.

and perioperatively.[151] It is effective for afterload reduction in the setting of severe heart failure.[151] Sodium nitroprusside is administered by continuous intravenous infusion, with the dosage titrated to maintain the desired blood pressure and afterload (SVR) with a rapid onset of action. Prolonged administration with poor excretion via the kidneys can result in thiocyanate (cyanide) toxicity.[151] This rare event can be avoided by limiting the dose and duration of the nitroprusside infusion and switching to an alternative antihypertensive medication as soon as feasible. Cyanide toxicity symptoms may be absent or are nonspecific, such as restlessness, nausea, and delirium, and are easily missed or misdiagnosed.[151]

Nitroglycerin

Intravenous nitroglycerin causes both arterial and venous vasodilation, but its venous effect is more pronounced. It is used in the critical care setting for the treatment of acute heart failure because it reduces cardiac filling pressures, relieves pulmonary congestion, and decreases cardiac workload and oxygen consumption. Nitroglycerin dilates the coronary arteries and is a useful adjunct in the treatment of unstable angina and acute MI. The initial dosage is 5 mcg/min, and the infusion is titrated upward to achieve the desired clinical effect: a reduction or elimination of chest pain, decreased PAOP (wedge pressure), or a decrease in blood pressure. Nitroglycerin should be avoided in patients with head injury or stroke because the increase in cerebral blood flow can increase intracranial pressure.[152] The most common side effects from a nitroglycerin infusion are hypotension, reflex tachycardia, and headache. Nitroglycerin becomes less effective with prolonged infusions because tolerance develops within 24 to 48 hours.

Hydralazine

Hydralazine is a potent arterial vasodilator. It is administered in slow IV doses of 5 to 10 mg every 4 to 8 hours. Occasionally, hydralazine is given as an intermediate agent during the transition between weaning of a continuous infusion and initiation of oral antihypertensive medications. It is also used for management of acute hypertension in pregnancy. The major side effect is reflex tachycardia mediated by the sympathetic nervous system.

Calcium Channel Blockers to Manage Hypertension

Calcium channel blockers are a chemically diverse group of medications with differing pharmacologic effects based on their classification (Table 14.22). Calcium channel blockers are generally used in critical care for one of two indications.

- To treat hypertension—dihydropyridines category
- To treat tachyarrhythmias—nondihydropyridine category (described earlier)

Nifedipine (Procardia), nicardipine (Cardene), and clevidipine (Cleviprex) are dihydropyridines. Medications in this group of calcium channel blockers (with the suffix "-pine") are used primarily as arterial vasodilators to lower blood pressure and treat hypertension. These agents reduce the influx of calcium in the arterial resistance vessels. Coronary and peripheral arteries are affected.

Nicardipine

Nicardipine was the first available intravenous calcium channel blocker and can be titrated to control blood pressure. It is classified as a second-generation dihydropyridine calcium channel antagonist.[153] Because nicardipine has vasodilatory effects on coronary and cerebral vessels, it is beneficial in treating hypertension in patients with CAD, ischemic stroke, and other cerebrovascular conditions.[153] Side effects of nicardipine are related to vasodilation and include hypotension, reflex tachycardia, flushing, and headache.

Clevidipine

Clevidipine is a third-generation short-acting calcium channel blocker that allows for even more precise titration of blood pressure in the management of acute hypertension. Advantages of this agent include its short half-life (approximately 1 minute), rapid onset of action, predictable dose response, and minimal effect on heart rate.[154] It is considered a first-line agent for lowering blood pressure in acute ischemic stroke and neurocritical

TABLE 14.22 PHARMACOLOGIC MANAGEMENT

Calcium Channel Blockers

Medication	Dosage	Actions	Special Considerations
Dihydropyridines			
Nicardipine (Cardene)	5 mg/h IV, titrated to 15 mg/h	Short-term control of hypertension	Hypotension, reflex tachycardia, headache, flushing
Nifedipine (Procardia)	10–30 mg PO	Hypertension	Hypotension, reflex tachycardia, headache
Clevidipine (Cleviprex)	1–2 mg/h IV infusion, titrated to 32 mg/h	Short-term control of hypertension	Hypotension, reflex tachycardia, nausea, vomiting, rebound hypertension
Nondihydropyridines			
Diltiazem (Cardizem)	Bolus dose of 0.25 mg/kg IV over 2 min, followed by infusion of 5–15 mg/h	Treatment of SVT, AFib, AF, angina	Bradycardia, hypotension, atrioventricular block
Verapamil (Calan, Isoptin)	5–10 mg IV, may repeat in 15–30 min	Treatment of AFib, AF, PSVT	Hypotension, bradycardia, heart failure

AF, Atrial flutter; *AFib*, atrial fibrillation; *IV*, intravenous/intravenously; *PO*, by mouth; *PSVT*, paroxysmal supraventricular tachycardia; *SVT*, supraventricular tachycardia.

care. Recent clinical trials report that it is noninferior (equally effective) to nicardipine, but because clevidipine is more expensive, its adoption is limited.[152] Of note, clevidipine is mixed in a phospholipid emulsion and can cause allergic reactions in patients with allergies to soybeans or eggs.

Alpha-Adrenergic Blockers

Peripheral adrenergic blockers block alpha-receptors in arteries and veins, resulting in vasodilation. Orthostatic hypotension is a common side effect and may result in syncope. Long-term therapy also may be complicated by fluid and water retention.

Phentolamine

Phentolamine (Regitine) is a nonselective peripheral alpha-blocker that deceases blood pressure through arterial vasodilation. It is administered by slow intravenous push 1 to 5 mg every 6 hours to reduce blood pressure. Phentolamine is used only in very specific circumstances for catecholamine-induced hypertension or toxicities related to ingestion of illegal drugs such as cocaine. Phentolamine is the medication of choice to control blood pressure and sweating caused by *pheochromocytoma*, an epinephrine-secreting tumor that can arise from the adrenal medulla.[154]

Phentolamine also is used to treat the *extravasation of dopamine* or other vasopressors into peripheral tissues. If this occurs, 5 to 10 mg is diluted in 10 mL normal saline and administered intradermally into the infiltrated area as soon as possible after extravasation.

Labetalol

Medications can be developed with pharmacological properties from different classes to increase effectiveness. Labetalol (Normodyne) is a combined peripheral alpha-blocker and a noncardioselective beta-blocker used to decrease blood pressure in the treatment of acute stroke and other hypertensive emergencies.[152] The blockade of nonselective beta-receptors permits a decrease of blood pressure without the risk of reflexive tachycardia and increased cardiac output.[154]

NURSING MANAGEMENT OF VASOACTIVE MEDICATIONS

The titration of vasoactive agents is a fundamental skill in critical care and nurses have safely performed this task independently for decades. Specialized training, maintenance of competencies, clinical experience, and high-level critical thinking are all required when titrating these agents. In addition, the titration of vasoactive medications often relies on clinical judgment and nursing intuition. A strong understanding of pharmacology is paramount to safely manipulate these medications. The decision to increase vasoactive agents and augment hemodynamics with additional medications may often be less complicated.[155] As such, the majority of this section will focus on downward titration of vasoactive medications. Titration decisions should always be guided by clear endpoints and therapeutic goals. Examples of these include MAP, heart rate, cardiac output, SVR, urinary output, and mentation.

The number of vasoactive agents continues to expand although agreement on the most effective way to wean vasoactive agents remains unresolved.[156] Table 14.23 provides examples of titration-weaning dosages for vasopressors as well as the time intervals for safe titration. It is important to know that titration guideline norms can vary between hospitals and critical care settings, and it remains imperative to be aware of hospital protocols when titrating vasoactive medications.

Vasopressor Titration Strategies

In patients receiving multiple different vasopressors, the question of which medication to wean first is an important decision.

One of the most common considerations for determining which continuous infusion to wean first is an awareness of the adverse effects associated with one medication over the other.[157] Some case exemplars may be helpful to illustrate this situation in the absence of clear clinical guidelines and recognizing that robust evidence for selection of one vasopressor over another is often limited.

- **Exemplar 1:** A patient who was hypotensive is experiencing tachydysrhythmias while receiving both norepinephrine and phenylephrine infusions. Because of the tachydysrhythmias, the recommendation would be to wean the norepinephrine drip first given the sympathomimetic action on the beta-1 adrenergic receptors. Phenylephrine is less likely to contribute to dysrhythmias and would remain the agent of choice to support blood pressure in this scenario.
- **Exemplar 2:** A patient has experienced a decrease in cardiac output while on norepinephrine and phenylephrine. In this scenario, the recommendation would be to wean the phenylephrine first because of the strong effects on alpha-1 receptors (vasoconstriction), which increases afterload and reduces cardiac output.
- **Exemplar 3:** A patient with septic shock is receiving both epinephrine and norepinephrine infusions to maintain adequate hemodynamics.[146] When the decision is made to

TABLE 14.23 Vasopressor Dose and Titration Ranges

Vasopressor	Usual Dose Range	Side Effects	Titration Range
Phenylephrine	10–300 mcg/min	Reflex bradycardia, tissue and visceral ischemia	10–20 mcg/min every 3–5 minutes
Norepinephrine	0.5–30 mcg/min 0.01–3 mcg/kg/min	Tachycardia, arrhythmias, cardiac and tissue ischemia	2–5 mcg/min every 3–5 minutes
Epinephrine	0.5–10 mcg/min 0.01–1 mcg/kg/min	Tachycardia, arrhythmias, cardiac and tissue ischemia	0.5–2 mcg/min every 3–5 minutes
Dopamine	2–20 mcg/kg/min	Tachycardia, arrhythmias, cardiac and tissue ischemia	2–5 mcg/kg/min every 5–10 minutes
Vasopressin	0.01–0.1 U/min (fixed dose 0.04 U/min)	Arrhythmias, cardiac, tissue, visceral and splanchnic ischemia	0.01 U/min every 10–15 minutes
Angiotensin II	10 ng/kg/min-80 ng/kg/min	Tachycardia, tissue ischemia, thromboembolic events	10–15 ng/kg/min every 5–15 minutes

wean the vasopressors, epinephrine should be weaned first because, according to the Surviving Sepsis Guidelines, norepinephrine is the drug of choice for sepsis-induced hypotension and should remain as the primary vasopressor.[146]

- **Exemplar 4:** Clinical judgment may be utilized when determining the individual patient response to vasoactive agents. Patients may respond better to one medication than another, despite textbook knowledge of physiology and pharmacology. For example, if a patient shows marked improvement in hemodynamics after the addition of dopamine to the standard norepinephrine utilized for sepsis, the prioritization would be to wean norepinephrine to allow the medication that elicits the best response to remain.

Many clinical guidelines list the medications to use but do not provide definitive weaning instructions.[146] Overall, the research regarding weaning of vasoactive agents is limited, and titration of vasoactive agents is often driven by clinical nurses using clinical judgment, nursing intuition, and critical thinking.[158]

Titration Parameters

The final target for vasoactive agents is the eventual discontinuation of the medication while ensuring hemodynamic stability. Parameters for titration during titration of vasoactive agents are helpful, such as the examples listed in Table 14.24.

Clinical assessment to ensure the patient is not experiencing wide variations in hemodynamics is recommended before starting titration of vasoactive agents. In some cases, this will also include confirmation that the patient has received adequate fluid resuscitation. Before starting titration, discussion with the critical care team might include the following questions:

- Which vasoactive medications should be weaned/titrated first?
- What is the expected rate of titration?
- What are the blood pressure and heart rate parameters?
- Can monitor alarms be narrowed to increase reminders?

The goal is to avoid dramatic changes in hemodynamics during titration. The nurse collaborates with the critical care team to determine which vasoactive medication should be titrated first if the patient is receiving multiple medications. There can be a discussion about alteration of the bedside monitor alarms to narrow reminders and enhance aggressive titration.

Hemodynamic monitoring is utilized during the titration process. For example, an increased heart rate during rapid vasopressor weaning may be indicative of compensation and indicates a slower titration may be beneficial to prevent further hemodynamic compromise.

Close monitoring of patients receiving vasoactive agents is paramount. This may include the need for an arterial catheter or other hemodynamic monitoring. Close observation should continue even after vasoactive medications have been discontinued in case therapy needs to be resumed. Targeted alarm parameters on the bedside monitor can be used to alert the nurse of changes and may prevent adverse outcomes.[157]

Typically, vasopressors are administered using a central line, but if central venous access is not available, the Surviving Sepsis guidelines suggest administration of vasopressors via a peripheral access.[146]

Vasopressor Infusions in Peripheral Catheters

While most vasopressors are administered using a central venous catheter line, guidelines support administration of vasopressors via a peripheral intravenous catheter (PIVC) line for short periods, in an emergency.[146] A recent international survey of hospital pharmacists in five countries (132 hospitals) reported that 86% had infused norepinephrine via a PIVC, typically for 24 hours (median).[159] Other peripheral vasopressor infusions were phenylephrine, dopamine, and metaraminol.[159] Fortunately, the incidence of vasopressor PIVC infiltration was low.[160]

When norepinephrine or another vasopressor is infusing peripherally, the nurse is responsible for ensuring that the PIVC does not infiltrate and result in extravasation of the vasopressor, which could injure the surrounding tissues. Awareness of the potential risk and need for close observation of the PIVC site is important. If extravasation does occur the PIVC is removed and the alpha-blocker phentolamine is injected subcutaneously as an antidote (described previously).

PHARMACOLOGIC TREATMENT OF HEART FAILURE

The goals of treatment in heart failure include alleviating symptoms, slowing the progression of the disease, and improving survival. Findings from numerous randomly controlled clinical trials have resulted in guidelines for the pharmacologic treatment of heart failure.[33] More information about heart failure is available in Chapter 14. Table 14.23 reviews medications currently recommended for treatment of heart failure. Types of medications that have been found to worsen heart failure should be avoided, including most antidysrhythmics, calcium channel blockers, and NSAIDs.[33]

Angiotensin-Converting Enzyme Inhibitors

An angiotensin-converting enzyme inhibitor (ACEi) produces vasodilation by blocking the conversion of angiotensin I to angiotensin II. ACE inhibition is a mainstay of heart failure

TABLE 14.24 **PHARMACOLOGIC MANAGEMENT**

Heart Failure

Classification and Medications	Mechanism of Action	Effects	Special Considerations
ACEi			
Captopril (Capoten) Enalapril (Vasotec) Fosinopril (Monopril) Lisinopril (Prinivil) Perindopril (Aceon) Quinapril (Accupril) Ramipril (Altace) Trandolapril (Mavik)	Interfere with RAAS by preventing conversion of angiotensin I to angiotensin II	Decrease afterload Decrease preload Reverse ventricular remodeling	Agents appear equivalent in treatment of heart failure Monitor closely for hypotension when initiating therapy May be contraindicated in patients with elevated creatinine, indicating kidney failure Side effects may include cough and life-threatening angioedema
Angiotensin-Receptor Blockers			
Candesartan (Atacand) Losartan (Cozaar) Valsartan (Diovan)	Interfere with RAAS by blocking effect of angiotensin II at the angiotensin II receptor site	Decrease afterload Decrease preload Reverse ventricular remodeling	Used as primary therapy or as an alternative for patients who cannot tolerate ACEi because of side effects such as severe cough Can also be used in combination with ACEi for systolic dysfunction; monitor renal function and serum potassium levels
Angiotensin-Receptor–Neprilysin Inhibitor			
Valsartan/Sacubitril (Entresto)	Combines an ARB with an inhibitor of neprilysin, an enzyme that breaks down peptides with beneficial cardiovascular effects	Effects of ARBs (above) with vasodilation and natriuresis	Recommended in place of ACE or ACEi in patients with Stage C heart failure and low ejection fraction to reduce mortality and morbidity Contraindicated in patients with a history of angioedema Dual treatment with an ACEi or ARB is contraindicated
Beta-Blockers			
Metoprolol succinate (Toprol XL) Bisoprolol (Zebeta) Carvedilol (Coreg)	Counteract SNS response activated in heart failure by blocking receptor sites Metoprolol and bisoprolol are cardioselective beta-blockers, whereas carvedilol blocks alpha- and beta-receptor sites	Slow heart rate Prevent dysrhythmias Decrease blood pressure Reverse ventricular remodeling	Not initiated during decompensated stage of heart failure Use cautiously in patients with reactive airway disease, poorly controlled diabetes, bradydysrhythmias, or heart block Carvedilol dose is increased slowly, while monitoring for symptoms caused by vasodilation such as dizziness or hypotension
Selective Sinus Node Inhibitor			
Ivabradine (Corlanor)		Selectively inhibits the sinoatrial node to reduce heart rate without lowering blood pressure	Recommended for Class 3 heart failure patients with low ejection fraction who have a resting heart rate >70 beats/min on maximal beta blocker therapy
Aldosterone Antagonists			
Spironolactone (Aldactone) Eplerenone (Inspra)	Counteract effects of aldosterone, which include sodium and water retention	Decrease preload Decrease myocardial hypertrophy	May increase serum potassium
Inotropes			
Digoxin (Lanoxin)	Affects Na^+,K^+-ATPase pump in myocardial cells to increase the strength of contraction	Increases contractility Increases cardiac output Prevents atrial dysrhythmias	Risk of toxicity is increased with hypokalemia

ACEi, Angiotensin-converting enzyme inhibitor; ARB, angiotensin-receptor blocker; *Na^+,K^+-ATPase*, sodium-potassium adenosine triphosphatase; *RAAS*, renin-angiotensin-aldosterone system; *SNS*, sympathetic nervous system.

management.[33] Because angiotensin is a potent vasoconstrictor, limiting its production decreases vascular resistance. In contrast to the direct vasodilators, an ACEi does not cause reflex tachycardia or induce sodium and water retention. However, these medications may cause a profound fall in blood pressure, especially in patients who are volume depleted. Blood pressure must be monitored carefully, especially at the initiation of therapy.

ACEi is used in patients with heart failure to decrease SVR (afterload) and filling pressures (preload).[33] Most of these medications are available only in an oral form. Enalaprilat is available in an IV form and may be used to decrease afterload in emergent situations.

Angiotensin-Receptor Blockers

An angiotensin-receptor blocker (ARB) prevents the vasoconstrictive effects of angiotensin II through direct blockade at the receptor site, producing hemodynamic effects that are similar to an ACEi. ARB agents may be used as an alternative in patients who cannot tolerate an ACEi because of side effects, such as cough.[33] At the present time, ARBs are available only in oral form.

Digoxin

Current heart failure guidelines recommend digoxin only in patients with heart failure who remain symptomatic after maximizing other heart failure therapies.[33] Similarly, in rapid atrial fibrillation, digoxin is considered only when beta-blockers or nondihydropyridine calcium channel blockers are ineffective or contraindicated.[9] See Tables 14.17 and 14.18.

ADDITIONAL RESOURCES

See Box 14.25 for Internet resources related to cardiovascular therapeutic management

BOX 14.25 Internet Resources

Cardiovascular Therapeutic Management

- American Heart Association Guidelines and statements https://professional.heart.org/en/guidelines-and-statements
- National Heart, Lung, and Blood Institute Health Information for the Public: Heart and Vascular Diseases: www.nhlbi.nih.gov/health/resources/heart
- Centers for Disease Control and Prevention Heart Disease: https://www.cdc.gov/heartdisease/
- Medtronic Academy (Pacemakers and ICD education): www.medtronicacademy.com

BOX 14.26 Abbreviations—Summary List

AAA	Abdominal aortic aneurysm
ABI	Ankle-brachial index
ACEi	Angiotensin-converting enzyme inhibitor
ACS	Acute coronary syndrome
ACLS	Advanced cardiac life support
AKI	Acute kidney injury
ARB	Angiotensin-receptor blocker
ARDS	Acute respiratory distress syndrome
AV	Atrioventricular
BMS	Bare metal stent
BTT	Bridge to transplantation (for heart transplant)
BHV	Bioprosthetic heart valve
CABG	Coronary artery bypass surgery
CAD	Coronary artery disease
CAS	Carotid artery stent
CEA	Carotid endarterectomy
CIED	Cardiac implantable electronic device
CI-AKI	Contrast-induced acute kidney injury
CPB	Cardiopulmonary bypass
CRT	Cardiac resynchronization therapy
CRT-P	Cardiac resynchronization therapy with pacing
CRT-D	Cardiac resynchronization therapy with defibrillation
CSA-AKI	Cardiac surgery–associated acute kidney injury
CT	Computed tomography
CVP	Central venous pressure
CABG	Coronary artery bypass graft
DAOC	Direct-acting oral anticoagulant
DAPT	Dual antiplatelet therapy
DCB	Drug-coated balloon
DES	Drug-eluting stents
DDD	Dual chamber synchronous pacing
DOO	Dual chamber asynchronous pacing
DT	Destination therapy (ventricular assist devices)
ECG	Electrocardiogram
ECMO	Extracorporeal membrane oxygenation
EF	Ejection fraction
EHR	Electronic health record
EMI	Electromagnetic interference
EPS	Electrophysiology study
EVAR	Endovascular aneurysm repair
FDA	United States Food and Drug Administration
IAB	Intra-aortic balloon
IABP	Intra-aortic balloon pump
ICD	Implantable cardioverter defibrillator
ITA	Internal thoracic artery
IV	Intravenous
IVUS	Intravascular ultrasound
LAA	Left atrial appendage
LV	Left ventricle
LVAD	Left ventricular assist device
mA	milliampere
MAP	Mean arterial pressure
MCS	Mechanical circulatory support
MHV	Mechanical heart valves
MIDCAB	Minimally invasive direct CABG
MRI	Magnetic resonance imaging
mcg/kg/min	Micrograms per kilogram per minute
Ms	Millisecond
mV	Millivolt
NSAID	Nonsteroidal antiinflammatory drugs
NSTEMI	Non-ST elevation myocardial infarction
OP-CABG	Off-pump coronary artery bypass graft
PA	Pulmonary artery
PAD	Peripheral arterial disease
PAOP	Pulmonary artery occlusion pressure
PCA	Patient-controlled analgesia
PMBC	Percutaneous mitral balloon commissurotomy
PCI	Percutaneous coronary intervention
PIVC	Peripheral intravenous catheter
PTCA	Percutaneous transluminal coronary angioplasty
PVI	Pulmonary vein isolation
P wave	Atrial depolarization waveform visible on the ECG
QRS	Ventricular depolarization waveform visible on the ECG
RA	Right atrium
RCT	Randomized controlled trial
RV	Right ventricle
RF	Radiofrequency
SCD	Sudden cardiac death
S-ICD	Subcutaneous implantable cardioverter defibrillator (no leads)
STEMI	ST elevation myocardial infarction
SVG	Saphenous vein graft
SVR	Systemic vascular resistance
SVT	Supraventricular tachycardia
TAVI	Transcatheter aortic valve implantation
TAVR	transcatheter aortic valve replacement
TEE	Transoesophageal echocardiogram
TEER	Transcatheter edge-to-edge repair
TECAB	Totally endoscopic coronary artery bypass
TIMI	Thrombolysis in myocardial infarction
T wave	Ventricular repolarization waveform visible on the ECG
TENS	Transcutaneous electrical nerve stimulation
VAD	Ventricular assist device
VA ECMO	Venoarterial extracorporeal membrane oxygenation
VF	Ventricular fibrillation
VT	Ventricular tachycardia
VVECMO	Venovenous extracorporeal membrane oxygenation
VVI	Ventricular synchronous (demand) pacing
VOO	Ventricular asynchronous (fixed rate) pacing

CASE STUDY 14.1 Patient With a Cardiac Problem

Brief Patient History

Mrs. G is a 54-year-old African American woman who has been having intermittent indigestion for the past month. She has a history of hypertension and hyperlipidemia. She was admitted as an inpatient on a medical floor for management of her blood pressure and is scheduled to undergo endoscopy tomorrow. Mrs. G suddenly becomes diaphoretic and complains of nausea and epigastric pain.

Clinical Assessment

The rapid response team is called to evaluate Mrs. G. When the team arrives at her bedside, she continues to complain of pain, which now radiates to her neck and back. She has some slight shortness of breath and is vomiting.

Diagnostic Procedures

The admission electrocardiogram shows ST segment elevation in leads II, III, and AVF. Baseline vital signs are as follows: blood pressure of 160/90 mm Hg, heart rate of 98 beats/min (sinus rhythm), respiratory rate of 18 breaths/min, temperature of 99°F, and oxygen saturation of 94%.

Medical

Mrs. G is diagnosed with an inferior myocardial infarction.

Questions

1. What major outcomes do you expect to achieve for this patient?
2. What problems or risks must be managed to achieve these outcomes?
3. What interventions must be initiated to monitor, prevent, manage, or eliminate the problems and risks identified?
4. What interventions could be initiated to promote optimal functioning, safety, and well-being of the patient?
5. What technology can be used to monitor this patient and prevent complications?
6. What other interprofessional team members are needed to assist with the management of this patient?
7. What possible learning needs do you anticipate for this patient?
8. What cultural and age-related factors may have a bearing on the patient's plan of care?

KEY POINTS

Pacemakers

- Pacemakers are electronic devices that can be used to initiate a heartbeat when the heart's intrinsic electrical system cannot generate a rate adequate to support cardiac output.
- The goal of therapy with either a temporary (external) or a permanent (implanted) pacemaker is to simulate normal physiologic cardiac depolarization and conduction.
- Nursing responsibilities for patients with pacemakers include assessment and prevention of pacemaker malfunction, protection against microshock, surveillance for complications, and patient education.

Implantable Cardioverter Defibrillators

- An ICD is a cardiac implantable electronic device (CIED) that is used to terminate life-threatening ventricular dysrhythmias through pacing, cardioversion, or defibrillation.
- Nursing management of a patient with an ICD includes assessing for dysrhythmias, monitoring for complications, and patient education.

Fibrinolytic Therapy

- Fibrinolytic therapy is used to restore blood flow through an occluded coronary artery in patients with an acute ST segment elevation MI.
- Nursing care for patients receiving fibrinolytic agents includes identifying appropriate candidates for therapy, administering the fibrinolytic agent, assessing for evidence of reperfusion, and monitoring for bleeding complications.

Catheter-Based Interventions for Coronary Artery Disease

- Percutaneous coronary intervention (PCI) refers to a variety of catheter-based procedures to open blocked or narrowed coronary arteries using angioplasty, atherectomy, and stent implantation.
- Antiplatelet therapy is considered an essential adjunct to PCIs to help maintain vessel patency during and after the procedure.
- Complications associated with PCIs include coronary artery spasm, dissection, and thrombosis; contrast-induced kidney injury; and bleeding at the vascular access site.

Catheter-Based Interventions for Cardiac Valvular Disease

- Percutaneous valve repair offers an alternative to surgery for mitral and aortic valves.

Cardiac Surgery

- CABG surgery provides myocardial revascularization by using a conduit to bypass an occluded coronary artery.
- Valvular surgery is used either to repair a cardiac valve or to replace it with a mechanical or biologic valve.
- Cardiopulmonary bypass (CPB) is an extracorporeal circuit used to circulate and oxygenate a patient's blood during some cardiac surgical procedures.
- Complications associated with CPB include intravascular fluid deficits, myocardial depression, coagulopathy, pulmonary dysfunction, hemolysis, hyperglycemia, electrolyte disturbances, neurologic dysfunction, and hypertension.
- Postoperative nursing management for cardiac surgery patients includes optimizing cardiac function (heart rate, preload, afterload, and contractility), temperature regulation, control of bleeding, and monitoring for complications.

Mechanical Circulatory Assist Devices

- Mechanical circulatory assist devices are used in the treatment of heart failure to decrease myocardial workload and maintain adequate perfusion to vital organs.
- Indications for an intra-aortic balloon pump (IABP) include failure to wean from CPB, unstable or recurrent angina, post-STEMI complications, hemodynamic support for high-risk interventions, cardiogenic shock, and as a bridge to definitive therapy.
- Nursing interventions for patients with an IABP include monitoring for and preventing complications, assessing for proper timing, evaluating hemodynamic changes, and providing patient education.
- Ventricular assist devices (VADs) can be used on a temporary basis as a bridge to recovery or transplant or as permanent destination therapy.
- Nursing management for a patient with a VAD consists of monitoring for hemodynamic changes and complications related to device failure, bleeding, infection, and thromboembolism.

Vascular Surgery

- Vascular surgery may be performed to treat arterial occlusive disease or to correct structural abnormalities such as aneurysms.
- Many patients with vascular disease can be effectively treated with percutaneous procedures (i.e., angioplasty, atherectomy, endovascular stents) rather than open surgical repair.
- Nursing care focuses on observing for vascular complications such as hematoma or reocclusion and the prompt recognition and treatment of complications arising from comorbidities such as cardiac, pulmonary, and kidney disease.

Effects of Cardiovascular Medications

- Multiple medications are used in the treatment of critically ill patients, and the nurse is responsible for administration, titration, and monitoring for side effects.
- Antidysrhythmic medications are used to terminate or prevent abnormal cardiac rhythms and are classified according to their primary effect on the action potential of cardiac cells.
- Inotropic agents increase myocardial contractility, resulting in improved cardiac output, more complete emptying of the ventricles, and decreased filling pressures.
- Vasodilators have varying effects on arterial and venous dilation and can be used to reduce preload, afterload, or both.
- Vasopressors mediate peripheral vasoconstriction, which results in an increase in SVR and elevates blood pressure.
- Goals of pharmacologic treatment of heart failure include alleviating symptoms, slowing the progression of the disease, and improving survival.
- Nursing management of titratable drugs requires knowledge of the medication actions, side effects, and parameters for titration.

Visit the Evolve site at http://evolve.elsevier.com/Urden/CriticalCareNursing for additional study materials.

REFERENCES

1. Steffen MM, Osborn JS, Cutler MJ. Cardiac implantable electronic device therapy: permanent pacemakers, implantable cardioverter defibrillators, and cardiac resynchronization devices. *Med Clin North Am.* 2019;103(5):931–943. https://doi.org/10.1016/j.mcna.2019.04.005.
2. Chung MK, Patton KK, Lau CP, et al. 2023 HRS/APHRS/LAHRS guideline on cardiac physiologic pacing for the avoidance and mitigation of heart failure. *J Arrhythm.* 2023;39(5):681–756. https://doi.org/10.1002/joa3.12872.
3. Cronin B, Dalia A, Goh R, Essandoh M, Orestes O, Brien E. Temporary epicardial pacing after cardiac surgery. *J Cardiothorac Vasc Anesth.* 2022;36(12):4427–4439. https://doi.org/10.1053/j.jvca.2022.08.017.
4. Gillham MJ, Barr TM. Temporary epicardial pacing after cardiac surgery. *BJA Educ.* 2023;23(9):337–349. https://doi.org/10.1016/j.bjae.2023.05.003.
5. Tjong FVY, de Ruijter UW, Beurskens NEG, Knops RE. A comprehensive scoping review on transvenous temporary pacing therapy. *Neth Heart J.* 2019;27(10):462–473. https://doi.org/10.1007/s12471-019-01307-x.
6. Suarez K, Banchs JE. A review of temporary permanent pacemakers and a comparison with conventional temporary pacemakers. *J Innov Card Rhythm Manag.* 2019;10(5):3652–3661. https://doi.org/10.19102/icrm.2019.100506.
7. Kusumoto FM, Schoenfeld MH, Barrett C, et al. 2018 ACC/AHA/HRS guideline on the evaluation and management of patients with bradycardia and cardiac conduction delay: Executive summary: a report of the American College of Cardiology/American Heart Association Task Force on Clinical Practice Guidelines and the Heart Rhythm Society. *J Am Coll Cardiol.* 2019;74(7):932–987. https://doi.org/10.1016/j.jacc.2018.10.043.
8. January CT, Wann LS, Calkins H, et al. 2019 AHA/ACC/HRS focused update of the 2014 AHA/ACC/HRS guideline for the management of patients with atrial fibrillation: a report of the American College of Cardiology/American Heart Association Task Force on Clinical Practice Guidelines and the Heart Rhythm Society in collaboration with the society of thoracic surgeons. *Circulation.* 2019;140(2). https://doi.org/10.1161/CIR.0000000000000665.
9. Joglar JA, Chung MK, Armbruster AL, et al. 2023 ACC/AHA/ACCP/HRS guideline for the diagnosis and management of atrial fibrillation: a report of the American College of Cardiology/American Heart Association Joint Committee on Clinical Practice Guidelines. *Circulation.* 2024;149(1):e1–e156. https://doi.org/10.1161/CIR.0000000000001193.
10. Peotter AM, Brown DR, Kalscheur MR, Von Bergen NH. Atrial Electrography for postoperative tachyarrhythmia analysis in patients. *J Innov Card Rhythm Manag.* 2021;12(10):4726–4743. https://doi.org/10.19102/icrm.2021.121003.
11. Glikson M, Nielsen JC, Kronborg MB, et al. 2021 ESC Guidelines on cardiac pacing and cardiac resynchronization therapy. *Eur Heart J.* 2021;42(35):3427–3520. https://doi.org/10.1093/eurheartj/ehab364.
12. Özkartal T, Demarchi A, Caputo ML, Baldi E, Conte G, Auricchio A. Perioperative management of patients with cardiac implantable electronic devices and utility of magnet application. *J Clin Med.* 2022;11(3):691. https://doi.org/10.3390/jcm11030691.
13. Adams A, Adams C. Transcutaneous pacing: an emergency nurse's guide. *J Emerg Nurs.* 2021;47(2):326–330. https://doi.org/10.1016/j.jen.2020.11.003.
14. Fox WE, Marshall M, Walters SM, et al. Bedside Clinician's guide to pulmonary artery catheters. *Crit Care Nurse.* 2023;43(4):9–18. https://doi.org/10.4037/ccn2023133.
15. Bernstein AD, Daubert JC, Fletcher RD, et al. The revised NASPE/BPEG generic code for antibradycardia, adaptive-rate, and multisite pacing. North American Society of Pacing and Electrophysiology/British Pacing and Electrophysiology Group. *Pacing Clin Electrophysiol.* 2002;25(2):260–264. https://doi.org/10.1046/j.1460-9592.2002.00260.x.
16. Arcinas LA, Sheldon RS. Complications related to pacemakers and other cardiac implantable electronic devices: essentials for internists and emergency physicians. *Intern Emerg Med.* 2023;18(3):851–862. https://doi.org/10.1007/s11739-023-03227-6.
17. Khurshid S, Frankel DS. Pacing-induced cardiomyopathy. *Card Electrophysiol Clin.* 2021;13(4):741–753. https://doi.org/10.1016/j.ccep.2021.06.009.
18. Stanley A, Athanasuleas C, Buckberg G. How His bundle pacing prevents and reverses heart failure induced by right ventricular pacing. *Heart Fail Rev.* 2021;26(6):1311–1324. https://doi.org/10.1007/s10741-020-09962-8.
19. Blomström-Lundqvist C, Traykov V, Erba PA, et al. European Heart Rhythm Association (EHRA) international consensus document on how to prevent, diagnose, and treat cardiac implantable electronic device infections-endorsed by the Heart Rhythm Society (HRS), the Asia Pacific Heart Rhythm Society (APHRS), the Latin American Heart Rhythm Society (LAHRS), International Society For Cardiovascular Infectious Diseases (ISCVID), and the European Society of Clinical Microbiology and Infectious Diseases (ESCMID) in collaboration with the European Association for Cardio-Thoracic Surgery (EACTS). *Eur Heart J.* 2020;41(21):2012–2032. https://doi.org/10.1093/eurheartj/ehaa010.
20. Baddour LM, Esquer Garrigos Z, Rizwan Sohail M, et al. Update on cardiovascular implantable electronic device infections and their prevention, diagnosis, and management: a scientific statement from the American heart association. *Circulation.* 2023. https://doi.org/10.1161/CIR.0000000000001187. Published online December 4.
21. Phillips P, Krahn AD, Andrade JG, et al. Treatment and prevention of Cardiovascular Implantable Electronic Device (CIED) infections. *CJC Open.* 2022;4(11):946–958. https://doi.org/10.1016/j.cjco.2022.07.010.
22. Crossley GH, Piccini JP, Longacre C, Higuera L, Stromberg K, El-Chami MF. Leadless versus transvenous single-chamber ventricular pacemakers: 3 year follow-up of the Micra CED study. *J Cardiovasc Electrophysiol.* 2023;34(4):1015–1023. https://doi.org/10.1111/jce.15863.

23. El-Chami MF, Bonner M, Holbrook R, et al. Leadless pacemakers reduce risk of device-related infection: review of the potential mechanisms. *Heart Rhythm*. 2020;17(8):1393–1397. https://doi.org/10.1016/j.hrthm.2020.03.019.
24. Huang J, Bhatia NK, Lloyd MS, et al. Outcomes of leadless pacemaker implantation after cardiac surgery and transcatheter structural valve interventions. *J Cardiovasc Electrophysiol*. 2023;34(11):2216–2222. https://doi.org/10.1111/jce.16074.
25. Gupta SK, Ya'qoub L, Wimmer AP, Fisher S, Saeed IM. Safety and clinical impact of MRI in patients with non-MRI-conditional cardiac devices. *Radiol Cardiothorac Imaging*. 2020;2(5):e200086. https://doi.org/10.1148/ryct.2020200086.
26. Peshock RM. Clearing the path to optimal care in patients with non-MRI-conditional cardiac devices. *Radiol Cardiothorac Imaging*. 2020;2(5):e200560. https://doi.org/10.1148/ryct.2020200560.
27. Prinzen FW, Auricchio A, Mullens W, Linde C, Huizar JF. Electrical management of heart failure: from pathophysiology to treatment. *Eur Heart J*. 2022;43(20):1917–1927. https://doi.org/10.1093/eurheartj/ehac088.
28. Boriani G, Ziacchi M, Nesti M, et al. Cardiac resynchronization therapy: how did consensus guidelines from Europe and the United States evolve in the last 15 years? *Int J Cardiol*. 2018;261:119–129. https://doi.org/10.1016/j.ijcard.2018.01.039.
29. Ferrick AM, Raj SR, Deneke T, et al. 2023 HRS/EHRA/APHRS/LAHRS expert consensus statement on practical management of the remote device clinic. *J Arrhythm*. 2023;39(3):250–302. https://doi.org/10.1002/joa3.12851.
30. López-Liria R, López-Villegas A, Leal-Costa C, et al. Effectiveness and safety in remote monitoring of patients with pacemakers five years after an implant: the poniente study. *Int J Environ Res Public Health*. 2020;17(4):1431. https://doi.org/10.3390/ijerph17041431.
31. White WB, Berberian JG. Pacemaker malfunction-review of permanent pacemakers and malfunctions encountered in the emergency department. *Emerg Med Clin North Am*. 2022;40(4):679–691. https://doi.org/10.1016/j.emc.2022.06.007.
32. Al-Khatib SM, Stevenson WG, Ackerman MJ, et al. 2017 AHA/ACC/HRS guideline for management of patients with ventricular arrhythmias and the prevention of sudden cardiac death: a report of the American College of Cardiology/American Heart Association Task Force on Clinical Practice Guidelines and the Heart Rhythm Society. *Circulation*. 2018;138(13). https://doi.org/10.1161/CIR.0000000000000549.
33. Heidenreich PA, Bozkurt B, Aguilar D, et al. 2022 AHA/ACC/HFSA guideline for the management of heart failure: a report of the American College of Cardiology/American Heart Association Joint Committee on Clinical Practice Guidelines. *Circulation*. 2022;145(18). https://doi.org/10.1161/CIR.0000000000001063.
34. Tankut S, Goldenberg I, Kutyifa V, et al. Cardiac resynchronization therapy and ventricular tachyarrhythmia burden. *Heart Rhythm*. 2021;18(5):762–769. https://doi.org/10.1016/j.hrthm.2020.12.034.
35. Fong KY, Ng CJR, Wang Y, Yeo C, Tan VH. Subcutaneous versus transvenous implantable defibrillator therapy: a systematic review and meta-analysis of randomized trials and propensity score-matched studies. *J Am Heart Assoc*. 2022;11(11):e024756. https://doi.org/10.1161/JAHA.121.024756.
36. Alsamman M, Prashad A, Abdelmaseih R, Khalid T, Prashad R. Update on wearable cardioverter defibrillator: a comprehensive review of literature. *Cardiol Res*. 2022;13(4):185–189. https://doi.org/10.14740/cr1387.
37. Berger JM, Sengupta JD, Bank AJ, et al. Causes and clinical consequences of inappropriate shocks experienced by patients wearing a cardioverter-defibrillator. *Heart Rhythm*. 2023;20(7):970–975. https://doi.org/10.1016/j.hrthm.2023.03.1604.
38. Duffett S, El Hajjaji I, Manlucu J, Yee R. Implantable cardioverter defibrillator implantation with or without defibrillation testing. *Card Electrophysiol Clin*. 2018;10(1):119–125. https://doi.org/10.1016/j.ccep.2017.11.012.
39. Healey JS, Hohnloser SH, Glikson M, et al. Cardioverter defibrillator implantation without induction of ventricular fibrillation: a single-blind, non-inferiority, randomised controlled trial (SIMPLE). *Lancet*. 2015;385(9970):785–791. https://doi.org/10.1016/S0140-6736(14)61903-6.
40. Milman A, Nof E, Rav AM, et al. Outcome and safety of intraoperative defibrillation testing during device replacement: the simpler trial. *Europace*. 2023;25(3):956–960. https://doi.org/10.1093/europace/euac282.
41. Friedman P, Murgatroyd F, Boersma LVA, et al. Efficacy and safety of an extravascular implantable cardioverter-defibrillator. *N Engl J Med*. 2022;387(14):1292–1302. https://doi.org/10.1056/NEJMoa2206485.
42. Dichtl W, De Sousa J, Rubin Lopez JM, et al. Low rates of inappropriate shocks in contemporary real-world implantable cardioverter defibrillator patients: the CARAT observational study. *Europace*. 2023;25(9):euad186. https://doi.org/10.1093/europace/euad186.
43. Cronin EM, Bogun FM, Maury P, et al. 2019 HRS/EHRA/APHRS/LAHRS expert consensus statement on catheter ablation of ventricular arrhythmias. *J Interv Card Electrophysiol*. 2020;59(1):145–298. https://doi.org/10.1007/s10840-019-00663-3.
44. Lawton JS, Tamis-Holland JE, Bangalore S, et al. 2021 ACC/AHA/SCAI guideline for coronary artery revascularization: a report of the American College of Cardiology/American Heart Association Joint Committee on Clinical Practice Guidelines. *Circulation*. 2022;145(3). https://doi.org/10.1161/CIR.0000000000001038.
45. Yildiz M, Wade SR, Henry TD. STEMI care 2021: addressing the knowledge gaps. *Am Heart J Plus*. 2021;11:100044. https://doi.org/10.1016/j.ahjo.2021.100044.
46. Bhatt DL, Lopes RD, Harrington RA. Diagnosis and treatment of acute coronary syndromes: a review. *JAMA*. 2022;327(7):662–675. https://doi.org/10.1001/jama.2022.0358.
47. O'Gara PT, Kushner FG, Ascheim DD, et al. 2013 ACCF/AHA guideline for the management of ST-elevation myocardial infarction: a report of the American College of Cardiology Foundation/American Heart Association Task Force on Practice Guidelines. *Circulation*. 2013;127(4). https://doi.org/10.1161/CIR.0b013e3182742cf6.
48. Harrington DH, Stueben F, Lenahan CM. ST-elevation myocardial infarction and non-ST-elevation myocardial infarction: medical and surgical interventions. *Crit Care Nurs Clin North Am*. 2019;31(1):49–64. https://doi.org/10.1016/j.cnc.2018.10.002.
49. Amsterdam EA, Wenger NK, Brindis RG, et al. 2014 AHA/ACC guideline for the management of patients with non–ST-elevation acute coronary syndromes: Executive summary: a report of the American College of Cardiology/American Heart Association Task Force on Practice Guidelines. *Circulation*. 2014;130(25):2354–2394. https://doi.org/10.1161/CIR.0000000000000133.
50. Krittanawong C, Hahn J, Kayani W, Jneid H. Fibrinolytic therapy in patients with acute ST-elevation myocardial infarction. *Interv Cardiol Clin*. 2021;10(3):381–390. https://doi.org/10.1016/j.iccl.2021.03.011.
51. Byrne RA, Stone GW, Ormiston J, Kastrati A. Coronary balloon angioplasty, stents, and scaffolds. *Lancet*. 2017;390(10096):781–792. https://doi.org/10.1016/S0140-6736(17)31927-X.
52. Protty MB, Gallagher S, Sharp ASP, et al. The impact of intracoronary imaging on PCI outcomes in cases utilising rotational atherectomy: an analysis of 8,417 rotational atherectomy cases from the British cardiovascular intervention society database. *J Interv Cardiol*. 2022;2022:5879187. https://doi.org/10.1155/2022/5879187.
53. Dong P, Colmenarez J, Lee J, et al. Load-sharing characteristics of stenting and post-dilation in heavily calcified coronary artery. *Sci Rep*. 2023;13(1):16878. https://doi.org/10.1038/s41598-023-43160-4.
54. Shlofmitz E, Shlofmitz R, Lee MS. Orbital atherectomy: a comprehensive review. *Interv Cardiol Clin*. 2019;8(2):161–171. https://doi.org/10.1016/j.iccl.2018.11.006.
55. Ahadi F, Azadi M, Biglari M, Bodaghi M, Khaleghian A. Evaluation of coronary stents: a review of types, materials, processing techniques, design, and problems. *Heliyon*. 2023;9(2):e13575. https://doi.org/10.1016/j.heliyon.2023.e13575.
56. Forrestal B, Case BC, Yerasi C, Musallam A, Chezar-Azerrad C, Waksman R. Bioresorbable scaffolds: current technology and future perspectives. *Rambam Maimonides Med J*. 2020;11(2):e0016. https://doi.org/10.5041/RMMJ.10402.

57. Widmer RJ, Pollak PM, Bell MR, Gersh BJ, Anavekar NS. The evolving face of myocardial reperfusion in acute coronary syndromes: a primer for the internist. *Mayo Clin Proc.* 2018;93(2):199–216. https://doi.org/10.1016/j.mayocp.2017.11.016.
58. Di Santo P, Simard T, Wells GA, et al. Transradial versus transfemoral access for percutaneous coronary intervention in ST-segment-elevation myocardial infarction: a systematic review and meta-analysis. *Circ Cardiovasc Interv.* 2021;14(3):e009994. https://doi.org/10.1161/CIRCINTERVENTIONS.120.009994.
59. Mehran R, Dangas GD, Weisbord SD. Contrast-associated acute kidney injury. *N Engl J Med.* 2019;380(22):2146–2155. https://doi.org/10.1056/NEJMra1805256.
60. Mason PJ, Shah B, Tamis-Holland JE, et al. An update on radial artery access and best practices for transradial coronary angiography and intervention in acute coronary syndrome: a scientific statement from the American Heart Association. *Circ Cardiovasc Interv.* 2018;11(9):e000035. https://doi.org/10.1161/HCV.0000000000000035.
61. Shroff AR, Gulati R, Drachman DE, et al. SCAI expert consensus statement update on best practices for transradial angiography and intervention. *Catheter Cardiovasc Interv.* 2020;95(2):245–252. https://doi.org/10.1002/ccd.28672.
62. Noori VJ, Eldrup-Jørgensen J. A systematic review of vascular closure devices for femoral artery puncture sites. *J Vasc Surg.* 2018;68(3):887–899. https://doi.org/10.1016/j.jvs.2018.05.019.
63. Reich R, Helal L, Mantovani VM, Rabelo-Silva ER. Hemostasis control after femoral percutaneous approach: a systematic review and meta-analysis. *Int J Nurs Stud.* 2023;137:104364. https://doi.org/10.1016/j.ijnurstu.2022.104364.
64. Sohal S, Mathai SV, Nagraj S, et al. Comparison of suture-based and collagen-based vascular closure devices for large bore arteriotomies-A meta-analysis of bleeding and vascular outcomes. *J Cardiovasc Dev Dis.* 2022;9(10):331. https://doi.org/10.3390/jcdd9100331.
65. Davidson LJ, Davidson CJ. Transcatheter treatment of valvular heart disease: a review. *JAMA.* 2021;325(24):2480–2494. https://doi.org/10.1001/jama.2021.2133.
66. Bavaria JE, Tommaso CL, Brindis RG, et al. 2018 AATS/ACC/SCAI/STS expert consensus systems of care document: operator and institutional recommendations and requirements for transcatheter aortic valve replacement: a Joint report of the American Association for Thoracic Surgery, American College of Cardiology, Society for Cardiovascular Angiography and Interventions, and Society of Thoracic Surgeons. *J Am Coll Cardiol.* 2019;73(3):340–374. https://doi.org/10.1016/j.jacc.2018.07.002.
67. Ganatra R, Smith R. Transcatheter mitral valve intervention. *Br J Cardiol.* 2021;28(4):51. https://doi.org/10.5837/bjc.2021.051.
68. Otto CM, Nishimura RA, Bonow RO, et al. 2020 ACC/AHA guideline for the management of patients with valvular heart disease: executive summary: a report of the American College of Cardiology/American Heart Association Joint Committee on Clinical Practice Guideline. *Circulation.* 2021;143(5):e35–e71. https://doi.org/10.1161/CIR.0000000000000932.
69. Turi ZG. The 40th Anniversary of percutaneous balloon valvuloplasty for mitral stenosis: current status. *Struct Heart.* 2022;6(5):100087. https://doi.org/10.1016/j.shj.2022.100087.
70. Otto CM, Kumbhani DJ, Alexander KP, et al. 2017 ACC expert consensus decision pathway for transcatheter aortic valve replacement in the management of adults with aortic stenosis: a report of the American College of Cardiology Task Force on Clinical Expert Consensus Documents. *J Am Coll Cardiol.* 2017;69(10):1313–1346. https://doi.org/10.1016/j.jacc.2016.12.006.
71. Aldea GS, Bakaeen FG, Pal J, et al. The Society of Thoracic Surgeons Clinical Practice Guidelines on Arterial Conduits for Coronary Artery Bypass Grafting. *Ann Thorac Surg.* 2016;101(2):801–809. https://doi.org/10.1016/j.athoracsur.2015.09.100.
72. Baddour LM, Wilson WR, Bayer AS, et al. Infective endocarditis in adults: diagnosis, antimicrobial therapy, and management of complications: a scientific statement for healthcare professionals from the American Heart Association. *Circulation.* 2015;132(15):1435–1486. https://doi.org/10.1161/CIR.0000000000000296.
73. Shore-Lesserson L, Baker RA, Ferraris VA, et al. The Society of Thoracic Surgeons, The Society of Cardiovascular Anesthesiologists, and The American Society of ExtraCorporeal Technology: Clinical Practice Guidelines-Anticoagulation During Cardiopulmonary Bypass. *Ann Thorac Surg.* 2018;105(2):650–662. https://doi.org/10.1016/j.athoracsur.2017.09.061.
74. Bakaeen FG, Svensson LG. Off-pump CABG fails to EXCEL in surgical revascularization of left main disease. *J Am Coll Cardiol.* 2019;74(6):741–743. https://doi.org/10.1016/j.jacc.2019.06.036.
75. Quin JA, Wagner TH, Hattler B, et al. Ten-year outcomes of off-pump vs on-pump coronary artery bypass grafting in the Department of Veterans Affairs: a randomized clinical trial. *JAMA Surg.* 2022;157(4):303–310. https://doi.org/10.1001/jamasurg.2021.7578.
76. Benedetto U, Puskas J, Kappetein AP, et al. Off-pump versus on-pump bypass surgery for left main coronary artery disease. *J Am Coll Cardiol.* 2019;74(6):729–740. https://doi.org/10.1016/j.jacc.2019.05.063.
77. Chyou JY, Barkoudah E, Dukes JW, et al. Atrial fibrillation occurring during acute hospitalization: a scientific statement from the American Heart Association. *Circulation.* 2023;147(15):e676–e698. https://doi.org/10.1161/CIR.0000000000001133.
78. McIntyre WF. Post-operative atrial fibrillation after cardiac surgery: challenges throughout the patient journey. *Front Cardiovasc Med.* 2023;10:1156626. https://doi.org/10.3389/fcvm.2023.1156626.
79. O'Brien B, Burrage PS, Ngai JY, et al. Society of cardiovascular anesthesiologists/European association of cardiothoracic anaesthetists practice advisory for the management of perioperative atrial fibrillation in patients undergoing cardiac surgery. *J Cardiothorac Vasc Anesth.* 2019;33(1):12–26. https://doi.org/10.1053/j.jvca.2018.09.039.
80. Gaudino M, Dangas GD, Angiolillo DJ, et al. Considerations on the management of acute postoperative ischemia after cardiac surgery: a scientific statement from the American Heart Association. *Circulation.* 2023;148(5):442–454. https://doi.org/10.1161/CIR.0000000000001154.
81. Carson JL, Stanworth SJ, Guyatt G, et al. Red blood cell transfusion: 2023 AABB international guidelines. *JAMA.* 2023;330(19):1892–1902. https://doi.org/10.1001/jama.2023.12914.
82. McIlroy D, Murphy D, Kasza J, Bhatia D, Marasco S. Association of postoperative blood pressure and bleeding after cardiac surgery. *J Thorac Cardiovasc Surg.* 2019;158(5):1370–1379.e6. https://doi.org/10.1016/j.jtcvs.2019.01.063.
83. Lobdell KW, Engelman DT. Chest tube management: past, present, and future directions for developing evidence-based best practices. *Innovations (Phila).* 2023;18(1):41–48. https://doi.org/10.1177/15569845231153623.
84. McCarthy C, Fletcher N. Early extubation in enhanced recovery from cardiac surgery. *Crit Care Clin.* 2020;36(4):663–674. https://doi.org/10.1016/j.ccc.2020.06.005.
85. Sankar A, Rotstein AJ, Teja B, et al. Prolonged mechanical ventilation after cardiac surgery: substudy of the Transfusion Requirements in Cardiac Surgery III trial. *Can J Anaesth.* 2022;69(12):1493–1506. https://doi.org/10.1007/s12630-022-02319-9.
86. Chen H, Mo L, Hu H, Ou Y, Luo J. Risk factors of postoperative delirium after cardiac surgery: a meta-analysis. *J Cardiothorac Surg.* 2021;16(1):113. https://doi.org/10.1186/s13019-021-01496-w.
87. Deininger MM, Schnitzler S, Benstoem C, et al. Standardized pharmacological management of delirium after on-pump cardiac surgery reduces ICU stay and ventilation in a retrospective pre-post study. *Sci Rep.* 2023;13(1):3741. https://doi.org/10.1038/s41598-023-30781-y.
88. von Groote T, Sadjadi M, Zarbock A. Acute kidney injury after cardiac surgery. *Curr Opin Anaesthesiol.* 2023. https://doi.org/10.1097/ACO.0000000000001320. Published online October 6.
89. Zarbock A, Küllmar M, Ostermann M, et al. Prevention of cardiac surgery-associated acute kidney injury by implementing the KDIGO guidelines in high-risk patients identified by biomarkers: the PrevAKI-multicenter randomized controlled trial. *Anesth Analg.* 2021;133(2):292–302. https://doi.org/10.1213/ANE.0000000000005458.
90. Society of Thoracic Surgeons Task Force on Resuscitation After Cardiac Surgery. The society of thoracic surgeons expert consensus

for the resuscitation of patients who arrest after cardiac surgery. *Ann Thorac Surg*. 2017;103(3):1005–1020. https://doi.org/10.1016/j.athoracsur.2016.10.033.
91. Ley SJ. Cardiac surgical resuscitation: state of the science. *Crit Care Nurs Clin North Am*. 2019;31(3):437–452. https://doi.org/10.1016/j.cnc.2019.05.010.
92. Calkins H, Hindricks G, Cappato R, et al. 2017 HRS/EHRA/ECAS/APHRS/SOLAECE expert consensus statement on catheter and surgical ablation of atrial fibrillation. *Heart Rhythm*. 2017;14(10):e275–e444. https://doi.org/10.1016/j.hrthm.2017.05.012.
93. Badhwar V, Rankin JS, Damiano RJ, et al. The society of thoracic surgeons 2017 clinical practice guidelines for the surgical treatment of atrial fibrillation. *Ann Thorac Surg*. 2017;103(1):329–341. https://doi.org/10.1016/j.athoracsur.2016.10.076.
94. Whitlock RP, Belley-Cote EP, Paparella D, et al. Left atrial appendage occlusion during cardiac surgery to prevent stroke. *N Engl J Med*. 2021;384(22):2081–2091. https://doi.org/10.1056/NEJMoa2101897.
95. Rosati F, de Maat GE, Valente MAE, Mariani MA, Benussi S. Surgical clip closure of the left atrial appendage. *J Cardiovasc Electrophysiol*. 2021;32(10):2865–2872. https://doi.org/10.1111/jce.15181.
96. Andrade JG, Deyell MW, Macle L, et al. Progression of atrial fibrillation after cryoablation or drug therapy. *N Engl J Med*. 2023;388(2):105–116. https://doi.org/10.1056/NEJMoa2212540.
97. Rottner L, Bellmann B, Lin T, et al. Catheter ablation of atrial fibrillation: state of the art and future perspectives. *Cardiol Ther*. 2020;9(1):45–58. https://doi.org/10.1007/s40119-019-00158-2.
98. Gopinathannair R, Chen LY, Chung MK, et al. Managing atrial fibrillation in patients with heart failure and reduced ejection fraction: a scientific statement from the American Heart Association. *Circ Arrhythm Electrophysiol*. 2021;14(6):HAE0000000000000078. https://doi.org/10.1161/HAE.0000000000000078.
99. Salter BS, Gross CR, Weiner MM, et al. Temporary mechanical circulatory support devices: practical considerations for all stakeholders. *Nat Rev Cardiol*. 2023;20(4):263–277. https://doi.org/10.1038/s41569-022-00796-5.
100. Pahuja M, Yerasi C, Lam PH, et al. Review of pathophysiology of cardiogenic shock and escalation of mechanical circulatory support devices. *Curr Cardiol Rep*. 2023;25(4):213–227. https://doi.org/10.1007/s11886-023-01843-4.
101. González LS, Chaney MA. Intraaortic balloon pump counterpulsation, Part I: history, technical aspects, physiologic effects, contraindications, medical applications/outcomes. *Anesth Analg*. 2020;131(3):776–791. https://doi.org/10.1213/ANE.0000000000004954.
102. González LS, Chaney MA. Balloon pump counterpulsation Part II: perioperative hemodynamic support and new directions. *Anesth Analg*. 2020;131(3):792–807. https://doi.org/10.1213/ANE.0000000000004999.
103. Botti G, Gramegna M, Burzotta F, et al. Impella RP for patients with acute right ventricular failure and cardiogenic shock: a subanalysis from the IMP-IT registry. *J Pers Med*. 2022;12(9):1481. https://doi.org/10.3390/jpm12091481.
104. Maybauer MO, Koerner MM, Swol J, El Banayosy A, Maybauer DM. The novel ProtekDuo ventricular assist device: configurations, technical aspects, and present evidence. *Perfusion*. 2023;38(5):887–893. https://doi.org/10.1177/02676591221090607.
105. Brewer JM, Capoccia M, Maybauer DM, Lorusso R, Swol J, Maybauer MO. The ProtekDuo dual-lumen cannula for temporary acute mechanical circulatory support in right heart failure: a systematic review. *Perfusion*. 2023;38(1_suppl):59–67. https://doi.org/10.1177/02676591221149859.
106. Combes A, Schmidt M, Hodgson CL, et al. Extracorporeal life support for adults with acute respiratory distress syndrome. *Intensive Care Med*. 2020;46(12):2464–2476. https://doi.org/10.1007/s00134-020-06290-1.
107. Schmidt M, Hajage D, Lebreton G, et al. Prone positioning during extracorporeal membrane oxygenation in patients with severe ARDS: the PRONECMO randomized clinical trial. *JAMA*. 2023. https://doi.org/10.1001/jama.2023.24491. Published online December 1.
108. Worku E, Brodie D, Ling RR, Ramanathan K, Combes A, Shekar K. Venovenous extracorporeal CO2 removal to support ultraprotective ventilation in moderate-severe acute respiratory distress syndrome: a systematic review and meta-analysis of the literature. *Perfusion*. 2023;38(5):1062–1079. https://doi.org/10.1177/02676591221096225.
109. Mehra MR, Cleveland JC, Uriel N, et al. Primary results of long-term outcomes in the MOMENTUM 3 pivotal trial and continued access protocol study phase: a study of 2200 HeartMate 3 left ventricular assist device implants. *Eur J Heart Fail*. 2021;23(8):1392–1400. https://doi.org/10.1002/ejhf.2211.
110. Mehra MR, Goldstein DJ, Cleveland JC, et al. Five-year outcomes in patients with fully magnetically levitated vs axial-flow left ventricular assist devices in the MOMENTUM 3 randomized trial. *JAMA*. 2022;328(12):1233–1242. https://doi.org/10.1001/jama.2022.16197.
111. Gopinathannair R, Cornwell WK, Dukes JW, et al. Device therapy and arrhythmia management in left ventricular assist device recipients: a scientific statement from the American Heart Association. *Circulation*. 2019;139(20):e967–e989. https://doi.org/10.1161/CIR.0000000000000673.
112. Noly PE, Wu X, Hou H, et al. Association of days alive and out of the hospital after ventricular assist device implantation with adverse events and quality of life. *JAMA Surg*. 2023;158(4):e228127. https://doi.org/10.1001/jamasurg.2022.8127.
113. Rich K, Treat-Jacobson D, DeVeaux T, et al. Society for Vascular Nursing-Carotid endarterectomy (CEA) updated nursing clinical practice guideline. *J Vasc Nurs*. 2017;35(2):90–111. https://doi.org/10.1016/j.jvn.2017.03.004.
114. Krawisz AK, Carroll BJ, Secemsky EA. Risk stratification and management of extracranial carotid artery disease. *Cardiol Clin*. 2021;39(4):539–549. https://doi.org/10.1016/j.ccl.2021.06.007.
115. AbuRahma AF, Avgerinos ED, Chang RW, et al. Society for Vascular Surgery clinical practice guidelines for management of extracranial cerebrovascular disease. *J Vasc Surg*. 2022;75(1S):4S–22S. https://doi.org/10.1016/j.jvs.2021.04.073.
116. Kleindorfer DO, Towfighi A, Chaturvedi S, et al. 2021 guideline for the prevention of stroke in patients with stroke and transient ischemic attack: a guideline from the American Heart Association/American Stroke Association. *Stroke*. 2021;52(7):e364–e467. https://doi.org/10.1161/STR.0000000000000375.
117. Kakisis JD, Antonopoulos CN, Mantas G, Moulakakis KG, Sfyroeras G, Geroulakos G. Cranial nerve injury after carotid endarterectomy: incidence, risk factors, and time trends. *Eur J Vasc Endovasc Surg*. 2017;53(3):320–335. https://doi.org/10.1016/j.ejvs.2016.12.026.
118. Halliday A, Bulbulia R, Bonati LH, et al. Second Asymptomatic Carotid Surgery Trial (ACST-2): a randomised comparison of carotid artery stenting versus carotid endarterectomy. *Lancet*. 2021;398(10305):1065–1073. https://doi.org/10.1016/S0140-6736(21)01910-3.
119. Müller MD, Lyrer P, Brown MM, Bonati LH. Carotid artery stenting versus endarterectomy for treatment of carotid artery stenosis. *Cochrane Database Syst Rev*. 2020;2(2):CD000515. https://doi.org/10.1002/14651858.CD000515.pub5.
120. Vilacosta I, San Román JA, di Bartolomeo R, et al. Acute aortic syndrome revisited: JACC state-of-the-art review. *J Am Coll Cardiol*. 2021;78(21):2106–2125. https://doi.org/10.1016/j.jacc.2021.09.022.
121. Isselbacher EM, Preventza O, Hamilton Black J, et al. 2022 ACC/AHA guideline for the diagnosis and management of aortic disease: a report of the American heart association/American College of cardiology Joint committee on clinical practice guidelines. *Circulation*. 2022;146(24):e334–e482. https://doi.org/10.1161/CIR.0000000000001106.
122. Kohlman-Trigoboff D, Rich K, Foley A, et al. Society for Vascular Nursing endovascular repair of abdominal aortic aneurysm updated nursing clinical practice guideline. *J Vasc Nurs*. 2020;38(2):36–65. https://doi.org/10.1016/j.jvn.2020.01.004.
123. Chaikof EL, Dalman RL, Eskandari MK, et al. The Society for Vascular Surgery practice guidelines on the care of patients with an abdominal aortic aneurysm. *J Vasc Surg*. 2018;67(1):2–77.e2. https://doi.org/10.1016/j.jvs.2017.10.044.
124. Kinio A, Ramsay T, Jetty P, Nagpal S. Declining institutional memory of open abdominal aortic aneurysm repair. *J Vasc Surg*. 2021;73(3):889–895. https://doi.org/10.1016/j.jvs.2020.06.125.

125. Sharma A, Sethi P, Gupta K. Endovascular abdominal aortic aneurysm repair. *Interv Cardiol Clin.* 2020;9(2):153–168. https://doi.org/10.1016/j.iccl.2019.12.005.
126. Meertens MM, Tenorio ER, Lemmens CC, et al. Safety of percutaneous femoral access for endovascular aortic aneurysm repair through previously surgically exposed or repaired femoral arteries. *J Endovasc Ther.* 2023;30(5):730–738. https://doi.org/10.1177/15266028221092980.
127. Yei K, Mathlouthi A, Naazie I, Elsayed N, Clary B, Malas M. Long-term outcomes associated with open vs endovascular abdominal aortic aneurysm repair in a medicare-matched database. *JAMA Netw Open.* 2022;5(5):e2212081. https://doi.org/10.1001/jamanetworkopen.2022.12081.
128. McGinigle KL, Spangler EL, Pichel AC, et al. Perioperative care in open aortic vascular surgery: a consensus statement by the Enhanced Recovery After Surgery (ERAS) society and society for vascular surgery. *J Vasc Surg.* 2022;75(6):1796–1820. https://doi.org/10.1016/j.jvs.2022.01.131.
129. Abramson BL, Al-Omran M, Anand SS, et al. Canadian cardiovascular society 2022 guidelines for peripheral arterial disease. *Can J Cardiol.* 2022;38(5):560–587. https://doi.org/10.1016/j.cjca.2022.02.029.
130. McGinigle KL, Spangler EL, Ayyash K, et al. A framework for perioperative care for lower extremity vascular bypasses: a consensus statement by the Enhanced Recovery After Surgery (ERAS®) society and society for vascular surgery. *J Vasc Surg.* 2023;77(5):1295–1315. https://doi.org/10.1016/j.jvs.2023.01.018.
131. Gerhard-Herman MD, Gornik HL, Barrett C, et al. 2016 AHA/ACC guideline on the management of patients with lower extremity peripheral artery disease: a report of the American Cardiology/American Heart Association Task Force on Clinical Practice Guidelines. *Circulation.* 2017;135(12):e726–e779. https://doi.org/10.1161/CIR.0000000000000471.
132. Feldman DN, Armstrong EJ, Aronow HD, et al. SCAI guidelines on device selection in aorto-iliac arterial interventions. *Catheter Cardiovasc Interv.* 2020;96(4):915–929. https://doi.org/10.1002/ccd.28947.
133. Beckman JA, Schneider PA, Conte MS. Advances in revascularization for peripheral artery disease: revascularization in PAD. *Circ Res.* 2021;128(12):1885–1912. https://doi.org/10.1161/CIRCRESAHA.121.318261.
134. The Joint Commission. The Joint Commission. The Joint Commission clarifies expectations for implementing medication titration orders. *Joint Commission Perspectives.* 2020;40(6):7. https://www.jointcommission.org.
135. Joseph R, Lee SW, Anderson SV, Morrisette MJ. Impact of interoperability of smart infusion pumps and an electronic medical record in critical care. *Am J Health Syst Pharm.* 2020;77(15):1231–1236. https://doi.org/10.1093/ajhp/zxaa164.
136. Mankad P, Kalahasty G. Antiarrhythmic drugs: risks and benefits. *Med Clin North Am.* 2019;103(5):821–834. https://doi.org/10.1016/j.mcna.2019.05.004.
137. Safi S, Sethi NJ, Korang SK, et al. Beta-blockers in patients without heart failure after myocardial infarction. *Cochrane Database Syst Rev.* 2021;11(11):CD012565. https://doi.org/10.1002/14651858.CD012565.pub2.
138. Tednes P, Marquardt S, Kuhrau S, Heagler K, Rech M. Keeping it "current": a review of treatment options for the management of supraventricular tachycardia. *Ann Pharmacother.* 2023:10600280231199136. https://doi.org/10.1177/10600280231199136. Published online September 24.
139. Ray L, Geier C, DeWitt KM. Pathophysiology and treatment of adults with arrhythmias in the emergency department, part 2: ventricular and bradyarrhythmias. *Am J Health Syst Pharm.* 2023;80(17):1123–1136. https://doi.org/10.1093/ajhp/zxad115.
140. Tisdale JE, Chung MK, Campbell KB, et al. Drug-induced arrhythmias: a scientific statement from the American Heart Association. *Circulation.* 2020;142(15):e214–e233. https://doi.org/10.1161/CIR.0000000000000905.
141. Vora P, Morgan Stewart H, Russell B, Asiimwe A, Brobert G. Time trends and treatment pathways in prescribing individual oral anticoagulants in patients with nonvalvular atrial fibrillation: an observational study of more than three million patients from Europe and the United States. *Int J Clin Pract.* 2022;2022:6707985. https://doi.org/10.1155/2022/6707985.
142. van Es N, De Caterina R, Weitz JI. Reversal agents for current and forthcoming direct oral anticoagulants. *Eur Heart J.* 2023;44(20):1795–1806. https://doi.org/10.1093/eurheartj/ehad123.
143. Margraf DJ, Brown SJ, Blue HL, Bezdicek TL, Wolfson J, Chapman SA. Comparison of 3-factor versus 4-factor prothrombin complex concentrate for emergent warfarin reversal: a systematic review and meta-analysis. *BMC Emerg Med.* 2022;22(1):14. https://doi.org/10.1186/s12873-022-00568-x.
144. Gustafsson F, Damman K, Nalbantgil S, et al. Inotropic therapy in patients with advanced heart failure. A clinical consensus statement from the Heart Failure Association of the European Society of Cardiology. *Eur J Heart Fail.* 2023;25(4):457–468. https://doi.org/10.1002/ejhf.2814.
145. Panchal AR, Berg KM, Hirsch KG, et al. 2019 American Heart Association focused update on advanced cardiovascular life support: use of advanced airways, vasopressors, and extracorporeal cardiopulmonary resuscitation during cardiac arrest: an update to the American Heart Association guidelines for cardiopulmonary resuscitation and emergency cardiovascular care. *Circulation.* 2019;140(24):e881–e894. https://doi.org/10.1161/CIR.0000000000000732.
146. Evans L, Rhodes A, Alhazzani W, et al. Executive summary: surviving sepsis campaign: international guidelines for the management of sepsis and septic shock 2021. *Crit Care Med.* 2021;49(11):1974–1982. https://doi.org/10.1097/CCM.0000000000005357.
147. Jentzer JC, Hollenberg SM. Vasopressor and inotrope therapy in cardiac critical care. *J Intensive Care Med.* 2021;36(8):843–856. https://doi.org/10.1177/0885066620917630.
148. Johnson AJ, Tidwell W, McRae A, Henson CP, Hernandez A. Angiotensin-II for vasoplegia following cardiac surgery. *Perfusion.* 2023;13:2676591231215920. https://doi.org/10.1177/02676591231215920. Published online November.
149. Klijian A, Khanna AK, Reddy VS, et al. Treatment with angiotensin II is associated with rapid blood pressure response and vasopressor sparing in patients with vasoplegia after cardiac surgery: a post-Hoc analysis of Angiotensin II for the Treatment of High-Output Shock (ATHOS-3) study. *J Cardiothorac Vasc Anesth.* 2021;35(1):51–58. https://doi.org/10.1053/j.jvca.2020.08.001.
150. Lambden S, Creagh-Brown BC, Hunt J, Summers C, Forni LG. Definitions and pathophysiology of vasoplegic shock. *Crit Care.* 2018;22(1):174. https://doi.org/10.1186/s13054-018-2102-1.
151. Hottinger DG, Beebe DS, Kozhimannil T, Prielipp RC, Belani KG. Sodium nitroprusside in 2014: a clinical concepts review. *J Anaesthesiol Clin Pharmacol.* 2014;30(4):462–471. https://doi.org/10.4103/0970-9185.142799.
152. Stewart MH. Hypertensive crisis: diagnosis, presentation, and treatment. *Curr Opin Cardiol.* 2023;38(4):311–317. https://doi.org/10.1097/HCO.0000000000001049.
153. Saldana S, Breslin J, Hanify J, et al. Comparison of clevidipine and nicardipine for acute blood pressure reduction in hemorrhagic stroke. *Neurocrit Care.* 2022;36(3):983–992. https://doi.org/10.1007/s12028-021-01407-w.
154. Brathwaite L, Reif M. Hypertensive emergencies: a review of common presentations and treatment options. *Cardiol Clin.* 2019;37(3):275–286. https://doi.org/10.1016/j.ccl.2019.04.003.
155. Teja B, Bosch NA, Walkey AJ. How we escalate vasopressor and corticosteroid therapy in patients with septic shock. *Chest.* 2023;163(3):567–574. https://doi.org/10.1016/j.chest.2022.09.019.
156. Davidson JE, Doran N, Petty A, et al. Survey of nurses' experiences applying the Joint commission's medication management titration standards. *Am J Crit Care.* 2021;30(5):365–374. https://doi.org/10.4037/ajcc2021716.
157. Arellano DL, Hanneman SK. Vasopressor weaning in patients with septic shock. *Crit Care Nurs Clin North Am.* 2014;26(3):413–425. https://doi.org/10.1016/j.ccell.2014.04.001.
158. Hunter S, Considine J, Manias E. Nurse decision-making when managing noradrenaline in the intensive care unit: a naturalistic observational study. *Intensive Crit Care Nurs.* 2023;77:103429. https://doi.org/10.1016/j.iccn.2023.103429.
159. Abu SA, Penm J, Oliver M, et al. International pharmacy survey of peripheral vasopressor infusions in critical care (INFUSE). *J Crit Care.* 2023;78:154376. https://doi.org/10.1016/j.jcrc.2023.154376.
160. Owen VS, Rosgen BK, Cherak SJ, et al. Adverse events associated with administration of vasopressor medications through a peripheral intravenous catheter: a systematic review and meta-analysis. *Crit Care.* 2021;25(1):146. https://doi.org/10.1186/s13054-021-03553-1.

15

Pulmonary Anatomy and Physiology

Kathleen M. Stacy

http://evolve.elsevier.com/Urden/CriticalCareNursing

The pulmonary system consists of the thorax, conducting airways, respiratory airways, and pulmonary blood and lymph supply. The primary functions of the pulmonary system are ventilation and respiration. *Ventilation* is the movement of air in and out of the lungs. *Respiration* is the process of gas exchange by means of movement of oxygen from the atmosphere into the bloodstream and movement of carbon dioxide from the bloodstream into the atmosphere. The anatomic structures that constitute the pulmonary system are intimately related to function, and structural abnormalities can readily translate into pulmonary disorders. Applicable knowledge of anatomy and physiology is imperative in caring for a patient with pulmonary dysfunction.

ANATOMY

Thorax

The thorax contains the major organs of respiration and consists of the thoracic cage, lungs, pleura, and muscles of ventilation. Together, these structures form the ventilatory pump, which performs the work of breathing.

Thoracic Cage

The thoracic cage is a cone-shaped structure that is rigid but flexible to protect the underlying structures and to accommodate inhalation and exhalation. The cage consists of 12 thoracic vertebrae, each with a pair of ribs. Posteriorly, each rib is attached to its own vertebra, but anteriorly, attachment varies (Fig. 15.1). The first seven pairs of ribs are attached directly to the sternum. The 8th, 9th, and 10th pairs are attached by cartilage to the ribs above. Because the 11th and 12th ribs have no anterior attachment, they sometimes are referred to as *floating ribs*. The second rib is attached to the sternum at the angle of Louis, which is the raised ridge that can be felt just below the suprasternal notch.[1]

Lungs

The lungs are cone-shaped organs that have a total volume of approximately 3.5 to 8.5 L. The superior portion is known as the *apex*, and the inferior portion is known as the *base*. The apical portion of each lung rises a few centimeters above the clavicle (see Fig. 15.1). Each lung is firmly attached to the thoracic cavity at the hilum and at the pulmonary ligament.[2]

Lobes and segments. The lungs are divided into lobes and segments (Fig. 15.2), with the lobes being separated by pleural membrane–covered fissures. The right lung, which is larger and heavier than the left, is divided into upper, middle, and lower lobes. The left lung is divided into only an upper and a lower lobe.[2] A portion of the left lung, the lingula, corresponds anatomically with the right middle lobe. The horizontal fissure divides the right upper lobe from the right middle lobe. The oblique fissure divides the right upper and middle lobes from the lower lobe and the left upper lobe from the lower lobe. The lobes are divided into 18 segments, each of which has its own bronchus branching immediately off a lobar bronchus. There are 10 segments in the right lung and 8 in the left lung.[1]

Mediastinum. The area between the two lungs, the mediastinum, contains the heart, great vessels, lymphatics, and esophagus. A portion of the mediastinal area contains the root of the lungs, also known as the hilum, in which the visceral and parietal pleural membranes form a sheath around the main stem bronchi, the major blood vessels, and the nerves that enter and exit the lungs.[2]

Pleura

The pleura is a thin membrane that lines the outside of the lungs and the inside of the chest wall. The visceral pleura adheres to the lungs, extending onto the hilar bronchi and into the major fissures. The parietal pleura lines the inner surface of the chest wall and mediastinum.[2] The two pleural surfaces are separated by an airtight space that contains a thin layer of lubricating fluid. Pleural fluid allows the visceral and parietal pleural membranes to glide against each other during inhalation and exhalation.[1,3] The pleural space has the capacity to hold much more fluid than its normal volume of a few milliliters.[1]

Intrapleural pressure. The pleural space has a pressure within it called *intrapleural pressure*, which differs from intrapulmonary (pressure within the lungs) and atmospheric pressures.[4] Under normal conditions, intrapleural pressure is less than intrapulmonary pressure and less than atmospheric pressure, with a normal range of −4 to −10 cm H_2O during exhalation and inhalation, respectively.[3] A deep inhalation can generate intrapleural pressures of −12 to −18 cm H_2O. This negative intrapleural pressure results from forces within the chest wall that exert pressure to pull the parietal pleura outward and away

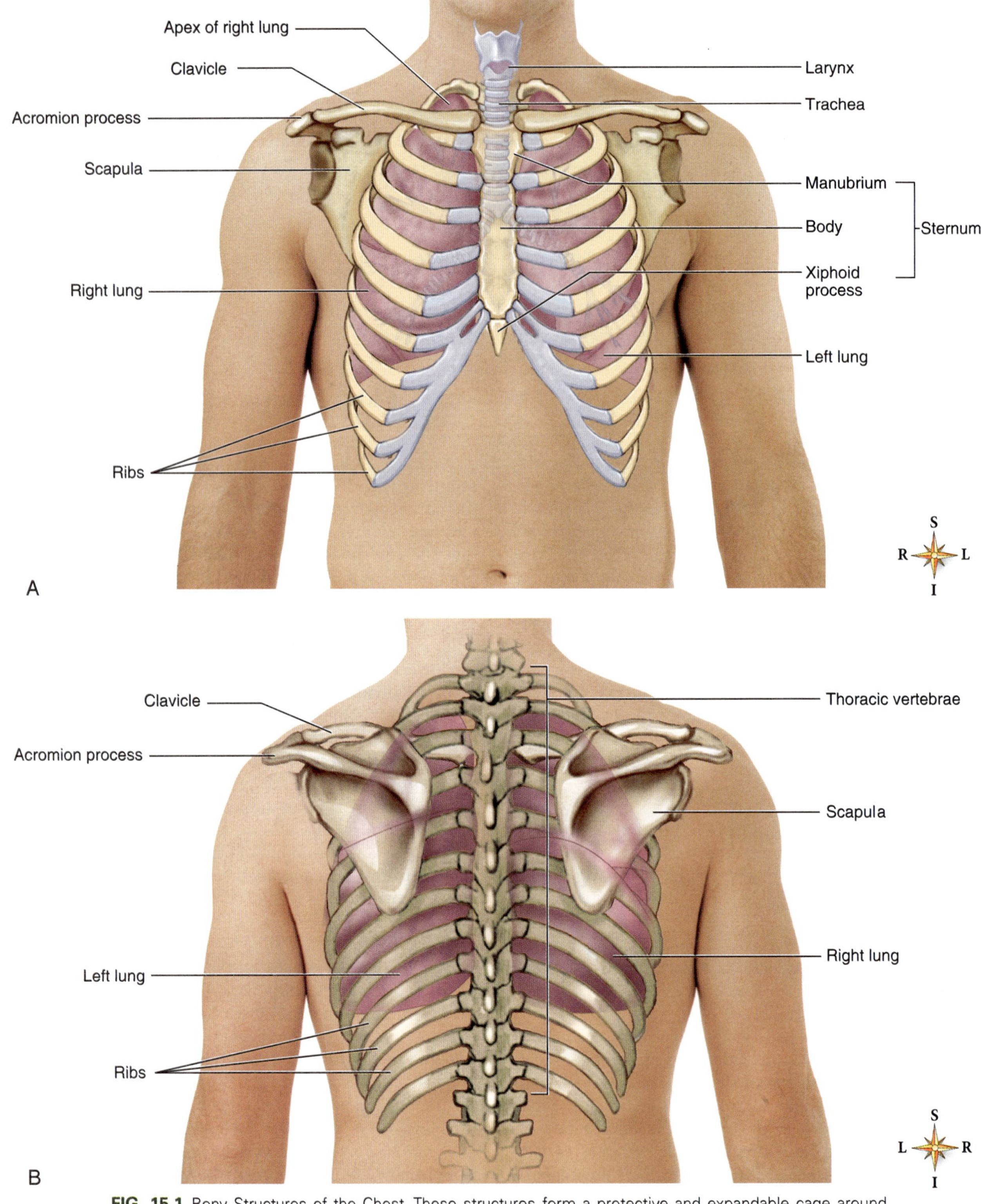

FIG. 15.1 Bony Structures of the Chest. These structures form a protective and expandable cage around the lungs and heart. (A) Anterior view. (B) Posterior view. (Adapted from Thompson JM, Wilson SF. *Health Assessment for Nursing Practice*. Mosby; 1996. In Patton KT, Bell F, Thompson T, Williamson P. *Anatomy and Physiology*. 11th ed. Elsevier; 2022.)

from the visceral pleura, whereas the elastic fibers within the lungs exert pressure to pull the visceral pleura inward away from the parietal pleura. The constant pull of the two pleural membranes in opposite directions causes the pressure within the space to be subatmospheric.[4] The negative pressure in the pleural space keeps the lungs inflated (Box 15.1). If atmospheric pressure enters the pleural space, all or part of a lung will collapse, producing a pneumothorax.[1]

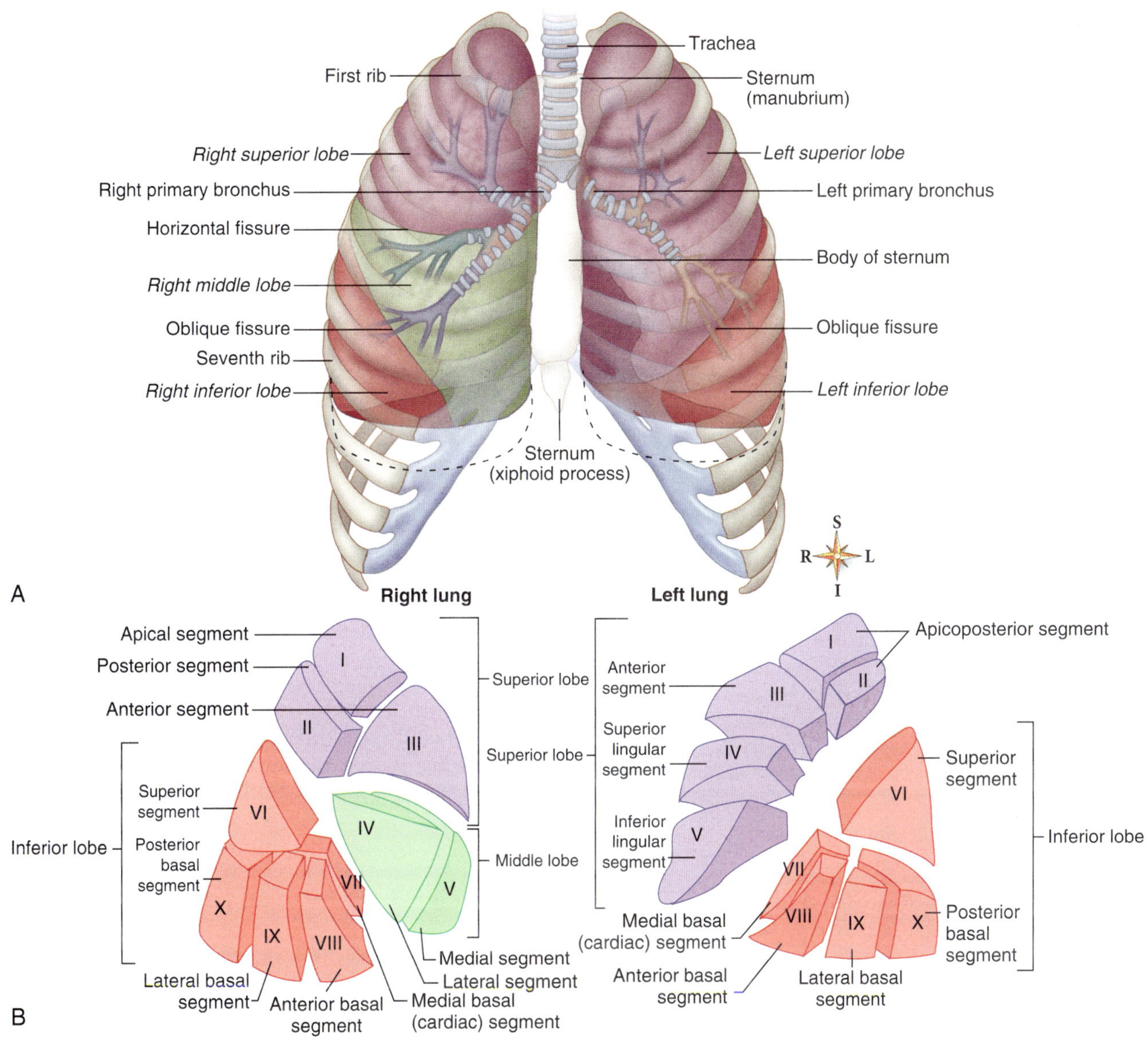

FIG. 15.2 Lobes and Segments of the Lungs. (A) Anterior view of the lungs, bronchi, and trachea. (B) Expanded diagram showing the bronchopulmonary segments. (From Patton KT, Bell F, Thompson T, Williamson P. *Anatomy and Physiology*. 11th ed. Elsevier; 2022.)

Muscles of Ventilation

The muscles of ventilation (Fig. 15.3) are governed by the regulatory activity of the central nervous system, which sends messages to the muscles to stimulate contraction and relaxation. This muscular activity controls inhalation and exhalation. Muscles that increase the size of the chest are called *muscles of inhalation;* muscles that decrease the size of the chest are called *muscles of exhalation*.[5]

Inhalation. The main muscle of inhalation is the diaphragm. The diaphragm is a dome-shaped, fibromuscular septum that separates the thoracic and abdominal cavities and is connected to the sternum, ribs, and vertebrae. During normal, quiet breathing, the diaphragm does approximately 80% of the work of breathing. On inhalation, the diaphragm contracts and flattens, pushes down on the viscera, and displaces the abdomen outward. Diaphragmatic contraction also lifts and expands the rib cage to some extent.[1,5,6]

The action of the diaphragm is governed by the medulla, which sends its impulses through the phrenic nerve. The phrenic nerve arises from the cervical plexus through the fourth cervical nerve, with secondary contributions by the third and fifth cervical nerves. For this reason and because the diaphragm does most of the work of inhalation, trauma involving levels C3 to C5 causes ventilatory dysfunction.[5]

Muscles that lift the rib cage are other muscles of inhalation. The most important of these are the external intercostal muscles, which elevate the ribs and expand the chest cage outward. The scalene, anterior serratus, and sternocleidomastoid muscles also participate to elevate the first two ribs and sternum.[1,5,6]

Exhalation. Exhalation in the healthy lung is a passive event requiring very little energy. Exhalation occurs when the diaphragm relaxes and moves back up toward the lungs. The intrinsic elastic recoil of the lungs assists with exhalation.

Because exhalation is a passive act, there are no true muscles of exhalation other than the internal intercostal muscles, which assist the inward movement of the ribs. However, exhalation becomes a more active event during exercise, requiring some participation of the accessory muscles of ventilation. Several muscles of the abdomen are thought to contribute to active exhalation.[4,5]

BOX 15.1 Why Do the Lungs Stay Inflated?

The lungs stay inflated because the pressure surrounding them (intrapleural) is always less than the pressure within them (intrapulmonary).

Why Is the Intrapleural Pressure Less Than the Intrapulmonary Pressure?

The intrapleural pressure is always (1) less than intrapulmonary pressure, (2) less than atmospheric pressure, and (3) considered negative because of the pull of the two pleural membranes in opposite directions. The parietal pleura is pulled outward by forces within the chest wall, whereas the visceral pleura is pulled inward by the force of the elastic fibers within the lungs.

Why Do the Two Pleural Membranes Pull in Opposite Directions?

The parietal pleura, attached to the chest, is pulled outward because the elastic fibers within the intercostal muscles exert outward pressure on the ribs. These fibers are in a relaxed state when the rib cage is fully expanded, such as during a deep inhalation. The visceral pleura is attached to the lungs and is pulled inward because the elastic fibers within the lungs that are responsible for elastic recoil exert pressure to make the lungs smaller. Elastic fibers in the lung are in a relaxed position only when the lung is at its smallest configuration, as occurs with a pneumothorax. Because of the opposite pull of the chest wall and the lung and because the pleural membranes are attached to these structures, there is a constant pull of the two membranes in opposite directions. The subatmospheric pressure that results within the pleural space and the greater-than-atmospheric intrapulmonary pressure within the lungs allows the lungs to remain inflated. Anything that causes the pressure within the pleural space to rise to atmospheric pressure or above will cause the lung to collapse: a pneumothorax.

Accessory muscles. The accessory muscles of ventilation usually are considered muscles that enhance chest expansion during exercise but that are not active during normal, quiet breathing. These muscles include the scalene, sternocleidomastoid, and other chest and back muscles, such as the trapezius and the pectoralis major.[1,5,6]

Conducting Airways

The conducting airways consist of the upper airways, the trachea, and the bronchial tree. The conducting airways warm and humidify the inhaled air, act as a protective mechanism that prevents the entrance of foreign matter into the gas-exchange areas, and serve as a passageway for air entering and leaving the gas-exchange regions of the lungs.[1–3]

Upper Airways

The upper airways consist of the nasal and oral cavities, the pharynx, and the larynx (Fig. 15.4). Their main contribution to ventilation is the conditioning of inspired air. *Conditioned air* is air that has been warmed, humidified, and cleansed of some irritants. Warming and humidifying, which are essential to prevent irritation of the lower airways, occur mainly within the nose by means of a dense vascular network that lines the nasal passages. The air is cleansed by the coarse hairs that line the nasal passages and filter large inhaled particles.[1,3]

Epiglottis. The epiglottis is located in the upper airways. The epiglottis protects the lower airways by closing the opening to the trachea during swallowing so that food passes into the esophagus and not the trachea. The epiglottis is a thin,

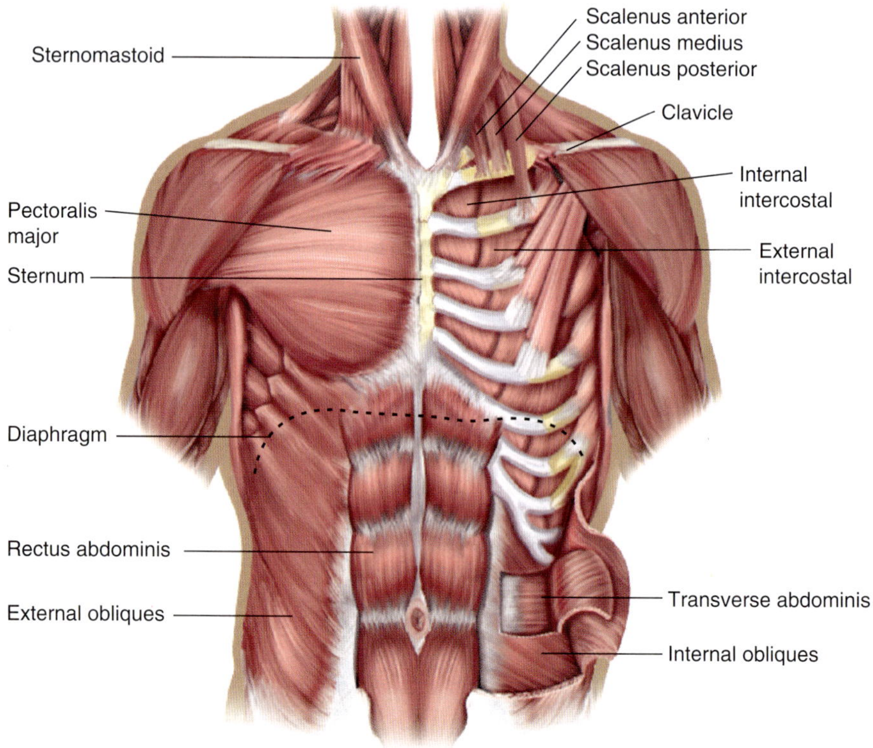

FIG. 15.3 Muscles of Ventilation. (From Wilkins RL, Stoller JK, Scanlan CL, eds. *Egan's Fundamentals of Respiratory Care.* 8th ed. Mosby; 2003.)

leaf-shaped, elastic cartilage that is located directly posterior to the root of the tongue and attached to the thyroid cartilage (see Fig. 15.4). The epiglottis opens widely during inhalation, permitting air to pass through the trachea into the lower airways.[1]

Trachea

The trachea is a hollow tube approximately 11 cm (4.5 inches) long and 2.5 cm (1 inch) in diameter (Fig. 15.5). The trachea begins at the cricoid cartilage and ends at the bifurcation (major carina) from which the two main stem bronchi arise. The carina is positioned approximately at the level of the aortic arch, the fifth thoracic vertebra,[7] or just below the level of the angle of Louis.[1] The trachea consists of smooth muscle supported anteriorly by 16 to 20 C-shaped, cartilaginous rings. They prevent tracheal collapse during bronchoconstriction and strong coughing. The posterior wall of the trachea lies contiguous with the anterior wall of the esophagus. Having no cartilaginous support, this wall is composed only of muscle tissue, which is separated from the anterior esophageal wall by loose connective tissue (see Fig. 15.5).[1]

Bronchial Tree

The two main stem bronchi are structurally different (see Fig. 15.5). The left bronchus is slightly narrower than the right, and because of its position above the heart, the left bronchus angles directly toward the left lung at approximately 45 to 55 degrees from the midline. The right bronchus is wider and angles at 20 to 30 degrees from the midline. Because of this angulation and the forces of gravity, the most common site of aspiration of foreign objects is through the right main stem bronchus into the lower lobe of the right lung.[2,3]

Bronchi. Each branching of the tracheobronchial tree produces a new generation of tubes (Fig. 15.6A,B). The main stem bronchi are the first generation; the next branch, the five lobar bronchi, is the second generation. The third generation includes the 18 segmental bronchi. The fourth through approximately the ninth generations are referred to as the small bronchi, beginning with the subsegmental bronchi. In these bronchi, diameters decrease; however, because the number of bronchi increases with each generation, the total cross-sectional area increases with each generation. This great increase in the cross-sectional area of the lung is significant, because it allows easy ventilation despite decreasing airway lumens.[1]

Bronchioles. The final subdivision of the conducting airways is the bronchioles. These tubes have a diameter less than 1 mm and have no connective tissue and cartilage within their walls. However, their walls do contain smooth muscle.[2] When smooth muscle constriction occurs, these airways may close completely

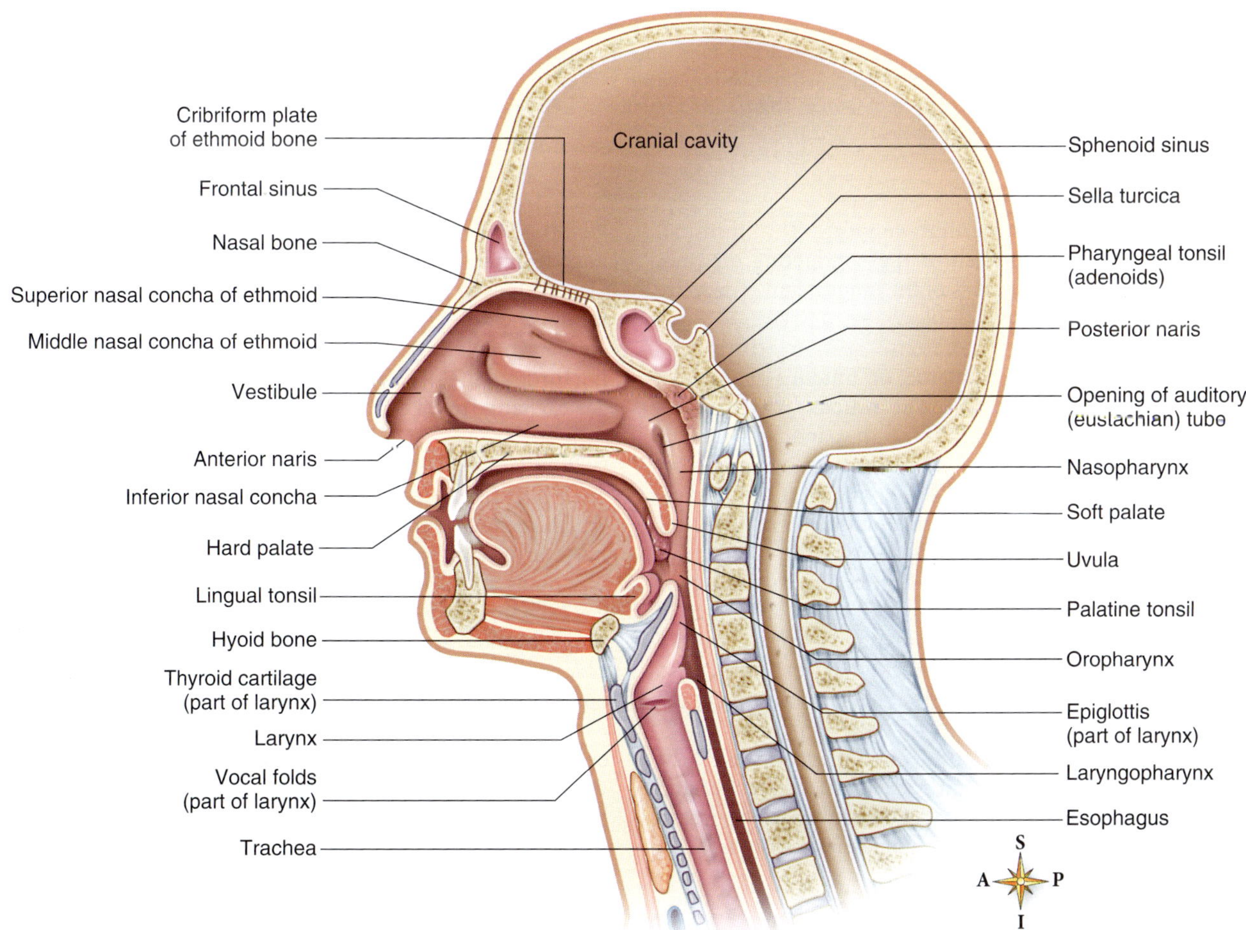

FIG. 15.4 Upper Respiratory Tract. In this midsagittal section through the upper respiratory tract, the nasal septum has been removed to reveal the turbinates (nasal conchae) of the lateral wall of the nasal cavity. The three divisions of the pharynx (nasopharynx, oropharynx, and laryngopharynx) are also visible. (From Patton KT, Bell F, Thompson T, Williamson P. *Anatomy and Physiology.* 11th ed. Elsevier; 2022.)

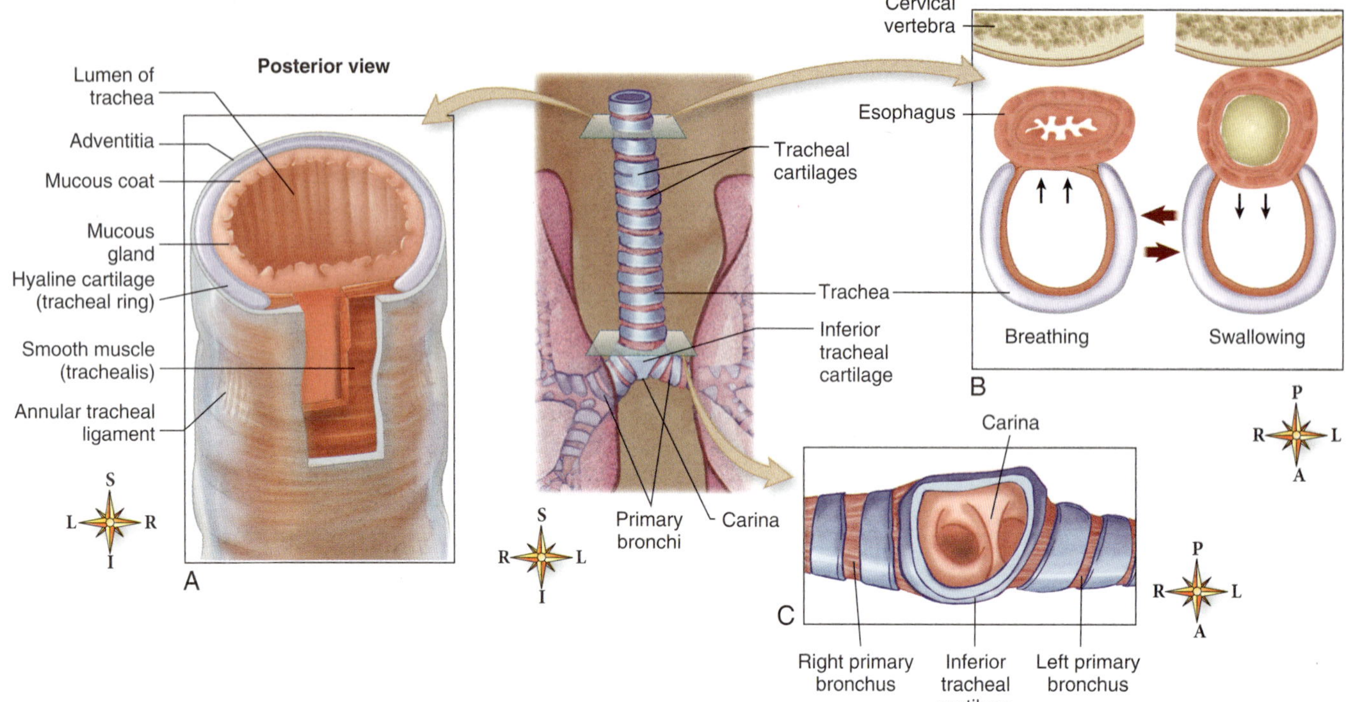

FIG. 15.5 Cross Section of the Trachea. The middle image with the trachea and parts of each lung shows where the section of the trachea was cut. (A) Structure of the trachea. (B) Incomplete tracheal rings and elasticity of posterior tracheal wall allow the esophagus to expand during swallowing. (C) The inferior tracheal cartilage has a middle portion called the carina, which has an internal ridge covered with sensory mucosa that detects the presence of foreign objects. (From Patton KT, Bell F, Thompson T, Williamson P. *Anatomy and Physiology*. 11th ed. Elsevier; 2022.)

because of the lack of structural support. The terminal bronchioles form the last branch of the conducting airways, after which the gas-exchange areas of the lungs begin. There are more than 32,000 terminal bronchioles.[1]

Defense system. The main defense system within the airways is the mucociliary escalator, or mucous blanket, a combination of mucus and cilia. The mucus, which floats atop the cilia (Fig. 15.7), traps foreign particles. Ciliary movement propels the entire mucous blanket and any trapped particles upward toward the pharynx at an average speed of 1 mm/min in the smaller bronchioles and 12 mm/min in the larger airways and trachea. After the pharynx is reached, the mucus is swallowed or cleared. The submucous glands of the airways produce approximately 100 mL of mucus per day, with all but approximately 10 mL resorbed through the bronchial lining. The mucociliary escalator is so efficient that almost no particles larger than 3 microns reach the alveoli.[8]

The cough reflex is another protective mechanism in the lungs. Excessive amounts of foreign particles in the trachea and bronchi can initiate the cough reflex. Once initiated, the rapid expulsion of air carries away any foreign particles with it.[9]

Respiratory Airways

The respiratory airways consist of the respiratory bronchioles and the alveoli. The respiratory airways also are known as the *terminal respiratory units*, or the *acini*. Gas exchange takes place in these areas of the lungs.

Respiratory Bronchioles

Each terminal bronchiole gives rise to two respiratory bronchioles, with each branching two to four more times.[2] The respiratory bronchioles form the transition zone of the lungs, acting as conducting airways and gas-exchange units. While air is moving through them, alveolar outpouchings on their surfaces allow gas exchange to take place (see Fig. 15.6).[1]

Alveoli

Each respiratory bronchiole gives rise to several alveolar ducts, which terminate in clusters of 10 to 16 alveoli (see Fig. 15.6). Each terminal respiratory unit contains approximately 100 alveolar ducts and 2000 alveoli.[2] The alveolus is the primary site of gas exchange and the endpoint in the respiratory tract. The two lungs contain approximately 300 million alveoli. The alveoli comprise several types of cells, including type I and II alveolar epithelial cells and alveolar macrophages.[1,3]

Type I alveolar epithelial cells. Type I alveolar epithelial cells constitute approximately 90% of the total alveolar surface within the lungs (Fig. 15.8). They are the chief structural cells of the alveolar wall and play a major role in the maintenance of the gas-blood barrier and gas exchange. Type I cells are extremely susceptible to injury and become inflamed when exposed to inhaled toxins.[1]

Collateral air passages. A variety of collateral air passages are located within the lower regions of the lungs. Within the walls of the type I cells are the pores of Kohn (see Fig. 15.6C), which allow collateral movement of air between alveoli. The

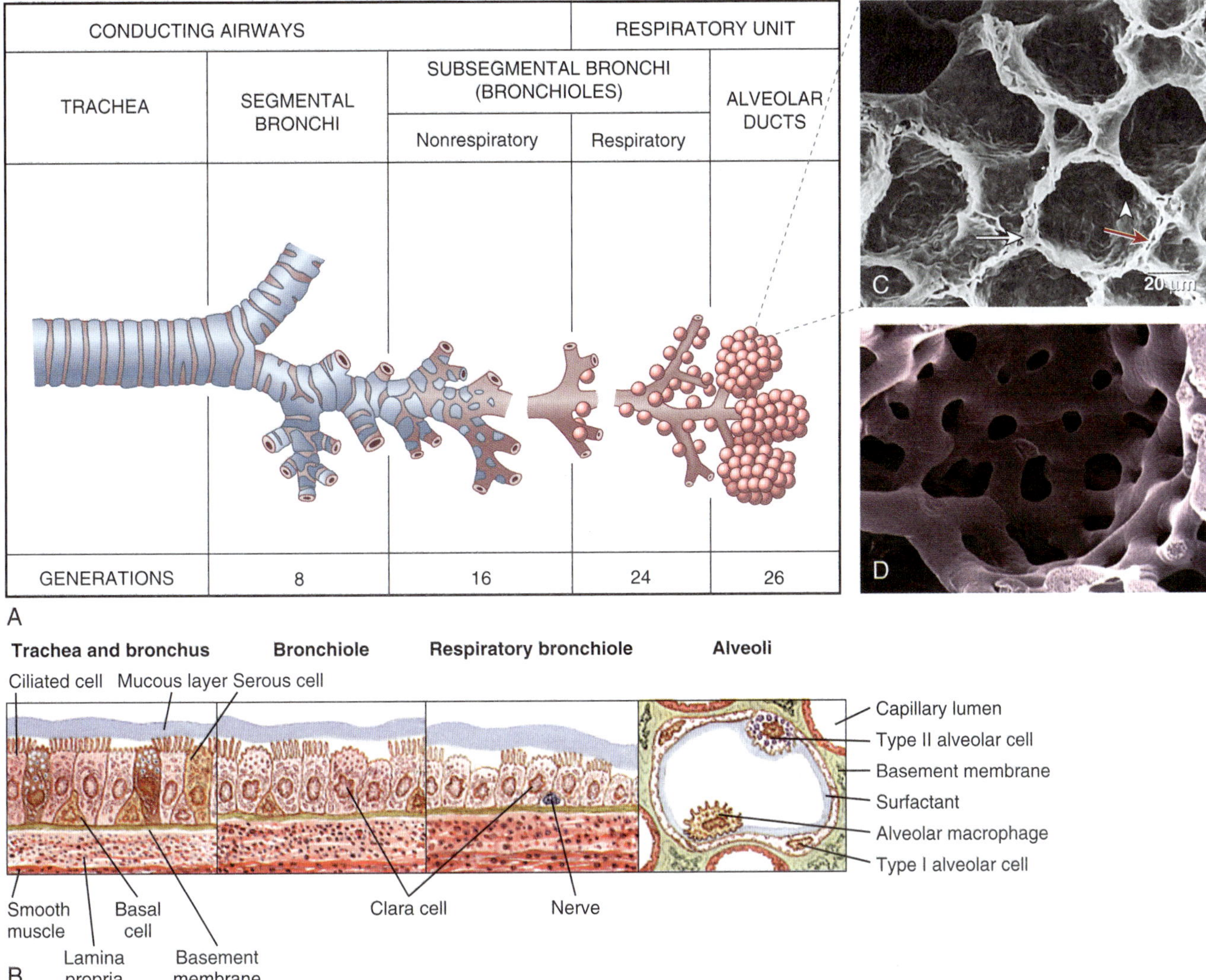

FIG. 15.6 Conducting Airways and Respiratory Unit. (A) Structures of respiratory airways. (B) Changes in the bronchial wall with progressive branching. (C) Electron micrograph of alveoli: *long white arrow* identifies type II alveolar cells (pneumocytes—secretes surfactant); *short white arrowhead* identifies pores of Kohn; *red arrow* identifies alveolar capillary. (D) Plastic cast of pulmonary capillaries at high magnification. (A, redrawn from Thompson JM, McFarland GK, Hirsch, JE, et al. *Mosby's Clinical Nursing*. 5th ed. Mosby; 2002. B, from Wilson SF, Thompson JM. *Respiratory Disorders*. Mosby; 1990. C, from Mason RJ, Broaddus VC, Martin T, et al: *Murray and Nadel's Textbook of Respiratory Medicine*. 5th ed. Saunders; 2010. D, courtesy A. Churg, MD, and J. Wright, MD, Vancouver, Canada. From Leslie KO, Wick MR. *Practical Pulmonary Pathology: A Diagnostic Approach*. 2nd ed. Saunders; 2011. In McCance KL, Huether SE, eds. *Pathophysiology: The Biologic Basis for Disease in Adults and Children*. 8th ed. Elsevier; 2019.)

canals of Lambert are collateral air pathways that exist between the alveoli and the respiratory and terminal bronchioles. They are of particular benefit when a respiratory bronchiole is blocked or collapsed because they allow gas to pass into alveoli distal to the blockage. Collateral air passages are of significant benefit in any pathologic condition of the lung that results in obstruction of airflow into a portion of the lungs. However, these pores and canals also allow the movement of microorganisms through lung tissue.[1,2]

Type II alveolar epithelial cells. Type II alveolar epithelial cells occur in much greater numbers than type I cells, but because of their minute size, they constitute a smaller portion of the total alveolar wall. After an injury to the alveolar wall, type II cells rapidly divide to line the surface; later, they transform into type I cells. The most important function of the type II cells is their ability to produce, store, and secrete pulmonary surfactant (see Fig. 15.6C).[1,3]

Surfactant. Surfactant is a phospholipid composed of fatty acids bound to lecithin. Similar to other surfactants, such as detergents and soaps, pulmonary surfactant functions to lower the surface tension of the alveoli. With detergents and soaps, this decrease in surface tension cleans clothes, whereas within the lungs, surfactant stabilizes the alveoli, increases lung compliance, and eases the work of breathing. When pulmonary disease disrupts the normal synthesis and storage of surfactant, the lungs become less compliant, and the work of breathing increases. Severe loss of surfactant results in alveolar instability and collapse and impairment of gas exchange.[10]

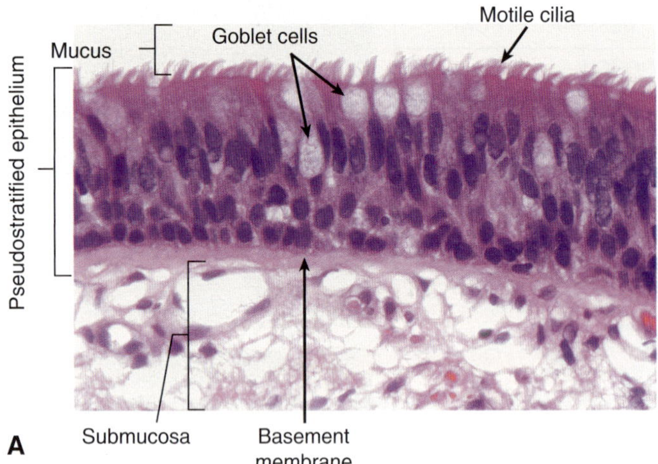

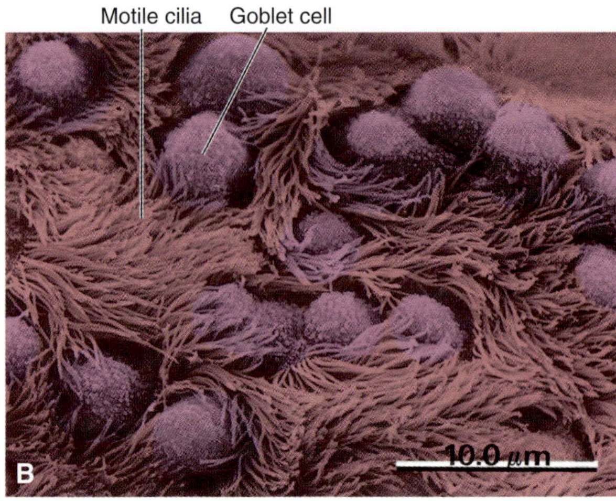

FIG. 15.7 Respiratory Mucosa. (A) Light micrograph (×200). (B) Scanning electron micrograph (×2000) of respiratory mucosa. Note the numerous motile (moving) cilia and mucus-producing goblet cells. (From Patton KT, Bell F, Thompson T, Williamson P. *Anatomy and Physiology*. 11th ed. Elsevier; 2022.)

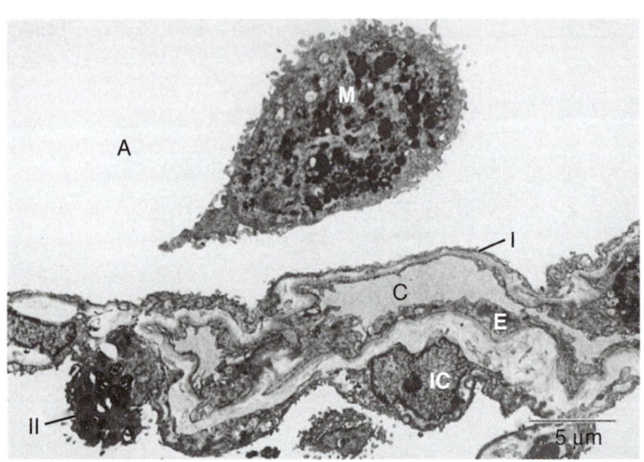

FIG. 15.8 Cells of the Terminal Respiratory Unit. An alveolar macrophage (M) is located in an alveolus (A). Alveolar macrophages are the air space scavengers that are cleared either up the mucociliary escalator or into the interstitium. These cells can be activated to express and secrete cytokines, which may interact with other cells. Cells of the alveolar wall are the lining alveolar type I and II cells (I and II, respectively) and the enclosed capillary (C), endothelial cells (E), and interstitial cells (IC). (Human lung surgical specimen, transmission electron microscopy.) (From Broaddus VC, ed. *Murray and Nadel's Textbook of Respiratory Medicine*. 7th ed. Elsevier; 2022.)

Defense system. Alveolar macrophages are monocytes that originate in bone marrow and are released into the bloodstream (see Fig. 15.8).[1–3] On entering the pulmonary capillary circulation, they move through the capillary membrane wall into the interstitial space and through to the alveoli. In the alveoli, the monocytes transform into macrophages and assume a phagocytic role. They move from alveolus to alveolus through the pores of Kohn, keeping the alveoli clean and sterile through phagocytosis and microbial killing activity, which includes the secretion of hydrogen peroxide, lysozyme, and other substances that kill microorganisms.[2,3]

Pulmonary Blood and Lymph Supply

Two vascular systems and one lymphatic system make up the pulmonary blood and lymph supply. The pulmonary circulation is the vascular system that forms the gas-exchange network surrounding the alveoli. The bronchial circulation is the vascular system that perfuses the tracheobronchial tree.[1]

Pulmonary Circulation

The pulmonary circulatory system begins at the pulmonary artery, which receives venous blood from the right side of the heart. The pulmonary artery then divides into left and right branches and continues to branch until it forms the capillaries that surround the alveoli (Fig. 15.9). After gas exchange takes place, the blood is returned to the left side of the heart through the pulmonary veins.[1,2]

Pulmonary artery pressures. The pulmonary circulation is by far the largest vascular bed within the body, and it is the only one that receives the entire cardiac output. Just as the systemic circulation has a systolic and a diastolic blood pressure, so does the pulmonary circulation. However, because of the relative lack of smooth muscle within the vessels of the pulmonary circulation, the pressures are vastly lower than within the systemic circulation.[1,3] Pulmonary artery systolic pressure ranges from 15 to 30 mm Hg, pulmonary artery diastolic pressure ranges from 4 to 12 mm Hg, and pulmonary artery mean pressure ranges from 9 to 18 mm Hg.[11] Because of the low pulmonary artery pressures, right ventricular wall thickness needs to be only approximately one-third of left ventricular wall thickness. However, just as hypertension can occur within the systemic circulation, hypertension also can occur within the pulmonary circulation.[12]

Alveolar-Capillary Membrane

The vessels of the alveolar-capillary membrane form a network around each alveolus that is so dense it forms an almost continuous sheet of blood covering the alveoli.[2] The interior diameter of each capillary segment is just large enough to allow red blood cells to squeeze by in single file so that their cell membranes touch the capillary walls (Fig. 15.10).[3] In this way, oxygen and carbon dioxide need not pass through significant amounts of plasma when diffusing into and out of the alveoli, making a highly efficient vehicle for gas exchange. Each red blood cell spends approximately three-fourths of a second in the alveolar-capillary network and is exposed to the alveolar gas of two or

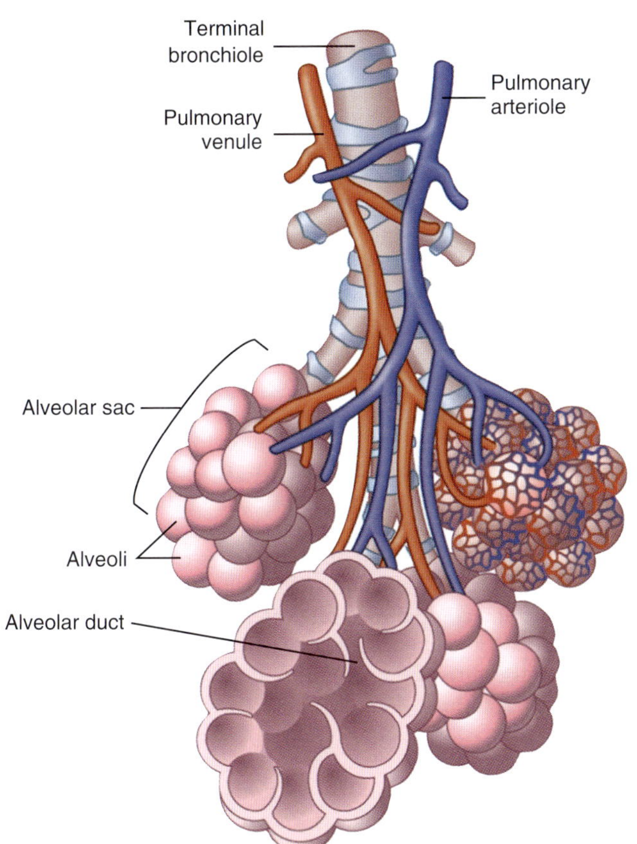

FIG. 15.9 Terminal Ventilation and Perfusion Units of the Lung. Respiratory bronchioles subdivide to form tiny tubes called alveolar ducts, which end in clusters of alveoli called alveolar sacs. Note the alveolar pores. (From Patton KT, Bell F, Thompson T, Williamson P. *Anatomy and Physiology*. 11th ed. Elsevier; 2022.)

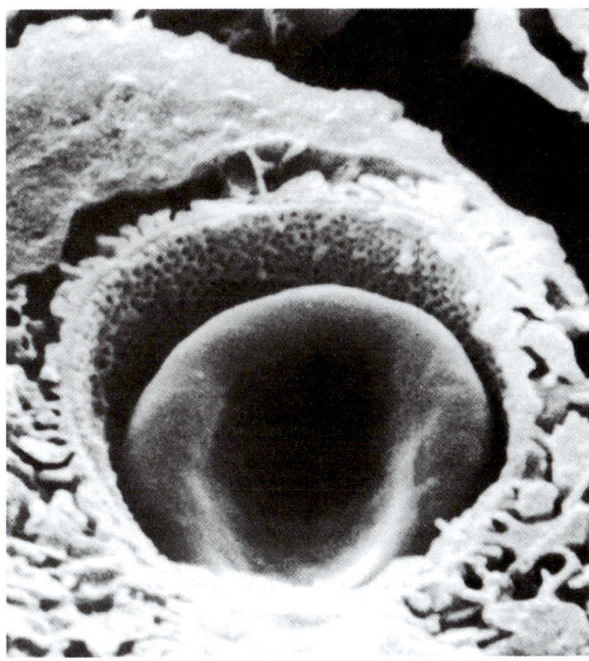

FIG. 15.10 Scanning Electron Micrograph of a Red Blood Cell in a Capillary. Note the diameters of both are similar. In many instances, the red blood cells course through even smaller capillaries, often through capillaries that are one-half of the diameter of the red blood cell. This is possible because the cells are pliable, mainly as a result of their biconcave disk shape. (From Martin DE. *Respiratory Anatomy and Physiology*. Mosby; 1988.)

three alveoli.[1] In that short time, hemoglobin is brought from its normal venous blood saturation level of 75% to its arterial saturation of more than 96%.[3] Hemoglobin levels have been shown to reach normal within only a 0.25-second exposure to alveolar gas; under conditions such as in tachycardia, in which the red blood cells spend less time within the pulmonary capillary network, normal oxygenation can still occur.[3]

Membrane layers. The alveolar-capillary membrane is less than 0.5 mcm thick[13] and is composed of several layers of cells: alveolar epithelium, alveolar basement membrane, interstitial space, capillary basement membrane, and capillary endothelium (Fig. 15.11). Oxygen and carbon dioxide traverse easily across these layers, which present no barrier to diffusion because the membrane is very thin.[3]

Bronchial Circulation

Bronchial circulation, also known as the *systemic blood supply to the lungs*, is the system that perfuses the tracheobronchial tree, the visceral pleura, interstitial and connective tissue, some arteries and veins, lymph nodes, and the nerves within the thoracic cavity. The bronchial arteries that perfuse structures in the left side of the thorax branch off the aorta, and the arteries that perfuse the right-sided structures branch from the intercostal, subclavian, or internal mammary artery. After perfusing the specific lung structures, most of the venous blood returns to the right side of the heart; however, some venous blood from the bronchial circulation returns directly into the pulmonary veins and the left atrium.[14]

Physiologic Shunting

The left atrium normally contains pure oxygenated blood, with a hemoglobin saturation level of 100%. The mixing of venous blood from the bronchial circulation with the oxygenated blood in the left atrium decreases the saturation of left atrial blood to 96% to 99%. For this reason, while a person is breathing room air, the oxygen saturation of arterial blood is less than 100%. The dumping of venous blood into the left atrium is known as an *anatomic shunt*. The thebesian veins, which drain the right coronary circulation, are also responsible for the addition of venous blood to the left atrium. These two systems constitute the normal anatomic shunt, which accounts for approximately 3% to 5% of the total cardiac output.[15]

Lymphatic Circulation

The lungs are more richly supplied with lymphatic tissue than any other organ, perhaps because of their constant exposure to the external environment. The lymphatic vessels parallel much of the pulmonary vasculature and the tracheobronchial tree to the level of the terminal and respiratory bronchioles. Lymphatic vessels also are located within the connective tissue of lung parenchyma and within the pleural membranes. These vessels eventually drain into the primary lymph nodes located at the hila of the lungs. The lymphatic system in the lungs serves two purposes. As part of the immune system, the lymphatic system is responsible for removing foreign particles and cell debris from the lungs and for producing antibody-mediated and cell-mediated immune responses. The lymphatic system also is responsible for removing fluid from the lungs and for keeping the alveoli clear.[1–3]

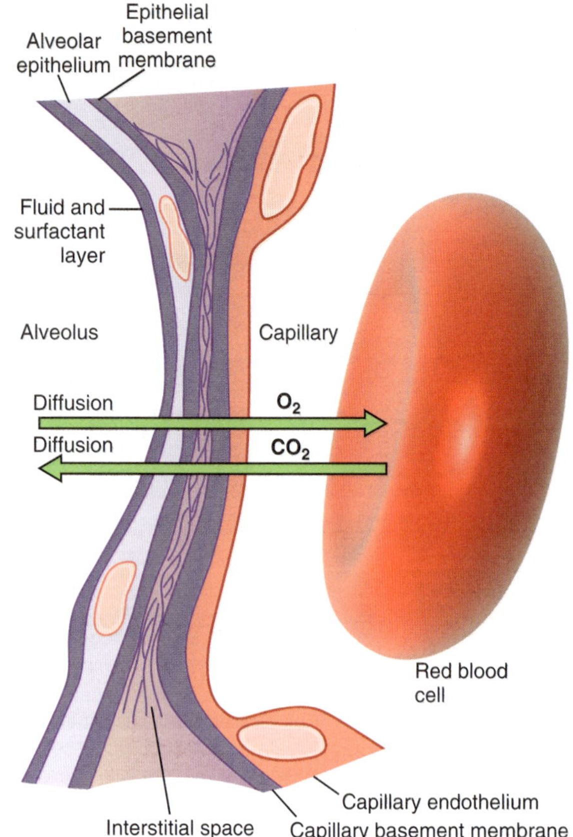

FIG. 15.11 Layers of the Alveolar–Capillary Membrane. (From Hall JE, Hall ME, eds. *Guyton and Hall Textbook of Medical Physiology*. 14th ed. Elsevier; 2021.)

PHYSIOLOGY

Ventilation

Air moves into and out of the lungs because of the difference between intrapulmonary pressure (pressure inside the lungs) and atmospheric pressure. The movement of air into the lungs is known as *inhalation* (Fig. 15.12), and the movement of air out of the lungs is known as *exhalation* (Fig. 15.13). At the command of the central nervous system, the muscles of ventilation contract, the thorax and lungs expand, and intrapulmonary pressure decreases. When the pressure falls below atmospheric pressure, air enters the lungs, and inhalation occurs. At the end of inhalation, the muscles of ventilation relax, the thorax contracts and the lungs are compressed, and intrapulmonary pressure increases. When the pressure rises above atmospheric pressure, air exits the lungs, and exhalation occurs.[4,16]

Work of Breathing

The work of breathing is the amount of work that must be performed to overcome the elastic and resistive properties of the lungs. The elastic properties are determined by lung recoil, chest wall recoil, and the surface tension of the alveoli. The resistive properties are determined by airway resistance.[1,16,17] Normally, the work of breathing occurs during inhalation, but even exhalation can be a strain when lung recoil, chest wall recoil, or airway resistance is abnormal.[4,16]

During normal, quiet ventilation, only 1% to 2% of basal oxygen consumption is required by the pulmonary system.[17] During heavy exercise, the amount of energy required by the pulmonary system can become progressively greater. The work of breathing can be a factor that limits exercise in a patient with pulmonary disease. Pathologic conditions of the pulmonary system can drastically change the energy requirement for ventilation. Pulmonary diseases that decrease lung compliance (e.g., atelectasis, pulmonary edema), decrease chest wall compliance (e.g., kyphoscoliosis), increase airway resistance (e.g., bronchitis, asthma), or decrease lung recoil (e.g., emphysema) can increase the work of breathing so much that one-third or more of the total body energy is used for ventilation (Box 15.2).[4,16]

Pulmonary Volumes and Capacities

Pulmonary ventilation can be described in terms of volumes and capacities (Fig. 15.14). Tidal volume (V_T) is the amount of air inhaled and exhaled with each breath. Inspiratory reserve volume (IRV) is the maximum amount of air that can be inhaled over and above the normal V_T. Expiratory reserve volume (ERV) is the maximum amount of air that can be exhaled beyond the normal V_T. The residual volume (RV) is the amount of air left in the lungs after a complete exhalation. Inspiratory capacity is the sum of the V_T and the inspiratory reserve. Functional residual capacity is the sum of the ERV and the RV. Vital capacity is the sum of the IRV, the V_T, and the ERV. Total lung capacity is the sum of all four volumes and represents the maximal amount of air that can be inhaled.[3,16]

Physiologic dead space. The portion of total ventilation that participates in gas exchange is known as *alveolar ventilation*. The portion of ventilation that does not participate in gas exchange is known as *wasted ventilation*. The areas in the lungs that are ventilated but in which no gas exchange occurs are known as *dead space regions*. The conducting airways are referred to as *anatomic dead space* because they are ventilated but not perfused and therefore are unable to participate in gas exchange. Some ventilation goes to unperfused alveoli. Without perfusion, gas exchange cannot take place, and the ventilation is wasted. These unperfused alveoli are known as *alveolar dead space*. Anatomic dead space plus alveolar dead space is called *physiologic dead space*.[3,15,16]

Regulation of Ventilation

Regulation of ventilation by the brain is complex and not completely understood. Ventilation is regulated by a triad comprising a controller (located within the central nervous system), a group of effectors (muscles of ventilation), and various sensors that include chemoreceptors (central and peripheral) and mechanoreceptors (located in chest wall and lungs). Efferent nerve fibers convey impulses from the controller to the effectors, whereas afferent nerve fibers carry impulses from some of the sensors to the controller (Fig. 15.15).[18]

Controller. The central nervous system houses what is known as the *controller of ventilation*. The controller is not located in one specific area; rather, it is in several areas that work together to provide coordinated ventilation. The brainstem regulates automatic ventilation, the cerebral cortex allows voluntary ventilation, and neurons housed in the spinal cord process information from the brain and from the peripheral receptors, allowing them to send final information to the muscles of ventilation.[18]

Brainstem. In the brainstem, the medulla oblongata and the pons are involved in ventilation. Four different groups of neurons are thought to participate in the regulation of

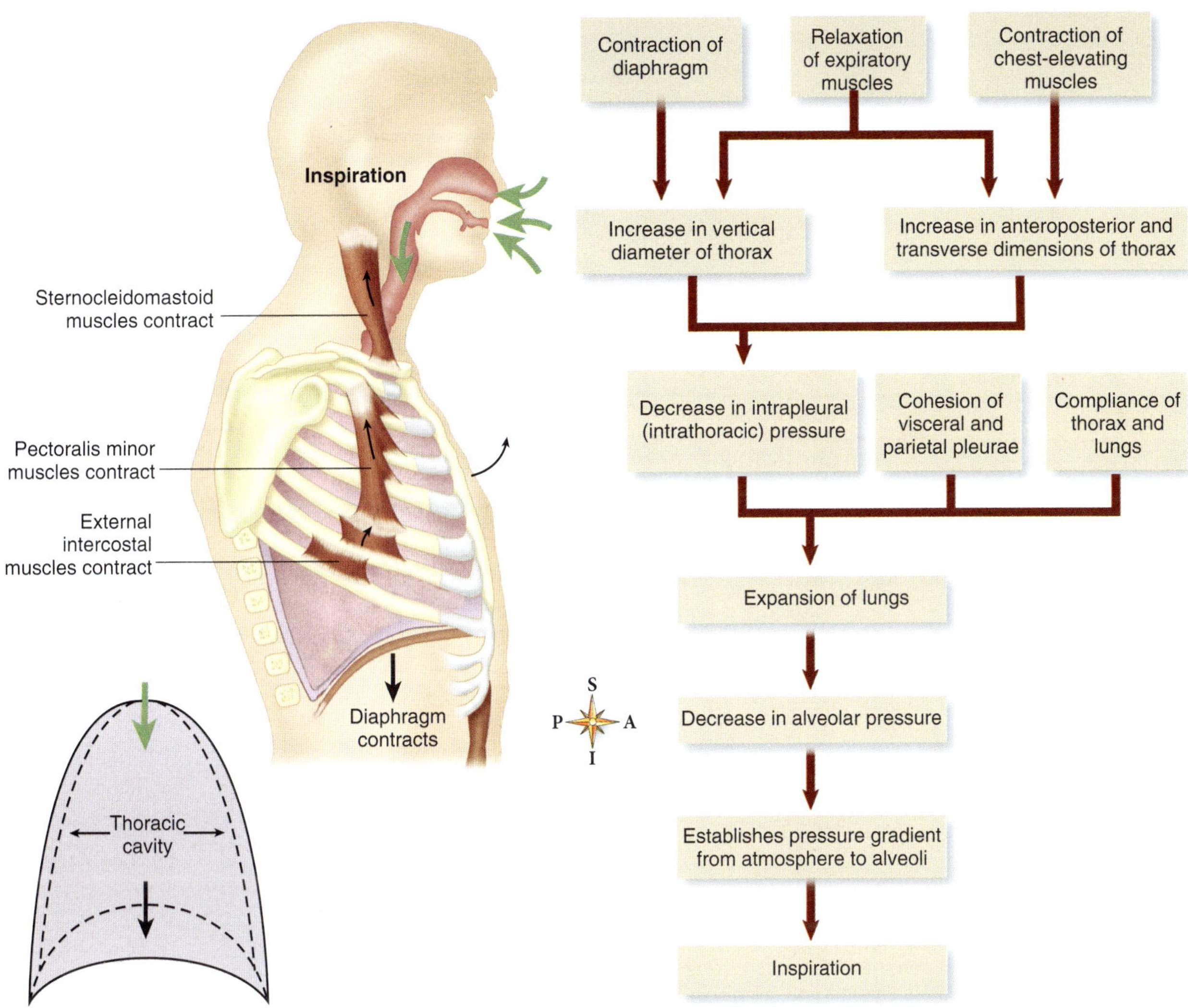

FIG. 15.12 Mechanism of Inspiration. Note the role of the diaphragm and the chest-elevating muscles (pectoralis minor and external intercostals) in increasing thoracic volume, which decreases pressure in the lungs and draws air inward. (From Patton KT, Bell F, Thompson T, Williamson P. *Anatomy and Physiology*. 11th ed. Elsevier; 2022.)

inhalation and exhalation. The dorsal respiratory group, located in the medulla, is responsible for the basic rhythm of ventilation. Cells in this area are thought to fire automatically and trigger inhalation. The pneumotaxic center in the pons is responsible for limiting inhalation and triggering exhalation. This response also facilitates control of the rate and pattern of respiration. The ventral respiratory group, located in the medulla, is responsible for inspiration and expiration during periods of increased ventilation. The apneustic center in the lower pons is thought to work with the pneumotaxic center to regulate the depth of inspiration.[18]

Cerebral cortex. The cerebral cortex functions by allowing voluntary ventilation to override the automatic controls of the medulla and pons. Voluntary ventilatory control is most important during behavioral states such as crying, laughing, singing, and talking. During these states, voluntary control may override the automatic control, which responds chiefly to chemical stimuli and to changes in lung inflation.[3,18]

Effectors. The effectors of ventilation are the muscles of ventilation (see Fig. 15.3). In considering their function in the control of ventilation, the most important issue is that they function in a coordinated fashion. The central nervous system regulates this function.[18]

Sensors. The main sensors for the regulation of ventilation are the central and peripheral chemoreceptors (see Fig. 15.15). These chemoreceptors respond to changes in the chemical composition of the blood or other fluid around them. Other sensors that are found in the lung include the irritant receptors, stretch receptors, and the juxtacapillary receptors (J-receptors).[3,18]

Central chemoreceptors. The central chemoreceptors are located near the ventral surface of the medulla in the chemosensitive area (see Fig. 15.15). These chemoreceptors are surrounded by cerebral extracellular fluid and respond primarily to changes in the hydrogen ion concentration of that fluid. Ventilation increases when the hydrogen ion concentration rises and decreases when the hydrogen ion concentration falls. A rise in the partial pressure of carbon dioxide ($Paco_2$) causes the movement of carbon dioxide across the blood-brain barrier into the cerebrospinal fluid, stimulating the movement of hydrogen ions into the extracellular fluid of the brain. These hydrogen ions then

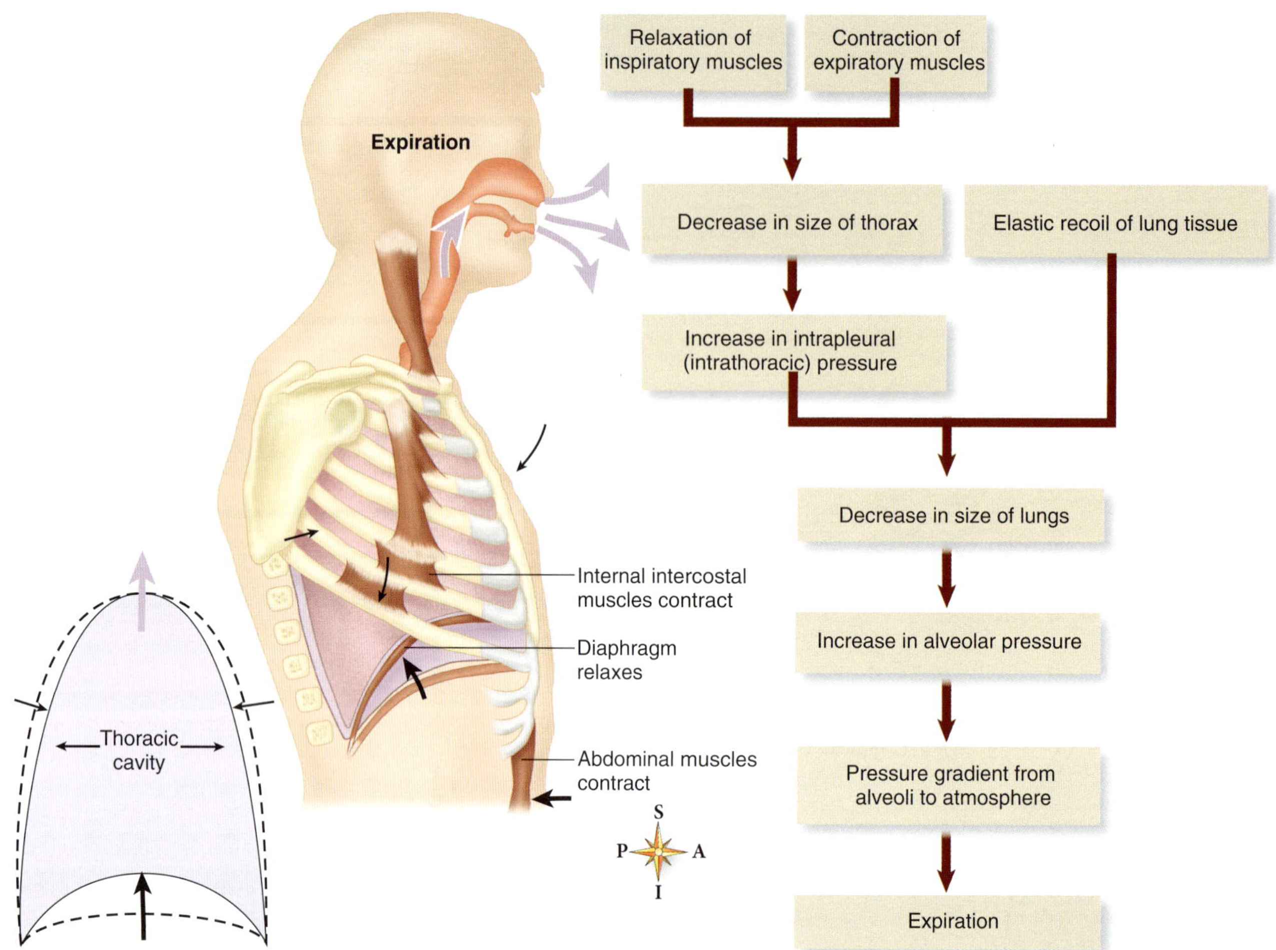

FIG. 15.13 Mechanism of Expiration. Note that relaxation of the diaphragm plus contraction of chest-depressing muscles (internal intercostals) reduces thoracic volume, which increases pressure in the lungs and pushes air outward. (From Patton KT, Bell F, Thompson T, Williamson P. *Anatomy and Physiology*. 11th ed. Elsevier; 2022.)

BOX 15.2 How Can Lung Disease Alter Ventilation?

Normal muscular action of the diaphragm, flexibility of the rib cage, elasticity of the lungs, and airway diameter are instrumental in allowing easy inhalation and exhalation. Any interference with these actions impairs normal ventilation. Pulmonary diseases can be categorized as obstructive or restrictive, depending on how the underlying cause affects normal ventilation.

Restrictive diseases limit lung or chest wall movement and include diffuse interstitial lung fibrosis, atelectasis, kyphoscoliosis, and severe chest wall pain. These conditions can be acute or chronic, and because they restrict lung or chest wall expansion or both, patients have smaller V_Ts but an increased ventilatory rate to maintain minute ventilation.

Obstructive diseases impede normal airflow. Classic examples are emphysema, in which airflow is decreased because of a decrease in lung recoil, and asthma, in which airflow is decreased because of diffuse airway narrowing. Emphysema results in lungs that inflate easily but, lacking the normal elastic recoil, do not compress to assist with exhalation. Patients with emphysema may have little difficulty inhaling but struggle to exhale.

stimulate the chemoreceptors, and ventilation is increased. The increase in ventilation causes exhalation of excess carbon dioxide, the $PaCO_2$ decreases, and ventilation returns to normal. Central chemoreceptors are not affected by changes in the partial pressure of oxygen (PaO_2).[18]

Peripheral chemoreceptors. The peripheral chemoreceptors are located above and below the aortic arch and at the bifurcation of the common carotid arteries (see Fig. 15.15). The most important action of the peripheral chemoreceptors is their response to changes in the PaO_2 because they are the primary receptors that increase ventilation in response to arterial hypoxemia. Immediate hyperventilation, one of the principal compensatory mechanisms in response to hypoxemia, is governed by these chemoreceptors. The peripheral chemoreceptors also respond to changes in $PaCO_2$ and hydrogen ion concentration. An increase in either $PaCO_2$ or hydrogen ion concentration results in an increase in ventilation. Studies indicate that the peripheral chemoreceptors probably are more involved with the short-term response to carbon dioxide, whereas the central chemoreceptors are responsible for the long-term response to carbon dioxide.[18]

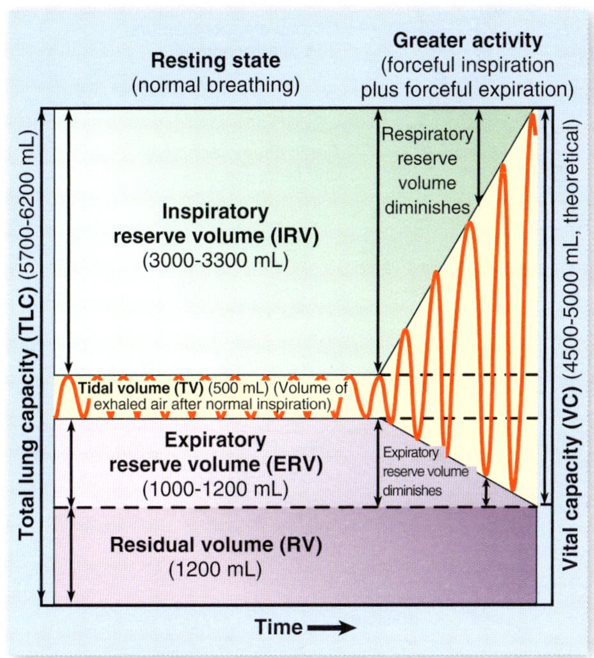

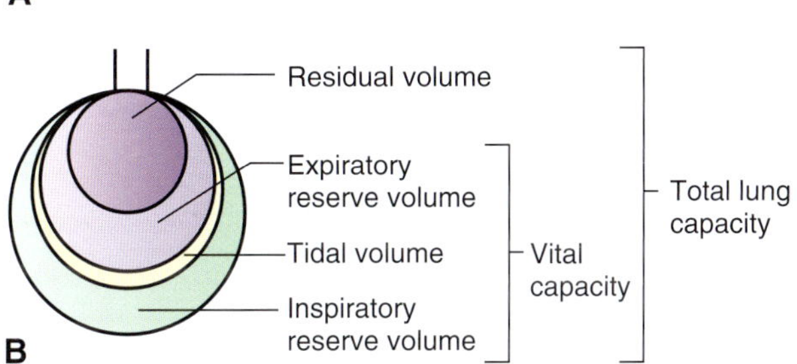

FIG. 15.14 Pulmonary Ventilation Volumes and Capacities. (A) Spirogram. (B) Pulmonary volumes (at rest) represented as relative proportions of an inflated balloon. During normal, quiet respirations, the atmosphere and lungs exchange approximately 500 mL of air *(TV)*. With forcible inspiration, approximately 3300 mL more air can be inhaled *(IRV)*. After a normal inspiration and normal expiration, approximately 1000 mL more air can be forcibly expired *(ERV)*. Vital capacity is the amount of air that can be forcibly expired after a maximal inspiration and indicates the largest amount of air that can enter and leave the lungs during respiration. Residual volume is the air that remains trapped in the alveoli. (From Patton KT, Bell F, Thompson T, Williamson P, eds. *The Human Body in Health & Disease*. 8th ed. Elsevier; 2024.)

Other receptors. Irritant receptors lie between airway epithelial cells, and they stimulate bronchoconstriction and hyperpnea in response to inhaled irritants. Stretch receptors, which are located in the airways, are stimulated by changes in lung volume. They inhibit inhalation and are thought to protect the lung from overinflation (Hering-Breuer reflex). J-receptors lie in the alveolar walls close to the capillaries. They are stimulated by engorgement of the pulmonary capillaries and an increase in the interstitial fluid volume. Stimulation of the J-receptors is thought to cause rapid, shallow breathing.[19]

Respiration

Respiration refers to the movement of oxygen and carbon dioxide. Gas exchange that takes place at the lung level through the alveolar-capillary membrane is referred to as *external respiration*. The diffusion of gases in and out of the cells at the tissue level is referred to as *internal respiration*.[3]

Diffusion

Oxygen and carbon dioxide move throughout the body by diffusion. Diffusion moves molecules from an area of high concentration to an area of low concentration. The difference in the concentrations of the gases is referred to as the *driving pressure*. The greater the driving pressure of the gas through the membrane, the greater the rate of diffusion.[3] Within the lungs, diffusion occurs because of the difference in the driving pressure between the pulmonary capillaries and the alveoli. Oxygen is in high concentration within the alveoli and exerts a higher driving pressure compared with the pulmonary capillaries; therefore oxygen moves by diffusion from the alveoli into the pulmonary capillaries. Carbon dioxide is in higher concentration and has a higher driving pressure within the pulmonary capillaries compared with the alveoli; therefore carbon dioxide diffuses out of the capillaries into the alveoli, where carbon dioxide is exhaled (Fig. 15.16). The driving pressure of oxygen is lower at higher altitudes because the effects of gravity on the gases are lessened,[20] and the driving pressure of oxygen is higher when supplemental oxygen is administered.[21]

In addition to the driving pressure of gases, several other factors affect the rate of diffusion, such as the thickness of the alveolar-capillary membrane,[3] the surface area of the membrane,[21] and the diffusion coefficient of the gas.[21] An increase in the thickness of the alveolar-capillary membrane (e.g., pulmonary edema, fibrosis)[3] or a decrease in the surface area of the membrane (e.g., pneumonectomy, lobectomy, pulmonary embolus, emphysema)[21] decreases the rate of diffusion. The diffusion coefficient of each gas is determined by its solubility. The higher the diffusion coefficient, the faster the gas diffuses. Carbon dioxide has a much higher diffusion coefficient than oxygen, and carbon dioxide diffuses 20 times more rapidly than oxygen.[21]

Ventilation/Perfusion Relationships

Ventilation ($\dot{V}$) and perfusion ($\dot{Q}$) should be equally matched at the alveolar-capillary membrane level for optimal gas exchange to take place, but because of normal regional variations in the distribution of ventilation and perfusion, this is not the case. Normally, alveolar ventilation is approximately 4 L/min, and pulmonary capillary perfusion is approximately 5 L/min. The normal ventilation/perfusion ratio ($\dot{V}/\dot{Q}$) is 4:5, or 0.8.[15,21]

Distribution of Ventilation

The distribution of ventilation throughout the lungs is uneven as a result of a variety of factors, including the configuration of the thorax and the effects of gravity on intrapleural pressure. The thorax allows more lung expansion at the base than at the apex, which permits more ventilation to the base and limits ventilation to the apex. Gravity also produces regional variations in intrapleural pressure. At rest, the negative intrapleural pressure at the apex is greater than at the base, and alveoli in the apexes are larger and have more air left in them at the end of expiration. Because the alveoli are larger, they are less compliant and more difficult to inflate. On inhalation, the alveoli at the base expand more because they have less pressure to overcome.[3,15,16] In an upright person, the base of the lung receives approximately

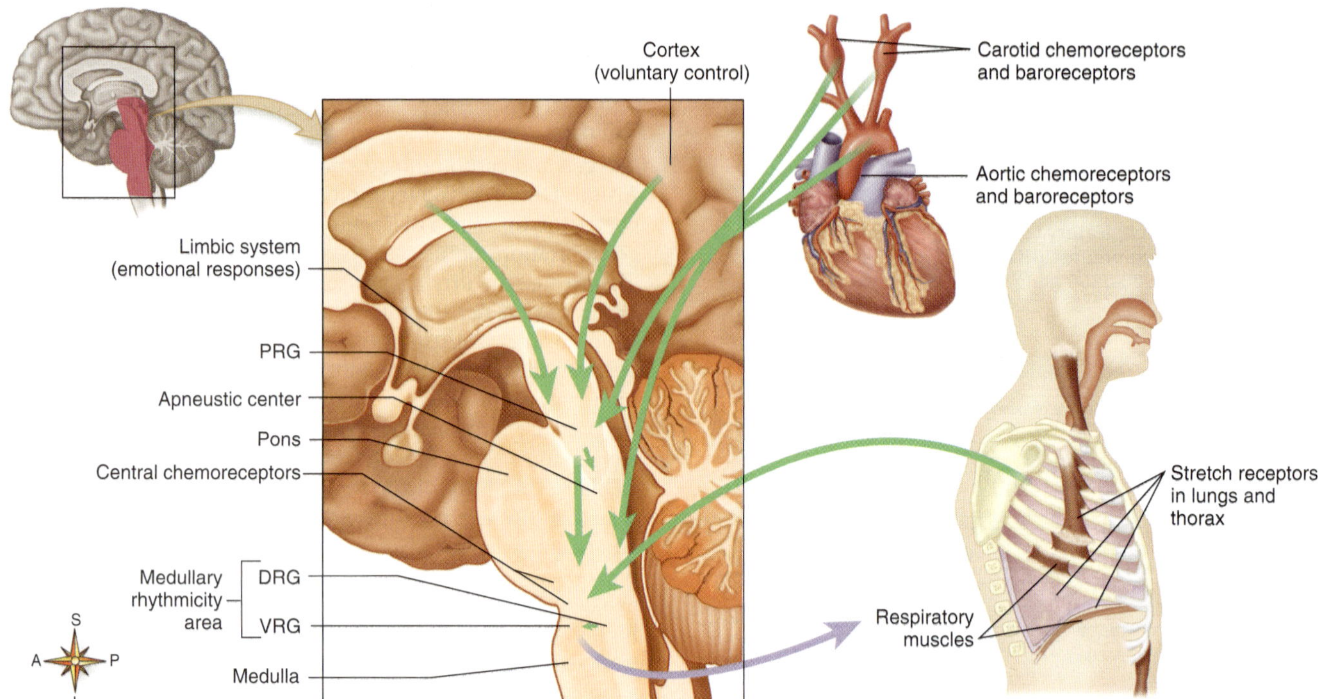

FIG. 15.15 Regulation of Breathing. The dorsal respiratory group (DRG) and ventral respiratory group (VRG) of the medulla represent the medullary rhythmicity area. The pontine respiratory group (PRG, or pneumotaxic center) and apneustic center of the pons influence the basic respiratory rhythm by means of neural input to the medullary rhythmicity area. The brainstem also receives input from other parts of the body; information from chemoreceptors, baroreceptors, and stretch receptors can alter the basic breathing pattern, as can emotional (limbic) and sensory input. Despite these subconscious reflexes, the cerebral cortex can override the "automatic" control of breathing to some extent to do such activities as sing or blow up a balloon. *Green arrows* show the flow of information to the respiratory control centers. The *purple arrow* shows the flow of information from the control centers to the respiratory muscles that drive breathing. (From Patton KT, Bell F, Thompson T, Williamson P, eds. *The Human Body in Health & Disease*. 8th ed. Elsevier; 2024.)

four times more ventilation than the apex.[16] In a supine person, gravity produces the same effects in the dependent zones of the lungs (posterior regions).[3,15,16]

Distribution of Perfusion

The distribution of perfusion through the lungs is related to gravity and intraalveolar pressures. Because of the effects of gravity, the pressure in the capillaries in the lungs is higher in the bases than in the apexes. This promotes preferential blood flow to the gravity-dependent areas of the lungs. Intraalveolar pressures also vary throughout the different regions of the lungs, with the highest pressure in the apexes and the lowest pressure in the bases. In some areas of the lungs, the intraalveolar pressure has the potential of exceeding capillary hydrostatic pressure, resulting in an absence of blood flow to these areas. On the basis of this concept, the lung can be divided into three zones. Zone 1 is the nondependent portion of the lung, which has the potential of no perfusion. Zone 2 is the middle portion of the lung, which receives various degrees of blood flow. Zone 3 is the gravity-dependent area of the lung, which receives a constant blood flow (Fig. 15.17).[3,15]

Ventilation/Perfusion Mismatch

Various factors can affect the matching of ventilation to perfusion in the lungs, and their relationship can be considered as a continuum (Fig. 15.18). At one end of the continuum, the alveolus is receiving ventilation but is not receiving any perfusion and is unable to participate in gas exchange. This situation is referred to as *alveolar dead space*. On the other end of the continuum, the alveolus is receiving perfusion but is not receiving any ventilation and is unable to participate in gas exchange. This situation is referred to as *intrapulmonary shunting*. In this case the blood is returned to the left side of the heart unoxygenated.[21] An infinite number of ventilation/perfusion mismatches exist between these two extremes. Situations in which ventilation exceeds perfusion ($\dot{V}/\dot{Q}$ >0.8) are considered to be *dead space producing*, whereas situations in which perfusion exceeds ventilation ($\dot{V}/\dot{Q}$ <0.8) are considered to be *shunt producing*. Although minor mismatching of ventilation may not significantly affect gas exchange, significant alterations in the relationship result in hypoxemia.[15,21]

Hypoxic vasoconstriction. The distribution of perfusion is affected by the amount of oxygen in the alveoli. Although most blood vessels in the body dilate in response to hypoxia, the pulmonary vessels constrict when the PaO_2 is less than 60 mm Hg. This event, known as *hypoxic vasoconstriction*, usually occurs when a portion of the pulmonary capillaries perfuses unventilated or underventilated alveoli. Hypoxic vasoconstriction is thought to be a compensatory response used to limit the return of unoxygenated blood to the left side of the heart. If the response is prolonged and generalized throughout the lungs, pulmonary hypertension results.[3]

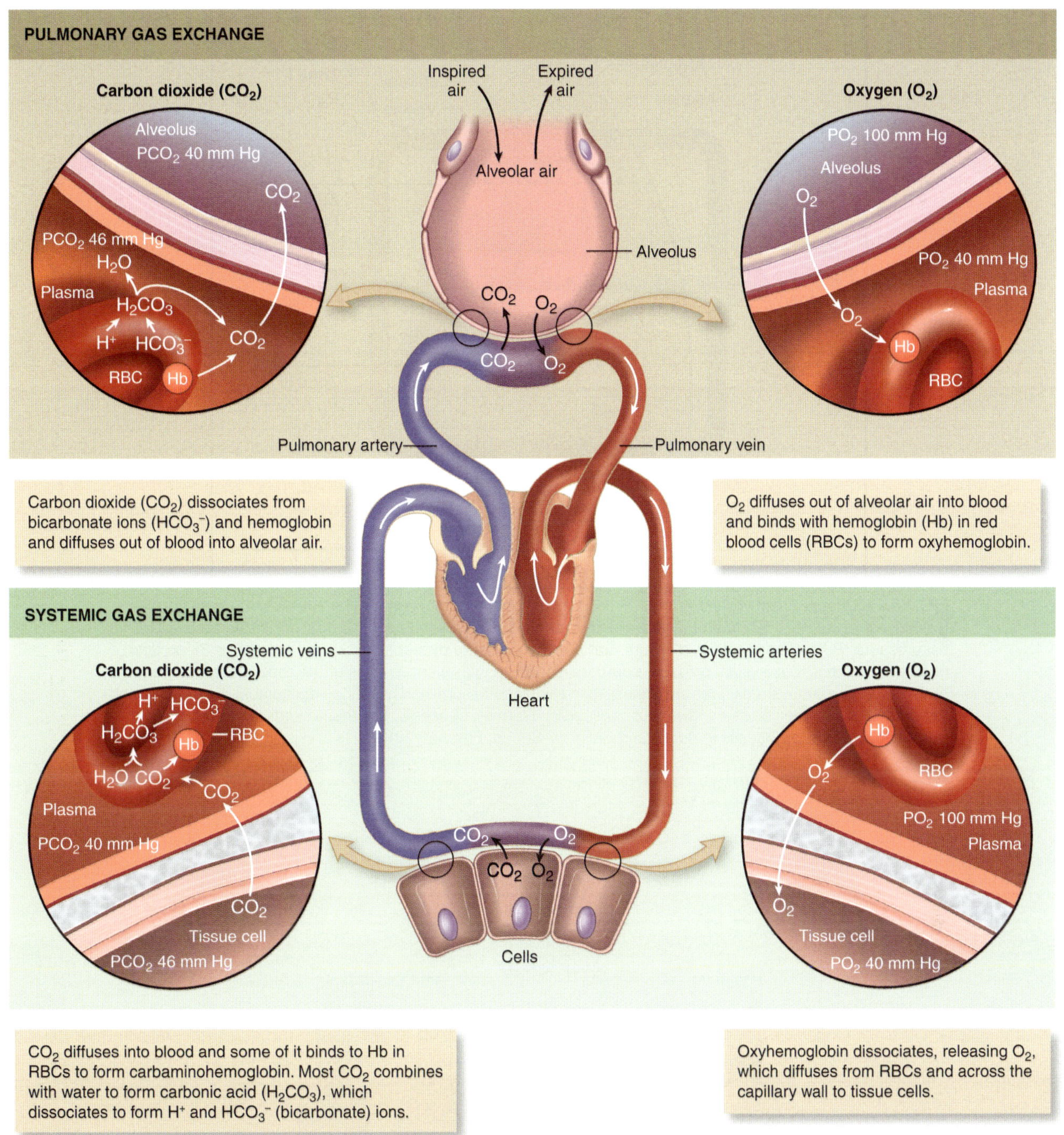

FIG. 15.16 Exchange and Transport of Gases. The *top panel* of the diagram shows pulmonary gas exchange, and the *bottom panel* shows systemic gas exchange. In each, the *left inset* shows the transport and movement of carbon dioxide (CO_2), and the *right inset* shows the transport and movement of oxygen (O_2). (From Patton KT, Bell F, Thompson T, Williamson P, eds. *The Human Body in Health & Disease*. 8th ed. Elsevier; 2024.)

Gas Transport

Gas transport refers to the movement of oxygen and carbon dioxide to and from the tissue cells. The transportation vehicle is the bloodstream, which is moved by the pumping action of the heart (cardiac output). At the tissue level, oxygen and carbon dioxide move into and out of the cell by diffusion. Oxygen diffuses into the cell because of the pressure gradient that exists between oxygen in the capillary and oxygen in the cell (Fig. 15.19A). Carbon dioxide diffuses into the capillary because of the pressure gradient that exists between carbon dioxide in the cell and carbon dioxide in the capillary (Fig. 15.19B).[3]

Oxygen Content

Oxygen is transported to the tissues by the blood in two ways: dissolved in plasma (PaO_2) or bound to hemoglobin molecules (oxygen saturation). Most of the oxygen is transported by hemoglobin, with the portion of oxygen dissolved in plasma equal to approximately 3% of the total oxygen within

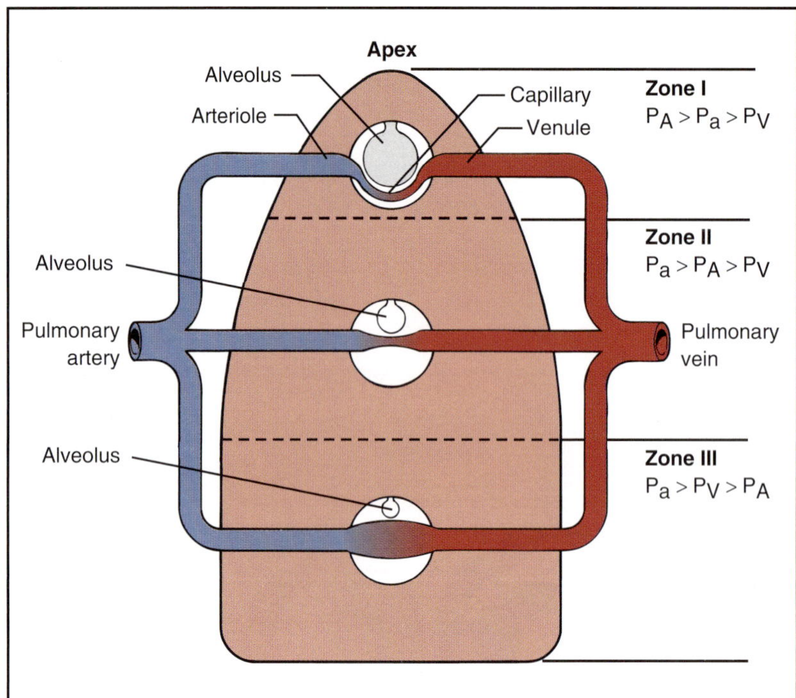

FIG. 15.17 Effects of Gravity and Alveolar Pressure on Pulmonary Blood Flow. Note three lung zones. In zone I, alveolar pressure *(P_A)* is greater than arterial and venous pressure, and no blood flow occurs. In zone II, arterial pressure *(P_a)* exceeds alveolar pressure, but alveolar pressure exceeds venous pressure *(P_V)*. Blood flow occurs in this zone, but alveolar pressure compresses the venules (venous ends of the capillaries). In zone III, both arterial and venous pressures are greater than alveolar pressure, and blood flow fluctuates, depending on the difference between arterial and venous pressures. (From McCance KL, Huether SE, eds. *Pathophysiology: The Biologic Basis for Disease in Adults and Children.* 8th ed. Elsevier; 2019.)

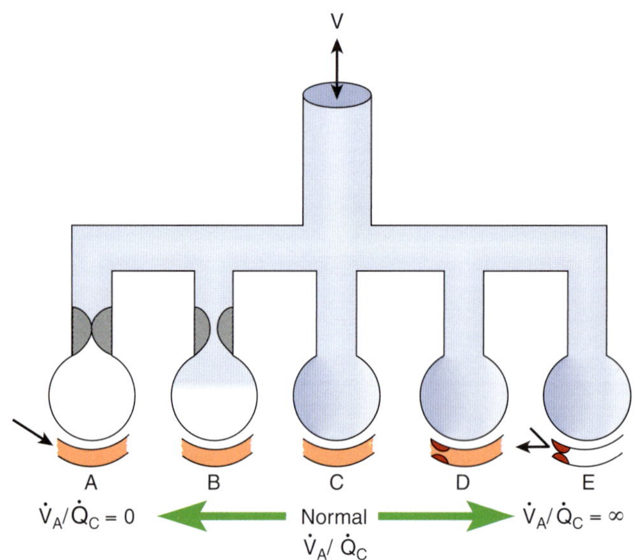

FIG. 15.18 Continuum of Ventilation/Perfusion ($\dot{V}/\dot{Q}$) Relationships. (A) Intrapulmonary shunting. (B) ($\dot{V}/\dot{Q}$) mismatching is a shunt-producing situation. (C) Normal ($\dot{V}/\dot{Q}$) ratio. (D) ($\dot{V}/\dot{Q}$) mismatching is a dead space–producing situation. (E) Alveolar dead space. (Redrawn from Misasi RS, Keyes JL. Matching and mismatching ventilation and perfusion in the lung. *Crit Care Nurse.* 1996;16(3):23.)

the blood.[22] The pressure exerted by the oxygen dissolved in plasma is important, because this oxygen diffuses across the capillary membrane into the cells first and serves as the vehicle for the unloading of the oxygen from the hemoglobin molecule. As dissolved oxygen leaves the plasma and diffuses into the cells, the molecules of oxygen move off the hemoglobin molecule, dissolve into the plasma, and diffuse into the cells.[20] For this process to begin, a pressure gradient must exist between the oxygen level in the capillary and the oxygen level in the cell.

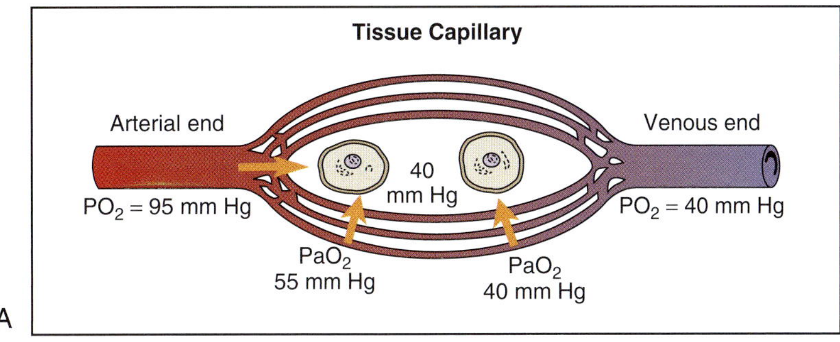

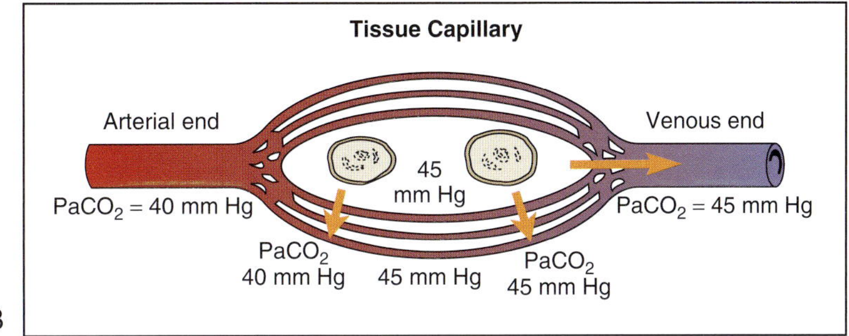

FIG. 15.19 Internal Respiration. (A) Diffusion of oxygen from a tissue capillary into a tissue cell. (B) Diffusion of carbon dioxide from a tissue cell into a tissue capillary.

Oxygen content formula. The amount of oxygen in the arterial blood can be calculated using the arterial oxygen content (CaO_2) formula. The amount of oxygen in the venous blood can be calculated using the venous oxygen content (CvO_2) formula (see Appendix B).[22]

Oxyhemoglobin dissociation curve. The relationship between dissolved oxygen and hemoglobin-bound oxygen is plotted as the oxyhemoglobin dissociation curve (Fig. 15.20). The sigmoid shape of the oxyhemoglobin dissociation curve illustrates several essential points about the relationship between the two ways oxygen is carried. The steep lower portion of the curve, at PaO_2 levels of 10 to 60 mm Hg, shows that the peripheral tissues can withdraw large amounts of oxygen from the hemoglobin molecule with only a small change in PaO_2, preserving the gradient for the continued unloading of hemoglobin.[20,22] The area at PaO_2 levels of 60 to 100 mm Hg is called the *flat upper portion* of the curve. This portion shows that the saturation of hemoglobin remains high, even as the PaO_2 declines. For example, in a healthy person, a PaO_2 of 60 mm Hg yields an oxygen saturation level of 89%, whereas a PaO_2 of 100 mm Hg yields an oxygen saturation level of 98%. The large drop in PaO_2 (from 100 to 60 mm Hg) causes only a small drop in oxygen saturation (from 98% to 89%).[21,22]

Shifts in the oxyhemoglobin dissociation curve. Under normal circumstances, hemoglobin has a steady and predictable affinity for oxygen. The combination of oxygen and hemoglobin based on this affinity is responsible for the position of the oxyhemoglobin dissociation curve in which a given PaO_2 yields a predictable oxygen saturation.[20,22] Occasionally, events occur that alter the affinity hemoglobin has for oxygen. These events include changes in pH, $PaCO_2$, temperature, and 2,3-diphosphoglycerate (2,3-DPG) levels (Box 15.3). When this affinity is altered, the position of the oxyhemoglobin dissociation curve shifts (Fig. 15.20). Shifts in the position of the curve mean there is a change in the way oxygen is taken up by the hemoglobin molecule at the alveolar level and a change in the way oxygen is delivered at the tissue level.[21,22]

Shift to the right. When the curve is shifted to the right (see Fig. 15.20, curve C), there is a lower oxygen saturation level for any given PaO_2; in other words, hemoglobin has less affinity for oxygen. Although the saturation level is lower than expected, a right shift enhances oxygen delivery at the tissue level because hemoglobin unloads more readily. Factors that cause this change in oxygen-hemoglobin affinity and shift the curve to the right include fever, increased $PaCO_2$, acidosis, and increased 2,3-DPG levels.[21,22]

Shift to the left. When the curve is shifted to the left (see Fig. 15.20, curve A), the reverse occurs. There is a higher arterial saturation for any given PaO_2 because hemoglobin has an increased affinity for oxygen. Although the saturation level is higher, oxygen delivery to the tissues is impaired because hemoglobin does not unload as easily. Factors that contribute to this effect include hypothermia, alkalemia, decreased $PaCO_2$, and decreased 2,3-DPG levels.[21,22]

Abnormalities of hemoglobin. Hemoglobin carries approximately 97% of the total amount of oxygen held within the bloodstream. This great carrying capacity depends on hemoglobin that is normal in amount and molecular structure. Most hemoglobin abnormalities affect the oxygen-carrying capability of this molecule. The most common abnormality involving hemoglobin is a decrease in the amount of hemoglobin. This can be an acute or chronic (anemia) situation. Abnormal hemoglobin structure also can pose problems, such as hemoglobin S, which is responsible for sickle cell anemia. Hemoglobin S has less affinity for oxygen than normal hemoglobin. Normal hemoglobin can become abnormal hemoglobin under certain conditions. Methemoglobin and carboxyhemoglobin are two examples. Methemoglobin occurs when the iron atoms within the hemoglobin molecule are oxidized from the ferrous state to the ferric state. Methemoglobin

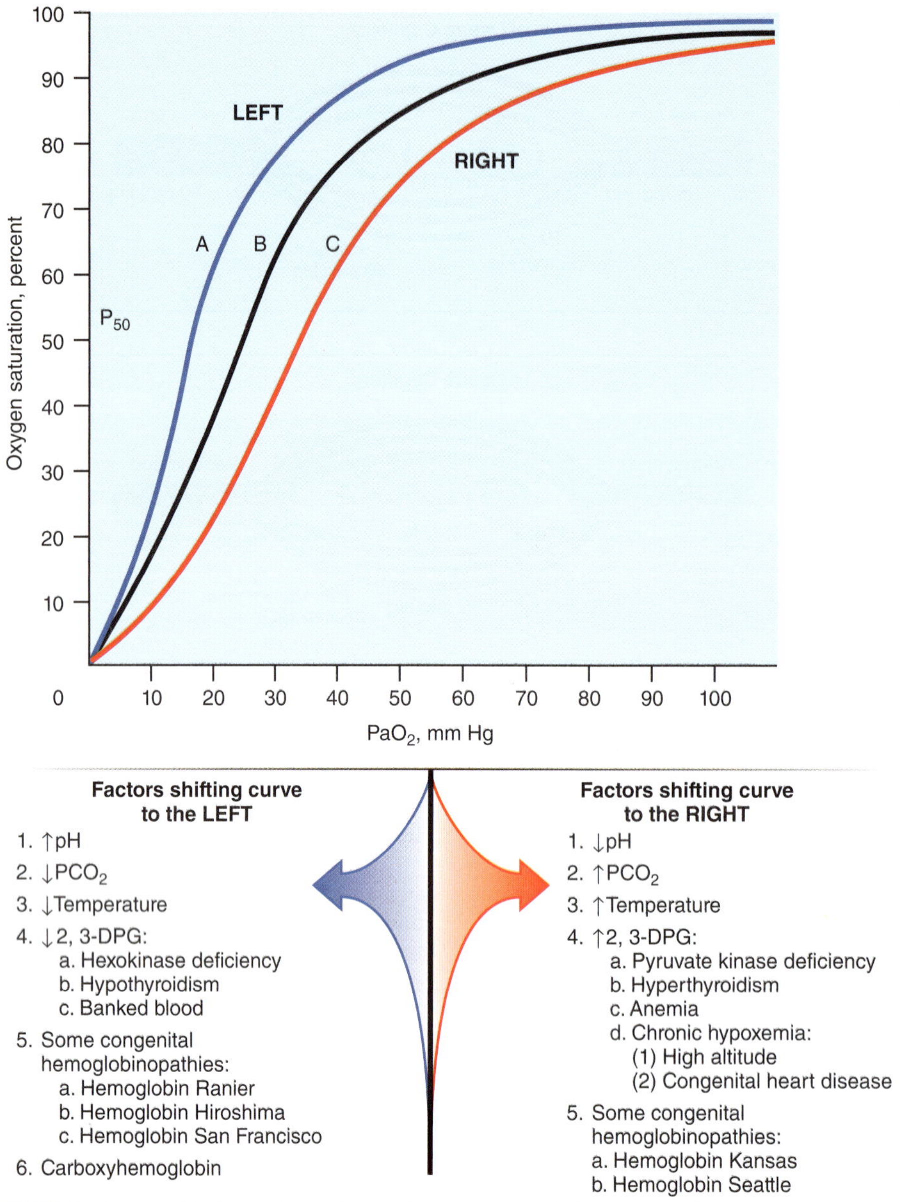

FIG. 15.20 Oxyhemoglobin Dissociation Curve. (A) The curve is shifted to the left because of hemoglobin's increased affinity for oxygen. (B) Standard oxyhemoglobin dissociation curve. (C) The curve is shifted to the right because of hemoglobin's decreased affinity for oxygen.

does not carry oxygen. Carboxyhemoglobin occurs when carbon monoxide combines with hemoglobin. Carbon monoxide uses the same binding site as oxygen and has a much greater affinity for hemoglobin.[21]

Carbon Dioxide Content

Carbon dioxide, one of the end products of aerobic cellular metabolism, is produced continuously within the cells. On its way from the cells to the lungs, carbon dioxide is transported within the plasma and the erythrocytes. Carbon dioxide is transported, physically dissolved as the $PaCO_2$ (5%), bound to blood proteins (including hemoglobin) in the form of carbaminohemoglobin compounds (5% to 1%), and combined with water to form carbonic acid (8% to 9%), some of which dissociates into hydrogen ions and bicarbonate. In the lungs, these methods of carbon dioxide carriage are reversed as the carbon dioxide leaves the plasma and erythrocytes for exhalation.[21]

KEY POINTS

Anatomy

- The pulmonary system consists of the thorax, conducting airways, respiratory airways, and pulmonary blood and lymph supply.
- The thorax consists of the thoracic cage, lungs, pleura, and muscles of ventilation, and its major function is to form the ventilatory pump and perform the work of breathing.
- The conducting airways consist of the upper airways, the trachea, and the bronchial tree, and their major functions are to warm and humidify the inhaled air, to prevent the entrance of foreign matter into the gas-exchange areas, and to serve as a passageway for air entering and leaving the gas-exchange regions of the lungs.
- The respiratory airways consist of the respiratory bronchioles and the alveoli, and their major function is gas exchange.

BOX 15.3 What Is 2,3-DPG?

2,3-diphosphoglycerate (2,3-DPG), an organic phosphate found primarily in red blood cells, has the ability to alter the affinity of hemoglobin for oxygen. When the level of 2,3-DPG increases within the red blood cells, hemoglobin's affinity for oxygen is decreased (a shift in the oxyhemoglobin curve to the right), making more oxygen available to the tissues. Increased synthesis of 2,3-DPG is an important component of the adaptive responses in healthy individuals to an acute need for more tissue oxygen. Tissue hypoxia stimulates the production of 2,3-DPG, and increased amounts have been found in patients with anemia, right-to-left shunts, or acute heart failure and in individuals residing at high altitudes.

A decrease in the amount of 2,3-DPG is detrimental to tissue oxygenation because it causes hemoglobin's affinity for oxygen to increase (a shift in the oxyhemoglobin curve to the left). Decreased 2,3-DPG levels occur with hypophosphatemia, septic shock, and the use of banked blood. Blood preserved with acid citrate dextrose loses most of its red cell 2,3-DPG within several days. Blood preserved with citrate phosphate dextrose maintains its 2,3-DPG levels for several weeks. Transfusion of blood with a low level of 2,3-DPG cannot be beneficial for tissue oxygenation until the 2,3-DPG level is restored, which may take 18 to 24 hours.

- The pulmonary circulation is the vascular system that forms the gas-exchange network surrounding the alveoli, and the bronchial circulation is the vascular system that perfuses the tracheobronchial tree.
- The lymphatic system is responsible for removing foreign particles and cell debris from the lungs for producing antibody-mediated and cell-mediated immune responses, for removing fluid from the lungs, and for keeping the alveoli clear.

Physiology

- The primary functions of the pulmonary system are ventilation and respiration.
- Ventilation is the movement of air in (inhalation) and out (exhalation) of the lungs.
- The work of breathing is the amount of work that must be performed to overcome the elastic and resistive properties of the lungs.
- Respiration is the process of gas exchange.
- External respiration takes place at the lung level through the alveolar-capillary membrane.
- Internal respiration is the diffusion of gases in and out of the cells at the tissue level.

Visit the Evolve site at http://evolve.elsevier.com/Urden/CriticalCareNursing for additional study materials.

REFERENCES

1. Rodriguez NE, Silva S. The respiratory system. In: Kacmarek RM, Stoller JK, Heuer AJ, eds. *Egan's Fundamentals of Respiratory Care*. 12th ed. St Louis: Elsevier; 2021.
2. Albertine KH, Ramirez MI, Morty RE. Anatomy. In: Broaddus VC, ed. *Murray and Nadel's Textbook of Respiratory Medicine*. 7th ed. Philadelphia: Elsevier; 2022.
3. Brashers VL. Structure and function of the pulmonary system. In: McCance KL, Huether SE, eds. *Pathophysiology: The Biologic Basis for Disease in Adults and Children*. 8th ed. St. Louis: Elsevier; 2019.
4. Charalampidis C, Youroukou A, Lazaridis G, et al. Pleura space anatomy. *J Thorac Dis*. 2015;7(Suppl 1):S27–S32. https://doi.org/10.3978/j.issn.2072-1439.2015.01.48.
5. Ricoy J, Rodríguez-Núñez N, Álvarez-Dobaño JM, et al. Diaphragmatic dysfunction. *Pulmonology*. 2019;25(4):223–235. https://doi.org/10.1016/j.pulmoe.2018.10.008.
6. McCool FD, Hilbert JH, Wolfe LF, Benditt JO. The respiratory system and neuromuscular diseases. In: Broaddus VC, ed. *Murray and Nadel's Textbook of Respiratory Medicine*. 7th ed. Philadelphia: Elsevier; 2022.
7. Mehran RJ. Fundamental and practical aspects of airway anatomy: from glottis to segmental bronchus. *Thorac Surg Clin*. 2018;28(2):117–125. https://doi.org/10.1016/j.thorsurg.2018.02.003.
8. Whitsett JA. Airway epithelial differentiation and mucociliary clearance. *Ann Am Thorac Soc*. 2018;15(Suppl 3):S143–S148. https://doi.org/10.1513/AnnalsATS.201802-128AW.
9. Sykes DL, Morice AH. The cough reflex: the Janus of respiratory medicine. *Front Physiol*. 2021;12:684080. https://doi.org/10.3389/fphys.2021.684080.
10. Pérez-Gil J. A recipe for a good clinical pulmonary surfactant. *Biomed J*. 2022;45(4):615–628. https://doi.org/10.1016/j.bj.2022.03.001.
11. Bootsma IT, Boerma EC, de Lange F, Scheeren TWL. The contemporary pulmonary artery catheter. Part 1: Placement and waveform analysis. *J Clin Monit Comput*. 2022;36(1):5–15. https://doi.org/10.1007/s10877-021-00662-8.
12. Poch D, Mandel J. Pulmonary hypertension. *Ann Intern Med*. 2021;174(4):ITC49–ITC64. https://doi.org/10.7326/AITC202104200.
13. Mccormack MC, West JD. Ventilation, blood flow, and gas exchange. In: Broaddus VC, ed. *Murray and Nadel's Textbook of Respiratory Medicine*. 7th ed. Philadelphia: Elsevier; 2022.
14. Kandathil A, Chamarthy M. Pulmonary vascular anatomy & anatomical variants. *Cardiovasc Diagn Ther*. 2018;8(3):201–207. https://doi.org/10.21037/cdt.2018.01.04.
15. Hopkins SR. Ventilation/perfusion relationships and gas exchange: Measurement approaches. *Compr Physiol*. 2020;10(3):1155–1205. https://doi.org/10.1002/cphy.c180042.
16. Mireles-Cabodevila E. Ventilation. In: Kacmarek RM, Stoller JK, Heuer AJ, eds. *Egan's Fundamentals of Respiratory Care*. 12th ed. St. Louis: Elsevier; 2021.
17. Kidson KM, Ayas NT, Henderson WR. Respiratory system mechanics and energetics. In: Broaddus VC, ed. *Murray and Nadel's Textbook of Respiratory Medicine*. 7th ed. Philadelphia: Elsevier; 2022.
18. Chowdhuri S, Badr MS. Control of ventilation in health and disease. *Chest*. 2017;151(4):917–929. https://doi.org/10.1016/j.chest.2016.12.002.
19. Hainsworth R. Cardiovascular control from cardiac and pulmonary vascular receptors. *Exp Physiol*. 2014;99(2):312–319. https://doi.org/10.1113/expphysiol.2013.072637.
20. Mallet RT, Burtscher J, Richalet JP, et al. Impact of high altitude on cardiovascular health: Current Perspectives. *Vasc Health Risk Manag*. 2021;17:317–335. https://doi.org/10.2147/VHRM.S294121.
21. Cohen Z. Gas exchange and transport. In: Kacmarek RM, Stoller JK, Heuer AJ, eds. *Egan's Fundamentals of Respiratory Care*. 12th ed. St. Louis: Elsevier; 2021.
22. Mallat J, Rahman N, Hamed F, et al. Pathophysiology, mechanisms, and managements of tissue hypoxia. *Anaesth Crit Care Pain Med*. 2022;41(4):101087. https://doi.org/10.1016/j.accpm.2022.101087.

16

Pulmonary Clinical Assessment

Darlene M. Burke

http://evolve.elsevier.com/Urden/CriticalCareNursing

Assessment of a patient with pulmonary dysfunction is a systematic process that incorporates an inquiry into the chronology of the present illness, better known as the *history*, and an investigation of the current physical manifestations, better known as the *focused physical assessment*. The purpose of the assessment is twofold: first, to recognize changes in the patient's pulmonary status that necessitate nursing or medical intervention, and second, to determine how the patient's pulmonary dysfunction is interfering with their self-care activities. After completion, the assessment serves as the foundation for developing the management plan for the patient. The assessment process can be brief or involve a detailed history and examination, depending on the nature and immediacy of the patient's situation. Whatever the setting, the nurse should develop and practice a sequential pattern of assessment to avoid omitting portions of the examination.

HISTORY

A thorough and accurate history is essential to the assessment process. The patient's history provides the foundation and direction for the rest of the assessment. The overall goal of the patient interview is to expose key clinical manifestations that will facilitate the identification of the underlying cause of the illness. This information then assists in the development of an appropriate management plan.

Initial Presentation

The patient's initial presentation determines the interview's rapidity and direction. For a patient in acute distress, the history is curtailed to just a few questions about the patient's chief complaint and precipitating events. For a patient in no apparent distress, the history focuses on five areas: (1) review of the patient's present illness, (2) overview of the patient's general respiratory status, (3) examination of the patient's general health status, (4) survey of the patient's family and social background, and (5) description of the patient's current symptoms. Specific items included in each of these areas are outlined in Box 16.1.

Common Symptoms

Symptoms common in a patient with a pulmonary disorder include dyspnea, cough, wheezing, edema, palpitations, fatigue, chest pain, hemoptysis, and sputum abnormalities. Information is elicited regarding the location, onset and duration, characteristics, setting, aggravating and alleviating factors, associated symptoms, and efforts to treat the symptoms. If the cough is productive, the patient is asked questions about the sputum's color, amount, odor, and consistency.[1]

FOCUSED PHYSICAL ASSESSMENT

Four techniques are used in physical assessment: inspection, palpation, percussion, and auscultation. *Inspection* is the process of looking intently at the patient. *Palpation* is touching the patient to judge the size, shape, texture, and temperature of the body surface or underlying structures. *Percussion* creates sound waves on the body's surface to determine the abnormal density of any underlying areas. *Auscultation* is the process of concentrated listening with a stethoscope to assess characteristics of body functions.

Inspection

Inspection of the patient focuses on three areas: (1) observation of the tongue and sublingual area, (2) assessment of chest wall configuration, and (3) evaluation of respiratory effort. If possible, patients are positioned upright.[2] Inspection usually begins during the interview.

Tongue and Sublingual Area

The patient's tongue and sublingual area are observed for a blue, gray, or dark purple tint or discoloration, indicating the presence of central cyanosis. *Central cyanosis* is a sign of hypoxemia, or inadequate blood oxygenation, and is life threatening. Central cyanosis occurs when reduced hemoglobin (unsaturated hemoglobin) exceeds 5 g/dL. The fingers and toes may also appear discolored, an indication of the presence of peripheral cyanosis.[3]

Chest Wall Configuration

The size and shape of the patient's chest wall are assessed for an increase in the anteroposterior diameter and structural deviations (Fig. 16.1). The ratio of anteroposterior diameter to lateral diameter ranges from 1:2 to 5:7 normally.[1] An increase in the anteroposterior diameter suggests chronic obstructive pulmonary disease.[1] The shape of the chest is inspected for any structural deviations. Some more frequently seen abnormalities are pectus excavatum, pectus carinatum, barrel chest, and spinal deformities. In *pectus excavatum* (funnel chest), the sternum and lower ribs are displaced posteriorly, creating a funnel or pit-shaped depression in the chest. This abnormality causes a decrease in the anteroposterior diameter of the chest and may interfere with respiratory function. In *pectus carinatum* (pigeon breast), the sternum projects forward, causing an increase in

BOX 16.1 **DATA COLLECTION**

Pulmonary History Common Pulmonary Symptoms

Cough

- Onset and duration
- Sudden or gradual
- Episodic or continuous
- Characteristics
- Dry or wet
- Hacking, hoarse, barking, or congested
- Productive or nonproductive
- Sputum
- Present or absent
- Frequency of production
- Appearance—color (e.g., clear, mucoid, purulent, bloodtinged, mostly bloody), foul odor, frothy
- Amount
- Pattern
- Paroxysmal
- Related to time of day, weather, activities, talking, or deep breathing
- Change over time
- Severity
- Causes fatigue
- Disrupts sleep or conversation
- Produces chest pain
- Associated symptoms
- Shortness of breath
- Chest pain or tightness with breathing
- Fever
- Upper respiratory tract signs (e.g., sore throat, congestion, increased mucus production)
- Noisy respirations or hoarseness
- Gagging or choking
- Anxiety, stress, or panic reactions
- Efforts made to treat
- Prescription or nonprescription medications
- Vaporizers
- Effective or ineffective

Shortness of Breath or Dyspnea on Exertion

- Onset and duration
- Sudden or gradual
- Gagging or choking episode a few days before onset
- Pattern
- Related to position—improves when sitting up or with head elevated; number of pillows used to alleviate problems
- Related to activity—exercise or eating; extent of activity that produces dyspnea
- Related to other factors—time of day, season, or exposure to something in the environment
- Harder to inhale or harder to exhale
- Severity
- Extent activity is limited
- Breathing itself causes fatigue
- Anxiety about getting enough air
- Associated symptoms
- Pain or discomfort—exact location in respiratory tree
- Cough, diaphoresis, swelling of ankles, or cyanosis
- Efforts made to treat
- Prescription or nonprescription medications
- Oxygen
- Effective or ineffective

Chest Pain

- Onset and duration
- Gradual or sudden
- Associated with trauma, coughing, or lower respiratory tract infection
- Associated symptoms
- Shallow breathing
- Uneven chest expansion
- Fever
- Cough
- Radiation of pain to neck or arms
- Anxiety about getting enough air
- Efforts made to treat
- Heat, splinting, or pain medication
- Effective or ineffective
- Pulmonary Risk Factors
- Tobacco use—current and past
- Type of tobacco—cigarettes, cigars, pipes, or smokeless
- Duration and amount—age started, inhale when smoking, amount used in the past and present
- Pack years—number of packs per day multiplied by number of years patient has smoked
- Efforts to quit—previous attempts and current interest
- Work environment
- Nature of work
- Environmental hazards—chemicals, vapors, dust, pulmonary irritants, or allergens
- Use of protective devices
- Home environment
- Location
- Possible allergens—pets, house plants, plants and trees outside the home, or other environmental hazards
- Type of heating
- Use of air conditioning or humidifier
- Ventilation
- Stairs to climb

Medical History

Child

- Infectious respiratory diseases
- Strep throat
- Mumps
- Tonsillitis
- Asthma
- Cystic fibrosis
- Immunizations

Adult

- Previous diagnosis of pulmonary disorders—dates of hospitalization
- Chronic pulmonary disease—date, treatment, and compliance with therapy
- Tuberculosis
- Bronchitis
- Emphysema
- Bronchiectasis
- Asthma
- Sinus infection
- Other chronic disorders—cardiovascular, cancer, musculoskeletal, neurologic, immune
- Obstruction of one or both nares
- Mouth breathing often necessary (especially at night)
- History of nasal discharge
- Compromised immune system function
- Nosebleed

Continued

BOX 16.1 DATA COLLECTION—cont'd

Pulmonary History Common Pulmonary Symptoms

- Sleep apnea
- Obstructive
- Central
- Previous tests
- Allergy testing
- Pulmonary function tests
- Tuberculin and fungal skin tests
- Chest radiographs

Surgical
- Thoracic trauma
- Thoracic surgery
- Nasal surgery or injury

Family History
- Tuberculosis
- Cystic fibrosis
- Emphysema
- Allergies
- Asthma
- Atopic dermatitis
- Smoking by household members
- Malignancy

Current Medication Use
- Inhalators
- Steroids
- Antibiotics
- Immunizations
- Pneumococcal (Pneumovax)
- Influenza

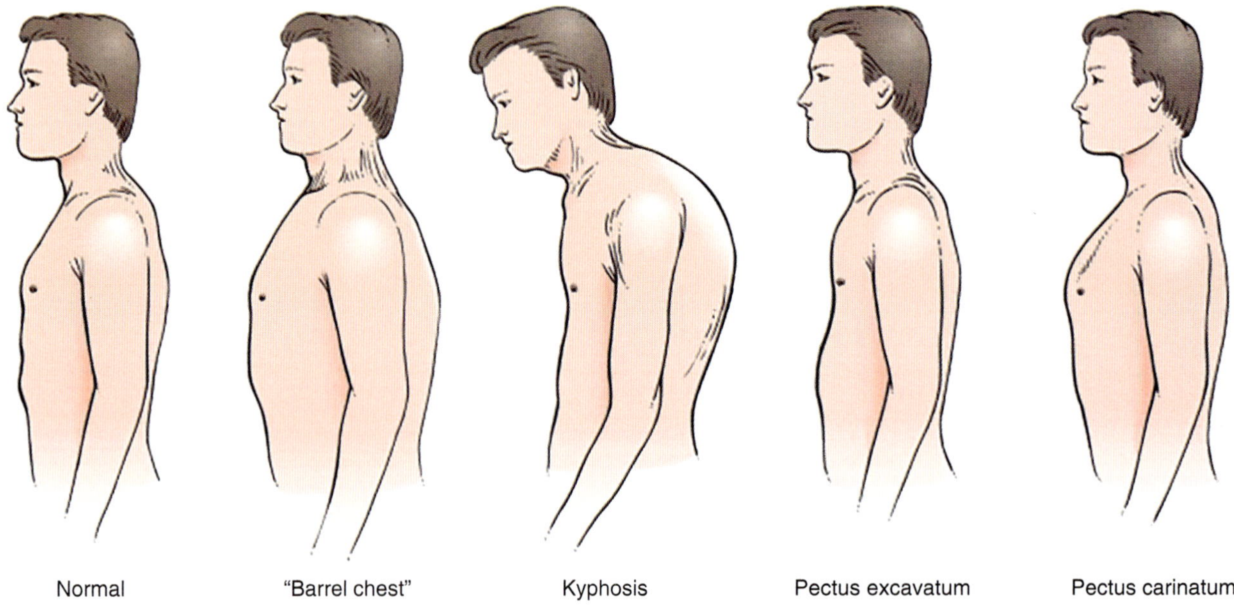

FIG. 16.1 Common Chest Wall Configurations. (From Schwartz MH. *Textbook of Physical Diagnosis*. 8th ed. Elsevier; 2021.)

the anteroposterior diameter of the chest. The *barrel chest* also increases the anteroposterior diameter of the chest and is characterized by displacement of the sternum forward and the ribs outward). Spinal deformities, such as *kyphosis, lordosis*, and *scoliosis*, also may be present and can interfere with respiratory function.[4]

Respiratory Effort

Respirations should be even, unlabored, and regular at a rate of 12 to 20 breaths per minute.[2] An imbalance between respiratory effort, muscle capacity, and ventilatory demand may lead to muscle fatigue or deconditioning, abnormal gas exchange, or abnormal breathing patterns.[5] There are various respiratory patterns (Fig. 16.2). Some more commonly seen patterns in patients with pulmonary dysfunction are tachypnea, hyperventilation, and air trapping. *Tachypnea* is manifested by an increase in the rate and a decrease in the depth of ventilation. *Hyperventilation* is manifested by an increase in the rate and depth of ventilation. Patients with chronic obstructive pulmonary disease often experience obstructive breathing or *air trapping*. As the patient breathes, air becomes trapped in the lungs and ventilations become progressively shallower until the patient actively and forcefully exhales.[6]

Additional Assessment Areas

Other areas assessed are the use of accessory muscles, the presence of intercostal retractions, unequal chest wall movement, and flaring of nares.[2] The presence of iatrogenic features, such as chest tubes, central venous lines, artificial airways, and nasogastric tubes, is identified because these features may affect assessment findings.

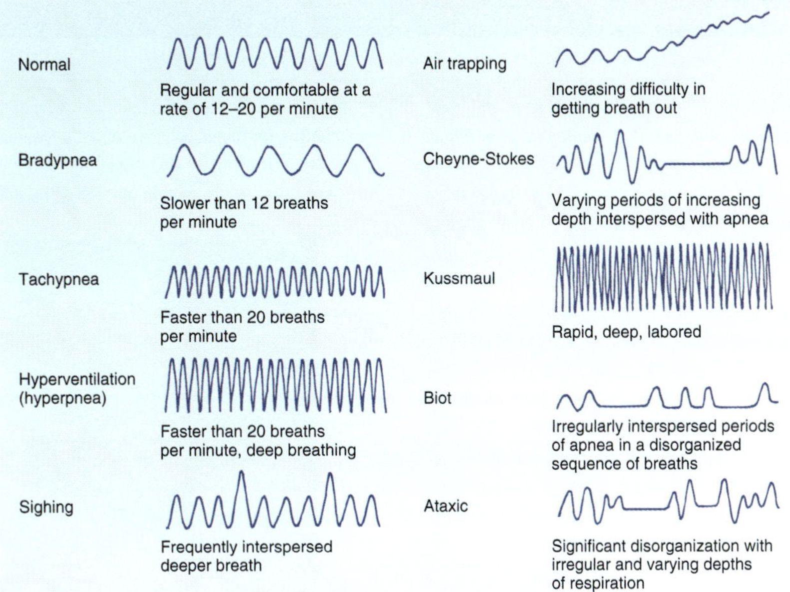

FIG. 16.2 Patterns of Respiration. (From Ball JW, Dains J, Flynn J, et al. *Seidel's Guide to Physical Examination: An Interprofessional Approach*. 10th ed. Elsevier; 2023.)

Palpation

Palpation of the patient focuses on three areas: (1) confirmation of the position of the trachea, (2) assessment of thoracic expansion, and (3) evaluation of fremitus. The thorax is assessed for tenderness, lumps, or bony deformities.

Position of the Trachea

The position of the patient's trachea is confirmed at midline and is assessed by placing the fingers in the suprasternal notch and moving upward (Fig. 16.3).[6] Deviation of the trachea to either side may indicate a pneumothorax, unilateral pneumonia, diffuse pulmonary fibrosis, a large pleural effusion, or severe atelectasis. With atelectasis, the trachea shifts to the same side as the problem; with pneumothorax, the trachea shifts to the opposite side of the problem.[4]

Thoracic Expansion

The patient's thoracic expansion is assessed for the degree and symmetry of movement[3] and is evaluated by placing the hands on the anterolateral chest with the thumbs extended along the costal margin, pointing to the xiphoid process, or on the posterolateral chest with the thumbs on either side of the spine at the level of the 10th rib (Fig. 16.4). The patient is instructed to take a few normal breaths and then a few deep breaths. Chest movement is assessed for equality, which signifies symmetry of thoracic expansion.[4,6]Asymmetry is an abnormal finding that can occur with pneumothorax, pneumonia, or other disorders that interfere with lung inflation. The degree of chest movement is felt to ascertain the extent of lung expansion. The thumbs should separate 3 to 5 cm during deep inspiration.[1,6] Lung expansion of a hyperinflated chest is less than normal chest expansion.[1,6]

Tactile Fremitus

The patient is assessed for tactile fremitus to identify, describe, and localize areas of increased or decreased fremitus. Tactile fremitus refers to the palpable vibrations felt through the chest wall when the patient speaks and is assessed by placing the palmar surface of the hands against opposite sides of the chest wall and having the patient repeat the word "ninety-nine" (Fig. 16.5). The hands are moved systematically around the thorax until the anterior, posterior, and both lateral areas have been assessed.[4,6] If only one hand is used, the hand is moved from one side of the chest to the corresponding area on the other side of the chest until all areas have been assessed.[6]

Tactile fremitus varies from patient to patient and depends on the pitch and intensity of the voice. Fremitus is described as normal, decreased, or increased. With normal fremitus, vibrations can be felt over the trachea but are barely palpable over the periphery.[7] With decreased fremitus, there is interference with the transmission of vibrations. Examples of disorders that decrease fremitus include pleural effusion, pneumothorax, bronchial obstruction, pleural thickening, and emphysema. With increased fremitus, there is an increase in the transmission of vibrations. Examples of disorders that increase fremitus include pneumonia, lung cancer, and pulmonary fibrosis.[1]

Percussion

Percussion of the patient focuses on two areas: (1) evaluation of the underlying lung structure and (2) assessment of diaphragmatic excursion. Although the technique is not used often, percussion helps confirm suspected abnormalities.

Underlying Lung Structure

The patient's underlying lung structure is evaluated to estimate the amounts of air, liquid, or solid material present. This assessment is performed by placing the middle finger of the nondominant hand on the chest wall. The distal portion, between the last joint and the nail bed, is then struck with the middle finger of the dominant hand. The hands are moved systematically and side to side around the thorax to compare similar areas until the anterior, posterior, and both lateral areas have been assessed (Fig. 16.6). Five tones can be elicited: resonance, hyperresonance, tympany, dullness, and flatness. Differences in intensity, pitch, duration, and quality distinguish these tones. Table 16.1

SUPPORTING NURSE WELL-BEING

Emotional Wellness

I have been an RN for almost 4 years, most of it worked in critical care, and I was recently promoted to day shift supervisor. Although it is exciting to be in a new role, it has also been challenging to be now a supervisor to nurses with whom I was previously "one of them." Most of them have been great and happy that I took on this new position. I have found that the new role has been demanding as I have so many responsibilities and duties that I have had to learn and accomplish. I do have a supportive manager who has helped me a lot. Lately, I feel drained after my shift—differently than when I provided direct nursing care. The outcomes of my work are often not seen immediately, and there seem to be so many things left unfinished. I'm really at a loss for whether I will succeed in this role. Recently, I discovered a method called mindfulness and have been practicing it. In addition, my RN cousin recommended getting into some form of exercise to relieve some of my stress. I am beginning to see a positive difference now!

The example described above describes a new role's stress on a nurse, even though there was support and encouragement from the manager and co-workers. According to the Centers for Disease Control, an increasing number of U.S. adults are dealing with stress that can lead to mental health problems. In 2022, more than 32% of U.S. adults reported having symptoms of anxiety or depression.[1] Sadness, fear, worry, and other emotions can negatively affect persons during and after challenging and troublesome times. In addition to daily influences, grief, and loss of family members or close friends, worsening health problems and experiences related to diversity, equity, and inclusion can further contribute to stress. Persons who are emotionally well have fewer negative emotions and can bounce back from difficulties much faster. Building resilience is an essential component of being emotionally well. Emotional wellness is the ability to handle life's stressors and adapt to challenging times successfully. There are several elements to achieving emotional wellness: building resilience; reducing stress; being mindful; coping with loss; strengthening social connections; and getting quality sleep.[2] Another critical factor is social connectedness, which is deeply personal. Even small acts of connection lay the groundwork for building supported, valued, inclusive, and meaningful relationships. One must establish and maintain social connections and consider the support you give, receive, and have available. Strategies to strengthen social bonds and inhibit barriers to social connection include:

- Develop healthy physical habits
- Take time for yourself each day; set priorities
- Look at problems from different angles and learn from your mistakes
- Show compassion for yourself
- Relax before bedtime and limit the use of electronics
- Find and use mindfulness resources
- Take care of yourself in times of loss and grief; talk to a caring friend or relative; try not to make any crucial decisions right away
- Join a group focused on a favorite hobby or something new you want to learn
- Volunteer for things you care about in your community
- Expand and diversify your social network by making a new acquaintance or friend, especially someone who might be different from you.

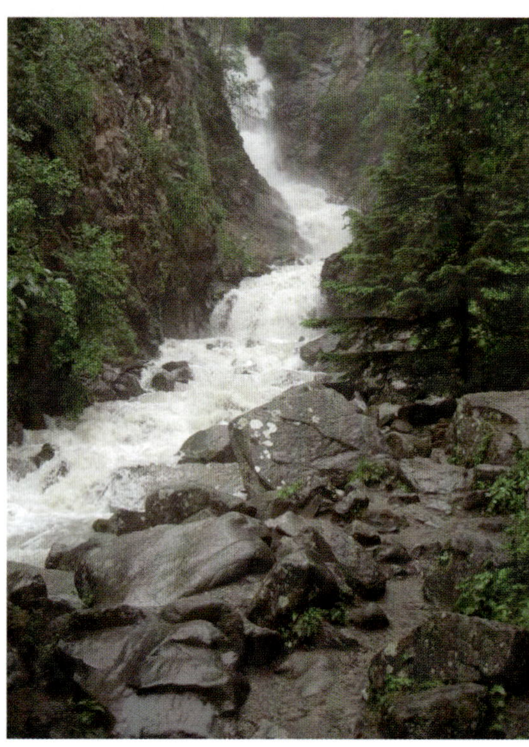

Each person deserves a day in which no problems are confronted, no solutions searched for. Each of us needs to withdraw from cares which will not withdraw from us.

Maya Angelou

References

1. *Emotional Well-Being.* Centers for Disease Control and Prevention; 2023. Reviewed February 10. https://www.cdc.gov/emotional-wellbeing/. Accessed August 8, 2023.
2. *Your Healthiest Self: Wellness Toolkits.* National Institutes of Health; 2023. Reviewed May 19. https://www.nih.gov/wellnesstoolkits. Accessed August 8, 2023.

describes the different percussion tones and their associated conditions.[4]

Diaphragmatic Excursion

The patient is assessed for diaphragmatic excursion to evaluate the movement of the diaphragm. This assessment is accomplished by measuring the difference in the level of the diaphragm on inspiration and expiration. It is performed by instructing the patient to inhale and hold the breath. The posterior chest is percussed downward, over the intercostal spaces, until the dull sound produced by the diaphragm is heard. The spot is marked. The patient is then instructed to take a few breaths in and out, exhale completely, and then hold their breath. The posterior chest is percussed again, and the new area of dullness over the diaphragm is located and marked. The difference between the two spots is identified and measured (Fig. 16.7). Normal diaphragmatic excursion is 3 to 5 cm.[6] Diaphragmatic excursion is decreased in ascites, pregnancy, hepatomegaly, and emphysema and is increased in pleural effusion and disorders that elevate the diaphragm, such as atelectasis or paralysis.[4]

Auscultation

Auscultation of the patient focuses on three areas: (1) evaluation of normal breath sounds, (2) identification of abnormal breath sounds, and (3) assessment of voice sounds. Auscultation requires a quiet environment, proper patient positioning, and a bare chest.[8] Breath sounds are best heard with the patient in the upright position.[1]

Normal Breath Sounds

The patient's breath sounds are auscultated to evaluate the quality of air movement through the lungs and identify abnormal sounds. This assessment is performed by placing the diaphragm of the stethoscope against the chest wall and instructing the patient to breathe in and out slowly with their mouth open.[2] Breath sounds are assessed during both inspiration and expiration. Auscultation is done systematically: side to side, top to bottom, posteriorly, laterally, and anteriorly (Fig. 16.8).[1] Normal breath sounds are different, depending on their location. There are three categories: vesicular, bronchovesicular, and bronchial. Fig. 16.9 describes the characteristics of normal breath sounds and their associated conditions.[1,2,8]

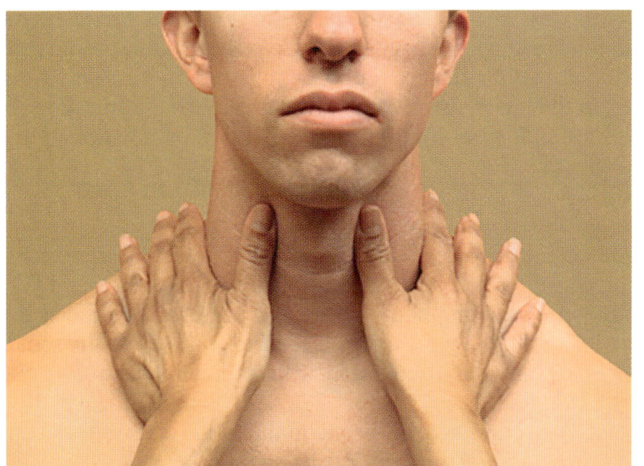

FIG. 16.3 Position of the Trachea. (From Wilson SF, Giddens JF. *Health Assessment for Nursing Practice.* 7th ed. Elsevier; 2022.)

Abnormal Breath Sounds

Abnormal breath sounds are identified after normal breath sounds have been delineated. There are three categories of abnormal breath sounds: absent or diminished breath sounds, displaced bronchial breath sounds, and adventitious breath sounds. Table 16.2 describes the various abnormal breath sounds and their associated conditions.[1,2,8]

An *absent* or *diminished breath sound* indicates little or no airflow to a particular portion of the lung (a small segment or an entire lung). *Displaced bronchial breath sounds* are normal bronchial sounds heard in the peripheral lung fields instead of over the trachea. This condition is usually indicative of fluid or exudate in the alveoli.[8] *Adventitious breath sounds* are extra or added sounds heard in addition to the other sounds previously discussed. They are classified as crackles, rhonchi, wheezes, and friction rubs.

Adventitious breath sounds. *Crackles*, also called *rales*, are short, discrete popping or crackling sounds produced by fluid in the small airways or alveoli or by the snapping open of collapsed airways during inspiration. They can be heard on inspiration and expiration and may clear with coughing.[8]

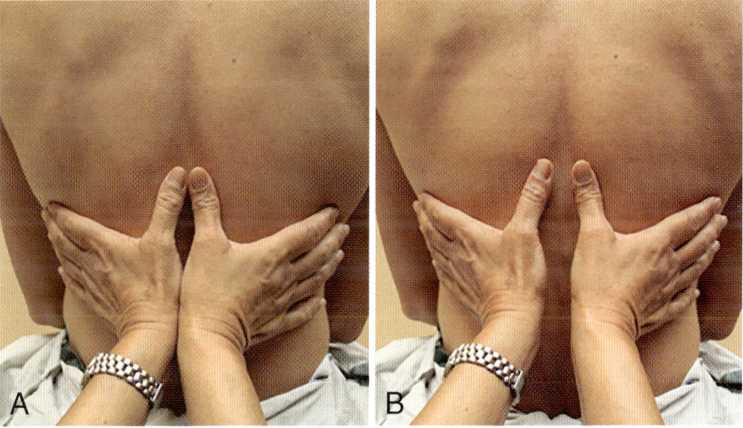

FIG. 16.4 Thoracic Expansion. (A) Position of the hands for palpation of posterior thorax excursion. (B) As the patient inhales, movement of chest excursion separates the nurse's thumbs. (From Wilson SF, Giddens JF. *Health Assessment for Nursing Practice.* 7th ed. Elsevier; 2022.)

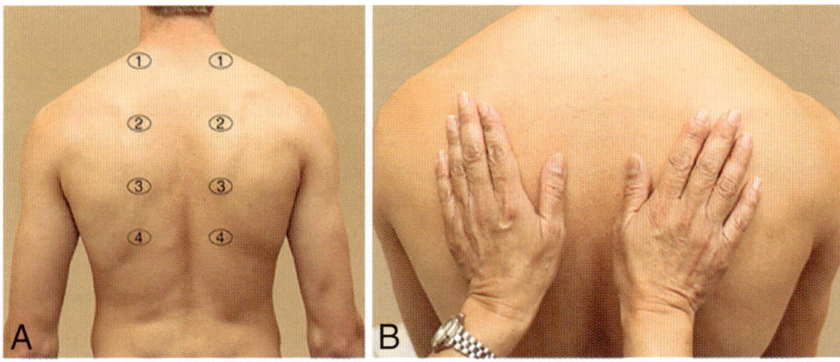

FIG. 16.5 Tactile Fremitus. (A) Hand position for assessment. (B) Simultaneous application of the fingertips of both hands to compare sides. (From Wilson SF, Giddens JF. *Health Assessment for Nursing Practice.* 7th ed. Elsevier; 2022.)

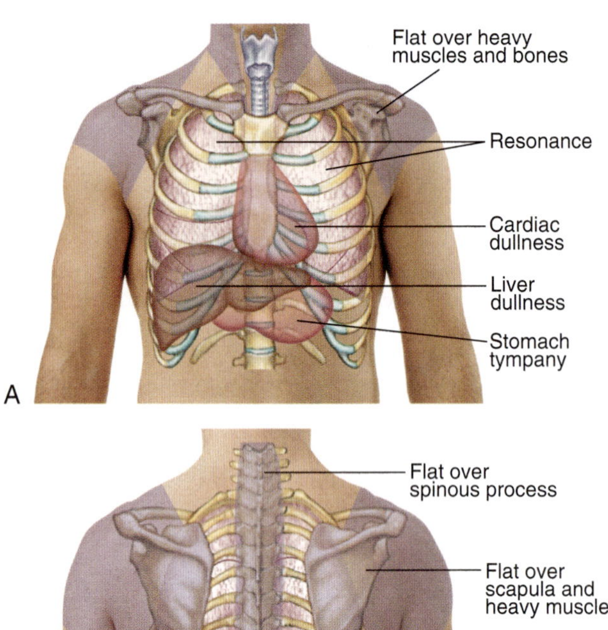

FIG. 16.6 Percussion Tones of Underlying Lung Structures. (A) Anterior view. (B) Posterior view. (From Ball JW, Dains J, Flynn J, et al. *Seidel's Guide to Physical Examination: An Interprofessional Approach.* 10th ed. Elsevier; 2023.)

TABLE 16.1 Percussion Tones

Tone	Description	Condition
Resonance	Intensity: Loud Pitch: Low Duration: Long Quality: Hollow	Normal lung Bronchitis
Hyperresonance	Intensity: Very loud Pitch: Very low Duration: Long Quality: Booming	Asthma Emphysema Pneumothorax
Tympany	Intensity: Loud Pitch: Musical Duration: Medium Quality: Drumlike	Large pneumothorax Emphysematous blebs
Dullness	Intensity: Medium Pitch: Medium-high Duration: Medium Quality: Thudlike	Atelectasis Pleural effusion Pulmonary edema Pneumonia Lung mass
Flatness	Intensity: Soft Pitch: High Duration: Short Quality: Extremely dull	Massive atelectasis Pneumonectomy

Crackles can be further classified as fine, medium, or coarse, depending on pitch.[8] *Rhonchi* are coarse, rumbling, low-pitched sounds produced by airflow over secretions in the larger airways or narrowing of the large airways. They are heard mainly on expiration and sometimes can be cleared with coughing. Rhonchi can be further classified as bubbling, gurgling, or sonorous, depending on the characteristics of the sound.[8] *Wheezes* are high-pitched, squeaking, whistling sounds produced by airflow through narrowed small airways. They are heard mainly on expiration but may be heard throughout the ventilatory cycle. Depending on their severity, wheezes can be further classified as mild, moderate, or severe.[8] A *pleural friction rub* is a creaking, leathery, loud, dry, coarse sound produced by irritated pleural surfaces rubbing together. It is usually heard best in the lower anterolateral chest area during inspiration and expiration. Pleural friction rubs are caused by inflammation of the pleura.[1]

Voice Sounds

Assessment of voice sounds is particularly helpful in detecting lung consolidation or lung compression. Three abnormal voice sounds are bronchophony, whispering pectoriloquy, and egophony.[8] *Bronchophony* describes a condition in which the spoken voice is heard on auscultation with higher intensity and clarity than usual. Usually, the spoken word is muffled when heard through the stethoscope. Bronchophony is assessed by placing the diaphragm of the stethoscope against the posterior side of the patient's chest and instructing the patient to say "ninety-nine." When the sound heard is clear, distinct, and loud, bronchophony is present.[8]

Whispering pectoriloquy describes a condition of unusually clear transmission of the whispered voice on auscultation. Typically, the whispered word is unintelligible when heard through the stethoscope. Whispering pectoriloquy is assessed by placing the stethoscope against the posterior side of the chest and instructing the patient to whisper "one, two, three." When the sound heard is clear and distinct, whispering pectoriloquy is present.[8] *Egophony* describes a condition in which the voice sounds increase in intensity and develop a nasal bleating quality on auscultation. Egophony is assessed by placing the stethoscope against the posterior side of the patient's chest and instructing the patient to say "e-e-e." Egophony is present when the "e" sound changes to an "a" sound.[1,8]

ASSESSMENT FINDINGS OF COMMON DISORDERS

Table 16.3 presents various common pulmonary disorders and their associated assessment findings.

KEY POINTS

History

- A review of the patient's current illness and symptoms, including the presence or absence of shortness of breath, chest pain, and cough, is essential to the patient's medical history.
- As the patient's condition permits, additional information is obtained regarding their general respiratory status; general health status; and family and social background, including tobacco use, work environment, and home environment.

Focused Physical Assessment

- Inspection focuses on the tongue and sublingual area, chest wall configuration, and respiratory effort.
- Palpation focuses on the position of the trachea, thoracic expansion, and fremitus (normal, decreased, or increased).

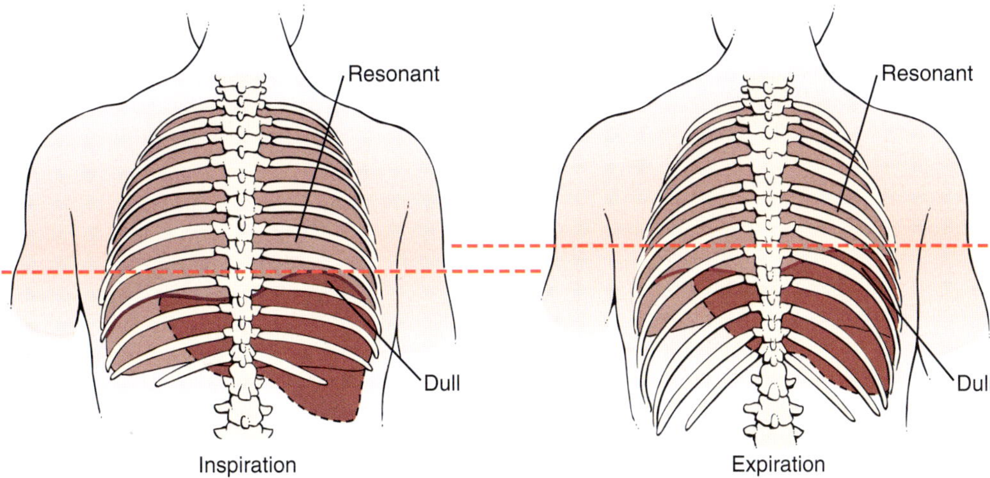

FIG. 16.7 Diaphragmatic Excursion. During inspiration *(left figure)*, percussion in the right seventh posterior interspace at the midscapular line would be resonant due to the presence of the underlying lung. During expiration *(right figure)*, the liver and diaphragm move up. Percussion in the same area would now be dull because of the presence of the underlying liver. (From Schwartz MH. *Textbook of Physical Diagnosis*. 8th ed. Elsevier; 2021.)

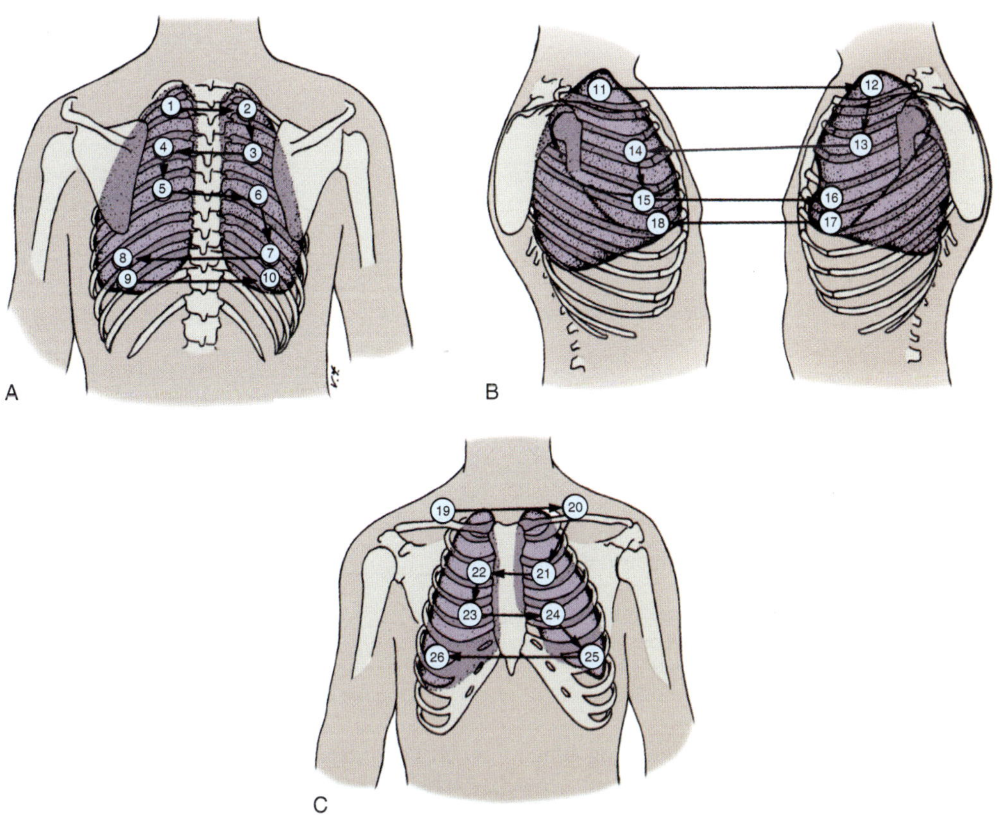

FIG. 16.8 Auscultation Sequence. (A) Posterior. (B) Lateral. (C) Anterior. (From Perry AG, Potter PA, Ostendorf WR, et al. *Clinical Nursing Skills and Techniques*. 10th ed. Elsevier; 2022.)

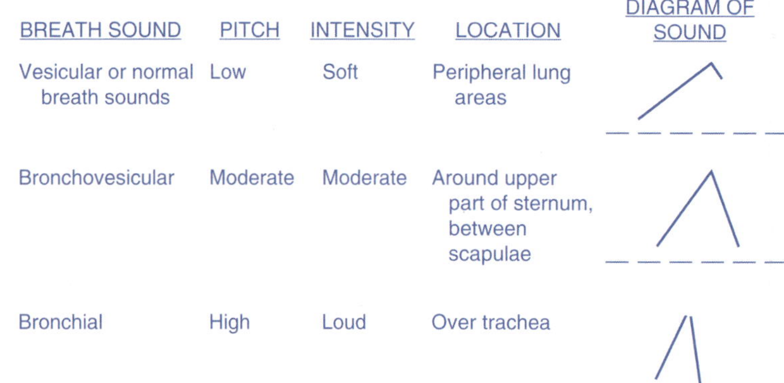

FIG. 16.9 Characteristics of Normal Breath Sounds. (From Kacmarek RM, Stoller JK, Heuer AJ, eds. *Egan's Fundamentals of Respiratory Care.* 12th ed. Elsevier; 2021.)

TABLE 16.2 Abnormal Breath Sounds

Abnormal Sound	Description	Condition
Absent breath sounds	No airflow to a particular portion of the lung	Pneumothorax Pneumonectomy Emphysematous blebs Pleural effusion Lung mass Massive atelectasis Complete airway obstruction
Diminished breath sounds	Little airflow to a particular portion of the lung	Emphysema Pleural effusion Pleurisy Atelectasis Pulmonary fibrosis
Displaced bronchial sounds	Bronchial sounds heard in peripheral lung fields	Atelectasis with secretions Lung mass with exudates Pneumonia Pleural effusion Pulmonary edema
Crackles (rales)	Short, discrete popping or crackling sounds	Pulmonary edema Pneumonia Pulmonary fibrosis Atelectasis Bronchiectasis
Rhonchi	Coarse, rumbling, low-pitched sounds	Pneumonia Asthma Bronchitis Bronchospasm
Wheezes	High-pitched, squeaking, whistling sounds	Asthma Bronchospasm
Pleural friction rub	Creaking, leathery, loud, dry, coarse sounds	Pleural effusion Pleurisy

- Percussion (when performed) focuses on underlying lung structure and diaphragmatic excursion.
- Auscultation focuses on the presence or absence of normal breath sounds (vesicular, bronchovesicular, and bronchial), abnormal breath sounds (diminished or absent breath sounds, displaced bronchial breath sounds, and adventitious breath sounds), and voice sounds (bronchophony, whispering pectoriloquy, and egophony).
- Adventitious breath sounds are classified as crackles, rhonchi, wheezes, and friction rubs.
- Auscultation is done systematically: side to side, top to bottom, posteriorly, laterally, and anteriorly.

Visit the Evolve site at http://evolve.elsevier.com/Urden/CriticalCareNursing for additional study materials.

TABLE 16.3 Assessment Findings With Associated Lung Conditions

Condition[a]	Breath Sounds	Description	Inspection	Palpation	Percussion	Auscultation
Normal Lung	Inspiration > expiration Pitch: Low Intensity: Soft Adventitious sounds: None	Tracheobronchial tree and alveoli are clear; pleurae are thin and close together; chest wall is mobile	Good, symmetric rib and diaphragmatic movement Anteroposterior diameter < transverse diameter Respirations 12–20 breaths/min and regular	Trachea: Midline Expansion: Adequate, symmetric Tactile fremitus: Moderate and symmetric No lesions or tenderness	Resonant Diaphragmatic excursion: 3–5 cm	Breath sounds: Vesicular Vocal resonance: Muffled Adventitious sounds: None except for a few transient crackles at bases
Asthma Bronchospasm	Inspiration = Expiration Pitch: Moderate Intensity: Soft Adventitious sounds: Expiratory sibilant wheezes	Asthma is characterized by intermittent episodes of airway obstruction caused by bronchospasm, excessive bronchial secretion, or edema of bronchial mucosa; resultant airway resistance, especially during expiration, produces symptoms of wheezing, dyspnea, and chest tightness	Cyanosis Air trapping with audible wheezing Use of accessory muscles of respiration Increased respiratory rate	Tactile fremitus: Decreased	Hyperresonant	Breath sounds: Distant Vocal resonance: Decreased Adventitious sounds: Wheezes

Continued

TABLE 16.3 **Assessment Findings With Associated Lung Conditions—cont'd**

Atelectasis 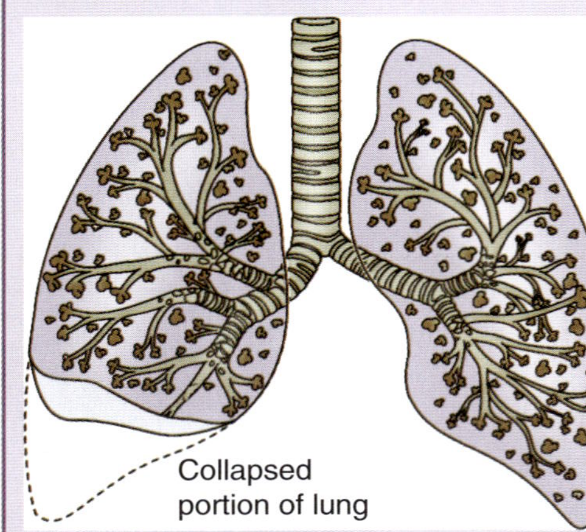 	Over empty area: Inspiration > expiration Pitch: Low or absent Intensity: Soft or absent Adventitious sounds: Fine, high-pitched crackles over terminal portion of inspiration if bronchus patent **Note**: Over consolidated lung: Bronchial breath sounds, crackles, and wheezes 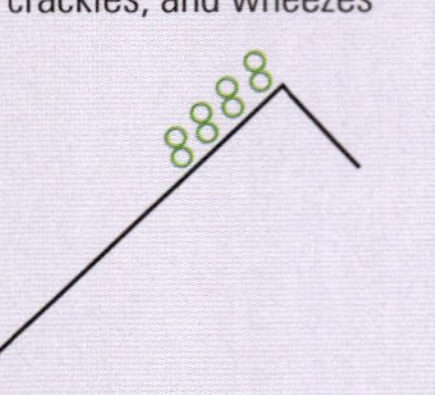	Atelectasis is collapse of alveolar lung tissue, and findings reflect presence of small, airless lung; this condition is caused by complete obstruction of draining bronchus by tumor, thick secretions, or aspirated foreign body or by compression of lung	Less chest motion on affected side Affected side retracted, with ribs appearing close together Cough Rapid, shallow breathing	Trachea: Shifted to affected side Expansion: Decreased on affected side Tactile fremitus: Decreased or absent	Dull to flat over collapsed lung Hyperresonant over remainder of affected hemithorax	Breath sounds: Decreased or absent Vocal resonance: Varies in intensity, usually reduced or absent in affected area Adventitious sounds: Fine, high-pitched crackles may be heard over terminal portion of inspiration
Bronchiectasis 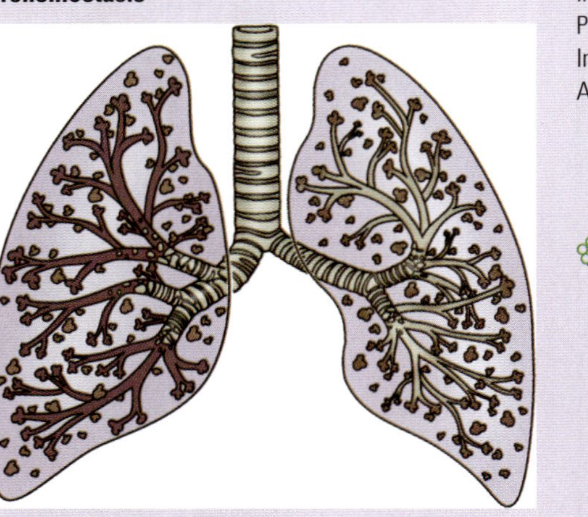	Inspiration > expiration Pitch: Low Intensity: Soft Adventitious sounds: Crackles (sometimes disappear after) 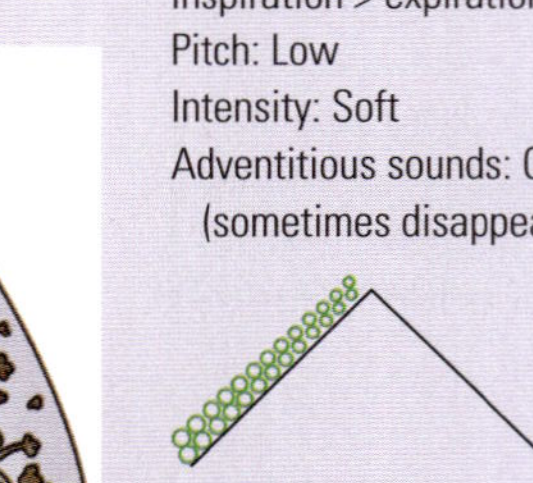	Bronchiectasis is abnormal dilation of bronchi or bronchioles, or both (coughing)	If mild, respirations are normal If severe, tachypnea Less expansion of affected side Cough with purulent sputum	Trachea: Midline or deviated toward affected side Expansion: Decreased on affected side Tactile fremitus: Increased	Resonant or dull	Breath sounds: Usually vesicular Vocal resonance: Usually muffled Adventitious sounds: Crackles

TABLE 16.3 Assessment Findings With Associated Lung Conditions—cont'd

Condition[a]	Breath Sounds	Description	Inspection	Palpation	Percussion	Auscultation
Bronchitis, Acute 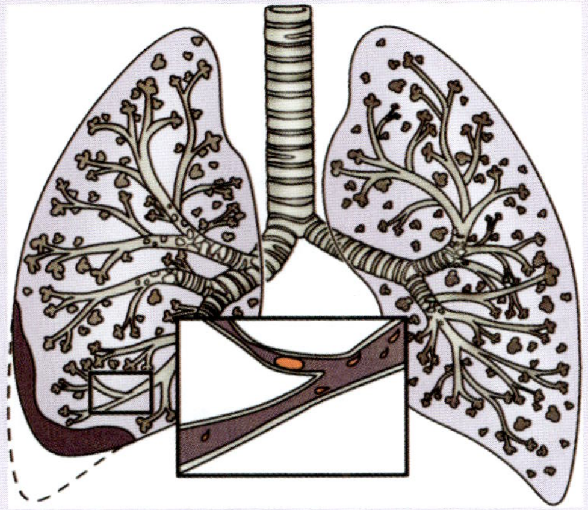	Inspiration ≥ expiration Pitch: Low Intensity: Soft Adventitious sounds: Localized crackles, expiratory sibilant wheezes 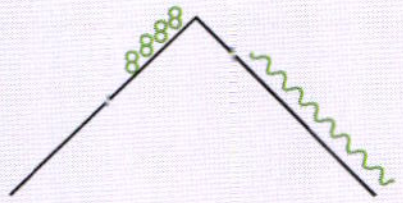	Acute bronchitis is inflammation of bronchial tree characterized by partial bronchial obstruction and secretions or constrictions; it results in abnormally deflated portions of lung	If severe, tachypnea and cyanosis Rasping cough with mucoid sputum	Tactile fremitus: Normal to increased	Resonant	Breath sounds: Vesicular Vocal resonance: Moderate Adventitious sounds: Localized crackles, sibilant wheezes
Emphysema 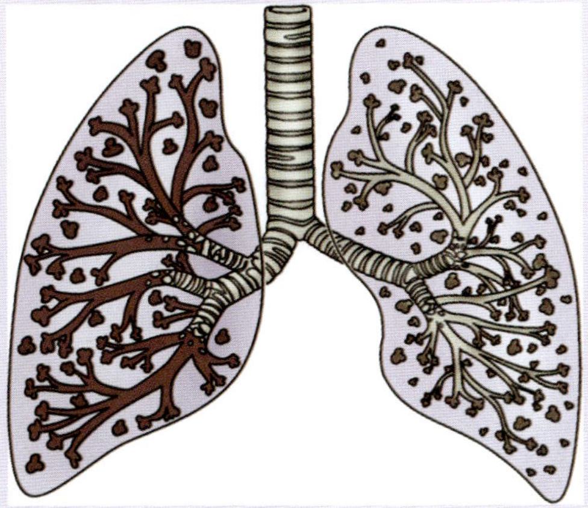	Inspiration = expiration Pitch: Low to very low Intensity: Soft to very soft Adventitious sounds: Occasional rhonchi and/or sibilant wheezes; fine inspiratory crackles 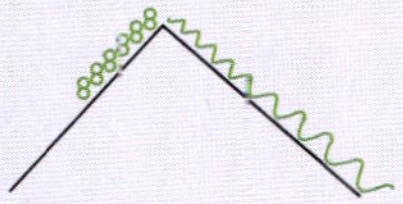	Emphysema is a permanent hyperinflation of lung beyond terminal bronchioles, with destruction of alveolar walls; airway resistance is increased, especially on expiration	Dyspnea with exertion Barrel chest Tachypnea Use of accessory muscles of respiration	Expansion: Limited Tactile fremitus: Decreased	Resonant to hyperresonant Diaphragmatic excursion: Decreased	Breath sounds: Decreased intensity; often prolonged expiration Vocal resonance: Muffled or decreased Adventitious sounds: Occasional wheezes; often fine crackles in late inspiration

Continued

TABLE 16.3 Assessment Findings With Associated Lung Conditions—cont'd

Pleural Effusion and Thickening 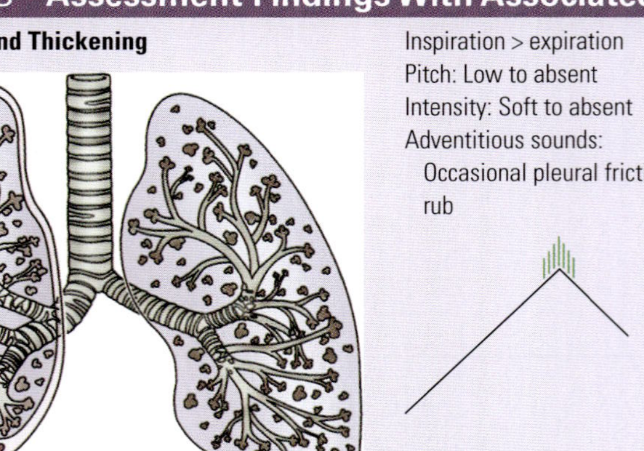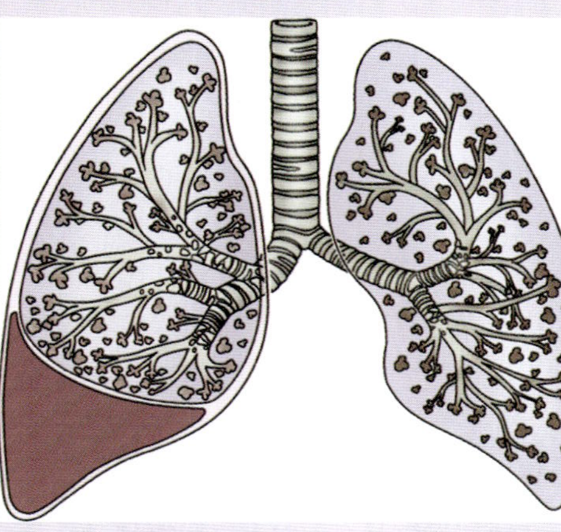	Inspiration > expiration Pitch: Low to absent Intensity: Soft to absent Adventitious sounds: Occasional pleural friction rub	Pleural effusion is collection of fluid in pleural space; if pleural effusion is prolonged, fibrous tissue may also accumulate in pleural space; clinical picture depends on amount of fluid or fibrosis present and rapidity of development; fluid tends to gravitate to most dependent areas of thorax, and adjacent lung is compressed	Tachypnea Decrease in definition of intercostal spaces on affected side Dyspnea	Trachea: Deviation toward normal side Expansion: Decreased on affected side Tactile fremitus: Decreased or absent	Dull to flat No diaphragmatic excursion on affected side	Breath sounds: Decreased or absent Vocal resonance: Muffled or absent; if fluid compresses lung, sounds may be bronchial over compression, and bronchophony, egophony, and whisper pectoriloquy may be present Adventitious sounds: Pleural friction rub sometimes present
Pneumonia With Consolidation 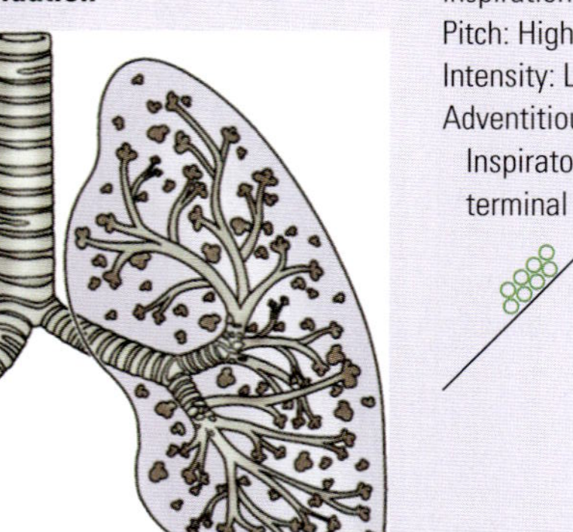	Inspiration = expiration Pitch: High Intensity: Loud Adventitious sounds: Inspiratory crackles in terminal third of inspiration	Pneumonia with consolidation occurs when alveolar air is replaced by fluid or tissue; physical findings depend on amount of parenchymal tissue involved	Tachypnea Guarding and less motion on affected side	Expansion: Limited on affected side Tactile fremitus: Usually increased, but may be weak if bronchus leading to affected area is plugged	Dull to flat	Breath sounds: Increased in intensity; bronchovesicular or bronchial breath sounds over affected area Vocal resonance: Increased bronchophony, egophony, whisper pectoriloquy present Adventitious sounds: Inspiratory crackles in terminal third of inspiration

TABLE 16.3 Assessment Findings With Associated Lung Conditions—cont'd

Condition[a]	Breath Sounds	Description	Inspection	Palpation	Percussion	Auscultation
Pneumothorax	Inspiration > expiration Pitch: Low to absent Intensity: Soft to absent Adventitious sounds: None	Pneumothorax implies air in pleural space 1. Closed type: Air in pleural space does not communicate with air in lung 2. Open type: Air in pleural space freely communicates with air in lung; air in pleural space is atmospheric 3. Tension type: Air in pleural space communicates with air in lungs only on inspiration; air pressure in pleural space is greater than atmospheric pressure Physical signs depend on degree of lung collapse and presence or absence of pleural effusion	Restricted lung expansion on affected side If large, tachypnea Bulging in intercostal spaces on affected side Cyanosis	Trachea: Deviated toward normal side Expansion: Decreased on affected side Tactile fremitus: Absent	Hyperresonant Decreased diaphragmatic excursion	Breath sounds: Usually decreased or absent; if open pneumothorax, have amorphous quality Vocal resonance: Decreased or absent Adventitious sounds: None
Pulmonary Fibrosis, Diffuse	Inspiration = expiration Pitch: Low to absent Intensity: Soft to absent Adventitious sounds: Crackles	Pulmonary fibrosis is presence of excessive amount of connective tissue in lungs; consequently, lungs are smaller than normal and less compliant; lower lobes are usually affected most	Dyspnea on exertion Tachypnea Thoracic expansion diminished Cyanosis	Trachea: Deviated to most affected side	Resonant to dull	Breath sounds: Reduced or absent, bronchovesicular or bronchial Vocal resonance: Increased, whisper pectoriloquy may be present Adventitious sounds: Crackles on inspiration

[a]Although some disease conditions are bilateral, one diseased lung and one normal lung are illustrated for each condition to provide contrast. When an abnormality is illustrated, the pathologic condition is illustrated on the left side, and the normal lung is illustrated on the right side.

From Barkauskas V, Baumann L, Darling-Fisher CS. *Health and Physical Assessment*. 3rd ed. Mosby; 2002.

REFERENCES

1. Heuer AJ. Bedside assessment of the patient. In: Stoller JK, Heuer AJ, Chatburn RL, Mireles-Cabodevila E, Vines DL, eds. *Egan's Fundamentals of Respiratory Care*. 13th ed. St. Louis: Elsevier; 2025.
2. Morgan S. Respiratory assessment: undertaking a physical examination of the chest in adults. *Nurs Stand*. 2022;37(3):75–82. https://doi.org/10.7748/ns.2021.e11602.
3. Smith J, Rushton M. How to perform respiratory assessment. *Nurs Stand*. 2015;30(7):34–36. https://doi.org/10.7748/ns.30.7.34.s45.
4. Davis JL, Murray JF. History and physical examination. In: Broaddus VC, ed. *Murray and Nadel's Textbook of Respiratory Medicine*. 7th ed. Philadelphia: Elsevier; 2022.
5. Scott JB, Kaur M. Monitoring breathing frequency, pattern, and effort. *Respir Care*. 2020;65(6):793–806. https://doi.org/10.4187/respcare.07439.
6. Ball JW, Dains JE, Flynn JA, et al. *Seidel's Guide to Physical Examination: An Interprofessional Approach*. 10th ed. St. Louis: Elsevier; 2023.
7. Massey D, Meredith T. Respiratory assessment 1: why do it and how to do it? *Brit J Cardiac Nurs*. 2010;5(11):1–11. https://doi.org/10.12968/bjca.2010.5.11.79634.
8. Bohadana A, Izbicki G, Kraman SS. Fundamentals of lung auscultation. *N Engl J Med*. 2014;370(8):744–751. https://doi.org/10.1056/NEJMra1302901.

17

Pulmonary Diagnostic Procedures

Darlene M. Burke

http://evolve.elsevier.com/Urden/CriticalCareNursing

The patient's laboratory studies and diagnostic tests are reviewed to complete the assessment of a critically ill pulmonary patient. Although many procedures exist for diagnosing pulmonary disease, their application in a critically ill patient is limited. Only studies and tests used in the critical care setting are presented here. Bedside monitoring devices are also discussed.

LABORATORY STUDIES

Arterial Blood Gases

Interpreting arterial blood gas (ABG) levels can be challenging, especially if the nurse is pressured to do it quickly and accurately. One method that can help ensure accuracy when analyzing ABG levels is to follow the same interpretation steps each time. A specific method to be used each time blood gas values must be interpreted is presented here (Box 17.1).

Steps for Interpretation of Blood Gas Levels

Step 1. *Look at the PaO_2 level, and answer this question: Does the PaO_2 show hypoxemia?* PaO_2 measures the partial pressure (P) of oxygen dissolved in arterial (a) blood plasma. Sometimes, PaO_2 is shortened to PO_2. It is reported in millimeters of mercury (mm Hg). The PaO_2 reflects 3% of the total oxygen in the blood.[1]

The PaO_2 level is analyzed before the levels of other blood gas components. The normal range of PaO_2 values for individuals breathing room air at sea level is 80 to 100 mm Hg. However, the normal range is age dependent for infants and adults 60 years or older. The normal level for infants breathing room air is 50 to 70 mm Hg.[1] The normal level for adults 60 years or older decreases with age as changes occur in the ventilation/perfusion (V/Q) matching in the aging lung.[1,2] The correct PaO_2 for older adults can be ascertained as follows: 80 mm Hg (the lowest normal value) minus 1 mm Hg for every year of age more than 60 years. Using this formula, a 65-year-old individual can have a PaO_2 of 75 mm Hg (80 mm Hg − 5 mm Hg = 75 mm Hg) and still be within the normal range. An acceptable range for an 80-year-old person (20 years older than 60 years) is 60 mm Hg (80 mm Hg − 20 mm Hg = 60 mm Hg). A PaO_2 value less than the predicted lowest value indicates hypoxemia (i.e., a lower-than-normal amount of oxygen is dissolved in plasma)[1] and requires intervention.

Step 2. *Look at the pH level, and answer this question: Is the pH on the acid or alkaline side of 7.40?* The pH is the hydrogen ion (H^+) concentration of plasma. PH is calculated using the arterial partial pressure of carbon dioxide ($PaCO_2$) and the plasma bicarbonate level (HCO_3^-). The formula used is the Henderson-Hasselbalch equation.[1]

The normal pH of arterial blood is 7.35 to 7.45, and the mean is 7.40. If the pH level is less than 7.40, it is on the acid side of the mean. A pH of less than 7.35 is known as *acidemia*, and the overall condition is called *acidosis*. If the pH level is greater than 7.40, it is on the alkaline side of the mean. A pH level greater than 7.45 is known as *alkalemia*, and the overall condition is called *alkalosis*.[1]

Step 3. *Look at the $PaCO_2$ level, and answer this question: Does the $PaCO_2$ show respiratory acidosis, alkalosis, or normalcy?* $PaCO_2$ is a measure of the partial pressure of carbon dioxide dissolved in arterial blood plasma, and it is reported in mm Hg. The $PaCO_2$ is the acid–base component that reflects the effectiveness of ventilation in relation to the metabolic rate.[1] In other words, the $PaCO_2$ value indicates whether the patient can ventilate well enough to rid the body of the carbon dioxide produced due to metabolism.

The normal range for $PaCO_2$ is 35 to 45 mm Hg. This range does not change as a person ages. A $PaCO_2$ value greater than 45 mm Hg defines *respiratory acidosis*, which is caused by alveolar hypoventilation. Hypoventilation can result from chronic obstructive pulmonary disease (COPD), oversedation, head trauma, anesthesia, drug overdose, neuromuscular disease, or hypoventilation with mechanical ventilation.[3]

Ventilatory failure results when the $PaCO_2$ level exceeds 50 mm Hg. Acute ventilatory failure occurs when the $PaCO_2$ level is greater than 50 mm Hg and the pH level is less than 7.30. Ventilatory failure is referred to as *acute* because the pH is abnormal, not allowing enough time for the body to compensate by returning the pH to the normal range. Chronic ventilatory failure is defined as a $PaCO_2$ value greater than 50 mm Hg and a pH level greater than 7.30.[1]

A $PaCO_2$ value less than 35 mm Hg defines *respiratory alkalosis*, which is caused by alveolar hyperventilation. Hyperventilation can result from hypoxia, anxiety, pulmonary embolism, pregnancy, and hyperventilation with mechanical ventilation or as a compensatory mechanism for metabolic acidosis.[3,4]

Step 4. *Look at the HCO_3^- level and answer this question: Does the HCO_3^- show metabolic acidosis, alkalosis, or normalcy?* Bicarbonate (HCO_3^-) is the acid–base component that reflects kidney function. The HCO_3^- level is reduced or increased in the plasma by renal mechanisms. The normal range is 22 to 26 mEq/L.[3,4]

An HCO_3^- level of less than 22 mEq/L defines *metabolic acidosis*, which can result from ketoacidosis, lactic acidosis, renal failure, or diarrhea. The cumulative effect is a gain of acids or a loss of base. An HCO_3^- level that is greater than 26 mEq/L defines *metabolic alkalosis*, which can result from fluid loss

BOX 17.1 Interpretation of Arterial Blood Gases

Step 1
Look at the arterial partial pressure of oxygen (PaO_2) level and answer this question: Does the PaO_2 level show hypoxemia?

Step 2
Look at the pH level and answer this question: Is the pH level on the acid or alkaline side of 7.40?

Step 3
Look at the arterial partial pressure of carbon dioxide ($PaCO_2$) level and answer this question: Does the $PaCO_2$ level show respiratory acidosis, alkalosis, or normalcy?

Step 4
Look at the bicarbonate (HCO_3^-) level and answer this question: Does the HCO_3^- level show metabolic acidosis, alkalosis, or normalcy?

Step 5
Look again at the pH level, and answer this question: Does the pH show a compensated or an uncompensated condition?

BOX 17.2 Uncompensated Arterial Blood Gas Values

Example 1		Example 2	
PaO_2	mm Hg	PaO_2	90 mm Hg
pH	7.25	pH	7.25
$PaCO_2$	50 mm Hg	$PaCO_2$	40 mm Hg
HCO_3^-	22 mEq/L	HCO_3^-	17 mEq/L

Interpretation: Uncompensated respiratory acidosis (Example 1)

Interpretation: Uncompensated metabolic acidosis (Example 2)

from the upper gastrointestinal tract (vomiting or nasogastric suction), diuretic therapy, severe hypokalemia, alkali administration, or steroid therapy.[3,4]

Step 5. *Look again at the pH level, and answer this question: Does the pH show a compensated or an uncompensated condition?* If the pH level is abnormal (less than 7.35 or greater than 7.45), the $PaCO_2$ value or the HCO_3^- level, or both, will also be abnormal. This situation is an *uncompensated* condition because the body has not had enough time to return the pH to its normal range.[3,5] Box 17.2 provides two examples of uncompensated ABG values. If the pH level is within normal limits and the $PaCO_2$ value and the HCO_3^- level are abnormal, the condition is *compensated* because the body has had enough time to restore the pH to its normal range.[3,5]

Differentiating the primary disorder from the compensatory response can be difficult. The primary disorder is the abnormality that caused the pH level to shift initially and is determined according to the pH level; the primary disorder is considered the one on whichever side of 7.40 the pH level occurs.[4] Box 17.3 provides two examples of compensated ABG values. Partial compensation may be present and is evidenced by abnormal pH, $PaCO_2$, and HCO_3^- levels, indications that the body is attempting to return the pH to its normal range.[3,4]

Table 17.1 summarizes the changes in the acid–base components accompanying various acid–base disorders.[4,5] In addition to the parameters previously discussed, other factors must be considered when reviewing a patient's ABG levels, including oxygen saturation, oxygen content, base excess and deficit, and anion gap analysis. Table 17.2 summarizes conditions that may potentiate acid–base abnormalities.[3,5]

BOX 17.3 Compensated Arterial Blood Gas Values

Example 1		Example 2	
PaO_2	90 mm Hg	PaO_2	90 mm Hg
pH	7.37	pH	7.42
$PaCO_2$	60 mm Hg	$PaCO_2$	48 mm Hg
HCO_3^-	38 mEq/L	HCO_3^-	35 mEq/L

Interpretation: Compensated respiratory acidosis with metabolic alkalosis. (Acidosis is considered the primary disorder, and alkalosis is the compensatory response because the pH is on the acid side of 7.40.) (Example 1)

Interpretation: Compensated metabolic alkalosis with respiratory acidosis. (Alkalosis is considered the primary disorder, and acidosis is the compensatory response because the pH is on the alkaline side of 7.40.) (Example 2)

TABLE 17.1 Arterial Blood Gas Assessment

Disorder	pH	$PaCO_2$ (mm Hg)	HCO_3^- (mEq/L)
Respiratory Acidosis			
Uncompensated	<7.35	>45	22–26
Partially compensated	<7.35	>45	>26
Compensated	7.35–7.39	>45	>26
Respiratory Alkalosis			
Uncompensated	>7.45	<35	22–26
Partially compensated	>7.45	<35	<22
Compensated	7.41–7.45	<35	<22
Metabolic Acidosis			
Uncompensated	<7.35	35–45	<22
Partially compensated	<7.35	<35	<22
Compensated	7.35–7.39	<35	<22
Metabolic Alkalosis			
Uncompensated	>7.45	35–45	>26
Partially compensated	>7.45	>45	>26
Compensated	7.41–7.45	>45	>26
Combined (or mixed) respiratory and metabolic acidosis	<7.35	>45	<22
Combined (or mixed) respiratory and metabolic alkalosis	>7.45	<35	>26

HCO_3^-, Bicarbonate; *$PaCO_2$*, arterial partial pressure of carbon dioxide.

Oxygen Saturation

Oxygen saturation measures the amount of oxygen bound to hemoglobin compared with the maximal capability of hemoglobin for binding oxygen. It can be assessed as a component of the ABGs (SaO_2) or measured noninvasively using a pulse oximeter (SpO_2).[1] Oxygen saturation is reported as a percentage or decimal; normal values are greater than 95% when the patient is on room air. Usually, the saturation level cannot reach 100% (on room air) because of physiologic shunting.[1] However, when supplemental oxygen is administered, oxygen saturation may approach 100% so closely that it is reported as 100%.

TABLE 17.2 Acid–Base Disorders

Disorders	Potential Cause
Respiratory acidosis	Chronic obstructive pulmonary disease
	Acute airway obstruction
	Central nervous system depression
	Sedatives
	Anesthetics
	Opioids
	Trauma
	Spinal cord
	Brain
	Chest wall
	Neuromuscular disease
	Poliomyelitis
	Myasthenia gravis
	Guillain-Barré syndrome
	Hypoventilation with mechanical ventilation
Respiratory alkalosis	Hypoxia
	Anxiety
	Fear
	Pain
	Stimulants
	Pulmonary embolism
	Hyperventilation with mechanical ventilation
Metabolic acidosis	Lactic acidosis
	Ketoacidosis
	Renal failure (uremia)
	Rhabdomyolysis
	Ingestion of acids (methanol, salicylates, ethylene glycol)
	Diarrhea
	Renal tubular acidosis
	Ileostomy
	Pancreatic fistula
Metabolic alkalosis	Steroid therapy
	Vomiting
	Gastrointestinal suction
	Diuretic therapy
	Hypokalemia
	Hypovolemia
	Hypochloremia
	Sodium bicarbonate intake

Proper evaluation of the oxygen saturation level is vital. For example, a SaO_2 of 97% means that 97% of the available hemoglobin is bound with oxygen. The word *available* is essential to evaluating the SaO_2 level because the hemoglobin level is not always within normal limits, and oxygen can bind only with what is available. A 97% saturation level associated with 10 g/dL of hemoglobin does not deliver as much oxygen to the tissues as does a 97% saturation level associated with 15 g/dL of hemoglobin. Assessing only the SaO_2 level and finding it within normal limits does not ensure the patient's oxygenation status is normal. The hemoglobin level must also be evaluated before a decision on oxygenation status can be made.[1,5]

Oxygen Content

Oxygen content (CaO_2) is a measure of the total amount of oxygen carried in the blood, including the amount dissolved in plasma (measured by the PaO_2) and the amount bound to the hemoglobin molecule (measured by the SaO_2). CaO_2 is reported in milliliters of oxygen carried per 100 mL of blood. The normal value is 20 mL of oxygen per 100 mL of blood. To calculate the oxygen content, the PaO_2, the SaO_2, and the hemoglobin level are used (see Appendix B). A change in any one of these parameters affects the CaO_2.[1,5]

TABLE 17.3 Oxygenation Status

Patient	PaO_2 Level (mm Hg)	SaO_2 Level (%)	Hgb (g/dL)	CaO_2 (mL/dL)
A	100	97	15	19.8
B	100	97	10	13.3

CaO_2, Arterial oxygen content; *Hgb*, hemoglobin; *PaO_2*, arterial partial pressure of oxygen; *SaO_2*, arterial oxygen saturation.

The examples in Table 17.3 best illustrate the value of assessing the CaO_2. The ABG parameters that are used most to evaluate oxygenation status (PaO_2 and SaO_2) are both normal. Considering only the PaO_2 and the SaO_2 would lead to the invalid conclusion that Patient B's oxygenation status is normal. However, consideration of the hemoglobin level and the CaO_2 reveals that the oxygenation of Patient B's blood is significantly abnormal.

Base Excess and Base Deficit

Base excess and base deficit reflect the nonrespiratory contribution to acid–base balance and are reported in milliequivalents per liter (mEq/L) above or below the normal range of −2 mEq/L to +2 mEq/L. A negative base level is reported as a *base deficit*, which correlates with *metabolic acidosis*, whereas a positive base level is reported as a *base excess*, which correlates with *metabolic alkalosis*.[1,4,5]

Classic Shunt Equation and Oxygen Tension Indices

The efficiency of oxygenation can be assessed by measuring the degree of intrapulmonary shunting that occurs in a patient at any one time using the classic shunt equation and oxygen tension indices. *Intrapulmonary shunting* (QS/QT [the portion of cardiac output not exchanging with alveolar blood divided by the total cardiac output]) refers to venous blood that flows to the lungs without being oxygenated because of nonfunctioning alveoli.[1] Other names for this condition include shunt effect, low V/Q, wasted blood flow, and venous admixture.[1,5]

Direct determination of intrapulmonary shunting requires using the classic shunt equation (see Appendix B), which is invasive and cumbersome. A shunt greater than 10% is considered abnormal and indicative of a shunt-producing disorder. A shunt greater than 30% is a severe and potentially life-threatening condition that requires pulmonary intervention.[1]

Often, intrapulmonary shunting is estimated by using the oxygen tension indices. One advantage to these methods is the ease of performance, although they are unreliable in critically ill patients.[1] An estimate of intrapulmonary shunting can be determined by computing the difference between the alveolar and arterial oxygen concentrations. Normally, alveolar (A) and arterial (a) PO_2 values are approximately equal. When they are not, it indicates that venous blood is passing malfunctioning alveoli and returning unoxygenated to the left side of the heart.[1] The most common oxygen tension indices used to estimate intrapulmonary shunting are the PaO_2/FiO_2 ratio, the PaO_2/PaO_2 ratio, and the A–a gradient ($P[A - a]O_2$).

PaO_2/FiO_2 Ratio

The PaO_2/FiO_2 ratio is the easiest formula to calculate because this formula does not call for the computation of the alveolar PO_2. Normally, the PaO_2/FiO_2 ratio is greater than 286; the lower the value, the worse the lung function.[1,5]

PaO_2/PAO_2 Ratio

The PaO_2/PAO_2 ratio (arterial/alveolar oxygen ratio) is normally greater than 60%. The disadvantage to using this formula is that this formula calls for the computation of the alveolar PO_2 (see Appendix B), but the advantage is that this formula is unaffected by changes in the FiO_2 as long as the underlying lung condition is stable.[1,5]

Alveolar–Arterial Gradient

The A–a gradient ($P[A - a]O_2$) is usually less than 20 mm Hg on room air for patients younger than 61 years. This estimate of intrapulmonary shunting is the least reliable clinically, but it is often used in clinical decision making. A significant disadvantage to using this formula is that it is greatly influenced by the amount of oxygen the patient is receiving.[1,5] Serial determinations of the estimates of intrapulmonary shunting provide the provider with objective data on which to base clinical decisions.[1] Table 17.4 shows the change in intrapulmonary shunting in hypoxemic patients using the previously described oxygen tension indices to estimate the severity of shunting.

Dead Space Equation

The efficiency of ventilation can be measured using the clinical dead space (Vd/Vt) equation (see Appendix B). The formula measures the fraction of tidal volume not participating in gas exchange. A dead space value greater than 0.6 indicates a dead space–producing disorder and is considered abnormal. The major limitations to using this formula are that it requires the measurement of exhaled carbon dioxide to complete and that the work of breathing by patients must remain stable during the collection.[1,6]

Sputum Studies

Careful analysis of sputum specimens is crucial for rapidly identifying and treating pulmonary infections. The most difficult aspect of sputum examination is the proper collection of the specimen. Collection of a good sputum sample requires a conscious, cooperative, and sufficiently hydrated patient.[7] When the patient has difficulty producing sputum, heated, nebulized saline may help loosen secretions for expectoration.[7] Chest physiotherapy combined with nebulization improves the success rate. Collection of a sputum specimen is best done in the morning because a greater volume of secretions is present as a result of nighttime pooling. Brushing the teeth and rinsing the oropharyngeal airway is recommended to reduce contamination before collecting a sample.[7,8] Many critically ill patients cannot cough effectively, and sputum collection by other means is required. These methods include tracheobronchial aspiration, transtracheal aspiration, and fiberoptic bronchoscopy with a protected brush catheter. Because each method has benefits and risks, the patient's clinical condition determines the appropriate technique. Many critically ill patients have endotracheal or tracheostomy tubes already in place. Collecting sputum specimens from these patients requires special attention to technique (Box 17.4). Deep specimens are obtained to avoid collecting specimens that contain resident upper airway flora that may have migrated down the tube. Colonization of the lower airways with upper airway flora can occur within 48 hours of intubation.[7–9] After obtaining a sputum specimen, the sputum is examined for volume, physical properties, mucopurulence, and color (Table 17.5). Next, a microscopic examination is done to identify the source of the specimen. If a bacterial infection is suspected, a Gram stain is performed, followed by culture and sensitivity assessments.[7–9]

TABLE 17.4 Calculation of Intrapulmonary Shunting

FiO_2	PaO_2 Level (mm Hg)	PAO_2 Level (mm Hg)	PaO_2/FiO_2	A/a Ratio (%)	A-a Gradient (mm Hg)
0.21	40	97	190	41	57
0.50	80	300	160	27	220
1.0	150	610	150	25	460

A, Alveolar; *a*, arterial; *FiO_2*, fraction of inspired oxygen; *PaO_2*, arterial partial pressure of oxygen.

Modified from Murray JF, Nadel JA, eds. *Textbook of Respiratory Medicine*. Saunders; 1988.

DIAGNOSTIC PROCEDURES

Bronchoscopy

Indications

Fiberoptic bronchoscopy is a relatively safe procedure done at the bedside; it is most often used as a diagnostic and therapeutic tool (Fig. 17.2). Diagnostic indications include hemoptysis, infectious pneumonia, difficult intubation, pulmonary injury after chest trauma, acute burn inhalation injury, aspiration lung injuries, and acute upper airway obstruction. Therapeutic indications include aspiration of foreign bodies; removal of obstructing secretions; atelectasis; difficult intubation; and resection of small, benign growths from the airway.[10]

Procedural Considerations

Before bronchoscopy, a complete medical history is obtained, and a thorough examination, including a chest x-ray examination, is performed. Preprocedural patient evaluation includes clotting studies (prothrombin time, partial thromboplastin

BOX 17.4 Procedure for Sputum Specimen Collection

Clear the endotracheal or tracheostomy tube of all local secretions, avoiding deep airway penetration.

Attach a sputum trap to a sterile suction catheter and advance the catheter into the trachea while avoiding contact with the endotracheal tube or tracheostomy tube (Fig. 17.1).

After fully advancing the catheter, apply suction until secretions return to the sputum trap. When enough secretions are collected, discontinue suctioning, and remove the catheter.

Do not apply suction while the catheter is withdrawn because this can contaminate the sample with sputum from the upper airway. Do not flush the catheter with sterile water because this dilutes the sample.

If the catheter becomes plugged with secretions, place it in a sterile container, and send it to the laboratory. The specimen must be transported immediately or refrigerated if a delay is necessary.

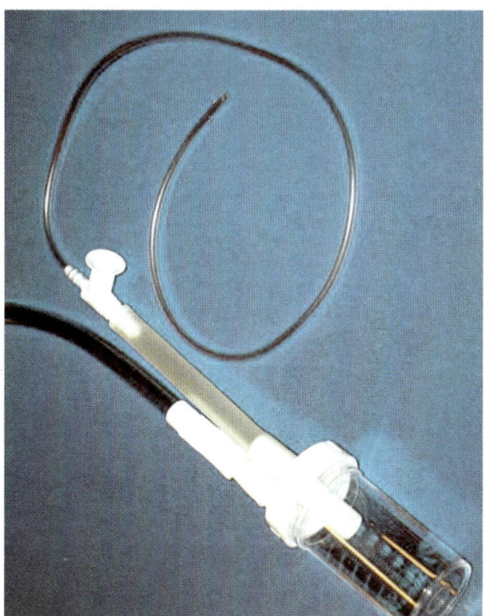

FIG. 17.1 Specimen Container. (From Kacmarek RM, Stoller JK, Heuer AJ, eds. *Egan's Fundamentals of Respiratory Care*. 12th ed. Elsevier; 2021.)

TABLE 17.5 Sputum Appearance and Possible Causes

Appearance	Possible Causes
Mucoid	Asthma, tumors, tuberculosis, emphysema, pneumonia
Mucopurulent	Asthma, tumors, tuberculosis, emphysema, pneumonia
Yellow-green, purulent	Bronchiectasis, chronic bronchitis
Rust-colored, purulent	Pneumococcal pneumonia
Red currant jelly	*Klebsiella pneumoniae* infection
Foul odor	Lung abscess
Pink, blood-tinged	Streptococcal or staphylococcal pneumonia
Gravel	Broncholithiasis
Pink, frothy	Pulmonary edema
Profuse, colorless (also known as *bronchorrhea*)	Alveolar cell carcinoma
Bloody	Pulmonary emboli, bronchiectasis, abscess, tuberculosis, tumor, cardiac causes, bleeding disorders

From Schwartz, MH. *Textbook of Physical Diagnosis*. 8th ed. Elsevier, 2021.

time, and platelet count) and evaluation of the ABG levels. Hypoxemic patients need supplemental oxygen during the procedure. The patient is generally instructed to have no oral intake for at least 6 hours before bronchoscopy to reduce the risk of aspiration.[11]

Although a topical anesthetic can be used alone, the anesthetic is usually supplemented by an intravenous sedative, analgesic, or both. A benzodiazepine for sedative effects and an opioid analgesic are administered intravenously during the procedure.[10] Preprocedural medications for a diagnostic bronchoscopy may include atropine and intramuscular codeine. Atropine lessens the vasovagal response and reduces the secretions, whereas codeine decreases the cough reflex. When bronchoscopy is performed therapeutically to remove secretions, the patient has decreased cough and gag reflexes, which may impair secretion clearance.[10] Maintenance of the airway is essential to prevent complications.

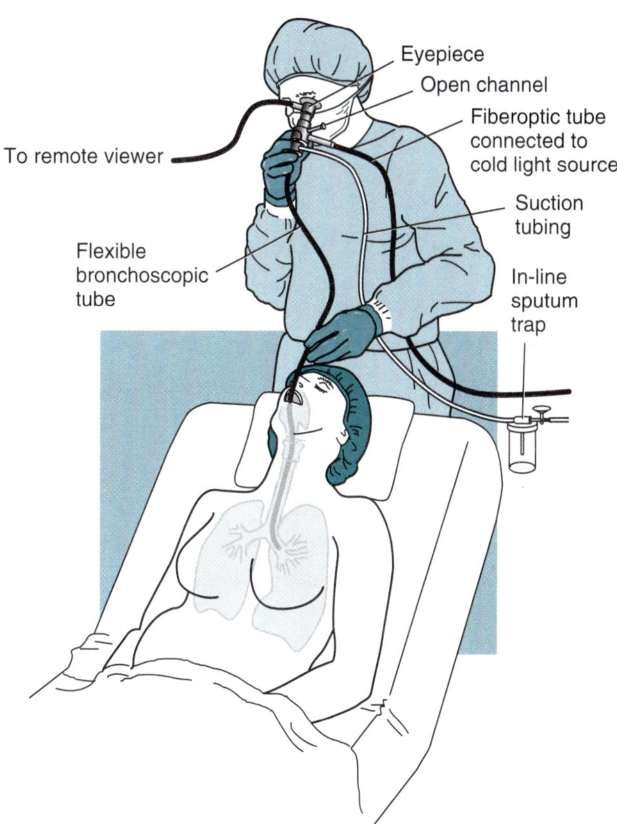

FIG. 17.2 Flexible Fiberoptic Bronchoscopy. The catheter is introduced into a small airway. Bronchial alveolar lavage is performed by injecting and withdrawing small amounts of sterile normal saline solution, gently aspirating after each instillation. Specimens are sent to the laboratory for analysis. (From Malarkey LM, McMorrow ME. *Saunders Nursing Guide to Laboratory and Diagnostic Tests*. 2nd ed. Saunders; 2012.)

Complications

Complications of the procedure may be related to the procedure itself, the anesthetic, or an ancillary procedure (e.g., biopsy), including laryngospasm, bronchospasm, epistaxis, fever, vomiting, and transient hypotension. More severe but rarer complications include anaphylaxis, infection, cardiac dysrhythmias, pneumothorax, bleeding, respiratory failure, hypoxemia, hemodynamic instability, and cardiopulmonary arrest.[10]

Thoracentesis

Indications

Thoracentesis is a simple, usually uncomplicated procedure done at the bedside for the removal of fluid or air from the pleural space (Fig. 17.3). A thoracentesis is used most often as a diagnostic measure; it may also be performed therapeutically for the drainage of a pleural effusion or empyema.[11] No absolute contraindications to thoracentesis exist, although some risks may contraindicate the procedure in all but emergency situations. These risk factors include unstable hemodynamics, coagulation defects, mechanical ventilation, the presence of an intra-aortic balloon pump, and uncooperative patients. In most clinical situations, diagnostic thoracentesis can be delayed until these risk factors are mitigated or eliminated.[11]

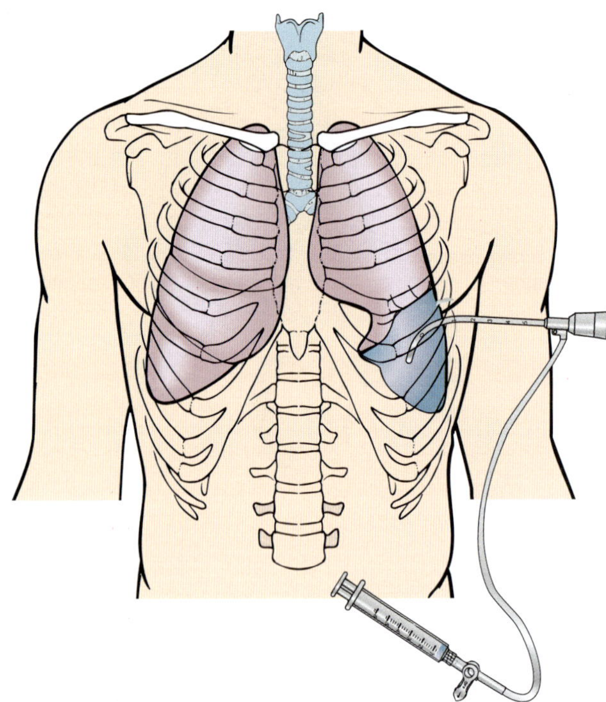

FIG. 17.3 Thoracentesis. The needle has penetrated the fluid-filled pleural space to remove the fluid. (From Harding MM, Kwong J, Hagler D, Reinisch C, eds. *Lewis's Medical-Surgical Nursing: Assessment and Management of Clinical Problems*. 12th ed. Elsevier; 2023.)

Procedural Considerations

The patient is placed in a sitting position with legs over the side of the bed and with hands and arms supported on a padded overbed table. If the patient's condition precludes sitting, the side-lying position with the back flush with the edge of the bed and the affected side down can be used.[11] The patient is cautioned not to move or cough during the procedure.[11] During the thoracentesis, the needle insertion site is usually determined using ultrasonography. A local anesthetic minimizes the patient's discomfort during the insertion of the thoracentesis needle.[11]

Complications

Complications associated with thoracentesis include pain, pneumothorax, and reexpansion pulmonary edema. Pneumothorax can occur because of the introduction of air into the pleural space, lung puncture, or visceral pleura rupture.[11] Reexpansion pulmonary edema can occur when a large amount of effusion fluid (approximately 1000 to 1500 mL) is removed from the pleural space. Removal of the fluid increases the negative intrapleural pressure, which can lead to edema when the lung does not reexpand to fill the space. The patient experiences severe coughing and shortness of breath. The onset of these symptoms is an indication to discontinue the thoracentesis.[12]

Bedside Pulmonary Function Tests

Indications

Pulmonary function tests (PFTs) are designed to quantify respiratory function and are essential to a thorough pulmonary evaluation. PFTs are used for various purposes, including monitoring occupational exposures, assessing surgical risk, providing data to support the diagnosis of lung disease, quantifying the severity level of lung disease, monitoring the lung disease, and evaluating response to treatment. Results are individualized according to age, gender, and body size.[6,13]

A complete PFT consists of four components: lung volumes, breathing mechanics, diffusion, and ABGs. PFTs may take 2 hours to complete. Because of the severity of illness encountered in the critical care area, all four components are rarely completed. Most often, pulmonary function measurements in a critically ill patient are limited to areas that provide information about the patient's risk for respiratory failure and need for intubation and mechanical ventilation or their readiness for extubation and liberation from mechanical ventilation. This section covers the areas tested most often at the bedside of critically ill patients.

Measuring lung volumes and capacities (Box 17.5) provides valuable information about the origin of a disease process. Four lung volumes and four lung capacities can be measured. Measurement of volumes at the bedside is limited to tidal volume and vital capacity. A vital capacity of 10 to 15 mL/kg usually is a minimally accepted value for weaning, with a respiratory rate of less than 24 breaths/min.[6]

BOX 17.5 Lung Volumes and Capacities[a]

Tidal volume (Vt): The volume of air inhaled or exhaled with each normal breath. The normal value is 500 mL. (V_T × respiratory rate = minute ventilation)

Inspiratory reserve volume (IRV): The maximum volume of air that can be inhaled after a normal inhalation. The normal value is 3000 to 3100 mL.

Expiratory reserve volume (ERV): The maximum volume of air that can be exhaled after a normal exhalation. The normal value is 1100 to 1200 mL.

Residual volume (RV): The volume of air remaining in the lungs after maximal exhalation. The normal value is 1200 to 1300 mL.

Total lung capacity (TLC): The volume of air in the lungs at the end of a maximal inhalation. The normal value is 5800 to 6000 mL. *(RV+ Vt + ERV + IRV = TC)*

Functional residual capacity (FRC): The volume of air remaining in the lungs after a normal exhalation. The normal value is 2300 to 2400 mL. *(RV + ERV = FRC)*

Inspiratory capacity (IC): The maximum volume of air that can be inhaled after a normal exhalation. The normal value is 3500 to 3600 mL. *(IR + Vt = IC)*

Vital capacity (VC): The maximum volume of air that can be exhaled after a maximal inhalation. The normal value is 4600 to 4800 mL. *(IC + Vt + ERV = VC)*

[a] The normal values for these measures vary with the height of the individual, gender, age, and race.

Static and Dynamic Compliance

Assessment of the mechanics of breathing includes measurement of the gas flow, lung and chest compliance, respiratory muscle strength, and tissue resistance. In the critical care area, dynamic and static compliance are measured at the bedside. *Compliance* measures the distensibility of the lungs (how easily they are inflated). Dynamic compliance is measured during the breathing cycle. A value of 46 to 66 mL/cm H_2O is normal (see Appendix B). Measurement of dynamic compliance does not differentiate among resistance forces. Conditions that increase resistance alter the dynamic compliance value. Dynamic compliance decreases with any reduction in lung compliance or increase in airway resistance, as occurs with bronchospasm and retained secretions. Static compliance is measured under no-flow conditions so that resistance forces are removed. Static compliance decreases with any decrease in lung compliance, as occurs with pneumothorax, atelectasis, pneumonia, pulmonary edema, and chest wall restrictions. A normal range is 57 to 85 mL/cm H_2O (see Appendix B).[13]

Inspiratory Muscle Strength

Assessment of inspiratory muscle strength can be evaluated through the measurement of maximal inspiratory pressure (MIP) and negative inspiratory pressure. Both should be more negative than −20 to −25 cm H_2O. Other names for these tests are negative inspiratory effort, peak inspiratory pressure (PIP), and peak inspiratory force. Assessing the maximal inspiratory pressure and negative inspiratory pressure requires a cooperative patient, and the values can provide useful information about spontaneous breathing ability. Maximal expiratory pressure (MEP) can be measured to test coughing ability in patients with neuromuscular dysfunction. Other common methods to assess respiratory muscle strength are maximum voluntary ventilation (MVV), minute ventilation (Ve), and breathing pattern.[13]

Spirometry

Dynamic PFTs are designed to evaluate the function of the respiratory muscles, thorax, and lungs. These tests are timed breathing studies that assess the degree of respiratory impairment and include forced vital capacity (FVC), peak expiratory flow rate (PEFR), forced expiratory volume in 1 second (FEV_1), and forced expiratory volume divided by forced vital capacity (FEV_1/FVC). Forced expiratory flow ($FEF_{25\%-75\%}$) is the mean rate of airflow over the middle half of the FVC and is a good index of airway resistance. When these studies are performed at the bedside, they require spirometry for volume measurement. The tests can be achieved with intubated or nonintubated patients. In an intubated patient, the spirometer is attached to the end of the endotracheal tube. In a nonintubated patient, a nose clip is placed on the patient and the patient is instructed to breathe through a spirometer tube. The patient is seated on the side of the bed if possible.[6,13] Each of these parameters is described in Table 17.6.

Ventilation/Perfusion Scanning

Indications

V/Q scanning is indicated when a serious alteration of the normal V/Q relationship is suspected. V/Q studies are often ordered to diagnose and follow a suspected pulmonary embolus. V/Q scanning is approximately 90% accurate in determining this diagnosis. Comparing the perfusion scan with the clinical examination results may improve this percentage.[14]

Procedure

The V/Q scan consists of a ventilation scan and a perfusion scan. The ventilation scan is performed by having the patient inhale a radiolabeled gas and air mixture through a mask. The perfusion scan is performed by giving the patient an intravenous radioisotope injection. Scintillation cameras record the gamma radiation images produced by the isotope as it is breathed or perfused into the lung. When an obstruction of the isotope's flow into an area of the lung occurs, the diminished radioactivity is reflected in the camera image of that zone.[14]

Results

Because the results are less than 100% accurate in predicting pulmonary emboli, most V/Q scans are interpreted in one of four ways. The scan is interpreted as normal when the perfusion scan is normal and the probability of pulmonary embolism approaches zero. A low probability interpretation is given when there are small V/Q mismatches when there are focal V/Q matches with no corresponding radiographic abnormalities, or when the perfusion defects are considerably smaller than the radiographic abnormalities. This finding is associated with a 12% chance of pulmonary embolus.[14] An intermediate or indeterminate probability is assigned when there are severe diffuse airflow obstructions; perfusion defects corresponding in size and position to radiographic abnormalities; and a single, moderate V/Q mismatch without a corresponding radiographic abnormality. A high probability interpretation is used when the perfusion defects are substantially larger than the radiographic abnormalities or when there are one or more large or two or more moderate V/Q mismatches with no corresponding radiographic abnormalities. This finding is seen infrequently but has a highly predictive value.[14]

Chest Radiography

Chest radiography is an essential diagnostic procedure for any critically ill patient. Chest x-ray examinations aid in diagnosing various disorders and complications and assist in evaluating treatment.[15,16] When interpreting a chest radiograph, a systematic method is used for viewing (Box 17.6). Areas of the radiographic film that are assessed include bones, mediastinum, diaphragm, pleural space, and lung tissue. Fig. 17.4 provides an example of a normal chest radiograph.

TABLE 17.6 Bedside Pulmonary Function Tests

Test	Description
Respiratory rate (f)	The number of breaths per minute
Tidal volume (Vt)	The volume of air exhaled after a normal resting inhalation
Minute ventilation (Ve)	The volume of air expired per minute (tidal volume respiratory rate = minute ventilation)
Maximal voluntary ventilation (MVV)	The maximum amount of air that can be moved into and out of the lungs in 1 minute
Forced vital capacity (FVC)	The maximum amount of air that can be forcefully exhaled from the lungs after maximal inhalation
Maximal inspiratory pressure (MIP)	The maximum negative pressure generated on inhalation
Maximal expiratory pressure (MEP)	The maximum positive pressure generated on exhalation
Peak expiratory flow rate (PEFR)	The maximum flow rate achieved during forced exhalation
Forced expiratory flow at midpoint of vital capacity ($FEF_{25\%-75\%}$)	The measure of average flow rate during the middle 50% of exhalation
Forced expiratory flow at 1 second (FEV_1)	The volume of air exhaled during the first second of forced exhalation

Bones

The clavicles, ribs, thoracic and cervical spine, and scapulas are assessed. The clavicles should be symmetric and the ribs should be an equal distance apart. Intervertebral disk spaces should be evident, indicating an adequately exposed inspiratory film.[15,16] The thoracic and cervical spine should be straight, without signs of curvature. The scapulas usually appear as areas of added density in the upper lung fields. There should be no evidence of fractures, calcification and lesions (increased density), or demineralization (decreased density).[15,16]

BOX 17.6 Chest Radiograph Interpretation

Step 1
Look at the different densities (black, gray, and white) and answer this question: What is air, fluid, tissue, and bone?

Step 2
Look at the shape or form of each density and answer this question: What normal anatomic structure is this?

Step 3
Look at the right and left sides and answer this question: Are the findings the same on both sides or are there physiologic and pathophysiologic differences?

Step 4
Look at all the structures (bones, mediastinum, diaphragm, pleural space, and lung tissue) and answer this question: Are any abnormalities present?

Step 5
Look for all tubes, wires, and lines and answer this question: Are the tubes, wires, and lines in the proper place?

Mediastinum

The structures assessed in the mediastinal area are the aortic knob and the trachea. The trachea should be positioned in the midline, with a slight deviation to the right as the trachea approaches the carina.[14] Shifting of the mediastinal structures can occur with atelectasis and removal of all or a portion of a lung (toward the area of involvement), pneumothorax (away from the area of involvement), pleural effusion, and tumors.[15,16]

Diaphragm

The diaphragm should be clearly visible, with sharp costophrenic angles seen where the chest wall and the tapered edges of the diaphragm meet.[16] The level of the diaphragm (on deep inspiration) should appear at the 10th or 11th rib,[16] with the right side 1 to 2 cm higher than the left side.[16] A gastric air bubble may be found under the left side of the diaphragm.[15,16] An elevated diaphragm may be seen in pregnancy, obesity, conditions that cause air or fluid accumulation in the peritoneal space, and intestinal obstruction.[16] An elevated hemidiaphragm is associated with several conditions, including phrenic nerve injury, previous chest surgery, subphrenic abscess, trauma, stroke, tumor, pneumonia, and radiation therapy.[16] Flattening

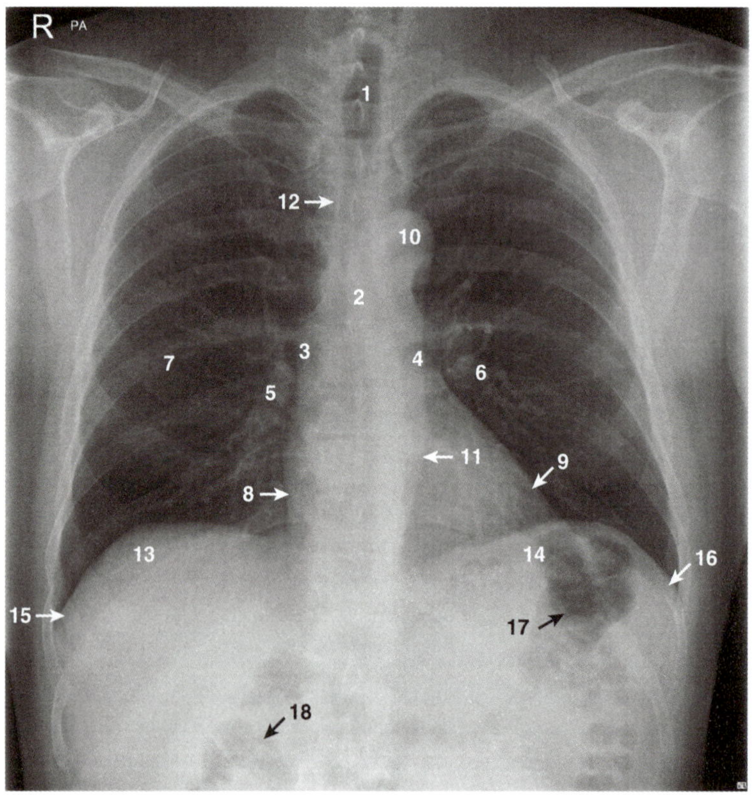

FIG. 17.4 Normal Chest Radiograph. *1,* Trachea; *2,* carina; *3,* right main bronchi; *4,* left main bronchi; *5,* right hilar structure; *6,* left hilar structure; *7,* right horizontal fissure; *8,* right cardiac border formed by the right atrium; *9,* left cardiac border formed by the left ventricle; *10,* aortic knob; *11,* descending thoracic aorta *12,* right paratracheal line; *13,* right hemidiaphragm; *14,* left hemidiaphragm; *15,* right costophrenic angle; *16,* left costophrenic angle; *17,* gastric air bubble; *18,* gas in the colon. (From Corne J, Au-Yong J. *Chest X Ray Made Easy.* 5th ed. Elsevier; 2023.)

of the diaphragm can indicate increased air in the lungs, as occurs with chronic COPD or pleural effusion.[16] Obliteration or "blunting" of the costophrenic angle can occur with pleural effusion, atelectasis, or pneumothorax.[16]

Pleural Space

Identification of the pleural space on a chest radiograph is an abnormal finding. The pleural space is not visible unless air (pneumothorax) or fluid (pleural effusion) enters the space. As fluid accumulates in the pleural space, it surrounds the lung and eventually compresses it. With a pleural effusion, blunting of the costophrenic angle may be evident first, with flattening of the diaphragm and obscuring of the heart borders occurring as the effusion grows.[16] With a pneumothorax, the pleural edges become evident as the examiner looks through and between the images of the ribs on the film. A thin line appears just parallel to the chest wall, indicating where the lung markings have pulled away from the chest wall.[16] The collapsed lung manifests as an area of increased density separated by an area of radiolucency (blackness).

Lung Tissue

The lung tissue is viewed for areas of increased density or radiolucency that may indicate an abnormality. Increased density can result from fluid accumulation in the lungs (water, pus, blood, edema fluid) or collapse of lung tissue (with atelectasis or pneumothorax). Increased radiolucency is caused by increased air in the lungs, as may occur with COPD.[16] In some patients, a fine line may be present on the right side at approximately the level of the sixth rib in the midlung field. This situation is a normal finding and represents the horizontal fissure, which separates the right upper lobe from the right middle lobe.[16]

Tubes, Wires, and Lines

The chest radiograph is assessed for proper placement of all tubes, wires, and lines (Fig. 17.5). When properly positioned, an endotracheal tube is 2 to 3 cm above the carina, and a nasogastric tube runs the length of the esophagus, with the tip in the stomach.[16] The origin of a central venous catheter is observed as a thin, continuous, radiopaque line at the level of the jaw, progressing toward the superior vena cava in an internal jugular approach. In contrast, a subclavian approach originates in the clavicular area. A pulmonary artery catheter is viewed running through the right atrium and right ventricle into the pulmonary artery.[16] Additional items that may be present include temporary or permanent pacing wires, a permanent pacing generator, an implantable cardioverter defibrillator, a peripherally inserted central catheter, chest tubes (pleural or mediastinal), electrocardiographic electrodes, and surgical markers and clips.[16]

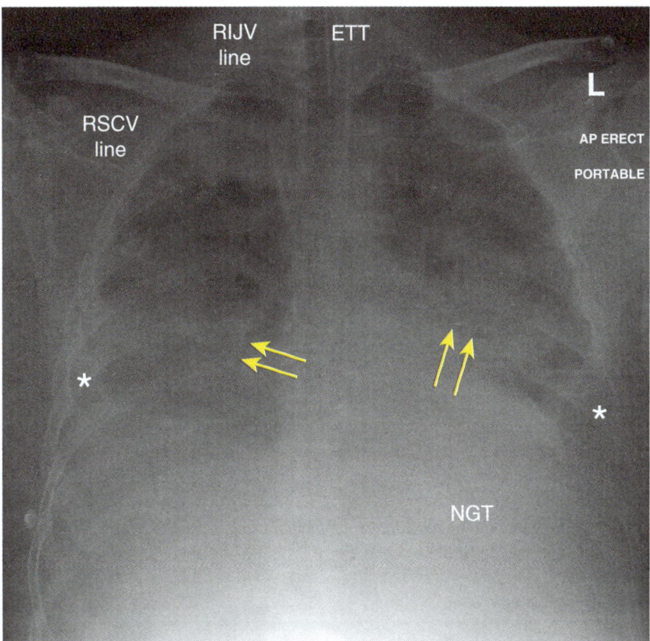

FIG. 17.5 Chest Radiograph with Lines and Tubes. Note the placement of the endotracheal tube (*ETT*), a nasogastric tube (*NGT*), and two central lines (right internal jugular [*RIJV*] and right subclavian [RSCV]). The *yellow arrows* point to the air bronchograms associated with bilateral alveolar infiltrates. The *stars* (*) depict the location of bilateral pleural effusions. (From Acute Respiratory Distress Syndrome (ARDS) – Chest X-Ray. Radiology St. Vincent's University Hospital. http://www.svuhradiology.ie/case-study/adult-respiratory-distress-syndrome-ards-chest-x-ray/ Accessed August 9, 2023.)

Other Diagnostic Procedures

Table 17.7 presents an overview of several other diagnostic procedures that may be used to evaluate the critically ill patient with pulmonary dysfunction.

Nursing Management

Nursing management of a patient undergoing a diagnostic procedure involves various interventions, including preparing the patient psychologically and physically for the procedure, monitoring the patient's responses to the procedure, and assessing the patient after the procedure. Preparing the patient includes teaching the patient about the procedure, answering any questions, and positioning the patient for the procedure. Monitoring the patient's responses to the procedure includes observing the patient for signs of pain, anxiety, or respiratory decompensation (Box 17.7) and monitoring vital signs, lung sounds, and oxygen saturation. Assessing the patient after the procedure includes observing for complications and medicating the patient for any postprocedural discomfort.

BEDSIDE MONITORING

Capnography

- Capnography measures exhaled carbon dioxide (CO_2) gas and is also known as *end-tidal CO_2* monitoring.

Basic Principles

Normally, alveolar and arterial carbon dioxide concentrations are equal in the presence of normal V/Q relationships. In a hemodynamically stable patient, the partial pressure of end-tidal CO_2 ($PETCO_2$) can be used to estimate the $PaCO_2$, with $PETCO_2$ levels 1 to 5 mm Hg less than $PaCO_2$ levels. However, a normal V/Q relationship must be established before the correlation of $PETCO_2$ and $PaCO_2$ can be assumed.[17] Causes of increased $PETCO_2$ include conditions in which carbon dioxide production is increased, such as hyperthermia, sepsis, and seizures, or in which alveolar ventilation is decreased, such as respiratory depression. Causes of decreased $PETCO_2$ include conditions in which carbon dioxide production is decreased, such as hypothermia, cardiac arrest, and pulmonary embolism, or in which alveolar ventilation is increased, such as hyperventilation.[17]

TABLE 17.7 Other Pulmonary Diagnostic Procedures

Diagnostic Procedure	Description
Computed tomography (CT) scan	This procedure is performed to diagnose suspicious lesions that are difficult to assess (e.g., mediastinum, hilum, pleura) by conventional x-ray. Common types are helical or spiral CT (contrast medium is usually used) and high-resolution CT scan (contrast medium is not used). CT pulmonary angiography (CTPA) is used to diagnose a pulmonary embolism.
Magnetic resonance imaging (MRI)	This procedure is used for in-depth diagnosis of lesions challenging to assess by CT scan (e.g., lung apex) and differentiating vascular from nonvascular structures.
Pulmonary angiogram	This procedure is used to visualize pulmonary vasculature and locate obstruction or pathologic conditions (e.g., pulmonary embolus). Contrast medium is injected through a catheter threaded into the pulmonary artery or right side of the heart. A series of x-rays are taken after the contrast medium is administered. Chest CT is replacing angiography because it is less invasive.
Positron emission tomography (PET) scan	This procedure is used to distinguish benign from malignant pulmonary nodules. Because malignant lung cells have an increased glucose uptake, the PET scan, which uses an IV radioactive glucose preparation, can demonstrate increased glucose uptake in malignant lung cells.
Lung biopsy	This procedure is used to obtain specimens for laboratory analysis. Specimens may be obtained by transbronchial or percutaneous biopsy or via transthoracic needle aspiration (TTNA), video-assisted thoracoscopic surgery (VATS), or open lung biopsy.

Modified from Harding MM, Kwong J, Hagler D, Reinisch C, eds. *Lewis's Medical-Surgical Nursing: Assessment and Management of Clinical Problems.* 12th ed. Elsevier; 2023.

BOX 17.7 Patient Safety Clinical Manifestations of Respiratory Decompensation

Inadequate Airway

Stridor
Noisy respirations
Supraclavicular and intercostal retractions
Flaring of nares
Labored breathing with the use of accessory muscles

Inadequate Ventilation

Absence of air exchange at nose and mouth (breathlessness)
Minimal/absent chest wall motion
Manifestations of an obstructed airway
Central cyanosis
Decreased or absent breath sounds (bilateral, unilateral)
Restlessness, anxiety, confusion
Paradoxical motion involving a significant portion of the chest wall
Decreased PaO_2, increased $PaCO_2$, decreased pH

Inadequate Gas Exchange

Tachypnea
Decreased PaO_2
Increased dead space
Central cyanosis
Chest infiltrates on radiographic evaluation

Use in Critical Care

In the critical care area, continuous capnography is used to assess and monitor the patient's ventilatory status in various situations, including weaning from mechanical ventilation and undergoing procedural sedation. Changes in physiologic dead space can be evaluated with $PETCO_2$ monitoring, based on the degree of difference between $PaCO_2$ and $PETCO_2$. As the severity of pulmonary impairment increases, so does the disparity between $PaCO_2$ and $PETCO_2$, as indicated by an increased gradient. A gradient greater than 5 mm Hg is evident with underperfused alveolar–capillary units (dead space–producing situations) and nonperfused alveolar–capillary units (alveolar dead space). Increased dead space ventilation results from decreased pulmonary blood flow, cardiac output, and lung disease. This situation leads to an abnormality in the transfer of carbon dioxide from the blood to the lung. The result is a $PETCO_2$ level that is lower than the $PaCO_2$ level because of the mixing of carbon dioxide between perfused and nonperfused units. The result is an increased or widened $PaCO_2/PETCO_2$ gradient.[17]

The noninvasive measurement of $PETCO_2$ enables assessment of the adequacy of cardiopulmonary resuscitation and endotracheal tube placement. Decreased pulmonary blood flow is associated with lower $PETCO_2$ values, reflected clinically by decreased cardiac output, as in the case of cardiopulmonary resuscitation. During endotracheal intubation, a low $PETCO_2$ reading indicates that the tube is positioned in the stomach because the amount of carbon dioxide in the esophagus is expected to be low.[17]

Types

There are two primary forms of capnography: mainstream and side-stream. All forms can be used in intubated patients, but side-stream capnography can also be used in nonintubated patients, broadening the application of $PETCO_2$ monitoring.

Mainstream capnography. Mainstream capnography directly measures the carbon dioxide level by a sensor in the exhalation port of the ventilator tubing. Gas passes over the sensor during exhalation and an electrical cable transfers the information to the display unit. The display unit produces a waveform called a *capnogram* (Fig. 17.6) and a numeric recording ($PETCO_2$). Disadvantages to this form of capnography include the weight of the sensor on the ventilator tubing and possible obstruction of the sensor by secretions and condensation.

Side-Stream capnography. In side-stream capnography, the carbon dioxide gas is continuously aspirated through a side port in the ventilator tubing or nasal cannula. It is measured and analyzed by a side unit. Disadvantages of this type of capnography include obstruction of the sampling tube with secretions and slow response time. Proximal diverting capnography is a newer and improved version of side-stream capnography that transports gas a short distance from the airway to a site where the sensor is located, reducing the bulkiness of the airway.[17]

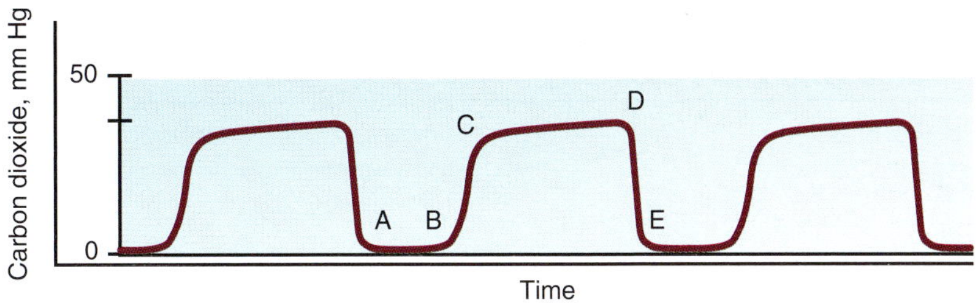

FIG. 17.6 Capnogram. Normal findings on a capnogram. *A → B* indicates the baseline; *B → C*, the expiratory upstroke; *C → D*, the alveolar plateau; *D*, the partial pressure of end-tidal carbon dioxide; and *D → E*, the inspiratory downstroke. (From Frakes M. Measuring end-tidal carbon dioxide: clinical applications and usefulness. *Crit Care Nurse*. 2001;21[5]:23.)

Caution

Capnography and $PETCO_2$ analysis have many diverse applications in the critical care area, but the practitioner must never assume that the $PETCO_2$ values reflect $PaCO_2$ values without waveform analysis. Any change in the waveform can indicate a change in the patient's pulmonary status and warrants further evaluation. Loss of the waveform may signal loss of effective respirations.[17]

Pulse Oximetry

Pulse oximetry is a noninvasive method for monitoring peripheral oxygen saturation (SpO_2) and is indicated in any situation in which the patient's oxygenation status requires continuous observation.

Basic Principles

A conventional pulse oximeter comprises a microprocessor and a transmission or reflectance probe. The probe consists of light-emitting diodes and a photodetector. With transmission pulse oximetry (Fig. 17.7), the probe is placed on a digit, earlobe, lip, or nasal alar, and the diodes transmit red and infrared light wavelengths through the pulsating arterial vascular bed to the photodetector on the other side. The percentage of oxygen saturation is determined by the difference in absorbance of the red and infrared light caused by the difference in color between oxygen bound (bright red) and oxygen unbound (dark red) hemoglobin. The photodetector converts the light signals into an electric signal that is sent to the microprocessor, which converts the electric signal into a digital reading. With reflectance pulse oximetry, the photodetector lies adjacent to the light source on a flat surface and captures the reflection of light from a site such as the forehead.[18]

Limitations

Pulse oximeters are usually calibrated to a range of saturation from 70% to 100%, with an accuracy of 2% to 4% compared to SaO_2, when the SpO_2 is greater than or equal to 70%.[18,19] However, several physiologic and technical factors impact the accuracy of the measurement and may limit the effective use of the monitoring system.[17]

Physiologic. Physiologic limitations of pulse oximetry include elevated levels of abnormal hemoglobins, the presence of vascular dyes, and conditions that impair peripheral perfusion. The pulse oximeter cannot differentiate between normal and abnormal hemoglobin. Elevated abnormal hemoglobin levels (e.g., carboxyhemoglobin associated with carbon monoxide poisoning or smoking tobacco) falsely elevate the SpO_2. Intravascular dyes color the serum in the blood and may interfere with the light absorption spectrum, resulting in falsely low readings.[18] Impaired peripheral perfusion from hypotension, hypothermia, pharmacologic vasoconstrictors, peripheral vascular disease, or peripheral edema leads to loss of pulsatile flow and signal failure.[17]

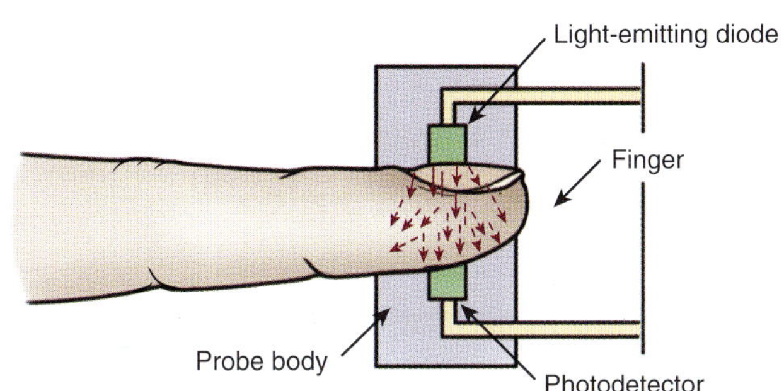

FIG. 17.7 Pulse Oximeter Finger Probe. (From Wilkins RL, Stoller JK, Scanlan CL, eds. *Egan's Fundamentals of Respiratory Care*. 8th ed. Mosby; 2006.)

Technical. Technical limitations of pulse oximetry include bright lights, excessive motion, and incorrect probe placement. Bright lights may interfere with the photodetector and cause inaccurate results. The probe must be covered to limit optical interference. Excessive motion can mimic arterial pulsations and can lead to false readings. Incorrect probe placement can lead to inaccurate results because part of the light can reach the photodetector without passing through blood (optical shunting). Interventions to limit these problems include using the probe in the appropriate spot (e.g., not using a finger sensor on the ear), applying the probe according to the directions, and ensuring that the monitored area has adequate perfusion.[17] Dark fingernail polish, long artificial nails, thick skin, and dark skin pigmentation also limit the accuracy of pulse oximeters.[18] Patients with dark skin may have their oxygen saturation overestimated as much as 2%,[18,19] especially at lower saturation (<80%).[20] These findings vary depending on which device is used[18] and the level of skin pigmentation.[19]

Caution

In a critically ill patient, pulse oximetry is reliable only for monitoring the patient's oxygenation status. Pulse oximetry is an unreliable method for monitoring the patient's ventilatory status. The ability of a pulse oximeter to detect hypoventilation is accurate only when the patient is breathing room air. Because most critically ill patients require some form of oxygen therapy, pulse oximetry is unreliable for detecting hypercapnia and should not be used for this purpose.[17]

SOCIAL DETERMINANTS OF HEALTH

Health Disparities Associated with Pulse Oximetry

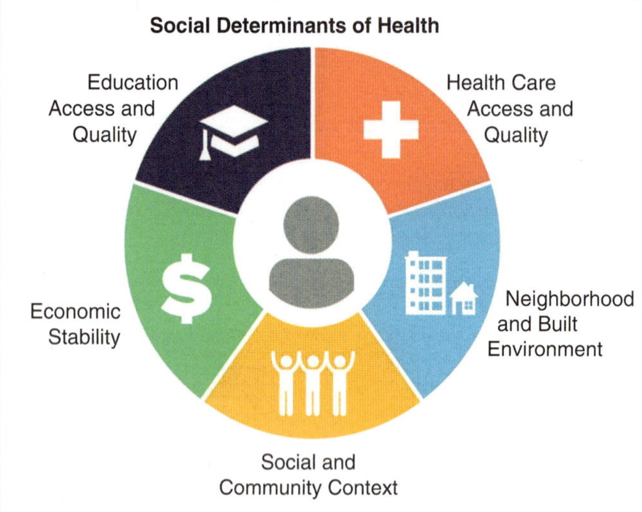

Several studies have indicated that racial and ethnic minorities, particularly people with darker skin tones, may experience inaccuracies or lower readings when using standard pulse oximeters.[1] This discrepancy is primarily due to how these devices work, which relies on the differential absorption of light by oxygenated and deoxygenated hemoglobin. Darker skin contains more melanin, which can absorb more light and potentially lead to inaccurate readings.

Melanin, the pigment responsible for skin, hair, and eye color, can absorb light at specific wavelengths. Higher melanin levels can lead to increased light absorption in people with darker skin, potentially resulting in less accurate readings. This absorption can make it challenging for pulse oximeters to accurately distinguish between oxygenated and deoxygenated blood, particularly at lower oxygen saturation levels.

This issue gained significant attention during the COVID-19 pandemic when it was observed that pulse oximeters might underestimate oxygen levels in individuals with darker skin tones. Inaccurate readings from pulse oximeters can have implications for medical care, as they may lead to delayed recognition of low oxygen levels or incorrect assessments of a patient's condition. Since low oxygen saturation is a critical indicator of severe pulmonary dysfunction, this discrepancy raised concerns about delayed medical interventions for individuals not accurately identified as at risk.

Health care professionals have called for increased awareness of this issue and the need for improved technology and standards in pulse oximetry. Some proposed solutions include developing pulse oximeters designed to account for different skin tones or using alternative methods to monitor oxygen levels, especially in populations with darker skin tones. It's important to note that while advancements are being made to address these issues, further research and development are needed to ensure accurate and reliable oxygen saturation monitoring for individuals of all skin colors.[2]

References

1. Jamali H, Castillo LT, Morgan CC, et al. Racial disparity in oxygen saturation measurements by pulse oximetry: Evidence and implications. *Ann Am Thorac Soc.* 2022;19(12):1951–1964. https://doi.org/10.1513/AnnalsATS.202203-270CME.
2. Okunlola OE, Lipnick MS, Batchelder PB, et al. Pulse oximeter performance, racial inequity, and the work ahead. *Respir Care.* 2022;67(2):252–257. https://doi.org/10.4187/respcare.09795.

Illustration from Healthy People 2030, U.S. Department of Health and Human Services, Office of Disease Prevention and Health Promotion. Retrieved September 8, 2022, from https://health.gov/healthypeople/objectives-and-data/social-determinants-health.

BOX 17.8 Internet Resources

Pulmonary Diagnostic Procedures

- American Association of Critical-Care Nurses (AACN): www.aacn.org
- American Association of Respiratory Care (AARC): www.aarc.org
- American College of Chest Physicians (ACCP): www.chestnet.org/accp
- American College of Physicians (ACP): www.acponline.org
- American Lung Association: www.lung.org
- American Medical Association (AMA): www.ama-assn.org
- American Thoracic Society (ATS): www.thoracic.org
- Centers for Disease Control and Prevention (CDC): www.cdc.gov
- National Institutes for Health (NIH): www.nih.gov
  Office of Disease Prevention and Health Promotion: healthfinder.gov
  Respiratory Nursing Society and Interprofessional Collaborative (RNSIC): respiratorynursingsociety.org
- Society for Critical Care Medicine (SCCM): www.sccm.org

ADDITIONAL RESOURCES

See Box 17.8 for additional resources for the diagnosis of the patient with pulmonary dysfunction.

KEY POINTS

Laboratory Studies

- Interpretation of ABG levels involves looking at the PaO_2 (normal range, 80 to 100 mm Hg), the pH (normal range, 7.35 to 7.45), the $PaCO_2$ (normal range, 35 to 45 mm Hg), and HCO_3^- (normal range, 22 to 26 mEq/L).
- The efficiency of oxygenation can be assessed by measuring the degree of intrapulmonary shunting using the classic shunt equation and oxygen tension indices (PaO_2/FiO_2 ratio, PaO_2/PAO_2 ratio, and A–a gradient).
- Sputum specimens are crucial for rapid identification and treatment of pulmonary infections.

Diagnostic Procedures

- Fiberoptic bronchoscopy and thoracentesis are often used as diagnostic and therapeutic procedures.
- PFTs are used for preoperative assessment, evaluating lung mechanics, diagnosing and tracking pulmonary diseases, and monitoring therapy.
- V/Q scanning is indicated when a severe alteration of the normal V/Q relationship is suspected, such as with a pulmonary embolus.
- Chest x-ray examination aids in the diagnosis of various pulmonary disorders and assists in the evaluation of treatments.

Bedside Monitoring

- Capnography is a noninvasive method used to monitor a patient's ventilatory status by measurement of exhaled carbon dioxide gas.
- Pulse oximetry is a noninvasive method used to monitor a patient's oxygenation status by measurement of oxygen saturation.

Visit the Evolve site at http://evolve.elsevier.com/Urden/CriticalCareNursing for additional study materials.

REFERENCES

1. Cohen Z. Gas exchange and transport. In: Stoller JK, Heuer AJ, Chatburn RL, Mireles-Cabodevila E, Vines DL, eds. *Egan's Fundamentals of Respiratory Care*. 13th ed. St. Louis: Elsevier; 2025.
2. Yeager JJ. Laboratory and diagnostic tests. In: Meiner SE, Yeager JJ, eds. *Gerontology Nursing*. 6th ed. St. Louis: Elsevier; 2019.
3. Tucker AM, Johnson TN. Acid-base disorders: a primer for clinicians. *Nutr Clin Pract*. 2022;37(5):980–989. https://doi.org/10.1002/ncp.10881.
4. Mirza SH. Acid base balance. In: Stoller JK, Heuer AJ, Chatburn RL, Mireles-Cabodevila E, Vines DL, eds. *Egan's Fundamentals of Respiratory Care*. 13th ed. St. Louis: Elsevier; 2025.
5. Heuer AJ, Havard J. Interpretation of blood gases. In: Heuer AJ, ed. *Wilkin's Clinical Assessment in Respiratory Care*. 9th ed. St. Louis: Elsevier; 2022.
6. Venkateshiah L, Jerusalem Z, Mireles-Cabodevila E. Ventilation. In: Stoller JK, Heuer AJ, Chatburn RL, Mireles-Cabodevila E, Vines DL, eds. *Egan's Fundamentals of Respiratory Care*. 13th ed. St. Louis: Elsevier; 2025.
7. Mehta R, Bulger J, Elshikh A. Solutions, body fluids and electrolytes. In: Stoller JK, Heuer AJ, Chatburn RL Mireles-Cabodevila E, Vines DL, eds. *Egan's Fundamentals of Respiratory Care*. 13th ed. St. Louis: Elsevier; 2025.
8. Sputum Culture, Bacterial. Testing. Update January 24. https://www.testing.com/tests/sputum-culture-bacterial/#.Vg1PEsfMrak.gmail; 2020. Accessed August 8, 2023.
9. Tetteh ES. Interpreting clinical and laboratory data. In: Stoller JK, Heuer AJ, Chatburn RL, Mireles-Cabodevila E, Vines DL, eds. *Egan's Fundamentals of Respiratory Care*. 13th ed. St. Louis: Elsevier; 2025.
10. Scott JB. Airway management. In: Stoller JK, Heuer AJ, Chatburn RL, Mireles-Cabodevila E, Vines DL, eds. *Egan's Fundamentals of Respiratory Care*. 13th ed. St. Louis: Elsevier; 2025.
11. Cicenia J, Low SW. Pleural diseases. In: Stoller JK, Heuer AJ, Chatburn RL, Mireles-Cabodevila E, Vines DL, eds. *Egan's Fundamentals of Respiratory Care*. 13th ed. St. Louis: Elsevier; 2025.
12. Park SJ, Herren JL, Gaba RC. Lessons in IR: Re-expansion pulmonary edema following therapeutic thoracentesis. *J Vasc Interv Radiol*. 2023;34(8):1467–1468. https://doi.org/10.1016/j.jvir.2023.02.017.
13. Cohen Z. Pulmonary function testing. In: Stoller JK, Heuer AJ, Chatburn RL, Mireles-Cabodevila E, Vines DL, eds. *Egan's Fundamentals of Respiratory Care*. 13th ed. St. Louis: Elsevier; 2025.
14. Tonelli AR, Dweik RA. Pulmonary vascular disease. In: Stoller JK, Heuer AJ, Chatburn RL, Mireles-Cabodevila E, Vines DL, eds. *Egan's Fundamentals of Respiratory Care*. 13th ed. St. Louis: Elsevier; 2025.
15. Azok JT, Stoller JK. Review of thoracic imaging. In: Stoller JK, Heuer AJ, Chatburn RL, Mireles-Cabodevila E, Vines DL, eds. *Egan's Fundamentals of Respiratory Care*. 13th ed. St. Louis: Elsevier; 2025.
16. Corne J, Au-Yong J. *Chest X Ray Made Easy*. 5th ed. London: Elsevier; 2023.
17. Shaikh H, Littleton S, Laghi F. Analysis and monitoring of gas exchange. In: Stoller JK, Heuer AJ, Chatburn RL, Mireles-Cabodevila E, Vines DL, eds. *Egan's Fundamentals of Respiratory Care*. 13th ed. St. Louis: Elsevier; 2025.
18. Torp KD, Modi P, Simon LV. Pulse oximetry. In: *StatPearls NCBI Bookshelf Version*. StatPearls Publishing; 2022. https://www.ncbi.nlm.nih.gov/books/NBK470348/. Accessed August 9, 2023.
19. Shi C, Goodall M, Dumville J, et al. The accuracy of pulse oximetry in measuring oxygen saturation by levels of skin pigmentation: A systematic review and meta-analysis. *BMC Med*. 2022;20(1):267. https://doi.org/10.1186/s12916-022-02452-8.
20. Cabanas AM, Fuentes-Guajardo M, Latorre K, et al. Skin pigmentation influence on pulse oximetry accuracy: a systematic review and bibliometric analysis. *Sensors*. 2022;22(9):3402. https://doi.org/10.3390/s22093402.

18

Pulmonary Disorders

Kathleen M. Stacy

http://evolve.elsevier.com/Urden/CriticalCareNursing

Understanding the pathology of a disease, the areas of assessment on which to focus, and the usual medical management allows the critical care nurse to more accurately anticipate and plan nursing interventions. This chapter focuses on pulmonary disorders commonly seen in the critical care environment.

ACUTE RESPIRATORY FAILURE

Description and Etiology

Acute respiratory failure (ARF) is a clinical condition in which the pulmonary system fails to maintain adequate gas exchange.[1–3] It is the most common type of organ dysfunction seen in the critical care unit. ARF results from a deficiency in the performance of the pulmonary system. It usually occurs secondary to another disorder that has altered the normal function of the pulmonary system in such a way as to decrease the ventilatory drive, decrease muscle strength, decrease chest wall elasticity, decrease the lung's capacity for gas exchange, increase airway resistance, or increase metabolic oxygen requirements.[1,3]

ARF can be classified as hypoxemic normocapnic respiratory failure (type I) or hypoxemic hypercapnic respiratory failure (type II), depending on the analysis of the patient's arterial blood gases (ABGs). In type I respiratory failure, the patient presents with a low arterial oxygen pressure (PaO_2) and a normal arterial carbon dioxide pressure ($PaCO_2$); in type II respiratory failure, the patient presents with a low PaO_2 and a high $PaCO_2$.[1,2,4] Fig. 18.1 summarizes the key concepts for managing the patient with ARF.

Etiology

The causes of ARF may be classified as *extrapulmonary* or *intrapulmonary*, depending on the origin of the patient's primary disorder. Extrapulmonary causes include disorders that affect the brain, the spinal cord, the neuromuscular system, the thorax, the pleura, and the upper airways.[1] Intrapulmonary causes include disorders that affect the lower airways and alveoli, the pulmonary circulation, and the alveolar-capillary membrane.[3-6] Table 18.1 lists ARF's different etiologies and associated disorders.

Pathophysiology

Hypoxemia results from impaired gas exchange and is the hallmark of ARF. Hypercapnia may be present, depending on the underlying cause of the problem. The main causes of hypoxemia are alveolar hypoventilation, ventilation/perfusion ($\dot{V}/\dot{Q}$) mismatching, and intrapulmonary shunting.[1–3] Type I respiratory failure usually results from $\dot{V}/\dot{Q}$ mismatching and intrapulmonary shunting, whereas type II respiratory failure usually results from alveolar hypoventilation, which may or may not be accompanied by $\dot{V}/\dot{Q}$ mismatching and intrapulmonary shunting.[2]

Alveolar Hypoventilation

Alveolar hypoventilation occurs when the amount of oxygen brought into the alveoli is insufficient to meet the body's metabolic needs. This situation can result from increasing metabolic oxygen needs or decreasing ventilation. Decreasing ventilation can occur secondary to failure of the ventilatory pump or failure of ventilatory drive. Patients with failure of the ventilatory pump often present with tachypnea, whereas patients with failure of ventilatory drive usually present with bradypnea. The development of alveolar hypoventilation is often secondary to an extrapulmonary disorder. Regardless of the underlying cause, hypoxemia ensues due to insufficient oxygenation.[1,7]

Ventilation/Perfusion Mismatching

$\dot{V}/\dot{Q}$ mismatching occurs when ventilation and blood flow are mismatched in various lung regions in excess of what is normal. Blood passes through alveoli that are underventilated for the given amount of perfusion, leaving these areas with a lower than normal amount of oxygen. $\dot{V}/\dot{Q}$ mismatching is the most common cause of hypoxemia and is usually the result of alveoli that are partially collapsed or partially filled with fluid.[8]

Intrapulmonary Shunting

Intrapulmonary shunting, the extreme form of $\dot{V}/\dot{Q}$ mismatching, occurs when blood reaches the arterial system without participating in gas exchange. The mixing of unoxygenated (shunted) blood and oxygenated blood lowers the average level of oxygen present in the blood. Intrapulmonary shunting occurs when blood passes through a portion of a lung that is not ventilated. This situation may result from (1) alveolar collapse secondary to atelectasis or (2) alveolar flooding with pus, blood, or fluid.[8]

Tissue Hypoxia

If allowed to progress, hypoxemia can result in a deficit of oxygen at the cellular level. As the tissue demands for oxygen continue and the supply diminishes, an oxygen supply/demand imbalance occurs and tissue hypoxia develops. Decreased oxygen to the cells contributes to impaired tissue perfusion and the development of lactic acidosis and multiple-organ dysfunction syndrome.[7]

Acute Respiratory Failure		
Clinical and diagnostic assessments	**Signs**	**Nursing interventions**

• History and risk factors
  • Tobacco use
  • Chronic pulmonary disease
• Obtain vital signs
  • O_2 saturation
• Clinical assessment
  • Inspect thorax
  • Auscultate breath sounds
  • Palpate chest wall
• Laboratory studies
  • Obtain ABGs
• Diagnostic procedures
  • Assist with bronchoscopy
  • Verify chest x-ray
  • Verify chest CT
	Type I ARF
	• Low PaO_2
	• Normal $PaCO_2$
	• Low O_2 saturation
	• Tachypnea
	• Shortness of breath
	• Abnormal breath sounds
	
	Type II ARF
	• Low PaO_2
	• Elevated $PaCO_2$
	• Low O_2 saturation
	• Tachypnea
	• Shortness of breath
	• Abnormal breath sounds
		• Assist with identifying the underlying cause
		• Administer O_2 therapy
		• Initiate NIV as appropriate
		• Assist with intubation as needed
		• Maintain MV
		• Administer medications
		• Initiate nutritional support
		• Position patient to optimize ventilation/perfusion matching
		• Promote secretion clearance
		• Prevent desaturation
		• Maintain surveillance for complications
		• Provide comfort and emotional support
		• Provide patient and family education

FIG. 18.1 Summary of Key Concepts Related to Acute Respiratory Failure. *ABGs,* Arterial blood gases; *ARF,* acute respiratory failure, *CT,* computed tomography; *MV,* mechanical ventilation; *NIV,* noninvasive ventilation; *O_2,* oxygen; *$PaCO_2$,* partial pressure of carbon dioxide in arterial blood; *PaO_2,* partial pressure of oxygen in arterial blood; *X-ray,* radiograph.

Assessment and Diagnosis

Assessment

A patient with ARF may experience a variety of clinical manifestations, depending on the underlying cause and the extent of tissue hypoxia. The clinical manifestations commonly seen in patients with ARF are usually related to the development of hypoxemia, hypercapnia, and acidosis.[1] Because the clinical symptoms are so varied, they are not considered reliable in predicting the degree of hypoxemia or hypercapnia or the severity of ARF.[6]

Diagnosis

Diagnosing and following the course of respiratory failure is best accomplished by ABG analysis. ABG analysis confirms the level of $PaCO_2$, PaO_2, and blood pH. ARF is generally accepted as being present when the PaO_2 is less than 60 mm Hg. If the patient is also experiencing hypercapnia, the $PaCO_2$ will be greater than 45 mm Hg. In patients with chronically elevated $PaCO_2$ levels, these criteria must be broadened to include a pH less than 7.35.[6]

Various additional tests are performed depending on the patient's underlying condition. These include bronchoscopy for airway surveillance or specimen retrieval, chest radiography, thoracic ultrasound, thoracic computed tomography (CT), and selected lung function studies.[4]

Medical Management

Medical management of a patient with ARF aims to treat the underlying cause, promote adequate gas exchange, correct acidosis, initiate nutrition support, and prevent complications. Medical interventions to facilitate gas exchange are aimed at improving oxygenation and ventilation.

Oxygenation

Actions to improve oxygenation include supplemental oxygen administration, with either a low-flow system or a high-flow system, and the use of positive pressure ventilation.[4,9,10] The purpose of oxygen therapy is to correct hypoxemia, although the absolute level of hypoxemia varies in each patient. Most treatment approaches aim to keep the arterial hemoglobin oxygen saturation between 96% and 98% for young adults, 94% and 98% for older adults, and 88% and 92% for patients at risk for hypercapnia. The goal is to satisfy the tissues' needs but not produce hypoxemia or hyperoxemia.[9]

Supplemental oxygen administration is effective in treating hypoxemia related to alveolar hypoventilation and $\dot{V}/\dot{Q}$ mismatching. When intrapulmonary shunting exists, supplemental oxygen alone may be ineffective. In this situation, positive pressure may be necessary to open collapsed or clear fluid-filled alveoli to facilitate their participation in gas exchange. Positive pressure is delivered via invasive and noninvasive mechanical ventilation. Positive pressure is usually administered noninvasively via a mask to avoid intubation.[4]

A recent systematic review comparing low-flow oxygen, high-flow oxygen, and noninvasive ventilation found that high-flow oxygen therapy may be superior to low-flow oxygen therapy and noninvasive ventilation in treating ARF. The review also found that high-flow oxygen therapy is better tolerated and more comfortable than noninvasive ventilation. It also concluded that more studies are needed for more definitive recommendations.[10] For further information on supplemental oxygen therapy and noninvasive ventilation, see Chapter 19.

Ventilation

Interventions to improve ventilation include the use of noninvasive and invasive mechanical ventilation. Depending on the underlying cause and the severity of the ARF, the patient may be treated initially with noninvasive ventilation.[11] Current guidelines recommend that patients with hypercapnic respiratory failure be given a trial on noninvasive ventilation unless the patient is rapidly deteriorating.[12]

TABLE 18.1 Etiologies of Acute Respiratory Failure

Affected Area	Disorders[a]
Extrapulmonary	
Brain	Oversedation Central alveolar hypoventilation syndrome Brain trauma or lesion Postoperative general anesthesia depression
Spinal cord	Guillain-Barré syndrome Poliomyelitis Amyotrophic lateral sclerosis Spinal cord trauma or lesion
Neuromuscular system	Myasthenia gravis Multiple sclerosis Neuromuscular-blocking agents Organophosphate poisoning Muscular dystrophy Critical illness polyneuropathy
Thorax	Massive obesity Chest trauma
Pleura	Pleural effusion Pneumothorax Malignancy
Upper airways	Sleep apnea Tracheal obstruction Epiglottitis Vocal cord paralysis
Intrapulmonary	
Lower airways and alveoli	Chronic obstructive pulmonary disease Asthma Bronchiolitis Cystic fibrosis Pneumonia
Pulmonary circulation	Pulmonary emboli
Alveolar–capillary membrane	Acute respiratory distress syndrome Inhalation of toxic gases Near-drowning

[a]Not an exhaustive list.

If the patient is deteriorating, the patient should be intubated and invasive mechanical ventilation initiated.[13] The selection of ventilatory mode and settings depends on the patient's underlying condition, severity of respiratory failure, and body size. Initially, the patient is started on volume ventilation in the assist/control mode. In a patient with chronic hypercapnia, the settings are adjusted to keep the ABG values within the parameters expected to be maintained by the patient after extubation.[1] For further information on mechanical ventilation, see Chapter 19.

Pharmacology

Medications to facilitate dilation of the airways may also be beneficial in treating ARF. Bronchodilators, such as beta-2 agonists and anticholinergic agents, aid in smooth muscle relaxation and are of particular benefit to patients with airflow limitations.[14,15] Methylxanthines, such as aminophylline, are no longer recommended as a first-line treatment because of their adverse side effects.[14] Steroids also are often administered to decrease airway inflammation and enhance the effects of beta-2 agonists.[14,15] Mucolytics may be used to decrease sputum viscosity and facilitate secretion clearance. Expectorants are also no longer used because they have been found to be of no benefit in this patient population.[15]

Sedation is necessary in many patients to assist with maintaining adequate ventilation. Sedation can be used to comfort the patient and decrease the work of breathing, particularly if the patient is experiencing ventilator dyssynchrony. Analgesics are administered for pain control.[16,17] In some patients, sedation does not decrease spontaneous respiratory efforts enough to allow adequate ventilation. Neuromuscular paralysis may be necessary to facilitate optimal ventilation if sedation does not achieve the desired outcome. Paralysis may also be required to decrease oxygen consumption in severely compromised patients.[17]

Acidosis

Acidosis may occur in a patient for many reasons. Hypoxemia causes impaired tissue perfusion, leading to the production of lactic acid and the development of metabolic acidosis. Impaired ventilation leads to the accumulation of carbon dioxide and the development of respiratory acidosis. The acidosis should correct itself once the patient is adequately oxygenated and ventilated. The use of sodium bicarbonate to correct metabolic acidosis has been shown to be of minimal benefit to the patient and is no longer recommended as first-line treatment.[18] Bicarbonate therapy shifts the oxygen-hemoglobin dissociation curve to the left and can worsen tissue hypoxia. Sodium bicarbonate may be used if metabolic acidosis is severe (pH less than 7.2), refractory to therapy, and causing dysrhythmias or hemodynamic instability.[19]

Nutrition Support

Initiating nutrition support is of utmost importance in managing a patient with ARF. The goals of nutrition support are to meet the overall nutrition needs of the patient while avoiding overfeeding, to prevent nutrition delivery-related complications, and to improve patient outcomes.[20] Failure to provide the patient with adequate nutrition support leads to malnutrition. Both malnutrition and overfeeding can interfere with the performance of the pulmonary system, further perpetuating ARF. Malnutrition decreases the patient's ventilatory drive and muscle strength, whereas overfeeding increases carbon dioxide production, which increases the patient's ventilatory demand, resulting in respiratory muscle fatigue.[21]

The enteral route is the preferred method of nutrition administration. If the patient cannot tolerate enteral feedings or cannot receive enough nutrients enterally, they will be started on parenteral nutrition. Because the parenteral route is associated with a higher rate of complications, the goal is to switch to enteral feedings as soon as the patient can tolerate them. Nutrition support is initiated before the third day of mechanical ventilation for well-nourished patients and within 24 hours for malnourished patients.[20,21]

Complications

Patients with ARF are at risk for several complications, including delirium, venous thromboembolism (VTE), and stress ulcers. These patients may also experience complications associated with artificial airways, mechanical ventilation, enteral and parenteral nutrition, and vascular access devices.

Delirium. Delirium is a form of acute brain dysfunction that results from various factors, including hypoxemia, sepsis, sedation, and metabolic derangements. It has been reported in

60% to 80% of mechanically ventilated patients[22] Additional information about delirium and delirium management can be found in Chapter 8.

Venous thromboembolism. VTE is precipitated by venous stasis resulting from immobility and places the patient at risk of developing a pulmonary embolism (PE). Current guidelines recommend early initiation of prophylaxis using intermittent pneumatic compression devices and low-dose unfractionated heparin or low-molecular-weight heparin (LMWH).[23]

Stress ulcers. Stress ulcers are gastrointestinal tract erosions secondary to hypoperfusion. They can be prevented using histamine receptor antagonists and proton pump inhibitors. In the past, there have been some concerns that the use of stress ulcer prophylaxis increased the risk of ventilator-associated pneumonia (VAP) and *Clostridioides difficile* infection. However, the latest literature indicates that stress ulcer prophylaxis is safe and does not increase the risk for these complications.[24]

Nursing Management

The patient care management plan for a patient with ARF incorporates a variety of patient problems (Box 18.1). Nursing actions are driven by the specific cause of the respiratory failure, although there are some common interventions that are appropriate for all patients with ARF. The nurse has a significant role in optimizing oxygenation and ventilation, providing comfort and emotional support, maintaining surveillance for complications, and educating the patient and family.

Optimize Oxygenation and Ventilation

Nursing interventions to optimize oxygenation and ventilation include positioning, preventing desaturation, and promoting secretion clearance.

Positioning. Positioning of a patient with ARF depends on the type of lung injury and the underlying cause of hypoxemia. For patients with $\dot{V}/\dot{Q}$ mismatching, positioning is used to facilitate better matching of ventilation with perfusion to optimize gas exchange. Because gravity normally facilitates preferential ventilation and perfusion to the dependent areas of the lungs, the best gas exchange would take place in the dependent areas of the lungs. Thus, positioning aims to place the least affected area of the patient's lung in the most dependent position. Patients with unilateral lung disease are positioned with the healthy lung in a dependent position. Patients with diffuse lung disease may benefit from being positioned with the right lung down because it is larger and more vascular than the left lung.[25] For patients with alveolar hypoventilation, positioning aims to facilitate ventilation. These patients benefit from nonrecumbent positions such as sitting or a semierect position.[26] Elevating the head of the bed 30 to 45 degrees has also been shown to decrease the risk of aspiration[27] and VAP[28]; however, it also has been shown to increase the risk of pressure injuries.[29] Frequent repositioning is beneficial in optimizing the patient's ventilatory pattern and $\dot{V}/\dot{Q}$ matching.

Preventing desaturation. Numerous activities can prevent desaturation, including performing procedures only as needed, hyperoxygenating the patient before suctioning, providing adequate rest and recovery time between procedures, and minimizing oxygen consumption. Interventions to minimize oxygen consumption include limiting the patient's physical activity, administering sedation to control anxiety, and providing measures to control fever. The patient is continuously monitored with a pulse oximeter to warn of signs of desaturation.

Promoting secretion clearance. Interventions to promote secretion clearance in the patient who is intubated include providing adequate systemic hydration, oxygen humidification, and suctioning. These therapies are further discussed in Chapter 19. Postural drainage and chest percussion and vibration are of little benefit in critically ill patients and are not discussed here.[30,31] Once the patient is extubated, airway clearance therapy may be needed depending on the patient's underlying condition. It is essential to collaborate with the patient's pulmonary practitioner and respiratory care practitioner to determine the best treatment for the patient.

Educate the Patient and Family

Early in the patient's hospital stay, the patient and family are taught about ARF, its causes, and its treatment. Closer to discharge, patient and family education focuses on the interventions necessary to prevent the precipitating disorder's reoccurrence (Box 18.2). If the patient uses tobacco, they are encouraged to stop using tobacco products (Box 18.3) and are referred to a tobacco cessation program (Box 18.4).[32] In addition, the importance of participating in a pulmonary rehabilitation program is stressed.[33]

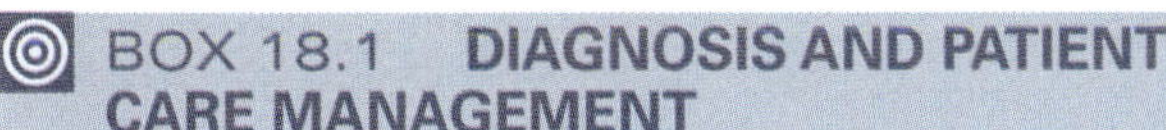
BOX 18.1 DIAGNOSIS AND PATIENT CARE MANAGEMENT

Acute Respiratory Failure

- Impaired Gas Exchange due to alveolar hypoventilation
- Impaired Gas Exchange due to ventilation-perfusion mismatching or intrapulmonary shunting
- Impaired Breathing due to musculoskeletal fatigue or neuromuscular impairment
- Risk for Aspiration
- Impaired Nutritional Intake due to lack of exogenous nutrients and increased metabolic demand
- Risk for Infection
- Impaired Breathing due to respiratory muscle fatigue or metabolic factors
- Delirium due to sensory overload, sensory deprivation, and sleep pattern disturbance
- Anxiety due to threat to biological, psychological, or social integrity
- Impaired Family Coping due to critically ill family member
- Lack of Knowledge of Treatment Regime due to lack of previous exposure to information (see Box 18.2, Patient and Family Education Plan: Acute Respiratory Failure)

Patient Care Management Plans are located in Appendix A.

ACUTE RESPIRATORY DISTRESS SYNDROME

Description and Etiology

Acute respiratory distress syndrome (ARDS) is a complex clinical condition that manifests as the severest form of ARF.[34] It is characterized by severe hypoxemia due to noncardiac pulmonary edema as a result of disruption of the alveolar-capillary membrane.[34-36] Even though management of ARDS has improved significantly over the past 2 decades, it continues to be a leading cause of death in critically ill patients. The mortality rates remain consistently around 30% to 40%.[37]

Many different diagnostic criteria have been used to identify ARDS, which has led to confusion, particularly among researchers. In 2012, in an attempt to address the limitations

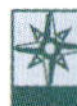

BOX 18.2 PATIENT AND FAMILY EDUCATION PLAN

Acute Respiratory Failure

Before discharge, the patient should be able to teach back the following topics:

- Pathophysiology of disease
- Specific etiology
- Modification of precipitating factors
- Importance of taking medications
- Breathing techniques (e.g., pursed-lip breathing, diaphragmatic breathing)
- Energy conservation techniques
- Measures to prevent pulmonary infections (e.g., proper nutrition, handwashing, immunization against *Streptococcus pneumoniae* and influenza viruses)
- Signs and symptoms of pulmonary infections (e.g., sputum color change, shortness of breath, fever)
- Cough enhancement techniques (e.g., cascade cough, huff cough, end-expiratory cough, augmented cough)

BOX 18.3 Tobacco Products

- Cigarettes (i.e., cigs, ciggies)
- Cigarette tobacco (i.e., roll-your-own, roll-ups, hand rolled)
- Smokeless tobacco (i.e., dip, snuff, snus, spit tobacco, chew, chewing tobacco)
- Kreteks (i.e., clove cigarettes)
- Pipe tobacco
- Hookah tobacco (i.e., waterpipe, maassel, shisha or sheesha, narghile, argileh or argileh)
- Cigars, cigarillos, and little filtered cigars
- Nicotine gels
- Dissolvable tobacco (i.e., dissolvables)
- Electronic nicotine delivery systems
  - Vape pens (i.e., vapes)
  - Vaporizers
  - Hookah pens
  - E-cigarettes (i.e., e-cigs)
  - E-pipes
  - E-cigars

Data from *U.S. Food and Drug Administration*. Tobacco Products. https://www.fda.gov/tobacco-products.

of the existing definition of ARDS, the ARDS Definition Task Force drafted a new definition (known as the *Berlin Definition*) of ARDS. This definition eliminated the term "acute lung injury" and proposed three distinct categories (mild, moderate, and severe) of ARDS based on the severity of hypoxemia. The Berlin Definition of ARDS is as follows:

- Timing: Within 1 week of known clinical insult or new or worsening respiratory symptoms
- Chest imaging: Bilateral opacities not fully explained by effusions, lobar/lung collapse, or nodules
- Origin of edema: Respiratory failure not fully explained by heart failure or fluid overload; objective assessment needed to exclude hydrostatic edema if no risk factor present
- Oxygenation: Mild (200 mm Hg less than PaO_2/fraction of inspired oxygen [FiO_2] less than or equal to 300 mm Hg with positive end-expiratory airway pressure [PEEP] or continuous positive airway pressure [CPAP] greater than or equal to

BOX 18.4 Evidence-Based Practice

Tobacco Cessation Guidelines

The following are the key recommendations of the updated guideline *Treating Tobacco Use and Dependence*, based on the literature review and expert panel opinion

- Tobacco dependence is a chronic disease that often requires repeated intervention and multiple attempts to quit. However, effective treatments exist that can significantly increase long-term abstinence rates.
- It is essential that clinicians and health care delivery systems consistently identify and document tobacco use status and treat every tobacco user seen in a health care setting.
- Tobacco dependence treatments are effective across a broad range of populations. Clinicians should encourage every patient willing to make a quit attempt to use the counseling treatments and medications recommended in this guideline.
- Brief tobacco dependence treatment is effective. Clinicians should offer every patient who uses tobacco at least the brief treatments shown to be effective in this guideline.
- Individual, group, and telephone counseling are effective, and their effectiveness increases with treatment intensity. Two components of counseling are especially effective, and clinicians should use these when counseling patients making a quit attempt:
  - Practical counseling (problem solving/skills training)
  - Social support delivered as part of treatment
- Numerous effective medications are available for tobacco dependence, and clinicians should encourage their use by all patients attempting to quit smoking, except when medically contraindicated or with specific populations for which there is insufficient evidence of effectiveness (e.g., pregnant women, smokeless tobacco users, light smokers, and adolescents).
- Seven first-line medications (five nicotine and two nonnicotine) reliably increase long-term smoking abstinence rates:
  - Bupropion SR
  - Nicotine gum
  - Nicotine inhaler
  - Nicotine lozenge
  - Nicotine nasal spray
  - Nicotine patch
  - Varenicline
- Clinicians also should consider using certain combinations of medications identified as effective in this guideline.
- Counseling and medication are effective when used by themselves for treating tobacco dependence. However, the combination of counseling and medication is more effective than either alone. Thus clinicians should encourage all individuals making a quit attempt to use both counseling and medication.
- Telephone quitline counseling is effective with diverse populations and has broad reach. Therefore clinicians and health care delivery systems should both ensure patient access to quitlines and promote quitline use.
- If a tobacco user currently is unwilling to make a quit attempt, clinicians should use the motivational treatments shown in this guideline to be effective in increasing future quit attempts.
- Tobacco dependence treatments are both clinically effective and highly cost effective relative to interventions for other clinical disorders. Providing coverage for these treatments increases quit rates. Insurers and purchasers should ensure that all insurance plans include the counseling and medication identified as effective in this guideline as covered benefits.

From Tobacco Use and Dependence Guideline Panel. Treating Tobacco Use and Dependence: 2008 Update. Health and Human Service Website. 2008. https://www.ahrq.gov/sites/default/files/wysiwyg/professionals/clinicians-providers/guidelines-recommendations/tobacco/clinicians/update/treating_tobacco_use08.pdf.

5 cm H_2O); moderate (100 mm Hg less than PaO_2/FiO_2 less than or equal to 200 mm Hg with PEEP greater than or equal to 5 cm H_2O); or severe (PaO_2/FiO_2 less than or equal to 100 mm Hg with PEEP greater than or equal to 5 cm H_2O).[38]

Etiology

A wide variety of clinical conditions is associated with the development of ARDS. These are categorized as *direct* or *indirect*, depending on the primary site of injury (Fig. 18.2). Direct injuries are injuries in which the lung epithelium sustains a direct insult.[39] The recent coronavirus disease-2019 (COVID-19) pandemic, which resulted from Severe Acute Respiratory Syndrome Coronavirus-2 (SARS-CoV-2) infection, is an example of a virus causing direct injury to the lung epithelium (Box 18.5).[40] Indirect injuries are injuries where the insult occurs elsewhere in the body, and mediators are transmitted via the bloodstream to the lungs.[39] Sepsis, pancreatitis, aspiration of gastric contents, diffuse pneumonia, and trauma were found to be major risk factors for the development of ARDS.[39] Several risk factors have been identified that increase susceptibility to ARDS, including tobacco use, alcohol abuse, air pollution, and hypoalbuminaemia.[34,41]

Pathophysiology

ARDS is a dysregulated inflammatory response that starts with stimulation of the inflammatory-immune system secondary to an injury to the alveolar-capillary membrane (Fig. 18.3).[34,42]

Exudative Phase

The exudative or acute phase ensues within 72 hours after the initial insult. During this phase, alveolar macrophages are activated, leading to the recruitment of neutrophils and other circulating macrophages to the site, further stimulating the release of proinflammatory mediators. These mediators cause damage to the pulmonary capillary endothelium and alveolar epithelium, impairing the integrity of the alveolar-capillary membrane. The damage allows protein-rich fluid, blood cells, and fibrin to escape into the interstitial space from the damaged capillaries. The volume of fluid quickly overwhelms the lymphatic drainage system, resulting in the development of interstitial edema. The fluid then moves from the interstitial space into the damaged alveoli, resulting in alveolar edema. Damage to the type I alveolar epithelial cells allows hyaline membranes to form secondary to proteins, fibrin, and cellular debris deposition. Interstitial edema also causes compression of the alveoli and small airways. Damage to the pulmonary capillaries also causes the development of microthrombi and elevation of pulmonary artery pressures. Eventually, the type II alveolar epithelial cells are damaged, leading to impaired surfactant production. Injury to the alveolar epithelial cells and the loss of surfactant lead to further alveolar collapse. This phase may last 7 to 10 days.[34,35,40]

Hypoxemia occurs as a result of intrapulmonary shunting and $\dot{V}/\dot{Q}$ mismatching secondary to compression, collapse, and flooding of the alveoli and small airways. Increased work of breathing occurs due to increased airway resistance, decreased functional residual capacity (FRC), and decreased lung compliance secondary to atelectasis and compression of the small airways. Hypoxemia and the increased work of breathing lead to patient fatigue and the development of alveolar hypoventilation.[41] Pulmonary hypertension occurs as a result of damage to the pulmonary capillaries, microthrombi, and hypoxic vasoconstriction, leading to the development of increased alveolar dead

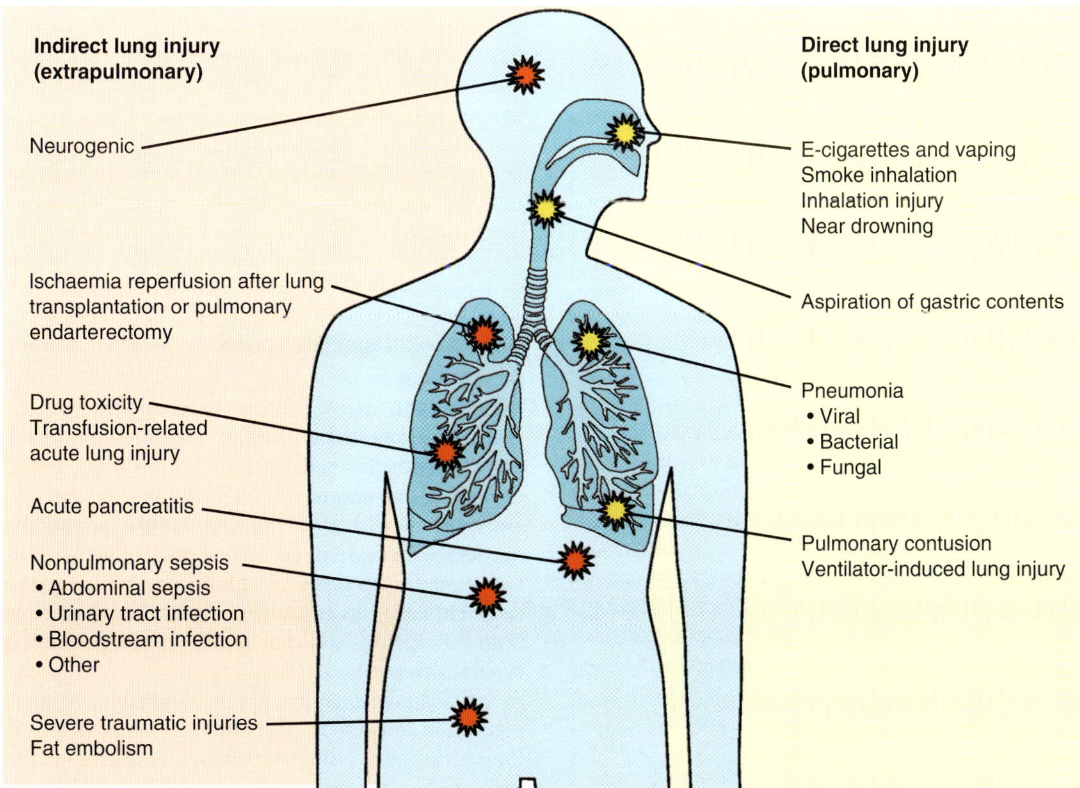

FIG. 18.2 Causes of Acute Respiratory Distress Syndrome. (From Bos LDJ, Ware LB. Acute respiratory distress syndrome: causes, pathophysiology, and phenotypes. *Lancet.* 2022;400(10358):1145–1156.)

BOX 18.5 Coronaviruses and COVID-19

Coronaviruses

The global COVID-19 coronavirus pandemic has focused worldwide attention on viral infectious disease transmission and mortality risk. According to the Centers for Disease Control and Prevention, there are seven known types of infectious coronavirus.[1]

Four coronavirus types cause mild upper respiratory infections similar to the common cold and do not pose a serious health risk:[1]

- Alpha coronaviruses 229E and NK63
- Beta coronaviruses OC43 and HKU1

Three coronaviruses are known to be highly infectious for humans and associated with high mortality. Coronaviruses are present in both animals and humans, and the following three have evolved to infect humans:[1]

- MERS-CoV: a beta coronavirus that causes Middle East Respiratory Syndrome (MERS)
- SARS-CoV: a beta coronavirus that causes severe acute respiratory syndrome (SARS)
- SARS-CoV-2: a novel coronavirus that causes coronavirus disease 2019 (COVID-19)

The mortality for SARS is reported at 9.5%.[2] The mortality for MERS is much higher and is reported as 34%.[2] The absolute mortality rate for COVID-19 is still uncertain as the pandemic continues. What is known is that COVID-19 has a higher mortality rate in older adults and those with underlying medical conditions or comorbidities. In addition, COVID-19 is more easily transmitted from person to person than either SARS or MERS.[2]

COVID-19 Clinical Features

The clinical features associated with COVID-19 are highly variable. Some individuals may contract the virus and be asymptomatic. Others may have a high temperature, cough, dyspnea, muscle aches, and extreme fatigue but can recover at home. Other individuals develop severe ARF/ARDS and end-organ damage and are admitted to a critical care unit.

Patients with severe COVID-19 admitted to a critical care unit often have respiratory distress and low oxygen saturation that requires high-flow oxygen or intubation and mechanical ventilation. COVID-19 can also impair the neurologic, cardiovascular, gastrointestinal, and dermatologic systems.[3]

COVID-19 Clinical Management

The clinical management of COVID-19 depends on the specific manifestations of the infection. Critical care management is individualized to signs and symptoms, and treatments evolve as new medications with proven effectiveness are approved. Examples of treatment for severe COVID-19 are the use of the antiviral medication Remdesivir and the corticosteroid dexamethasone.[4] Many other medications are undergoing clinical trials.

COVID-19 Environmental Management

Because COVID-19 is highly transmissible, it poses unique risks for health care workers caring for patients who are positive for COVID-19. Optimal use of personal protective equipment (PPE) continues to evolve as more is learned about the virus. Environmental protection can include a negative-flow pressure room (if available) and limiting family visitors to decrease transmission. Health care personnel may use N95 masks, eye goggles/face shields, disposable protective gowns, gloves, head-covering hats, and shoe covers, depending on the situation. There have been controversies about optimal PPE, especially due to shortages at the beginning of the pandemic. The CDC has some guidance about optimizing the supply of PPE during shortages and the correct procedures for donning and doffing PPE.[5]

References

1. Centers for Disease Control and Prevention. Coronavirus types. https://www.cdc.gov/coronavirus/types.html; 2020.
2. Malik P, Patel K, Akrmah M, et al. COVID-19: A disease with a potpourri of histopathologic findings-a literature review and comparison to the closely related SARS and MERS. *SN Compr Clin Med.* 2021:1–28. https://doi.org/10.1007/s42399-021-01029-5.
3. Long B, Carius BM, Chavez S, et al. Clinical update on COVID-19 for the emergency clinician: Presentation and evaluation. *Am J Emerg Med.* 2022;54:46–57. https://doi.org/10.1016/j.ajem.2022.01.028.
4. Bai C, Chotirmall SH, Rello J, et al. Updated guidance on the management of COVID-19: From an American Thoracic Society/European Respiratory Society coordinated International Task Force (29 July 2020). *Eur Respir Rev.* 2020;29(157):200287. https://doi.org/10.1183/16000617.0287-2020.
5. Centers for Disease Control and Prevention. Optimizing supply of PPE and other equipment during shortages. https://www.cdc.gov/coronavirus/2019-ncov/hcp/ppe-strategy/index.html; 2020.

space and right ventricular afterload.[43] Hypoxemia worsens due to alveolar hypoventilation and increased alveolar dead space.[41] Right ventricular afterload increases and leads to right ventricular dysfunction and a decrease in cardiac output (CO).[43]

Proliferative Phase

The proliferative or subacute phase begins as healing is initiated to restore the alveolar-capillary membrane. Antiinflammatory mediators neutralize inflammatory mediators. Fibroblasts form a provisional matrix to facilitate repair. The type II alveolar epithelial cells multiply, some of which differentiate into type I alveolar epithelial cells, facilitating the restoration of the alveolus. Alveolar macrophages remove cellular debris. Pulmonary capillaries are reestablished. The hyaline membranes are cleared, and intraalveolar fluid is transported from the alveoli into the interstitium. This phase occurs over 2 to 3 weeks and is the recovery point for some patients.[35,40]

Fibrotic Phase

In some patients, ARDS does not resolve, and they enter a fibrotic or chronic phase. Resolution failure can occur for several reasons, including ongoing inflammation and an imbalance between profibrotic and antifibrotic mediators. This situation can lead to reabsorption failure of the provisional matrix and collagen deposition. Persistent fibroblast activation leads to interstitial and intraalveolar fibrosis and microvascular damage. This state leads to stiffening of the lungs, ongoing pulmonary hypertension, and continued hypoxemia. The patient ends up with residual fibrosis and persistent pulmonary dysfunction.[35,41]

Assessment and Diagnosis

Assessment

Patients with ARDS initially may be seen with various clinical manifestations, depending on the precipitating event. As the disorder progresses, the patient will exhibit signs and symptoms of respiratory failure. Initially, the patient may report dyspnea and present with tachypnea, restlessness, apprehension, and a moderate increase in accessory muscle use. ARDS must be differentiated from acute heart failure (AHF) as part of the diagnosis.[35] However, in some situations, the patient may experience both ARDS and AHF, particularly if the patient has a history of cardiac disease.[44]

ABG analysis shows a low PaO_2 despite increases in supplemental oxygen administration (refractory hypoxemia). The $PaCO_2$ initially is low secondary to tachypnea but eventually increases as the patient fatigues. The pH is high initially but decreases as respiratory acidosis develops.

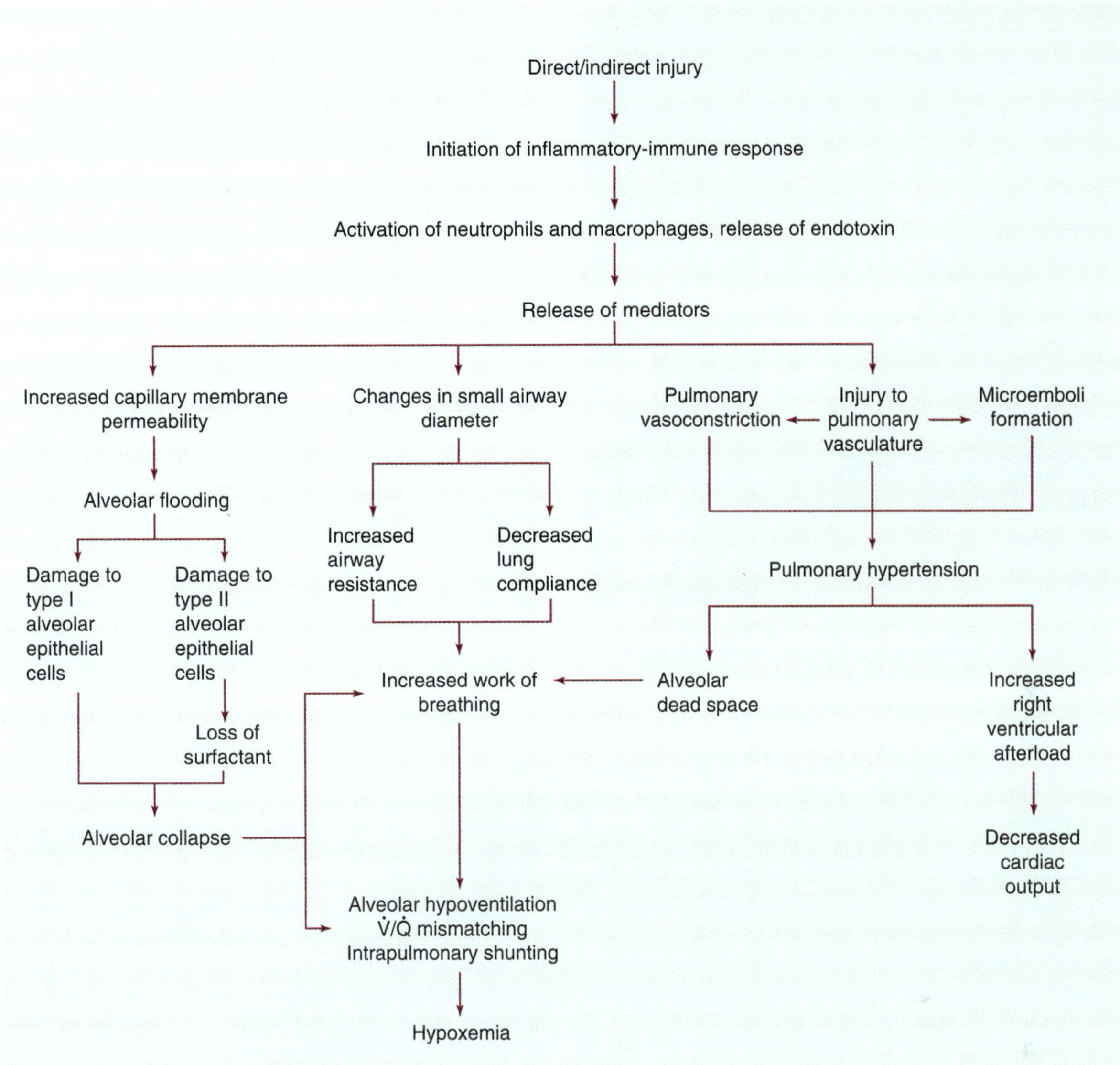

FIG. 18.3 Pathophysiology of Acute Respiratory Distress Syndrome.

Initially, the chest radiograph may be normal because lung changes may not become evident for 24 hours. As the pulmonary edema becomes apparent, diffuse, patchy interstitial and alveolar infiltrates appear (Fig. 18.4). This progresses to multifocal consolidation of the lungs, which appears as a "whiteout" on the chest radiograph.[44]

Diagnosis

There is no specific laboratory test or diagnostic procedure for identifying ARDS. The diagnosis is made based on the patient's clinical signs and symptoms. Different tests and procedures are used to identify the underlying cause and will vary depending on the suspected cause. The diagnosis is made using the Berlin criteria. However, this definition has some limitations and may miss certain patients. This situation became evident during the COVID-19 pandemic as patients were being treated with high-flow nasal oxygen (HFNO) therapy (instead of CPAP), which is not part of the Berlin definition.[44] A proposal has been put forth to revise the Berlin definition to include treatment with HFNO of at least 30 L/min to be included in the definition.[45]

Medical Management

Medical management of a patient with ARDS involves a multifaceted approach. This strategy includes treating the underlying cause, promoting gas exchange, supporting tissue oxygenation, initiating nutritional support, and preventing complications. The patient is at risk for VTE and stress ulcers and should be started on prophylaxis to prevent these complications.[35] Patients with mild ARDS may benefit from noninvasive ventilation or HFNO. However, most patients require intubation and mechanical ventilation to facilitate adequate gas exchange, given the severity of hypoxemia.[35]

Ventilation

Volume-control or pressure-control ventilation can be used to ventilate the patient with ARDS.[46] With volume-controlled ventilation, gas is delivered at a preset tidal volume, while pressure-controlled ventilation gas is delivered at a preset pressure. For more information on mechanical ventilation, see Chapter 19. Current guidelines strongly recommend not using high-frequency oscillatory ventilation, as research has

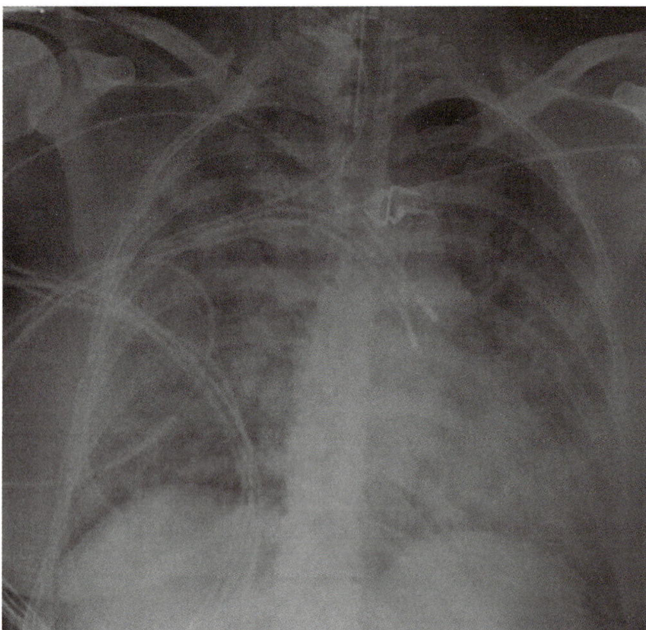

FIG. 18.4 Chest Radiograph. Bilateral alveolar infiltrates on chest radiograph. (From Janz DR, Ware LB. Approach to the patient with the acute respiratory distress syndrome. *Clin Chest Med.* 2014;35(4):685–696.)

demonstrated that this mode of ventilation does not provide any additional benefit over conventional ventilation and may even be harmful.[40,47]

Regardless of the ventilation mode used, the goal is to avoid further lung injury. It is now known that repeated opening and closing of the alveoli cause injury to the lung units (atelectrauma), resulting in inhibited surfactant production and increased inflammation (biotrauma), resulting in the release of mediators and an increase in pulmonary capillary membrane permeability. In addition, excessive pressure in the alveoli (barotrauma) or excessive volume in the alveoli (volutrauma) leads to excessive alveolar wall stress and damage to the alveolar-capillary membrane, resulting in air escaping into the surrounding spaces.[40] Thus, a couple of different approaches have been developed to facilitate the mechanical ventilation of patients with ARDS. The goal is to keep the patient's plateau pressure (end-inspiratory static pressure) lower than 30 cm H_2O.[46]

Low tidal volume. Low tidal volume ventilation uses smaller tidal volumes (4 to 8 mL/kg) to ventilate the patient in an attempt to limit the effects of barotrauma and volutrauma.[47] The goal is to provide the maximum tidal volume possible while maintaining an end-inspiratory plateau pressure of less than 30 cm H_2O.[47] To allow for adequate carbon dioxide elimination, the respiratory rate may be increased up to 35 breaths/min.[35,36,48]

Permissive hypercapnia. Permissive hypercapnia uses low tidal volume ventilation in conjunction with normal respiratory rates in an attempt to limit the effects of atelectrauma and biotrauma.[48] To maintain normocapnia, the patient's respiratory rate normally would have to be increased to compensate for the small tidal volume. In ARDS, increasing the respiratory rate can lead to worsening alveolar damage. Thus, the patient's carbon dioxide level is allowed to increase, and the patient becomes hypercapnic. As a rule, the patient's $PaCO_2$ should not exceed 50 mm Hg. Because of the negative cardiopulmonary effects of severe acidosis, the arterial pH is generally maintained at 7.30 or greater.[35] To maintain the pH, adjustments may need to be made to the respiratory rate or tidal volume.[35]

Oxygen Therapy

Oxygen is administered at the lowest level possible to support tissue oxygenation. Continued exposure to high oxygen levels can lead to oxygen toxicity, which perpetuates the entire process. The goal of oxygen therapy is to maintain PaO_2 between 55 mm Hg and 80 mm Hg oxygen saturation between 88% to 95%.[48]

Positive end-expiratory pressure. Because the hypoxemia that develops with ARDS is often refractory or unresponsive to oxygen therapy, it is necessary to facilitate oxygenation with PEEP. PEEP is used in a patient with ARDS to improve oxygenation while reducing FiO_2 to less toxic levels.[36] PEEP has several positive effects on the lungs, including opening collapsed alveoli, stabilizing flooded alveoli, and increasing FRC.[47] Thus, PEEP decreases intrapulmonary shunting and increases compliance. PEEP has several adverse effects, including (1) decreasing CO due to decreasing venous return secondary to increased intrathoracic pressure and (2) barotrauma due to gas escaping into the surrounding spaces secondary to alveolar rupture.[36] The most commonly used method is to match the PEEP to the FiO_2 using an algorithm. The higher the FiO_2, the higher the PEEP.[36] In patients with moderate to severe ARDS, a PEEP greater than 12 cm H_2O is associated with a lower mortality.[35] If PEEP is too high, it can result in overdistention of the alveoli, which can impede pulmonary capillary blood flow, decrease surfactant production, and worsen intrapulmonary shunting.[47] If PEEP is too low, it allows the alveoli to collapse during expiration, which can result in more damage to the alveoli.

Extracorporeal membrane oxygenation. Extracorporeal membrane oxygen (ECMO) is a technique used in the treatment of severe ARDS when conventional therapy has failed. ECMO allows the lungs to rest by facilitating carbon dioxide removal and providing oxygen external to the lungs through an "artificial lung" or membrane/fiber oxygenator. ECMO is similar to cardiopulmonary bypass in that blood is removed from the body and pumped through a membrane oxygenator, where CO_2 is removed, O_2 is added and then returned to the body. Extracorporeal carbon dioxide removal is a variation of ECMO in which the primary focus is the removal of CO_2.[35,41]

Tissue Perfusion

Adequate tissue perfusion depends on an adequate supply of oxygen being transported to the tissues. An adequate CO and hemoglobin level is critical to oxygen transport. CO depends on heart rate, preload, afterload, and contractility. Various fluids and medications are used to manipulate these parameters. The goal is to decrease the amount of fluid leakage into the lungs while maintaining an adequate CO.[42] Currently, there is no ideal fluid strategy, and different approaches may be needed depending on the severity of ARDS and the underlying cause.[49]

Nursing Management

The patient care management plan for a patient with ARDS incorporates a variety of patient problems (Box 18.6). The nurse has a significant role in optimizing oxygenation and ventilation, providing comfort and emotional support, and maintaining surveillance for complications.

BOX 18.6 DIAGNOSIS AND PATIENT CARE MANAGEMENT

Acute Respiratory Distress Syndrome

- Impaired Gas Exchange due to ventilation/perfusion mismatching or intrapulmonary shunting
- Impaired Cardiac Output due to alterations in preload
- Impaired Nutritional Intake due to lack of exogenous nutrients or increased metabolic demand
- Risk for Aspiration
- Risk for Infection
- Anxiety due to biological, psychological, and/or social integrity
- Impaired Family Coping due to critically ill family member

Patient Care Management plans are located in Appendix A.

Optimize Oxygenation and Ventilation

Nursing interventions to optimize oxygenation and ventilation include positioning, preventing desaturation, and promoting secretion clearance. For further discussion of these interventions, see Nursing Management of Acute Respiratory Failure earlier in this chapter. One additional nursing intervention that can be used to improve the oxygenation and ventilation of a patient with ARDS is prone positioning.

Prone positioning. Numerous studies have shown that prone positioning of a patient with ARDS results in an improvement in oxygenation. Although many theories propose how prone positioning improves oxygenation, the discovery that with ARDS there is greater damage to the dependent areas of the lungs probably provides the best explanation. It was initially thought that ARDS was a diffuse homogeneous disease that affected all areas of the lungs equally. It is now known that the dependent lung areas are more heavily damaged than the nondependent lung areas. Turning the patient prone improves perfusion to less damaged parts of the lungs and improves $\dot{V}/\dot{Q}$ matching and decreases intrapulmonary shunting. Prone positioning appears more effective when initiated during the early phases of ARDS and applied for at least 16 hours a day.[42] For more information on prone positioning, see Chapter 19.

Interprofessional collaborative management of a patient with ARDS is outlined in Box 18.7.

BOX 18.7 Teamwork and Collaboration

Acute Respiratory Distress Syndrome

- Intubate the patient and initiate mechanical ventilation.
  - Low tidal volume ventilation
  - Permissive hypercapnia
  - Positive end-expiratory pressure (PEEP)
- Administer medications.
  - Bronchodilators
  - Sedatives
  - Analgesics
  - Neuromuscular blocking agents
- Maximize tissue perfusion.
  - Preload
  - Afterload
  - Contractility
- Position patient prone.
- Suction as needed.
- Provide rest and recovery time between procedures.
- Initiate nutrition support.
- Maintain surveillance for complications.
  - Delirium
  - Venous thromboembolism
  - Stress ulcers
  - Ventilator-induced lung injury
  - Oxygen toxicity
- Provide comfort and emotional support.

PNEUMONIA

Description and Etiology

Pneumonia is an acute inflammation of the lung parenchyma that is caused by an infectious agent that can lead to alveolar consolidation.[50] Pneumonia can be classified as community-acquired pneumonia (CAP), hospital-acquired pneumonia (HAP), or VAP.[51] Pneumonia is referred to as community acquired when it occurs outside of the hospital or within 48 hours of admission to the hospital.[51] Severe CAP requires admission to the critical care unit and accounts for approximately 19% of all patients with pneumonia.[52] The mortality for this patient group is approximately 30%,[53] with increasing age as a major risk factor.[54] Pneumonia is referred to as hospital acquired when it occurs while the patient is in the hospital for at least 48 hours and is not associated with mechanical ventilation.[51] VAP refers to the development of pneumonia occurring at least 48 hours after the insertion of an artificial airway.[55] Approximately 10% of patients requiring mechanical ventilation develop VAP,[55] and the mortality rate in VAP may be as high as 30% to 70%.[56]

The spectra of etiologic pathogens of pneumonia vary with the type of pneumonia, as do the risk factors for the disease. Pathogens that can cause pneumonia include bacteria, viruses, and fungi. Fig. 18.5 summarizes the key concepts for managing a patient with severe pneumonia.

Severe Community-Acquired Pneumonia

Bacterial pathogens associated with CAP include *Streptococcus pneumoniae*, *Legionella* species, *Haemophilus influenzae*, *Moraxella catarrhalis*, *Staphylococcus aureus*, *Mycoplasma pneumoniae*, *Chlamydia pneumoniae*, *Klebsiella pneumoniae*, and *Pseudomonas aeruginosa*.[2] Viral pathogens include SARS-CoV-2, influenza, parainfluenza viruses, adenoviruses, and respiratory syncytial virus (RSV).[54] Two common fungal pathogens are Histoplasma and Coccidioides.[52]

Numerous factors increase the risk of developing CAP, including lifestyle influences such as tobacco and alcohol misuse and comorbid conditions such as respiratory, cardiovascular, liver, kidney, and neurologic disease, diabetes, and malignancy.[57] Impaired swallowing and altered mental status also contribute to the development of CAP because they result in increased exposure to various pathogens related to chronic aspiration of oropharyngeal secretions.[2,58] Box 18.8 highlights the management of adult patients with a history of cystic fibrosis.

Hospital-Acquired Pneumonia

Bacterial pathogens associated with HAP include *S. pneumoniae*, *S. aureus*, *K. pneumoniae*, *P. aeruginosa*, and *Enterobacter*

Severe Pneumonia

Clinical and diagnostic assessments	Signs	Nursing interventions

• History and risk factors - CAP
  • Chronic pulmonary disease
  • Diabetes
  • Impaired swallowing
• History and risk factors - HAP
  • Impaired host defenses
  • Invasive treatments
  • Inadequate handwashing
• Obtain vital signs
  • O_2 saturation
• Clinical assessment
  • Inspect thorax
  • Auscultate breath sounds
  • Palpate chest wall
  • Percuss chest wall
• Laboratory studies
  • Obtain ABGs
  • Sputum gram stain and C&S
• Diagnostic procedures
  • Assist with bronchoscopy
  • Verify chest x-ray
	• Confusion/Disorientation
	• Shortness of breath
	• Fever
	• Cough
	  • Productive
	  • Nonproductive
	• Tachypnea
	• Crackles on auscultation
	• Dullness to percussion
	• Low PaO_2
	• Elevated $PaCO_2$
	• Low O_2 saturation
	• Pulmonary infiltrates on x-ray
		• Administer O_2 therapy
		• Initiate NIV as appropriate
		• Assist with intubation as needed
		• Maintain MV
		• Administer antibiotics
		• Position patient to optimize ventilation/perfusion matching
		• Promote secretion clearance
		• Prevent desaturation
		• Prevent the spread of infection
		• Maintain surveillance for complications
		• Provide comfort and emotional support
		• Monitor patient response to antibiotics

FIG. 18.5 Summary of Key Concepts Related to Severe Pneumonia. *ABGs,* Arterial blood gases; *C&S,* culture and sensitivity; *MV,* mechanical ventilation; *NIV,* noninvasive ventilation; *O_2,* oxygen; *$PaCO_2$,* partial pressure of carbon dioxide in arterial blood; *PaO_2,* partial pressure of oxygen in arterial blood; *X-ray,* radiograph.

species. Risk factors for HAP can be categorized as host related, treatment related, and infection-control related (Box 18.9).[51]

Ventilator-Associated Pneumonia

VAP is a misleading term because it is not really related to mechanical ventilation but to the presence of an artificial airway.[52] The types of pathogens that can cause VAP vary with the time of onset, geographic areas, specific patient characteristics, and risk factors for multidrug-resistant (MDR) organisms, such as prior antibiotic exposure.[59] Bacterial pathogens include *S. aureus, P. aeruginosa, Escherichia coli, K. pneumoniae,* and *Acinetobacter* species.[60] While early-onset (within 4 days of hospitalization) VAP is usually associated with oropharyngeal organisms, late-onset (occurring after 4 days of hospitalization) VAP is associated with MDR organisms.[60]

Pathophysiology

Development of acute pneumonia implies a defect in host defenses, a particularly virulent organism, or an overwhelming inoculation event. Bacterial invasion of the lower respiratory tract can occur by inhalation of aerosolized infectious particles, aspiration of organisms colonizing the oropharynx, migration of organisms from adjacent sites of colonization, direct inoculation of organisms into the lower airway, spread of infection to the lungs from adjacent structures, spread of infection to the lung through the blood, and reactivation of latent infection (usually in the setting of immunosuppression). The most common mechanism appears to be aspiration of oropharyngeal organisms.[61] Disruption of the gag and cough reflexes, altered consciousness, and abnormal swallowing can predispose the patient to aspiration and colonization of the lungs and subsequent infection. Table 18.2 lists the precipitating conditions that can facilitate the development of pneumonia.

Fig. 18.6 depicts the pathophysiology of HAP. Colonization of the patient's oropharynx with infectious organisms is a major contributor to the development of HAP. The oropharynx normally has a stable population of resident flora that may be anaerobic or aerobic. Pathogenic organisms replace normal resident flora when stress occurs, such as with illness, surgery, or infection. Previous antibiotic therapy also affects the resident flora population, making replacement by pathologic organisms more likely. The pathogens are then able to invade the sterile lower respiratory tract.[61]

Infection results in pulmonary inflammation with or without significant exudates. Increased capillary permeability occurs, leading to increased interstitial and alveolar fluid. $\dot{V}/\dot{Q}$ mismatching and intrapulmonary shunting occur, resulting in hypoxemia as lung consolidation progresses. Untreated pneumonia can result in ARF, initiation of the inflammatory-immune response, and the development of ARDS.[2,54]

In addition, the patient may develop a pleural effusion. This condition results from the vascular response to inflammation, whereby capillary permeability is increased, and fluid from the pulmonary capillaries diffuses into the pleural space.[62]

Assessment and Diagnosis

Assessment

The clinical manifestations of severe pneumonia vary with the offending pathogen. Symptoms are acute in onset, usually developing over 24 to 48 hours.[57] The patient initially presents with a fever, cough (productive or nonproductive), fatigue, headache, myalgia, and arthralgia. Mucopurulent sputum is suggestive of a bacterial organism as the cause. As the pneumonia progresses, the patient develops dyspnea, tachypnea,

BOX 18.8 Management of Pneumonia in the Adult Patient With Cystic Fibrosis

Cystic fibrosis (CF) is an autosomal recessive genetic disorder characterized by altered cellular sodium and chloride ions transport, affecting the exocrine glands. This life-limiting multisystem disorder affects various body systems, including the lungs, pancreas, biliary tract, and reproductive tract.[1]

The initial signs and symptoms of CF usually appear during childhood; however, given the variation in the severity and progression of the disorder, some patients are diagnosed as adults. The prognosis for patients with CF has significantly improved over the past several decades due to improvements in diagnosis and management. Fifty years ago, the median age of survival was 16 years. Today, patients are living for 40 years or longer.[2] These improvements have also resulted in more adult patients with a history of CF being admitted to the critical care unit.

CF's lung effects make the airway secretions thick and sticky, making them difficult to clear. Eventually, the secretions obstruct the small airways and promote infection, leading to chronic infections, tissue destruction, and, ultimately, the development of bronchiectasis.[3] Patients with CF often present with respiratory failure secondary to pneumonia. Patients with CF may also experience pancreatic insufficiency, chronic pancreatitis, cirrhosis, malabsorption syndrome, chronic sinusitis, and infertility. These conditions can also lead to diabetes, pneumothorax, portal hypertension, and pulmonary hypertension.[3]

- Nursing management of the patient with pneumonia secondary to CF focuses on airway clearance techniques.
- Chest physiotherapy to include:
  - Postural drainage, percussion, and vibration to mobilize lung secretions.
  - Oscillating positive expiratory pressure devices (i.e., flutter valves) to promote clearance of excess secretions and reduce air trapping.
  - High-frequency chest wall oscillation vests to help loosen secretions.
- Breathing exercises.
- Metered-dose inhalers and ultrasonic nebulizers to administer:
  - Beta-2 adrenergic receptor agonists to dilate airways.
  - Inhaled glucocorticoids to reduce lung inflammation.
  - Hypertonic saline to loosen and liquefy thickened mucus.
  - Mucolytics (e.g., dornase alfa [specifically for patients with CF]) to decrease mucus viscosity.
  - Inhaled antibiotics to treat pulmonary infections.

Additional information can be found on the CF Foundation website (www.cff.org).

References

1. Shteinberg M, Haq IJ, Polineni D, et al. Cystic fibrosis. *Lancet.* 2021;397(10290):2195–2211. https://doi.org/10.1016/S0140-6736(20)32542-3.
2. Bergeron C, Cantin AM. Cystic fibrosis: Pathophysiology of lung disease. *Semin Respir Crit Care Med.* 2019;40(6):715–726. https://doi.org/10.1055/s-0039-1694021.
3. Brown SD, White R, Tobin P. Keep them breathing: Cystic fibrosis pathophysiology, diagnosis, and treatment. *JAAPA.* 2017;30(5):23–27. https://doi.org/10.1097/01.JAA.0000515540.36581.92.

tachycardia, and signs of hypoxemia. The patient may also experience pleuritic chest pain, which is a sharp, stabbing, or burning pain in the chest when inhaling, coughing, or sneezing.[54,57] Coarse crackles on auscultation and dullness to percussion may also be present.

Diagnosis

Chest radiography is used to evaluate a patient with suspected pneumonia. The presence of a new pulmonary infiltrate establishes the diagnosis. The radiographic pattern of the infiltrates varies with the organism.[63] In addition, chest CT may be needed to aid in the diagnosis of complex cases of pneumonia or complications related to pneumonia.[54]

Given the recent pandemic, polymerase chain reaction (PCR) testing for SARS-CoV-2 is usually one of the first laboratory studies obtained.[52] A sputum Gram stain and culture are also done to facilitate the identification of the infectious pathogen.[64] In some cases, a causative agent may not be identified. A diagnostic bronchoscopy may be needed, particularly if the diagnosis is unclear, current therapy is not working, or the patient cannot produce sputum.[51] However, if the patient cannot produce sputum, endotracheal aspiration should be

BOX 18.9 Risk Factors for Hospital-Acquired Pneumonia

Host Related

- Advanced age
- Altered level of consciousness
- Chronic obstructive pulmonary disease
- Altered immune system
- Severity of illness
- Poor nutrition
- Hemodynamic compromise
- Trauma
- Tobacco use
- Dental plaque

Infection Control Related

- Poor handwashing practices

Treatment Related

- Mechanical ventilation
- Endotracheal intubation
- Unintentional extubation
- Bronchoscopy
- Nasogastric tube
- Previous antibiotic therapy
- Elevated gastric pH secondary to histamine receptor antagonists, proton pump inhibitors, and enteral feedings
- Upper abdominal surgery
- Thoracic surgery
- Supine position

TABLE 18.2 Precipitating Conditions of Pneumonia

Condition	Etiologies
Depressed epiglottal and cough reflexes	Unconsciousness, neurologic disease, endotracheal or tracheal tubes, anesthesia, aging
Decreased cilia activity	Smoke inhalation, tobacco use history, oxygen toxicity, hypoventilation, intubation, viral infections, aging, chronic obstructive pulmonary disease (COPD)
Increased secretion	COPD, viral infections, bronchiectasis, general anesthesia, endotracheal intubation, tobacco use
Atelectasis	Trauma, foreign body obstruction, tumor, splinting, shallow ventilations, general anesthesia
Decreased lymphatic flow	Heart failure, tumor
Fluid in alveoli	Heart failure, aspiration, trauma
Abnormal phagocytosis and humoral activity	Neutropenia, immunocompetent disorders, patients receiving chemotherapy
Impaired alveolar macrophages	Hypoxemia, metabolic acidosis, tobacco use history, hypoxia, alcohol use, viral infections, aging

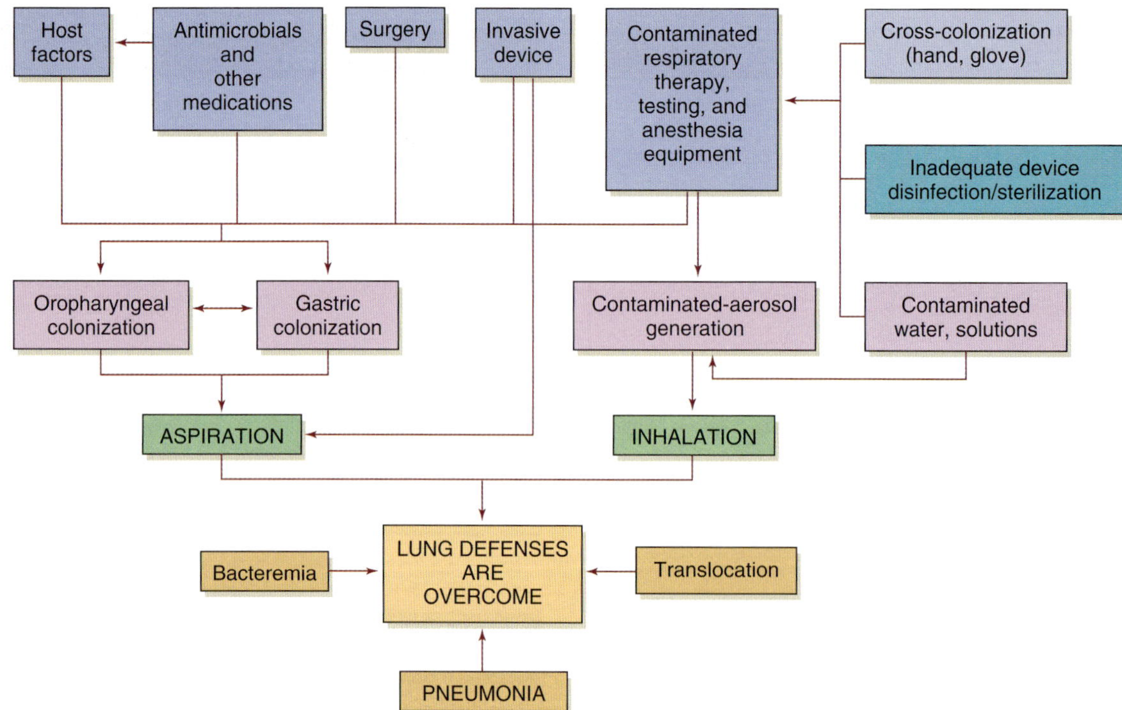

FIG. 18.6 Pathophysiology of Hospital-Acquired Pneumonia. (From Tablan OC, Anderson LJ, Arden NH, Breiman RF, Butler JC, McNeil MM. Guideline for prevention of nosocomial pneumonia. The Hospital Infection Control Practices Advisory Committee, Centers for Disease Control and Prevention. *Am J Infect Control.* 1994;22[4]:247–292.)

attempted before a bronchoscopy to decrease the risk to the patient.[55] In addition, a complete blood count with differential, chemistry panel, blood cultures, and ABGs is obtained.[51] During influenza season, PCR testing may be done to identify respiratory viruses.[64]

Medical Management

Medical management of a patient with pneumonia includes antibiotic or antiviral therapy,[64] oxygen therapy for hypoxemia, mechanical ventilation if ARF develops, fluid management for hydration, nutrition support, and treatment of associated medical problems and complications. For patients having difficulty mobilizing secretions, a therapeutic bronchoscopy may be necessary.[51]

Antibiotic Therapy

Although pathogen-specific antibiotic therapy is the goal, this may not be initially possible because of difficulties in identifying the organism and the seriousness of the patient's condition. The time involved in obtaining a sputum culture is balanced against the need to begin treatment. Antibiotics should be started as soon as possible to slow the progression of the infection,[54] so empiric therapy has become a generally acceptable approach.[56,64] In this approach, the choice of antibiotic treatment is based on the most likely etiologic organism while avoiding toxicity, superinfection, and unnecessary cost.[56,64] If available, Gram stain results are used to guide the choice of antibiotics. Antibiotics that offer broad coverage of the usual pathogens in the hospital or community are chosen.[56,64] Failure to respond to such therapy may indicate that the chosen antibiotic regimen does not appropriately cover all the etiologic pathogens or that a new source of infection has developed.[51] Optimal timing for the initiation of antibiotics has been an ongoing issue. A recent systematic review concluded that antibiotic therapy should be initiated in patients with community-acquired pneumonia within 4 to 8 hours of hospital arrival.[65]

Independent Lung Ventilation

In patients with unilateral pneumonia or severely asymmetric pneumonia, independent lung ventilation, an alternative mode of mechanical ventilation, may be necessary to facilitate oxygenation. As the alveoli in the affected lung become flooded with pus, the lung becomes less compliant and difficult to ventilate. This condition results in a shifting of ventilation to the good lung without an accompanying shift in perfusion and, thus, an increase in $\dot{V}/\dot{Q}$ mismatching. Independent lung ventilation allows each lung to be ventilated separately, controlling the flow, volume, and pressure each lung receives. A double-lumen endotracheal tube is inserted, and each lumen is usually attached to a separate mechanical ventilator. The ventilator settings are then customized to the needs of each lung to facilitate optimal oxygenation and ventilation.[66]

Nursing Management

The patient care management plan for a patient with pneumonia incorporates a variety of patient problems (Box 18.10). The nurse has a significant role in optimizing oxygenation and ventilation, preventing the spread of infection, providing comfort and emotional support, and maintaining surveillance for complications. The patient's response to antibiotic therapy is monitored for adverse effects.

BOX 18.10 DIAGNOSIS AND PATIENT CARE MANAGEMENT

Pneumonia

- Impaired Airway Clearance due to excessive secretions or abnormal viscosity of mucus
- Impaired Gas Exchange due to ventilation/perfusion mismatching or intrapulmonary shunting
- Impaired Nutritional Intake due to lack of exogenous nutrients or increased metabolic demand
- Risk for Aspiration
- Risk for Infection
- Anxiety due to threat to biological, psychological, or social integrity
- Powerlessness due to lack of control over current situation or disease progression
- Impaired Family Coping due to critically ill family member

Patient Care Management Plans are located in Appendix A.

Optimize Oxygenation and Ventilation

Nursing interventions to optimize oxygenation and ventilation include positioning, preventing desaturation, and promoting secretion clearance. For further discussion of these interventions, see Nursing Management of Acute Respiratory Failure earlier in this chapter.

Prevent Spread of Infection

Prevention is directed at eradicating pathogens from the environment and interrupting the spread of organisms from person to person. Significant progress has been made in removing contaminants from the patient environment through proper disinfection of respiratory equipment and increased use of disposable supplies. Other possible environmental sources of pathogens include suctioning equipment and indwelling lines. These invasive tools must be given proper aseptic care.

Proper hand hygiene is the most essential measure available to prevent the spread of bacteria from person to person (Box 18.11). Hand hygiene is performed before and after touching a patient or their surroundings, before a procedure, and after exposure to body fluids.[67] In addition, meticulous oral care, including suctioning of the secretions pooling above the cuff of the artificial airway, is critical to decreasing the bacterial colonization of the oropharynx.[68] Prevention of ventilator-associated pneumonia and oral hygiene are discussed further in Chapter 19.

BOX 18.11 Safety

Quality Improvement

Hand Hygiene Guidelines

The following are key recommendations from the Hand Hygiene Task Force, based on the literature review and expert panel opinion:

- Wash hands with soap and water when visibly dirty or contaminated with blood and other body fluids.
- When washing hands with soap and water, wet hands first with water, apply an amount of product recommended by the manufacturer to hands, and rub hands together vigorously for at least 15 seconds, covering all surfaces of the hands and fingers. Rinse hands with water and dry thoroughly with a disposable towel. Use a towel to turn off the faucet. Avoid using hot water because repeated exposure to hot water may increase the risk of dermatitis.
- If hands are not visibly soiled, use an alcohol-based hand rub for routinely decontaminating hands.
- When decontaminating hands with an alcohol-based hand rub, apply product to the palm of one hand and rub hands together, covering all surfaces of hands and fingers until hands are dry (follow the manufacturer's recommendations regarding the volume of product to use).
- Decontaminate hands before and after having direct contact with patients.
- Decontaminate hands before and after donning gloves.
- Wear gloves when contact with blood or other potentially infectious materials, mucous membranes, or nonintact skin could occur.
- Change gloves during patient care if moving from a contaminated body site to a clean one.
- Remove gloves after caring for a patient. Do not wear the same pair of gloves for the care of more than one patient, and do not wash gloves between uses with different patients.
- Decontaminate hands after contact with inanimate objects (including medical equipment).
- Do not wear artificial fingernails or extenders when having direct contact with patients at high risk (e.g., those in critical care units or operating rooms).
- Keep natural nail tips less than one-fourth inch long.

From Boyce JM, Pittet D; Healthcare Infection Control Practices Advisory Committee; HICPAC/SHEA/APIC/IDSA Hand Hygiene Task Force. Guideline for hand hygiene in health care settings: Recommendations of Healthcare Infection Control Practices Advisory Committee, and the HICPAC/SHEA/APIC/IDSA Hand Hygiene Task Force. Society for Healthcare Epidemiology of America/Association for Professionals in Infection Control/Infectious Diseases Society of America. *MMWR Recomm Rep.* 2002;51(RR16):1–45.

ASPIRATION PNEUMONITIS

Description and Etiology

Aspiration pneumonitis is caused by an inflammatory response to aspirated material. This condition can be the precipitating event that brings the patient to the critical care unit, or it can happen to a patient already in the unit. The most common aspirates are sterile gastric contents and bacterial-laden oropharyngeal secretions.[69] The inhalation of a large volume of gastric contents into the lungs is referred to as *aspiration pneumonitis*. The inhalation of oropharyngeal bacteria into the lungs is referred to as *aspiration pneumonia*. With aspiration pneumonitis, the injury to the lungs is due to the chemical characteristics of the aspirate, while with aspiration pneumonia, the injury to the lungs is due to the infectious process.[70] Unfortunately, it can be difficult to distinguish between the two disorders, and the patient may be unnecessarily treated with antibiotics.[70] Aspiration pneumonitis is also referred to as *chemical pneumonitis* and *Mendelson syndrome*[71] and can be a precursor to ARDS.[69] Aspiration pneumonia is further discussed under the Pneumonia section earlier in this chapter.

Etiology

Not all aspiration events will result in an adverse outcome, as several protective airway mechanisms can prevent the aspirate from entering the lungs. However, numerous factors have been identified in critically ill patients that place them at risk for aspiration (Table 18.3). If the patient aspirates, gastric contents' effects on the lungs will vary based on the pH of the fluid and the presence of particulates and digestive enzymes.[72] If the pH is less than 2.5, the patient will develop severe chemical pneumonitis, resulting in acute hypoxemia. If the pH is greater than 2.5, the immediate damage to the lungs will be lessened, but the elevated pH may have promoted bacterial overgrowth in the

TABLE 18.3 **Risk Factors for Aspiration**

Risk Factor	Rationale
Decreased LOC from either CNS problems or the use of sedatives	Decreased ability to protect the airway from oropharyngeal secretions and regurgitated gastric contents Cough and gag reflexes diminish as LOC diminishes, whether from CNS disorder or sedation Slowed gastric emptying Decreased tone of lower esophageal sphincter
Supine position	Increases probability of gastroesophageal reflux
Presence of nasogastric tube	Interferes with closure of lower esophageal sphincter Biofilm on tube predisposes to aspiration of pathogenic organisms
Vomiting	Sudden and forceful entry of gastric contents into the oropharynx predisposes to aspiration Predisposes to displacement of feeding tube ports into the esophagus
Feeding tube ports positioned in the esophagus	Infused feedings reflux into the oropharynx
Tracheal intubation	Reduction in upper airway defense related to ineffective cough, desensitization of oropharynx and larynx, disuse atrophy of laryngeal muscles, and esophageal compression by an inflated cuff
Mechanical ventilation	Positive abdominal pressure predisposes to aspiration of gastric contents, probably by increasing gastroesophageal reflux
Accumulation of subglottic secretions above the endotracheal cuff	Subglottic secretions can leak around the cuff into the lower respiratory tract, especially when the cuff is deflated
Inadequate cuff inflation of tracheal devices	Persistent low cuff pressure predisposes to aspiration of oropharyngeal secretions and refluxed gastric contents
Gastric feeding site when gastric emptying significantly impaired	Accumulation of formula and gastrointestinal secretions predisposes to gastroesophageal reflux and aspiration
High GRVs	High GRVs predispose to gastroesophageal reflux and aspiration
Bolus feedings	Volume of infused formula may exceed the tolerance of patients who have poor cough and gag reflexes
Poor oral health	Colonized oropharyngeal secretions may be aspirated into the respiratory tract
Advanced age	Older patients tend to have reduced swallowing ability and are more likely to have neurologic disorders that increase aspiration risks There is a strong association between advanced age and the probability of developing pneumonia once aspiration has occurred
Hyperglycemia	Mild hyperglycemia can cause delayed gastric emptying by disrupting postprandial antral contractions

CNS, Central nervous system; *GRVs*, gastric residual volumes; *LOC*, level of consciousness.
From Metheny NA. Strategies to prevent aspiration-related pneumonia in tube-fed patients. *Respir Care Clin N Am.* 2006;12(4):603–617.

stomach.[73,74] In this case, the normally sterile gastric contents may be full of bacteria, which are then aspirated into the lungs, resulting in the development of bacterial pneumonia.[74,75]

Pathophysiology

The type of lung injury that develops after aspiration is determined by many factors, including the quality and pH of the aspirate and the status of the patient's respiratory defense mechanisms.[74]

Acid Liquid Gastric Contents

Aspiring acid (pH less than 2.5) liquid gastric contents cause a chemical burn of the airway epithelium and lung parenchyma. Bronchospasm occurs almost immediately.[74,75] Over the next 2 hours, cell damage causes increased alveolar-capillary permeability, interstitial edema, alveolar flooding, and hemorrhage. Severe hypoxemia develops as a result of intrapulmonary shunting and $\dot{V}/\dot{Q}$ mismatching.[76] The inflammatory response is initiated within 4 to 6 hours, and proinflammatory mediators are released.[76] The severity of the response is increased if small nonobstructing food particles are present in the gastric liquid.[77]

Nonacid Liquid Gastric Contents

The aspiration of nonacid (pH greater than 2.5) liquid gastric contents is similar to acid-liquid aspiration initially, but minimal structural damage occurs. Intrapulmonary shunting and $\dot{V}/\dot{Q}$ mismatching usually start to reverse within 4 hours, and hypoxemia clears within 24 hours. The severity of the response is increased if small nonobstructing food particles are present in the gastric liquid.[77]

Outcome

Depending on the severity of the damage, the patient's underlying health, and the extent of hypoxemia, the ensuing clinical course may progress in various ways. Cellular regeneration usually starts 3 days after the injury so that the patient can experience rapid improvement in 1 week. If the patient experiences severe hypoxemia, ARF may occur. If the inflammatory response becomes dysregulated, ARDS can occur. If bacteria enters the damaged lungs, pneumonia can develop.[72,74,76,77]

Assessment and Diagnosis

Assessment

Clinically, patients present with signs of acute respiratory distress, and gastric contents may be present in the oropharynx. Patients have shortness of breath, coughing, wheezing, cyanosis, and signs of hypoxemia. Tachypnea, tachycardia, hypotension, fever, and crackles also are present.[74] Copious amounts of bloody or frothy sputum are produced as alveolar edema develops.[75]

Diagnosis

ABGs reflect severe hypoxemia. Changes on chest radiography appear 12 to 24 hours after the initial aspiration,[70] with no one pattern being diagnostic of the event. Infiltrates appear in various distribution patterns depending on the patient's position during aspiration and the volume of the aspirate.[74] If bacterial infection becomes established, leukocytosis and positive sputum cultures occur.[77]

Medical Management

Management of a patient with aspiration pneumonitis includes both emergency and follow-up treatment. When aspiration is witnessed, emergency treatment is instituted to secure the airway and minimize pulmonary damage. The patient's head is turned to the side, and the oral cavity and upper airway are suctioned immediately to remove the gastric contents.[77] Direct visualization by bronchoscopy is indicated to remove large particulate aspirate or to confirm an unwitnessed aspiration event.[71,75] Bronchoalveolar lavage is not recommended because this practice disseminates the aspirate in the lungs and increases damage.[75]

After airway clearance, attention is given to supporting oxygenation and hemodynamics.[74] Hypoxemia is corrected with supplemental oxygen, high-flow oxygen therapy, or mechanical ventilation with PEEP, if necessary.[71] Hemodynamic changes result from fluid shifts into the lungs that can occur after massive aspirations. Monitoring intravascular volume is essential, and judicious amounts of replacement fluids are instituted to maintain adequate urinary output and vital signs.

Empiric antibiotic therapy is usually not indicated after aspiration of gastric contents. However, antibiotic therapy is considered if pneumonia is suspected or the aspiration event occurs in the presence of small bowel obstruction or colonized gastric contents.[74] Corticosteroids have not been demonstrated to be beneficial in treating aspiration pneumonitis and are not recommended.[71]

Nursing Management

The patient care management plan for a patient with aspiration pneumonitis incorporates a variety of patient problems (Box 18.12). The nurse has a significant role in optimizing oxygenation and ventilation, preventing further aspiration events, providing comfort and emotional support, and maintaining surveillance for complications.

Optimize Oxygenation and Ventilation

Nursing interventions to optimize oxygenation and ventilation include positioning, preventing desaturation, and promoting secretion clearance. For further discussion of these interventions, see Nursing Management of Acute Respiratory Failure earlier in this chapter.

Prevent Aspiration

One of the most critical interventions for preventing aspiration is identifying patients at risk for aspiration (Box 18.13). Actions to prevent aspiration include confirming feeding tube placement, checking for signs and symptoms of feeding intolerance, elevating the head of the bed at least 30 to 45 degrees, feeding the patient via a small-bore feeding tube or gastrostomy tube, avoiding the use of a large-bore nasogastric tube, ensuring proper inflation of artificial airway cuffs, and frequent suctioning of the oropharynx of an intubated patient to prevent secretions from pooling above the cuff of the tube. The feeding tube is placed in the small bowel for patients at risk for aspiration or intolerance of gastric feedings.

Interprofessional collaborative management of a patient with aspiration pneumonitis is outlined in Box 18.14.

ACUTE PULMONARY EMBOLISM

Description and Etiology

A PE occurs when a clot (thrombotic embolus) or other matter (nonthrombotic embolus) lodges in the pulmonary arterial system, disrupting blood flow to a region of the lungs

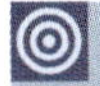

BOX 18.12 DIAGNOSIS AND PATIENT CARE MANAGEMENT

Aspiration Pneumonitis

- Impaired Gas Exchange due to ventilation/perfusion mismatching or intrapulmonary shunting
- Impaired Airway Clearance due to excessive secretions or abnormal viscosity of mucus
- Risk for Aspiration
- Risk for Infection
- Anxiety due to biological, psychological, or social integrity
- Impaired Adaptation due to situational crisis and personal vulnerability
- Impaired Family Coping due to critically ill family member

Patient Care Management Plans are located in Appendix A.

BOX 18.13 Evidence-Based Practice

Aspiration Prevention Guidelines

The following are the key recommendations from the AACN Practice Alert: Preventing Aspiration:

1. Maintain head-of-bed elevation at an angle of 30 to 45 degrees unless contraindicated.
2. Use sedatives as sparingly as feasible.
3. For patients receiving gastric tube feedings, assess for gastrointestinal intolerance to the feedings at 4-hour intervals.
4. For tube-fed patients, avoid bolus feedings in those at high risk for aspiration.
5. Consult with a practitioner about obtaining a swallowing assessment before oral feedings are started for recently extubated patients who have experienced prolonged intubation.
6. Maintain endotracheal cuff pressures at an appropriate level and ensure that secretions are cleared from above the cuff before it is deflated.

Data from American Association of Critical-Care Nurses: AACN Practice Alert: Prevention of aspiration in adults. *Crit Care Nurse.* 2016;38(1):e20–e24 (updated 2018).

BOX 18.14 Teamwork and Collaboration

Aspiration Pneumonitis

- Administer oxygen therapy.
- Secure the patient's airway.
- Suction patient's oropharyngeal area.
- Initiate mechanical ventilation as required.
- Maintain surveillance for complications:
  - Pneumonia
  - Acute respiratory failure
  - Acute respiratory distress syndrome
- Provide comfort and emotional support.

(Fig. 18.7).[78] The American Heart Association has developed a classification schema for acute PE, stratifying patients into one of three categories: massive, submassive, or low risk. A massive PE is defined as an acute PE with sustained hypotension (systolic blood pressure less than 90 mm Hg) for more than 15 minutes, the need for inotropes not based on other causes or signs of shock. A submassive PE is defined as an acute PE with evidence of right ventricular dysfunction or myocardial necrosis. A patient with none of these conditions is defined as low risk.[79]

Etiology

Most thrombotic emboli arise from the pelvic and deep leg veins, particularly the iliac, femoral, and popliteal veins. Other sources include the right ventricle and the upper extremities.[80] Nonthrombotic emboli arise from fat, tumors, amniotic fluid, air, foreign bodies, and infectious vegetations.[78] Thrombus formation is enabled by hypercoagulability, injury to vascular endothelium, and venous stasis (Virchow triad).[80] Numerous predisposing factors and precipitating conditions put a patient at risk for developing PE (Box 18.15). However, about 30% of the patients will not present with a known risk factor.[78] This section focuses on PE secondary to thrombotic emboli. Fig. 18.8 summarizes the key concepts for managing a patient with an acute PE.

Pathophysiology

A PE occurs when a clot detaches from its original location, referred to as an *embolus*, and travels through the venous system through the right side of the heart into the pulmonary arterial tree.

Depending on the size of the embolus, it may occlude one or more pulmonary arteries.[81] A massive PE occurs with the blockage of a lobar or larger artery, resulting in pulmonary vascular bed occlusion. Blockage of the pulmonary arterial system has both pulmonary and hemodynamic consequences. The effects on the pulmonary system are increased alveolar dead space, bronchoconstriction, and compensatory shunting. Hemodynamic effects include an increase in pulmonary vascular resistance and right ventricular workload.[82,83]

Increased Dead Space

An increase in alveolar dead space occurs because an area of the lung receives ventilation without being perfused. The ventilation in this area is known as *wasted ventilation* because it does not participate in gas exchange. This effect leads to alveolar dead space ventilation and an increase in the work of breathing. To limit the amount of dead space ventilation, localized bronchoconstriction occurs.[82,83]

Bronchoconstriction

Bronchoconstriction develops due to alveolar hypocarbia, hypoxia, and the release of mediators. Alveolar hypocarbia occurs due to decreased carbon dioxide in the affected area. It leads to constriction of the local airways, increased airway resistance, and redistribution of ventilation to perfused areas of the lungs. Various mediators are released from the site of the injury, either from the clot or the surrounding lung tissue, which further causes constriction of the airways. Bronchoconstriction promotes the development of atelectasis.[82,83]

Compensatory Shunting

Compensatory shunting occurs due to the unaffected areas of the lungs having to accommodate the entire CO. A situation results in which perfusion exceeds ventilation, and blood is returned to the left side of the heart without participating in gas exchange. This change leads to the development of hypoxemia.[82,83]

Hemodynamic Consequences

The major hemodynamic consequence of PE is the development of pulmonary hypertension secondary to the blockage in the pulmonary arterial system. In addition, the mediators released at the injury site and the development of hypoxia cause pulmonary vasoconstriction, which further exacerbates pulmonary hypertension. As the pulmonary vascular resistance increases, so does the workload of the right ventricle, as reflected by an increase in pulmonary artery pressures. Consequently, right

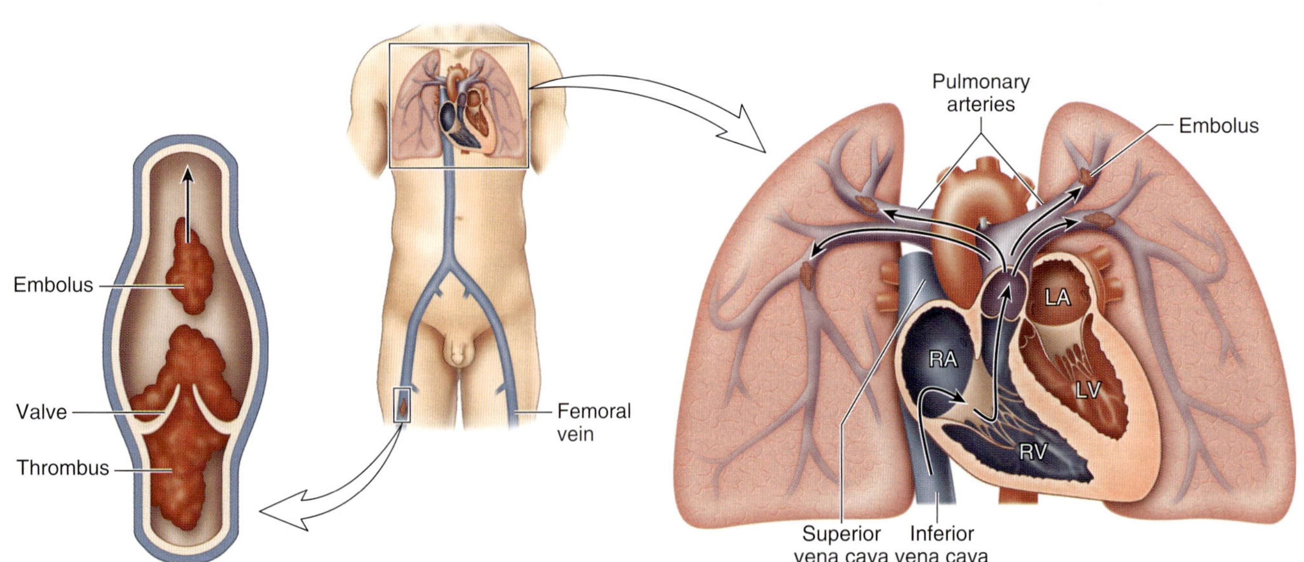

FIG. 18.7 Pathophysiology of Pulmonary Embolism. Thromboemboli travel through the right side of the heart to reach the lungs. *LA*, Left atrium; *LV*, left ventricle; *RA*, right atrium; *RV*, right ventricle.

BOX 18.15 Risk Factors for Pulmonary Thromboembolism

Predisposing Factors

- Venous stasis
  - Atrial fibrillation
  - Decreased cardiac output
  - Immobility
- Injury to vascular endothelium
  - Local vessel injury
  - Infection
  - Incision
  - Atherosclerosis
- Hypercoagulability
  - Polycythemia
  - Thrombocytopenia
  - Older age
  - Obesity

Precipitating Conditions

- Previous history of venous thromboembolism
- Family history of venous thromboembolism
- Autoimmune disease
- Sickle cell disease
- Cardiovascular disease
  - Heart failure
  - Right ventricular infarction
  - Cardiomyopathy
  - Cor pulmonale
- Surgery
  - Orthopedic
  - Vascular
  - Abdominal
- Cancer
  - Ovarian
  - Pancreatic
  - Stomach
  - Extrahepatic bile duct system
- Trauma (injury or burns)
  - Lower extremities
  - Pelvis
  - Hips
- Gynecologic status
  - Pregnancy
  - Postpartum
  - Birth control pills
  - Estrogen replacement therapy
  - Presence of intravenous catheters or devices
- Hereditary conditions
  - Factor V Leiden
  - Antithrombin deficiency
  - Protein C deficiency
  - Protein S deficiency

ventricular failure occurs, leading to decreased left ventricular preload, CO, and blood pressure and shock.[78,82,83]

Assessment and Diagnosis

Assessment

A patient with PE may have numerous presenting signs and symptoms, with the most common being dyspnea, pleuritic or substernal chest pain, and tachycardia.[84] Additional signs and symptoms that may be present include syncope, hemoptysis, evidence of deep vein thrombosis (DVT),[84] fever, cough, and signs of respiratory distress.[78] Hemoptysis is indicative of a lung infarction.[85] Hypoxemia and hemodynamic instability, as evidenced by hypotension and tachycardia, can occur as a result of right ventricular failure.[78]

Diagnosis

Initial laboratory studies and diagnostic procedures that may be done include ABG analysis, D-dimer, electrocardiogram (ECG), chest radiography, and echocardiography. ABGs may show a low PaO_2, indicating hypoxemia; a low $PaCO_2$, indicating hypocarbia; and a high pH, indicating respiratory alkalosis.[85] The hypocarbia with resulting respiratory alkalosis is caused by tachypnea. An elevated d-dimer occurs with PE and many other disorders. A normal d-dimer does not occur with a PE and can be used to rule out a PE as the diagnosis.[85]

An ECG is done to assist with a differential diagnosis. The most common ECG finding among patients with PE is sinus tachycardia.[85] The classic ECG pattern associated with a PE, S wave in lead I and Q wave with inverted T wave in lead III occurs in less than 25% of patients[78] and is only found in severe cases. Other ECG findings associated with a PE include right bundle branch block, new-onset atrial fibrillation, T wave inversion, and p-pulmonale.[85]

A chest x-ray is also done to assist with a differential diagnosis. Findings vary from normal to abnormal and are of little value in confirming the presence of a PE. Abnormal findings include cardiomegaly, pleural effusion, elevated hemidiaphragm, enlargement of the right descending pulmonary artery (Palla sign), a wedge-shaped density above the diaphragm (Hampton hump), and the presence of atelectasis.[85]

Transthoracic or transesophageal echocardiography is helpful in the identification of a PE because it can provide visualization of any embolus in the central pulmonary arteries.[85] In addition, it can be used for assessing the hemodynamic consequences of PE on the right side of the heart.[78]

Differentiating PE from other illnesses can be difficult because many clinical manifestations of PE are found in various other disorders. The gold standard diagnostic procedure for identifying a PE, which also provides information regarding the degree and severity of the PE, is commuted tomography pulmonary angiography (CTPA). If CTPA is unavailable or the patient is unable to tolerate contrast, then a ventilation-perfusion ($\dot{V}/\dot{Q}$) scintigraphy can be done.[78] A Doppler ultrasound of the lower extremities may also be performed to look for a DVT.[2]

Medical Management

Medical management of a patient with a PE involves both prevention and treatment strategies. Prevention measures focus on VTE prophylaxis. Two interventions for all hospitalized patients are early and frequent ambulation and mechanical prophylaxis.[86] Pneumatic compression is an effective method of prophylaxis in low-risk patients.[87] For patients at higher risk for VTE, subcutaneous injections of unfractionated heparin (UFH) or LMWH may be added to the regimen.[86]

Treatment strategies include preventing the recurrence or extension of the thrombus, facilitating clot dissolution, reversing the effects of pulmonary hypertension, promoting gas exchange, and preventing complications.

Acute Pulmonary Embolism

Clinical and diagnostic assessments

- History and risk factors
  - Venous stasis
  - Injury to vascular endothelium
  - Hypercoagulability
- Obtain vital signs
  - O_2 saturation
- Clinical assessment
  - Inspect lower extremities
  - Auscultate breath sounds
- Laboratory studies
  - Obtain ABGs
  - Obtain d-dimer
- Diagnostic procedures
  - Verify chest x-ray
  - Obtain ECG
  - Verify echocardiogram
  - Verify CTPA or $\dot{V}/\dot{Q}$ scan

Signs

- Dyspnea
- Pleuritic/substernal chest pain
- Tachycardia
- Tachypnea
- Syncope
- Hemoptysis
- Evidence of a DVT
- Fever
- Cough
- Hypotension
- Crackles on auscultation
- Low PaO_2
- Low $PaCO_2$
- Low O_2 saturation
- Elevated d-dimer
- Sinus tachycardia

Nursing interventions

- Administer O_2 therapy
- Assist with intubation as needed
- Maintain MV
- Administer medications
  - Fibrinolytic
  - Anticoagulant
  - Inotropic agents
- Administer fluids
- Promote secretion clearance
- Prevent desaturation
- Maintain surveillance for complications
- Monitor patient response to fibrinolytic and anticoagulant
- Provide comfort and emotional support
- Educate the patient and family

FIG.18.8 Summary of Key Concepts Related to Acute Pulmonary Embolism. *ABGs,* Arterial blood gases; *CTPA,* commuted tomography pulmonary angiography; *DVT,* deep vein thrombosis; *ECG,* electrocardiogram; *MV,* mechanical ventilation; *O_2,* oxygen; *$PaCO_2$,* partial pressure of carbon dioxide in arterial blood; *PaO_2,* partial pressure of oxygen in arterial blood; $\dot{V}/\dot{Q}$, ventilation/perfusion; *X-ray,* radiograph.

Medical interventions to promote gas exchange include supplemental oxygen administration, intubation, and mechanical ventilation.[85]

Prevention of Recurrence or Extension of the Thrombus

Interventions to prevent the recurrence or extension of the thrombus include the administration of parenteral and oral anticoagulants. Prevention strategies include the use of prophylactic anticoagulation with LMWH, vitamin-K antagonists (VKAs), and direct oral anticoagulants (DOACs).[84] A parenteral anticoagulant is administered to prevent further clots from forming; however, this treatment has no effect on the existing clot. An oral anticoagulant is started, overlapping with the parenteral anticoagulant. Once the appropriate level of anticoagulation is achieved with the oral anticoagulant, the parenteral anticoagulant is discontinued. The patient remains on the oral anticoagulant for at least 3 months, depending on their risk for thromboembolic disease.[86]

Interruption of the inferior vena cava is reserved for patients in whom anticoagulation is contraindicated.[88] The procedure involves the placement of a percutaneous venous filter (e.g., Greenfield filter) into the vena cava, usually below the renal arteries. The filter prevents further thrombotic emboli from migrating into the lungs. Depending on the type of filter, it may be permanent or it may be retrievable. The risks associated with prolonged implantation of the filter, including perforation, thrombosis, and migration, make placement of the retrievable filter more desirable.[89]

Clot Dissolution

The administration of fibrinolytic agents in treating PE has had some success. At present, fibrinolytic therapy is recommended for patients with PE and concomitant hemodynamic instability.[88] The U.S. Food and Drug Administration has approved three different thrombolytics for treating PE: (1) urokinase administered as a 4400-IU/kg intravenous (IV) bolus, followed by a 4400-IU/kg/h infusion over 12 to 24 hours; (2) streptokinase administered as a 250,000-IU IV loading dose over 30 minutes, followed by 100,000 IU/h over 12 to 24 hours; and (3) alteplase administered as a 100-mg IV infusion over 2 hours. The therapeutic window for using fibrinolytic therapy is up to 14 days, although the most benefit is usually obtained when given within 48 hours.[90] The fibrinolytic agent may be administered systemically via an intravenous infusion or locally via a catheter in the pulmonary artery. In addition, ultrasound may be added to the catheter-directed system to allow for better penetration of the fibrinolytic agent into the thrombus.[84]

If fibrinolytic therapy is contraindicated, a surgical embolectomy or a catheter-directed embolectomy may be performed, depending on the patient's underlying condition and the location of the embolus.[84] A surgical pulmonary embolectomy is performed while the patient is on cardiopulmonary bypass. The chest is opened, an incision is made in the pulmonary artery, and the clot is extracted.[91] A catheter-directed embolectomy involves the insertion of an embolectomy catheter into the pulmonary artery, mechanical fragmentation of the embolus, and aspiration of the dispersed particles.[89]

Reversal of Pulmonary Hypertension

Additional measures may be taken to reverse the hemodynamic effects of pulmonary hypertension, including administering vasoactive agents and fluid. Fluids are administered to increase right ventricular preload, which stretches the right ventricle and increases contractility, overcoming elevated pulmonary arterial pressures. The patient needs to be monitored closely as excessive fluid administration may overload the already stressed right ventricle, leading to AHF and cardiogenic shock. Vasopressor agents should be administered to treat hypotension. Inotropic agents should be administered to increase contractility to facilitate an increase in CO. ECMO should be considered for patients in shock.[85]

BOX 18.16 Evidence-Based Practice

Venous Thromboembolism Prevention Guidelines

The following are key recommendations from the AACN Practice Alert: Preventing Venous Thromboembolism in Adults:

1. Assess all patients on admission to the critical care unit for risk factors of venous thromboembolism (VTE) and anticipate orders for VTE prophylaxis based on the risk assessment.
2. For patients at risk for VTE prophylaxis:
   - For acutely ill medical patients, use low-molecular-weight heparin (LMWH), low-dose unfractionated heparin (LDUH), or fondaparinux.
   - For acutely ill general surgery patients, use LMWH, LDUH, or mechanical prophylaxis (graduated compression stockings or intermittent pneumatic compression devices).
   - For critically ill patients, use LMWH or LDUN.
   - For patients at high risk for bleeding, use mechanical prophylaxis.
   - The use of mechanical prophylaxis should be anticipated in conjunction with anticoagulant-based prophylaxis regimens.
3. Review the patient's current risk factors daily during multidisciplinary rounds. Risk factors include the patient's current clinical status and response to treatment, the need for central venous access devices, and the patient's current VTE prophylaxis regimen and risk for bleeding.
4. Maximize the patient's mobility whenever possible. Implement measures to reduce the amount of time the patient is immobile. Mobilizing the patient does not negate the need for chemical prophylaxis because the patient may still be at risk for VTE.
5. Ensure that mechanical prophylaxis devices are always fitted correctly and in use except when removed for skin cleaning or inspection.

Data from American Association of Critical-Care Nurses: AACN Practice Alert: Preventing venous thromboembolism in adults. *Crit Care Nurse.* 2016;36(5):e20–e23 (updated 2018).

Nursing Management

Prevention of PE is a significant nursing focus because most critically ill patients are at risk for this disorder. Nursing actions are aimed at preventing the development of DVT (Box 18.16), which is a major complication of immobility and a leading cause of PE. These measures include using pneumatic compression devices, active/passive range-of-motion exercises involving foot extension, adequate hydration, and progressive ambulation.

The patient care management plan for a patient with a PE incorporates a variety of patient problems (Box 18.17). The nurse has a significant role in optimizing oxygenation and ventilation, monitoring for bleeding, providing comfort and emotional support, maintaining surveillance for complications, and educating the patient and family.

Optimize Oxygenation and Ventilation

Nursing interventions to optimize oxygenation and ventilation include preventing desaturation and promoting secretion clearance. For further discussion of these interventions, see Nursing Management of Acute Respiratory Failure earlier in this chapter.

Monitor for Bleeding

Patients receiving anticoagulant or fibrinolytic therapy are observed for signs of bleeding. The patient's gums, skin, urine, stool, and emesis are monitored for signs of overt or covert bleeding. In addition, monitoring the patient's international normalized ratio or activated partial thromboplastin time is critical to managing the anticoagulation therapy.

BOX 18.17 DIAGNOSIS AND PATIENT CARE MANAGEMENT

Acute Pulmonary Embolism

- Impaired Gas Exchange due to ventilation/perfusion mismatching or intrapulmonary shunting
- Acute Pain due to transmission and perception of cutaneous, visceral, muscular, or ischemic impulses
- Risk for Aspiration
- Anxiety due to threat to biological, psychological, or social integrity
- Powerlessness due to lack of control over current situation or disease progression
- Impaired Family Coping due to critically ill family member
- Lack of Knowledge of Treatment Regime due to lack of previous exposure to information (see Box 18.18, Patient and Family Education Plan: Acute Pulmonary Embolism)

Patient Care Management Plans are located in Appendix A.

BOX 18.18 PATIENT AND FAMILY EDUCATION PLAN

Acute Pulmonary Embolism

Before discharge, the patient should be able to teach back the following topics:

- Pathophysiology of disease
- Specific etiology
- Modification of precipitating factors
- Measures to prevent deep vein thrombosis (DVT) (e.g., avoid tight-fitting clothes, crossing legs, and prolonged sitting or standing; elevate legs when sitting; exercise)
- Signs and symptoms of DVT (e.g., redness, swelling, sharp or deep leg pain)
- Importance of taking medications
- Signs and symptoms of anticoagulant complications (e.g., excessive bruising, discoloration of skin, changes in color of urine or stools)
- Measures to prevent bleeding (e.g., use a soft-bristle toothbrush, caution when shaving)

Educate the Patient and Family

Early in the patient's hospital stay, the patient and family are taught about pulmonary embolus, its causes, and its treatment (Box 18.18). Closer to discharge, the patient's education plan focuses on the interventions necessary for preventing the reoccurrence of DVT and subsequent emboli, signs and symptoms of DVT and anticoagulant complications, and measures to prevent bleeding. Patients who use tobacco products are encouraged to stop using them and are referred to a tobacco cessation program.

CRITICAL ASTHMA SYNDROME

Description and Etiology

Asthma is a form of chronic obstructive pulmonary disease[92] that is characterized by partially reversible airflow obstruction, airway inflammation, and bronchial hyperresponsiveness to a variety of stimuli.[93] *Critical asthma syndrome* is an overarching term that describes various forms of acute asthma exacerbations that can lead to ARF and death. It encompasses several types of (or different terms for) asthma, including acute severe asthma, refractory asthma, status asthmaticus, life-threatening asthma, brittle asthma, and near-fatal asthma.[94,95] In each of these conditions, physical fatigue secondary to increased work of breathing leads to severe hypoxemia and hypercapnia, respiratory failure, and death.[94] Of those patients admitted for a severe asthma exacerbation, 10% of the patients require care in the critical care unit, with 2% of those patients requiring intubation and mechanical ventilation.[92,96]

Etiology

The precipitating cause of a severe asthma exacerbation is usually an upper respiratory infection, allergen exposure,[93,97] or poor symptom control.[95] Other factors that have been implicated include cold air,[97] exercise,[93,97] irritant inhalation (e.g., paint, perfume, smoke, cleaning solutions),[98] environmental pollutants,[97] lack of access to health care,[92] inadequate use of inhaled or oral corticosteroids,[98] and poor compliance with the treatment regimen.[98] Medications such as beta-blockers and aspirin have also been identified as triggers.[99]

Pathophysiology

An acute asthma exacerbation is initiated when exposure to an irritant or trigger occurs, stimulating the inflammatory response in the airways. Airway hyperresponsiveness ensues secondary to the release of eosinophils, mast cells, and CD4 cells.[93] Bronchospasm occurs along with increased vascular permeability and increased mucus production. Mucosal edema and thick, tenacious mucus further increase airway responsiveness. The combination of bronchospasm, airway inflammation, and hyperresponsiveness results in the narrowing of the airways and airflow obstruction.[93,99] These changes have significant effects on the pulmonary and cardiovascular systems.

Pulmonary Effects

As the diameter of the airways decreases, airway resistance increases, resulting in increased residual volume, hyperinflation of the lungs, increased work of breathing, and abnormal ventilation distribution. $\dot{V}/\dot{Q}$ mismatching occurs, which results in hypoxemia. Alveolar dead space also increases as hypoxic vasoconstriction occurs, resulting in hypercapnia.[93]

Cardiovascular Effects

Inspiratory muscle force also increases in an attempt to ventilate the hyperinflated lungs. This results in a significant increase in negative intrapleural pressure, leading to an increase in venous return and pooling of blood in the right ventricle. The stretched right ventricle causes the intraventricular septum to shift, impinging on the left ventricle. In addition, the left ventricle must work harder to pump blood from the markedly negative pressure in the thorax to elevated pressure in the systemic circulation. This situation leads to a decrease in CO and a fall in systolic blood pressure on inspiration (pulsus paradoxus).[100]

Assessment and Diagnosis

Assessment

The patient with an acute asthma exacerbation may initially present with coughing, wheezing, chest tightness, and shortness of breath.[93,97,99] As the exacerbation of asthma continues, the patient develops agitation,[92] tachypnea,[99] tachycardia,[96,99] increased accessory muscle use,[96,97] prolonged expiration,[96] tripoding,[96] the inability to complete sentences,[99] air hunger,[92] and an oxygen saturation less than 90%.[92] Altered level of consciousness,[97,99] exhaustion,[99] inability to speak,[93,96] significantly diminished or absent breath sounds,[97,99] and inability to lie supine[92] herald the onset of ARF.

Diagnosis

Initial ABGs indicate hypocapnia and respiratory alkalosis caused by hyperventilation.[92,97] As the exacerbation continues and the patient starts to fatigue, hypoxemia and hypercapnia develop.[92,97] Lactic acidosis may also occur due to lactate overproduction by the respiratory muscles. The end result is the development of respiratory and metabolic acidosis.[101]

Deterioration of pulmonary function tests despite aggressive bronchodilator therapy is diagnostic of a severe asthma exacerbation and indicates the potential need for intubation. A peak expiratory flow rate (PEFR) less than 50% of the patient's normal best[99] or the predicted value[98] or forced expiratory volume in 1 second (FEV1) less than 60% of the predicted value[95] indicates severe airflow obstruction, and the need for intubation with mechanical ventilation may be imminent.

Medical Management

Medical management of a patient with critical asthma syndrome is directed toward supporting oxygenation and ventilation. Bronchodilators, corticosteroids, oxygen therapy, noninvasive ventilation, and intubation and mechanical ventilation are the mainstays of therapy.

Bronchodilators

Inhaled short-acting beta-2 agonists and anticholinergics (antimuscarinics) are the bronchodilators of choice for a severe acute asthma exacerbation. Short-action beta-2 agonists promote bronchodilation and are usually administered by nebulizer. Albuterol and salbutamol are usually used as they are rapid-acting with a half-life of 4 to 6 hours. Anticholinergics that inhibit bronchoconstriction are not very effective by themselves, but in conjunction with beta-2 agonists, they have a synergistic effect and produce a greater improvement in airflow. They can be administered via nebulizer or metered-dose inhaler (MDI). Ipratropium is the medication mainly used in this situation.[95]

If a patient is refractory to conventional therapies, ketamine may be administered to reduce bronchoconstriction. Ketamine decreases airway inflammation and bronchial hyperreactivity, subsequently decreasing bronchospasm. Ketamine also increases bronchial secretions, which decreases mucus plugs. Studies regarding the use of ketamine have found that the patient has improved pulmonary function, decreased oxygen requirement, and decreased need for invasive ventilation.[93]

Many studies have focused on the bronchodilator abilities of magnesium. Although it has been demonstrated that magnesium is inferior to beta-2 agonists as a bronchodilator, it may be beneficial in patients who are refractory to conventional treatment. A bolus of 2 g of intravenous magnesium over 20 minutes has been reported to produce desirable effects.[95]

Many other studies are evaluating the effects of leukotriene inhibitors, such as zafirlukast and montelukast, in the treatment of critical asthma syndromes. Leukotrienes are inflammatory mediators known to cause bronchoconstriction and airway inflammation. Research suggests that these agents may be beneficial as bronchodilators in patients who are refractory to beta-2 agonists. However, more research is needed to prove the clinical efficacy of these medications.[95]

SOCIAL DETERMINANTS OF HEALTH

Health Disparities Associated With Asthma

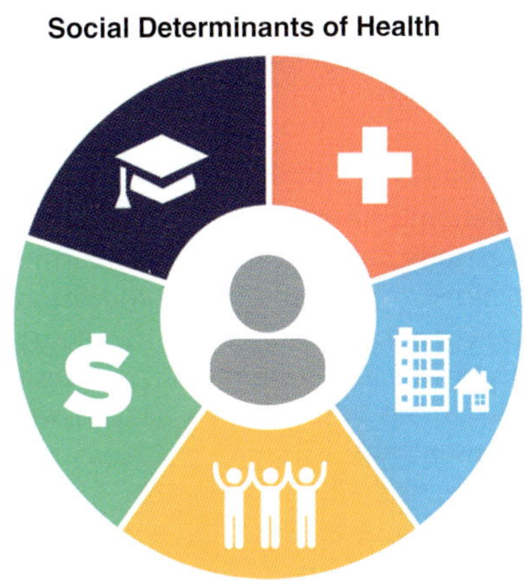

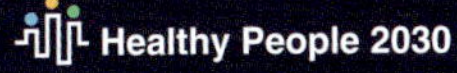

Severe asthma does not respond well to standard asthma treatments, and the symptoms are more intense than typical asthmatic symptoms. They can last for extended periods, resulting in admission to the critical care unit. However, significant disparities exist in mortality among patients who experience severe asthma, particularly among African-American, Hispanic, American Indian, and Native Alaska populations. Various social determinants exist for these differences, including poverty, lack of employment, education, environmental conditions, poor housing, lack of access to health care, lower quality of health care, and poor health literacy. These issues are further compounded by inherent structural causes such as racism and discrimination, behavioral issues such as nonadherence to treatment and mistrust of the health care system, and biological factors such as susceptibility to asthma. These factors are depicted in Figure 18.B.

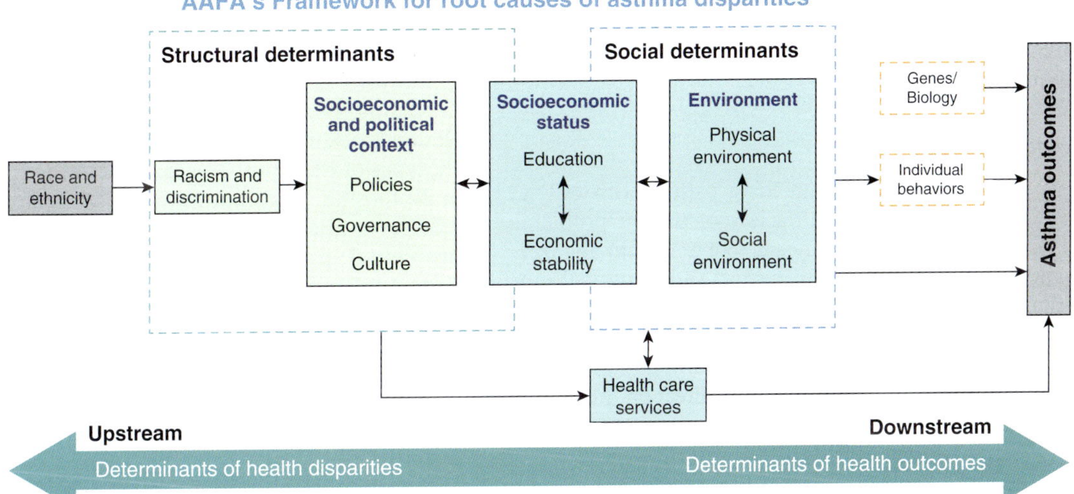

(From Asthma and Allergy Foundation of America. (2020). *Asthma disparities in America: A roadmap to reducing burden on racial and ethnic minorities: Executive summary*. https://www.aafa.org/media/2709/asthma-disparities-in-america-burden-by-race-ethnicity-executive-summary.pdf.)

Strategies to improve these disparities include the development of:

- Public policies to expand access to care, increase economic stability, improve education, and enhance the physical environment.
- Interventions to enhance culturally competent clinical management, expanded adoption of asthma education programs, and initiation of community-based partnerships.
- Research to better understand the disease in these patient populations.

Reference

1. Asthma and Allergy Foundation of America. (2020). Asthma disparities in America: A roadmap to reducing burden on racial and ethnic minorities: Executive summary. https://www.aafa.org/media/2709/asthma-disparities-in-america-burden-by-race-ethnicity-executive-summary.pdf.

Illustration from Healthy People 2030, U.S. Department of Health and Human Services, Office of Disease Prevention and Health Promotion. https://health.gov/healthypeople/objectives-and-data/social-determinants-health.

Systemic Corticosteroids

Intravenous or oral corticosteroids also are used in the treatment of an acute asthma exacerbation. Their antiinflammatory effects limit mucosal edema, decrease mucus production, and potentiate beta-2 agonists.[95] It usually takes 6 to 12 hours for the effects of the corticosteroids to become evident.[98] The use of inhaled corticosteroids for treating critical asthma syndrome is undecided at the present time. Initial studies indicate they may be beneficial in certain patient populations.[98]

Oxygen Therapy

The initial treatment of hypoxemia is with supplemental oxygen.[93] High-flow oxygen therapy is administered to keep the patient's oxygen saturation greater than 92%.[93] Another therapy currently under investigation is the use of heliox. Heliox, a mixture of helium and oxygen, has a lower density and higher viscosity than an oxygen and air mixture. Heliox is believed to reduce the work of breathing and improve gas exchange because it flows more easily through constricted areas. Studies have shown that it reduces air trapping and carbon dioxide and helps relieve respiratory acidosis.[93]

Ventilation

Interventions to improve ventilation include the use of noninvasive and invasive mechanical ventilation. Depending on the severity of the asthma exacerbation, the patient may be treated initially with noninvasive ventilation.[102] Current guidelines recommend that patients with acute severe asthma exacerbations be given a trial on noninvasive ventilation unless the patient is rapidly deteriorating.[103] The patient must be closely monitored with particular attention to the work of breathing. If the patient is deteriorating, the patient should be intubated, and invasive mechanical ventilation initiated.[93]

Indications for mechanical ventilation include cardiac or respiratory arrest, disorientation, failure to respond to bronchodilator therapy, and exhaustion. A large endotracheal tube (8 mm) is used to decrease airway resistance and facilitate secretions suctioning.[104] Ventilating a patient with critical asthma syndrome can be very difficult. High inflation pressures are avoided because they can result in barotrauma. The use of PEEP is monitored closely because the patient is prone to developing air trapping. Patient–ventilator asynchrony can also be a major problem. Sedation and neuromuscular paralysis may be necessary to allow for adequate ventilation of the patient.[93]

Nursing Management

The patient care management plan for a patient with critical asthma syndrome incorporates a variety of patient problems (Box 18.19). The nurse has a significant role in optimizing oxygenation and ventilation, providing comfort and emotional support, maintaining surveillance for complications, and educating the patient and family. A systematic review examined the effect of severe asthma on the quality of life and found that the symptoms and activity limitations had a negative effect on the quality of life for these patients.[105]

Optimize Oxygenation and Ventilation

Nursing interventions to optimize oxygenation and ventilation include positioning, preventing desaturation, and promoting secretion clearance. For further discussion of these interventions, see Nursing Management of Acute Respiratory Failure earlier in this chapter.

Educate the Patient and Family

Early in the patient's hospital stay, the patient and family are taught about asthma, its triggers, and its treatment (Box 18.20). Closer to discharge, patient and family education focuses on the interventions necessary for preventing the recurrence of asthma exacerbations, early warning signs of worsening airflow obstruction, correct use of an inhaler and a peak flowmeter, measures to prevent pulmonary infections, and signs and symptoms of a pulmonary infection. Patients who use tobacco products are encouraged to stop using them and are referred to a tobacco cessation program. In addition, the importance of participating in a pulmonary rehabilitation program is stressed. Pulmonary rehabilitation has been shown to improve functional exercise capacity and quality of life in adult patients with asthma.[106]

Interprofessional collaborative management of a patient with critical asthma syndrome is outlined in Box 18.21.

PNEUMOTHORAX

Description and Etiology

A pneumothorax occurs with the accumulation of air in the pleural space, resulting in partial or total lung collapse.[2] Different types of pneumothoraces are described in Table 18.4.

A tension pneumothorax is a medical emergency that requires immediate intervention. It develops when air enters the pleural space on inhalation and cannot exit on exhalation. As the pressure inside the pleural space increases, it results in the collapse of the lung and shifting of the mediastinum and trachea to the unaffected side (Fig. 18.9). The resultant effect

BOX 18.19 DIAGNOSIS AND PATIENT CARE MANAGEMENT

Critical Asthma Syndrome

- Impaired Gas Exchange due to alveolar hypoventilation
- Impaired Gas Exchange due to ventilation/perfusion mismatching or intrapulmonary shunting
- Impaired Breathing Pattern due to musculoskeletal fatigue or neuromuscular impairment
- Impaired Airway Clearance due to excessive secretions or abnormal viscosity of mucus
- Risk for Infection
- Anxiety due to threat to biological, psychological, or social integrity
- Disturbed Body Image due to actual change in body structures, function, or appearance
- Impaired Family Coping due to critically ill family member
- Lack of Knowledge of Treatment Regime due to lack of previous exposure to information (see Box 18.20, Patient and Family Education Plan: Critical Asthma Syndrome)

Patient Care Management Plans are located in Appendix A.

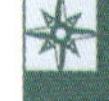

BOX 18.20 PATIENT AND FAMILY EDUCATION PLAN

Critical Asthma Syndrome

Before discharge, the patient should be able to teach back the following topics:

- Pathophysiology of disease
- Specific etiology
- Early warning signs of worsening airflow obstruction (20% decrease in peak expiratory flow rate below predicted or personal best, increase in cough, shortness of breath, chest tightness, wheezing)
- Treatment of exacerbations
- Importance of taking prescribed medications and avoidance of over-the-counter asthma medications
- Correct use of an inhaler (with and without spacer device)
- Correct use of a peak flowmeter
- Removal or avoidance of environmental triggers (e.g., pollen; dust; mold spores; cat and dog dander; cold, dry air; strong odors; household aerosols; tobacco smoke; air pollution)
- Measures to prevent pulmonary infections (e.g., proper nutrition and handwashing, immunization against *Streptococcus pneumoniae* and influenza viruses)
- Signs and symptoms of pulmonary infection (e.g., sputum color change, shortness of breath, fever)
- Importance of participating in a pulmonary rehabilitation program

BOX 18.21 Teamwork and Collaboration

Critical Asthma Syndrome

- Administer oxygen therapy.
  - Low-flow oxygen therapy
  - High-flow oxygen therapy
- Initiate ventilation.
  - Noninvasive ventilation
  - Intubation
  - Mechanical ventilation
- Administer medications.
  - Bronchodilators
  - Corticosteroids
  - Sedatives
- Maintain surveillance for complications.
  - Acute respiratory failure
- Provide comfort and emotional support.

TABLE 18.4 Types of Pneumothoraces

Type	Description
Tension	Occurs when air is allowed to enter the pleural space but not to exit it; as pressure increases inside the pleural space, the lung collapses and the mediastinum shifts to the unaffected side; it may result from a spontaneous or traumatic pneumothorax
Spontaneous	
Primary	Disruption of the visceral pleura that allows air from the lung to enter the pleural space; occurs spontaneously in patients *without* underlying lung disease
Secondary	Disruption of the visceral pleura that allows air from the lung to enter the pleural space; occurs spontaneously in patients *with* underlying lung disease
Traumatic	
Open	Laceration in the parietal pleura that allows atmospheric air to enter the pleural space; occurs as a result of penetrating chest trauma
Closed	Laceration in the visceral pleura that allows air from the lung to enter the pleural space; occurs as a result of blunt chest trauma
Iatrogenic	Laceration in the visceral pleura that allows air from the lung to enter the pleural space; occurs as a result of therapeutic or diagnostic procedures, such as central line insertion, thoracentesis, and needle aspiration

is compression of the vena cava, decreased venous return, and compression of the unaffected lung.[107]

Etiology

The two main causes of a pneumothorax are (1) disruption of the parietal or visceral pleura[2] and (2) rupture of alveoli.[107]

Parietal or visceral pleura disruption. Disruption of the parietal pleura occurs as the result of penetrating trauma to the chest wall, which allows atmospheric air to enter the pleural space (traumatic open pneumothorax).[107] This can be secondary to a knife or a gunshot wound to the chest. Disruption of the visceral pleura allows air to enter the pleural space from the lung. This condition may be caused by blunt chest wall trauma (traumatic closed pneumothorax),[2,107]

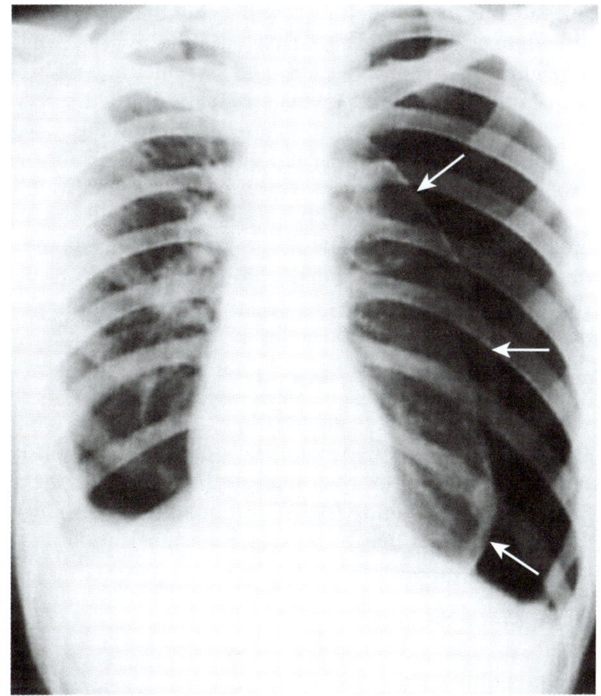

FIG. 18.9 Left-Sided Tension Pneumothorax. Notice the shift of the heart and mediastinum to the right. Arrows point out the edge of the lung showing the amount of lung collapse. (From Des Jardin T, Burton GC. *Clinical Management and Assessment of Respiratory Disease.* 3rd ed. Mosby; 1995.)

diagnostic or therapeutic procedures (traumatic iatrogenic pneumothorax),[2,107] diseases of the pulmonary system (secondary spontaneous pneumothorax),[2,108] or ruptured subpleural blebs (primary spontaneous pneumothorax).[2,108]

Alveolar rupture. Rupture of alveoli occurs because of a change in the pressure gradient between the alveoli and the surrounding interstitial space. An increase in alveolar pressure or a decrease in interstitial pressure can lead to overdistention of the alveoli, rupture, and air leakage into the interstitial space. This situation can occur secondary to external chest trauma or mechanical ventilation.[107] When this happens secondary to mechanical ventilation, it is known as *ventilator-induced lung injury*. Alveolar rupture secondary to mechanical ventilation can be the result of excessive pressure in the alveoli (barotrauma), excessive volume in the alveoli (volutrauma), or shearing caused by repeated opening and closing of the alveoli (atelectrauma).[109] Ventilator-induced lung injury is discussed further in Chapter 19.

Pathophysiology

Regardless of the cause, air entering the pleural space compresses the affected lung. As the lung collapses, the alveoli become underventilated, causing $\dot{V}/\dot{Q}$ mismatching and intrapulmonary shunting. If the pneumothorax is large, hypoxemia ensues, and ARF quickly develops. Increased pressure within the chest can lead to shifting of the mediastinum, compression of the great vessels, and decreased CO.[107]

Assessment and Diagnosis

Assessment

The clinical manifestations of a pneumothorax depend on the degree of lung collapse and can range from asymptomatic to impending respiratory failure. The patient may present with shortness of breath and chest discomfort.[108] If the pneumothorax is large, the patient will exhibit tachypnea, decreased or absent breath sounds on the affected side, and asymmetric lung expansion. Decreased respiratory excursion on the affected side with bulging intercostal muscles and decreased tactile fremitus may also be present. If the patient experiences alveolar rupture, subcutaneous emphysema may be evident. This situation will be manifested by crepitus, usually around the face, neck, and upper chest. If the patient has a tension pneumothorax, they will exhibit all the signs previously discussed, along with tracheal deviation away from the affected side, hyperresonance to percussion, tachycardia, hypotension, jugular venous distension, and signs of hypoxemia.[107]

Diagnostic Procedures

If the patient has a large pneumothorax, ABG analysis demonstrates hypoxemia and hypercapnia. A chest radiograph confirms the pneumothorax with increased translucency evident on the affected side (Fig. 18.9). In addition, increased sharpness of the affected border may be present. If it is unclear, a chest CT may be done.[107]

Medical Management

Medical management of a pneumothorax varies depending on the degree of collapse and the severity of symptoms. A tension pneumothorax requires immediate attention. Treatment comprises administering supplemental oxygen and inserting a large-bore needle or catheter into the second intercostal space at the midclavicular line of the affected side. This action relieves the pressure within the chest. The needle remains in place until the patient is stabilized, and a chest tube is inserted.[107]

A small pneumothorax usually requires no treatment other than supplemental oxygen administration unless complications occur or underlying lung disease or injury is present. A large pneumothorax requires inserting a chest tube (also called a *tube thoracostomy*) to evacuate the air from the pleural space and facilitate the reexpansion of the collapsed lung.[108,110] Surgical intervention may be necessary in patients with a persistent air leak or failure of the lung to expand within 5 to 7 days. The preferred procedure is a video-assisted thoracoscopic surgery.[111]

Chest Tube Placement

Interventions include placement of a small-bore (12 to 20 Fr) or large-bore (24 to 40 Fr) chest tube. Chest tubes are inserted into the pleural space to remove fluid or air, reinstate the negative intrapleural pressure, and reexpand a collapsed lung.[112] The trend appears to be toward placing a small-bore tube, as the smaller tubes are more comfortable for the patient and just as effective as large-bore tubes.[108] A recent study found that a 28 Fr catheter is the ideal size for most pneumothoraces.[113]

Chest tubes are usually inserted in the fourth or fifth intercostal space on the midaxillary line.[112] After the tube is inserted, it is attached to a Heimlich valve or a chest drainage system. The Heimlich valve is a small one-way valve device that allows air to exit from the pleural space but not enter it (Fig. 18.10). It can be used alone or attached to a drainage bag.[112] Complications of chest tube insertion include malposition of the chest tube, hemothorax, and injury to the lung tissue, thoracic duct, diaphragm, great vessels, or abdominal organs.[112]

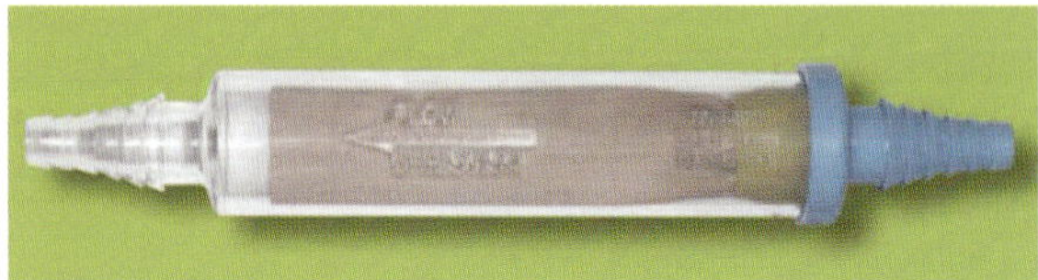

FIG. 18.10 Heimlich Valve. (Courtesy and © Becton, Dickinson and Company.)

Chest Drainage Systems

A chest drainage system is a disposable plastic unit with three separate chambers: a water-seal or dry-seal chamber, a suction-control chamber, and a drainage-collection chamber (Fig. 18.11). In a system with a water-seal chamber, the chamber is filled to the 2-cm level. The water-seal chamber acts as a one-way valve, allowing air to escape from the chest but not to enter it. In a system with a dry-seal chamber, a mechanical one-way valve replaces the water seal. The suction-control chamber is adjusted to the desired level of suction. After the chest tubes are placed, the suction-control chamber is attached to an external suction regulator, which is adjusted until the desired suction level (usually 20 cm H_2O) is established as measured on the chest drainage system. Any fluid draining from the chest will be evident in the collection chamber. Connection points of the drainage tubing are sealed with tape, and an occlusive dressing is applied over the chest tube insertion site. After the tubes are inserted and connected to either device, a chest radiograph is obtained to confirm the reexpansion of the lung.[112]

Nursing Management

The patient care management plan for a patient with a pneumothorax incorporates a variety of patient problems (Box 18.22). The nurse has a significant role in optimizing oxygenation and ventilation, maintaining the chest drainage system, providing comfort and emotional support, and maintaining surveillance for complications.

Optimize Oxygenation and Ventilation

Nursing interventions to optimize oxygenation and ventilation include positioning, preventing desaturation, and promoting secretion clearance. For further discussion of these interventions, see Nursing Management of Acute Respiratory Failure earlier in this chapter.

Maintain Chest Drainage System

Maintaining the chest drainage system involves careful attention to the suction applied and the maintenance of unobstructed drainage tubes. Kinks and large loops of tubing must be avoided because they impede drainage and air evacuation, which may prevent timely lung reexpansion or may result in a tension pneumothorax. Retained drainage also becomes an excellent medium for bacterial growth. The system is routinely observed for air leaks.

Air Leak in chest drainage system. If an air leak is present, the source must be identified. To determine whether the source is within the system or the patient, systematic brief clamping of the drainage tube is performed. A padded clamp is placed on the drainage tubing as close to the chest dressing as possible. If the air leak stops, the leak is located between the patient and the clamp. The air leak can be within the patient or at the insertion site. The clamp is then removed, and the chest tube site is exposed. The tube is inspected at the site where it enters the chest to ensure all eyelets are within the patient. If an eyelet port is outside the chest, it can be a

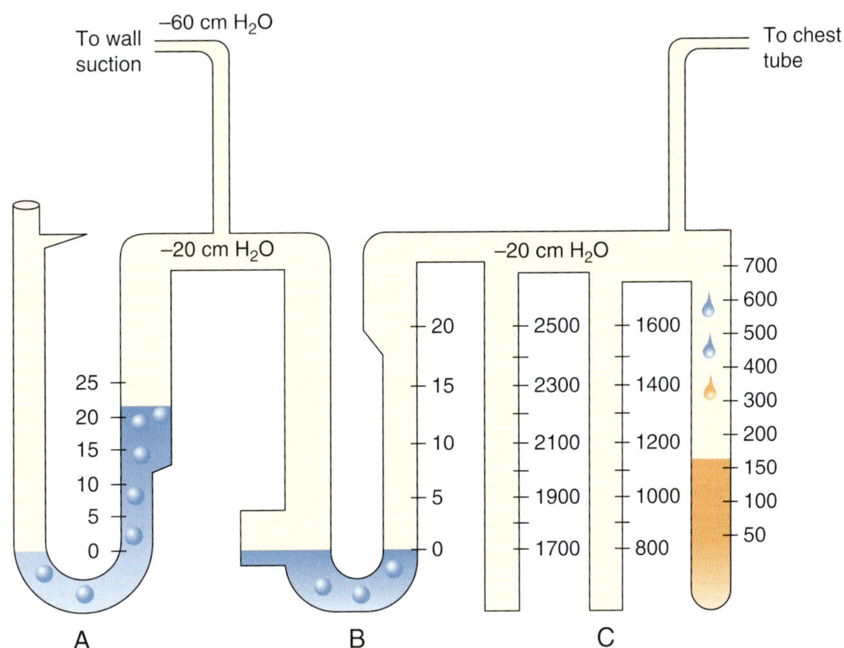

FIG. 18.11 Three-Chamber Underwater-Seal Drainage System. *A*, water-seal chamber; *B*, suction-control chamber; *C*, drainage-collection chamber (From Kacmarek RM, Stoller JK, Heuer AJ, eds. *Egan's Fundamentals of Respiratory Care*. 12th ed. Elsevier; 2021.)

BOX 18.22 DIAGNOSIS AND PATIENT CARE MANAGEMENT

Pneumothorax

- Impaired Gas Exchange due to ventilation/perfusion mismatching or intrapulmonary shunting
- Ineffective Breathing Pattern due to decreased lung expansion
- Acute Pain due to transmission and perception of cutaneous, visceral, muscular, or ischemic impulses
- Anxiety due to threat to biological, psychological, or social integrity
- Disturbed Body Image due to actual change in body structures, function, or appearance
- Impaired Family Coping due to critically ill family member

Patient Care Management plans are located in Appendix A.

BOX 18.23 Teamwork and Collaboration

Pneumothorax

- Administer oxygen therapy.
- Intubate patient as needed.
- Initiate mechanical ventilation as needed.
- Evacuate air from the pleural space.
  - Percutaneous catheter attached to Heimlich valve
  - Chest tube to a chest drainage system
- Maintain surveillance for complications.
  - Acute respiratory failure
- Maintain chest drainage system.
- Provide comfort and emotional support.

source of an air leak and must be occluded, which may require the practitioner's attention. After the insertion site has been eliminated as a leakage source, the chest dressing is reapplied, securely covering the site. If the air leak does not stop when a clamp is placed on the chest tube, the leak must be located between the clamp and the drainage collector. It can be found by releasing the clamp and moving it down the tubing a few inches at a time until the bubbling stops. After the area of the leak is located, it can be taped to reestablish a seal, or the system can be replaced.

Disruption of the chest drainage system. A sterile occlusive dressing and a bottle of sterile water should always be available at the patient's bedside. If the chest drainage system is inadvertently interrupted, the chest tube is placed a few centimeters into the bottle of water while the drainage system is reestablished. If the chest tube is inadvertently dislodged at the insertion site, a sterile dressing is placed on the site and taped on three sides. The fourth side should be left open to allow air to escape from the chest to avoid causing a tension pneumothorax. Immediate implementation of these techniques minimizes or prevents the formation of a pneumothorax and avoids greater complications.

Periodic assessments. Throughout the duration of chest tube placement, the patient is assessed periodically for reexpansion of the lung and complications associated with the chest drainage system. The thorax and lungs are assessed, paying particular attention to any tracheal deviation, asymmetric chest movement, presence of subcutaneous emphysema, characteristics of breathing, quality of lung sounds, and presence of tympany or percussion sounds, which are indicative of pneumothorax.

Interprofessional collaborative management of a patient with an air leak disorder is outlined in Box 18.23.

LONG-TERM MECHANICAL VENTILATOR DEPENDENCE

Description

Long-term mechanical ventilator dependence (LTMVD) is a secondary disorder that occurs when a patient requires assisted ventilation longer than expected, given the patient's underlying condition. It is the result of complex medical problems that do not allow the weaning process to take place in a normal and timely manner. Generally, the patient has failed multiple weaning attempts. A literature review reveals a great deal of confusion regarding an exact definition of LTMVD, mainly regarding an actual time frame. The WIND classification is a standardized tool to classify the stages of weaning from mechanical ventilation.[114] It provides a systematic way to document and communicate a patient's progress through the weaning process. The WIND classification divides patients into categories based on the duration and success of their weaning attempts:

- No Weaning (Category 0): Patients who are not ready for any weaning attempts due to critical illness, sedation, or other reasons.
- Short-Term Weaning (Category 1): For patients who successfully separate from mechanical ventilation within 1 day. This stage often includes patients who pass an initial spontaneous breathing trial (SBT) and are extubated shortly after.
- Intermediate Weaning (Category 2): For patients who require more than one day but less than 7 days to be successfully weaned from the ventilator. This group may include patients who initially fail the SBT but can progress to extubation with a few more trials over the course of several days.
- Prolonged Weaning (Category 3): For patients who require more than 7 days to successfully wean from mechanical ventilation. This may include patients with complex medical conditions, severe respiratory dysfunction, or other complicating factors that extend the duration of their weaning.

Etiology and Pathophysiology

Approximately 10% of patients requiring mechanical ventilation develop LTMVD.[115] A wide variety of physiologic and psychological factors contribute to the development of LTMVD. Physiological factors include conditions that result in decreased gas exchange, increased ventilatory workload, increased ventilatory demand, decreased ventilatory drive, and increased respiratory muscle fatigue (Box 18.24).[116] Psychological factors include conditions that result in loss of breathing pattern control, lack of motivation and confidence, and delirium (Box 18.24).[116] The development of LTMVD is also affected by the severity and duration of the patient's current illness and any underlying chronic health problems.

BOX 18.24 Physiological and Psychological Factors Contributing to LTMVD

Physiological Factors

Decreased Gas Exchange
- Ventilation/perfusion mismatching
- Intrapulmonary shunting
- Alveolar hypoventilation
- Anemia
- Acute heart failure

Increased Ventilatory Workload
- Decreased lung compliance
- Increased airway resistance
- Small endotracheal tube
- Decreased ventilatory sensitivity
- Improper positioning
- Abdominal distention
- Dyspnea

Increased Ventilatory Demand
- Increased pulmonary dead space
- Increased metabolic demands
- Improper ventilator mode/settings
- Metabolic acidosis
- Overfeeding

Decreased Ventilatory Drive
- Respiratory alkalosis
- Metabolic alkalosis
- Hypothyroidism
- Sedatives
- Malnutrition

Increased Respiratory Muscle Fatigue
- Increased ventilatory workload
- Increased ventilatory demand
- Malnutrition
- Hypokalemia
- Hypomagnesemia
- Hypophosphatemia
- Hypothyroidism
- Critical illness polyneuropathy
- Inadequate muscle rest

Psychological Factors

Loss of Breathing Pattern Control
- Anxiety
- Fear
- Dyspnea
- Pain
- Ventilator asynchrony
- Lack of confidence in the ability to breathe

Lack of Motivation and Confidence
- Inadequate trust in staff
- Depersonalization
- Hopelessness
- Powerlessness
- Depression
- Inadequate communication

Delirium
- Sensory overload
- Sensory deprivation
- Sleep deprivation
- Pain
- Medications

LTMVD, Long-term mechanical ventilator dependence

Medical and Nursing Management

The goal of medical and nursing management of patients with LTMVD is successful weaning. The management of a patient with LTMVD is described in three stages: (1) preweaning stage, (2) weaning process stage, and (3) weaning outcome stage. In addition, the common patient problems for this patient population are listed in Box 18.25.

Preweaning Stage

For a patient with LTMVD, the preweaning phase consists of resolving the precipitating event that necessitated ventilatory assistance and preventing the physiologic and psychological factors that can interfere with weaning. Before any attempts at weaning, the patient is assessed for weaning readiness, an approach is determined, and a method is selected.

Weaning preparedness. The patient should be physiologically and psychologically prepared to initiate the weaning process by addressing factors that can interfere with weaning. Aggressive medical management to prevent and treat $\dot{V}/\dot{Q}$ mismatching, intrapulmonary shunting, anemia, heart failure, decreased lung compliance, increased airway resistance, acid-base disturbances, hypothyroidism, abdominal distention, and electrolyte imbalances should be initiated. In addition, interventions to decrease the work of breathing should be implemented, such as replacing a small endotracheal tube with a larger tube or a tracheostomy, suctioning airway secretions, administering bronchodilators, optimizing the ventilator settings and trigger sensitivity, initiating early mobilization, and positioning the patient in straight alignment with the head of the bed elevated at least 30 degrees. Enteral nutrition is started, and the patient's nutrition state is optimized. Physical

BOX 18.25 DIAGNOSIS AND PATIENT CARE MANAGEMENT

Long-Term Mechanical Ventilation Dependence

- Impaired Ventilatory Weaning due to physical, psychosocial, or situational factors
- Risk for Aspiration
- Impaired Nutritional Intake due to lack of exogenous nutrients or increased metabolic demand
- Risk for Infection
- Delirium due to sensory overload, sensory deprivation, and sleep pattern disturbance
- Relocation Stress due to transfer out of intensive care unit
- Powerlessness due to lack of control over current situation or disease progression
- Impaired Family Coping due to critically ill family member

Patient Care Management Plans are located in Appendix A.

therapy is initiated because increased mobility facilitates weaning. A means of communication should be established with the patient. Sedatives can be administered to provide anxiety control, but it is critical to avoid respiratory depression.

Weaning readiness. Although various methods for assessing weaning readiness have been developed, none has proven accurate in predicting weaning success in a patient with LTMVD. Because so many variables can affect the patient's ability to wean, any assessment of weaning readiness should incorporate these variables. Cardiac function, gas exchange, pulmonary mechanics, nutrition status, electrolyte and fluid balance, and motivation are considered when deciding to wean. This assessment is ongoing to reflect the dynamic nature of the process.[116,117]

Weaning approach. Although weaning patients requiring short-term mechanical ventilation is a relatively simple process that can usually be accomplished with a nurse and respiratory therapist, weaning a patient with LTMVD is a much more complex process that usually requires a multidisciplinary team approach.

PATIENT-CENTERED CRITICAL CARE

Pet Visitors in Critical Care

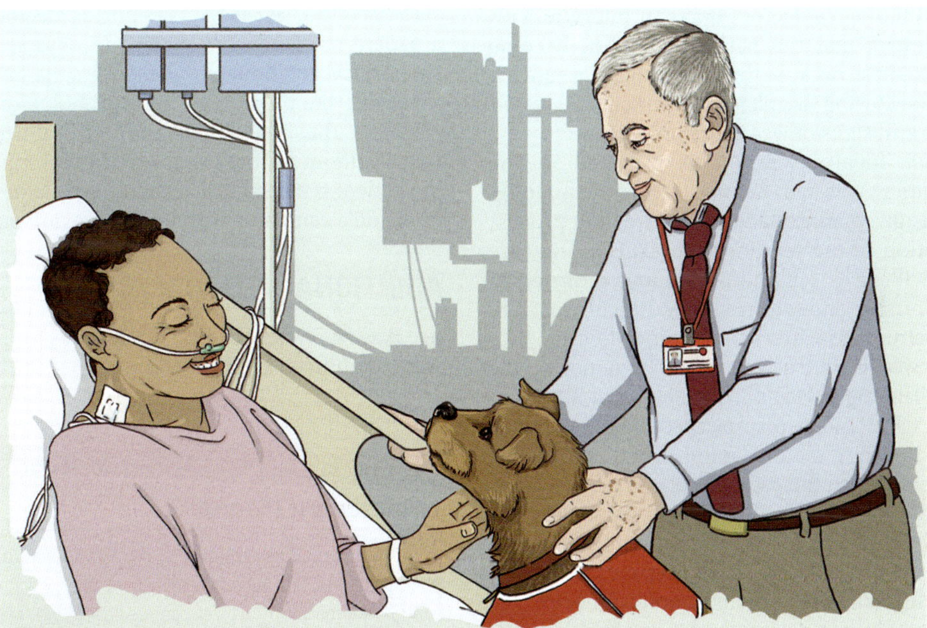

Pet visitation is a relatively new intervention to relieve patient stress in the critical care unit. Dogs, with their owners, are the most common animals that participate. This visit is a hospital-wide program, and there are guidelines to make the pet visit a positive experience.

The pet must be bathed 24 to 48 hours before coming to the hospital to minimize any risk of infection. Also, the pet must have a calm temperament and not become excited by the hospital environment or by being stroked by strangers. Both the pet owner and the dog will have photo-identification badges, and both must check in at the hospital department in charge of the pet visitor program before visiting patient units, including critical care units. This department might be called volunteer services/guest services or similar.

Patients and families often ask for a visit from a pet visitor, especially if their own pet cannot visit. The dog always remains on a leash, and their human handler must wash or sanitize their hands before and after meeting any patient. This visit is not a therapy session but a short social visit.

Not all people like dogs, and some people have allergies or other concerns about animal visitation in hospitals. Therefore, it is essential to ask the patient's and family's permission to ensure the pet visit will be welcomed. Pet visitation is a novel distraction for those who like animals and are sufficiently alert to enjoy the visit.

Multidisciplinary weaning teams that use a coordinated and collaborative approach have demonstrated improved patient outcomes and decreased weaning times. The team ideally consists of a practitioner, nurse, respiratory therapist, dietitian, physical therapist, social worker or case manager, and clinical nurse specialist. Additional members, if possible, include an occupational therapist, a speech therapist, and a discharge planner. Working together, the team members develop a comprehensive plan of care for the patient that is efficient, consistent, progressive, and cost effective. Several studies have demonstrated successful weaning through the use of nurse and respiratory therapist–managed protocols.[118]

Weaning method. Various weaning methods are available; no one method has consistently proven superior to the others. These methods include T-tube (T-piece), CPAP, pressure support ventilation (PSV), and synchronized intermittent mandatory ventilation (SIMV). One multicenter study lends evidence to support the use of PSV for weaning over T-tube or SIMV weaning. Often, these weaning methods are used in combination with each other, such as SIMV with PSV, CPAP with PSV, or SIMV with CPAP.[116]

Weaning Process Stage

For a patient with LTMVD, the weaning process phase consists of initiating the selected weaning method and minimizing the physiological and psychological factors that can interfere with weaning. It is imperative that the patient does not become exhausted during this phase because this can result in a setback in the weaning process. During this phase, the patient is assessed for weaning progress and signs of weaning intolerance.[116]

Weaning initiation. Ideally, weaning is initiated in the morning while the patient is rested. Before starting the weaning process, the patient is given an explanation of how the process works and a description of the sensations to expect. They are reassured that they will be closely monitored and returned to the original ventilator mode and settings if any difficulty occurs. This information is reinforced with each weaning attempt.

T-tube and CPAP weaning are accomplished by removing the patient from the ventilator and placing the patient on a T-tube or placing the patient on CPAP mode for a specified duration of time, known as a weaning trial, for a specified number of times per day. When the weaning trial is over, the patient is placed on the assist-control mode or similar mode and allowed to rest to prevent respiratory muscle fatigue. The duration of time spent weaning is gradually increased, as is the frequency, until the patient can breathe spontaneously for 24 hours. If PSV is used in conjunction with CPAP, the PSV is initially set to provide the patient with an assisted tidal volume of 10 to 12 mL/kg, and this is gradually weaned until a level of 6 to 8 cm H_2O of pressure support is achieved. Weaning with SIMV and PSV is accomplished by gradually decreasing the number of breaths or the amount of pressure support the patient receives by a specified amount until the patient can breathe spontaneously for 24 hours.[116]

Weaning progress. Weaning progress can be evaluated using various methods. Evaluation of weaning progress when using a weaning method that gradually withdraws ventilatory support, such as SIMV or PSV, can be accomplished by measuring the percentage of the minute ventilation requirement provided by the ventilator. If the percentage steadily decreases, weaning is progressing. Evaluation of weaning progress when using a weaning method that removes ventilatory support, such as T-tube or CPAP, can be accomplished by measuring the amount of time the patient remains free from support. If the time steadily increases, weaning is progressing.

Weaning intolerance. Once the weaning process has begun, the patient is continuously assessed for signs of intolerance. When present, these signs indicate when to place the patient back on the ventilator or to return the patient to the previous ventilator settings. Commonly used indicators include dyspnea, accessory muscle use, restlessness, anxiety, change in facial expression, changes in heart rate and blood pressure, rapid, shallow breathing, and discomfort.[116] See the patient management plan Impaired Ventilatory Weaning in Appendix A for specific interventions to manage these issues.

Facilitative therapies. Additional therapies may be needed to facilitate weaning in a patient who is having difficulty making weaning progress. These therapies include ventilatory muscle training and biofeedback. Inspiratory muscle training enhances the strength and endurance of the respiratory muscles. Biofeedback can be used to promote relaxation and assist in the management of dyspnea and anxiety.

Weaning Outcome Stage

Two outcomes are possible for a patient with LTMVD: weaning completed and incomplete weaning.

Weaning completed. Weaning is deemed successful when a patient can breathe spontaneously for 24 hours without ventilatory support. When this occurs, the patient may be extubated or decannulated at any time, although this is not necessary for weaning to be considered successful.

Incomplete weaning. Weaning is deemed incomplete when a patient has reached a plateau (5 days at the same ventilatory support level without any changes) in the weaning process despite managing the physiologic and psychological factors that impede weaning. Thus, the patient cannot breathe spontaneously for 24 hours without full or partial ventilatory support. Once this occurs, the patient is placed in a subacute ventilator facility or discharged home on a ventilator with home care nursing follow-up.[115]

ADDITIONAL RESOURCES

See Box 18.26 for additional resources for managing the patient with pulmonary dysfunction.

BOX 18.26 Internet Resources

Pulmonary Disorders

- American Lung Association: https://www.lung.org/
- ARDS Foundation: https://ardsglobal.org/
- Smokefree.gov: https://smokefree.gov/
- American Association of Critical-Care Nurses (AACN): https://www.aacn.org/
- American Association of Respiratory Care (AARC): https://www.aarc.org/
- American College of Chest Physicians (ACCP): https://www.chestnet.org/
- American College of Physicians (ACP): https://www.acponline.org/
- American Medical Association (AMA): https://www.ama-assn.org/
- American Society for Parenteral and Enteral Nutrition (ASPEN): http://www.nutritioncare.org/
- American Thoracic Society (ATS): https://www.thoracic.org/
- Centers for Disease Control and Prevention (CDC): https://www.cdc.gov/
- National Institutes for Health (NIH): https://www.nih.gov/
- Office of Disease Prevention and Health Promotion (ODPHP): https://health.gov/myhealthfinder
- Respiratory Nursing Society and Interprofessional Collaborative (RNSIC): https://www.respiratorynursingsociety.org/
- Society for Critical Care Medicine (SCCM): https://www.sccm.org/Home
- Society for Vascular Surgery: https://vascular.org/
- Asthma and Allergy Foundation of America (AAFA): https://www.aafa.org/

KEY POINTS

Acute Respiratory Failure

- ARF is a clinical condition in which the pulmonary system fails to maintain adequate gas exchange; it results from a deficiency in the performance of the pulmonary system.
- Hypoxemia is the hallmark of ARF and is the result of impaired gas exchange as a result of alveolar hypoventilation, V̇/Q̇ mismatching, or intrapulmonary shunting.
- Medical management focuses on treating the underlying cause, promoting adequate gas exchange, correcting acidosis, initiating nutrition support, and preventing complications (i.e., ischemic-anoxic encephalopathy, cardiac dysrhythmias, VTE, and gastrointestinal bleeding).
- Nursing actions include optimizing oxygenation and ventilation (by positioning, preventing desaturation, and promoting secretion clearance), providing comfort and emotional support, maintaining surveillance for complications, and educating the patient and family.

Acute Respiratory Distress Syndrome

- ARDS is characterized by noncardiac pulmonary edema and disruption of the alveolar-capillary membrane because of injury to the pulmonary vasculature or the airways.
- The hallmark of ARDS is refractory hypoxemia.
- Medical management focuses on treating the underlying cause, promoting gas exchange, supporting tissue oxygenation, and preventing complications.
- Nursing actions include optimizing oxygenation and ventilation, providing comfort and emotional support, and maintaining surveillance for complications.

Pneumonia

- Pneumonia is an acute inflammation of the lung parenchyma caused by an infectious agent that can lead to alveolar consolidation and can be classified as community acquired or hospital acquired.
- Medical management focuses on initiating antibiotic therapy, administering oxygen and mechanical ventilation, managing fluids and nutrition support, and treating complications.
- Nursing actions include optimizing oxygenation and ventilation, preventing the spread of infection, providing comfort and emotional support, and maintaining surveillance for complications.

Aspiration Pneumonitis

- Aspiration pneumonitis is the presence of abnormal toxic substances in the airways and alveoli, resulting in injury to the lungs.
- Medical management focuses on removing toxic substances from the airways, supporting oxygenation, and maintaining hemodynamics.
- Nursing actions include optimizing oxygenation and ventilation, preventing further aspiration events, providing comfort and emotional support, and maintaining surveillance for complications.

Pulmonary Embolism

- A PE occurs when a clot (thrombotic embolus) or other matter (nonthrombotic embolus) lodges in the pulmonary arterial system, disrupting the blood flow to a region of the lungs.
- Medical management focuses on preventing the recurrence of PE, initiating clot dissolution, reversing the effects of pulmonary hypertension, promoting gas exchange, and preventing complications.
- Nursing actions include optimizing oxygenation and ventilation, monitoring for bleeding, providing comfort and emotional support, maintaining surveillance for complications, and educating the patient and family.

Critical Asthma Syndrome

- Critical asthma syndrome is an overarching term that describes various forms of acute asthma exacerbations that can lead to ARF and death.
- Medical management focuses on support of oxygenation (by bronchodilators, corticosteroids, and oxygen therapy) and ventilation.
- Nursing actions include optimizing oxygenation and ventilation, providing comfort and emotional support, maintaining surveillance for complications, and educating the patient and family.

Pneumothorax

- A pneumothorax occurs with the accumulation of air in the pleural space, resulting in partial or total lung collapse.
- A tension pneumothorax is a medical emergency that requires immediate intervention.
- Medical management varies depending on the degree of collapse and the severity of symptoms.
- Nursing actions include optimizing oxygenation and ventilation, maintaining the chest drainage system, providing comfort and emotional support, and maintaining surveillance for complications.

Long-Term Mechanical Ventilation Dependence

- LTMVD is a secondary disorder that occurs when a patient requires assisted ventilation for longer than expected, given the patient's underlying condition.
- Weaning can be divided into three stages: preweaning, weaning process, and weaning outcome.
- The preweaning phase consists of resolving the precipitating event that necessitated ventilatory assistance and preventing the physiologic and psychological factors that can interfere with weaning.
- The weaning process phase consists of initiating the selected weaning method and minimizing the physiological and psychological factors that can interfere with weaning.
- Weaning is deemed successful when the patient can breathe spontaneously for 24 hours without ventilatory support.

Visit the Evolve site at http://evolve.elsevier.com/Urden/CriticalCareNursing for additional study materials.

REFERENCES

1. Hill NS, Garpestad G, Schumaker GL. Acute ventilatory failure. In: Broaddus VC, ed. *Murray and Nadel's Textbook of Respiratory Medicine*. 7th ed. Philadelphia: Elsevier; 2022.
2. Villgran VD, Lyons C, Nasrullah A, et al. Acute respiratory failure. *Crit Care Nurs Q*. 2022;45(3):233–247. https://doi.org/10.1097/CNQ.0000000000000408.

3. Lamba TS, Sharara RS, Singh AC, et al. Pathophysiology and classification of respiratory failure. *Crit Care Nurs Q*. 2016;39(2):85–93. https://doi.org/10.1097/CNQ.0000000000000102.
4. Prasad S, O'Neill S. Respiratory failure. *Surgery (Oxford)*. 2021;39(10):654–659. https://doi.org/10.1016/j.mpsur.2021.08.007.
5. Kapil S, Wilson JG. Mechanical ventilation in hypoxemic respiratory failure. *Emerg Med Clin North Am*. 2019;37(3):431–444. https://doi.org/10.1016/j.emc.2019.04.005.
6. Weinberger SE, Cockrill BA, Mandel J. Classification and pathophysiologic aspects of respiratory failure. In: Weinberger SE, Cockrill BA, Mandel J, eds. *Principles of Pulmonary Medicine*. 8th ed. Philadelphia: Elsevier; 2024.
7. Mallat J, Rahman N, Hamed F, et al. Pathophysiology, mechanisms, and managements of tissue hypoxia. *Anaesth Crit Care Pain Med*. 2022;41(4):101087. https://doi.org/10.1016/j.accpm.2022.101087.
8. Aboussouan LS. Respiratory failure and the need for ventilatory support. In: Stoller JK, Heuer AJ, Chatburn RL, Mireles-Cabodevila E, Vines DL, eds. *Egan's Fundamentals of Respiratory Care*. 13th ed. St. Louis: Elsevier; 2025.
9. O'Driscoll BR, Smith R. Oxygen use in critical illness. *Respir Care*. 2019;64(10):1293–1307. https://doi.org/10.4187/respcare.07044.
10. Baldomero AK, Melzer AC, Greer N, et al. Effectiveness and harms of high-flow nasal oxygen for acute respiratory failure: an evidence report for a clinical guideline from the American College of Physicians. *Ann Intern Med*. 2021;174(7):952–966. https://doi.org/10.7326/M20-4675.
11. Popowicz P, Leonard K. Noninvasive ventilation and oxygenation strategies. *Surg Clin North Am*. 2022 Feb;102(1):149–157. https://doi.org/10.1016/j.suc.2021.09.012.
12. Rochwerg B, Brochard L, Elliot MW, et al. Official ERS/ATS clinical practice guidelines: Noninvasive ventilation for acute respiratory failure. *Eur Respir J*. 2017;50(2):1602426. https://doi.org/10.1183/13993003.02426-2016.
13. Weinberger SE, Cockrill BA, Mandel J. Management of respiratory failure. In: Weinberger SE, Cockrill BA, Mandel J, eds. *Principles of Pulmonary Medicine*. 8th ed. Philadelphia: Elsevier; 2024.
14. Johnston C, Nixon P. Asthma and chronic obstructive pulmonary disease in the intensive care unit. *Anaesth Intensive Care Med*. 2022;23(10):628–634. https://doi.org/10.1016/j.mpaic.2022.07.006.
15. Brand J, Arrowsmith JE. Respiratory system: Applied pharmacology. *Anaesth Intensive Care Med*. 2021;22(3):151–155. https://doi.org/10.1016/j.mpaic.2021.01.007.
16. Devlin JW, Skrobik Y, Gélinas C, et al. Clinical practice guidelines for the prevention and management of pain, agitation/sedation, delirium, immobility, and sleep disruption in adult patients in the ICU. *Crit Care Med*. 2018;46(9):e825–e873. https://doi.org/10.1097/CCM.0000000000003299.
17. Welhengama C, Hall A, Hunter JM. Neuromuscular blocking drugs in the critically ill. *BJA Educ*. 2021;21(7):258–263. https://doi.org/10.1016/j.bjae.2021.02.002.
18. Lo KB, Garvia V, Stempel JM, et al. Bicarbonate use and mortality outcome among critically ill patients with metabolic acidosis: a meta analysis. *Heart Lung*. 2020;49(2):167–174. https://doi.org/10.1016/j.hrtlng.2019.10.007.
19. Rudnick MR, Blair GJ, Kuschner WG, Barr J. Lactic acidosis and the role of sodium bicarbonate: a narrative opinion. *Shock*. 2020;53(5):528–536. https://doi.org/10.1097/SHK.0000000000001415.
20. McClave SA, Taylor BE, Martindale, et al. Society of critical care medicine; American society for parenteral and enteral nutrition: guidelines for the provision and assessment of nutrition support therapy in the adult critically ill patient: society of critical care medicine (SCCM) and American+Society for parenteral and enteral nutrition (ASPEN). *J Parenter Enteral Nutr*. 2016;40(2):159–211. https://doi.org/10.1177/0148607115621863.
21. Hill A, Elke G, Weimann A. Nutrition in the intensive care unit-A narrative review. *Nutrients*. 2021;13(8):2851. https://doi.org/10.3390/nu13082851.
22. Stollings JL, Kotfis K, Chanques G, et al. Delirium in critical illness: clinical manifestations, outcomes, and management. *Intensive Care Med*. 2021 Oct;47(10):1089–1103. https://doi.org/10.1007/s00134-021-06503-1.
23. Kahn SR, Lim W, Dunn AS, et al. Prevention of VTE in nonsurgical patients: antithrombotic therapy and prevention of thrombosis, 9th ed, American college of chest physicians evidence-based clinical practice guidelines. *Chest*. 2012;141(suppl 2):e195S–e226S. https://doi.org/10.1378/chest.11-2296.
24. Saeed M, Bass S, Chaisson NF. Which ICU patients need stress ulcer prophylaxis? *Cleve Clin J Med*. 2022;89(7):363–367. https://doi.org/10.3949/ccjm.89a.21085.
25. Mezidi M, Guérin C. Effects of patient positioning on respiratory mechanics in mechanically ventilated ICU patients. *Ann Transl Med*. 2018;6(19):384. https://doi.org/10.21037/atm.2018.05.50.
26. Katz S, Arish N, Rokach A, et al. The effect of body position on pulmonary function: a systematic review. *BMC Pulm Med*. 2018 Oct;18(1):159. https://doi.org/10.1186/s12890-018-0723-4.
27. Tatsumi H. Enteral tolerance in critically ill patients. *J Intensive Care*. 2019;7:30. https://doi.org/10.1186/s40560-019-0378-0.
28. Güner CK, Kutlutürkan S. Role of head-of-bed elevation in preventing ventilator-associated pneumonia bed elevation and pneumonia. *Nurs Crit Care*. 2022;27(5):635–645. https://doi.org/10.1111/nicc.12633.
29. Zhuo X, Pan L, Zeng X. The effects of the 45° semi-recumbent position on the clinical outcomes of mechanically ventilated patients: a systematic review and meta-analysis study. *Ann Palliat Med*. 2021;10(10):10643–10651. https://doi.org/10.21037/apm-21-2359.
30. Goñi-Viguria R, Yoldi-Arzoz E, Casajús-Sola L, et al. Respiratory physiotherapy in intensive care unit: bibliographic review. *Enferm Intensiva (Engl Ed)*. 2018;29(4):168–181. https://doi.org/10.1016/j.enfi.2018.03.003.
31. Chen X, Jiang J, Wang R, et al. Chest physiotherapy for pneumonia in adults. *Cochrane Database Syst Rev*. 2022;9(9):CD006338. https://doi.org/10.1002/14651858.CD006338.pub4.
32. Montes de Oca M. Smoking cessation/vaccinations. *Clin Chest Med*. 2020;41(3):495–512. https://doi.org/10.1016/j.ccm.2020.06.013.
33. Troosters T, Blondeel A, Janssens W, et al. The past, present and future of pulmonary rehabilitation. *Respirology*. 2019;24(9):830–837. https://doi.org/10.1111/resp.13517.
34. Huppert LA, Matthay MA, Ware LB. Pathogenesis of acute respiratory distress syndrome. *Semin Respir Crit Care Med*. 2019;40(1):31–39. https://doi.org/10.1055/s-0039-1683996.
35. Saguil A, Fargo MV. Acute respiratory distress syndrome: diagnosis and management. *Am Fam Physician*. 2020;101(12):730–738.
36. Meyer NJ, Gattinoni L, Calfee CS. Acute respiratory distress syndrome. *Lancet*. 2021;398(10300):622–637. https://doi.org/10.1016/S0140-6736(21)00439-6.
37. Williams GW, Berg NK, Reskallah A, et al. Acute respiratory distress syndrome. *Anesthesiology*. 2021;134(2):270–282. https://doi.org/10.1097/ALN.0000000000003571.
38. The ARDS Definition Task Force. Acute respiratory distress syndrome: the Berlin definition. *JAMA*. 2012;307(23):2526–2533. https://doi.org/10.1001/jama.2012.5669.
39. Bos LDJ, Ware LB. Acute respiratory distress syndrome: causes, pathophysiology, and phenotypes. *Lancet*. 2022;400(10358):1145–1156. https://doi.org/10.1016/S0140-6736(22)01485-4.
40. Swenson KE K, Swenson ER. Pathophysiology of acute respiratory distress syndrome and COVID-19 lung injury. *Crit Care Clin*. 2021;37(4):749–776. https://doi.org/10.1016/j.ccc.2021.05.003.
41. Matthay MA, Zemans RL, Zimmerman GA, et al. Acute respiratory distress syndrome. *Nat Rev Dis Primers*. 2019;5(1):18. https://doi.org/10.1038/s41572-019-0069-0.
42. Powers M. K. Acute respiratory distress syndrome. *JAAPA*. 2022;35(4):29–33. https://doi.org/10.1097/01.JAA.0000823164.50706.27.
43. Cortes-Puentes GA L, Oeckler RA, Marini JJ. Physiology-guided management of hemodynamics in acute respiratory distress syndrome. *Ann Transl Med*. 2018;6(18):353. https://doi.org/10.21037/atm.2018.04.40.
44. Kotas ME I, Thompson BT. Toward optimal acute respiratory distress syndrome outcomes: recognizing the syndrome and identifying its causes. *Crit Care Clin*. 2021;37(4):733–748. https://doi.org/10.1016/j.ccc.2021.05.011.

45. Matthay MA N, Thompson BT, Ware LB. The Berlin definition of acute respiratory distress syndrome: should patients receiving high-flow nasal oxygen be included? *Lancet Respir Med.* 2021;9(8):933–936. https://doi.org/10.1016/S2213-2600(21)00105-3.
46. Banavasi H, Nguyen P, Osman H, et al. Management of ARDS—what works and what does not. *Am J Med Sci.* 2021;362(1):13–23. https://doi.org/10.1016/j.amjms.2020.12.019.
47. Fan E, Del Sorbo L, Goligher EC, et al. An official American thoracic society/European society of intensive care medicine/society of critical care medicine clinical practice guideline: mechanical ventilation in adult patients with acute respiratory distress syndrome. *Am J Respir Crit Care Med.* 2017;195(9):1253–1263. https://doi.org/10.1164/rccm.201703-0548ST. [published correction appears in Am J respir crit care med. 2017 Jun 1;195(11):1540].
48. Gragossian A, Siuba MT. Acute respiratory distress syndrome. *Emerg Med Clin North Am.* 2022;40(3):459–472. https://doi.org/10.1016/j.emc.2022.05.002.
49. Vignon P, Evrard B, Asfar P, et al. Fluid administration and monitoring in ARDS: which management? *Intensive Care Med.* 2020;46(12):2252–2264. https://doi.org/10.1007/s00134-020-06310-0.
50. Quinton LJ A, Walkey AJ, Mizgerd JP. Integrative physiology of pneumonia. *Physiol Rev.* 2018;98(3):1417–1464. https://doi.org/10.1152/physrev.00032.2017.
51. Lanks CW, Musani AL, Hsia DW. Community-acquired pneumonia and hospital-acquired pneumonia. *Med Clin North Am.* 2019;103(3):487–501. https://doi.org/10.1016/j.mcna.2018.12.008.
52. Decker BK, Forrester LA, Henderson DK. Management of unique pneumonias seen in the intensive care unit. *Infect Dis Clin North Am.* 2022;36(4):825–837. https://doi.org/10.1016/j.idc.2022.07.003.
53. Rafeq R, Igneri LA. Infectious pulmonary diseases. *Emerg Med Clin North Am.* 2022;40(3):503–518. https://doi.org/10.1016/j.emc.2022.05.005.
54. Delijani K, Price MC, Little BP. Community and hospital acquired pneumonia. *Semin Roentgenol.* 2022;57(1):3–17. https://doi.org/10.1053/j.ro.2021.10.006.
55. Modi AR, Kovacs CS. Hospital-acquired and ventilator-associated pneumonia: diagnosis, management, and prevention. *Cleve Clin J Med.* 2020;87(10):633–639. https://doi.org/10.3949/ccjm.87a.19117.
56. Kalil AC, Metersky ML, Klomplas M, et al. Management of adults with hospital-acquired and ventilator-associated pneumonia: 2016 clinical practice guidelines by the Infectious Diseases Society of America and the American Thoracic Society. *Clin Infect Dis.* 2016;63(5):e61–e111. https://doi.org/10.1093/cid/ciw353.
57. Perry M. Community-acquired pneumonia in adults. *JCN.* 2022;36(3):51–55.
58. Neill S, Dean N. Aspiration pneumonia and pneumonitis: a spectrum of infectious/noninfectious diseases affecting the lung. *Curr Opin Infect Dis.* 2019;32(2):152–157. https://doi.org/10.1097/QCO.0000000000000524.
59. Luyt CE, Hékimian G, Koulenti D, et al. Microbial cause of ICU-acquired pneumonia: hospital-acquired pneumonia versus ventilator-associated pneumonia. *Curr Opin Crit Care.* 2018;24(5):332–338. https://doi.org/10.1097/MCC.0000000000000526.
60. Papazian L, Klompas M, Luyt CE. Ventilator-associated pneumonia in adults: a narrative review. *Intensive Care Med.* 2020;46(5):888–906. https://doi.org/10.1007/s00134-020-05980-0.
61. Mandell LA, Niederman MS. Aspiration pneumonia. *N Engl J Med.* 2019;380(7):651–663. https://doi.org/10.1056/NEJMra1714562.
62. Jany B, Welte T. Pleural effusion in adults-etiology, diagnosis, and treatment. *Dtsch Arztebl Int.* 2019;116(21):377–386. https://doi.org/10.3238/arztebl.2019.0377.
63. Cook AE, Garrana SH, Martínez-Jiménez S, et al. Imaging patterns of pneumonia. *Semin Roentgenol.* 2022;57(1):18–29. https://doi.org/10.1053/j.ro.2021.10.005.
64. Metlay JP, Waterer GW, Long AC, et al. Diagnosis and treatment of adults with community-acquired pneumonia. An official clinical practice guideline of the American thoracic society and infectious diseases society of America. *Am J Respir Crit Care Med.* 2019;200(7):e45–e67. https://doi.org/10.1164/rccm.201908-1581ST.
65. Lee LS, Giesler DL, Gellad WF, et al. Antibiotic therapy for adults hospitalized with community-acquired pneumonia: a systematic review. *JAMA.* 2016;315(6):593–602. https://doi.org/10.1001/jama.2016.0115.
66. Berg S, Bittner EA, Berra L, et al. Independent lung ventilation: Implementation strategies and review of literature. *World J Crit Care Med.* 2019;8(4):49–58. https://doi.org/10.5492/wjccm.v8.i4.49.
67. Glowicz JB, Landon E, Sickbert-Bennett EE, et al. SHEA/IDSA/APIC Practice Recommendation: strategies to prevent healthcare-associated infections through hand hygiene: 2022 Update. *Infect Control Hosp Epidemiol.* 2023:1–22. https://doi.org/10.1017/ice.2022.304.
68. Coppadoro A, Bellani G, Foti G. Non-pharmacological interventions to prevent ventilator-associated pneumonia: a literature review. *Respir Care.* 2019;64(12):1586–1595. https://doi.org/10.4187/respcare.07127.
69. Lee AS, Ryu JH. Aspiration pneumonia and related syndromes. *Mayo Clin Proc.* 2018;93(6):752–762. https://doi.org/10.1016/j.mayocp.2018.03.011.
70. Almirall J, Boixeda R, de la Torre MC, et al. Aspiration pneumonia: a renewed perspective and practical approach. *Respir Med.* 2021;185:106485. https://doi:10.org/1016/j.rmed.2021.106485.
71. Neill S, Dean N. Aspiration pneumonia and pneumonitis: a spectrum of infectious/noninfectious diseases affecting the lung. *Curr Opin Infect Dis.* 2019;32(2):152–157. https://doi.org/10.1097/QCO.0000000000000524.
72. Hunt EB, Sullivan A, Galvin J, et al. Gastric aspiration and its role in airway inflammation. *Open Respir Med J.* 2018 Jan 23;12:1–10. https://doi.org/10.2174/1874306401812010001.
73. Niederman MS, Cilloniz C. Aspiration pneumonia. *Rev Esp Quimioter.* 2022;35(Suppl 1):73–77. https://doi.org/10.37201/req/s01.17.2022.
74. Moore A. Aspiration pneumonia and pneumonitis. *Hosp Med Clin.* 2017;6(1):16–27. https://doi.org/10.1016/j.ehmc.2016.07.002.
75. Košutova P, Mikolka P. Aspiration syndromes and associated lung injury: Incidence, pathophysiology and management. *Physiol Res.* 2021;70(Suppl4):S567–S583. https://doi.org/10.33549/physiolres.934767.
76. Ashford A, Eastaugh-Waring T. Regurgitation and aspiration. *Anaesth Intensive Care Med.* 2021;22(10):621–624. https://doi.org/10.1016/j.mpaic.2021.07.014.
77. Son YG, Shin J, Ryu HG. Pneumonitis and pneumonia after aspiration. *J Dent Anesth Pain Med.* 2017;17(1):1–12. https://doi:10.org/17245/jdapm.2017.17.1.1.
78. Trott T, Bowman J. Diagnosis and management of pulmonary embolism. *Emerg Med Clin North Am.* 2022;40(3):565–581. https://doi.org/10.1016/j.emc.2022.05.008.
79. Jaff MR, McMurtry MS, Archer SL, et al. American heart association council on cardiopulmonary, critical care, perioperative and resuscitation; American heart association council on peripheral vascular disease; American heart association council on arteriosclerosis, thrombosis and vascular biology: management of massive and submassive pulmonary embolism, iliofemoral deep vein thrombosis, and chronic thromboembolic pulmonary hypertension: a scientific statement from the American heart association. *Circulation.* 2011;123(16):1788–1830. https://doi.org/10.1161/CIR.0b013e318214914f.
80. Freund Y, Cohen-Aubart F, Bloom B. Acute pulmonary embolism: a review. *JAMA.* 2022;328(13):1336–1345. https://doi.org/10.1001/jama.2022.16815.
81. Wenger N, Sebastian T, Engelberger RP, et al. Pulmonary embolism and deep vein thrombosis: Similar but different. *Thromb Res.* 2021;206:88–98. https://doi.org/10.1016/j.thromres.2021.08.015.
82. Francis S, Kabrhel C. Current controversies in caring for the critically ill pulmonary embolism patient. *Emerg Med Clin North Am.* 2020;38(4):931–944. https://doi.org/10.1016/j.emc.2020.06.012.
83. Baram M, Awsare B, Merli G. Pulmonary embolism in intensive care unit. *Crit Care Clin.* 2020;36(3):427–435. https://doi.org/10.1016/j.ccc.2020.02.001.
84. Roy PM, Douillet D, Penaloza A. Contemporary management of acute pulmonary embolism. *Trends Cardiovasc Med.* 2022;32(5):259–268. https://doi.org/10.1016/j.tcm.2021.06.002.
85. Giritharan D, Mora JC. The management of pulmonary embolism. *Anaesth Intensive Care Med.* 2023;24(2):115–122. https://doi.org/10.1016/j.mpaic.2022.12.001.

86. Blitzer RR, Eisenstein S. Venous thromboembolism and pulmonary embolism: strategies for prevention and management. *Surg Clin North Am.* 2021;101(5):925–938. https://doi.org/10.1016/j.suc.2021.06.015.
87. Sachdeva A, Dalton M, Lees T. Graduated compression stockings for prevention of deep vein thrombosis. *Cochrane Database Syst Rev.* 2018;11(11):CD001484. https://doi.org/10.1002/14651858.CD001484.pub4.
88. Stevens SM, Woller SC, Baumann Kreuziger L, et al. Executive summary: antithrombotic therapy for VTE disease: second update of the CHEST guideline and expert panel report. *Chest.* 2021;160(6):2247–2259. https://doi.org/10.1016/j.chest.2021.07.056.
89. Ruohoniemi DM, Sista AK. Interventional radiology therapy: Inferior vena cava filter and catheter-based therapies. *Crit Care Clin.* 2020;36(3):481–495. https://doi.org/10.1016/j.ccc.2020.02.005.
90. Ucar EY. Update on thrombolytic therapy in acute pulmonary thromboembolism. *Eurasian J Med.* 2019;51(2):186–190. https://doi.org/10.5152/eurasianjmed.2019.19291.
91. Deas DS, Keeling B. Surgical pulmonary embolectomy. *Crit Care Clin.* 2020;36(3):497–504. https://doi.org/10.1016/j.ccc.2020.02.009.
92. Long B, Lentz S, Koyfman A, Gottlieb M. Evaluation and management of the critically ill adult asthmatic in the emergency department setting. *Am J Emerg Med.* 2021;44:441–451. https://doi.org/10.1016/j.ajem.2020.03.029.
93. Long B, Rezaie SR. Evaluation and management of asthma and chronic obstructive pulmonary disease exacerbation in the emergency department. *Emerg Med Clin North Am.* 2022;40(3):539–563. https://doi.org/10.1016/j.emc.2022.05.007.
94. Kenyon N, Zeki AA, Albertson TE, Louie S. Definition of critical asthma syndromes. *Clin Rev Allergy Immunol.* 2015;48(1):1–6. https://doi.org/10.1007/s12016-013-8395-6.
95. Vatrella A, Maglio A, Pelaia C, et al. Pharmacotherapeutic strategies for critical asthma syndrome: a look at the state of the art. *Expert Opin Pharmacother.* 2020;21(12):1505–1515. https://doi.org/10.1080/14656566.2020.1766023.
96. Garner O, Ramey JS, Hanania NA. Management of life-threatening asthma: severe asthma series. *Chest.* 2022;162(4):747–756. https://doi.org/10.1016/j.chest.2022.02.029.
97. Johnston C, Nixon P. Asthma and chronic obstructive pulmonary disease in the intensive care unit. *Anaesth Intensive Care Med.* 2022;23(10):628–634. https://doi.org/10.1016/j.mpaic.2019.09.014.
98. Agnihotri NT, Saltoun C. Acute severe asthma (status asthmaticus). *Allergy Asthma Proc.* 2019;40(6):406–409. https://doi.org/10.2500/aap.2019.40.4258.
99. Carlsson JA, Bayes HK. Acute severe asthma in adults. *Medicine.* 2020;48(5):297–302.
100. Bosi A, Tonelli R, Castaniere I, et al. Acute severe asthma: management and treatment. *Minerva Med.* 2021;112(5):605–614. https://doi.org/10.23736/S0026-4806.21.07372-9.
101. Vasileiadis I, Alevrakis E, Ampelioti S, et al. Acid-base disturbances in patients with asthma: a literature review and comments on their pathophysiology. *J Clin Med.* 2019;8(4):563. https://doi.org/10.3390/jcm8040563.
102. Althoff MD, Holguin F, Yang F, et al. Noninvasive ventilation use in critically ill patients with acute asthma exacerbations. *Am J Respir Crit Care Med.* 2020;202(11):1520–1530. https://doi.org/10.1164/rccm.201910-2021OC.
103. Global Initiative for Asthma (GINA). Global Strategy for Asthma Management and Prevention (2022 Update). Available online: https://ginasthma.org/gina-reports/.
104. Kashiouris MG, Chou CD, Sedhai YR, et al. Endotracheal tube size is associated with mortality in patients with status asthmaticus. *Respir Care.* 2022;67(3):283–290. https://doi.org/10.4187/respcare.09609.
105. Likhar N, Mothe RK, Esam H, et al. The impact of severe asthma on the quality of life: a systematic review. *Value Health.* 2015;18(7):A710. https://doi.org/10.1016/j.jval.2015.09.2673.
106. Osadnik CR, Gleeson C, McDonald VM, et al. Pulmonary rehabilitation versus usual care for adults with asthma. *Cochrane Database Syst Rev.* 2022;8(8):CD013485. https://doi.org/10.1002/14651858.CD013485.pub2.
107. Tran J, Haussner W, Shah K. Traumatic pneumothorax: a review of current diagnostic practices and evolving management. *J Emerg Med.* 2021;61(5):517–528. https://doi.org/10.1016/j.jemermed.2021.07.006.
108. Hallifax R, Janssen JP. Pneumothorax-time for new guidelines? *Semin Respir Crit Care Med.* 2019;40(3):314–322. https://doi.org/10.1055/s-0039-1693499.
109. Cruz FF, Ball L, Rocco PRM, et al. Ventilator-induced lung injury during controlled ventilation in patient with acute respiratory distress syndrome: Less is probably better. *Expert Rev Respir Med.* 2018;12(5):403–414. https://doi.org/10.1080/17476348.2018.1457954.
110. Park BC, Mallemat H. Special procedures for pulmonary disease in the emergency department. *Emerg Med Clin North Am.* 2022;40(3):583–602. https://doi.org/10.1016/j.emc.2022.05.009.
111. DeMaio A, Semaan R. Management of pneumothorax. *Clin Chest Med.* 2021;42(4):729–738. https://doi.org/10.1016/j.ccm.2021.08.008.
112. Porcel JM. Chest tube drainage of the pleural space: a concise review for pulmonologists. *Tuberc Respir Dis (Seoul).* 2018;81(2):106–115. https://doi.org/10.4046/trd.2017.0107.
113. Chestovich PJ, Jennings CS, Fraser DR, et al. Too big, too small or just right? Why the 28 French chest tube is the best size. *J Surg Res.* 2020;256:338–344. https://doi.org/10.1016/j.jss.2020.06.048.
114. Béduneau G, Pham T, Schortgen F, et al. Epidemiology of weaning outcome according to a new definition. The WIND study. *Am J Respir Crit Care Med.* 2017;195(6):772–783. https://doi.org/10.1164/rccm.201602-0320OC.
115. Sahetya S, Allgood S, Gay PC, Lechtzin N. Long-term mechanical ventilation. *Clin Chest Med.* 2016;37(4):753–763. https://doi.org/10.1016/j.ccm.2016.07.014.
116. Cairo J. Weaning and discontinuation from mechanical ventilation. In: Cairo J, ed. *Pilbeam's Mechanical Ventilation, Physiological and Clinical Applications.* 8th ed. St. Louis: Elsevier; 2024.
117. Ward D, Fulbrook P. Nursing strategies for effective weaning of the critically ill mechanically ventilated patient. *Crit Care Nurs Clin North Am.* 2016;28(4):499–512. https://doi.org/10.1016/j.cnc.2016.07.008.
118. Borges LGA, Savi A, Teixeira C, et al. Mechanical ventilation weaning protocol improves medical adherence and results. *J Crit Care.* 2017;41:296–302. https://doi.org/10.1016/j.jcrc.2017.07.014.

19

Pulmonary Therapeutic Management

Kathleen M. Stacy

http://evolve.elsevier.com/Urden/CriticalCareNursing

OXYGEN THERAPY

Normal cellular function depends on the delivery of an adequate supply of oxygen to the cells to meet their metabolic needs. The goal of oxygen therapy is to provide a sufficient concentration of inspired oxygen to permit full use of the oxygen-carrying capacity of the arterial blood; this ensures adequate cellular oxygenation, provided that the cardiac output and hemoglobin concentration are adequate.[1,2]

Principles of Therapy

Oxygen is an atmospheric gas that must also be considered a medication because, similar to most other medications, it has detrimental as well as beneficial effects. Oxygen is one of the most commonly used and misused medications. As a medication, oxygen must be administered for a good reason and in a proper, safe manner.[1] Oxygen is usually ordered in liters per minute (L/min), as a concentration of oxygen expressed as a percentage (e.g., 40%), or as a fraction of inspired oxygen (FiO_2; e.g., 0.4).

Indications

The primary indication for oxygen therapy is hypoxemia.[3] The amount of oxygen administered depends on the pathophysiologic mechanisms affecting the patient's oxygenation status. The current clinical practice guidelines from the American Association for Respiratory Care recommend maintaining an SpO_2:[4]

- 94% to 98% for acutely and critically ill adults
- 88% to 92% for critically ill adults with CO_2 retention and/or COPD
- 88% to 93% for critically ill patients requiring FiO_2 of 0.70 or higher who are not invasively ventilated with a high positive end-expiratory pressure (PEEP) strategy

The concentration of oxygen given to an individual patient is a clinical judgment based on the many factors that influence oxygen transport, such as hemoglobin concentration, cardiac output, and arterial oxygen tension.

Monitoring

After oxygen therapy has begun, the patient is continuously assessed for level of oxygenation and the factors affecting it. The patient's oxygenation status is evaluated several times daily until the desired oxygen level has been reached and has stabilized. If the desired response to the amount of oxygen delivered is not achieved, the oxygen supplementation is adjusted and the patient's condition is reevaluated. It is important to use this dose-response method so that the lowest possible level of oxygen is administered that will still achieve a satisfactory PaO_2 or SaO_2.[2,3]

Methods of Delivery

Oxygen therapy can be delivered by many different devices (Table 19.1). Common problems with these devices include system leaks and obstructions, device displacement, and skin irritation. These devices are classified as low-flow, reservoir, or high-flow systems.[3]

Low-Flow Systems

A low-flow oxygen delivery system provides supplemental oxygen directly into the patient's airway at a flow of 8 L/min or less. Because this flow is insufficient to meet the patient's inspiratory volume requirements, this method of oxygen delivery results in a variable FiO_2 as the supplemental oxygen is mixed with room air. The patient's ventilatory pattern affects the FiO_2 of a low-flow system: As this pattern changes, differing amounts of room air gas are mixed with the constant flow of oxygen. A nasal cannula is an example of a low-flow device.[3]

Reservoir Systems

A reservoir system incorporates some type of device to collect and store oxygen between breaths. When the patient's inspiratory flow exceeds the oxygen flow of the oxygen delivery system, the patient can draw from the reservoir of oxygen to meet their inspiratory volume needs. Less mixing of the inspired oxygen occurs with room air than in a low-flow system. A reservoir oxygen delivery system can deliver a higher FiO_2 than a low-flow system. Examples of reservoir systems are simple face masks, partial rebreathing masks, and nonrebreathing masks.[3]

High-Flow Systems

With a high-flow system, the oxygen flows out of the device and into the patient's airways in an amount sufficient to meet all inspiratory volume requirements. This type of system is not affected by the patient's ventilatory pattern. A high-flow system uses either an air-entrainment system or a blending system to mix air and oxygen to achieve the desired FiO_2. An air-entrainment mask is an example of a high-flow system that delivers precisely controlled oxygen at the lower FiO_2 range.[3]

High-flow nasal cannula. One newer high-flow system is the high-flow nasal cannula (HFNC) (Fig 19.1). With this system, warmed and humidified oxygen is delivered to the patient via a nasal cannula using a blending system. This system has been shown to improve oxygenation and ventilation and decrease the

TABLE 19.1 Oxygen Therapy Systems

Category	Device	Flow	FiO_2 Range (%)	FiO_2 Stability	Advantages	Disadvantages	Best Use
Low-flow	Nasal cannula	0.25–8 L/min (adults) ≤2 L/min (infants)	22–45	Variable	Use on adults, children, infants; easy to apply; disposable, low cost; well tolerated	Unstable, easily dislodged; high flows uncomfortable; can cause dryness or bleeding; polyps, deviated septum may block flow	Stable patient needing low FiO_2; home care patient requiring long-term therapy
	Nasal catheter	0.25–8 L/min	22–45	Variable	Use on adults, children, infants; good stability; disposable, low cost	Difficult to insert; high flows increase back-pressure; needs regular changing; polyps, deviated septum may block insertion; may provoke gagging, air swallowing, aspiration	Procedures in which cannula is difficult to use (bronchoscopy); long-term care for infants
	Transtracheal catheter	0.25–4 L/min	22–35	Variable	Lower oxygen usage/cost; eliminates nasal/skin irritation; improved compliance; increased exercise tolerance; increased mobility; enhanced image	High cost; surgical complications; infection; mucus plugging; lost tract	Home care or ambulatory patients who need increased mobility or who do not accept nasal oxygen
Reservoir	Reservoir cannula	0.25–4 L/min	22–35	Variable	Lower oxygen usage/cost; increased mobility; less discomfort because of lower flows	Unattractive, cumbersome; poor compliance; must be regularly replaced; breathing pattern affects performance	Home care or ambulatory patients who need increased mobility
	Simple mask	5–12 L/min	35–50	Variable	Use on adults, children, infants; quick, easy to apply; disposable, inexpensive	Uncomfortable; must be removed for eating; prevents radiant heat loss; blocks vomitus in unconscious patients	Emergencies; short-term therapy requiring moderate $_2$2
	Partial rebreathing mask	6–10 L/min (prevent bag collapse on inspiration)	35–60	Variable	Same as simple mask; moderate to high FiO_2	Same as simple mask; potential suffocation hazard	Emergencies; short-term therapy requiring moderate to high FiO_2
	Nonrebreathing mask	6–10 L/min (prevent bag collapse on inspiration)	55–70	Variable	Same as simple mask; high FiO_2	Same as simple mask; potential suffocation hazard	Emergencies; short-term therapy requiring high FiO_2
	Nonrebreathing circuit (closed)	3× Ve (prevent bag collapse on inspiration)	21–100	Fixed	Full range of FiO_2	Potential suffocation hazard; requires 50 psi air or oxygen; blender failure common	Patients requiring precise FiO_2 at any level (21%–100%)
High-flow	Air-entrainment mask	Varies; should provide output flow >60 L/min	24–50	Fixed	Easy to apply; disposable, inexpensive; stable, precise FiO_2	Limited to adult use; uncomfortable, noisy; must be removed for eating; FiO_2 >0.40 not ensured; FiO_2 varies with back-pressure	Unstable patients requiring precise low FiO_2
	Air-entrainment nebulizer	10–15 L/min input; should provide output flow of at least 60 L/min	28–100	Fixed	Provides temperature control and extra humidification	FiO2 <28% or >0.40 not ensured; FiO_2 varies with back-pressure; high infection risk	Patients with artificial airways requiring low to moderate FiO_2
	Blending system (open)	Should provide output flow of at least 60 L/min	21–100	Fixed	Full range of FiO_2	Requires 50 psi air + oxygen; blender failure or inaccuracy common	Patient with high Ve who needs high FiO_2
	High-flow cannula system	Up to 40 L/min (depending on system)	35–90	Variable or fixed depending on system and input flow	Wide range of FiO_2 and relative or absolute humidity; use on adults, children, infants	FiO_2not ensured depending on input flow and patient breathing pattern; infection risk	Patients of all ages with high or variable Ve who need supplemental oxygen, positive pressure, or humidity

FiO_2, Fraction of inspired oxygen; Ve, minute volume.

Modified from Kacmarek RM, Stoller JK, Heuer AJ, eds. *Egan's Fundamentals of Respiratory Care.* 12th ed. Elsevier; 2021.

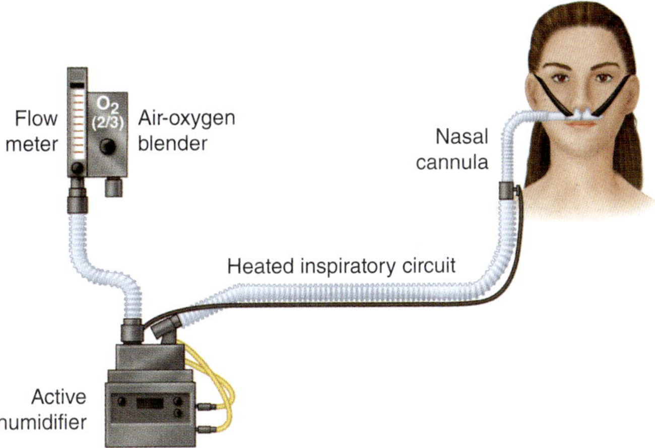

FIG. 19.1 High-Flow Oxygen Delivery System. (From Ignatavicius DD, Workman ML, Rebar C, Heimgartner M, eds. *Medical-Surgical Nursing: Concepts for Interprofessional Collaborative Care.* 10th ed. Elsevier; 2021.)

work of breathing in a patient with acute respiratory failure. A high-flow nasal cannula also is more comfortable and better tolerated than similar therapies.[5]

Complications of Oxygen Therapy

Oxygen, like most medications, has adverse effects and complications resulting from its use. The adage "If a little is good, a lot is better" does not apply to oxygen. The lung is designed to handle a concentration of 21% oxygen, with some adaptability to higher concentrations, but adverse effects and oxygen toxicity can result if a high concentration is administered for too long.[5]

Oxygen Toxicity

The most detrimental effect of breathing a high concentration of oxygen is the development of oxygen toxicity. Oxygen toxicity can occur in any patient who breathes oxygen concentrations of greater than 50% for longer than 24 hours. Oxygen toxicity is most likely to develop in patients who require intubation, mechanical ventilation, and high oxygen concentrations for extended periods.[3]

Hyperoxia, or the administration of higher-than-normal oxygen concentrations, produces an overabundance of oxygen free radicals. These radicals are responsible for the initial damage to the alveolar–capillary membrane. Oxygen-free radicals are toxic metabolites of oxygen metabolism. Normally, enzymes neutralize the radicals, preventing any damage from occurring. During the administration of high levels of oxygen, the large number of oxygen-free radicals produced exhausts the supply of neutralizing enzymes. Damage to the lung parenchyma and vasculature occurs, resulting in the initiation of acute respiratory distress syndrome (ARDS).[2,6]

Many clinical manifestations are associated with oxygen toxicity. The first symptom is substernal chest pain that is exacerbated by deep breathing. A dry cough and tracheal irritation follow. Eventually, definite pleuritic pain occurs on inhalation, followed by dyspnea. Upper airway changes may include a sensation of nasal stuffiness, sore throat, and increased pressure sensation in the ears. Chest radiographs and pulmonary function tests show no abnormalities until symptoms are severe. Complete, rapid reversal of these symptoms occurs as soon as normal oxygen concentrations are restored.[6]

Carbon Dioxide Retention

In patients with severe chronic obstructive pulmonary disease (COPD), carbon dioxide (CO_2) retention may occur as a result of administration of oxygen in high concentrations. Numerous theories have been proposed for this phenomenon. One states that the normal stimulus to breathe (i.e., increasing CO_2 levels) is muted in patients with COPD and that decreasing oxygen levels become the stimulus to breathe. If hypoxemia is corrected by the administration of oxygen, the stimulus to breathe is abolished; hypoventilation develops, resulting in a further increase in the arterial partial pressure of carbon dioxide ($PaCO_2$).[2,3] Another theory is that the administration of oxygen abolishes the compensatory response of hypoxic pulmonary vasoconstriction. This results in an increase in perfusion of underventilated alveoli and the development of dead space, producing ventilation/perfusion ($\dot{V}/\dot{Q}$) mismatch. As alveolar dead space increases, so does CO_2 retention.[2,3] One further theory states that the increase in CO_2 is related to the ratio of deoxygenated to oxygenated hemoglobin (Haldane effect). Deoxygenated hemoglobin carries more CO_2 compared with oxygenated hemoglobin. Administration of oxygen increases the proportion of oxygenated hemoglobin, which causes increased release of CO_2 at the lung level.[6] Because of the risk of CO_2 accumulation, all patients who are chronically hypercapnic require careful low-flow oxygen administration.[3]

Absorption Atelectasis

Another adverse effect of high concentrations of oxygen is absorption atelectasis. Breathing high concentrations of oxygen washes out the nitrogen that normally fills the alveoli and helps hold them open (residual volume). As oxygen replaces the nitrogen in the alveoli, the alveoli start to shrink and collapse. This occurs because oxygen is absorbed into the bloodstream faster than it can be replaced in the alveoli, particularly in areas of the lungs that are minimally ventilated.[3]

Nursing Management

Nursing management of the patient receiving oxygen focus on (1) ensuring the oxygen is being administered as ordered and (2) observing for complications of the therapy. Confirming that the oxygen therapy device is properly positioned and replacing it after removal is important. During meals, an oxygen mask is changed to a nasal cannula if the patient can tolerate one. A patient receiving oxygen therapy is also transported with the oxygen. In addition, oxygen saturation is periodically monitored using a pulse oximeter.

ARTIFICIAL AIRWAYS

Pharyngeal Airways

Pharyngeal airways are used to maintain airway patency by keeping the tongue from obstructing the upper airway. The two types of pharyngeal airways are oropharyngeal and nasopharyngeal airways. Complications of these airways include trauma to the oral or nasal cavity, obstruction of the airway, laryngospasm, gagging, and vomiting.[7]

Oropharyngeal Airway

An oropharyngeal airway is made of plastic and is available in various sizes. The proper size is selected by holding the airway against the side of the patient's face and ensuring that it extends from the corner of the mouth to the angle of the jaw. If the airway is improperly sized, it will occlude the airway. An oral airway is placed by inserting a tongue depressor into the patient's mouth to displace the tongue downward and then passing the airway into the patient's mouth, slipping it over the patient's tongue (Fig. 19.2) When properly placed, the tip of the airway lies above the epiglottis at the base of the tongue. An oropharyngeal airway is used only in an unconscious patient who has an absent or diminished gag reflex.[7]

Nasopharyngeal Airway

A nasopharyngeal airway is usually made of plastic or rubber and is available in various sizes. The proper size is selected by holding the airway against the side of the patient's face and ensuring that the nasopharyngeal airway extends from the tip of the nose to the ear lobe. A nasal airway is placed by lubricating the tube and inserting it midline along the floor of the naris into the posterior pharynx. When properly placed, the tip of the airway lies above the epiglottis at the base of the tongue.[7]

Endotracheal Tubes

An endotracheal tube (ETT) is the most used artificial airway for providing short-term airway management. Indications for endotracheal intubation include maintenance of airway patency, protection of the airway from aspiration, application of positive-pressure ventilation, facilitation of pulmonary hygiene, and use of high oxygen concentrations.[8] An ETT may be placed through the orotracheal route via direct laryngoscopy, video laryngoscopy, or flexible fiberoptic bronchoscopy or the nasotracheal route via blind nasal intubation, direct laryngoscopy, video laryngoscopy or flexible fiberoptic bronchoscopy.[9] In most situations involving emergency placement, the orotracheal route is used, because this route is simpler and allows the use of a larger diameter ETT. Nasotracheal intubation provides greater patient comfort over time and is preferred in patients with a jaw fracture.[8] The advantages of orotracheal and nasotracheal intubation are presented in Table 19.2.

ETTs are available in various sizes, which are based on the inner diameters of the tubes and have a radiopaque marker that runs the length of the tube. On one end of the tube is a cuff that is inflated with the use of the pilot balloon. Because of the high incidence of cuff-related problems, low-pressure, high-volume cuffs are preferred. On the other end of the tube is a 15-mm adapter that facilitates connection of the tube to a manual resuscitation bag (MRB), T-tube, or ventilator (Fig. 19.3).[9,10]

Rapid Sequence Intubation

Rapid sequence intubation (RSI) is a seven-step process that is often used to intubate a critically ill patient. This method is considered safer for the patient because it decreases the risk of aspiration.[11-14]

Step 1: preparation. Before intubation, the necessary equipment is gathered and organized to facilitate the procedure. Readily available equipment includes a suction system with catheters and tonsil suction, an MRB with a mask connected to 100% oxygen, a laryngoscope handle with assorted blades, ETTs in various sizes, and a stylet or introducer. Before the procedure is started, all equipment is inspected to ensure that the equipment is in working order.[11-14] The patient is prepared for the procedure, if possible, with an intravenous catheter in place and monitored with a pulse oximeter.[12,14] Ideally end-tidal carbon dioxide ($EtCO_2$) should also be used during the procedure;[14] however, this type of monitoring may not be available during an emergent intubation. Consideration should be given to initiating airborne precautions depending on the patient's condition and the presence of endemic diseases.[12]

Step 2: preoxygenation. Once everything is ready, the patient is preoxygenated with 100% oxygen for 3 to 5 minutes via a tight-fitting face mask, MRB, HFNC, or noninvasive ventilation (NIV). If the patient is at high risk for aspiration, they should be carefully ventilated with the MRB as to avoid gastric insufflation that increases the chances of gastric distention and the risk of aspiration.[11-14]

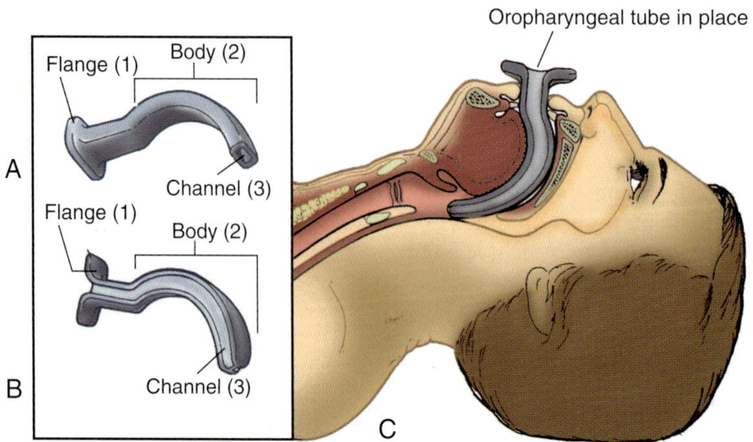

FIG. 19.2 Oropharyngeal Airways. (A) Guedel airway. (B) Berman airway. (C) Airway in place. (From Kacmarek RM, Stoller JK, Heuer AJ, eds. *Egan's Fundamentals of Respiratory Care.* 12th ed. Elsevier, 2021.)

TABLE 19.2 Advantages of Orotracheal, Nasotracheal, and Tracheostomy Tubes

Orotracheal Tubes	Nasotracheal Tubes	Tracheostomy Tubes

• Easier access
• Avoids nasal and sinus complications
• Allows for larger diameter tube, which facilitates:
  • Work of breathing
  • Suctioning
  • Fiberoptic bronchoscopy
	• Easily secured and stabilized
	• Reduces risk of unintentional extubation
	• Well tolerated by patient
	• Enables swallowing and oral hygiene
	• Facilitates communication
	• Avoids need for bite block
		• Easily secured and stabilized
		• Reduces risk of unintentional decannulation
		• Well tolerated by patient
		• Enables swallowing, speech, and oral hygiene
		• Avoids upper airway complications
		• Allows for larger diameter tube, which facilitates:
		  • Work of breathing
		  • Suctioning
		  • Fiberoptic bronchoscopy

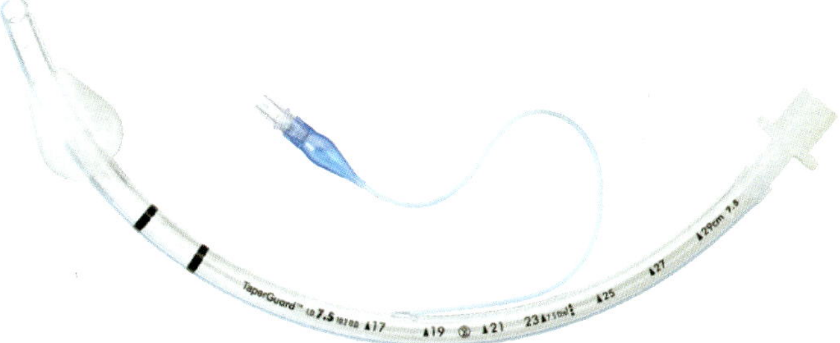

FIG. 19.3 Endotracheal Tube. (©2024 Medtronic. All rights reserved. Used with the permission of Medtronic.)

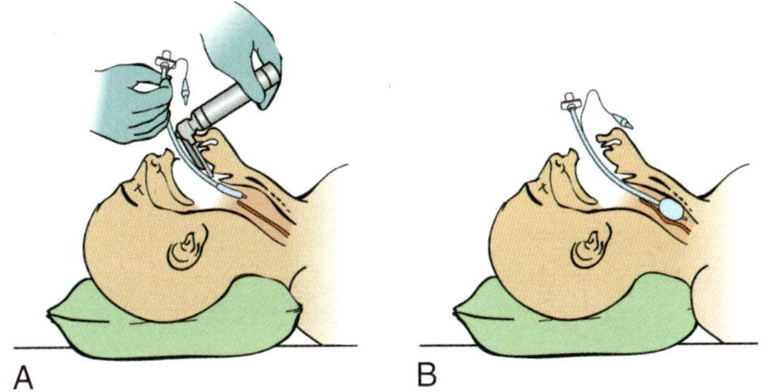

FIG. 19.4 Insertion of Tube With Laryngoscope in Place. (A) Insert tube with the tip initially against the right buccal mucosa so that a clear view of the vocal cords can be always maintained. As it advances, watch the tube pass through the cord. (B) Tube is correctly placed when the tip is 2 to 3 cm beyond the vocal cords. (From Fowler GC, ed. *Pfenninger and Fowler's Procedures for Primary Care.* 4th ed. Elsevier; 2020.)

Step 3: pretreatment. While the patient is being preoxygenated, the patient is pretreated with adjunct medications to decrease the physiologic response to intubation. These medications include atropine, fentanyl, and atropine. A very low dose of a paralytic agent may be administered to prevent fasciculations. The use of these medications depends on the patient's underlying condition. If possible, pretreatment occurs 3 minutes before the next step.[12–14]

Step 4: paralysis with induction. A sedative agent and a paralytic agent are administered in "rapid sequence" to achieve induction and paralysis. Various sedative agents, including etomidate, midazolam, ketamine, and propofol, are used to facilitate rapid loss of consciousness. Induction dosages for these medications are usually slightly higher than the typical dosages used for sedation. The two most commonly administered neuromuscular blocking agents used to facilitate skeletal muscle relaxation are succinylcholine and rocuronium.[11–14]

Step 5: protection and positioning. The procedure is initiated by positioning the patient with the neck flexed and head slightly extended in the "sniff" position.[11–13] Patients who are obese may be positioned in the "ramp" position.[11,12,14] To place the patient in this position, the head of the bed is elevated 25 degrees and the patient's head is positioned at the top of the mattress, so the face is horizontal to the floor.[11] The goal is to achieve horizontal alignment of the external auditory meatus with sternal notch.[14] The oral cavity and pharynx are suctioned, and any dental devices are removed.

Step 6: placement of endotracheal tube. The ETT is inserted into the trachea (Fig. 19.4), and placement is confirmed.[12,13] Each intubation attempt is limited to 30 seconds to prevent hypoxemia. After the ETT is inserted, the patient is assessed for bilateral breath sounds and chest movement. The absence of breath sounds is indicative of esophageal intubation, whereas breath sounds heard over only one side of the chest is indicative of a mainstem intubation. A disposable end-tidal CO_2 detector (Fig. 19.5) is used to initially verify correct airway placement, after which the cuff of the tube is inflated, and the tube is secured. Finally, a chest radiograph is obtained to confirm placement. The tip of the ETT should be approximately 3 to 4 cm above the carina when the patient's head is in the neutral position.[8]

Step 7: postintubation management. After final adjustment of the ETT position is complete, the level of insertion (marked in centimeters on the side of the tube) at the teeth is noted. The ETT is then secured to the patient's face using tape or a commercial tube holder (Fig. 19.6). Securing the tube stabilizes it to prevent movement and potential dislodgment.[8]

Complications

Numerous complications can occur during the intubation procedure, including nasal and oral trauma, pharyngeal and hypopharyngeal trauma, vomiting with aspiration, and cardiac arrest.[15] Tracheal rupture is a rare and often fatal complication that is associated with emergent intubation.[16] Hypoxemia and hypercapnia can also occur, resulting in bradycardia, tachycardia, dysrhythmias, hypertension, and hypotension.[8,15]

Several complications can occur while the ETT is in place, including nasal and oral inflammation and ulceration, sinusitis and otitis, laryngeal and tracheal injuries, and tube obstruction and displacement. Other complications can occur days to weeks after the ETT is removed, including laryngeal and tracheal stenosis and a cricoid abscess (Box 19.1). Delayed complications usually require some form of surgical intervention.[17,18]

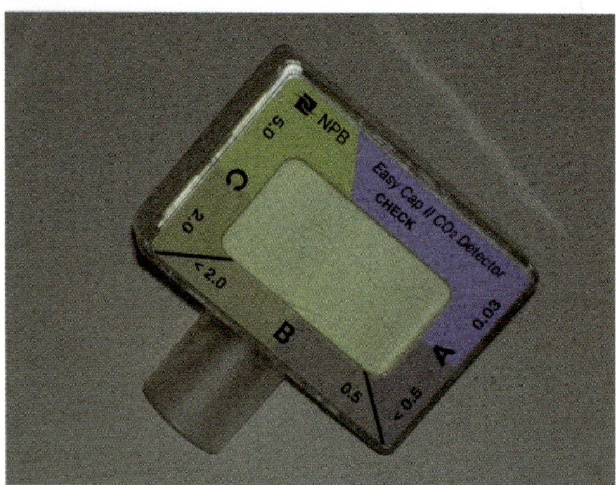

FIG. 19.5 Carbon Dioxide Detector. Disposable colorimetric CO_2 detector for confirming tracheal intubation. (From Kacmarek RM, Stoller JK, Heuer AJ, eds. *Egan's Fundamentals of Respiratory Care*. 12th ed. Elsevier; 2021.)

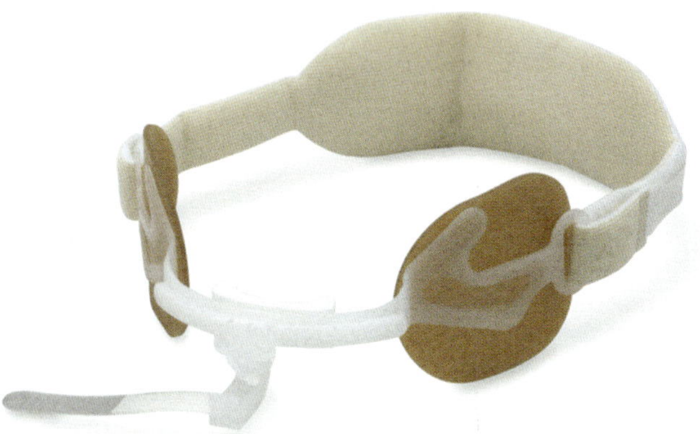

FIG. 19.6 Commercial Tube Holder. Anchor Fast oral endotracheal tube fastener. (Courtesy Hollister Incorporated, Libertyville, IL.)

Tracheostomy Tubes

A tracheostomy tube is the preferred method of airway maintenance in a patient who requires long-term intubation. Although no ideal time to perform the procedure has been identified, it is commonly accepted that if a patient has been intubated or is anticipated to be intubated for longer than 7 days, a tracheostomy should be performed.[19] A tracheostomy is also indicated in several other situations such as the presence of an upper airway obstruction secondary to trauma, tumors, or swelling and the need to facilitate airway clearance secondary to spinal cord injury, neuromuscular disease, or severe debilitation.[20,21]

A tracheostomy tube provides the best route for long-term airway maintenance, because this route avoids the oral, nasal, pharyngeal, and laryngeal complications associated with an ETT. The tube is shorter, has a wider diameter, and is less curved than an ETT; the resistance to airflow is less; and breathing is easier. Additional advantages of a tracheostomy tube include ease with secretion removal, increased patient acceptance and comfort, capability of the patient to eat and talk if possible, and easier ventilator weaning.[8,20] See Table 19.2 for a list of the advantages of a tracheostomy tube.

Tracheostomy tubes are made of plastic or metal and may have one or two lumens. Single-lumen tubes consist of the tube; a built-in cuff, which is connected to a pilot balloon for inflation purposes; and an obturator, which is used during tube insertion. Double-lumen tubes consist of the tube with the attached cuff, the obturator, and an inner cannula that can be removed for cleaning and then reinserted or, if disposable, replaced by a new sterile inner cannula. The inner cannula can be removed quickly if the cannula becomes obstructed, making the system safer for patients with significant secretion problems. Single-lumen tubes provide a larger internal diameter for airflow, so airflow resistance is reduced, and the patient can ventilate through the tube with greater ease. Plastic tracheostomy tubes also have a 15-mm adapter on the end (Fig. 19.7).[20,21]

Tracheostomy Procedure

A tracheostomy tube is inserted by an open procedure or a percutaneous procedure. An open procedure is usually performed in the operating room, whereas a percutaneous procedure can be done at the patient's bedside.[21,22]

Complications

Numerous complications can occur during the tracheostomy procedure, including misplacement of the tracheal tube, hemorrhage, laryngeal nerve injury, pneumothorax, pneumomediastinum, and cardiac arrest.[17,20,23] Several complications can occur while the tracheostomy tube is in place, including stomal infection, hemorrhage, tracheomalacia, tracheoesophageal fistula, tracheoinnominate artery fistula, and tube obstruction and displacement.[20,23] Many complications can occur days to weeks after the tracheostomy tube is removed, including tracheal stenosis and tracheocutaneous fistula (Box 19.2). Delayed complications usually require some form of surgical intervention.[23]

Nursing Management

Nursing management of a patient with an endotracheal or tracheostomy tube requires some additional measures to address the effects associated with tube placement on the respiratory and other body systems. Nursing interventions for the patient with an artificial airway focus on providing humidification, managing the cuff, suctioning, establishing a method of communication, and providing oral hygiene. Because the tube bypasses the upper airway system, warming and humidifying the air must be performed by external means. Because the cuff of the tube can cause damage to the walls of the trachea, proper cuff inflation and management are imperative. In addition, the normal defense mechanisms are impaired, and secretions may accumulate; thus suctioning may be needed to promote secretion clearance. Because the tube does not allow airflow over the vocal cords, developing a method of communication is also very important. Last, observing the patient to ensure proper placement of the tube and patency of the airway is essential. Patient safety interventions for the patient with an artificial airway are discussed in Box 19.3.

One study examined patients' perception of ETT-related discomforts. Of the patients, 46% reported remembering having the ETT while in the critical care unit. Most of these patients found the discomfort associated with the ETT and the inability to speak very stressful. In addition, some patients continued to have problems with hoarseness, sore throat, and voice changes days to months later.[24]

Humidification

Humidification of air normally is performed by the mucosal layer of the upper respiratory tract. When this area is bypassed, as occurs with ETT and tracheostomy tubes or when supplemental

BOX 19.1 Safety

Complications of Endotracheal Tubes

Complications	Causes	Prevention and Treatment
Tube obstruction	Patient biting tube Tube kinking during repositioning Cuff herniation Dried secretions, blood, or lubricant Tissue from tumor Trauma Foreign body	**Prevention:** Place bite block. Sedate patient PRN. Suction PRN. Humidify inspired gases. **Treatment:** Replace tube.
Tube displacement	Movement of patient's head Movement of tube by patient's tongue Traction on tube from ventilator tubing Self-extubation	**Prevention:** Secure tube to upper lip. Sedate patient PRN. Ensure that only 2 inches of tube extend beyond lip. Support ventilator tubing. **Treatment:** Replace tube.
Sinusitis and nasal injury	Obstruction of paranasal sinus drainage Pressure necrosis of nares	**Prevention:** Avoid nasal intubations. Cushion nares from tube and tape or ties. **Treatment:** Remove all tubes from nasal passages. Administer antibiotics.
Tracheoesophageal fistula	Pressure necrosis of posterior tracheal wall, resulting from overinflated cuff and rigid nasogastric tube	**Prevention:** Inflate cuff with minimal amount of air necessary. Monitor cuff pressures every 8 hours. **Treatment:** Position cuff of tube distal to fistula. Place gastrostomy tube for enteral feedings. Place esophageal tube for secretion clearance proximal to fistula.
Mucosal lesions	Pressure at tube and mucosal interface	**Prevention:** Inflate cuff with minimal amount of air necessary. Monitor cuff pressures every 8 hours. Use appropriate size tube. **Treatment:** May resolve spontaneously. Perform surgical intervention.
Laryngeal or tracheal stenosis	Injury to area from end of tube or cuff, resulting in scar tissue formation and narrowing of airway	**Prevention:** Inflate cuff with minimal amount of air necessary. Monitor cuff pressures every 8 hours. Suction area above cuff frequently. **Treatment:** Perform tracheostomy. Place laryngeal stent. Perform surgical repair.
Cricoid abscess	Mucosal injury with bacterial invasion	**Prevention:** Inflate cuff with minimal amount of air necessary. Monitor cuff pressures every 8 hours. Suction area above cuff frequently. **Treatment:** Perform incision and drainage of area. Administer antibiotics.

PRN, As needed.

oxygen is used, humidification by external means is necessary. Various humidification devices add water to inhaled gas to prevent drying and irritation of the respiratory tract, to prevent undue loss of body water, and to facilitate secretion removal.[25,26] The humidification device provides inspired gas conditioned (heated) to body temperature and saturated with water vapor.[27]

Cuff Management

Because the cuff of the ETT or tracheostomy tube is a major source of the complications associated with artificial airways, proper cuff management is essential. To prevent the complications associated with cuff design, only low-pressure, high-volume cuffed tubes are used in clinical practice.[8–10] Even with these tubes, cuff pressures can be generated that are high enough to lead to tracheal ischemia and injury. Proper cuff inflation techniques and cuff pressure monitoring are critical components of the care of a patient with an artificial airway.[8]

Cuff pressure monitoring. Cuff pressures are monitored at a minimum of every shift with a cuff pressure manometer (Fig. 19.8). Cuff pressures are maintained within 20 to 30 cm H_2O because greater pressures decrease blood flow to the capillaries in the tracheal wall and lesser pressures increase the risk of aspiration. Pressures greater than 30 cm H_2O should be reported to the practitioner. Cuffs are not routinely deflated, because this increases the risk of aspiration.[8]

Foam cuff tracheostomy tubes. One tracheostomy tube on the market has a cuff made of foam that is self-inflating (Fig. 19.9). The cuff is deflated during insertion, after which the pilot port is opened to atmospheric pressure (room air) and the cuff self-inflates. After inflation, the foam cuff conforms to the size and shape of the patient's trachea, reducing the pressure against the tracheal wall. The pilot port can be left open to atmospheric pressure or attached to the mechanical ventilator tubing, allowing the cuff to inflate and deflate with the cycling of the ventilator. Routine maintenance of a foam cuff tracheostomy tube includes aspirating the pilot port every 8 hours to measure cuff volume, to remove any condensation from the cuff area, and to assess the integrity of the cuff. Removal is accomplished by deflating the cuff; this can be complicated if the plastic sheath covering the foam is perforated. If perforation occurs, the foam may not be deflatable, because the air cannot be totally aspirated.[23]

Subglottic secretion removal. The cuff has also been implicated in the development of ventilator-associated pneumonia (VAP). Fluids can leak around the cuff into the airway, resulting in microaspiration. Bacteria-laden oral secretions trickle down

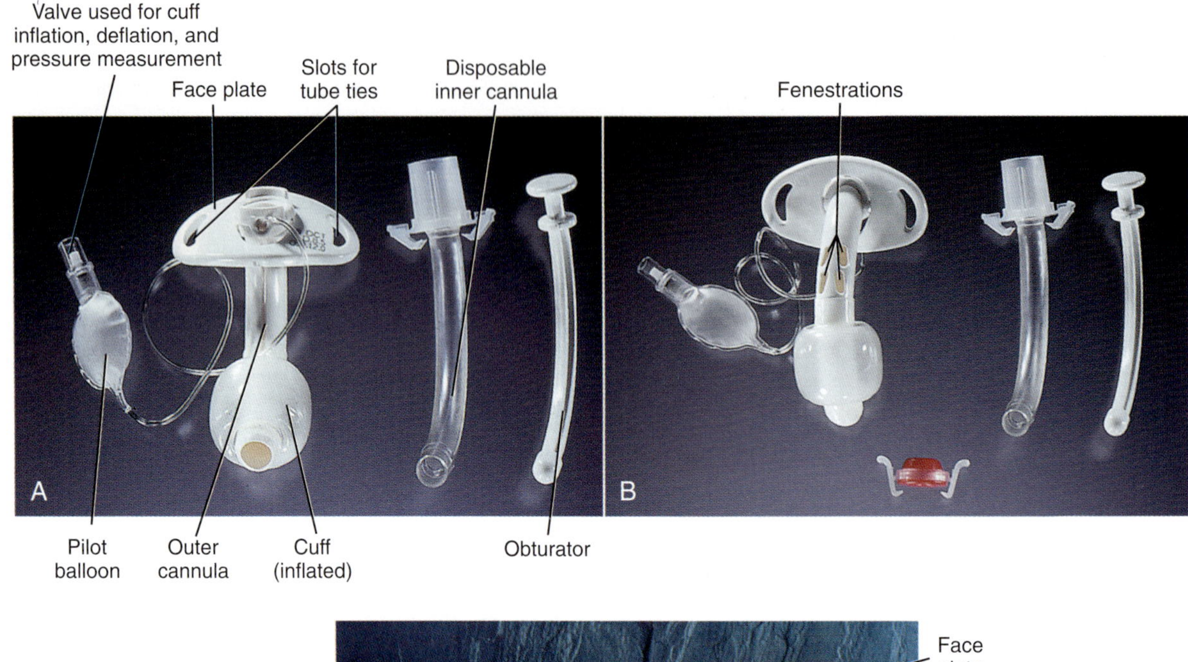

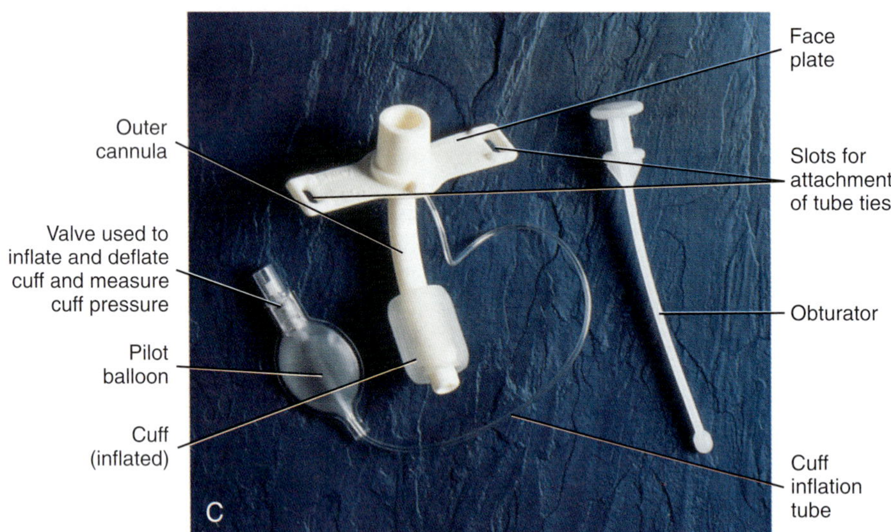

FIG. 19.7 Tracheostomy Tubes. (A) Dual-lumen cuffed tracheostomy tube with disposable inner cannula. (B) Dual-lumen cuffed fenestrated tracheostomy tube. (C) Single-lumen cannula cuffed tracheostomy tube. (From Ignatavicius DD, Workman ML, Rebar C, Heimgartner M, eds. *Medical-Surgical Nursing: Concepts for Interprofessional Collaborative Care.* 10th ed. Elsevier; 2021.)

the larynx and pool above the cuff of the artificial airway. These secretions are referred to as *subglottic secretions.* Subglottic secretions can then leak into the lower airways around the cuff via the longitudinal folds that form in the cuff as it accommodates to the shape of the airway, when an underinflated cuff fails to form a proper seal in the airway, or in the event of inadvertent movement of the ETT within the airway. The use of established cuff inflation techniques, monitoring of cuff pressures, using an appropriate method of tube stabilization, and oral hygiene are important interventions for preventing this problem.[28]

Deep oropharyngeal suctioning to remove subglottic secretions with routine oral care has been suggested as an intervention to decrease microaspiration of the secretions and potentially decrease the incidence of VAP. However, there is very little evidence to support this intervention.[29]

Specialized tubes are available to allow for the continuous removal of subglottic secretions. These tubes have an additional lumen, with an opening above the cuff, which is connected to continuous (−20 to −30 cm H_2O) suction (Fig. 19.10).[30] These tubes are recommended for patients who are expected to be intubated for longer than 48 to 72 hours.[31] One issue with these tubes is that the aspiration lumen can become clogged, and a small amount of air needs to be injected into the aspiration port every few hours.[30]

Suctioning

Suctioning is often required to maintain a patent airway in a patient with an ETT or tracheostomy tube. Suctioning is a sterile procedure that is performed only when the patient needs it and not on a routine schedule.[32] Indications for suctioning include the presence of coarse crackles over the trachea on auscultation, visible secretions in the airway, and a sawtooth pattern on the flow-volume loop on the ventilator monitor.[32]

Types of suction catheters. There are two different methods for suctioning based on the type of catheter. The open suction method requires disconnecting the patient from the ventilator

 BOX 19.2 **Safety**

Complications of Tracheostomy Tubes

Complications	Causes	Prevention and Treatment
Hemorrhage	Vessel opening after surgery Vessel erosion caused by tube	**Prevention:** Use appropriate size tube. Treat local infection. Suction gently. Humidify inspired gases. Position tracheal window not lower than third tracheal ring. **Treatment:** Pack lightly. Perform surgical intervention.
Wound infection	Colonization of stoma with hospital flora	**Prevention:** Perform routine stoma care. **Treatment:** Remove tube, if necessary. Perform aggressive wound care and débridement. Administer antibiotics.
Subcutaneous emphysema	Positive-pressure ventilation Coughing against tight, occlusive dressing or sutured or packed wound	**Prevention:** Avoid suturing or packing wound closed around tube. **Treatment:** Remove any sutures or packing, if present.
Tube obstruction	Dried blood or secretions False passage into soft tissues Opening of cannula positioned against tracheal wall Foreign body Tissue from tumor	**Prevention:** Suction PRN. Humidify inspired gases. Use tube with removable inner cannula. Position tube so that opening does not press against tracheal wall. **Treatment:** Remove or replace inner cannula. Replace tube.
Tube displacement	Patient movement Coughing Traction on ventilatory tubing	**Prevention:** Use commercial tube holder. Use tubes with adjustable neck plates for patients with short necks. Support ventilatory tubing. Sedate patient PRN. Restrain patient PRN. **Treatment:** Cover stoma and manually ventilate patient by mouth. Replace tube.
Tracheal stenosis	Injury to area from end of tube or cuff, resulting in scar tissue formation and narrowing of airway	**Prevention:** Inflate cuff with minimal amount of air necessary. Monitor cuff pressures every 8 hours. **Treatment:** Perform surgical repair.
Tracheoesophageal fistula	Pressure necrosis of posterior tracheal wall, resulting from overinflated cuff and rigid nasogastric tube	**Prevention:** Inflate cuff with minimal amount of air necessary. Monitor cuff pressures every 8 hours. **Treatment:** Perform surgical repair.
Tracheoinnominate artery fistula	Direct pressure from elbow of cannula against innominate artery Placement of tracheal stoma below fourth tracheal ring High-lying innominate artery	**Prevention:** Position tracheal window not lower than third tracheal ring. **Treatment:** Hyperinflate cuff to control bleeding. Remove tube and replace with ETT, and apply digital pressure through stoma against sternum. Perform surgical repair.
Tracheocutaneous fistula	Failure of stoma to close after removal of tube	**Treatment:** Perform surgical repair.

ETT, Endotracheal tube; *PRN*, as needed.

 BOX 19.3 **Safety**

Unintentional Extubation or Decannulation

Patient safety is of paramount importance when caring for a patient with an artificial airway because loss of the tube can result in loss of the patient's airway. In the event of unintentional extubation or decannulation, the patient's airway is opened with the head tilt–chin lift maneuver and maintained with an oropharyngeal or nasopharyngeal airway. If the patient is not breathing, they are manually ventilated with an manual resuscitation bag and face mask with 100% oxygen. In the case of a tracheostomy, the stoma is covered to prevent air from escaping through it. If the tracheostomy remains open, consideration is given to ventilating the patient through the stoma instead of the mouth. To facilitate reinsertion of a tracheostomy tube, it is important to maintain a same-sized sterile tracheostomy tube and a one-size smaller sterile tracheostomy tube at the bedside along with a spare securement device.

and inserting a single-use, disposable, suction catheter into the artificial airway. This is commonly used to suction a patient with a tracheostomy tube who is not requiring mechanical ventilation. The closed suction method requires a sterile, closed tracheal suction system (CTSS) (Fig. 19.11) and allows the patient to be suctioned while remaining on the ventilator.[8] The CTSS consists of a multiple-use sterile suction catheter, protected in a transparent plastic sheath, that is connected in-line with the ventilator circuit. Advantages of the CTSS include maintenance of oxygenation and PEEP during suctioning, reduction of hypoxemia-related complications, and protection of staff members from the patient's secretions.[33] The CTSS is convenient to use, requiring only one person to perform the procedure. Current evidence suggests that either method can be used to safely suction an artificial airway in an adult patient.[32]

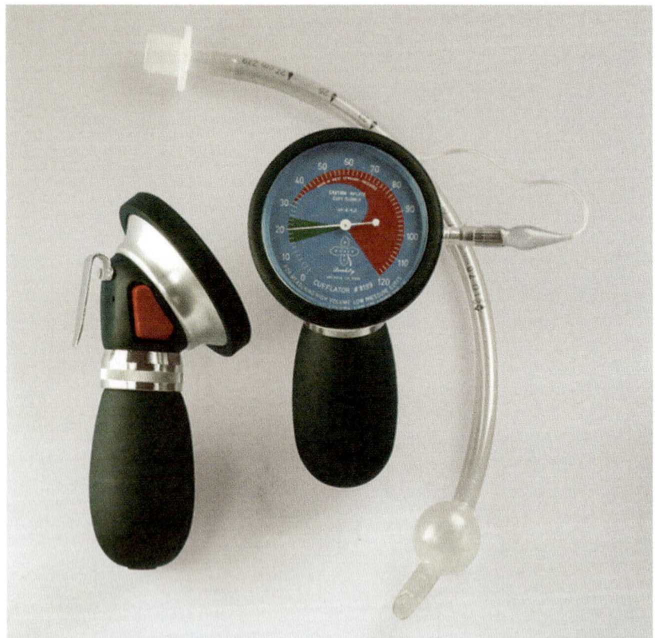

FIG. 19.8 Cuff Pressure Manometer. Aneroid pressure manometer for cuff inflation and measuring cuff pressures. (From Ignatavicius DD, Workman ML, Rebar C, Heimgartner M, eds. *Medical-Surgical Nursing: Concepts for Interprofessional Collaborative Care*. 10th ed. Elsevier; 2021.)

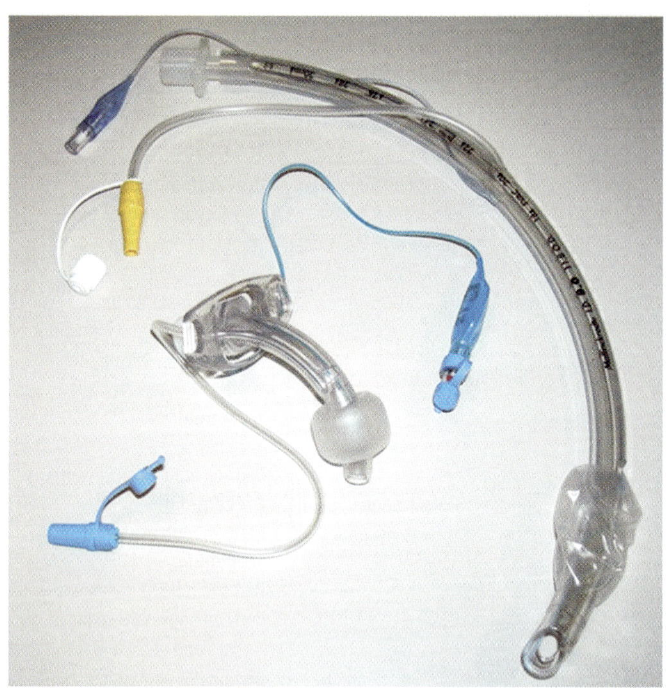

FIG. 19.10 Endotracheal and Tracheostomy Tubes With Subglottic Suction Ports. (From Kacmarek RM, Stoller JK, Heuer AJ, eds. *Egan's Fundamentals of Respiratory Care*. 12th ed. Elsevier; 2021.)

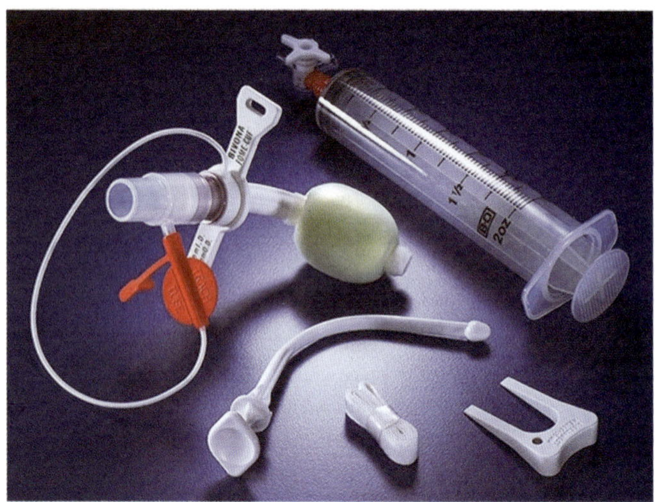

FIG. 19.9 Foam Cuff Tracheostomy Tube. (Courtesy Smiths Medical, Inc., London, United Kingdom.)

Suction depth. There are two different techniques for suctioning depending on how deeply the suction catheter is inserted into the trachea: shallow suctioning and deep suctioning. For shallow suctioning, the suction catheter is inserted to the end of the ETT or tracheostomy tube, and then the suction is applied. For deep suctioning, the suction catheter is inserted until resistance is met, the catheter is pulled back approximately 1 cm, and then suction is applied. Evidence suggests that shallow suctioning is as effective as deep suctioning for secretion removal and is associated with fewer complications. Deep suctioning should only be used when shallow suctioning is ineffective.[8,32]

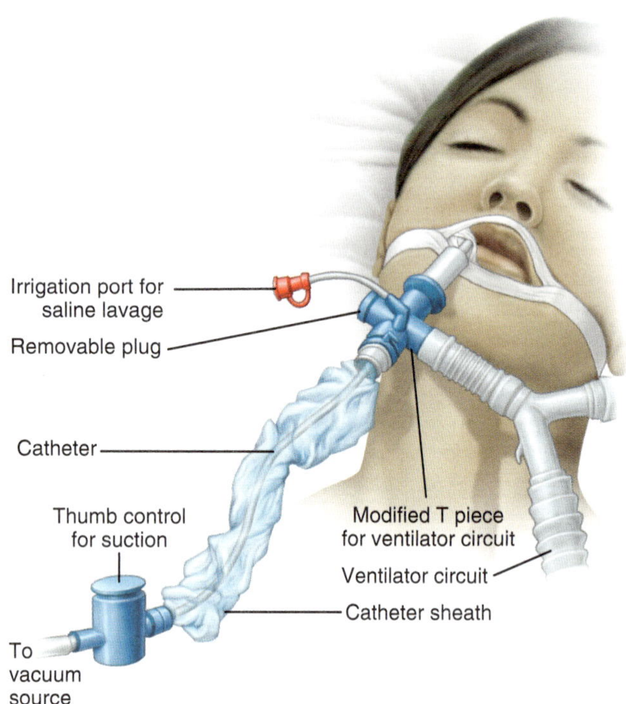

FIG. 19.11 Closed Tracheal Suction System. (Modified from Sills JR. *Entry-level Respiratory Therapist Exam Guide*. Mosby; 2000.)

Complications. Complications associated with suctioning include hypoxemia, dysrhythmia, hypertension, hypotension, atelectasis, airway trauma, bacterial colonization of the lower airways, and increased intracranial pressure.[8,32] Hypoxemia can result because the oxygen source is disconnected from the patient, or the oxygen is removed from the patient's airways when the suction is applied. Atelectasis is thought to occur secondary to use of a suction catheter that is more than 50% larger than the diameter of the ETT,[8,32] prolonged suctioning, and excessive negative suction pressure.[8] Cardiac dysrhythmias, particularly bradycardias, are attributed to vagal stimulation. Tachycardia can occur due to hypoxemia or agitation.[8] Airway trauma occurs with impaction of the catheter in the airways and excessive negative pressure applied to the catheter.[8] Bacterial colonization of the lower airway has been associated with the instillation of normal saline to help remove secretions. This practice has not been proved to be of any benefit, and it may contribute to the development of hypoxemia and VAP.[32,34]

Suctioning recommendations. Several practices have been found to be helpful in limiting the complications of suctioning and are currently recommended.

- Preoxygenate the patient with 100% oxygen[8,32] for 30 to 60 seconds before suctioning and for at least 60 seconds after suctioning to minimize hypoxemia and tachycardia.[8]
- Use a suction catheter with an external diameter of less than one-half of the internal diameter of the ETT[8,32] to minimize atelectasis.[8]
- Use 200 mm Hg or less of negative pressure for suction[32] to decrease the chance of hypoxemia, atelectasis, and airway trauma.[8]
- Limit the duration of each suction pass to less than 15 seconds[8,32] to minimize hypoxemia, airway trauma, and cardiac dysrhythmias.[8]
- Apply continuous suction instead of intermittent suction, as intermittent suction has been shown to be of no benefit.[35]

Communication

Impaired communication is a major stressor for a patient with an artificial airway. This stress is related to the inability to speak, insufficient explanations from staff members, inadequate understanding, fear of being unable to communicate, and difficulty with communication methods.[36,37] Many interventions can facilitate communication for a patient with an ETT or tracheostomy tube. These include establishing an environment that fosters communication, performing a complete assessment of the patient's ability to communicate, anticipating the patient's needs, teaching the patient and family how to communicate, using a variety of methods to communicate, and facilitating the patient's ability to communicate by providing the patient with their eyeglasses or hearing aid.[38]

Methods to facilitate communication in this patient population include the use of verbal and nonverbal language and various devices to assist the patient on short-term and long-term ventilator assistance. Nonverbal communication may include the use of sign language, gestures, lip reading, pointing, facial expressions, or eye blinking. Simple devices include pencil and paper; Magic Slates; magnetic boards with plastic letters; picture, alphabet, or symbol boards; and flash cards. More sophisticated devices include typewriters, computers, talking ETT and tracheostomy tubes, and external handheld vibrators. Regardless of the method selected, the patient must be taught how to use the device.[38]

Passy-Muir valve. The Passy-Muir valve is a device used to assist a mechanically ventilated patient with a tracheostomy to speak. This one-way valve opens on inhalation, allowing air to enter the lungs through the tracheostomy tube, and closes on exhalation, forcing air over the vocal cords and out the mouth, permitting the patient to speak (Fig. 19.12). Before the valve can be placed on a tracheostomy tube, the cuff must be deflated to allow air to pass around the tube, and the tidal volume of the ventilator must be increased to compensate for the air leak. In addition to aiding communication, the Passy-Muir valve can assist a ventilator-dependent patient with relearning normal breathing patterns. The valve is contraindicated in patients with laryngeal or pharyngeal dysfunction, excessive secretions, or poor lung compliance.[8]

Oral Hygiene

Patients with artificial airways are extremely susceptible to developing VAP because of microaspiration of subglottic secretions. These secretions are full of microorganisms from the patient's mouth. Because the cuff of the artificial airway does not form a tight seal in the patient's airway, these secretions seep around the cuff into the patient's lungs, promoting the development of VAP.[30,39] Although bacteria are normally present in a patient's mouth, increased amounts of bacteria and more resistant bacteria are present in critically ill patients. Decreased salivary flow, poor mucosal status, and dental plaque all contribute to this problem.[40]

Proper oral hygiene has been shown to decrease the incidence of VAP.[40,41] However, studies have shown that oral care is not routinely performed for a variety of reasons.[40,42] No evidence-based protocol exists for oral care at the present time. Research studies are lacking, particularly regarding the

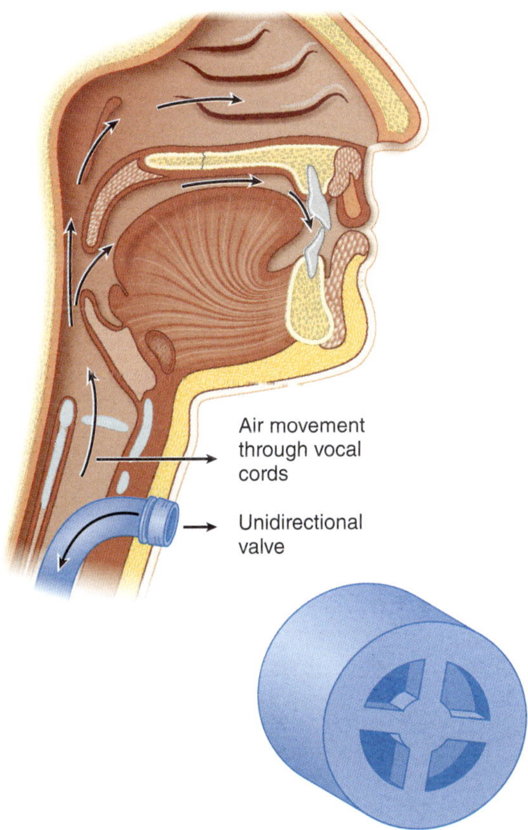

FIG. 19.12 Passy-Muir Valve. (Redrawn from Manzano JL, Subillo S, Henríquez D, Martín JC, Pérez MC, Wilson DJ. Verbal communication of ventilator dependent patients. *Crit Care Med.* 1992;21(4):512–517; with permission.)

frequency and effectiveness of different products and procedures. The current recommendation for oral care is simply daily toothbrushing without chlorhexidine. Chlorhexidine solution is no longer recommended as it has been shown to be of no benefit to the patient.[31] A large randomized controlled trial found that the use of chlorhexidine with oral care did not affect the rate of VAP, intensive care mortality, or time to extubation.[43] This area of nursing care needs additional research.

Extubation and Decannulation

An artificial airway is removed when it is no longer needed. Extubation, the process of removing an ETT, is a simple procedure that can be done at the bedside. Before the cuff of an ETT or tracheostomy tube is deflated in preparation for removal, it is important to ensure that secretions are cleared from above the tube cuff. Complications of extubation include sore throat, stridor, hoarseness, odynophagia, vocal cord immobility, pulmonary aspiration, and cough.[44] Decannulation is the process of removing a tracheostomy tube.[20] Once it is determined that the patient no longer needs the tube, the patient may be weaned from the tube, or the tube simply removed. There are a variety of methods for weaning a tracheostomy tube including switching to a smaller tube, switching to an uncuffed tube, and/or capping the tube and observing the patient for signs of respiratory distress.[45] It is a simple process to remove the tube and it can be performed at the bedside. After removal the stoma is usually covered with a dry dressing with the expectation that it will close within several days.[20,45] Difficulty removing the tracheostomy tube because of a tight stoma is usually the only complication associated with decannulation.

INVASIVE MECHANICAL VENTILATION

Indications

Mechanical ventilation is the process of using an apparatus to facilitate the transport of oxygen and CO_2 between the atmosphere and the alveoli for the purpose of enhancing pulmonary gas exchange. Mechanical ventilation is indicated for physiologic and clinical reasons. Physiologic objectives include supporting cardiopulmonary gas exchange (alveolar ventilation and arterial oxygenation), increasing lung volume (end expiratory lung inflation and functional residual capacity), and reducing the work of breathing. Clinical objectives include reversing hypoxemia and acute respiratory acidosis, relieving respiratory distress, preventing or reversing atelectasis and respiratory muscle fatigue, permitting sedation and neuromuscular blockade, decreasing oxygen consumption, reducing intracranial pressure, and stabilizing the chest wall.[46–48]

Use of Mechanical Ventilators

Types of Ventilators

The two main types of ventilators available at the present time are (1) positive-pressure ventilators and (2) negative pressure ventilators. Negative pressure ventilators are applied externally to the patient and decrease the atmospheric pressure surrounding the thorax to initiate inspiration. They generally are not used in the critical care environment. Positive-pressure ventilators use a mechanical drive mechanism to force air into the patient's lungs through an ETT or tracheostomy tube.[47]

Ventilator Mechanics

To properly ventilate the patient, the ventilator must complete four phases of ventilation: (1) change from exhalation to inspiration, (2) inspiration, (3) change from inspiration to exhalation, and (4) exhalation. The ventilator uses four different variables to begin, sustain, and terminate each of these phases. These variables are described in terms of *volume, pressure, flow*, and *time*.[47,49]

Trigger. The phase variable that initiates the change from exhalation to inspiration is called the *trigger*. Breaths may be pressure triggered or flow triggered, depending on the sensitivity setting of the ventilator and the patient's inspiratory effort, or they may be time triggered, depending on the rate setting of the ventilator. A breath that is initiated by the patient is known as a *patient-triggered* or *patient-assisted* breath, whereas a breath that is initiated by the ventilator is known as a *machine-triggered* or *machine-controlled* breath.[47,49]

A *time-triggered breath* is a machine-controlled breath that is initiated by the ventilator after a preset length of time has elapsed and is controlled by the rate setting on the ventilator (e.g., a rate of 10 breaths/min yields 1 breath every 6 seconds). *Flow-triggered* and *pressure-triggered* breaths are patient-assisted breaths that are initiated by decreased flow or pressure, respectively, within the breathing circuit. Flow triggering (also known as *flow-by*) is controlled by adjusting the flow-sensitivity setting of the ventilator, whereas pressure triggering is controlled by adjusting the pressure-sensitivity setting. Many ventilators offer the various types of triggers in combination. For example, a breath may be time triggered and flow triggered, depending on the patient's ability to interact with the ventilator and initiate a breath.[47,49]

Limit. The variable that maintains inspiration is called the *limit* or *target*. Inspiration can be pressure limited, flow limited, or volume limited. A *pressure-limited breath* is one in which a preset pressure is attained and maintained during inspiration. A *flow-limited breath* is one in which a preset flow is reached before the end of inspiration. A *volume-limited breath* is one in which a preset volume is delivered during the inspiration. However, the limit variable does not end inspiration; it only sustains it.[47,49]

Cycle. The variable that ends inspiration is called the *cycle*. The classification of positive-pressure ventilators is based on this variable: volume-cycled, pressure-cycled, flow-cycled, and time-cycled ventilators. Volume-cycled ventilators are designed to deliver a breath until a preset volume is delivered. Pressure-cycled ventilators deliver a breath until a preset pressure is reached within the patient's airways. Flow-cycled ventilators deliver a breath until a preset inspiratory flow rate is achieved. Time-cycled ventilators deliver a breath over a preset time interval.[47,49]

Baseline. The variable that is controlled during exhalation is called the *baseline*. Pressure is almost always used to adjust this variable. The patient exhales to a certain baseline pressure that is set on the ventilator. The baseline variable may be set at zero (i.e., atmospheric pressure) or above atmospheric pressure (i.e., PEEP).[47,49]

Modes of Ventilation

The term *ventilator mode* refers to how the machine ventilates the patient. Selection of a particular mode of ventilation determines how much the patient will participate in their own ventilatory pattern. The choice depends on the patient's situation and the goals of treatment. The mode is determined by the combination of phase variables selected. Many modes are available (Table 19.3), and some may be used in conjunction with

TABLE 19.3 **Modes of Mechanical Ventilation**

Mode of Ventilation	Clinical Application	Nursing Implications
Continuous mandatory (volume or pressure) ventilation (CMV), also known as assist/control (AC) ventilation: Delivers gas at preset tidal volume or pressure (depending on selected cycling variable) in response to patient's inspiratory efforts and initiates breath if patient fails to do so within preset time.	Volume-controlled (VC) CMV is used as primary mode of ventilation in spontaneously breathing patients with weak respiratory muscles. Pressure-controlled (PC) CMV is used in patients with decreased lung compliance or increased airway resistance, particularly when patient is at risk for volutrauma.	Hyperventilation can occur in patients with increased respiratory rates. Sedation may be necessary to limit number of spontaneous breaths. Patient on VC-CMV is monitored for volutrauma. Patient on PC-CMV is monitored for hypercapnia.
Pressure-regulated volume control ventilation (PRVCV): Variation of CMV that combines volume and pressure features; delivers preset tidal volume using lowest possible airway pressure; airway pressure will not exceed preset maximum pressure limit.	PRVCV is used in patients with rapidly changing pulmonary mechanics (airway resistance and lung compliance), limiting potential complications.	
Pressure-controlled inverse ratio ventilation (PC-IRV): PC-CMV mode in which inspiratory-to-expiratory (I:E) time ratio is >1 : 1.	PC-IRV is used in patients with hypoxemia refractory to PEEP; longer inspiratory time increases functional residual capacity and improves oxygenation by opening collapsed alveoli, and shorter expiratory time induces auto-PEEP that prevents alveoli from recollapsing.	Requires sedation and/or pharmacologic paralysis because of discomfort. Increased intrathoracic pressure can result in excessive air trapping and decreased cardiac output.
Intermittent mandatory (volume or pressure) ventilation (IMV), also known as synchronous intermittent mandatory ventilation (SIMV): Delivers gas at preset tidal volume or pressure (depending on selected cycling variable) and rate, while allowing patient to breathe spontaneously; ventilator breaths are synchronized to patient's respiratory effort.	VC-IMV is used as primary mode of ventilation in many clinical situations and as weaning mode. PC-IMV is used in patients with decreased lung compliance or increased airway resistance when the need to preserve the patient's spontaneous efforts is important.	May increase work of breathing and promote respiratory muscle fatigue. Patient is monitored for hypercapnia, particularly with PC-IMV.
Adaptive support ventilation (ASV): Ventilator automatically adjusts settings to maintain 100 mL/min/kg of minute ventilation; pressure support.	ASV is a computerized mode of ventilation that increases or decreases ventilatory support based on patient needs; can be used with any patient requiring volume-controlled ventilation.	Not intended as a weaning mode. Adapts to changes in patient position.
Continuous positive airway pressure (CPAP): Positive pressure applied during spontaneous breaths; patient controls rate, inspiratory flow, and tidal volume.	CPAP is spontaneous breathing mode used in patients to increase functional residual capacity and improve oxygenation by opening collapsed alveoli at end expiration; it is also used for weaning.	Side effects include decreased cardiac output, volutrauma, and increased intracranial pressure. No ventilator breaths are delivered in PEEP or CPAP mode unless used with CMV or IMV.
Airway pressure release ventilation (APRV): Two different levels of CPAP (inspiratory and expiratory) are applied for set periods of time, allowing spontaneous breathing to occur at both levels.	APRV is spontaneous breathing mode used to maintain alveolar recruitment without imposing additional peak inspiratory pressures that could lead to barotrauma	Patient needs to be monitored for hypercapnia.
Pressure support ventilation (PSV): Preset positive pressure used to augment patient's inspiratory efforts; patient controls rate, inspiratory flow, and tidal volume.	PSV is spontaneous breathing mode used as primary mode of ventilation in patients with stable respiratory drive to overcome any imposed mechanical resistance (e.g., artificial airway). PSV can also be used with IMV to support spontaneous breaths.	Patient is monitored for hypercapnia. Advantages include reduced patient work of breathing and improved patient–ventilator synchrony.
Volume-assured pressure support ventilation (VAPSV), also known as pressure augmentation (PA): Variation of PSV with set tidal volume to ensure that patient receives minimum tidal volume with each pressure support breath.	VAPSV is spontaneous breathing mode used to treat acute respiratory illness and to facilitate weaning.	Advantages include increased patient comfort, decreased work of breathing, decreased respiratory muscle fatigue, and promotion of respiratory muscle conditioning.
Neurally adjusted ventilatory assist (NAVA): Partial ventilatory support mode that uses electrical activity of diaphragm to control patient ventilator interaction.	NAVA delivers assisted breath in proportion to and in synchrony with patient's respiratory effort.	Requires esophageal catheter (similar to nasogastric tube) that measures electrical signal to diaphragm.
Independent lung ventilation (ILV): Each lung is ventilated separately.	ILV is used in patients with unilateral lung disease, bronchopleural fistulas, or bilateral asymmetric lung disease.	Requires double-lumen ETT, two ventilators, sedation, and pharmacologic paralysis.

Continued

TABLE 19.3 Modes of Mechanical Ventilation—cont'd

Mode of Ventilation	Clinical Application	Nursing Implications
High-frequency ventilation (HFV): Delivers small volume of gas at rapid rate. • High-frequency positive-pressure ventilation (HFPPV): Delivers 60–100 breaths/min • High-frequency jet ventilation (HFJV): delivers 100–600 cycles/min • High-frequency oscillation (HFO): delivers 900–3000 cycles/min	HFV is used in situations in which conventional mechanical ventilation compromises hemodynamic stability, in patients with bronchopleural fistulas, during short-term procedures, and with diseases that create risk of volutrauma.	Patients require sedation and/or pharmacologic paralysis. Inadequate humidification can compromise airway patency. Assessment of breath sounds is difficult.

ETT, Endotracheal tube; *PEEP*, positive end-expiratory pressure.

TABLE 19.4 Ventilator Settings

Parameter	Description	Typical Settings
Respiratory rate or frequency	Number of breaths ventilator delivers per minute	6–20 breaths/min
Vt	Volume of gas delivered to patient during each ventilator breath	6–10 mL/kg 4–8 mL/kg in ARDS
Oxygen concentration (FiO_2)	FiO_2 delivered to patient	May be set between 21% and 100%; adjusted to maintain PaO_2 level >60 mm Hg or SpO_2 level >92%
PEEP	Positive pressure applied at end of expiration of ventilator breaths	3–5 cm H_2O
PS	Positive pressure used to augment patient's inspiratory efforts	5–10 cm H_2O
Inspiratory flow rate and time	Speed with which Vt is delivered	40–80 L/min Time: 0.8–1.2 seconds
I:E ratio	Ratio of duration of inspiration to duration of expiration	1:2 to 1:1.5 unless inverse ratio ventilation is desired
Sensitivity	Determines amount of effort patient must generate to initiate a ventilator breath; it may be set for pressure triggering or flow triggering	Pressure trigger: 0.5–1.5 cm H_2O below baseline pressure Flow trigger: 1–3 L/min below baseline flow
High-pressure limit	Regulates maximal pressure ventilator can generate to deliver Vt; when pressure limit is reached, ventilator terminates breath and spills undelivered volume into atmosphere	10–20 cm H_2O above peak inspiratory pressure

ARDS, Acute respiratory distress syndrome; *FiO_2*, fraction of inspired oxygen; *I:E*, inspiratory to expiratory; *PaO_2*, arterial oxygen pressure; *PEEP*, positive end-expiratory time; *PS*, pressure support; *SpO_2*, oxygen saturation as measured by pulse oximetry; *Vt*, tidal volume.

others.[46–48,50,51] Because brands of ventilators vary in their ability to perform certain functions, not all modes are available on all ventilators.[49]

Ventilator Settings

Settings on the ventilator allow the ventilator parameters to be individualized to the patient and allow selection of the desired ventilation mode (Table 19.4). Each ventilator has a patient-monitoring system that allows all aspects of the patient's ventilatory pattern to be assessed, monitored, and displayed.[46,48,50,52]

Complications

Mechanical ventilation is often lifesaving, but, like other interventions, it is not without complications. Some complications are preventable, whereas others can be minimized but not eradicated. Physiologic complications associated with mechanical ventilation include ventilator-induced lung injury, cardiovascular compromise, patient-ventilator dyssynchrony, and VAP.

Ventilator-Induced Lung Injury

Mechanical ventilation can cause two different types of injury to the lungs: (1) air leaks and (2) biotrauma.[53,54] Air leaks related to mechanical ventilation are the result of excessive pressure in the alveoli (barotrauma), excessive volume in the alveoli (volutrauma), or shearing caused by repeated opening and closing of the alveoli (atelectrauma).[53–55] Barotrauma, volutrauma, and atelectrauma can lead to excessive alveolar wall stress and damage to the alveolar–capillary membrane, resulting in air leakage into the surrounding spaces. The air then travels out through the hilum and into the mediastinum (pneumomediastinum), pleural space (pneumothorax), subcutaneous tissues (subcutaneous emphysema), pericardium (pneumopericardium), peritoneum (pneumoperitoneum), and retroperitoneum (pneumoretroperitoneum). The resultant disorders vary from benign to potentially lethal—the most lethal of which is a pneumothorax or pneumopericardium resulting in cardiac tamponade.[56]

Barotrauma, volutrauma, and atelectrauma can also cause the release of cellular mediators and initiation of the inflammatory-immune response. This type of ventilator-induced injury is known as *biotrauma*.[54,57] Biotrauma can result in the development of ARDS.[55] To limit ventilator-induced lung injury, the plateau pressure (pressure needed to inflate the alveoli) is kept at less than 28 cm H_2O, the driving pressure (the difference in pressure from end-expiration to end-inspiration) is kept less than 15 cm H_2O, the tidal volume is set between 4 to 10 mL/kg, and PEEP is used to avoid end expiratory collapse and reopening.[52]

Cardiovascular Compromise

Positive-pressure ventilation increases intrathoracic pressure, which decreases venous return to the right side of the heart. Impaired venous return decreases preload, which results in a decrease in cardiac output. As a secondary consequence, hepatic and renal dysfunction may occur. Positive-pressure ventilation impairs cerebral venous return. In patients with impaired autoregulation, positive-pressure ventilation can result in increased intracranial pressure.[58]

Patient-Ventilator Dyssynchrony

Because the ventilatory pattern is normally initiated by the establishment of negative pressure within the chest, the application of positive pressure can lead to patient difficulties in breathing while on the ventilator. To achieve optimal ventilatory assistance, the patient should breathe in synchrony with the machine. The selected mode of ventilation, the settings, and the type of ventilatory circuitry used can increase the work of breathing and lead to breathing out of synchrony with the ventilator. Patient–ventilator dyssynchrony can result in decreased effectiveness of mechanical ventilation, the development of auto-PEEP, and psychological distress. Patients who are not breathing in synchrony with the ventilator appear to be fighting or "bucking" the ventilator. To minimize this problem, the ventilator is adjusted to accommodate the patient's spontaneous breathing pattern and to work with the patient. If this is not possible, the patient may need to be sedated or pharmacologically paralyzed.[47,57]

Ventilator-Associated Pneumonia

VAP is an infection of the pulmonary parenchyma in patients requiring invasive mechanical ventilation for at least 48 hours. It is a subtype of hospital-acquired pneumonia.[59] However, it is the presence of the artificial airway (versus the ventilator) that places the patient at risk for developing pneumonia either though aspiration or inhalation (see Fig 18.3). The severity of the patient's illness, advanced age, the presence of chronic lung disease or kidney disease, alcoholism, malnutrition, and prior antibiotic exposure significantly increase the likelihood that an infection will ensue.[60] Additional information on managing a patient with pneumonia is provided in Chapter 18. Prevention of VAP is crucial; strategies to prevent VAP are listed in Box 19.4.

BOX 19.4 Evidence-Based Practice

Ventilator-Associated Pneumonia Prevention Strategies

- Use high-flow nasal oxygen or noninvasive ventilation, when possible, to avoid intubation.
- Minimize the use of sedation.
- Use a ventilator liberation protocol.
- Maintain or enhance physical conditioning.
- Elevate the head of the bed 30 to 45 degrees.
- Change ventilator circuits only when visibly soiled, malfunctioning, or per the manufacturers' recommendations.
- Perform routine oral care with a toothbrush and without chlorhexidine.
- Provide early enteral nutrition.

Modified from Klompas M, Branson R, Cawcutt K, et al. Strategies to prevent ventilator-associated pneumonia, ventilator-associated events, and nonventilator hospital-acquired pneumonia in acute-care hospitals: 2022 Update. *Infect Control Hosp Epidemiol.* 2022;43(6):687–713.

Aspiration and inhalation. Aspiration can occur when bacteria-laden oral secretions trickle down the larynx and pool above the cuff of the artificial airway. These subglottic secretions can leak around the cuff into the lower airway, resulting in microaspiration. Leakage can occur via the longitudinal folds that form in the cuff as it accommodates to the shape of the airway, when an underinflated cuff fails to form a proper seal in the airway, or in the event of inadvertent movement of the ETT within the airway.[28,30]

A number of alternative ETT cuff designs have been proposed to decrease the incidence of VAP by limiting leakage around the cuff. Two examples of alternative cuffs are ultrathin polyurethane cuffs and tapered cuffs. Polyurethane cuffs are much thinner than the traditional polyvinyl cuffs and do not form folds when they are inflated thus theoretically limiting leakage around the cuff. A taper-shaped cuff appears to be better for preventing fluid leakage compared with a cylindrical cuff commonly found on most tubes.[39] However, the research supporting these cuff designs has been inconsistent and they are not currently recommended.[31]

Therapeutic measures such as nasogastric intubation and gastric alkalization with enteral feedings or medications can also facilitate the development of pneumonia. Nasogastric tubes promote aspiration by acting as a wick for stomach contents, whereas enteral feedings, antacids, histamine inhibitors, and proton pump inhibitors increase the pH level of the stomach, promoting the growth of bacteria that can then be aspirated (Fig. 19.13).[61]

Lower airway contamination can occur via inhalation particularly as the artificial airway bypasses or impairs many of the normal defense mechanisms of the lung. The use of respiratory therapy devices (e.g., ventilators, nebulizers, aerosol generating devices) can increase the risk of pneumonia particularly if they are inadequately disinfected. In addition, poor hygiene practices and frequent circuit changes had also been implicated.[60]

Silver-coated ETTs have also been used to reduce the incidence of VAP by decreasing biofilm formation. The silver coating limits bacterial colonization by decreasing biofilm formation. Biofilm is formed when bacteria cling to the inner lumen of the ETT and then secrete an exopolysaccharide substance. This substance forms a gelatinous matrix that allows bacteria to thrive on a nonbiologic surface.[39] However, the research supporting silver-coated ETTs has be inconsistent and they are not currently recommended.[31]

Semirecumbency. Positioning of a patient who requires mechanical ventilation is very important. Semirecumbent positioning (elevation of the head of the bed 30 to 45 degrees) reduces the incidence of gastroesophageal reflux and subsequent aspiration of oropharyngeal secretions and decreases the incidence of VAP. The head of the patient's bed is always elevated to 30 to 45 degrees unless contraindicated (e.g., hemodynamic instability, presence of intra-aortic balloon pump, practitioner's order to the contrary).[39,62] However, this intervention increases the risk of skin shear on the coccyx, and extra surveillance is mandatory for prevention of pressure injuries.[63]

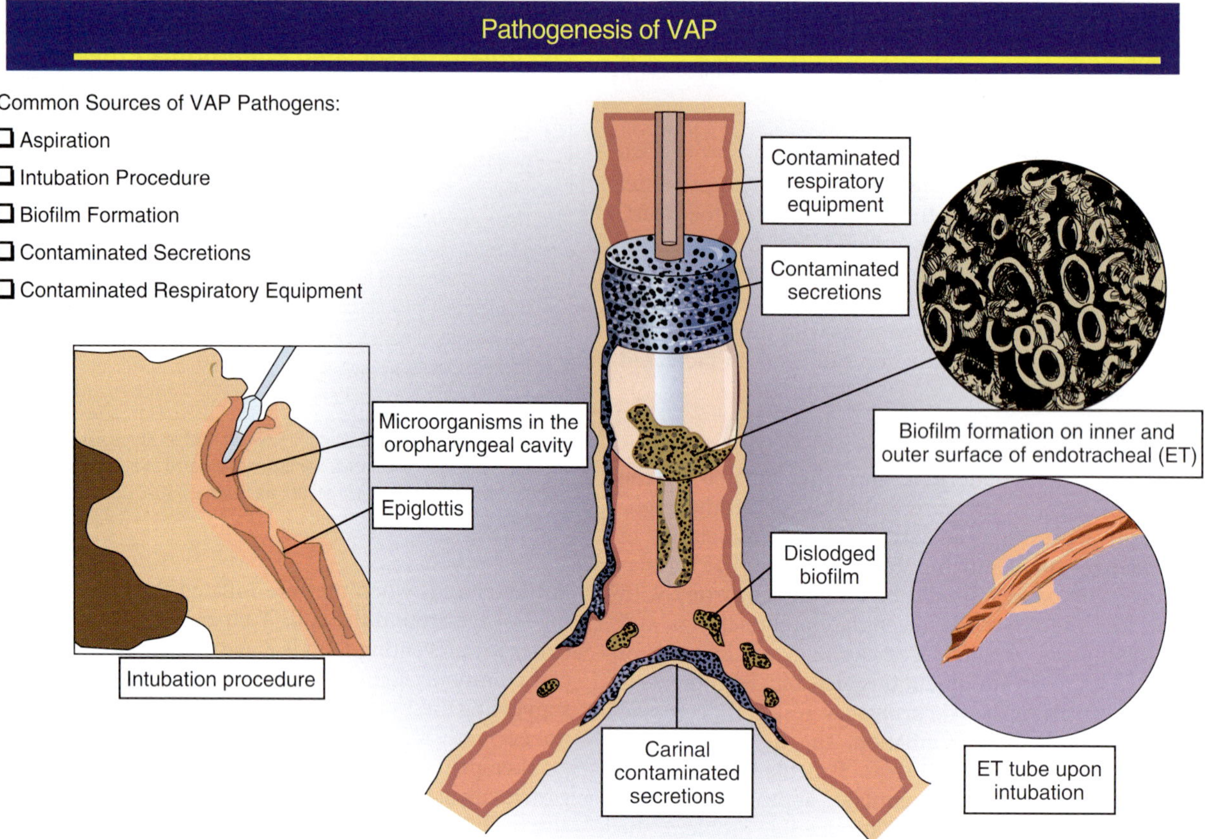

FIG. 19.13 Pathogenesis of Ventilator-Associated Pneumonia. (Redrawn from Sachdev G, Napolitano LM. Postoperative pulmonary complications: pneumonia and acute respiratory failure. *Surg Clin North Am.* 2012;92(2):321–344.)

Sedation vacation. Many patients receiving mechanical ventilation require sedation to ameliorate symptoms of anxiety and stress associated with critical illness. However, the prolonged use of sedation has been shown to contribute to the development of complications, including oversedation, prolonged mechanical ventilation, and delirium. To decrease the incidence of these complications, the concept of a "sedation vacation" has been developed. A "sedation vacation" is simply the daily interruption of sedation to evaluate the patient and their need for continued sedation and mechanical ventilation.[64] Not every patient is a candidate for this procedure. Contraindications include hemodynamic instability, increased intracranial pressure, ongoing agitation, seizures, alcohol withdrawal, and use of neuromuscular blocking agents. If the patient is able to tolerate being off the sedation for a predetermined amount of time (this number varies depending on the protocol being used), the sedation is discontinued. Signs of intolerance include ongoing agitation, increased respiratory rate, decreasing oxygen saturation, cardiac dysrhythmias, and signs of respiratory distress.[65]

Weaning

Weaning is the withdrawal of the mechanical ventilator and the re-establishment of spontaneous breathing. In the past, weaning was the gradual withdrawal of mechanical ventilation; however, newer approaches use a more abrupt discontinuation and transition to spontaneous breathing.[66] Weaning is begun only after the original process for which ventilator support was required has been corrected and patient stability has been achieved. Other factors to consider when weaning are length of time on ventilator, sleep deprivation, and nutritional status. Major factors that affect the patient's ability to wean include the ability of the lungs to participate in ventilation and respiration, cardiovascular performance, and psychological readiness.[66] This discussion focuses on weaning of a patient from short-term (3 days or less) mechanical ventilation. Management of weaning in a patient on long-term mechanical ventilation is discussed in Chapter 18.

Readiness to Wean

Patients are screened every day for their readiness to be weaned. The screen includes an evaluation of the patient's level of consciousness, physiologic and hemodynamic stability, adequacy of oxygenation and ventilation, spontaneous breathing capability, and respiratory rate and pattern.[66] Parameters that may be assessed are presented in Table 19.5.

The rapid shallow breathing index (RSBI) is often used to predict weaning success. To calculate an RSBI, the patient's respiratory rate and minute ventilation are measured for 1 minute during spontaneous breathing. The measured respiratory rate is then divided by the tidal volume (expressed in liters). An RSBI of less than 105 is considered predictive of weaning success. If the patient is receiving sedation, the medication is discontinued at least 1 hour before the RSBI is measured. If the patient meets criteria for weaning readiness and has an RSBI of less than 105, a spontaneous breathing trial (SBT) can be performed.[67] A recent meta-analysis found that the RSBI has moderate sensitivity and poor specificity for predicting extubation success.[68] In other words, the RSBI is a moderate predictor of which patients can be successfully weaned but a poor predictor of which patient cannot be successfully weaned. Thus, it is important that this parameter not be used as the sole predictor of weaning success. Fig. 19.14 outlines one approach commonly used in the critical care setting.

TABLE 19.5 Conventional Weaning Parameters

Parameters	Weanable Values	Normal Ranges
NIF (cm H_2O)	<−20	<−50
VC (mL/kg)	>10	>65–75
Vt (mL/kg)	<5	>5–7
RR (breaths/min)	<32	12–20
Ve (L/min)	>10	>10
RSBI (RR/Vt)	<105	<40

NIF, Negative inspiratory force; *RR,* respiratory rate; *RSBI,* rapid shallow breathing index; *VC,* vital capacity; *Ve,* minute ventilation; *Vt,* tidal volume.
From Benjamin IJ, ed. *Andreoli and Carpenter's Cecil Essentials of Medicine.* 9th ed. Elsevier; 2016.

Weaning Trial

After the patient's readiness to be weaned has been established, the patient is prepared for a weaning trial.[69] The patient is positioned upright to facilitate breathing and suctioned to ensure airway patency. The process is explained to the patient, and the patient is offered reassurance and diversional activities. The patient is assessed immediately before the start of the trial and frequently during the weaning period for signs of weaning intolerance (Box 19.5).[69]

Numerous methods can be used for conducting a weaning. The three main methods that are used are (1) SBT, (2) pressure support ventilation (PSV) trial, and (3) synchronized intermittent

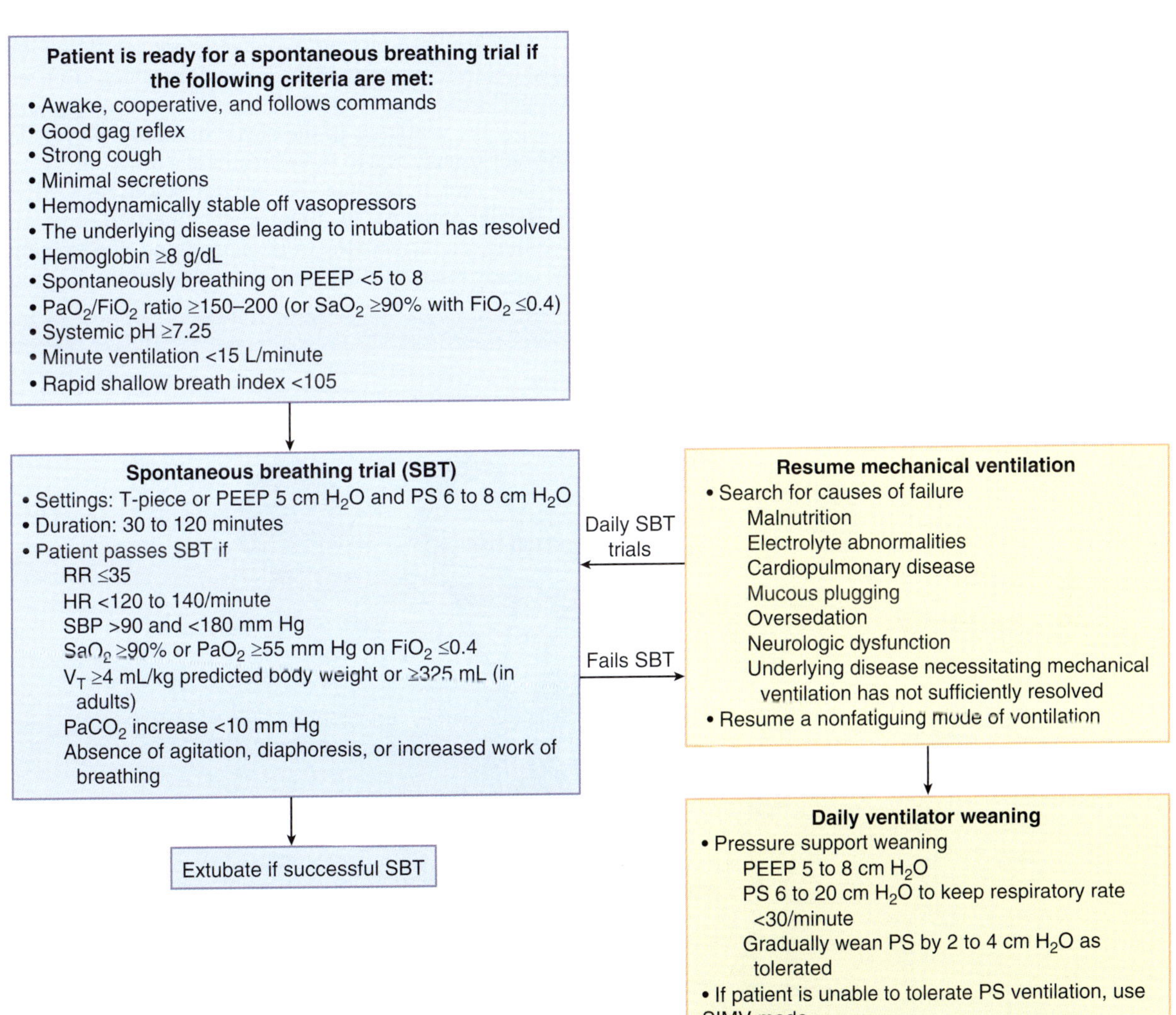

FIG. 19.14 Weaning and Liberation Algorithm. Weaning and liberation from mechanical ventilators. *FiO_2,* Fraction of inspired oxygen; *HR,* heart rate; *$PaCO_2$,* partial pressure of arterial carbon dioxide; *PaO_2,* partial pressure of arterial oxygen; *PEEP,* positive end-expiratory pressure; *PS,* pressure support; *RR,* respiratory rate; *SaO_2,* arterial oxygen saturation; *SBP,* systolic blood pressure; *SIMV,* synchronized intermittent mandatory ventilation; *V_T,* tidal volume. (Modified from MacIntyre NR, Cook DJ, Ely EW Jr, et al. Evidence-based guidelines for weaning and discontinuing ventilatory support. *Chest.* 2001;120[6 Suppl]:375S–395S. [From Goldman L, Scharfer AI, eds. *Goldman-Cecil Medicine.* 26th ed. Elsevier; 2020.])

mandatory ventilation (SIMV) trial.[66] The method selected depends on the patient, their pulmonary status, and length of time on the ventilator. Regardless of the method selected, evidence shows that using a standardized approach decreases weaning time and length of stay in the critical care unit.[70]

BOX 19.5 Weaning Intolerance Indicators

- Decrease in level of consciousness
- Systolic blood pressure increased or decreased by 20 mm Hg
- Diastolic blood pressure greater than 100 mm Hg
- Heart rate increased by 20 beats/min
- Premature ventricular contractions greater than 6 per minute, couplets, or runs of ventricular tachycardia
- Changes in ST segment (usually elevation)
- Respiratory rate greater than 30 breaths/min or less than 10 breaths/min
- Respiratory rate increased by 10 breaths/min
- Spontaneous tidal volume less than 250 mL
- $PaCO_2$ increased by 5 to 8 mm Hg and/or pH less than 7.30
- SpO_2 less than 90%
- Use of accessory muscles of ventilation
- Complaints of dyspnea, fatigue, or pain
- Paradoxical chest wall motion or chest abdominal asynchrony
- Diaphoresis
- Severe agitation or anxiety unrelieved by reassurance

$PaCO_2$, Arterial carbon dioxide pressure; *SpO_2*, oxygen saturation as measured by pulse oximetry.

Spontaneous breathing trials. A SBT can be done with the patient either on or off the ventilator. One method is to remove the patient from the ventilator, placing them on a T-piece oxygen delivery system via the ETT or tracheostomy tube, and have the patient breathe spontaneously. Another method is to leave the patient on the ventilator and discontinue the mandatory breaths. When this is done, continuous positive airway pressure (CPAP) may be added to prevent atelectasis and improve oxygenation or pressure support may be added to augment inspiration.[69,71] One recommendation for the initial SBT for patients who have been mechanically ventilated for longer than 24 hours is the addition of 5 to 8 cm H_2O of pressure support.[72] A single daily SBT usually lasts from 30 minutes to 2 hours. During the weaning process, the patient is observed closely for respiratory muscle fatigue. If the trial is successful, extubation is considered. If the trial is unsuccessful, a period of rest is provided before another trial is attempted.[66,67,69] If the patient has been receiving mechanical ventilation for longer than 24 hours and is at high risk for extubation failure, the patient should be extubated and placed on NIV.[72]

Synchronized intermittent mandatory ventilation trials. The goal of SIMV weaning is the gradual transition from ventilatory support to spontaneous breathing. SIMV weaning is initiated by placing the ventilator in the SIMV mode and slowly decreasing the rate, usually one to three breaths at a time, until a rate of zero or near-zero is reached. An arterial blood gas (ABG) sample is usually obtained 30 minutes after the trial. This method of weaning can increase the work of breathing, and the patient must be closely monitored for signs of respiratory muscle fatigue.[66]

PATIENT-CENTERED CRITICAL CARE

Early Mobility on a Ventilator in the Critical Care Unit

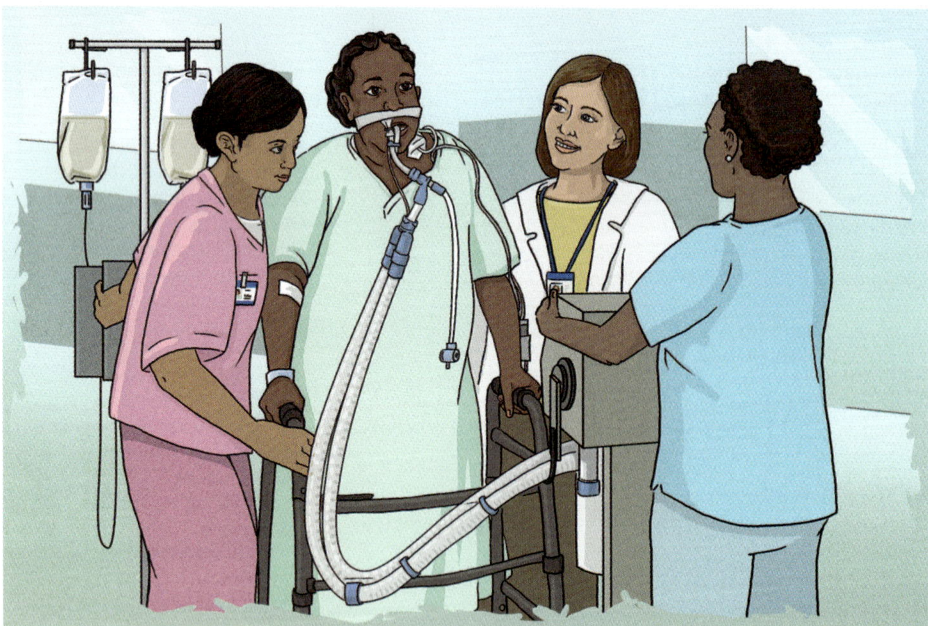

Exercise or "early mobility" is part of the ABCDEF program, which promotes an evidence-based approach to ventilator weaning. The letters stand for **A**irway; **B**reathing; Coordination of **C**are; **D**elirium prevention; **E**xercise, and **F**amily involvement.

Nurses should encourage patients to get out of bed to prevent loss of muscle mass and to prevent weakness related to immobility. Because of all the equipment, lines, and tubes, walking with a patient who is ventilated requires coordination by the bedside nurse and other health care professionals. This is always a cooperative team effort involving the skills of respiratory therapy, physiotherapy, nursing, and often family members.

There are many safety concerns to consider when walking with a patient who has an endotracheal tube or tracheostomy tube. The goal is to provide gradual exercise while avoiding adverse events such as a fall or self-extubation. Another benefit is that exercise during the day will promote better sleep at night and potentially reduce the risk of delirium for patients who are ventilator dependent.

Pressure support ventilation trials. PSV weaning consists of placing the patient on the pressure support mode and setting the pressure support at a level that facilitates the patient's achieving a spontaneous tidal volume of 10 to 12 mL/kg. PSV augments the patient's spontaneous breaths with a positive pressure boost during inspiration. During the weaning process, the level of pressure support is gradually decreased in increments of 3 to 6 cm H_2O, while the tidal volume is maintained at 10 to 15 mL/kg until a level of 5 cm H_2O is achieved. If the patient is able to maintain adequate spontaneous respirations at this level, extubation is considered. PSV also can be used with SIMV weaning to help overcome the resistance in the ventilator system.[66]

Nursing Management

Routine assessment of patients requiring mechanical ventilation includes monitoring for patient-related and ventilator-related complications.

Patient Assessment

Assessment of a patient requiring mechanical ventilation focuses on the pulmonary system, placement of the ETT or tracheostomy tube, and monitoring for the development of subcutaneous emphysema and dyssynchrony with the ventilator. Bedside evaluation of vital capacity, minute ventilation, ABG values, and other pulmonary function tests may be warranted, according to the patient's condition. The use of pulse oximetry can facilitate continuous, noninvasive assessment of oxygenation. The use of capnography may facilitate continuous noninvasive assessment of ventilation. Static and dynamic compliance are also monitored to assess for changes in lung compliance (see Appendix B).[73]

Symptom Management

Patients requiring mechanical ventilation may present with a variety of disturbing symptoms, including anxiety, pain, shortness of breath, confusion and agitation, and sleep disturbances. These symptoms are often managed with sedation and analgesic medications. As discussed earlier, these medications could contribute to prolonged mechanical ventilation and delirium. Nonpharmacologic interventions have been shown to be of benefit to these patients. These interventions include promoting a healing environment, promoting sleep, and interventions to lessen anxiety (e.g., music therapy, guided imagery, nursing presence, and animal-assisted therapy). Nursing activities to promote a healing environment include minimizing noise levels, ensuring the patient has access to natural light, establishing a method of communication with the patient, and providing the patient with explanations of what is occurring around them.[74] Referral to a complementary and alternative therapy specialist (if one is available) is also appropriate.

ABCDEF Bundle

Another bundle that has been proposed is the Awakening and Breathing Coordination, Delirium Monitoring, Early Mobility, and Family Engagement and Empowerment (ABCDEF) bundle. This bundle focuses on enhancing communication between team members in the critical care unit, standardizing patient care processes, and decreasing the incidence of delirium and prolonged weakness associated with critical illness.[75] The ABCDEF bundle activities are presented in Box 19.6. To facilitate the implementation of the ABCDEF bundle, the patient must be allowed to sleep. Box 19.7 discusses issues surrounding sleep disturbance in the critically ill patient.

Ventilator Assessment

Assessment of the ventilator includes a review of all the ventilator settings and alarms. A clear understanding of the alarms and their related problems is important (Box 19.8). Peak inspiratory pressure, exhaled tidal volume, and ABGs are also monitored.

Patient Safety

Several measures are required to maintain a trouble-free ventilator system. These include maintaining a functional MRB connected to oxygen at the bedside, ensuring that the ventilator tubing is free of water, positioning the ventilator tubing to avoid kinking, maintaining the patency of ventilator tubing and connections, changing ventilator tubing per hospital policy, and monitoring the temperature of the inspired air. If the ventilator malfunctions, the patient is removed from the ventilator and ventilated manually with an MRB. Alarms should be sufficiently audible with respect to distance and competing noise within the unit.

NONINVASIVE VENTILATION

NIV is an alternative method of ventilation that uses a mask instead of an ETT to deliver the therapy. Advantages of this type of ventilation include decreased frequency of hospital-acquired pneumonia; increased comfort; and the noninvasive nature of the procedure, which allows easy application and removal. NIV is indicated in type I and type II acute respiratory failure, cardiogenic pulmonary edema, and other situations in which intubation is not an option. Contraindications to NIV include hemodynamic instability; dysrhythmias; apnea; uncooperativeness; intolerance of the mask; recent upper airway or esophageal surgery; and inability to maintain a patent airway, clear secretions, or properly fit the mask.[76]

NIV can be applied with a full-face, nasal, or face mask and ventilator or with a bilevel positive airway pressure (BiPAP) machine. A recent meta-analysis found that 25% of the patients will develop pressure injuries secondary to the mask.[77] This type of ventilation uses a combination of PSV and PEEP supplied by a ventilator or inspiratory and expiratory positive airway pressure supplied by a BiPAP machine to assist the spontaneously breathing patient with ventilation. On inspiration, the patient receives PSV or inspiratory positive airway pressure to increase tidal volume and minute ventilation, resulting in increased alveolar ventilation, a decreased $PaCO_2$ level, relief of dyspnea, and reduced accessory muscle use. On expiration, the patient receives PEEP or expiratory positive airway pressure to increase functional residual capacity, resulting in an increased PaO_2 level. Humidified supplemental oxygen is administered to maintain a clinically acceptable PaO_2 level, and timed breaths may be added, if necessary.[78]

Nursing Management

Nursing interventions for the patient with noninvasive mechanical ventilation focus on evaluating the patient for patient-related complications and monitoring the patient for ventilator-related complications. Routine assessment of these patients includes monitoring for patient-related and ventilator-related complications. As with invasive mechanical ventilation, the patient must be closely monitored. Respiratory rate, accessory muscle use,

BOX 19.6 Patient-Centered Care

ABCDEF Bundle

Bedside Treatments for ABCDEF Protocol
Awakening & Breathing Coordination

ABC

SAT Safety Screen If passed the SAT safety screen, perform SAT	If passed the SAT, perform SBT safety screen If fail SAT → Restart sedatives if needed at ½ dose & titrate	If passed the SBT safety screen, perform SBT	If passed the SBT, team should consider extubation If fail → Return ventilator support to previous settings

D

Delirium Nonpharm Interventions

Pain: Monitor and/or manage pain using an objective scale

Orientation: Talk about day, date, place; discuss current events; provide caregiver names; use clock and calendar in room

Sensory: Determine need for hearing aids and/or eyeglasses

Sleep: Noise reduction, day-night variation, "time-out" to minimize interruptions of sleep, promoting comfort & relaxation (e.g., massage, daytime bath, back care, wash face/hands, oral care)

E

Early Exercise & Mobility

Perform Exercise Safety Screen. If passed, perform therapy at patient's highest level of ability.

1. Active range of motion exercises in bed and sitting position in bed
2. Dangling
3. Transfer to chair (active), includes standing without marching in place
4. Ambulation (marching in place, walking in room/hall)

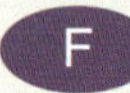

Family Engagement & Empowerment

1. Use simplified speech – Patients experiencing either delirium or other forms of cognitive impairment best understand both simple (noncomplex) sentences and basic (nonmedical) vocabulary.
2. Be concrete – Effective verbal communication with cognitively impaired patients should involve the use of concrete, readily understood language and an avoidance of abstract vocabulary, complicated metaphors, and colloquialisms.
3. Take your time – Rapid communication often prevents patients from comprehending what is being communicated, although communicating with patients in a way that fosters comprehension should be a primary goal.

SAT, Spontaneous awakening trial; *SBT*, spontaneous breathing trial.
Modified from ICU Delirium and Cognitive Impairment Study Group. Bedside treatments for ABCDE protocol. https://www.icudelirium.org/docs/ABCDEF_Pocket_Reference.pdf.

BOX 19.7 Patient-Centered Care

Sleep Promotion

Sleep disturbance in critically ill patients stems from various factors, including stress associated with critical illness and the critical care environment, pain, and muscular and joint discomfort resulting from bed rest. Bright nocturnal light, excessive noise, and frequent interruptions for care procedures may also disturb sleep in critically ill patients. Because a primary cause of sleep pattern disturbance in patients in the critical care unit is a state of heightened anxiety and discomfort, nursing interventions such as massage that promote relaxation and comfort may be effective. Providing a relaxed, caring environment that encourages confidence in care providers may also assist the patient to relax. Allowing close family members to sit quietly at the bedside while the patient rests may comfort the family and the patient and allow the patient to rest better. Nurses should limit interruptions for care procedures and should coordinate the care among other disciplines to allow patients time for consolidated nocturnal sleep and a daytime nap. Draperies or blinds should be opened during the day to allow patients to receive bright natural light and to help orient them to time of day; lights should be dimmed at night. Noise from staff, squeaky carts, alarms, televisions, slamming doors, and ringing phones should be minimized. Offering the patient earplugs or eye shields may help decrease noise, limit the effects of light, and promote sleep.

and oxygenation status are continually assessed to ensure that the patient is tolerating this method of ventilation. Continuous pulse oximetry is also used.[78]

The key to ensuring adequate ventilatory support is a properly fitted mask. A nasal mask, face mask, or full-face mask may be used, depending on the patient. A properly fitted mask minimizes air leakage and discomfort for the patient. Transparent dressings placed over the pressure points of the face help minimize air leakage and prevent facial pressure injuries caused by the mask.[79] The BiPAP machine can compensate for air leaks.[78]

The patient is positioned with the head of the bed elevated at 45 degrees to minimize the risk of aspiration and to facilitate breathing. Insufflation of the stomach is a complication of this mode of therapy and places the patient at risk for aspiration. The patient is closely monitored for gastric distention, and a nasogastric tube is placed for decompression, as necessary. Patients are often very anxious and have high levels of dyspnea before the initiation of noninvasive mechanical ventilation. After adequate ventilation has been established, anxiety and dyspnea are usually sufficiently relieved. Heavy sedation is avoided, but if it is needed, it would constitute the need for intubation and invasive mechanical ventilation. It is important to spend 30 minutes with the patient after initiation of

BOX 19.8 **Safety**

Troubleshooting Ventilator Alarms

Problem	Causes	Interventions
Low exhaled Vt	Altered settings; any condition that triggers high- or low-pressure alarm; patient stops spontaneous respirations; leak in system preventing Vt from being delivered; cuff insufficiently inflated; leak through chest tube; airway secretions; decreased lung compliance; spirometer disconnected or malfunctioning	Check settings; evaluate patient, check respiratory rate; check all connections for leaks; suction patient's airway; check cuff pressure; calibrate spirometer.
Low inspiratory pressure	Altered settings; unattached tubing or leak around ETT; ETT displaced into pharynx or esophagus; poor cuff inflation or leak; tracheoesophageal fistula; peak flows that are too low; low Vt; decreased airway resistance resulting from decreased secretions or relief of bronchospasm; increased lung compliance resulting from decreased atelectasis; reduction in pulmonary edema; resolution of ARDS; change in position	Reset alarm; reconnect tubing; modify cuff pressures; tighten humidifier; check chest tube; adjust peak flow to meet or exceed patient demand and correct for patient's Vt; reposition or change ETT.
Low exhaled minute volume	Altered settings; leak in system; airway secretions; decreased lung compliance; malfunctioning spirometer; decreased patient-triggered respiratory rate resulting from medications, sleep, hypocapnia, alkalosis, fatigue, change in neurologic status	Check settings; assess patient's respiratory rate, mental status, work of breathing; evaluate system for leaks; suction airway; assess patient for changes in disease state; calibrate spirometer.
Low PEEP/CPAP pressure	Altered settings; increased patient inspirator/flows; leak; decreased expiratory flows from ventilator	Check settings and correct; observe for leaks in system; if unable to correct problem, increase PEEP settings.
High respiratory rate	Increased metabolic demand; medication administration; hypoxia; hypercapnia; acidosis; shock; pain; fear; anxiety	Evaluate ABGs; assess patient; calm and reassure patient.
High-pressure limit	Improper alarm setting; airway obstruction resulting from patient fighting ventilator (holding breath as ventilator delivers Vt); patient circuit collapse; tubing kinked; ETT in right mainstem bronchus or against carina; cuff herniation; increased airway resistance resulting from bronchospasm, airway secretions, plugs, and coughing; water from humidifier in ventilator tubing; decreased lung compliance resulting from tension pneumothorax, change in patient position, ARDS, pulmonary edema, atelectasis, pneumonia, or abdominal distention	Reset alarms; clear obstruction from tubing; unkink and reposition patient off of tubing; empty water from tubing; check breath sounds; reassure patient and sedate if necessary; check ABGs for hypoxemia; observe for abdominal distention that would put pressure on diaphragm; check cuff pressures; obtain chest radiograph and evaluate for ETT position, pneumothorax, and pneumonia; reposition ETT; give bronchodilator therapy.
Low-pressure oxygen inlet	Improper oxygen alarm setting; oxygen not connected to ventilator; dirty oxygen intake filter	Correct alarm setting; reconnect or connect oxygen line to 50-psi source; clean or replace oxygen filter.
I:E ratio	Inspiratory time longer than expiratory time; use of an inspiratory phase that is too long with a fast rate; peak flow setting too low, whereas rate too high; machine too sensitive	Change inspiratory time or adjust peak flow; check inspiratory phase, or hold; check machine sensitivity.
Temperature	Sensor malfunction; overheating resulting from too low or no gas flow; sensor picking up outside airflow (from heater, open door or window, air conditioner); improper water levels	Test or replace sensor; check gas flow; protect sensor from outside source that would interfere with readings; check water levels.

ABGs, Arterial blood gases; *ARDS,* acute respiratory distress syndrome; *CPAP,* continuous positive airway pressure; *ETT,* endotracheal tube; *I:E,* inspiratory to expiratory; *PEEP,* positive end-expiratory pressure; *Vt,* tidal volume.
Modified from Flynn JBM, Bruce NP. *Introduction to Critical Care Nursing Skills.* Mosby; 1993.

NIV, because the patient needs reassurance and must learn how to breathe on the machine.[78] The patient who requires NIV with a face mask should never be restrained. The patient must be able to remove the mask if it becomes displaced or the patient vomits. A displaced mask can force the patient's bottom jaw inward and occlude the patient's airway.

POSITIONING THERAPY

Positioning therapy can help match ventilation and perfusion through the redistribution of oxygen and blood flow in the lungs, which improves gas exchange. On the basis of the concept that preferential blood flow occurs to the gravity-dependent areas of the lungs, positioning therapy is used to place the least damaged portion of the lungs into a dependent position. The least damaged portions of the lungs receive preferential blood flow, resulting in less $(\dot{V}/\dot{Q})$ mismatch. Two approaches to position therapy are (1) prone positioning and (2) rotation therapy.

Prone Positioning

Prone positioning is a therapeutic modality that is used to improve oxygenation in patients with ARDS.[80–82] It involves turning the patient completely over onto their stomach in the face-down position. Although numerous theories have been proposed to explain how prone positioning improves oxygenation, the discovery that ARDS causes greater damage to the dependent areas of the lungs probably provides the best explanation. It was originally thought that ARDS was a diffuse, homogeneous disease that affected all areas of the lungs equally. It is now known that the dependent lung areas are more heavily damaged than the nondependent lung areas. Turning the patient to the prone position improves perfusion to the less damaged areas of the lungs, improves $(\dot{V}/\dot{Q})$ match, and decreases intrapulmonary shunting.[80–82] Prone positioning can be used to facilitate the mobilization of secretions[80] and provide pressure relief. Prone positioning is contraindicated in patients with increased intracranial pressure, hemodynamic instability, spinal cord injuries, or abdominal surgery. Patients who are unable to tolerate the face-down position are also not appropriate candidates for this type of therapy.[80]

No standard has been established for the length of time a patient should remain in the prone position. A review of the research on this subject revealed a wide variation ranging from 6 to 20 hours.[82] However, a recent meta-analysis found that prone positioning is likely to decrease mortality in patients with severe ARDS when applied for at least 12 hours daily.[83] The positioning schedule (length of time in the prone position and frequency of turning) is usually based on the patient's tolerance of the procedure, the success of the procedure in improving the patient's PaO_2, and whether the patient is able to sustain improvements in PaO_2 when turned back to the supine position. Prone positioning is discontinued when the patient no longer demonstrates a response to the position change.

The biggest limitation to prone positioning is the actual mechanics of turning the patient. Numerous methods have been discussed in the literature, including manually turning the patient and positioning with pillows to support the patient and use of the RotoProne therapy system (ArjoHuntleigh, Sweden) (Fig. 19.15). Regardless of the method used, the abdomen must be allowed to hang free to facilitate diaphragmatic descent.[80]

Before the patient is turned to the prone position, their eyes are lubricated and taped closed, tubes and drains are secured, and the procedure is explained to the patient and family (Box 19.9). A team is organized to implement the turning procedure, and one member is positioned at the head of the bed to maintain the patient's airway. Complications of the procedure include dislodgment or obstruction of tubes and drains, hemodynamic instability, massive facial edema, pressure injuries (Box 19.10), aspiration, and corneal ulcerations.[80,81,84]

Rotation Therapy

Automated turning beds to provide rotation therapy are often used in the critical care setting. Kinetic therapy and continuous lateral rotation therapy (CLRT) are two forms of rotation therapy. The patient is continuously turned from side to side with a rotation of 40 degrees or greater (kinetic therapy) or with a rotation of less than 40 degrees (CLRT).[85] Two types of beds can perform this type of therapy: (1) an oscillation bed, in which the mattress inflates and deflates to provide rotation, and (2) a kinetic bed, in which the entire platform of the bed rotates.

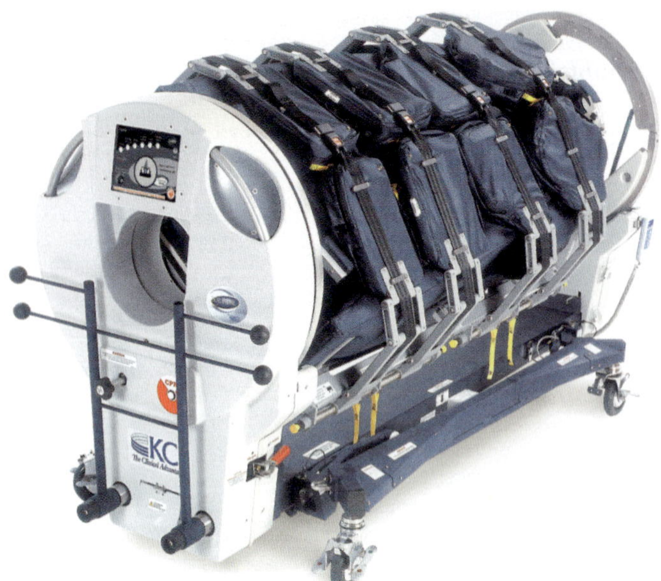

FIG. 19.15 RotoProne Therapy System. (Courtesy Kinetic Concepts, Inc., San Antonio, TX. RotoProne is a trademark of the Arjo Huntleigh group of companies.)

Rotation therapy is thought to improve oxygenation through better matching of ventilation to perfusion and to prevent pulmonary complications associated with bed rest and mechanical ventilation.[85] However, there is very limited evidence to support this supposition[85] and currently this therapy is not recommended for the prevention of VAP.[31]

Complications of the procedure include dislodgment or obstruction of tubes, drains, and lines; hemodynamic instability; and pressure injuries. Lateral rotation does not replace manual repositioning to prevent pressure injuries. Repositioning changes the relationship of the patient's posterior surface to the mattress. This gives the skin a chance to reperfuse and to ventilate. Repositioning shifts weight-bearing points. To prevent pressure injuries, the patient is positioned 30 degrees from the surface of the mattress regardless of the degree of rotational turn.

THORACIC SURGERY

The term *thoracic surgery* refers to numerous surgical procedures that involve opening the thoracic cavity (thoracotomy), the organs of respiration, or both. Indications for thoracic surgery range from tumors and abscesses to repair of the esophagus and thoracic vessels.[86] Table 19.6 describes various thoracic surgical procedures and their indications. This discussion focuses only on the surgical procedures that involve the removal of lung tissue.

Preoperative Care

Before surgery, a complete evaluation of the patient is needed to determine the appropriateness of surgery as a treatment and to determine whether lung tissue can be removed without jeopardizing respiratory function. This is especially important when

BOX 19.9 Safety

ABCDEFG of Prone Positioning

		Before Prone Positioning	After Prone Positioning
A	Attachments	Disconnect attachments such as ECG electrodes, oxygen saturation probe, end-tidal carbon dioxide probe, temperature probe, and noninvasive blood pressure cuff.	Reattach the disconnected attachments.
B	Bedding	Keep another bed sheet ready for replacement.	Check the bedding for any inappropriate item that might hurt, for example, an inappropriate fold in the sheet, bumps, needle caps.
C	Catheters	The horizontal movement should be to the side with central venous catheters, detach infusions if necessary. Be careful with dialysis and arterial catheters. Ensure adequate slack in infusion lining.	Check position, reattach infusions.
D	Dependent regions	Pad-dependent regions, which are common sites of pressure sores, such as forehead, chin, and knee, with adhesive pads.	Padding may get displaced while rotating; ensure position after prone positioning.
E	Endotracheal tube	Mark the position of the endotracheal tube. Secure the tube throughout the movement. Ensure adequate slack in the ventilator tubings.	Confirm position by noting down the mark.
F	Foley Catheter	Foley catheter with the urine bag should be detached from the side of the bed and should be kept between the legs.	Attach on either side.
G	Genitals	Genitals need special attention, as these can be an ignored site of pressure sores.	

ECG, Electrocardiogram.
From Baldi, M, Sehgal IS, Dhorria S, Agarwal R. Prone positioning? Remember ABCDEFG. *Chest*. 2017;151(5):1184–1185.

a lobectomy or pneumonectomy is being considered. When resection is being undertaken for tumor treatment, preoperative care includes evaluation of the type and extent of the tumor and the physical condition of the patient.[87]

The evaluation of the patient's physical status focuses on the adequacy of cardiopulmonary function. The preoperative evaluation includes pulmonary function tests to determine the patient's ability to manage with less lung tissue. Cardiac function is also evaluated. Uncontrolled dysrhythmias, acute myocardial infarction, severe chronic heart failure, and unstable angina all are contraindications to surgery.[88]

BOX 19.10 Quality Improvement

Prevention of Hospital-Acquired Pressure Injury in the Prone Patient

Patients undergoing prone positioning are at risk for several complications, including hospital-acquired pressure injuries. Once the patient is placed in the prone position, they may remain there for 18 hours or longer, depending on the proning protocol. Sustained periods in this position place the patient at risk of pressure damage. Areas at high risk include the patient's head (i.e., forehead, nose, cheeks, and chin), torso (i.e., clavicle, breasts, iliac crests, ischium, symphysis pubis, and genitalia), and arms and legs (i.e., shoulders, elbows, knees, feet, and toes).[1]

Assessment is vital in preventing pressure injuries, particularly watching for uneven pressure redistribution. The patient's skin should be assessed regularly and before turning either supine or prone. It is important to document a comprehensive skin assessment at regular intervals. The patient's skin should be kept clean and moisturized.

If manually proning the patient, a pressure redistribution surface (e.g., mattress or overlay) should be used along with positioning devices to offload pressure to high-risk areas. While in the prone position, minor position adjustments can be performed. The patient's arms and head should be placed in the freestyle swim position. In this position, one arm is placed at the patient's side and the other is placed next to the head. The patient's head is then turned toward the arm. The position of the patient's arms and head is routinely alternated at least every 4 hours, allowing for pressure relief. Additional prophylactic measures that can be taken include the application of:[1]

- Soft silicone multi-layered form dressings to the high-risk pressure areas.
- Thin foam dressings under medical devices
- Liquid skin sealants on the face to protect from excessive moisture and oral secretions
- Foam positioning devices to offload pressure to the patient's head and feet

It is essential to follow the manufacturer's instructions when using positioning devices, dressings, and other products. For more information about pressure injuries, check out the National Pressure Injury Advisory Panel (NPIAP) website (www.npiap.com).

Reference

1. National Pressure Injury Advisory Panel. *Pressure Injury Prevention: PIP Tips for Prone Positioning*; 2020. https://cdn.ymaws.com/npiap.com/resource/resmgr/press_releases/npiap_pip_tips_-_proning_202.pdf.

Surgical Considerations

The type and location of surgery dictate the type of surgical approach that is used. The most common approach is the posterolateral thoracotomy, which allows for exposure of both the lung and the mediastinum. Other approaches that are used include anterolateral thoracotomy and median sternotomy.[86]

Special care is taken to avoid drainage of blood or secretions into the unaffected lung during surgery (Fig. 19.16), because such an occurrence could cause hypoxemia and cardiac dysfunction. A double-lumen ETT is used during surgery to protect the unaffected lung from secretions and necrotic tumor fragments. To decrease the incidence of hypoxemia during the procedure, 5 to 10 cm H_2O of PEEP is maintained to the deflated lung. In addition, the deflated lung is intermittently ventilated during the procedure.[89]

Complications and Medical Management

Many complications are associated with a lung resection, including acute respiratory failure, bronchopleural fistula, hemorrhage, cardiovascular disturbances, and mediastinal shift.

TABLE 19.6 Thoracic Surgeries

Procedure	Definition	Indications
Pneumonectomy 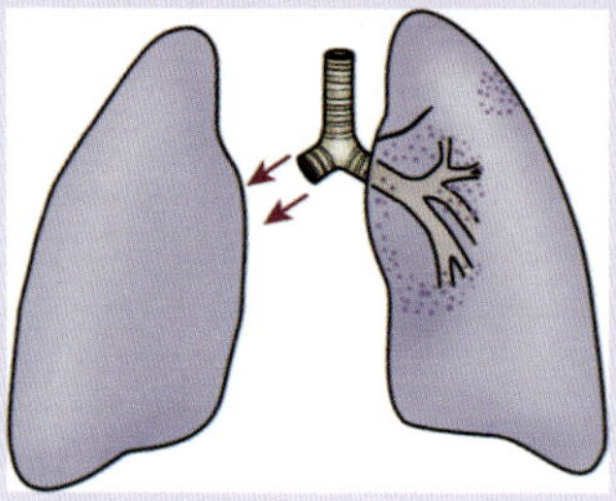	Removal of entire lung with or without resection of mediastinal lymph nodes	Malignant lesions Unilateral tuberculosis Extensive unilateral bronchiectasis Multiple lung abscesses Massive hemoptysis Bronchopleural fistula
Lobectomy 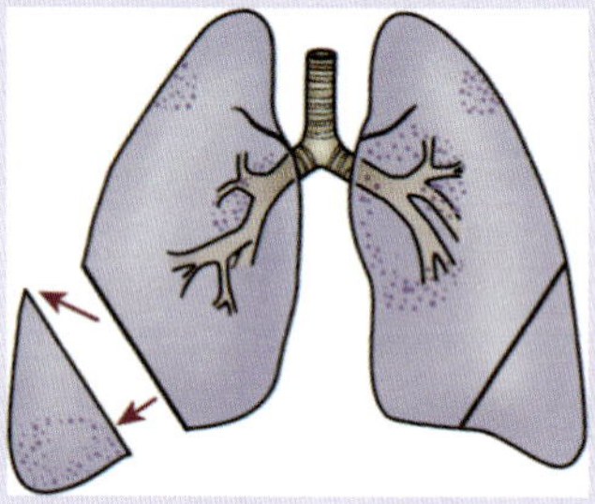	Resection of one or more lobes of lung	Lesions confined to single lobe Pulmonary tuberculosis Bronchiectasis Lung abscesses or cysts Trauma
Segmental resection 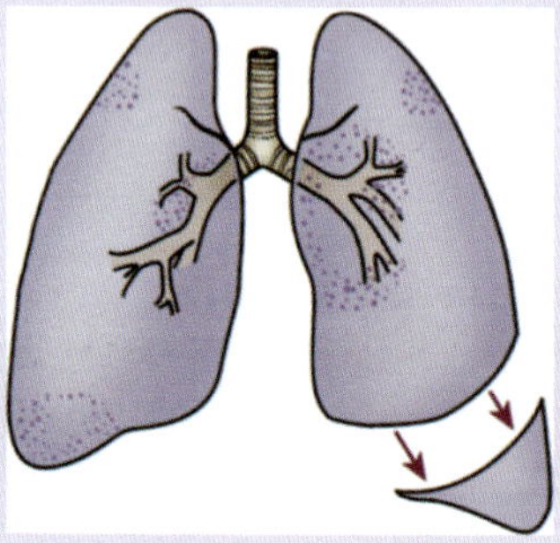	Resection of bronchovascular section of lung lobe	Small peripheral lesions Bronchiectasis Congenital cysts or blebs
Wedge resection 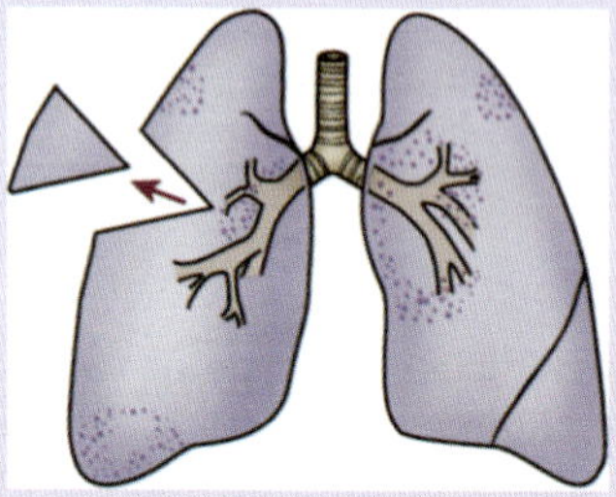	Removal of small wedge-shaped section of lung tissue	Small, peripheral lesions (without lymph node involvement) Peripheral granulomas Pulmonary blebs
Bronchoplastic reconstruction (also called *sleeve resection*) 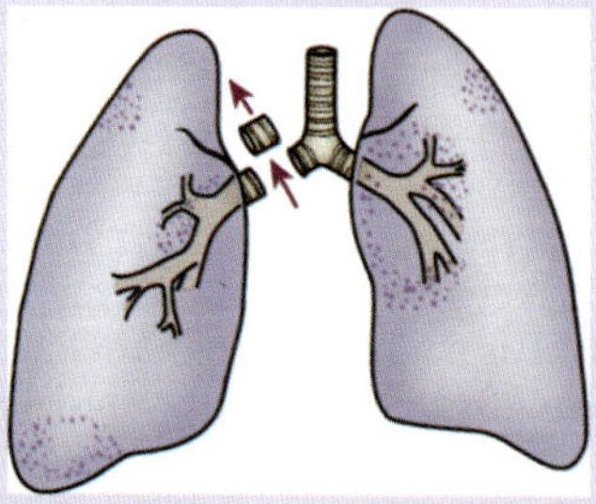	Resection of lung tissue and bronchus with end-to-end reanastomosis of bronchus	Small lesions involving carina or major bronchus without evidence of metastasis May be combined with lobectomy
Lung volume reduction surgery	Resection of most damaged portions of lung tissue, allowing more normal chest wall configuration	Severe emphysema

TABLE 19.6 Thoracic Surgeries—cont'd

Procedure	Definition	Indications
Bullectomy	Resection of large bulla (airspace that is >1 cm in diameter that formed as a result of pulmonary tissue destruction)	Severe emphysema with large bullae compressing surrounding tissue
Open lung biopsy	Resection of small portion of lung for biopsy	Failure of closed lung biopsy Removal of small lesions
Decortication	Removal of fibrous membrane from pleural surface of lung	Fibrothorax resulting from hemothorax or empyema
Drainage of empyema	Drainage of pus in pleural space	Acute and chronic infections
Partial rib resection	Removal of one or more ribs to allow healing of underlying lung tissue	Chronic empyemic infections
VATS	Endoscopic procedure performed through small incisions in chest	Evaluation of pulmonary, pleural, mediastinal, or pericardial conditions Biopsy of lung, pleural, or mediastinal lesions Recurrent spontaneous pneumothorax Evacuation of emphysema, hemothorax, pleural effusion, or pericardial effusion Blebectomy or bullectomy Pleurodesis Sympathectomy Closure of bronchopleural fistula Lysis of adhesions

VATS, Video-assisted thoracoscopy.

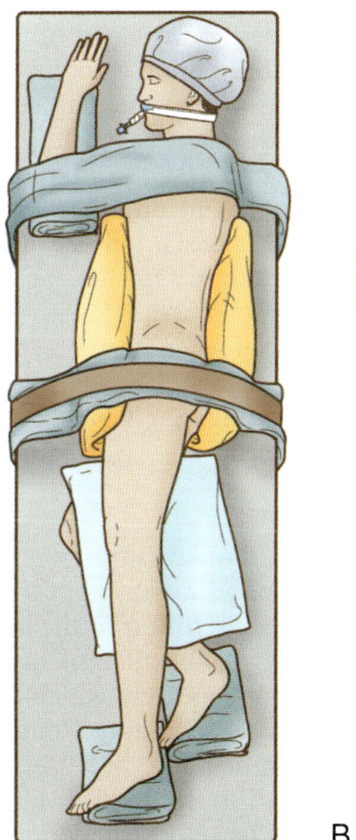

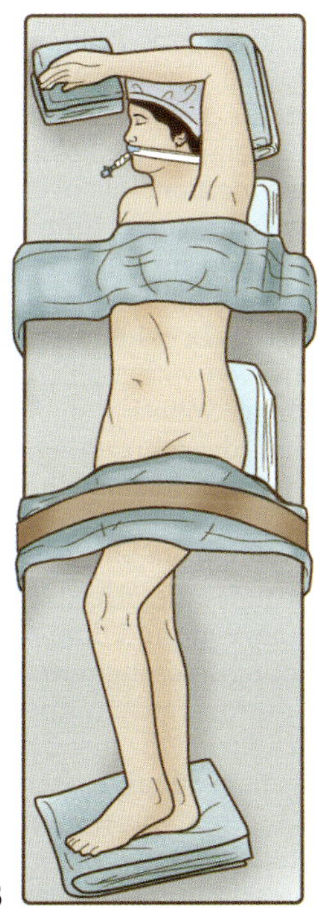

FIG. 19.16 Positions for Thoracotomy Incisions. (A) Lateral position for posterolateral incision. (B) Semilateral position for axillary or anterolateral position. (From Rothrock JC, ed. *Alexander's Care of the Patient in Surgery*. 16th ed. Elsevier; 2019.)

Acute Respiratory Failure

In the postoperative period, acute respiratory failure may result from atelectasis or pneumonia. Atelectasis can occur because of anesthesia, the surgical procedure, immobilization, and pain. Treatment is aimed at correcting the underlying problems and supporting gas exchange. Supplemental oxygen and mechanical ventilation with PEEP may be necessary.[90]

Bronchopleural Fistula

Development of a postoperative bronchopleural fistula is a major cause of mortality after a lung resection. A bronchopleural fistula develops when the suture line fails to secure occlusion of the bronchial stump and an opening develops into the pleural space.[91] This can result from an imperfect stump closure, perforation of the stump (e.g., with a suction catheter), high pressure within the airways (e.g., caused by mechanical ventilation), or infection.[92] During surgery, careful attention is given to isolating and closing the bronchus in an attempt to secure a lasting seal with subsequent stump healing.[86] In addition, early extubation is encouraged to eliminate the possibility of perforation of the stump and high airway pressures.[92] Clinical manifestations of a bronchopleural fistula include shortness of breath and coughing up serosanguineous sputum. Immediate surgery is usually necessary to close the stump and prevent flooding of the remaining lung with fluid from the residual space. If this occurs, the patient is placed with the operative side down (remaining lung up), and a chest tube is inserted to drain the residual space.[86]

Hemorrhage

Hemorrhage is an early, life-threatening complication that can occur after a lung resection and can result from bronchial or intercostal artery bleeding or disruption of a suture or clip around a pulmonary vessel.[92] Excessive chest tube drainage can signal the presence of this complication. During the immediate postoperative period, chest tube drainage is measured every 15 minutes; this frequency is decreased as the patient stabilizes. If chest tube drainage is greater than 100 mL/h, fresh blood is noted, or a sudden increase in drainage occurs, hemorrhage should be suspected.

Cardiovascular Disturbances

Cardiovascular complications after thoracic surgery include dysrhythmias and pulmonary edema. Resections of a large lung area or a pneumonectomy may be followed by an increase in central venous pressure. With the loss of one lung, the right ventricle must empty its stroke volume into a vascular bed that has been reduced by 50%. This means a higher pressure system is created, which increases right ventricular workload and precipitates right ventricular failure. Depending on previous heart function, acute decompensation of both ventricles can result. Measures are aimed at supporting cardiac function and avoiding intravascular volume excess. These measures include optimizing preload, afterload, and contractility with vasoactive agents.

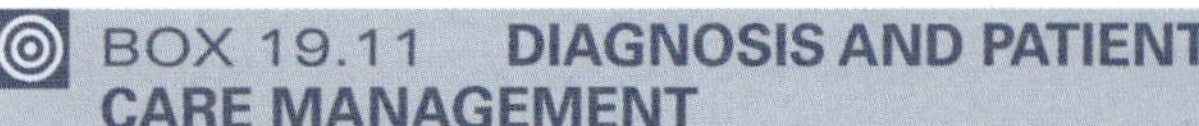

BOX 19.11 DIAGNOSIS AND PATIENT CARE MANAGEMENT

Thoracic Surgery

- Impaired Breathing due to decreased lung expansion
- Impaired Gas Exchange due to ventilation-perfusion mismatching or intrapulmonary shunting
- Impaired Gas Exchange due to alveolar hypoventilation
- Acute Pain due to transmission and perception of cutaneous, visceral, muscular, or ischemic impulses
- Anxiety due to threat to biologic, psychological, or social integrity

Patient Care Management plans are located in Appendix A.

Postoperative Nursing Management

Nursing care of a patient who has had thoracic surgery incorporates many patient problems (Box 19.11). Nursing interventions include optimizing oxygenation and ventilation, preventing atelectasis, maintaining the chest tube system, assisting the patient to return to an adequate activity level, providing comfort and emotional support, and maintaining surveillance for complications.

Optimizing Oxygenation and Ventilation

Nursing interventions to optimize oxygenation and ventilation include positioning, preventing desaturation during procedures, and promoting secretion clearance.

Preventing Atelectasis

Nursing interventions to prevent atelectasis include proper patient positioning and early ambulation, deep-breathing exercises, incentive spirometry, and pain management. The goal is to promote maximal lung ventilation and prevent hypoventilation.

Patient positioning and early ambulation. When positioning the patient, the nurse considers the surgical incision site and the type of surgery. After a lobectomy, the patient is turned onto the nonoperative side to promote ($\dot{V}/\dot{Q}$) matching. When the good lung is dependent and blood flow is greater to the area with better ventilation, ($\dot{V}/\dot{Q}$) matching is better. ($\dot{V}/\dot{Q}$) mismatching results when the affected lung is positioned down because of the increase in blood flow to an area with less ventilation. The patient is turned frequently to promote secretion removal but should have the affected lung dependent as little as possible. A patient who has had a pneumonectomy is positioned supine or on the operative side during the initial period. Turning onto the operative side promotes splinting of the incision and facilitates deep-breathing exercises. Tilting the patient slightly toward the unaffected side is possible, but the surgeon should indicate when free side-to-side positioning is safe.

When sitting at the bedside or ambulating, patients must be encouraged to keep the thorax in straight alignment while they breathe deeply. This position best accommodates diaphragmatic descent and intercostal muscle action. The sitting or standing position provides enhanced ventilation to areas of the lung that are dependent in the supine position, accommodating maximal inflation and promoting gas exchange. Ambulation is essential in restoring lung function and is initiated as soon as possible.[90]

Deep breathing and incentive spirometry. Deep breathing and incentive spirometry are performed regularly by patients who have undergone a thoracotomy. Deep breathing involves having the patient take a deep breath and holding the breath for approximately 3 seconds or longer. Incentive spirometry involves having the patient take at least 10 deep, effective breaths per hour using an incentive spirometer. These activities help reexpand collapsed lung tissue, promoting early resolution of the pneumothorax in patients with partial lung resections. The chest is auscultated during inflation to ensure that all dependent parts of the lung are well ventilated and to help the patient understand the depth of breath necessary for optimal effect. Coughing, which is encouraged only when secretions are present, assists in mobilizing secretions for removal.[93]

Pain management. Pain can be a significant problem after thoracic surgery. Pain can increase the workload of the heart, precipitate hypoventilation, and inhibit mobilization of secretions. Clinical manifestations of pain include tachypnea, tachycardia, elevated blood pressure, facial grimacing, splinting of the incision, hypoventilation, moaning, and restlessness. Several alternatives for pain management after thoracic surgery can be used including epidural anesthesia, topical anesthetics, and oral antiinflammatory medications. Opioids are generally avoided.[90] In addition, the patient is assisted with splinting the incision with a pillow or blanket when deep breathing and coughing. Splinting stabilizes the area and reduces pain when moving, deep breathing, or coughing. See Chapter 7 for in-depth discussion of pain management.

Maintaining the Chest Tube System

Chest tubes are placed after most thoracic surgery procedures to remove air and fluid. The drainage initially appears bloody, becoming serosanguineous and then serous over the first 2 to 3 days postoperatively. Approximately 100 to 300 mL of drainage occurs during the first 2 hours postoperatively, which decreases to less than 50 mL/h over the next several hours. Routine stripping of chest tubes is not recommended, because excessive negative pressure can be generated in the chest. If blood clots are present in the drainage tubing or an obstruction is present, the chest tubes may be carefully milked. The chest tube may be placed to suction or water seal.[94]

During auscultation of the lungs, air leaks are evaluated. In the early phase, an air leak is commonly heard over the affected area because the pleura has not yet tightly sealed. As healing occurs, this leak should disappear. An increase in an air leak or the appearance of a new air leak warrants prompt investigation of the chest drainage system to discover whether air is leaking into the system from outside or whether the leak is originating from the incision. Increased air leaks not related to the thoracic drainage system may indicate disruption of sutures.[90]

Assisting the Patient to Return to Adequate Activity Level

Within a few days after surgery, range-of-motion exercises for the shoulder on the operative side are performed. The patient frequently splints the operative side and avoids shoulder movement because of pain. If immobility is allowed, stiffening of the shoulder joint can result. This is referred to as *frozen shoulder* and may require physical therapy and rehabilitation to regain satisfactory range of motion of the shoulder joint.

The patient is usually able to sit in a chair the day after surgery. Activity is systematically increased, with attention to the patient's activity tolerance. With adequate pulmonary function before surgery and a surgical approach designed to preserve respiratory function, full return to previous activity levels is possible. This may take 6 months to 1 year, depending on the tissue resected and the patient's general condition.

PHARMACOLOGY

Numerous pharmacologic agents are used in the care of a critically ill patient with pulmonary dysfunction. Table 19.7 reviews these agents and the special considerations necessary for administering them.

TABLE 19.7 PHARMACOLOGIC MANAGEMENT

Pulmonary Disorders

Medication	Dosage	Actions	Special Considerations
NMBAs			
Vecuronium (Norcuron)	Loading dose: 0.08–0.1 mg/kg IV IV infusion: 0.8–1.2 mcg/kg/min	Used to paralyze patient to decrease oxygen demand and avoid ventilator dyssynchrony	*Boxed Warning From FDA:* Risk of anaphylactic and anaphylactoid-type adverse reactions, including fatalities reported in association with use of neuromuscular blockers. Administer sedative and analgesic agents concurrently, because NMBAs have no sedative or analgesic properties. Evaluate level of paralysis q4h using peripheral nerve stimulator. Protect patients from environment because they are unable to respond. Prolonged muscle paralysis may occur after discontinuation of paralytic agent.
Pancuronium (Pavulon)	Loading dose: 0.06–0.1 mg/kg IV IV infusion: 0.02–0.04 mg/kg/h		
Rocuronium (Zemuron)	Loading dose: 0.6–1.2 mg/kg IV IV infusion: 10–12 mcg/kg/min		
Atracurium (Tracrium)	Loading dose: 0.30–0.50 mg/kg IV IV infusion: 4–12 mcg/kg/min		
Cisatracurium (Nimbex)	Loading dose: 0.15–0.2 mg/kg IV IV infusion: 0.5–10.2 mcg/kg/min		
Mucolytics			
Acetylcysteine (Mucomyst)	Nebulizer, 20% solution: 3–5 mL tid-qid Nebulizer, 10% solution: 6–10 mL tid-qid	Used to decrease viscosity and elasticity of mucus by breaking down disulfide bonds within mucus	May be administered with a bronchodilator because medication can cause bronchospasms and inhibit ciliary function. Treatment considered effective when bronchorrhea develops and coughing occurs. Antidote for acetaminophen overdose.
Beta-2 Agonists			
Epinephrine (Adrenalin)	Nebulizer, 1% solution: 2.5–5 mg (0.25–0.5 mL) qid	Used to relax bronchial smooth muscle and dilate airways to prevent bronchospasms	May cause skeletal muscle tremors.
Racemic epinephrine	Nebulizer, 2.25% solution: 5.625–11.25 mg (0.25–0.5 mL) qid		Higher doses may cause tachycardia, palpitations, increased blood pressure, dysrhythmias, and angina.
Isoetharine 1% (Bronkosol)	Nebulizer, 1% solution: 2.5–5 mg (0.25–0.5 mL) qid		May increase serum glucose and decrease serum potassium levels.
Terbutaline	MDI, 340 mcg/puff: 1–2 puffs qid MDI, 200 mcg/puff: 2 puffs q4–6 h		Treatment considered effective when breath sounds improve and dyspnea is lessened.
Metaproterenol (Alupent, Metaprel)	Nebulizer, 5% solution: 15 mg (0.3 mL) tid-qid MDI, 650 mcg/puff: 2–3 puffs tid-qid		Only approximately 10% of administered dose reaches the site of action within the lungs.
Albuterol (Proventil, Ventolin)	Nebulizer, 5% solution: 2.5 mg (0.5 mL) tid-qid MDI, 90 mcg/puff: 2 puffs tid-qid		
Levalbuterol (Xopenex)	Nebulizer: 0.63 mg q6–8 h		

Continued

TABLE 19.7 PHARMACOLOGIC MANAGEMENT—cont'd

Pulmonary Disorders

Medication	Dosage	Actions	Special Considerations
Anticholinergic Agents			
Ipratropium (Atrovent)	Nebulizer, 0.02% solution: 0.5 mg (2.5 mL) q6–8 h	Used to block constriction of bronchial smooth muscle and reduce mucus production	There are relatively few adverse effects, because systemic absorption is poor.
Xanthines			
Theophylline	Loading dose: 4.6 mg/kg IV IV infusion: 0.4–0.8 mg/kg/h	Used to dilate bronchial smooth muscle and reverse diaphragmatic muscle fatigue	Administer loading dose over 30 minutes. Monitor serum blood levels; therapeutic level is 10–20 mg/dL.
Aminophylline	Loading dose: 5.7 mg/kg IV IV infusion: 0.5–1 mg/kg/h		Administer with caution to patients with cardiac, renal, or hepatic disease. Signs of toxicity include central nervous system excitation, seizures, confusion, irritability, hyperglycemia, headache, nausea, hypotension, and dysrhythmias.
Inhaled Corticosteroids			
Beclomethasone (Vanceril, Beclovent)	MDI, 42 mcg/puff: 2 puffs tid-qid	Used to decrease airway inflammation and enhance effectiveness of beta agonists	Suppresses inflammatory response and interferes with ability to fight infection.
Flunisolide (AeroBid)	MDI, 250 mcg/puff: 2 puffs bid		Oral candidiasis is a side effect that can be minimized by having patients rinse their mouths after treatment.
Triamcinolone (Azmacort)	MDI, 100 mcg/puff: 2 puffs tid-qid		

FDA, U.S. Food and Drug Agency; *IV*, intravenous/intravenously; *MDI*, metered-dose inhaler; *NMBAs*, neuromuscular blocking agents; *qid*, four times a day; *tid*, three times a day.
Data from ClinicalKey Drug Monographs.

Bronchodilators and Adjuncts

Medications to facilitate removal of secretions and dilate airways are of major benefit in the treatment of pulmonary disorders. Mucolytics are administered to help liquefy mucus secretions, which facilitates their removal. Bronchodilators such as $beta_2$ agonists and anticholinergic agents aid in smooth muscle relaxation and are of particular benefit to patients with airflow limitations. Steroids are often used in conjunction with $beta_2$ agonists to enhance their effects and to decrease airway inflammation.[95-97]

Neuromuscular Blocking Agents

Sedation is necessary in many patients to assist with maintaining adequate ventilation. Sedation can be used to comfort the patient and to decrease the work of breathing, particularly if the patient is fighting the ventilator. More information about sedation is provided in Chapter 8. In some patients, sedation does not decrease spontaneous respiratory efforts enough to allow adequate ventilation, and patient–ventilator dyssynchrony may develop. Neuromuscular paralysis may be necessary to facilitate optimal ventilation. Paralysis also may be necessary to decrease oxygen consumption in a patient who is severely compromised.[99,100]

The nursing management plan for a patient receiving a neuromuscular blocking agent incorporates many additional interventions. Because paralytic agents only halt skeletal muscle movement and do not inhibit pain or awareness, they must be administered with a sedative or anxiolytic agent. Pain medication is administered if the patient has a pain-producing illness or surgery. Providing reorientation and explanations for all procedures is crucial because the patient can still hear but cannot move or see. The patient is also at high risk for developing the complications of immobility, so interventions related to the prevention of skin breakdown, atelectasis, and deep vein thrombosis are also implemented. Patient safety is another concern because the patient cannot react to the environment. Special precautions are taken to protect the patient at all times.[101]

Peripheral Nerve Stimulator

Long-term use of neuromuscular blocking agents can result in prolonged neuromuscular blockade and skeletal muscle weakness. To avoid this complication, the patient's level of paralysis is carefully monitored with the use of a peripheral nerve stimulator (PNS). The PNS delivers an electrical stimulus (single twitch, posttetanic count, double-burst stimulation, or train-of-four [TOF]) to a preselected nerve (ulnar, facial, posterior tibial, or peroneal) by electrodes (needle, ball, or pregelled), and the response is monitored to gauge the level of paralysis.[101]

In most cases, the ulnar nerve is used, with pregelled electrodes placed 2 to 3 inches proximal to the crease of the wrist (Fig. 19.17). The TOF stimulation test, which delivers four electrical stimuli in a row, is the most common test used. When the ulnar nerve is stimulated with TOF, the expected response is four twitches (adduction) of the thumb medially across the palm of the hand. The number of twitches correlates with the level of paralysis: four twitches indicate less than 75% blockade; three twitches, approximately 75% blockade; two twitches, approximately 80% blockade; one twitch, approximately 90% blockade; and no twitch, 100% blockade. The neuromuscular blocking agent usually is titrated to maintain an 80% blockade

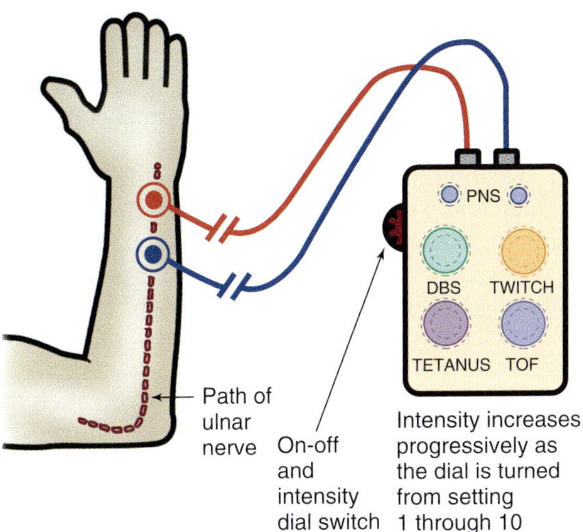

FIG. 19.17 Peripheral Nerve Stimulator (PNS). Note placement of electrodes along the ulnar nerve. *DBS*, Double-burst stimulation; *TOF*, train-of-four.

BOX 19.12 Internet Resources

Pulmonary Therapeutic Management

- American Association of Critical-Care Nurses (ACCN): www.aacn.org
- American Association of Respiratory Care (AARC): www.aarc.org
- American College of Chest Physicians (ACCP): www.chestnet.org
- American College of Physicians (ACP): www.acponline.org
- American College of Surgeons (ACS): www.facs.org
- American Holistic Nurses Association (AHNA): www.ahna.org
- American Lung Association: www.lung.org
- American Medical Association (AMA): www.ama-assn.org
- American Thoracic Society (ATS): www.thoracic.org
- Centers for Disease Control and Prevention (CDC): www.cdc.gov
- Critical Illness, Brain Dysfunction, and Survivorship (CIBS) Center: www.icudelirium.org/index.html
- National Heart, Lung, and Blood Institute: www.nhlbi.nih.gov
- Respiratory Nursing Society and Interprofessional Collaborative (RNSIC): www.respiratorynursingsociety.org
- Society for Critical Care Medicine (SCCM): www.sccm.org

(two twitches). The goal is to administer the smallest dose possible of the paralytic agent to avoid prolonged weakness after the therapy is discontinued.[101]

Use of the PNS for estimating the degree of paralysis is not without problems. Poor skin contact, improper electrode placement, edema in the extremity being monitored, and malfunction of the device can lead to overestimation of the degree of blockade. The patient appears to have a zero-twitch TOF response, but evidence of muscle movement is present. More problematic is underestimation of the degree of blockade. Direct stimulation of the muscle or mistaking finger responses for responses of the thumb can result in a false-positive twitch response. This can result in unnecessary administration of additional doses of the paralytic agent. It is imperative that the patient's twitch response be correlated with clinical observations of patient movement.[101]

ADDITIONAL RESOURCES

See Box 19.12 for Internet resources pertaining to pulmonary therapeutic management.

CASE STUDY 19.1 Patient With Acute Respiratory Failure

Brief Patient History

Mr. B is a 63-year-old man who is clinically obese. He has a long history of chronic obstructive pulmonary disease (COPD) associated with smoking two packs of cigarettes a day for 40 years. During the past week, Mr. B has experienced a flu-like illness with fever, chills, malaise, anorexia, diarrhea, nausea, vomiting, and a productive cough with thick, brownish, purulent sputum.

Clinical Assessment

Mr. B is admitted to the intermediate care unit from the emergency department with acute respiratory insufficiency. He is sitting up in bed, leaning forward, with his elbows resting on the over-the-bed table. Mr. B is breathing through his mouth, taking rapid shallow breaths, using his accessory muscles to ventilate. On inhalation, his nostrils flare and his accessory muscles retract. During exhalation, Mr. B uses pursed-lip breathing, and his intercostal muscles bulge. He appears anxious and irritable and is able to speak only one or two barely audible words between each breath. Auscultation reveals crackles posteriorly over the right and left lower lung fields.

Diagnostic Procedures

His admission chest radiograph reveals infiltrates in the right lower lobe and left lower lobe. Gram stain of a sputum sample shows numerous gram-positive diplococci. His baseline vital signs are as follows: blood pressure of 110/60 mm Hg, heart rate of 108 beats/min (sinus tachycardia), respiratory rate of 30 breaths/min, and temperature of 101.3°F. His baseline arterial blood gas values on a 28% Venturi face mask are as follows: PaO_2 of 58 mm Hg, $PaCO_2$ of 33 mm Hg, pH of 7.52, HCO_3^- level of 28, and oxygen saturation of 88%.

Medical Diagnosis

Mr. B is diagnosed with community-associated pneumococcal pneumonia.

Questions

1. What major outcomes do you expect to achieve for this patient?
2. What problems or risks must be managed to achieve these outcomes?
3. What interventions could be initiated to monitor, prevent, manage, or eliminate the problems and risks identified?
4. What interventions could be initiated to promote optimal functioning, safety, and well-being of the patient?
5. What technology can be used to monitor this patient and prevent complications?
6. What other interprofessional team members are needed to assist with the management of this patient?
7. What possible learning needs would you anticipate for this patient?
8. What cultural and age-related factors might have a bearing on the patient's plan of care?

KEY POINTS

Oxygen Therapy

- Oxygen is a medication, and the primary indication for its use is hypoxemia.
- Oxygen can be delivered by various methods, including low-flow systems, reservoir systems, and high-flow systems.
- Complications of oxygen therapy include oxygen toxicity, CO_2 retention, and absorption atelectasis.

Artificial Airways

- Artificial airways (oropharyngeal and nasopharyngeal) are used to maintain airway patency by keeping the tongue from obstructing the upper airway.

- ETTs (oral and nasal) are used to maintain airway patency, to protect the airway from aspiration, to facilitate access to invasive positive-pressure ventilation, and to aid in secretion removal.
- Complications of ETTs include tube obstruction, tube displacement, sinusitis and nasal injury, tracheoesophageal fistula, mucosal lesions, laryngeal or tracheal stenosis, and cricoid abscess.
- Tracheostomy tubes provide the best method of long-term airway maintenance.
- Complications of tracheostomy tubes include hemorrhage, wound infection, subcutaneous emphysema, tube obstruction, tube displacement, tracheal stenosis, tracheoesophageal fistula, tracheoinnominate artery fistula, and tracheocutaneous fistula.
- Cuff pressure is monitored every shift and is maintained at 20 to 30 cm H_2O).
- Humidification is required for all ETTs and tracheostomy tubes.
- Complications associated with suctioning can be minimized if hyperoxygenation is initiated before the start of the procedure, each suction pass is limited to 10 to 15 seconds, and normal saline is not instilled.
- The current recommendation for oral care is simply daily toothbrushing without chlorhexidine.
- An artificial airway is removed when it is no longer needed.

Invasive Mechanical Ventilation

- Indications for mechanical ventilation include supporting cardiopulmonary gas exchange (alveolar ventilation and arterial oxygenation), increasing lung volume (end expiratory lung inflation and functional residual capacity), and reducing the work of breathing.
- Complications associated with mechanical ventilation include ventilator-induced lung injury, cardiovascular compromise, patient–ventilator dyssynchrony, and VAP.
- Strategies to prevent VAP ("VAP Bundle") include elevation of the head of the bed, daily "sedation vacations" and assessment of readiness to extubate, peptic ulcer disease prophylaxis, deep vein thrombosis prophylaxis, and daily oral care with chlorhexidine.
- Weaning is the gradual withdrawal of the mechanical ventilator and the reestablishment of spontaneous breathing; weaning begins only after the original process for which ventilator support was required has been corrected and patient stability has been achieved.

Noninvasive Mechanical Ventilation

- Noninvasive mechanical ventilation uses a mask instead of an ETT to administer positive-pressure ventilation and is indicated in type I and type II acute respiratory failure, cardiogenic pulmonary edema, and other situations in which intubation is not an option.
- Respiratory rate, accessory muscle use, and oxygenation status are continually assessed to ensure that the patient is tolerating this method of ventilation.

Positioning Therapy

- On the basis of the concept that preferential blood flow occurs to the gravity-dependent areas of the lungs, positioning therapy is used to place the least damaged portion of the lungs into a dependent position.
- Prone positioning involves turning the patient completely over onto their stomach in the face-down position; prone positioning is used to improve oxygenation in ARDS.
- Kinetic therapy (continuous turning of a patient from side to side with a 40-degree or greater rotation) and CLRT (continuous turning with a less than 40-degree rotation) are two forms of rotation therapy.
- Rotation therapy is thought to improve oxygenation through better matching of ventilation to perfusion and to prevent pulmonary complications associated with bed rest and mechanical ventilation.

Thoracic Surgery

- The term *thoracic surgery* refers to numerous surgical procedures that involve opening the thoracic cavity (thoracotomy) or the organs of respiration, or both; indications for thoracic surgery range from tumors and abscesses to repair of the esophagus and thoracic vessels.
- Before surgery, a complete evaluation of the patient is needed to determine the appropriateness of surgery as a treatment and whether lung tissue can be removed without jeopardizing respiratory function.
- The most common approach is the posterolateral thoracotomy, which allows for exposure of the lung and the mediastinum.
- Complications of a lung resection include acute respiratory failure, bronchopleural fistula, hemorrhage, cardiovascular disturbances, and mediastinal shift.
- Nursing actions include optimizing oxygenation and ventilation, preventing atelectasis, monitoring chest tubes, assisting the patient to return to an adequate activity level, providing comfort and emotional support, and maintaining surveillance for complications.

Pharmacology

- Mucolytics are administered to help liquefy mucus secretions, which facilitates removal.
- Bronchodilators, such as beta-2 agonists and anticholinergic agents, aid in smooth muscle relaxation and are of particular benefit to patients with airflow limitations.
- Steroids are often used in conjunction with beta-2 agonists to enhance their effects and to decrease airway inflammation.
- Sedation is necessary in many patients to assist with maintaining adequate ventilation; sedation can be used to comfort the patient and to decrease the work of breathing, particularly if the patient is fighting the ventilator.
- Neuromuscular paralysis may be necessary to facilitate optimal ventilation and to decrease oxygen consumption in a severely compromised patient.
- To avoid prolonged neuromuscular blockade, the patient's level of paralysis is carefully monitored by means of a PNS.

Visit the Evolve site at http://evolve.elsevier.com/Urden/CriticalCareNursing for additional study materials.

REFERENCES

1. Rolfe S, Paul F. Oxygen therapy in adult patients. Part 1: Understanding the relevant physiology and pathophysiology. *Br J Nurs*. 2018;27(14):798–804. https://doi.org/10.12968/bjon.2018.27.14.798.
2. Rolfe S, Paul F. Oxygen therapy in adult patients. Part 2: Promoting safe and effective practice in patients' care and management. *Br J Nurs*. 2018;27(17):988–995. https://doi.org/10.12968/bjon.2018.27.17.988.
3. Heuer AJ, Lombardo G. Medical gas therapy. In: Stoller JK, Heuer AJ, Chatburn RL, Mireles-Cabodevila E, Vines DL, eds. *Egan's Fundamentals of Respiratory Care*. 13th ed. St. Louis: Elsevier; 2025..
4. Piraino T, Madden M, J Roberts K, et al. AARC clinical practice guideline: Management of adult patients with oxygen in the acute care setting. *Respir Care*. 2022;67(1):115–128. https://doi.org/10.4187/respcare.09294.
5. Lewis SR, Baker PE, Parker R, Smith AF. High-flow nasal cannulae for respiratory support in adult intensive care patients. *Cochrane Database Syst Rev*. 2021;3(3):CD010172. https://doi.org/10.1002/14651858.CD010172.pub3.
6. Young PJ, Frei D. Oxygen therapy for critically Ill and post-operative patients. *J Anesth*. 2021;35(6):928–938. https://doi.org/10.1007/s00540-021-02996-8.
7. Tola DH, Rojo A, Morgan B. Basic airway management for the professional nurse. *Nurs Clin North Am*. 2021;56(3):379–388. https://doi.org/10.1016/j.cnur.2021.04.005.
8. Scott JB. Airway management. In: Stoller JK, Heuer AJ, Chatburn RL, Mireles-Cabodevila E, Vines DL, eds. *Egan's Fundamentals of Respiratory Care*. 13th ed. St. Louis: Elsevier; 2025.
9. Laurie A, Macdonald J. Equipment for airway management. *Anaesth Intensive Care Med*. 2021;22(9):535–543. https://doi.org/10.1016/j.mpaic.2021.06.019.
10. Colice GL. Technical standards for tracheal tubes. *Clin Chest Med*. 1991;12(3):433–448.
11. Scott JA, Heard SO, Zayaruzny M, Walz JM. Airway management in critical illness: an update. *Chest*. 2020;157(4):877–887. https://doi.org/10.1016/j.chest.2019.10.026.
12. Karamchandani K, Wheelwright J, Yang AL, et al. Emergency airway management outside the operating room: current evidence and management strategies. *Anesth Analg*. 2021;133(3):648–662. https://doi.org/10.1213/ANE.0000000000005644.
13. Admass BA, Endalew NS, Tawye HY, et al. Evidence-based airway management protocol for a critical ill patient in medical intensive care unit: systematic review. *Ann Med Surg (Lond)*. 2022;80:104284. https://doi.org/10.1016/j.amsu.2022.104284.
14. Edelman D, Brewster D. Airway management in the intensive care unit. *Anaesth Intensive Care Med*. 2022;23(10):589–593. https://doi.org/10.1016/j.mpaic.2022.07.012.
15. Kabrhel C, Thomsen TW, Setnick GS, et al. Videos in clinical medicine. Orotracheal intubation. *N Eng J Med*. 2007;356(17):e15.
16. Schaeffer C, Galas T, Teruzzi B, et al. Iatrogenic tracheal rupture caused by endotracheal intubation: a case report. *J Emerg Med*. 2018;55(1):e15–e18. https://doi.org/10.1016/j.jemermed.2018.02.014.
17. Cooper JD. Tracheal injuries complicating prolonged intubation and tracheostomy. *Thorac Surg Clin*. 2018;28(2):139–144. https://doi.org/10.1016/j.thorsurg.2018.01.001.
18. Tikka T, Hilmi OJ. Upper airway tract complications of endotracheal intubation. *Br J Hosp Med (Lond)*. 2019;80(8):441–447. https://doi.org/10.12968/hmed.2019.80.8.441.
19. Adly A, Youssef TA, El-Begermy MM, et al. Timing of tracheostomy in patients with prolonged endotracheal intubation: a systematic review. *Eur Arch Otorhinolaryngol*. 2018;275(3):679–690. https://doi.org/10.1007/s00405-017-4838-7.
20. Avery B, Jankowski S. Management of and indications for tracheostomy in care of the critically ill patient. *Surg (Oxford)*. 2021;39(1):37–47. https://doi.org/10.1016/j.mpsur.2020.11.008.
21. Patton J. Tracheostomy care. *Br J Nurs*. 2019;28(16):1060–1062. https://doi.org/10.12968/bjon.2019.28.16.1060.
22. Ghattas C, Alsunaid S, Pickering EM, et al. State of the art: percutaneous tracheostomy in the intensive care unit. *J Thorac Dis*. 2021;13(8):5261–5276. https://doi.org/10.21037/jtd-19-4121.
23. Bontempo LJ, Manning SL. Tracheostomy emergencies. *Emerg Med Clin North Am*. 2019;37(1):109–119. https://doi.org/10.1016/j.emc.2018.09.010.
24. Samuelson KA. Adult intensive care patients' perception of endotracheal tube-related discomforts: a prospective evaluation. *Heart Lung*. 2011;40(1):49–55. https://doi.org/10.1016/j.hrtlng.2009.12.009.
25. American Association for Respiratory Care, Restrepo RD, Walsh BK. AARC clinical practice guidelines. Humidification during invasive and noninvasive mechanical ventilation: 2012. *Respir Care*. 2012;57(5):782–788. https://doi.org/10.4187/respcare.01766.
26. Li J, Lin HL. Humidity and bland aerosol therapy. In: Stoller JK, Heuer AJ, Chatburn RL, Mireles-Cabodevila E, Vines DL, eds. *Egan's Fundamentals of Respiratory Care*. 13th ed. St. Louis: Elsevier; 2025..
27. Al Dorzi HM, Ghanem AG, Hegazy MM, et al. Humidification during mechanical ventilation to prevent endotracheal tube occlusion in critically ill patients: a case control study. *Ann Thorac Med*. 2022;17(1):37–43. https://doi.org/10.4103/atm.atm_135_21.
28. Rouzé A, Martin-Loeches I, Nseir S. Airway devices in ventilator-associated pneumonia pathogenesis and prevention. *Clin Chest Med*. 2018;39(4):775–783. https://doi.org/10.1016/j.ccm.2018.08.001.
29. Sole ML, Talbert S, Yan X, et al. Impact of deep oropharyngeal suctioning on microaspiration, ventilator events, and clinical outcomes: a randomized clinical trial. *J Adv Nurs*. 2019;75(11):3045–3057. https://doi.org/10.1111/jan.14142.
30. Dexter AM, Scott JB. Airway management and ventilator-associated events. *Respir Care*. 2019;64(8):986–993. https://doi.org/10.4187/respcare.07107.
31. Klompas M, Branson R, Cawcutt K, et al. Strategies to prevent ventilator-associated pneumonia, ventilator-associated events, and nonventilator hospital-acquired pneumonia in acute-care hospitals: 2022 Update. *Infect Control Hosp Epidemiol*. 2022;43(6):687–713. https://doi.org/10.1017/ice.2022.88.
32. Blakeman TC, Scott JB, Yoder MA, et al. AARC Clinical practice guidelines: artificial airway suctioning. *Respir Care*. 2022;67(2):258–271. https://doi.org/10.4187/respcare.09548.
33. Imbriaco G, Monesi A. Closed tracheal suctioning systems in the era of COVID-19: is it time to consider them as a gold standard? *J Infect Prev*. 2021;22(1):44–45. https://doi.org/10.1177/1757177420963775.
34. Wang CH, Tsai JC, Chen SF, et al. Normal saline instillation before suctioning: a meta-analysis of randomized controlled trials. *Aust Crit Care*. 2017;30(5):260–265. https://doi.org/10.1016/j.aucc.2016.11.001.
35. Czarnik RE, Stone KS, Everhart CC, et al. Differential effects of continuous versus intermittent suction on tracheal tissue. *Heart Lung*. 1991;20(2):144–151.
36. Modrykamien AM. Strategies for communicating with conscious mechanically ventilated critically ill patients. *Proc (Bayl Univ Med Cent)*. 2019;32(4):534–537. https://doi.org/10.1080/08998280.2019.1635413.
37. Jenabzadeh NE, Chlan L. A nurse's experience being intubated and receiving mechanical ventilation. *Crit Care Nurse*. 2011;31(6):51–54. https://doi.org/10.4037/ccn2011182.
38. Hoom T, Elbers PW, Girbes AR, et al. Communicating with conscious and mechanically ventilated critically ill patients: a systematic review. *Crit Care*. 2016;20(1):333. https://doi.org/10.1186/s13054-016-1483-2.
39. Coppadoro A, Bellani G, Foti G. Non-pharmacological interventions to prevent ventilator-associated pneumonia: a literature review. *Respir Care*. 2019;64(12):1586–1595. https://doi.org/10.4187/respcare.07127.
40. Lombardo L, Ferguson C, George A, et al. Interventions to promote oral care regimen adherence in the critical care setting: a systematic review. *Aust Crit Care*. 2022;35(5):583–594. https://doi.org/10.1016/j.aucc.2021.08.010.
41. Haghighi A, Shafipour V, Bagheri-Nesami M, et al. The impact of oral care on oral health status and prevention of ventilator-associated pneumonia in critically ill patients. *Aust Crit Care*. 2017;30(2):69–73. https://doi.org/10.1016/j.aucc.2016.07.002.

42. Andersson M, Wilde-Larsson B, Persenius M. Intensive care nurses fail to translate knowledge and skills into practice: a mixed-methods study on perceptions of oral care. *Intensive Crit Care Nurs.* 2019;52:51–60. https://doi:.org/10.1016/j.iccn.2018.09.006.
43. Dale CM, Rose L, Carbone S, et al. Effect of oral chlorhexidine de-adoption and implementation of an oral care bundle on mortality for mechanically ventilated patients in the intensive care unit (CHORAL): a multi-center stepped-wedge cluster-randomized controlled trial. *Intensive Care Med.* 2021;47(11):1295–1302. https://doi.org/10.1007/s00134-021-06475-2.
44. Artime CA, Hagberg CA. Tracheal extubation. *Respir Care.* 2014;59(6):991–1005. https://doi.org/10.4187/respcare.02926.
45. Singh RK, Saran S, Baronia AK. The practice of tracheostomy decannulation-a systematic review. *J Intensive Care.* 2017;5:38. https://doi.org/10.1186/s40560-017-0234-z.
46. Pham T, Brochard LJ, Slutsky AS. Mechanical ventilation: state of the art. *Mayo Clin Proc.* 2017;92(9):1382–1400. https://doi.org/10.1016/j.mayocp.2017.05.004.
47. Ward J, Noel C. Basic modes of mechanical ventilation. *Emerg Med Clin North Am.* 2022;40(3):473–488. https://doi.org/10.1016/j.emc.2022.05.003.
48. Chatburn RL, Garnero AJ. Mechanical ventilators. In: Stoller JK, Heuer AJ, Chatburn RL, Mireles-Cabodevila E, Vines DL, eds. *Egan's Fundamentals of Respiratory Care.* 13th ed. St. Louis: Elsevier; 2025..
49. Cairo JM. How a breath is delivered. In: Cairo JM, ed. *Pilbeam's Mechanical Ventilation: Physiological and Clinical Applications.* 8th ed. St. Louis: Elsevier; 2024.
50. Walter JM, Corbridge TC, Singer BD. Invasive mechanical ventilation. *South Med J.* 2018;111(12):746–753. https://doi.org/10.14423/SMJ.0000000000000905.
51. Cawley MJ. Advanced modes of mechanical ventilation: introduction for the critical care pharmacist. *J Pharm Pract.* 2019;32(2):186–198. https://doi.org/10.1177/0897190017734766.
52. Vines DL. Initiating and adjusting invasive ventilatory support. In: Stoller JK, Heuer AJ, Chatburn RL, Mireles-Cabodevila E, Vines DL, eds. *Egan's Fundamentals of Respiratory Care.* 13th ed. St. Louis: Elsevier; 2025..
53. Beitler JR, Malhotra A, Thompson BT. Ventilator-induced lung injury. *Clin Chest Med.* 2016;37(4):633–646. https://doi.org/10.1016/j.ccm.2016.07.004.
54. Curley GF, Laffey JG, Zhang H, et al. Biotrauma and ventilator-induced lung injury: clinical implications. *Chest.* 2016;150(5):1109–1117. https://doi.org/10.1016/j.chest.2016.07.019.
55. Cruz FF, Ball L, Rocco PRM, et al. Ventilator-induced lung injury during controlled ventilation in patient with acute respiratory distress syndrome: less is probably better. *Expert Rev Respir Med.* 2018;12(5):403–414. https://doi.org/10.1080/17476348.2018.1457954.
56. Chatburn RL, Kacmarek RM. Physiology of ventilatory support. In: Stoller JK, Heuer AJ, Chatburn RL, Mireles-Cabodevila E, Vines DL, eds. *Egan's Fundamentals of Respiratory Care.* 13th ed. St. Louis: Elsevier; 2025..
57. Chen L, Xia HF, Shang Y, Yao SL. Molecular mechanisms of ventilator-induced lung injury. *Chin Med J (Engl).* 2018;131(10):1225–1231. https://doi.org/10.4103/0366-6999.226840.

57a. Davies JD, Kneyber MCJ. Optimizing patient-ventilator synchrony in adult and pediatric populations. In: Cheifetz I, MacIntyre N, Marini JJ, eds. *Mechanical Ventilation: Essentials for Current Adult and Pediatric Practice.* Mount Prospect, IL: Society of Critical Care Medicine; 2017.

58. Marini JJ, Prodhan P. Cardiopulmonary interactions. In: Cheifetz I, MacIntyre N, Marini JJ, eds. *Mechanical Ventilation: Essentials for Current Adult and Pediatric Practice.* Mount Prospect, IL: Society of Critical Care Medicine; 2017.

58a. De Oliveira B, Aljaberi N, Taha A, et al. Patient-ventilator dyssynchrony in critically ill patients. *J Clin Med.* 2021;10(19):4550. https://doi.org/10.3390/jcm10194550.

59. Spalding MC, Cripps MW, Minshall CT. Ventilator-associated pneumonia: new definitions. *Crit Care Clin.* 2017;33(2):277–292. https://doi.org/10.1016/j.ccc.2016.12.009.
60. Jenkins-Lonidier L. Pulmonary infections, including ventilator-associated pneumonia. *Crit Care Nurs Clin North Am.* 2021;33(4):381–393. https://doi.org/10.1016/j.cnc.2021.08.002.
61. Modi AR, Kovacs CS. Hospital-acquired and ventilator-associated pneumonia: diagnosis, management, and prevention. *Cleve Clin J Med.* 2020;87(10):633–639. https://doi.org/10.3949/ccjm.87a.19117.
62. Güner CK, Kutlutürkan S. Role of head-of-bed elevation in preventing ventilator-associated pneumonia bed elevation and pneumonia. *Nurs Crit Care.* 2022;27(5):635–645. https://doi.org/10.1111/nicc.12633.
63. Grap MJ, Munro CL, Wetzel PA, et al. Backrest elevation and tissue interface pressure by anatomical location during mechanical ventilation. *Am J Crit Care.* 2016;25(3):e56–e63. https://doi.org/10.4037/ajcc2016317.
64. Vagionas D, Vasileiadis I, Rovina N, et al. Daily sedation interruption and mechanical ventilation weaning: a literature review. *Anaesthesiol Intensive Ther.* 2019;51(5):380–389. https://doi.org/10.5114/ait.2019.90921.
65. Lima JT, Silva RFAD, Assis AP, Silva A. Checklist for managing critical patients' daily awakening. *Rev Bras Ter Intensiva.* 2019;31(3):318–325. https://doi.org/10.5935/0103-507X.20190057.
66. Ramandeep K, Vines DL. Discontinuing ventilatory support. In: Stoller JK, Heuer AJ, Chatburn RL, Mireles-Cabodevila E, Vines DL, eds. *Egan's Fundamentals of Respiratory Care.* 13th ed. St. Louis: Elsevier; 2025..
67. Penuelas O, Thille AW, Esteban A. Discontinuation of ventilator support: new solutions to old dilemmas. *Curr Opin Crit Care.* 2015;21(1):74–81. https://doi.org/10.1097/MCC.0000000000000169.
68. Trivedi V, Chaudhuri D, Jinah R, et al. The usefulness of the rapid shallow breathing index in predicting successful extubation: a systematic review and meta-analysis. *Chest.* 2022;161(1):97–111. https://doi.org/10.1016/j.chest.2021.06.030.
69. Ward D, Fulbrook P. Nursing strategies for effective weaning of the critically ill mechanically ventilated patient. *Crit Care Nurs Clin N Am.* 2016;28(4):499–512. https://doi.org/10.1016/j.cnc.2016.07.008.
70. Jordan J, Rose L, Dainty KN, et al. Factors that impact on the use of mechanical ventilation weaning protocols in critically ill adults and children: a qualitative evidence-synthesis. *Cochrane Database Syst Rev.* 2016;10(10):CD011812. https://doi.org/10.1002/14651858.CD011812.pub2.
71. Akella P, Voigt LP, Chawla S. To wean or not to wean: a practical patient focused guide to ventilator weaning. *J Intensive Care Med.* 2022;37(11):1417–1425. https://doi.org/10.1177/08850666221095436.
72. Schmidt G, Girard TD, Kress JP, et al. Official executive summary of an American Thoracic Society/American College of Chest Physicians clinical practice guideline: liberation from mechanical ventilation in critically ill adults. *Am J Resp Crit Care Med.* 2017;195(1):115–119. https://doi.org/10.1164/rccm.201610-2076ST.
73. Grasselli G, Brioni M, Zanella A. Monitoring respiratory mechanics during assisted ventilation. *Curr Opin Crit Care.* 2020;26(1):11–17. https://doi.org/10.1097/MCC.0000000000000681.
74. Tronstad O, Flaws D, Lye I, et al. The intensive care unit environment from the perspective of medical, allied health and nursing clinicians: a qualitative study to inform design of the 'ideal' bedspace. *Aust Crit Care.* 2021;34(1):15–22. https://doi.org/10.1016/j.aucc.2020.06.003.
75. ABCDEF (A2F) overview. *Critical Illness, Brain Dysfunction, and Survivorship CIBS Center Website*; 2023. www.icudelirium.org/medicalprofessionals.html.
76. Gill HS, Marcolini EG. Noninvasive mechanical ventilation. *Emerg Med Clin North Am.* 2022;40(3):603–613. https://doi.org/10.1016/j.emc.2022.05.010.
77. Wei Y, Pei J, Yang Q, et al. The prevalence and risk factors of facial pressure injuries related to adult non-invasive ventilation equipment: a systematic review and meta-analysis. *Int Wound J.* 2023;20(3):621–632. https://doi.org/10.1111/iwj.13903.
78. Scott JB. Noninvasive ventilation. In: Stoller JK, Heuer AJ, Chatburn RL, Mireles-Cabodevila E, Vines DL, eds. *Egan's Fundamentals of Respiratory Care.* 13th ed. St. Louis: Elsevier; 2025.
79. Alqahtani JS, Al Ahmari MD. Evidence based synthesis for prevention of noninvasive ventilation related facial pressure ulcers. *Saudi Med J.* 2018;39(5):443–452. https://doi.org/10.15537/smj.2018.5.22058.

80. Papazian L, Munshi L, Guérin C. Prone position in mechanically ventilated patients. *Intensive Care Med.* 2022;48(8):1062–1065. https://doi.org/10.1007/s00134-022-06731-z.
81. Banavasi H, Nguyen P, Osman H, et al. Management of ARDS - What works and what does not. *Am J Med Sci.* 2021;362(1):13–23. https://doi.org/10.1016/j.amjms.2020.12.019.
82. Gattinoni L, Busana M, Giosa L, et al. Prone positioning in acute respiratory distress syndrome. *Semin Respir Crit Care Med.* 2019;40(1):94–100. https://doi.org/10.1055/s-0039-1685180.
83. Munshi L, Del Sorbo L, Adhikari NKJ, et al. Prone position for acute respiratory distress syndrome. A systematic review and meta-analysis. *Ann Am Thorac Soc.* 2017;14(Supplement_4):S280–S288. https://doi:.org/10.1513/AnnalsATS.201704-343OT.
84. Morata L, Vollman K, Rechter J, et al. Manual prone positioning in adults: Reducing the risk of harm through evidence-based practices. *Crit Care Nurse.* 2023;43(1):59–66. https://doi.org/10.4037/ccn2023174.
85. Hewitt N, Bucknall T, Faraone NM. Lateral positioning for critically ill adult patients. *Cochrane Database Syst Rev.* 2016;2016(5):CD007205. https://doi.org/10.1002/14651858.CD007205.pub2.
86. McGrath R. Thoracic surgery. In: Rothrock JC, ed. *Alexander's Care of the Patient in Surgery.* 17th ed. St. Louis: Elsevier; 2023.
87. Hanley C, Donahoe L, Slinger P. Fit for surgery? What's new in preoperative assessment of the high-risk patient undergoing pulmonary resection. *J Cardiothorac Vasc Anesth.* 2021;35(12):3760–3773. https://doi.org/10.1053/j.jvca.2020.11.025.
88. Roy PM. Preoperative pulmonary evaluation for lung resection. *J Anaesthesiol Clin Pharmacol.* 2018;34(3):296–300. https://doi.org/10.4103/joacp.JOACP_89_17.
89. Odor PM, Bampoe S, Gilhooly D, et al. Perioperative interventions for prevention of postoperative pulmonary complications: systematic review and meta-analysis. *BMJ.* 2020;368:m540. https://doi.org/10.1136/bmj.m540.
90. Hoy H, Lynch T, Beck M. Surgical treatment of lung cancer. *Crit Care Nurs Clin North Am.* 2019;31(3):303–313. https://doi.org/10.1016/j.cnc.2019.05.002.
91. Keshishyan S, Revelo AE, Epelbaum O. Bronchoscopic management of prolonged air leak. *J Thora Dis.* 2017;9(suppl 10):S1034–S1046. https://doi.org/10.21037/jtd.2017.05.47.
92. Bribriesco A, Patterson GA. Management of postpneumonectomy bronchopleural fistula: From thoracoplasty to transsternal closure. *Thorac Surg Clin.* 2018;28(3):323–335. https://doi.org/10.1016/j.thorsurg.2018.05.008.
93. Gardner DD, Vines DL. Airway clearance therapy. In: Stoller JK, Heuer AJ, Chatburn RL, Mireles-Cabodevila E, Vines DL, eds. *Egan's Fundamentals of Respiratory Care.* 13th ed. St. Louis: Elsevier; 2025.
94. Sasa RI. Evidence-based update on chest tube management. *Am Nurse Today.* 2019;14(4):10–14.
95. Brand J, Arrowsmith JE. Respiratory system: Applied pharmacology. *Anaesthe. Intensive Care Med.* 2021;22(3):151–155. https://doi.org/10.1016/j.mpaic.2021.01.007.
96. Gardenhire DS. Airway pharmacology. In: Stoller JK, Heuer AJ, Chatburn RL, Mireles-Cabodevila E, Vines DL, eds. *Egan's Fundamentals of Respiratory Care.* 13th ed. St. Louis: Elsevier; 2025.
97. Kerstjens HAM, Upham JW, Yang IA. Airway pharmacology: Treatment options and algorithms to treat patients with chronic obstructive pulmonary disease. *J Thora Dis.* 2019;11(Suppl 17):S2200–S2209. https://doi.org/10.21037/jtd.2019.10.57.
98. Taggart K. Pharmacology focus: Neuromuscular blocking agents: A basic overview. *S D Med.* 2020;73(12):588–590.
99. deBacker J, Hart N, Fan E. Neuromuscular blockade in the 21st century management of the critically ill patient. *Chest.* 2017;151(3):697–706. https://doi.org/10.1016/j.chest.2016.10.040.
100. Smetana KS, Roe NA, Doepker BA, et al. Review of continuous infusion neuromuscular blocking agents in the adult intensive care unit. *Crit Care Nurs Q.* 2017;40(4):323–343. https://doi.org/10.1097/CNQ.0000000000000171.
101. Rodríguez-Blanco J, Rodríguez-Yanez T, Rodríguez-Blanco JD, et al. Neuromuscular blocking agents in the intensive care unit. *J Int Med Res.* 2022;50(9):3000605221128148. https://doi.org/10.1177/03000605221128148.

20

Neurologic Anatomy and Physiology

Kathleen M. Stacy

http://evolve.elsevier.com/Urden/CriticalCareNursing

The nervous system is the "executive suite" of the human body. It directs all other systems and provides the unique ability for thought, emotion, understanding of complex information, and integration of numerous stimuli. As the recipient of all sensory information for analysis, the nervous system generates intellectual and motor responses aimed at maintaining the integrity of life structures. Critical care nurses must attain a basic understanding of the anatomy and physiology of this complex system because the nervous system serves as the basis for innervation and proper functioning of all other systems. This chapter reviews the anatomic divisions and functions of the central nervous system (CNS), including the cellular microstructure, protective encasement, networked functions, and mechanisms aimed at maintenance of structural and physiologic integrity. The cranial nerves, a component of the peripheral nervous system (PNS), are presented in tabular form.

DIVISIONS OF THE NERVOUS SYSTEM

The nervous system is the most highly organized system of the body, with all its parts functioning as an inseparable unit. This system is usually classified by anatomic function.

ANATOMIC DIVISIONS

The CNS comprises the brain and the spinal cord. The PNS comprises 12 pairs of cranial nerves, 31 pairs of spinal nerves, and all other nerves serving a variety of functions throughout the body.

Physiologic Divisions

The somatic, or voluntary, nervous system is composed of fibers that connect the CNS with structures of the skeletal muscles and the skin. The autonomic, or involuntary, nervous system is composed of fibers that connect the CNS with smooth muscle, cardiac muscle, internal organs, and glands. The autonomic nervous system includes sympathetic and parasympathetic branches.

Most activities of the nervous system originate from sensory receptors such as visual, auditory, or tactile receptors. This sensory information is transmitted to the CNS by afferent fibers (sensory fibers). Efferent fibers (motor fibers) transmit the CNS response to the periphery to produce a motor response, such as contraction of skeletal muscles, contraction of the smooth muscles of organs, or secretion by endocrine glands. To better understand the macrostructure and functions of the nervous system, it helps to study the microstructure, or the cellular level.

MICROSTRUCTURE OF THE NERVOUS SYSTEM

Two types of cells make up the nervous system: (1) neurons and (2) neuroglia.[1] Neurons are the cells primarily charged with the functional work of the nervous system, including receipt of information, integration, and transmission or conduction of nerve impulses to recipient cells. Neuroglial cells serve as the support infrastructure of the nervous system, providing protection and a structural foundation for neurons and participating in neuronal repair.

Neuroglia

In the nervous system, 6 to 10 times more neuroglial cells exist than do neurons. Neuroglial cells consist of four types: (1) astroglia (astrocytes), (2) oligodendroglia, (3) ependyma, and (4) microglia (Fig. 20.1).[1] These cells provide the neuron with structural support, nourishment, and protection (Table 20.1). They retain the ability to replicate, but they can replicate abnormally and are the primary source of CNS neoplasms.[2]

Neurons

Neurons are the basic functional unit within the CNS, and they are charged with the highly specialized task of data integration and signal transmission. The CNS is made up of more than 10 billion neurons. The cellular appearance of neurons varies, but each cell contains three basic components: (1) the cell body, (2) dendrites, and (3) an axon (Fig. 20.2). Neurons are structurally classified as *unipolar*, a cell body with one process that divides into a central branch (one axon) and a peripheral branch (one dendrite); as *bipolar*, a cell body with two processes (one axon and one dendrite); or as *multipolar*, a cell body with one axon and several dendrites.

Cell Body

The cell body (soma) controls the metabolic activity of the neuron and contains the organelles, such as the nucleus, mitochondria, endoplasmic reticulum, Golgi apparatus, and liposomes, which are necessary for cellular metabolism and maintenance. Compared

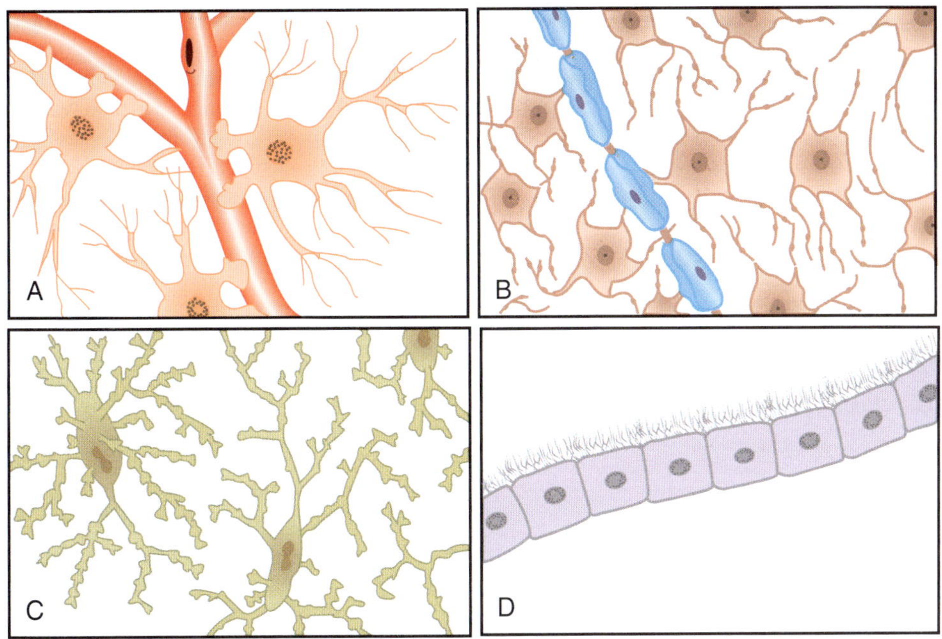

FIG. 20.1 Neuroglial Cells. (A) Astrocytes along the capillary. (B) Oligodendrocytes along the nerves. (C) Microglia (phagocytes). (D) Ependymal cells form a sheet that lines fluid cavities in the brain. (From Black JM, Hawks JH. *Medical-Surgical Nursing: Clinical Management for Positive Outcomes*. 8th ed. Saunders; 2009.)

TABLE 20.1 Neuroglial Cells

Cell Type	Function
Astroglia (astrocyte)	Supplies nutrients to neuron structure and to support framework for neurons and capillaries; forms part of blood-brain barrier
Oligodendroglia	Forms myelin sheath in central nervous system
Ependyma	Lines ventricular system; forms choroid plexus, which produces cerebrospinal fluid
Microglia	Occurs mainly in white matter; phagocytizes waste products from injured neurons

with other body cells, the neuron's protein-embedded membrane with its phospholipid bilayer is unique, consisting of specialized pores that work as ion-specific channels or pumps to promote passage of ions through an otherwise impermeable plasma membrane.[3]

The neuronal cell body is the life support unit of the neuron. The metabolic demands of these specialized units necessitate uninterrupted perfusion with glucose and oxygen to maintain neuronal life and optimal functioning. Originally, it was believed that CNS neuronal repair was impossible, but research has validated that neurons are more plastic than was previously thought, although rates of repair (plasticity) or restoration of neuronal function are driven by factors that remain largely unknown.[4] Within the brain and the spinal cord, neuronal cell bodies make up regions of gray matter. Outside the CNS, ganglia are cell bodies within the PNS that reside near and work closely with CNS neurons.

Dendrites

Dendrites form the receptive component of the neuron; they are branched fibers extending only a short distance from the cell body. Each neuron may have several dendrites, which function as impulse receivers for the cell body. The axon is the part of the neuron concerned with transmission of impulses away from the cell body to other neurons, muscle cells, endocrine glands, or some other effector organ. Neurons contain only one axon, whose length may be microscopic or, in some cases, may extend up to 4 feet. Some axons are protected by a myelin sheath, a white phospholipid complex laid down by Schwann cells in the PNS and by oligodendroglia in the CNS. The myelin sheath protects neuronal axons and provides insulation for the conduction of nerve impulses. Fibers enclosed in the sheath are called *myelinated fibers;* fibers that are not enclosed are called *unmyelinated fibers*. The white matter of the CNS is composed of myelinated fiber tracts.

Saltatory Conduction

Myelinated fibers use a process called *saltatory conduction* to support rapid axonal transmission of nerve impulses. Structurally, axons participating in this form of impulse transmission are laid out with a noncontinuous myelin cover, interrupted with 2-micron bare segments called the *nodes of Ranvier*. These nodes are packed with sodium channels, making them extremely sensitive to membrane depolarization. Because segments of the axon covered by myelin are impervious to sodium influx, impulse transmission is pulled down the length of the axon to the next node of Ranvier.[5] Saltatory conduction increases transmission velocity up to 100-fold, allowing transmission at rates of 130 m/s.[6]

Neuronal Function

Neuronal function is driven by depolarization-repolarization cycles, similar to that described for cardiac physiology (see Chapter 10), but what makes the nervous system so exceptional is its ability to undergo the depolarization-repolarization cycle up to 1000 times per second to ensure optimal receipt, integration, and transmission of information throughout the body. The movement of ions across the neuronal membrane generates electrical action potentials. Neuronal resting membrane potential (RMP) is −70 mV, approximating the equilibrium potential for potassium; on depolarization, sodium channels open, shifting the equilibrium potential in the positive direction (Fig. 20.3).

Neuronal Channels

Mechanisms for ionic movement involve two types of neuronal channels: (1) voltage-gated and (2) transmitter-gated (also

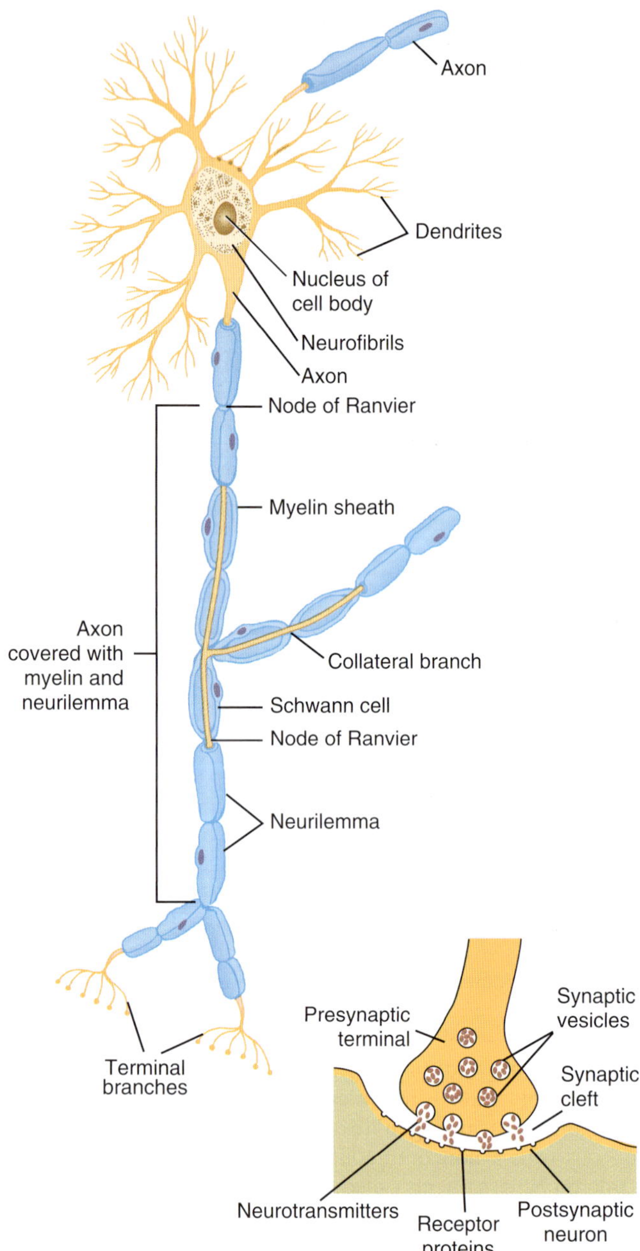

FIG. 20.2 Neuron. A neuron (the basic element of the nervous system) and a chemical synapse. (From Black JM, Hawks JH. *Medical-Surgical Nursing: Clinical Management for Positive Outcomes*. 8th ed. Saunders; 2009.)

referred to as *ligand-gated*). Many pharmaceutical and therapeutic agents currently in use or undergoing testing manipulate these ionic transport mechanisms. Voltage-gated channels become activated with changes in transmembrane electrical potential, promoting sodium and calcium influx and potassium efflux. These channels are the primary drivers of cellular action potentials.[7] Transmitter-gated channels are primarily concerned with mitigating the response of a postsynaptic neuron to synapse and are discussed in more detail later.

Action Potentials

After an action potential reaches the axon terminal, the action potential initiates a cascade of events that promote interneuronal communication, or *synapse*. Two types of synapse exist: (1) electrical and (2) chemical. In an electrical synapse, gap junctions made up of narrow bridges allow cytoplasm and intracellular metabolites to pass in an essentially continuous fashion between neurons, facilitating impulse conduction from one neuron to the next. In a chemical synapse, which is involved in most synaptic events, no physical bridge exists between neurons. Instead, a large synaptic cleft of 20 to 30 nm prevents direct action potential transmission from one neuron to another. When the wave of depolarization reaches the presynaptic terminal, it signals the release of neurotransmitters into the synaptic cleft.[6]

Neurotransmitters

The two classifications of neurotransmitters are (1) small-molecule transmitters and (2) neuroactive peptides. Examples of small-molecule transmitters include acetylcholine, dopamine, norepinephrine, epinephrine, serotonin, histamine, gamma-aminobutyric acid (GABA), glycine, and glutamate.[8] Neuroactive peptides include pituitary peptides, hypothalamic-releasing hormones, and neurohypophyseal hormones. This chapter is primarily concerned with the small-molecule transmitters, which are stored in vesicles within the axon terminal and released into the synapse through a process called *exocytosis*. Exocytosis is stimulated by arrival of the action potential in the axon terminal and results in release of neurotransmitters into the synaptic cleft, where these molecules rapidly diffuse to interact with postsynaptic receptors.[8]

Channel Receptors

Transmitter-gated channels are activated by binding of transmitter agonists to receptors on the postsynaptic neuron. Ions passing through transmitter-gated channels promote an excitatory or inhibitory response within postsynaptic neurons.[8] The most prevalent excitatory transmitter-gated channel receptors in the brain and spinal cord are ionotropic glutamate receptors, which are primarily concerned with gating sodium, potassium, and calcium ions. Examples of inhibitory transmitter-gated channel receptors include GABA receptors, glycine receptors, and nicotinic acetylcholine receptors. Most GABA receptors are found in the brain, where GABA serves as the primary inhibitory neurotransmitter, whereas glycine serves as the primary postsynaptic inhibitory neurotransmitter of the spinal cord. GABA and glycine channels gate chloride ions, which inhibit by promoting repolarization to the chloride equilibrium potential (−60 mV) and by short-circuiting incoming excitatory potentials by gating anions and clamping the membrane shut to excitatory cations.[9] In other words, when inhibitor neurotransmitters are released, the neuron's internal charge becomes more negative, and the resistance to depolarization is increased. Metabotropic receptors contribute to impulse transmission, promoting sustained effects of postsynaptic excitation or inhibition. Examples of metabotropic receptors include catecholamine receptors, neuropeptide receptors, and muscarinic receptors.[8]

Synaptic Termination

Termination of the synapse reaction is most commonly accomplished through reuptake, in which transporter proteins embedded in neuron and glial cell membranes direct neurotransmitter molecules within the cleft to move back to the intracellular compartment for vesicle repackaging. Neurotransmitters may also go through enzyme degradation, with their component parts taken up for further neurotransmitter synthesis and storage. Ultimately, remaining neurotransmitter diffuses away from the synaptic cleft.[9]

The response in the postsynaptic neuron to synapse is an excitatory or inhibitory potential. Membrane potentials are not strong enough by themselves to generate a complete action potential within the postsynaptic neuron, but they are instead summarized

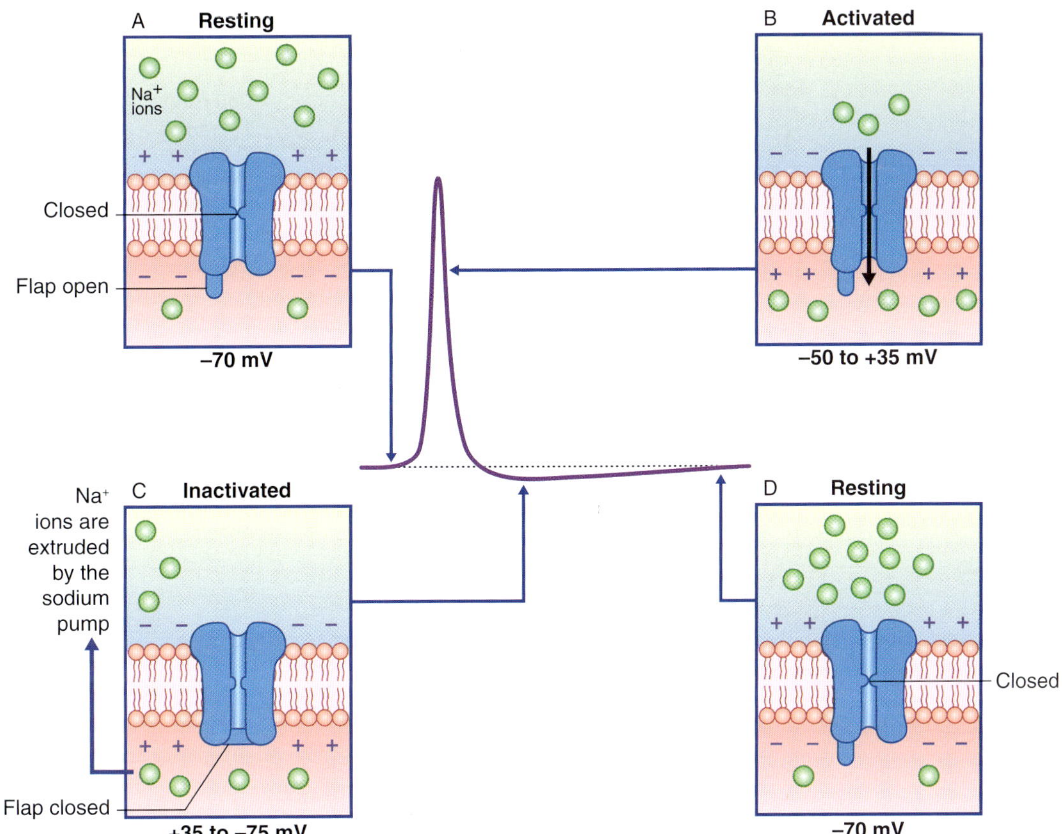

FIG. 20.3 Action Potentials. Voltage-gated Na^+ channel behavior during various phases of an action potential. (A) During the resting phase prior to onset, the activation gate is closed and the inactivation gate is open. (B) When the threshold level is crossed, the activation gate opens, and the channel is open completely. (C) The channel is closed by the inactivation gate. (D) Restoration of the resting potential causes the activation gate to close and the inactivation gate to open, thus resetting the channel. (From Mtui E, Gruener G, Dockery P. *Fitzgerald's Clinical Neuroanatomy and Neuroscience*. 8th ed. Elsevier; 2021.)

or integrated by the neuronal cell body in the process of information transmission. When the postsynaptic neuron is bombarded with excitatory potentials, they may combine (summation) to become capable of stimulating an action potential.[9]

Examples of disease-induced or chemically induced mechanisms that alter neuronal transmission are provided in Fig. 20.4.

CENTRAL NERVOUS SYSTEM

The CNS consists of the brain and the spinal cord. Serving as the control unit for all body systems, the remarkably delicate CNS requires significant protection to preserve normal function. This section addresses the anatomy and physiology of the brain and the spinal cord, supporting the critical care nurse's understanding of pathophysiologic changes that contribute to clinical examination findings.

Cranial Protective Mechanisms

Cranium

The outermost protective measures underneath the integument are the bony structures that encase the CNS. The skull, or cranium, surrounds the brain and is composed of eight flat, irregular bones fused at sutures during early childhood (Fig. 20.5). The skull protects the brain from direct force and superficial trauma, although excessive force may fracture the skull, destroying this protective mechanism and driving bony fragments into fragile brain tissue.

If the skull is seen from the inside, the superior surfaces form a smooth inner wall, whereas the basilar skull contains ridges and folds with sharp edges. Traumatic impact to the head often results in fracture of the basilar skull as a result of gravitational forces that displace energy in a downward fashion toward the skull base.[10]

The cranium is a solid, nonexpanding bony vault with only one large opening at the base called the *foramen magnum*, through which the brainstem projects and connects to the spinal cord. Several other very small openings in the base of the skull allow entrance and exit of blood vessels and nerve fibers.

Meninges

The meninges lie directly beneath the skull, forming another source of protection for the CNS. The meninges consist of three layers: (1) the dura mater, (2) the arachnoid mater, and (3) the pia mater (Fig. 20.6).

Dura mater. The outermost layer of meninges directly beneath the skull is the dura mater. *Dura* is the Latin term for "tough," and true to its name, this layer is made up of fibrous tissue that is double folded to support the CNS, nerves, and vascular structures. Within the double layers of the dura mater lie venous sinuses that collect blood from intracranial and meningeal veins for drainage into the internal jugular veins.

Four extensions of the dura mater directly support and separate specific areas of the brain: (1) the falx cerebri, (2) the tentorium cerebelli, (3) the falx cerebelli, and (4) the diaphragma sellae. The falx cerebri divides the right and left hemispheres of the brain vertically through the longitudinal fissures extending

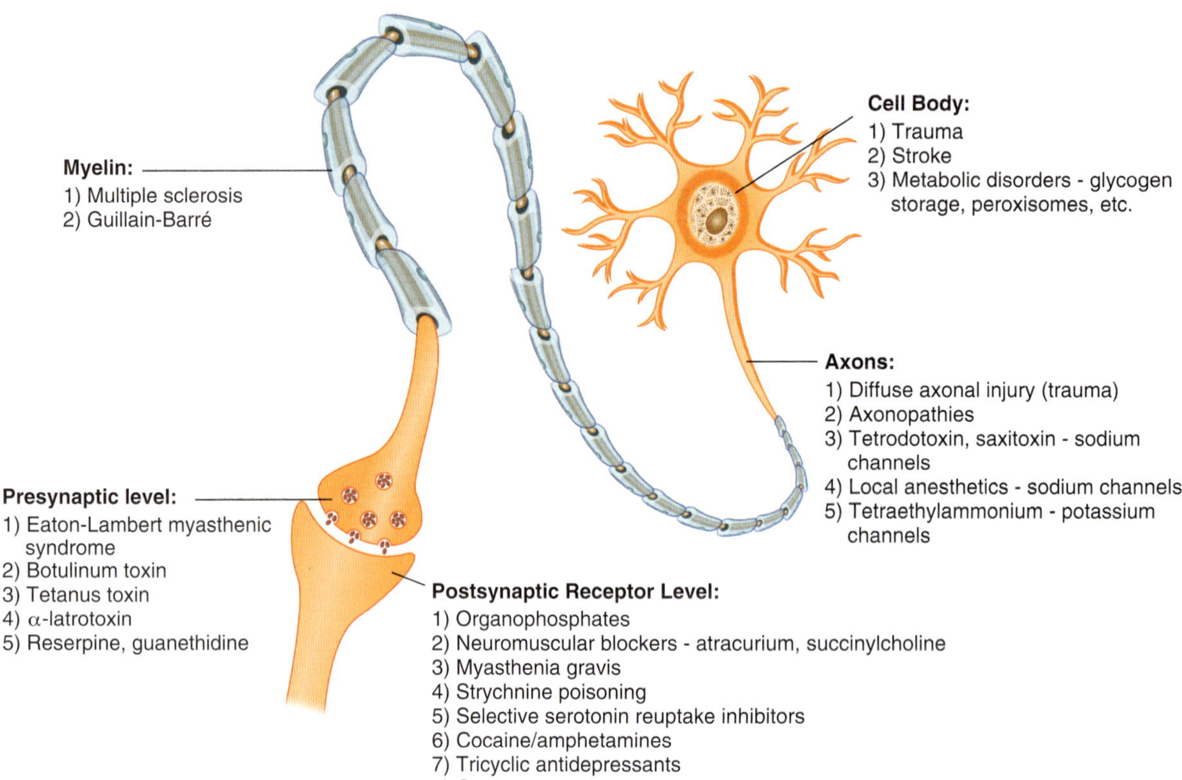

FIG. 20.4 Neuronal Pathophysiology. (Modified from Layon AJ, Gabrielli A, Friedman WA. *Textbook of Neuro-intensive Care.* Saunders; 2004.)

from the frontal lobe to the occipital lobe. The tentorium cerebelli forms a tent between the occipital lobes and the cerebellum and separates the cerebral hemispheres from the brainstem and the cerebellum. Structures within the brain that are located above the tentorium are often referred to as *supratentorial*, whereas structures located below the tentorium are referred to as *infratentorial* and make up the region of the brain called the *posterior fossa*. The falx cerebelli forms the division between the two lateral lobes of the cerebellum, and the diaphragma sellae forms a roof over the sella turcica, which houses the pituitary gland.

Blood supply. The main blood supply for the dura mater is the middle meningeal artery. This artery lies on the surface of the dura in the epidural space and within grooves formed on the inside of the parietal bone. Traumatic disruption of the parietal bone may result in tearing of the middle meningeal artery and development of an epidural hematoma.[11] A potential space exists between the dura mater and the arachnoid mater. This area contains numerous unsupported small veins that may become disrupted and torn when traumatic head injury occurs, leading to development of a subdural hematoma.[11]

Arachnoid mater. The arachnoid membrane is a delicate, fragile membrane that loosely surrounds the brain. Fine threads of elastic tissue called *trabeculae* connect the arachnoid to the pia mater, creating a spongy, weblike structure called the *subarachnoid space*. Cerebrospinal fluid (CSF) circulates freely in the subarachnoid space, which also contains the origins of the brain's large arteries where they enter the skull and differentiate into anterior and posterior circulatory branches. Rupture of an artery within the subarachnoid space allows for blood to mix with CSF, producing a subarachnoid hemorrhage.[12]

Cisterns. At the base of the brain, widened areas of subarachnoid space form cisterns, or spaces, that are filled with CSF. The largest of these cisterns, the cisterna magna, lies between the medulla and the cerebellum, and it communicates with the fourth ventricle.

Arachnoid villi. Tufts of arachnoid membrane, called *arachnoid villi*, or granulations, project into the superior sagittal and transverse venous sinuses. Absorption of CSF by arachnoid villi allows its removal by the venous drainage system. The delicate structure of the arachnoid villi places them at risk for obstruction by blood in subarachnoid hemorrhage, resulting in obstructive hydrocephalus.[13]

Pia mater. The pia mater adheres directly to brain tissue. Rich in small blood vessels that supply a large volume of arterial blood to the CNS, this membrane closely follows all folds and convolutions of the brain's surface. Tufts or folds of the pia mater in the lateral, third, and fourth ventricles form a portion of the choroid plexus that is responsible for the production of CSF.

Ventricular System

The ventricular system consists of four CSF-filled canals lined with ependymal cells, a type of neuroglial cell (Fig. 20.7). This system is made up of two large lateral ventricles that each lie within a hemisphere of the cerebral cortex. Extending from the frontal lobes to the occipital lobe, the lateral ventricles consist of a body; an atrium; and frontal, temporal, and occipital horns. When cannulation of the ventricular system is required for intracranial pressure monitoring, CSF drainage, or placement of a CSF shunt, the frontal horn of the lateral ventricle on the nondominant side of the brain is most often selected.[14]

The foramen of Monro connects the two lateral ventricles with a central cavity, the third ventricle. Located directly above

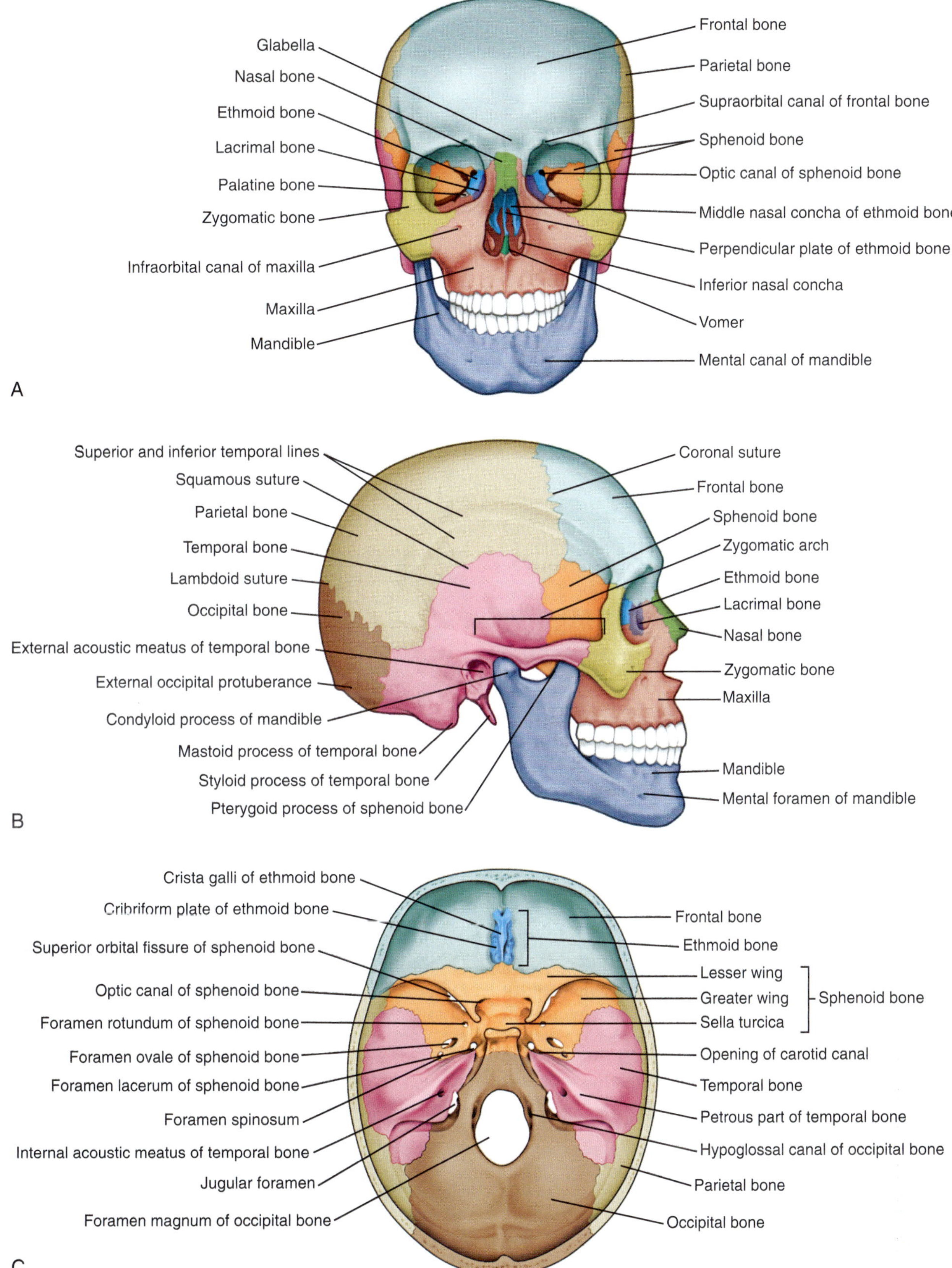

FIG. 20.5 Skull. (A) Anterior view. (B) Skull viewed from the right side. (C) Floor of the cranial cavity viewed from above. (From Patton KT, Bell F, Thompson T, Williamson P. *Anatomy and Physiology*. 11th ed. Elsevier; 2022.)

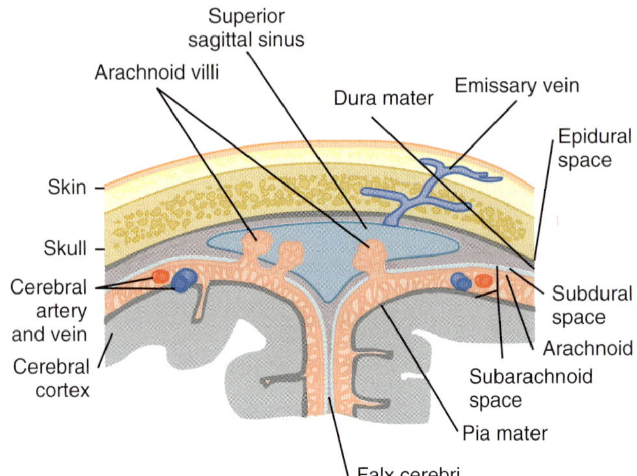

FIG. 20.6 Meninges. Coronal section of the meninges through the superior sagittal sinus. (From Black JM, Hawks JH. *Medical-Surgical Nursing: Clinical Management for Positive Outcomes*. 8th ed. Saunders; 2009.)

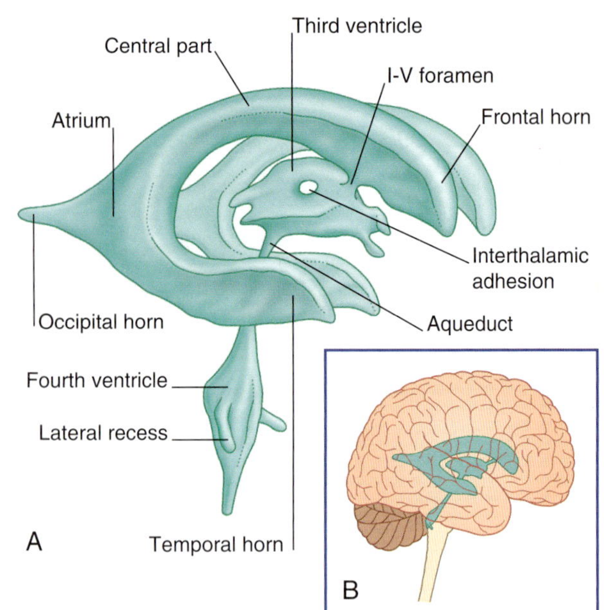

FIG. 20.7 Ventricular System. (A) Isolated cast. (B) Ventricular system in situ. (From Mtui E, Gruener G, Dockery P. *Fitzgerald's Clinical Neuroanatomy and Neuroscience*. 8th ed. Elsevier; 2021.)

the midbrain, the walls of the third ventricle are formed by the thalami. The cerebral aqueduct (aqueduct of Sylvius) is the canal between the third ventricle and fourth ventricle, which lies between the brainstem and the cerebellum. At the base of the fourth ventricle, two openings—the foramen of Luschka and the foramen of Magendie—open into the subarachnoid space. Blockage of CSF flow occurring within the ventricular system obstructs the normal circulation of CSF, causing dilation of the ventricles, a condition called *obstructive hydrocephalus*.[13]

Cerebrospinal Fluid

CSF fills the ventricular system and surrounds the brain and spinal cord in the subarachnoid space. Protection of the CNS is further provided by CSF, which acts as a shock absorber when energy is displaced in traumatic injury. CSF is normally clear, colorless, and odorless. CSF is secreted by the choroid plexuses of the ventricular system, although small amounts are also synthesized by capillaries of the pia mater. Believed to be a filtrate of blood, CSF contains some unique properties that make its synthesis a mystery (Table 20.2).

Production and resorption. The production of CSF occurs at a rate of approximately 20 mL/h, or 500 mL/day.[15] With a circulating volume of approximately 140 mL, CSF must be regularly resorbed to prevent development of hydrocephalus.[16] Resorption through intact arachnoid villi is favored by increased hydrostatic pressure mechanics that maintain CSF volume within normal limits. The flow of CSF begins in the lateral ventricles, moves through the foramina of Monro into the third ventricle, moves through the cerebral aqueduct into the fourth ventricle, and moves out the foramen of Magendie and the foramina of Luschka into the subarachnoid space of the brain and spinal cord (Fig. 20.8).

TABLE 20.2 Normal Values for Cerebrospinal Fluid

Property	Values
pH	7.35–7.45
Specific gravity	1.007
Appearance	Clear and colorless
Cells	0 WBCs/mm^3; 0 RBCs/mm^3; 0–10 lymphocytes/mm^3
Glucose	50–75 mg/dL (two-thirds of blood sugar value)
Protein	5–25 mg/dL
Volume	135–150 mL
Pressure	70–200 mm H_2O (lumbar puncture); 3–15 mm Hg (ventricular)

RBCs, Red blood cells; *WBCs*, white blood cells.

Blood-Brain Barrier

The blood-brain barrier is a physiologic mechanism that helps maintain the delicate metabolic balance in the CNS. The blood-brain barrier regulates the transport of nutrients, ions, water, and waste products through selective permeability. Stabilization of the physical and chemical environment surrounding the neurons of the CNS is the task of the blood-brain barrier. Many substances such as metabolites or toxic compounds cannot cross the blood-brain barrier. Other substances such as antibiotics cross slowly, resulting in lower concentrations of them in the brain than in other areas of the body.

Tight junctions. The blood-brain barrier operates on the concept of tight junctions between adjacent cells and consists of three separate barriers. The vascular endothelial barrier is formed by tight junctions between the endothelial cells of cerebral blood vessels. The blood-CSF barrier consists of tight junctions between the epithelial cells of the choroid plexus. The arachnoid barrier is created by tight junctions between the cells that form the outermost layer of the arachnoid mater. The selective permeability of the blood-brain barrier keeps out toxic or harmful compounds and protects neuronal function.

The blood-brain barrier exists only in certain areas of the CNS. The areas in which it does not exist—the pineal region, the basal hypothalamus, and the floor of the fourth

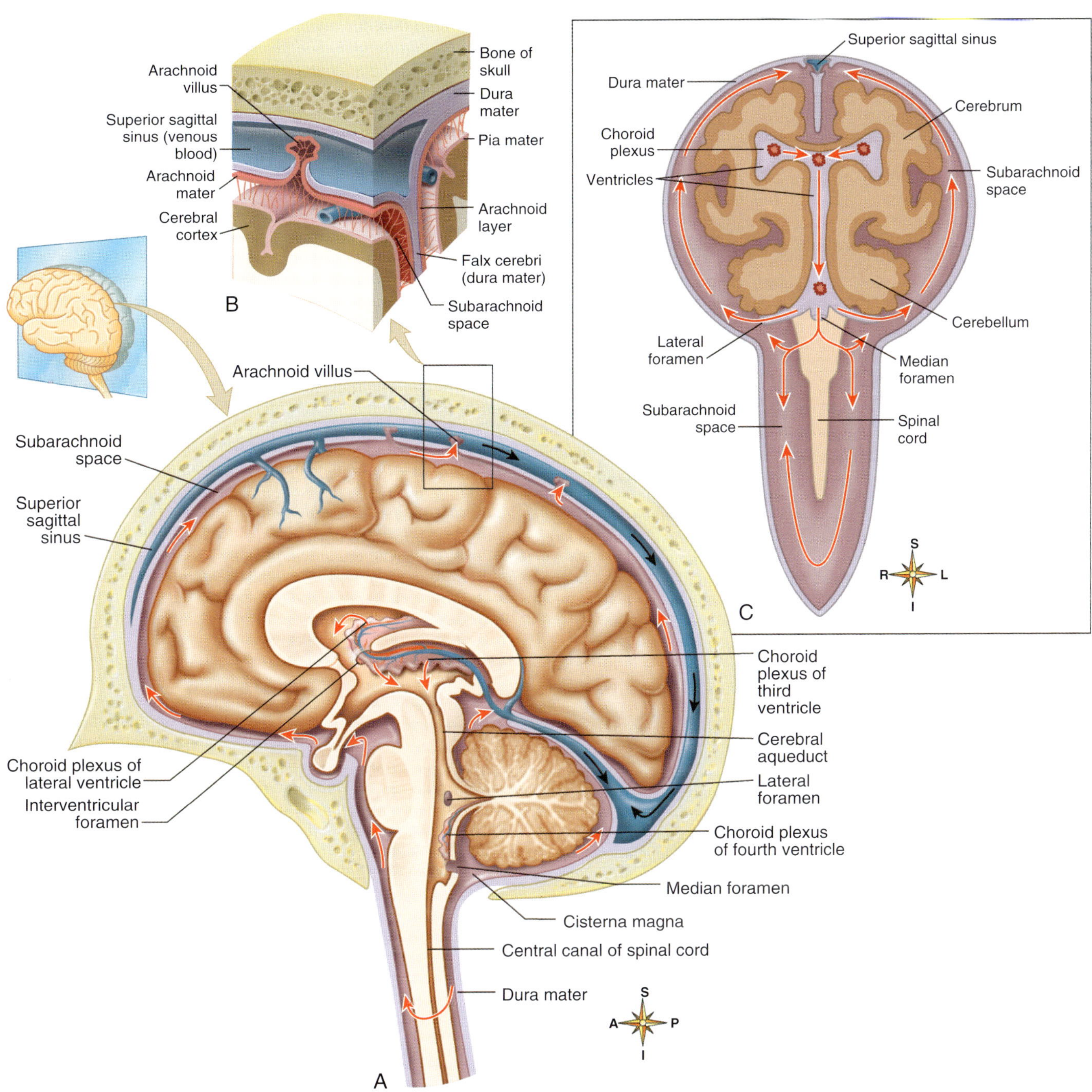

FIG. 20.8 Flow of Cerebrospinal Fluid. (A) Fluid produced by filtration of blood by the choroid plexus of each ventricle flows inferiorly through the lateral ventricles, interventricular foramen, third ventricle, cerebral aqueduct, fourth ventricle, and subarachnoid space and to blood. (B) Inset showing arachnoid villus, where CSF is reabsorbed into the blood of the superior sagittal sinus. (C) Simplified diagram showing flow of CSF. (From Patton KT, Bell F, Thompson T, Williamson P. *Anatomy and Physiology*. 11th ed. Elsevier; 2022.)

ventricle—require contact with plasma to sense changes in concentration of glucose and carbon dioxide and changes in serum osmolality. Initiation of feedback mechanisms by the hypothalamus in response to these changes regulates the internal environment of the remainder of the body.

Permeability. Passage of substances across the blood-brain barrier is a function of particle size, lipid solubility, and protein-binding potential. Most medications or compounds that are lipid soluble and stable at body pH rapidly cross the blood-brain barrier. The blood-brain barrier is also highly permeable to water, oxygen, carbon dioxide, and glucose.[17] Of clinical significance, disruption or alteration of blood-brain barrier permeability occurs with injury to brain tissue from trauma, toxic insults, and ischemic injury.[18]

Cerebrum

The cerebrum is the largest portion of the brain, constituting 80% of its weight, and is composed of two cerebral hemispheres (right and left), separated by the longitudinal fissure and connected at the base by the corpus callosum (Fig. 20.9B). The

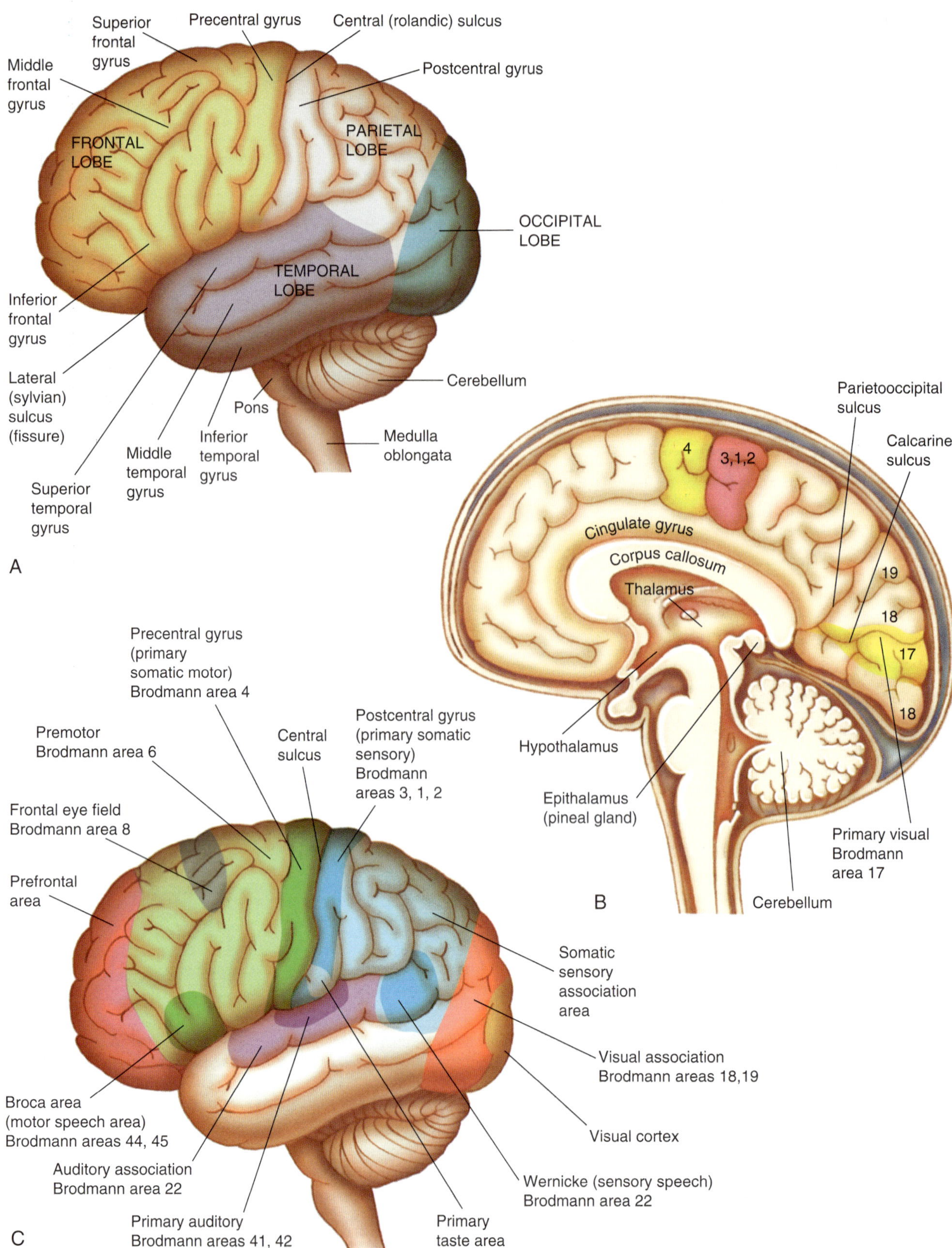

FIG. 20.9 Cerebral Hemispheres. (A) Left hemisphere of cerebrum, lateral view. (B) Functional areas of the cerebral cortex, midsagittal view. (C) Functional areas of the cerebral cortex, lateral view. (From Huether SE, McCance KL, Brashers VL, eds. *Understanding Pathophysiology*. 7th ed. Elsevier; 2020.)

outermost aspect of the cerebrum is called the cerebral cortex and is made up of gray matter, consisting of neuronal cell bodies. Directly below the cerebral cortex lies white matter, consisting of myelinated axons, which communicate impulses from the cerebral cortex to other areas of the brain. White matter tracts consist of three types of fibers: (1) commissural (transverse), (2) projection, and (3) association. Commissural fibers are tracts that communicate between the two cerebral hemispheres, and the corpus callosum is the largest commissural tract. Projection fibers communicate between the cerebral cortex and the lower regions of the brain and the spinal cord. Association fibers communicate between various regions of the same hemisphere.

The cerebral hemispheres are divided into the frontal, parietal, temporal, and occipital lobes (Fig. 20.9A). The rhinencephalon is often labeled the fifth lobe of the cerebral cortex. Lying deep inside the cerebrum and anatomically associated with the temporal lobe, the rhinencephalon is sometimes referred to as the limbic lobe.

Function

The primary functions of the cerebral cortex include sensory, motor, and intellectual (cognitive) functions, making this area of the brain vital to normal human functioning and providing capabilities that make humans unique as a species. Brodmann's classification of cerebral cortical cytoarchitecture identifies more than 100 unique areas and provides a useful way to localize specific cortical functions within the brain (Fig. 20.9C). This section covers the areas within Brodmann's classification that are commonly assessed in relation to the development of specific neurologic pathology.

Frontal Lobe

The frontal lobe lies underneath the frontal bone of the skull and is separated posteriorly from the parietal lobe by the central sulcus (fissure of Rolando) and inferiorly from the temporal lobe by the lateral fissure (sylvian fissure) (see Fig. 20.9A). The major functions of the frontal lobe are voluntary motor function, cognitive function (orientation, memory, insight, judgment, arithmetic, and abstraction), and expressive language (verbal and written).

Prefrontal area. The prefrontal areas (see Fig. 20.9C), located just behind the frontal bone's distribution over the forehead, are concerned with cognition. These areas work in concert with other areas of the brain to intellectually appraise and respond to environmental information or stimuli. They augment the intellect with socially trained emotional responses learned over the course of childhood and young adulthood, and they participate in triggering autonomic nervous system responses such as tachycardia in relation to situational needs. The location of the prefrontal cortex makes it vulnerable to traumatic injury, often resulting in profound changes in cognitive capacity and social responses to environmental stimuli after brain injury.[19]

Motor strip. The motor strip of the frontal cortex is represented by Brodmann area 4 (see Fig. 20.9C) and consists of cell bodies for neurons associated with voluntary (pyramidal) motor functions. Because most voluntary motor tracts cross over to the opposite side as they descend through the brainstem, the right motor strip represents voluntary motor function for the left side of the body, and vice versa. The motor homunculus (Fig. 20.10B) is a graphic representation of the distribution of voluntary motor function throughout area 4. Appearing as an upside-down man, the foot of the homunculus is illustrated on the superior medial aspects of the frontal lobes, with the knees, hips, trunk, and shoulders extending along the lateral surfaces and with the hands, thumb, head, face, and tongue represented in a lateral inferior distribution extending to the sylvian fissure. The homunculus demonstrates larger body part size to denote areas with greater representation because of the amount of dexterity associated with the part's function. The large surface area of the trunk occupies a relatively small part of the motor strip, whereas smaller body areas such as the thumb or tongue, which involve a great deal of dexterity and fine motor movement, occupy a larger area of the motor strip. Damage to the motor strip results in compromise of motor function on the opposite side of the body.[20]

Broca area. The Broca area (Brodmann areas 44 and 45) is located at the inferior frontal gyrus close to the motor strip's facial distribution (see Fig. 20.9C). Most commonly, the Broca area is located on the left side of the frontal lobe, although it occasionally is located in the right frontal hemisphere. The Broca area is responsible for expressive language and is used in the formation of verbal and written communication. Damage occurring to this area results in disability ranging from difficulties with word finding to an expressive or nonfluent aphasia, in which verbal and written communication are significantly compromised, although verbal language reception and comprehension may remain intact.[21]

Parietal Lobe

The parietal lobe lies directly behind the frontal lobe on the opposite side of the central sulcus. The posterior border of the parietal lobe is the parieto-occipital fissure, which separates the parietal lobe from the occipital lobe (see Fig. 20.9A). The parietal lobes are primarily concerned with sensory functions, including integration of sensory information; awareness of body parts; interpretation of touch, pressure, and pain; and recognition of object size, shape, and texture.

Sensory strip. The parietal lobe contains a sensory strip (Brodmann areas 1, 2, and 3) that lies opposite the motor strip of the frontal lobe (see Fig. 20.9C). Similar to the homunculus of the motor strip, a sensory homunculus recreates a caricature of an upside-down man (see Fig. 20.10A) representing areas that account for receipt and initial analyses of sensory information from different areas of the body. Areas of the body with greater sensory needs occupy larger areas on the sensory strip, which is concerned with deep or internal sensations and with cutaneous sensations such as touch, pressure, position, and vibration. Injury to these areas may result in tactile sensory loss on the opposite side of the body.[20]

Somatic sensory associative area. The somatic sensory associative area of the parietal lobe (see Fig. 20.9C) facilitates further assessment of sensory stimuli, promoting an ability to determine size, shape, texture, locality of stimuli, temperature, vibration, and precise purpose of familiar objects based solely on tactile discrimination. Interpretive aspects of the response of the parietal lobe to stimuli include awareness of body parts, perceptual orientation in space, and recognition of environmental spatial relationships. Injury to these areas may result in perceptual neglect or inattention.[21]

Wernicke area. The Wernicke area (Brodmann area 22) is partially located within the parietal lobe and partially in the temporal lobe, most commonly on the left side of the cerebral cortex (see Fig. 20.9C). This area is concerned with reception of written and verbal language and includes many intricate connections to other parts of the brain associated with auditory and visual functions, cognitive appraisal, and expressive language. Injury to this area of the brain may result in disability ranging from minor receptive language dysfunction to receptive or fluent aphasia, in which expressive language function remains but is illogical in content, or a "word salad." When brain injury includes the areas important to language reception

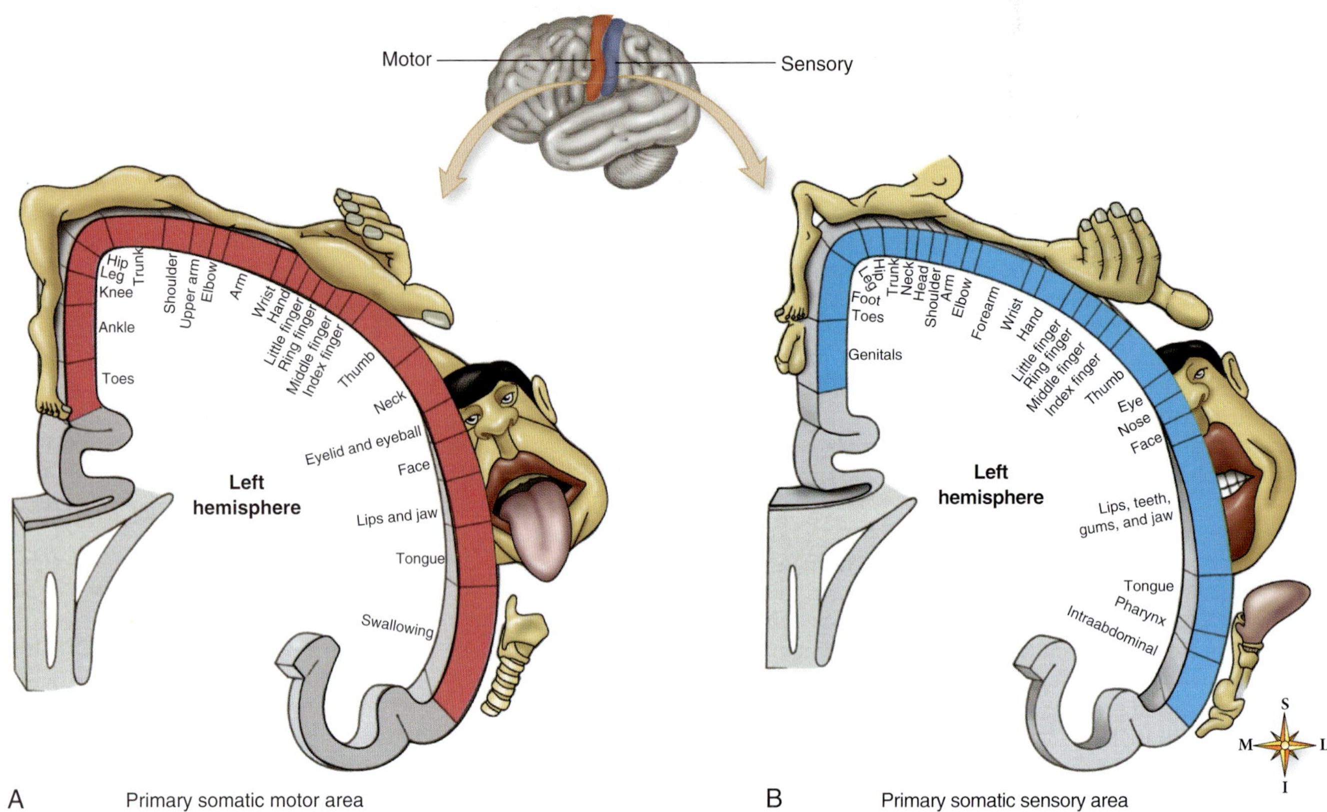

FIG. 20.10 Sensory and Motor Cortex. Primary somatic sensory (A) and motor (B) areas of the cortex. (From Patton KT, Bell F, Thompson T, Williamson P. *Anatomy and Physiology.* 11th ed. Elsevier; 2022.)

and expression, global aphasia may result, significantly limiting receipt and expression of language.[22]

Temporal Lobe

The temporal lobe lies beneath the temporal bone in the lateral portion of the cranium (see Fig. 20.9A). The anterior, lower border of the temporal lobe is encased in the sphenoid wing. With a strong blow to the head, the temporal lobe is easily contused and lacerated as it moves against this hard, irregular surface. Separated from the frontal and parietal lobes by the lateral fissure, this lobe has the primary functions of hearing, speech, behavior, and memory.

Auditory areas. The primary auditory areas (Brodmann areas 41 and 42) receive sound impulses and assist in determining the source and meaning of sound (see Fig. 20.9C). Injury to these areas may result in auditory perceptual loss.[23] Auditory centers in the temporal lobe are closely linked with the Wernicke area. In the superior portion of the temporal lobe, where the frontal, parietal, and temporal lobes meet, is an essential interpretive area in which auditory, visual, and somatic association areas are integrated into complex thought and memory. Seizures in this region of the temporal lobe cause auditory, visual, and sensory hallucinations.[24]

Occipital Lobe

The occipital lobe forms the most posterior aspects of the cerebral cortex (see Fig. 20.9A) and is concerned with interpretation of visual stimuli. The primary visual cortex (see Fig. 20.9C) receives impulses from projections of the optic nerve (cranial nerve II). These impulses are then referred to the visual associative areas (Brodmann areas 18 and 19) for interpretation and integration (see Fig. 20.9C). Injury to the occipital lobes may result in cortical blindness, in which the eye structures remain intact but the ability to receive and interpret visual stimuli is lost.[25]

Limbic Lobe

The rhinencephalon, or limbic lobe, lies medially along the inner aspects of the temporal lobe. The core of the limbic system consists of the hippocampus and the amygdaloid nucleus. Compared with animals living in the wild, the limbic lobe is poorly developed in humans as a result of the sophisticated cognitive capabilities of the frontal lobe, which mediate many of the protective strategies used by humans in everyday life.

Function. The limbic lobe's primary functions are related to self-preservation and include functions such as recall of pleasurable and unpleasant or potentially dangerous events, modification of mood and emotional responses in relation to perceived events, interpretation of smell, and augmentation of visceral processes (e.g., heart rate, respiration) associated with emotion. When the injured prefrontal cortex results in cognitive disability, this controversial area of the brain may take on increased control to support self-preservation needs. This may result in significantly aberrant behavior that is typically judged as socially unacceptable.[26]

Internal Capsule

Fiber tracts from many portions of each half of the cerebrum converge in the area of the brain known as the *internal capsule* as they progress toward the brainstem and the spinal cord. The internal capsule contains afferent and efferent fibers (Fig. 20.11).

Function

Afferent (sensory) impulses destined for the cortex travel through the internal capsule in the following succession: brainstem to thalamus to internal capsule to cerebral cortex. Efferent (motor) fibers leaving the cortex also pass through the internal capsule. Injury to a portion of the internal capsule may result in pure sensory loss, motor loss, or both on the opposite side of the body with preservation of cortical function.[27]

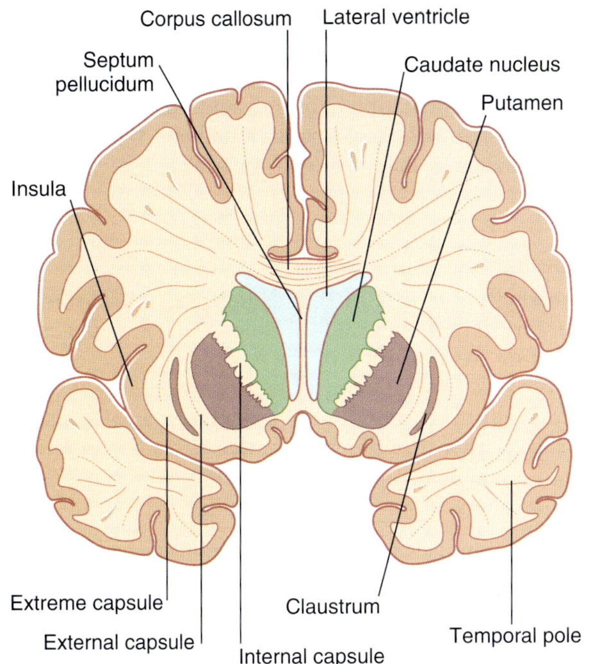

FIG. 20.11 Internal Capsule. Coronal section through the anterior limb of the internal capsule. (From Mtui E, Gruener G, Dockery P. *Fitzgerald's Clinical Neuroanatomy and Neuroscience*. 8th ed. Elsevier; 2021.)

Basal Ganglia

The basal ganglia participate in regulating extrapyramidal (involuntary) motor function. Located deep within the white matter of the cerebral hemispheres, the basal ganglia consist of four nuclei: (1) the corpus striatum (caudate nucleus and putamen), (2) the globus pallidus, (3) the substantia nigra, and (4) the subthalamic nucleus (see Fig. 20.11). The basal ganglia are considered a telencephalic, or cerebral, structure, and they are embryologically separate from the thalamus, which is considered a diencephalic structure.

Function

Although the basal ganglia play a major role in regulating voluntary motor function, they do not provide direct input to motor tracts through the spinal cord. Instead, input from the cerebral cortex stimulates basal ganglia output, which is sent to the brainstem and the thalamus for relay back to the frontal cortex. Ultimately, the basal ganglia integrate associated movements and postural adjustments with voluntary motor movement, suppressing skeletal muscle tone as needed to provide fluid, smooth motor function. Dysfunction of the basal ganglia may result in tremor or other involuntary movements; rigid, nonfluid muscle tone; and slowness of movement without paralysis.[28]

Diencephalon

The diencephalon lies below the cerebral cortex and consists of two structures: (1) the thalamus and (2) the hypothalamus (Fig. 20.12). Although structurally wedded to the hypothalamus, the pituitary gland is considered an endocrine organ and is not a

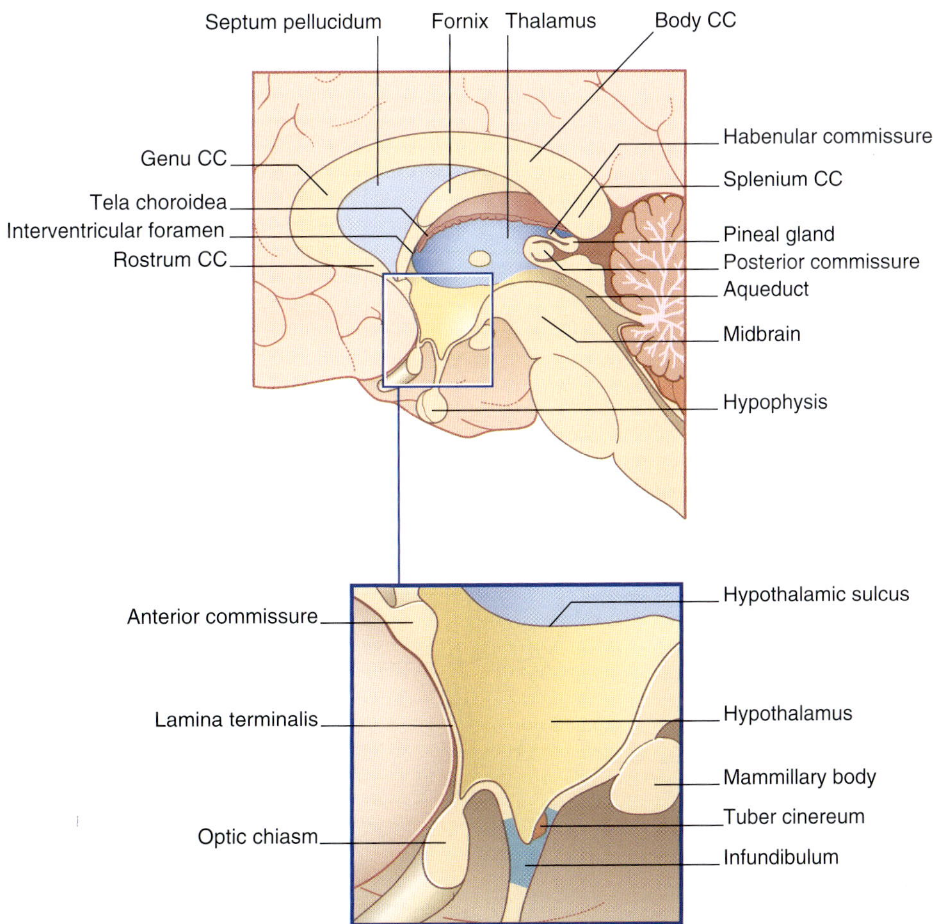

FIG. 20.12 Diencephalon. The diencephalon and its boundaries. *CC*, Corpus callosum. (From Mtui E, Gruener G, Dockery P. *Fitzgerald's Clinical Neuroanatomy and Neuroscience*. 8th ed. Elsevier; 2021.)

part of the CNS. Pituitary gland anatomy and physiology are discussed in detail in Chapter 29.

Thalamus

The thalamus consists of two connected ovoid masses of gray matter and forms the lateral walls of the third ventricle (see Fig. 20.12). The two thalami serve as a relay station and gatekeeper for motor and sensory stimuli, preventing or enhancing transmission of impulses based on the behavioral needs of the person.

Function. More than 50 nuclei support thalamic function and are divided into specific relay nuclei and nonspecific diffusely projecting nuclei. Relay nuclei have a specific relationship or trajectory within the cerebral cortex, whereas diffusely projecting nuclei are thought to mediate cortical arousal. Thalamic injury may result in sensory or motor dysfunction, or both, when normal impulse pathways are interrupted.[29]

Hypothalamus

The hypothalamus is located below the thalamus and is connected to the pituitary gland by the hypothalamic or pituitary stalk (see Fig. 20.12). Neural control of emotion involves many regions of the brain, including the amygdala and limbic associations with the prefrontal cortex, but to ensure homeostasis, these systems all work through the hypothalamus to coordinate the body's behavioral responses to emotion.

Function. The hypothalamus maintains internal homeostasis through its ability to stimulate autonomic nervous system response and endocrine system function in relation to body needs, giving the hypothalamus a role in temperature regulation, regulation of food and water intake, control of pituitary hormone release, and augmentation of overall autonomic nervous system output to a sympathetic or parasympathetic state. Damage to the hypothalamus may result in a variety of neuroendocrine disorders.[30]

Cerebellum

The cerebellum (Fig. 20.13), or hindbrain, is separated from the cerebrum by the dural fold called the *tentorium cerebelli*. Accounting for one-fifth of the brain's size, the cerebellum consists of two lateral hemispheres connected by the vermis. The cerebellum is composed of an outer layer of gray matter, or cortex, with a core of white matter tracts lying beneath.

Function

Cerebellar impulses are communicated to descending motor pathways to integrate spatial orientation and equilibrium with posture and muscle tone, ensuring synchronized adjustments in movement that maintain overall balance and motor coordination (see Fig. 20.13). Cerebellar monitoring and adjustment of motor activity occurs simultaneously with movement, enabling significant control of fine motor function. The cerebellum is bombarded with information related to the goals of movement and disparities between actual and intended movements. Axons projecting into the cerebellum are 40 times more numerous than the axons leaving the

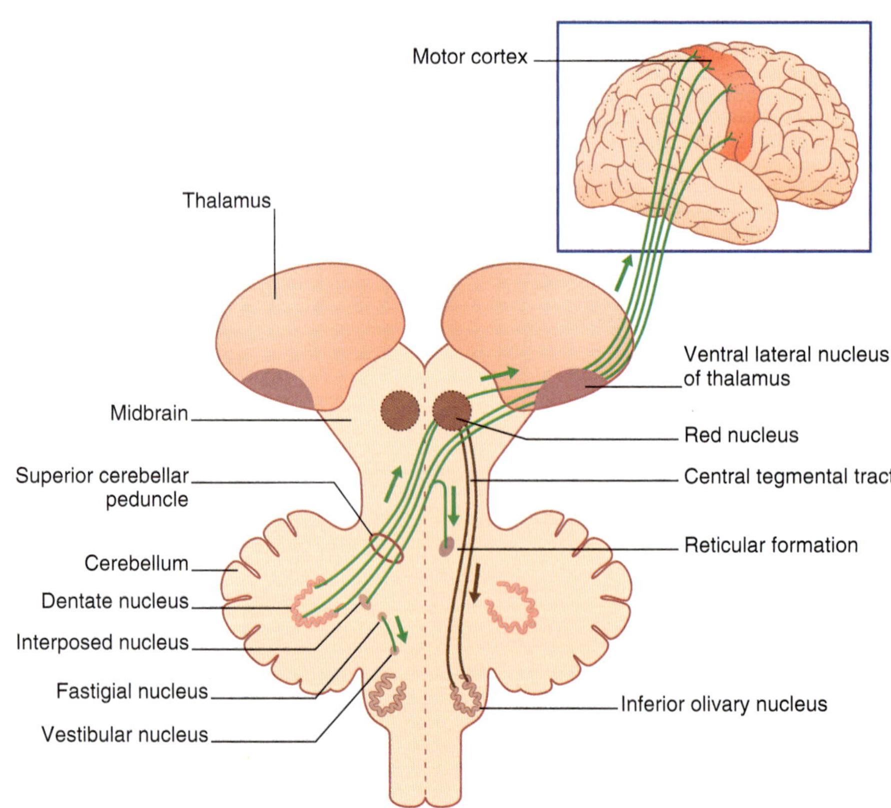

FIG. 20.13 Principal Cerebellar Efferents. *Arrows* indicate directions of impulse conduction. (From Mtui E, Gruener G, Dockery P. *Fitzgerald's Clinical Neuroanatomy and Neuroscience*. 8th ed. Elsevier; 2021.)

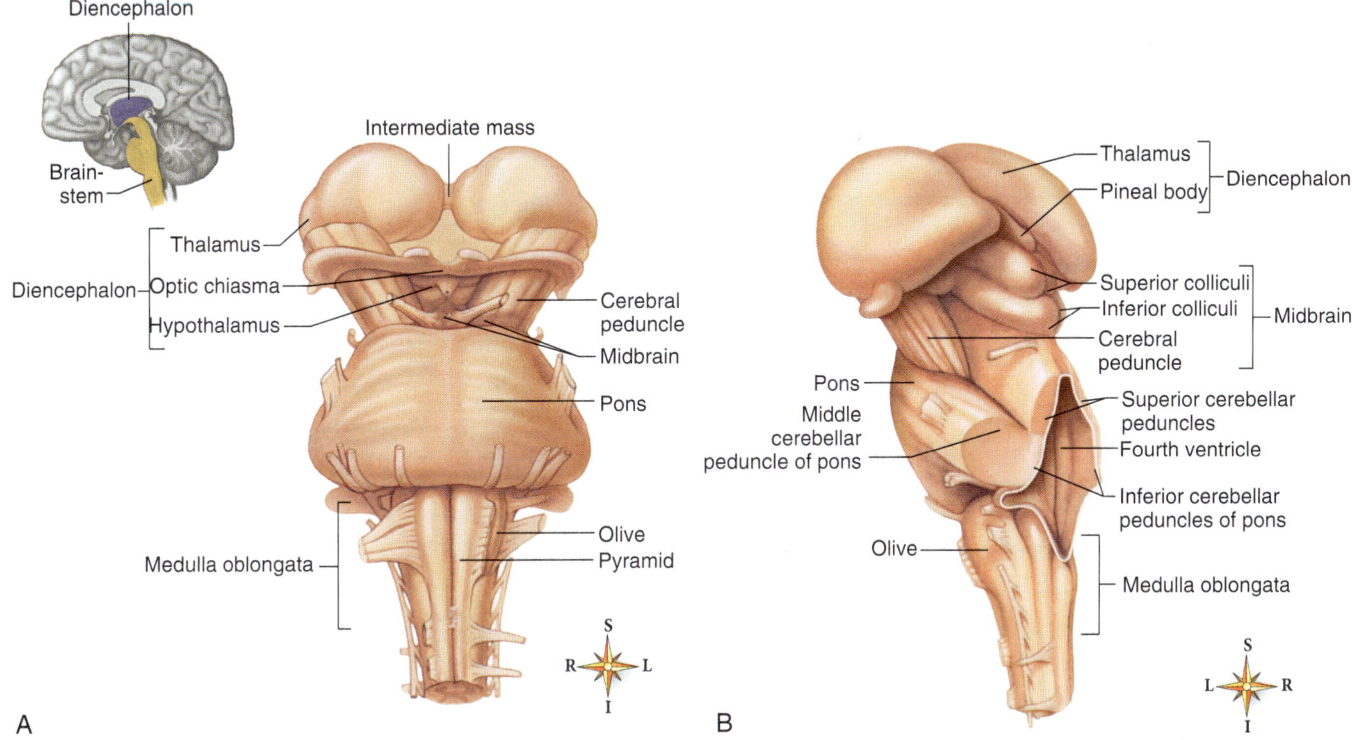

FIG. 20.14 Brainstem and Diencephalon. (A) Anterior aspect. (B) Posterior aspect (shifted slightly to lateral). (From Patton KT, Bell F, Thompson T, Williamson P. *Anatomy and Physiology.* 11th ed. Elsevier; 2022.)

cerebellum to ensure adequate receipt of motor information. Injury to the cerebellum produces ataxia, defined as preservation of motor strength with lack of control (coordination) over fine motor function.[31]

Brainstem

The brainstem consists of three major divisions: (1) the midbrain, (2) the pons, and (3) the medulla oblongata. The brainstem is packed with sensory and motor pathways traveling between the spinal cord and the brain and contains numerous centers that regulate vital mechanisms throughout the body.

Midbrain

The midbrain forms the junction between the pons and the diencephalon. The cell bodies of cranial nerves III and IV originate in the midbrain. The midbrain is divided by a sagittal plane into the two cerebral peduncles (Fig. 20.14) and anatomically constitutes the location of the aqueduct of Sylvius. The major function of the midbrain is to relay stimuli to and from the brain through ascending sensory tracts and descending motor pathways.

Pons

Located above the medulla, the pons relays information to and from the brain through sensory and motor pathways. The posterior aspects of the pons make up the upper surface of the fourth ventricle (see Fig. 20.14). Two respiratory control centers are located in the pons: the apneustic and pneumotaxic centers. The apneustic center controls the length of inspiration and expiration, whereas the pneumotaxic center controls respiratory rate.

The cell bodies of cranial nerves V (trigeminal), VI (abducens), VII (facial), and VIII (acoustic) are located in the pons. The medial longitudinal fasciculus is an important fiber tract in the pons that connects cranial nerves III, IV, and VI with the vestibular portion of the acoustic nerve and pontine paramedian reticular formation (RF), allowing coordinated and appropriate movements of the eyes in response to noise, motion, position, and arousal. The structural integrity of the brainstem may be assessed through clinical stimulation of the medial longitudinal fasciculus in caloric testing.

Medulla Oblongata

The medulla oblongata forms the last section of the brainstem, situated between the pons and the spinal cord (see Fig. 20.14). In the pyramids of the medulla, decussation (crossing) of voluntary motor fibers occurs, lending the name *pyramidal* to voluntary motor function (Box 20.1). Below the point of decussation, stimuli from the right side of the brain control movement for the left side of the body and vice versa.

BOX 20.1 Decussation of Voluntary Motor Fibers

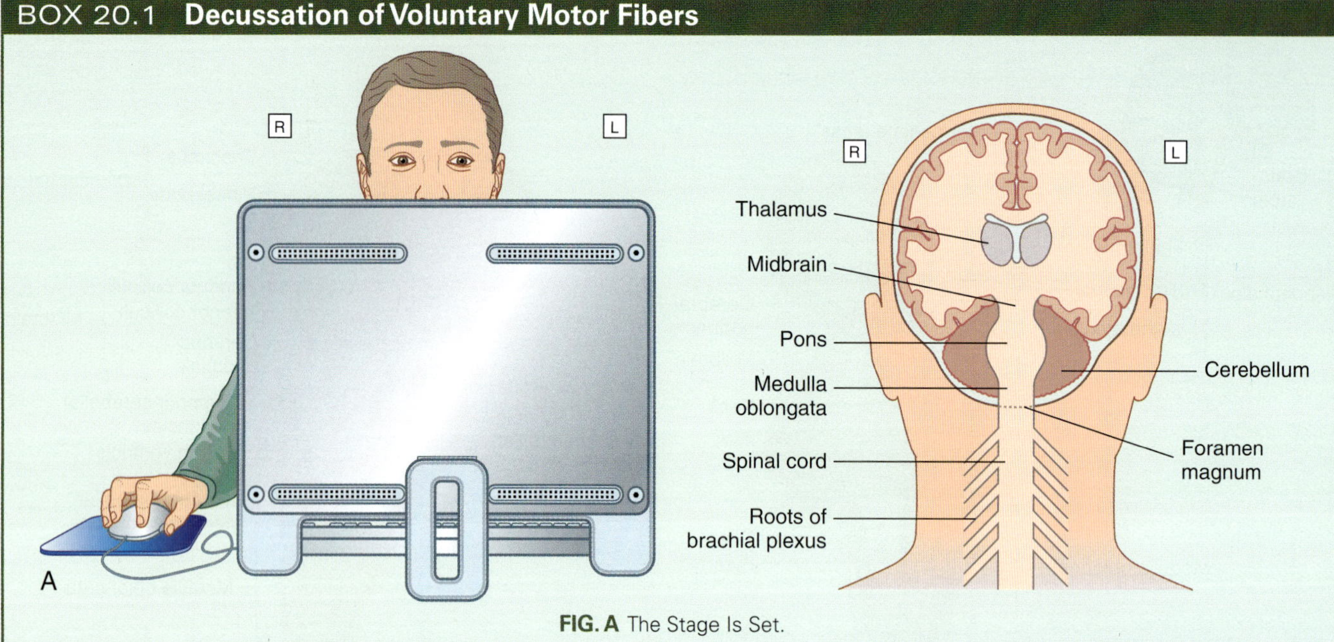

FIG. A The Stage Is Set.

The subject's right hand is about to click the mouse while the eyes are directed elsewhere. The coronal section identifies key structures.

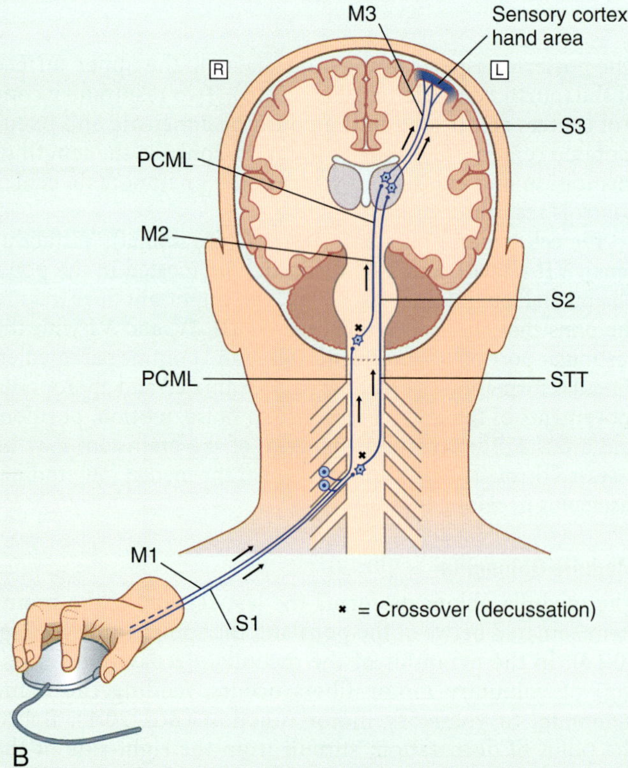

FIG. B Afferents.

The left parietal lobe constructs a map of the right hand in relation to the mouse, based on information sent to the left somatic sensory cortex (postcentral gyrus) from the skin and deep tissues. The information is relayed by three successive sets of neurons from the skin and by another set of three neurons from the deep tissues. The first set in each case is composed of first-order or primary afferent neurons. These neurons are called unipolar, because each axon emerges from a single point (or pole) of the cell body and divides in a T-shaped manner to provide continuity of impulse conduction from tissue to central nervous system. The primary afferent neurons terminate by forming contacts known as *synapses* on the multipolar (more or less star-shaped) cells of the second-order (secondary) set. The axons of the second-order neurons project across the midline before turning up to terminate on third-order (tertiary) multipolar neurons projecting to the postcentral gyrus.

Primary afferents activated by contacts with the skin of the hand (S1) terminate in the posterior horn of the gray matter of the spinal cord. Second-order cutaneous afferents (S2) cross the midline in the anterior white commissure and ascend to the thalamus within the spinothalamic tract (STT), to be relayed by third-order neurons to the hand area of the sensory cortex.

The most significant deep tissue sensory organs are neuromuscular spindles (muscle spindles) contained within skeletal muscles. The primary afferents supplying the muscle spindles of the intrinsic muscles of the hand belong to large unipolar neurons whose axons (labeled M1) ascend ipsilaterally (on the same side of the spinal cord) within the posterior funiculus. They synapse in the nucleus cuneatus in the medulla oblongata. The multipolar second-order neurons send their axons across the midline in the sensory decussation. The axons ascend (M2) through pons and midbrain before synapsing on third-order neurons (M3) projecting from thalamus to sensory cortex. *PCML*, Posterior column–medial lemniscal pathway; *STT*, spinothalamic tract.

BOX 20.1 **Decussation of Voluntary Motor Fibers—cont'd**

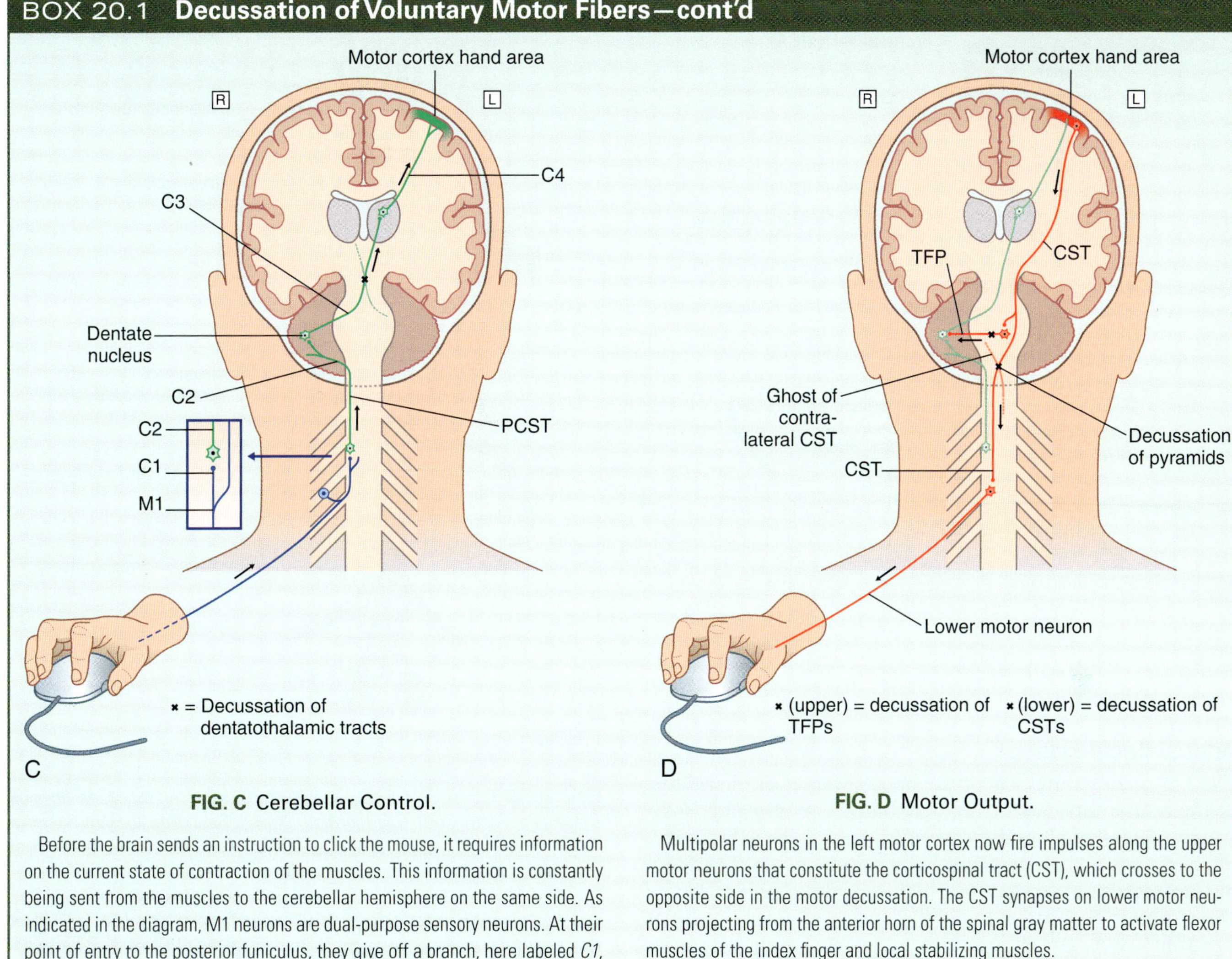

FIG. C Cerebellar Control.

Before the brain sends an instruction to click the mouse, it requires information on the current state of contraction of the muscles. This information is constantly being sent from the muscles to the cerebellar hemisphere on the same side. As indicated in the diagram, M1 neurons are dual-purpose sensory neurons. At their point of entry to the posterior funiculus, they give off a branch, here labeled *C1*, to a spinocerebellar neuron that projects *(C2)* to the ipsilateral cerebellum. From here, a cerebellothalamic neuron *(C3)* is shown projecting across the midbrain to the contralateral thalamus, where a further neuron *(C4)* relays information to the hand area of the motor cortex in the precentral gyrus.

FIG. D Motor Output.

Multipolar neurons in the left motor cortex now fire impulses along the upper motor neurons that constitute the corticospinal tract (CST), which crosses to the opposite side in the motor decussation. The CST synapses on lower motor neurons projecting from the anterior horn of the spinal gray matter to activate flexor muscles of the index finger and local stabilizing muscles.

Note that a copy of the outgoing message is sent to the right cerebellar hemisphere by way of transverse fibers of the pons (TFP) originating in multipolar neurons located on the left side of the pons.

Modified from Mtui E, Gruener G, Dockery P. *Fitzgerald's Clinical Neuroanatomy and Neuroscience*. 7th ed. Elsevier; 2016.

Involuntary functions. Centers for control of involuntary functions such as swallowing, vomiting, hiccupping, coughing, heart rate, arterial vasoconstriction, and respiration are located within the medulla oblongata. The medullary respiratory center works in conjunction with the apneustic and pneumotaxic centers in the pons to control respiratory function and is responsible for the rhythm of respiration. The cell bodies of cranial nerves IX (glossopharyngeal), X (vagus), XI (spinal accessory), and XII (hypoglossal) are located in the medulla oblongata (see Fig. 20.14).

Reticular Formation

The RF of the brainstem is located at the core of the brainstem and is active in modulating sensation, movement, consciousness, reflexive behaviors, and the activities of the cranial nerves arising from the brainstem (III through XII). The RF extends from the upper pons to the diencephalon. The ascending RF is referred to as the *reticular activating system (RAS)* and is responsible for increasing wakefulness, vigilance, and responsiveness of cortical and thalamic neurons to sensory stimuli. In the thalamus, the RAS activates relay and diffuse projection nuclei to increase distribution of sensory stimuli throughout the cerebral cortex. The RAS also works through activation of the hypothalamus, which results in diffuse cortical stimulation and autonomic stimulation. Damage to the thalamic or hypothalamic RAS pathways results in impaired consciousness.[32]

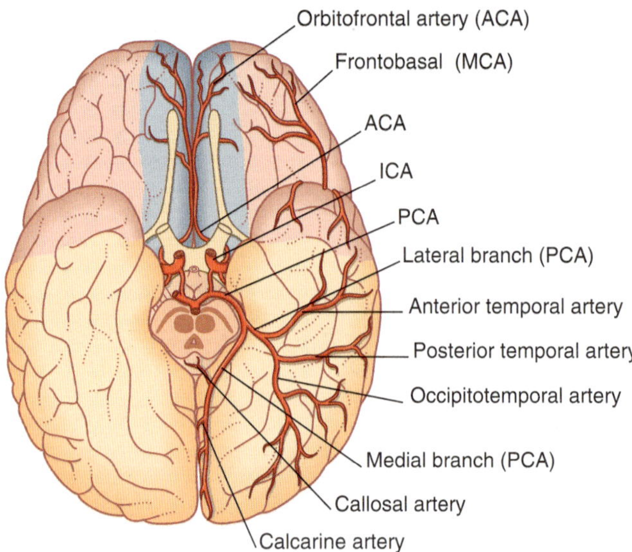

FIG. 20.15 Cerebral Arteries. View from below the cerebral hemispheres, showing the cortical branches and territories of the three cerebral arteries. *ACA*, Anterior cerebral artery; *ICA*, internal carotid artery; *MCA*, middle cerebral artery; *PCA*, posterior cerebral artery. (From Mtui E, Gruener G, Dockery P. *Fitzgerald's Clinical Neuroanatomy and Neuroscience*. 8th ed. Elsevier; 2021.)

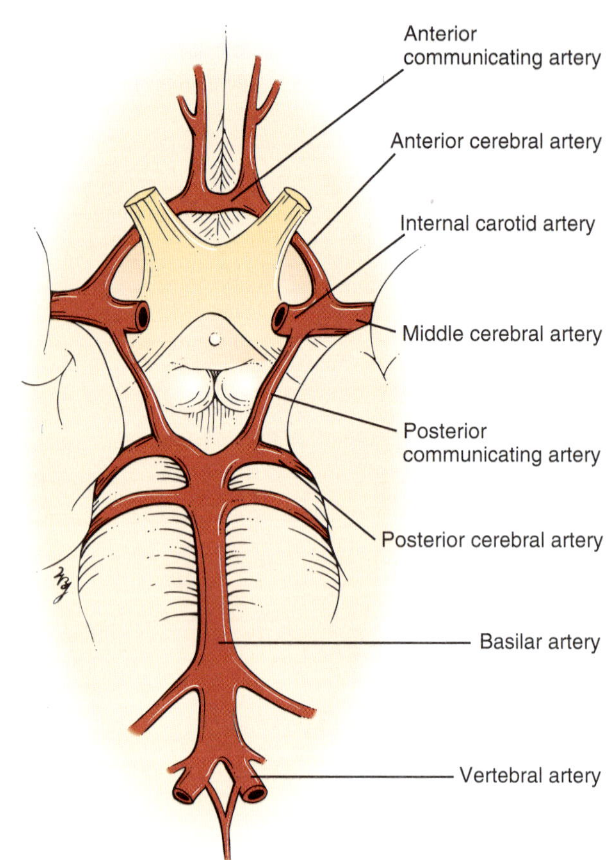

FIG. 20.16 Circle of Willis. (From Swartz MH. *Textbook of Physical Diagnosis: History and Examination*. 8th ed. Saunders; 2021.)

Arterial Circulation

The brain constitutes 2% of the body's weight but uses 20% of the body's total resting cardiac output, requires approximately 750 mL of blood flow per minute, and can extract 45% of arterial oxygen to meet normal metabolic needs. The brain has no reserve of oxygen or glucose, making reductions of these substances critical to the disruption of normal cellular function. Two pairs of arteries, the internal carotid arteries and the vertebral arteries, provide blood to the brain and are anatomically separated into the anterior and posterior circulations that connect at the base of the brain to form the circle of Willis (Figs. 20.15 and 20.16). Knowledge of the brain's arterial supply as it correlates to neurologic function is an essential aspect of neuroscience critical care nursing, especially in the care of patients who had experienced a stroke.

Anterior Circulation

The anterior circulation of the brain is supplied by the right and left internal carotid arteries and their branches (Fig. 20.16). Originating as the common carotids, the left common carotid takes off from the arch of the aorta, whereas the right common carotid originates from the innominate artery. At the level of the cricothyroid junction, the common carotid splits to form the external and internal carotid arteries. The external carotid feeds the face, the scalp, and the skull and includes the branch called the *middle meningeal artery*, which lies between the skull and the dura mater.

The internal carotid artery continues upward through the carotid siphon and enters the base of the skull through an opening in the petrous bone. At the base of the brain, the internal carotid gives off the right and left middle cerebral arteries; the right and left anterior cerebral arteries (ACAs), which are connected by the anterior communicating artery (ACoA); and the two posterior communicating arteries (PCoAs). The anterior circulation provides 80% of the blood flow to the cerebral hemispheres, covering the needs of the frontal lobes and most of the parietal and temporal lobes and supplying the subcortical structures residing above the brainstem. The internal carotid artery gives rise to the ophthalmic artery at the siphon before bifurcating into the anterior cerebral and middle cerebral arteries. The ophthalmic artery supplies blood to the optic nerve and eye and may reverse its course to supplement the arterial blood volume of the anterior circulation in the case of internal carotid artery occlusion.

Posterior Circulation

The posterior circulation begins with the two vertebral arteries (Fig. 20.17), which originate from the subclavian arteries and travel posteriorly through small openings in the lateral spinous processes of the cervical spine. They enter the skull through the foramen magnum, and at the level of the pons, the two vertebral arteries fuse to form the basilar artery. The terminal portion of the vertebral arteries gives rise to two important arterial branches before basilar artery fusion: the posterior inferior cerebellar arteries. Two major infratentorial branches of the basilar artery include the anterior inferior cerebellar arteries and the superior cerebellar arteries, which together with the posterior inferior cerebellar arteries supply

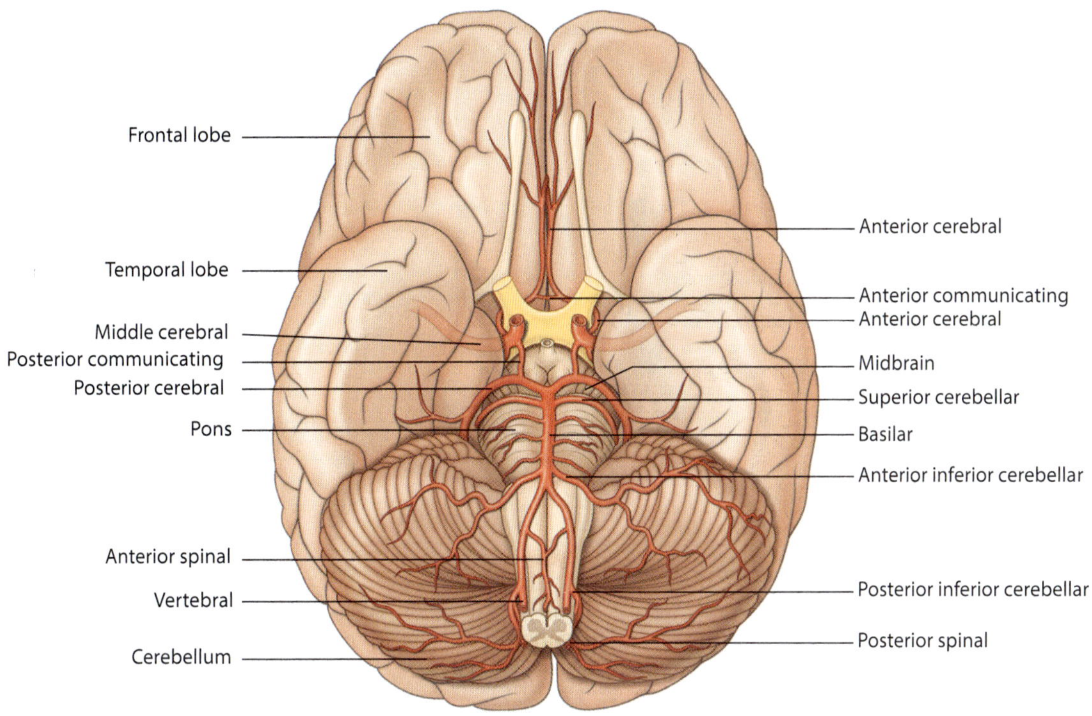

FIG. 20.17 Posterior Arterial Distribution. Arteries at the base of the brain. (From Drake RL, Vogl AW, Mitchell AWM. *Gray's Anatomy for Students*, 4th ed. Elsevier; 2020.)

the cerebellum. The distal basilar artery gives rise to the two posterior cerebral arteries, which emerge in the supratentorial region to supply the posterior aspects of the cerebral cortex.

Circle of Willis

The circle of Willis is a vascular supply system unique to the brain's circulation (see Figs. 20.15 and 20.16). Located above the optic chiasm in the subarachnoid space, the circle is fed by branches of the internal carotid and basilar arteries. The anterior circulation is connected between the two ACAs by the ACoA and to the posterior circulation by the two PCoAs. Approximately 50% of the population has a complete or "ideal" circle of Willis. In others, atretic (small and nonfunctional or hypoplastic) segments often are found in the first branch of the ACAs, called A1; in the first branch of the posterior cerebral arteries, called P1; and in the PCoAs. When complete, the circle of Willis is capable of supporting some degree of collateral blood flow in the case of arterial occlusion, although a sufficient arterial supply in the face of arterial obstruction is not guaranteed.[33]

Venous Circulation

Venous drainage occurs through venous sinuses, many of which are housed in the double-folded membrane of the dura mater (Fig. 20.18). Capillaries drain into venules, which then flow into cerebral veins, ultimately emptying into sinuses located throughout the cranium. Blood from these sinuses empties into the internal jugular vein, which empties into the superior vena cava (Fig. 20.19). Cerebral veins have thinner walls relative to veins in the general circulation and lack a muscular layer or valves.

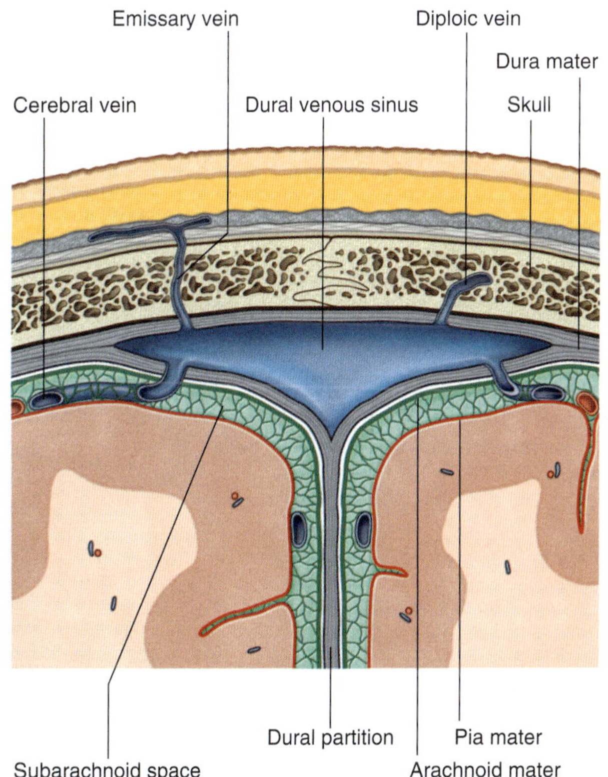

FIG. 20.18 Dural Venous Sinuses. (From Drake RL, Vogl AW, Mitchell AWM. *Gray's Anatomy for Students*, 4th ed. Elsevier; 2020.)

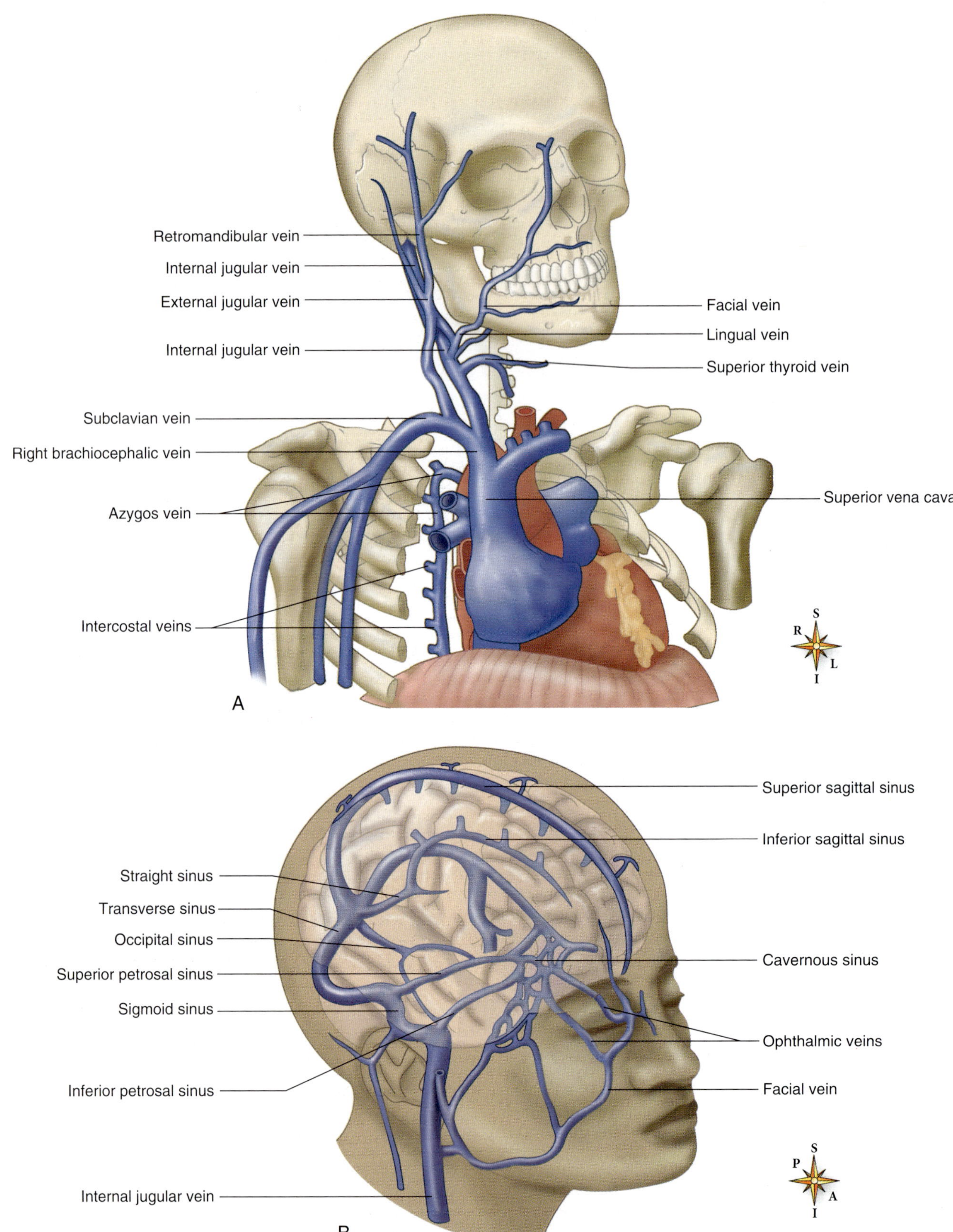

FIG. 20.19 Major Veins of the Head and Neck. (A) Anterior view showing veins on the right side of the head and neck. (B) Lateral, superior view showing the position of major veins relative to the brain. The venous sinuses shown here are within the dura mater and are thus called *dural sinuses*. (From Patton KT, Bell F, Thompson T, Williamson P. *Anatomy and Physiology*. 11th ed. Elsevier; 2022.)

Spinal Cord

The spinal cord, one division of the CNS, extends from the medulla below the foramen magnum. Similar to the brain, the spinal cord is composed of gray and white matter, although gray matter in the spinal cord is located internally, and the white matter is on its surface. The distal end of the spinal cord tapers to the conus medullaris, which is situated at the level of the first or second lumbar vertebra. Exiting from the spinal cord are 31 pairs of spinal nerves, which exit through intervertebral foramina. Because the spinal cord ends at vertebrae L1 and the final nerve roots do not exit until the coccyx, long lengths of nerves, called the *cauda equina*, extend below the conus medullaris toward their associated intervertebral foramina to exit the spinal canal (Fig. 20.20).

Spinal Protective Mechanisms

Protective mechanisms similar to those listed for the brain provide protection to the spinal cord.

Vertebral Column

The bony structure that encases the spinal cord is the vertebral column. Comprising 33 vertebrae and 24 intervertebral disks, this column is held together by ligaments and tendons. The vertebral column provides support and protection for the spinal cord and the structure and flexibility required for body movement. The vertebrae are divided into sections in relation to their appearance (Fig. 20.21). There are 7 cervical vertebrae, 12 thoracic vertebrae, 5 lumbar vertebrae, 5 sacral vertebrae (fused together as one), and 4 coccygeal vertebrae (fused together as one). Although differences in vertebral appearance exist, the basic structure includes a vertebral body connected by two pedicles to the transverse processes. Two laminae connect the transverse processes to the posterior segment of the vertebra, the spinous process, forming a ring. The center of the spinal foramen is the canal housing the spinal cord.

Intervertebral Disks

Vertebral bodies are separated by an intervertebral disk. These fibrocartilaginous structures lie between each vertebral body, extending from the cervical vertebra to the beginning of the sacrum. Intervertebral disks are composed of two layers. The inner core, called the *nucleus pulposus*, is a soft, gelatinous material that assists in shock absorbency. Surrounding the nucleus pulposus is the anulus fibrosus, a thick, tough outer layer. The diagnosis of herniated disk refers to dislocation of the normal anatomic position of an intervertebral disk that compromises or puts pressure on a spinal nerve.[34]

Meninges

The meninges of the spinal cord are similar to the meninges in the cranium (Fig. 20.22). The dura mater is a continuation of the intracranial dura mater and encases the cord, the nerve roots, and the spinal nerves until they exit from the vertebral column. The dura extends to the level of the second sacral vertebra, even though the spinal cord itself ends at the L1 or L2 level.

The arachnoid mater provides the same weblike, delicate structure as in the cranium, with CSF flow within the subarachnoid space. Because the spinal cord terminates at L2 and the meninges continue to S2, a volume of CSF is contained in the lumbar cistern and constitutes the site targeted for a lumbar

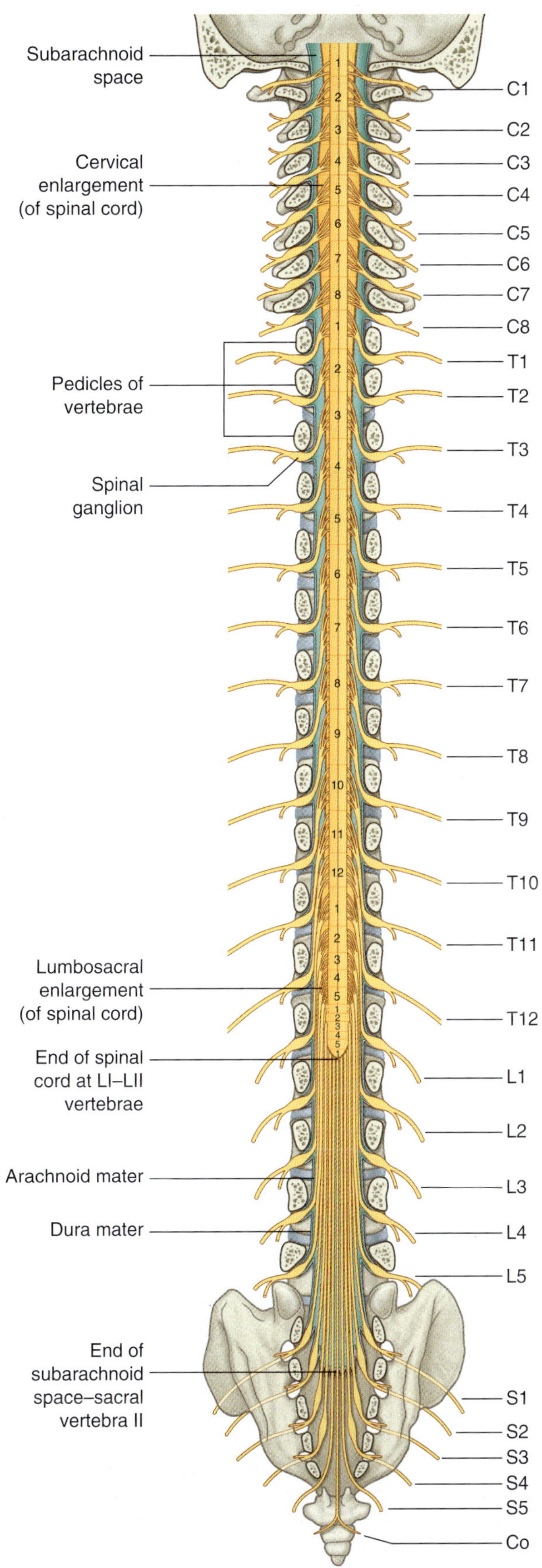

FIG. 20.20 Vertebral Canal, Spinal Cord, and Spinal Nerves. (From Drake RL, Vogl AW, Mitchell AWM. *Gray's Anatomy for Students*, 4th ed. Elsevier; 2020.)

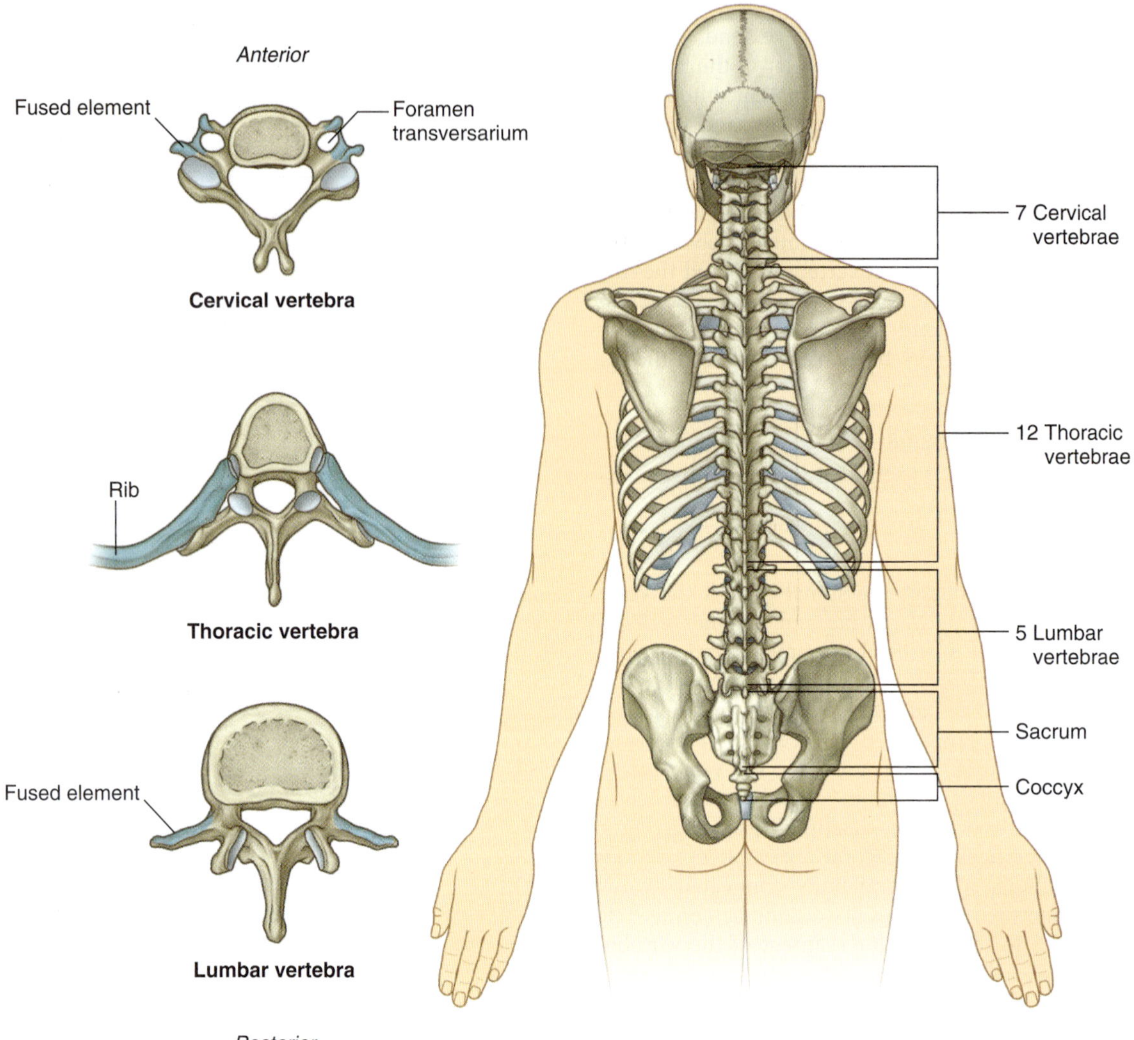

FIG. 20.21 Vertebrae. (From Drake RL, Vogl AW, Mitchell AWM. *Gray's Anatomy for Students*, 4th ed. Elsevier; 2020.)

puncture. The pia mater of the spinal cord is a thicker, firmer, less vascular membrane than that in the cranium.

Vascular Supply

Arterial blood supply to the spinal cord is provided by branches of the vertebral arteries and small radicular arteries that enter through intervertebral foramina. They combine to form the anterior spinal and two posterior spinal arteries. These three arteries, along with some additional radicular arterial flow from cervical, intercostal, lumbar, and sacral arteries, feed the entire length of the spinal cord (Fig. 20.23).

Arterial supply to the spinal cord is segmented at best, making portions of the spinal cord that receive blood supply from two separate sources vulnerable to low-flow states. The most vulnerable of these areas are C2 to C3, T1 to T4, and L1 to L2. Evidence of this tenuous blood supply is occasionally evident after surgical procedures that involve cross-clamping of the aorta, resulting in spinal cord infarction.[35]

PERIPHERAL NERVOUS SYSTEM

The PNS comprises the spinal nerves, the cranial nerves, and all other nerves serving a variety of functions throughout the body. Nerves that originate from the brain are referred to as *cranial nerves*, whereas nerves that originate from the spinal cord are referred to as *spinal nerves*.

Spinal Nerves

The 31 pairs of spinal nerves include 8 cervical, 12 thoracic, 5 lumbar, 5 sacral, and 1 coccygeal (see Fig. 20.20). In the cervical region, the first seven pairs of nerves exit the cord above the corresponding vertebrae. The C8 nerve pair exits the spinal cord below the C7 vertebra. From this point on, all thoracic, lumbar, and sacral nerves exit below the corresponding vertebrae. In other words, spinal cord segments associated with each spinal nerve and the corresponding vertebra do not directly line up.

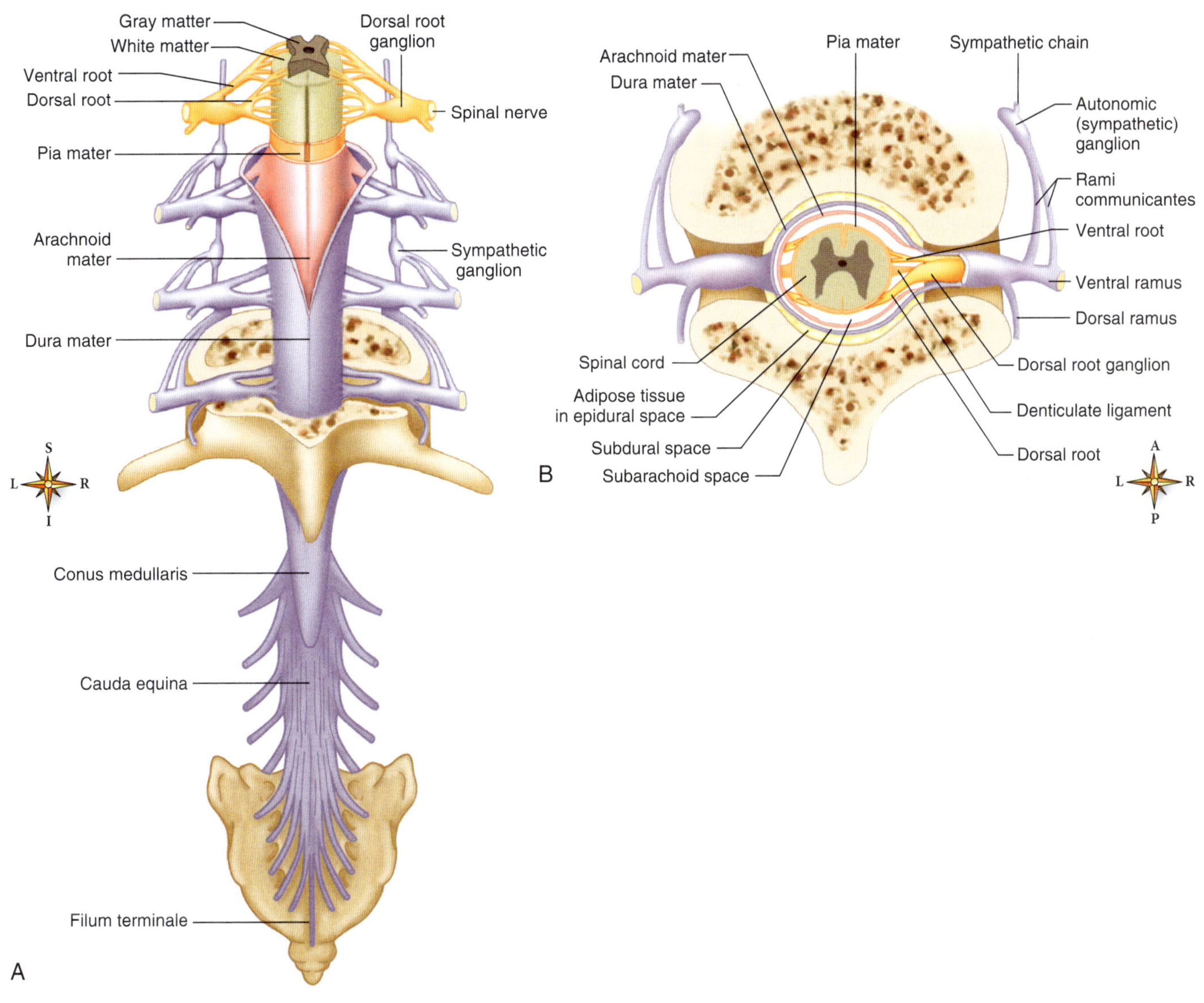

FIG. 20.22 Coverings of the Spinal Cord. The dura mater is shown in *purple*. Note how it extends to cover the spinal nerve roots and nerves. The arachnoid is highlighted in *dark pink*, and the pia mater is highlighted in *light pink*. (Patton KT, Bell F, Thompson T, Williamson P. *Anatomy and Physiology*. 11th ed. Elsevier; 2022.)

Spinal Roots

The spinal nerve has two roots: (1) the dorsal root and (2) the ventral root. The dorsal root is an afferent pathway that carries sensory impulses from the body into the spinal cord. The ventral root is an efferent pathway that carries motor information from the spinal cord to the body. The dorsal and ventral roots join together as they exit the spinal foramen and become a spinal nerve (see Fig. 20.22). Distribution of the sensory components of each spinal nerve are illustrated as dermatomes. Dermatome diagrams facilitate identification of sensory innervation throughout the body (Fig. 20.24).

Gray and White Matter

The spinal cord is composed of gray matter and white matter. The central gray matter, which appears in the shape of an "H," consists of cell bodies, small projection fibers, and glial support cells. The gray matter of the spinal cord has been divided into areas based on cell body type and location. The three main divisions are (1) the anterior horn, (2) the lateral horn, and (3) the posterior horn. The anterior horn contains motor neurons and is the final junction for motor information before exiting the CNS. The lateral horn contains preganglionic fibers of the autonomic nervous system: sympathetic fibers T1 to L2 and parasympathetic fibers S2 to S4. The posterior horn contains sensory

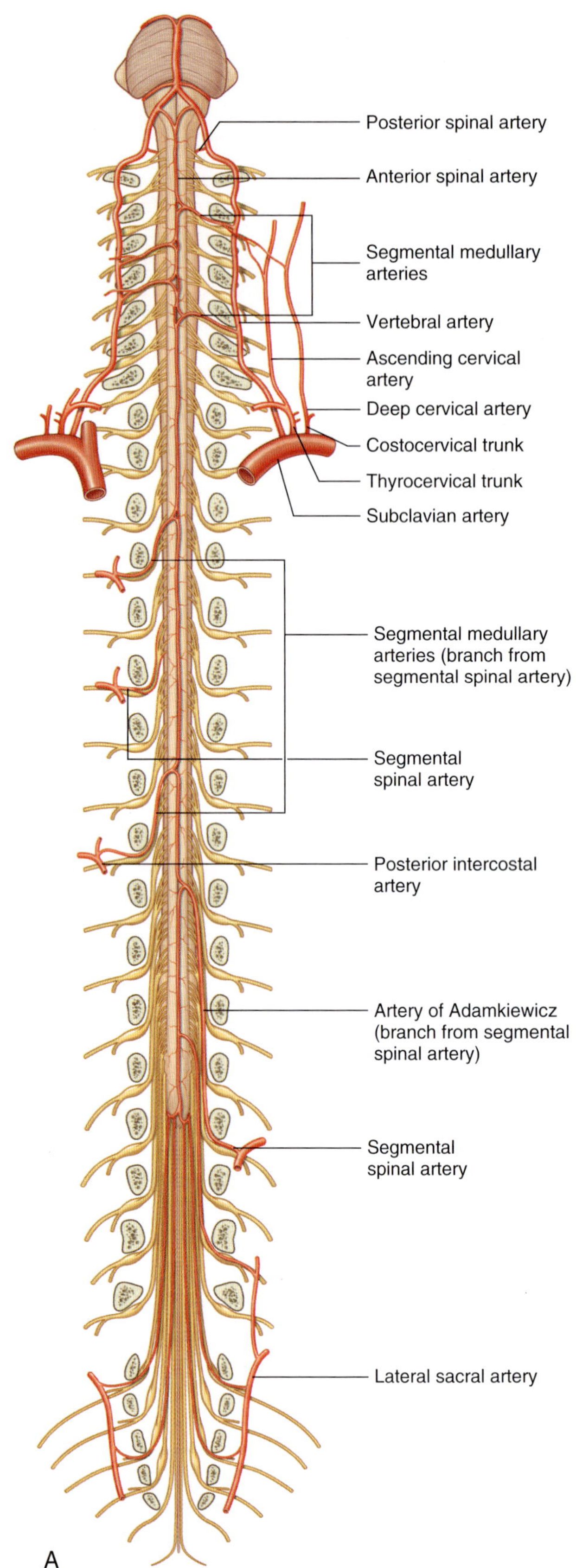

FIG. 20.23 Arteries That Supply the Spinal Cord. (A) Anterior view of spinal cord (not all segmental spinal arteries are shown).

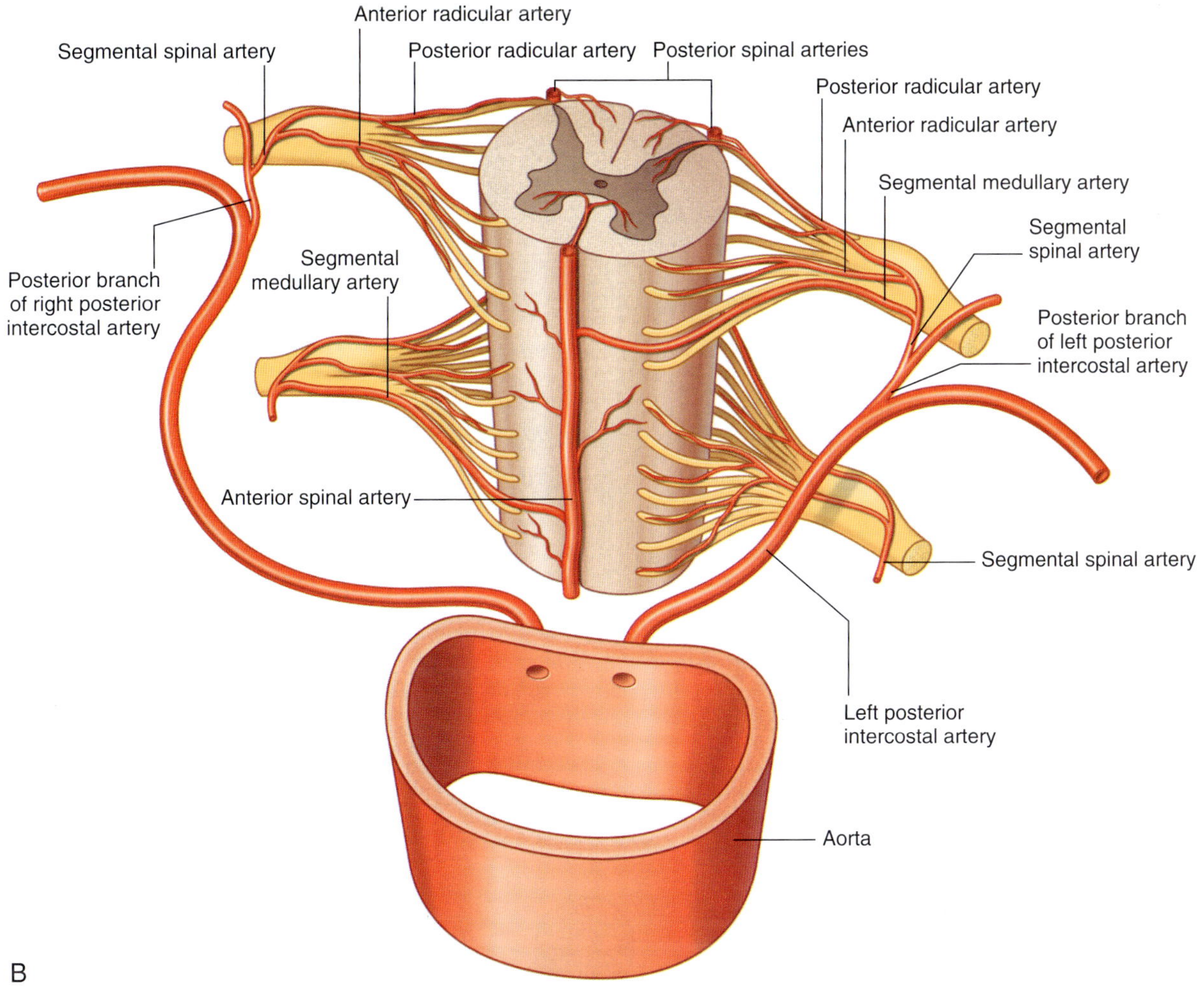

FIG. 20.23, cont'd (B) Segmental supply of spinal cord. (From Drake RL, Vogl AW, Mitchell AWM. *Gray's Anatomy for Students*, 4th ed. Elsevier; 2020.)

neurons and becomes the entry point for afferent impulses to the CNS.

The white matter, which surrounds the gray matter, contains the myelinated ascending and descending tracts, which carry information to and from the brain (Fig. 20.25). Spinal tracts are named in such a way that the prefix denotes the origin of the tract, and the suffix is the destination, promoting easy identification of sensory or motor tracts. Sensory tracts begin with the prefix *spino-*, and motor tracts end with the suffix *-spinal* (Tables 20.3 and 20.4). The complexity of spinal cord tracts is beyond the scope of this chapter, which is limited to the tracts that are most clinically significant and easily tested.

Cranial Nerves

There are 12 pairs of cranial nerves (Fig. 20.26) that arise from the nervous tissue of the brain. They exit through the openings in the cranium (thus the origin of the name *cranial nerves*). The origin and function of each of them is presented in Table 20.5.

AUTONOMIC NERVOUS SYSTEM

The autonomic nervous system consists of two main divisions, the sympathetic nervous system (SNS) and the PNS (Fig. 20.27). The function of each division is presented in Table 20.6.

KEY POINTS

Anatomy

- Nervous tissue is composed of neurons and neuroglial cells.
- The CNS comprises the brain and spinal cord.
- The somatic nervous system is composed of fibers that connect the CNS with structures of the skeletal muscles and the skin.
- The autonomic nervous system (sympathetic and parasympathetic) is composed of fibers that connect the CNS with smooth muscle, cardiac muscle, internal organs, and glands.
- The brain is contained within the cranial vault, the spinal cord is contained within the vertebral column, and both are surrounded by the meninges (dura mater, arachnoid mater, and pia mater).

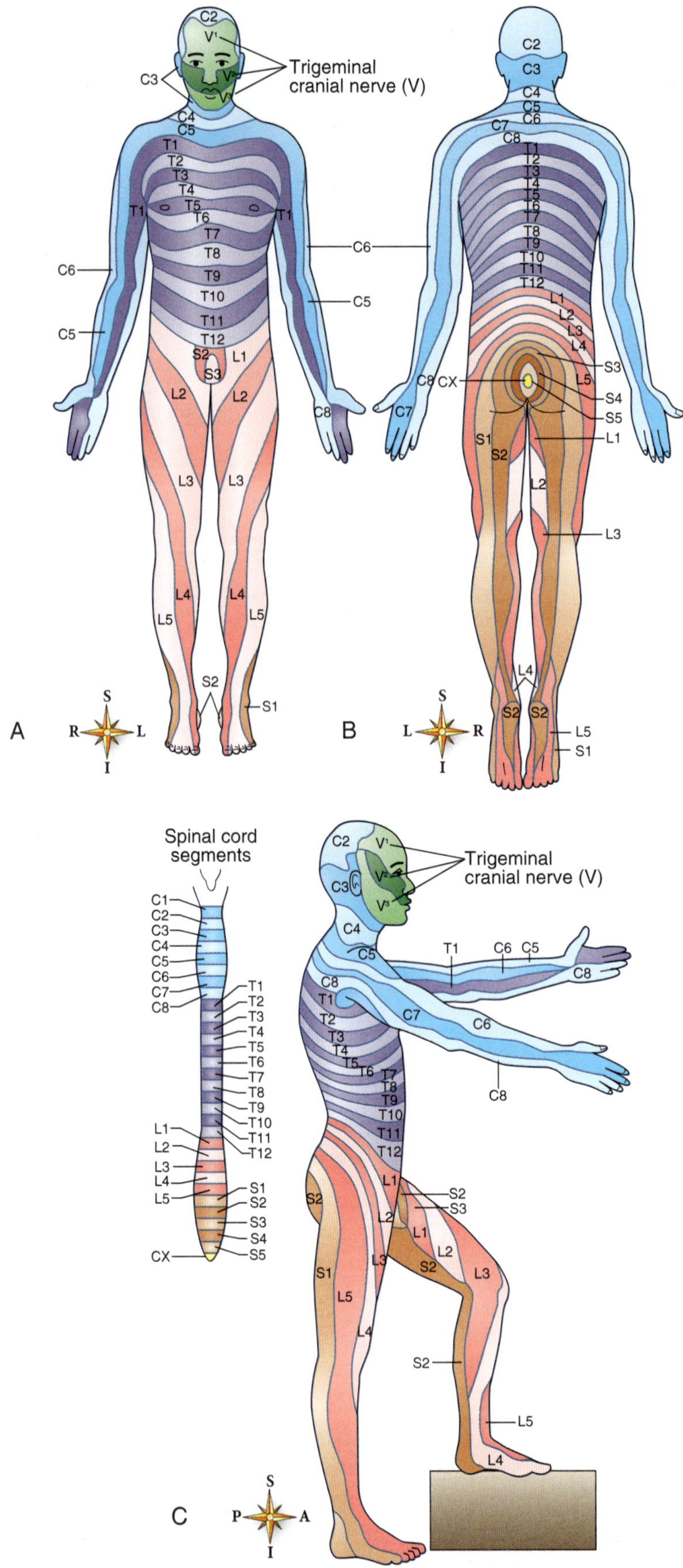

FIG. 20.24 Dermatome Distribution of Spinal Nerves. (A) The front of the body's surface. (B) The back of the body's surface. (C) The side of the body's surface. The *inset* shows the segments of the spinal cord connected with each of the spinal nerves associated with the sensory dermatomes shown. *C*, Cervical segments and spinal nerves; *L*, lumbar segments and spinal nerves; *S*, sacral segments and spinal nerves; *T*, thoracic segments and spinal nerves. (Patton KT, Bell F, Thompson T, Williamson P., eds. *Anatomy and Physiology*. 11th ed. Elsevier; 2022.)

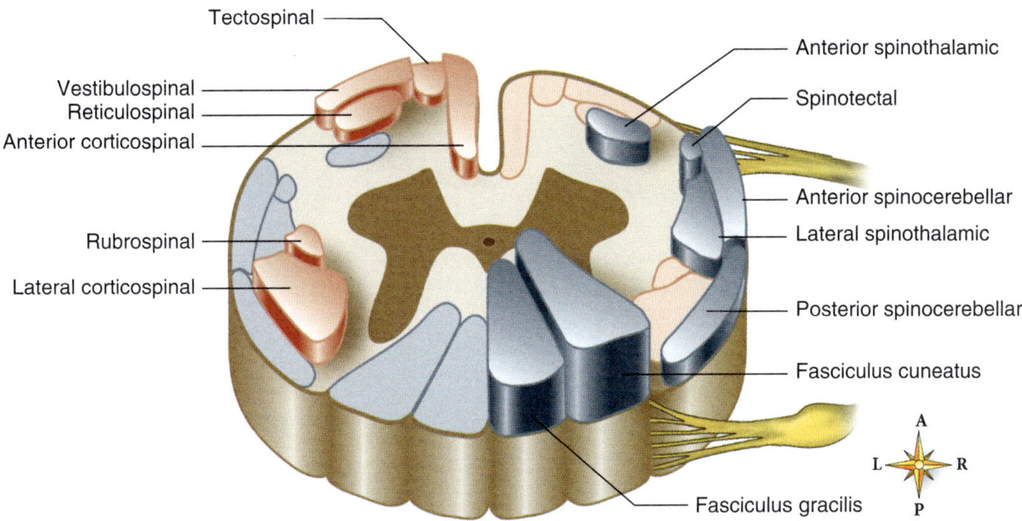

FIG. 20.25 Major Tracts of the Spinal Cord. The major ascending (sensory) tracts are highlighted in *blue*. The major descending (motor) tracts are highlighted in *red*. (From Patton KT, Bell F, Thompson T, Williamson P. *Anatomy and Physiology*. 11th ed. Elsevier; 2022.)

TABLE 20.3 Major Ascending Tracts of Spinal Cord

Name	Function	Location	Origin[a]	Termination[b]
Lateral spinothalamic	Pain, temperature, and crude touch on opposite side	Lateral white columns	Posterior gray column on opposite side	Thalamus
Anterior spinothalamic	Crude touch and pressure	Anterior white columns	Posterior gray column on opposite side	Thalamus
Fasciculi gracilis and cuneatus	Discriminating touch and pressure sensations, including vibration, stereognosis, and 2-point discrimination; also conscious kinesthesia	Posterior white columns	Spinal ganglia on same side	Medulla
Anterior and posterior spinocerebellar	Unconscious kinesthesia	Lateral white columns	Anterior or posterior gray column	Cerebellum
Spinotectal	Touch related to visual reflexes	Lateral white columns	Posterior gray columns	Superior colliculus (midbrain)

[a]Location of cell bodies of neurons from which axons of tract arise.
[b]Structure in which axons of tract terminate.
From Patton KT, Bell F, Thompson T, Williamson P. *Anatomy and Physiology*. 11th ed. Elsevier; 2022.

TABLE 20.4 Major Descending Tracts of Spinal Cord

Name	Function	Location	Origin[a]	Termination[b]
Lateral corticospinal (or crossed pyramidal)	Voluntary movement, contraction of individual or small groups of muscles, particularly muscles moving hands, fingers, feet, and toes of opposite side	Lateral white columns	Motor areas or cerebral cortex of opposite side from tract location in cord	Lateral or anterior gray columns
Anterior corticospinal (direct pyramidal)	Same as lateral corticospinal except mainly muscles of same side	Anterior white columns	Motor cortex but on same side as location in cord	Lateral or anterior gray columns
Reticulospinal	Maintain posture during movement	Anterior white columns	Reticular formation (midbrain, pons, medulla)	Anterior gray columns
Rubrospinal	Coordination of body movement and posture	Lateral white columns	Red nucleus (of midbrain)	Anterior gray columns
Tectospinal	Head and neck movement during visual reflexes	Anterior white columns	Superior colliculus (midbrain)	Medulla and anterior gray columns
Vestibulospinal	Coordination of posture or balance	Anterior white columns	Vestibular nucleus (pons, medulla)	Anterior gray columns

[a]Location of cell bodies of neurons from which axons of tract arise.
[b]Structure in which axons of tract terminate.
From Patton KT, Bell F, Thompson T, Williamson P. *Anatomy and Physiology*. 11th ed. Elsevier; 2022.

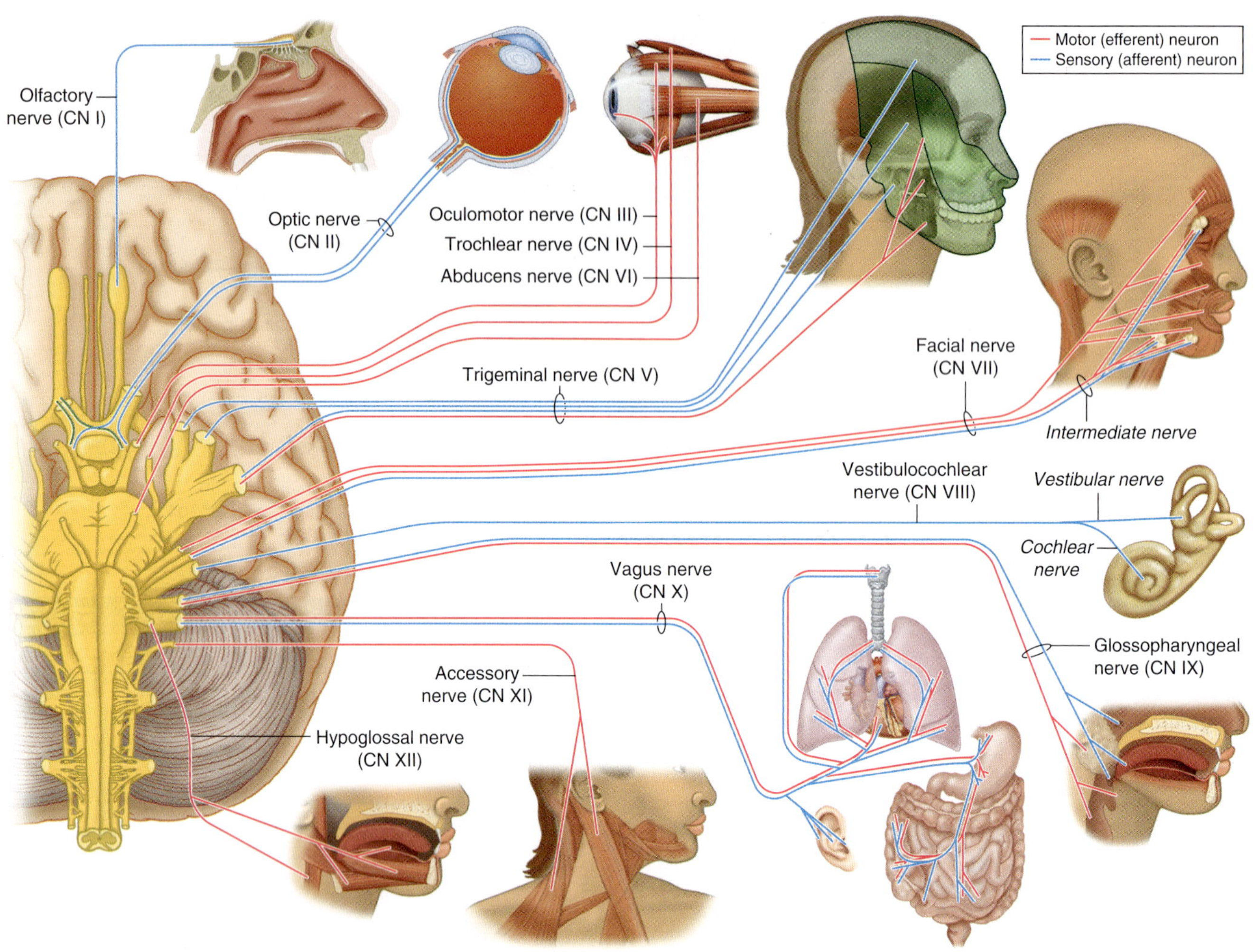

FIG. 20.26 Cranial Nerves. Ventral surface of the brain showing attachment of the cranial nerves. (Patton KT, Bell F, Thompson T, Williamson P. *Anatomy and Physiology.* 11th ed. Elsevier; 2022.)

- CSF fills the ventricular system and surrounds the brain and spinal cord in the subarachnoid space.
- Two pairs of arteries (internal carotid arteries and vertebral arteries) provide blood to the brain and are anatomically separated into the anterior (right and left ACAs and the ACoA) and posterior (right and left PCoAs) circulations that connect at the base of the brain to form the circle of Willis.
- The PNS comprises the cranial nerves, the spinal nerves, and all other nerves serving a variety of functions throughout the body.

Physiology

- Neurons perform the functional work of the nervous system, including receipt of information, integration, and transmission of nerve impulses to recipient cells.
- Neuroglial cells (astrocytes, oligodendroglia, ependyma, and microglia) serve as the support infrastructure of the nervous system, providing protection, structural support, and neuronal repair.
- Most activities of the nervous system originate from sensory receptors such as visual, auditory, or tactile receptors and are transmitted to the CNS by afferent fibers (sensory fibers).
- Efferent fibers (motor fibers) transmit the CNS response to the periphery to produce a motor response, such as contraction of skeletal muscles, contraction of the smooth muscles of organs, or secretion by endocrine glands.
- The flow of CSF begins in the lateral ventricles, moves through the foramina of Monro into the third ventricle, moves through the cerebral aqueduct into the fourth

TABLE 20.5 Cranial Nerves

Cranial Nerve	Origin and Course	Function
I: Olfactory		
Sensory	Found in the mucosa of the nasal cavity; only cranial nerves with a cell body are located in the peripheral structure (nasal mucosa). It passes through the cribriform plate of the ethmoid bone and goes on to olfactory bulbs at the floor of the frontal lobe. Final interpretation is in the temporal lobe.	Smell. However, the system is more than receptor and interpreter for odors; perception of smell also sensitizes other body systems and responses, such as salivation, peristalsis, and sexual stimulus. Loss of sense of smell is called *anosmia*.
II: Optic		
Sensory	Ganglion cells of the retina converge to the optic disc and form the optic nerve. Nerve fibers pass to the optic chiasm, which is above the pituitary gland. Some fibers decussate; others do not. The two tracts go to the lateral geniculate body near the thalamus and then on to the end station for interpretation in the occipital lobe.	Vision
III: Oculomotor		
Motor	Originates in the midbrain and emerges from the brainstem at the upper pons.	Extraocular movement of eyes
Motor	Motor fibers go to superior, medial, and inferior recti and to the inferior oblique for eye movement and levator muscle of the eyelid.	Raising of eyelid
Parasympathetic	Parasympathetic fibers go to ciliary muscles and iris of eye.	Constriction of pupil; changing shape of lens
IV: Trochlear		
Motor	Midbrain origin near oculomotor nerve, emerges at upper pons near cerebral peduncle; motor fibers go to superior oblique muscle of the eyeball.	Extraocular movement of eyes
V: Trigeminal		
Sensory	Originates in the fourth ventricle and emerges at lateral parts of the pons; has three branches to face: ophthalmic, maxillary, and mandibular.	*Ophthalmic branch:* Sensation to cornea, ciliary body, iris, lacrimal gland, conjunctiva, nasal mucosal membranes, eyelids, eyebrows, forehead, and nose *Maxillary branch:* Sensation to skin of cheek, lower lid, side of nose and upper jaw, teeth, mucosa of mouth, sphenopalatine-pterygoid region, and maxillary sinus *Mandibular branch:* Sensation to skin of lower lip, chin, ear, mucous membrane, teeth of lower jaw, and tongue
Motor	Goes to temporalis, masseter, pterygoid gland, and anterior part of digastric muscles (all for mastication) and tensor tympani and tensor veli palatine muscles (clench jaw).	Supplies muscles for chewing (mastication) and opening jaw
VI: Abducens		
Motor	Posterior part of pons goes to lateral rectus muscle for eye movement. Lateral rectus tested by gaze directed outward away from nose (lateral).	Extraocular eye movement; rotates eyeball outward
VII: Facial		
Sensory	Lower portion of pons goes to anterior two-thirds of tongue and soft palate.	Taste in anterior two-thirds of tongue; sensation to soft palate
Motor	Pons to muscles of forehead, eyelids, checks, lips, ears, nose, and neck.	Movement of facial muscles to produce facial expressions, close eyes
Parasympathetic	Pons to salivary gland and lacrimal glands.	Secretory for salivation and tears
VIII: Acoustic		
Sensory	Nerve has two divisions. *Cochlear division* originates in spinal ganglia of the cochlea, with peripheral fibers to the organ of Corti in the internal ear. It goes to the pons, and impulses are transmitted to the temporal lobe.	Hearing

Continued

TABLE 20.5 Cranial Nerves—cont'd

Cranial Nerve	Origin and Course	Function
	Vestibular division originates in the otolith organs of the semicircular canals in the inner ear and in the vestibular ganglion. It terminates in the pons, with some fibers continuing to the cerebellum. It is the only cranial nerve that originates wholly within a bone, the petrous portion of the temporal bone.	Equilibrium
IX: Glossopharyngeal		
Sensory	Posterior one-third of tongue for taste sensation and sensations from soft palate, tonsils, and opening to mouth in back of oral pharynx (fauces). Fibers go to the medulla and then to the temporal lobe for taste and sensory cortex for other sensations.	Taste in posterior one-third of tongue; sensation in back of throat; stimulation elicits gag reflex
Motor	Medulla to constrictor muscles of pharynx and stylopharyngeal muscles.	Voluntary muscles for swallowing and phonation
Parasympathetic	Medulla to parotid salivary gland through the otic ganglia.	Secretory, salivary glands; carotid reflex
X: Vagus		
Sensory	Sensory fibers in back of the ear and posterior wall of the external ear go to the medulla oblongata and on to the sensory cortex.	Sensation behind ear and part of external ear meatus
Motor	Fibers go from the medulla oblongata through the jugular foramen with glossopharyngeal nerve and on to the pharynx, larynx, esophagus, bronchi, lungs, heart, stomach, small intestine, liver, pancreas, and kidneys.	Voluntary muscles for phonation and swallowing; involuntary activity of visceral muscles of heart, lungs, and digestive tract
Parasympathetic	Medulla oblongata to the larynx, trachea, lungs, aorta, esophagus, stomach, small intestines, and gallbladder.	Carotid reflex; autonomic activity of respiratory tract and digestive tract, including peristalsis and secretion from organs
XI: Spinal Accessory		
Motor	The nerve has two roots: cranial and spinal. Cranial portion arises at several rootlets at the side of medulla, runs below the vagus, and is joined by the spinal portion from motor cells in the cervical cord. Some fibers go along with vagus nerve to supply motor impulse to pharynx, larynx, uvula, and palate. Major portion goes to the sternomastoid and trapezius muscles, branches to cervical spinal nerves C2–C4.	Some fibers for swallowing and phonation; turning head and shrugging shoulders
XII: Hypoglossal		
Motor	Arises in the medulla oblongata and goes to the muscles of the tongue.	Movement of tongue necessary for swallowing and phonation

ventricle, and moves out the foramen of Magendie and the foramina of Luschka into the subarachnoid space of the brain and spinal cord.

- The primary functions of the cerebral cortex include sensory, motor, and cognitive functions.
- The primary functions of the cerebellum include balance and motor coordination.
- The primary function of the brainstem (midbrain, pons, and medulla) is the regulation of vital functions such as breathing.
- Voluntary motor movement is controlled by the motor strip in the frontal cortex, and as the tracts descend through the brainstem, they cross over to the opposite side. The right motor strip controls the left side of the body, and vice versa.
- The Broca area is located in the left frontal lobe and is responsible for expression of written and verbal language. Damage to the area can result in expressive aphasia.
- The Wernicke area is located in the left parietal lobe and is responsible for reception of written and verbal language. Damage to the area can result in receptive aphasia.
- The circle of Willis provides collateral blood flow to the brain.

Visit the Evolve site at http://evolve.elsevier.com/Urden/CriticalCareNursing for additional study materials.

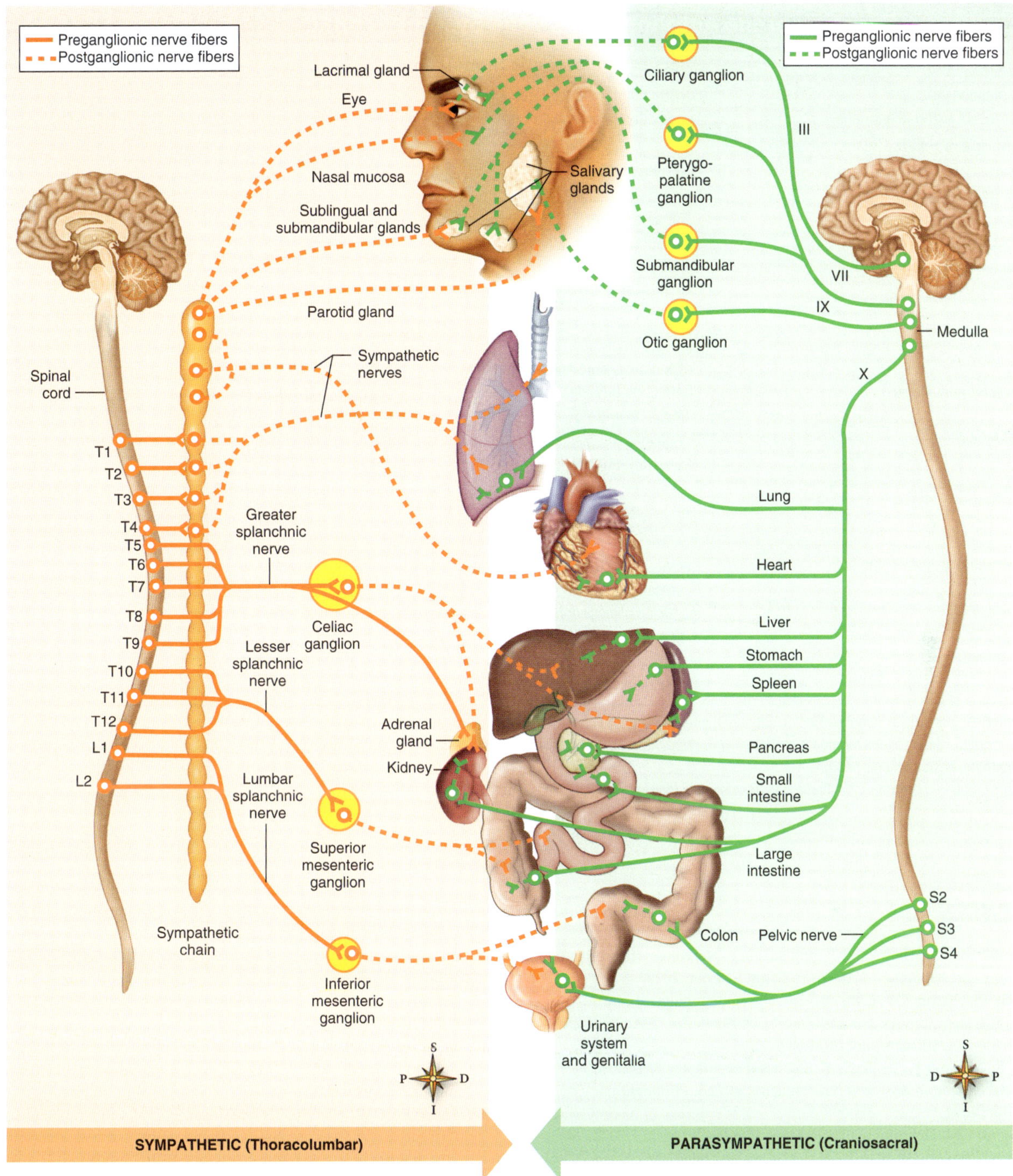

FIG. 20.27 Autonomic Nervous System. (Patton KT, Bell F, Thompson T, Williamson P. *Anatomy and Physiology*. 11th ed. Elsevier; 2022.)

TABLE 20.6 Function of the Autonomic Nervous System

Autonomic Effector	Effect of Sympathetic Stimulation	Effect of Parasympathetic Stimulation
Cardiac Muscle	Increased rate and strength of contraction (beta receptors)	Decreased rate and strength of contraction
Smooth Muscle of Blood Vessels		
Skin blood vessels	Constriction (alpha receptors)	No effect
Skeletal muscle blood vessels	Dilation (beta receptors)	No effect
Coronary blood vessels	Constriction (alpha receptors) Dilation (beta receptors)	Dilation

Continued

TABLE 20.6 Function of the Autonomic Nervous System—cont'd

Autonomic Effector	Effect of Sympathetic Stimulation	Effect of Parasympathetic Stimulation
Abdominal blood vessels	Constriction (alpha receptors)	No effect
Blood vessels of external genitalia	Constriction (alpha receptors)	Dilation of blood vessels causing erection
Smooth Muscle of Hollow Organs and Sphincters		
Bronchioles	Relaxation (dilation)	Constriction
Digestive tract, except sphincters	Decreased peristalsis	Increased peristalsis
Sphincters of digestive tract	Contraction	Relaxation
Urinary bladder	Relaxation	Contraction
Urinary sphincters	Contraction	Relaxation
Reproductive ducts	Constriction	Relaxation
Eye		
Iris	Contraction of radial muscle; dilated pupil	Contraction of circular muscle; constricted pupil
Ciliary	Relaxation; accommodates for far vision	Contraction; accommodates for near vision
Hairs (arrector pili muscles)	Contraction produces goose pimples, or piloerection (alpha receptors)	No effect
Skeletal Muscle[a]	During intense exercise, regulates contractility to prevent fatigue (beta receptors)	No effect
Glands		
Sweat	Increased sweat	No effect
Lacrimal	No effect	Increased secretion of tears
Digestive (salivary, gastric, etc.)	Decreased secretion of saliva; not known for others	Increased secretion of saliva
Pancreas, including islets	Decreased secretion	Increased secretion of pancreatic juice and insulin
Liver	Increased glycogenolysis (beta receptors); increased blood sugar level	No effect
Adrenal medulla[b]	Increased epinephrine secretion	No effect
Adipose	Increased lipolysis	No effect

[a]Skeletal muscle is primarily a somatic effector, but during intense exercise subconscious autonomic stimulation also occurs.
[b]Sympathetic preganglionic axons terminate in contact with secreting cells of the adrenal medulla. Thus the adrenal medulla functions, to quote someone's descriptive phrase, as a "giant sympathetic postganglionic neuron."
From Patton KT, Bell F, Thompson T, Williamson P. *Anatomy and Physiology*. 11th ed. Elsevier; 2022.

REFERENCES

1. Patton KT, Bell F, Thompson T, Williamson P. Nervous system cells. In: *Anatomy and Physiology*. 11th ed. St. Louis: Elsevier; 2022.
2. Francis SS, Ostrom QT, Cote DJ, et al. The epidemiology of central nervous system tumors. *Hematol Oncol Clin North Am*. 2022;36(1):23–42. https://doi.org/10.1016/j.hoc.2021.08.012.
3. Mtui E, Gruener G, Dockery P. Electrical events. In: *Fitzgerald's Clinical Neuroanatomy and Neuroscience*. 8th ed. Philadelphia: Elsevier; 2021.
4. Innocenti GM. Defining neuroplasticity. *Handb Clin Neurol*. 2022;184:3–18. https://doi.org/10.1016/B978-0-12-819410-2.00001-1.
5. Stadelmann C, Timmler S, Barrantes-Freer A, et al. Myelin in the central nervous system: structure, function, and pathology. *Physiol Rev*. 2019;99(3):1381–1431. https://doi.org/10.1152/physrev.00031.2018.
6. Patton KT, Bell F, Thompson T, Williamson P. Nerve signaling. In: *Anatomy and Physiology*. 11th ed. St. Louis: Elsevier; 2022.
7. Xu L, Ding X, Wang T, et al. Voltage-gated sodium channels: structures, functions, and molecular modeling. *Drug Discov Today*. 2019;24(7):1389–1397. https://doi.org/10.1016/j.drudis.2019.05.014.
8. Mtui E, Gruener G, Dockery P. Transmitters and receptors. In: *Fitzgerald's Clinical Neuroanatomy and Neuroscience*. 8th ed. Philadelphia: Elsevier; 2021.
9. Fletcher A. Nerve cell function and synaptic mechanisms. *Anaesth Intensive Care Med*. 2019;20(4):238–242. https://doi.org/10.1016/j.mpaic.2019.01.015.
10. Gordts F, Foulon I, Hachimi-Idrissi S. Basilar skull fractures: the petrous bone. *B-ENT*. 2016;26(1):193–201.
11. Aromatario M, Torsello A, D'Errico S, et al. Traumatic epidural and subdural hematoma: epidemiology, outcome, and dating. *Medicina (Kaunas)*. 2021;57(2):125. https://doi.org/10.3390/medicina57020125.
12. Muehlschlegel S. Subarachnoid hemorrhage. *Continuum (Minneap Minn)*. 2018;24(6):1623–1657. https://doi.org/10.1212/CON.0000000000000679.
13. Ellenbogen JR, Mallucci C. Management of cerebrospinal fluid disorders. *Surgery (Oxford)*. 2018;36(11):646–654. https://doi.org/10.1016/j.mpsur.2018.09.003.
14. Hawryluk GWJ, Citerio G, Hutchinson P, et al. Intracranial pressure: current perspectives on physiology and monitoring. *Intensive Care Med*. 2022;48(10):1471–1481. https://doi.org/10.1007/s00134-022-06786-y.
15. Mtui E, Gruener G, Dockery P. Meninges. In: *Fitzgerald's Clinical Neuroanatomy and Neuroscience*. 8th ed. Philadelphia: Elsevier; 2021.
16. Patton KT, Bell F, Thompson T, Williamson P. Central nervous system. In: *Anatomy and Physiology*. 11th ed. St. Louis: Elsevier; 2022.
17. Langen UH, Ayloo S, Gu C. Development and cell biology of the blood-brain barrier. *Annu Rev Cell Dev Biol*. 2019;35:591–613. https://doi.org/10.1146/annurev-cellbio-100617-062608.
18. Profaci CP, Munji RN, Pulido RS, et al. The blood-brain barrier in health and disease: important unanswered questions. *J Exp Med*. 2020;217(4):e20190062. https://doi.org/10.1084/jem.20190062.
19. Reber J, Tranel D. Frontal lobe syndromes. *Handb Clin Neurol*. 2019;163:147–164. https://doi.org/10.1016/B978-0-12-804281-6.00008-2.
20. Bakalkin G. The left-right side-specific endocrine signaling in the effects of brain lesions: questioning of the neurological dogma. *Cell Mol Life Sci*. 2022;79(11):545. https://doi.org/10.1007/s00018-022-04576-9. 11.

21. Grossman M, Irwin DJ. Primary progressive aphasia and stroke aphasia. *Continuum (Minneap Minn)*. 2018;24(3, Behavioral Neurology and Psychiatry):745–767. https://doi.org/10.1212/CON.0000000000000618.
22. Nasios G, Dardiotis E, Messinis L. From Broca and Wernicke to the neuromodulation era: insights of brain language networks for neurorehabilitation. *Behav Neurol*. 2019;2019:9894571. https://doi.org/10.1155/2019/9894571.
23. Miceli G, Caccia A. Cortical disorders of speech processing: pure word deafness and auditory agnosia. *Handb Clin Neurol*. 2022;187:69–87. https://doi.org/10.1016/B978-0-12-823493-8.00005-5.
24. Vinti V, Dell'Isola GB, Tascini G, et al. Temporal lobe epilepsy and psychiatric comorbidity. *Front Neurol*. 2021;12:775781. https://doi.org/10.3389/fneur.2021.775781.
25. Sen N. An insight into the vision impairment following traumatic brain injury. *Neurochem Int*. 2017;111:103–107. https://doi.org/10.1016/j.neuint.2017.01.019.
26. Brewer-Smyth K, Burgess AW. Neurobiology of female homicide perpetrators. *J Interpers Violence*. 2021;36(19–20):8915–8938. https://doi.org/10.1177/0886260519860078.
27. Hiraga A. Pure motor monoparesis due to ischemic stroke. *Neurologist*. 2011;17(6):301–308. https://doi.org/10.1097/NRL.0b013e318220c690.
28. Kamble N, Pal PK. Tremor syndromes: a review. *Neurol India*. 2018;66(suppl):S36–S47. https://doi.org/10.4103/0028-3886.226440.
29. Habas C, Manto M, Cabaraux P. The cerebellar thalamus. *Cerebellum*. 2019;18(3):635–648. https://doi.org/10.1007/s12311-019-01019-3.
30. Schultz BA, Bellamkonda E. Management of medical complications during the rehabilitation of moderate-severe traumatic brain injury. *Phys Med Rehabil Clin N Am*. 2017;28(2):259–270. https://doi.org/10.1016/j.pmr.2016.12.004.
31. Marsden JF. Cerebellar ataxia. *Handb Clin Neurol*. 2018;159:261–281. https://doi.org/10.1016/B978-0-444-63916-5.00017-3.
32. Luppi PH, Fort P. Sleep-wake physiology. *Handb Clin Neurol*. 2019;160:359–370. https://doi.org/10.1016/B978-0-444-64032-1.00023-0.
33. Jones JD, Castanho P, Bazira P, et al. Anatomical variations of the circle of Willis and their prevalence, with a focus on the posterior communicating artery: a literature review and meta-analysis. *Clin Anat*. 2021;34(7):978–990. https://doi.org/10.1002/ca.23662.
34. Benzakour T, Igoumenou V, Mavrogenis AF, et al. Current concepts for lumbar disc herniation. *Int Orthop*. 2019;43(4):841–851. https://doi.org/10.1007/s00264-018-4247-6.
35. Arora L, Hosn MA. Spinal cord perfusion protection for thoraco-abdominal aortic aneurysm surgery. *Curr Opin Anaesthesiol*. 2019;32(1):72–79. https://doi.org/10.1097/ACO.0000000000000670.

21

Neurologic Clinical Assessment and Diagnostic Procedures

Lauren Malinowski-Falk

http://evolve.elsevier.com/Urden/CriticalCareNursing

Assessment of a critically ill patient with neurologic dysfunction includes a review of the patient's health history, a focused physical assessment, and an analysis of laboratory data. Numerous invasive and noninvasive diagnostic procedures may also be performed to identify the patient's disorder. A thorough patient assessment is imperative for the early identification and treatment of neurologic disorders. It also serves as a source of comparison for ongoing patient assessments. Change is the most critical finding in any neurologic assessment, which should be reported promptly. Early identification of neurologic deterioration is vital to preventing secondary brain injury and leads to improved outcomes.[1] Other medical conditions, and the administration of various medications, can affect the clinical assessment and should be considered when the neurologic examination results are abnormal. This chapter focuses on clinical assessments, laboratory studies, and diagnostic procedures for critically ill patients with neurologic dysfunction.

HISTORY

Common to all neurologic assessments is the need to obtain a comprehensive history. An adequate neurologic history includes information about the patient's normal baseline status, manifestation of neurologic symptoms, events preceding the onset of symptoms, precipitating factors, progression of symptoms, current medication use, substance use and abuse, and familial occurrences (Box 21.1).[2,3] The ideal historian for recounting this information is someone able to provide a detailed description and chronology of events. If the patient cannot serve as the historian, family members or significant others, who frequently interact with the patient, should be queried. The information obtained from the history often informs the priorities of the physical examination.[3]

FOCUSED PHYSICAL ASSESSMENT

The focused physical assessment helps establish baseline data regarding the patient's condition. The neurologic evaluation of a critically ill patient comprises five major components: (1) level of consciousness, (2) motor function, (3) pupillary function, (4) respiratory function, and (5) vital signs. A complete neurologic examination requires an assessment of all five components.[4]

Level of Consciousness

Assessment of the level of consciousness is the most essential aspect of the neurologic examination. In most situations, a patient's level of consciousness deteriorates before any other neurologic changes are noticed. These deteriorations often are subtle and must be monitored carefully. Arousal and awareness are the fundamental constituents of consciousness and should be evaluated and documented repeatedly for trend analysis.[3]

Evaluation of Arousal

Assessment of the arousal component of consciousness is an evaluation of the reticular activating system and its connection to the thalamus and the cerebral cortex. Arousal is the lowest level of consciousness, and observation centers on the patient's ability to respond to verbal or noxious stimuli in the appropriate manner expected in the waking state.[5] To stimulate the patient, begin with verbal stimuli in a normal tone. Eye opening in response to name indicates that the patient's reticular activating center (brainstem) functioning is intact. However, it does not provide evidence that the patient is awake or aware.[3] If the patient does not respond, increase the stimuli by talking very loudly to the patient. If there is still no response, further increase the stimuli by gently shaking the patient.

If previous attempts to arouse the patient are unsuccessful, noxious stimuli should be employed using central stimulation techniques.[5] Central stimulation produces an overall body response and is more reliable than peripheral stimulation.[5] The sternal rub and the trapezius muscle pinch are two standard central stimulation techniques. A sternal rub is conducted by applying pressure to the center of the sternum with the knuckles of a clenched fist.[4] A trapezius muscle squeeze involves pitching or squeezing the trapezius muscle located at the angle of the shoulder and the neck muscle.[4] If the patient does not respond to verbal stimulus but moves spontaneously in a purposeful manner, the patient is *localizing*. Painful stimulus is not required if spontaneous localization has been observed. Localizing is purposeful and intentional movement intended to eliminate a noxious stimulus, whereas *withdrawal* is a smaller movement used to escape the noxious stimulus.[3] The symmetry and pattern of the motor response to noxious stimuli and associated neurologic symptoms should be documented for all patients suspected of having a neurologic dysfunction.[5]

Appraisal of Awareness

If a patient is arousable, an assessment of awareness should follow. As a higher level function, awareness means that the cerebral cortex is working in conjunction with the reticular activating system (arousal) and that the patient can interact with and interpret their environment.[3] Appraisal of awareness involves assessment of the patient's orientation to person, place, time, and situation and requires the patient to give appropriate

BOX 21.1 DATA COLLECTION

Neurologic History

Common Neurologic Symptoms

- Fainting
- Dizziness
- Blackouts
- Seizures
- Headache
- Memory loss
- Weakness
- Fatigue
- Paralysis
- Tremors or other involuntary movements
- Lack of coordination
- Pain
- Numbness
- Tingling
- Speech disturbances
- Vision disturbances

Events Preceding Onset of Symptoms

- Travel
- Animal contact
- Falls, recent trauma
- Infection
- Dental problems or procedures
- Sinus or middle ear infections
- Prodromal symptoms
- Food or medications ingested

Progression of Symptoms

- Initial onset
- Evolution
- Frequency
- Severity
- Duration
- Associated activities or aggravating factors
- Any relieving factors

Family History

- Stroke (arteriovenous malformation, aneurysm)
- Diabetes mellitus
- Hypertension
- Seizures
- Tumors
- Headaches
- Emotional problems or depression

Medical History

Child

- Birth injuries, congenital defects, encephalitis, meningitis, bedwetting, fainting, seizures, trauma

Adult

- Diabetes; hypertension; cardiovascular, pulmonary, kidney, liver, or endocrine disease; tuberculosis; tropical infection; sinusitis; visual problems; tumors; psychiatric disorders

Surgical History

- Neurologic, ear-nose-throat, dental, eye surgery

Traumatic History

- Motor vehicle accidents; falls; blows to head, neck, or back; loss of consciousness

Allergies

- Medications, food, environment

Patient Profile

- Personal habits
- Use of alcohol, recreational drugs, over-the-counter medications, smoking, dietary habits, sleeping patterns, elimination patterns, exercise habits
- Recent life changes
- Living conditions
- Working conditions
- Exposure to toxins, chemicals, and fumes; occupational duties
- General temperament

Current Medication Use and Compliance

- Sedatives, tranquilizers
- Pain medications
- Anticonvulsants
- Psychotropics
- Anticoagulants
- Antibiotics
- Calcium channel blockers
- Beta-blockers
- Nitrates
- Oral contraceptives
- Natural, over-the-counter supplements

answers to various questions.[6] Changes in the patient's answers that reflect increasing confusion and disorientation may be the first sign of neurologic deterioration.[1]

TABLE 21.1 Glasgow Coma Scale

Category	Score	Response
Eye opening	4	Spontaneous: Eyes open spontaneously without stimulation
	3	To speech: Eyes open with verbal stimulation but not necessarily to command
	2	To pain: Eyes open with noxious stimuli
	1	None: No eye opening regardless of stimulation
Verbal response	5	Oriented: Accurate information about person, place, time, reason for hospitalization, and personal data
	4	Confused: Answers not appropriate to questions, but use of language is correct
	3	Inappropriate words: Disorganized, random speech, with no sustained conversation
	2	Incomprehensible sounds: Moans, groans, and incomprehensible mumbles
	1	None: No verbalization despite stimulation
Best motor response	6	Obeys commands: Performs simple tasks on command; able to repeat performance
	5	Localizes to pain: Organized attempt to localize and remove painful stimuli
	4	Withdraws from pain: Withdraws extremity from source of painful stimuli
	3	Abnormal flexion: Decorticate posturing spontaneously or in response to noxious stimuli
	2	Extension: Decerebrate posturing spontaneously or in response to noxious stimuli
	1	None: No response to noxious stimuli; flaccid

Glasgow Coma Scale

Introduced in 1974, the Glasgow Coma Scale (GCS) is the most widely recognized tool for assessing level of consciousness.[6] This scored scale is based on the evaluation of three categories: (1) eye opening, (2) verbal response, and (3) best motor response (Table 21.1). The three components can be scored separately or combined in a sum score ranging from 3 to 15. A score of 7 or less usually indicates coma. Evidence suggests that the GCS score can assess neurological state and trend clinical progress.[7] However, the GCS has additional shortcomings. These include inconsistent interobserver reliability, concerns over its ability to predict the extent of the brain damage, the impracticality of verbal response assessment in intubated patients or patients with dysphasia, the exclusion of brainstem functions and the measurement of pupillary response from the GCS, and the inability to detect subtle changes in neurologic status.[6–9]

Full Outline of UnResponsiveness Score

The Full Outline of UnResponsiveness (FOUR) score may be a suitable alternative or complementary tool for the GCS.[10] Since its introduction in 2005, the FOUR score has been compared with the GCS and was found to have equivalent interrater reliability and a similar, if not higher, predication of mortality and poor neurologic outcome in the general critical care unit population, traumatic brain injury (TBI) patients, and stroke patients.[8,9,] It is a 17-point scale to assess four domains of neurologic functions: eye responses, motor responses, brainstem reflexes, and breathing pattern (Fig. 21.1).[11] Each domain carries five parameters with total points ranging from 0 to 4, with

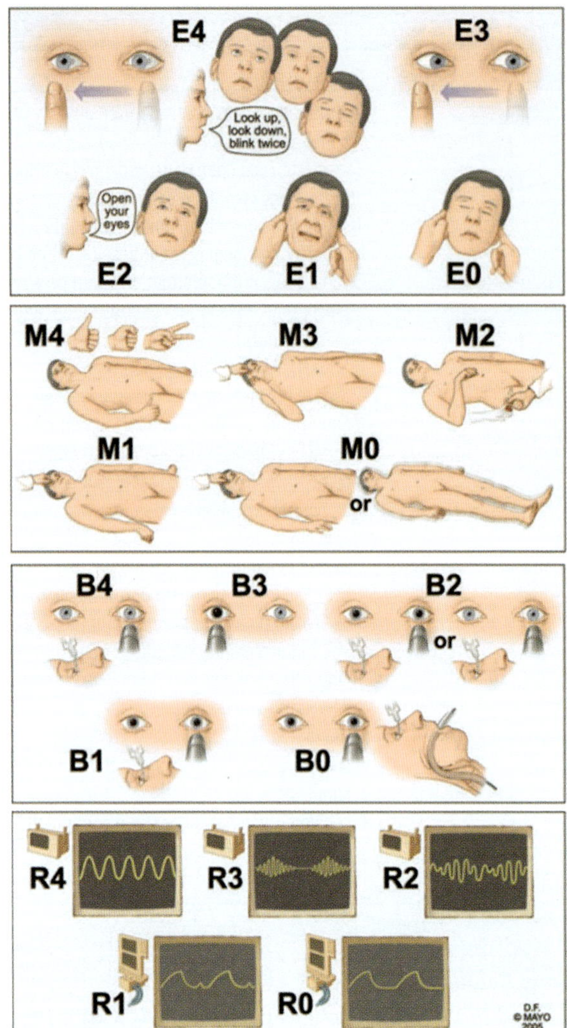

FIG. 21.1 Description of Full Outline of UnResponsiveness (FOUR) Score. Eye response: E4 = eyelids open or opened, tracking, or blinking to command; E3 = eyelids open but not tracking; E2 = eyelids closed but open to loud voice; E1 = eyelids closed but open to pain; E0 = eyelids remain closed with pain. Motor response: M4 = thumbs-up, fist, or peace sign; M3 = localizing to pain; M2 = flexion response to pain; M1 = extension response to pain; M0 = no response to pain or generalized myoclonus status. Brainstem reflexes: B4 = pupil and corneal reflexes present; B3 = one pupil wide and fixed; B2 = pupil or corneal reflexes absent; B1 = pupil and corneal reflexes absent; B0 = absent pupil, corneal, and cough reflex. Respiration pattern: R4 = not intubated, regular breathing pattern; R3 = not intubated, Cheyne-Stokes breathing pattern; R2 = not intubated, irregular breathing; R1 = breathes above ventilatory rate; R0 = breathes at ventilator rate or apnea. (From Iyer VN. Validity of the FOUR Score Coma Scale in the medical intensive care unit. *Mayo Clin Proc.* 2009;84(8):694–701.)

a potential sum score ranging from 0 to 16. The FOUR score is applicable for both traumatic and nontraumatic brain injuries.[8]

Motor Function

Assessment of motor function provides valuable information about the patient with neurologic dysfunction. This process includes assessing the patient's muscle size and tone, muscle strength, response to peripheral tactile stimuli, and abnormal motor responses.[3] Each side of the body is assessed individually and compared with the other.[10]

Evaluation of Muscle Size and Tone

Initially, muscles are inspected for size and shape. The presence of atrophy is noted. Muscle tone is assessed by evaluating opposition to passive movement. The patient is instructed to relax the extremity while passive range-of-motion movements are performed, and the degree of resistance is evaluated. Muscle tone is appraised for signs of flaccidity (no resistance), hypotonia (little resistance), hypertonia (increased resistance), spasticity, or rigidity.[12] If tone is absent in an unconscious patient, the hand is lifted approximately 30 cm above the bed and carefully dropped while protecting the limb from injury. The test is repeated with all extremities. Typically, the lower the level of consciousness, the closer to flaccid the limb(s) will be. An asymmetric examination may indicate a lesion in the contralateral hemisphere or brainstem.[3]

Estimation of Muscle Strength

Having the patient perform movements against resistance assesses muscle strength. The strength of the movement is graded on a six-point scale (Box 21.2). The patient is asked to extend both arms with the palms turned upward and hold that position with closed eyes. If the patient has a weaker side, that arm will drift downward and pronate. The lower extremities are tested by asking the patient to contract the muscle by extending or flexing the joint, then push and pull the feet against resistance.[12]

Peripheral Tactile Response

The peripheral reflex response is the response to tactile stimuli peripherally and usually elicits a reflex response rather than a central or brain response.[3] To elicit a response, progressively apply stimuli using the least noxious stimuli necessary. Each extremity is assessed individually. Noxious stimuli is used if there is no light or firm pressure response. The typical technique for asserting a peripheral noxious stimulus involves applying pressure on the nail beds.[3]

Abnormal Motor Responses

Patients may experience abnormal motor responses spontaneously or to stimuli. Noxious stimuli are necessary to determine motor responses if the patient cannot comprehend and follow a simple command. The stimulus is applied to each extremity separately to allow evaluation of individual extremity function. The *triple-flexion response* is a withdrawal of the limb in a straight line with flexion of the wrist–elbow–shoulder or the ankle–knee–hip. This response is considered a spinal reflex and does not indicate brain involvement in the movement. The triple-flexion response is typical in patients with severe neurologic dysfunction.[3] *Decorticate (flexor) posturing* is seen when there is damage to a cerebral hemisphere and the brainstem (Fig. 21.2A). It is characterized by adduction of the shoulder and arm, elbow flexion, and pronation and flexion of the wrist while the legs extend. *Decerebrate (extensor) posturing* is seen with severe metabolic disturbances or upper brainstem lesions (Fig. 21.2B). It is characterized by extension and pronation of the arm(s) and extension of the legs.[3] Additionally, it is possible for the patient to exhibit abnormal flexion on one side of the body and abnormal extension on the other (Fig. 21.2C).[4] Onset of posturing, or a change from abnormal flexion to abnormal extension, requires immediate health care practitioner notification.

BOX 21.2 Muscle Strength Grading Scale

0/5	No movement or muscle contraction
1/5	Trace contraction
2/5	Active movement with gravity eliminated
3/5	Active movement against gravity
4/5	Active movement with some resistance
5/5	Active movement with full resistance

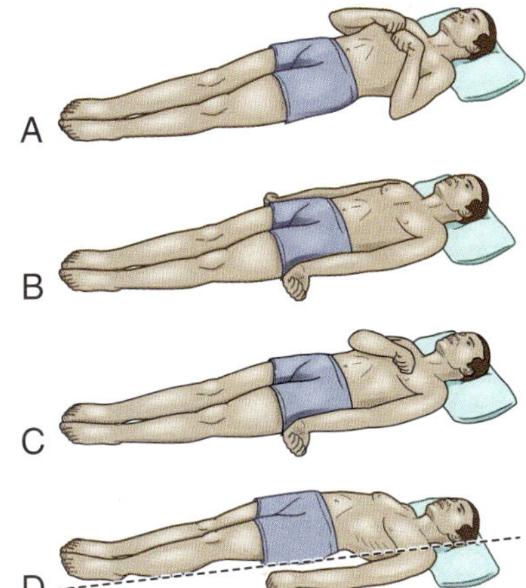

FIG. 21.2 Abnormal Motor Responses. Decorticate and decerebrate posturing. (A) Decorticate response. Flexion of arms, wrists, and fingers with adduction in upper extremities. Extension, internal rotation, and plantar flexion in lower extremities. (B) Decerebrate response. All four extremities in rigid extension, with hyperpronation of forearms and plantar flexion of feet. (C) Decorticate response on right side of body and decerebrate response on left side of body. (D) Opisthotonic posturing. (From Harding MM, Kwong J, Hagler D, Reinisch C, eds. *Lewis's Medical-Surgical Nursing: Assessment and Management of Clinical Problems*. 12th ed. Elsevier; 2023.)

Evaluation of Reflexes

A health care practitioner usually evaluates reflexes when performing a complete neurologic evaluation. Deep tendon reflexes (DTRs) and superficial reflexes are typically tested.

Deep tendon reflexes. DTRs are tested by tapping the appropriate tendon using a reflex or percussion hammer. For reflex testing to be accurate, the muscle needs to be relaxed, the joint needs to be at midposition, and the patient should not be thinking about what is being tested. The four reflexes tested are (1) Achilles (ankle jerk), (2) quadriceps (knee jerk), (3) biceps, and (4) triceps. DTRs are graded on a scale from 0 (absent) to 4 (hyperactive). A DTR grade of 2 is normal (Fig. 21.3). Hyperreflexia occurs with hyperactive or repeating reflexes, and hyporeflexia is an absent or diminished reflex response.[12] Hyperreflexia is associated with upper motor neuron interruption. Hyporeflexia is associated with lesions of the lower motor neurons.[13]

Superficial reflexes. Superficial reflexes are tested by stimulating cutaneous receptors of the skin, cornea, or mucous membrane. Superficial reflexes are normal if present and abnormal if absent. Stroking, scratching, or touching can be used as the stimulus (Table 21.2). The corneal reflex is present if the eyelids quickly close when the cornea is lightly stroked with a wisp of cotton.[13] An alternative approach is to drop a small amount of water or saline onto the cornea.[4] The pathway for the corneal reflex is formed by the trigeminal nerve (cranial nerve [CN] V), the facial nerve (CN VII), and the pons. The pharyngeal reflex is present if retching or gagging occurs with stimulation of the back of the pharynx, along with upward movement of the palate.[13]

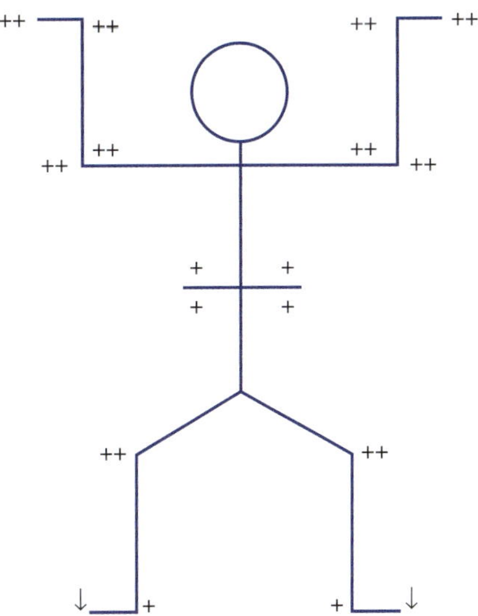

Scoring Deep Tendon Reflexes

Grade	Deep Tendon Reflex Response
0	No response
1+	Sluggish or diminished
2+	Active or expected response
3+	More brisk than expected, slightly hyperactive
4+	Brisk, hyperactive, with intermittent or transient clonus

FIG. 21.3 Reflex Scoring. The patient's reflex scores are recorded by entering the correct scores at the right location on the stick figure. (From Barker E. *Neuroscience Nursing: A Spectrum of Care*. 3rd ed. Mosby; 2008.)

TABLE 21.2 Superficial Reflexes

Reflex	Nerves Involved	Normal Reaction
Corneal	CN V and VII	Prompt closure of both eyelids when cornea touched with a wisp of cotton
Pharyngeal	CN IX and X	Gagging response to pharyngeal stimulation
Abdominal	Epigastric (T6–T9); midabdominal (T9–T11); hypogastric (T11–L1)	Contraction of abdominal muscle when stroked so that a brief, brisk movement of the umbilicus toward stimulus occurs
Cremasteric	L1, L2	Elevation of testicle when the inner aspect of thigh stroked
Anal		Contraction of the anal ring as the perineum is stroked or scratched
Bulbocutaneous	S4, S5	
Anocutaneous	S5	
Plantar	L5, S1	Flexion of toes from stimulation of the sole of the foot

CN, Cranial nerve.
From Barker E. *Neuroscience Nursing: A Spectrum of Care*. 3rd ed. Mosby; 2008.

Pathologic reflexes. The presence of pathologic reflexes is an abnormal neurologic finding. The grasp reflex is present when tactile stimulation of the palm of the hand produces a grasp response that is not a conscious voluntary act. The grasp reflex is a primitive reflex that usually disappears with maturational development. The presence of the grasp reflex in an adult indicates cortical damage. The Babinski reflex is a pathologic sign in individuals older than 2 years. The presence of this reflex is tested by slow, deliberate stroking of the lateral half of the sole of the foot. A sustained extensor response of the big toe indicates a positive Babinski reflex. This response is sometimes accompanied by the fanning out of the other four toes. Flexor response of all the toes in response to the same stimulus is a normal finding and indicates the absence of the Babinski reflex (Fig. 21.4). The Babinski reflex is a significant neurologic finding because it indicates an upper motor neuron lesion in the brain, brainstem, or spinal cord.[14] The disease may be degenerative, neoplastic, inflammatory, vascular, or posttraumatic. The Babinski reflex may also become positive during transtentorial herniation.[4]

Pupillary Function

Assessment of pupillary function focuses on three areas: (1) estimation of pupil size and shape, (2) evaluation of pupillary reaction to light, and (3) assessment of eye movements. Pupillary function is an extension of the autonomic nervous system. Parasympathetic control of the pupil occurs through innervation of the oculomotor nerve (CN III), which exits from the brainstem in the midbrain area. When the parasympathetic fibers are stimulated, the pupil constricts. Sympathetic control originates in the hypothalamus and travels down the entire length of the brainstem. When the sympathetic fibers are stimulated, the pupil dilates. Pupillary changes provide a valuable assessment tool because of pathway locations. The oculomotor nerve lies at the junction of the midbrain and the tentorial notch. Any increase of pressure that exerts force down through the tentorial notch compresses the oculomotor nerve. Oculomotor nerve compression results in a dilated, nonreactive pupil. Sympathetic pathway disruption occurs with involvement in the brainstem. Loss of sympathetic control leads to pinpoint, nonreactive pupils. Control of eye movements occurs with the interaction of three cranial nerves: (1) oculomotor (CN III), (2) trochlear (CN IV), and (3) abducens (CN VI). The pathways for these cranial nerves provide integrated function through the internuclear pathway of the medial longitudinal fasciculus (MLF) located in the brainstem. The MLF provides coordination of eye movements with the vestibular nerve (CN VIII) and the reticular formation.[15]

Estimation of Pupil Size and Shape

Pupil size. Diameter of the pupil is documented in millimeters with a pupillometer to reduce the subjectivity of the description. Most individuals have pupils of equal size, between 2 and 5 mm. A discrepancy up to 1 mm between the two pupils is normal; it is called *anisocoria* and occurs in 15% to 17% of humans without any known clinical significance.[16] Change or inequality in pupil size, especially in patients who previously have not shown this discrepancy, is a significant neurologic sign. It may indicate impending danger of herniation and should be reported immediately. With the location of CN III at the notch of the tentorium, pupil size and reactivity play a vital role in the physical assessment of intracranial pressure (ICP) changes and herniation syndromes. Changes in pupil size occur for other reasons besides CN III compression. Large pupils can result from the instillation of cycloplegic agents, such as atropine or scopolamine, or can indicate extreme stress. Extremely small pupils can indicate opioid/narcotic overdose, lower brainstem compression, or bilateral damage to the pons.[16,17]

Pupil shape. Pupil shape is included in the assessment of pupils. Although the pupil is normally round, an irregularly shaped or oval pupil may be observed in patients who have undergone eye surgery. Initial stages of CN III compression from elevated ICP can also cause the pupil to have an oval shape.[4,16]

Evaluation of Pupillary Reaction to Light

The pupillary light reflex depends on the optic nerve (CN II), which relays visual signals to the brain, and the oculomotor nerve (CN III), which controls the parasympathetic response of the pupil (Fig. 21.5).[18] Each pupil is evaluated for direct light response and consensual response.

Direct light response. The technique for evaluating the pupillary light response involves using a narrow-beamed bright light shone into the pupil from the outer canthus of the eye. If the light is shone directly onto the pupil, glare or reflection of the light may prevent the assessor's proper visualization. Pupillary reaction to light is identified as brisk, sluggish, nonreactive, or fixed.[4]

Consensual light response. The consensual pupillary response is constriction in response to a light shining into the opposite eye.[18] This reflex occurs due to nerve fibers crossing at the optic chiasm.[4] Evaluation of consensual response is necessary to rule out optic nerve dysfunction as a cause for the lack of a direct light reflex. Because the optic

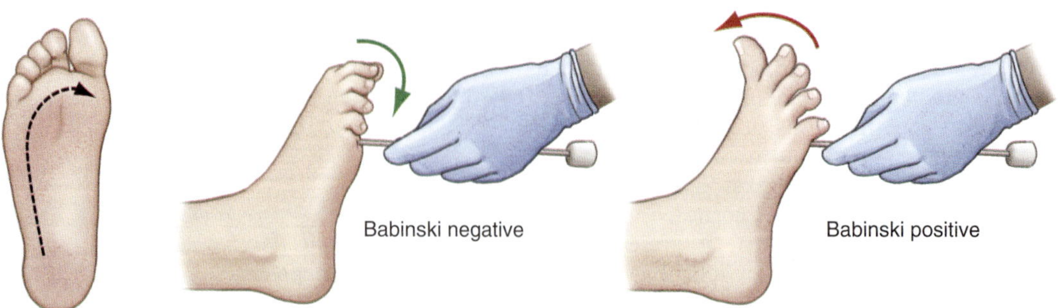

FIG. 21.4 Babinski Reflex. Test maneuver: Using a blunt point, scratch the sole of the foot as shown. Normal response (absence of the Babinski response) is plantar flexion of the toes. Abnormal response (presence of the Babinski response) is dorsiflexion of the big toe and often a fanning of the other toes. (From Stein LNM, Hollen CJ. *Concept-Based Clinical Nursing Skills.* 2nd ed. Elsevier, 2024.)

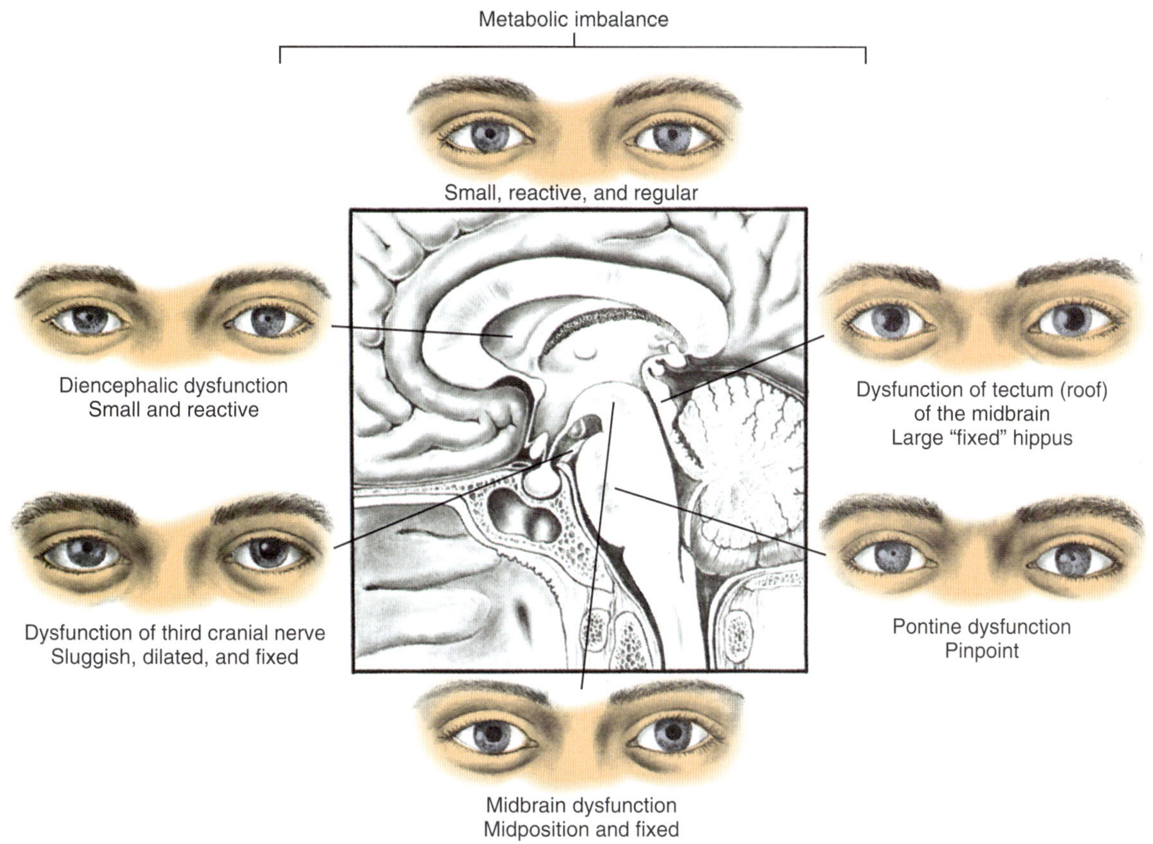

FIG. 21.5 Abnormal Pupillary Responses.

nerve is the afferent pathway for the light reflex, shining a light into a blind eye produces neither a direct light response in that eye nor a consensual response in the opposite eye. A consensual response in a blind eye, produced by shining a light into the opposite functional eye, demonstrates an intact oculomotor nerve. Oculomotor compression, associated with transtentorial herniation and increased ICP, affects the affected pupil's direct light response and consensual response.[16]

Assessment of Eye Movement

In a conscious patient, the function of the three cranial nerves of the eye and their MLF innervation can be assessed by asking the patient to follow a finger through the full range of eye motion. Extraocular movements are intact if the eyes move together into all six fields (Fig. 21.6).[15]

Doll's eye reflex. In an unconscious patient, ocular function and MLF innervation is assessed by eliciting the doll's eye reflex. If the patient is unconscious due to trauma, the absence of a cervical injury and the presence of neck stability must be ascertained before performing this examination.[11] To assess the oculocephalic reflex, hold the patient's eyelids open and briskly turn the head to one side, observing the eye movement, and then briskly turn the head to the other side, again observing the eye movement. If the eye movement deviates to the opposite direction in which the head is turned, the doll's eye reflex is present, and the oculocephalic reflex arc is intact (Fig. 21.7A). If the oculocephalic reflex arc is not intact, the reflex is absent. This lack of response, in which the eyes remain midline and move with the head, indicates significant brainstem injury (Fig. 21.7C). The reflex may also be absent in severe metabolic coma. An abnormal oculocephalic reflex is present when the eyes rove or move in opposite directions from each other (Fig. 21.7B). An abnormal oculocephalic reflex indicates some degree of brainstem injury.[4,5]

Oculovestibular reflex. The oculovestibular reflex is performed by a health care practitioner often as one of the final physical assessments of brainstem function. After confirmation that the tympanic membrane is intact, the patient's head is raised to a 30-degree angle, and 20 to 100 mL of ice water is injected into the external auditory canal. The normal eye movement response is a conjugate, slow, tonic nystagmus, deviating toward the irrigated ear and lasting 30 to 120 seconds. This response indicates brainstem integrity. In a conscious patient with cortical functioning, rapid nystagmus returns the eye position back to the midline when the irrigation stops (Fig. 21.8).[10,19] An abnormal response is disconjugate eye movement, which indicates a brainstem lesion, or no response, which indicates little or no brainstem function. The oculovestibular reflex may be temporarily absent in reversible metabolic encephalopathy. This test is a highly noxious stimulation and may produce a decorticate or decerebrate posturing response in an unconscious patient. In a conscious patient, the eyes will deviate towards the irrigated ear and cause horizontal nystagmus that beats towards the opposite eye, resulting in nausea and vertigo.[19]

Respiratory Function

Assessment of respiratory function focuses on two areas: (1) observation of respiratory pattern and (2) evaluation of airway

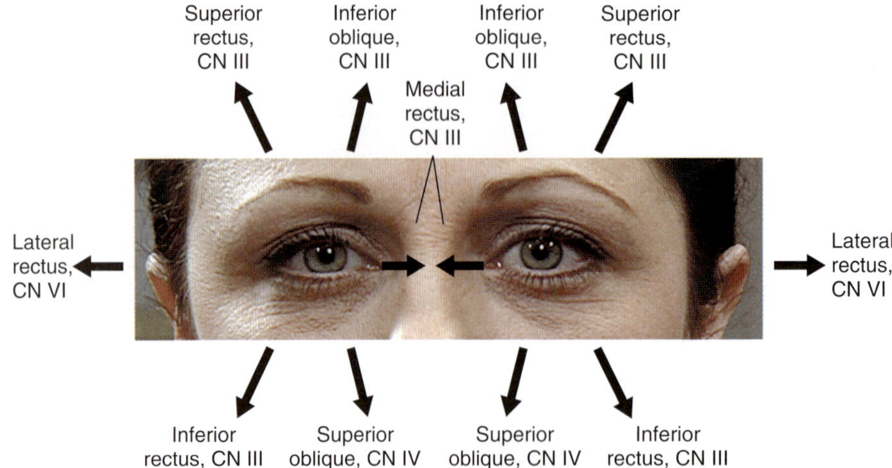

FIG. 21.6 Extraocular Eye Movements. (From Ball JW, Dains JE, Flynn JA, et al. *Seidel's Guide to Physical Examination: An Interprofessional Approach.* 10th ed. Elsevier; 2023.)

status. The activity of respiration is a highly integrated function that receives input from the cerebrum, brainstem, and metabolic mechanisms. Correlations exist among altered levels of consciousness, the level of brain or brainstem injury, and the patient's respiratory pattern. Under the influence of the cerebral cortex and the diencephalon, three brainstem centers control respirations. The lowest center, the *medullary respiratory center*, sends impulses through the vagus nerve to innervate muscles of inspiration and expiration. The *apneustic* and *pneumotaxic centers of the pons* are responsible for the length of inspiration and expiration and the underlying respiratory rate.[10]

Observation of Respiratory Pattern

Changes in respiratory patterns assist in identifying the level of brainstem dysfunction or injury (Fig. 21.9 and Table 21.3). Evaluation of the respiratory pattern must include assessment of the effectiveness of gas exchange in maintaining adequate oxygen and carbon dioxide levels. Hypoventilation is common in patients with altered level of consciousness. Alterations in oxygenation or carbon dioxide levels can result in further neurologic dysfunction.[10] ICP increases with hypoxemia or hypercapnia.[4]

Evaluation of Airway Status

Evaluation of respiratory function in a patient with a neurologic deficit must include assessment of airway maintenance and secretion control. Cough, gag, and swallow reflexes responsible for airway protection may be absent or diminished.[20]

Vital Signs

Assessment of vital signs focuses on two areas: (1) evaluation of blood pressure and (2) observation of heart rate and rhythm. As a result of the brain and brainstem influences on cardiac, respiratory, and body temperature functions, changes in vital signs could be signs of deterioration in neurologic status.[4]

Evaluation of Blood Pressure

A common manifestation of intracranial injury is systemic hypertension. Cerebral autoregulation, responsible for controlling cerebral blood flow (CBF), is frequently lost with any intracranial injury.[20] After a cerebral injury, the body often is in a hyperdynamic state (increased heart rate, blood pressure, and cardiac output) as part of a compensatory response.[21] With the loss of autoregulation as blood pressure increases, CBF and cerebral blood volume increase and ICP increases. Control of systemic hypertension is necessary to stop this cycle, but caution must be exercised. The mean arterial pressure must be maintained at a level sufficient to produce adequate CBF in the presence of elevated ICP.[21] Attention must also be paid to the pulse pressure (systolic BP-diastolic BP) because widening of this value may occur in the late stages of intracranial hypertension.[22]

Observation of Heart Rate and Rhythm

The medulla and the vagus nerve provide parasympathetic control to the heart. When stimulated, this lower brainstem system produces bradycardia. Sympathetic stimulation increases the heart rate and contractility.[23] Various intracranial pathologies and abrupt ICP changes can produce bradycardia, premature ventricular contractions, Q–T interval changes, and myocardial damage.[24]

Cushing triad. Cushing triad is a set of three clinical manifestations (systolic hypertension with widening pulse pressure, bradycardia, and bradypnea) related to pressure on the medullary area of the brainstem. These signs may occur in response to intracranial hypertension or a herniation syndrome. The appearance of Cushing triad is a late finding and may be absent in patients with severe neurologic deterioration. Once this pattern of vital signs occurs, it may be too late to completely reverse intracranial hypertension.[25]

RAPID NEUROLOGIC ASSESSMENT

A neurologic assessment should be organized, thorough, and simple to perform accurately and efficiently at each assessment point. A complete neurologic assessment covers all significant areas of neurologic control. Any abnormalities identified can be further evaluated and investigated in a more focused and rapid manner. Findings are always considered with respect to the results of previous examinations. One critical assessment point is the hand-off between nurses caring for the patient.

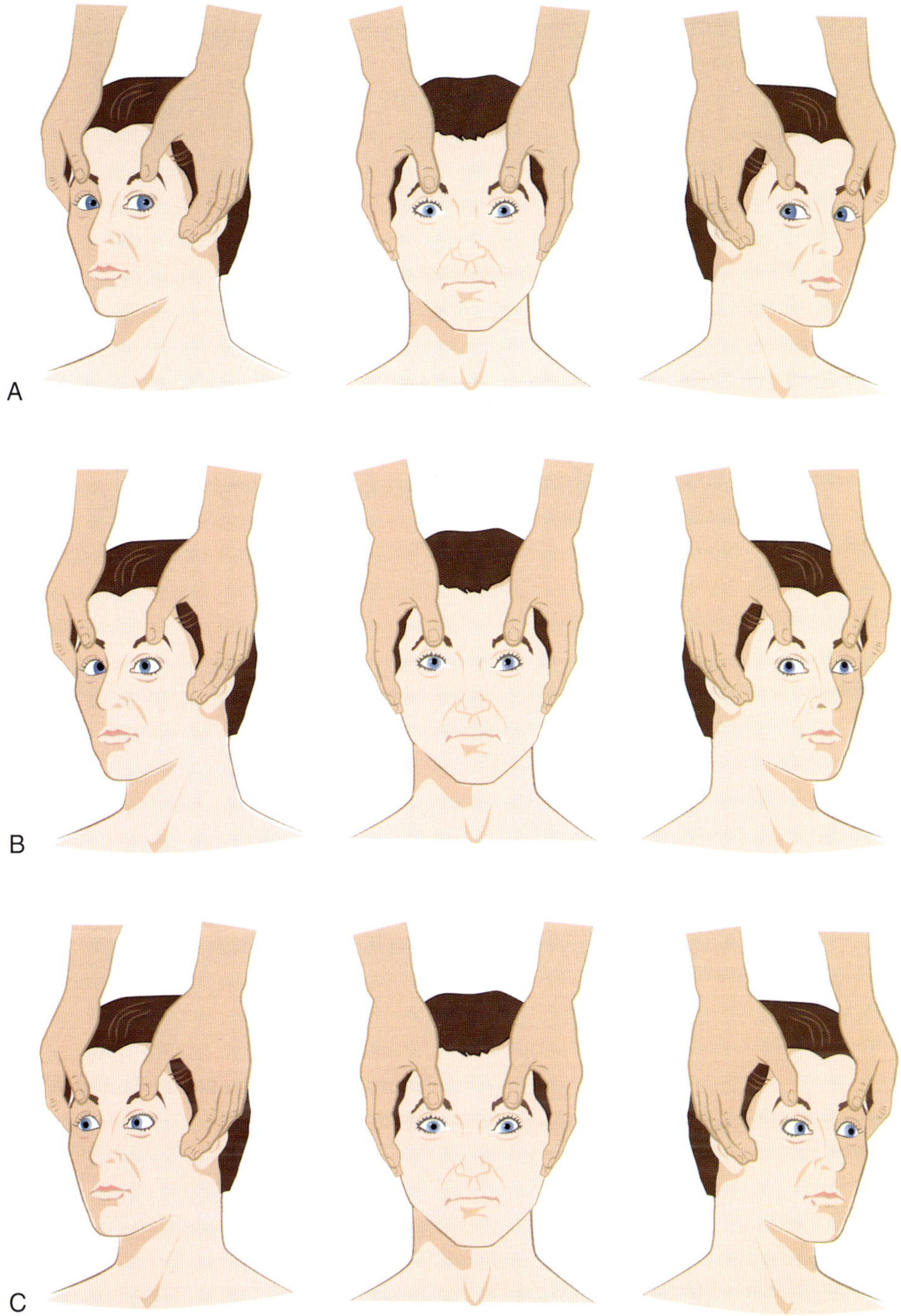

A

B

C

FIG. 21.7 Oculocephalic Reflex (Doll's Eye Reflex). (A) Normal. (B) Abnormal. (C) Absent.

A

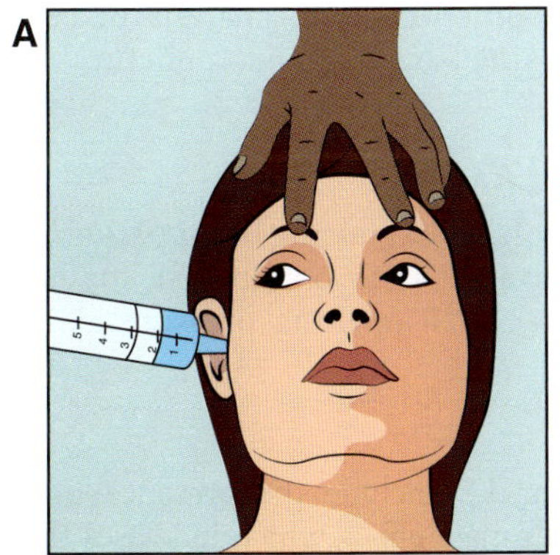

B

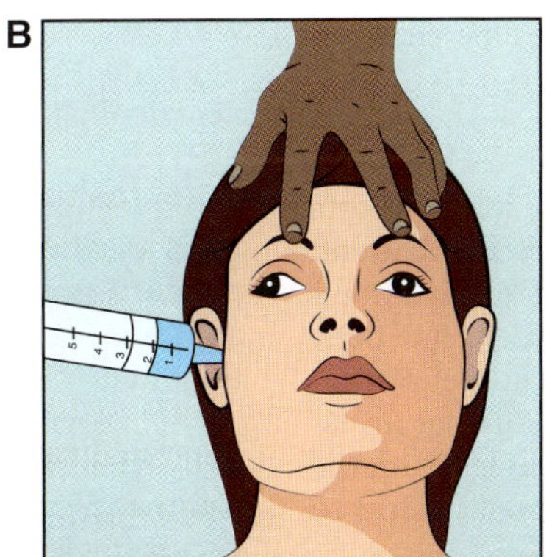

C

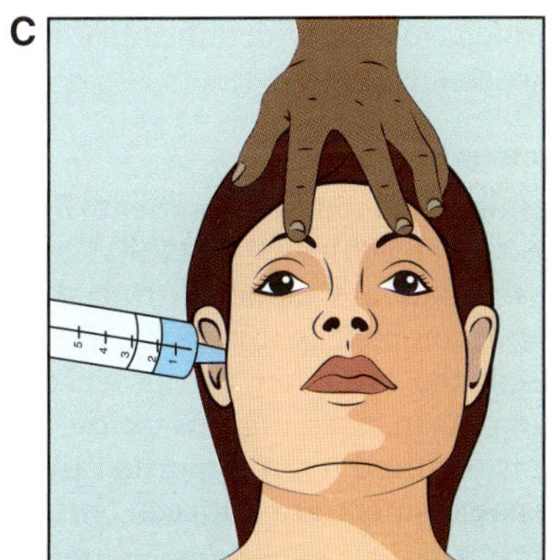

FIG. 21.8 Oculovestibular Reflex (Cold Caloric Test). (A) Normal. (B) Abnormal. (C) Absent.

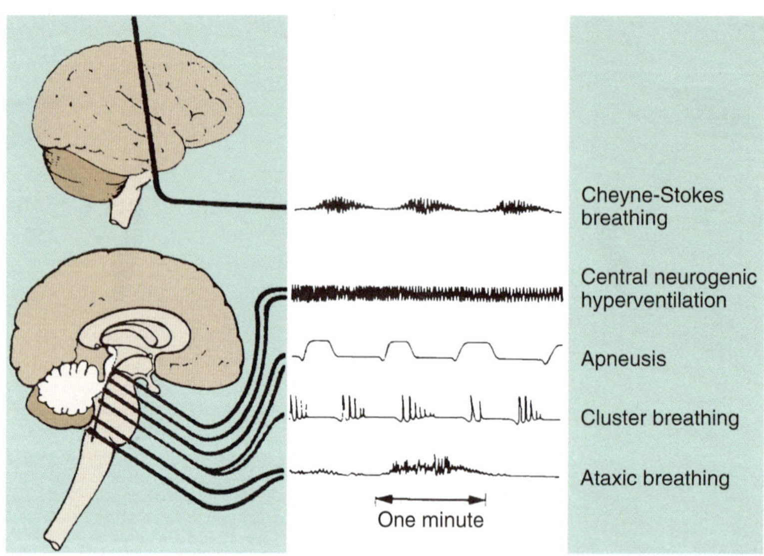

FIG. 21.9 Abnormal Respiratory Patterns. Abnormal respiratory patterns with corresponding levels of central nervous system activity.

TABLE 21.3 Respiratory Patterns

Pattern of Respiration	Description of Pattern	Significance
Cheyne-Stokes breathing	Rhythmic crescendo and decrescendo of rate and depth of respiration; includes brief periods of apnea	Usually seen with bilateral deep cerebral lesions or some cerebellar lesions
Central neurogenic hyperventilation	Very deep, very rapid respirations with no apneic periods	Usually seen with lesions of the midbrain and upper pons
Apneustic breathing	Prolonged inspiratory or expiratory pause of 2–3 seconds	Usually seen in lesions of middle to lower pons
Cluster breathing	Clusters of irregular, gasping respirations separated by long periods of apnea	Usually seen in lesions of the lower pons or upper medulla
Ataxic respirations	Irregular, random pattern of deep and shallow respirations with irregular apneic periods	Usually seen in lesions of the medulla

It is essential that the off-going nurse perform a neurologic assessment with the on-coming nurse. This action ensures the reliability of the assessment and decreases variability between nurses.

Conscious Patient

Box 21.3 outlines an example of a rapid neurologic assessment that can be performed during the hand-off of a conscious patient with a known or potential neurologic deficit. This assessment usually takes less than 4 minutes and provides a starting point. More detailed attention must be focused on that abnormality if any neurologic deficit is identified that is new or different from the last assessment.

Unconscious Patient

In assessing an unconscious patient (Box 21.4), initial efforts are directed at achieving maximal arousal of the patient. Calling the patient's name, patting the chest, or shaking a shoulder accomplishes this task. After the patient has been stimulated, the examiner can proceed with the neurologic evaluation. As in assessing a conscious patient, further investigation is required if any abnormalities or changes from the previous assessment are noticed. This assessment takes 3 to 4 minutes.

Neurologic Changes Associated With Intracranial Hypertension

Assessing a patient for signs of increasing ICP is an essential responsibility of the critical care nurse. Increasing ICP can be identified by changes in the level of consciousness, pupillary reaction, motor response, vital signs, and respiratory patterns (Fig. 21.10).[10,26]

LABORATORY STUDIES

The primary laboratory study performed on a patient with neurologic dysfunction is an analysis of cerebrospinal fluid (CSF) obtained by a lumbar puncture (LP) or a ventriculostomy.

Cerebrospinal Fluid Analysis

LP is an essential tool for diagnosing brain pathology.[27] The primary purpose of a LP is to obtain CSF for laboratory analysis (Table 21.4). CSF opening pressure also may be obtained.

Contraindications

Contraindications for LP include the presence of a space-occupying lesion with mass effect, which increases the risk for

BOX 21.3 Teamwork and Collaboration

Rapid Neurologic Assessment of the Conscious Patient

This outline should be used for the hand-off of a critically ill conscious patient with neurologic dysfunction:

1. *Level of consciousness:* Address the patient and ask a variety of orientation questions; avoid obvious, overused questions about name, date, and place, and focus on questions about recent and past events from the patient's experiences, such as spouse's name, home address, or what was eaten at the previous meal. As an examiner, you should know the correct answers to all questions.
2. *Facial movements:* During the assessment of level of consciousness, observe the patient's facial movements for symmetry, and listen to speech patterns for evidence of slurred speech.
3. *Pupillary function and eye movements:* Perform pupil check and assess extraocular eye movements.
4. *Motor assessment:* Assess movement and strength in the upper and lower extremities.
5. *Sensory:* With a finger, stroke the patient bilaterally on the face and upper aspect of the arm, hand, leg, and foot; ask the patient to identify what is touched and any difference in sensation between the two sides.
6. *Vital signs:* Observe alterations in blood pressure, heart rate or rhythm, respiratory pattern, or temperature.
7. *Change in status:* Ask the patient if they feel any differences between this and the previous examination.

BOX 21.4 Teamwork and Collaboration

Rapid Neurologic Assessment of the Unconscious Patient

This outline should be used for the hand-off of a critically ill unconscious patient with neurologic dysfunction:

1. *Level of consciousness:* Perform Glasgow Coma Scale assessment.
2. *Pupillary assessment:* Perform pupillary assessment with particular attention to pupil size, reactivity, and shape compared with the opposite eye.
3. *Motor examination:* Assess each extremity individually using a predetermined coding score of motor movement.
4. *Respiratory pattern:* If the patient is not receiving mechanical ventilation, observe respiratory patterns for evidence of deteriorating level of function.
5. *Vital signs:* Include comparing preassessment vital signs with vital signs after assessment, paying particular attention to arterial blood pressure and intracranial pressure if these parameters are being monitored.

cerebral herniation if the patient undergoes an LP; increased ICP caused by increased CSF pressure and Arnold–Chiari malformation; increased bleeding risk (thrombocytopenia, coagulopathies, anticoagulant medications); and local infections at the puncture site.[28]

Preprocedure Preparation

Before the procedure is initiated, the patient's coagulation status and platelet count should be assessed for abnormalities.[27,28] A computed tomography (CT) or magnetic resonance imaging (MRI) scan should be obtained before an LP if the patient has an abnormal clinical neurologic examination, papilledema, reduced level of consciousness, previous CNS disease, or experienced recent seizures. An intracranial space-occupying lesion with mass effect or a posterior fossa mass can lead to brain herniation during an LP.[28]

Procedure

A LP involves the introduction of a 25-gauge hollow needle into the subarachnoid space of the lumbar sac at L3 to L4 or L4 to L5, below the level of the spinal cord, using aseptic technique. For the procedure, a patient is most commonly placed in a flexed lateral recumbent position and must remain still (Fig. 21.11). If the patient is not fully alert and cooperative, the patient may need assistance maintaining the proper position for the LP. Collection of up to 30 mL of CSF is passively withdrawn and placed in designated laboratory specimen containers.[28] The patient's neurologic and respiratory status is monitored during and after the procedure and compared to the patient's preprocedural baseline.

DIAGNOSTIC PROCEDURES

The nursing management of a patient undergoing a neurodiagnostic procedure involves a variety of interventions. Nursing activities are directed toward preparing the patient psychologically and physically for the procedure, monitoring the patient's responses during the procedure, and assessing the patient afterward. Preparation includes teaching the patient about the procedure, answering questions, transporting the patient, and positioning the patient for the procedure. During the procedure, the patient is observed for signs of pain, anxiety, or bleeding and vital signs monitored. After the procedure, the patient is observed for complications and medicated for postprocedure discomfort. Any evidence of increasing ICP should be immediately reported to the practitioner, and emergency measures to maintain circulation must be initiated.

Radiologic Procedures

The following discussion focuses on the more commonly performed radiologic procedures used to diagnose a critically ill patient with neurologic dysfunction.

Skull and Spine Films

The purpose of radiographs of the skull or spine is to identify fractures, anomalies, or possible tumors. The role of skull radiographs in trauma has diminished with the advent of CT. If the patient is to undergo a CT scan during the initial assessment process, a skull radiograph may be unnecessary.[29]

Skull series. The procedure for obtaining skull and spine radiographs is relatively painless. In many situations, a single lateral view of the skull is adequate, but a complete skull series is required in some cases. A skull series consists of four different views: (1) lateral, (2) posteroanterior, (3) half-axial (Towne), and (4) submentovertical (base) views.[29] A cervical spine series consists of four views: (1) atlas and axial, (2) anteroposterior, (3) lateral, and (4) oblique. A thoracic and lumbar spine series consists of two views: (1) anteroposterior and (2) lateral.[29]

Spine series. Proper patient positioning is essential, especially for radiographs of the spine. Nursing care involves positioning the patient to obtain adequate radiographs. Spinal precautions (e.g., cervical collar, strict maintenance of head alignment) must be maintained until lateral radiographs confirm the integrity of the cervical structures. The patient should maintain strict body

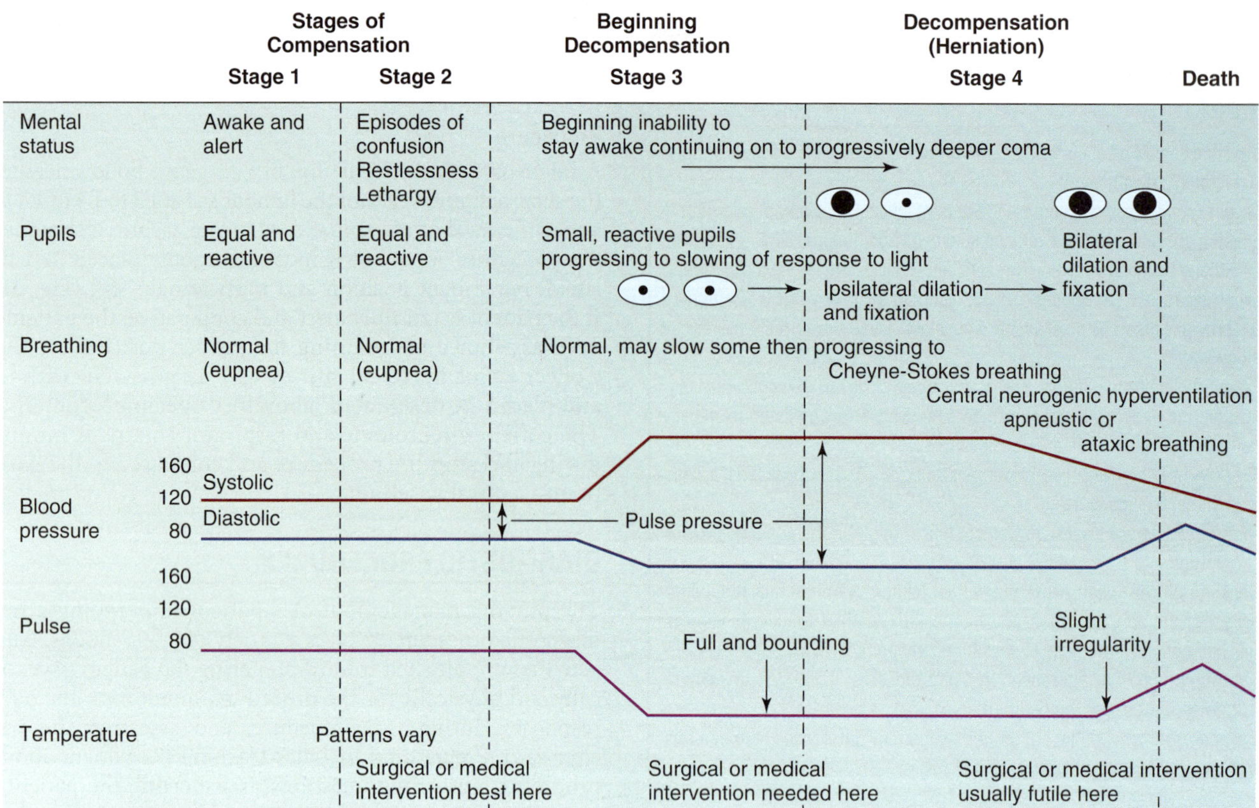

FIG. 21.10 Signs and Symptoms of Intracranial Hypertension. Clinical correlates of compensated and decompensated phases of intracranial hypertension. (From Beare PG, Myers JL, eds. *Principles and Practice of Adult Health Nursing*. 3rd ed. Mosby; 1998.)

alignment, and the cervical spine must be treated as unstable until proven otherwise in any situation in which traumatic injury, especially head injury, is the cause of the patient's admission to the critical care unit.

Computed Tomography

CT, which uses a computer to digitally construct an image based on measuring the absorption of x-rays through the brain, is the primary neuroimaging technique in the initial evaluation of the acute brain injury patient. The degree of x-ray absorption by the various tissues is expressed and displayed as shades of gray in the CT image. The denser the substance through which an x-ray beam passes, the whiter it appears on the finished film. The less dense a substance is, the blacker it appears. With normal findings for a CT scan of the head, bone and other dense tissue appear white, blood appears off-white, brain tissue appears shaded gray, CSF appears off-black, and air appears black (Fig. 21.12).[30,31]

Procedure. CT offers rapid, convenient, noninvasive visualization of structures and is the diagnostic study of choice for an acute head injury. Serial evaluations may be obtained to verify a midline shift and increasing ICP.[31] CT also diagnoses space-occupying lesions, hemorrhage, vascular abnormalities, skull fractures, cerebral edema, hydrocephalus, and severe headache. CT can be performed with and without the use of a contrast medium. Without a contrast medium, the scan is noninvasive, requires no patient premedication, and is effective for analyzing and locating normal brain structures. Using an intravenously injected contrast medium enhances the vascular areas, thus enabling the detection of vascular lesions or further definition of lesions identified on a non–contrast-enhanced scan. As a result, CT perfusion (CTP) studies in ischemic stroke have become an important adjunct, along with CT angiography (CTA), to conventional unenhanced CT brain imaging and aid in determining potential further treatment.[32] Before a patient is scheduled for a CT scan with contrast, a patient history should be obtained regarding allergies, asthma, and previous reactions to the contrast medium. Risk factors for contrast reactions include multiple medication allergies and asthma.[33] If a patient has had a previous minor reaction to an IV iodinated contrast agent, precontrast administration of a corticosteroid and antihistamine may decrease the risk of a subsequent reaction. A history of anaphylactic reaction would preclude IV contrast except in extreme emergencies.[33]

Nursing management. Nursing management of a patient undergoing CT can be divided into two areas of focus: (1) observation of the patient's tolerance of the procedure and (2) monitoring for a possible reaction to the radiocontrast medium. Because of the associated activity and positioning, transporting and scanning a critically ill patient with known or suspected intracranial hypertension can cause deterioration in the patient's condition. During the CT scan, the patient's neurologic status, vital signs, and, if monitored, ICP are closely observed.

During infusion of the contrast medium and 10 to 30 minutes afterward, the patient should be observed closely for an anaphylactic reaction, such as hives, flushing, or stridor, and emergency equipment should be readily available. Another

SUPPORTING NURSE WELL-BEING

Career Wellness

I have been a nurse for 10 years and have spent most of my career in the intensive care unit. Over the last several months, many of my colleagues have either left the profession or gotten "easier" jobs. The pandemic has taken quite a toll on the staff in this unit. We now have many new nurses who are both new to nursing and the intensive care unit. I want to start a nurse retention program in our unit to help the new nurses adjust to their new careers. While I am not against nurses moving on to new jobs, it pains me when they leave the profession. I want to help them develop good habits to maintain their enthusiasm for their new careers.

Nursing career wellness refers to nurses' overall well-being and health in their professional roles. It encompasses various aspects, including physical, emotional, social, and mental well-being, work–life balance, and job satisfaction. Prioritizing nursing career wellness is essential for the individual nurse's benefit, patient care quality, and the overall health care system.

Here are some actions that can facilitate career wellness:

- Prioritize self-care, including regular exercise, healthy eating habits, and sufficient rest. Taking care of physical health provides the stamina required for demanding work.
- Develop healthy coping mechanisms, access to support networks, and opportunities for debriefing or counselling when needed. Dealing with patients' suffering and challenging situations can be emotionally taxing.
- Maintain a healthy balance between work and personal life. Long and irregular shifts can be physically and emotionally draining, so seeking ways to ensure time for families, hobbies, and relaxation is essential.
- Engage in continuous learning and professional development to stay updated on the latest advancements and improve skills. These activities can provide opportunities for career advancement.
- Foster a positive and supportive work environment through respectful communication and recognition of others' contributions.
- Engage with mentors and supportive colleagues, especially when new to the profession. Mentorship can guide and encourage, while peer support fosters camaraderie and a sense of belonging.
- Develop effective stress management techniques, such as mindfulness, meditation, or engaging in hobbies outside of work.
- Actively advocate for health and safety at work, including adherence to safety protocols, proper use of personal protective equipment (PPE), and reporting unsafe conditions.
- Recognize the efforts of others, as this can boost morale and job satisfaction. Feeling valued and appreciated for hard work and dedication is essential for career wellness.
- Set achievable short-term and long-term goals, as this can give a sense of purpose and direction to a career. Accomplishing these goals can bring a sense of fulfilment and motivation to continue growing professionally.

By focusing on career wellness, health care organizations can promote a positive and thriving nursing workforce, improving patient outcomes and the overall effectiveness of health care systems.[1]

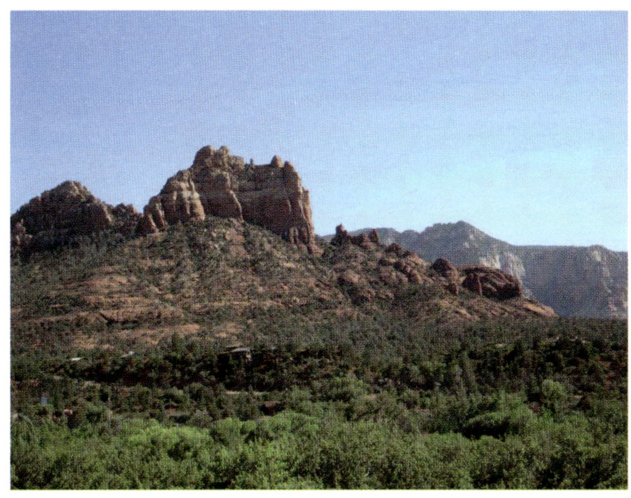

We need to do a better job of putting ourselves higher on our own to-do list.

Michelle Obama

Reference

1. National Academy of Medicine. *National Plan for Health Workforce Well-Being.* The National Academies Press; 2022. https://doi.org/10.17226/26744.

potential complication of contrast medium administration is contrast-induced nephropathy (CIN). Two measures reported to reduce the incidence and severity of CIN are (1) limiting the amount of contrast and (2) adequate hydration before and after the study.[34]

Magnetic Resonance Imaging

MRI produces images with greater detail than CT and provides views of several planes (sagittal, coronal, axial, and oblique) that cannot be obtained with CT. No ionizing radiation is used. For MRI, the patient is placed in a large magnetic field that stimulates the nuclei of the body's atoms. Introducing radiofrequency waves causes resonance of the nuclei, which is emitted as the nuclei relax. A computer then constructs an image of the tissue (Fig. 21.13). Intravenous administration of a non–iodine-based contrast medium enhances the images by influencing the magnetic environment and signal intensity.[29,30]

With MRI, small tumors, whose tissue densities are different from the densities of the surrounding cells, can be identified before they can be visualized through any other radiographic test. MRI also can detect cerebral infarct areas within minutes of stroke and identify small hemorrhages deep in the brain that are invisible on CT. MRI with contrast is the preferred study for detecting infectious and inflammatory processes of the central nervous system (CNS), malignancy and metastatic lesions, cervical spine imaging, and postoperative evaluation of tumor recurrence. MRI is also the diagnostic study of choice in evaluating spinal cord injury.[31]

Nursing management. As with CT scanning, nursing management for a patient undergoing MRI is focused on concerns related to the transport of a patient with neurologic dysfunction, the patient's tolerance of the procedure, and, if contrast medium is used, monitoring for a possible patient reaction. Teaching and preparation of the patient are essential for the successful performance of an MRI. The procedure is lengthy and requires the patient to lie motionless in a tight, enclosed cylinder (closed MRI) or in a cylinder open on two sides (open MRI). Patients in a closed MRI may experience anxiety, panic, and an acute

TABLE 21.4 Analysis of Cerebrospinal Fluid

Characteristic	Normal Findings	Abnormal Findings	Possible Causes and Comments
Pressure	<200 mm H_2O	<60 mm H_2O	Faulty needle placement Dehydration Spinal block along subarachnoid space Block of the foramen magnum Hydrocephalus
		>200 mm H_2O	Muscle tension Abdominal compression Brain tumor Subdural hematoma Brain abscess Brain cyst Cerebral edema (any cause)
Color	Clear, colorless	Cloudy	Cloudy as a result of microorganisms (e.g., WBCs)
		Turbid	Turbid as a result of increased cell count
		Yellow (xanthochromic)	Breakdown of RBCs with RBC pigments, high protein count
		Smoky	RBCs
Blood	None	Red blood cells: Blood tinged	Traumatic tap: Blood in the first sample
		Grossly bloody	Traumatic tap: Bloody in all samples
Volume	150 mL	Increase	Hydrocephalus
Specific gravity	1.007	Increase	Infection, presence of cells or protein
WBCs	0–5 cells/mm^3	<500 cells/mm^3	Bacterial or viral infections of meninges, neurosyphilis, subarachnoid hemorrhage, infarction, abscess, tuberculous meningitis, metastatic lesions
		>500 cells/mm^3	Purulent infection
Glucose	50–75 mg/dL or 60%–70% of blood glucose	<40 mg/dL	Bacterial meningitis, tuberculosis, parasitic, fungal carcinomatous, subarachnoid hemorrhage
		>80 mg/dL	May not be of neurologic significance
Chloride	700–750 mg/dL	Decreased (<625 mg/dL)	Meningeal infection, tuberculosis meningitis, hypochloremia
		Increased (>800 mg/dL)	May not be of neurologic significance; correlated with blood levels of chloride and not routine; done only on request
Culture and sensitivity	No organisms present	*Neisseria* or *Streptococcus*	Identify organisms to begin therapy; Gram stain for some cultures may take several weeks
Serology for syphilis	Negative	Positive	Syphilis
Protein[a]	15–50 mg/dL	Increased (>60 mg/dL)	Bacterial meningitis, brain tumors (benign and malignant), complete spinal block, ALS, Guillain-Barré syndrome, subarachnoid hemorrhage, infarction, CNS trauma, CNS degenerative diseases, herniated disk, DM with polyneuropathy
		Decreased (<10 mg/dL)	May not be of neurologic significance
Osmolality	295 mOsm/L	Increased	Protein, WBCs, microorganisms, RBCs
Lactate	10–20 mg/dL	Increased	Bacterial, seizure activity, fungal meningitis, CNS trauma, coma related to toxic or metabolic causes

[a]Blood in CSF will increase the protein level.

ALS, Amyotrophic lateral sclerosis; *CNS*, central nervous system; *CSF*, cerebrospinal fluid; *DM*, diabetes mellitus; *RBC*, red blood cell; *WBC*, white blood cell.

From Barker E. *Neuroscience Nursing: A Spectrum of Care*. 3rd ed. Mosby; 2008.

sense of claustrophobia. Mild sedation, a blindfold, or music may make the procedure tolerable. A patient with neurologic impairment may be unable to comprehend the instructions, and sedation, possibly combined with neuromuscular blockade, may be necessary. Removal of all metal from the patient's body and clothing is essential because the basis of MRI is a strong magnetic field. Transdermal medication patches should also be removed to prevent burns to the patient's skin.

Cerebral Angiography

The following discussion focuses on more commonly performed angiography procedures used to diagnose a critically ill patient with neurologic dysfunction.

Conventional angiography. Conventional angiography involves the injection of a radiopaque contrast medium into the intracranial or extracranial vasculature (Fig. 21.14). Using serial radiologic filming, an angiogram traces blood flow from the arterial circulation, through the capillary bed, to the venous circulation. Cerebral angiography allows visualization of the lumen of vessels to provide information about patency, size (narrowing or dilation), irregularities, or occlusion. Angiography is used to diagnose cerebral aneurysms, vasospasm, arteriovenous malformation (AVM), carotid artery disease, and some vascular tumors. Angiography also is used to evaluate cerebral vasculature in patients with stroke. Information obtained from the angiogram guides the surgeon in choosing the operative approach or provides information to aid in making medical management decisions other than surgery.[35]

Procedure. The procedure involves the placement of a catheter in the femoral or radial artery, which is threaded up

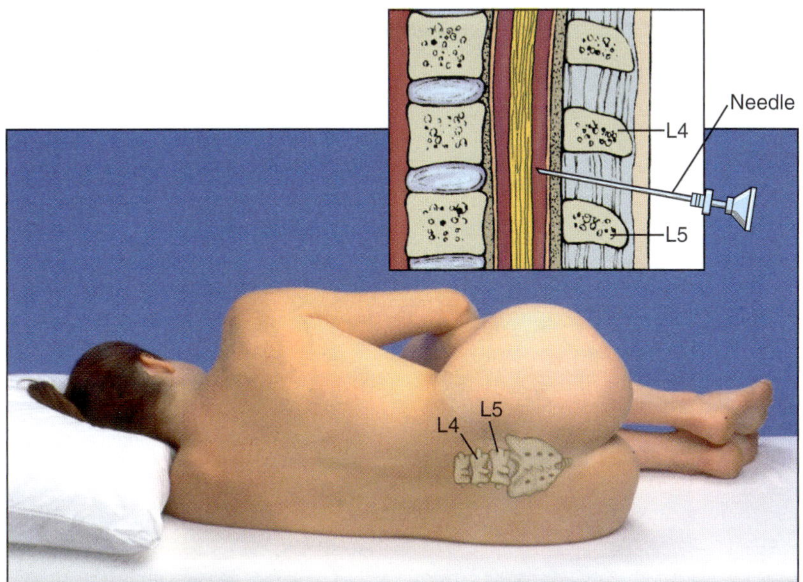

FIG. 21.11 Lumbar Puncture. With the patient in a flexed position to maximize the space between vertebrae, the lumbar puncture needle is inserted between L4 and L5 to gain entry to the subarachnoid space. (From Monahan FD, Sands J, Neighbors M, et al., eds. *Phipps' Medical-Surgical Nursing: Health and Illness Perspectives*. 8th ed. Mosby; 2007.)

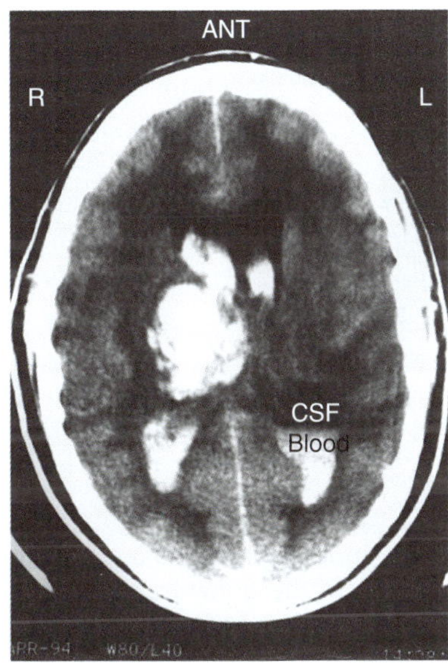

FIG. 21.12 Computed Tomography Scan of the Brain Demonstrating an Intracerebral Hemorrhage. In this patient with hypertension and an acute severe headache, a noncontrast computed tomography scan shows a large area of fresh blood in the region of the right thalamus. Blood also is seen in the anterior and posterior horns of the lateral ventricles. Because blood is denser than cerebrospinal fluid, it is layered dependently. (From Mettler FA. *Essentials of Radiology*. 4th ed. Elsevier; 2019.)

the aorta and into the cerebral circulation. Other less commonly used injection sites include direct carotid or vertebral artery puncture or catheter placement in the brachial, axillary, or subclavian artery. Several views of vessels can be studied using angiography. A four-vessel angiogram involves injections into the right and left internal carotid arteries and the right and left vertebral arteries. If the area of suspected disease has already been identified, a single-vessel study may be all that is required. This situation is particularly true when angiography is used as a follow-up in evaluating intracranial vascular surgery. If carotid artery disease is a working diagnosis, the angiographic study may include views of the aorta arch and external and internal carotid arteries.[29] After the catheter is appropriately placed, the contrast medium is injected. A rapid succession of radiographs is taken as the contrast medium progresses through the cerebral circulation. This study provides the gold standard look at cerebral blood vessels with a level of detail beyond that of the other modalities. Since pictures are taken multiple times per second, blood flow can be evaluated.[32]

Nursing management. Nursing management associated with this invasive procedure is comprehensive. Renal insufficiency, bleeding, and cardiac instability are contraindications to cerebral angiography and must be assessed before the procedure. As with other contrast-enhanced imaging studies, the patient must be assessed for allergies and possible sensitivity to the contrast medium. Patient education is essential to patient preparation. The patient's complete understanding of the process and its role in diagnosis relieves anxiety about the unknown and ensures cooperation in what is commonly an uncomfortable procedure.

In preparation for the procedure, the patient should abstain from oral intake (NPO status) for at least 4 hours. Sedation is administered immediately before the procedure, and a local anesthetic is injected at the catheter insertion site. There is a possibility that the patient will feel discomfort upon catheter insertion and from lying still on a hard table. The patient also may experience a hot, burning sensation when the contrast medium is injected. Following the procedure, enhanced hydration is necessary to assist the kidneys in clearing the heavy contrast load. Hemostasis of the catheter insertion site is obtained via handheld pressure or by applying a vascular closure device. If a femoral approach is used, the patient is instructed to remain supine with the involved leg kept straight for 2 to 6 hours.[36] Postprocedure assessment involves measurement of vital signs, neurologic evaluation, monitoring of kidney function,

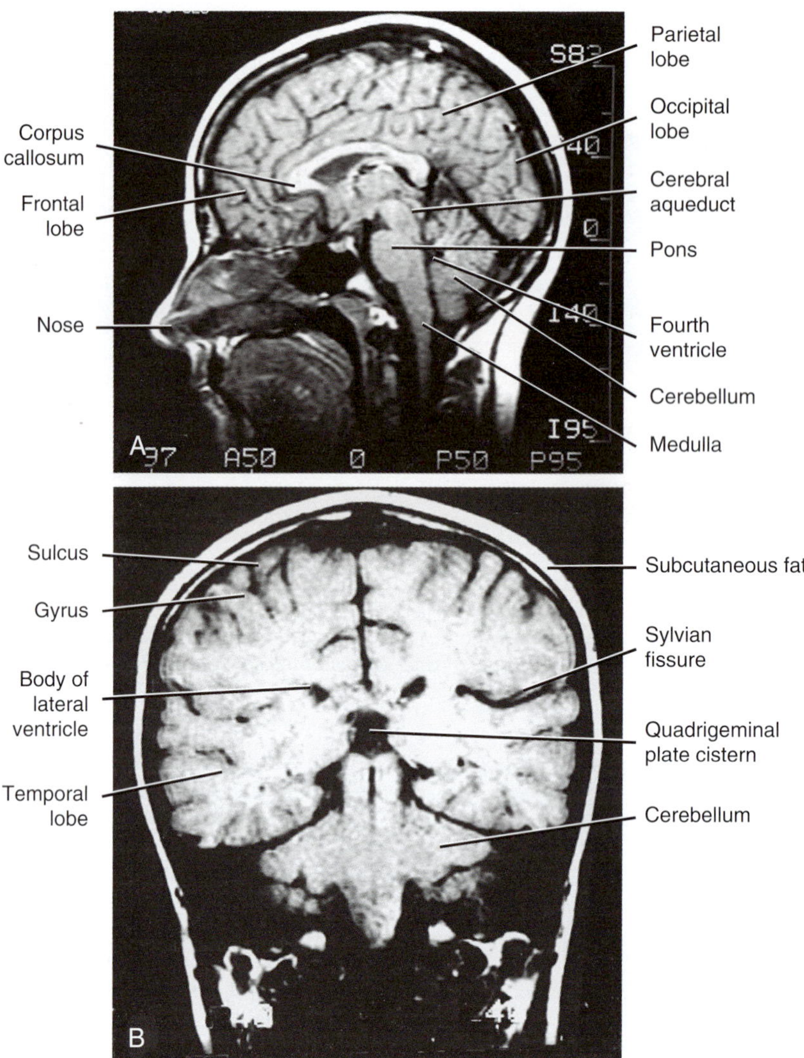

FIG. 21.13 Normal Magnetic Resonance Imaging Anatomy of the Brain. (A) Coronal projection. (B) Sagittal projection. (From Mettler FA. *Essentials of Radiology*. 4th ed. Elsevier; 2019.)

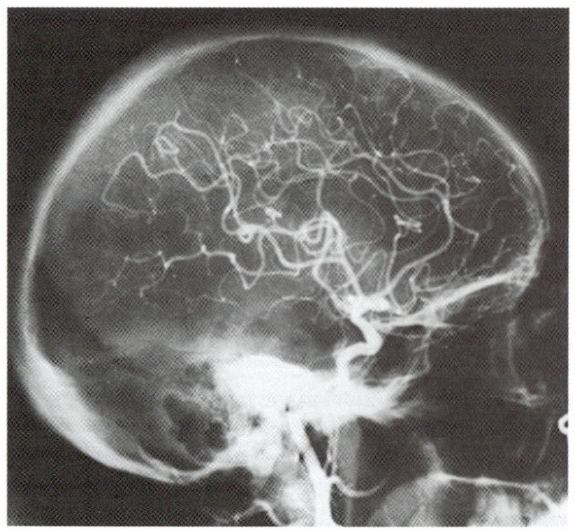

FIG. 21.14 Cerebral Angiography. (From Ehrlich RA, Coakes DM. *Patient Care in Radiography*. 10th ed. Elsevier; 2021.)

observation of the puncture site, and assessment of neurovascular integrity distal to the puncture site. Any abnormalities should be reported immediately. Complications associated with cerebral angiography include (1) cerebral embolus caused by the catheter dislodging a segment of atherosclerotic plaque in the vessel; (2) hemorrhage or hematoma formation at the insertion site; (3) vasospasm of a vessel caused by the irritation of catheter placement; (4) thrombosis of the extremity distal to the injection site; and (5) allergic or adverse reaction to the contrast medium, including renal impairment.[29]

Digital subtraction angiography. Digital subtraction angiography (DSA) is a medical imaging technique used to visualize blood vessels in detail, particularly within the arteries and veins of the body. It is commonly used to diagnose and evaluate vascular conditions, such as aneurysms, stenosis (narrowing), AVMs, and other vascular abnormalities.[37] DSA has been essential in diagnosing and guiding treatment for various vascular conditions. However, medical imaging technology has evolved, and alternatives such as CTA and magnetic resonance angiography (MRA) have become more prevalent due to their noninvasive nature and advanced imaging capabilities. These alternatives have often reduced the need for invasive procedures like DSA.

Procedure. The procedure involves injecting a contrast dye into the blood vessels of interest, typically through a catheter inserted into an artery or vein. This contrast agent is radiopaque, which absorbs x-rays, making the blood vessels more visible on x-ray images. The catheter is usually threaded through the vasculature to the specific area being examined.

X-ray images are taken before and after the contrast dye is injected. The initial images, called "mask" images, provide a baseline view of the blood vessels without the contrast agent. These images are subtracted from the subsequent images taken after the contrast injection. The images taken after the contrast injection are subtracted from the mask images. This subtraction eliminates the bones and tissues in the initial images, leaving only the contrast-filled blood vessels behind.

Advantages. This process results in a more precise visualization of the vasculature without the superimposed anatomical structures. DSA is often performed in real-time, allowing the physician to monitor the flow of contrast dye through the blood vessels as it happens. This real-time visualization can help detect abnormalities in blood flow, such as blockages or irregularities.

Limitations. DSA is an invasive procedure requiring catheter insertion, which carries certain risks, such as infection, bleeding, or damage to blood vessels. Some patients may be allergic to the contrast dye used in DSA, which can lead to adverse reactions. While DSA may offer reduced radiation exposure compared to other angiography methods, it still involves ionizing radiation, which carries some risk.

Magnetic resonance angiography. MRA offers a noninvasive visualization of the cerebrovascular system.[31] It uses MRI technology to evaluate CBF and provide details about cerebral vessels. MRA of the carotid arteries has become an established complement to preoperative ultrasound evaluation. MRA also identifies intracranial aneurysms, stroke, arteriovenous malformations, and vasospasm.[31] Contrast-enhanced MRA may be performed to improve image resolution and enhance visualization of venous flow. The most commonly used agent is gadolinium, a noniodinated contrast medium that is injected intravenously.[30]

Computed tomography angiography. CT angiography is a technique that uses high-speed spiral CT technology, with the administration of a contrast medium, to visualize the cerebrovascular system. With its three-dimensional reconstructions, CT angiography can simultaneously demonstrate the bony skull base and its related vasculature, making it a valuable diagnostic tool for managing patients with cerebrovascular disease. The use of ionizing radiation and an iodine-based intravascular contrast medium with CT angiography is a disadvantage compared with MRA, but it is quicker and requires less patient cooperation than MRA.[38]

Myelography

Myelography is a radiographic examination of the spinal cord and vertebral column that occurs after injection of contrast medium into the subarachnoid space through the lumbar region of the spine between L2 and L3 or L3 and L4 or by cisternal puncture. Myelography allows visualization of the spinal canal, the subarachnoid space around the spinal cord, and the spinal nerve roots. MRI has often replaced myelography, but myelography may be necessary for postoperative patients with multiple clips or metallic hardware. Possible risks involved in using myelography include accidental injection of the contrast medium outside the subarachnoid space, arachnoiditis due to irritation of the arachnoid membranes from foreign material, and allergic reaction. Other adverse reactions include bleeding, infection, CSF leak, headache, and seizures.[39] Postprocedure care includes keeping the patient's head elevated 30 to 45 degrees for 3 to 4 hours, monitoring neurologic status, and encouraging intake of oral fluids.

Cerebral Blood Flow and Metabolism Imaging

Measurement of CBF provides valuable information for the clinical management of critically ill patients with neurologic dysfunction.[40] The average CBF in a human is 50 mL/100 g of brain per minute, but actual values may vary, with lower values seen in the white matter (~20 mL/100 g of brain per minute) and higher values seen in the gray matter (~80 mL/100 g of brain per minute).[41] The ischemic threshold for CBF is approximately 15 to 20 mL/100 g per minute, with 15 mL/100 g per minute often considered the threshold for irreversible injury.[42] CBF is influenced by mean arterial pressure, ICP, and the partial pressure of carbon dioxide and oxygen.[43] The measurements of CBF and cerebral perfusion pressure (CPP) do not address the brain's metabolic need for oxygen, as neuronal demand for oxygen is governed by the metabolic rate. The rate at which the brain consumes oxygen is known as the cerebral metabolic rate of oxygen ($CMRO_2$), the normal average value of which is 3.0 mL/100 g per minute.[44] Measurement of $CMRO_2$ is a valuable tool for assessing brain vitality and function and is a better marker of injury severity in hypoxia–ischemia than CBF alone.[44]

The following discussion focuses on the more commonly performed imaging studies that assess CBF and cerebral metabolism in critically ill patients with neurologic dysfunction.

Perfusion Computed Tomography

CTP allows rapid evaluation of cerebral perfusion. In addition to revealing the structure of brain tissue, CTP measures CBF, cerebral blood volume, and mean transit time. This study is performed by scanning the patient several times every few seconds before, during, and after intravenous delivery of a contrast agent that absorbs the x-rays. CTP was initially developed to evaluate ischemic stroke but has utility after TBI for identifying secondary hypoperfusion.[45] Besides using an iodinated contrast medium, another drawback of this technique is that poor spatial resolution limits the evaluation of the posterior circulation and definition of the brain volume at risk for ischemic damage.[45]

Xenon Computed Tomography

Xenon CT (Xe-CT) is used to study regional CBF. The execution of a baseline CT scan precedes the acquisition of this study. After inhaling xenon gas, which can cross the blood-brain barrier and reach deep brain tissue, serial CT scans and end-tidal gas samples are obtained. Xe-CT provides a quick assessment of quantitative CBF data during many pathologic conditions, with limited radiation exposure for the patient.[46] It also has higher resolution in blood flow measurements than other techniques, such as positron emission tomography (PET). The scan takes roughly 10 minutes but is sensitive to motion artifact, so measurements may not be reliable in patients that cannot remain still.[46] Xe-TC may be performed at the bedside with a portable scanner.

Perfusion Magnetic Resonance Imaging

Perfusion-weighted MRI (PW-MRI) is a specific type of MRI that focuses on visualizing and quantifying the blood flow and perfusion characteristics within tissues, particularly in the brain. It is commonly used to study cerebral perfusion in neuroimaging. PW-MRI involves using a contrast agent, typically a gadolinium-based contrast agent, which is injected into the bloodstream. The contrast agent enhances the signal in MRI images, allowing for the visualization of blood flow dynamics over time. PW-MRI sequences acquire multiple images rapidly after the injection of the contrast agent, capturing the passage of blood through the tissue being examined. The acquired data are then used to calculate several perfusion-related parameters, providing insights into tissue perfusion and vascular characteristics. However, as with all MRI imaging, movement artifact, claustrophobia, contraindications, and challenging patient monitoring during execution may limit its use.[45] The main applications are the identification of vascular pathologies (e.g., ischemic strokes, vasospasm) and tumoral pathologies.[47]

Carotid Ultrasonography

Although ultrasound technology does not provide an absolute measure of CBF, it is a noninvasive technique that provides information about blood flow velocity through the carotid vessels. A carotid duplex study is a routine screening procedure for intraluminal narrowing of the common and internal carotid arteries, often due to atherosclerotic plaques. A Doppler probe is placed externally over the vessel, high-frequency sound waves (ultrasound) are generated, and blood flow velocities are calculated. As the diameter of the vessel changes, the velocity of blood flow through the vessel changes; the higher the flow velocity, the narrower the vessel. Carotid duplex studies are noninvasive, painless, quick, and can be performed at the bedside. When changes in flow velocities are identified on ultrasonography, which may indicate significant occlusion of the vessel, CT angiography has been used, often as an alternative to MRA, to verify the degree of severity of the narrowed vessel, depict the length of the stenotic segment, or evaluate the degree of plaque ulceration. This severe complication can lead to intraplaque hemorrhage.[48]

Emission Tomography Studies

The following discussion focuses on two nuclear medicine studies that may be used to evaluate critically ill patients with neurologic dysfunction.

Positive emission tomography. A PET scan is a functional and molecular imaging technique used to study cerebral blood flow (CBF) and glucose metabolism of the brain. It allows for three-dimensional mapping of positron-emitting radiopharmaceuticals administered in minuscule quantities without causing significant physiologic or pharmacologic effects.[49] Oxygen-15 (^{15}O) labeled water is injected into the patient. The PET camera measures the amount of the radiotracer as it flows through the brain, which allows for the measurement of CBF, the fraction of oxygen extracted from the arterial blood by the cerebral tissue, and $CMRO_2$.[50] When the measurement of the oxygen extraction fraction is elevated it can indicate hemodynamic failure and early ischemia.[51] Clinically, a PET scan can show acute occlusion of the middle cerebral artery territory in 76% of cases of stroke within the first 5 hours and perfusion deficits that transcranial Doppler (TCD) failed to show in patients with subarachnoid hemorrhage (SAH) developing delayed cerebral ischemia.[45] The amount of radiation the patient is exposed to is very small. During the procedure, the patient must remain motionless in an enclosed space for 1 to 3 hours, as a movement of more than 1 cm may blur the resulting pictures. Major disadvantages are that a patient must be physiologically stable enough to travel to the location of the scanner and remain stable throughout the scan and that the scan provides an assessment of brain perfusion and CBF only at specific points in time.[51] Other drawbacks are the high cost and the common unavailability of this technique.[45]

Single-photon emission computed tomography. Single-photon emission computed tomography (SPECT) is another nuclear medicine scanning procedure that integrates CT and a radioactive tracer to produce a three-dimensional measurement of regional CBF. This test differs from PET in that tracer stays in the bloodstream rather than being absorbed by surrounding tissue, limiting the images to areas where blood flows. SPECT is less expensive and more readily available than higher-resolution PET.[45] The primary clinical uses of SPECT are to detect cerebrovascular disease, seizures, and tumors.[52]

Electrophysiology Studies

The following discussion focuses on two frequently performed electrophysiology studies used in diagnosing and managing critically ill patients with neurologic dysfunction.

Electroencephalography

EEG records electrical impulses generated by the brain, commonly called *brain waves*. The purpose of EEG is to detect and localize abnormal electrical activity. EEG alterations correlate to CBF reduction in critical care units and surgical settings.[45] This abnormal activity can be defined as *slowing*, which occurs in areas of injury or infarct, or as *spikes* and *waves*, seen in irritated tissue. Indications for using EEG include suspected seizure activity, cerebral infarction, metabolic encephalopathies, altered consciousness, infectious disease, some head injuries, and confirmation of brain death.[53] During an EEG, noninvasive electrodes are placed on the head, and the electrical impulses detected are transferred to a central recording device that records the information in a waveform.

Types of brain waves. Six types of waves or rhythms may be present (Table 21.5). Intermittent slowing with triphasic wave morphology is associated with metabolic encephalopathy. Continuous, generalized slowing in the delta or theta range is associated with anoxic damage. The combination of alpha waves that do not change with stimulation and a coma state is called *alpha coma*, and it is associated with a poor prognosis.[54] Other EEG abnormalities associated with poor prognosis are *burst suppression* (occasional generalized bursts of activity with intervening inactivity or severe voltage depression) and *periodic patterns* (generalized spikes at fixed intervals of one to two per second). The absence of electrical activity on EEG termed *electrocerebral silence* can occur transiently in the period immediately after cardiopulmonary resuscitation, severe hypothermia, and CNS depressant overdose. Enduring electrocerebral silence provides evidence for the clinical determination of brain death.[54]

Limitations. EEG has significant limitations. Only electrical activity involving large areas of the cortex is recorded on EEG. The accuracy of EEG depends on the location of electrophysiologic activity. Abnormal EEG findings are not

TABLE 21.5 Types of Electrical Brain Waves

Wave	Duration	Description
Delta	1–4 cycles/s	Normal; seen in stages 3 and 4 of sleep
Alpha	8–13 cycles/s	Normal; relaxed state with eyes closed; often seen in occipital leads
Theta	4–7 cycles/s	Less common in adults than in children; characteristic of coma in brain injury
Beta	12–40 cycles/s	Fast waves indicating mental or physical activity
Sleep spindles	12–14 cycles/s	Seen in stage 2 sleep, not rapid eye movement
Spike and slow waves	Variable	Seen in irritable brain tissue (e.g., seizure)

cause specific. Similar EEG changes occur with a variety of conditions. The EEG result can be normal even when significant pathology and neurologic impairment is present.[53]

Nursing management. In preparing the patient for an EEG, the noninvasive aspects of this procedure are stressed to the patient. During the procedure, the awake patient may be asked to perform simple physical tasks, such as blinking, closing the eyes, or swallowing, or recordings may be made during sleep.

Evoked Potentials

Evoked potentials are cerebral electrical impulses generated in response to a sensory stimulus. Impulses are recorded as they travel through the brainstem and into the cerebral cortex. Measuring evoked potentials is a sophisticated way of observing the status of sensory pathways as they enter the CNS, travel through the brainstem, and reach the cerebral cortex. Evoked potential studies are used to determine coma prognosis and the extent of brainstem or spinal cord injury in a traumatically injured patient. Evaluation of evoked potentials is valuable during therapeutically induced comas, such as barbiturate coma, since these sensory pathways are unaffected by the depressive activity of such medications. Evoked potentials are monitored intraoperatively during spinal surgery and cerebral tumor dissection to detect the functional integrity of the brain and spinal cord.[53]

Types of tests. The four types of evoked potential tests are (1) visual evoked responses (VERs), (2) brainstem auditory evoked responses (BAERs), (3) somatosensory evoked responses (SSERs), and (4) motor evoked potentials (MEPs). VERs involve monitoring the visual pathways through the brainstem and cortex in response to the patient viewing a shifting geometric pattern on a screen or a flashing light stimulus emitted from a mask placed over the eye.[53] BAERs involve monitoring the auditory pathway through the brainstem and cortex in response to a rhythmic clicking sound sent through earphones placed over the patient's ears. BAERs help assess brainstem integrity in the critical care unit when cranial nerve testing cannot be performed or is inconclusive.[53] SSERs involve monitoring the sensory pathways from the extremities and the intensity and time the signal takes to ascend the spinal cord, go through the brainstem, and deliver information to the cortex. This test is performed by administering a small electrical shock to a nerve root in the periphery, such as the ulnar or radial nerve. SSERs can be used to evaluate cortical functioning after cardiac arrest or head trauma. SSERs also are routinely used during spinal surgery.[53] MEPs assess the functional integrity of descending motor pathways. The motor cortex is stimulated by direct high-voltage electrical stimulation through the scalp or by using a magnetic field to induce an electrical current within the brain. Electrical stimulation is a painful procedure and must be reserved for anesthetized patients. Magnetic coil stimulation is painless.[53]

BEDSIDE MONITORING

Monitoring for secondary brain injury is fundamental to caring for critically ill patients with neurologic dysfunction. By using multiple monitoring techniques, the observer is more likely to determine whether a genuine change in cerebral physiology has occurred and what the most appropriate intervention should be. The following discussion focuses on multimodal techniques to monitor ICP, CPP, brain oxygenation, CBF, cerebral metabolism, and brain function.

Intracranial Pressure Monitoring

Based on clinical or imaging features, ICP monitoring is recommended as a part of protocol-driven care in patients at risk of elevated ICP.[55] In general, indications for ICP monitoring include TBI, intracranial hemorrhage, SAH, hydrocephalus, hepatic failure with encephalopathy, acute ischemic stroke with large infarction, and meningitis.[56] A contraindication for ICP monitoring is coagulopathy.[56] The appropriate threshold for ICP has not been defined.[55] However, the normal range for ICP in adults is generally 5 to 15 mm Hg,[57,58] and the threshold for intracranial hypertension is considered to be greater than 20 to 25 mm Hg.[55] It is recommended that ICP monitoring be used in conjunction with other intracranial monitoring devices to enhance clinical decision-making.[55] The duration of ICP monitoring varies according to the clinical context.[55]

Both noninvasive and invasive methods of monitoring ICP are available. Noninvasive techniques for measuring ICP include TCD, tympanic membrane displacement, optic nerve sheath diameter, CT/MRI, and fundoscopy.[58] Noninvasive techniques do not have complications related to invasive techniques. However, the noninvasive techniques have yet to measure ICP accurately enough to be used as alternatives to invasive measurement.[58]

Types of Intracranial Pressure Monitoring Devices

There are several different invasive methods of ICP monitoring. Depending on the location and type of brain injury and the monitoring technique, ICP monitoring can be undertaken in other intracranial anatomic locations: intraventricular, intraparenchymal, epidural, subdural, and subarachnoid (Fig. 21.15).[58] The most commonly used ICP monitoring devices use the intraventricular and intraparenchymal locations.

Intraventricular catheter monitoring device. The most common method for placement of an intraventricular catheter is a coronal burr hole approach at Kocher point, with the tip of the catheter placed in the third ventricle. Once CSF flow is visualized, the catheter can be transduced to obtain an opening ICP. The mean opening pressure has significant prognostic implications and influences medical management strategies, including the height of the collection chamber.[59] The catheter is then tunneled through the skin, sutured in place, and connected to an external drainage system.[59] The combination of a ventriculostomy with a closed drainage system is also known as an external ventricular drain (EVD). The underlying condition of the patient and the ICP are considered when determining the prescribed level of

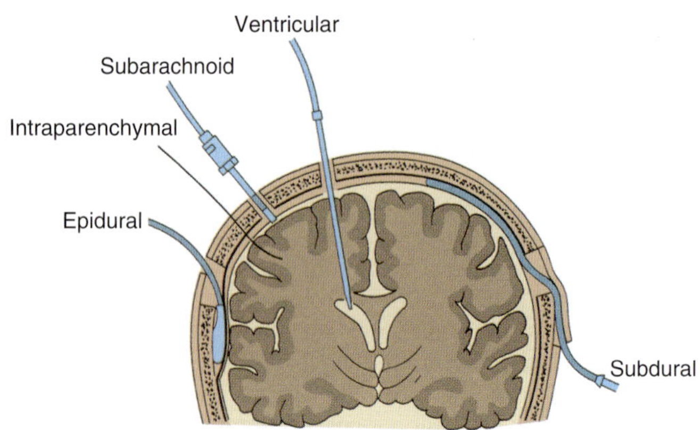

FIG. 21.15 Intracranial Pressure Monitoring Sites. (From Harding MM, Kwong J, Hagler D, Reinisch C, eds. *Lewis's Medical-Surgical Nursing: Assessment and Management of Clinical Problems.* 12th ed. Elsevier; 2023.)

the EVD drainage point. Drainage can be continuous at a set level, fixed volume per desired time, or as needed according to ICP elevations.[59] Drawbacks of ICP monitoring by open EVD include undetected increases in ICP above thresholds and less reliable assessment of cerebrovascular autoregulation.[60] An EVD requires repeated zeroing and leveling so that the pressure transducer is in line with the foramen of Monro (which falls at the level of the external auditory meatus of the ear when the patient is supine). Decreased CSF drainage also requires frequent nursing interventions, as it may lead to dangerously high ICPs and neurologic deterioration.[56]

Complications with this device include inadvertent catheter placement, obstruction and mechanical failure, post-procedural hemorrhage, and ventriculostomy-associated infections.[57,59,61] Imaging guidance systems may improve the likelihood of optimal placement.[61] An antibiotic-impregnated or silver-coated catheter may decrease the risk of infection.[57,58] Nevertheless, further research is needed regarding the ideal method of placement for intracranial monitoring devices, the timing of DVT prophylaxis as it relates to bleeding, and infection prevention.[61]

Intraparenchymal microsensor monitoring device. ICP monitors inserted into brain parenchyma work through fiberoptic, strain gauge, or pneumatic technologies. Fiberoptic devices transmit light via a fiberoptic cable toward a displaceable mirror. Changes in ICP move the mirror, and the differences in intensity of the reflected light are translated to an ICP value.[58] Another parameter that may be measured with the fiberoptic transducer-tipped catheter is brain temperature.[56] With strain gauge device technology, ICP is calculated when the ICP bends the transducer and changes the level of resistance.[58] Pneumatic sensor technology measures ICP by using a small balloon in the distal end of the catheter to register changes in pressure.[58] Pneumatic sensors also allow for quantitative measurement of intracranial compliance.[58]

The catheter can be easily placed via a cranial access device, a burr hole, or during a craniotomy. The device's accuracy depends on the placement relative to the injury site. Intraparenchymal pressure probes placed in the hemisphere contralateral to an intracerebral hematoma may dramatically underestimate ICP.[62] ICP values should be interpreted carefully and in conjunction with clinical and radiological assessments of patients, as episodic events, such as rises in ICP due to coughing or suctioning, may not truly reflect the intracranial volume-buffering reserve, and responding to such events may unnecessarily prolong invasive ICP monitoring.[62] Additional disadvantages of intraparenchymal microsensor devices are that microtransducer systems can encounter drift when used for more than 5 days, in vivo calibration. CSF drainage is impossible, and transducer-tipped catheters are not MRI compatible.[56] An error message or loss of waveform on the ICP monitor may indicate a broken catheter or malposition of the catheter.[56]

Combination intraventricular/fiberoptic catheter. The intraventricular/fiberoptic catheter combines the capability of CSF's EVD with ICP monitoring. This hybrid device can monitor ICP intermittently or continuously and drain CSF intermittently or continuously.[63] There are advantages and disadvantages to using the combination catheter. A disadvantage is that the catheter can be zeroed only before insertion. However, because the transducer is in the tip of the fiberoptic catheter, there is no external strain gauge transducer and no repetitive zeroing and leveling of a transducer with the anatomic reference point for the foramen of Monro.[63] An advantage of the catheter is that it allows for CSF drainage. To prevent underdrainage or overdrainage of CSF, attention must be paid to the level of the reference point of the drip chamber to the anatomic reference point for the foramen of Monro and the setting of the pressure level at the top of the graduated burette (drip chamber).[63] Consequences of CSF underdrainage include headache, neurologic deterioration, hydrocephalus, increased ICP, secondary neuronal injury, herniation, and death.[63] Consequences of CSF overdrainage include headache, subdural hematoma, pneumocephalus, ventricular collapse, herniation, and death.[63]

Intracranial Pressure Waves

ICP waveform analysis provides information that may identify patients with decreased adaptive capacity who are at risk for increases in ICP and decreases in CPP, which may contribute to secondary brain injury and have a negative impact on neurologic outcomes.[64] ICP pulse waveform is observed on a continuous, real-time pressure display, and it corresponds to each heartbeat.[65] The amplitude of the ICP waveform is directly related to craniospinal elasticity.[66] The complex interaction of the arterial input, intracranial contents, and venous outflow determines the shape of the waveform.[67] Although a systolic and diastolic component to the ICP waveform is evident, ICP is read as a mean value.[56]

Normal intracranial pressure waveform. The normal ICP wave has three or more defined peaks (Fig. 21.16). The first peak (P1) is called the *percussion wave*. Originating from the pulsations of the choroid plexus, it has a sharp peak and is relatively constant in its amplitude.[66] The second peak (P2) is called the *tidal wave*. The tidal wave varies in shape and amplitude, ending on the dicrotic notch. The P2 portion of the pulse waveform has been most directly linked to decreased compliance. When the P2 component is equal to or higher than P1, decreased compliance occurs (Fig. 21.17). Immediately after the dicrotic notch is the third wave (P3), called the *dicrotic wave*. After the dicrotic wave, the pressure usually tapers down to the diastolic position unless retrograde venous pulsations add a few more peaks.[67] When ICP increases, the amplitude of the ICP waveform increases. In performing basic checks of whether the ICP signal is truly representative of the ICP, it is essential to ensure that there is

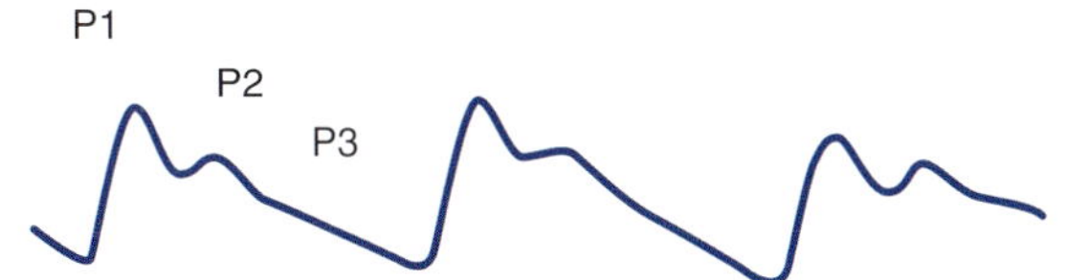

FIG. 21.16 Normal Intracranial Pressure Waveform. (From Bader MK, Littlejohns LR, eds. *AANN Core Curriculum for Neuroscience Nursing*. 4th ed. Mosby; 2004.)

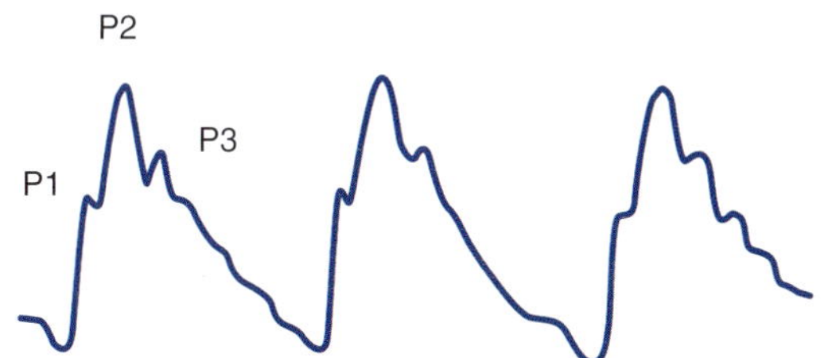

FIG. 21.17 Abnormal Intracranial Pressure Waveform. (From Bader MK, Littlejohns LR, eds. *AANN Core Curriculum for Neuroscience Nursing*. 4th ed. Mosby; 2004.)

an oscillating pressure curve with the progressively decreasing P1, P2, and P3 notches present, indicating propagation of the cardiac pulse pressure signal.[58] Loss of the ICP waveform may indicate blockage, loose system connections, or possibly transducer failure. A numeric value without a corresponding waveform is of no value.[56]

Abnormal intracranial pressure waveforms. A, B, and C pressure waves are not true waveforms (Fig. 21.18). Instead, they are the graphically displayed trend data of ICP over time. These waves reflect spontaneous alterations in ICP associated with respiration, systemic blood pressure, and deteriorating neurologic status.

A waves. Also called *plateau waves* because of their distinctive shape, A waves are the most clinically significant of the three types. They usually occur in an already elevated baseline ICP (>20 mm Hg). They are characterized by sharp increases in ICP of 30 to 69 mm Hg, which plateau for 2 to 20 minutes and then return to baseline. The cause of A waves is unknown, but they may result from vasodilation and increased CBF, decreased venous outflow (and increased cerebral blood volume), fluctuations in arterial partial pressure of carbon dioxide ($PaCO_2$) (and changes in cerebral blood volume), or decreased CSF absorption. Plateau waves indicate decreased intracranial compliance and are considered significant because of the reduced CPP associated with ICP in the 50 to 100 mm Hg range. Transient signs of intracranial hypertension, such as a decreased level of consciousness, bradycardia, pupillary changes, or respiratory changes, may accompany these waves. Sustained increases in ICP associated with plateau waves may be disabling or deadly, leading to brain herniation, cerebral perfusion arrest, and cerebral ischemia.[68]

B waves. B waves are sharp, rhythmic oscillations with a sawtooth appearance that occur every 30 seconds to 2 minutes and can increase the ICP from 5 to 70 mm Hg. B waves often precede A waves. They are a normal physiologic phenomenon that can occur in any patient, but they are amplified in states of low intracranial compliance. B waves appear to reflect fluctuations in cerebral blood volume and suggest low brain compliance.[65]

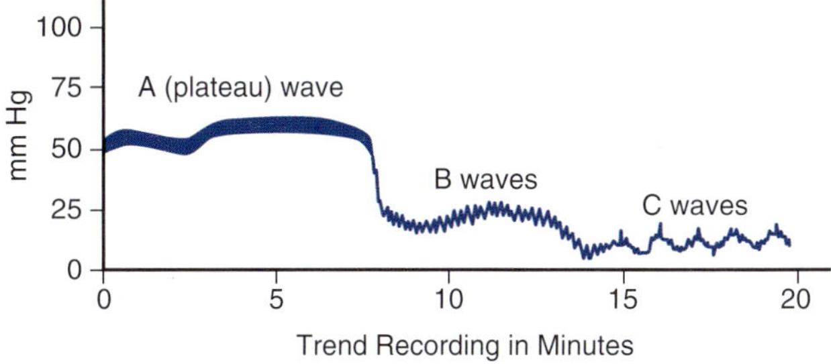

FIG. 21.18 Intracranial Pressure Waves. Composite diagram of A waves (plateau waves), B waves (sawtooth waves), and C waves (small rhythmic waves). (From Barker E: *Neuroscience Nursing: A Spectrum of Care*. 3rd ed. Mosby; 2008.)

C waves. C waves are small, rhythmic waves that occur every 4 to 8 minutes at normal levels of ICP. They are nonpathological and related to normal fluctuations in respiration and systemic arterial pressure.[65]

Pupillometry

Automated infrared pupillometry enables the quantitative assessment of basic fundamental neurologic tests, such as pupillary symmetry and reactivity, using a handheld pupillometer (Fig. 21.19) and the Neurological Pupil index (NPi).[69] The pupillometer is a handheld infrared system that automatically tracks and analyzes pupil dynamics, including fluctuations in size, over 3 seconds, without altering pupil size or movement.[69] A detachable headrest facilitates the correct and consistent placement of the pupillometer in front of the eye. The device has been designed to minimize interobserver variability in the pupillary evaluation.[69] The NPi classifies pupil reactivity using an algorithm. An inverse relationship between decreasing pupil reactivity and increasing ICP has been identified using pupillometry and the NPi.[69] Pupillometry is used to trend increased ICP in patients with TBI, aneurysmal SAH, cerebral infarction, or intracerebral hemorrhage.[69]

Cerebral Perfusion Pressure Monitoring

Measurement of ICP allows for an estimation of CPP. CPP is the driving force responsible for adequate brain perfusion and oxygenation.[66] It is calculated as the difference between the incoming MAP and the opposing ICP on the arteries: CPP = MAP − ICP. CPP is related to CBF and is modifiable through its relationship with MAP and ICP.[57] Following a significant increase in ICP, CPP decreases, resulting in inadequate brain tissue perfusion and oxygenation. The consequent ischemia induces further cytotoxic edema, resulting in an even higher ICP.[66] Adequate CPP provides some protection against secondary ischemia; however, the requisite CPP for each patient is unknown. Evidence-based guidelines, such as the Brain Trauma Foundation Guidelines for the Management of Severe Traumatic Brain Injury, support a CPP range of 60 to 70 mm Hg for adults to promote survival and favorable outcomes.[70] The CPP threshold may vary from patient to patient depending on factors like variation of how the MAP is measured, the patient's disease state, autoregulatory status, and intracranial compliance.[55] Intracranial compliance is defined as a change in ICP in relationship to the change in intracranial volume. Cerebral autoregulation is the intrinsic ability of the cerebral vessels to constrict and dilate as needed to maintain adequate cerebral perfusion.[57] A CPP threshold likely exists individually, and that optimal CPP can be identified by multimodality monitoring.[57]

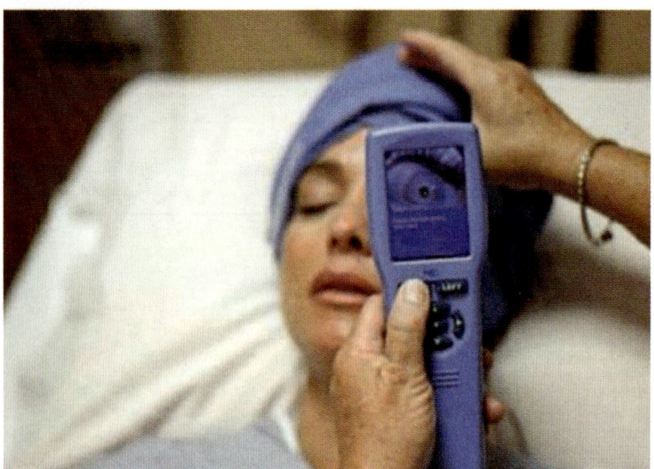

FIG. 21.19 Pupillometer. (Courtesy Neuroptics, Inc.)

Cerebral autoregulation is impaired with brain injury, and the CBF becomes passively dependent on the systemic blood flow. The cerebral blood vessels can no longer react to maintain CPP in response to a change in blood pressure. Continuous bedside monitoring of autoregulatory efficiency is possible through online calculation of derived indices, such as the pressure reactivity index. It may be helpful in broad targeting of cerebral perfusion management goals and prognostication in acute brain injury.[55,57]

Cerebral Blood Flow Monitoring

CBF monitoring provides an understanding of the perfusion status of the brain.[45] Tools used in the clinical and research setting for the assessment of CBF are TCD, transcranial color-coded duplex sonography (TCCS), thermal diffusion flowmetry (TDF), and laser Doppler flowmetry (LDF).

Transcranial Doppler

TCD is an established noninvasive technique for assessing cerebral hemodynamics in real-time. CBF velocity is measured through the skull's cranial windows (thinned areas). Three areas commonly used are (1) the temporal bone (transtemporal), (2) the eye (transorbital), and (3) the foramen magnum (transoccipital). Depending on the angle of the Doppler probe, flow velocities can be measured in the anterior, middle, or posterior cerebral arteries and the vertebral and basilar arteries.[71] Soundwaves emitted by the probe are reflected by the red blood cells moving inside the vessels, and the transducer captures this reflection. The obtained signal is proportional to the velocity of the blood.[45]

The noninvasive technique, speed, and portability of the equipment allow frequent bedside monitoring of flow velocity and vascular diameter. Using serial TCD studies to detect cerebral vasospasm greatly reduces the need for cerebral angiograms and imaging studies to verify and follow post-SAH vasospasm.[71] Additional uses of TCD include the identification of intracranial lesions in a patient with stroke, detection of arteriovenous malformations and venous sinus thrombosis, evaluation of flow-velocity changes during carotid endarterectomy, and detection of reduced CBF and impaired autoregulation associated with increased ICP in patients with TBI.[71,72] There are limitations associated with the use of TCD. Its accuracy is operator dependent. The correct location and angle of the probe are essential. Patient age, female sex, and other factors affecting bone thickness can make exploration through the temporal window difficult or impossible for 10% of patients.[71] Because only the larger basal arteries can be studied with this technique, the values estimate global CBF. Because of the soundwaves' low penetration, it is impossible to examine the artery's diameter. Consequently, the given values are not absolute flow parameters but rather relative speed values.[45] A normal TCD study does not entirely rule out the presence of vasospasm because vasospasm may not be evident in the particular vessel examined. TCD results should always be evaluated with clinical assessment findings and other diagnostic modalities.[71]

Transcranial Color-Coded Duplex Sonography

TCCS is a method of TCD recording that displays a two-dimensional color-coded image of the large cerebral arteries, outlining parenchymal structures and flow directionality information.[72] TCCS can detect narrowing or occlusion of cerebral arteries, screen for vasospasm, and monitor changes in intracranial dynamics.[55] Current recommendations for TCCS include predicting (1) angiographic vasospasm after aneurysmal SAH, (2) delayed ischemic neurologic deficits caused by vasospasm after aneurysmal SAH, and (3) vasospasm after traumatic SAH.[55]

Thermal Diffusion Flowmetry

TDF is an invasive technique that uses thermal clearance to estimate brain perfusion.[45] It allows for the quantitative measurement of regional CBF, an essential upstream monitoring parameter indicative of tissue viability.[45] TDF has also been used to diagnose delayed cerebral ischemia in patients with SAH. For the procedure, a thermal diffusion regional CBF microprobe is placed 20 to 25 mm below the cortical surface via a small burr hole and is secured by tightening a metal bolt.[73] When the microprobe is in place, it is attached to the perfusion monitor cable for calibration.[74] The microprobe includes a heated distal thermistor and a proximal thermistor. The distal thermistor measures blood flow via heat transfer to the capillaries. A microprocessor then converts this information into a measure of CBF in mL per 100 g per minute, representing the K value on the monitor. Generally, mean thermal diffusion regional CBF values range from 18 to 35 mL/100 g per minute.[74]

It is essential to consider that CBF values measured by thermal diffusion regional CBF vary depending on the placement of the probe.[73] Another important consideration with TDF is that the monitor provides CBF parameters only within a temperature range of 25°C to 39.5°C.[74] Therefore, patient cooling should be considered if the brain's temperature is greater than 38.5°C.[74] Another consideration with TDF is that the probe can be viewed on CT or with radiography but is not compatible with MRI. Also, because the TDF monitor does not run on battery power, the probe must be disconnected from the umbilical cord and secured to the patient's head dressing before patient transport. Additionally, if the probe is used with a microdialysis catheter, the two catheters must be separated by 2 mm for accurate results.[74]

Laser Doppler Flowmetry

LDF is an invasive indirect technique that continuously measures red blood cell velocity in the cerebral capillaries, thus real-time microcirculation monitoring.[45,56] It has been used to map microvascular blood flow intraoperatively and to help manage severe TBI and aneurysmal SAH vasospasm.[56] The laser diffusion flowmetry probe is inserted into the brain parenchyma or placed on

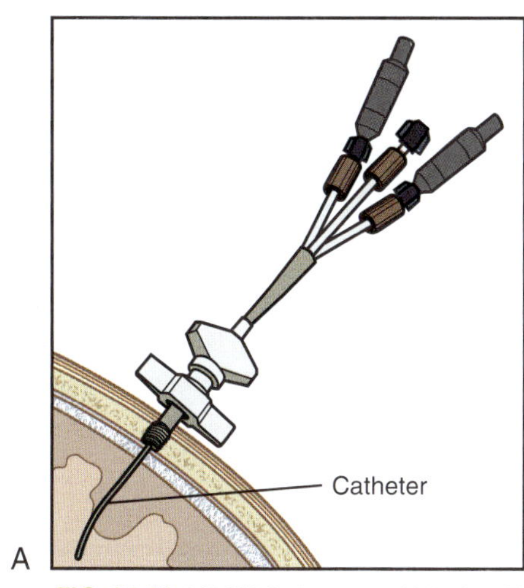

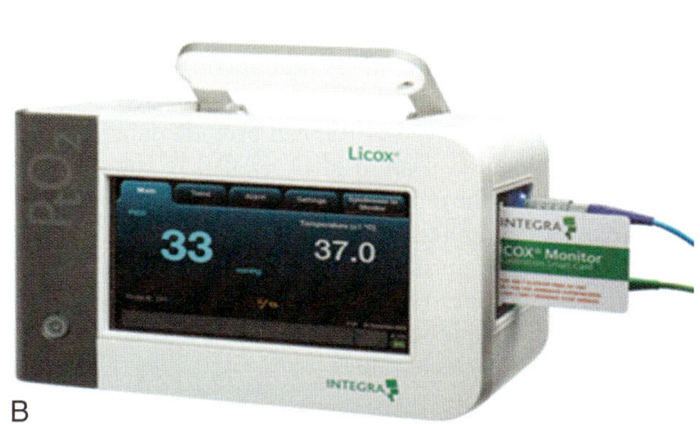

FIG. 21.20 LICOX Catheter and Monitor. The LICOX brain tissue oxygen system involves a catheter inserted through an intracranial bolt (A). The system measures oxygen in the brain, brain tissue temperature, and intracranial pressure (B). (A From Harding MM, Kwong J, Hagler D, Reinisch C, eds. *Lewis's Medical-Surgical Nursing: Assessment and Management of Clinical Problems.* 12th ed. Elsevier; 2023. B Courtesy Integra LifeSciences Corporation, Plainsboro, NJ.)

the cerebral cortex. In contrast to TDF, LDF does not quantify CBF absolutely but provides a measure of relative change in flow. Several limitations affect the usefulness of LDF. The main drawback is that the small volume of the brain wherein the flow is assessed reflects only local microcirculation. Movement artifacts from the patient or the probe can result in inaccurate values. Finally, the CBF is only evaluated by qualitative means.[56]

Cerebral Oxygenation and Metabolic Monitoring

Maintaining adequate brain tissue oxygenation and key brain energy substrates is a critical objective in managing critically ill patients with neurologic disorders. The following methods may be used in the critical care unit to monitor the patient's cerebral oxygenation status and cerebral metabolic state.

Partial Brain Tissue Oxygen Pressure

Monitoring partial brain parenchymal oxygen tension ($PbtO_2$) is a reliable and sensitive diagnostic method to monitor cerebral oxygenation. $PbtO_2$ allows continuous monitoring of regional tissue oxygenation and identifies areas of high ischemic risk.[56,75] The device consists of a monitoring probe on the end of a catheter, which is inserted into the brain parenchyma and attached to a bedside monitor (Fig. 21.20). The probe may be inserted into the damaged portion of the brain to measure regional oxygenation or inserted into the undamaged part of the brain to measure global oxygenation. Placement of the catheter itself causes some microtrauma, and values obtained in that area may not be valid from 30 minutes up to 2 hours after placement.[56]

Normal $PbtO_2$ is estimated to be 23 to 35 mm Hg.[55] A $PbtO_2$ threshold of less than 20 mm Hg represents compromised brain oxygen and is a threshold to consider intervention.[55] $PbtO_2$ values below 20 mm Hg carry a high risk of poor outcomes. In contrast, a $PbtO_2$ of less than 10 mm Hg for more than 30 minutes has a higher risk of unfavorable outcomes and death.[76] Lower $PbtO_2$ values and the longer time spent at the lower $PbtO_2$ levels correlate with poorer outcomes.[45,76] Observational studies suggest a potential benefit when $PbtO_2$-guided therapy is added to a management protocol for severe TBI and SAH.[55,75] However, it is recommended that brain oxygen monitors be used with clinical indicators and other monitoring modalities for accurate prognostication.[55] Drawbacks related to $PbtO_2$ monitoring include the requirement of a brain CT scan to confirm the positioning of the electrode, and typical risks of any invasive brain monitoring system (infections, bleeding, etc.).[45]

Retrograde Jugular Bulb Oxygen Saturation

Oxygen levels in the cerebral venous outflow may inversely correlate with global brain oxygen consumption.[45] Therefore, oxygen saturation in the jugular bulb ($SjvO_2$) may be used for indirect estimation of cerebral oxygen consumption and a bedside measurement of global oxygenation status of the brain.[45,75]

Sampling and measuring $SjvO_2$ intermittently or continuously using fiberoptic oximetry requires the tip of the catheter to be placed retrograde through the internal jugular into the jugular bulb above the level of C2/C3, and placement must be confirmed by skull/neck radiography.[45,75] Normal $SjvO_2$ is 55% to 70%.[56] $SjvO_2$ of less than 50% represents global cerebral ischemia, and $SjvO_2$ of greater than 75% represents an absolute or relative global hyperemia that exceeds the brain's metabolic demand. Both $SjvO_2$ less than 50% and $SjvO_2$ greater than 75% have been associated with unfavorable outcomes.[56] Indications for $SjvO_2$ monitoring include risk for global hypoxia, severe TBI, and aneurysmal SAH.[56]

A limitation of $SjvO_2$ monitoring is that it cannot detect focal ischemia.[75] Also, $SjvO_2$ readings are affected by the position and movement of the patient's head, and the monitoring system requires frequent calibration.[77] Technical difficulties and inaccuracies with $SjvO_2$ monitoring can also include catheter misplacement, contamination with extracerebral blood when the catheter abuts the blood vessel wall, poor sampling technique, and thrombosis occurring around the catheter tip.[55]

Near-Infrared Spectroscopy

Brain oxygenation also can be assessed using transcranial near-infrared spectroscopy (NIRS).[56] A noninvasive monitor of cerebral oxygenation, NIRS quantifies the relative concentrations of oxygenated and deoxygenated hemoglobin through reliance on the transmission and absorption of near-infrared light as it passes through tissue.[57] NIRS has many potential advantages over other monitoring techniques. It is a noninvasive technique, has high temporal and spatial resolution, and provides simultaneous measurements over multiple regions of interest.[57] Algorithms based on multiple detectors (spatially resolved NIRS) can provide data that give a value of the regional saturation of O_2 (rSO_2).[45] The main shortcomings of NIRS are the unknown contribution to the signal from extracranial tissues, and the given values are relative. In the critical care unit setting, scalp and facial traumas may prevent the application of the optodes (sensors placed on various positions on the scalp), and brain lesions, like intraparenchymal hematomas, may lead to unpredictable values.[45]

Cerebral Microdialysis

Cerebral microdialysis is a tool for investigating the metabolic status of the injured brain at the bedside.[3] A catheter with a 10-mm semipermeable distal membrane is inserted into the brain parenchyma (ideally placed in the frontal lobe) via a twist drill hole or transcranial bolt.[3,74,78] Here, substances in the extracellular fluid surround the semipermeable membrane at the tip of the catheter. Following diffusion, the dialysate can then be analyzed hourly for glucose, lactate, and pyruvate (as indicators of hypoxia and ischemia) and interstitial glycerol (as an indicator of lipolysis or cell damage) to detect neurochemical changes indicative of primary and secondary brain injury.[3,79] The ratio of lactate to pyruvate, a product of glucose metabolism, is becoming more clinically significant than looking only at lactate, as an increasing ratio can indicate worsening brain injury.[78] Monitoring cerebral microdialysis is recommended in patients with TBI or SAH who are at risk for cerebral ischemia, hypoxia, energy failure, and glucose deprivation.[55,78]

Continuous Electroencephalography Monitoring

Continuous EEG (cEEG) has the advantage of being noninvasive and has the potential to detect alterations in brain physiology at a reversible stage, which may trigger treatment before permanent brain injury occurs.[3,80] The main applications of cEEG are diagnosing nonconvulsive status epilepticus, monitoring and guiding the treatment of status epilepticus, and detecting delayed cerebral ischemia from vasospasm in SAH patients.[3] In 10% to 20% of comatose patients with poor-grade SAH, nonconvulsive seizures may be detected on continuous EEG.[81] However, while many epileptic abnormalities can be captured using short-term recording, c-EEG for 24 hours or more can detect the severity of epileptiform activity and should be considered in patients who fail to improve neurologically or have neurologic deterioration of undetermined etiology.[80,81] Clinically unrecognized electrographic seizures and periodic epileptiform discharges are often frequent and associated with poor outcomes in patients with severe brain injury from different etiologies, including TBI, ischemic and hemorrhagic strokes, and CNS infection.[3] EEG sensitivity to ischemia allows its use in situations where cerebral perfusion is at risk. Changes over time can trigger focused neurologic examination, imaging studies, and early treatment.[3]

There are several challenges related to cEEG implementation, including the requirement for continuous access to technicians and neurophysiologists for preparation and interpretation and difficulties in data storage.[82] Other drawbacks to using cEEG are that it is expensive, labor intensive, and subject to artifact from the critical care unit environment.[80,82] More recently, EEG training courses have improved the accuracy of quantitative EEG reading by general intensivists.[83] Also, the development of spectral analysis (quantitative EEG) and software enabling artifact elimination have made cEEG use in the critical care unit more practical and reliable.

BOX 21.5 Internet Resources

Neurologic Clinical Assessment and Diagnostic Procedures

- American Academy of Neurology: www.aan.com
- American Association of Critical-Care Nurses: www.aacn.org
- American Association of Neurological Surgeons: www.aans.org
- American Association of Neuroscience Nurses: www.aann.org
- American College of Physicians: www.acponline.org
- American College of Surgeons: www.facs.org
- American Medical Association: www.ama-assn.org
- American Stroke Association: www.stroke.org
- National Institutes of Health: www.nih.gov
- Society for Critical Care Medicine: www.sccm.org
- Society for Neuroscience: www.sfn.org

ADDITIONAL RESOURCES

See Box 21.5 for Internet resources pertaining to neurologic assessment and diagnostic procedures.

KEY POINTS

History

- A neurologic history includes information about clinical manifestations, associated complaints, precipitating factors, progression of symptoms, familial occurrences, and events preceding the onset of symptoms.
- If the patient's condition permits, additional information is gathered regarding the patient's personal and social status, general health status, and family history.

Focused Physical Assessment

- The five major components of a neurologic examination are the evaluation of (1) level of consciousness, (2) motor function, (3) pupillary function, (4) respiratory function, and (5) vital signs.
- Assessment of the level of consciousness focuses on evaluating arousal and appraisal of awareness.
- Assessment of motor function focuses on the evaluation of muscle size and tone and the estimation of muscle strength.
- Assessment of pupillary function focuses on the estimation of pupil size and shape, evaluation of pupillary reaction to light, and appraisal of eye movements.
- Assessment of respiratory functions focuses on the observation of respiratory patterns and evaluation of airway status.
- Assessment of vital signs focuses on evaluating blood pressure and observing heart rate.
- Increasing ICP can be identified by changes in the level of consciousness, pupillary reaction, motor response, vital signs, and respiratory patterns.

Diagnostic Procedures

- Radiologic procedures are often performed to identify abnormalities of the brain, spinal cord, and surrounding bone and tissue. These tests include skull and spine radiography, CT, MRI, cerebral angiography, and myelography.
- Imaging of CBF and metabolism can help define the cause and extent of brain injury, identify appropriate treatments, and predict the outcome. These tests include CTP, Xe-CT, PW-MRI, carotid duplex sonography, PET, and SPECT.
- Electrophysiology studies are often performed to evaluate the electrical impulses of the brain. These tests include EEG, VERs, BAERs, SSERs, and MEPs.

Laboratory Studies

- CSF analysis is performed, by LP or ventriculostomy placement, to look for the presence of blood or infection in the subarachnoid space.

Bedside Monitoring

- ICP monitoring is used in patients with suspected intracranial hypertension. Measurement of ICP allows for an estimation of CPP, which is the blood pressure gradient across the brain. ICP and CPP monitoring are recommended as a part of protocol-driven care and should be used in conjunction with other intracranial monitors to guide medical and surgical interventions and detect life-threatening imminent herniation.
- CBF monitoring is essential in neurologic care because the brain depends on continuous blood flow to supply glucose and oxygen. TCD, TCCS, TDF, and LDF are techniques to monitor CBF.
- Brain oxygenation and metabolism measurements provide insight into understanding acute brain injury and ways to manage secondary brain injury. Techniques to monitor brain oxygenation, metabolism, or both include $PbtO_2$, $SjvO_2$, NIRS, and cerebral microdialysis.
- The primary applications of cEEG are diagnosing nonconvulsive status epilepticus, monitoring and guiding, the treatment of status epilepticus, and detecting delayed cerebral ischemia from vasospasm in SAH patients.

Visit the Evolve site at http://evolve.elsevier.com/Urden/CriticalCareNursing for additional study materials.

REFERENCES

1. Sheetz LJ, Horst MA, Arbour RB. Early neurological deterioration in older adults with traumatic brain injury. *Int Emerg Nurs*. 2018;37:29–34. https://doi.org/10.1016/j.ienj.2016.11.003.
2. Jankovic J, Mazziotta JC, Newman NJ, et al. Diagnosis of neurological disease. In: Jankovic J, Mazziotta JC, Pomeroy SC, et al., eds. *Bradley and Daroff's Neurology in Clinical Practice*. 8th ed. Philadelphia: Elsevier; 2022.
3. Chamberlain D, Kuzmiuk L. Neurological assessment and monitoring. In: Aitken L, Marshall A, Chaboyer W, eds. *ACCCN's Critical Care Nursing*. 4th ed. St. Louis: Elsevier; 2019.
4. Barker E. The adult neurologic assessment. In: Barker E, ed. *Neuroscience Nursing: A Spectrum of Care*. 3rd ed. St. Louis: Mosby; 2008.
5. Cavanna AE, Shah S, Eddy CM, et al. Consciousness: a neurological perspective. *Behav Neurol*. 2011;24:107–116. https://doi.org/10.3233/BEN-2011-0322.
6. Teasdale G, Jennett B. Assessment of coma and impaired consciousness—a practical scale. *Lancet*. 1974;2(7872):81–84. https://doi.org/10.1016/s0140-6736(74)91639-0.
7. Le Roux P, Menon DK, Citerio G, et al. Consensus summary statement of the international multidisciplinary consensus conference on multimodality monitoring in neurocritical care: a statement for healthcare professionals from the neurocritical care society and the European society of intensive care medicine. *Neurocrit Care*. 2014;21(suppl 2):1–26. https://doi.org/10.1007/s12028-014-0041-5.
8. Khanal K, Bhandari SS, Shrestha N, et al. Comparison of outcome predictions by the Glasgow Coma Scale and the Full Outline of UnResponsiveness score in the neurological and neurosurgical patients in the intensive care unit. *Indian J Crit Care Med*. 2016;20(8):473–476. https://doi.org/10.4103/0972-5229.188199.
9. Kornbluth J, Bhardwaj A. Evaluation of coma: a critical appraisal of popular scoring systems. *Neurocrit Care*. 2011;14(1):134–143. https://doi.org/10.1007/s12028-010-9409-3.
10. Berger JR, Price R. Stupor and coma. In: Jankovic J, Mazziotta JC, Pomeroy SC, et al., eds. *Bradley and Daroff's Neurology in Clinical Practice*. 8th ed. Philadelphia: Elsevier; 2022.
11. Iyer VN. Validity of the FOUR Score Coma Scale in the medical intensive care unit. *Mayo Clin Proc*. 2009;84(8):694–701. https://doi.org/10.4065/84.8.694.
12. Musculoskeletal system. In: Ball JW, Dains JE, Flynn JA, et al., eds. *Seidel's Guide to Physical Examination: An Interprofessional Approach*. 10th ed. St. Louis: Elsevier; 2023.
13. Neurologic system. In: Ball JW, Dains JE, Flynn JA, et al., eds. *Seidel's Guide to Physical Examination: An Interprofessional Approach*. 10th ed. St. Louis: Elsevier; 2023.
14. McGee S. Examination of the motor system: approach to weakness. In: McGee S, ed. *Evidence-Based Physical Diagnosis*. 5th ed. Philadelphia: Elsevier; 2022.
15. Rucker JC, Lavin PJM. Neuro-ophthalmology: ocular motor system. In: Jankovic J, Mazziotta JC, Pomeroy SC, et al., eds. *Bradley and Daroff's Neurology in Clinical Practice*. 8th ed. Philadelphia: Elsevier; 2022.
16. Adoni A, McNett M. The pupillary response in traumatic brain injury: a guide for trauma nurses. *J Trauma Nurs*. 2007;14(4):191–196. https://doi.org/10.1097/01.jtn.0000318921.90627.fe.
17. Bouffard MA. The pupil. *Continuum (Minneap Minn)*. 2019;25(5):1194–1214. https://doi.org/10.1212/CON.0000000000000771.
18. Yoo H D, Mihalia DM. Neuroanatomy, pupillary light reflexes and pathway. In: *StatPearls. NCBI Bookshelf Version*. StatPearls Publishing; 2022. https://www.ncbi.nlm.nih.gov/books/NBK553169/. Accessed August 11, 2023.
19. Morgan B. Oculomotor nerve (cranial nerve III). Critical Care Trauma Centre. Updated April 12, 2022. Accessed August 11, 2023. https://www.lhsc.on.ca/critical-care-trauma-centre/oculomotor-nerve-cranial-nerve-iii.
20. Marehbian J, Muehlschlegel S, Edlow BL, et al. Medical management of the severe traumatic brain injury patient. *Neurocrit Care*. 2017;27(3):430–446. https://doi.org/10.1007/s12028-017-0408-5.
21. Robinson CP. Moderate and severe traumatic brain injury. *Continuum (Minneap Minn)*. 2021;27(5):1278–1300. https://doi.org/10.1212/CON.0000000000001036.
22. Kahraman S, Dutton RP, Hu P, et al. Heart rate and pulse pressure variability are associated with intractable intracranial hypertension after severe traumatic brain injury. *J Neurosurg Anesthesiol*. 2010;22(4):296–302. https://doi.org/10.1097/ANA.0b013e3181e25fc3.
23. Silvani A, Calandra-Buonaura G, Dampney RA, et al. Brain-heart interactions: physiology and clinical implications. *Philos Trans A Math Phys Eng Sci*. 2016;374(2067). https://doi.org/10.1098/rsta.2015.0181.
24. Keller C, Williams A. Cardiac dysrhythmias associated with central nervous system dysfunction. *J Neurosci Nurs*. 1993;25(6):349–355. https://doi.org/10.1097/01376517-199312000-00005.
25. Dinallo S, Waseem M. Cushing reflex. In: *StatPearls. NCBI Bookshelf Version*. StatPearls Publishing; 2023. https://www.ncbi.nlm.nih.gov/books/NBK549801/. Accessed August 11, 2023.

26. Marcoline E, Stretz C, DeWitt KM. Intracranial hemorrhage and intracranial hypertension. *Emeg Med Clin North Am*. 2019;37(3):529–544. https://doi.org/10.1016/j.emc.2019.04.001.
27. Engelborghs S, Niemantsverdriet E, Stuyfs H, et al. Consensus guidelines for lumbar puncture in patients with neurological diseases. *Alzheimers Dement (Amst)*. 2017;8:111–126. https://doi.org/10.1016/j.dadm.2017.04.007.
28. Euerle BD. Spinal puncture and cerebrospinal fluid examination. In: Roberts JR, ed. *Roberts and Hedges' Clinical Procedures in Emergency Medicine and Acute Care*. 7th ed. Philadelphia: Elsevier; 2019.
29. Van Thielen T, van den Hauwe L, Van Goethem JW, et al. Current status of imaging of the spine and anatomical features. In: Adam A, Dixon AK, Gillard JH, et al., eds. *Grainger & Allison's Diagnostic Radiology: A Textbook of Medical Imaging*. London: Elsevier Churchill Livingstone; 2021.
30. Cogbill TH, Ziegelbein KJ. Computed tomography, magnetic resonance, and ultrasound imaging: basic principles, glossary of terms, and patient safety. *Surg Clin North Am*. 2011;91(1):1–14. https://doi.org/10.1016/j.suc.2010.10.006.
31. Masdeu JC, Ajtai B, Faridar A. Structural imaging using magnetic resonance imaging and computed tomography. In: Jankovic J, Mazziotta JC, Pomeroy SC, et al., eds. *Bradley and Daroff's Neurology in Clinical Practice*. ed 8. Philadelphia: Elsevier; 2022.
32. Gigliotti M, Simon S. Cerebralvascular imaging. American Association of Neurological Surgeons. Accessed August 12, 2023. https://www.aans.org/Patients/Neurosurgical-Conditions-and-Treatments/Cerebrovascular-Imaging.
33. Rawson JV, Pelletier AL. When to order a contrast-enhanced CT. *Am Fam Physician*. 2013;88(5):312–316.
34. Zhang F, Lu Z, Wang F. Advances in the pathogenesis and prevention of contrast-induced nephropathy. *Life Sci*. 2020;259:118379. https://doi.org/10.1016/j.lfs.2020.118379.
35. McInnis LA, Parsons, Krau SD. Angiography: from a patient's perspective. *Crit Care Nurs Clin North Am*. 2010;22(1):51–60. https://doi.org/10.1016/j.ccell.2009.10.007.
36. Zuckerman SL, Bhatia R, Tsujiara C, et al. Prospective series of two hours supine rest after 4fr sheath-based diagnostic cerebral angiography: outcomes, productivity and cost. *Interv Neuroradiol*. 2015;21(1):114–119. https://doi.org/10.15274/INR-2014-10102.
37. Rindler RS, Allen JW, Barrow JW, et al. Neuroimaging of intracerebral hemorrhage. *Neurosurgery*. 2020;86(5):E414–E423. https://doi.org/10.1093/neuros/nyaa029.
38. *National Imaging Associates: 2023 Magellan Clinical Guidelines For Medical Necessity Review: Advanced Imaging Guidelines*. Maryland Heights: Magellan Healthcare; 2022. https://www1.radmd.com/media/1014041/2023-magellan-advanced-imaging-guidelines.pdf. Accessed August 12, 2023.
39. Price DB, Ortiz AO. Myelography from lipid-based to gadolinium-based contrast agents. *Magnetic resonance imaging clinics*. 2017;25(4):713–724. https://doi.org/10.1016/j.mric.2017.06.005.
40. Kim N, Durduran T, Frangos S, et al. Noninvasive measurement of cerebral blood flow and blood oxygenation using near-infrared and diffuse correlation spectroscopies in critically brain-injured adults. *Neurocrit Care*. 2010;12(2):173–180. https://doi.org/10.1007/s12028-009-9305-x.
41. Fantini S, Sassaroli A, Tgavalekos KT, et al. Cerebral blood flow and autoregulation: current measurement techniques and prospects for noninvasive optical methods. *Neurophotonics*. 2016;3(3):1–33. https://doi.org/10.1117/1.NPh.3.3.031411.
42. von Kummer R, Dzialowski I. Imaging of cerebral ischemic edema and neuronal death. *Neuroradiology*. 2017;59(6):545–553. https://doi.org/10.1007/s00234-017-1847-6.
43. Grüne F, Klimek M. Cerebral blood flow and its autoregulation – when will there be some light in the black box? *Br J Anaesth*. 2017;119(6):1077–1079. https://doi.org/10.1093/bja/aex355.
44. Lin W, Powers WJ. Oxygen metabolism in acute ischemic stroke. *J Cereb Blood Flow Metab*. 2018;38(9):1481–1499. https://doi.org/10.1177/0271678X17722095.
45. Rasulo F, Matta B, Varanini N. Cerebral blood flow monitoring. In: Prabhakar H, ed. *Neuromonitoring Techniques: Quick Guide for Clinicians and Residents*. London: Academic Press; 2018.
46. Moradi S, Ferdinando H, Zienkiewicz A, et al. Measurement of cerebral circulation in human. In: Scerrati A, Ricciardi L, Dones F, eds. *Cerebral Circulation-Updates on Models, Diagnostics and Treatments of Related Diseases*. London: IntechOpen; 2022. https://doi.org/10.5772/intechopen.102383. Accessed August 12, 2023.
47. Tong E, Sugrue L, Wintermark M. Understanding the neurophysiology and quantification of brain perfusion. *Top Mag Reson Imaging*. 2017;26(2):57–65. https://doi.org/10.1097/RMR.0000000000000128.
48. Adamczyk P, Liebeskind DS. Vascular imaging: computed tomographic angiography, magnetic resonance angiography, and ultrasound. In: Jankovic J, Mazziotta JC, Pomeroy SC, et al., eds. *Bradley and Daroff's Neurology in Clinical Practice*. 8th ed. Philadelphia: Elsevier; 2022.
49. Lameka K, Farwell MD, Ichise M. Positron emission tomography. *Handb Clin Neurol*. 2016;135:209–227. https://doi.org/10.1016/B978-0-444-53485-9.00011-8.
50. Herholz K, Teipel S, Hellwig S, et al. Functional and molecular neuroimaging. In: Jankovic J, Mazziotta JC, Pomeroy SC, et al., eds. *Bradley and Daroff's Neurology In Clinical Practice*. 8th ed. Philadelphia: Elsevier; 2022.
51. Rabinstein A, Braksick SA. Neurointensive care. In: Jankovic J, Mazziotta JC, Pomeroy SC, et al., eds. *Bradley and Daroff's Neurology in Clinical Practice*. 8th ed. Philadelphia: Elsevier; 2022.
52. Wang D, Gilmore D, Zukotynski K. Central nervous system. In: Gilmore D, Waterstram-Rich KM, eds. *Nuclear Medicine and Molecular Imaging*. 9th ed. St. Louis: Elsevier; 2023.
53. Hahn CD, Emercon RG. Electroencephalography and evoked potentials. In: Jankovic J, Mazziotta JC, Pomeroy SC, et al., eds. *Bradley and Daroff's Neurology in Clinical Practice*. 8th ed. Philadelphia: Elsevier; 2022.
54. Walter U, Fernández-Torre JL, Kirschstein T, et al. When is "brainstem death" brain death? The case for ancillary testing in primary infratentorial brain lesion. *Clin Neurophysiol*. 2018;129(11):2451–2465. https://doi.org/10.1016/j.clinph.2018.08.009.
55. Le Roux P, Menon DK, Citerio G, et al. Consensus summary statement of the international multidisciplinary consensus conference on multimodality monitoring in neurocritical care: a statement for healthcare professionals from the neurocritical care society and the European society of intensive care medicine. *Neurocrit Care*. 2014;21(suppl 2):S1–S26. https://doi.org/10.1007/s12028-014-0081-x.
56. Blisset PA. Hemodynamic and intracranial dynamic monitoring in neurocritical care. In: Lough ME, ed. *Hemodynamic Monitoring: Evolving Technologies and Clinical Practice*. St. Louis: Elsevier; 2016.
57. Kirkman MA, Smith M. Intracranial pressure monitoring, cerebral perfusion pressure estimation, and ICP/CPP-guided therapy: a standard of care or optional extra after brain injury? *Br J Anesth*. 2014;112(1):3–46. https://doi.org/10.1093/bja/aet418.
58. Raboel PH, Barteck J, Andresen BBM. Intracranial pressure monitoring: invasive versus non-invasive methods—a review. *Crit Care Res Pract*. 2012;2012:950393. https://doi.org/10.1155/2012/950393.
59. Muralidharan R. External ventricular drains: management and complications. *Surg Neurol Int*. 2015;6(suppl 6):6S271–S274. https://doi.org/10.4103/2152-7806.157620.
60. Hockel K, Schuhmann MU. ICP monitoring by open extraventricular drainage: common practice but not suitable for advanced neuromonitoring and prone to false negativity. *Acta Neurochir Suppl*. 2018;126:281–286. https://doi.org/10.1007/978-3-319-65798-1_55.
61. Tavakoli S, Peitz G, Ares W, et al. Complications of invasive intracranial pressure monitoring devices in neurocritical care. *Neurosurg Focus*. 2017;43(5):1–9. https://doi.org/10.3171/2017.8.FOCUS17450.
62. Lavinio A, Menon DK. Intracranial pressure: why we monitor it, how to monitor it, what to do with the number and what's the future? *Curr Opin Anaesthesiol*. 2011;24(2):117–123. https://doi.org/10.1097/ACO.0b013e32834458c5.

63. Rogers MS. Intracranial pressure monitoring, nursing care, troubleshooting, and removal. In: Johnson KL, ed. *AACN Procedure Manual for Critical Care*. 8th ed. St. Louis: Elsevier; 2024.
64. Lavinio A, Menon DK. Intracranial pressure: why we monitor it, how to monitor it, what to do with the number and what's the future? *Curr Opin Anaesthesiol*. 2011;24(2):117–123. https://doi.org/10.1097/ACO.0b013e32834458c5.
65. Elwishi M, Dinsmore J. Monitoring the brain. *BJA Education*. 2019;19(2):54–59. https://doi.org/10.1016/j.bjae.2018.12.001.
66. Rabba C. Intracranial pressure monitoring. In: Prabhakar H, ed. *Neuromonitoring Techniques: Quick Guide for Clinicians and Residents*. London: Academic Press; 2018.
67. Kirkness CJ, Mitchell PH, Burr RL, et al. Intracranial pressure waveform analysis: clinical and research implications. *J Neurosci Nurs*. 2000;32(5):271–277.
68. Rosengart AJ, Park SM, Segal AZ, et al. Recognition and management of intracranial hypertension. *J Neurocrit Care*. 2008;1:87–100.
69. Lussier BL, Olson DM, Aiyagari V. Automated pupillometry in neurocritical care: research and practice. *Curr Neurol Neurosci Rep*. 2019;19(10):71. https://doi.org/10.1007/s11910-019-0994-z.
70. Carney N, Totten AM, O'Reilly C, et al. *Guidelines for the Management of severe traumatic brain injury. 17. Cerebral perfusion thresholds.* Brain trauma foundation 2016. *Neurosurgery*. 2017;80(1):6–15. https://braintrauma.org/uploads/03/12/Guidelines_for_Management_of_Severe_TBI_4th_Edition.pdf. Accessed August 12, 2023.
71. Bouzat P, Oddo M, Payen JF. Transcranial Doppler after traumatic brain injury: is there a role? *Curr Opin Crit Care*. 2014;20(2):153–160. https://doi.org/10.1097/MCC.0000000000000071.
72. Marshall SA, Nyquist P, Ziai WC. The role of transcranial Doppler ultrasonography in the diagnosis and management of vasospasm after aneurysmal subarachnoid hemorrhage. *Neurosurg Clin N Am*. 2010;21(2):291–303. https://doi.org/10.1016/j.nec.2009.10.010.
73. Vajkoczy P, Schomacher M, Czabanka M, et al. Monitoring cerebral blood flow in neurosurgical intensive care. *US Neurological Disease*. 2007;7:19–22.
74. Cecil S, Chen PM, Callaway SE. Traumatic brain injury: advanced multimodal neuromonitoring from theory to clinical practice. *Crit Care Nurse*. 2011;31(2):25–36. https://doi.org/10.4037/ccn2010226.
75. Oddo M, Bösel J, Participants in the International Multidisciplinary Consensus Conference on Multimodality Monitoring. Monitoring of brain and systemic oxygenation in neurocritical care patients. *Neurocrit Care*. 2014;21:103–120. https://doi.org/10.1007/s12028-014-0024-6.
76. Hirschi R, Hawryluk GWJ, Nielson JL, et al. Analysis of high-frequency $PbtO_2$ measures in traumatic brain injury: insights into the treatment threshold. *J Neurosurg*. 2018:1–11. https://doi.org/10.3171/2018.4.JNS172604.
77. Rasulo F, Matta B, Varanini N. Cerebral blood flow monitoring. In: Prabhakar H, ed. *Neuromonitoring Techniques: Quick Guide for Clinicians and Residents*. London: Academic Press; 2018.
78. McLawhorn M, James ML. Brain microdialysis. In: Prabhakar H, ed. *Neuromonitoring Techniques: Quick Guide for Clinicians and Residents*. London: Academic Press; 2018.
79. Barazangi N, Hemphill IIIJC. Advanced cerebral monitoring in neurocritical care. *Neurol India*. 2008;56(4):405–414. https://doi.org/10.4103/0028-3886.44628.
80. Vulliemoz S, Perrig S, Pellise D, et al. Imaging compatible electrodes for continuous electroencephalogram monitoring in the intensive care unit. *J Clin Neurophysiol*. 2009;26(4):236–243. https://doi.org/10.1097/WNP.0b013e3181af1c95.
81. Diringer MN, Bleck TP, Claude Hemphill J, et al. Critical care management of patients following aneurysmal subarachnoid hemorrhage: recommendations from the Neurocritical Care Society's multidisciplinary consensus conference. *Neurocrit Care*. 2011;15(2):211–240. https://doi.org/10.1007/s12028-011-9605-9. Available from:.
82. Kubota Y, Nakamoto H, Egawa S, et al. Continuous EEG monitoring in ICU. *J Intensive Care*. 2018;6:39. https://doi.org/10.1186/s40560-018-0310-z.
83. Abid S, Papin G, Vellieus G, et al. A simplified electroencephalography montage and interpretation for evaluation of comatose patients in the ICU. *Crit Care Explor*. 2022;4(11):e0781. https://doi.org/10.1097/CCE.0000000000000781.

22

Neurologic Disorders and Therapeutic Management

Allison M. Lang

http://evolve.elsevier.com/Urden/CriticalCareNursing

To accurately anticipate and plan nursing interventions for patients with neurologic disorders, the critical care nurse must understand the disease pathology, determine the areas of focused assessment, and be well acquainted with the medical management of the patient. Despite a wide array of neurologic disorders, only a few disorders routinely require care in the critical care environment.

STROKE

Stroke is a descriptive term for the sudden onset of acute neurologic deficit persisting for more than 24 hours and caused by the interruption of blood flow to the brain. Stroke is the fifth leading cause of death in the United States, preceded by heart disease, cancer, COVID-19, and accidental injury. Each year, approximately 795,000 people have a stroke; 610,000 strokes annually are first attacks, and 185,000 are recurrent attacks.[1,2]

Strokes are classified as ischemic and hemorrhagic. Hemorrhagic strokes can be categorized as subarachnoid hemorrhages (SAHs) and intracerebral hemorrhages (ICHs). Approximately 87% of all strokes are ischemic, 10% are ICHs, and 3% are SAHs.[1] Although less common, hemorrhagic strokes (ICHs and SAHs) have a higher mortality rate than ischemic strokes.[1] Between 2018 and 2019, the annual cost for care and loss of productivity was estimated to be $56.5 billion.[1]

The national concern for the incidence and effects of stroke is illustrated by the inclusion of emergent stroke care in the American Heart Association guidelines for basic and advanced life support. Major public education programs, stroke appraisal screening programs, the development of stroke centers, and algorithms for stroke management are based on the success these approaches have had with coronary artery disease.

Ischemic Stroke

Description and Etiology

Ischemic stroke results from interruption of blood flow to the brain, accounting for 87% of strokes.[1] The interruption can be the result of a thrombotic or embolic event. Thrombosis can form in large vessels (large-vessel thrombotic strokes) or small vessels (small-vessel thrombotic strokes). Embolic sources include the heart (cardioembolic strokes) and atherosclerotic plaques in larger vessels (atheroembolic strokes). In 25% of the cases, the underlying cause of the stroke is unknown (cryptogenic strokes).[3] Fig. 22.1 summarizes the key concepts for managing a patient with an ischemic stroke.

Etiology. Strokes are preventable. Most thrombotic strokes result from the accumulation of atherosclerotic plaque in the vessel lumen, especially at the bifurcations or curves of the vessel. The pathogenesis of cerebrovascular disease is identical to the pathogenesis of coronary vasculature. The most significant risk factor for ischemic stroke is hypertension.[4] Other risk factors are dyslipidemia, diabetes, smoking, and carotid atherosclerotic disease.[1] Common sites of atherosclerotic plaque are the bifurcation of the common carotid artery, the origins of the middle and anterior cerebral arteries, and the origins of the vertebral arteries.[4] Ischemic strokes resulting from vertebral artery dissection have been reported after chiropractic manipulation of the cervical spine.[5]

An embolic stroke occurs when an embolus from the heart or lower circulation travels distally and lodges in a small vessel, obstructing the blood supply. At least 20% of ischemic strokes are attributed to a cardioembolic phenomenon.[4] The most common cause of cardiac emboli is atrial fibrillation. It is responsible for approximately 50% of all cardiac emboli.[6] Other cardiac emboli sources are mitral stenosis, mechanical valves, atrial myxoma, endocarditis, and recent myocardial infarction.[6] Researchers hypothesize that a patent foramen ovale or atrial septal aneurysm may cause a cryptogenic stroke.[3]

Pathophysiology

Ischemic stroke is a cerebral hemodynamic insult. Ischemic injury occurs when cerebral blood flow (CBF) is insufficient to maintain neuronal viability. In focal stroke, an area of hypoperfused tissue, the ischemic penumbra, surrounds a core of ischemic cells. The ischemic penumbra can be salvaged with the return of blood flow. However, sustained anoxic insult initiates a chain of biochemical events leading to apoptosis or cellular death.[7]

The phenomenon of a focal ischemic stroke is identical to myocardial infarction, which is why the term *brain attack* is used in public education strategies. Often, a history of transient ischemic attacks, brief episodes of neurologic symptoms that last less than 24 hours, offer a warning that stroke is likely to occur. Sudden onset indicates embolism as the final insult to flow.[2] The stroke's size depends on the occluded vessel's size and location and the availability of collateral blood flow. Global ischemia results when severe hypotension or cardiopulmonary arrest provokes a transient decrease in blood flow to all areas of the brain.[7]

Cerebral edema sufficient to produce clinical deterioration develops in 10% to 20% of patients with ischemic stroke and can result in intracranial hypertension. The edema results from a loss of normal metabolic function of the cells and peaks at 4 days.[4] This process is commonly the cause of death during the first week after a stroke.[8] Secondary hemorrhage at the site of the stroke lesion, known as *hemorrhagic conversion*, and seizures are the two other major acute neurologic complications of ischemic stroke.[8]

Acute Ischemic Stroke

Clinical and diagnostic assessments	Signs*	Nursing interventions

• History and risk factors
  • Atrial fibrillation
  • Hypertension
  • Dyslipidemia
  • Diabetes
  • Smoking
  • Atherosclerotic disease
• Obtain vital signs
  • O_2 saturation
• Clinical assessment
  • NIH stroke scale
  • Neurologic
  • Musculoskeletal
  • Respiratory
• Laboratory studies
  • Obtain ABGs
• Diagnostic procedures
  • Noncontrast CT
  • MRI
	• Facial drooping/numbness – on one side
	• Arm weakness/numbness – on one side
	• Leg weakness/numbness – on one side
	• Difficulty speaking
	• Difficulty understanding speech
	• Confusion
	• Changes in LOC
	• Loss of balance
	• Severe headache
	• Vision changes
	• Nausea and vomiting
	
	*Signs will vary depending on the area of the brain affected by the interruption of blood flow.
		• Prepare patient for thrombectomy or administer fibrinolytic therapy
		• Administer medications for blood pressure control
		• Protect the patient's airway
		• Administer O_2
		• Provide ventilatory assistance as required.
		• Perform frequent neurologic assessments.
		• Maintain surveillance for complications
		• Provide comfort and emotional support
		• Implement appropriate rehabilitation program
		• Educate the patient and family

FIG. 22.1 Summary of Key Concepts Related to Ischemic Stroke. *ABGs,* Arterial blood gases; *CT,* computed tomography; *LOC,* level of consciousness; *MRI,* magnetic resonance imaging; *NIH,* National Institutes of Health; O_2, oxygen.

Assessment and Diagnosis

Assessment. The characteristic sign of an ischemic stroke is the sudden onset of focal neurologic signs persisting for more than 24 hours.[4] These signs usually occur in combination. Table 22.1 lists common patterns of neurologic symptoms associated with an ischemic stroke. Hemiparesis, aphasia, and hemianopia are common. Changes in the level of consciousness (LOC) usually occur only with brainstem or cerebellar involvement, seizure, hypoxia, hemorrhage, or elevated intracranial pressure (ICP). These changes may be exhibited as stupor, coma, confusion, and agitation. The reported frequency of seizures in patients with ischemic stroke is approximately 11%. If seizures occur, they are usually seen within the first 2 weeks of an insult.[8]

NIH stroke scale. The National Institutes of Health Stroke Scale (NIHSS) is often used as the basis of the focused neurologic examination.[9] The score ranges from 0 to 42 points; the higher the score, the more neurologically impaired the patient is. A change of four points on the scale indicates significant neurologic change. The components of the NIHSS include LOC; LOC questions; LOC commands; gaze; visual fields; face, arm, and leg strength; sensation; limb ataxia; and language function. A copy of the NIHSS with complete instructions is available at https://www.ninds.nih.gov/sites/default/files/documents/NIH_Stroke_Scale_508C.pdf.

Diagnosis. Confirmation of the diagnosis of ischemic stroke is the first step in the emergent evaluation of these patients. Differentiation from intracranial hemorrhage is vital. In most instances, noncontrast computed tomography (CT) scanning is the method of choice for this purpose, and it is considered the most critical initial diagnostic study. In addition to excluding intracranial hemorrhage, CT can assist in identifying early neurologic complications and the cause of the insult. Magnetic resonance imaging (MRI) can demonstrate infarction of cerebral tissue earlier than CT and is an appropriate alternative to a noncontrast CT scan for excluding ICH.[9,10]

Because of the strong correlation between acute ischemic stroke and heart disease, 12-lead electrocardiography and continuous cardiac monitoring are suggested to detect a cardiac cause or coexisting condition. A chest radiograph is obtained if lung disease is suspected. However, getting these studies should not delay the administration of fibrinolysis.[9] Echocardiography is valuable in identifying a cardioembolic phenomenon when a sufficient index of suspicion warrants its use.[4] Laboratory studies to evaluate hematologic and renal function, coagulation, electrolyte and glucose levels, and troponin are also recommended. Arterial blood gas analysis is performed if hypoxia is suspected. A lumbar puncture may be performed if a SAH is suspected and the CT scan is normal.[9]

Medical Management

Rapid diagnosis of stroke and initiation of treatment are essential to maximize recovery, prevent stroke recurrence, and prevent complications (Box 22.1). Definitive management of a patient with an ischemic stroke focuses on revascularization of the affected area of the brain with either fibrinolytic therapy or mechanical thrombectomy before neurons die of ischemia.[9] The goal is to reverse or minimize the effects of stroke.

Fibrinolytic therapy. Fibrinolytic therapy with intravenous recombinant tissue plasminogen activator (rtPA) is recommended to facilitate clot dissolution within 3 hours of ischemic stroke onset.[9] The exclusion criteria for patients who should be considered for fibrinolysis are listed in Box 22.2. The time frame for rtPA can be extended to 4.5 hours, with some additional exclusions including patients older than 80 years of age, patients taking oral anticoagulants, patients with a baseline NIHSS score greater than 25, patients with evidence of ischemic injury involving more than one-third of the middle cerebral artery territory, and patients with a history of both stroke and diabetes.[9] The diagnosis must be confirmed with a CT scan before rtPA administration.[9]

TABLE 22.1 Stroke Syndromes Secondary to Occlusion or Stenosis

Location/Vessel	Area of Brain Infarcted	Signs and Symptoms Noted
Anterior and Central Circulation		
Note: The internal carotid artery enters the circle of Willis and supplies the lateral anterior and central portions of the cerebral hemispheres through the middle cerebral artery and the paramedial frontal lobe superior to the corpus callosum through the anterior cerebral artery; penetrating branches serve the deeper layers of the hemispheres.		
Internal carotid	If collateral circulation is intact, there is commonly no infarction; if infarcted, it is in the same area of the middle cerebral artery	• Arterial pressure may be low in the retina • Bruits over the internal carotid artery • Possible retinal emboli • History of transient ischemic attacks (TIAs) • Positive noninvasive studies
Middle cerebral artery (MCA) (most common area); either stem or branches of MCA	Cortical motor area (face, arm, leg) or posterior limb, internal capsule, corona radiata	• **Motor:** contralateral hemiparesis or hemiplegia, greater in face and arm than leg
	Cortical sensory area (face, arm, leg) or posterior limb of the internal capsule	• **Sensation:** contralateral loss in the same distribution as motor loss
	Broca area and deep fibers in the dominant hemisphere	• **Speech:** expressive (motor) disorder with anomia (left hemisphere most commonly affected) with nonfluent aphasia and some comprehension defects
	Broca area and deep fibers in the nondominant hemisphere	• **Speech:** dysarthria
	Optic radiations deep in the temporal lobe	• **Vision:** contralateral homonymous hemianopsia or quadranopsia
	Location not known	• **Motor:** mirror movements • **Respirations:** Cheyne–Stokes respirations, contralateral hyperhidrosis, occasional mydriasis
	Posterior limb or internal capsule and adjacent corona radiate	• **Motor:** pure motor hemiplegia
	Penetrating branches of MCA (lenticulostriate branches) into the basal nuclei	• **Motor:** varying degrees of contralateral weakness of the face, arm, or leg • **Sensory:** little or no loss; if present, contralateral following the motor distribution • **Speech:** transcortical sensory aphasia (communicating pathways are interrupted) • **Perception:** transient visual and sensory neglect on the left if a right lesion
Anterior cerebral artery (ACA) (least common)	Proximal segment: corona radiata (rarely)	• **Motor:** when present, a mild contralateral hemiparesis, greater in the leg; with bilateral occlusion of ACA, cerebral paraplegia in both legs can occur
	Main stem (complete occlusion is uncommon; thus areas affected differ and collateral circulation may alleviate signs or symptoms); medial aspect of frontal lobes, caudate nucleus, and corpus callosum are supplied by the ACA	• **Motor:** contralateral paralysis or paresis (greater in foot and thigh); mild upper extremity weakness • **Sensory:** mild contralateral lower extremity deficiency with loss of vibratory or position sense, loss of two-point discrimination • **Speech:** may have transcortical motor and sensory aphasia if the left hemisphere • Frontal lobe releasing signs (grasp, snout, root, and suck reflexes) • Apraxia
Posterior Circulation		
Note: The posterior circulation includes the posterior cerebral artery, the vertebral arteries, and the basilar artery; the anatomic territory covered includes the posterior aspects of the hemispheres, the central areas of the thalamus and midbrain, and the brainstem; occlusion of the vessels is most commonly by emboli; effects of infarct in these vessels and their penetrating vessels can be specific or devastatingly global; many complex syndromes have been identified.		
Vertebral arteries	Medulla and spinal cord tracts, anterior spinal artery and penetrating branches (medial medullary syndrome)	• **Motor:** contralateral hemiparesis (face spared) or impaired contralateral proprioception; flaccid weakness or paralysis of the tongue or dysarthria
Basilar artery (three sets of branches)	Midline structures of pons (paramedian branches); three general areas of infarction are common: (1) medial inferior pontine syndrome, (2) medial midpontine syndrome, and (3) medial superior pontine syndrome	• **Motor:** contralateral hemiparesis or hemiplegia, ipsilateral lower motor neuron facial palsy, "locked-in syndrome" • **Sensory:** contralateral loss of vibratory sense, sense of position with dysmetria, loss of two-point discrimination, impaired rapid alternating movements • **Visual:** inferior pontine: diplopia; impaired abduction of the ipsilateral eye: internuclear ophthalmoplegia; medial superior; diplopia, internuclear ophthalmoplegia, skewed deviation
	Corticospinal and corticobulbar tracts in the pons, sensory tracts of medial and lateral lemnisci, vestibular nuclei, inferior and middle cerebellar peduncles, cranial nerve nuclei or fibers, cerebellar connections in tectum, descending sympathetic pathways, central brainstem, pontine tegmentum (vertebrobasilar syndrome)	• **Motor:** upper motor neuron type of weakness: paralysis in combinations involving face, tongue, throat, and extremities; dysphagia, facial weakness, dysmetria, ataxia (either trunk or extremities), weak mastication muscles • **Sensation:** combinations of impaired sensation (vibratory, two-point, position sense, pain, temperature), facial hypesthesia, anesthesia of cranial nerve V

TABLE 22.1 **Stroke Syndromes Secondary to Occlusion or Stenosis—cont'd**

Location/Vessel	Area of Brain Infarcted	Signs and Symptoms Noted
Posterior cerebral artery (PCA)	Central territory (thalamic area, dentatothalamic tract, cerebral peduncle, red nucleus, subthalamic nucleus, and cranial nerve III)	• **Motor:** contralateral hemiplegia with possible dysmetria, dyskinesia, hemiballism or choreoathetosis, dystaxia, cerebellar ataxia, and tremor; contralateral upper motor neuron palsy; several syndromes are associated: (1) Weber: cranial nerve III palsy and contralateral hemiplegia; (2) thalamoperforate syndrome: superior crossed cerebellar ataxia or inferior crossed cerebellar ataxia with cranial nerve III palsy (Claude syndrome); (3) decerebrate attacks • **Sensory:** contralateral sensory loss of all modalities without agraphia • **Function:** prosopagnosia (inability to recognize familiar faces), topographic disorientation, memory deficits, alexia, inability to read, color anomia • **Level of consciousness:** in bilateral PCA syndromes, coma with absent doll's eyes reflex or loss of alertness may occur; if the tegmentum of the midbrain near the hypothalamus and third ventricle is damaged, akinetic mutism may occur
Small Vessel Disease		
Note: Small penetrating vessels in brain parenchyma that supply areas near the basal ganglia are most vulnerable to infarction, although any small vessels can occlude deep in the brain and cause injury, producing neurologic signs or symptoms; such infarcts are commonly called *lacunes* (small pit or hollow), a term that is changing in meaning; they can be caused by emboli but are most commonly associated with microatheromas; although they can be found in otherwise healthy people, those with concurrent atherosclerosis, arterial hypertension, or diabetes have a higher incidence of this type of infarct.		
	Internal capsule, most commonly	• **Motor:** contralateral hemiparesis on a single side, with an equal deficit in face, arm, and leg; often unaccompanied by detectable signs of sensory, visual, and speech loss, depending on location; the old term is *pure motor stroke*, although evidence suggests that other neurologic signs are present but overlooked because of low intensity
	Thalamus, most commonly	• **Sensory:** complete or partial loss in face, arm, trunk, and leg that appears exactly midline; may be accompanied by pain, hyperesthesias, and uncomfortable sensations (hemisensory stroke)
	Pons	Dysarthria, clumsy hand
	Pons, midbrain, capsule or parietal white matter	Hemiparesis, ataxia on same side

Modified from Barker E. *Neuroscience Nursing.* Mosby; 1994.

Fibrinolytic agents. The most common fibrinolytic agent used is alteplase. The recommended dosage is 0.9 mg/kg, up to a maximum dosage of 90 mg; 10% of the total dose is administered as an initial intravenous bolus, and the remaining 90% is administered by intravenous infusion over 60 minutes.[9] Tenecteplase is an alternative in patients with minor neurologic impairment without major intracranial occlusions. The recommended dosage is 0.4 mg/kg, administered as a single intravenous bolus.[9] Bleeding, especially intracranial hemorrhage, is the major risk and complication of rtPA therapy. In contrast to fibrinolytic protocols for acute myocardial infarction, subsequent treatment with anticoagulant or antiplatelet agents is not recommended after rtPA administration in ischemic stroke. Patients receiving fibrinolytic therapy for stroke should not receive aspirin, heparin, warfarin, ticlopidine, or other antithrombotic or antiplatelet medications for at least 24 hours after treatment.[9]

Thrombectomy. Mechanical thrombectomy is a newer therapy for treating ischemic stroke in selected patients.[11] Current guidelines recommend that the device be employed within 6 hours of the onset of symptoms; under certain circumstances, the treatment window can be increased to 24 hours.[9,11] A mechanical thrombectomy is the endovascular retrieval of a thrombus from a sizeable intracranial vessel with a catheter. Although several different types of devices are available, current guidelines recommend using a stent retrieval system. A stent retrieval system uses a self-expanding stent that can be deployed and retrieved. When the device is deployed into a cerebral vessel across a thrombus, it pushes the thrombus against the vessel wall, reestablishing blood flow to the area downstream from the clot. The thrombus is then ensnared in the struts of the stent, and the stent is retrieved.[11,12]

Blood pressure management. Hypertension is often present in the early period as a compensatory response, and in most cases, blood pressure must not be lowered. This action is sometimes referred to as permissive hypertension.[9,13] For patients who have not received fibrinolytic therapy, antihypertensive therapy is considered only if the diastolic blood pressure is greater than 120 mm Hg or the systolic blood pressure is greater than 220 mm Hg.[9] Criteria are different for patients who have received rtPA. Their blood pressure is maintained at less than 180/105 mm Hg to prevent intracranial hemorrhage. Intravenous labetalol or nicardipine is used to achieve blood pressure management. If these agents are ineffective, nitroprusside should be considered.[9]

Adjunct care. Other emergent care for a patient with ischemic stroke must include airway protection and ventilatory assistance to maintain adequate tissue oxygenation.[9] Supplemental oxygen should be provided to maintain oxygen saturation above 94%.[9] Body temperature and glucose levels also must be normalized.[9] Medical management also includes identifying and treating acute complications such as cerebral edema or seizure activity. Prophylaxis for these complications is not recommended. However, deep vein thrombosis (DVT) prophylaxis should be initiated to decrease the risk of pulmonary embolism.[9]

Treatment delays. The significant barriers to the effective application of definitive therapy for ischemic stroke are

BOX 22.1 Teamwork and Collaboration

Acute Stroke Teams

Given the short time available to restore blood flow to the brain after a stroke, an organized approach must be taken to provide the patient with the best chance of a positive outcome. To meet this challenge, many health care organizations have developed acute stroke teams. An acute stroke team comprises transdisciplinary health care professionals with experience and training in the definitive management of a patient experiencing a stroke. The team aims to reduce in-hospital delays in obtaining appropriate medical care for these patients.

Members will vary depending on the health care organization; however, the acute stroke team usually includes an emergency room practitioner, a neurologist, an interventional radiologist, a pharmacist, a laboratory technician, and one or more registered nurses. The team is available 24 hours a day and is notified via a specialized notification system (e.g., "Stroke Code"). The acute stroke team is responsible for stabilizing the patient, performing initial testing to determine the type of stroke, and initiating the selected treatment regimen to help the patient achieve the best possible functional outcome.[1]

Teamwork and collaboration are essential for the success of these teams. They often have to learn to work together as a team as they come together with a common shared goal. Many teams use crew resource management tools to facilitate team development. Crew resource tools focus on the non-clinical aspects of the team, including team communication, leadership, and organization. Many teams use ongoing stroke-specific simulation training to enhance team knowledge and cohesiveness.[2]

References

1. Tahtali D, Bohmann F, Rostek P, Wagner M, Steinmetx H, Pfeilschifter W. Setting up a stroke team algorithm and conducting simulation-based training in the emergency department—a practical guide. *J Vis Exp.* 2017;(119):55138. https://doi.org/10.3791/55138.
2. Willems LM, Kurka N, Bohmann F, Rostek P, Pfeilschifter W. Tools for your stroke team: adapting crew-resource management for acute stroke care. *Pract Neurol.* 2019;19(1):36–42. https://doi.org/10.1136/practneurol-2018-001966.

BOX 22.2 Exclusion Criteria for Intravenous Recombinant Tissue Plasminogen Activator

- Age ≤18 years
- Onset of symptoms <3 or 4.5 hours (see text for more information)
- Stroke in previous 3 months
- Intracranial or intraspinal surgery in the previous 3 months
- Severe head trauma in previous 3 months
- Subarachnoid hemorrhage
- Intracranial hemorrhage—acute and prior history
- Intracranial neoplasm
- Aortic arch dissection
- Infective endocarditis
- Gastrointestinal malignancy
- Gastrointestinal hemorrhage in previous 21 days
- Uncontrolled severe hypertension
- Active internal bleeding
- Coagulopathy (platelets <100,000/mm^3, INR >1.7, aPTT >40 s, or PT >15)
- Low molecular weight heparin within the previous 24 hours

aPTT, Activated partial thromboplastin time; *INR,* international normalized ratio; *PT,* protime.

Data from Powers WJ, Rabinstein AA, Ackerson T, et al. Guidelines for the early management of patients with acute ischemic stroke: 2019 update to the 2018 guidelines for the early management of acute ischemic stroke: A guideline for healthcare professionals from the American Heart Association/American Stroke Association. *Stroke* 2019;50(12):e344-e418.

BOX 22.3 Hunt and Hess Classification of Subarachnoid Hemorrhage

- *Grade I:* Asymptomatic or minimal headache and slight nuchal rigidity
- *Grade II:* Moderate to severe headache, nuchal rigidity, but no neurologic deficit other than cranial nerve palsy
- *Grade III:* Drowsiness, confusion, or mild focal deficit
- *Grade IV:* Stupor, moderate to severe hemiparesis, possible early decerebrate rigidity, and vegetative disturbances
- *Grade V:* Deep coma, decerebrate rigidity, moribund appearance

From Hunt WE, Hess RM. Surgical risks as related to time of intervention in the repair of intracranial aneurysms. *J Neurosurg.* 1968;28:14–20. https://doi.org/10.3171/jns.1968.28.1.0014.

prehospital and in-hospital delays. To help decrease delays, the public needs to be educated about stroke symptoms and the activation of the emergency medical system. Emergency medical system responders need adequate education and training on managing a patient with an acute ischemic stroke, focusing on stabilization and transport of the patient quickly to the emergency department. The receiving hospital should ideally have certification for primary stroke treatment and have expert staff and the infrastructure to care for a patient with a complex stroke.[9,14] Box 22.3 discusses the benefits of informatics in care of stroke patients particularly the effect on treatment delays.

Subarachnoid Hemorrhage

Description and Etiology

SAH is due to bleeding into the subarachnoid space.[15] Cerebral aneurysm rupture accounts for approximately 80% of all cases of spontaneous nontraumatic SAH.[15] Other causes of SAH include arteriovenous malformations (AVMs), moyamoya, vasculitis, amyloid angiopathy, and intracranial artery dissections.[15–18] Known risk factors for SAH include prior history or family history of SAH, hypertension, smoking, heavy alcohol use, and sympathomimetic drugs such as cocaine.[15–18]

Cerebral aneurysm. An aneurysm is an outpouching of the wall of a blood vessel that results from the weakening of the vessel's wall (Table 22.2).[16] Most aneurysms are congenital—the cause of which is unknown. Other causes include traumatic injury (that stretches and tears the muscular middle layer of the arterial vessel), infectious material (most often from infectious vegetation on valves of the left side of the heart after bacterial endocarditis) that lodges against a vessel wall and erodes the muscular layer, atherosclerosis, radiation, neoplasms, and connective tissue disorders.[19] The overall prevalence of cerebral aneurysms ranges from 0.5% to 6.0%, depending on the patient population.[12] SAH is associated with a 30-day mortality rate of 45%, with 25% of the patients dying within 24 hours of the insult.[15]

Arteriovenous malformations. AVM rupture is responsible for approximately 6% of all SAHs.[19] An AVM is a tangled mass of arterial and venous blood vessels that shunt blood directly from the arterial side into the venous side, bypassing the capillary system. AVMs may be small, focal, or large, diffuse lesions that occupy almost an entire hemisphere. They are always congenital, although the exact embryonic cause for these malformations is unknown. They also occur in the spinal cord and the renal, gastrointestinal, and integumentary systems.[19] Small, superficial

TABLE 22.2 **Classification of Aneurysms**

Types of Aneurysms	Characteristics
Berry or saccular	• **Shape:** Have a sac or pouch-like form, resembling a small berry attached to the side of a blood vessel; shape distinguishes them from other types of aneurysms. • **Location:** Commonly found at arterial bifurcations or branch points in the brain's blood vessels; most common site is along the circle of Willis • **Risk Factors:** Several factors contribute to the development of saccular aneurysms, including genetic predisposition, high blood pressure (hypertension), smoking, and certain connective tissue disorders.
Fusiform	• **Shape:** Have a cylindrical or spindle-like shape, stretching the artery uniformly along a segment; dilation of the artery affects its entire circumference, making the vessel appear elongated and widened. • **Location:** Can occur in various arteries throughout the body, including the aorta and its branches, as well as other major arteries. • **Risk Factors:** Several factors contribute to the development of fusiform aneurysms, including atherosclerosis, hypertension, trauma, and connective tissue disorders
Mycotic	• **Shape:** Can assume different shapes, including saccular, fusiform, or irregular shapes, similar to aneurysms caused by other factors. • **Location:** Can occur in various arteries throughout the body; more commonly found in larger arteries • **Risk Factors:** Due to bacterial infections, most commonly bacterial endocarditis (infection of the heart valves) or septicemia (bloodstream infection). The infection spreads to the arterial wall, weakening it and leading to the formation of an aneurysm.
Charcot–Bouchard or Microaneurysms	• **Shape:** Charcot–Bouchard aneurysms are typically small, ranging in size from a few millimeters to a few centimeters in diameter. • **Location:** Commonly found in the small blood vessels of deep brain structures, particularly in areas where blood vessels branch or bifurcate. • **Risk Factors:** Primary risk factor is chronic hypertension; high blood pressure exerts increased pressure on the walls of small arteries, leading to weakening and bulging.

AVMs are seen as port wine stains on the skin. In contrast to SAH from an aneurysm in middle-aged patients, SAH from an AVM usually occurs in the second to fourth decades of life.[19,20] Hemorrhage from AVM rupture has a better chance of survival and is associated with an overall mortality rate of 10% to 15%.[20]

Pathophysiology

The pathophysiologies of the two most common causes of SAH, cerebral aneurysm, and AVM, are distinctly different.

Cerebral aneurysm. As an individual with a congenital cerebral aneurysm ages, blood pressure increases, and more stress is placed on the poorly developed thin vessel wall. Ballooning of the vessel occurs, giving the aneurysm a berrylike appearance. Most cerebral aneurysms are saccular or berrylike, with a stem or neck. Aneurysms are usually small, are 2 to 7 mm in diameter, and often occur at the base of the brain on the circle of Willis.[15] Fig. 22.2 illustrates the usual distribution between the vessels. Most cerebral aneurysms occur at the bifurcation of blood vessels.[15]

The aneurysm becomes clinically significant when the vessel wall becomes so thin that it ruptures, sending arterial blood at high pressure into the subarachnoid space. For a moment after the aneurysm ruptures, ICP is thought to approach mean arterial pressure, and cerebral perfusion decreases.[19] In other situations, the unruptured aneurysm expands and places pressure on surrounding structures. This situation is particularly true with posterior communicating artery aneurysms because they put pressure on the oculomotor nerve (cranial nerve III), causing ipsilateral pupil dilation and ptosis.[19]

Arteriovenous malformation. The pathophysiologic features of an AVM are related to the size and location of the malformation. One or more cerebral arteries, known as *feeders*, supply an AVM. These feeder arteries tend to enlarge over time, increasing the volume of blood shunted through the malformation and the overall mass effect. Large, dilated, tortuous draining veins develop due to increasing arterial blood flow delivered at a higher than normal pressure. Normal vascular flow has a mean arterial pressure of 70 to 80 mm Hg, a mean arteriole pressure of 35 to 45 mm Hg, and a mean capillary pressure that decreases from 35 to 10 mm Hg as it connects with the venous side. Lack of this capillary bridge allows blood with a mean pressure of 35 to 45 mm Hg to flow into the venous system. In contrast to arteries, veins have no muscular layer and become extremely engorged and rupture easily. Some patients with AVMs also have cerebral atrophy, which results from chronic ischemia secondary to the shunting of blood through the AVM and away from normal cerebral circulation.[19]

Assessment and Diagnosis

A patient with a SAH characteristically has an abrupt onset of pain, described as the "worst headache of my life." A brief loss of consciousness, nausea, vomiting, focal neurologic deficits, photophobia, and a stiff neck may accompany the headache.[15–18] The SAH may result in coma or death.

Assessment. The patient's history may reveal one or more incidences of sudden onset of headache with vomiting in the weeks preceding a major SAH. These are small "warning leaks" of an aneurysm in which small amounts of blood ooze from the aneurysm into the subarachnoid space. The presence of blood irritates the meninges, particularly the arachnoid membrane, and the irritation causes headaches, stiff neck, and photophobia. These warning leaks seldom are detected because the condition is not severe enough for the patient to seek medical attention. If a neurologic deficit such as third cranial nerve palsy develops before the aneurysm ruptures, medical intervention is sought, and the aneurysm may be surgically secured before the

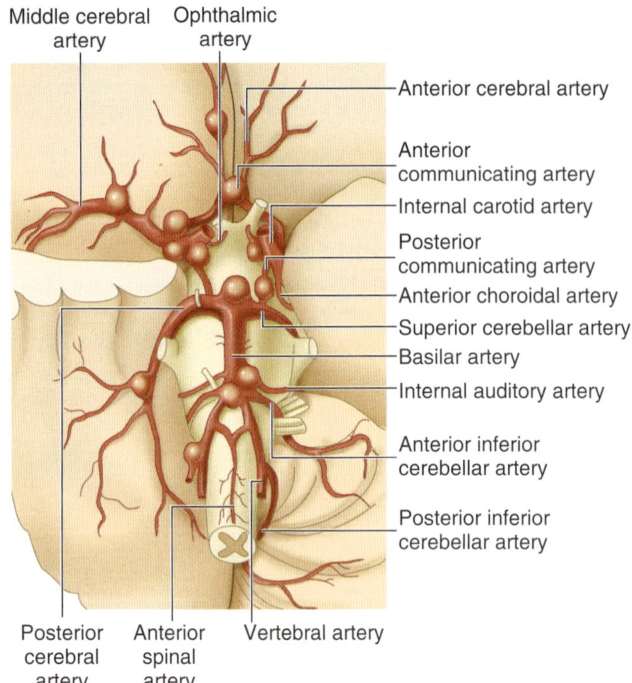

FIG. 22.2 Common Sites of Berry Aneurysms. The size of the aneurysm in the drawing is proportional to the frequency of occurrence at the various sites. (From Goldman L, Schafer AI, eds. *Goldman-Cecil Medicine*. 26th ed. Elsevier; 2020.)

devastation of a rupture can occur. Symptoms of unruptured AVM, such as headaches with dizziness or syncope or fleeting neurologic deficits, also may be found in the history.[15–17]

Diagnosis. SAH diagnoses are based on clinical presentation, CT findings, and lumbar puncture results. Noncontrast CT is the cornerstone of a definitive SAH diagnosis.[21] In 93% of the cases, CT demonstrates blood in the subarachnoid space if performed within the first hours of the hemorrhage.[22] Based on the SAH's appearance and location, diagnosis of the cause—aneurysm or AVM—may be made from the CT scan. MRI is not routinely used, but it may provide greater sensitivity for detecting the areas of SAH clot and the potential location of the bleeding.[22]

Lumbar puncture. If the initial CT finding is negative, a lumbar puncture is performed to obtain cerebrospinal fluid (CSF) for analysis. After SAH, CSF appears bloody and has a red blood cell count greater than 1000 cells/mm^3. If the lumbar puncture is performed more than 12 hours after the SAH, the CSF fluid may appear xanthochromic (dark amber) because the blood products have started to break down.[22] Cloudy CSF usually indicates some type of infectious process, such as bacterial meningitis, not SAH.[19]

Pinpointing the underlying cause. After the SAH has been documented, cerebral digital subtraction angiography or CT angiography is necessary to identify the exact cause of the hemorrhage (Fig. 22.3).[22] If a cerebral aneurysm rupture is the cause, angiography is essential for identifying the exact location of the aneurysm in preparation for surgery. After the aneurysm has been located, it is graded using the Hunt and Hess classification scale.[23] This scale categorizes the patient based on the severity of the neurologic deficits associated with the hemorrhage (Box 22.4).[16–18] If AVM rupture is the cause, angiography is necessary to identify the malformation's feeding arteries and draining veins.[19]

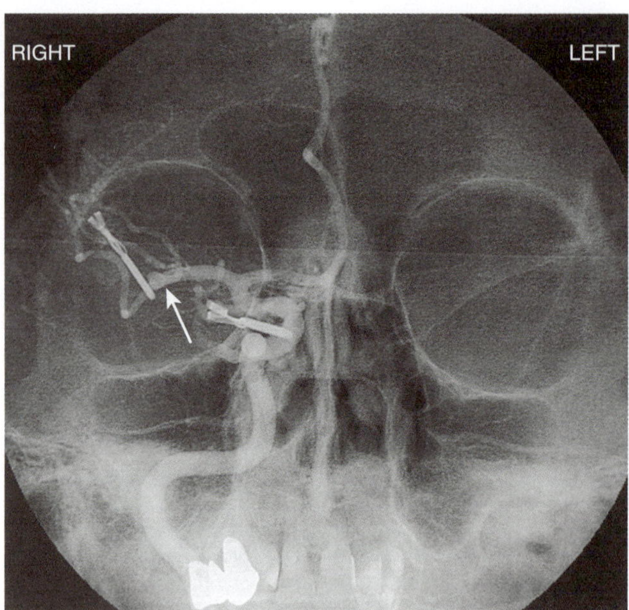

FIG. 22.3 Cerebral Angiogram. Cerebral angiography shows the location of an aneurysm *(arrow)* at the posterior communicating artery. (From Tortorici M. *Fundamentals of Angiography*. Mosby; 1982.)

Medical Management

SAH is a medical emergency, and timely diagnosis and treatment are essential to preserve neurologic function. Initial treatment must always support vital functions. Airway management and ventilatory assistance may be necessary.[16] If intubation is required, rapid-sequence induction is recommended using a combination of rocuronium, fentanyl, and propofol.[18] A ventriculostomy may be performed to manage ICP if the patient's LOC is depressed.[16,24] After the initial intervention has provided the necessary support for vital physiologic functions, medical management of acute SAH is aimed primarily at preventing and treating the complications of SAH, which may produce further neurologic damage and death.

After initial stabilization, the focus of medical management is directed toward the prevention of rebleeding. Rebleeding is the occurrence of a second SAH in an unsecured aneurysm or, less commonly, an AVM. Most rebleeding episodes occur during the first 6 hours after the first bleed. The mortality rate associated with rebleeding is approximately 20% to 60%.[22,25] Current guidelines for managing patients with SAH are addressed in Box 22.5.

Blood pressure management. Conservative measures to prevent rebleeding have historically included blood pressure management and SAH precautions (see Nursing Management). An elevation in blood pressure is a normal compensatory response to maintain adequate cerebral perfusion after a neurologic insult. In the belief that hypertension contributes to rebleeding, continuous intravenous antihypertensive medications, such as nicardipine, clevidipine, or labetalol, are used to maintain a systolic blood pressure less than 160 mm Hg.[16,21,22] Evidence suggests that rebleeding has more to do with variations or fluctuations in blood pressure than maintaining blood pressure below an absolute value.[22] This is why continuous intravenous antihypertensive medications are preferred over intermittent administration of antihypertensive medications. Individualized guidelines must be determined based on the patient's clinical condition and preexisting

BOX 22.4 Informatics

Informatics in Stroke Patient Care

Health care informatics, the integration of technology and health care, plays a crucial role in the care of stroke patients. Stroke is a complex condition that requires timely and coordinated interventions. Informatics tools and technologies enhance the efficiency, accuracy, and quality of stroke care by facilitating communication, data analysis, and decision-making across the care continuum.

Key Applications of Informatics in Stroke Care:

- Electronic Health Records (EHRs):
  - EHRs allow health care practitioners across different specialties (neurologists, radiologists, rehabilitation specialists) to access and update relevant patient information, enabling coordinated care and better continuity.
- Telestroke and Telemedicine:
  - Telestroke programs use telemedicine technology to connect patients with acute stroke in underserved areas with stroke specialists at designated stroke centers.
  - This facilitates rapid diagnosis and treatment decisions, such as administering fibrinolytic therapy or performing thrombectomy.
- Imaging Informatics:
  - Picture archiving and communication systems (PACS) and radiology information systems (RIS) play a critical role in stroke care by allowing prompt and secure sharing of medical images, such as CT scans and MRIs, among healthcare practitioners.
  - This process accelerates the interpretation and decision-making process.
- Clinical Decision Support Systems:
  - Informatics tools provide health care professionals with evidence-based guidelines and protocols for stroke treatment.
  - These decision support systems help guide timely interventions, such as administering fibrinolytic therapy within the appropriate window.
- Mobile Apps and Wearable Devices:
  - Stroke patients may benefit from mobile apps and wearable devices that track physical activity, monitor vital signs, and provide medication reminders.
  - These tools help patients and caregivers manage their recovery and stay connected to healthcare practitioners.
- Data Analytics for Outcome Assessment:
  - Informatics enables data collection, analysis, and interpretation to assess stroke treatment outcomes.
  - This data-driven approach helps health care teams adjust treatment plans based on real-time insights and benchmarks.
- Communication and Care Coordination:
  - Informatics tools, such as secure messaging platforms, facilitate communication among interdisciplinary stroke teams.
  - This collaboration ensures that all team members are informed and involved in decision-making.

The benefits of informatics in stroke care include timely intervention, data-driven decision-making, interprofessional collaboration, remote access to expertise, and patient engagement and self-management. There are several considerations to using this type of technology, including data security, privacy concerns, interoperability, training and adoption of health care practitioners, and equity of access. Not all stroke patients may have access to the necessary technology, potentially leading to disparities in care. Informatics in stroke care optimizes patient outcomes and empowers patients and practitioners with tools to improve the quality, efficiency, and coordination of stroke care across the continuum—from acute interventions to rehabilitation and long-term management.

BOX 22.5 Evidence-Based Practice

Subarachnoid Hemorrhage Management Guidelines

The current recommendations from the American Heart Association and American Stroke Association for managing the patient with a subarachnoid hemorrhage (DAH) are located here: https://www.ahajournals.org/doi/epub/10.1161/STR.0000000000000436.

blood pressure values.[22] It is essential that the patient's blood pressure is not kept too low because this increases the risk of cerebral infarction.[18] Antifibrinolytic medications may also be administered on a short-term basis (less than 72 hours) to prevent rebleeding.[16,22]

Definitive management. Definitive management of a ruptured cerebral aneurysm or AVM should be performed as early as possible.[21] Early intervention eliminates the risk of rebleeding and allows more aggressive therapy to treat vasospasm in the postoperative period.[21] Endovascular coiling and surgical clipping are the two primary approaches used for treating a ruptured cerebral aneurysm.[15,17] The two primary approaches used for treating a ruptured AVM are surgical resection and embolization.[20]

Endovascular coiling of aneurysms. Endovascular coiling involves the placement of one or more detachable coils into an aneurysm to produce an endovascular thrombus (Fig. 22.4). This method is preferred over surgical clipping.[15] There are several different methods available. A microcatheter is inserted into the femoral artery and is advanced into the affected cerebral artery. Once the microcatheter is in place at the base of the aneurysm, tiny platinum coils are threaded through a microcatheter and pushed into the aneurysm, where they conform to the shape of the aneurysm. Once the aneurysm is filled in with coils, blood flow into the aneurysm is obstructed, and a thrombus forms, occluding the aneurysm and preventing future bleeding. Recovery is usually shorter and easier.[26]

Surgical clipping of aneurysms. Surgical clipping is necessary if endovascular coiling is unavailable or the aneurysm is not appropriate for coiling. The surgical procedure involves a craniotomy to expose and isolate the aneurysm area. A clip is placed over the neck of the aneurysm to eliminate the area of weakness (Fig. 22.5).[19] This is a technically challenging procedure requiring an experienced neurosurgeon's skill. It is not uncommon, particularly in early surgery, for the clot to break away from the aneurysm as it is surgically exposed. Extensive hemorrhage into the craniotomy site results, causing increased neurologic deficits. Deficits also may occur due to surgical manipulation to gain access to the aneurysm site. Early surgery allows the neurosurgeon to flush out the excess blood and clots from the basal cisterns (reservoir of CSF around the base of the brain and circle of Willis) to reduce the risk of vasospasm. Careful consideration of the patient's clinical situation is necessary to determine the optimal surgery time.

Surgical resection of arteriovenous malformations. Management of AVM has traditionally involved surgical excision or conservative management of symptoms such as seizures and headaches. The decision for surgical excision depends on the location and size of the AVM. Some malformations are so deep in the cerebral structures (thalamus or midbrain) that attempts to remove the AVM would cause severe neurologic deficits.

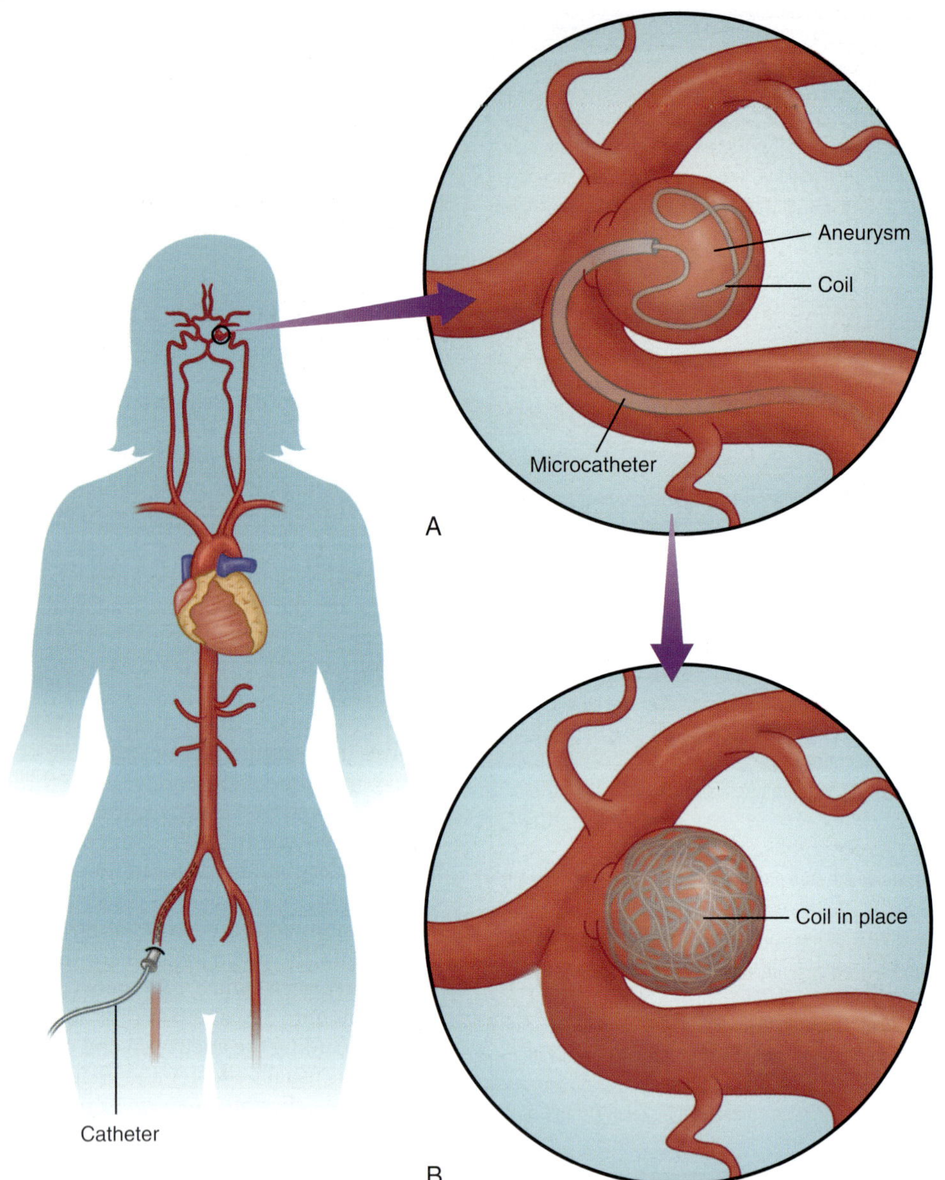

FIG. 22.4 Endovascular Occlusion of a Posterior Communicating Artery Aneurysm. (A) Insertion of the microcatheter into the aneurysm through the right femoral artery, aorta, and left carotid artery. (B) Occlusion of the aneurysm with coils.

History of a previous hemorrhage and the patient's age and overall condition are also considered when deciding on surgical intervention.[20]

Surgical excision of large AVMs includes the risk of reperfusion bleeding. As feeding arteries of the AVM are clamped off, the arterial blood that usually flows into the AVM is diverted into the surrounding circulation. In many cases, the surrounding tissue has been in a state of chronic ischemia, and the arterial vessels feeding these areas are maximally dilated. As arterial blood begins to flow at a higher volume and pressure into these dilated arteries, blood may seep from the vessels. Evidence of reperfusion bleeding in the operating room indicates that no more arterial blood can be diverted from the AVM without risk of serious ICH. Low blood pressure is maintained in the postoperative phase to prevent further reperfusion bleeding. For large AVMs, two to four stages of surgery may be required over 6 to 12 months.[20]

Embolization of arteriovenous malformations. Embolization is used to secure an AVM that is surgically inaccessible because of the size or location of the AVM or the medical instability of the patient. Although there are a variety of interventional neuroradiology techniques used for embolization, all methods use a percutaneous transfemoral approach in a manner like angiography. Under fluoroscopy, the catheter is threaded up to the internal carotid artery. Specially developed microcatheters are then manipulated into the area of the vascular anomaly, and embolic materials are placed endovascularly. Three embolization techniques are used, depending on the underlying pathologic derangement.[23]

The first type of embolization is used for an AVM. Small polymeric silicone (Silastic) beads or glue are slowly introduced into the vessels feeding the AVM. Blood flow carries the material to the site, and embolization is achieved. This procedure may be used in combination with surgery. One to three sessions of

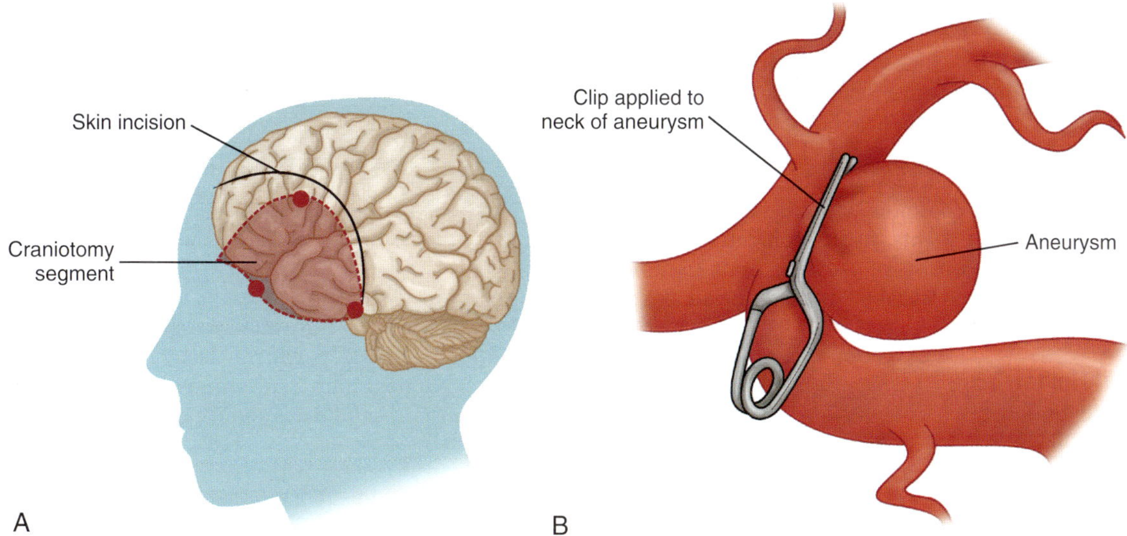

FIG. 22.5 Clipping of a Posterior Communicating Artery Aneurysm. (A) *Solid curved line* shows the typical skin incision and *dashed lines* show the craniotomy location. (B) Application of the clip to the aneurysm.

embolization of the feeding vessels are performed to reduce the lesion size before a craniotomy is performed for total excision. The primary risk of this procedure is lodging the embolic substance in a vessel that feeds normal tissue, creating an embolic stroke with the immediate onset of neurologic symptoms.[23]

Delayed cerebral ischemia. Delayed cerebral ischemia (DCI) is a disabling complication of SAH that occurs in up to 30% of patients within 2 weeks after the hemorrhage that is not associated with the initial bleed or other complications. It presents as a new focal neurologic impairment or deterioration in LOC lasting for more than 1 hour and is associated with poor clinical outcomes. DCI is thought to occur due to arterial vasospasm, microthrombosis, inflammation, microcirculation dysfunction, and cortical ischemia.[28,29]

The presence or absence of cerebral vasospasm significantly affects the outcome of aneurysmal SAH. This complication does not occur with SAH resulting from AVM rupture. Cerebral vasospasm is a narrowing of the lumen of the cerebral arteries, possibly in response to subarachnoid blood clots coating the outer surface of the blood vessels. Because aneurysms usually occur at the circle of Willis, the major vessels responsible for feeding the cerebral circulation are affected by vasospasm. Depending on the arterial vessels involved in the vasospasm reaction, decreased arterial flow occurs in large areas of the cerebral hemispheres.[30] The onset of vasospasm is usually 3 to 10 days after the initial hemorrhage.[29] The three recommended vasospasm management treatments are normovolemic-induced hypertension, oral nimodipine, and transluminal cerebral angioplasty.

Normovolemic-induced hypertension. Normovolemic-induced hypertension therapy involves increasing the patient's blood pressure and cardiac output with vasoactive medications—the increase in pressure forces blood through the vasospastic area at higher pressures. The first step is to ensure the patient is not hypovolemic; normal saline should be administered to maintain euvolemia. Next, intravenous norepinephrine, dopamine, or phenylephrine is administered to augment the patient's blood pressure. Based on the patient's clinical response, blood pressure is raised slowly to a maximum systolic target of 220 mm Hg or a mean arterial target of 140 mm Hg. Once the desired response is achieved, the therapy is continued for 24 to 48 hours.[28,29]

The obvious deterrent to normovolemic-induced hypertension is the risk of rebleeding in an unsecured aneurysm. Surgical clipping or endovascular coiling of the aneurysm before starting the therapy is preferred. Cerebral edema, elevated ICP, heart failure, and electrolyte imbalance are risks of hemodynamic augmentation therapy. Careful monitoring of the patient's neurologic status, hemodynamic parameters, ICP, and serum electrolytes is necessary.[30]

Nimodipine. Nimodipine is strongly recommended to reduce the poor outcomes associated with vasospasm. The exact nature of the effect of nimodipine is unclear. Still, the medication has demonstrated consistently positive effects on outcomes without any demonstrable effect on the incidence or severity of vasospasm.[21,29] Sixty mg of nimodipine is given orally every 4 hours for 21 days. Nimodipine may produce hypotension, especially when administered concurrently with other antihypertensive agents.[29]

Cerebral angioplasty. Cerebral angioplasty is used when pharmacologic management of cerebral vasospasm has failed. It is performed only when CT or MRI proves infarction has not occurred. An interventional neuroradiologist performs the procedure, and the patient is placed under procedural sedation. The technique of cerebral angioplasty is very similar to the method used in the coronary vasculature. Risks include intimal perforation or rupture; cerebral artery thrombosis or embolism; recurrence of stenosis; and severe, diffuse vasospasm unresponsive to therapy. Bleeding at the femoral site also may occur. This procedure is recommended when conventional therapy is unsuccessful.[21,29]

Hyponatremia. Hyponatremia develops in up to 50% of patients with SAH due to central salt-wasting syndrome of inappropriate secretion of antidiuretic hormone (SIADH). It usually occurs during the same period as vasospasm, several days after the initial hemorrhage.[22] Sodium is replenished with isotonic fluids in patients with SAH; using fluid restriction to treat hyponatremia is associated with a poor outcome.[15,29]

Hydrocephalus. Hydrocephalus is a complication that occurs in approximately 30% of patients after SAH,[15] with 20% of patients developing acute symptomatic hydrocephalus within days after the initial event.[22] Blood that has circulated in the subarachnoid space and has been absorbed by the arachnoid villi may obstruct the villi and reduce the rate of CSF absorption. Over time, increasing volumes of CSF in the intracranial space produce communicating hydrocephalus and increased ICP. In 30% of patients, hydrocephalus will resolve spontaneously. Treatment consists of placing a drain to remove CSF. This therapy can be accomplished by inserting an external ventricular or lumbar drain.[18,22]

Intracerebral Hemorrhage

Description and Etiology

ICH is bleeding directly into cerebral tissue.[31] ICH destroys cerebral tissue, causes cerebral edema, and increases ICP. The source of intracerebral bleeding is usually a small artery. It also can occur secondary to an AVM or aneurysm rupture, a brain tumor, or a cerebral infarct.[31] The most common cause of spontaneous ICH is chronic hypertension,[31,32] and this section concentrates on spontaneous hypertensive ICH.

Spontaneous intracerebral hemorrhage. Spontaneous ICH accounts for at least 15% of all strokes.[31,32] The likelihood of death or disability is higher with ICH than with ischemic stroke or SAH. The mortality rate for hemorrhagic stroke is 50% within 1 month. Only 20% of patients with ICH return to a functional life at 6 months.[33] The critical risk factors for ICH are age and hypertension.[31,32]

ICH is most often caused by the rupture of a cerebral vessel resulting from a long-standing history of hypertension.[31] Risk factors include cigarette smoking, anticoagulation or fibrinolytic therapy, coagulation disorders, drug and alcohol abuse, diabetes, chronic kidney disease, and older age.[31,34] Often, on questioning, a patient with a hypertensive hemorrhage admits to having discontinued antihypertensive medication 2 to 3 weeks before the bleeding. Cerebral amyloid angiopathy is a major cause in older adults.[32]

Pathophysiology

The pathophysiology of ICH is caused by continued elevated blood pressure exerting force against smaller arterial vessels that have become damaged from arteriosclerotic changes. Eventually, these arteries break, and blood bursts from the vessels into the surrounding cerebral tissue, creating a hematoma. ICP rises precipitously in response to the increase in overall intracranial volume.[34]

Assessment and Diagnosis

The initial assessment usually reveals a critically ill patient who often is unconscious and requires ventilatory support. History from a relative or significant other describes a sudden onset of focal deficit often accompanied by severe headache, nausea, vomiting, and rapid neurologic deterioration. Signs and symptoms vary depending on the location of the ICH.[34] Approximately 50% of patients sustain an early loss of consciousness, a key feature differentiating ICH from ischemic stroke. More than one-half of patients with ICH present with a smooth progression of neurologic symptoms, an uncommon finding in cases of ischemic stroke or SAH.[35] One-third of patients have maximal symptoms at onset. Assessment of vital signs usually reveals a severely elevated blood pressure (200/100 to 250/150 mm Hg).

 **BOX 22.6 Evidence-Based Practice**

Spontaneous Intracerebral Hemorrhage Management Guidelines

The current recommendations from the American Heart Association and American Stroke Association for managing the patient with a spontaneous intracerebral hemorrhage (ICH) are located here: https://www.ahajournals.org/doi/full/10.1161/STR.0000000000000407.

Signs of increased ICP are often present when the patient arrives in the emergency department. Diagnosis is established easily with CT. Angiography is recommended only in patients considered surgical candidates and if a clear cause of bleeding is not evident.[33–35]

Medical Management

ICH is a medical emergency. Initial management requires attention to the airway, breathing, and circulation. Intubation is usually necessary. Anticoagulant medications should be reversed, and coagulopathies should be corrected. Current guidelines for managing patients with ICH are addressed in Box 22.6.

Blood pressure management. Blood pressure management must be based on individual factors. Reduction in blood pressure is usually necessary to decrease ongoing bleeding, but lowering blood pressure too much or too rapidly may compromise cerebral perfusion pressure (CPP), especially in a patient with elevated ICP. National guidelines recommend that in patients presenting with systolic blood pressure between 150 mm Hg and 220 mm Hg, lowering the systolic blood pressure to 140 mm Hg is safe and can effectively improve functional outcomes.[35]

Adjunct therapies. Increased ICP is common with ICH and is a significant contributor to mortality. Recommended management includes mannitol, when indicated; hyperventilation; and neuromuscular blockade with sedation. Steroids are avoided. CPP must be maintained at greater than 70 mm Hg.[33]

The goal for fluid management is euvolemia. Body temperature is maintained at less than 38.5°C using acetaminophen or cooling blankets. Euglycemia, a blood glucose level less than 140 mg/dL, is supported by insulin therapy, but hypoglycemia should be avoided. Short-acting benzodiazepines or propofol are recommended to treat agitation or hyperactivity (which would increase ICP). Pneumatic compression devices are used to decrease the risk of pulmonary embolism. Prophylactic anticonvulsant therapy is sometimes used.[31,35]

Surgical management. The benefit of surgical treatment for spontaneous ICH is unclear. Recommendations for surgical removal of the clot depend on the size and location of the hematoma, the patient's ICP, and other neurologic symptoms.[35] Medical treatment is recommended if the hemorrhage is small (less than 10 cm) or the neurologic deficit is minimal.[35] Likewise, surgery offers no improvement in outcome for patients with a Glasgow Coma Scale (GCS) score of 4 or less. Surgical evacuation of the clot is recommended for patients with cerebellar hemorrhage greater than 3 cm with neurologic deterioration or hydrocephalus with brainstem compression and young patients with moderate or large lobar hemorrhage with clinical deterioration.[35] Numerous techniques are being investigated to lessen the risk of brain damage associated with craniotomy for ICH.

BOX 22.7 DIAGNOSIS AND PATIENT CARE MANAGEMENT

Stroke

- Ineffective Tissue Perfusion due to decreased cerebral blood flow
- Unilateral Neglect due to perceptual disruption
- Impaired Verbal Communication due to cerebral speech center injury
- Impaired Swallowing due to neuromuscular impairment, fatigue, and limited awareness
- Risk for Aspiration
- Risk for Infection
- Anxiety due to threat to biological, psychological, or social integrity
- Disturbed Body Image due to actual change in body structure, function, or appearance
- Impaired Family Coping due to critically ill family member
- Lack of Knowledge of Treatment Regime due to lack of previous exposure to information (see Box 22.8, Patient and Family Education Plan for Stroke)

Patient Care Management plans are located in Appendix A.

Nursing Management

The patient care management plan for a patient with stroke incorporates a variety of problems (Box 22.7). The nurse has a significant role in monitoring for changes in neurologic and hemodynamic status, maintaining surveillance for complications, providing comfort and emotional support, and educating the patient and family.

Monitor for Changes in Neurologic and Hemodynamic Status

The goal of frequent assessments is early recognition of neurologic or hemodynamic deterioration. Close monitoring of the patient's neurologic and vital signs is essential and requires almost continuous observation. Automatic noninvasive devices such as a blood pressure cuff and a pulse oximeter are helpful. Seizure activity must be identified and treated immediately. It is essential that all personnel working with the patient be aware of the desired hemodynamic and neurologic parameters set by the practitioner and that the practitioner be notified at the first sign of any changes.[35,36]

Maintain Surveillance for Complications

A patient with a stroke should be monitored closely for signs of bleeding, vasospasm, and increased ICP. Other stroke complications include aspiration, malnutrition, pneumonia, DVT, pulmonary embolism, pressure injuries, contractures, and joint abnormalities.[19,36] Nursing measures to prevent these complications are well known.

Additional complications that may be seen in a patient with stroke are related to the area of the brain that has been damaged. Damage to the temporoparietal area can create disturbances affecting the patient's ability to interpret sensory information. Damage to the dominant hemisphere (usually left) produces problems with speech and language and abstract and analytic skills. Damage to the nondominant hemisphere (usually right) produces problems with spatial relationships. The resulting deficits include agnosia, apraxia, and visual field defects. Perceptual deficits are not as readily noticeable as motor deficits, but they may be more debilitating and lead to the inability to perform skilled or purposeful tasks.[37] The patient also may experience impaired swallowing.[8,9]

Bleeding and vasospasm. In a patient with a cerebral aneurysm, sudden onset of, or an increase in, headache and nausea and vomiting, increased blood pressure, and changes in respiration herald the onset of rebleeding. The first indication of vasospasm is usually the appearance of new focal or global neurologic deficits.[16,17,38]

Subarachnoid hemorrhage precautions. SAH precautions must be implemented to prevent any stress or strain that could precipitate rebleeding. Precautions include blood pressure management; bed rest; a dark, quiet environment; and stool softeners. Short-acting analgesics and sedatives are used to relieve pain and anxiety. The patient must be kept calm. Limb restraints cause straining and must be avoided. The head of the bed should always be elevated to 35 to 45 degrees. The patient is taught to avoid any activities that involve the performance of the Valsalva maneuver, such as pushing with the legs to move up in bed, straining for a bowel movement, or holding their breath during procedures or discomfort. DVT precautions are routinely implemented. Caregivers collaborate with the patient and family to establish a visitation plan to meet patient and family needs. Family members at the bedside can assist the patient to remain calm.[17]

Increased intracranial pressure. Numerous signs and symptoms of increased ICP can be observed. A change in the LOC is the most sensitive indicator. Others include unequal pupil size, decreased pupillary response to light, headache, projectile vomiting, altered breathing patterns, Cushing triad (bradycardia, systolic hypertension, and bradypnea), diminished brainstem reflexes, papilledema, and abnormal extension (decerebrate posturing) or flexion (decorticate posturing).

Damage to nondominant hemisphere. Patients with pathologic conditions affecting the nondominant hemisphere may exhibit emotional lability, with periods of euphoria, impulsiveness, and inattention. A short attention span, lack of insight, and poor judgment may lead to injuries as the patient attempts to perform activities beyond their capabilities. These patients also may experience agnosia, visual field defects, and apraxia.[37]

Agnosia. Agnosia is a disturbance in the perception of familiar sensory (e.g., verbal, tactile, visual) information. Unilateral neglect is a form of agnosia characterized by an unawareness or denial of the affected half of the body. This denial may range from inattention to refusing to acknowledge a paralysis by neglecting the involved side of the body or denying ownership of the side, attributing the paralyzed arm or leg to someone else. The neglect also may extend to extrapersonal space. This defect often results from right hemispheric brain damage that causes left hemiplegia.[37]

Other types of agnosia exist in addition to unilateral neglect. Some patients are unable to recognize objects visually (visual object agnosia). In contrast, others cannot recognize faces (prosopagnosia) and may have to rely on a familiar person's voice or characteristic mannerisms to identify that person. Tactile agnosia is a perceptual disorder in which a patient cannot recognize an object in their hand by touch alone. This disorder may occur even in an intact sense of touch. If allowed to see or hear the object, the patient usually recognizes it.[37]

Spatial orientation is affected, interfering with the patient's ability to judge position, distance, movement, form, and the relationship of their body parts to surrounding objects. Patients may confuse "up and down" or "forward and backward." They may have difficulty following a route from one place to another and get lost in once-familiar areas. Patients with stroke may also experience reading and writing problems related to visual perception and visuospatial deficits. One type of spatial dyslexia is related to unilateral spatial neglect. The patient may not look at the beginning of a line of written material that appears on the left. Instead, the patient fixes attention on a point to the right of the beginning of the line and reads to the end. If asked to draw a design, the person completes only half of a design or drawing.[39]

Visual field defects. Visual field defects may accompany agnosia, although they do not cause it. A hemispheric lesion can interrupt the visual pathways, with the resulting visual defect dependent on the location and extent of the lesion. At the optic chiasm, nerve fibers from each retina's nasal half cross to the opposite side, whereas fibers from the temporal half of each retina do not cross. This partial crossing allows binocular vision. In the optic chiasm, fibers from the nasal half of each retina join the uncrossed fibers from the temporal half of the retina to form the optic tract. Impulses conducted to the right hemisphere by the right optic tract represent the left field of vision, and impulses conducted to the left hemisphere by the left optic tract represent the right field of vision. Optic radiations extend back to the occipital lobes. Visual defects restricted to a single field, right or left, are called *homonymous hemianopsia.*[40]

The nurse may be the first to notice the patient has this defect. A patient with hemianopsia may neglect all sensory input from the affected side and initially may appear unresponsive if approached from the affected side. If the nurse approaches the patient from the healthy side, the patient may be quite alert. The patient eating food only from one-half of the tray is another clue to hemianopsia. Hemianopsia may recede gradually with time. Many patients can learn to scan their environment visually to compensate for the defect. However, in the acute stage of stroke, the patient may be too lethargic to follow instructions in methods of visual scanning. This visual defect can lead to fear and confusion and can present a risk to the patient's safety.[40]

Apraxia. Lesions in the parietal lobe and other cortical structures can result in apraxia, an inability to perform a learned movement voluntarily. Although a patient may understand the task and have intact motor ability, the patient cannot perform the task and often fumbles and makes mistakes. For example, a patient experiencing dressing apraxia may be unable to orient clothing in space, becoming tangled in their clothes when attempting to dress.[39]

Damage to dominant hemisphere. Damage to the dominant hemisphere produces problems with speech and language. Impaired communication is a condition that results from a patient's difficulty in expressing and exchanging thoughts, ideas, or desires. The posterior temporoparietal area contains the receptive speech center, known as the *Wernicke area*. The center for the perception of written language lies anterior to the visuoreceptive areas. Located at the base of the motor strip of the frontal lobe and slightly anterior to it is the *Broca area*, also known as the *motor speech center*. A large bundle of nerve fibers connects these sensory and motor areas. Rather than receptive and motor language functions being entirely within discrete areas, language is considered an integrated sensorimotor process, the management of which is roughly located in the dominant cerebral hemisphere. It also is recognized that the elaborately complex functions of speech and language depend on other associative areas of the cerebrum and their thalamic connections. Consequently, much inconsistency exists in the degree of communication impairment among patients with lesions in the same brain area.[39]

Aphasia is a loss of language abilities caused by brain injury, usually to the dominant hemisphere. It involves more than just understanding speech or expressing oneself through verbal means. *Language* is a broader term referring to the individual's attempts to interpret or convey through listening, speaking, reading, writing, and gesturing. Most cases of aphasia are partial rather than complete. The severity of the disorder depends on the area and the extent of the cerebral damage.[39]

Receptive aphasia. Receptive aphasia, also called *sensory, Wernicke*, or *fluent aphasia*, occurs when the connection between the primary auditory cortex in the temporal lobe and the angular gyrus in the parietal lobe is destroyed. The patient's speech comprehension is impaired, but they can still talk if the motor area for speech (Broca area) is intact. The patient may excessively speak, with many errors in the use of words. The patient can hear the examiner but cannot comprehend what is being said and cannot repeat the examiner's words. These patients may talk nonsensically, with a rambling speech that gives little information. Patients with receptive aphasia also cannot read words, although they can see them.[39]

Expressive aphasia. Expressive aphasia, also known as *motor, Broca*, or *nonfluent aphasia*, is primarily a deficit in language output or speech production. Depending on the size and exact location of the lesion, wide variation in the motor deficit can result. Expressive aphasia can range from mild dysarthria (imperfect articulation due to weakness or lack of coordination of speech musculature) to incorrect intonation and phrasing and, in its most severe form, to complete loss of ability to communicate through verbal and written means. In this severe form of aphasia, the patient also experiences a loss of ability to communicate through conventional gestures such as nodding or shaking the head for "yes" or "no." In most cases of expressive aphasia, the muscles of articulation are intact. If speech is possible, the words "yes" and "no" are occasionally uttered, sometimes appropriately. Some patients may sing the words of well-known songs. Other patients, when excited or angered, may utter expletives. Some patients with expressive aphasia struggle or hesitate in trying to express words. They struggle to form words while using motor musculature (*verbal apraxia*), an articulatory disorder that is a feature of some expressive types of aphasia. All these difficulties lead to exasperation and despair in the patient. Most patients with expressive aphasia also have severely impaired writing ability. Although penmanship may be intact, they cannot express themselves through writing—a deficit called *agraphia*. If the right hand is paralyzed, as is often the case, the patient still cannot write or print with the left hand. In the recovery phase of severe expressive aphasia, patients can speak aloud to some degree, although words are uttered slowly and laboriously. However, many patients can learn to communicate ideas to some extent.[39]

Global aphasia. Global aphasia results when a massive lesion affects the motor and sensory speech areas. The patient cannot transform sounds into words or comprehend spoken words. All language modalities are affected, and impairment may be so severe that the patient cannot communicate on any level. These patients usually have severe hemiplegia and homonymous hemianopsia. Their language function rarely recovers to a significant degree unless some transient disorder, such as cerebral edema or metabolic derangement, causes the lesion.[39]

Impaired swallowing. Normal swallowing occurs in four phases that are controlled by the cranial nerves. Damage

BOX 22.8 PATIENT AND FAMILY EDUCATION PLAN

Stroke

Before discharge, the patient should be able to teach back the following topics:

- Pathophysiology of disease
- Specific cause
- Risk factor modification
- Importance of taking medications
- Activities of daily living
- Measures to prevent injuries of impaired limbs
- Measures to compensate for residual deficits
- Basic rehabilitation techniques
- Importance of participating in a neurologic rehabilitation program or support group

to the brain, brainstem, or cranial nerves may result in various swallowing deficits that could place the patient at risk for aspiration. A patient with stroke is observed for signs of dysphagia, including drooling; difficulty handling oral secretions; absence of gag, cough, or swallowing reflexes; moist, gurgling voice quality; decreased mouth and tongue movements; and dysarthria. A speech therapy consultation is initiated if any of these signs are present. The patient must not be orally fed. In the absence of these warning signs, the patient may be fed, as ordered by the practitioner, although they must be continually monitored for signs of aspiration.[35,36]

Educate the Patient and Family

Rehabilitation starts in the critical care area, with a multidisciplinary team designing and implementing an individualized plan for maximizing the patient's potential for neurologic rehabilitation. Early in the patient's hospital stay, the patient and family must be taught about stroke, its causes, and its treatment (Box 22.8). Closer to discharge, teaching focuses on the interventions necessary for preventing the recurrence of the event and on maximizing the patient's rehabilitation potential. The patient's family must be encouraged to participate in the patient's care; learn how to feed, dress, and bathe the patient; and learn some basic rehabilitation techniques. The importance of participating in a neurologic rehabilitation program, support group, or both must be stressed.

Interprofessional collaborative management of a patient with stroke is outlined in Box 22.9.

BOX 22.9 Teamwork and Collaboration

Stroke

- Distinguish the cause of the stroke:
  - Ischemic
  - Subarachnoid hemorrhage
  - Cerebral aneurysm
  - Arteriovenous malformation
  - Intracerebral bleed
- Implement treatment according to the cause of the bleed:
  - Ischemic
    - Fibrinolytic therapy
    - Mechanical thrombectomy
    - Blood pressure management
  - Subarachnoid hemorrhage
    - Surgical aneurysm clipping or arteriovenous malformation excision
    - Embolization
  - Intracerebral bleed
    - Blood pressure management
- Protect the patient's airway.
- Administer oxygen.
- Provide ventilatory assistance as required.
- Perform frequent neurologic assessments.
- Maintain surveillance for complications:
  - Cerebral edema and intracranial hypertension
  - Cerebral vasospasm and ischemia
  - Rebleeding
  - Impaired swallowing
  - Neurologic deficits
  - Hyponatremia
  - Hydrocephalus
- Provide comfort and emotional support.
- Implement a rehabilitation program.
- Educate the patient and family.

COMA

Description and Etiology

Normal consciousness requires awareness and arousal. Awareness is the combination of cognition (mental and intellectual) and affect (mood) that can be construed based on the patient's interaction with the environment. Alterations of consciousness may result from deficits in awareness, arousal, or both. The four discrete disorders of consciousness are (1) coma, (2) vegetative state, (3) minimally conscious state, and (4) locked-in syndrome. Coma is characterized by the absence of both wakefulness and awareness, whereas a *vegetative state* is characterized by the presence of wakefulness with the absence of awareness. In a *minimally conscious state*, wakefulness is present, and awareness is severely diminished but not absent. *Locked-in syndrome* is characterized by wakefulness and awareness but with quadriplegia and the inability to communicate verbally; thus, the patient appears unconscious.[41] Box 22.10 lists the disorders of consciousness in descending order of wakefulness.

Coma is the deepest state of unconsciousness; arousal and awareness are lacking.[41,42] The patient cannot be aroused and does not demonstrate any purposeful response to the surrounding environment.[37] Coma is a symptom rather than a disease due to some underlying process.[42] The incidence of coma is challenging to ascertain because various conditions can induce coma.[42] This state of unconsciousness is commonly encountered in the critical care unit and is the focus of the following discussion.

Etiology

The causes of coma can be divided into two general categories: structural or surgical and metabolic or medical. Structural causes of coma include ischemic stroke, ICH, trauma, and brain tumors.[42] Metabolic causes of coma include drug overdose, infectious diseases, endocrine disorders, and poisonings.[42] The three most common causes of nontraumatic coma are stroke, anoxia, and poisonings.[42] Coma demands immediate attention, resulting in a high percentage of admissions to all hospital services.[43] Box 22.11 lists the possible causes of coma.

BOX 22.17 Operative Terms

- *Burr hole:* Hole made into the skull using a special drill
- *Craniotomy:* Surgical opening of the skull
- *Craniectomy:* Removal of a portion of the skull without replacing it
- *Cranioplasty:* Plastic repair of the skull
- *Supratentorial:* Above the tentorium, separating the cerebrum from the cerebellum
- *Infratentorial:* Below the tentorium, includes the brainstem and the cerebellum; an infratentorial surgical approach may be used for temporal or occipital lesions
- *Stereotactic:* Minimally invasive surgical intervention that uses a three-dimensional coordinate system to localize a specific area of the brain for ablation, biopsy, dissection, or radiosurgery

risk for complications because of underlying cardiopulmonary dysfunction or the surgical approach used.[58] Box 22.17 provides definitions of common neurosurgical terms.

Preoperative Care

Protection of the integrity of the CNS is a major priority of care for a patient awaiting neurosurgery. Optimal arterial oxygenation, hemodynamic stability, and cerebral perfusion are essential for adequate cerebral oxygenation. Management of seizure activity is critical for controlling metabolic needs.[60]

Detailed assessment and documentation of the patient's preoperative neurologic status are imperative for accurate postoperative evaluation. Attention is focused on identifying and describing the nature and extent of any preoperative neurologic deficits. When pituitary surgery is planned, a thorough assessment of endocrine function is necessary to prevent major intraoperative and postoperative complications.[60]

Trends in health care demand judicious use of routine preoperative studies. Depending on the type of surgery to be performed and the general health of the patient, preoperative screening may include a complete blood cell count; tests for blood urea nitrogen, creatinine, and fasting blood sugar; chest radiography; and electrocardiography. A blood type and crossmatch may also be ordered.[61]

Preoperative Teaching

Preoperative teaching is necessary to prepare the patient and family for what to expect in the postoperative period. A description of the intravascular lines and intracranial catheters used during the postoperative period allows the family to focus on the patient and not be overwhelmed by masses of tubing. Some or all of the patient's hair is shaved off in the operating room, and a large, bulky, turban-like craniotomy dressing is applied. Most patients experience some degree of postoperative eye or facial swelling and periorbital ecchymosis. An explanation of these temporary changes in appearance helps alleviate the shock and fear many patients and families experience in the immediate postoperative period.[61]

All patients who undergo craniotomy require instruction to avoid activities that provoke sudden changes in ICP. These activities include bending, lifting, straining, and the Valsalva maneuver. Patients commonly elicit the Valsalva maneuver during repositioning in bed by holding their breath and straining with a closed epiglottis. This action is prevented effectively by teaching the patient to continue to breathe deeply through the mouth during all position changes.[61]

Patients undergoing transsphenoidal surgery require preparation for the sensations associated with nasal packing. Patients often awaken with alarm because of the inability to breathe through the nose. Preoperative instruction in mouth breathing and avoidance of coughing, sneezing, or blowing of the nose facilitates postoperative cooperation.[60]

Psychosocial Preparation

The psychosocial issues associated with the prospect of neurosurgery cannot be overemphasized. Few procedures are as threatening as procedures involving the brain or spinal cord. For some patients, the fear of permanent neurologic impairment may be as ominous or more ominous than the fear of death. Steps to meet the needs of the patient and the family include collaboration with religious and social services personnel, patient-managed visitation, and provision of as much privacy as the patient's condition permits. The patient and family must be allowed to express their fears and concerns jointly and apart from each other.[58]

Surgical Considerations

Although the emphasis in the surgical approach is to gain adequate exposure to the surgical site, the neurosurgeon must select a route that also produces the least amount of disruption to the intracranial contents. Neural tissue is unforgiving. A significant portion of neurologic trauma and postoperative deficits is related to the surgical pathway through the brain tissue rather than the procedure performed at the site of pathology. Depending on the location of the lesion and the surgical route chosen, a transcranial or a transsphenoidal approach is used to open the skull.

Transcranial Approach

In the transcranial approach, a scalp incision is made, and a series of burr holes are drilled into the skull to form an outline of the area to be opened (Fig. 22.7). A special saw is used to cut between the holes. In most cases, the bone flap is left attached to the muscle to create a hinge effect. Sometimes, the bone flap is removed completely, placed in the abdomen for later retrieval and implantation, or discarded and replaced with synthetic material. Next, the dura mater is opened and retracted. After the intracranial procedure, the dura mater and the bone flap are closed, the muscles and scalp are sutured, and a turban-like dressing is applied.[58]

Transsphenoidal Approach

The transsphenoidal approach is the technique of choice for removing a pituitary tumor without extension into the intracranial vault (Fig. 22.8).[60,61] This approach creates a microsurgical entrance into the cranial vault through the nasal cavity. The sphenoid sinus is entered to reach the anterior wall of the sella turcica. The sphenoid bone and the dura mater are opened to gain intracranial access. After removing the tumor, the surgical bed is packed with a small section of adipose tissue taken from the patient's abdomen or thigh. After the closure of the intranasal structures, nasal splints and soft packing or nasal tampons impregnated with antibiotic ointment are placed in the nasal cavities. Occasionally, epistaxis balloons are used instead. A nasal drip pad or mustache-type dressing is placed at the base of the nose to catch surgical drainage.[58]

Positioning

The patient may be placed in the supine, prone, or sitting position for a craniotomy procedure. A skull clamp connected to skull pins positions and secures the patient's head throughout the operation.

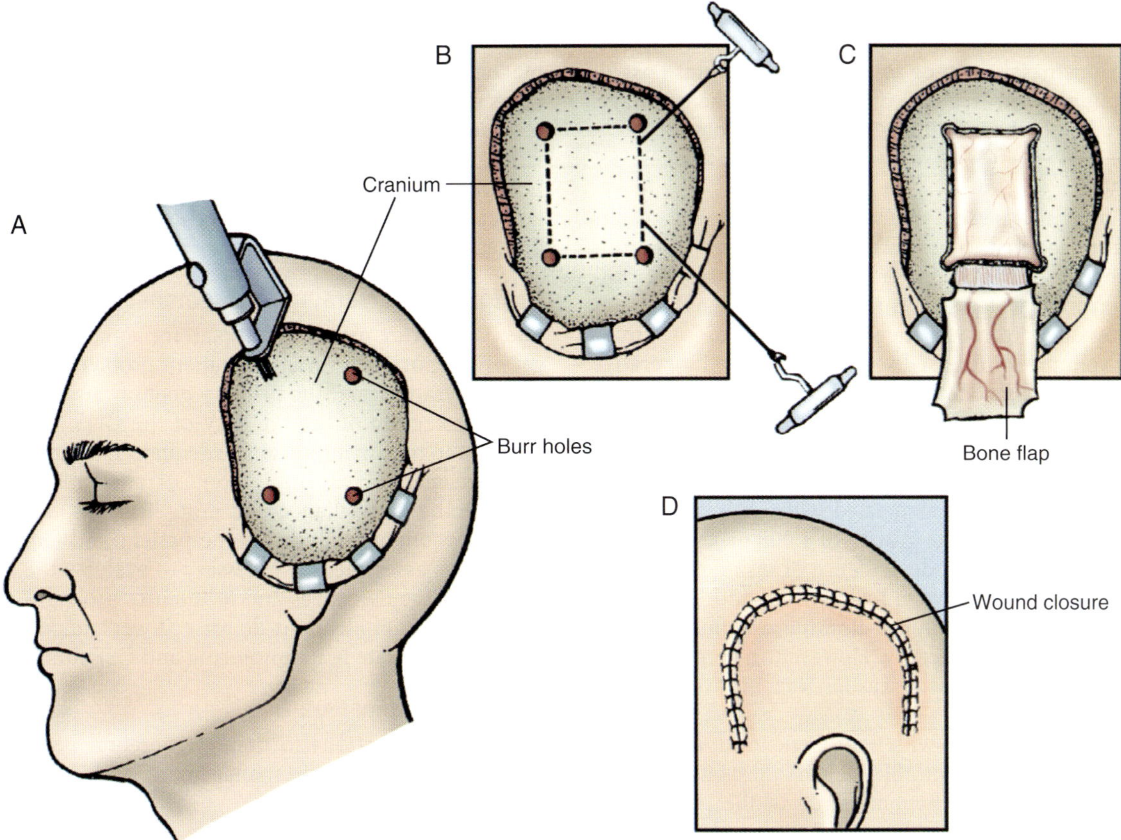

FIG. 22.7 Craniotomy Procedure. (A) Burr holes are drilled into the skull. (B) The skull is cut between burr holes with a surgical saw. (C) The bone flap is turned back to expose cranial contents. (D) After surgery, the bone flap is replaced and the wound is closed. (From Monahan FD, Sands J, Neighbors M, et al. eds. *Phipps' Medical-Surgical Nursing: Health and Illness Perspective*. 8th ed. Mosby; 2007.)

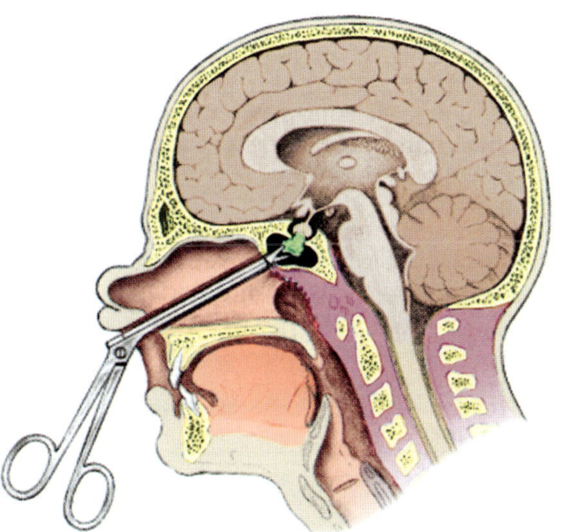

FIG. 22.8 Transsphenoidal Hypophysectomy.

During a transsphenoidal or transcranial approach into the infratentorial area, the patient's head is elevated during surgery. This position places the patient at risk for an air embolism. Air can enter the vascular system through the edges of the dura mater or a venous opening. Continuous monitoring of the patient's heart sounds by Doppler signal allows immediate recognition of this complication. If air embolism occurs, an attempt may be made to withdraw the embolus from the right atrium through a central line. Flooding the surgical field with irrigation fluid and placing a moistened sterile surgical sponge over the surgical site creates an immediate barrier to any further air entrance.[58]

Postoperative Medical Management

Definitive management of a postoperative neurosurgical patient varies depending on the underlying reason for the craniotomy. During the initial postoperative period, management is usually directed toward preventing complications. Complications associated with a craniotomy include intracranial hypertension, surgical hemorrhage, fluid imbalance, CSF leak, and DVT.

Intracranial Hypertension

Postoperative cerebral edema is expected to peak 48 to 72 hours after surgery. If the bone flap is not replaced during surgery, intracranial hypertension will produce bulging at the surgical site. Close monitoring of the surgical site is important to ensure the integrity of the incision can be maintained. Management of intracranial hypertension after craniotomy is usually accomplished through CSF drainage, patient positioning, and steroid administration.[62]

Surgical Hemorrhage

After a transcranial procedure, surgical bleeding can occur in the intracranial vault and manifests as signs and symptoms of increasing ICP. Bleeding after a transsphenoidal craniotomy may be evident from external drainage, the patient's complaint of persistent postnasal drip, or excessive swallowing. Loss of vision after pituitary surgery indicates an evolving hemorrhage. Postoperative hemorrhage requires surgical reexploration.[62]

Fluid Imbalance

Fluid imbalance in a patient after craniotomy usually results from a disturbance in the production or secretion of antidiuretic hormone (ADH). ADH is secreted by the posterior pituitary (neurohypophysis) gland. It stimulates the renal tubules and collecting ducts to retain water in response to low circulating blood volume or increased serum osmolality. Inoperative trauma or postoperative edema of the pituitary gland or hypothalamus can result in insufficient ADH secretion. The outcome is unabated renal water loss even when blood volume is low, and serum osmolality is high. This condition is known as *diabetes insipidus* (DI). The polyuria associated with DI is often more than 200 mL/h. Urine specific gravity of 1.005 or less and elevated serum osmolality provide evidence of insufficient ADH. The loss of volume may provoke hypotension and inadequate cerebral perfusion. DI is usually self-limiting, and fluid replacement is the only required therapy. However, in some cases, it may be necessary to administer vasopressin intravenously to manage fluid loss.[63]

SIADH commonly occurs with neurologic insult and results from excessive ADH secretion. SIADH manifests as inappropriate water retention with hyponatremia in the presence of normal renal function. Urine specific gravity is elevated, and urine osmolality is greater than serum osmolality. The dangers associated with SIADH include circulating volume overload and electrolyte imbalance, both of which may impair neurologic functioning. SIADH is usually self-limiting, with the mainstay of treatment being fluid restriction.[63]

Cerebrospinal Fluid Leak

Leakage of CSF results from an opening in the subarachnoid space, as evidenced by clear fluid draining from the surgical site. When this complication occurs after transsphenoidal surgery, it is evidenced by excessive, clear drainage from the nose or persistent postnasal drip.[64] A specimen is tested for glucose content to differentiate CSF drainage from postoperative serous drainage. A CSF leak is confirmed by glucose values of 30 mg/dL or greater. Management of a patient with a CSF leak includes bed rest and head elevation. Lumbar puncture or placement of a lumbar subarachnoid catheter may be used to reduce CSF pressure until the dura mater heals. The risk of meningitis associated with CSF leak often necessitates surgical repair to reseal the opening.[65]

Deep Vein Thrombosis

Patients who have undergone neurosurgery are at particularly high risk for developing DVT. Research has demonstrated that these patients have a variety of additional risk factors, including preoperative leg weakness, longer preoperative and postoperative stay in the critical care unit, longer operative procedure time, prone positioning on frames with flexion of the hips or knees, longer time in the postanesthesia care unit, more days on bed rest, lengthy operative procedures, and delay of postoperative mobility and activity.[66,67] Clinical manifestations of DVT include leg or calf pain and erythema, warmth, and swelling of the affected limb. However, a patient with a DVT is often asymptomatic, and the diagnosis is not made until the patient experiences a pulmonary embolus.[68] The primary treatment for DVT is mechanical and pharmacological prophylaxis. After neurosurgery, sequential (intermittent) pneumatic compression sleeves are effective in reducing the incidence of DVT. Effectiveness is enhanced when these devices are initiated in the preoperative period. Low-molecular-weight heparin may also be used prophylactically in high-risk patients when the risk of bleeding has decreased.[69]

Postoperative Nursing Management

The patient care management plan for a patient after neurosurgery incorporates a variety of patient problems (Box 22.18). As in preoperative care, the primary goal of nursing management is the protection of the integrity of the CNS. The nurse has a significant role in preserving adequate CPP, promoting arterial oxygenation, providing comfort and emotional support, maintaining surveillance for complications, initiating early rehabilitation, and educating the patient and family. Frequent neurologic assessment is necessary to evaluate the accomplishment of these objectives and to identify problems and quickly intervene if complications do arise. A ventriculostomy often is placed to facilitate ICP monitoring and CSF drainage.

Preserve Cerebral Perfusion

Nursing interventions to preserve cerebral perfusion include patient positioning, fluid management, and avoiding postoperative vomiting and fever.

Positioning. Patient positioning is an essential component of care after craniotomy. The head of the bed should always be elevated to 30 to 45 degrees (unless otherwise ordered) to reduce the incidence of bleeding, facilitate venous drainage, and manage ICP. Other positioning measures to control ICP include always maintaining the patient's head in a neutral position and avoiding neck or hip flexion. These positioning rules must be followed throughout all nursing activities, including linen changes and patient transporting for diagnostic evaluation. Most patients after craniotomy can be turned from side to side within these restrictions, using pillows for support, except in some cases of extensive tumor removal, cranioplasty, and when the bone flap is not replaced. Specific orders from the surgeon must be obtained in these instances. A patient with an infratentorial incision may be restricted to only a very small pillow under the head to prevent strain on the incision. Avoidance of anterior or lateral neck flexion also protects the integrity of this type of incision.

BOX 22.18 DIAGNOSIS AND PATIENT CARE MANAGEMENT

Neurosurgery

- Decreased Intracranial Adaptive Capacity due to failure of normal intracranial compensatory mechanisms
- Ineffective Tissue Perfusion due to decreased cerebral blood flow
- Acute Pain due to transmission and perception of cutaneous, visceral, muscular, or ischemic impulses
- Disturbed Body Image due to actual change in body structure, function, or appearance
- Lack of Knowledge of Treatment Regime due to lack of previous exposure to information (See Box 22.19, Patient and Family Education Plan for Craniotomy)

Patient Care Management plans are located in Appendix A.

Fluid management. Fluid management is another important component of postcraniotomy care. Hourly monitoring of fluid intake and output facilitates early identification of fluid imbalance. Urine-specific gravity must be measured if DI is suspected. Fluid restriction may be ordered as a routine measure to lessen the severity of cerebral edema or as a treatment for the fluid and electrolyte imbalances associated with SIADH.[63]

Avoidance of vomiting and fever. Experiencing nausea and vomiting after a craniotomy is not uncommon and can be attributed to various factors related to the surgery, anesthesia, and the body's response to the procedure. Postoperative vomiting must be avoided to prevent sharp spikes in ICP and possibly surgical hemorrhage. Antiemetics are administered as soon as nausea is apparent. Using medications that target different chemoreceptors in the vomiting center of the brain is recommended. Ondansetron and dexamethasone are the most frequently used.[70] Early nutrition in the patient is beneficial. If the patient cannot eat, enteral hyperalimentation delivered through a feeding tube is the preferred method of nutrition support and can be initiated 24 hours after surgery. Postoperative fever may also adversely affect ICP and increase the brain's metabolic needs. Acetaminophen is administered orally, rectally, or through a feeding tube. External cooling measures such as a hypothermia blanket may be necessary.

Promote Arterial Oxygenation

Routine pulmonary care is used to maintain airway clearance and prevent pulmonary complications. To avert dangerous elevations in ICP, this care measure must be performed using proper technique and at time intervals that are adequately spaced from other patient care activities. If pulmonary complications arise, consideration must be given to maintaining adequate oxygenation during repositioning. It may be necessary to restrict turning to only the side that places the good lung down.

Provide Comfort and Emotional Support

Pain management in patients after craniotomy primarily involves the management of headaches. Traditionally small doses of intravenous opioids are used with the goal of starting oral analgesics as soon as they can be tolerated. Nonopioid analgesics may be used as an adjunct medication. Because opioid analgesics cause constipation, administering stool softeners and initiating a bowel program are important components of postcraniotomy care. Constipation is hazardous because straining to have a bowel movement can create significant elevations in blood pressure and ICP. However, newer approaches are being evaluated because of the side effects of opioid analgesics. Intraoperative dexmedetomidine, preoperative and postoperative gabapentin and acetaminophen, and scalp blocks are some of the alternative pain modalities being researched.[71]

Maintain Surveillance for Complications

Following neurosurgery, patients are at risk for infection, corneal abrasions, and injury from falls or seizures.

Infection. After neurosurgery, patients are at risk for various infections, including meningitis, cerebral abscesses, bone flap infections, and subdural empyema.[72] Care of the incision and surgical dressings is specific to the institution and the practitioner. The rule of thumb for a craniotomy dressing is to reinforce it as needed and change it only on a practitioner's order. A drain is often left in place to facilitate decompression of the surgical site. If a ventriculostomy is present, it is treated as a component of the surgical site. All drainage devices must be secured to the dressing to prevent unintentional displacement with patient movement. Sterile technique is required to prevent infection. Postoperatively, an infection should be suspected if the patient exhibits signs of mental status changes, headache, fever, purulent drainage, and swelling around the incision site.[72]

Corneal abrasions. Routine eye care may be necessary to prevent corneal drying and ulceration. Periorbital edema interferes with normal blinking and eyelid closure, which is essential to adequate corneal lubrication. Saline drops are instilled to maintain lubrication. Covering the eyes with a polyethylene film extending over the orbits and eyebrows may be beneficial if the patient remains comatose.[49]

Injury. After craniotomy, the patient may experience periods of altered mentation. Protection from injury may require the use of restraint devices. The bed's side rails must be padded to protect the patient from harm. Having a family member stay at the bedside or using music therapy is often helpful to keep the patient calm during periods of restlessness. In rare circumstances, continuous sedation with or without neuromuscular blockade may be necessary to manage patient activity and metabolic needs on a short-term basis.

Initiate Early Rehabilitation

Increased activity, including ambulation, is begun as soon as tolerated by the patient in the postoperative period. Rehabilitation measures and discharge planning may start in the critical care unit, but discussion is beyond the scope of this chapter. Transfer to a general care or rehabilitation unit is usually accomplished as soon as the patient is deemed stable and free of complications.

Educate the Patient and Family

Preoperatively, the patient and family should be taught about the precipitating event necessitating the craniotomy and its expected outcome (Box 22.19). The severity of the disease and the need for critical care management postoperatively must be stressed. As the patient moves toward discharge, teaching

BOX 22.19 PATIENT AND FAMILY EDUCATION PLAN

Neurosurgery

Before discharge, the patient should be able to teach back the following topics:

Before Surgery

- Pathophysiology and the expected outcome of underlying disease
- Need for critical care management after surgery
- Routine preoperative surgical care

After Surgery

- Routine postoperative surgical care
- Discharge medications—purpose, dosage, and side effects
- Incisional care
- Signs and symptoms of infection
- Signs and symptoms of increased intracranial pressure
- Measures to compensate for residual deficits
- Basic rehabilitation techniques
- Importance of participating in a neurologic rehabilitation program

CPP, Cerebral perfusion pressure; *ICP,* intracranial pressure; *$PaCO_2$,* arterial partial pressure of carbon dioxide.

focuses on medication instructions, incisional care, including the signs of infection, and the signs and symptoms of increased ICP. If the patient has neurologic deficits, teaching focuses on the interventions to maximize the patient's rehabilitation potential, and the patient's family members must be encouraged to participate in the patient's care and learn some basic rehabilitation techniques. The importance of participating in a neurologic rehabilitation program must be stressed.

INTRACRANIAL HYPERTENSION

Pathophysiology

The intracranial space comprises three components: (1) brain substance (80%), (2) CSF (10%), and (3) blood (10%). Under normal physiologic conditions, the mean ICP is maintained at less than 15 mm Hg.[73–75] Essential to understanding the pathophysiology of ICP, the Monro–Kellie hypothesis proposes that an increase in the volume of one intracranial component must be compensated by a decrease in one or more of the other components so that total volume remains fixed. This compensation, although limited, includes displacing CSF from the intracranial vault to the lumbar cistern, increasing CSF absorption, and compressing the low-pressure venous system.[75,76] Pathophysiologic alterations that can elevate ICP are outlined in Table 22.4.

Volume-Pressure Curve

When capable of compliance, the brain can tolerate significant increases in intracranial volume without increasing ICP. However, the amount of intracranial compliance has a limit. After this limit has been reached, a state of decompensation with increased ICP results. As the ICP increases, the relationship between volume and pressure changes, and small increases in volume may cause major elevations in ICP (Fig. 22.9).[73,74] The exact configuration of the volume-pressure curve and the point at which the steep increase in pressure occurs vary among patients. The configuration of this curve is also influenced by the cause, and the rate of volume increases within the intracranial vault; for example, neurologic deterioration occurs more rapidly in a patient with an acute epidural hematoma than in a patient with a meningioma of the same size. Regardless of how fast the pressure increases, intracranial hypertension occurs when ICP is greater than 20 mm Hg.[73,74]

TABLE 22.4 Mechanisms of Intracranial Pressure Elevation

Pathophysiology	Examples
Disorders of CSF	
Overproduction of CSF	Choroid plexus tumors (papilloma or carcinoma)
Communicating hydrocephalus	Obstructed arachnoid villi Old subarachnoid hemorrhage
Noncommunicating hydrocephalus	Posterior fossa tumor obstructing aqueduct Aqueductal stenosis
Interstitial edema	Any of above
Disorders of Intracranial Blood Flow	
Intracranial hemorrhage	Epidural hematoma Subdural hematoma Intraparenchymal hematoma
Vasospasm	Subarachnoid hemorrhage
Vasodilation	Elevated $PaCO_2$
Increasing cerebral blood volume	Hypoxia
Disorders of Brain Substance	
Expanding mass lesion with local vasogenic edema	Brain tumor Abscess Brain injury Ischemic stroke
Ischemic brain injury with cytotoxic edema	Anoxic brain injury Hypoxic encephalopathy
Increased cerebral metabolic rate increasing CBF	Seizures Hyperthermia

CBF, Cerebral blood flow; CSF, cerebrospinal fluid; $PaCO_2$*, arterial partial pressure of carbon dioxide.*

Cerebral Blood Flow and Autoregulation

CBF corresponds to the brain's metabolic demands and is normally 50 mL/100 g of brain tissue/min. Although the brain makes up only 2% of body weight, it requires 15% to 20% of the resting cardiac output and 15% of the body's oxygen demands. The normal brain has a complex capacity to maintain constant CBF, despite wide ranges in systemic arterial pressure—an effect known as *autoregulation*. A mean arterial pressure of 50 to 150 mm Hg does not alter CBF when autoregulation is functioning. Outside the limits of this autoregulation, CBF becomes passively dependent on the perfusion pressure.[75]

Factors other than arterial blood pressure that affect CBF are conditions that result in acidosis, alkalosis, and changes in metabolic rate. Conditions that cause acidosis (e.g., hypoxia, hypercapnia, ischemia) result in cerebrovascular dilation. Conditions causing alkalosis (e.g., hypocapnia) result in cerebrovascular constriction. Usually, a reduction in metabolic rate (e.g., from hypothermia or barbiturates) decreases CBF, and increases in metabolic rate (e.g., from hyperthermia) increase CBF.[76]

Arterial blood gases exert a profound effect on CBF. Carbon dioxide, which affects the pH of the blood, is a potent vasoactive substance. Carbon dioxide retention (hypercapnia) leads

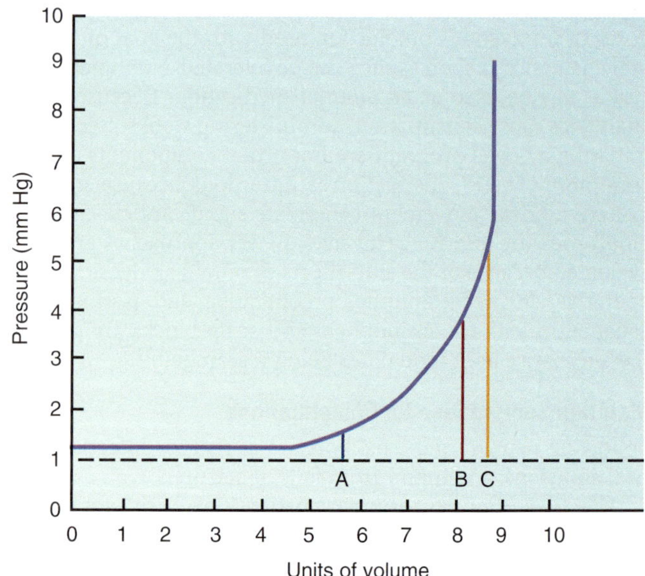

FIG. 22.9 Intracranial Volume-Pressure Curve. *A*, Pressure is normal, and increases in intracranial volume are tolerated without increases in intracranial pressure. *B*, Volume increases may cause pressure increases. *C*, Small increases in volume may cause larger increases in pressure.

Intracranial Hypertension

Clinical and diagnostic assessments	Signs	Nursing interventions
• History and risk factors • Disorders of CSF • Disorders of intracranial blood flow • Disorders of brain tissue • Obtain vital signs • O_2 saturation • Clinical assessment • LOC • Pupils • Motor function • Respiratory function • Laboratory studies • Obtain ABGs • Diagnostic procedures • Noncontrast CT • MRI	• Decreased LOC • Confusion → Coma • Pupillary changes • Unequal pupils → Bilateral fixed and dilated • Headache • Unresponsive to pain medication • Changes in breathing pattern • Cheyne-stokes → Ataxic • Nausea and vomiting • Projectile vomiting • Extremity weakness or paralysis • Slurred speech • Cushing's triad: (Late sign) • Systolic hypertension with widening pulse pressure • Bradycardia • Bradypnea	• Position the patient to achieve maximal ICP reduction • Reduce environmental stimulation • Maintain normothermia • Management ventilation to ensure normal $PaCO_2$ level (35mm Hg ± 2) • Administer diuretic agents, anticonvulsants, sedation, analgesia, paralytic agents, and vasoactive medications to ensure CPP >70 mm Hg • Drain cerebrospinal fluid for ICP >20 mm Hg • Protect the patient's airway • Perform frequent neurologic assessments. • Maintain surveillance for complications • Provide comfort and emotional support • Implement appropriate rehabilitation program • Educate the patient and family

FIG. 22.10 Summary of Key Concepts Related to Intracranial Hypertension. *ABGs*, Arterial blood gases; *CPP*, cerebral perfusion pressure; *CSF*, cerebrospinal fluid; *CT*, computed tomography; *ICP*, intracranial pressure; *LOC*, level of consciousness; *MRI*, magnetic resonance imaging; O_2, oxygen. $PaCO_2$, partial pressure of carbon dioxide in arterial blood.

to cerebral vasodilation, with increased cerebral blood volume, whereas hypocapnia leads to cerebral vasoconstriction and reduced cerebral blood volume. However, prolonged hypocapnia can lead to cerebral ischemia, especially at an arterial partial pressure of carbon dioxide ($PaCO_2$) levels less than 20 mm Hg. Low arterial partial pressure of oxygen (PaO_2) levels, especially less than 40 mm Hg, lead to cerebral vasodilation, which increases the intracranial blood volume and can contribute to increased ICP. High PaO_2 levels have not been shown to affect CBF in either direction.[76]

Assessment and Diagnosis

The numerous signs and symptoms of increased ICP include decreased LOC, Cushing triad (bradycardia, systolic hypertension, and widening pulse pressure), diminished brainstem reflexes, papilledema, decerebrate posturing (abnormal extension), decorticate posturing (abnormal flexion), unequal pupil size, projectile vomiting, decreased pupillary reaction to light, altered breathing patterns, and headache.[77] Patients may exhibit one or all of these symptoms, depending on the underlying cause of the elevation in ICP. One of the earliest and most important signs of increased ICP is decreased LOC. This change must be reported immediately to the practitioner.[76,77]

Monitoring Devices

A monitoring device may be placed within the skull to quantify ICP in a patient with suspected intracranial hypertension. Under normal physiologic conditions, the mean ICP is maintained at less than 15 mm Hg. The device monitors serial ICPs and assists with managing intracranial hypertension. An increase in ICP can decrease blood flow to the brain, causing brain damage. The monitoring device can also provide sterile access for draining excess CSF. The four sites for monitoring ICP are the intraventricular space, the subarachnoid space, the epidural space, and the parenchyma. Each site has advantages and disadvantages for monitoring ICP. The type of monitor chosen depends on the suspected pathologic condition and the practitioner's preferences.[75–78] Chapter 21 provides a more detailed discussion of ICP monitoring.

Medical and Nursing Management

After intracranial hypertension is observed, therapy must be prompt to prevent secondary insults. Although the exact pressure level denoting intracranial hypertension is uncertain, most current evidence suggests that ICP generally must be treated when it exceeds 20 mm Hg.[76] All therapies are directed toward reducing the volume of one or more components (e.g., blood, brain, CSF) within the intracranial vault. A primary goal of therapy is to determine the cause of the elevated pressure and, if possible, to remove the reason.[76] In the absence of a surgically treatable mass lesion, intracranial hypertension is treated medically. Nurses are essential in rapidly assessing and implementing appropriate therapies for reducing ICP. Fig. 22.10 summarizes the key concepts for managing a patient with intracranial hypertension.

Positioning and Other Nursing Activities

Positioning of the patient is a significant factor in the prevention and treatment of intracranial hypertension. Head elevation has long been advocated as a conventional nursing intervention to management ICP, presumably by increasing venous return; however, this may decrease CPP. Close monitoring of ICP and

CPP should be done with positioning, customizing positioning to maximize CPP and minimize ICP.[75]

Positions that impede venous return from the brain cause elevations in ICP. Obstruction of jugular veins or increased intrathoracic or intraabdominal pressure is communicated as increased pressure throughout the open venous system, impeding drainage from the brain and increasing ICP. Positions that decrease venous return from the head (e.g., Trendelenburg, prone, extreme flexion of the hips, and angulation of the neck) must be avoided if possible. If changes to positions such as Trendelenburg are necessary to provide adequate pulmonary care, critical care nurses must closely monitor ICP and vital signs.

Some routine nursing activities affect ICP and may be harmful. Positive end-expiratory pressures greater than 20 cm H_2O, coughing, suctioning, tight tracheostomy tube ties, and Valsalva maneuver have been associated with increased ICP. Cumulative increases in ICP have been reported when care activities are performed one after another. Conversely, family contact and gentle touch have been associated with decreases in ICP.

Hyperventilation

Managed hyperventilation has been an essential therapy adjunct for patients with increased ICP. The rationale employed in hyperventilation is that if $PaCO_2$ can be reduced from its normal level of 35 to 40 mm Hg to a range of 25 to 30 mm Hg in a patient with intracranial hypertension, vasoconstriction of cerebral arteries, reduction of CBF, and increased venous return will result. This practice is being reexamined. Additional research has indicated that severe or prolonged hyperventilation can reduce cerebral perfusion and lead to cerebral ischemia and infarction.[79] The current trend is maintaining $PaCO_2$ levels on the lower side of normal (35 mm Hg ± 2) by carefully monitoring arterial blood gas measurements and adjusting ventilator settings.[75–78]

Although hypoxemia must be avoided, excessively high oxygen levels offer no benefits, and increasing inspired oxygen concentrations to greater than 60% may lead to toxic changes in lung tissue. Pulse oximetry has led to greater awareness of the circumstances, such as pain and anxiety, that can cause oxygen desaturation and elevate ICP.

Temperature Management

Directly proportional to body temperature, cerebral metabolic rate increases by 7% per 1°C of increase in body temperature.[76,77] This fact is significant because blood flow to the brain must increase as the cerebral metabolic rate increases to meet the tissue demands. To avoid the increased blood volume associated with an increased cerebral metabolic rate, nurses must prevent hyperthermia in a patient with a brain injury. Antipyretics and cooling devices must be used when appropriate while the source of the fever is being determined.[76,77]

Blood Pressure Management

Maintenance of arterial blood pressure in the high-normal range is essential in patients with brain injury. Inadequate perfusion pressure decreases the supply of nutrients and oxygen requirements for cerebral metabolic needs. However, a blood pressure that is too high increases cerebral blood volume and may increase ICP.[76] Fig. 22.11 shows the relationship between blood pressure and ICP.

Hypertension. Management of systemic hypertension may require nothing more than administering a sedative agent. Small, frequent doses may be sufficient to blunt noxious stimuli

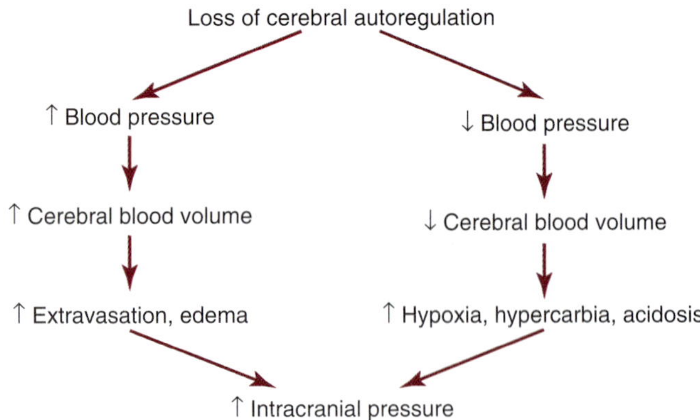

FIG. 22.11 Loss of Pressure Autoregulation.

and prevent them from triggering increases in blood pressure. When sedation proves inadequate in managing systemic arterial hypertension, antihypertensive agents are used. Care must be taken in choosing these agents because many peripheral vasodilators (e.g., nitroprusside, nitroglycerin) are also cerebral vasodilators. All antihypertensives are believed to cause some degree of cerebral vasodilation. To reduce this vasodilating effect, concurrent treatment with beta-blockers (e.g., metoprolol, labetalol) may be beneficial.[76]

Hypotension. Systemic hypotension should be treated aggressively with fluids to maintain a systolic blood pressure greater than 90 mm Hg. Depending on the patient's condition, crystalloids, colloids, and blood products can be used. Studies have demonstrated a positive effect on ICP and CPP with hypertonic saline.[80,81] If fluids fail to elevate the patient's blood pressure adequately, inotropic agents may be necessary.

Seizure Management

The incidence of posttraumatic seizures in patients with head injuries has been estimated to be 15% to 20%. Because of the risk of a secondary ischemic insult associated with seizures, many practitioners prescribe anticonvulsant medications prophylactically. Seizures cause metabolic requirements to increase, which results in the elevation of CBF, cerebral blood volume, and ICP, even in paralyzed patients. If blood flow cannot match demand, ischemia develops, cerebral energy stores are depleted, and irreversible neuronal destruction occurs.[75] Fast-acting, short-duration agents such as lorazepam may be indicated for breakthrough seizures until therapeutic medication levels can be achieved.[82]

Cerebrospinal Fluid Drainage

CSF drainage for intracranial hypertension may be used with other treatment modalities (Figs. 22.12 and 22.13). CSF drainage is accomplished by inserting a pliable catheter into the anterior horn of the lateral ventricle (ventriculostomy), preferably on the nondominant side. This drainage can help support the patient through cerebral edema periods by controlling ICP spikes. A major advantage of ventriculostomy is its dual role as a monitoring device and a treatment modality.[83] Care should be taken to avoid infection. However, cleansing ointment such as bacitracin or povidone is not recommended. Ventriculitis occurs in 10% to 20% of patients with a ventriculostomy.[84]

Hyperosmolar Therapy

Osmotic diuretics and hypertonic saline have also been used to reduce increased ICP. Hyperosmolar therapy draws water

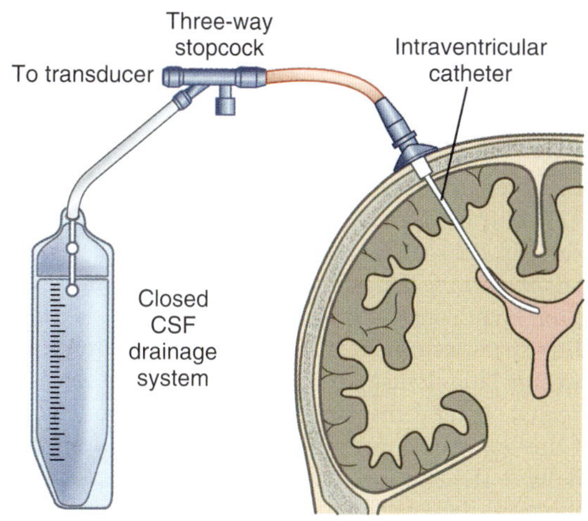

FIG. 22.12 Intermittent Drainage System. Intermittent drainage involves draining cerebrospinal fluid (CSF) through a ventriculostomy when intracranial pressure exceeds the upper pressure parameter set by the practitioner. Intermittent drainage is achieved by opening the three-way stopcock to allow CSF to flow into the drainage bag for brief periods (30 to 120 seconds) until the pressure is below the upper pressure parameter. (From Harding MM, Kwong J, Hagler D, Reinisch C, eds. *Lewis's Medical-Surgical Nursing: Assessment and Management of Clinical Problems*. 12th ed. Elsevier; 2023.)

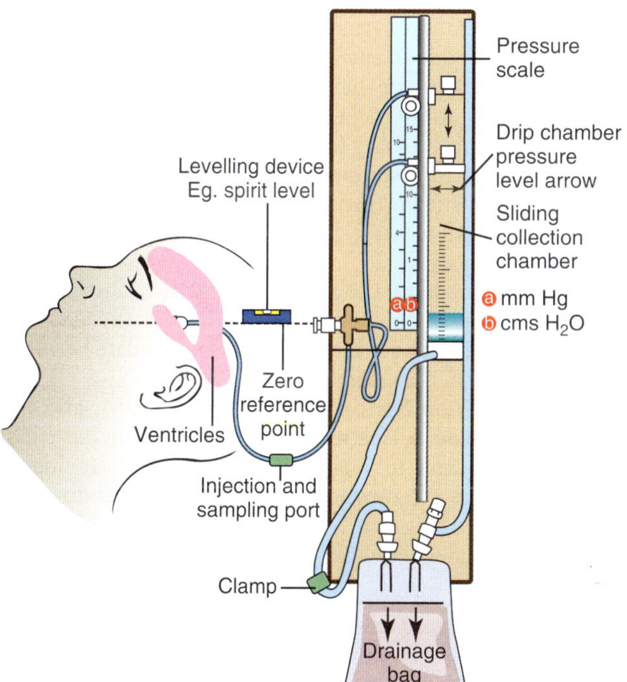

FIG. 22.13 Continuous Drainage System. Continuous drainage involves placing the drip chamber of the drainage system at a specified level above the foramen of Monro (usually 15 cm). The system is left open to allow continuous cerebrospinal fluid drainage into the chamber (which drains into a collection bag) against a pressure gradient that prevents excessive drainage and ventricular collapse.

from brain tissue into the intravascular compartment in the presence of an intact blood-brain barrier. The flow direction is from the hypoconcentrated tissue to the hyperconcentrated cerebral vasculature. If the situation becomes reversed and the tissue becomes hyperconcentrated in relation to the cerebral vasculature, a rebound phenomenon may occur. These agents have a little direct effect on edematous cerebral tissue situated in an area of a defective blood-brain barrier; instead, they require an intact blood-brain barrier for osmosis to occur.[81] The most widely used osmotic diuretic is mannitol, a large-molecule agent that is retained almost entirely in the extracellular compartment and has little of the rebound effect observed with other osmotic diuretics. Administration of mannitol increases CBF and induces cerebral vasoconstriction as part of the brain's autoregulatory response to keep blood flow constant.[80,85]

Perhaps the most common difficulty associated with using osmotic agents is the provocation of electrolyte disturbances. Careful attention must be paid to body weight and fluid and electrolyte stability. Serum osmolality must be kept between 300 and 320 mOsm/L. Hypernatremia and hypokalemia often are associated with repeated administration of osmotic agents. Central venous pressure readings must be monitored to prevent hypovolemia. Smaller doses of mannitol simplify fluid and electrolyte management, and their use is encouraged whenever possible.[80] Hypertonic 3% saline can also be used to treat increased ICP. Hypertonic saline is equally as effective as mannitol for reducing increased ICP.[85] Adverse effects include electrolyte abnormalities, hypotension, pulmonary edema, acute kidney injury, hemolysis, central pontine myelinolysis, coagulopathy, and dysrhythmias.

Management of Metabolic Demand

Any treatment modality that increases the incidence of noxious stimulation to the patient can potentially increase ICP. Noxious stimuli include pain, the presence of an endotracheal tube, coughing, suctioning, repositioning, bathing, and many other routine nursing interventions. Agents used to reduce metabolic demands include the use of benzodiazepines such as midazolam and lorazepam, intravenous sedative-hypnotics such as propofol, opioids such as fentanyl and morphine, and neuromuscular blocking agents such as vecuronium and atracurium. These agents may be administered separately or in combination via continuous drip or as an intravenous bolus on an as-needed basis.

The preferred treatment regimen begins with administering benzodiazepines for sedation and opioids for analgesia. Propofol or a neuromuscular blocking agent is added if these agents fail to blunt the patient's response to noxious stimuli. These medications are recommended only in patients with an ICP monitor because sedatives, opioids, and neuromuscular blocking agents affect the reliability of neurologic assessment. Using neuromuscular blocking agents without sedation is not recommended. These agents cause skeletal muscle paralysis but have no analgesic effect and do not adequately protect the patient from pain and the physiologic responses that can occur from pain-producing procedures.[76] If these agents fail to management ICP, barbiturate therapy is considered.

Barbiturate therapy. Barbiturate therapy is a treatment protocol for managing uncontrolled intracranial hypertension that has not responded to the previously described conventional treatments.[76] The most commonly used medication in high-dose barbiturate therapy is pentobarbital. The goal is a reduction of ICP to 15 to 20 mm Hg while a mean arterial pressure of 70 to 80 mm Hg is maintained. Patients are maintained on high-dose barbiturate therapy until ICP has been controlled within the normal range for 24 hours. Barbiturates must never be stopped abruptly; they are tapered slowly over approximately 4 days. Despite the theoretical reasons for barbiturate use, clinical trials of its use have not shown improved outcomes.[82]

Complications of high-dose barbiturate therapy can be disastrous unless a specific and organized approach is used. The most common complications are hypotension, hypothermia, and myocardial depression. If any complications occur and are allowed to persist unchecked, they may cause secondary insults to an already damaged brain. Hypotension, the most common complication, results from peripheral vasodilation and can be compounded in an already dehydrated patient who has received large doses of an osmotic diuretic to management ICP. Careful monitoring of fluid status by central venous pressure or a pulmonary artery catheter can help prevent this complication. Myocardial depression results from cardiac muscle suppression and can be avoided by frequently monitoring fluid status, cardiac output, and serum medication levels. If an adequate cardiac output cannot be maintained in the presence of normothermia, barbiturates must be reduced, regardless of serum levels.[85,86]

Herniation Syndromes

The goal of neurologic evaluation, ICP monitoring, and treatment of increased ICP is to prevent herniation. Herniation of intracerebral contents results in tissue shifting from one compartment of the brain to another and places pressure on cerebral vessels and vital function centers of the brain. If unchecked, herniation rapidly causes death as a result of the cessation of CBF and respirations.[82]

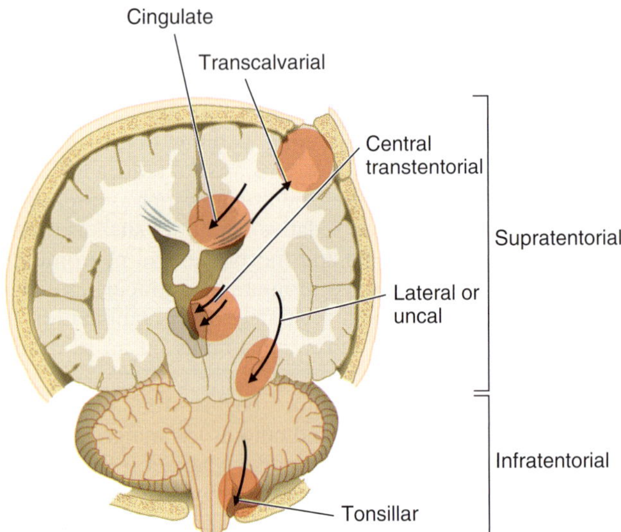

FIG. 22.14 Types of Intracranial Herniation. (From Black JM, Hawks JH. *Medical-Surgical Nursing: Clinical Management for Positive Outcomes*, 8th ed. Saunders; 2009.)

Supratentorial Herniation

The four types of supratentorial herniation syndrome are (1) uncal; (2) central or transtentorial; (3) cingulate; and (4) transcalvarial (Fig. 22.14) (Table 22.5).

Uncal herniation. Uncal herniation is the most common herniation syndrome. In uncal herniation, a unilateral, expanding mass lesion, usually of the temporal lobe, increases ICP, causing lateral displacement of the tip of the temporal lobe (uncus). Lateral displacement pushes the uncus over the edge of the tentorium, puts pressure on the oculomotor nerve (cranial nerve III) and the posterior cerebral artery ipsilateral to the lesion, and flattens the midbrain against the opposite side. Clinical manifestations of uncal herniation include ipsilateral pupil dilation, decreased LOC, respiratory pattern changes leading to respiratory arrest, and contralateral hemiplegia leading to abnormal flexion (decorticate) or abnormal extension (decerebrate) posturing. If no intervention occurs, uncal herniation results in fixed and dilated pupils, flaccidity, and respiratory arrest.[82]

Central herniation. In central or transtentorial herniation, an expanding mass lesion of the midline, frontal, parietal, or occipital lobe results in the downward displacement of the hemispheres, basal ganglia, and diencephalon through the tentorial notch. Central herniation often is preceded by uncal and cingulate herniation. Clinical manifestations of central herniation include loss of consciousness; small, reactive pupils progressing to fixed, dilated pupils; respiratory changes leading to respiratory arrest; and abnormal flexion (decorticate) posturing progressing to flaccidity. In the late stages, uncal and central herniation syndromes affect the brainstem similarly.[82]

Cingulate herniation. Cingulate herniation occurs when an expanding lesion of one hemisphere shifts laterally and forces the cingulate gyrus under the falx cerebri. Cingulate herniation occurs often. When a lateral shift is observed on a CT scan, cingulate herniation has occurred. Little is known about the effects of cingulate herniation, and no accompanying clinical manifestations exist to assist in its diagnosis. A cingulate herniation is not life threatening, but if the expanding mass lesion that caused cingulate herniation is not managed, uncal or central herniation will follow.[82]

TABLE 22.5 Herniation Syndromes

Herniation	Pathophysiology	Presentation
Uncal subtype: Kernohan notch	• Parasympathetic fibers of cranial nerve III compression • Pyramidal tract compression • Compression of cerebral peduncle in uncal herniation • Secondary condition caused by primary injury on the opposite hemisphere	• Ipsilateral fixed and dilated pupil • Contralateral motor paralysis • Ipsilateral hemiplegia/hemiparesis, called Kernohan sign • False localizing sign
Central transtentorial	• Midline lesion with compression of midbrain	• Bilateral nonresponsive midpoint pupils, bilateral Babinski, increased muscular tone
Cerebellotonsillar	• Cerebellar tonsil herniation through the foramen magnum	• Pinpoint pupils, flaccid paralysis, sudden death
Upward posterior fossa/ transtentorial	• Cerebellar and midbrain movement upward through the tentorial opening	• Pinpoint pupils, downward conjugate gaze, irregular respirations • Death

From Long G, Koyfman A. Secondary gains: Advances in neurotrauma management. *Emerg Med Clin North Am.* 2018;36(1):107–133. https://doi.org/10.1016/j.emc.2017.08.007.

Transcalvarial herniation. Transcalvarial herniation is the extrusion of cerebral tissue through the skull. In severe cerebral edema, transcalvarial herniation occurs through an opening from a skull fracture or craniotomy site.[82]

Infratentorial Herniation

The two infratentorial herniation syndromes are upward transtentorial herniation and downward cerebellar herniation.

Upward transtentorial herniation. Upward transtentorial herniation occurs when an expanding mass lesion of the cerebellum causes protrusion of the vermis (central area) of the cerebellum and the midbrain upward through the tentorial notch. Compression of the third cranial nerve and diencephalon occurs. Blockage of the central aqueduct and distortion of the third ventricle obstruct CSF flow. Deterioration progresses rapidly.[82]

Downward cerebellar herniation. Downward cerebellar herniation occurs when an expanding cerebellum lesion exerts pressure downward, sending the cerebellar tonsils through the foramen magnum. Compression and displacement of the medulla oblongata occur, rapidly resulting in respiratory and cardiac arrest.[82]

TABLE 22.6 PHARMACOLOGIC MANAGEMENT

Neurologic Disorders

Medication	Dosage	Action	Special Considerations
Anticonvulsants			
Phenytoin (Dilantin)	Loading dose: 10–20 mg/kg IV	Prevents influx of sodium at the cell membrane	Monitor serum levels closely; therapeutic level is 10–20 mg/L (if hypoalbuminemia, monitor free phenytoin serum levels: therapeutic level of 0.1–0.2 mg/L)
	Maintenance dose: 100 mg q6–8 h IV		Infuse phenytoin no faster than 50 mg/min; administer with normal saline only because it precipitates with other solutions
Fosphenytoin (Cerebyx)	Loading dose: 15–20 mg/kg IV	Prevents influx of sodium at the cell membrane	Monitor serum levels closely; the therapeutic level is 10–20 mg/L
	Maintenance dose: 4–6 mg/kg/24 h IV		Dosage, concentration, and infusion rate of fosphenytoin expressed as FE
Barbiturates			
Phenobarbital	Loading dose: 6–8 mg/kg IV	Produces CNS depression and reduces the spread of epileptic focus	It may depress cardiac and respiratory function
	Maintenance dose: 1–3 mg/kg/24 h IV		Administer phenobarbital at a rate of 60 mg/min; monitor serum level closely; therapeutic level is 15–40 mcg/mL
Pentobarbital	Loading dose: 3–10 mg/kg over 30 min Maintenance dose: 0.5–3 mg/kg/h IV	Induces barbiturate coma	Monitor the serum level of pentobarbital closely; the therapeutic level for coma is 15–40 mg/L
Osmotic Diuretics			
Mannitol	1–2 g/kg IV	Treats cerebral edema by pulling fluid from extravascular space into intravascular space; requires intact blood-brain barrier	Side effects include hypovolemia and increased serum osmolality Monitor serum osmolality and notify the practitioner if >310 mOsm/L Warm and shake before administering to ensure crystals are dissolved
Calcium Channel Blockers			
Nimodipine (Nimotop)	60 mg q4h NG or PO for 21 days	Decreases cerebral vasospasm	Side effects include hypotension, palpitations, headache, and dizziness Monitor blood pressure frequently when implementing therapy
Local Anesthetics			
Lidocaine	50–100 mg IV or 2 mL of 4% solution	Blunts effects of tracheal stimulation on intracranial pressure	Must be administered not longer than 5 min before suctioning
Fibrinolytics			
tPA	0.9 mg/kg total, with 10% of the dose administered as IV bolus over 1 min and 90% of the dose administered as continuous IV infusion over 1 h	Converts plasminogen to plasmin to dissolve the clot	Treatment must start within 4.5 h of the onset of symptoms Do not exceed 90 mg Do not use anticoagulants during the first 24 h Monitor patient for bleeding

CNS, Central nervous system; *FE*, phenytoin sodium equivalents; *IV*, intravenous/intravenously; *NG*, nasogastric; *PO*, by mouth; *tPA*, tissue-type plasminogen activator.
Data from Gold Standard (www.clinicalkey.com).

BOX 22.20 Internet Resources

Neurologic Disorders and Therapeutic Management

- American Academy of Neurology: https://www.aan.com/
- American Association of Critical-Care Nurses: https://www.aacn.org/
- American Association of Neurological Surgeons: https://www.aans.org/
- American Association of Neuroscience Nurses: https://aann.org/
- American College of Physicians: https://www.acponline.org/
- American College of Surgeons: https://www.facs.org/
- American Medical Association: https://www.ama-assn.org/
- American Stroke Association: https://www.stroke.org/
- The Internet Stroke Center: https://www.strokecenter.org/
- National Institutes of Health: https://www.nih.gov/
- Society for Critical Care Medicine: https://www.sccm.org/Home
- Society for Neuroscience: https://www.sfn.org/

PHARMACOLOGIC AGENTS

Many pharmacologic agents are used in the care of patients with neurologic disorders. Table 22.6 reviews the agents used and any special considerations necessary for administering them.

ADDITIONAL RESOURCES

See Box 22.20 for Internet resources pertaining to neurologic disorders and therapeutic management.

KEY POINTS

Stroke

- A stroke is the sudden onset of an acute neurologic deficit persisting for more than 24 hours, and it is caused by the interruption of blood flow to the brain.
- Strokes are classified as ischemic or hemorrhagic. Hemorrhagic strokes can be further categorized as SAHs (cerebral aneurysms and AVMs) and ICHs.
- Nursing interventions focus on monitoring for changes in neurologic status, maintaining surveillance for complications, providing comfort and emotional support, initiating rehabilitation measures, and educating the patient and family.

Ischemic Stroke

- The two leading causes of ischemic stroke are thrombosis and embolism, resulting in a neuronal tissue injury from decreased or absent blood flow.
- The characteristic sign of an ischemic stroke is the sudden onset of focal neurologic signs persisting for more than 24 hours. The signs depend on the affected portion of the brain.
- Medical management focuses on preserving brain tissue through fibrinolytic therapy, managing blood pressure, and treating complications.

Subarachnoid Hemorrhage

- SAH is bleeding into the subarachnoid space, usually caused by a cerebral aneurysm rupture or AVM.
- Medical management focuses on preserving neurologic function, supporting vital functions, and treating complications (rebleeding, vasospasm, hyponatremia, and hydrocephalus).

Intracerebral Hemorrhage

- ICH is bleeding directly into cerebral tissue and is usually caused by a rupture of a small artery in the brain resulting from hypertension.
- Medical management focuses on preserving neurologic function, managing blood pressure, supporting vital functions, and managing intracranial hypertension.

Coma

- The two leading causes of coma are structural (e.g., ischemic stroke, ICH, trauma, brain tumors) and metabolic (e.g., drug overdose, infectious diseases, endocrine disorders, poisonings).
- Coma is the deepest state of unconsciousness; arousal and awareness are lacking due to diffuse dysfunction of both cerebral hemispheres or diffuse or focal dysfunction of the RAS.
- Medical management focuses on identifying and treating the condition's underlying cause and supporting vital functions.
- Nursing interventions focus on supporting all body functions, maintaining surveillance for complications, providing comfort and emotional support, initiating rehabilitation measures, and educating the patient and family.

Guillain-Barré Syndrome

- Guillain-Barré syndrome involves a rapidly progressive, ascending peripheral nerve dysfunction leading to paralysis that may produce respiratory failure.
- Medical management focuses on supporting vital functions and administering treatments to limit the duration of the syndrome.
- Nursing interventions focus on maintaining surveillance for complications, initiating rehabilitative measures, providing comfort and emotional support, and educating the patient and family about the disorder.

Neurosurgery

- Neurosurgery is performed to access portions of the CNS inside the skull for tumor resection or removal, cerebral decompression, evacuation of hematoma or abscess, or repair of an aneurysm or AVM.
- Postoperative medical management focuses on preventing complications, including intracranial hypertension, bleeding, fluid imbalances, CSF leaks, and DVT.
- Nursing interventions focus on positioning the patient's head per the practitioner's orders, monitoring the patient's intake and output, administering medications to manage vomiting and fever, promoting postoperative pulmonary care, providing comfort and emotional support, maintaining surveillance for complications, initiating rehabilitative measures, and education of the patient and family.

Intracranial Hypertension

- One of the earliest signs of increased ICP is a decrease in LOC.
- ICP can be measured using an ICP monitor and should be treated when it exceeds 20 mm Hg.
- Medical and nursing management is directed toward reducing the volume of one or more components (e.g., blood, brain, CSF) within the intracranial vault.
- Herniation of intracerebral contents results in tissue shifting from one compartment of the brain to another and places pressure on cerebral vessels and vital function centers of the brain. If unchecked, it rapidly causes death.

CASE STUDY 22.1 Patient With a Neurologic Problem

Brief Patient History

Mr. P is a 74-year-old man who is a retired engineer. He has a history of hypertension, hyperlipidemia, and type 2 diabetes. He reports occasional smoking, moderate alcohol consumption, and a sedentary lifestyle. He lives with his wife, who helps with daily activities.

Presenting Complaint

His wife brought Mr. P to the emergency department after suddenly experiencing weakness and numbness on the right side of his body. He was also unable to speak clearly and appeared confused. The symptoms began approximately 45 minutes before arrival.

Clinical Assessment:

Upon arrival, Mr. P was assessed by the Stroke Team. They noted the following:

- Right-sided weakness (hemiparesis) and numbness
- Difficulty speaking (aphasia)
- Confusion and disorientation
- Mild drooping of the left side of the face (facial droop)
- Blood pressure: 170/100 mmHg

Diagnostic Tests:

CT Scan: A noncontrast CT scan of the brain revealed a hypodense area in the left middle cerebral artery territory. This result indicated an ischemic stroke.

Diagnosis:

Mr. P was diagnosed with an acute ischemic stroke, likely due to an occlusion of the left middle cerebral artery. His risk factors, including hypertension, hyperlipidemia, and diabetes, increased his susceptibility to stroke.

Questions:

1. What major outcomes do you expect to achieve for this patient?
2. What problems or risks must be managed to achieve these outcomes?
3. What interventions could be initiated to monitor, prevent, manage, or eliminate the problems and risks identified?
4. What interventions could be initiated to promote optimal functioning, safety, and well-being of the patient?
5. What technology can be used to monitor this patient and prevent complications?
6. What other interprofessional team members are needed to assist with the management of this patient?
7. What possible learning needs would you anticipate for this patient?
8 What cultural and age-related factors might have a bearing on the patient's plan of care?

Visit the Evolve site at http://evolve.elsevier.com/Urden/CriticalCareNursing for additional study materials.

REFERENCES

1. Tsao CW, Aday AW, Almarzooq ZI, et al. Heart disease and stroke statistics—2023 Update: a report from the American Heart Association. *Circulation*. 2023;147(8):e93–e621. https://doi.org/10.1161/CIR.0000000000001123.
2. Xu J, Murphy SL, Kochanek KD, et al. Mortality in the United States; 2021. https://doi.org/10.15620/cdc:122516. . Accessed August 19, 2023. Published 2022.
3. Mac Grory B, Flood SP, Apostolidou E, et al. Cryptogenic stroke: diagnostic workup and management. *Curr Treat Options Cardiovasc Med*. 2019;21(11):77. https://doi.org/10.1007/s11936-019-0786-4.
4. Biller J, Ruland S, Schneck MJ. Ischemic cerebrovascular disease. In: Daroff RB, Jankovic J, Massiotta JC, Newman NJ, eds. *Bradley's Neurology in Clinical Practice*. 8th ed. Philadelphia: Elsevier; 2021.
5. Swait G, Finch R. What are the risks of manual treatment of the spine? A scoping review for clinicians. *Chiropr Man Therap*. 2017;25:37. https://doi.org/10.1186/s12998-017-0168-5.
6. O'Carroll CB, Barrett KM. Cardioembolic stroke. *Continuum (Minneap Minn)*. 2017;23(1, Cerebrovascular Disease):111–132. https://doi.org/10.1212/CON.0000000000000419.
7. Powers J, Hubner KE. Alterations of the brain, spinal cord, and peripheral nerves. In: Rogers J, ed. *McCance & Huether's Pathophysiology: The Biologic Basis for Disease in Adults and Children*. 9th ed. St. Louis: Elsevier; 2023.
8. Bustamante A, Garcia-Berrocoso T, Rodrieguez N, et al. Ischemic stroke outcome: a review of the influence of post-stroke complications within the different scenarios of stroke care. *Eur J Intern Med*. 2016;29:9–21. https://doi.org/10.1016/j.ejim.2015.11.030.
9. Powers WJ, Rabinstein AA, Ackerson T, et al. Guidelines for the early management of patients with acute ischemic stroke: 2019 update to the 2018 guidelines for the early management of acute ischemic stroke: a guideline for healthcare professionals from the American Heart Association/American Stroke Association. *Stroke*. 2019;50(12):e344–e418. https://doi.org/10.1161/STR.0000000000000211.
10. Yang Y, Yang J, Feng J, Wang Y. Early Diagnosis of acute ischemic stroke by brain computed tomography perfusion imaging combined with head and neck computed tomography angiography on deep learning algorithm. *Contrast Media Mol Imaging*. 2022;2022:5373585. https://doi.org/10.1155/2022/5373585.
11. Pratit P, Yavagal D, Khadelwal P. Hyperacute management of ischemic stroke. *J Am Coll Cardiol*. 2020;75(15):1844–1856. https://doi.org/10.1016/j.jacc.2020.03.006.
12. Sacks D, Baxter B, Campbell BCV, et al. Multisociety consensus quality improvement revised consensus statement for endovascular therapy of acute ischemic stroke. *J Vasc Interv Radiol*. 2017;29(4):441–453. https://doi.org/10.1016/j.jvir.2017.11.026.
13. Shelton S, Rose J, Melo C, et al. What duration of permissive hypertension leads to best outcomes after an ischemic stroke? *Evidence-Based Practice*. 2023;26(3):13–15. https://doi.org/10.1097/EBP.0000000000001811.
14. White CJ. Acute stroke intervention: the role of interventional cardiologists. *J Am Coll Cardiol*. 2019;73(12):1491–1493. https://doi.org/10.1016/j.jacc.2018.12.071.
15. Long B, Koyfman A, Runyon MS. Subarachnoid hemorrhage: updates in diagnosis and management. *Emer Med Clin N Am*. 2017;35(4):803–824. https://doi.org/10.1016/j.emc.2017.07.001.
16. Abraham MK, Chang WW. Subarachnoid hemorrhage. *Emerg Med Clin North Am*. 2016;34(4):901–916. https://doi.org/10.1016/j.emc.2016.06.011.
17. Wilson SE, Ashcraft S, Troiani L. Aneurysmal subarachnoid hemorrhage: management by the advanced practice provider. *J Nurse Pract*. 2019;15(8):553–558. https://doi.org/10.1016/j.nurpra.2019.05.017.
18. Boling B, Groves TR. Management of subarachnoid hemorrhage. *Crit Care Nurse*. 2019;39(5):58–67. https://doi.org/10.4037/ccn2019882.
19. Szeder V, Tateshima S, Duckwiler GR. Intracranial aneurysms and subarachnoid hemorrhage. In: Daroff RB, Jankovic J, Massiotta JC, Newman NJ, eds. *Bradley's Neurology in Clinical Practice*. 8th ed. Philadelphia, PA: Elsevier; 2021.
20. Rutledge C, Cooke DL, Hetts SW, Abla AA. Brain arteriovenous malformations. *Handb Clin Neurol*. 2021;176:171–178. https://doi.org/10.1016/B978-0-444-64034-5.00020-1.
21. Hoh BL, Ko NU, Amin-Hanjani S, et al. 2023 guideline for the management of patients with aneurysmal subarachnoid hemorrhage: a guideline from the American Heart Association/American Stroke Association. *Stroke*. 2023;54(7):e314–e370. https://doi.org/10.1161/STR.0000000000000436.
22. Chou SHY. Subarachnoid hemorrhage. *Continuum (Minneap Minn)*. 2021;27(5):1201–1245. https://doi.org/10.1212/CON.0000000000001052.

23. Hunt WE, Hess RM. Surgical risks as related to time of intervention in the repair of intracranial aneurysms. *J Neurosurg.* 1968;28(1):14–20.
24. Marcolini E, Hine J. Approach to the diagnosis and management of subarachnoid hemorrhage. *West J Emerg Med.* 2019;20(2):203–211. https://doi.org/10.5811/westjem.2019.1.37352.
25. Lu VM, Graffeo CS, Perry A, et al. Rebleeding drives poor outcome in aneurysmal subarachnoid hemorrhage independent of delayed cerebral ischemia: a propensity-score matched cohort study. *J Neurosurg.* 2019;133(2):360–369. https://doi.org/10.3171/2019.4.JNS19779.
26. Claassen J, Park S. Spontaneous subarachnoid haemorrhage. *Lancet.* 2022;400(10355):846–862. https://doi.org/10.1016/S0140-6736(22)00938-2.
27. Musmar B, Adeeb N, Ansari J, et al. Endovascular management of hemorrhagic stroke. *Biomedicines.* 2022;10(1):100. https://doi:10.3390/biomedicines10010100.
28. Francoeur CL, Mayer SA. Management of delayed cerebral ischemia after subarachnoid hemorrhage. *Crit Care.* 2016;20(1):277. https://doi.org/10.1186/s13054-016-1447-6.
29. Rouanet C, Sampaio G. Aneurysmal subarachnoid hemorrhage: current concepts and updates. *Arq Neuropsiquiatr.* 2019;77(11):806–814. https://doi.org/10.1590/0004-282X20190112.
30. Li K, Barras CD, Chandra RV, et al. A review of the management of cerebral vasospasm after aneurysmal subarachnoid hemorrhage. *World Neurosurg.* 2019;126:513–527. https://doi.org/10.1016/j.wneu.2019.03.083.
31. Sheth KN. Spontaneous intracerebral hemorrhage. *N Engl J Med.* 2022;387(17):1589–1596. https://doi.org/10.1056/NEJMra2201449.
32. Schrag M, Kirshner H. Management of intracerebral hemorrhage: JACC focus seminar. *J Am Coll Cardiol.* 2020;75(15):1819–1831. https://doi.org/10.1016/j.jacc.2019.10.066.
33. Godoy DA, Pinera GR, Koller P, et al. Steps to consider in the approach and management of critically ill patient with spontaneous intracerebral hemorrhage. *World J Crit Care Med.* 2015;4(3):213–229. https://doi.org/10.5492/wjccm.v4.i3.213.
34. Chaturvedi S, Selim M. Hemorrhagic cerebrovascular disease. In: Goldman L, Cooney KA, eds. *Goldman-Cecil Medicine.* 27th. St. Louis: Elsevier; 2024.
35. Greenberg SM, Ziai WC, Cordonnier C, et al. 2022 guideline for the management of patients with spontaneous intracerebral hemorrhage: a guideline from the American Heart Association/American Stroke Association. *Stroke.* 2022;53(7):e282–e361. https://doi.org/10.1161/STR.0000000000000407.
36. Amatangelo MP, Thomas SB. Priority nursing interventions caring for the stroke patient. *Crit Care Nurs Clin North Am.* 2020;32(1):67–84. https://doi.org/10.1016/j.cnc.2019.11.005.
37. Grow WA. The cerebral cortex. In: Haines DE, Mihailoff GA, eds. *Fundamental Neuroscience for Basic and Clinical Applications.* Philadelphia, PA: Elsevier; 2018.
38. Morad AE, Massoud M, Botros M, et al. Clinical and radiological predictors for early detection of cerebral vasospasm after subarachnoid haemorrhage. *Benha Med J.* 2019;36(2):32–41. https://doi.org/10.21608/bmfj.2019.14473.1008.
39. Aravind G, Lamontagne A. Effect of visuospatial neglect on spatial navigation and heading after stroke. *Ann Phys Rehabil Med.* 2018;61(4):198–206. https://doi.org/10.1016/j.rehab.2017.05.002.
40. Goodwin D. Homonymous hemianopia: challenges and solutions. *Clin Ophthalmol.* 2014;8:1919–1927. https://doi.org/10.2147/OPTH.S59452.
41. Eapen BC, Georgekutty J, Subbarao B, et al. Disorders of consciousness. *Phys Med Rehabil Clin N Am.* 2017;28(2):245–258. https://doi.org/10.1016/j.pmr.2016.12.003.
42. Traub SJ, Wijdicks EF. Initial diagnosis and management of coma. *Emerg Med Clin North Am.* 2016;34(4):777–793. https://doi.org/10.1016/j.emc.2016.06.017.
43. Horsting MW, Franken MD, Meulenbelt J, et al. The etiology and outcome of non-traumatic coma in critical care: a systematic review. *BMC Anesthesiol.* 2015;15:65. https://doi.org/10.1186/s12871-015-0041-9.
44. Edlow JA, Rabinstein A, Traub SJ, et al. Diagnosis of reversible causes of coma. *Lancet.* 2014;384(9959):2064–2076. https://doi.org/10.1016/S0140-6736(13)62184-4.
45. Roy K, Huether SE. Alteration in cognitive systems, cerebral hemodynamics, and motor function. In: Rogers J, ed. *McCance & Huether's Pathophysiology: The Biologic Basis for Disease in Adults and Children.* 9th ed. St. Louis: Elsevier; 2023.
46. Hocker S, Rabinstein AA. Management of the patient with diminished responsiveness. *Neurol Clin.* 2012;30(1):1–9. https://doi.org/10.1016/j.ncl.2011.09.009.
47. Kondzille D, Bender A, Diserens K, et al. European Academy of Neurology guideline on the diagnosis of coma and other disorders of consciousness. *Eur J Neurol.* 2020;27(5):741–756. https://doi.org/10.1111/ene.14151.
48. Bruno MA, Vanhaudenhuyse A, Thibaut A, et al. From unresponsive wakefulness to minimally conscious PLUS and functional locked-in syndromes: recent advances in our understanding of disorders of consciousness. *J Neurol.* 2011;258(7):1373–1384. https://doi.org/10.1007/s00415-011-6114-x.
49. Nikseresht T, Abdi A, Khatony A. Effectiveness of polyethylene cover versus polyethylene cover with artificial tear drop to prevent dry eye in critically ill patients: a randomized controlled clinical trial. *Clin Ophthalmol.* 2019;13:2203–2210. https://doi.org/10.2147/OPTH.S233404.
50. Sudulagunta RS, Sodalagunta MB, Sepehrar M, et al. Guillain-Barré syndrome: clinical profile and management. *Ger Med Sci.* 2015;13. https://doi.org/10.3205/000220.
51. van den Berg B, Walgaard C, Drenthen J, et al. Guillain-Barré syndrome: pathogenesis, diagnosis, treatment and prognosis. *Nat Rev Neurol.* 2014;10(8):469–482. https://doi.org/10.1038/nrneurol.2014.121.
52. Willison HJ, Jacobs BC, van Doorn PA. Guillain-Barré syndrome. *Lancet.* 2016;388(10045):717–727. https://doi.org/10.1016/S0140-6736(16)00339-1.
53. Esposito S, Longo MR. Guillain-Barré syndrome. *Autoimmun Rev.* 2017;16(1):96–101. https://doi.org/10.1016/j.autrev.2016.09.022.
54. Cortese I, Chaudhry V, So YT, et al. Evidence-based guideline update: Plasmapheresis in neurologic disorders: report of the therapeutics and technology assessment subcommittee of the American Academy of Neurology. *Neurology.* 2011;76(3):294–300. https://doi.org/10.1212/WNL.0b013e318207b1f6.
55. Patwa HS, Chaudhry V, Katzberg H, et al. Evidence-based guideline: intravenous immunoglobulin in the treatment of neuromuscular disorders: report of the therapeutics and technology assessment subcommittee of the American Academy of Neurology. *Neurology.* 2012;78(13):1009–1015. https://doi.org/10.1212/WNL.0b013e31824de293.
56. Novak P, Smid S, Vidmar G. Rehabilitation of Guillain-Barré syndrome patients: an observational study. *Int J Rehabil Res.* 2017;40(2):158–163. https://doi.org/10.1097/MRR.0000000000000225.
57. Sulli S, Scala L, Berardi A, et al. The efficacy of rehabilitation in people with Guillain-Barrè syndrome: a systematic review of randomized controlled trials. *Expert Rev Neurother.* 2021;21(4):455–461. https://doi.org/10.1080/14737175.2021.1890034.
58. Murphy MP, Whitmore DM, Germanovich SJ. Neurosurgery. In: Rothrock JC, ed. *Alexander's Care of the Patient in Surgery.* 17th ed. St. Louis: Elsevier; 2023.
59. Weston J, Greenhalgh J, Marson AG. Antiepileptic drugs as prophylaxis for post-craniotomy seizures. *Cochrane Database Syst Rev.* 2015;(3). https://doi.org/10.1002/14651858.CD007286.pub3. CD007286.
60. Miller BA, Loachimescu AG, Oyesiku NM. Contemporary indications for transsphenoidal pituitary surgery. *World Neurosurg.* 2014;82(6 Suppl):S147–S151. https://doi.org/10.1016/j.wneu.2014.07.037.
61. Yuan W. Managing the patient with transsphenoidal pituitary tumor resection. *J Neurosurg Nurs.* 2013;45(2):101–107. https://doi.org/10.1097/JNN.0b013e3182828e28.
62. Fugate JE. Complications of neurosurgery. *Continuum (Minneap Minn).* 2015;21(5 Neurocritical Care):1425–1444. https://doi.org/10.1212/CON.0000000000000227.
63. Hannon MJ, Finucane FM, Sherlock M, et al. Clinical review: disorders of water homeostasis in neurosurgical patients. *J Clin Endocrinol Metab.* 2012;97(5):1423–1433. https://doi.org/10.1210/jc.2011-3201.
64. Ausiello JC, Bruce JN, Freda PU. Postoperative assessment of the patient after transsphenoidal pituitary surgery. *Pituitary.* 2008;11(4):391–401. https://doi.org/10.1007/s11102-008-0086-6.

65. Daele JJ, Goffart Y, Machiels S. Traumatic, iatrogenic, and spontaneous cerebrospinal fluid (CSF) leak: endoscopic repair. *B-ENT.* 2011;7(Suppl 17):47–60.
66. Ganau M, Prisco L, Cebula H, et al. Risk of deep vein thrombosis in neurosurgery: state of the art on prophylaxis protocols and best clinical practices. *J Clin Neurosci.* 2017;45:60–66. https://doi.org/10.1016/j.jocn.2017.08.008.
67. Schneck MJ. Venous thromboembolism in neurologic disease. *Handb Clin Neurol.* 2014;119:289–304. https://doi.org/10.1016/B978-0-7020-4086-3.00020-5.
68. O'Brien A, Redley B, Wood B, et al. STOPDVTs: development and testing of a clinical assessment tool to guide nursing assessment of postoperative patients for deep vein thrombosis. *J Clin Nurs.* 2018;27(9–10):1803–1811. https://doi.org/10.1111/jocn.14329.
69. Anderson DR, Morgano GP, Bennett C, et al. American Society of Hematology 2019 guidelines for management of venous thromboembolism: prevention of venous thromboembolism in surgical hospitalized patients. *Blood Adv.* 2019;3(23):3898–3944. https://doi.org/10.1182/bloodadvances.2019000975.
70. Uribe AA, Stoicea N, Echeverria-Villalobos M, et al. Postoperative nausea and vomiting after craniotomy: an evidence-based review of general considerations, risk factors, and management. *J Neurosurg Anesthesiol.* 2021;33(3):212–220. https://doi.org/10.1097/ANA.0000000000000667.
71. Ban VS, Bhoja R, McDonagh DL. Multimodal analgesia for craniotomy. *Curr Opin Anaesthesiol.* 2019;32(5):592–599. https://doi.org/10.1097/ACO.0000000000000766.
72. Dashti SR, Baharvahdat H, Spetzler RF, et al. Operative intracranial infection following craniotomy. *Neurosurg Focus.* 2008;24(6):E10. https://doi.org/10.3171/FOC/2008/24/6/E10.
73. Robinson JD. Management of refractory intracranial pressure. *Crit Care Nurs Clin North Am.* 2016;28(1):67–75. https://doi.org/10.1016/j.cnc.2015.09.004.
74. Oswal A, Toma AK. Intracranial pressure and cerebral haemodynamics. *Anesthesia and Intensive Care Medicine.* 2017;18(5):259–263. https://doi.org/10.1016/j.mpaic.2017.03.002.
75. Blissitt PA. Hemodynamic and intracranial dynamic monitoring in neurocritical care. In: Lough ME, ed. *Hemodynamic Monitoring: Evolving Technologies and Clinical Practice.* St Louis: Elsevier; 2016.
76. Perez-Barcena J, Llompart-Pou JA, O'Phelan KM. Intracranial pressure monitoring and management of intracranial hypertension. *Crit Care Clin.* 2014;30(4):735–750. https://doi.org/10.1016/j.ccc.2014.06.005.
77. Latorre JG, Greer DM. Management of acute intracranial hypertension: a review. *Neurologist.* 2009;15(4):193–207. https://doi.org/10.1097/NRL.0b013e31819f956a.
78. Bhatia A, Gupta AK. Neuromonitoring in the intensive care unit. I. Intracranial pressure and cerebral blood flow monitoring. *Intens Care Med.* 2007;33(7):1263–1271. https://doi.org/10.1007/s00134-007-0678-z.
79. Curley G, Kavanagh BP, Laffey JG. Hypocapnia and the injured brain: more harm than benefit. *Crit Care Med.* 2010;38(5):1348–1359. https://doi.org/10.1097/CCM.0b013e3181d8cf2b.
80. Farrokh S, Cho SM, Suarez JI. Fluids and hyperosmolar agents in neurocritical care: an update. *Curr Opin Crit Care.* 2019;25(2):105–109. https://doi.org/10.1097/MCC.0000000000000585.
81. Abdelmalik PA, Draghic N, Ling GSF. Management of moderate and severe brain injury. *Transfusion.* 2019;59(S2):1529–1538. https://doi.org/10.1111/trf.15171.
82. Long G, Koyfman A. Secondary gains: advances in neurotrauma management. *Emerg Med Clin North Am.* 2018;36(1):107–133. https://doi.org/10.1016/j.emc.2017.08.007.
83. Hepburn-Smith M, Dynkevich I, Spektor M. Establishment of an external ventricular drain best practice guideline: the quest for a comprehensive, universal standard for external ventricular drain care. *J Neurosci Nurs.* 2016;48(1):54–65. https://doi.org/10.1097/JNN.0000000000000174.
84. Atkinson RA, Fikrey L, Vail A, et al. Silver-impregnated external-ventricular-drain-related cerebrospinal fluid infections: a meta-analysis. *J Hosp Infect.* 2016;92(3):263–272. https://doi.org/10.1016/j.jhin.2015.09.014.
85. Stevens RD, Shoykhet M, Cadena R. Emergency neurological life support: intracranial hypertension and herniation. *Neurocrit Care.* 2015;23(Suppl 2):S76–S82. https://doi.org/10.1007/s12028-015-0168-z.
86. Sacco TL, Delibert SA. Management of intracranial pressure: Part 1: pharmacologic interventions. *Dimens Crit Care Nurs.* 2018;37(3):120–129. https://doi.org/10.1097/DCC.0000000000000293.

23

Kidney Anatomy and Physiology

Kathrine Anne Winnie and Kimberly Sanchez

http://evolve.elsevier.com/Urden/CriticalCareNursing

The kidneys are complex organs responsible for numerous functions necessary to maintain homeostasis. The primary roles of the kidneys are urine formation, metabolic waste elimination, hemodynamic regulation, fluid–electrolyte balance, acid–base balance, erythrocyte production, and vitamin D activation. When a patient experiences kidney dysfunction, some or all of the functions of the kidneys may be decreased or absent, leading to altered homeostasis.

This chapter provides an overview of the anatomy and physiologic processes of the kidneys. An understanding of normal kidney function is essential to understanding the pathophysiology, symptoms, and therapeutic management of kidney disorders.

ANATOMY

Macroscopic Anatomy

The kidneys are paired organs located retroperitoneally, one on each side of the vertebral column between T12 and L3.[1] The right kidney is slightly lower than the left because of the position of the liver.[1] Each kidney is approximately 12 cm long, 7 cm wide, and 3 cm thick in an adult.[1] Kidney size and weight vary between men and women: 125 to 170 g in men and 115 to 155 g in women.[1] The kidneys are protected anteriorly and posteriorly by the rib cage and by a tough fibrous capsule that encloses each kidney.[2] Additional protection is provided by a cushion of perirenal fat and the support of the kidney fascia.[3]

Internally, the kidneys are made up of two distinct areas: the cortex and the medulla.[1] The kidney *cortex* is the outer layer and contains the glomeruli, proximal tubules, cortical portions of the loops of Henle, distal tubules, and cortical collecting ducts[3] (Fig. 23.1). The kidney cortex is approximately 1 cm in thickness.[1] The kidney *medulla* is within the inner kidney (Fig. 23.1) and is divided into an outer layer that contains an inner stripe and outer stripe, and a deeper inner layer (Fig. 23.2A).[1] The medulla is made up of *pyramids*,[1] which contain the medullary portions of the loops of Henle, the vasa recta vasculature, and the medullary portions of the collecting

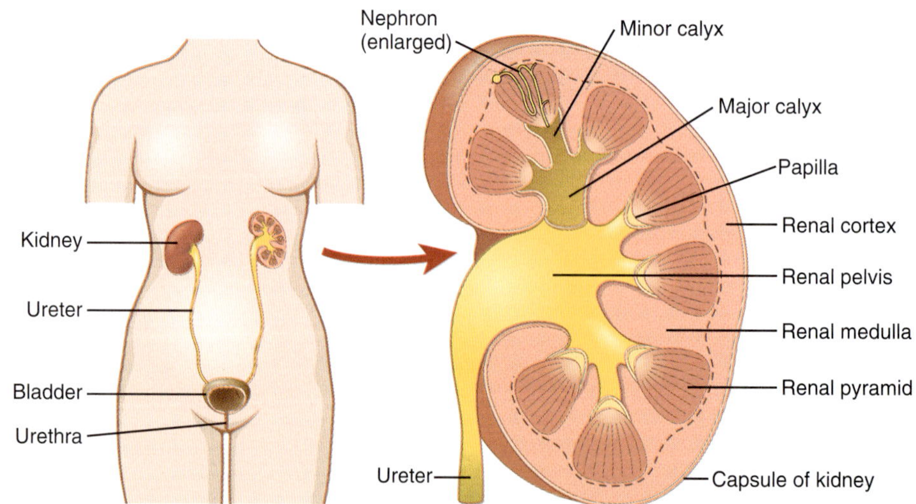

FIG. 23.1 Position of the Kidneys in the Abdomen, With a Schematic of the Kidney Cortex, Kidney Medulla, Kidney Pyramids, Calyces, Kidney Pelvis, and Ureter. (From Hall ME, Hall JE. *Guyton and Hall Textbook of Medical Physiology*. 14th ed. Elsevier; 2021.)

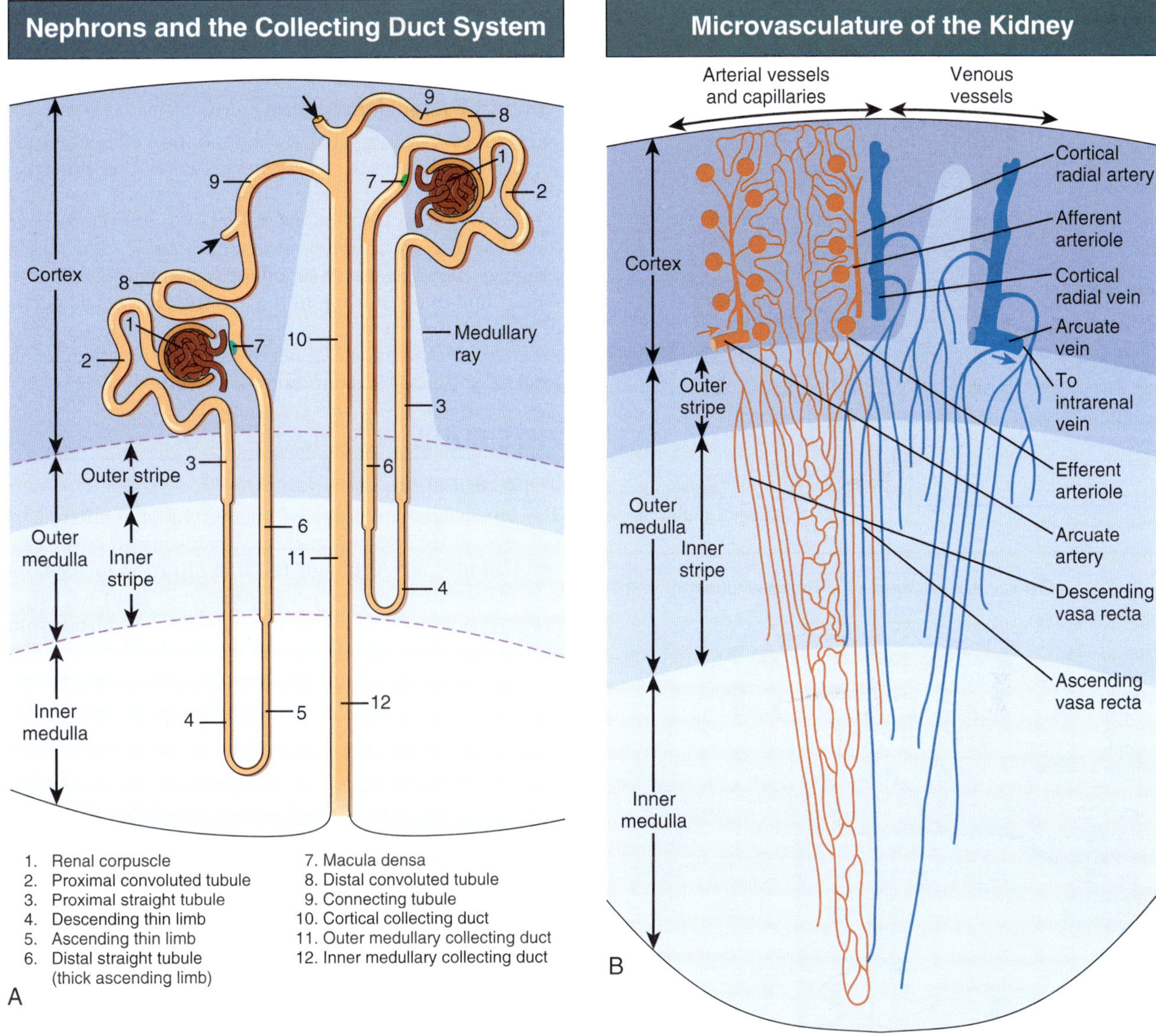

FIG. 23.2 (A) Nephron anatomy in detail; (B) Nephron vasculature in detail. (Adapted from Feehally J, Floege J, Tonelli M, Johnson RJ. *Comprehensive Clinical Nephrology*. 6th ed. Elsevier; 2019.)

ducts.[3] Numerous pyramids taper and join to form a minor calyx; several minor calyces join to form a major calyx.[2] The major calyces then join and enter the funnel-shaped kidney *pelvis*,[2] a 5- to 10-mL conduit that directs urine into the ureter[3] (Fig. 23.1).

The kidney system also includes the urinary drainage system comprising the ureters, bladder, and urethra (Fig. 23.1). [2] The ureters are fibromuscular tubes that exit the central part of the kidney pelvis.[2] The ureters are 28 to 34 cm in length[1] and enter the urinary bladder at an oblique angle.[2] Urine flows through the ureters by peristalsis.[2] The peristaltic action of the ureters and the angle at which the ureters enter the bladder help prevent reflux of urine from the bladder back up into the kidneys.[2] The bladder is a muscular sac within the pelvis and has a capacity of 280 to 500 mL. Urine leaves the bladder through the urethral orifice and is excreted from the body through the urethra. The male urethra is approximately 20 cm long; the female urethra is 3 to 5 cm long.

Microscopic Anatomy

The nephron is often described as the *functional unit* of the kidneys.[1] On average, each kidney is made up of approximately 1 million nephrons.[1] Because of the vast number of nephrons, the kidneys can continue to function even when several thousand nephrons are damaged or destroyed by disease or injury. Each nephron has the ability to perform all the individual functions of the kidneys. Two types of nephrons make up each kidney: the cortical nephrons and the juxtamedullary nephrons (Figs. 23.3 and 23.4).[2] Most are cortical nephrons. Cortical nephrons have glomeruli located in the outer cortex and have short loops of Henle that penetrate only the cortex and outer medulla.[2] Juxtamedullary nephrons have glomeruli located deep in the cortex and extend into the inner medullary layer of the kidney.[2] The juxtamedullary nephrons have long loops of Henle.[2] The nephron is made up of several distinct structures: the glomerulus, Bowman capsule, proximal tubule, loop of Henle, distal tubule, and collecting duct (Fig. 23.3 and Table 23.1).[2]

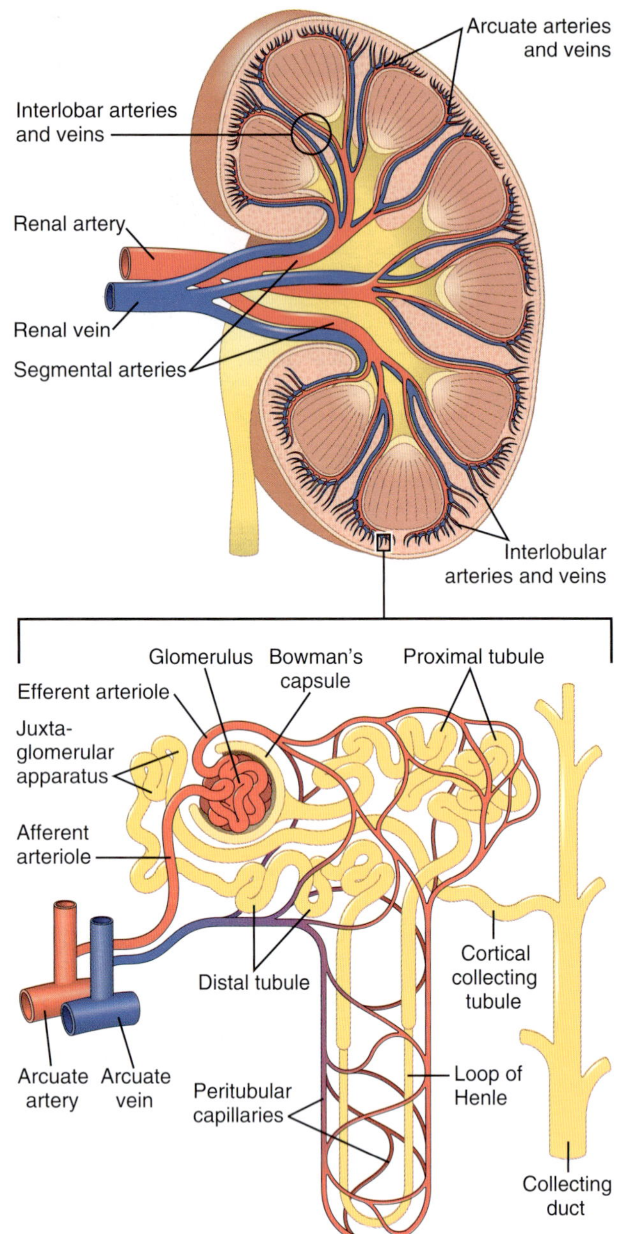

FIG. 23.3 Major Arterial and Venous Blood Supply to the Kidney With a Schematic of the Microcirculation to a Nephron. (From Hall ME, Hall JE. *Guyton and Hall Textbook of Medical Physiology*. 14th ed. Elsevier; 2021.)

Vascular Anatomy

The kidneys are highly vascular and receive about 20% of the cardiac output—approximately 1 to 1.2 L/min of blood flow.[4] Blood enters the kidneys through the renal arteries, which branch bilaterally from the abdominal aorta.[4] The renal artery divides into arterial branches that become progressively smaller vessels, eventually leading to the afferent arterioles. A single *afferent arteriole* supplies blood to each glomerulus (Fig. 23.4).[4] Blood exits the glomerulus by the *efferent arteriole*, delivering blood to the postglomerular capillary circulation.[4] Cortical nephrons are surrounded by peritubular capillaries and juxtamedullary nephrons have specialized peritubular capillaries known as the *vasa recta* (straight vessels) that parallel the long loops of Henle[2,5] (Fig 23.4). The capillaries then rejoin and form gradually enlarging vessels until the blood leaves each kidney through the renal vein and returns to the general circulation by the inferior vena cava.

Nervous System Innervation

The kidney is innervated by autonomic (efferent) and sensory (afferent) nerves.[6] These nerves enter the kidneys along the path of the renal arteries.[1] The sympathetic nerve fibers to the kidneys stem from paravertebral and prevertebral ganglia, including the aorticorenal, splanchnic, celiac, and mesenteric ganglia.[1] The vagus nerve supplies parasympathetic fibers to the kidney and upper portion of the ureters.[6] The pelvic nerve supplies parasympathetic fibers to the bladder and lower portion of the ureters.[6] The pudendal nerve supplies somatic fibers to the external sphincter surrounding the urethra.[6]

PHYSIOLOGY

Urine Formation

The entire blood volume of an individual is filtered by the kidneys 60 to 70 times each day, resulting in approximately 180 L of filtrate.[2] Although 180 L of filtrate is formed, 99% of it is reabsorbed, and only 1% is excreted as urine. The three processes necessary for changing the 180 L of filtrate into 1 to 2 L of urine are glomerular filtration, tubular reabsorption, and tubular secretion.[2] The glomerular filtration rate (GFR), or the amount of filtrate formed in the nephrons, is approximately 125 mL/min or 180 L/day.[7]

Glomerular Filtration

The first process in urine formation is glomerular filtration, which depends on glomerular blood flow and the sum of all pressures across the glomerular capillaries.[4,7] The kidneys have an intrinsic feedback mechanism, called autoregulation, maintaining a relatively constant renal blood flow and glomerular filtration rate even with large fluctuations in arterial blood pressure.[7]

In order for this autoregulatory mechanism to maintain kidney blood flow and perfusion at a constant level, arterial pressure needs to be between 80 mm Hg and 170 mm Hg.[7] The afferent and efferent arterioles of the glomeruli have the ability to increase or decrease the glomerular filtration through selective dilation and constriction. GFR is decreased if there is increased resistance of the afferent arterioles (e.g., arteriole constriction) and if constriction of efferent arterioles decreases renal blood flow.[7] GFR is increased with reduced resistance in the afferent arterioles (e.g., arteriole dilation) and if constriction of efferent arterioles doesn't decrease renal blood flow.[7]

The glomerulus has a complex filtration structure with multiple layers.[7] The first layer is the fenestrated capillary endothelium, followed by the basement membrane layer, and the outer layer the epithelial cells called podocytes.[7] This complex filtration structure is described as the glomerular filtration barrier and it controls filtration according size,[3,7] shape of the molecules,[3,8] rigidity of the molecule,[3] electrical charge,[3,7,8] and protein-binding capability.[3] It is freely permeable to water and small or midsized molecules, but large molecules such as albumin and red blood cells are prevented from entering the filtrate.[7]

After blood is filtered through the glomerular filtration barrier, the initial filtrate of fluid, solutes, and other substances enters the Bowman space. An increase in pressure in this space decreases filtration,[7] because the increased pressure resists the

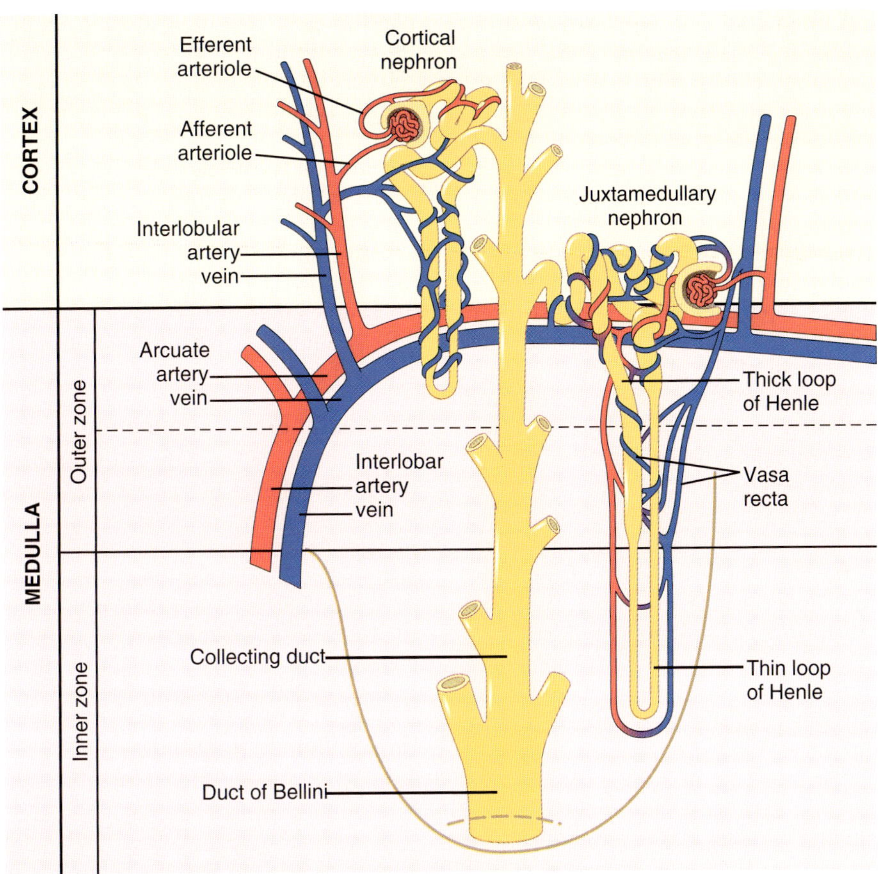

FIG. 23.4 Structure of Cortical Nephrons and Juxtamedullary Nephrons. (From Hall ME, Hall JE. *Guyton and Hall Textbook of Medical Physiology*. 14th ed. Elsevier; 2021.)

TABLE 23.1 Nephron Structures and Descriptions

Nephron Structure	Structure Description
Glomerulus	The first structure of each nephron is the glomerulus, a high-pressure capillary bed lined by a thin layer of endothelial cells.[1]
Bowman's Capsule	The glomerulus is covered by the Bowman's capsule,[2] a tough, membranous layer of epithelial cells. The Bowman space is located between the capillary walls of the glomerulus and the inner layer of the Bowman capsule.[1]
Proximal Tubule	The first portion of the nephron's tubular system is the proximal tubule, extending from the continuous structure that is the Bowman's capsule.[2] The proximal tubule is located in the cortex of the kidney.[2]
Loop of Henle	Depending on if the nephron has a short or long loop, the loop of Henle consists of a thin descending limb, a thin ascending limb, and a thick ascending limb[1] (Fig. 23.2A) and is surrounded by a dense capillary network (Fig. 23.2B). The nephrons with short loops of Henle do not have a thin ascending limb.[1] The thin descending limbs of short loops of Henle have flat, simple squamous epithelium.[5] The nephrons with long loops of Henle have a thin ascending limb with heavily interlaced, simple squamous epithelium[5] (Fig. 23.2A). The juxtamedullary nephrons have long loops of Henle.[2] The thick ascending limb of the loop of Henle is made of thicker, cuboidal epithelium.[2]
Juxtaglomerular Apparatus	The juxtaglomerular apparatus is located on the vascular side of the glomerulus not enclosed by the Bowman's capsule.[1] The juxtaglomerular apparatus contains specialized, columnar epithelial cells, known as the macula densa.[1] The macula densa is located at the end of the thick ascending limb and the beginning of the distal tubule[1] (Figs. 23.2A and 23.5).
Distal Tubule	The distal tubule extends from the thick ascending limb of the loop of Henle.[5] The distal tubule is located in the cortex of the kidney.[2]
Collecting Duct	The last portion of the nephron's tubular system is the collecting duct, beginning in the cortex and extending to the medulla.[2] The collecting ducts lead to calyces and ultimately the kidney pelvis.

movement of solutes and water from the capillaries into the space. For example, if the tubules of the nephrons are blocked by cellular debris or if the urinary tract is obstructed, backward pressure is exerted on the Bowman space, the GFR decreases, and urine output decreases. Conversely, a decrease in pressure in this space increases filtration.[7]

Tubular Reabsorption

The second process in the formation of urine is tubular reabsorption—the movement of a substance from the tubular lumen (filtrate) into the peritubular capillaries (blood).[8] Most tubular reabsorption occurs in the proximal tubule.[8] The proximal tubule reabsorbs (takes back) all of the glucose[9]; most of the bicarbonate,[9] sodium,[9] chloride[9]; much of the potassium[9] and phosphate[8]; some of the calcium[8]; and half of the urea.[9] The thin descending limb is very permeable to water but fairly impermeable to urea, sodium, and other solutes.[9] As a result, water (but not solute) is reabsorbed into the general circulation, and a more concentrated filtrate is produced. The filtrate then moves up the ascending limb, and both the thin and thick portions of the ascending limb are impermeable to water.[9] The thick ascending limb allows reabsorption of sodium, chloride, potassium, calcium, bicarbonate, and magnesium.[9] The distal tubule is impermeable to water and transports solutes such as sodium, chloride, potassium, bicarbonate, calcium.[3] Tubular reabsorption occurs by passive and active transport processes.[8]

Passive transport. Passive transport of substances depends on changes in concentration gradients and only requires kinetic energy.[10] Diffusion and osmosis are the primary passive transport processes.[10] Diffusion is the spontaneous movement of molecules or solutes from an area of higher concentration to an area of lower concentration across a semipermeable membrane (not all substances cross, particularly large molecules).[10] For example, when water is reabsorbed by the tubules, the concentration of urea in the tubules is increased. Urea then diffuses across the semipermeable membrane of the tubule and reenters the plasma to achieve balance in the concentration gradient.

Osmosis is the movement of water from an area of lower solute concentration to an area of higher solute concentration across a semipermeable membrane.[10] For example, when the solute concentration of the filtrate is greater in the tubular lumen than the peritubular capillaries, water passively moves from the capillaries into the tubular lumen to balance the concentration gradient.

Active transport. Active transport of substances requires energy in the form of adenosine triphosphate (ATP) to move against an electrochemical gradient.[10] In active transport, the substance combines with a carrier protein and is then moved across the semipermeable membrane using additional sources of energy besides kinetic energy.[10] Substances that are reabsorbed via active transport include glucose, amino acids, calcium, potassium, sodium, and chloride.[10] The rate at which substances can be actively reabsorbed depends on the availability of the carriers, saturation of the carriers, and availability of energy.[9] There is a transport maximum rate at which substances can be reabsorbed and varies according to each substance.[9]

Tubular Secretion

The third process in urine formation is tubular secretion[2]—the movement of a substance from the peritubular capillaries (blood) into the tubular lumen (filtrate).[3] Tubular secretion plays a lesser role than tubular reabsorption in changing the filtrate into urine, but tubular secretion is important in determining the amounts of substances that are excreted in the urine.[2] Tubular secretion allows the body to remove excess substances; it occurs by diffusion and by active transport, and it depends on the needs of the body.[3] Simply, if it isn't reabsorbed in the tubules, it is then secreted. The final composition of the urine occurs in the collecting duct. Acidification of the urine is accomplished by the transport of bicarbonate and hydrogen ions in the collecting duct. After the urine leaves the collecting duct, no change in the composition of the filtrate occurs. Box 23.1 summarizes urine formation in the various structures of the nephron.

Metabolic Waste Elimination

Metabolic processes in the body produce waste products that are selectively filtered out of the circulation by the kidneys. These waste products include urea, creatinine, uric acid, bilirubin, and metabolites of various hormones.[2] Urea is a byproduct of amino acid metabolism in the liver.[2] Urea is filtered by the glomerulus and about half is then reabsorbed back into the bloodstream by the tubules.[9] Creatinine is a byproduct of muscle metabolism.[2] Creatinine is normally completely filtered and minimally reabsorbed by the kidneys because it is larger molecule than urea.[9]

Hemodynamic Regulation

Renin-Angiotensin-Aldosterone System

The kidneys regulate arterial blood pressure by altering peripheral vascular resistance and by maintaining the circulating blood volume through the renin-angiotensin-aldosterone system (RAAS).[8] *Renin* is synthesized, stored, and released in the *juxtaglomerular apparatus*[8] (Fig. 23.5). Renin is released into circulation in response to reduced stretch of the afferent arteriole from decreased renal blood flow, *macula densa* detection of reduced sodium chloride delivery to the distal tubule, and

BOX 23.1 Urine Formation

Glomerulus
- Filters fluid and solutes from blood[3,7]

Proximal Tubule
- Reabsorbs glucose, bicarbonate, sodium, chloride, potassium, phosphate, calcium, urea[9]

Thin Descending Limb of Loop of Henle
- Very permeable to water[9]

Thin Ascending Limb of Loop of Henle
- Impermeable to water[9]

Thick Ascending Limb of Loop of Henle
- Reabsorbs magnesium, bicarbonate, sodium, chloride, potassium, calcium[9]
- Impermeable to water[9]

Distal Tubule
- Reabsorbs bicarbonate, sodium, chloride, potassium, calcium[3]
- Impermeable to water[3]

Collecting Duct
- Reabsorbs less than 5% of solutes[9]
- Hydrogen and bicarbonate ions reabsorbed or secreted to acidify urine

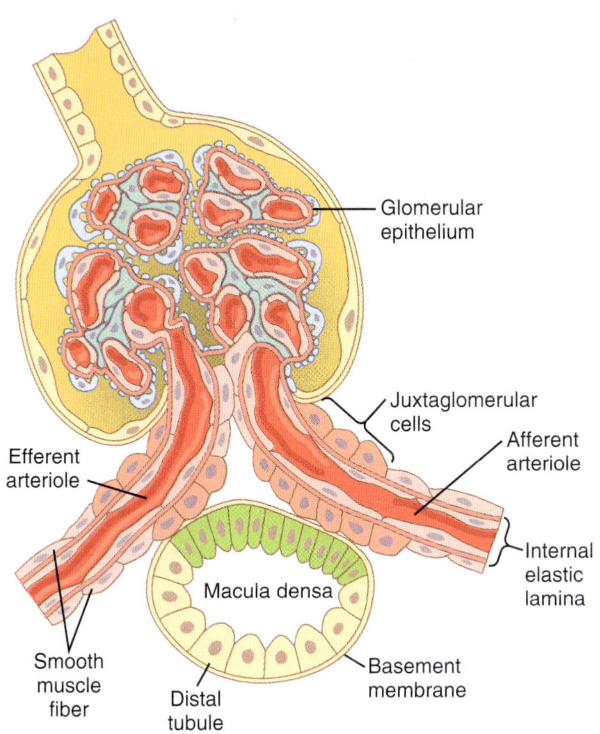

FIG. 23.5 Structure of Juxtaglomerular Apparatus. (From Hall ME, Hall JE. *Guyton and Hall Textbook of Medical Physiology*. 14th ed. Elsevier; 2021.)

increased sympathetic stimulation of the kidneys from low circulatory volume.[3,8] Renin converts angiotensinogen to *angiotensin I*.[8] In the lungs, angiotensin I is converted to *angiotensin II* by the angiotensin converting enzyme.[3] Angiotensin II is a powerful vasoconstrictor, increasing afferent and efferent arteriole vasoconstriction, increasing systemic vascular resistance, and increasing arterial blood pressure.[8] Additionally, angiotensin II binds to receptors in the adrenal cortex to stimulate release of *aldosterone*.[3,8] Aldosterone acts on the distal tubule to facilitate sodium and water reabsorption, resulting in an expanded circulating blood volume and increased blood pressure.[8] When the arterial blood pressure increases, the juxtaglomerular apparatus reduces the release of renin, and the RAAS is less active. Fig. 23.6 summarizes the major aspects of the renin-angiotensin-aldosterone system.

Prostaglandins

Eicosanoids are a vasoactive metabolite that include prostaglandins.[11] Some prostaglandins have a local vasodilatory effect and act primarily on the afferent arterioles to maintain blood flow, glomerular perfusion, and glomerular filtration.[3] These prostaglandins maintain blood flow to the kidneys despite systemic vasoconstriction from angiotensin II and increased sympathetic stimulation of the kidneys.[3]

Fluid Balance

A balance of the total amount and composition of water in the body is vital for homeostasis.[12]

A state of equilibrium is established when physiologic forces move fluid between compartments and solute composition in the fluid compartments are tightly regulated. Fluid balance is achieved by passive and active transport processes as discussed in the Urine Formation section.

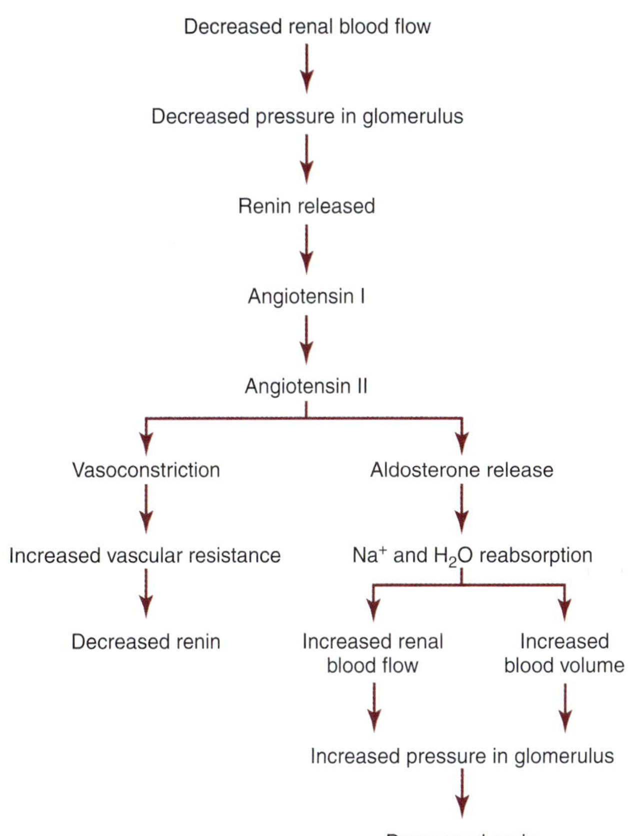

FIG. 23.6 Renin-Angiotensin-Aldosterone System.

In an average 70-kg man, total body water is about 42 liters, accounting for about 60% of the body weight.[12] The percent of body weight will vary based on age, sex, and adipose tissue.[12] The body has two main fluid compartments: intracellular and extracellular.[12] The *intracellular compartment* is the fluid inside each of the body's cells and accounts for 28 liters or 40% of the body weight.[12] The remaining fluid is outside the body's cells and makes up the *extracellular compartment*.[12] The extracellular compartment is composed of two distinct subcompartments: *intravascular* and *interstitial*.[12] The intravascular compartment, referring to the fluid within the blood vessels, accounts for 3 liters or 4% of the body weight.[12] The interstitial compartment is composed of fluid in the tissue spaces outside of the body cells and the blood vessels.[12] The interstitial compartment accounts for 11 liters or 16% of the body weight.[12] Approximate amounts of fluid contained in each compartment are shown in Fig. 23.7A. The composition of the intracellular, intravascular, and interstitial compartments is shown in Fig. 23.7B.

Intracellular fluid balance is influenced by tonicity and osmolality.[12] Tonicity affects the composition of the cell through movement of water in and out of the cell based on the osmolality differences between the intracellular and extracellular compartments.[12] Fig. 23.8 summarizes the effects of tonicity on the cell. Osmolality is the measure of the number of solutes in water, and the value is stated in milliosmoles per kilogram of water.[12] Osmolality affects fluid volume by moving water based on concentration gradients across body fluid compartments.

Intravascular and interstitial fluid balance is influenced by opposing hydrostatic and oncotic pressures.[13] Hydrostatic

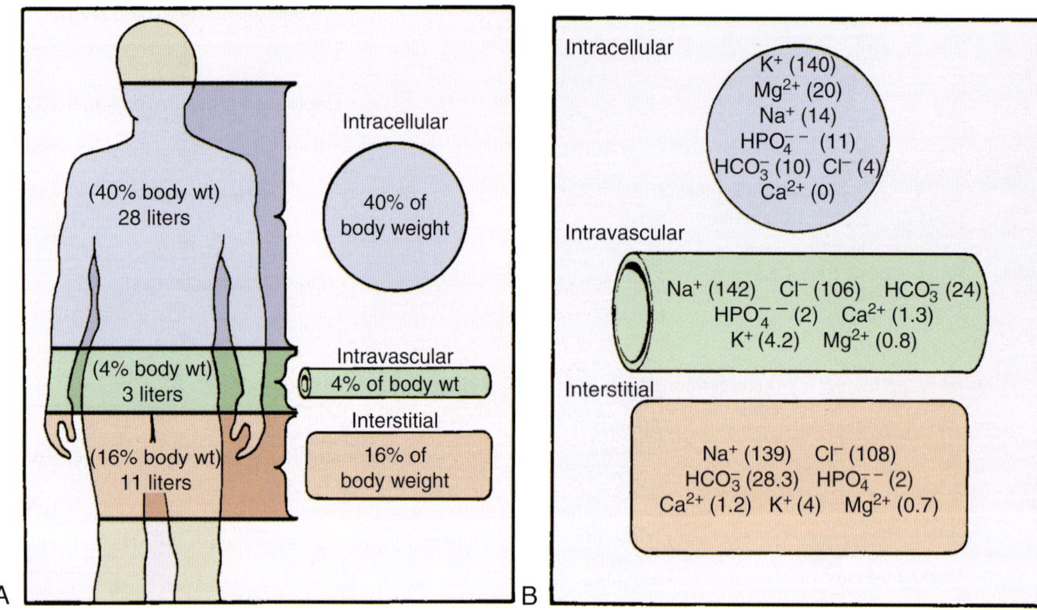

FIG. 23.7 (A) Fluid compartments. The values shown are for an average 70-kg man. (B) Electrolytes by fluid compartment. The values shown are in milliosmoles per liter of water.

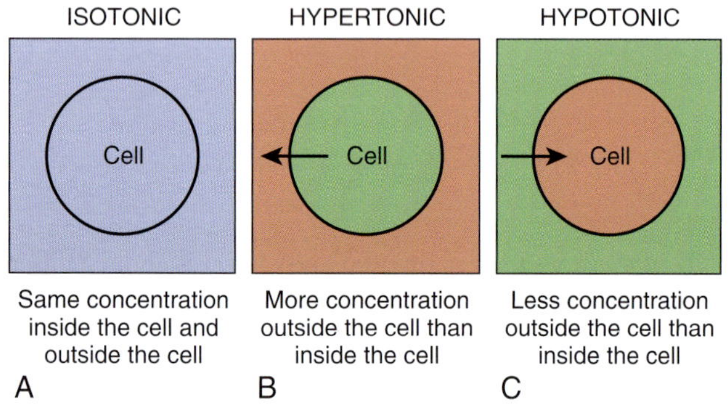

FIG. 23.8 (A) Isotonic solution. The extracellular solute concentration is the same as the intracellular concentration, with no movement of water into or out of the cell. (B) Hypertonic solution. The extracellular solute concentration is greater than the intracellular concentration. Water moves from the cell into the extracellular compartment. (C) Hypotonic solution. The extracellular solute concentration is less than the intracellular concentration. Water moves from the extracellular compartment into the cell.

pressure is the force of fluid against vessel walls, creating the tendency for fluids and solutes to move into the interstitial compartment by filtration (movement of fluid and substances from an area of high pressure to one of low pressure).[14] Oncotic pressure is the pull exerted by plasma proteins to retain fluid in the intravascular compartment.[14] This force is maintained because proteins are large and cannot move or be transported across the semipermeable membrane.[14] Without the oncotic pressure counteracting the hydrostatic pressure, fluid would leave the intravascular space until the space was depleted. Although hydrostatic pressure favors fluid and solute movement out of the intravascular compartment, the oncotic pressure of the plasma holds the fluid and substances in the intravascular compartment. When a decrease in serum protein lessens the oncotic pressure in the intravascular space so that the interstitial oncotic pressure is greater than the intravascular oncotic pressure, fluid is then moved from the vascular space into the interstitial space, causing edema.

The kidneys contribute to fluid balance through their ability to concentrate and dilute urine.

The key factors in concentration and dilution of urine are (1) sodium and water permeability in the nephron (see Urine Formation section), (2) osmolality gradients in the kidney cortex and medulla, and (3) neural and hormonal signals.[3]

Osmolality Gradients in the Kidney Cortex and Medulla

The osmolality of the interstitial fluid increases from the kidney cortex to the kidney medulla.[15] The countercurrent mechanism in the nephron is an important part of concentration and dilution of urine.[15] The countercurrent mechanism is the exchange of water and solutes between the loop of Henle and the peritubular capillaries known as the vasa recta.[15] The thin ascending limb of the loop of Henle, present in juxtamedullary and not cortical nephrons, is impermeable to water, adding to the high osmolality in the kidney medulla.[15] The osmolality of the filtrate changes as it goes through the nephron.[3] Because of the large number of solutes in the glomerular filtrate, the filtrate leaves the glomerulus hyperosmotic.[3] When the filtrate leaves the proximal tubule, it is isosmotic (equivalent to plasma).[3] Because of the concurrent mechanism in the loop of Henle, the filtrate leaves the thin ascending limb hypoosmotic (more dilute than plasma).[3] Lastly, filtrate leaves the distal tubule and collecting duct hypoosmotic until acted on by a neural or hormonal signal.[3] For example, when antidiuretic hormone (ADH) is present, filtrate becomes hyperosmotic.[3]

Neural and Hormonal Signals Affecting Concentration and Dilution of Urine

Antidiuretic hormone and aquaporins. ADH, also known as *vasopressin*, is secreted by the posterior pituitary gland.[15] As serum osmolality increases above normal (e.g., states of hypovolemia or hypernatremia), ADH is released and carried through the circulation to the nephrons.[15] It functions primarily on the water channels, called *aquaporins*, in the distal tubule and collecting duct to concentrate urine.[15] Water permeability, independent of solute excretion, is determined by the absence or presence of ADH.[15] In the absence of ADH or with small amounts of ADH, the urine becomes dilute, whereas larger amounts of ADH result in concentrated urine.

Atrial natriuretic peptide. Atrial natriuretic peptide (ANP) is secreted primarily by the cells in the atria of the heart.[3] As the atria stretch due to increased atrial distention and pressure, ANP is released and carried through the circulation to the nephrons.[15] It increases GFR by vasodilation of the afferent arteriole and vasoconstriction of the efferent arteriole.[3] ANP also influences sodium and water regulation by suppressing aldosterone release from the adrenal cortex,[16] inhibiting the RAAS,[16] and counterbalancing ADH secretion through a negative feedback mechanism.[17] Sodium and water excretion occurs in the proximal tubule, distal tubule, and collecting duct.[17] The overall effects of ANP are reduced peripheral and kidney vasoconstriction and decreased circulating volume.[3]

Electrolyte Balance

Electrolytes are elements or compounds that, when dissolved in water, dissociate into ions, electrically charged atomic particles. Ions in solution in the fluid allow the fluid to conduct an electrical current. A balance exists between cations (positively charged ions), anions (negatively charged ions), and other substances in the fluid compartments. Maintaining this balance, through passive and active transport across cell membranes, is important to the normal function of all body systems. Electrolytes exist in differing amounts in each of the fluid compartments. The primary electrolytes and other substances of importance in fluid and electrolyte balance are shown by fluid compartment in Fig. 23.7B. Normal serum values and select physiologic functions of potassium, sodium, chloride, phosphate, calcium, and magnesium are summarized in Table 23.2.

Potassium

Potassium (K^+) is the primary intracellular electrolyte[19] and is responsible for numerous physiologic functions[18] (Table 23.2). Intracellular and extracellular potassium concentrations are influenced by many factors, as listed in Box 23.2. The gastrointestinal (GI) tract and skin excrete small amounts of potassium, but the major regulators of potassium stores are the kidneys.[18] Potassium is filtered by the glomerulus, and most is immediately reabsorbed back into the bloodstream at the proximal tubule[28] (Fig. 23.9). Reabsorption and secretion of potassium are influenced by many factors, as listed in Box 23.3. Potassium and sodium are both cations, one intracellular and one extracellular respectively, and must remain in balance to preserve electrical neutrality at the cell membrane.

Sodium

Sodium (Na^+) is the most abundant extracellular electrolyte in the body[29] and is key to many physiologic functions (Table 23.2). Sodium is filtered by the glomerulus and then reabsorbed back into the bloodstream at the proximal tubule, in the loop of Henle, in the distal tubule, and in the collecting duct[29] (Fig. 23.10). Sodium reabsorption in the distal tubule and collecting duct is increased by

TABLE 23.2 Electrolyte Normal Serum Values and Select Physiologic Functions

Electrolyte	Normal Serum Value	Select Physiologic Functions
Potassium	3.5–4.5 mEq/L	• Transmission of nerve impulses[18] • Myocardial, skeletal, and smooth muscle contractility[18] • Intracellular osmolality[19] • Acid–base balance[20]
Sodium	135–145 mEq/L	• Body fluid movement and retention[21] • Extracellular osmolality[22] • Active transport mechanism (with potassium) • Neuromuscular activity • Acid–base balance[20]
Chloride	97–110 mEq/L	• Extracellular osmolality[23] (with sodium) • Body water balance (with sodium) • Red blood cell oxygenation and carbon dioxide transport • Acidity of body fluids, especially gastric secretions • Acid–base balance
Phosphorus	2.5–4.5 mg/dL	• Intracellular energy production (adenosine triphosphate)[24] • Bone strength[24] • Structure of cellular membrane[24] • Enzyme regulation[25] • Oxygen delivery to tissues • Acid–base balance[24]
Calcium	8.5–10.5 mg/dL	• Bone structure[26] • Skeletal muscle contraction[26] • Blood coagulation[26] • Heart muscle contraction[26]
Magnesium	1.3–2.1 mEq/L	• Neuromuscular transmission[25] • Contraction of heart muscle[25] • Activation of enzymes for cellular metabolism[27] • Active transport at cellular level[27]

BOX 23.2 Factors Affecting Intracellular and Extracellular Potassium Concentrations

Increased intracellular potassium concentration (movement of potassium into the cell)[19]:
- Insulin
- Epinephrine
- Metabolic alkalosis
- Decreased extracellular fluid osmolarity

Increased extracellular potassium concentration (movement of potassium out of the cell)[19]:
- Cell lysis
- Muscle injury (e.g., exercise)
- Metabolic acidosis
- Increased extracellular fluid osmolarity

BOX 23.3 Factors Affecting Reabsorption and Secretion of Potassium in the Nephron

- Increased secretion of potassium[19]: increased extracellular potassium concentration, increased aldosterone, increased tubular flow rate (e.g., high sodium intake, volume expansion, diuretics), chronic acidosis
- Decreases secretion of potassium[19]: acute acidosis

aldosterone.[19] Diuretics inhibit sodium reabsorption in the thick ascending limb of the loop of Henle and in the distal tubule,[21] and consequently sodium is eliminated in the urine. The body contains a complex system of safeguards and feedback mechanisms to protect the level of sodium in the extracellular fluid.[29]

Chloride

Chloride (Cl^-) is predominantly found in the extracellular fluid[29] and its physiologic functions are summarized in Table 23.2. Along with sodium, chloride is filtered by the glomerulus and then reabsorbed back into the bloodstream at the proximal tubule, in the loop of Henle, in the distal tubule, and in the collecting duct.[29] Serum chloride levels usually change alongside serum sodium levels.[23]

Phosphate

Phosphate (PO_4^{3-}) is predominantly found in the intracellular fluid,[24] and its several physiologic functions are listed in Table 23.2. Approximately 80% of phosphate is found in bones.[24,30] The serum phosphate values represent a minute portion of the actual body stores (less than 1%).[30] Serum phosphate levels are influenced by GI tract absorption, but the major regulators of serum phosphate are the kidneys.[30] Phosphate is filtered by the glomerulus and then reabsorbed back into the bloodstream at the proximal tubule.[19] Phosphate excretion by the kidney is increased by parathyroid hormone[27] and parathyroid hormone is released in

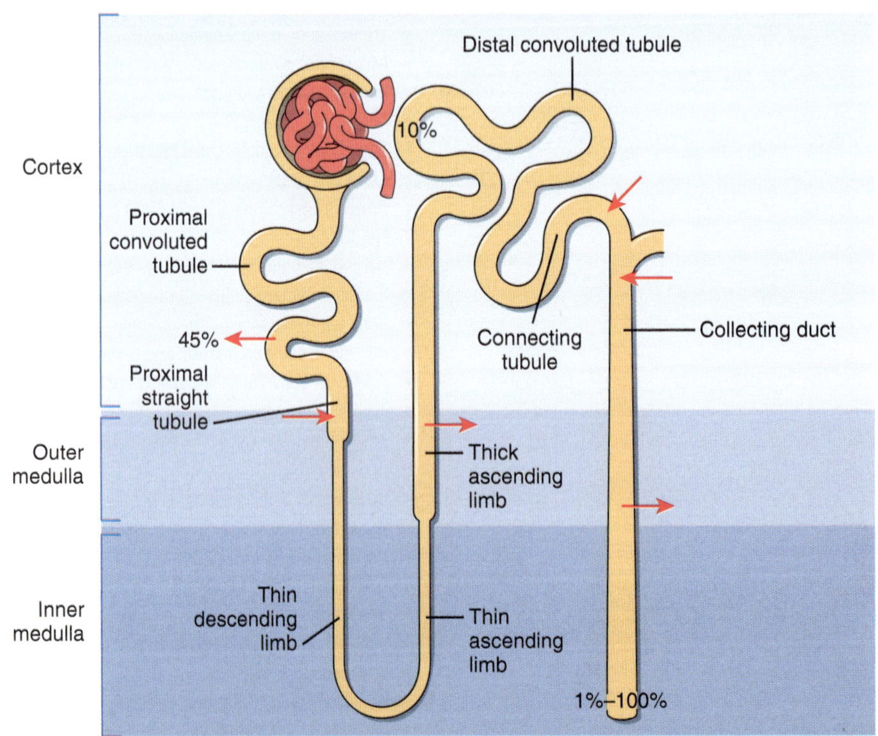

FIG. 23.9 Potassium Transport Along the Nephron. The percentages show the amount of potassium reabsorbed in the different areas: 45% reabsorption in the proximal convoluted tubule. Other factors also alter potassium reabsorption; potassium excreted in the urine is highly variable. (From Johnsen, RJ, Floege J, Tonelli M. *Comprehensive Clinical Nephrology*. 7th ed. Elsevier; 2024.)

response to low serum calcium levels.[26] This inverse relationship in kidney regulation of phosphate and calcium is also seen with vitamin D and its inhibition of phosphate excretion as it stimulates the reabsorption of calcium by the tubules.[27]

Calcium

Calcium (Ca^{2+}) is found in both intracellular and extracellular fluid.[25] The physiologic functions of calcium are outlined in Table 23.2. Almost all (99%) calcium is found in bones,[19,26] with only about 1% is in the intracellular fluid and 0.1% in the extracellular fluid.[19] Serum calcium levels are mainly influenced by GI tract absorption and secretion,[19] mobilization of calcium stores in bone,[25] and only minimally regulated by the kidneys in comparison.[19] Serum calcium exists in three forms: ionized (48%), protein bound (45%), and complexed (7%).[26] The kidneys filter ionized and complexed calcium in the glomerulus and reabsorb calcium back into the bloodstream at the proximal tubule[26] (Fig. 23.11). Parathyroid hormone and vitamin D decrease calcium excretion (increases calcium reabsorption).[19] The uptake of calcium is influenced by the levels of phosphate and regulated by the GI tract, bone, and kidneys in response to parathyroid hormone and vitamin D.[25]

Magnesium

Magnesium (Mg^{2+}) is the second most abundant intracellular electrolyte and is responsible for important physiologic functions[25] (Table 23.2). Magnesium is mainly found in bone, muscle, and soft tissue (99%), with only about 1% of magnesium in the extracellular fluid.[27] Though the GI tract and skin excrete magnesium, the primary route of magnesium elimination is through the kidneys.[25] Similar to calcium, serum magnesium is ionized (55%), protein bound (30%), and complexed (15%).[25] The kidneys filter ionized and complexed magnesium in the glomerulus and reabsorb magnesium back into the bloodstream at the loop of Henle, specifically the thick ascending limb[25] (Fig. 23.12). A rise or depletion of magnesium is the main factor influencing reabsorption in the kdney.[27]

Acid–Base Balance

The kidneys are actively involved in acid–base regulation by secreting hydrogen ions and by reabsorbing, producing, and excreting bicarbonate ions.[20] When a hydrogen ion is secreted, a bicarbonate ion is reabsorbed.[20] About 90% of hydrogen ion secretion and bicarbonate reabsorption occurs in the proximal tubule.[20] When excess hydrogen ions are secreted in the tubules, the ions combine with buffers to produce bicarbonate ions for reabsorption.[20] Bicarbonate, the principal extracellular buffer, performs the essential function of maintaining the acid–base balance.[20] In an alkalotic state, less hydrogen ions are secreted, less bicarbonate ions are reabsorbed, and more bicarbonate ions are excreted by the kidneys.[20] In contrast, when the body is in an acidotic state, secretion of hydrogen ions is increased, reabsorption of bicarbonate ions is increased, and production of additional bicarbonate ions for reabsorption is initiated by the

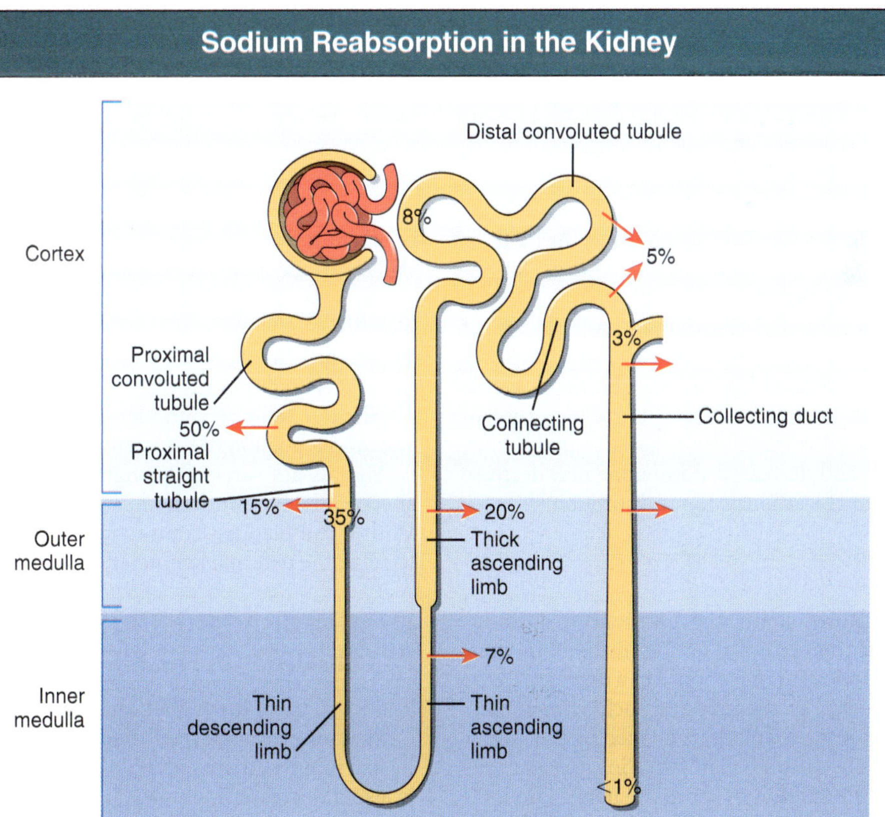

FIG. 23.10 Sodium Transport Along the Nephron. The percentages show the amount of sodium reabsorbed in the different areas: 50% reabsorption in the proximal convoluted tubule, 20% reabsorption in the thick ascending limb. Other factors also alter sodium reabsorption, as normally less than 1% of sodium is excreted in the urine. (From Johnsen, RJ, Floege J, Tonelli M. *Comprehensive Clinical Nephrology.* 7th ed. Elsevier; 2024.)

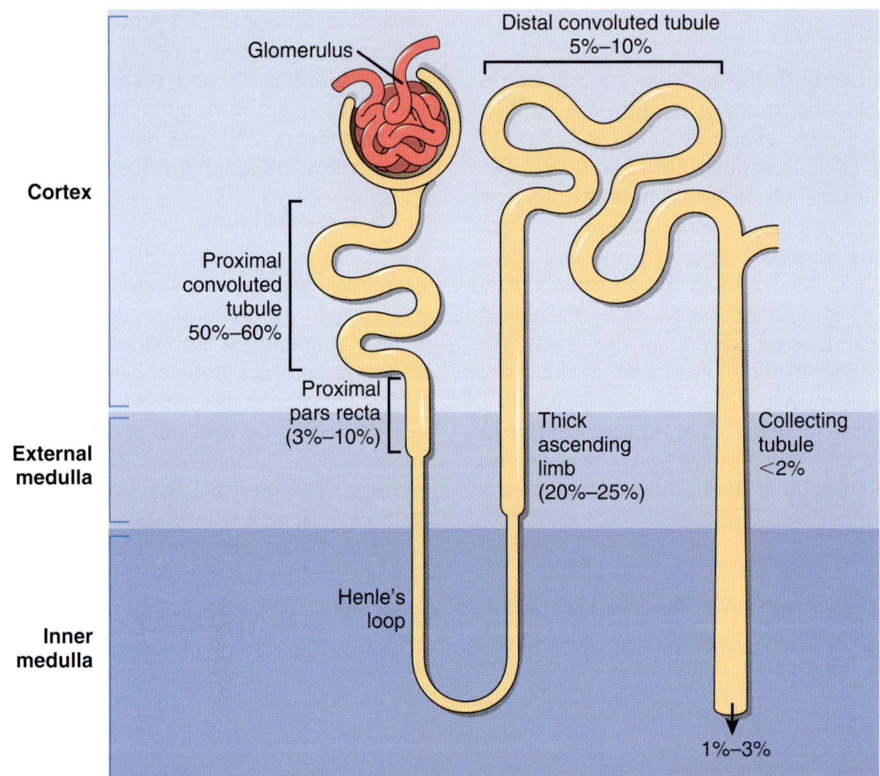

FIG. 23.11 Calcium Transport Along the Nephron. The percentages show the amount of calcium reabsorbed in the different areas: 50% to 60% reabsorption in the proximal convoluted tubule, 20% to 25% reabsorption in the thick ascending limb. Other factors also alter calcium reabsorption, as normally only 1% to 3% of calcium is excreted in the urine. (From Johnsen, RJ, Floege J, Tonelli M. *Comprehensive Clinical Nephrology.* 7th ed. Elsevier; 2024.)

kidneys.[20] The kidneys do not function as rapidly as the lungs in altering acid–base concentrations, but they are a potent day-to-day acid–base regulation system.[20]

The RAAS, as well as fluid and electrolyte imbalances, affect acid–base balance.[20] Decreased extracellular fluid volume, increased angiotensin II, increased aldosterone, and hypokalemia may increase hydrogen ion secretion and bicarbonate ion reabsorption.[20] Conversely, increased extracellular volume, hyperkalemia, decreased angiotensin II, and decreased aldosterone may decrease hydrogen ion secretion and bicarbonate ion reabsorption.[20]

Other Kidney Functions

Erythrocyte Production

The kidneys secrete erythropoietin, the hormone that stimulates erythrocyte (red blood cell) production in the bone marrow.[31] Erythropoietin is released in response to a decrease in the amount of oxygen delivered to the kidneys, such as in anemia or prolonged hypoxia.[31] Erythropoietin is formed by the kidney within minutes to hours of the body being in a low oxygen state and reaches maximum production in approximately 24 hours.[31]

Vitamin D Activation

The kidneys convert vitamin D from food sources into an active form, calcitriol, for use by the body.[27] Active vitamin D stimulates the absorption of calcium by the intestine and reabsorption of calcium by the tubules[27] so that calcium is available for bone and tooth metabolism and blood clotting functions.[26]

Urinary Drainage

When the bladder is full, it is emptied, and urine is released by a process called micturition.[2]

Bladder fullness stimulates stretch receptors in the bladder wall and a portion of the urethra.[2]

Signals are carried through nerves to contract the bladder, specifically the smooth muscle called the detrusor muscle.[2] With a full bladder, contractions usually are powerful enough to relax the external sphincter to release urine.[2]

EFFECTS OF AGING ON THE ANATOMY AND PHYSIOLOGY OF THE KIDNEY

The anatomy of the kidney changes with age. A decrease in size of the kidney can be seen after the age of 50 with the reduction in size mainly attributed to an atrophied kidney cortex.[32] There is also a decrease in glomeruli, and about 50% of nephrons are lost over the age of 50.[32] As a part of aging, the size of the kidney decreases, and kidney physiology is also altered.

Kidney function declines gradually with age. Glomerular filtration rate begins to decline, approximately 0.6 to 1 mL/min/1.73 m^2 per year, after the age of 40.[32,33] Comorbidities

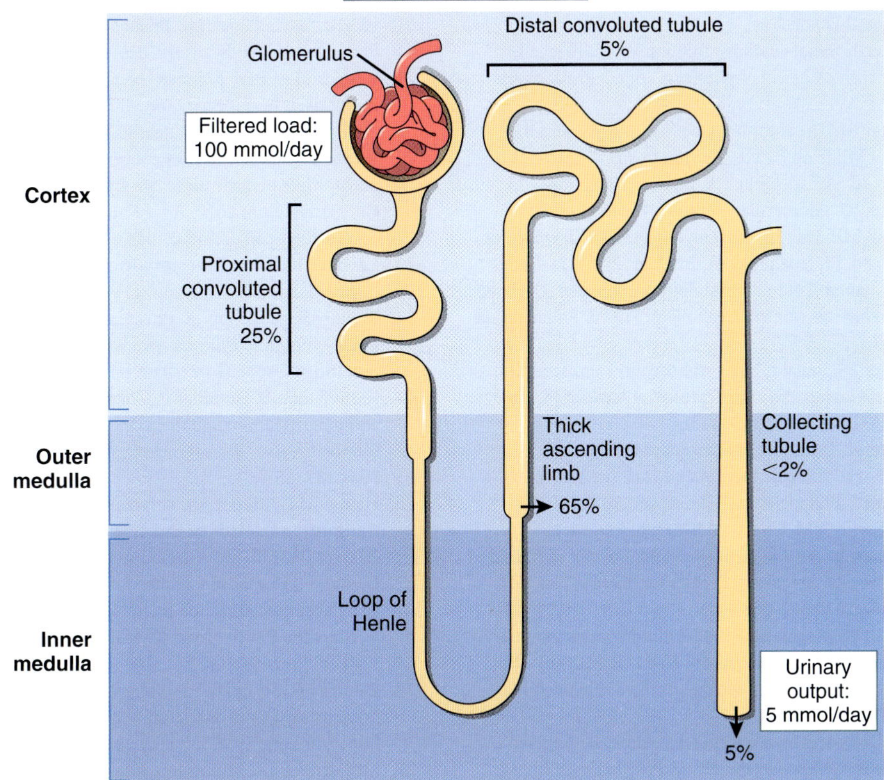

FIG. 23.12 Magnesium Transport Along the Nephron. The percentages show the amount of magnesium reabsorbed in the different areas: 65% reabsorption in the thick ascending limb, 25% reabsorption in the proximal convoluted tubule. Other factors also alter magnesium reabsorption, as normally only 5% of magnesium is excreted in the urine. (From Johnsen, RJ, Floege J, Tonelli M. *Comprehensive Clinical Nephrology*. 7th ed. Elsevier; 2024.)

prevalent among older adults, such as obesity and diabetes, contribute to unhealthy aging of the kidney and negatively impact GFR and lead to a faster decline.[32,33] However, despite a decrease in GFR and the associated reduction in creatinine clearance, the serum creatinine level may not rise. This occurs because the reduced muscle mass associated with aging produces less creatinine to be excreted by the kidneys, essentially masking the overall effects of aging on the kidneys.[32] Cystatin C may be a better indicator of GFR among older adults.[32,34] Other changes in kidney function during aging include decreased blood flow to the kidneys,[33] decreased capacity of the kidneys to dilute and concentrate urine,[32,33] decreased sodium and water reabsorption[33], and decreased potassium excretion.[33]

The kidneys carry out many functions. Although fluid balance is perhaps the most obvious function, an understanding of the numerous other roles of the kidneys provides crucial information for the care of any critically ill patient.

KEY POINTS

Anatomy

- The kidneys are paired organs located retroperitoneally, one on each side of the vertebral column between T12 and L3.
- The nephron is the functional unit of the kidney; it comprises the glomerulus, Bowman capsule, proximal tubule, loop of Henle, distal tubule, and collecting duct.

Physiology

- The kidneys play a major role in maintaining homeostasis.
- Important functions of the kidneys include urine formation, metabolic waste elimination, hemodynamic regulation, fluid–electrolyte balance, acid-base balance, erythrocyte production, and vitamin D activation.

Visit the Evolve site at http://evolve.elsevier.com/Urden/CriticalCareNursing for additional study materials.

REFERENCES

1. Verlander JW, Clapp WL. Chapter 2. Anatomy of the kidney. In: Yu ASL, Chertow GM, Luyckx V, Marsden PA, Skorecki K, Taal MW, eds. *Brenner & Rector's The Kidney*. 11th ed. Philadelphia, PA: Elsevier; 2020:38–79.
2. Hall JE, Hall ME. Chapter 26. The urinary system: functional anatomy and urine formation by the kidneys. In: Hall ME, Hall JE, eds. *Guyton and Hall Textbook of Medical Physiology*. 14th ed. Philadelphia, PA: Elsevier; 2021:321–330.

3. Russel S. Chapter 3. Physiology of the kidney. In: Bodin SM, ed. *Contemporary Nephrology Nursing*. 4th ed. Pitman, NJ: American Nephrology Nursing Association; 2022:63–82.
4. Navar LG, Maddox DA, Munger KA. Chapter 3. The renal circulations and glomerular filtration. In: Yu ASL, Chertow GM, Luyckx V, Marsden PA, Skorecki K, Taal MW, eds. *Brenner & Rector's the Kidney*. 11th ed. Philadelphia, PA: Elsevier; 2020:80–114.
5. Kriz W, Elger M. Chapter 1. Renal anatomy. In: Johnsen RJ, Floege J, Tonelli M, eds. *Comprehensive Clinical Nephrology*. 7th ed. Philadelphia, PA: Elsevier; 2024:1–12.
6. Hall JE, Hall ME. Chapter 61. The autonomic nervous system and the adrenal medulla. In: Hall ME, Hall JE, eds. *Guyton and Hall Textbook of Medical Physiology*. 14th ed. Philadelphia, PA: Elsevier; 2021:763–775.
7. Hall JE, Hall ME. Chapter 27. Glomerular filtration, renal blood flow, and their control. In: Hall ME, Hall JE, eds. *Guyton and Hall Textbook of Medical Physiology*. 14th ed. Philadelphia, PA: Elsevier; 2021:331–342.
8. Bailey MA, Unwin RJ. Chapter 2. Renal physiology. In: Johnsen RJ, Floege J, Tonelli M, eds. *Comprehensive Clinical Nephrology*. 7th ed. Philadelphia, PA: Elsevier; 2024:13–26.
9. Hall JE, Hall ME. Chapter 28. Renal tubular reabsorption and secretion. In: Hall ME, Hall JE, eds. *Guyton and Hall Textbook of Medical Physiology*. 14th ed. Philadelphia, PA: Elsevier; 2021:343–364.
10. Hall JE, Hall ME. Chapter 4. Transport of substances through cell membranes. In: Hall ME, Hall JE, eds. *Guyton and Hall Textbook of Medical Physiology*. 14th ed. Philadelphia, PA: Elsevier; 2021:51–62.
11. Harris RC, Zhang MZ, Breyer RM. Chapter 13. Arachidonic acid metabolites and the kidney. In: Yu ASL, Chertow GM, Luyckx V, Marsden PA, Skorecki K, Taal MW, eds. *Brenner & Rector's the Kidney*. 11th ed. Philadelphia, PA: Elsevier; 2020:357–388.
12. Hall JE, Hall ME. Chapter 25. Regulation of body fluid compartments: extracellular and intracellular fluids; Edema. In: Hall ME, Hall JE, eds. *Guyton and Hall Textbook of Medical Physiology*. 14th ed. Philadelphia, PA: Elsevier; 2021:305–320.
13. Ellison DH. Chapter 8. Disorders of extracellular volume. In: Johnsen RJ, Floege J, Tonelli M, eds. *Comprehensive Clinical Nephrology*. 7th ed. Philadelphia, PA: Elsevier; 2024:94–101.
14. Hall JE, Hall ME. Chapter 16. The microcirculation and lymphatic system: capillary fluid exchange, interstitial fluid, and lymph flow. In: Hall ME, Hall JE, eds. *Guyton and Hall Textbook of Medical Physiology*. 14th ed. Philadelphia, PA: Elsevier; 2021:193–204.
15. Hall JE, Hall ME. Chapter 29. Urine concentration and dilution; Regulation of extracellular fluid osmolarity and sodium concentration. In: Hall ME, Hall JE, eds. *Guyton and Hall Textbook of Medical Physiology*. 14th ed. Philadelphia, PA: Elsevier; 2021:365–381.
16. Fu S, Ping P, Wang F, Luo L. Synthesis, secretion, function, metabolism and application of natriuretic peptides in heart failure. *J Biol Eng*. 2018;12:2. https://doi.org/10.1186/s13036-017-0093-0.
17. Slotki IN, Skorecki K. Chapter 14. Disorders of sodium balance. In: Yu ASL, Chertow GM, Luyckx V, Marsden PA, Skorecki K, Taal MW, eds. *Brenner & Rector's the Kidney*. 11th ed. Philadelphia, PA: Elsevier; 2020:390–442.
18. Weiner ID, Linas SL, Wingo CS. Chapter 10. Disorders of potassium metabolism. In: Johnsen RJ, Floege J, Tonelli M, eds. *Comprehensive Clinical Nephrology*. 7th ed. Philadelphia, PA: Elsevier; 2024:125–136.
19. Hall JE, Hall ME. Chapter 30. Renal regulation of potassium, calcium, phosphate, and magnesium; Integration of renal mechanisms for control of blood volume and extracellular fluid volume. In: Hall ME, Hall JE, eds. *Guyton and Hall Textbook of Medical Physiology*. 14th ed. Philadelphia, PA: Elsevier; 2021:383–401.
20. Hall JE, Hall ME. Chapter 31. Acid-base regulation. In: Hall ME, Hall JE, eds. *Guyton and Hall Textbook of Medical Physiology*. 14th ed. Philadelphia, PA: Elsevier; 2021:403–420.
21. Kashkouli A, Berl T, Sands JM. Chapter 9. Disorders of water metabolism. In: Johnsen RJ, Floege J, Tonelli M, eds. *Comprehensive Clinical Nephrology*. 7th ed. Philadelphia, PA: Elsevier; 2024:108–124.
22. Winn SN, Lehrich RW, Greenberg A. Diagnosis and management of disorders of body tonicity – hyponatremia and hypernatremia: Core curriculum 2020. *Am J Kid Dis*. 2020;75(2):272–286. https://doi.org/10.1053/j.ajkd.2019.07.014.
23. Edwards JC. Chloride transport. *Compr Physiol*. 2012;2:1061–1092. https://doi.org/10.1002/cphy.c110027.
24. Rubio-Aliaga I, Krapf R. Phosphate intake, hyperphosphatemia, and kidney function. *Pflugers Arch*. 2022;474(8):935–947. https://doi.org/10.1007/s00424-022-02691-x.
25. Kestenbaum B, Houillier P. Chapter 11. Disorders of calcium, phosphate, and magnesium metabolism. In: Johnsen RJ, Floege J, Tonelli M, eds. *Comprehensive Clinical Nephrology*. 7th ed. Philadelphia, PA: Elsevier; 2024:137–153.
26. Hanna RM, Ahdoot RS, Kalantar-Zadeh K, Ghobry L, Kurtz I. Calcium transport in the kidney and disease processes. *Fron Endocrinol*. 2022;12:762130. https://doi.org/10.3389/fendo.2021.762130.
27. Berndt TJ, Kumar R. Chapter 7. The regulation of calcium, magnesium, and phosphate excretion by the kidney. In: Yu ASL, Chertow GM, Luyckx V, Marsden PA, Skorecki K, Taal MW, eds. *Brenner & Rector's the Kidney*. 11th ed. Philadelphia, PA: Elsevier; 2020:80–114.
28. Palmer BF, Clegg DJ. Physiology and pathophysiology of potassium homeostasis: Core curriculum 2019. *Am J Kid Dis*. 2019;74(5):682–695. https://doi.org/10.1053/j.ajkd.2019.03.427.
29. McCormick JA, Mount DB, Ellison DH. Chapter 6. Transport of sodium, chloride, and potassium. In: ASL Y, Chertow GM, Luyckx V, Marsden PA, Skorecki K, Taal MW, eds. *Brenner & Rector's the Kidney*. 11th ed. Philadelphia, PA: Elsevier; 2020:156–198.
30. Rubio-Aliaga J. Phosphate and kidney healthy aging. *Kidney Blood Press Res*. 2020;45:802–811. https://doi.org/10.1159/000509831.
31. Hall JE, Hall ME. Chapter 33. Red blood cells, anemia, and polycythemia. In: Hall ME, Hall JE, eds. *Guyton and Hall Textbook of Medical Physiology*. 14th ed. Philadelphia, PA: Elsevier; 2021:439–447.
32. Denic A, Rule AD, Glassock RJ. Healthy and unhealthy aging on kidney structure and function: human studies. *Curr Opin Nephrol Hypertens*. 2002;31:228–234. https://doi.org/10.1097/MNH.0000000000000780.
33. Narasaki Y, Rhee CM, Kramer H, Kalantar-Zadeh K. Protein intake and renal function in older adults. *Curr Opin Clin Nutr Metab Care*. 2021;24:10–17. https://doi.org/10.1097/MCO.0000000000000712.
34. Rosner MH, Zanella M, Kalantari K. Chapter 93. Geriatric nephrology. In: Johnsen RJ, Floege J, Tonelli M, eds. *Comprehensive Clinical Nephrology*. 7th ed. Philadelphia, PA: Elsevier; 2024:1046–1053.

Kidney Clinical Assessment and Diagnostic Procedures

Kathrine Anne Winnie and Kimberly Sanchez

http://evolve.elsevier.com/Urden/CriticalCareNursing

The body produces many clinical signs and symptoms that may be indicative of disorders in the kidneys. However, these signs and symptoms are often subtle, and although some symptoms point directly to the kidneys, many are exhibited by other body systems. A detailed history and careful physical assessment, along with diagnostic procedures, help focus on the kidneys as the source of symptoms and often uncover the cause of the problem.

HISTORY

A careful history that explores symptoms fully is an essential component of the clinical assessment. The history is structured to include patient identifiers, chief concern (CC), history of present illness or problem (HPI), past medical and surgical history (PMH), family history, personal and social history, and review of systems (ROS).[1] The patient, family member, or significant other should be encouraged to provide as much detail as possible during the history. During critical illness, a clinician may substitute a focused history for a complete history to tend to the patient's immediate, possibly life-threatening, needs.[1] Components of the history related to kidney disorders are outlined in Box 24.1.

FOCUSED PHYSICAL ASSESSMENT

Four techniques are used in the physical assessment of the kidney: inspection, auscultation, palpation, and percussion.[2] Visual *inspection* of the abdomen includes inspecting for bruises or localized discoloration, indicative of trauma or bleeding.[2] The renal arteries are *auscultated* for a bruit, a blowing or swishing sound.[2] The presence of a bruit is indicative of blood flow turbulence and may indicate vascular disease. Listen for bruits in the epigastric region and to the left and right of the umbilicus (Fig. 24.1).[2] A renal artery bruit usually indicates stenosis, which may lead to acute or chronic kidney dysfunction secondary to compromised blood flow to one or both kidneys. A bruit over the upper portion of the abdominal aorta may indicate an aneurysm or a stenotic area that can decrease blood flow to the kidneys. *Palpation* of the kidneys provides information about the size and shape of the kidneys.[2] Palpation of the kidneys is done through the bimanual capturing approach.[2] Capturing is accomplished by placing one hand posteriorly under the flank of a supine patient with fingers pointing to the midline and placing the opposite hand just below the rib cage anteriorly.[2] The patient is asked to inhale deeply while pressure is exerted to bring the hands together (Fig. 24.2).[2] As the patient exhales, the kidney may be felt between the hands.[2] After each kidney is palpated in this manner, the two kidneys should be compared for size and shape. Each kidney should be firm and smooth, and the two organs should be of equal size.[2] A normal left kidney may not palpable.[2] The right kidney is more easily palpated because of its lower position, caused by downward displacement by the liver.[2] Problems should be suspected if a mass (cancer) or an irregular surface (polycystic kidneys) is palpated or a size difference is detected.[2] *Percussion* is performed to detect size and density of the kidneys.[2] Additionally, percussion determine excess accumulation of air, fluid, or masses around the kidneys.[2] Percussion of a kidney is performed with the patient in a side-lying or sitting position, with a hand placed over the costovertebral angle (lower border of the rib cage on the flank).[2] Striking the back of the hand with the opposite fist produces a dull thud, which is normal.[2] Pain may indicate infection (e.g., urinary tract infection that has extended into the kidneys) or injury resulting from trauma.[2] In the critical care area, a nursing assessment does not routinely include a full physical assessment of the kidneys and urinary drainage system. However, the information gained through these physical assessment techniques can provide patient care data.

Fluid Volume Status

Determining fluid volume status in patients who are critically ill is a complex process that changes frequently.[3] Evaluating fluid volume status is necessary to prevent adverse outcomes.[3] Fluid volume overload is common in the critical care setting and is associated with adverse outcomes including increased mortality.[3] When used independent of other assessment methods, noninvasive physical assessment may be unreliable[3] because individual assessments lack specificity and/or because determining the compartmental distribution of fluid is challenging. The physical assessment should be used in conjunction with other diagnostic procedures to ensure accurate results and avoid inappropriate interventions. A general inspection of the patient is performed to note obvious signs of fluid volume overload or depletion that may signal kidney problems.

BOX 24.1 **DATA COLLECTION**

Kidney History

Common Kidney-Related Concerns
- Dyspnea
- Peripheral dependent edema
- Nocturia
- Nausea
- Metallic taste in mouth
- Loss of appetite
- Headache
- Rapid weight gain
- Itching
- Dry, scaly skin
- Weakness, fatigue
- Cognitive function changes
- Mental status change

History of Present Illness or Problem
- Current medication use

Past Medical and Surgical History
- Prior acute kidney injury
- Hypertension
- Diabetes mellitus
- Obstructive urologic problems (e.g., calculi)
- Frequent urinary tract infections
- Nephrotic syndrome
- Streptococcal infection
- Hypoplastic kidneys
- Vasculitis

Past Medication Use
- Use of over-the-counter medications, herbs, vitamins, and dietary supplements
- Nonsteroidal antiinflammatory medications
- Antibiotics, especially aminoglycosides
- Antihypertensives
- Diuretics

Past Kidney Studies
- Any diagnostic procedures performed using iodine-based radiopaque contrast media
- Kidney-ureters-bladder (KUB) radiograph
- Intravenous pyelogram
- Kidney ultrasound
- Renal arteriography
- Kidney biopsy
- Blood urea nitrogen (BUN)
- Creatinine
- Cystatin C
- BUN-to-creatine ratio
- Hemoglobin and hematocrit
- Anion gap
- Albumin and prealbumin
- Blood and urine osmolality
- Creatinine clearance
- Glomerular filtration rate (GFR)
- Urinalysis
- Urine toxicology screen

Family History
- Hypertension
- Diabetes mellitus
- Polycystic kidney disease
- Kidney disease
- Chronically swollen extremities

Personal and Social History
- Change in employment caused by illness
- Financial problems resulting from illness (financial cost, time off work)
- Sexual function (decreased libido, amenorrhea)
- Illicit drug use

Edema

Edema is caused by an intravascular problem and results in excess fluid in the interstitial space.[4] Inspect all areas of the body for a change in size or shape, focusing on dependent areas of the body, such as the feet and legs of an ambulatory person or the sacrum of an individual confined to bed.[4] Edema can be assessed by applying fingertip pressure for several seconds on the swollen area over a bony prominence, such as the ankles, pretibial areas (shins), and sacrum.[4] When no indentation is visible after applying fingertip pressure to a swollen area for several seconds, nonpitting edema is present.[4] If an indentation is present after applying fingertip pressure for several seconds, pitting edema exists.[4] One way of measuring the extent of pitting edema is by using a subjective scale of 1 to 4, with 1 indicating only minimal pitting and 4 indicating severe pitting (Table 24.1).[4] Edema may be present without fluid volume overload in patients with a compromised circulatory system[4] or hypoalbuminemia, common patient conditions in the critical care unit. In the presence of volume excess, edema may develop in the lungs. See Chapter 16 for pulmonary physical assessment information.

Skin Turgor

Assessment of skin turgor provides data for identifying fluid-related problems. To assess turgor, use the thumb and forefinger to gently pick up and release the skin over the forearm or sternal area.[5] Normal elasticity and fluid status allow an almost immediate return to shape after the skin is released.[5] In the presence of fluid volume deficit, the skin remains raised and does not return to its normal position for several seconds.[5] Because of the loss of skin elasticity in older persons, skin turgor assessment may not be an accurate fluid assessment measure for this age group.[5]

Oral Mucosa

Inspection of the oral cavity provides clues to fluid volume status. The most accurate way to assess the oral cavity is to inspect the mouth using a tongue blade and light.[6] The oral mucosa should be pinkish red, smooth, and moist.[6] When a fluid volume deficit exists, the mucous membranes of the mouth become dry.[7] However, mouth breathing and some medicines

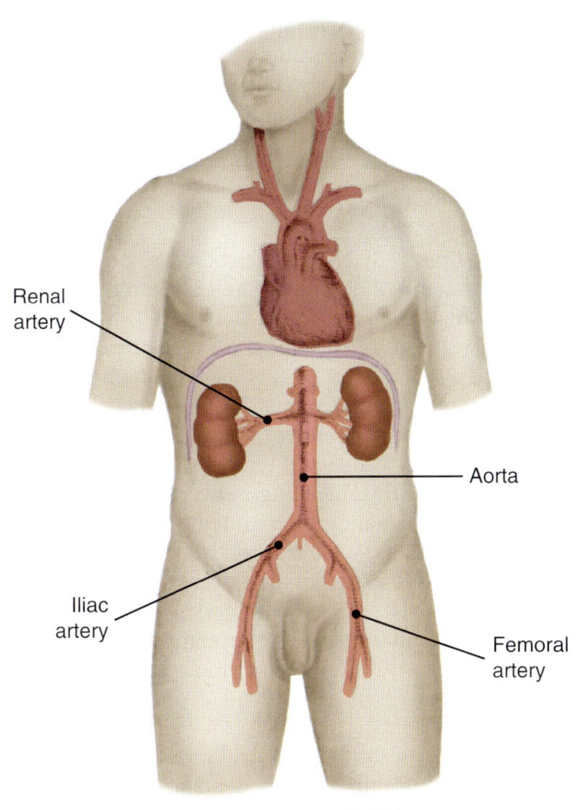

FIG. 24.1 Sites for Auscultation of Bruits.

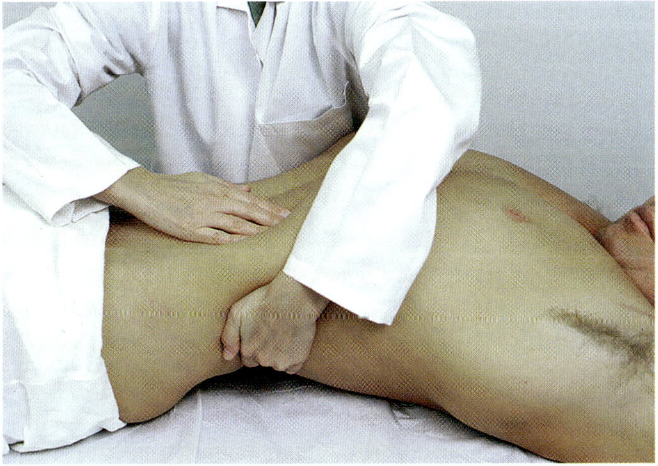

FIG. 24.2 Palpation of the Kidney. (From Ball JW, Dains, JE, Flynn JA, Solomon BS, Stewart RW. *Seidel's Guide to Physical Examination*. 10th ed. Elsevier; 2023.)

TABLE 24.1 Pitting Edema Scale[4]

Rating	Approximate Equivalent
+1	2-mm depth
+2	4-mm depth (lasting up to 15 seconds)
+3	6-mm depth (lasting up to 60 seconds)
+4	8-mm depth (lasting longer than 120 seconds)

(e.g., antihistamines) can also dry the mucous membranes temporarily.[6]

Relevant Cardiac Assessments

Heart rate, rhythm, sounds, and rubs may provide information about fluid volume status.

After performing relevant inspection, palpation, and percussion assessments of the heart (see Chapter 11), use the stethoscope for auscultation.[8] Assess the rate and rhythm for regularity in one of the five auscultatory areas of the heart using the diaphragm of the stethoscope.[8] Volume status may contribute to electrolyte imbalances (see Chapter 23). The effects of electrolyte imbalances on cardiac muscle contraction are discussed in Chapter 12. In a patient with heart issues, volume overload results in an audible S3, which is best heard with the bell of the stethoscope.[9] Although uncommon, patients with kidney disease may develop uremic pericarditis and may develop a pericardial friction rub.[10] See Chapter 11 for heart sounds.

Additional assessments are needed, along with a focused physical assessment of the kidneys and fluid volume status, to identify kidney disorders.

Additional Assessments

Hemodynamic Monitoring

Blood pressure and heart rate changes are considered when assessing fluid volume deficit. In a volume-depleted patient, blood pressure decreases due to an insufficient preload and the heart rate increases as a compensatory mechanism to maintain cardiac output and circulation. Assessment of heart rate, blood pressure, postural vital signs, and cardiac output are discussed in Chapters 11 and 12. Although changes in heart rate and blood pressure may indicate fluid volume status, effects from medications (e.g., beta-blockers) and neurologic disorders (e.g., loss of sympathetic tone) can result in changes unrelated to fluid volume status.

Central venous pressure (CVP) is the measurement of the pressure in the superior vena cava or right atrium and sometimes used as an estimate of fluid status.[11] Monitoring of CVP has its limitations and does not accurately predict fluid responsiveness.[11] CVP measurements are reviewed in Chapter 12.

Weight Monitoring

One of the most important assessments of kidney and fluid status is the patient's weight. Body weight should be measured serially.[12] Whenever possible, the patient should be weighed during admission to the critical care unit. Subsequent weights should occur for comparison with the previous weight measurement. In the critical care unit, weight is measured for each patient every day. The weight measurement should occur using the same scale at a consistent time in the day, with the patient wearing similar items as the previous weight measurement. A fluctuation in body weight of more than 1 kilogram per day usually indicates fluid rather than nutritional factors; 1 liter of fluid equals 1 kilogram, or approximately 2.2 pounds. It is recommended that patients on dialysis limit their weight gain between treatments to no more than 1 kilogram per day.[13] It is important to document whether the current weight differs from the usual weight,[12] before admission to the hospital. This can be documented as a percentage of their usual weight[12]:

Percent usual weight = (usual weight − current weight)/usual weight) × 100

Weight, as a component of body mass index (BMI), is an element of the nutrition assessment in patients with kidney disease.[12] Weight provides an indirect measure of body composition and should be obtained at routine intervals as fluid and electrolyte balance is continually altered throughout the day.[12] For example, for patients receiving dialysis, weight is best measured consistently after treatment when body fluid compartments are most balanced.[12] See Chapter 6 for more information on nutrition and kidney disease.

Intake and Output Monitoring

Similar to patient weight, intake and output is monitored for all patients in the critical care unit. Intake and output can be compared with the patient's weight to evaluate fluid gains or losses more accurately. Trends in daily intake and output volumes also assist in determining the extracellular fluid volume of the critically ill patient. Total water intake is usually about 2.3 liters per day, but it is highly variable among different people and even within the same person during different days, climate, and activities.[14] Total water output is the same (about 2.3 liters per day), with insensible losses accounting for about 900 mL.[14] When intake exceeds output (e.g., excessive intravenous fluid, decreased urine output), a positive fluid balance exists. With impaired kidney function, the positive fluid balance results in fluid volume overload. Conversely, if output exceeds intake (e.g., fever, increased respiration, profuse sweating, vomiting, diarrhea, gastric suction, diuretic therapy), a negative fluid balance exists and volume deficit results. In addition to an effect of fluid volume, an abnormal output may result in electrolyte and acid–base disturbances.

Individuals with acute kidney injury (AKI) often exhibit a decrease in urine output, or oliguria (less than 0.5 mL/kg per hour in adults for 6 hours).[15] Oliguria may be more pronounced in the presence of intact tubules still responsive to vasopressin and less pronounced with injured tubules unable to concentrate urine[15] (see Chapter 23 for detailed information on kidney physiology). Although urine output is a sensitive indicator, severity of kidney dysfunction cannot be accurately determined by urine output alone.[15] Monitoring urine output in the critical care unit may contribute to early detection of AKI and reduce 30-day mortality in patients with AKI.[16]

For additional information on AKI, see Chapter 25.

In maintaining daily records of intake and output, all measurable volumes must be recorded. A standard list of the fluid volume held in various containers (e.g., milk cartons, juice containers) expedites this process. Discussions about the importance of accurate recording of intake and output with the patient and family or friends are necessary and can improve the accuracy of assessment of intake and output volumes.

LABORATORY STUDIES

Common laboratory studies for patients with kidney disorders are those that contribute to diagnosis, categorize severity, identify declines or improvements in patient condition, and measure the associated alterations in fluid, electrolyte, and acid–base balance. Laboratory tests used to detect kidney dysfunction have limitations[17] but aid practitioners in recognizing changes or trends concerning the status of the kidneys.

Biomarkers

Blood Urea Nitrogen

Blood urea nitrogen (BUN) is a byproduct of protein metabolism[18] that enters the bloodstream and is excreted by the kidneys. The normal value for adults is 10 to 20 mg/dL but may be slightly elevated in older adults.[19] Excess urea in the blood is present when kidney excretion is inadequate; however, BUN lacks specificity as an indicator of kidney function and is not routinely used as an independent measure of kidney dysfunction.[19] Elevated BUN values not related to renal failure may be caused by gastrointestinal bleeding, dehydration, sepsis, congestive heart failure, pregnancy, high protein intake, protein catabolism, and medications, such as furosemide, antiinfectives, and methotrexate.[19] BUN values may be decreased in patients with a primary liver disease, low protein intake, and among patients taking other medications such as streptomycin.[19] It is common practice to measure BUN and creatinine together when assessing kidney function.[20]

Creatinine

Creatinine is a byproduct of muscle metabolism[18] that enters the bloodstream and is excreted by the kidneys. It is commonly used to diagnose kidney disease and determine disease severity.[20] In adults, serum creatinine values range from 0.5 to 1.3 mg/dL with slightly higher values considered normal in men and older adults.[19] Excess creatinine in the blood occurs when kidney excretion is inadequate.[19] Serum creatinine is used to estimate the glomerular filtration rate (GFR)[21] and although the serum creatinine value is considered a better measure of kidney function than the BUN value, there are limitations. Dehydration can also increase serum creatinine values.[19] The body's production of creatinine may be altered by differences in muscle mass.[19] Falsely low serum creatinine values are associated with cachexia, neuromuscular disease, other chronic conditions, older age, and female sex, and can lead to delayed diagnosis of kidney injury.[21] Additionally, an inaccurate measurement of kidney function may lead to underdosing or overdosing of medications cleared by the kidney.[21] Serum creatinine is routinely used for diagnosis of kidney disorders and to determine severity of kidney disease; however, the result is best used in combination with other laboratory tests to ensure accuracy.[19,21]

Blood Urea Nitrogen-to-Creatinine Ratio

The BUN-to-creatinine ratio is calculated to determine a possible cause of acute kidney injury. Normal values are range from 10:1 to 20:1.[22] Values greater than 20:1 may indicate a prerenal cause of kidney injury (e.g., hypovolemia, hypotension).[23] Values less than 10:1 may indicate an intrarenal cause (e.g., acute tubular necrosis).

Cystatin C

Cystatin C (CyC) is synthesized and released by nucleated cells in the body at a constant rate, excreted by glomerular filtration, with no secretion from the tubules.[18] Normal laboratory values for CyC range from 0.52 to 0.98 mg/L[19] with lab values being less affected by age, sex, or muscle mass.[18] In kidney dysfunction, the glomerular filtration of CyC is reduced, causing an increase in the blood.[18] High CyC values indicate kidney dysfunction.[18] The CyC value may be inaccurate in the presence of steroid therapy and untreated thyroid disorders.[24] Cystatin C is not currently drawn routinely but may be used more frequently in the future due to potential benefits in early detection of decreased GFR and a possible role in determining septic, nephrotoxic, or ischemic AKI.[20] Additionally, Kidney Disease Improving Global Outcomes (KDIGO) guidelines recommend measuring value in adults with eGFR of 45 to 59 mL/min/1.73 m^2 as a confirmatory test for chronic kidney disease.[25]

Other Biomarkers

Using current standard laboratory tests to signal kidney injury has proved unsatisfactory because either significant changes in GFR may occur before kidney injury is recognized[20] or there are other factors that affect the test results.[28] There is a need to identify an alternate test.[26] A superior marker would be naturally occurring, reliable, not be reabsorbed, secreted, synthesized, or metabolized in the tubule but would instead be fully (freely) filtered at the glomerulus.[26] Other current or potential biomarkers include upregulated proteins, low-molecular-weight proteins, and tubular enzymes.[20]

Glomerular Filtration Rate

The GFR is an estimate of the amount of filtrate moving through the glomerular capillaries into Bowman's space per unit of time.[26] An estimated glomerular filtration rate (eGFR) of 90 mL/min or greater is normal. An eGFR of 60 to 90 mL/min may indicate early-stage kidney disease, whereas an eGFR of 15 to 60 mL/min indicates kidney disease and an eGFR below 15 mL/min denotes kidney failure.[27] Serum creatinine is currently the most widely used marker for estimating GFR; however, it is not a precise measurement due to the small amount of creatinine that is secreted into the tubule.[26] Any inaccuracies in the creatinine value are then carried over to the GFR value. A common equation used to obtain the eGFR is based on the clearance of creatinine by the kidney and factors in age, sex, and race.[18] The use of race as a factor in the GFR equation has been questioned due to lack of evidence for the practice and may contribute additional inaccuracies in the GFR value.[26] Concerns of health inequities have led the nephrology community to propose GFR equations that do not adjust for race.[26] A more accurate method of measuring GFR requires the infusion of an exogenous substances such as inulin and then measuring clearance. The measured GFR is not routinely performed in clinical practice due to the time and cost constraints required to infuse the substance into the patient for testing.[18,26]

Creatinine Clearance

Creatinine clearance (CrCl) measures glomeruli and tubule function and is widely used to determine medication dosing in kidney dysfunction for medications excreted by the kidneys.[19] The value is calculated using the amount of creatinine in the excreted urine over 12 to 24 hours and the amount of creatinine in the blood during a single blood collection midway through the urine collection:

$$(\text{Urine creatinine} \times \text{Volume of urine})/\text{Serum creatinine}$$

Normal values for creatinine clearance in adult males less than 40 years old range from 107 to 139 mL/min and in adult females the range is 87 to 107 mL/min.[19] For each decade of life after the age of 20, it is expected that creatinine clearance values will decrease by approximately 6.5 mL/min.[19] Values less than 50 mL/min indicate significant kidney dysfunction.[19]

Additional Laboratory Studies

Additional urine and blood studies may be completed to evaluate kidney disorders, providing information on alterations in fluid, electrolyte, and acid–base balance, as well as kidney-associated conditions such as mineral bone disorders and malnutrition. Urine studies include urinalysis and urine electrolytes. Other select laboratory studies are summarized in Table 24.2.

Urine Studies

Urinalysis. Analysis of the urine may be performed as a routine screening test or to identify possible kidney disorders or extrarenal medical conditions.[30] The appearance of urine is expected to be amber yellow and clear.[30] Concentrated urine samples appear dark amber while dilute urine is very pale yellow.[30] Color may be affected by bleeding, medications, food consumed, or medical conditions.[30] Clarity of the urine may be affected by bacteria, WBCs, or urates. Normal fresh urine has an aromatic scent.[30] A strong odor may be caused by infection, medical conditions such as diabetic ketoacidosis,[30] medications, or foods consumed. Individual components of the urinalysis are presented in Tables 24.3 and 24.4. In a critically ill patient, the test may be performed when a urinary tract infection is suspected or to rule out the presence of protein or glucose in the urine.[30]

Urine electrolytes. Urine electrolyte measurement provides adjuvant diagnostic information but is not routinely performed in the critical care setting.[32] Results of common urine electrolyte tests may not be reliable in critically ill patients due to the multiple factors known to influence excretion and reabsorption including diuretic use, vasopressor use, acute changes in kidney function, decreased urine output, and suboptimal nutritional status.[32] These confounding factors should be considered if there are clinical circumstances in critical care where measurement is justified.[32] Urine sodium may be used to determine if AKI is due to prerenal causes or acute tubular necrosis and/or to assess effective circulating volume or volume status.[32] For example, in the presence of hypovolemia, the kidney tubules retain sodium (and water) and the amount of sodium in the urine is low. The opposite is true with volume overload and with kidney disorders that cause sodium excretion. The fractional excretion of sodium (FENa) is a calculation used to estimate sodium loss in the urine relative to sodium in the bloodstream to determine causes of prerenal and intrarenal AKI.[22] Urine chloride is also a measure of volume and additionally may provide further information on the etiology of metabolic alkalosis.[32]

TABLE 24.2 **Other Select Laboratory Studies**

Laboratory Test	Specimen Type	Normal Values	Notes
Electrolyte, sodium[22]	Blood	135–145 mEq/L	Measures the major cation that determines osmolality of the extracellular fluid Increased value: dehydration, osmotic diuresis, prolonged glucosuria, hyperaldosteronism, Cushing syndrome, diabetes insipidus Decreased value: burns, heart failure, diuretics or other salt-losing conditions, acute hyperglycemia, diarrhea, cirrhosis, pancreatitis
Electrolyte, chloride[22]	Blood	95–105 mEq/L	Measures the major anion that maintains the electrical and acid–base balance of body, and regulates renal tubular reabsorption of sodium and fluid Increased value: acidosis, compensatory respiratory alkalosis Decreased value: alkalosis, compensated respiratory acidosis, burns, heart failure, dehydration or other hyponatremic states
Electrolyte, phosphorus[22]	Blood	2.7–4.5 mg/dL	Measures the energy-rich phosphate used in metabolic reactions Increased value: renal failure, acidosis, vitamin D toxicity, tumor lysis syndrome, hypoparathyroidism, hyperthyroidism Decreased value: hypercalcemia, hypokalemia, hyperaldosteronism, GI losses, medications (e.g., steroids, phosphate binders, contraceptives, diuretics)
Electrolyte, other	Blood	See Chapter 12 for potassium, calcium, ionized calcium, magnesium	
Osmolality, blood[22]	Blood	275–295 mOsm/kg[a]	Measures the number of solutes in blood Increased value: dehydration, kidney failure with azotemia, hyperglycemia, mannitol therapy, alcohol, hypernatremia Decreased value: excess hydration, hyponatremia, inappropriate antidiuretic hormone secretion
Anion gap[22]	Blood	8–12 mEq/L[b]	Measures the difference between major positive and negative ions[c] Increased value: acidosis, renal failure, aspirin, methanol Decreased value: alkalosis, hypoalbuminemia, elevated potassium or magnesium or calcium, medications
Hemoglobin[22]	Blood	Males: 13.8–17.2 g/dL Females: 12.1–15.1 g/dL	Measures the major protein in erythrocytes Increased: volume depletion, hypoxia, polycythemia, high altitude living Decreased: fluid volume excess, blood loss, anemia, hemolytic reactions, liver damage
Alkaline phosphatase[22]	Blood	30–140 U/L	Measures the enzyme that is normally found in the liver, bones, intestine, and kidneys Increased value: bone resorption, osteomalacia, liver disease, rickets, hyperparathyroidism, hyperthyroidism, ulcerative colitis, bowel perforation Decreased value: vitamin D toxicity, fibrate therapy, malnutrition, pernicious anemia, hypothyroidism, celiac sprue
Parathyroid hormone[22]	Blood	10–65 pg/mL	Measures the hormone that is responsible for intestinal calcium absorption, bone resorption, and renal calcium and phosphate reabsorption Increased value: chronic kidney disease, calciphylaxis, extraskeletal calcification, hypersecretion or adenoma of parathyroid glands Decreased value: osteomalacia, low magnesium levels in blood, vitamin D toxicity, sarcoidosis, bone lesions
Vitamin D[19]	Blood	Males: 18–64 pg/mL Females: 18–78 pg/mL	Measures the fat-soluble vitamin that regulates calcium and phosphorus levels in the blood Increased value: vitamin D toxicity, Williams syndrome Decreased value: osteomalacia, liver disease, rickets, malabsorptive syndromes, inadequate exposure to light, inadequate dietary intake
Albumin[22]	Blood	3.5–5.0 g/dL	Measures the amount circulating carrier protein that assists with maintaining oncotic pressure Increased value: dehydration, shock Decreased value: malnutrition, proteinuric glomerular kidney disease, nephrotic syndrome, cirrhosis, autoimmune or genetic diseases, cancer
Prealbumin[19]	Blood	15–36 mg/dL	Measures the amount of protein made by the liver that is used to makes other proteins Low levels may be a sign of malnutrition but can also point to acute pathophysiological events
Micronutrients (zinc, selenium, copper)[19]	Blood	Depends on micronutrient	Patients receiving renal replacement therapies may have micronutrient loss
Urine toxicology screen[29]	Urine	None	Presence of alcohol, illegal drugs, prescription and nonprescription medications, and other substances excreted via the kidneys

[a]Simultaneous measurement with urine osmolality provides an accurate indication of fluid status. Urine osmolality may be inferred from urine specific gravity.
[b]Value range when using this calculation for anion gap: $[Na^+] - ([Cl^-] + [HCO_3^-])$.
[c]The measurement of the anion gap is a *rapid* method for identifying acid–base imbalance but cannot be used to pinpoint the source of the acid–base disturbance specifically.

TABLE 24.3 Urinalysis Results[31]

Test Component	Relevance to Kidney Function	Normal Values	Possible Causes of Low Values	Possible Causes of High Values
pH	Kidneys regulate acid–base balance Changes in metabolic function and kidney function produce changes in urinary pH	4.5–8.0 Average value is 6.0 Urine is normally acidic	• Systemic acidosis • High protein diets • Renal tubular acidosis (Type IV) • May indicate urinary calculi (cystine, uric acid, and calcium oxalate)	• Systemic alkalosis • Strict vegetarian diets • Infections • Renal tubular acidosis (Type I) • May indicate urinary calculi (calcium phosphate, and magnesium phosphate)
Specific gravity	Kidneys dilute and concentrate urine Test evaluates hydration status, fluid balance status, and/or ability of kidney to concentrate or dilute urine	1.001–1.035	• Excessive fluid intake • Diabetes insipidus • Psychogenic polydipsia	• Volume depletion • Syndrome of inappropriate antidiuretic hormone • Glucosuria • Administration of hyperosmotic solutions (e.g., albumin, dextran, iodinated contrast)
Protein	Kidneys do not freely filter proteins Test evaluates compromise of the glomerular membrane and intrinsic kidney damage	Negative reagent[a]	• Very dilute urine	• Highly concentrated urine • Iodinated contrast • Recent exercise • Hematuria • Alkaline urine • Infection
Glucose	Kidneys reabsorb glucose Test evaluates the reabsorbing capacity of the kidneys	Negative reagent	Negative is normal	• Diabetes • Cushing syndrome • Proximal tubular dysfunction (e.g., aminoglycosides, valproic acid, malignancies)
Ketones	Not applicable	Negative reagent	Negative is normal	• Diabetic ketoacidosis • Alcoholic acidosis • Starvation acidosis
Bilirubin	Not applicable	Negative reagent	Negative is normal	• Liver disease (hepatitis or cirrhosis) • Biliary tract obstruction
Urobilinogen	Not applicable	Small amounts	Small amounts are normal	• Hemolysis • Liver cirrhosis • Hepatitis • Excess unconjugated bilirubin
Leukocyte esterase	The kidney system also includes the urinary drainage system This test evaluates the presence of white blood cells	Negative reagent	Negative is normal	• Urinary tract infection
Nitrites	The kidney system also includes the urinary drainage system This test evaluates the presence of bacteria	Negative reagent	Negative is normal	• Urinary tract infection

[a]Positive reagent for protein should be followed up with an ACR or AER for further diagnosis of kidney disorders.

DIAGNOSTIC PROCEDURES

Imaging is used in the critical care areas when needed to identify or obtain further information related to kidney disorders. Imaging studies range from basic to more complex (Table 24.5). Artificial intelligence has been used more in health care and is currently being used in medical imaging interpretation. See Box 24.2 for other uses of artificial intelligence in health care.

Kidney Biopsy

Kidney biopsies are performed to diagnose kidney problems, evaluate existing kidney damage, determine kidney disorder progression, and to assist in treatment plans.[34] Percutaneous needle biopsy involves inserting a needle through the flank to obtain a specimen of cortical and medullary kidney tissue. An open biopsy is a surgical procedure. Biopsy is the last choice for diagnostic assessment in critically ill patients because of the periprocedural risks of bleeding, hematoma, and infection.

KEY POINTS

History

- The history is structured to include patient identifiers, chief concern (CC), history of present illness or problem (HPI),

TABLE 24.4 Microscopic Examination of Sediment[30,31]

Test Component	Normal Values	Possible Causes of Greater than Normal Values
White blood cells	0–4 per low power field	Urinary tract infection or inflammation, bacteriuria, interstitial nephritis, nephrolithiasis, genitourinary tuberculosis
Erythrocytes	0–2 per high power field	Hematuria (glomerular and nonglomerular), including trauma, tumor, and rhabdomyolysis
Epithelial cells	Less than 15–20 per high power field	Renal tubular damage, interstitial nephritis, sample contamination if squamous or transitional epithelial cells present
Leukocyte casts	None	Pyelonephritis, interstitial nephritis
Erythrocyte casts	None	Glomerulonephritis, interstitial nephritis, normal finding in healthy individuals after exercise
Epithelial casts	None	Acute tubular necrosis, interstitial nephritis, concentrated urine
Hyaline casts	None	Nonspecific; chronic kidney disease, fever, physical exertion, concentrated urine in healthy people
Granular casts	None	Acute tubular necrosis, glomerulonephritis, tubulointerstitial disease
Fatty casts	None	Nephrotic syndrome
Waxy casts	None	Nonspecific; advanced chronic kidney disease and acute kidney injury
Crystals (See pH for types)	None	Nephrolithiasis, cystinuria, high dietary oxalate, ethylene glycol ingestion, acute urate nephropathy, urinary tract infections

TABLE 24.5 Kidney Imaging Tests[33]

Test	Comments
Kidneys-ureters-bladder (KUB) Radiograph	An electrical device emits ionizing radiation that passes through the body and captures a picture of internal body structures; Useful for evaluating the presence of calculi, masses, and inflammation
Ultrasound	An electrical signal is generated from high-frequency sound wave transmissions and creates an image of tissues and organs; useful in identifying fluid accumulation or obstruction, calculi, transplant allograft, and differentiating solid or cystic masses
Computed tomography (CT)	Rotating ionizing radiation producing cross-sectional images that may be done with or without administration of an iodinated contrast; useful in evaluating vasculature, suspected kidney trauma, complications of obstruction (e.g., infection, atrophy), and further defining indeterminate results from radiograph and ultrasound
Magnetic resonance angiography (MRA)	A strong magnetic field and high-energy radiofrequency waves produce images of blood vessels with the administration of gadolinium contrast; useful in evaluating renal artery stenosis without nephrotoxic contrast agents or ionizing radiation, renal artery bypass grafts, transplant anastomosis, and mapping vasculature
Radionuclide kidney imaging	Radiotracers are administered intravenously, and gamma rays are detected to form an image of the organ; Useful in providing information on anatomy and function of kidney (e.g., measures individual kidney contribution to overall kidney function); useful in evaluating post–kidney transplant rejection, glomerular filtration rate, and renal plasma flow, acute pyelonephritis
Angiography	Insertion of a catheter and injection of a contrast agent into the arteries to highlight blood vessels as the contrast agent moves through them; useful in evaluating cystic renal artery diseases, preoperative transplant, and masses; useful in treatment of renal blood flow disorders

BOX 24.2 **Informatics**

Artificial Intelligence in Health Care

Artificial intelligence (AI) has been making significant advancements in health care and has the potential to revolutionize various aspects of the industry. Here are some key areas where AI is being utilized in health care:

- Medical Imaging Interpretation:
  - AI can detect subtle patterns and anomalies in radiologic imaging, aiding radiologists in diagnosing diseases more accurately and quickly.
- Diagnosis:
  - AI algorithms can analyze medical data, such as images, laboratory results, and patient records, to assist practitioners with diagnosing diseases such as cancer, cardiac disease, and neurological disorders.
- Personalized Treatment:
  - AI can analyze patient data to recommend personalized treatment plans based on a patient's genetic makeup, medical history, and other factors, leading to more effective and targeted treatments.
- Medication Development:
  - AI can predict the effectiveness and safety of medications, optimizing the development process.
- Natural Language Processing (NLP):
  - NLP allows computers to understand and generate human language, which can be used to transcribe medical records, extract information from clinical notes, and facilitate practitioner-patient communication.
- Virtual Health Assistants:
  - AI-powered chatbots and virtual assistants provide patients with medical information, answer basic health care questions, schedule appointments, and offer medication reminders.
- Remote Patient Monitoring:
  - AI-enabled devices can track patient vital signs and health metrics remotely, allowing health care practitioners to monitor patients with chronic conditions and intervene if necessary.
- Predictive Analytics:
  - AI can analyze historical patient data to predict disease outbreaks, patient admission rates, and resource requirements, helping health care organizations plan and allocate resources more effectively.
- Robotic Surgery:
  - AI-assisted robots can perform surgery with precision, aiding surgeons in complex procedures and minimizing the risk of human error.
- Epidemiology and Public Health:
  - AI can analyze large datasets to track disease outbreaks, monitor public health trends, and inform public health interventions.

While AI offers numerous benefits to health care, challenges remain, including data privacy concerns, regulatory hurdles, ethical considerations, and the need for rigorous validation of AI algorithms. Striking a balance between innovation and patient safety is crucial as AI transforms health care practices.[1]

Reference

1. Chen M, Decary M. Artificial intelligence in healthcare: an essential guide for health leaders. *Healthc Manage Forum.* 2020;33(1):10–18. https://do.org/10.1177/0840470419873123.

past medical and surgical history (PMH), family history, personal and social history, and review of systems (ROS).

Focused Physical Assessment

- Fluid volume overload is common in the critical care setting and is associated with adverse outcomes including increased mortality. Assessment of fluid volume status includes general inspection for edema, measurement of skin turgor, relevant cardiac assessment, hemodynamic monitoring, weight monitoring, and input and output monitoring.

Laboratory Studies

- An estimated glomerular filtration rate (eGFR) of 90 mL/min or greater is normal. An eGFR of 60 to 90 mL/min may indicate early-stage kidney disease, whereas an eGFR of 15 to 60 mL/min indicates kidney disease, and an eGFR below 15 mL/min denotes kidney failure. Serum creatinine is currently the most widely used marker for estimating GFR.
- Cystatin C is not currently drawn routinely but may be used more frequently in the future due to potential benefits.
- Additional laboratory studies include a urinalysis, urine electrolytes, and additional blood studies to evaluate kidney disorders, providing information on alterations in fluid, electrolyte, and acid–base balance, as well as kidney-associated conditions such as mineral bone disorders and malnutrition.

Diagnostic Procedures

- Imaging is used in the critical care areas when needed to identify or obtain further information related to kidney disorders. Some imaging studies include kidneys-ureters-bladder (KUB) radiograph, ultrasound, CT, magnetic resonance angiography (MRA), radionuclide kidney imaging, and angiography.

Visit the Evolve site at http://evolve.elsevier.com/Urden/CriticalCareNursing for additional study materials.

REFERENCES

1. Ball JW, Dains JE, Flynn JA, Solomon BS, Stewart RW. Chapter 2. The history and interviewing process. In: Ball JW, Dains JE, Flynn JA, Solomon BS, Stewart RW, eds. *Seidel's Guide to Physical Examination.* 10th ed. Philadelphia, PA: Elsevier; 2023:12–34.
2. Ball JW, Dains JE, Flynn JA, Solomon BS, Stewart RW. Chapter 18. Abdomen. In: Ball JW, Dains JE, Flynn JA, Solomon BS, Stewart RW, eds. *Seidel's Guide to Physical Examination.* 10th ed. Philadelphia, PA: Elsevier; 2023:303–447.
3. Bouchard J, Granado RC, Mehta RL. Chapter 134. Components of fluid balance and monitoring. In: Ronco C, Bellomo R, Kellum JA, Ricci Z, eds. *Critical Care Nephrology.* 3rd ed. Philadelphia, PA: Elsevier; 2019:816–821.
4. Ball JW, Dains JE, Flynn JA, Solomon BS, Stewart RW. Chapter 16. Blood vessels. In: Ball JW, Dains JE, Flynn JA, Solomon BS, Stewart RW, eds.

Seidel's Guide to Physical Examination. 10th ed. Philadelphia, PA: Elsevier; 2023:364–382.
5. Ball JW, Dains JE, Flynn JA, Solomon BS, Stewart RW. Chapter 9. Skin, hair, and nails. In: Ball JW, Dains JE, Flynn JA, Solomon BS, Stewart RW, eds. *Seidel's Guide to Physical Examination*. 10th ed. Philadelphia, PA: Elsevier; 2023:133–188.
6. Ball JW, Dains JE, Flynn JA, Solomon BS, Stewart RW. Chapter 13. Ears, nose, and throat. In: Ball JW, Dains JE, Flynn JA, Solomon BS, Stewart RW, eds. *Seidel's Guide to Physical Examination*. 10th ed. Philadelphia, PA: Elsevier; 2023:259–289.
7. Fukushima Y, Sano Y, Isozaki Y, et al. A pilot clinical evaluation of oral mucosal dryness in dehydrated patients using a moisture-checking device. *Clin Exp Dent Res*. 2019;5(2):116–120. https://doi.org/10.1002/cre2.145.
8. Ball JW, Dains JE, Flynn JA, Solomon BS, Stewart RW. Chapter 15. Heart. In: Ball JW, Dains JE, Flynn JA, Solomon BS, Stewart RW, eds. *Seidel's Guide to Physical Examination*. 10th ed. Philadelphia, PA: Elsevier; 2023:326–363.
9. Silverman ME. Chapter 24. The third heart sound. In: Walker HK, Hall WD, Hurst JW, eds. *Clinical Methods: The History, Physical, and Laboratory Examinations*. 3rd ed. Boston, MA: Butterworths; 1990. https://www.ncbi.nlm.nih.gov/books/NBK342/. Accessed September 17, 2023.
10. Chugh S, Singh J, Kichloo A, Gupta S, Katchi T, Solanki S. Uremic- and dialysis-associated pericarditis. *Cardiol Rev*. 2021;29(6):310–313. https://doi.org/10.1097/CRD.0000000000000381.
11. Hill B, Smith C. Central venous pressure monitoring in critical care settings. *Br J Nurs*. 2021;30(4):230–236. https://doi.org/10.12968/bjon.2021.30.4.230.
12. Ikizler TA, Burrowes JD, Byham-Gray LD, et al. KDOQI clinical practice guideline for nutrition in CKD: 2020 update. *Am J Kidney Dis*. 2020;76(3 Suppl 1):S1–S107. https://doi.org/10.1053/j.ajkd.2020.05.006.
13. *What Is Dry Weight?* National Kidney Foundation. 2023. https://www.kidney.org/atoz/content/dry-weight. Accessed September 17, 2023.
14. Hall JE, Hall ME. Chapter 25. Regulation of body fluid compartments: Extracellular and intracellular fluids; Edema. In: Hall ME, Hall JE, eds. *Guyton and Hall Textbook of Medical Physiology*. 14th ed. Philadelphia, PA: Elsevier; 2021:305–320.
15. Kidney Disease: Improving Global Outcomes (KDIGO) Acute Kidney Injury Work Group. KDIGO clinical practice guideline for acute kidney injury. *Kidney Inter Suppl*. 2012;2:1–138.
16. Jin K, Murugan R, Sileanu FE, et al. Intensive monitoring of urine output is associated with increased detection of acute kidney injury and improved outcomes. *Chest*. 2017;152(5):972–979. https://doi.org/10.1016/j.chest.2017.05.011.
17. Kashani K, Rosner MH, Ostermann M. Creatinine: from physiology to clinical application. *Eur J Intern Med*. 2020;72:9–14. https://doi.org/10.1016/j.ejim.2019.10.025.
18. Brooks DH. Chapter 6. Chronic kidney diseases: diagnosis, classification, and management. In: Bodin SM, ed. *Contemporary Nephrology Nursing*. 4th ed. Pitman, NJ: American Nephrology Nursing Association; 2022:121–159.
19. Chapter 2. Blood studies. In: Pagana KK, Pagana TJ, Pagana TN, eds. *Mosby's® Manual of Diagnostic and Laboratory Tests*. 7th ed. Philadelphia, PA: Elsevier; 2022.
20. Odom B, Lynch F. Chapter 37. Acute kidney injury. In: Bodin SM, ed. *Contemporary Nephrology Nursing*. 4th ed. Pitman, NJ: American Nephrology Nursing Association; 2022:913–982.
21. Ebert N, Bevc S, Bökenkamp A, et al. Assessment of kidney function: clinical indications for measured GFR. *Clin Kidney J*. 2021;14(8):1861–1870. https://doi.org/10.1093/ckj/sfab042.
22. Brown RS, Galdfarb-Rumyantzev A. Chapter 16. Laboratory values of nephrology. In: Brown RS, ed. *Clinical Handbook of Nephrology*. Philadelphia, PA: Elsevier; 2023:283–298.
23. Morley JE. Dehydration, hypernatremia, and hyponatremia. *Clin Geriatr Med*. 2015;31(3):389–399. https://doi.org/10.1016/j.cger.2015.04.007.
24. Cystatin C. *National Kidney Foundation*; 2023. from https://www.kidney.org/atoz/content/cystatinC. Accessed September 22, 2023.
25. Kidney Disease: Improving Global Outcomes (KDIGO). KDIGO 2012 clinical practice guideline for the evaluation and management of chronic kidney disease. *Kidney Inter Suppl*. 2013;3(1):1–163.
26. Russel S. Chapter 3. Physiology of the kidney. In: Bodin SM, ed. *Contemporary Nephrology Nursing*. 4th ed. Pitman, NJ: American Nephrology Nursing Association; 2022:63–82.
27. *Estimated Glomerular Filtration Rate (eGFR)*. National Kidney Foundation. 2023. https://www.kidney.org/atoz/content/gfr. Accessed August 30, 2023.
28. Gonyea JE. Chapter 7. Nutrition and chronic kidney disease. In: Bodin SM, ed. *Contemporary Nephrology Nursing*. 4th ed. Pitman, NJ: American Nephrology Nursing Association; 2022:161–185.
29. Moeller KE, Kissack JC, Atayee RS, Lee KC. Clinical interpretation of urine drug tests: what clinicians need to know about urine drug screens. *Mayo Clin Proc*. 2017;92(5):774–796. https://doi.org/10.1016/j.mayocp.2016.12.007.
30. Chapter 11. Urine studies. In: Pagana KK, Pagana TJ, Pagana TN, eds. *Mosby's® Manual of Diagnostic and Laboratory Tests*. 7th ed. Philadelphia, PA: Elsevier; 2022.
31. Haq K, Patel DM. Urinalysis: interpretation and clinical correlations. *Med Clin North Am*. 2023;107(4):659–679. https://doi.org/10.1016/j.mcna.2023.03.002.
32. Villeneuve P, Bagshaw SM. Chapter 55. Assessment of urine biochemistry. In: Ronco C, Bellamo R, Kellum JA, Ricci Z, eds. *Critical Care Nephrology*. 3rd ed. Philadelphia, PA: Elsevier; 2019:323–328.
33. Wymer DC, Wymer DT. Chapter 4. Kidney imaging techniques. In: Lerna EV, Sparks MA, Topf JM, eds. *Nephrology Secrets*. 4th ed. Philadelphia, PA: Elsevier; 2019:30–36.
34. Chapter 7. Microscopic studies and associated testing. In: Pagana KK, Pagana TJ, Pagana TN, eds. *Mosby's® Manual of Diagnostic and Laboratory Tests*. 7th ed. Philadelphia, PA: Elsevier; 2022.

25

Kidney Disorders and Therapeutic Management

Kathrine Anne Winnie and Kimberly Sanchez

http://evolve.elsevier.com/Urden/CriticalCareNursing

Kidney disease is an overarching term that is inclusive of both short-term and long-term kidney damage.[1] The term acute kidney diseases and disorders (AKD) describes structural and/or functional changes to the kidney that likely impact the health of the affected individual.[1] Acute kidney injury (AKI) is the most common AKD.[1] AKI can range from mild impairment of kidney function to acute kidney failure requiring renal replacement therapy (dialysis).[1] If the acute changes are unresolved after 3 months, the condition is then classified as chronic kidney disease (CKD), although not all CKD is preceded by AKD.[1] Criteria for AKD and CKD are not completely aligned.[1] This chapter describes both AKI and CKD and summarizes the therapeutic management of kidney disease.

ACUTE KIDNEY INJURY

Description and Etiology

AKI is a subgroup of AKD, often occurring concomitantly with other syndromes or emerging as a consequence of other medical conditions.[1] AKI is characterized by a sudden rise in serum creatinine and/or a decrease in urine output.[2] Current diagnostic criteria are listed in Box 25.1. Proposed diagnostic criteria are only slightly different: an increase in serum creatinine by 0.3 mg/dL within 2 days, increase in serum creatine by 50% in 7 days, or oliguria for greater than or equal to 6 hours.[3]

There have been inconsistencies in definitions and diagnostic criteria for kidney diseases and disorders. A multinational group of nephrologists standardized the criteria used to diagnose and stage AKI.[4] The acronym RIFLE stratifies AKI into three categories of increasing severity (risk, injury, failure) and two outcome categories (loss, end-stage kidney disease) (Fig. 25.1).[4] Measurements of urine output along with creatinine or estimated glomerular filtration rate (eGFR) values are used to assess severity of AKI.[4] Similar criteria were developed by the Acute Kidney Injury Network (AKIN).[4] The severity of kidney injury is categorized by urine output, creatinine values, and the need for renal replacement therapy (Fig. 25.1).[4] The severity of kidney injury is described in stages from 1 to 3, using serum creatinine level, urine output, use of renal replacement therapy, and eGFR.[4]

Typically, a patient is not admitted to the critical care unit with AKI alone. More than 50% of critically ill patients may have AKI in addition to a primary illness.[2] Patients admitted to a critical care unit with AKI have a higher mortality.[5] Mortality associated with AKI ranges from 15% to over 60%[6] and is influenced by the coexisting medical conditions and kidney recovery, with higher mortality-associated nonrecovery of the kidney.[2] The kidneys recover within 7 days in almost two-thirds of AKI cases[2]; if the kidneys do not recover, a diagnosis of kidney failure increases risk of death to 47%.[2]

Traditionally, AKI was classified by the location of the insult relative to kidney anatomy: prerenal (before), intrarenal (within), and postrenal (after), but emphasis on the physiological processes resulting in AKI (hypoperfusion, intrinsic kidney damage, or obstruction) may help increase understanding of how coexisting infections contribute to the development of AKI. AKI may be caused by hypoperfusion from reduced intravascular pressure and/or volume; intrinsic kidney damage from endogenous or exogenous nephrotoxic agents, inflammatory responses, or autoimmune diseases; or obstruction from masses, strictures (including neurologic dysfunction), or trauma.[5] Hemodynamic, cardiac, pulmonary, or liver compromise may lead to decreased organ perfusion, and subsequently AKI.[5] Sepsis also affects the kidneys and may contribute to the development of AKI.[5] A summary of causes of AKI is presented in Box 25.2. Hypoperfusion is the most common cause of AKI, accounting for up to 70% of AKI.[1] Key concepts related to acute kidney injury are summarized in Fig. 25.2.

Pathophysiology

AKI disrupts fluid volume equilibrium, electrolyte balance, and acid–base homeostasis. When arterial hypoperfusion secondary to low cardiac output, decreased intravascular volume, vasodilation, or obstruction of kidney blood vessels reduces the blood flow to the nephrons, the glomerular filtration decreases, and consequently, urine output decreases.[2] Intrinsic AKI from ischemic or toxic damage to the kidney tubules, glomeruli, interstitium, or kidney blood vessels also affects filtering, concentrating, or excreting functions of the kidneys.[6] Any obstruction that hinders the flow of urine from beyond the kidney through the remainder of the urinary tract may lead to AKI by increasing the pressure in the kidneys, resulting in a reduced GFR.[6]

Initially, the integrity of the kidney's nephron structure and function may be preserved.[6] If normal perfusion and cardiac output are restored quickly, the kidney recovers with no permanent injury.[6] However, if the cause is not corrected, the patient is at risk for significant kidney damage: GFR declines, blood urea nitrogen (BUN) concentration rises (prerenal azotemia), the patient develops oliguria, and consequently fluid volume overload.[6] Oliguria, defined as urine output less than 400 mL/day or urine output less than 0.5 mL/kg per hour, with an elevated serum creatinine, is a classic finding in AKI.[6]

Electrolyte imbalances (mainly increased value states) increase mortality with kidney failure.[7] Electrolyte levels require frequent observation, especially in the critical phases of AKI when potassium can quickly reach levels of 6.5 mEq/L or higher.[6] Specific electrocardiogram changes are associated with hyperkalemia, including peaked T waves, a widening of the QRS interval, and ultimately ventricular tachycardia or fibrillation.[8]

In AKI, the physiologic feedback mechanism regulating calcium and phosphorus levels, involving parathyroid hormone and fibroblast growth factor, is nonfunctional; the serum phosphorus level rises, and the serum calcium level falls.[6] Without adequate levels of serum calcium, a compensatory mechanism "steals" calcium from bones, making patients with kidney failure more vulnerable to fractures.[6]

Metabolic acidosis (pH less than 7.35) occurs as a result of the accumulation of waste products in the bloodstream and tissues. A low serum albumin has a slightly alkalizing effect but is not enough to offset the metabolic acidosis. Respiratory compensation and mechanical ventilatory support are rarely sufficient to reverse metabolic acidosis. Information on acidosis and arterial blood gas interpretation is presented in Chapter 17. Anion gap measurements are discussed in Chapter 24.

Assessment and Diagnosis

A physical assessment of fluid volume status, including edema, skin turgor, and inspection of the oral mucosa, in addition to hemodynamic monitoring (heart rate, blood pressure, cardiac output), daily weight monitoring, and intake and output monitoring, may provide information for medical management. Other signs of volume overload should also be assessed: pulmonary congestion, worsening heart failure, and changes in neurological status. When AKI is suspected, the degree of injury is assessed using blood analysis. Laboratory studies should also be ordered and trended over time to assist with management of AKI. See Chapter 24 for a comprehensive review of clinical assessments and diagnostic procedures.

BOX 25.1 Diagnostic Criteria for Acute Kidney Injury (AKI)[2]

AKI is defined by any one of the following:

- Serum creatinine increases by ≥0.3 mg/dL within 48 hours;
- Serum creatinine increases by ≥1.5 mg/dL from baseline within 7 days, which is known or presumed to have occurred in the last 7 days;
- Urine volume decreases to <0.5 mL/kg/h for 6 hours

Medical Management

Treatment goals for patients with AKI focus on prevention, along with fluid, electrolyte, and acid–base balance.[2] Patients with AKI may have related or coexisting conditions that have targeted treatment goals and are summarized in Table 25.1.

Prevention

The only truly effective remedy for AKI is prevention.[2] Effective prevention requires assessment of the patient's risk for AKI and avoiding the possible causes (see Box 25.2).[5] For patients at risk for hypoperfusion from reduced intravascular pressure and/or volume, fluid maintenance should be considered before hypotension, volume depletion, or ongoing losses occur.[17] Usually, maintenance fluids are administered at a weight-based rate: 1 mL/kg/hr.[18] Additional factors need to be considered when determining the rate of maintenance in a patient at risk for AKI, including cardiopulmonary reserve, adequacy of kidney function, urine output, fluid balance, and type of fluid replaced.[17] Patients at risk for kidney damage should have an interprofessional team collaborating to maintain fluid status and avoid nephrotoxic medications.

Fluid Balance

Replacement. The objectives of volume replacement are to replace fluid and electrolyte losses.[17] Patients who are fluid responsive may benefit from fluid replacement.[5] See Chapter 12 for information on fluid volume responsiveness.

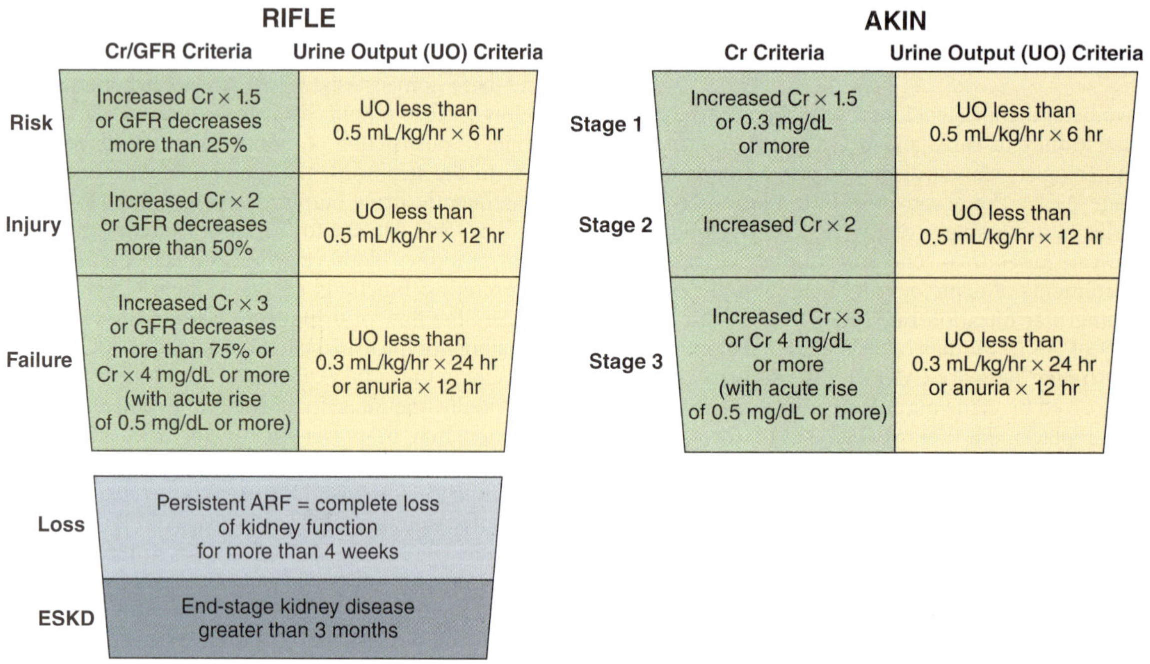

RIFLE

	Cr/GFR Criteria	Urine Output (UO) Criteria
Risk	Increased Cr × 1.5 or GFR decreases more than 25%	UO less than 0.5 mL/kg/hr × 6 hr
Injury	Increased Cr × 2 or GFR decreases more than 50%	UO less than 0.5 mL/kg/hr × 12 hr
Failure	Increased Cr × 3 or GFR decreases more than 75% or Cr × 4 mg/dL or more (with acute rise of 0.5 mg/dL or more)	UO less than 0.3 mL/kg/hr × 24 hr or anuria × 12 hr
Loss	Persistent ARF = complete loss of kidney function for more than 4 weeks	
ESKD	End-stage kidney disease greater than 3 months	

AKIN

	Cr Criteria	Urine Output (UO) Criteria
Stage 1	Increased Cr × 1.5 or 0.3 mg/dL or more	UO less than 0.5 mL/kg/hr × 6 hr
Stage 2	Increased Cr × 2	UO less than 0.5 mL/kg/hr × 12 hr
Stage 3	Increased Cr × 3 or Cr 4 mg/dL or more (with acute rise of 0.5 mg/dL or more)	UO less than 0.3 mL/kg/hr × 24 hr or anuria × 12 hr

FIG. 25.1 Diagnosis and Staging of Acute Kidney Injury. *ARF*, Acute renal failure; *Cr*, creatinine; *dL*, deciliter; *ESKD*, end-stage kidney disease; *GFR*, glomerular filtration rate; *hr*, hour; *kg*, kilogram; *mg*, milligram; *mL*, milliliter; *UO*, urine output.

Fluid replacement may be needed in patients with AKI also presenting with a fever, burn, and trauma as these conditions significantly increase fluid requirements. In patients with AKI, fluid replacement should cease once the patient is no longer fluid responsive or if there are clinical signs of fluid overload.[5,19]

BOX 25.2 Causes of Acute Kidney Injury[5]

Causes of Hypoperfusion
- Sepsis
- Shock
- Trauma
- Hemorrhage
- Cardiorenal syndrome
- Hepatorenal syndrome

Causes of Intrinsic Kidney Damage
- Acute tubular necrosis (ATN) from ischemic reperfusion injury and endogenous (Rhabdomyolysis) or exogenous nephrotoxic agents (chemotherapeutic agents, nonsteroidal antiinflammatory medications, illicit drugs, iodinated contrast)
- Acute interstitial nephritis (AIN) from infections, autoimmune, antibiotics, nonsteroidal antiinflammatory medications, elevated calcium or uric acid levels
- Acute glomerulonephritis (AGN) from infections and autoimmune or genetic disorder
- Vascular disease

Causes of Obstruction
- Benign or cancerous masses
- Kidney stones
- Neurogenic bladder
- Trauma

mg/dL, Milligrams per deciliter; *mL/kg/h*, milliliters per kilogram per hour.

The odds of mortality from fluid overload are two times higher in critically ill patients compared to not being fluid overloaded.[5] This outcome is similar in patients with AKI.[5]

Crystalloids and colloids are two different types of intravenous (IV) fluids used to increase intravascular volume in critically ill patients.[17] A crystalloid solution is an aqueous solution of mineral salts and other small, water-soluble molecules. Colloids are solutions containing oncotically active particles. Which IV replacement fluid to select to administer to hemodynamically unstable patients has been a controversial topic in critical care.[20] The debate often centers on the benefits of crystalloid versus colloid solutions for hypotension or hypovolemia (e.g., shock).[20,21] When comparing between crystalloids and colloids, there was no difference in mortality at 28 days.[21–23] When comparing within types of crystalloid solutions, balanced crystalloids (e.g., lactated Ringer solution, Normosol-R/PlasmaLyte) are associated with lower mortality at 28 days when compared to normal saline among critically ill patients.[20,24]

During fluid replacement, frequent monitoring of serum electrolyte levels is required, and strictly regulated intake and output are correlated with daily weight records. Composition of IV fluids should be evaluated prior to administration to patient with AKI. For example, lactated Ringer solution and Normosol-R/PlasmaLyte contain potassium (4–5 mEq/L). Frequently used intravenous solutions and their compositions are listed in Table 25.2.

Restriction. Fluid restriction constitutes a large part of medical management once AKI is established. Patients with kidney failure are usually restricted to 1 liter of fluid per 24 hours[17] if the urine output is 500 mL or less. Fluid restriction is used to prevent circulatory overload and the development of interstitial edema when the kidneys cannot remove excess volume.[17] Fluid requirements are calculated based on the daily intake and output measurement, as well as daily weight monitoring.

Acute Kidney Injury

Clinical and diagnostic assessments
- History and risk factors
  - Endogenous nephrotoxic agents (e.g., rhabdomyolysis)
  - Exogenous nephrotoxic agents (e g., radiopaque contrast medium)
  - Co-existing conditions (e.g., sepsis, organ failure)
- Obtain vital signs
  - Hypoperfusion (e g., decreased blood pressure, decreased CO, changes in heart rate)
- Clinical assessment
  - Edema
  - Skin turgor
  - Inspect oral mucosa
  - Daily weights
- Laboratory studies
  - Obtain blood and urine studies
- Diagnostic procedures
  - Assist with imaging studies

Signs
- Increased creatinine
- Increased BUN
- Decreased GFR
- Decreased UO
- Fluid overload
- Altered electrolytes

Nursing interventions
- Administer medications as ordered (e.g., diuretics)
- Manage treatment of co-existing conditions
- Administer fluids as ordered for maintenance replacement, or restriction
- Monitor intake and output
- Evaluate changes in weight
- Trend laboratory studies
- Perform renal replacement therapy as ordered

FIG. 25.2 Summary of Key Concepts Related to "Acute Kidney Injury." *CO*, Cardiac output; *BUN*, blood urea nitrogen; *GFR*, glomerular filtration rate; *UO*, urine output.

TABLE 25.1 Acute Kidney Injury: Related or Coexisting Conditions

Condition	Causes of Acute Kidney Injury	Pathophysiology	Treatment
Heart disease (cardiorenal syndrome)[9]	Hypoperfusion Intrinsic kidney damage	Decreased arterial pressure or volume from *heart failure* activates the kidney to increase venous pressure and volume that further stresses an already failing heart Increased venous pressure and volume and accumulation of metabolic waste may result from *kidney damage* and increases cardiac workload that can lead to heart failure and subsequent decreased arterial pressure and volume Cardiorenal syndrome subtypes are categorized by the primary organ dysfunction (types 1 and 2 originate from heart failure; types 3 and 4 originate from kidney diseases and disorder; and types 5 originates from other disease states that cause kidney and cardiac dysfunction)	Pharmacologic management Renal replacement therapy Treatment of underlying reversible cause if present
Liver disease with cirrhosis and ascites (hepatorenal syndrome)[10]	Hypoperfusion	Portal hypertension increases the risk of bacterial translocation, releasing inflammatory markers, that cause splanchnic and systemic arterial vasodilation and inadequate cardiac output Reduced circulatory volume to the kidneys contributes to kidney dysfunction	Pharmacologic management Treatment of underlying liver disease Liver transplantation
Pulmonary-renal syndrome[11]	Intrinsic kidney damage	Autoimmune diseases, particularly antineutrophil cytoplasmic antibodies (ANCA)-associated vasculitis and anti-glomerular basement membrane (anti-GBM) diseases, affect the pulmonary and glomerular capillaries, resulting in alveolar hemorrhage and rapidly progressing glomerulonephritis	Immunosuppression Plasmapheresis
Pulmonary disease[12]	Hypoperfusion	Accumulation of metabolic waste and increased production of inflammatory markers may result from kidney damage and may increase pulmonary congestion and may contribute to pulmonary hypertension Increased intrathoracic pressure from mechanical ventilation and pulmonary hypertension reduces cardiac output and that reduced flow to the kidney may result in damage	Organ support with lung protective mechanical ventilation and extracorporeal treatments Pharmacologic management
Sepsis[13]	Hypoperfusion	A microorganism stimulates the inflammatory/immune system, affecting clotting, the distribution of blood flow, capillary membrane permeability, and metabolism Reduced blood flow to the kidneys contributes to kidney dysfunction	Pharmacologic management Fluid replacement
Rhabdomyolysis[14]	Nephrotoxicity—Endogenous	Damaged muscle cells release creatine and myoglobin Increased creatine kinase (CK) indicates systemic muscle damage Increased circulating myoglobin is toxic to the kidneys Life-threatening hyperkalemia can occur as cell lysis results in intracellular potassium to be released into the bloodstream	Crystalloid fluid replacement Pharmacologic management
Iodinated contrast[15]	Nephrotoxicity—Exogenous	Contrast agents cause direct toxic damage to the kidney tubules and interstitium, ultimately leading to necrosis	Prevention should be the priority, focusing on (1) aggressive hydration prior to, during, and after the imaging study; (2) avoid dehydration; (3) discontinuation of other nephrotoxic medications prior to the imaging study if possible; (4) use of a lower quantity of contrast medium and use of nonionic low-osmolar or iso-osmolar contrast media that is less nephrotoxic The addition of acetylcysteine (Mucomyst, Mucosil) to reduce the risk of contrast-induced AKI is conflicting and more research is needed[16]
Hemorrhage	Hypoperfusion	Decreased intravascular volume from blood loss reduced blood flow to the kidney Reduced blood flow to the kidneys contributes to kidney dysfunction	Blood product replacement Pharmacologic management

AKI, Acute kidney injury.

TABLE 25.2 Frequently Used Intravenous Solutions

Solution	Composition
Crystalloids[a]	
Isotonic	
Normal saline solution (0.9% NaCl)	Sodium: 154 mEq/L Chloride: 154 mEq/L Osmolarity: 308 mOsm/L pH: 5
Lactated Ringer solution	Sodium: 130 mEq/L Potassium: 4 mEq/L Calcium: 3 mEq/L Chloride: 109 mEq/L Lactate: 28 mEq/L Osmolarity: 275 mOsm/L pH: 6.5
Normosol-R/PlasmaLyte	Sodium: 140 mEq/L Potassium: 5 mEq/L Magnesium: 3 mEq/L Chloride: 98 mEq/L Acetate: 27 mEq/L Gluconate: 23 mEq/L Osmolarity: 294 mOsm/L Normosol-R pH: 5.5 PlasmaLyte pH: 7.4
Hypotonic	
Dextrose in water (D_5W)[b]	Dextrose 5 g/L Osmolarity: 252 mOsm/L pH: 4
Half-normal saline solution (0.45% NaCl)	Sodium: 77 mEq/L Chloride: 77 mEq/L Osmolarity: 154 mOsm/L pH: 5.6
Hypertonic	
Dextrose in water (D5W) and Half-normal saline solution (0.45% NaCl)	Dextrose 5 g/L Sodium: 77 mEq/L Chloride: 77 mEq/L Osmolarity: 406 mOsm/L pH: 4.3
Hypertonic saline solution (3% NaCl)	Sodium: 513 mEq/L Chloride: 513 mEq/L Osmolarity: 1027 mOsm/L pH: 5
Colloids[c,d]	
5% Albumin	Albumin: 50 g/L Sodium: 130–160 mEq/L Potassium: <2 mEq/L Osmolality: 300 mOsm/L Oncotic pressure: 20 mm Hg pH: 6.4–7.4
25% Albumin	Albumin: 250 g/L Sodium: 130–160 mEq/L Potassium: <1 mEq/L Osmolality: 1500 mOsm/L pH: 6.4–7.4

[a]For crystalloid solutions that contain electrolytes, specific concentrations of electrolytes and pH vary according to the manufacturer.
[b]This solution is hypotonic at the time of infusion and becomes isotonic when dextrose is metabolized.
[c]Hetastarch, not listed in this table, has a boxed warning risk of mortality, kidney injury, and excess bleeding from the Food and Drug Administration and should not be used unless adequate alternative treatment is unavailable. (Accessed September 29, 2023, from https://www.fda.gov/vaccines-blood-biologics/safety-availability-biologics/labeling-changes-mortality-kidney-injury-and-excess-bleeding-hydroxyethyl-starch-products.)
[d]Dextran (dextran 40 or 70) is associated with severe, life-threatening anaphylaxis, and renal failure has been reported to occur after its use. (Accessed September 29, 2023, from https://www.pfizermedicalinformation.com/en-us/dextran/warnings.)
g, Gram; *L*, liter; *mEq*, Milliequivalent; *mm Hg*, millimeters of mercury; *mOsm*, milliosmole; *pH*, power of hydrogen.

Removal. Acute kidney injury results in retention of water, solutes, and potential toxins in the circulation, and prompt measures are needed to decrease their levels. Pharmacologic management may be needed to stimulate urine output and ultrafiltration may be accomplished with renal replacement therapy.

Electrolyte Balance

Electrolyte imbalances occur in patients with AKI. Serial electrolyte values should be monitored as hyperkalemia, hypocalcemia, hypo- or hypernatremia, and hyperphosphatemia may occur in AKI. The more likely imbalances are hyperkalemia and hypocalcemia, which can result in life-threatening cardiac dysrhythmias.

Acid–Base Balance

The acid–base imbalances that occur with AKI are monitored by arterial blood gas analyses. The goal of treatment is to maintain the pH within the normal range. See Chapter 17 for more information on arterial blood gases.

Nursing Management

The patient care plan for AKI involves a variety of patient problems (Box 25.3). All patients are evaluated for level of kidney function (fluid and electrolyte balance), readiness to learn, and need for education.

Hemodynamic Monitoring

Hemodynamic monitoring is important when assessing fluid volume status in a critically ill patient with AKI. Hemodynamic measures provide information of intravascular pressure and volume status in the presence or absence of edema. In critical illness, even though there is peripheral edema, and the patient may have gained 8 to 10 liters of fluid over their usual weight,

BOX 25.3 DIAGNOSIS AND PATIENT CARE MANAGEMENT

Acute Kidney Injury

- Ineffective Tissue Perfusion due to decreased kidney blood flow
- Hypervolemia due to renal dysfunction
- Anxiety due to threat to biological, psychological, or social integrity
- Impaired Cardiac Output due to alterations in preload
- Risk for Infection
- Disturbed Body Image due to functional dependence on life-sustaining technology

Lack of Knowledge of Treatment Regime due to lack of previous exposure to information (see Box 25.5, Patient and Family Education Plan for Acute Kidney Injury)

Patient Care Management plans are located in Appendix A.

BOX 25.4 Safety

Prevention of Catheter-Associated Urinary Tract Infections

Avoid Unnecessary Use of Indwelling Urinary Catheters

Critical Care Indications

- Accurate measurements of urinary output
- Prolonged immobilization (e.g., potentially unstable thoracic or lumbar spine, multiple traumatic injuries such as pelvic fractures)

Perioperative Indications

- Urologic or genitourinary tract surgery
- Prolonged duration of surgery (catheters inserted for this reason should be removed in the postanesthesia care unit)
- Large-volume infusions or diuretics administered during surgery
- Intraoperative monitoring of urinary output

Other Indications

- Acute urinary retention or bladder outlet obstruction
- Assist in healing of open sacral or perineal wounds in incontinent patients
- Improve comfort for end-of-life care if needed

Insert Urinary Catheters Using Aseptic Technique

Hand Hygiene

- Wash hands thoroughly before or after any patient care activity.

Aseptic Technique and Sterile Equipment

- Use standard supply kits that contain all necessary items: sterile gloves, drape, sponges, antiseptic solution for cleaning meatus, and single-use packet of lubricant jelly for insertion.
- Consider using urinary catheter systems with preconnected, sealed catheter-tubing junctions.
- Use as small a catheter as possible to minimize urethral trauma.

Adopt Evidence-Based Standards for Maintenance of Urinary Catheters

Maintenance of Closed Drainage System

- Maintain closed drainage system.
- Maintain unobstructed urine flow.
- Keep drainage bag below the level of the bladder at all times.
- Do not allow drainage bag to touch the floor.
- Use standard precautions during any manipulation of the catheter or collecting system.
- Empty collection bag regularly, using a separate container for each patient.
- Do not allow drainage spigot to touch the collection container.
- Collect from sampling port in the tubing drainage system, disinfecting the port and aspirating using aseptic technique.
- Avoid catheter irrigation except in the case of an anticipated obstructed catheter (e.g., blood clots).
- Routine scheduled replacement of catheters is not recommended.

Catheter Securement and Hygiene

- Keep urinary catheter secured to prevent catheter movement and urethral friction.
- Do not clean periurethral area with antiseptics. Urethral cleaning during a bath is appropriate.

Review Need for the Indwelling Urinary Catheter Daily and Remove Catheter Promptly

Documentation and Monitoring

- Document when catheter was inserted.
- Review the need for the urinary catheter for every patient every day.

Hospital Strategies to Ensure Early Removal of an Indwelling Urinary Catheter

- Ensure clinicians are aware that longer duration of catheter use increases catheter-associated urinary tract infection (CAUTI) risk. This awareness can be reinforced by:
  - Alerts in computerized ordering systems
  - Development of standardized nursing protocols that allow nurses to remove urinary catheters if predetermined criteria are met

Data from Gould CV, Umscheid CA, Agarwal RK, Kuntz G, Pegues DA; Healthcare Infection Control Practices Advisory Committee. Guideline for prevention of catheter-associated urinary tract infections 2009. *Infect Control Hosp Epidemiol.* 2010;31(4):319–326. doi:10.1086/651091

the patient may remain "intravascularly dry" and hemodynamically unstable because the retained fluid is not inside a vascular compartment and cannot contribute to maintenance of hemodynamic stability. Hemodynamic monitoring includes surveillance of changes in vital signs, including cardiac output. The range of monitoring devices has expanded, and assessment may be continuous or intermittent and be invasive, minimally invasive, or noninvasive, as described in Chapter 12.

Weight Monitoring

Daily weight is an important monitoring method. The daily weight, combined with accurate intake and output monitoring, is an indicator of fluid gains or losses over 24 hours. A 1-kg weight gain over 24 hours represents 1000 mL (1 liter) of additional fluid retention.

Intake and Output Monitoring

Monitoring of intake and output when caring for patients with AKI is important. For patients receiving renal replacement therapy, any fluid removed is included in the daily fluid balance. In patients with AKI, all measurable volumes should be recorded for accuracy, particularly urine output. Continent patients should be provided supplies for measurement (e.g., urinals, urine and stool collection pan). Incontinent patients should be provided external urinary collection devices (e.g., incontinent pads or wraps, external catheters).[25] If a patient presents with retention, consider intermittent catheterization before use of an indwelling urinary catheter.[25] If an indwelling urinary catheter is indicated, ensure infection prevention measures are in place (Box 25.4). It is important to continuously evaluate criteria for indwelling catheter removal to ensure prompt removal, leveraging external urinary collection devices for accurate output measurement.[25]

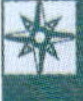

BOX 25.5 PATIENT AND FAMILY EDUCATION PLAN

Acute Kidney Injury

Before discharge, the patient should be able to teach back the following topics:

- Pathophysiology of acute kidney injury as a sudden decline in kidney function that caused an acute buildup of toxins in the blood.
- Explain diet and fluid restrictions.
- Emphasize need for exercise and rest.
- Describe medications and adverse effects.
- Explain need for ongoing follow-up with health care professional.
- Explain purpose of dialysis and importance of regular treatments.
- Describe complications associated with acute kidney injury.

Educate the Patient and Family

Accurate and uncomplicated information must be provided to the patient and family about AKI, including its pathophysiology, treatment, and possible complications (Box 25.5). When providing education, patients with an elevated BUN and creatinine may have an altered level of consciousness,[26] negatively affecting their readiness to learn. Encouraging the patient and family to voice concerns, frustrations, or fears and allowing the patient to control some aspects of the acute care environment and treatment are important. Specific topics related to their disease process should be covered. For example, patients with hyperphosphatemia may experience severe pruritus[27] and nursing education points should cover frequent skin care with emollients, discouraging scratching, and adhering to their medication regimen.

CHRONIC KIDNEY DISEASE

Description and Etiology

CKD is characterized by abnormalities of the structure and function of the kidney, for a duration of more than 3 months, that has health consequences.[28] Diagnostic criteria for CKD include a decreased eGFR and at least one indicator of kidney dysfunction, including albuminuria, that is present for more than 3 months.[28] First, an eGFR of <60 mL/min/1.73 m^2 must be present.[28] Second, there must be one or more indicators of kidney dysfunction: (1) albuminuria defined as an albumin excretion rate ≥30 mg/24 hours or an albumin-creatinine ratio ≥30 mg/g; (2) abnormalities in urine sediment; (3) abnormalities due to tubular disorders (e.g., electrolytes); (4) abnormalities detected by histology; (5) abnormalities detected by imaging; or (6) previous kidney transplantation.[28]

The patient's eGFR value and extent of albuminuria are used to grade the severity of CKD.[28] GFR classifications range from G1 to G5, with G1 being a normal to high eGFR (≥90 mL/min/1.73 m^2) and G5 being an eGFR <15 mL/min/1.73 m^2 (kidney failure).[28] Both G1 and G2 are only diagnosed as CKD if there is evidence of at least one indicator of kidney dysfunction.[28] Albuminuria classifications range from A1 to A3.[28] A1 denotes a normal or mildly increased amount of albumin in the urine, while A3 denotes a severely increased amount of albumin in the urine.[28] All patients with CKD should have routine assessments of eGFR and albuminuria because it is a risk factor for further decline.[28]

The causes of CKD may be classified into glomerular diseases (diabetes, amyloidosis), tubulointerstitial diseases (urinary tract infections, stone), vascular diseases (atherosclerosis, hypertension), cystic disease (polycystic or acquired cystic disease), and congenital disease (Alport syndrome, Fabry disease).[28]

The estimated incidence of CKD in the United States is 14%.[29] In the ICU, the percent of patient patients with CKD is low, but patients with CKD are at higher risk for end-stage renal disease, cardiovascular disease, and mortality.[30–32]

Pathophysiology

Chronic kidney disease disrupts the integrity of the kidney structures.[33] Each cause of CKD is an initial and sustained insult to the kidney.[33] These perpetuated insult damages the nephrons, ultimately leading to sclerosis and affecting filtering, concentrating, or excreting functions of the kidneys.[33]

Assessment and Diagnosis

Patients with lower CKD severity grades are often asymptomatic.[28] Symptoms present as the eGFR declines and are detected during routine assessments of coexisting conditions, like hypertension, anemia, bone and mineral disorders, dyslipidemia, diabetes, and malnutrition.[28] When CKD is suspected, the degree of severity is assessed with blood and urine studies.[28] See Chapter 24 for a comprehensive review of diagnostic procedures.

Medical Management

Blood Pressure Management

It is recommended that patients with CKD have a systolic blood pressure less than 120 mm Hg, when tolerated.[34] This recommendation is for CKD patients not receiving dialysis.[34] In patients with a kidney transplant, the recommended blood pressure parameter is a systolic less than 130 mm Hg and a diastolic less than 80 mm Hg.[34] Treatment to maintain this parameter includes prescribing angiotensin-converting enzyme inhibitors and angiotensin II receptor blockers for patients with hypertension, with or without diabetes, who have A2–3 albuminuria and G1–4 GFR classifications.[34] Considerations of the patient's entire medication profile should include exploring medication formulations, like generic or single pill combination for reduced pill burden and cost-effective care.[35]

Lifestyle interventions for lowering blood pressure include a low-sodium (<2 g per day) diet and 150 minutes of moderate to intense physical activity per week.[34]

Anemia Management

It is recommended that patients with CKD have a hemoglobin of greater than 12 g/dL.[36] Continual evaluation of anemia includes obtaining a CBC with differential, absolute reticulocyte count, serum ferritin, transferrin saturation, vitamin B12, and folate level.[36] Treatment for anemia depends on the cause.[36] Additionally, prescribing iron supplements and erythropoiesis-stimulating agents is recommended for the management of anemia.[36]

Mineral and Bone Disorder Management

In patients with G3–G5 GFR classifications, a bone mineral density scan is recommended.[37] Additionally, an abdominal radiograph or echocardiogram is recommended to evaluate for vascular calcification.[37] Continual evaluation of calcium, phosphate, parathyroid hormone, and alkaline phosphatase should occur for patient with G3–G5 GFR classifications.[37] Vitamin D should be evaluated based on the patient's baseline laboratory value and if they are on any treatment.[37] Treatment for mineral and bone disorders depends on trends in laboratory values, with a focus on managing phosphorus absorption, suppressing overactive parathyroid hormone, supplementing vitamin D, and replacing calcium.[37]

Lipid Management

An initial fasting lipid panel, including total cholesterol, low-density lipoprotein, high-density lipoprotein, and triglycerides,

SUPPORTING NURSE WELL-BEING

Financial Wellness

After finishing the new graduate RN orientation program and working as an ICU nurse for two years, my retired mom became ill, requiring frequent physician visits, hospitalizations, and at home care. It was hard to switch shifts to accommodate my mom's appointments. When she was in the hospital, it was nearly impossible to visit her before or after work with hospital-imposed visitation restrictions. I was a nurse at work and, on my days off, I was a nurse at home. After about a year of her declining health, I had exhausted my paid time off options, including sick and vacation time. Throughout the year, we had been receiving medical bills at a pretty regular cadence and these weren't $50 here, $100 there. To put things into perspective, the out-of-pocket expenses for one hospitalization was thousands of dollars, each individual medical service that was consulted during the hospitalization was additional several hundred dollars, and the diagnostic tests completed during the hospitalization were another few hundred dollars. Then, there were bills for post-discharge follow-up appointments. These medical bills, in addition to our necessary living expenses (mortgage, utilities, transportation, and food costs), became increasing difficult to pay off with only one income. It was hard to make ends meet.

The above vignette shows how one person is affected by financial stress, in addition to the physical, emotional, and psychological stress of keeping up with job requirements and caring for an ailing parent. Financial stress stems from an imbalance of income and expenses: an unforeseen expense, a foreseen expense whose amount was more than anticipated, an increase in expenses, or a loss of income. Trying to identify resources and options to address your situation while actively in the situation is another stressor. Financial stress can contribute to unhealthy behaviors, including picking up extra shifts when one is mentally and physically drained because "you need the money." Financial wellness encompasses an awareness of your current situation and a concerted effort to establish a financial infrastructure to support future needs. It is not needing to be "rich" or saving everything at the expense of a social life. Financial wellness is recognizing the need for and establishing a safety net for the unknown. That's the thing with the unknown—one doesn't know what it is or when it will happen.

Consider the following to maintain financial wellness:

- Determine your current financial state: What is your monthly net income? What are your monthly expenses?
- Save 3 to 6 months of expenses; if minimal expenses are accrued, save 3 to 6 months of income
- Establish and maintain a budget
- List what expenses you can reduce or eliminate should you have a loss of income or increase in expenses
- Evaluate your expenses quarterly to notice trends and attempt to reduce nonessential future spending. Look at the list of expenses you'd reduce or eliminate should you have a loss of income to help evaluate your expenses.
- Explore paid, unpaid, and partially paid leave benefits provided by your employer
- Consider professional resources for financial literacy

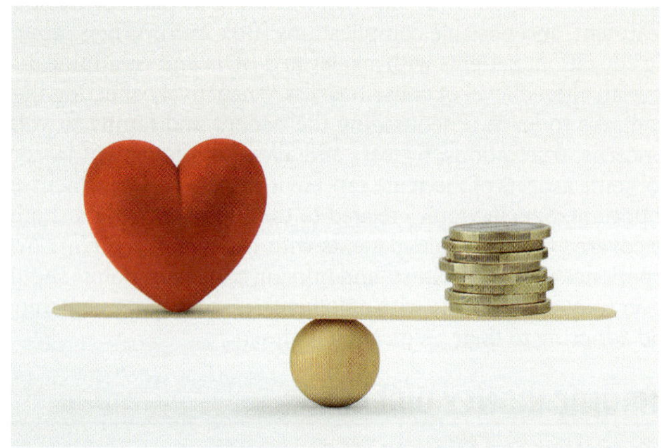

An investment in knowledge pays the best interest...

-Benjamin Franklin

is recommended for patients newly diagnosed with CKD.[38] Treatment with a statin is recommended for patients over the age of 18 with CKD with additional risk factors, such as coronary disease, diabetes, ischemic stroke, or any G1–G5 GFR classifications.[38] Initiation of statin treatment is not recommended if the patient is already on dialysis.[38] But statin treatments may be continued if the patient was already receiving statin treatments before initiating dialysis.[38]

Lifestyle interventions for lipid management include a low-fat (<15% of total calories) diet, reduced sugar and carbohydrate intake, weight reduction, increased physical activity, and reduced alcohol intake.[38]

Glycemic Management

It is recommended that patients with diabetes and CKD have a hemoglobin A1c less than 8%.[39] Hemoglobin A1c measurements may be obtained twice a year to monitor long-term glycemic control.[39] Patients with diabetes and CKD need a comprehensive treatment strategy to prevent progression of kidney and development of cardiovascular disease.[39] The first-line treatment for glycemic management in patients with diabetes and CKD is metformin.[39] Patients with diabetes, CKD, and an eGFR ≥20 mL/min/1.73 m^2 should be prescribed sodium–glucose cotransporter-2 inhibitors for kidney and cardiovascular protection.[39] Patients with diabetes, an eGFR ≥25 mL/min/1.73 m^2, normal serum potassium, and albuminuria ≥30 mg/g should be prescribed a nonsteroidal mineralocorticoid receptor antagonist, also for kidney and cardiovascular protection.[39]

Lifestyle interventions for glycemic management include avoiding or quitting tobacco products and at least 150 minutes of moderate to intense physical activity per week.[39] Dietary modifications for patients with diabetes and CKD include maintaining a protein intake of 0.8 g/kg/day for patients not treated with dialysis or up to 1.2 g/kg/day for patients treated with dialysis and eating a low-sodium (<2 g per day) diet.[39]

Nutrition Management

Nutrition recommendations for critically ill patients and patients with kidney disease are reviewed in Chapter 6.

Nursing Management

Educate the Patient and Family

Patient and family education should focus on lifestyle modifications and at home monitoring.

Education should focus on disease-related knowledge, self-management, and management of coexisting conditions. At-home monitoring equipment should be reviewed with patients to ensure consistent measurement for review with providers.

PHARMACOLOGY

An important part of pharmacologic management in patients with kidney disease includes ensuring all nephrotoxic medications are dose adjusted or stopped. Some pharmacologic principles and practices are discussed in the medical management section of AKI and CKD. In this section, diuretics along with potassium, phosphorus, and sodium management are reviewed. Collaboration among the interprofessional team is essential in promoting safe pharmacology practices.

Diuretics

Diuretics are used to stimulate urinary output in a patient with fluid overload.[40] Diuretics act on a specific site along the nephron where they inhibit transport.[40] Care must be taken to prevent the creation of secondary electrolyte abnormalities. Pharmacologic management with diuretics is outlined in Table 25.3. The pharmacologic site of action of diuretics in the nephron is depicted in Fig. 25.3.

Electrolyte Management

Electrolyte replacement is dependent on laboratory values and clinical presentation. Hyperkalemia is the most common electrolyte imbalance in patients with kidney disease. Management of hyperkalemia is outlined in Table 25.4.

Phosphorus Management

Phosphorus is present in many foods, especially foods with a high protein content such as meat, fish, and dairy.[37] Dietary

TABLE 25.3 PHARMACOLOGIC MANAGEMENT

Diuretic Medications

Medication	Dosage	Action	Special Considerations
Diuretics			
Osmotic Diuretics			
Mannitol	0.25–1.0 g/kg IV infusion as 15%–20% solution over 30–90 minutes	Increases glomerular filtration[41] Acts on proximal tubule to inhibit water reabsorption[41]	Monitor for hypotension Monitor electrolytes Monitor for worsening acute kidney injury Administer with filter and observe solution for crystal formation[42]
Carbonic Anhydrase Inhibitors			
Acetazolamide (Diamox)	250–500 mg/day PO or IV	Inhibits carbonic anhydrase to excrete bicarbonate ions in the urine[43] Acts on proximal tubule to inhibit sodium reabsorption[43]	Monitor acid–base balance (e.g., serum bicarbonate levels, arterial blood gas) Enhanced diuresis with loop diuretic[43]
Loop Diuretics			
Furosemide (Lasix)	20–80 mg/day PO or IV	Acts on loop of Henle to inhibit sodium and chloride reabsorption[40]	Monitor electrolytes Monitor for ototoxicity[44] Caution with sulfa allergy
Bumetanide (Bumex)	0.5–2 mg x1 PO, may be repeated 1 mg IV, may be repeated 1 mg IV bolus, then 0.5–2 mg/hr IV	Acts on loop of Henle to inhibit sodium and chloride reabsorption[40]	Monitor electrolytes Caution with sulfa allergy
Thiazide (Distal Convoluted Tubule) Diuretics			
Hydrochlorothiazide	25–100 mg/day PO	Acts on distal tubule to inhibit sodium and chloride reabsorption[40]	Monitor blood pressure Monitor electrolytes Caution with sulfa allergy. Synergistic effect with loop diuretics[40]
Metolazone (Zaroxolyn)	2.5–20 mg/day PO	Acts on distal tubule to inhibit sodium and chloride reabsorption[40]	Monitor electrolytes May be effective[45] when eGFR <20 mL/min/1.73 m^2
Potassium-Sparing Diuretics			
Spironolactone (Aldactone)	25–200 mg/day PO	Binds to mineralocorticoid receptors, antagonist to aldosterone, in collecting duct to promote sodium and water excretion and potassium retention[40]	Monitor for hyperkalemia
Vaptans			
Conivaptan (Vaprisol)	Loading dose: 20 mg IV as 30-min infusion Continuous IV infusion: 20 mg over 24 hr After first day, can be increased to 40 mg/24 hr Maximum infusion is 4 days	Acts on collecting duct to inhibit vasopressin to promote water excretion and sodium retention[46]	Monitor serum sodium levels Tolvaptan (Samsca) for oral dosing 15–60 mg/day

eGFR, Estimated glomerular filtration rate; *g*, gram; *hr*, hour; *IV*, intravenous/intravenously; *kg*, kilogram; *m*, meter; *mg*, milligram; *min*, minute; *mL*, milliliterl *PO*, by mouth.

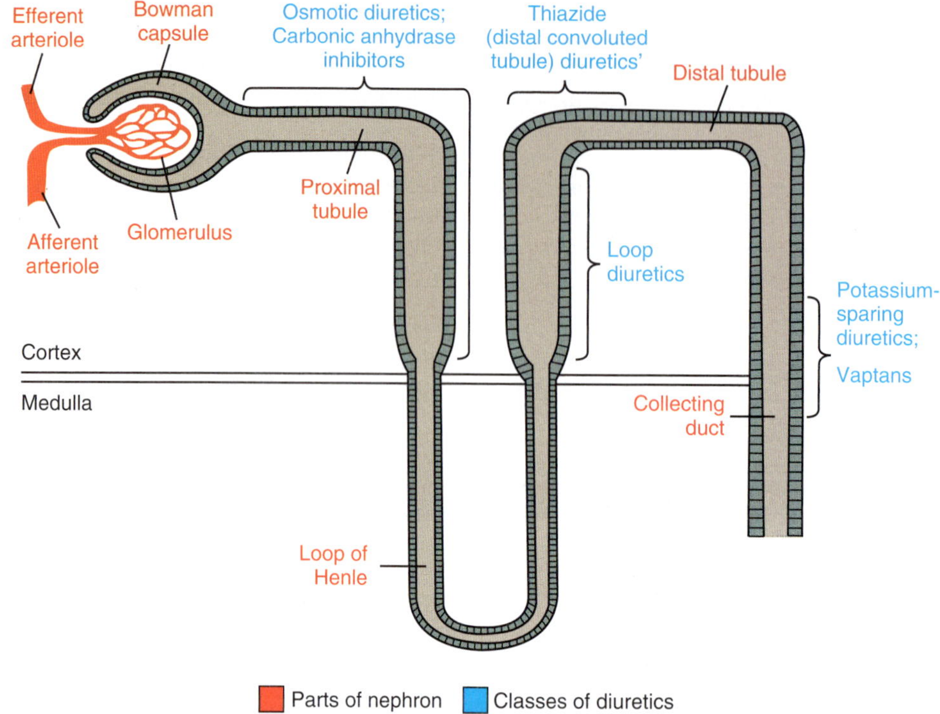

FIG. 25.3 Pharmacologic Site of Action of Diuretics in the Nephron.

TABLE 25.4 PHARMACOLOGIC MANAGEMENT

Electrolyte Management Medications

Medication	Dosage	Action	Special Considerations
Medications for Hyperkalemia			
Insulin and dextrose	5–10 units of insulin and 25–50 g of dextrose IV	Increases potassium transfer from the extracellular to the intracellular space[8] Dextrose is administered simultaneously because insulin results in hypoglycemia[8]	Monitor blood glucose 4–5 hours after administration[47] May need calcium gluconate or calcium chloride for myocardial protection[47]
Salbutamol (Albuterol)	10 mg nebulized	Increases potassium transfer from the extracellular to the intracellular space[8]	Monitor for tachycardia[8]
Sodium bicarbonate	100–250 mL of 8.4% sodium bicarbonate over 20 minutes IV	Increases potassium transfer from the extracellular to the intracellular space[48]	Monitor acid–base balance Monitor electrolytes Administer in patients with metabolic acidosis[48]
Cation-Exchange Resins			
Sodium zirconium cyclosilicate (Lokelma)	10 g one to three times per day PO	Exchanges sodium and potassium in the small and large intestine[8]	Monitor for gastrointestinal complications[8]
Patiromer (Veltassa)	8.4–25.2 g/d PO	Exchanges sodium and potassium in the large intestine[8]	Monitor electrolytes Monitor for gastrointestinal complications[8]
Sodium polystyrene sulfonate (Kayexalate)	15 g one to four times per day PO	Exchanges sodium and potassium in the large intestine[8]	Monitor electrolytes Monitor for gastrointestinal complications[8] Should not be administered with sorbitol[8]

d, Day; *g*, gram; *IV*, intravenous/intravenously; *mg*, milligram; *mL*, milliliter; *PO*, by mouth.

phosphate-binding medication is prescribed to manage hyperphosphatemia in patients with kidney disease.[49] These medications reduce the absorption of dietary phosphate in the gastrointestinal tract by exchanging phosphate with other ions (e.g., calcium, magnesium) and forming a compound that is excreted in feces.[49] The dietary phosphate binder is usually taken at the time of the meal.[49] If a calcium-based phosphate binder is taken between meals, it will increase only the level of calcium in the bloodstream and will not lower the serum phosphorus level.[50]

The types of dietary phosphorus binders used have changed over the years. The original binders were aluminum salts (aluminum hydroxide) that bound dietary phosphorus effectively in the gastrointestinal tract but conferred aluminum toxicity because some of the aluminum metal was also absorbed. For this reason, aluminum binders have been abandoned.[37] The second-generation dietary phosphorus–binding agents use calcium salts including calcium carbonate or calcium acetate to bind dietary phosphorus in the gastrointestinal tract. Calcium-based medications are safer, but elevated serum calcium levels and calcium deposits in other areas of the body (extraosseous calcification) are a problem.

A third generation of nonabsorbable dietary phosphorus–binding medications is available. These are nonaluminum-based and noncalcium-based and include sevelamer hydrochloride and lanthanum carbonate.[37] These medications have a better safety profile and are frequently prescribed to lower serum phosphorus levels in patients with kidney disease.[37]

Sodium Management

Patients with kidney disease may present with hypo- or hypernatremia.[51,52] The volume status is an important measure when deciding to treat sodium imbalance.[51,52] For example, patients who are hypervolemic/hyponatremic may receive vaptan medications for diuresis (Table 25.3) or hypertonic saline (Table 25.2).[52] When hypovolemia/hypernatremia is present, treatment may include enteral free water administration or intravenous administration of hypotonic solution (Table 25.2).[51]

RENAL REPLACEMENT THERAPY

Renal replacement therapy (RRT) removes toxins and corrects fluid, electrolyte, and acid–base imbalances by moving substances across a semipermeable membrane. Renal replacement therapies are performed continuously over 24 hours or intermittently for several hours, several days a week. The types of renal replacement therapies are summarized in Table 25.5.

Continuous Renal Replacement Therapy

Continuous renal replacement therapy (CRRT) is extracorporeal blood purification designed to take the place of kidney function over an extended amount of time.[53] CRRT provides controlled removal and replacement of fluid over many hours or days, maintaining hemodynamic stability.[53] This type of RRT is used for hemodynamically unstable patients with AKI requiring dialysis.[53] CRRT causes smaller, gentler fluid shifts and is indicated for patients with intracranial hypertension.[53] It may be considered for patients with other types of neurologic conditions.[53] Another indication for CRRT is for the removal of drugs and toxins.[53] Once ordered and initiated, CRRT runs constantly unless the filter needs to be changed or the patient's treatment interventions require disconnection from dialysis (e.g., some procedures, surgeries, or mobility activities). Organizational criteria should be developed to guide use of this therapy in time-limited episodes to evaluate response to treatment if the patient has a poor prognosis.[54] Additionally, organizations should develop criteria for discontinuation of the therapy.[54]

Access

A dialysis catheter may be placed in an internal jugular, femoral, or subclavian vein.[55] The site of choice is the right internal jugular vein.[55] When catheters are placed in the internal jugular vein, the tip of the catheter should rest at the junction of the superior vena cava and right atrium to enhance blood flow rates.[55] In patients who may require dialysis permanently, the subclavian veins should be avoided when possible due to the greater risk of central vein stenosis, limiting options for future dialysis access.[55] Different types of vascular catheters may be placed, but a double lumen catheter is preferred to ensure each lumen diameter is sufficiently sized to run therapy.[55] When compared to a double lumen catheter, a triple lumen catheter would have smaller lumen diameters.[55] Placing a double lumen dialysis catheter in the right internal jugular vein and ensuring the catheter tip is correctly positioned will help increase blood, rendering CRRT more effecting.[55]

TABLE 25.5 Comparison of Types of Renal Replacement Therapies

Type of Therapy	Usual Duration	Usual Access	Location	Ultrafiltration	Solute Removal	Mechanism of Solute Removal
Continuous renal replacement therapy (CRRT)	24 h	Central venous catheter	Hospital, in the ICU because of hemodynamic instability	Yes	Yes[a]	SCUF—N/A only ultrafiltration CVVH—Convection CVVHD—Diffusion CVVHDF—Convention and diffusion
Prolonged intermittent renal replacement therapy (PIRRT) (using CRRT equipment)	4–24 h	Central venous catheter	Hospital	Yes	Yes	Convention and diffusion
Sustained low efficiency dialysis (SLED) (using IHD equipment)	4–24 h	AV fistula AV graft Central venous catheter	Hospital	Yes	Yes	Diffusion
Intermittent hemodialysis (IHD)	3–4 h	AV fistula AV graft Central venous catheter	Hospital Clinic Home[b]	Yes	Yes	Diffusion
Peritoneal dialysis (PD)	8–12 h	Peritoneal catheter	Hospital Home	Yes	Yes	Diffusion and convection

[a]The CRRT mode of SCUF does not have a mechanism of solute removal.
[b]The availability of dialysis machines approved for home use and the potential for improved outcomes and cost savings for at-home therapy have led to home dialysis programs for appropriate individuals. In most cases, patients or family caregivers are trained to perform dialysis treatments.
AV, Arteriovenous; *h*, hour.

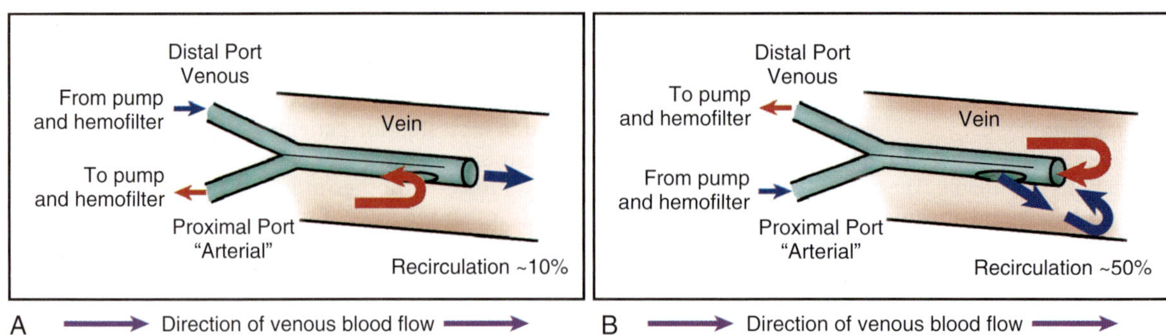

FIG. 25.4 Temporary Dialysis Venous Access Catheter. (A) Blood from pump and hemofilter connected to distal port on the dialysis venous access catheter and blood flows into vein with minimal recirculation, as blood is pumped from an opening that is proximal to the opening where blood is being returned. (B) Blood from pump and hemofilter connected to proximal port on the dialysis venous access catheter and blood returned into vein with higher recirculation, as blood is pumped from an opening that is distal to the opening where blood is being returned.

Once the dialysis catheter is in place and the patient is started on CRRT, a pump drives blood from the vein through an extracorporeal circuit that includes a filter.[53] The blood is then returned to the same vein.[53] The flow of blood through a temporary dialysis venous access catheter is depicted in Fig. 25.4.

Mechanism

In CRRT, different processes allow for ultrafiltration and solute transport.[53] Ultrafiltration is the transport of plasma water through a semipermeable membrane, driven by hydrostatic pressure. The excess fluid pulled from the blood is the ultrafiltrate.[56] The mechanisms of solute transport include diffusion and convection.[53] Diffusion describes the movement of solute along a concentration gradient from a high concentration to a low concentration across a semipermeable membrane.[57] Convection occurs when the pressure gradient is set up so that the fluid being pushed or pumped across the dialysis filter drags solutes from the bloodstream as it flows through the filter.[53] This method of solute removal is known as solvent drag and is commonly used in CRRT. Additionally, the filter attracts compounds that attach to the dialysis filter.[53]

Modes

Several modes of CRRT are available:

- Slow continuous ultrafiltration (SCUF)
- Continuous venovenous hemofiltration (CVVH)
- Continuous venovenous hemodialysis (CVVHD)
- Continuous venovenous hemodiafiltration (CVVHDF)

These modes have different mechanisms for ultrafiltration and solute transport (Fig. 25.5).[53] SCUF slowly removes fluid through ultrafiltration (Fig. 25.5A).[53] SCUF should only be used for patients with pathological and otherwise unmanageable volume overload.[58] Only a small amount of solutes will be removed from SCUF, so the therapy is not appropriate if solute clearance is needed.[58] CVVH uses ultrafiltration and convection for removal of small, medium, and large molecules (Fig. 25.5B).[53] Although no dialysis solution is used, replacement fluid is utilized to replace some or all of the ultrafiltrate.[53] Infusing replacement solution postfilter is more efficient but does not give the advantage of hemodilution of the blood prior to it entering the filter, and clotting is more likely than it would be if prefilter replacement solution is used.[56] CVVHD uses ultrafiltration and diffusion for small solute removal (Fig. 25.5C).[53] Dialysate solution is used in a countercurrent or co-current flow.[53] CVVHDF uses both hemodialysis and hemofiltration (Fig. 25.5D).[53] Dialysis solution and replacement solution are used.[53] Replacement solution can be given prefilter, postfilter, or both.[58] Convection and diffusion are used for removal of small, medium, and large molecules.[53]

The selection of a CRRT mode is often based on the equipment available and the prescribing practices of the health care team. Consistency in mode of therapy used may be more important to outcomes than the actual mode itself.[59] See Table 25.6 for a comparison of CRRT modes. See Table 25.7 for a review of molecule sizes and their mechanism of removal by CRRT.

Anticoagulation

Because the blood outside the body is in contact with artificial tubing and filters, the coagulation cascade and complement cascades are activated. To prevent the hemofilter from becoming obstructed by clotting, or clotting off, low-dose anticoagulation may be used but its use in practice is varied.[56] Typical anticoagulant choices include heparin and citrate.[56] Citrate is an effective prefilter anticoagulant, which has the side effect that it chelates (binds to and removes) calcium from the blood.[56] Consequently, ionized calcium levels are verified, and calcium is replaced per protocol when sodium citrate is the anticoagulant.

Nursing Management

Potential problems associated with CRRT and appropriate nursing interventions are listed in Box 25.6. The critical care nurse provides education about the disease process and treatment plan to the patient and family.

Intermittent Hemodialysis

Hemodialysis is an extracorporeal treatment that removes fluid and substances from the blood when the kidneys are damaged and not functioning normally. There are no set criteria for initiation of hemodialysis, but it should be considered after aggressive attempts at medical management and the patient persistently has signs and symptoms of kidney failure (Box 25.7).

Access

Ideally, initiation of hemodialysis is planned, allowing time for the creation of permanent vascular access for the patient approximately 6 months prior to the expected start of therapy.[61] The common feature in permanent vascular access devices is a conduit connection between the arterial circulation and the venous circulation.[62]

Temporary vascular access may be needed if a graft or fistula is nonfunctional or when hemodialysis is unplanned or needed before a permanent vascular access can be used. See earlier CRRT section for information on temporary access.

Arteriovenous Fistula. The arteriovenous fistula is created by surgically exposing a peripheral artery and vein and constructing a side-by-side opening in the artery and the vein to join the two vessels together.[62] High arterial flow causes enlargement of the area and results in a pseudoaneurysm.[61] Sufficient arterial flow to enlarge the access takes a minimum of 14 days, with AV maturation taking up to 6 weeks.[62] When the site is healed, a large-bore needle will be inserted to obtain arterial outflow

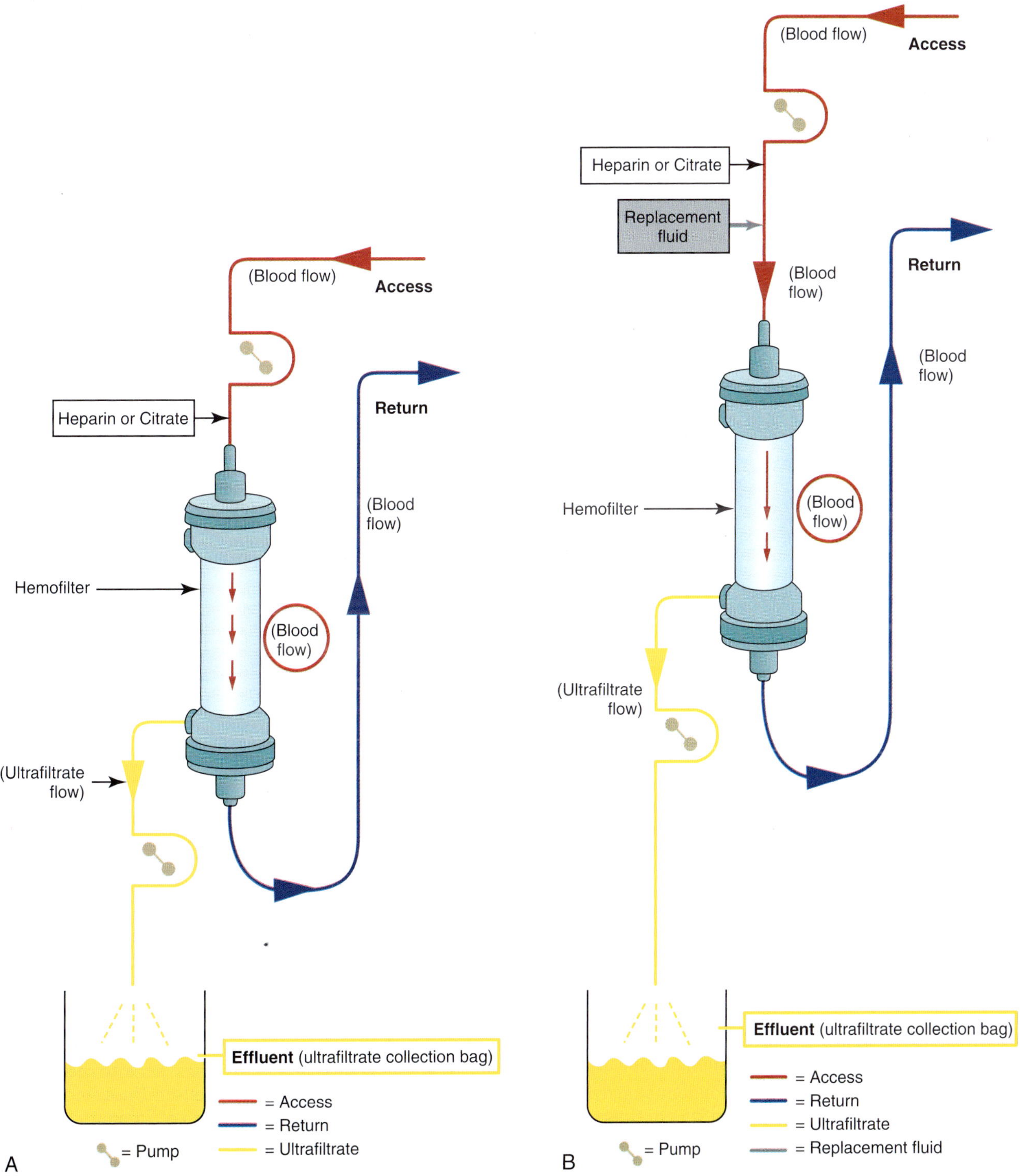

FIG. 25.5 Continuous Renal Replacement Therapy (CRRT) Systems. (A) Slow continuous ultrafiltration. (B) Continuous venovenous hemofiltration.

Continued

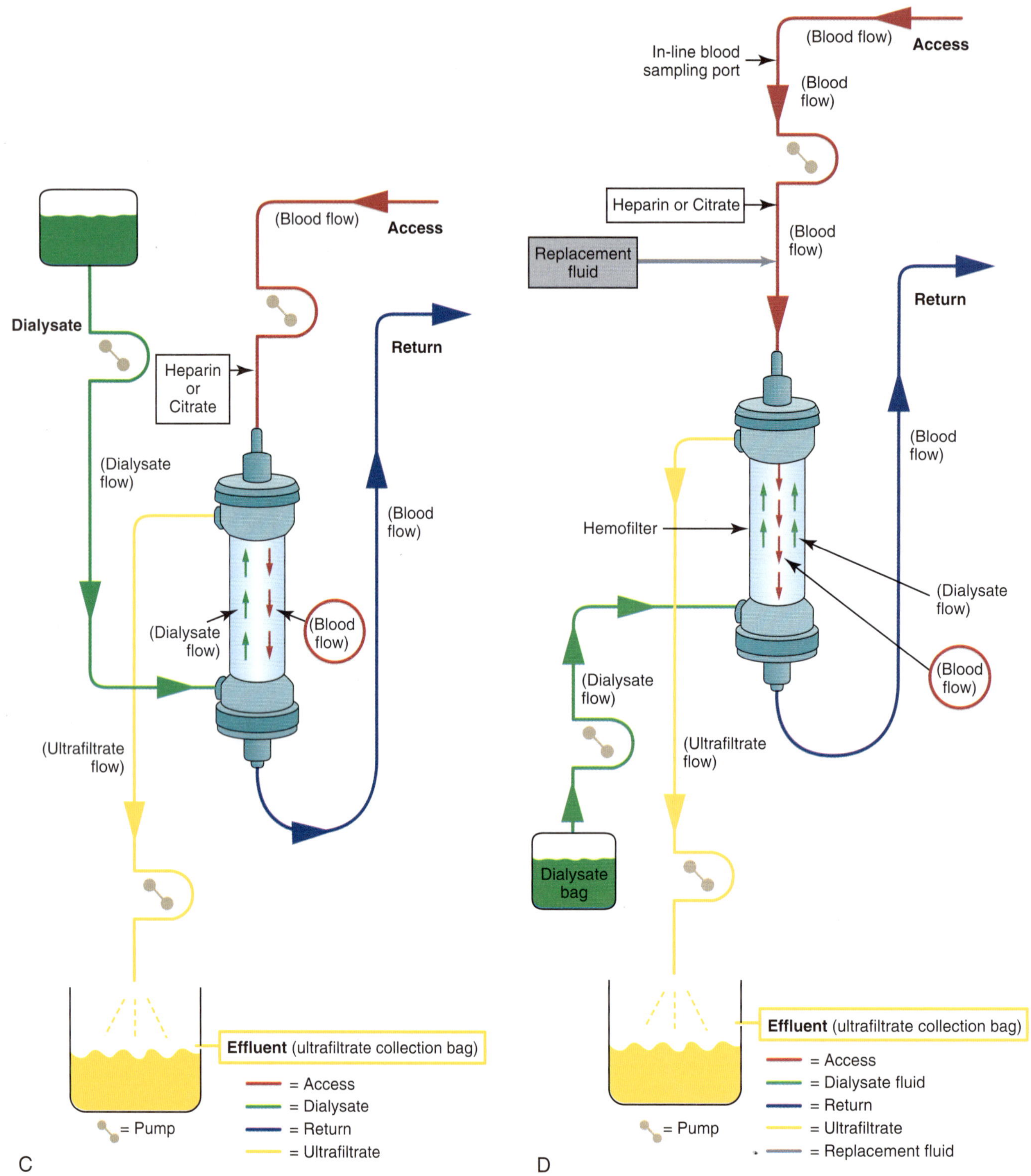

FIG. 25.5, cont'd (C) Continuous venovenous hemofiltration dialysis. (D) Continuous venovenous hemodiafiltration.

to the dialyzer. Inflow is accomplished through a second large-bore needle inserted into a peripheral vein distal to the fistula (Fig. 25.6A). Fistulas are the preferred mode of access over AV grafts because of the durability of blood vessels, relatively few complications, and less need for revision.[62]

Arteriovenous Graft. Arteriovenous grafts connect a vein and artery to allow vascular access for dialysis in chronic kidney failure.[62] The graft is a tube made of synthetic material that is surgically implanted inside the limb.[62] The area is surgically opened, and an artery and a vein are located.[63] A tunnel is created in the tissue where the graft is placed.[63] Anastomoses are made with the graft ends connected to the artery and vein.[62] The blood is allowed to flow through the graft, and the surgical area is closed.[62] The graft creates a raised area that looks like a

TABLE 25.6 Comparison of Continuous Renal Replacement Therapy Modes[53,58]

Modes	Fluid Replacement	Mechanism of Solute Removal	Goal of Therapy
SCUF	None	None	Fluid removal
CVVH	Predilution or postdilution, calculating hourly net loss	Convection	Fluid removal Small, medium, large molecule clearance
CVVHD	Predilution or postdilution, subtracting dialysate, then calculating hourly net loss	Diffusion	Fluid removal Small molecule clearance
CVVHDF	Predilution and/or postdilution, subtracting dialysate, then calculating hourly net loss	Convection and diffusion	Fluid removal Small, medium, large molecule clearance

CVVH, Continuous venovenous hemofiltration; *CVVHD*, continuous venovenous hemodialysis; *CVVHDF*, continuous venovenous hemodiafiltration; *SCUF*, slow continuous ultrafiltration.

TABLE 25.7 Size of Molecules and Mechanism of Removal by Continuous Renal Replacement Therapy

Type of Molecule	Size of Molecule	Solutes	Mechanism of Solute Removal
Small	<500 daltons	Urea, creatinine	Convection, diffusion
Medium	500–5000 daltons	Vancomycin, vitamin B	Convection better than diffusion
Low-molecular-weight (small) proteins	5000–50,000 daltons	Cytokines, complement	Convection or absorption onto hemofilter
Large proteins	>50,000 daltons	Albumin	Minimal removal

large peripheral vein just under the skin (Fig. 25.6B). Two large-bore needles are used for outflow from and inflow to the graft during dialysis.[63]

Mechanism

Hemodialysis works by circulating blood outside the body through synthetic tubing to a dialyzer, which consists of hollow-fiber tubes (Fig. 25.7).[64] While the blood flows through the membranes, which are semipermeable, a fluid (dialysate bath) bathes the membranes.[64] Through diffusion, fluid, electrolytes, and toxins from the blood are exchanged with the bath and toxins and dialysate then pass out of the dialyzer.[64] The fluid pulled from the blood is the ultrafiltrate.[64] The blood and the dialysate bath are shunted in opposite directions (countercurrent flow) through the dialyzer to match the osmotic and chemical gradients at the most efficient level for effective dialysis.[64] A schematic representation of the hemodialysis system is displayed in Fig. 25.8.

Medical Management

Medical management of dialysis first requires communication with the patient.[54] A goals-of-care discussion will guide the provider in determining if the patient is agreeable to routine dialysis, or if an alternate plan should be in place.[54] When a poor outcome is expected, the provider may discuss options including no dialysis, a time-limited trial of dialysis, or less frequent dialysis.[54] When hemodialysis is selected as a treatment, the provider will continue to evaluate kidney function by performing patient assessments and evaluating laboratory studies.[54]

Nursing Management

In caring for a patient with an AV fistula or graft, the critical care nurse frequently assesses the quality of blood flow.[63] The fistula or graft has a thrill when palpated gently with the fingers and has a bruit if auscultated with a stethoscope.[63] The extremity should be the patient's usual color and warm to the touch.[63] No blood pressure measurements, IV infusions, or laboratory phlebotomy procedures are performed on the arm with the AV fistula or graft.[61] Table 25.8 lists the focused assessment components of an AV fistula or graft.

Peritoneal Dialysis

Peritoneal dialysis is a treatment that uses the peritoneal cavity and membrane as a dialysis membrane for fluid and solute removal or exchange.[65] Prior to beginning peritoneal dialysis (PD) treatments, a single lumen dialysis catheter is placed in the lower abdomen.[65] Most catheters have four segments: an external segment outside the abdomen, a tunnel segment that passes through subcutaneous tissue and muscle, a cuff for stabilization at the peritoneal membrane, and an internal segment with numerous holes for fast delivery and drainage of dialysate (see Fig. 25.9).[65] When ready for use, the individual follows the PD process. The PD catheter is accessed and the cavity is filled with sterile dialysate solution.[65] The volume of dialysate instilled into the abdomen affects the clearance. The dialysate bathes the peritoneal membrane, which covers the abdominal organs and overlies the capillary beds that support the organs.[65] The dialysate then dwells in the peritoneal cavity for 4 to 6 hours. The dwell time affects the amount of fluid removed from the peritoneal capillaries.[65] By the processes of passive and active transport, excess fluid and solutes travel from the peritoneal capillary fluid through the capillary walls, through the peritoneal membrane, and into the dialyzing fluid.[65] The dialysate is then drained and the peritoneum is filled with new sterile dialysate (Fig. 25.9).[65] The process is then repeated at regular, prescribed intervals.[65] Continuous ambulatory peritoneal dialysis is a manual process.[65] Gravity is used to instill and remove fluid.[65] Continuous cycling peritoneal dialysis is automated.[65] Dialysis is delivered using a cycler, often overnight.[65] The PD process is relatively slow when compared to other renal replacement therapies.[65]

Nursing Management

Patients who use PD are knowledgeable partners in the maintenance of their health because of the huge commitment they

BOX 25.6 Safety

Complications Associated With Continuous Renal Replacement Therapy

Problem	Cause	Nursing Management
Patient		
Hypotension	Patient conditions (e.g., bleeding, air embolism)	Assess patient for possible patient factors
	Increased ultrafiltration (fluid removal) rate	Recommend fluid infusion or blood product administration or pressors, based on assessment
		Lower ultrafiltration (fluid removal) rate
Fluid and electrolyte changes	Too much or too little removal of fluid	Monitor vital signs and cardiac rhythm
	Composition of dialysate solution	Monitor electrolytes
		Administer electrolyte replacement
		Monitor intake and output
		Recommend changing of CRRT solutions
Bleeding	Patient condition	Assess patient for possible patient factors
	Anticoagulant	Recommend changing anticoagulant therapy
		Monitor coagulation studies
Hypothermia	No heating element used on extracorporeal circuit	Utilize heating element, if possible
		Perform warming measures
Circuit		
Increased access or return pressure	Kinked or clamped circuit or central venous catheter	Assess from patient to machine to unkink and unclamp, as needed
	Occlusion in circuit or central venous catheter	Assess for clotting in the circuit and change circuit without returning blood if clot present
	Patient movement or condition	Assess patency of central venous catheter and notify provider if line occluded
		If repeated access or pressure alarms, notify provider
Increased filter and transmembrane pressure	Clotting within the filter	Change circuit
		Recommend anticoagulation
Circuit disconnects	Connections not secured	Stop the machine and clamp the circuit and central venous catheter
		Change circuit

CRRT, Continuous renal replacement therapy.

make in daily management of their PD care. Normally, PD-dependent patients are well versed in the amount, type, and frequency of dialysate to be infused into the abdomen, with subsequent drainage into a waste bag. The infusion and removal of

BOX 25.7 Signs and Symptoms of Kidney Failure[60]

- Uncontrollable fluid volume status
- Uncontrollable blood pressure
- Unmanageable pruritis (e.g., uremia)
- Anorexia
- Worsening nutritional status unresponsive to diet modifications
- Weight loss with no other cause
- Neurological signs and symptoms due to:
  - Persistent electrolyte imbalance
  - Persistent acid–base abnormalities

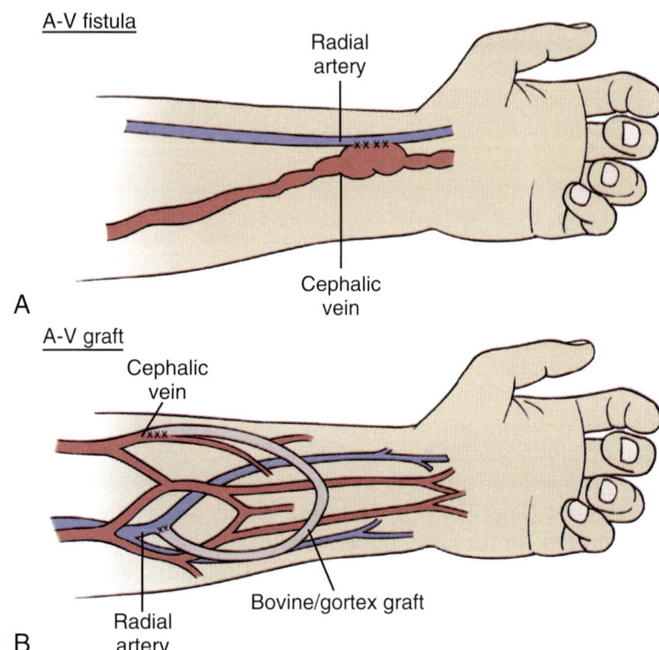

FIG. 25.6 Vascular Access for Hemodialysis. (A) Arteriovenous (AV) fistula between the vein and artery. (B) Internal synthetic graft connects the artery and vein.

the dialysate fluid are sterile procedures. The dialysate should be instilled at body temperature to be comfortable, provide some vasodilation, and provide increased solute transport in the peritoneum. The primary nursing consideration is to avoid contamination of the access point and monitor the patient's vital signs during this process. The most significant infection risk to the patient with the use of PD is development of peritonitis.[65] The nurse must remain vigilant and monitor for signs of localized catheter or abdominal infection manifested by catheter site redness, site swelling, cloudy dialysis effluent after the dwell time, and abdominal tenderness or pain.[65] The nurse should be aware of potential complications when caring for a patient receiving PD and these are listed in Box 25.8.

ADDITIONAL RESOURCES

Refer to Box 25.9 for Internet resources related to kidney disorders and therapeutic management.

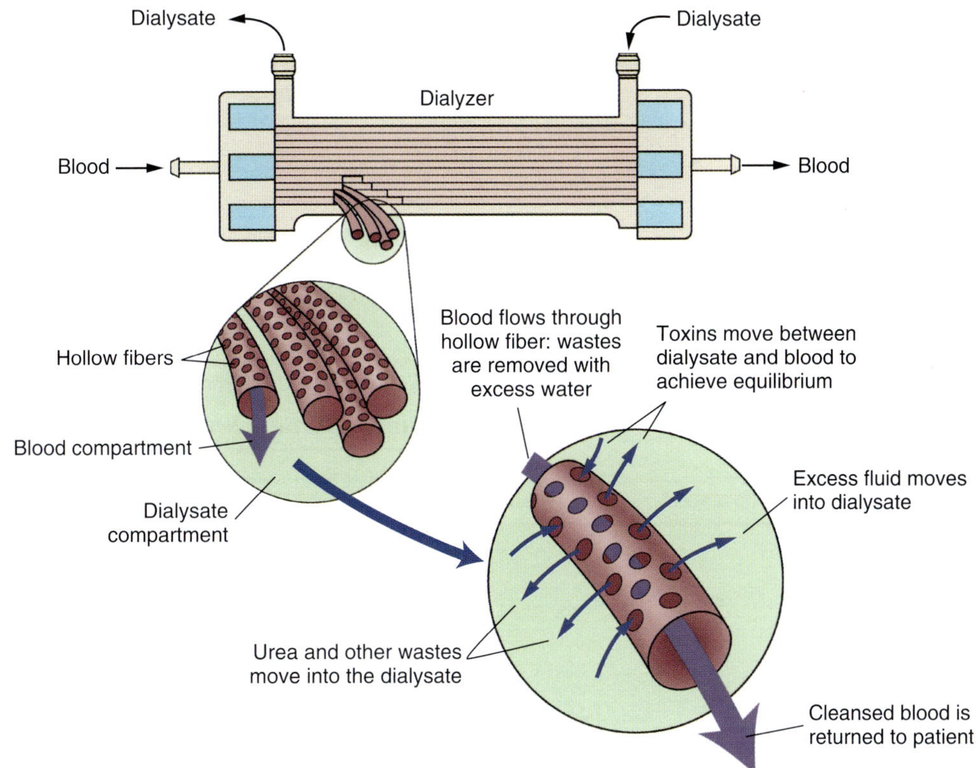

FIG. 25.7 Hemodialyzer.

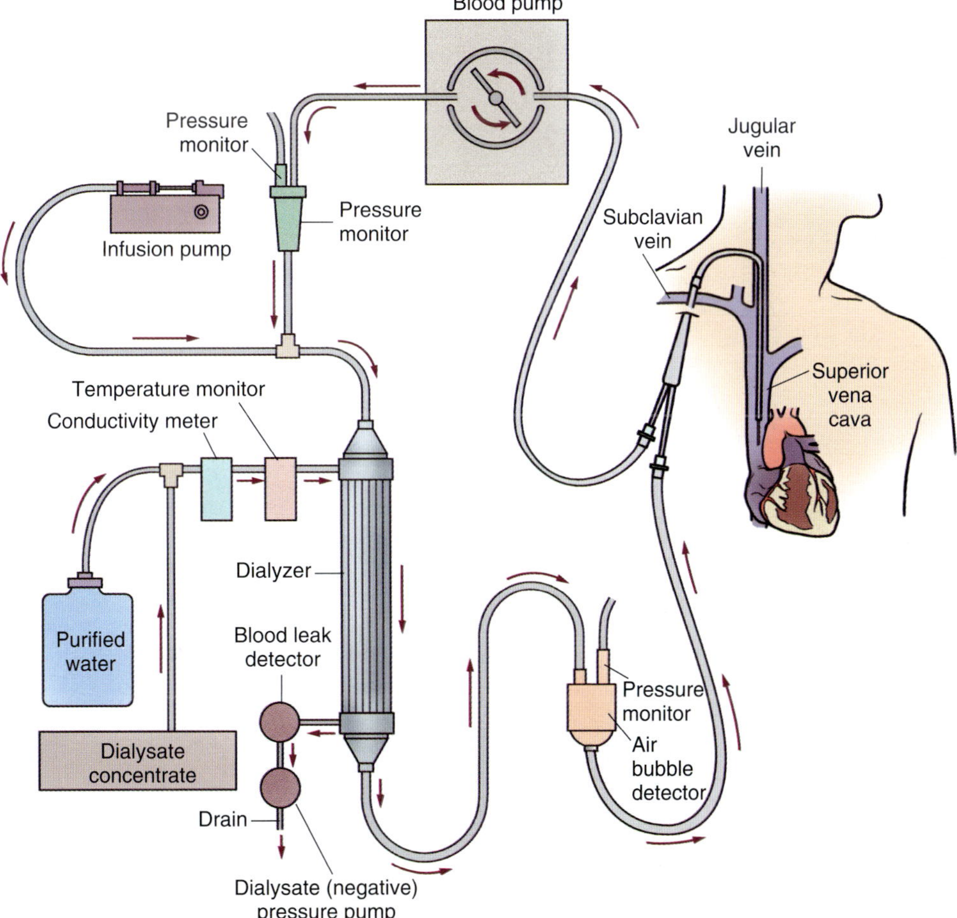

FIG. 25.8 Components of a Hemodialysis System.

TABLE 25.8 Focused Nursing Assessment of Arteriovenous Fistula or Graft[63]

Assessment Step	Normal Assessment Finding	Abnormal Assessment Finding
Inspect (Look)	Usual color for the patient Warm to touch Intact skin	Skin discoloration Cold and/or blue fingers Bruising Hematoma Skin bulges with shiny, bleeding, or peeling skin
Auscultate (Listen for a Bruit)	Low-pitched sound Continuous swooshing sound	Increasing pitch Discontinuous swooshing sound
Palpate (Feel for a Thrill)	Purring Vibrating	Pulsation No sensation

BOX 25.8 Safety

Potential Complications Associated With Peritoneal Dialysis

- Peritonitis
- Exit site infection
- Catheter flow dysfunction
- Catheter misplacement or pain from catheter position
- Hernia or abdominal pain
- Electrolyte imbalances

BOX 25.9 Internet Resources

Kidney Disorders and Therapeutic Management

- National Kidney Foundation: https://www.kidney.org
- Kidney Disease Improving Global Outcomes: https://kdigo.org/
- American Society of Nephrology: https://www.asn-online.org/
- American Association of Kidney Patients: https://aakp.org/

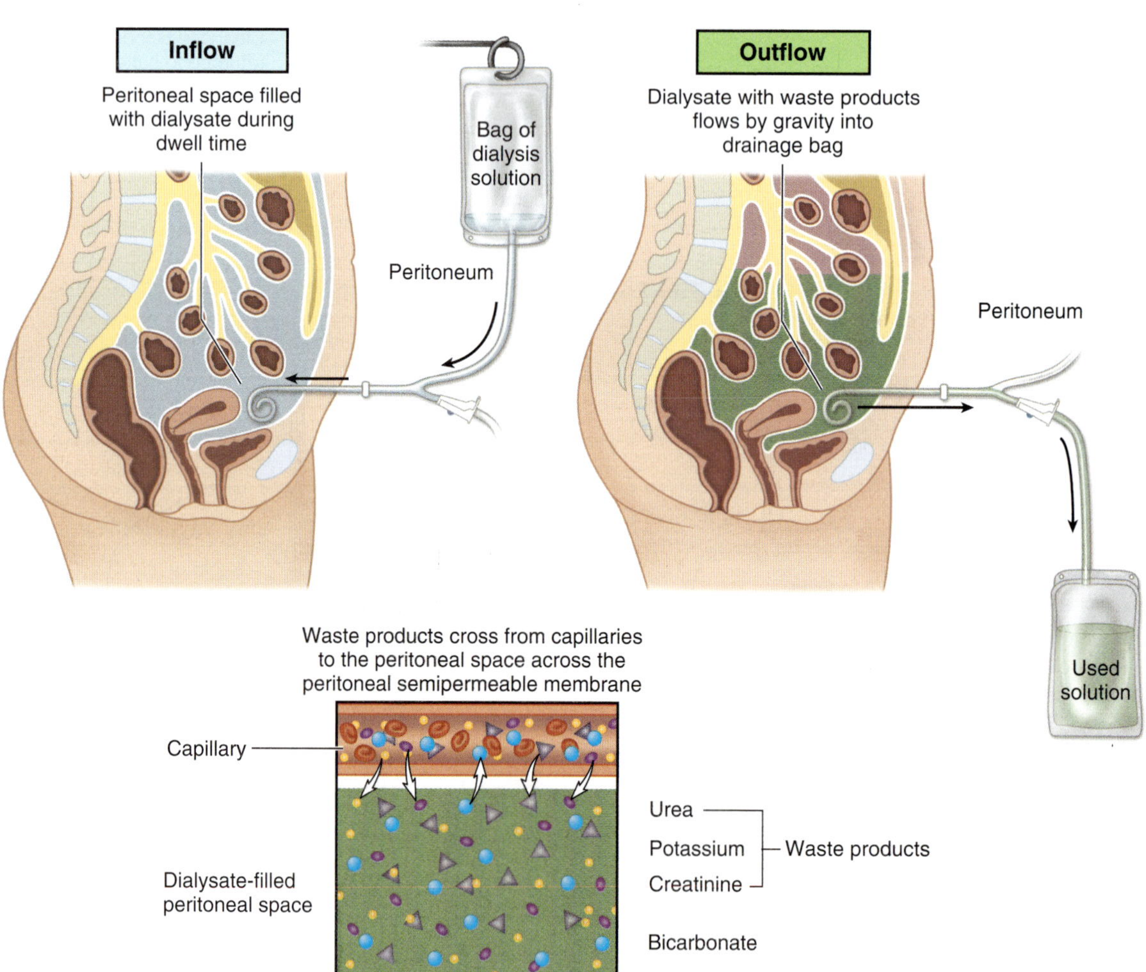

FIG. 25.9 Peritoneal Dialysis. In inflow, dialysate flows in by gravity or cycler. Waste products are "pulled" from the bloodstream across the peritoneal semipermeable membrane to mix with the intraperitoneal dialysate. In outflow, dialysate drains by gravity or cycler.

CASE STUDY 25.1 Patient With a Kidney Problem

Brief Patient History

Ms. L is a 32-year-old person who is transferred to the ICU with sepsis. She is awake but confused. She is unable to give any medical history and has no idea how long she has been in the hospital.

Clinical Assessment

Yesterday, Ms. L was admitted to the critical care unit with low urine output and edema. She continues to be confused, but her neurologic examination results are otherwise normal. She repeatedly tells the nurses that she is tired and feels sick. She is able to move all her extremities and has no signs of injury on skin examination.

Diagnostic Procedures

Today, laboratory tests show the following results: blood urea nitrogen 30 mg/dL (a slight increase from yesterday), creatinine 1.5 mg/dL (up from 1 mg/dL yesterday), serum sodium of 130 mEq/L, and serum potassium level of 4 mEq/L. Baseline vital signs are as follows: blood pressure of 85/60 mm Hg, heart rate of 128 beats/min (sinus tachycardia), respiratory rate of 18 breaths/min, temperature of 101.3°F, and oxygen saturation of 98%.

Medical Diagnosis

Ms. L is diagnosed with AKI.

Questions

1. What major outcomes do you expect to achieve for this patient?
2. What problems or risks must be managed to achieve these outcomes?
3. What interventions could be initiated to monitor, prevent, manage, or eliminate the problems and risks identified?
4. What interventions could be initiated to promote optimal functioning, safety, and well-being of the patient?
5. What technology can be used to monitor this patient and prevent complications?
6. What other interprofessional team members are needed to assist with the management of this patient?
7. What possible learning needs would you anticipate for this patient?
8. What cultural and age-related factors might have a bearing on the patient's plan of care?

KEY POINTS

Acute Kidney Injury

- AKI is characterized by a sudden rise in serum creatinine and/or a decrease in urine output
- AKI may be caused by hypoperfusion from reduced intravascular pressure and/or volume; intrinsic kidney damage from endogenous or exogenous nephrotoxic agents, inflammatory responses, or autoimmune diseases; or obstruction from masses, strictures (including neurologic dysfunction), or trauma.
- Treatment goals for patients with AKI focus on prevention, along with fluid, electrolyte, and acid–base balance
- The daily weight, combined with accurate intake and output monitoring, is an indicator of fluid gains or losses over 24 hours.

Chronic Kidney Disease

- Diagnostic criteria for CKD include a decreased eGFR and at least one indicator of kidney dysfunction, including albuminuria, that is present for more than 3 months.
- Each cause of CKD is an initial and sustained insult to the kidney, with this perpetuated insult damaging the nephrons, ultimately leading to sclerosis and affecting filtering, concentrating, or excreting functions of the kidneys.
- Medical management includes blood pressure, anemia, mineral and bone disorder, lipid, glycemic, and nutrition management.
- Patient and family education should focus on lifestyle modifications and at-home monitoring.

Pharmacology

- An important part of pharmacologic management in patients with kidney disease includes ensuring all nephrotoxic medications are dose adjusted or stopped.
- Collaboration among the interprofessional team is essential in promoting safe pharmacology practices.

Renal Replacement Therapy

- Renal replacement therapy (RRT) removes toxins and corrects fluid, electrolyte, and acid–base imbalances by moving substances across a semipermeable membrane.
- Renal replacement therapies are performed continuously over 24 hours or intermittently for several hours, several days a week.

Visit the Evolve site at http://evolve.elsevier.com/Urden/CriticalCareNursing for additional study materials.

REFERENCES

1. Odom B, Lynch F. Chapter 37. Acute kidney injury. In: Bodin SM, ed. *Contemporary Nephrology Nursing*. 4th ed. Pitman, NJ: American Nephrology Nursing Association; 2022:913–982.
2. Ronco C, Bellomo R, Kellum JA. Acute kidney injury. *Lancet*. 2019;394(10212):1949–1964. https://doi.org/10.1016/S0140-6736(19)32563-2.
3. Lameire NH, Levin A, Kellum JA, Conference Participants, et al. Harmonizing acute and chronic kidney disease definition and classification: report of a Kidney Disease: Improving Global Outcomes (KDIGO) consensus conference. *Kidney Int*. 2021;100(3):516–526. https://doi.org/10.1016/j.kint.2021.06.028.
4. Kidney Disease: Improving Global Outcomes (KDIGO) Acute Kidney Injury Work Group. KDIGO clinical practice guideline for acute kidney injury. *Kidney Inter Suppl*. 2012;2:1–138.
5. Moore PK, Hsu RK, Liu KD. Management of acute kidney injury: core curriculum 2018. *Am J Kidney Dis*. 2018;72(1):136–148. https://doi.org/10.1053/j.ajkd.2017.11.021.
6. Rogers JL. Alterations of renal and urinary tract function. In: McCance RJ, ed. *Huether's Pathophysiology: The Biologic Basis for Disease in Adults and Children*. 9th ed. Philadelphia, PA: Elsevier; 2023:1232–1269.
7. Woitok BK, Funk GC, Walter P, Schwarz C, Ravioli S, Lindner G. Dysnatremias in emergency patients with acute kidney injury: a cross-sectional analysis. *Am J Emerg Med*. 2020;38(12):2602–2606. https://doi.org/10.1016/j.ajem.2020.01.009.
8. Dépret F, Peacock WF, Liu KD, Rafique Z, Rossignol P, Legrand M. Management of hyperkalemia in the acutely ill patient. *Ann Intensive Care*. 2019;9(1):32. https://doi.org/10.1186/s13613-019-0509-8.
9. Kumar U, Wettersten N, Garimella PS. Cardiorenal syndrome: pathophysiology. *Cardiol Clin*. 2019;37(3):251–265. https://doi.org/10.1016/j.ccl.2019.04.001.
10. Angeli P, Garcia-Tsao G, Nadim MK, Parikh CR. News in pathophysiology, definition and classification of hepatorenal syndrome: a step beyond the International Club of Ascites (ICA) consensus document. *J Hepatol*. 2019;71(4):811–822. https://doi.org/10.1016/j.jhep.2019.07.002.

11. Saladi L, Shaikh D, Saad M, et al. Pulmonary renal syndrome: a case report of diffuse alveolar hemorrhage in association with ANCA negative pauci-immune glomerulonephritis. *Medicine (Baltimore)*. 2018;97(23):e10954. https://doi.org/10.1097/MD.0000000000010954.
12. Joannidis M, Forni LG, Klein SJ, et al. Lung-kidney interactions in critically ill patients: consensus report of the Acute Disease Quality Initiative (ADQI) 21 Workgroup. *Intensive Care Med*. 2020;46(4):654–672. https://doi.org/10.1007/s00134-019-05869-7.
13. Font MD, Thyagarajan B, Khanna AK. Sepsis and septic shock–basics of diagnosis, pathophysiology and clinical decision making. *Med Clin North Am*. 2020;104(4):573–585. https://doi.org/10.1016/j.mcna.2020.02.011.
14. Cabral BMI, Edding SN, Portocarrero JP, Lerma EV. Rhabdomyolysis. *Dis Mon*. 2020;66(8):101015. https://doi.org/10.1016/j.disamonth.2020.101015.
15. Zhang F, Lu Z, Wang F. Advances in the pathogenesis and prevention of contrast-induced nephropathy. *Life Sci*. 2020;259:118379. https://doi.org/10.1016/j.lfs.2020.118379.
16. Xu R, Tao A, Bai Y, Deng Y, Chen G. Effectiveness of N-acetylcysteine for the prevention of contrast-induced nephropathy: a systematic review and meta-analysis of randomized controlled trials. *J Am Heart Assoc*. 2016;5(9):e003968. https://doi.org/10.1161/JAHA.116.003968.
17. Kanbay M, Copur S, Mizrak B, Ortiz A, Soler MJ. Intravenous fluid therapy in accordance with kidney injury risk: when to prescribe what volume of which solution. *Clin Kidney J*. 2022;16(4):684–692. https://doi.org/10.1093/ckj/sfac270.
18. Oh TH. Formulas for calculating fluid maintenance requirements. *Anesthesiology*. 1980;53(4):351. https://doi.org/10.1097/00000542-198010000-00020.
19. Ogbu OC, Murphy DJ, Martin GS. How to avoid fluid overload. *Curr Opin Crit Care*. 2015;21(4):315–321. https://doi.org/10.1097/MCC.0000000000000211.
20. Hammond DA, Lam SW, Rech MA, et al. Balanced crystalloids versus saline in critically ill adults: a systematic review and meta-analysis. *Ann Pharmacother*. 2020;54(1):5–13. https://doi.org/10.1177/1060028019866420.
21. Annane D, Siami S, Jaber S, CRISTAL Investigators, et al. Effects of fluid resuscitation with colloids vs crystalloids on mortality in critically ill patients presenting with hypovolemic shock: the CRISTAL randomized trial. *JAMA*. 2013;310(17):1809–1817. https://doi.org/10.1001/jama.2013.280502.
22. Lewis SR, Pritchard MW, Evans DJ, et al. Colloids versus crystalloids for fluid resuscitation in critically ill people. *Cochrane Database Syst Rev*. 2018;8(8):CD000567. https://doi.org/10.1002/14651858.CD000567.pub7.
23. Heming N, Lamothe L, Jaber S, et al. Morbidity and mortality of crystalloids compared to colloids in critically ill surgical patients: a subgroup analysis of a randomized trial. *Anesthesiology*. 2018;129(6):1149–1158.
24. Semler MW, Self WH, Wanderer JP, et al. SMART investigators and the pragmatic critical care research group. Balanced crystalloids versus saline in critically ill adults. *N Engl J Med*. 2018;378(9):829–839. https://doi.org/10.1056/NEJMoa1711584. https://doi.org/10.1097/ALN.0000000000002413.
25. Gould CV, Umscheid CA, Agarwal RK, Kuntz G, Pegues DA, Healthcare Infection Control Practices Advisory Committee. Guideline for prevention of catheter-associated urinary tract infections 2009. *Infect Control Hosp Epidemiol*. 2010;31(4):319–326. https://doi.org/10.1086/651091.
26. Rosner MH, Husain-Syed F, Reis T, Ronco C, Vanholder R. Uremic encephalopathy. *Kidney Int*. 2022;101(2):227–241. https://doi.org/10.1016/j.kint.2021.09.025.
27. Cheng TY, Tarng DC, Liao YM, Lin PC. Effects of systematic nursing instruction on a low-phosphorus diet, serum phosphorus level and pruritus of patients on haemodialysis. *J Clin Nurs*. 2017 Feb;26(3–4):485–494. https://doi.org/10.1111/jocn.13471.
28. Kidney Disease: Improving Global Outcomes (KDIGO). KDIGO 2012 clinical practice guideline for the evaluation and management of chronic kidney disease. *Kidney Inter Suppl*. 2013;3(1):1–163.
29. CKD in the general population. National Institute of Diabetes and Digestive and Kidney Diseases: United States Renal Data System. From https://usrds-adr.niddk.nih.gov/2022/chronic-kidney-disease/1-ckd-in-the-general-population. Accessed September 30, 2023.
30. Tejera D, Varela F, Acosta D, et al. Epidemiology of acute kidney injury and chronic kidney disease in the intensive care unit. *Rev Bras Ter Intensiva*. 2017;29(4):444–452. https://doi.org/10.5935/0103-507X.20170061.
31. Fidalgo P, Bagshaw SM. Chronic kidney disease in the intensive care unit. *Management of Chronic Kidney Disease*. 2014 Mar;8:417–438. https://doi.org/10.1007/978-3-642-54637-2_32.
32. Huang ST, Ke TY, Chuang YW, Lin CL, Kao CH. Renal complications and subsequent mortality in acute critically ill patients without pre-existing renal disease. *CMAJ*. 2018;190(36):E1070–E1080. https://doi.org/10.1503/cmaj.171382.
33. Charles C, Ferris AH. Chronic kidney disease. *Prim Care*. 2020;47(4):585–595. https://doi.org/10.1016/j.pop.2020.08.001.
34. Kidney Disease: Improving Global Outcomes (KDIGO) Blood Pressure Work Group. KDIGO 2021 clinical practice guideline for the management of blood pressure in chronic kidney disease. *Kidney Int*. 2021;99(3S):S1–S87. https://doi.org/10.1016/j.kint.2020.11.003.
35. Parati G, Kjeldsen S, Coca A, Cushman WC, Wang J. Adherence to single-pill versus free-equivalent combination therapy in hypertension: a systematic review and meta-analysis. *Hypertension*. 2021;77(2):692–705. https://doi.org/10.1161/HYPERTENSIONAHA.120.15781.
36. Kidney Disease: Improving Global Outcomes (KDIGO) Anemia Work Group. KDIGO clinical practice guideline for anemia in chronic kidney disease. *Kidney Inter Suppl*. 2012;2:279–335.
37. Kidney Disease: Improving Global Outcomes (KDIGO) CKD-MBD Update Work Group. KDIGO 2017 clinical practice guideline update for the diagnosis, evaluation, prevention, and treatment of chronic kidney disease-mineral and bone disorder. *Kidney Inter Suppl*. 2017;7:1–59.
38. Kidney Disease: Improving Global Outcomes (KDIGO) Lipid Work Group. KDIGO clinical practice guideline for lipid management in chronic kidney disease. *Kidney Inter Suppl*. 2013;3:259–305.
39. Kidney Disease: Improving Global Outcomes (KDIGO) Diabetes Work Group. KDIGO 2022 clinical practice guideline for diabetes management in chronic kidney disease. *Kidney Int*. 2022;102(5S):S1–S127. https://doi.org/10.1016/j.kint.2022.06.008.
40. Ellison DH. Clinical pharmacology in diuretic use. *Clin J Am Soc Nephrol*. 2019;14(8):1248–1257. https://doi.org/10.2215/CJN.09630818.
41. Purnomo AF, Permana KR, Daryanto B. Acute kidney injury following mannitol administration in traumatic brain injury: a meta-analysis. *Acta Inform Med*. 2021;29(4):270–274. https://doi.org/10.5455/aim.2021.29.270-274.
42. Mannitol-mannitol injection, solution. B. Braun Medical Inc. 2023. From https://dailymed.nlm.nih.gov/dailymed/fda/fdaDrugXsl.cfm?setid=d12cc802-b538-4065-a264-f474ff3b3043&type=display#:~:text=Administer%20intravenously%20using%20sterile%2C%20filter,against%20infusion%20of%20mannitol%20crystals. Accessed September 30, 2023.
43. Malik BA, Nnodebe I, Fayaz A, et al. Effect of acetazolamide as add-on diuretic therapy in patients with heart failure: a meta-analysis. *Cureus*. 2023;15(4):e37792. https://doi.org/10.7759/cureus.37792.
44. Brummett RE, Bendrick T, Himes D. Comparative ototoxicity of bumetanide and furosemide when used in combination with kanamycin. *J Clin Pharmacol*. 1981;21(11):628–636. https://doi.org/10.1002/j.1552-4604.1981.tb05675.x.
45. Metolazone-metolazone tablet. Eons Labs Inc.; 2022. From https://dailymed.nlm.nih.gov/dailymed/fda/fdaDrugXsl.cfm?setid=0b619826-2567-49d7-8972-b6da5e4467df&type=display. Accessed October 1, 2023.
46. Seay NW, Lehrich RW, Greenberg A. Diagnosis and management of disorders of body tonicity-hyponatremia and hypernatremia: core curriculum 2020. *Am J Kidney Dis*. 2020;75(2):272–286. https://doi.org/10.1053/j.ajkd.2019.07.014.
47. Moussavi K, Fitter S, Gabrielson SW, Koyfman A, Long B. Management of hyperkalemia with insulin and glucose: pearls for the emergency clinician. *J Emerg Med*. 2019;57(1):36–42. https://doi.org/10.1016/j.jemermed.2019.03.043.

48. Geng S, Green EF, Kurz MC, Rivera JV. Sodium bicarbonate administration and subsequent potassium concentration in hyperkalemia treatment. *Am J Emerg Med*. 2021;50:132–135. https://doi.org/10.1016/j.ajem.2021.07.032.
49. Cozzolino M, Ketteler M, Wagner CA. An expert update on novel therapeutic targets for hyperphosphatemia in chronic kidney disease: preclinical and clinical innovations. *Expert Opin Ther Targets*. 2020;24(5):477–488. https://doi.org/10.1080/14728222.2020.1743680.
50. Haras MS, Cahill M. Chapter 19. Disorders of calcium and phosphorus metabolism. In: Bodin SM, ed. *Contemporary Nephrology Nursing*. 4th ed. Pitman, NJ: American Nephrology Nursing Association; 2022:489–515.
51. Yun G, Baek SH, Kim S. Evaluation and management of hypernatremia in adults: clinical perspectives. *Korean J Intern Med*. 2023;38(3):290–302. https://doi.org/10.3904/kjim.2022.346.
52. Lawless SJ, Thompson C, Garrahy A. The management of acute and chronic hyponatraemia. *Ther Adv Endocrinol Metab*. 2022;13:20420188221097343. https://doi.org/10.1177/20420188221097343.
53. Macedo E, Mehta RL. Continuous dialysis therapies: core curriculum 2016. *Am J Kidney Dis*. 2016;68(4):645–657. https://doi.org/10.1053/j.ajkd.2016.03.427.
54. Corbett CM. Chapter 8. Active medical management without dialysis. In: Bodin SM, ed. *Contemporary Nephrology Nursing*. 4th ed. Pitman, NJ: American Nephrology Nursing Association; 2022:187–217.
55. Huriaux L, Costille P, Quintard H, Journois D, Kellum JA, Rimmelé T. Haemodialysis catheters in the intensive care unit. *Anaesth Crit Care Pain Med*. 2017;36(5):313–319. https://doi.org/10.1016/j.accpm.2016.10.003.
56. Tandukar S, Palevsky PM. Continuous renal replacement therapy: who, when, why, and how. *Chest*. 2019;155(3):626–638. https://doi.org/10.1016/j.chest.2018.09.004.
57. Hall JE, Hall ME. Chapter 4. Transport of substances through cell membranes. In: Hall ME, Hall JE, eds. *Guyton and Hall Textbook of Medical Physiology*. 14th ed. Philadelphia, PA: Elsevier; 2021:51–62.
58. Meri N, Cerda J, Garzado F, Villa G, Ronco C. Chapter 3. Nomenclature for renal replacement therapy in acute kidney injury. In: Kellum JA, Bellomo R, Ronco C, eds. *Continuous Renal Replacement Therapy*. 2nd ed. New York, NY: Oxford University Press; 2016:21–34.
59. Bellomo R, Baldwin I. Chapter 13. The circuit and the prescription. In: Kellum JA, Bellomo R, Ronco C, eds. *Continuous Renal Replacement Therapy*. 2nd ed. New York, NY: Oxford University Press; 2016:111–115.
60. Kidney failure (ESRD) – symptoms, causes and treatment options. American Kidney Fund; 2022. From https://www.kidneyfund.org/all-about-kidneys/kidney-failure-symptoms-and-causes. Accessed October 2, 2023.
61. Arasu R, Jegatheesan D, Sivakumaran Y. Overview of hemodialysis access and assessment. *Can Fam Physician*. 2022;68(8):577–582. https://doi.org/10.46747/cfp.6808577.
62. Neyra NR, Wazir S. The evolving panorama of vascular access in the 21st century. *Front Nephrol*. 2022;2:917265. https://doi.org/10.3389/fneph.2022.917265.
63. Gilliand M. Chapter 14. Arteriovenous graft. In: Bodin SM, ed. *Contemporary Nephrology Nursing*. 4th ed. Pitman, NJ: American Nephrology Nursing Association; 2022:401–416.
64. Hellebrand A. Chapter 9. Hemodialysis. In: Bodin SM, ed. *Contemporary Nephrology Nursing*. 4th ed. Pitman, NJ: American Nephrology Nursing Association; 2022:219–283.
65. Teitelbaum I. Peritoneal dialysis. *N Engl J Med*. 2021;385(19):1786–1795. https://doi.org/10.1056/NEJMra2100152.

26 Gastrointestinal Anatomy and Physiology

Kathrine Anne Winnie and Kimberly Sanchez

http://evolve.elsevier.com/Urden/CriticalCareNursing

The gastrointestinal tract (GI) and accessory organs are responsible for numerous functions necessary to maintain homeostasis. The primary role of the GI tract is digestion, and this is supported by the pancreas, gallbladder, and liver. Disturbances of the GI system itself or of the complex hormonal and neural controls that regulate the GI tract can severely upset homeostasis and compromise the overall nutritional status of the patient.

This chapter provides an overview of the anatomy and physiologic processes of the GI tract and accessory organs. An understanding of normal GI function is essential to understanding the pathophysiology, symptoms, and therapeutic management of GI disorders.

ANATOMY

The GI tract consists of the mouth, esophagus, stomach, small intestine, and large intestine (Fig. 26.1).

Mouth

The mouth is the beginning of the alimentary canal and includes lips, gums, teeth, palate, tongue, salivary glands.[1]

Esophagus

The esophagus is a hollow muscular tube, lacking cartilage, that begins in the neck at the level of the C6 to T1 vertebrae and extends vertically through the mediastinum and diaphragm to the stomach at the level of T11.[2] In adults, the esophagus is 19 to 25 cm (7.5 to 10 inches) long[2] and 2 to 3 cm (1 inch) wide. The esophagus is the narrowest part of the digestive tract and lies posterior to the trachea and the heart, with attachments at the hypopharynx and at the lesser curvature of stomach below the diaphragm.[2] The esophagus has two sphincters: (1) the upper esophageal sphincter (also known as hypopharyngeal sphincter) and (2) the lower esophageal sphincter (also known as cardioesophageal or gastroesophageal sphincter).[2]

The arterial blood supply of the esophagus is provided by the thyroid and bronchial arteries for the upper third, descending thoracic aorta for the middle third, and gastric and phrenic arteries for the distal third of the esophagus.[3] Venous drainage of the esophagus is provided by the brachiocephalic veins for the upper portion of esophagus and the portal vein for the remaining portion of esophagus (Fig. 26.2).[3] Esophageal lymph drains into the deep cervical, trachea-bronchial, posterior mediastinal, and pre-aortic lymph nodes.[3] The esophagus is innervated by the autonomic nervous system. Sympathetic fibers arise from the esophageal plexus, and parasympathetic fibers arise from the vagus nerve.[3]

Stomach

The stomach is an elongated pouch with a 1.5-liter capacity, located under the lower part of the rib cage.[4] The stomach has

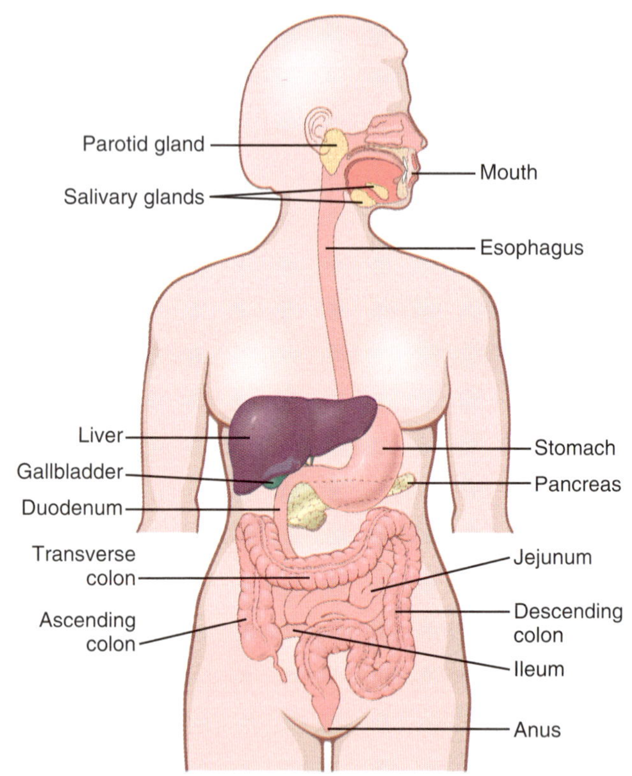

FIG. 26.1 Gastrointestinal System. Overall anatomy of the gastrointestinal system. (From Hall ME, Hall JE. *Guyton and Hall Textbook of Medical Physiology*. 14th ed. Elsevier; 2021.)

a variable size and shape depending on fullness of the stomach,[4] but it is approximately 25 to 30 cm (10 to 12 inches) long and 10 to 15 cm (4 to 6 inches) wide at the maximal transverse diameter (Fig. 26.3). The stomach is the widest part of the digestive tract and lies obliquely beneath the lower esophageal sphincter of the esophagus and above the small intestine at the pyloric sphincter.[4] The anatomic divisions of the stomach are the cardia (proximal end), the fundus (portion above and to the left of the cardiac sphincter), the body (middle portion), the antrum (elongated, constricted portion), and the pylorus (distal end connecting the antrum to the duodenum)[4] (Fig. 26.3). The greater curvature, which begins at the cardiac orifice and arches backward and upward around the fundus, is in contact with the transverse colon and the pancreas at the posterior edge.[4] The lesser curvature extends from the cardia to the pylorus.[4]

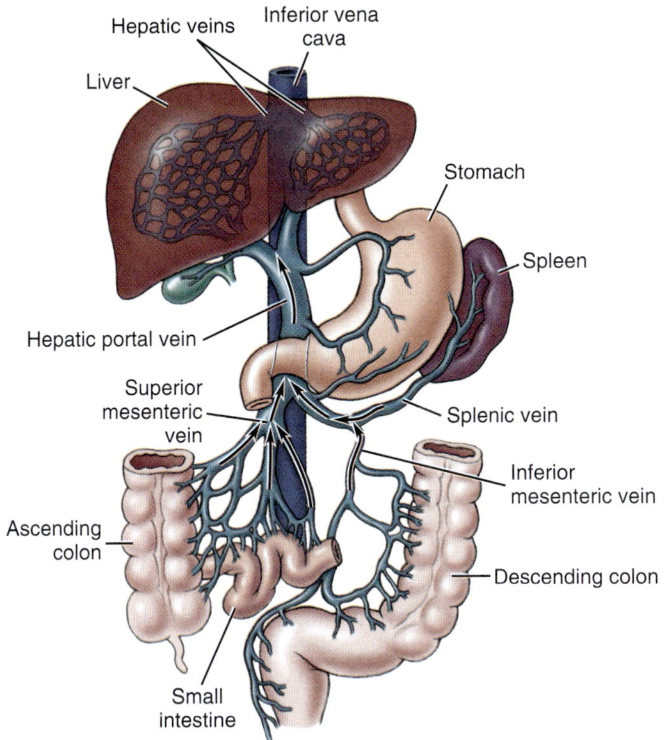

FIG. 26.2 Portal Circulation. (From Herlihy B. *The Human Body in Health and Illness.* 5th ed. Saunders; 2015.)

The stomach wall has four layers[5] (Fig. 26.4). The outermost layer, the serous layer (serosa),[5] consists of squamous epithelial tissue and continues as a double fold from the lower edge of the stomach to cover the intestine. The second layer, the muscular layer (muscularis),[5] extends from the fundus to the antrum and consists of three smooth muscle layers: the longitudinal layer, the circular layer, and the oblique layer. The third layer, the submucous layer (submucosa),[5] consists of connective tissue that contains blood vessels, lymphatics, and nerve plexuses. The innermost layer, the *mucous layer (mucosa)*,[5] consists of a muscular layer that is arranged in longitudinal folds, or rugae, that can expand as the stomach fills.

The celiac artery provides the blood supply to the stomach.[4] The splenic or superior mesenteric veins provide venous drainage for the stomach, and then those drain into the portal vein (Fig. 26.2).[4] Almost all lymph from the stomach will drain into the celiac lymph nodes.[4] The stomach is innervated by the autonomic nervous system. Sympathetic fibers arise from the celiac ganglia, and parasympathetic fibers arise from the vagus nerve.[4]

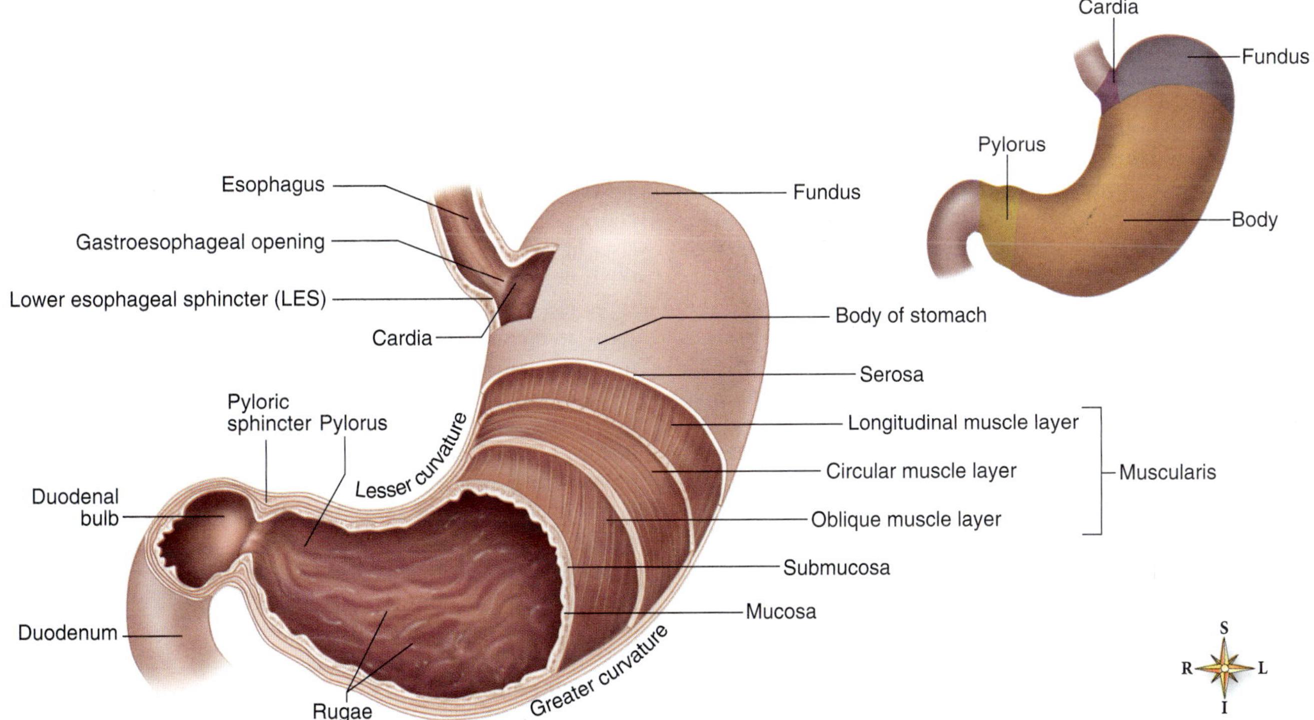

FIG. 26.3 Stomach. The gross anatomy of the stomach. (From Patton KT, Bell FB, Thompson T, Williamson PL. *Anatomy and Physiology.* 11th ed. Elsevier; 2022.)

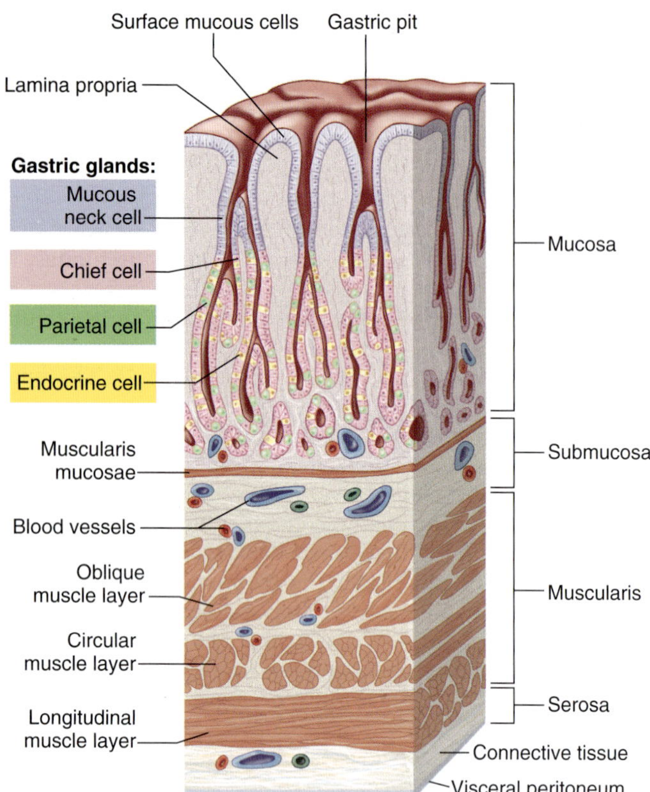

FIG. 26.4 Gastric Mucosa. The structure of the gastric mucosa. (From Patton KT, Bell FB, Thompson T, Williamson PL. *Anatomy and Physiology*. 11th ed. Elsevier; 2022.)

Small Intestine

The small intestine, a coiled, folded tube that is approximately 7 m (22 to 23 feet) long,[6] extends from the pyloric sphincter to the cecum and fills most of the abdominal cavity.[7] The small intestine has three anatomic divisions: (1) the duodenum, (2) the jejunum, and (3) the ileum.[7] The duodenum, which is shaped like the letter C, begins at the pyloric sphincter of the stomach and ends at the ligament of Treitz, a suspensory ligament of the duodenum.[7] The duodenum is about 25 cm (9–10 inches) long[7] and 4 cm (1–1.5 inches) wide. The jejunum, which is about 250 cm (8–9 feet) long[6] and 4 cm (1–1.5 inches) wide, lies in the left iliac and umbilical regions. The ileum, which is about 360 cm (11–12 feet) long[7] and 2.5 cm (1 inch) wide, lies in the hypogastric, right iliac, and pelvic regions. Although the demarcating line between the jejunum and the ileum is arbitrary, the ileum is narrower than the jejunum.[7] The ileocecal valve is located at the terminal end of the ileum at the junction of the cecum and colon[7] (Fig. 26.5).

The small intestine has four layers (Fig. 26.6).[6] The outermost layer, the serous layer (serosa), is a continuation of the serous coat surrounding the stomach.[6] The second layer, the muscular layer (muscularis), consists of two smooth muscle layers called the outer longitudinal and inner circular layers.[6] The third layer, the submucous layer (submucosa), consists of connective tissue that contains blood vessels, lymphatics, glands, and nerve plexuses.[6] The innermost layer, the mucous layer (mucosa), consists of simple columnar epithelium.[6] The mucosa and submucosa are arranged in circular folds (*plicae circulares*), which are largest and most numerous in the jejunum and upper ileum.[6] These folds are covered by a second series of projectile-like folds called *villi*,[6] which are in constant motion—constricting, lengthening, and shortening (villous movement). The 4 to 5 million villi (see Fig. 26.5) give the intestine a velvety appearance; they are more numerous and larger in the jejunum than in the ileum. Villi contain a network of capillaries and blind lymphatic vessels called *lacteals*.[6] The outer layer of the villus is composed of microvilli.[6] The circular folds (plicae circulares) of the small intestine, along with the villi and microvilli, increase the digestive-absorptive surface of the small intestine 600 times.[6]

Blood supply to the small intestine is primarily from the superior mesenteric artery, with the duodenum also receiving blood from the gastroduodenal artery.[6] The superior mesenteric vein provides for venous drainage of the small intestine.[6] Numerous lymphatic channels arise in the submucosa and drain into the mesenteric lymph nodes.[6] The small intestine is extrinsically innervated by the autonomic nervous system. Sympathetic fibers arise from the celiac and superior mesenteric ganglia, whereas parasympathetic fibers arise from the vagus nerve. Intrinsic innervation initiates motor functions and is located in the intestinal wall.[6] This intrinsic innervation is provided by Auerbach,[2] Meissner,[1] and subseroal[1] plexuses that are located in the intestinal wall.

Large Intestine

The large intestine, a tube-like structure that is approximately 150 cm (4 to 5 feet) long[8] and 4 to 6 cm (2 inches) in diameter, extends from the ileocecal valve to the anus.[8] The large intestine is divided into the ascending colon, transverse colon, descending colon, sigmoid colon, rectum, and anal canal (Fig. 26.7).[8] The ascending, transverse, descending, and sigmoid colon are directly on or suspended from the posterior abdominal wall.[8] The rectum and anal canal are in the perineum.[8] The ascending colon is about 15 cm (5–6 inches) long.[8] The transverse colon is about 45 cm (17–18 inches) in length.[8] The descending colon is about 25 cm (9–10 inches) long.[8] The sigmoid colon is approximately 35 to 40 cm (13–16 inches) in length.[8] The rectum begins at the midsacrum,[8] is 12 to 15 cm (5 inches) long, and is quite angulated. These angles are also known as *Houston valves*. The anal canal contains internal and external sphincters.[1]

The colon has four layers.[8] The outermost layer, the serous layer (serosa),[8] is formed from the visceral peritoneum and covers most of the large intestine, with the exclusion of the sigmoid colon. The second layer, the muscular layer (muscularis), consists of two smooth muscle layers: the outer longitudinal and the inner circular muscles.[8] The longitudinal muscle consists of three muscular bands that stretch from the cecum to the distal sigmoid colon.[1] This circular muscle separates the longitudinal muscular bands and creates sacculations of haustra.[1] The third layer, the submucous layer (submucosa),[8] consists of connective tissue that contains blood vessels, lymphatics, glands, and nerve plexuses. The innermost layer, the mucous layer (mucosa),[8] is lined with simple columnar epithelial cells and contains deep *crypts of Lieberkühn* that are lined with mucus-producing goblet cells.[1]

Arterial blood is supplied to the colon from branches of the superior and inferior mesenteric arteries.[8] Venous drainage occurs through the branches of the superior and inferior mesenteric veins into the portal vein (Fig. 26.2).[8] The lymph nodes draining the colon are the epicolic, paracolic, intermediate, and aortic lymph nodes.[8] The large intestine is extrinsically innerved by the autonomic nervous system. Sympathetic fibers arrive from the superior and inferior mesenteric ganglia,

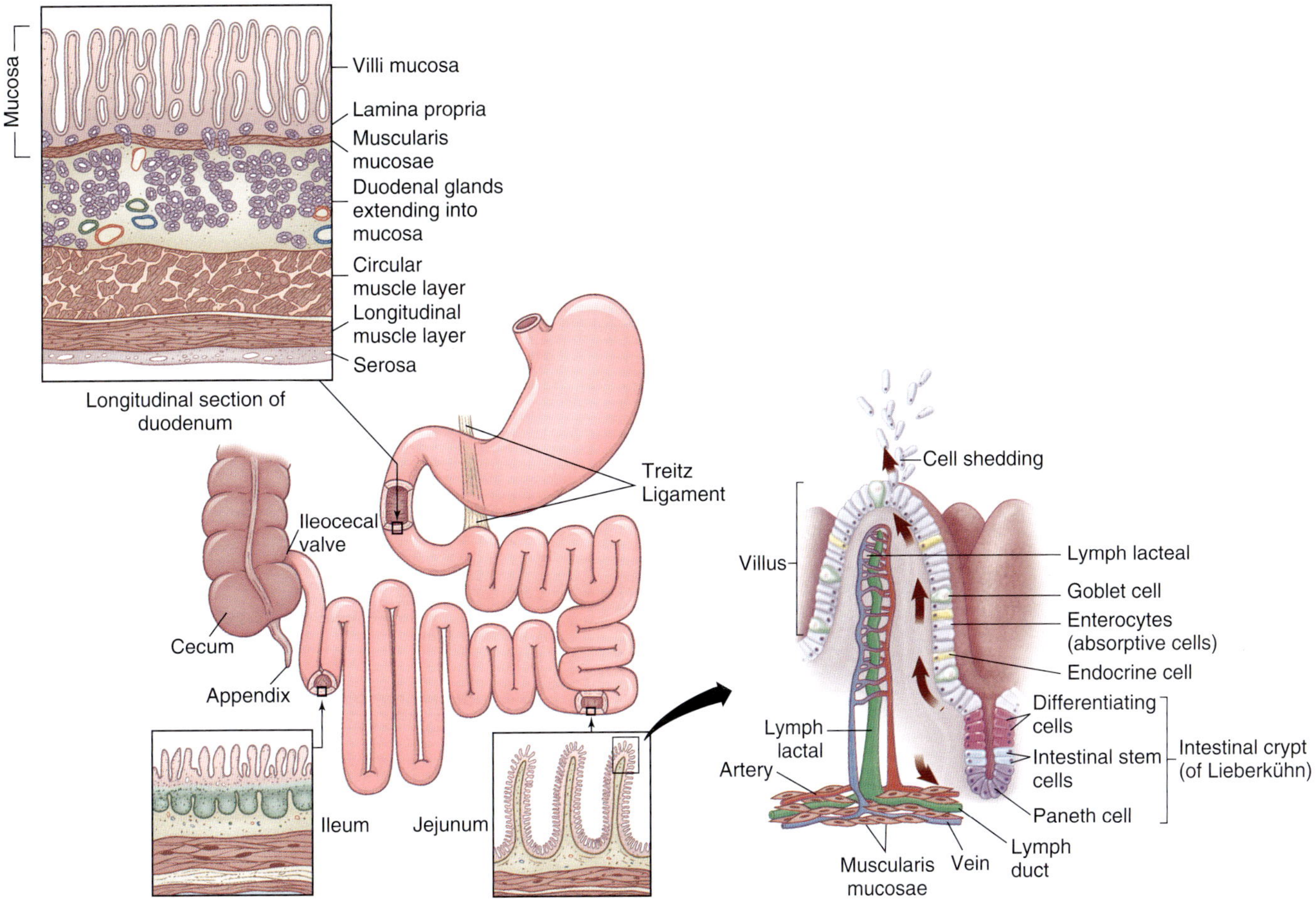

FIG. 26.5 Small Intestine. (From Rogers J. *McCance & Huether's Pathophysiology: The Biologic Basis for Disease in Adults and Children.* 9th ed. Elsevier; 2023.)

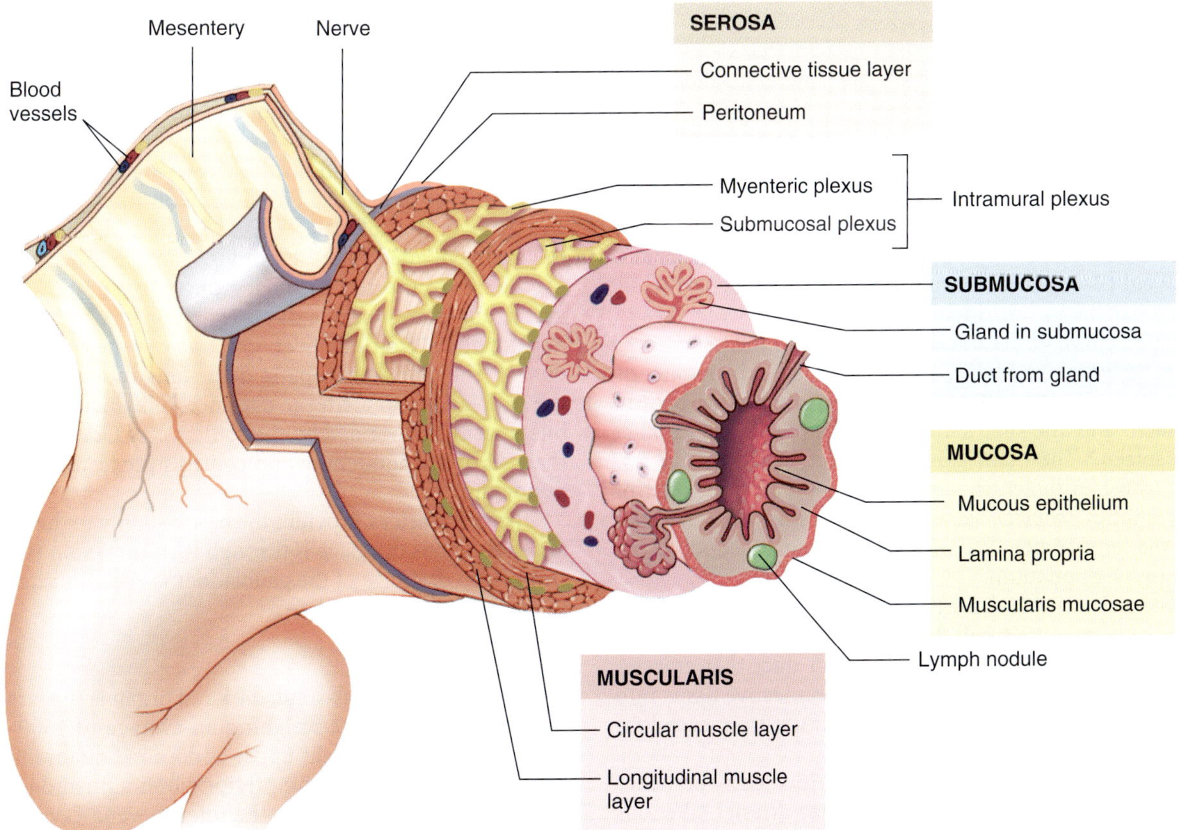

FIG. 26.6 Layers of Small Intestine. Cross-sectional view of the small intestine. (From Patton KT, Bell FB, Thompson T, Williamson PL. *Anatomy and Physiology.* 11th ed. Elsevier; 2022.)

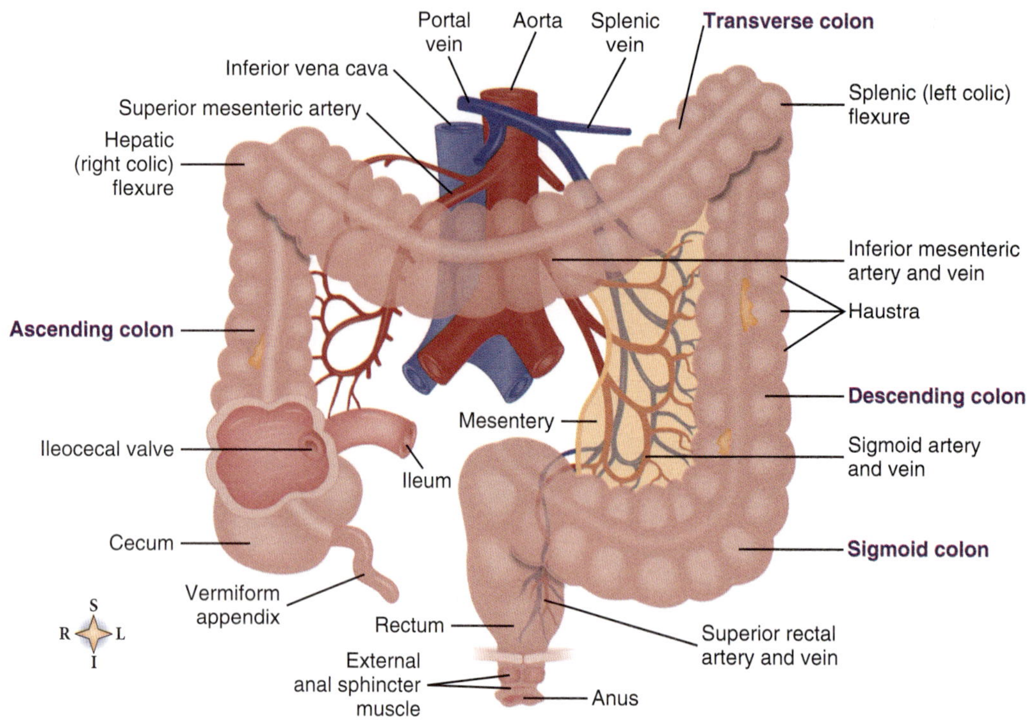

FIG. 26.7 Large Intestine. (From Patton KT, Bell FB, Thompson T, Williamson PL. *Anatomy and Physiology.* 11th ed. Elsevier; 2022.)

whereas parasympathetic fibers arise from the vagus and pelvic nerves. Intrinsic innervation initiates motor functions and is located in the intestinal wall.[6] The colon is intrinsically innervated by the Auerbach plexus.

Accessory Organs

The accessory organs of digestion are the pancreas, gallbladder, and liver (Fig. 26.8).

Pancreas

The pancreas is a soft, lobulated, fish-shaped gland (see Fig. 26.9) lying parallel to and beneath the stomach, duodenum, and spleen (see Fig. 26.8).[9,10] The pinkish yellow organ is approximately 20 cm (7–8 inches)[1] long and 5 cm (1–1.5 inches) wide. Its anatomic divisions include the head and neck, which lies in the C-shaped curve of the duodenum to which the pancreas is attached; the body, the main part of the gland, which extends horizontally across the abdomen and is largely hidden behind the stomach; and the tail, a thin, narrow portion in contact with the spleen.[9] The main pancreatic duct, called the *duct of Wirsung*, traverses the entire length of the organ.[9] The duct of Wirsung empties exocrine secretions into the ampulla of Vater, which is the same lumen draining the common bile duct, at the entrance to the duodenum.[9]

The internal structural unit of the pancreas is the lobule, consisting of numerous small ducts with secretory cells[9] called *tubuloacinar cells*. Each acinus has a small duct that empties into lobular ducts.[9] Lobules are joined by connective tissue into lobes, which unite to form the gland. The ducts from each lobule empty into the duct of Wirsung.

Arterial blood supply to the pancreas is provided by branches of the superior mesenteric artery and celiac arteries.[9] Venous drainage of the head of the pancreas occurs through the portal vein, and drainage of the body and tail occurs through the splenic vein (Fig. 26.2).[9] The pancreas is innervated by the autonomic nervous system. Sympathetic fibers arise from the celiac and superior mesenteric ganglia, and parasympathetic fibers arise from the vagus nerve.[1]

Gallbladder

The gallbladder, a pear-shaped organ, is attached to the liver by connective tissue, peritoneum, and blood vessels. The gallbladder is 7 to 10 cm (3–4 inches) long and 2.5 to 3.5 cm (approximately 1 inch), located on the underside of the liver between the right lobe and the quadrate lobe on the left (see Figs. 26.8 and 26.9).[11] The gallbladder has a storage capacity of about 50 mL and is divided into the fundus, body, and neck.[11] The gallbladder is connected to biliary ducts, including the hepatic, cystic, and common bile ducts (Fig. 26.9).[11] The right and left hepatic ducts, from the liver, join to form the common hepatic duct.[11] The common hepatic duct joins the cystic duct, from the gallbladder, to form the common bile duct.[11] The common bile duct is surrounded by the *sphincter of Oddi*, which pierces the wall of the duodenum and controls the flow of bile into the duodenum.[11]

The cystic artery provides the blood supply to the gallbladder and the venous drainage is through the portal vein (Fig. 26.2).[11] Lymphatic drainage of the gallbladder is accomplished through the cystic lymph node.[11]

Liver

The liver, a friable, soft-solid, dark red organ is the largest internal organ in the body, weighing an average of 1500 g (3 to 4 lb).[12] Located in the right upper abdominal quadrant, the liver fits snugly against the right interior diaphragm and is stabilized by hepatic veins attached to the inferior vena cava.[12] The liver is surrounded by connective tissue known as *Glisson capsule*, which is covered by serosa and contains blood vessels and lymphatics.[12] The peritoneum covering the liver forms the *falciform ligament*, which attaches the liver to the anterior portion of the abdomen between the diaphragm and umbilicus and divides the liver into two main lobes, right and left (Fig. 26.10A).[12] The right lobe, which is six times larger than the left, has three sections: the right lobe proper, the caudate lobe, and the quadrate lobe (Fig. 26.10B).[12]

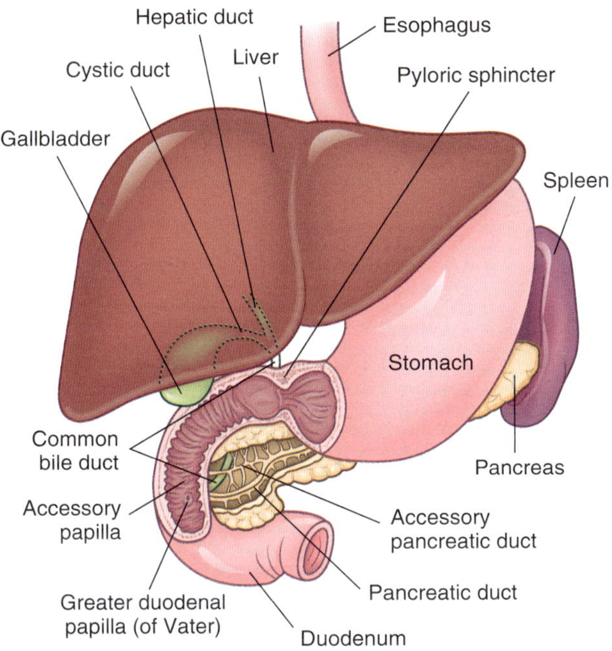

FIG. 26.8 Liver, Gallbladder, and Pancreas. (From Rogers J. *McCance & Huether's Pathophysiology: The Biologic Basis for Disease in Adults and Children*. 9th ed. Elsevier; 2023.)

The liver receives one-quarter of the total cardiac output from two major sources: (1) the hepatic artery, which provides oxygenated blood, and (2) the portal vein, which is supplied with nutrient-rich blood from the gut, pancreas, spleen, and stomach (Fig. 26.10B).[12] The portal vein, which accounts for 75% of the total liver blood flow, branches into sinusoids to transport blood to each lobule.[12] In contrast to capillaries, sinusoids lack a definite cell wall but contain a lining of phagocytic (*Kupffer*) cells[1] and some nonphagocytic cells of modified epithelium. Sinusoids empty blood into an intralobular vein in the center of the lobule. The hepatic artery also divides and subdivides between the lobules, supplying sinusoids with oxygenated blood before emptying into the hepatic vein. Venous drainage occurs through the right, middle, and left hepatic veins into the inferior vena cava (Fig. 26.10B).[12] The lymph nodes draining the liver are the hepatic and posterior mediastinal lymph nodes.[12]

PHYSIOLOGY

The major function of the GI tract is digestion, which is the conversion of ingested nutrients into simpler forms that can be transported from the lumen of the GI tract to the portal circulation and then used in metabolic processes. Digestion can be divided into mechanical and enzymatic processes.

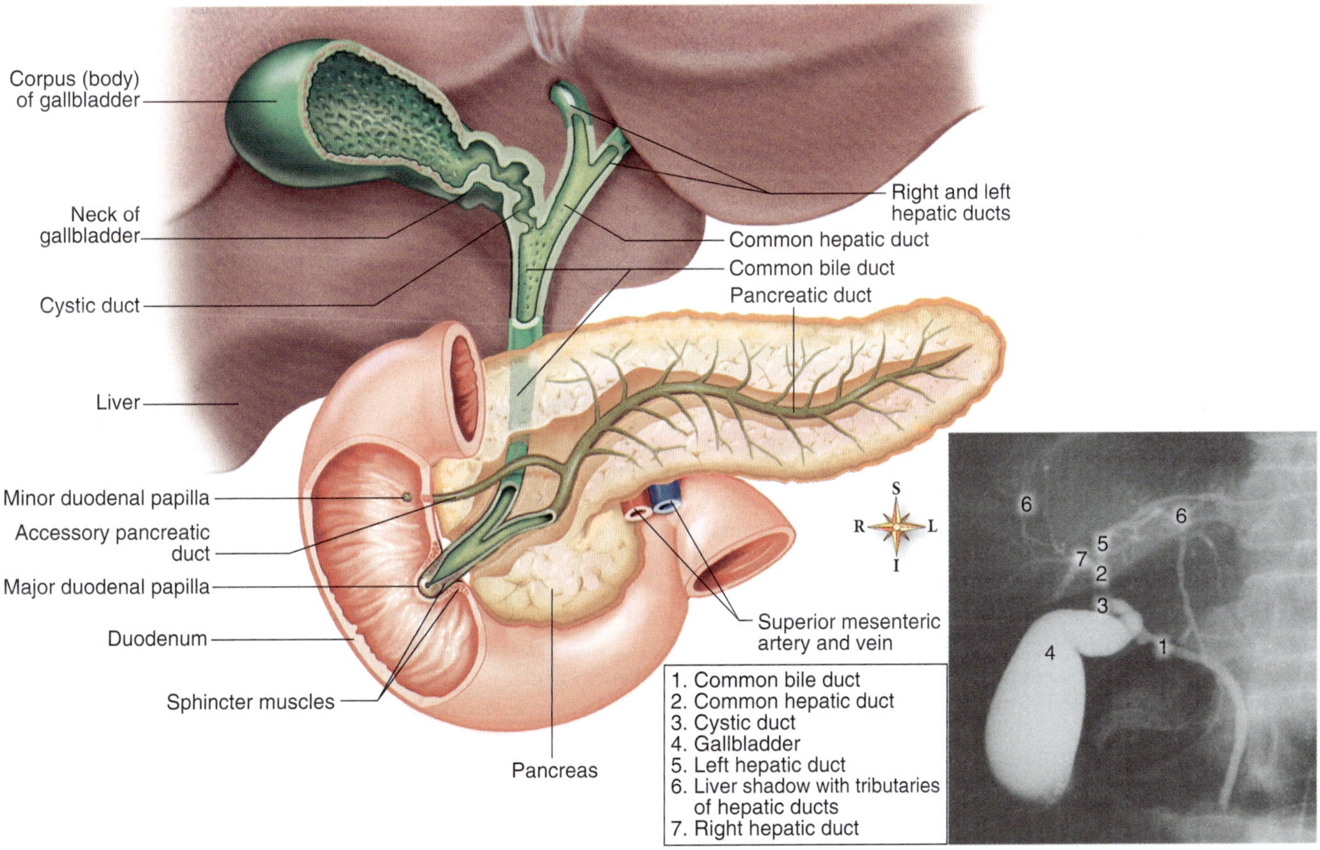

1. Common bile duct
2. Common hepatic duct
3. Cystic duct
4. Gallbladder
5. Left hepatic duct
6. Liver shadow with tributaries of hepatic ducts
7. Right hepatic duct

FIG. 26.9 Gallbladder and Pancreas. (From Patton KT, Bell FB, Thompson T, Williamson PL. *Anatomy and Physiology*. 11th ed. Elsevier; 2022.)

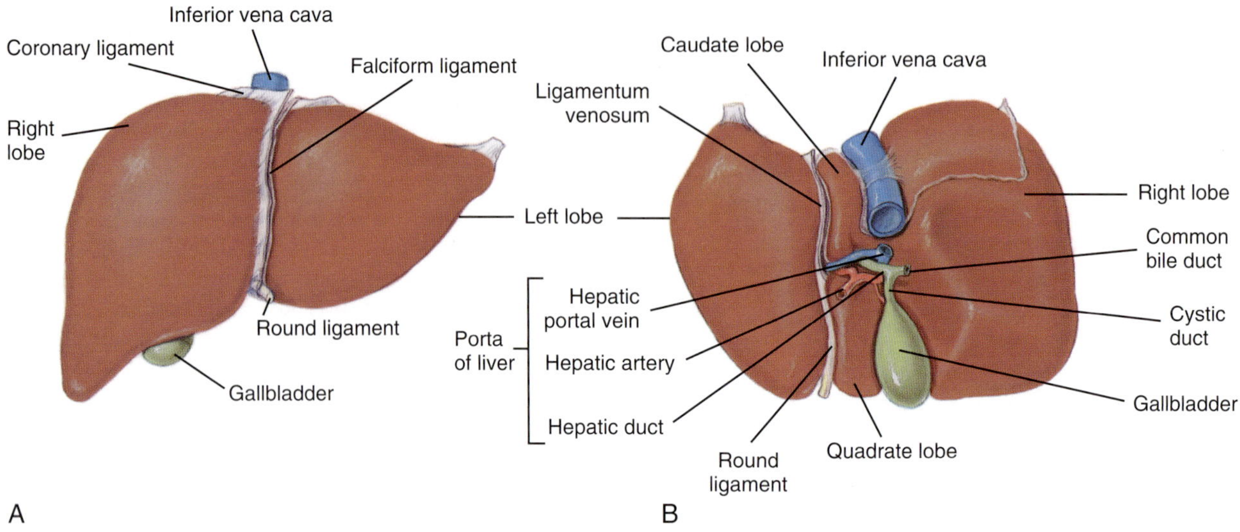

FIG. 26.10 Liver. (A) Anterior surface. (B) Visceral surface. (From Applegate E. *The Anatomy and Physiology Learning System*. 4th ed. Saunders; 2011.)

Mechanical Digestion for Propulsion and Segmentation

Mouth

The mouth performs the initial phases of mechanical digestion, which are ingestion, mastication, and salivation.[10,13] The mouth is the means for *ingestion* and the entry of nutrients.[13] Healthy dentition is vital for this process of *mastication*.[13] The teeth cut, grind, and mix food, transforming it into a form suitable for swallowing, called a bolus, and increasing the surface area of food available to mix with salivary secretions.[13] *Salivation* lubricates the mouth, facilitates the movement of the lips and the tongue during swallowing.[10] Approximately 800 to 1500 mL of saliva is produced each day by three pairs of major salivary glands: (1) the parotid glands, (2) the submandibular glands, and (3) the sublingual glands.[10] The mouth and pharynx also are lined with minor salivary glands that provide additional lubrication.[14] The salivary glands are regulated by the autonomic nervous system, with parasympathetic effects being predominant.[14] Increased parasympathetic stimulation results in profuse secretions of watery saliva, whereas decreased parasympathetic stimulation results in inhibition of salivation.[14]

Esophagus

The bolus of food, formed during mastication, is transported through the pharynx and into the esophagus.[15] The functions of the esophagus are to accept a bolus of food from the oropharynx, transport the bolus through the esophageal body by gravity and peristalsis, and release the bolus into the stomach through the lower esophageal sphincter. This process is known as *swallowing*.[15] Peristalsis consists of waves of circular muscle contractions and relaxations.[13] Peristalsis that is initiated by swallowing is known as *primary peristalsis*, whereas peristalsis that is initiated by esophageal distention is known as *secondary peristalsis*.[13] Peristaltic waves begin in the pharynx and move distally at a rate of 2 to 6 cm/s.[1] The upper esophageal sphincter inhibits air from entering the esophagus during respiration.[13] The lower esophageal sphincter controls the passage of food into the stomach and prevents reflux of gastric contents.[13]

Stomach

The stomach receives the bolus of food through the lower esophageal sphincter. The functions of the stomach include food storage, grinding, and emptying.[16] Food is stored in the stomach for a period and then ground into a semifluid consistency called *chyme*, which is delivered through the pylorus to the duodenum.[16] The movement of food through the stomach, called *gastric motility*, is regulated by the autonomic nervous system, digestive hormones (Table 26.1), and neural reflexes. Gastrin,[13] motilin,[16] and parasympathetic stimulation[16] increase gastric motility, whereas secretin,[13] cholecystokinin,[16] gastric inhibitory peptide,[13] and sympathetic stimulation[16] decrease gastric motility. The ileogastric reflex inhibits gastric motility when the ileum is distended.[1] Two sphincters control the rate of food passage: (1) the lower esophageal sphincter at the esophagogastric junction and (2) the pyloric sphincter at the gastroduodenal junction.[1]

Small Intestine

The small intestine becomes distended with chyme from the stomach.[13] The movement of chyme through the intestine, called *intestinal motility*, consists of two separate motions: (1) peristalsis and (2) haustral segmentation.[13] Peristalsis is sequential contraction and relaxation of short segments of the small intestine.[13] Peristaltic waves of the small intestine move distally at a rate of 0.5 to 2 cm/s.[13] Haustral segmentation is rhythmic contractions that facilitate the mixing and forward movement of chyme.[13] Intestinal motility is regulated by neural reflexes located along the length of the small intestine.[1] Motility is inhibited by the intestinointestinal reflex, which is activated by distention of the small intestine, and is stimulated by the gastroileal reflex, which is initiated by an increase in gastric motility.[1] The ileocecal valve controls the passage of chyme into the large intestine and prevents reflex of contents.[13]

Large Intestine

Chyme from the small intestine proceeds into the large intestine. The functions of the colon include forming solid feces

TABLE 26.1 **Digestive Hormones**[a]

Source	Hormone	Stimulus for Secretion	Action
Mucosa of stomach	Gastrin	Presence of partially digested proteins in stomach	Stimulates gastric glands to secrete hydrochloric acid, pepsinogen, and histamine; growth of gastric mucosa
	Histamine	Acid in stomach	Stimulates acid secretion
	Somatostatin	Acid in stomach	Inhibits acid, pepsinogen, and histamine secretion and release of gastrin
	Acetylcholine	Vagus and local nerves in stomach	Stimulates release of pepsinogen and acid secretion
	Gastrin-releasing peptide (bombesin)	Vagus and local nerves in stomach	Stimulates gastrin and release of pepsinogen and acid secretion
	Ghrelin	High during fasting	Stimulates growth hormone secretion and hypothalamus to increase appetite
Mucosa of small intestines	Motilin	Presence of acid and fat in duodenum	Increases gastrointestinal motility
	Secretin	Presence of chyme (acid, partially digested proteins, and fats) in duodenum	Stimulates pancreas to secrete alkaline pancreatic juice and liver to secrete bile; decreases gastrointestinal motility; inhibits gastrin and gastric acid secretion
	Serotonin (5-hydroxytryptamine)	Intestinal distention; vagal stimulation; presence of acids, amino acids, or hypertonic fluids; released from enterochromaffin cells throughout intestine	Stimulates intestinal secretion, motility and sensation (i.e., pain and nausea), vasodilation; activates gut immune responses
	Cholecystokinin	Presence of chyme (acid, partially digested proteins, and fats) in duodenum	Stimulates gallbladder to eject bile and pancreas to secrete alkaline fluid; decreases gastric motility; constricts pyloric sphincter; inhibits gastrin
	Enteroglucagon	Intraluminal fats and carbohydrates	Weakly inhibits gastric and pancreatic secretion and enhances insulin release, lipolysis, ketogenesis, and glycogenolysis
	Gastric inhibitory peptide	Fat and glucose in small intestine	Inhibits gastric secretion and gastric emptying; stimulates insulin release
	Peptide YY	Intraluminal fat and bile acids	Inhibits postprandial gastric acid and pancreatic secretion; delays gastric and small bowel emptying
	Pancreatic polypeptide	Protein, fat, and glucose in small intestine	Decreases pancreatic bicarbonate and enzyme secretion
	Vasoactive intestinal peptide	Intestinal mucosa and muscle	Relaxes intestinal smooth muscle

[a]The digestive hormones are not secreted into the gastrointestinal lumen, but rather into the bloodstream, where they travel to target tissues. Multiple peptide hormone genes and more than 100 hormonally active peptides are expressed in the gastrointestinal tract.

Modified from Johnson LR. *Gastrointestinal Physiology*. 8th ed. Mosby; 2014. Data from Feldman M, Friedman LS, Brandt LJ. *Sleisenger and Fordtran's Gastrointestinal and Liver Disease*. 10th ed. Saunders; 2015.

and storage of fecal matter.[13] Similar to the small intestine, the movement of chyme through the intestine consists of two separate motions: (1) peristalsis and (2) haustral segmentation.[13] The motility in the large intestine is sluggish in comparison, though, to the small intestine and it may take up to 15 hours for chyme to move from the ileocecal valve to the rectum.[13] The smooth muscle layers of the large intestine work together to propel fecal matter through the colon and to "knead" stool into a compact form. During this colonic motility, water and electrolytes are reabsorbed and solid feces are formed in the proximal half of the colon.[13] The fecal matter is stored in the distal half until the fecal matter is moved into the rectum via mass movements.[13] Mass movements, a type of peristalsis, occur when the colon undergoes a strong, slow contraction as a unit losing its haustrations, allowing for fecal matter to move *en masse* through the colon to the rectum.[13] The *Houston valves* are important in the defecation process because they tend to slow the passage of fecal matter in the rectal vault, assisting the continence mechanism. When fecal matter enters the rectum, defecation reflexes are triggered, contracting the rectum and relaxing the anal sphincters, to expel the fecal matter.[2] Mass movements are facilitated by gastrocolic and duodenocolic reflexes, resulting from distention of the stomach and duodenum.[13]

Enzymatic Digestion for Absorption

Enzymatic digestion, which involves breaking down large molecules into small ones, is essential for nutrient absorption (Fig. 26.11). Enzymatic digestion for absorption occurs in specific areas along the GI tract. Digestive hormones are summarized in Table 26.1.

Mouth and Esophagus

Salivation has an important role in the first stage of enzymatic digestion.[14] Salivation also helps promote oral health by washing away bacteria.[10] Parotid gland secretions are enzymatic, containing amylase (ptyalin), which begins the chemical breakdown of large polysaccharides into dextrins and sugars.[14] Saliva consists mostly of water and also contains mucus for lubrica tion, ions (such as bicarbonate, phosphate) for buffering acids, other electrolytes and proteins for taste, and immunoglobulin A and thiocyanate for antimicrobial actions.[14] When the bolus of food enters the esophagus, there is no enzymatic digestion; rather, the purpose of esophageal secretions is to coat the esophageal lining, protecting it from excoriation and ulceration from food before entering the stomach.[10]

Stomach

In addition to mechanical digestion, the function of the stomach is to produce digestive secretions.[10] The stomach has two types of glands, oxyntic (also known as gastric glands) and pyloric, that contain cells of various types that secrete about 1500 mL/day of gastric juice into the lumen.[10] *Oxyntic glands* are located in the proximal stomach and are composed of three types of cells: (1) mucous neck cells, secreting mucus[10]; (2) peptic, or chief, cells, secreting pepsinogen (necessary for the breakdown of protein when converted to its active form pepsin

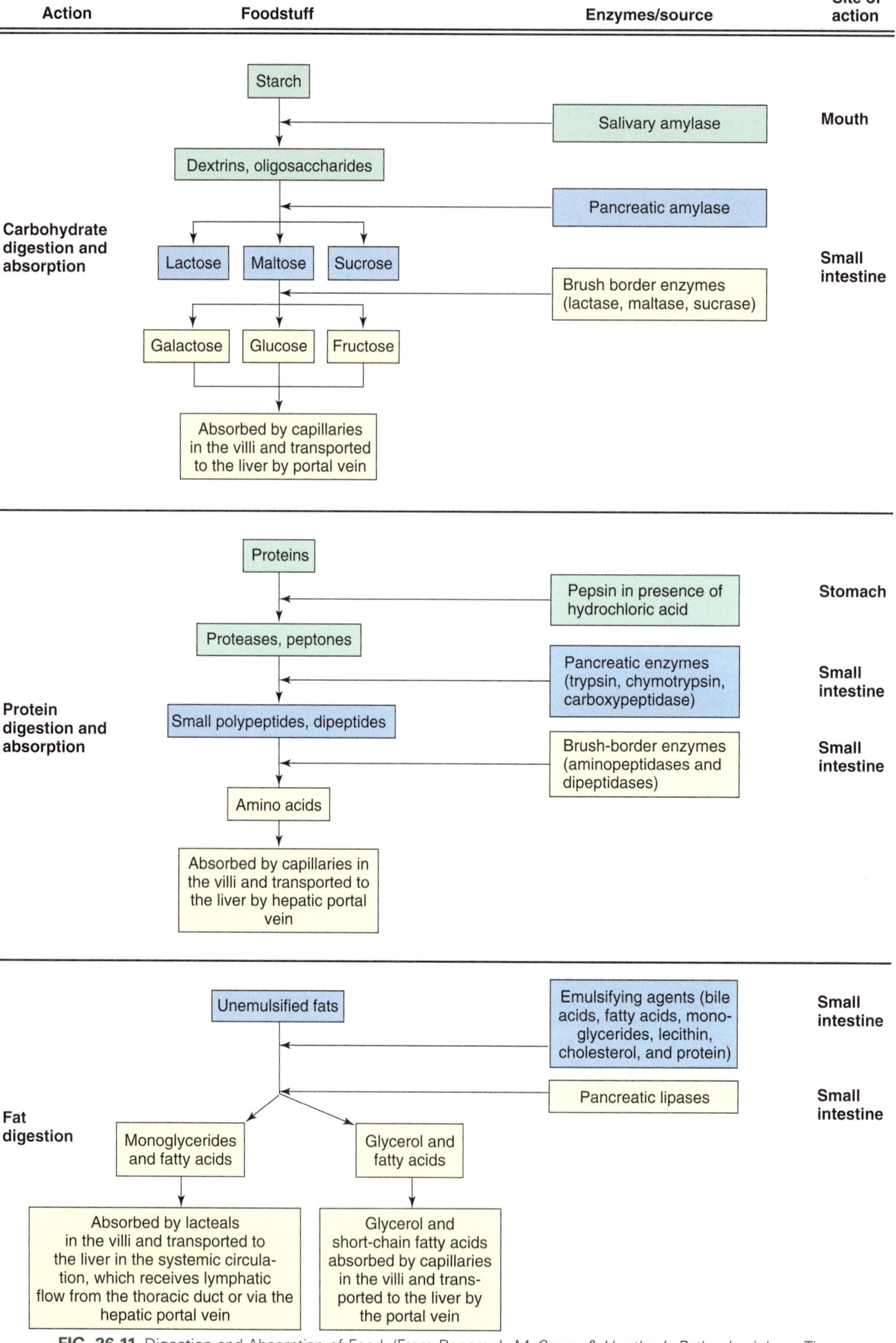

FIG. 26.11 Digestion and Absorption of Food. (From Rogers J. *McCance & Huether's Pathophysiology: The Biologic Basis for Disease in Adults and Children*. 9th ed. Elsevier; 2023.)

in the acidic environment of the stomach)[10]; and (3) parietal, or oxyntic, cells, secreting hydrochloric acid (necessary to dissolve food bolus and act as bactericide)[1] and intrinsic factor (necessary for vitamin B12 absorption in the ileum).[10] *Pyloric glands* are located in the distal stomach and are mainly composed of mucous neck cells, with only few peptic cells and gastrin cells, known as G cells.[10] As a result, pyloric glands protect the gastric mucosa from ulceration, secrete a small amount of pepsinogen, and secrete gastrin (necessary for gastric motility), respectively.[10]

The pH of gastric juice is 1.0 because of the secretion of hydrochloric acid by the parietal cells and the formation of a gastric barrier by tightly packed epithelial cells, preventing diffusion of hydrogen ions into the mucosa.[10] The gastric mucosa is protected from this extreme acidity by a layer of alkaline mucus produced by the epithelial cells.[10] Prostaglandins and nitric oxide protect the gastric mucosa by inhibiting the activation of parietal cells by histamine and stimulating mucus cells.[1] The gastric mucosa may be damaged by certain lipid-soluble substances such as alcohol and aspirin, resulting in mucosal ulceration from acid breaking through the mucosal barrier and penetrating the cells.[10]

Gastric glands are stimulated by the parasympathetic pathway.[10] Acetylcholine increases the secretion of oxyntic and pyloric glands.[10] Gastrin and histamine specifically increase secretion of parietal cells.[10] In contrast, secretin inhibits gastric secretions, as do other hormones like gastric inhibitory peptide and somatostatin, to slow the passage of chyme from the stomach into the small intestine.[10]

Small Intestine

In addition to mechanical digestion, the functions of the small intestine are enzymatic digestion and absorption.[10] The small intestine has two major types of glands: (1) Brunner glands and (2) intestinal glands.[10] *Brunner glands* lie in the mucosa of the duodenum and secrete mucus, an alkaline fluid that neutralizes chyme and protects the mucosa.[10] *Intestinal glands* are found in pits of the submucosa and are called the crypts of Lieberkühn. These crypts secrete 2 to 3 L/day of yellow fluid containing enzymes that assist in nutrient digestion while being absorbed through the epithelium.[10] These enzymes include peptidases (for breaking down peptides into amino acids); sucrase, maltase, isomaltase, and lactase (for breaking down disaccharides into monosaccharides); and intestinal lipase (for breaking down fats into glycerol and fatty acids).[10]

Gland secretion in the small intestine is stimulated by neural reflexes, initiated by stimuli from chyme in the intestinal lumen.[10] The entry of chyme into the duodenum stimulates the production of secretin, which stimulates the pancreas to secrete a highly alkaline fluid into the duodenum.[10] In the small intestine, chyme mixes with pancreatic enzymes, intestinal enzymes, and bile from the liver and gallbladder and is reduced to absorbable elements of proteins, fats, and carbohydrates.[10] The nutrients are absorbed through the villi and transported to the liver by the portal system for further processing.[10] In addition to nutrients, the small intestine absorbs up to 8 L/day of fluid, passing only a small part of this fluid into the large intestine.[10]

Pancreatic secretion into the small intestine. Exocrine functions of the pancreas are limited to enzymatic digestion.[1] Acinar cells of the pancreas produce enzymes and secrete alkaline fluid.[1] Enzymes produced in the pancreas include proteases (trypsin, chymotrypsin, carboxypeptidase, and elastase), amylases, and lipases.[1] With these enzymes, protein, carbohydrates, and fats can be metabolized for absorption.[1] The pancreas also produces a trypsin inhibitor that prevents activation of trypsinogen (inactive form of trypsin), which inhibits autodigestion.[1] The pancreatic juice, consists of water, sodium bicarbonate, and electrolytes at a highly alkaline pH to neutralize the acidic chyme from the stomach.[1] Pancreatic exocrine function is regulated by digestive hormones.[1] Cholecystokinin stimulates the production of pancreatic enzymes.[1] Secretin stimulates the secretion of this pancreatic juice.[1] The two hormones potentiate the effects of each other on the pancreas.[1]

Endocrine functions of the pancreas secrete hormones, such as insulin, glucagon, somatostatin, and pancreatic polypeptide, directly into the bloodstream and not the intestine.[10] These hormones are secreted from cells in spherical islets called *islets of Langerhans*, which are embedded within the lobules of acinar tissue throughout the pancreas, especially in the distal body and tail.[1] See Chapter 29 for more information on the endocrine functions of the pancreas.

Bile secretion into the small intestine. The production of bile makes the liver a vital organ in enzymatic digestion and absorption.[10] Bile is secreted by the liver into the common hepatic duct and enters the small intestine via the common bile duct.[10] If bile is diverted for storage, it enters the gallbladder via the cystic duct.[10]

In the small intestine, bile emulsifies fat globules and aids absorption of digested fat or fat-soluble vitamins.[10] Bile also serves as an excretion route for bilirubin and cholesterol.[10] The major components of bile are bile salts, lecithin, bilirubin, fatty acids, cholesterol, and water.[10] The principal electrolytes of bile are sodium, chloride, and bicarbonate.[10] Approximately 90% of bile salts are actively reabsorbed in the small intestine and are recycled to the liver through the enterohepatic circulation; only small amounts are lost in feces.[10] In the gallbladder, bile is collected, concentrated, and stored.[10] Once in the gallbladder, bile is concentrated up to 20-fold by absorption of almost all the water.[10] Cholesterol and pigment are likewise concentrated.[1] Bile, which is golden or orange-yellow in the liver, becomes dark brown when concentrated in the gallbladder.[1] Bile secretion is stimulated by secretin and elevated bile salt concentration in the blood.[10] Secretin stimulates the secretion of bile from the bile ducts and does not stimulate the liver to produce more bile.[10] Contraction of the gallbladder also facilitates the secretion of bile and is stimulated by cholecystokinin and the vagus nerve.[1] Relaxation of the sphincter of Oddi is coordinated with gallbladder contraction through the regulatory action of cholecystokinin.[1]

Bilirubin. The primary bile pigment, bilirubin, is formed from the heme portion of hemoglobin during the degradation of red blood cells by Kupffer cells.[1] When released into the bloodstream, bilirubin binds to albumin as fat-soluble, unconjugated bilirubin.[1] Taken up by liver hepatocytes, unconjugated bilirubin is conjugated with glucuronic acid to form water-soluble, conjugated bilirubin, which is excreted through hepatic ducts into the large intestine, and its derivatives cause the brown color of feces expelled by the large intestine.[1] The liver has other functions in that are summarized in Box 26.1.

Large Intestine

In addition to mechanical digestion, the major functions of the colon are absorption of water, sodium, chloride, glucose, and urea and putrefaction of contents by bacteria. Similar to the small intestine, the mucosa of the large intestine has crypts of Lieberkühn, but, unlike the small intestine, the large intestine

BOX 26.1 Functions of the Liver

- Secretion of bilirubin, bile salts, cholesterol, fatty acids, calcium, and other electrolytes into bile[10]
- Storage of glucose, vitamins (A, D, E, K, B_{12}), minerals (copper, iron), and blood[1]
- Conversion of complex sugars to simple sugars[17]
- Conversion of carbohydrates to fats[17]
- Conversion of glucose to glycogen (glycogenesis)[1]
- Conversion of amino acids and fats to glucose (gluconeogenesis)[1]
- Conversion of amino acids to fatty acids and triglycerides[1]
- Formation of phospholipids and cholesterol[1]
- Formation of lipoproteins from triglycerides and peptides[17]
- Conversion of amino acids to plasma proteins (e.g., albumin, globulins)[1]
- Phagocytosis of old red blood cells[1]
- Formation of clotting factors[1]
- Conversion of ammonia to urea[1]
- Conversion of vitamin D_3 to 25-hydroxycholecalciferol
- Detoxification of bacteria[17]
- Biotransformation of drugs to active and/or inactive metabolites[1]
- Deactivation of certain hormones (e.g., estrogen)[17]

contains no villi and the epithelial cells do not secrete digestive enzymes. Instead, the large intestine has mucous cells that only secrete mucus, protecting it from fecal excoriation, creating a barrier from the bacterial activity and acid formed in feces, and providing an adherent material for fecal matter.[10] The colon receives approximately 1000 to 2000 mL/day of chyme, and all but 50 to 250 mL of fluid and electrolytes is absorbed in the ascending and transverse colon.[18] The colon contains billions of anaerobic bacteria that putrefy remaining proteins and indigestible residue; synthesize folic acid, vitamin K, nicotinic acid, riboflavin, and some B vitamins; and convert urea salts to ammonium salts and ammonia for absorption into the portal circulation.[1] Common colonic bacteria include *Bacteroides* (gram negative) and *Firmicutes* (gram positive).[1]

EFFECTS OF AGING ON THE ANATOMY AND PHYSIOLOGY OF THE GASTROINTESTINAL SYSTEM

The mucosa of the GI tract changes with age.[19] A decrease in smooth muscle tone is found in older adults from a decrease in the number of nerve fibers.[19] Additionally, there is age-related atrophy.[19]

In older adults, GI function declines, affecting digestion.[19] In the mouth, taste is duller among older adults, reducing food intake.[19] Movement of food into the esophagus becomes more difficult as swallowing function declines.[19] There is also slowing of gastric emptying, which contributes to a reduced appetite from a feeling of fullness.[19] Additionally, there is a reduction of hydrochloric acid secretion that increases the risk of bacterial overgrowth.[19] The slowed gastric emptying limits entry of chyme into the small intestine for digestion and absorption, resulting in malnutrition being common in this population.[19] In the small intestine, there is also a reduction of Brunner glands that neutralize the pH of the chyme from the stomach.[19] Without this neutralization, pancreatic enzymes are not able to function.[19] The pancreas itself also undergoes structural changes that decrease its functional secretion of enzymes.[19] Lastly, the process of defecation is affected by decreased neural stimulation, contributing to constipation among older adults.[19]

An understanding of anatomy and physiology of the GI system provides crucial information for the care of any critically ill patient.

KEY POINTS

Anatomy

- The gastrointestinal tract consists of the mouth, esophagus, stomach, small intestine, and large intestine.
- The accessory organs of digestion are the pancreas, gallbladder, and liver.

Physiology

- The major function of the GI tract is digestion, which is the conversion of ingested nutrients into simpler forms that can be transported from the lumen of the GI tract to the portal circulation and then used in metabolic processes.
- Digestion can be divided into mechanical and enzymatic processes.
- The mouth performs the initial phases of mechanical digestion, which are ingestion, mastication, and salivation.
- The functions of the esophagus are to accept a bolus of food from the oropharynx, transport the bolus through the esophageal body by gravity and peristalsis, and release the bolus into the stomach through the lower esophageal sphincter.
- The functions of the stomach include food storage, grinding, and emptying. In addition to mechanical digestion, the function of the stomach is to produce digestive secretions.
- The movement of chyme through the intestine, called *intestinal motility*, consists of two separate motions: (1) peristalsis and (2) haustral segmentation. In addition to mechanical digestion, the functions of the small intestine are enzymatic digestion and absorption.
- Exocrine functions of the pancreas are limited to enzymatic digestion. Endocrine functions of the pancreas secrete hormones, such as insulin, glucagon, somatostatin, and pancreatic polypeptide, directly into the bloodstream and not the intestine.
- The production of bile makes the liver a vital organ in enzymatic digestion and absorption. If bile is diverted for storage, it enters the gallbladder.
- The functions of the colon include forming solid feces and storage of fecal matter. In addition to mechanical digestion, the major functions of the colon are absorption of water, sodium, chloride, glucose, and urea and putrefaction of contents by bacteria.

Visit the Evolve site at http://evolve.elsevier.com/Urden/CriticalCareNursing for additional study materials.

REFERENCES

1. Turner KC. Structure and function of the digestive system. In: McCance RJ, ed. *Huether's Pathophysiology: The Biologic Basis for Disease in Adults and Children*. 9th ed. Philadelphia, PA: Elsevier; 2023:1285–1317.
2. Oezcelik A, DeMeester SR. General anatomy of the esophagus. *Thorac Surg Clin*. 2011;21(2):289–297. https://doi.org/10.1016/j.thorsurg.2011.01.003.
3. Mahadevan V. Anatomy of the oesophagus. *Surg*. 2014;32(11):565–570. https://doi.org/10.1016/j.mpsur.2017.08.004.

4. Mahadevan V. Anatomy of the stomach. *Surg*. 2014;3(11):571–574. https://doi.org/10.1016/j.mpsur.2017.08.004.
5. Hall JE, Hall ME. Chapter 63. General principles of gastrointestinal function-Motility, nervous control, and blood circulation. In: Hall ME, Hall JE, eds. *Guyton and Hall Textbook of Medical Physiology*. 14th ed. Philadelphia, PA: Elsevier; 2021:787–796.
6. Volk N, Lacy B. Anatomy and physiology of the small bowel. *Gastrointest Endosc Clin N Am*. 2017;27(1):1–13. https://doi.org/10.1016/j.giec.2016.08.001.
7. Mahadevan V. Anatomy of the small intestine. *Surg*. 2020;38(6):283–288. https://doi.org/10.1016/j.mpsur.2020.03.012.
8. Mahadevan V. Anatomy of the caecum, appendix, and colon. *Surg*. 2020;38(1):1–6. https://doi.org/10.1016/j.mpsur.2019.10.017.
9. Bazira PJ, Mahadevan V. Anatomy of the pancreas and spleen. *Surg*. 2022;40(4):213–218. https://doi.org/10.1016/j.mpsur.2022.02.002.
10. Hall JE, Hall ME. Chapter 65. Secretory functions of the alimentary tract. In: Hall ME, Hall JE, eds. *Guyton and Hall Textbook of Medical Physiology*. 14th ed. Philadelphia, PA: Elsevier; 2021:807–822.
11. Ellis H. Anatomy of the gallbladder and bile ducts. *Surg*. 2011;29(12):593–596. https://doi.org/10.1016/j.mpsur.2011.09.011.
12. Mahadevan V. Anatomy of the liver. *Surg*. 2020;38(8):427–431. https://doi.org/10.1016/j.mpsur.2014.10.004.
13. Hall JE, Hall ME. Chapter 64. Propulsion and mixing of food in the alimentary tract. In: Hall ME, Hall JE, eds. *Guyton and Hall Textbook of Medical Physiology*. 14th ed. Philadelphia, PA: Elsevier; 2021:797–806.
14. Pedersen AML, Sørensen CE, Proctor GB, Carpenter GH, Ekström J. Salivary secretion in health and disease. *J Oral Rehabil*. 2018;45:730–746. https://doi.org/10.1111/joor.12664. 10.1111/nmo.13100.
15. Sasegbon A, Hamdy S. The anatomy and physiology of normal and abnormal swallowing in oropharyngeal dysphagia. *Neurogastroenterol Motil*. 2017;29(11):e13100.
16. Goyal RK, Guo Y, Mashimo H. Advances in the physiology of gastric emptying. *Neurogastroenterol Motil*. 2019;31(4):e13546. https://doi.org/10.1111/nmo.13546.
17. Hall JE, Hall ME. Chapter 71. The liver. In: Hall ME, Hall JE, eds. *Guyton and Hall Textbook of Medical Physiology*. 14th ed. Philadelphia, PA: Elsevier; 2021:871–876.
18. Hall JE, Hall ME. Chapter 66. Digestion and absorption in the gastrointestinal tract. In: Hall ME, Hall JE, eds. *Guyton and Hall Textbook of Medical Physiology*. 14th ed. Philadelphia, PA: Elsevier; 2021:823–832.
19. Soenen S, Rayner CK, Jones KL, Horowitz M. The ageing gastrointestinal tract. *Curr Opin Clin Nutr Metab Care*. 2016;19(1):12–18. https://doi.org/10.1097/MCO.0000000000000238.

27

Gastrointestinal Clinical Assessment and Diagnostic Procedures

Kathrine Anne Winnie and Kimberly Sanchez

http://evolve.elsevier.com/Urden/CriticalCareNursing

Assessments of critically ill patients with gastrointestinal (GI) dysfunction should be systematic, starting with a patient history, followed by a focused physical assessment, continued with an analysis of laboratory data, and including an interpretation of invasive and noninvasive diagnostic procedures. A detailed history and careful physical assessment, along with diagnostic procedures, may help identify GI disorders.

HISTORY

Taking a thorough and accurate history is extremely important to the assessment process. The patient's history provides the foundation and direction for the rest of the assessment. The overall goal of the patient interview is to expose key clinical manifestations that will facilitate the identification of the underlying cause of the illness. This information can assist in the development of an appropriate management plan.

The initial presentation of the patient determines the rapidity and direction of the interview.[1] For a patient in acute distress, the history should be curtailed to a few questions, focusing on the patient's chief concern and the precipitating events.[1] For a patient in no obvious distress, the complete history includes patient identifiers, chief concern (CC), history of present illness or problem (HPI), past medical and surgical history (PMH), family history, personal and social history, and review of systems (ROS).[1] Components of the history related to GI disorders are outlined in Box 27.1.

FOCUSED PHYSICAL ASSESSMENT

The abdomen is divided into four quadrants (left upper, right upper, left lower, and right lower), with the umbilicus as the middle point, to specify the location of examination findings (Fig. 27.1 and Box 27.2).[2] Four techniques are used in the physical assessment of the abdomen: inspection, auscultation, percussion, and palpation.[2] In the critical care area, a nursing assessment does not routinely include percussion or palpation. However, the information gained through these physical assessment techniques can provide data about the patient's condition.

Inspection

Inspection of the patient focuses on three areas: (1) observation of the oral cavity, (2) assessment of the skin over the abdomen, and (3) evaluation of the shape of the abdomen.

Observation of the Oral Cavity

Although assessment of the GI system classically begins with inspection of the abdomen, the patient's oral cavity should also be inspected to determine any unusual findings that may affect mechanical or enzymatic digestion. The most accurate way to inspect the oral cavity is with a tongue blade and light.[3] When inspecting the oral cavity, gums should not have inflammation, tenderness, or bleeding in the presence of natural teeth or dentures. Additionally, teeth should not be loose or missing.[3] If dentures are used, they should fit properly and not cause irritation.[3] Lastly, the oral mucosa should be moist from salivary production.[3]

Assessment of the Skin Over the Abdomen

Visual inspection of the abdomen includes observing color and surface characteristics.[2]

Abdominal color and characteristics should be consistent with other parts of the body.[2] The abdomen may be a lighter color than other sun-exposed areas of the skin.[2] The abdomen may have bruises or localized discoloration, indicative of jaundice, trauma, or bleeding.[2] A green bruising in the right flank (Grey Turner's sign) may suggest inflammation of the pancreas.[2] Bluish discoloration of the umbilicus (Cullen sign) may suggest intraabdominal bleeding.[2] Glistening of the skin may be from fluid accumulating in the abdomen (e.g., ascites), contributing to taut skin.[2]

Evaluation of the Shape of the Abdomen

The contour of the abdomen should be evaluated for symmetry.[2] The abdomen can be described as flat, rounded, or scaphoid.[2] Athletic, muscular adults may have flat abdomens; adults with increased subcutaneous fat or poor muscle tone may have rounded abdomens; underweight adults may have scaphoid (or concave) abdomens.[2] Marked distention is an abnormal finding. Ascites may cause generalized distention.[2] Asymmetric distention may indicate organ enlargement, large masses, hernia, or bowel obstruction.[2]

Auscultation

Auscultation of the patient focuses evaluation of bowel sounds and assessment of bruits.[2]

Evaluation of Bowel Sounds

Auscultation of the bowel sounds provides clinical data regarding the status of bowel motility.[2] Initially, listen with the diaphragm of the stethoscope below and to the right of the umbilicus (in the right lower quadrant).[2] The examination proceeds methodically through all four quadrants (Fig. 27.1). Normal bowel sounds include clicking or gurgling sounds that

BOX 27.1 DATA COLLECTION

Gastrointestinal History

Common Gastrointestinal Symptoms
- Oral lesions
- Digestion or indigestion (heartburn)
- Dysphagia
- Nausea
- Vomiting
- Hematemesis
- Change in stool color or contents (e.g., clay-colored, tarry, fresh blood, mucus, undigested food)
- Constipation
- Diarrhea
- Abdominal pain
- Jaundice
- Anal discomfort
- Fecal incontinence

History of Present Illness or Problem
- Current medication use
  - Laxatives
  - Stool softeners
  - Antiemetics
  - Antidiarrheals
  - Antacids
  - Aspirin
  - Acetaminophen
  - Nonsteroidal antiinflammatory drugs
  - Corticosteroids

Past Medical and Surgical History
- Chronic illnesses
- Previous weight gain or loss
- Tooth extractions or orthodontic work
- Gastrointestinal disorders (e.g., peptic ulcer, inflammatory bowel disease, polyps, cholelithiasis, diverticular disease, pancreatitis, intestinal obstruction, clostridia infections)
- Hepatitis or cirrhosis
- Abdominal surgery
- Abdominal trauma
- Cancer affecting gastrointestinal system
- Spinal cord injury
- Women: episiotomy or fourth-degree laceration during delivery
- Exposure to infectious agents (e.g., foreign travel, water source)
- Polyposis syndromes
- Cancer of GI tract
- Vascular diseases (e.g., portal hypertension, atherosclerotic disease)

Past Medication Use
- Nonsteroidal antiinflammatory drugs
- Corticosteroids
- Anticoagulants

Past Gastrointestinal Studies
- Esophagogastroduodenoscopy (EGD)
- Enteroscopy
- Colonoscopy
- Endoscopic retrograde cholangiopancreatography (ERCP)
- Plain abdominal series radiograph
- Abdominal ultrasound
- Computed tomography (CT) of the abdomen and pelvis
- Magnetic resonance imaging
- Radionuclide imaging (e.g., hepatobiliary scintigraphy, gastrointestinal bleeding scan)
- Angiography
- Liver biopsy
- Stool studies (occult blood, ova and parasites)
- Liver enzymes tests (alkaline phosphatase, aspartate aminotransferase [AST], alanine aminotransferase [ALT])
- Bilirubin
- Albumin
- Clotting studies (Prothrombin time [PT], partial thromboplastin time [PTT], international normalized ratio [INR])
- Pancreatic enzymes tests (amylase, lipase)

Family History
- Investigate for history of following disorders, and document (+ or −) responses
- Hirschsprung disease
- Obesity
- Metabolic disorders
- Inflammatory disorders
- Malabsorption syndromes
- Familial Mediterranean fever
- Rectal polyps

Personal and Social History
- Usual height and weight
- Dietary habits
- Usual number of meals or snacks per day
- Usual fluid intake per day
- Nutrient intake
- Types of food usually eaten at each meal or snack
- Food likes and dislikes
- Religious or medical food restrictions
- Food intolerances
- Patient's perceptions and concerns about adequacy of diet and appropriateness of weight
- Effects of lifestyle on food intake, weight gain or loss
- Vitamins or nutritional supplements (e.g., type, amount, frequency)
- Bowel elimination
- Usual frequency of bowel movements
- Usual consistency and color of stool
- Ability to control elimination of gas and stool
- Any changes in bowel elimination patterns
- Use of enemas or laxatives (e.g., reason for use, frequency, type, response)
- Alcohol intake (e.g., frequency, usual amounts)
- Exercise patterns

occur at a rate of 5 to 35 times per minute.[2] Hyper- and hypoactive bowel sounds indicate increased or decreased motility, respectively. Bowel sounds are absent if there are no sounds auscultated after 5 minutes of continuously listening and it requires immediate attention.[2]

Assessment of Bruits

Bruits are created by turbulent flow over a partially obstructed artery and are always considered an abnormal finding.[2] The abdomen should be auscultated for the presence of bruits using the bell of the stethoscope.[2] Listen for bruits in the epigastric region and to the left and right of the umbilicus (Fig. 27.2).[2] An increased venous hum, which is soft, lowpitched, and continuous, may indicate increased flow between the portal and systemic venous systems.[2]

Percussion

Percussion is performed to detect size and density of the organs in the abdomen, such as the liver.[2] Additionally, percussion may detect the presence of fluid, air, or masses.[2] Each abdominal quadrant is percussed for tympany and dullness, with tympany heard over air in the stomach or intestines and dullness heard over organs or masses.[2] Because the abdomen is a sensitive area, muscle tension may interfere with this part of the assessment.

Palpation

With the patient in a supine position, the abdomen should be palpated to provide information about organ size, shape, mobility, and consistency.[2] Light palpation, which has a palpation depth of approximately 1 cm, assesses to the depth of the skin and fascia.[2] The abdomen should feel smooth and that smoothness should be consistent in all quadrants or regions.[2] Deep palpation is performed bimanually by exerting pressure with the top hand but obtaining sensory information from the bottom hand.[2] Deep palpation is most helpful in detecting abdominal masses.[3] There should be no areas of tenderness, but if the patient complains of tenderness in a particular area, that quadrant or region should be palpated last. An expected finding with palpation is no tenderness or pain or hardened areas.[2]

LABORATORY STUDIES

Various laboratory studies may be used to diagnose and treat diseases of the GI system; however, no single study provides an overall picture of the functional state of the various organs, and no single value is predictive by itself. Select stool studies are

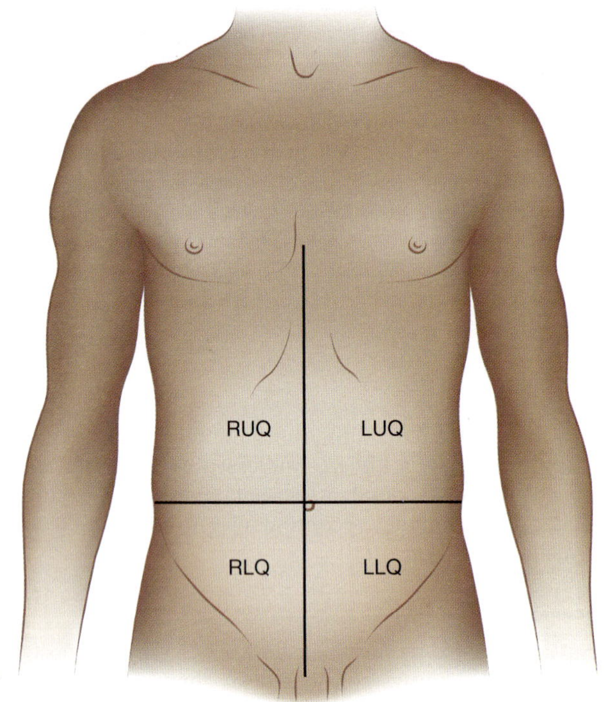

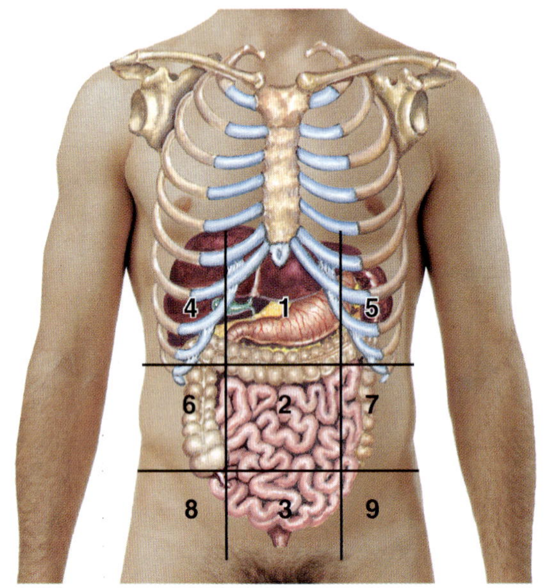

FIG. 27.1 Abdominal Quadrants and Regions. (A) Abdominal quadrants. *LLQ*, Left lower quadrant; *LUQ*, left upper quadrant; *RLQ*, right lower quadrant; *RUQ*, right upper quadrant. (B) Abdominal regions. *1*, Epigastric; *2*, umbilical; *3*, hypogastric; *4*, right hypochondriac; *5*, left hypochondriac; *6*, right lumbar; *7*, left lumbar; *8* right inguinal; and *9*, right and left inguinal. (From Ball JW, Dains, JE, Flynn JA, Solomon BS, Stewart RW. *Seidel's Guide to Physical Examination*. 10th ed. Elsevier; 2023.)

BOX 27.2 Anatomic Correlates of the Abdomen[2]

Right Upper Quadrant
- Liver and gallbladder
- Pylorus
- Duodenum
- Head of pancreas
- Right adrenal gland
- Portion of right kidney
- Hepatic flexure of colon
- Portion of ascending and transverse colon

Left Upper Quadrant
- Left lobe of liver
- Spleen
- Stomach
- Body of pancreas
- Left adrenal gland
- Portion of left kidney
- Splenic flexure of colon
- Portions of transverse and descending colon

Right Lower Quadrant
- Lower pole of right kidney
- Cecum and appendix
- Portion of ascending colon
- Bladder (if distended)
- Ovary and salpinx
- Uterus (if enlarged)
- Right spermatic cord
- Right ureter

Left Lower Quadrant
- Lower pole of left kidney
- Sigmoid colon
- Portion of descending colon
- Bladder (if distended)
- Ovary and salpinx
- Uterus (if distended)
- Left spermatic cord
- Left ureter

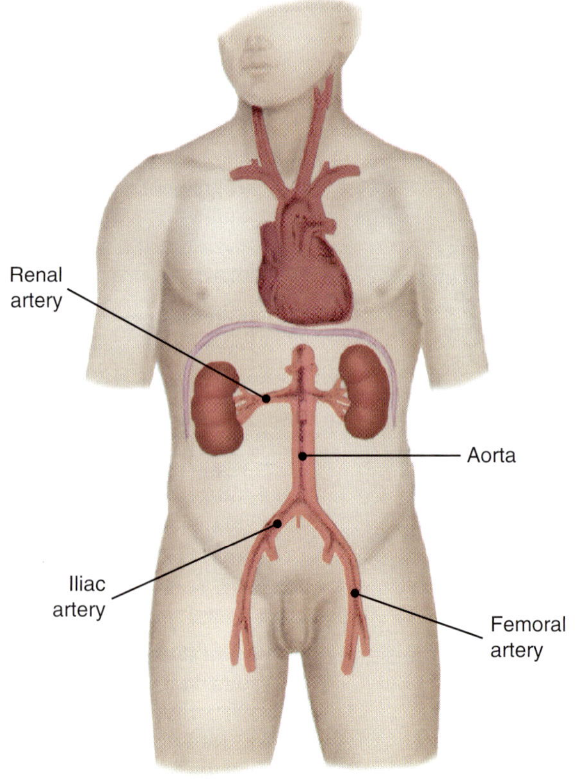

FIG. 27.2 Auscultation for Bruits.

listed in Table 27.1. Select laboratory studies used in the assessment of liver function and pancreatic function are presented in Tables 27.2 and 27.3.

DIAGNOSTIC PROCEDURES

In critically ill patients with GI dysfunction, several diagnostic procedures may be performed to identify or obtain further information related to structural or functional abnormalities of the GI tract and accessory organs.

Endoscopy

Endoscopy involves the use of a flexible or rigid tube-like instrument, called an endoscope, to visualize inside of an organ.[4] Endoscopy can provide information about lesions, mucosal changes,

SUPPORTING NURSE WELL-BEING

Social Wellness—Professional

I have been working on my unit for several years now and have really grown as a nurse. I am more confident in my knowledge and skills. I am more comfortable being assertive when advocating for my patients. Not every shift is smooth; sometimes, I leave all worked up. I usually tell my friends about work because we talk about all aspects of our lives. None of them are in health care and none of them are nurses. So, when I tell them my frustrations with not having scheduled medications readily available, or a provider not returning my page, or a resident response of "ok, I'll talk to my attending" when my patient is clinically deteriorating, I also have to explain to them the health care jargon and the workflows contributing to the frustration. With my coworkers, the situations I share with them are immediately relatable and I can vent "faster." We can discuss and validate our shared experiences and, often times, that leads to an exchange of tips for future similar situations. I am happy to have my friends and my coworkers as part of my social network.

The above vignette shows how one person attempts to leverage her social network to cope with inherent stressors in nursing practice environments, such as inefficient workflows, heavy assignments, and fragmented interprofessional communication. Social wellness, specifically in a professional setting, is having a network of people who have experienced the work you do in your role and share an understanding of the requirements needed to fulfill your professional responsibilities. The shared role and experiences allow for connectedness and support. The purpose of this network is not necessarily focused on professional development and career advancement. Because of the social aspect of this professional network, it is informal and unstructured. This group consists of your "nursing" friends, or to state it another way—your friends with whom you work or know through professional networking. This social network may not be solutions oriented but, in the sharing of experiences, individuals in the group learn from one another. That is the natural occurrence in social interactions. Having a social network among your peers creates a therapeutic community of individuals who can relate to workplace stressors to enhance emotional well-being.

Consider the following to maintain social wellness, specifically in a professional setting:

- Evaluate your current professional interactions: How do you contribute to your professional network? What feelings are evoked from interacting within your professional network?
- Determine your needs.
- Actively communicate and be intentional in that professional communication.
- Be genuine during and open to changes in professional circumstances.
- Embrace your need for professional growth.
- Attend nursing professional networking events.
- Join a local or national nursing professional organization.

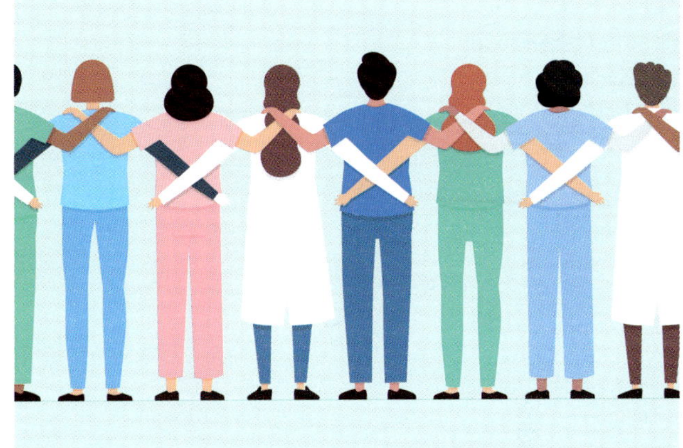

(Copyright (C) iStock.com/osker14)

Let us never consider ourselves finished nurses ... we must be learning all of our lives...

Florence Nightingale

TABLE 27.1 Selected Stool Studies

Test	Normal Findings	Interpretation
Stool studies	Resident microorganisms: clostridia, enterococci, *Pseudomonas*, a few yeasts	Detection of *Salmonella typhi* (typhoid fever), *Shigella* (dysentery), *Vibrio cholerae* (cholera), *Yersinia* (enterocolitis), *Escherichia coli* (gastroenteritis), *Staphylococcus aureus* (food poisoning), *Clostridium botulinum* (food poisoning), *Clostridium perfringens* (food poisoning), *Aeromonas* (gastroenteritis)
	Fat: 2–6 g/24 h	Steatorrhea (increased values) resulting from intestinal malabsorption or pancreatic insufficiency
	Pus: none	Large amounts of pus associated with chronic ulcerative colitis, abscesses, and anorectal fistula
	Occult blood: none (ortho-toluidine or guaiac test)	Positive test results associated with bleeding
	Ova and parasites: none	Detection of *Entamoeba histolytica* (amebiasis), *Giardia lamblia* (giardiasis), and worms
	Peak blood level: >30 mg/dL	

dL, Deciliter; *g*, gram; *h*, hour; *L*, liter; *mg*, milligram.
From Rogers J. *McCance & Huether's Pathophysiology: The Biologic Basis for Disease in Adults and Children.* 9th ed. Elsevier; 2023.

obstructions, and motility dysfunction, and a biopsy or removal of foreign objects may be performed during the procedure.[4] Different endoscopic procedures are available to examine the structure and function of the GI tract, as well as diagnose and treat GI disorders: esophagogastroduodenoscopy (EGD), enteroscopy, capsule endoscopy, colonoscopy, sigmoidoscopy, and endoscopic retrograde cholangiopancreatography (ERCP).[4] The main difference between the various diagnostic forms is the length of the anatomic area that can be examined. Complications of endoscopy include perforation, bleeding, and infection.[4]

Esophagogastroduodenoscopy

EGD permits viewing of the upper GI tract from the esophagus to the upper duodenum to explore complaints of dyspepsia, dysphagia, emesis, or other upper GI symptoms.[4] EGDs also allow for screening for disorders like Barrett's esophagus or ulcers and it is a treatment option for patients with a GI hemorrhage.[4]

Enteroscopy

An enteroscopy, and most recently capsule endoscopy, allows for visualization of the small intestine beyond the ligament of Treitz.[5]

TABLE 27.2 Selected Laboratory Studies of Liver Function

Test	Normal Value	Interpretation
Serum Enzymes		
Alkaline phosphatase	35–150 units/L	Increases with biliary obstruction and cholestatic hepatitis
Gamma-glutamyl transpeptidase	Male, 12–38 units/L Female, 9–31 units/L	Increases with biliary obstruction and cholestatic hepatitis
Aspartate aminotransferase (AST)	Male, 8–40 units/L Female, 6–34 units/L	Increases with hepatocellular injury and injury in other tissues (e.g., skeletal and cardiac muscle)
Alanine aminotransferase (ALT)	Male, 10–40 units/L Female, 9–32 units/L	Increases with hepatocellular injury and necrosis
Lactate dehydrogenase (LDH)	110–220 units/L	Isoenzyme lactate dehydrogenase (LD_5) is increased with hypoxic and primary liver injury
5′-Nucleotidase	2–11 units/L	Increases with elevated alkaline phosphatase and cholestatic disorders
Bilirubin Metabolism		
Serum Bilirubin		
Unconjugated (indirect)	0.1–1 mg/dL	Increases with hemolysis (lysis of red blood cells)
Conjugated (direct)	0.1–0.4 mg/dL	Increases with hepatocellular injury or obstruction
Total	<1 mg/dL	Increases with biliary obstruction
Urine bilirubin	0	Increases with biliary obstruction
Urine urobilinogen	0–4 mg/24 h	Increases with hemolysis or shunting or portal blood flow
Serum Proteins		
Albumin	3.5–5.5 g/dL	Decreases with hepatocellular injury
Globulin	2–4 g/dL	Increases with hepatitis
Total	6–7 g/dL	
Albumin/globulin (A/G) ratio	1.5–2.5:1	Ratio reverses with chronic hepatitis or other chronic liver disease
Transferrin	250–300 mcg/dL	Decreases with liver damage Increases with iron deficiency
Alpha-fetoprotein	6–20 ng/dL	Increases with primary hepatocellular carcinoma
Blood Clotting Functions		
Prothrombin time	10–13 s or 90%–100% of control	Increases with chronic liver disease (cirrhosis) or vitamin K deficiency
Partial thromboplastin time (PTT)	22–37 s	Increases with severe liver disease or heparin therapy
Bromsulphthalein (BSP) excretion	<6% retention in 45 min	Increased retention with hepatocellular injury

dL, Deciliter; *h*, hour; *L*, liter; *mcg*, microgram; *mg*, milligram; *min*, minute *ng*, nanogram; *s*, second.
From Rogers J. *McCance & Huether's Pathophysiology: The Biologic Basis for Disease in Adults and Children.* 9th ed. Elsevier; 2023.

TABLE 27.3 Selected Laboratory Studies of Pancreatic Function

Test	Normal Value	Interpretation
Serum amylase	25–125 units/mL	Increases with pancreatic inflammation
Serum lipase	20–240 units/mL	Increases with pancreatic inflammation (may be elevated with other conditions; differentiates with amylase isoenzyme study)
Urine amylase	35–260 Somogyi units/h	Increases with pancreatic inflammation
Secretin test	Volume 1.8 mL/kg/h Bicarbonate concentration: >80 mEq/L Bicarbonate output: >10 mEq/L/30 s	Decreases with pancreatic disease because secretin stimulates pancreatic secretion
Stool fat	2–5 g/24 h	Measures fatty acids: decreased pancreatic lipase increases stool fat
Fecal elastase	>200 mcg/g of stool	Decreases with pancreatic insufficiency

g, Gram; *h*, hour; *kg*, kilogram; *L*, liter; *mcg*, microgram.; *mEq*, milliequivalent; *mL*, milliliter; *s*, second.
From Rogers J. *McCance & Huether's Pathophysiology: The Biologic Basis for Disease in Adults and Children.* 9th ed. Elsevier; 2023.

The use of capsule endoscopy is limited to visualization at this time.[4] An enteroscopy is a more difficult diagnostic procedure to perform, but if performed may facilitate biopsy of the small intestine[4] and evaluate sources of GI bleeding that have not been identified previously with an EGD or lower GI endoscopy.

Colonoscopy and Sigmoidoscopy

Colonoscopies and sigmoidoscopies permit visualization of the lower GI tract from the rectum to the ileum, with the sigmoidoscopy examining up to the distal colon.[4] Lower GI endoscopies allow for exploration of patient complaints of GI signs and symptoms, such as changes in bowel habits or rectal bleeding.[4] Colorectal cancer screenings can also be done with lower GI endoscopies, and they aid in the removal of polyps or dilation of strictures.[4]

Endoscopic Retrograde Cholangiopancreatography

An ERCP uses an endoscope to enter the duodenum and the ampulla of Vater, where contrast is injected and radiographs are obtained to visualize the biliary and pancreatic ducts.[4]

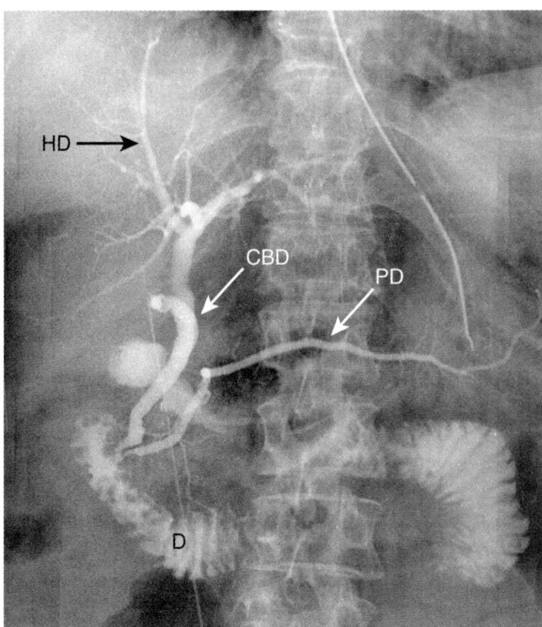

FIG. 27.3 Normal Endoscopic Retrograde Cholangiopancreatography. Placement of a fiberoptic gastroscope allows cannulation of the common bile duct *(CBD)* and pancreatic duct *(PD)* at the level of the ampulla of Vater. Retrograde injection of contrast also allows visualization of intrahepatic ducts *(HD)*. Contrast is seen spilling around the cannulation site into the duodenal sweep and proximal jejunum. *D*, Duodenum. (From Mettler FA. *Essentials of Radiology*. 4th ed. Elsevier; 2019.)

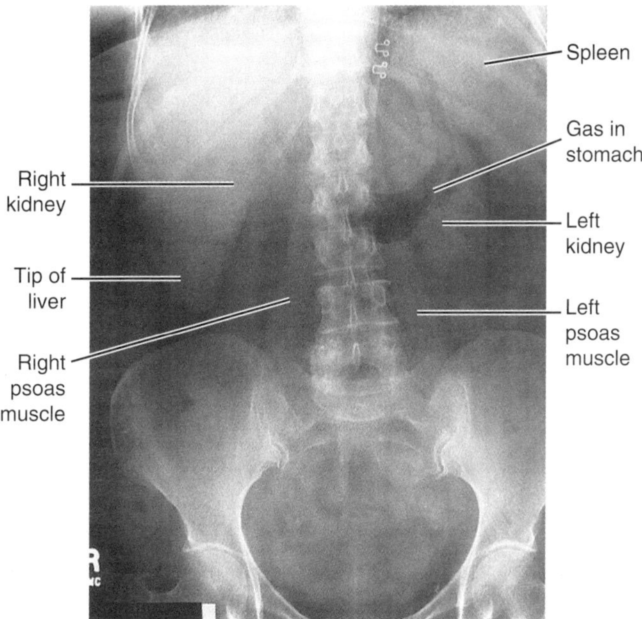

FIG. 27.4 Normal Plain Abdominal Radiograph in the Supine Position. (From Mettler FA. *Essentials of Radiology*. 4th ed. Elsevier; 2019.)

With an ERCP, obstructions may be identified and removal of obstructive material may be attempted. It may be used in the evaluation of pancreatitis. Additionally, strictures may be visualized and treated with stents. Lastly, biopsies may be obtained to differentiate benign or malignant masses.[4] A normal endoscopic retrograde cholangiopancreatography is depicted in Fig. 27.3.

Plain Abdominal Radiograph

In plain abdominal radiographs, an electrical device emits ionizing radiation that passes from the front to the back of the abdomen and captures a picture of internal body structures.[6] These radiographs are useful in evaluating bowel gas patterns, abdominal organs, calcifications (e.g., cholelithiasis), implanted devices (e.g., stents), or foreign bodies (e.g., metal, glass).[6] Plain abdominal radiographs may help identify pathologic patterns of bowel gas from an ileus, obstruction, volvulus, dilation, bowel inflammatory or ulcerative diseases, and fecal impaction.[6] Pathologic air outside of the abdomen may also be visualized, like a pneumothorax or pneumoperitoneum.[6] In addition to evaluating bowel gas or air patterns, plain abdominal radiographs may help visualize enlarged organs, like the liver, or fluid accumulations, like ascites.[6] Contrast may be administered for a plain abdominal radiograph to enhance the images of internal structure. When an abdominal radiograph is performed to evaluate the kidneys, ureters, and bladder, it is called a KUB. A normal plain abdominal radiograph in the supine position is depicted in Fig. 27.4.

Abdominal Ultrasound

An abdominal ultrasound generates an electrical signal from high-frequency sound wave transmissions and creates an image of tissues and organs. The ultrasound helps in identifying fluid accumulation (e.g., ascites), biliary obstruction or dilation, calculi (e.g., cholelithiasis), and masses.[7] The electrical signal may not penetrate air, present in the bowel, and hinder visualization of underlying pathology.[7]

Computed Tomography of the Abdomen and Pelvis

Computed tomography (CT) involves rotating ionizing radiation producing cross-sectional images that may be done with or without administration of an iodinated intravenous (IV) contrast or iodinated or barium-based oral or rectal contrast.[7] IV contrast enhances images of solid organs.[7] Oral contrast enhances the images of the stomach, small intestine, colon, and rectum.[7] For patients who are unable to tolerate oral contrast, a placement of a nasogastric tube (NGT) may be indicated for contrast administration. Rectal contrast, specifically, helps diagnose anastomotic leaks after surgery in patients who may not be able to have oral contrast due to an obstruction or ileus.[8] If ultrasound images are nondiagnostic, a computed tomography is usually needed.[7] If additional evaluation is needed after plain abdominal radiographs or if ultrasound images are nondiagnostic, a computed tomography is usually needed.[7] A normal computed tomography of the abdomen and pelvis is depicted in Fig. 27.5.

Magnetic Resonance Imaging

Magnetic resonance imaging (MRI) involves a strong magnetic field and high-energy radiofrequency waves to produce images of organs, masses, and blood vessels with or without the administration of gadolinium contrast.[7] An MRI provides information of inflammatory (e.g., Crohn's, infectious colitis) and oncological GI disorders (e.g., tumors of the GI tract and accessory organs).[9] Recent advances in MRI technology allow for a capture of organ movement, promoting research on the use of MRI to evaluate GI motility.[9] When magnetic resonance is used to assess blood vessels and blood flow, it is called a magnetic resonance angiography (MRA). When magnetic resonance is used to evaluate the biliary and pancreatic ducts, it is called a

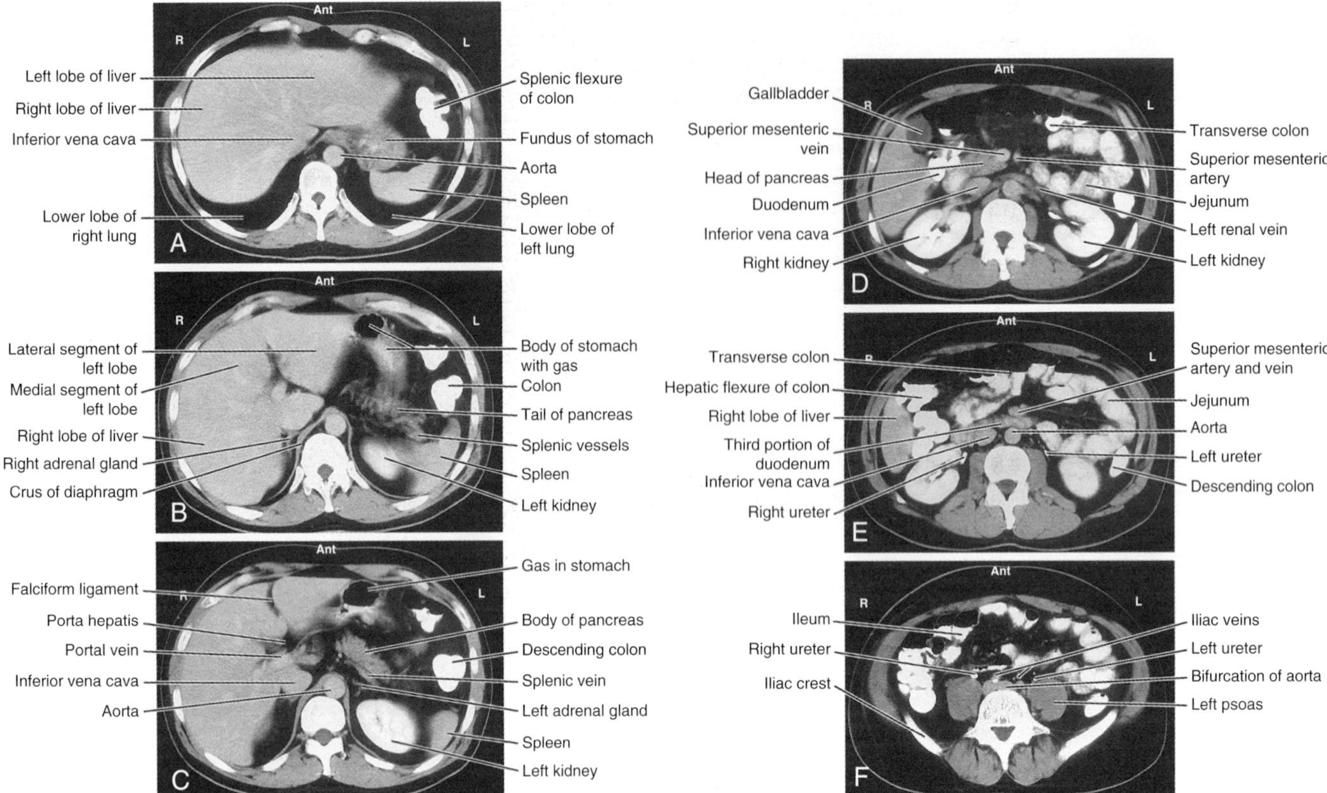

FIG. 27.5 Normal Computed Tomography of the Abdomen and Pelvis. (A–F) Cross-sectional images of abdominal and pelvis CT scan in a patient after receiving intravenous, oral, and rectal contrast. (From Mettler FA. *Essentials of Radiology*. 4th ed. Elsevier; 2019.)

magnetic resonance cholangiopancreatography (MRCP).[9] An MRCP is preferred over an ERCP if therapeutic intervention, like stents, is not needed.[9] Overall, an MRI is beneficial as it produces images without the need to use nephrotoxic iodinated contrast agents and without exposing the patient to ionizing radiation.[7,9]

MRIs require important safety considerations. The strong magnetic field of the MRI machine attracts ferromagnetic objects rapidly and forcefully toward the center of the MRI machine, making them projectiles with the potential to cause serious injury to patients and staff when these objects are near the MRI machine. For this reason, patients with metallic implants that are incompatible with MRI should not receive an MRI and metallic objects that are not permanently implanted should be removed before the procedure.

Radionuclide Imaging

In radionuclide imaging studies (also known as nuclear medicine scans), radiotracers are administered intravenously and gamma rays are detected to form an image of the organ.[7] There are a few nuclear medicine studies that are performed to diagnose GI disorders. The first study is a hepatobiliary scintigraphy in which the liver, gallbladder, and biliary ducts may be assessed for inflammation (e.g., cholecystitis), biliary obstruction, or biliary leaks.[7] A hepatobiliary scintigraphy is also known as a hepatobiliary iminodiacetic acid (HIDA) scan. The second study is a gastrointestinal bleeding scan in which red blood cells are labeled, or "tagged," with the radioactive material to detect movement of the blood and locate possible bleeding that was not found on endoscopy.[7] A bleeding scan helps localize low-flow *active* bleeding (as low as 0.5 mL/min) that would otherwise not be seen in an angiogram that detects bleeding at a flow of 4 mL/min.[7] Another nuclear medicine scan that helps with assessing GI function is one where food or liquid are tagged with radioactive material to quantify gastric emptying times or amount of gastroesophageal reflux.[7]

Angiography

Angiography involves the insertion of a catheter and injection of a contrast agent into the arteries to highlight blood vessels as the contrast agent moves through them. Angiography is used as a diagnostic and a therapeutic procedure. Diagnostically, it is used to evaluate the status of the GI and accessory organ circulation (Fig. 27.6). It may help identify the source of active bleeding at a flow rate of 4 mL/min if not localized on endoscopy.[7] Therapeutically, it is used to control of GI bleeding, with embolization, that was not managed with endoscopy.[10] Complications associated with angiography include hematomas and contrast-related complications.[10]

Liver Biopsy

Liver biopsy is a diagnostic procedure that is used to evaluate and stage liver disease.[11] There are different biopsy techniques and include percutaneous, transvenous, and laparoscopic.[11] Percutaneous liver biopsy involves inserting a needle through the abdomen to obtain a specimen from the liver. Transvenous liver biopsy involves inserting a needle through the veins to the liver to obtain a specimen. A laparoscopic biopsy is a surgical procedure. The two most common complications of a liver biopsy include pain and bleeding.[11]

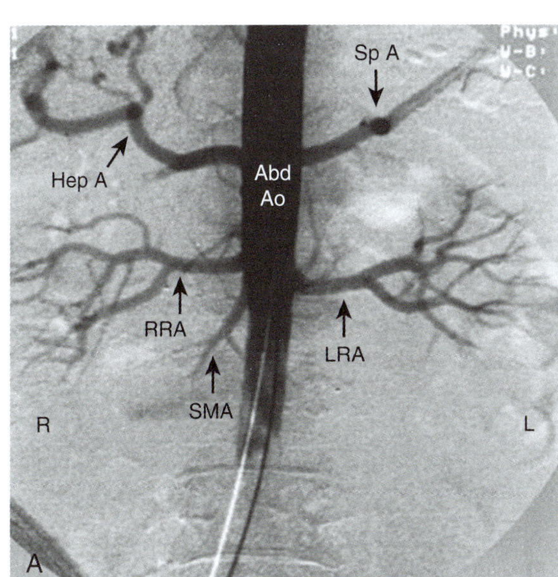

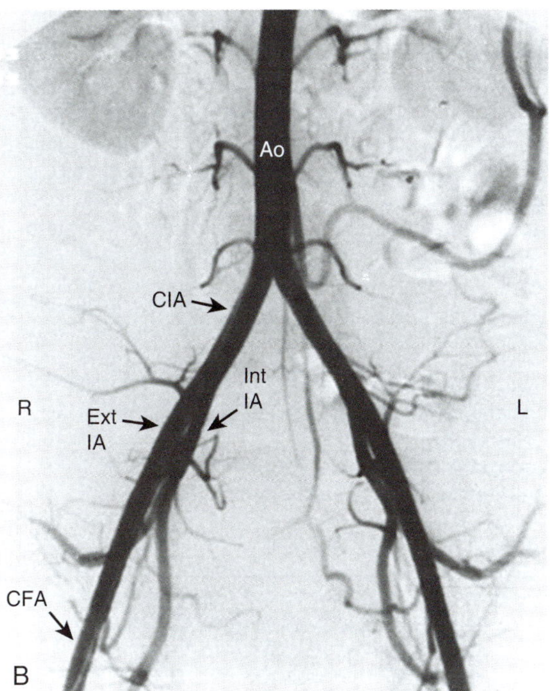

FIG. 27.6 Normal Vascular Anatomy of the Abdomen and Pelvis. (A) An angiogram in an anteroposterior projection of the upper abdomen shows the abdominal aorta *(Abd Ao)*, hepatic artery *(Hep A)* and splenic artery *(Sp A)*, right renal artery *(RRA)* and left renal artery *(LRA)*, and superior mesenteric artery *(SMA)*. (B) A subsequent image over the lower abdomen and pelvis taken a few seconds later shows the distal abdominal aorta with small lumbar branches, common iliac artery *(CIA)*, internal iliac artery *(Int IA)* and external iliac artery *(Ext IA)*, and common femoral artery *(CFA)*. *Ao,* Aorta. (From Mettler FA. *Essentials of Radiology*. 4th ed. Elsevier; 2019.)

KEY POINTS

History

- The history is structured to include patient identifiers, chief concern (CC), history of present illness or problem (HPI), past medical and surgical history (PMH), family history, personal and social history, and review of systems (ROS).

Focused Physical Assessment

- The abdomen is divided into four quadrants (left upper, right upper, left lower, and right lower), with the umbilicus as the middle point, to specify the location of examination findings.
- Inspection of the patient focuses on three areas: (1) observation of the oral cavity, (2) assessment of the skin over the abdomen, and (3) evaluation of the shape of the abdomen.
- Auscultation of the patient focuses on the evaluation of bowel sounds and assessment of bruits.
- Percussion is performed to detect size and density of the organs in the abdomen, such as the liver, and to detect the presence of fluid, air, or masses.
- With the patient in a supine position, the abdomen should be palpated to provide information about organ size, shape, mobility, and consistency.

Laboratory Studies

- No single laboratory study provides an overall picture of the functional state of the various organs in the GI tract.

Diagnostic Procedures

- In critically ill patients with GI dysfunction, several diagnostic procedures may be performed to identify or obtain further information related to structural or functional abnormalities of the GI tract and accessory organs, including endoscopy, plain abdominal radiograph, abdominal ultrasound, computed tomography (CT), magnetic resonance imaging (MRI), radionuclide imaging, angiography, and liver biopsy.
- Endoscopy can provide information about lesions, mucosal changes, obstructions, and motility dysfunction, and a biopsy or removal of foreign objects may be performed during the procedure.
- Plain abdominal radiographs are useful in evaluating bowel gas patterns, abdominal organs, calcifications (e.g., cholelithiasis), implanted devices (e.g., stents), or foreign bodies (e.g., metal, glass).
- The abdominal ultrasound helps in identifying fluid accumulation (e.g., ascites), biliary obstruction or dilation, calculi (e.g., cholelithiasis), and masses.
- During a CT, intravenous contrast enhances images of solid organs; oral contrast enhances the images of the stomach, small intestine, colon, and rectum; and rectal contrast helps diagnosis anastomotic leaks after surgery in patients who may not be able to have oral contrast due to an obstruction or ileus.
- An MRI provides information of inflammatory (e.g., Crohn's, infectious colitis) and oncological GI disorders (e.g., tumors of the GI tract and accessory organs)

- A hepatobiliary scintigraphy assesses the liver, gallbladder, and biliary ducts for inflammation (e.g., cholecystitis), biliary obstruction, or biliary leaks
- A gastrointestinal bleeding scan is when red blood cells are labeled, or "tagged," with the radioactive material to detect movement of the blood and locate possible bleeding that was not found on endoscopy.
- Diagnostically, an angiography is used to evaluate the status of the GI and accessory organ circulation.
- Therapeutically, an angiography is used to control GI bleeding, with embolization, that was not managed with endoscopy.
- Liver biopsy is a diagnostic procedure that is used to evaluate and stage liver disease.

Visit the Evolve site at http://evolve.elsevier.com/Urden/CriticalCareNursing **for additional study materials.**

REFERENCES

1. Ball JW, Dains JE, Flynn JA, Solomon BS, Stewart RW. Chapter 2. The history and interviewing process. In: Ball JW, Dains JE, Flynn JA, Solomon BS, Stewart RW, eds. *Seidel's Guide to Physical Examination.* 10th ed. Philadelphia, PA: Elsevier; 2023:12–34.
2. Ball JW, Dains JE, Flynn JA, Solomon BS, Stewart RW. Chapter 18. Abdomen. In: Ball JW, Dains JE, Flynn JA, Solomon BS, Stewart RW, eds. *Seidel's Guide to Physical Examination.* 10th ed. Philadelphia, PA: Elsevier; 2023:303–447.
3. Ball JW, Dains JE, Flynn JA, Solomon BS, Stewart RW. Chapter 13. Ears, nose, and throat. In: Ball JW, Dains JE, Flynn JA, Solomon BS, Stewart RW, eds. *Seidel's Guide to Physical Examination.* 10th ed. Philadelphia, PA: Elsevier; 2023:259–289.
4. Keen T, Brooks C. Principles of gastrointestinal endoscopy. *Surg.* 2023;41(2):100–105. https://doi.org/10.1016/j.mpsur.2022.11.005.
5. Oka P, McAlindon M, Sidhu R. Capsule endoscopy - a non-invasive modality to investigate the GI tract: out with the old and in with the new? *Expert Rev Gastroenterol Hepatol.* 2022;16(7):591–599. https://doi.org/10.1080/17474124.2022.2089113.
6. Loo JT, Duddalwar V, Chen FK, Tejura T, Lekht I, Gulati M. Abdominal radiograph pearls and pitfalls for the emergency department radiologist: a pictorial review. *Abdom Radiol (NY).* 2017;42(4):987–1019. https://doi.org/10.1007/s00261-016-0859-8.
7. Mettler FA. Chapter 6. Gastrointestinal system. In: Mettler FA, ed. *Essentials of Radiology.* 4th ed. Philadelphia, PA: Elsevier; 2019:125–167.
8. Marres CCM, Engelmann EWM, Buskens CJ, Haak HE, Bemelman WA, van de Ven AWH. The importance of rectal contrast in CT assessment to detect anastomotic leakage after colorectal surgery. *Colorectal Dis.* 2021;23(9):2466–2471. https://doi.org/10.1111/codi.15764.
9. Maccioni F, Busato L, Valenti A, Cardaccio S, Longhi A, Catalano C. Magnetic resonance imaging of the gastrointestinal tract: current role, recent advancements and future prospectives. *Diagnostics (Basel).* 2023;13(14):2410. https://doi.org/10.3390/diagnostics13142410.
10. Širvinskas A, Smolskas E, Mikelis K, Brimienė V, Brimas G. Transcatheter arterial embolization for upper gastrointestinal tract bleeding. *Wideochir Inne Tech Maloinwazyjne.* 2017;12(4):385–393. https://doi.org/10.5114/wiitm.2017.72319.
11. Khalifa A, Rockey DC. The utility of liver biopsy in 2020. *Curr Opin Gastroenterol.* 2020;36(3):184–191. https://doi.org/10.1097/MOG.0000000000000621.

28

Gastrointestinal Disorders and Therapeutic Management

Kathrine Anne Winnie and Kimberly Sanchez

http://evolve.elsevier.com/Urden/CriticalCareNursing

Understanding the pathology of gastric disorders, the areas of assessment on which to focus, and the usual medical management allows the critical care nurse to accurately anticipate and plan nursing interventions. This chapter focuses on gastrointestinal (GI) disorders commonly seen in the critical care environment.

ACUTE GASTROINTESTINAL HEMORRHAGE

Description and Etiology

GI hemorrhage is a manifestation of multiple GI disorders.[1] Because the manifestation is a potentially life-threatening emergency and a common complication of critical illness, the management of bleeding is the focus in critical care. GI hemorrhage is acute bleeding in the upper or lower GI tract. Bleeding proximal to the ligament of Treitz is considered to be from the upper GI tract, and bleeding distal to the ligament of Treitz is considered to be from the lower GI tract.[2] Anatomical differentiation between upper and lower GI tract is depicted in Fig. 28.1. The various causes of acute GI hemorrhage are listed in Box 28.1.[2,3] Most causes of GI hemorrhage occur in the upper GI tract.

Nonvariceal Upper Gastrointestinal Hemorrhage

Upper GI ulcers are a common cause of GI hemorrhage and develop from the breakdown of the gastric mucosal lining. The normal protective features of the gastric mucosal lining that prevent ulcerations (outlined in Chapter 26) are disrupted by an erosive process, such as hypersecretory disorders, use of nonsteroidal antiinflammatory medications, and the bacterial action of *Helicobacter pylori*. The ulcerations that develop extend through the mucosa and into the sub-mucosa, resulting in autodigestion when gastric secretions penetrate the mucosal layers. This may result in damaged blood vessels and subsequent gastrointestinal hemorrhage.[1] Acute stress-related gastric ulcers and peptic ulcers are two common types of upper GI ulcers that are present in patients in critical care units. Both peptic ulcers and acute-stress related gastric ulcers have the same pathological, erosive mechanisms that may lead to hemorrhage.[4]

Acute stress-related gastric ulcers. Acute stress-related gastric ulcers may develop with within hours to days of critical illness and range from superficial mucosal erosions to deep focal lesions. The primary causative factors in acute stress-related gastric ulcers are increased acid production and decreased blood flow, resulting in ischemia and degeneration of the mucosal lining. Patients at risk of stress-related gastritis are those in situations of high physiological stress, as occurs with mechanical ventilation, burns, severe trauma, major surgery, shock, sepsis, coagulopathy, or acute neurological disease.[5] Acute stress-related gastric ulcers are decreasing in incidence because of advances in therapeutic techniques and prevention of hypoperfusion of the mucosa.[6]

Peptic ulcers. The most common causes of peptic ulcers are increased acid production,[7] resulting in degeneration of the mucosal lining, or direct damage of the mucosal lining from an inflammatory response that can erode from contact with gastric acid.[8] Patients at risk for peptic ulcers are those who use nonsteroidal antiinflammatory medications or have an infection with *H. pylori*.[9] *H. pylori* identification and treatment along with proton pump inhibitors (PPIs) have been beneficial in decreasing incidence of peptic ulcers.[9]

Variceal Upper Gastrointestinal Hemorrhage

Varices are another common cause of GI hemorrhage. Varices are a manifestation of portal hypertension caused by hepatic cirrhosis, a chronic disease of the liver that results in damage to the liver sinusoids (Fig. 28.2).[10] Without adequate sinusoid function to transport blood to each lobule of the liver, resistance to the portal blood flow is increased and pressure within the liver is elevated. Increased vascular resistance is caused by anatomical structural distortion (e.g., fibrosis, vascular occlusion) and intrahepatic vasoconstriction. Blood flow increases due to splanchnic arteriolar vasodilation. Collateral circulation develops to divert portal blood from areas of high pressure within the liver to adjacent areas of low pressure outside the liver, such as into the veins of the esophagus, spleen, intestines, and stomach (Fig. 28.2).[11] The tiny, thin-walled submucosal vessels of the esophagus and proximal stomach that receive this diverted blood become engorged and dilated. Elevated intravariceal pressure and vessel wall tension may lead to vessel rupture and hemorrhage.[11] Key concepts related to acute GI hemorrhage are summarized in Fig. 28.3.

Pathophysiology

External erosion to or internal pressure of the blood vessels leads to vessel rupture and release of blood from the broken vessel. Blood may be retained inside the body or exit the body depending on the location of the hemorrhage, amount of blood lost, and rate of the loss. Circulating blood volume is decreased and, as a result, tissue oxygen demand is not met. Hypoperfusion of organs can lead to ischemia and organ failure.

Assessment and Diagnosis

The initial clinical presentation of a patient with acute GI hemorrhage depends on the amount of blood lost. Minimal

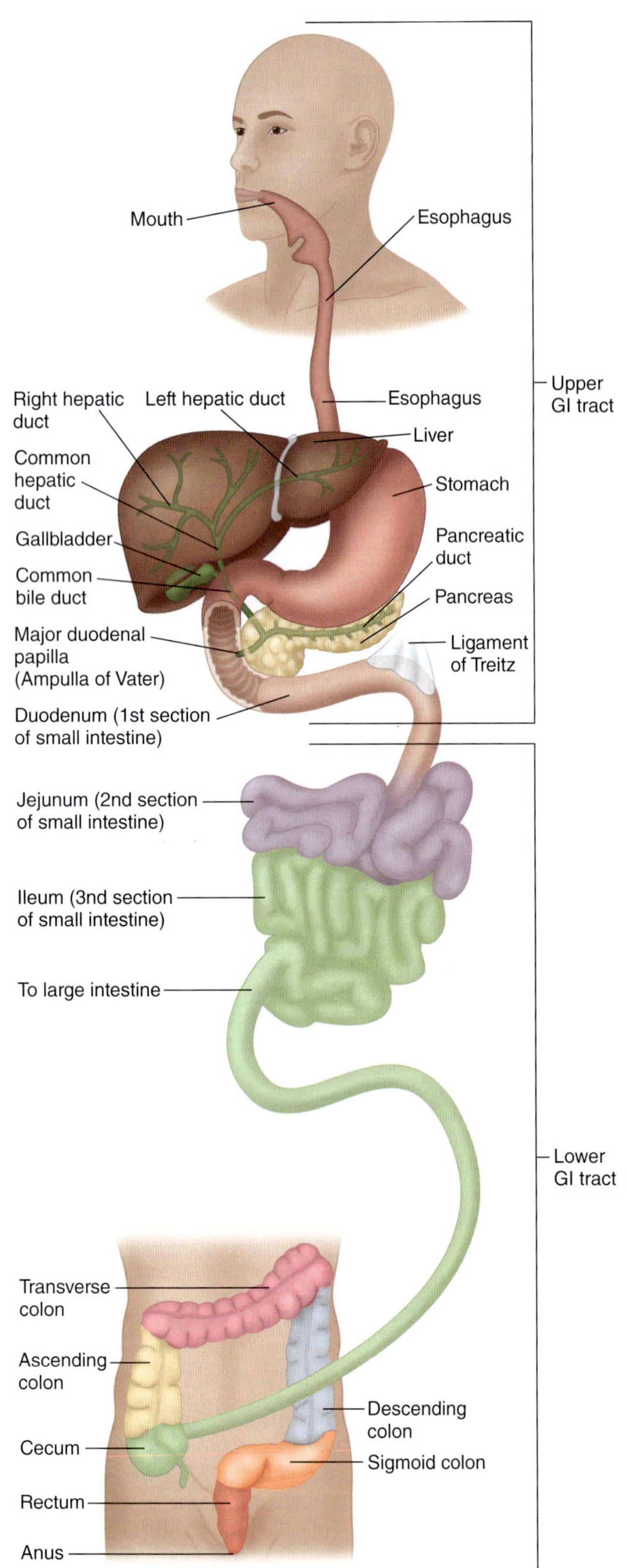

FIG. 28.1 Anatomy of Upper and Lower Gastrointestinal Tract. The ligament of Treitz is the anatomical division between the upper and lower GI tract. Bleeding proximal to the ligament of Treitz is classified as an upper GI bleed. Bleeding distal to the ligament of Treitz is classified as a lower GI bleed.

BOX 28.1 Causes of Acute Gastrointestinal Hemorrhage

Upper Gastrointestinal Tract
- Peptic ulcer disease
- Stress-related erosive syndrome
- Esophagogastric varices
- Mallory-Weiss tear
- Esophagitis
- Neoplasm
- Aortoenteric fistula
- Angiodysplasia

Lower Gastrointestinal Tract
- Diverticulosis
- Angiodysplasia
- Neoplasm
- Inflammatory bowel disease
- Trauma
- Infectious colitis
- Radiation colitis
- Ischemia
- Aortoenteric fistula
- Hemorrhoids

blood loss may be well tolerated; however, when blood loss is mild to severe, decreased blood pressure, increased heart rate, and mental status changes are likely present. Clinical signs and symptoms of hemorrhage are listed by amount of blood loss in Table 28.1. Hematemesis (bright red or brown, "coffee grounds" emesis), melena (black, tarry, or dark red stools), and hematochezia (bright red stools) are the hallmarks of GI hemorrhage.[1] A patient who is vomiting blood is usually bleeding from a source above the duodenojejunal junction;[3] reverse peristalsis is seldom enough to cause hematemesis if the bleeding point is below this area. The hematemesis may be bright red or look like coffee grounds, depending on the amount of gastric contents at the time of bleeding and the length of time the blood has been in contact with gastric secretions. Bright red emesis results from profuse bleeding with little contact with gastric secretions. Gastric acid converts bright red hemoglobin to brown hematin, accounting for the "coffee grounds" appearance of the emesis. The presence of blood in the GI tract results in increased peristalsis and diarrhea. Once blood passes the duodenojejunal junction and is digested throughout the GI tract, black tarry stools may be excreted by the patient; melena is indicative of an upper GI bleed[3] and may take several days to clear after the bleeding has stopped. Hematochezia occurs from massive lower GI hemorrhage and, if rapid enough, upper GI hemorrhage.[3]

Laboratory Studies

Laboratory tests can help determine the extent of bleeding. As whole blood is lost, plasma and red blood cells are lost in the same proportion.[1] The patient's hemoglobin level and hematocrit are poor indicators of the severity of blood loss if the bleeding is acute, but serial hemoglobin and hematocrit may be helpful.[12] A basic metabolic panel should also be collected[12] and an elevated BUN-to-creatinine ratio may indicate upper GI bleeding. Coagulation studies are helpful in selecting management strategies[12,13] and a type and crossmatch are required for transfusions.[12]

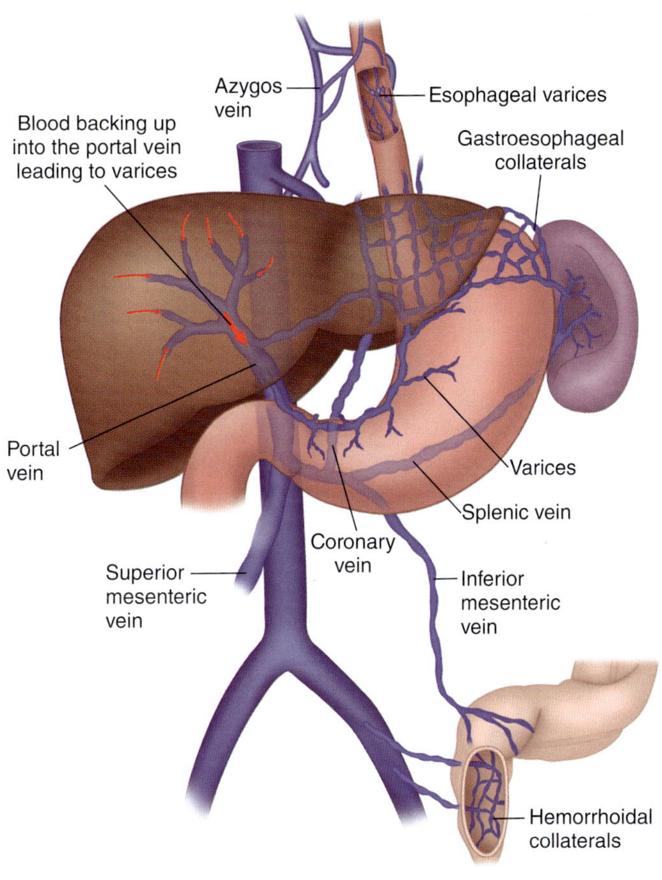

FIG. 28.2 Varices Related to Portal Hypertension. Portosystemic circulation is depicted, highlighting esophageal and gastroesophageal varices as a common site of gastrointestinal hemorrhage.

Acute Gastrointestinal Hemorrhage

Clinical and diagnostic assessments	Signs	Nursing interventions

• History and risk factors
  • Stressors (e.g., mechanical ventilation, coagulopathy, sepsis)
  • NSAID use
  • *H. pylori* infection
  • Portal hypertension
• Obtain vital signs
  • Hypoperfusion (e.g., decreased blood pressure, decreased CO, changes in heart rate)
• Clinical assessment
  • Any signs of bleeding
• Laboratory studies
  • Obtain CBC, BMP, type and screen
• Diagnostic procedures
  • Assist with endoscopy
	• Decrease in hemoglobin and hematocrit trend
	• Decreased UO
	• Increased BUN-to-Cr ratio
	• Altered electrolytes
	• Altered mental status
	• Fluid volume deficit
		• Administer fluids and blood products as ordered
		• Administer medications as ordered (e.g., PPI, octreotide)
		• Insert gastrointestinal tube as ordered
		• Maintain large bore IVs
		• Trend laboratory studies

FIG. 28.3 Summary of Key Concepts Related to "Acute Gastrointestinal Hemorrhage." *BMP*, Basic metabolic panel; *BUN*, blood urea nitrogen; *CBC*, complete blood count; *CO*, cardiac output; *Cr*, creatinine; *NSAID*, nonsteroidal antiinflammatory drug; *PPI*, proton pump inhibitor; *UO*, urine output.

TABLE 28.1 Clinical Signs and Symptoms of Hemorrhage by Amount of Blood Loss

Class	Blood Loss	Clinical Signs and Symptoms
1: Minimal blood loss	<15 % <750 mL	Mental status: slightly anxious or apprehensive Heart rate: normal or mild increase Blood pressure: normal Capillary refill: brisk (<2 s) Skin: warm and pink Respiratory rate: normal Urine output: >0.5 mL/kg/h (>30 mL/h)
2: Mild blood loss	15%–30% 750–1500 mL	Mental status: irritable and confused Heart rate: increased (≥100 beats/min) Blood pressure: normal Pulse pressure: decreased Peripheral pulses: diminished Capillary refill: delayed Skin: cool extremities, mottling Respiratory rate: mild increase Blood pressure: normal (supine) Urine output: mild oliguria (25–30 mL/h)
3: Moderate blood loss	30%–40% 2000 mL	Mental status: lethargic Heart rate: significantly increased (≥120 beats/min) Blood pressure: hypotension Peripheral pulses: thready Capillary refill: prolonged Skin: cool extremities, pale Respiratory rate: moderate increase Urine output: oliguria (5–15 mL/h)
4: Severe blood loss	>40 % >2000 mL	Mental status: lethargic, comatose Heart rate: severely increased (≥140 beats/min) Blood pressure: severe hypotension Central pulses: thready Skin: cold extremities, pallor, cyanosis Respiratory rate: severe increase Urine output: anuria

h, Hour; *min*, minute; *mL*, milliliter; *s*, seconds.

Medical Management

Prevention of GI hemorrhage is important to reduce the need for acute medical management. Priorities in the medical management of a patient with an acute GI hemorrhage include hemodynamic stability and bleeding control.[14]

Prevention

Management of a hospitalized patient at risk for GI hemorrhage may include prophylactic administration of pharmacologic agents for neutralization or suppression of gastric acids. Proton pump inhibitors and histamine-2 (H_2) antagonists are frequently used.[15] A meta-analysis suggested that patients who are receiving enteral feedings may not require stress ulcer prophylaxis.[15] Once a patient presents with bleeding, high-dose proton pump inhibitors are started immediately and treatment priorities focus on hemodynamic stability.

Hemodynamic Stability

The initial treatment priority is the restoration of adequate circulating blood volume to treat or prevent shock. This is accomplished with the administration of intravenous infusions of crystalloids, blood, and blood products.[12] A restrictive transfusion strategy is recommended for most patients, with acceptable hemoglobin levels greater than or equal to 8 g/dL. Patients with cardiac conditions should maintain a higher hemoglobin level, and the transfusion protocol for these patients is less restrictive. Patients in hypovolemic shock or with significant ongoing bleeding may be transfused to a higher hemoglobin level.[16] Two large-diameter peripheral intravenous catheters are needed to facilitate the rapid administration of intravenous fluids.[13]

A simultaneous treatment priority is maintaining a patent airway. If patients have active hematemesis or are unable to maintain a patent airway, tracheal intubation may be needed for stability and potential endoscopy.[10]

Bleeding Control (Nonvariceal)

Interventions to control bleeding are initiated after hemodynamic stability is achieved. Although nasogastric lavage has previously been routinely used prior to endoscopy to improve visualization during the procedure, there is no evidence to support the practice[12] and no evidence that it improves outcomes.[17] Prokinetic agents such as erythromycin intravenous infusion prior to endoscopy may improve visualization[12,17] but are not routinely recommended.[16]

Endoscopy is performed within 24 hours of presentation of acute bleeding.[16] Hemostatic therapy is recommended for actively bleeding ulcers, a visible vessel within an ulcer bed, or other high-risk circumstances.[16] Bleeding hemostasis may be accomplished by endoscopic injection therapy, thermal coagulation, or through-the-scope or over-the-scope hemostatic clips.[18] *Endoscopic injection therapy* involves the injection of a liquid agent in and around the ulcer, and often times the agent is epinephrine, to cause vasoconstriction and create a tamponade effect; however, it is a temporary solution to aid in the visualization of the ulcer and not an acceptable monotherapy. Other endoscopic injection agents are used for sclerosing of the bleed (e.g., ethanol), causing an inflammatory reaction that eventually produces a fibrous band.[19] *Thermal coagulation* uses heat or an electric current, causing coaptation of blood vessels. Risks include thermal injuries and risk of perforation.[18] *Through-the-scope* and *over-the-scope clips* provide mechanical hemostasis and thermal injury risk is minimal. Through-the-scope clips are used in patients with coagulopathies. Deploying these clips can be difficult in patients with fibrotic ulcers.[18] Over-the-scope clips are often used for refractory bleeding. Rare but severe complications include position deviation and intestinal obstruction.[18] If the source of the bleed is not localized during endoscopy, the patients will be monitored for continued bleeding or resolution.

The high-dose proton pump inhibitors that were started immediately upon bleeding presentation are continued for 72 hours after endoscopy due to the high risk of rebleeding. After 72 hours, doses are decreased to normal levels. A recent meta-analysis reported no difference in rebleeding, surgery, or mortality when proton pump inhibitors were administered orally versus intravenously.[12] When rebleeding occurs after endoscopy, a repeat endoscopy is recommended. When endoscopic therapy fails, the patient may require surgery or transarterial embolization (TAE).[14] Agents used during TAE include permanent (microspheres or platinum coils) or temporary materials (gelatin sponge).[20] The agent used during TAE is decided by the provider performing the procedure.[20]

Bleeding Control (Variceal)

Endoscopic intervention to control bleeding is initiated after hemodynamic stability is achieved and after octreotide has been infusing for at least 30 minutes. The use of octreotide, a sandostatin analog, is used to reduce pressure in blood vessels. An intravenous bolus dose of 50 mcg (repeated in first hour if patient continues to bleed) is followed by a continuous intravenous infusion at 50 mcg/hr for 2 to 5 days. It is recommended octreotide be discontinued after bleeding definitively stops. Octreotide will inhibit gastric secretions and concurrent use with a PPI is not necessary. Due to the high risk of infection and bacterial translocation in these patients, prophylactic antibiotics are administered for up to 7 days.

Once stability is achieved and octreotide has been infusing for 30 minutes, endoscopy is recommended within 12 hours. Intravenous erythromycin may be used for visualization prior to endoscopy.[10] Several endoscopic procedures may be performed to manage the bleeding. First, endoscopic variceal ligation (EVL) includes the use of elastic bands around the circumference of the bleeding varices to obstruct the varices to prevent further bleeding (Fig. 28.4). EVL is a common endoscopic treatment for varices. Although EVL requires several endoscopies, it destroys the varices, is easy to use, and is considered a better alternative than sclerotherapy.[18] Days after the procedure, the band and tissue naturally slough off after a scar forms around the EVL site. When performing an EVL, there is a risk of ulceration or stricture formation from the band used to obstruct the varices. Another endoscopic procedure to manage the bleeding is endoscopic injection therapy with glue. The glue solidifies the varices and has a high initial hemostasis rate. Complications with this endoscopic injection therapy are rare but severe and include pulmonary embolism and portal vein thrombosis. The next endoscopic procedure available for treatment is an endoscopic ultrasound-guided glue injection and coiling. The endoscopy allows visualization and the ultrasound provides information about blood flow. Once the bleeding is localized, embolization coils can be deployed. Though the technical skill required to complete this endoscopic ultrasound-guided procedure is increased, performing the procedure requires less glue and less endoscopies for the patient.[18] Complications of endoscopic ultrasound-guided glue injection and coiling are rare but include pulmonary embolism. Lastly, other endoscopic procedures use hemostasis powder or self-expanded metal stents. Not all facilities have the ability to use stents and their placement is technically demanding. However, when stenting is performed, the procedure has higher clinical success than balloon tamponade and lower risk for some complications, including esophageal tear, aspiration, and mucosal ischemia.[18]

When endoscopic treatment fails, the transjugular intrahepatic portosystemic shunt (TIPS) procedure may be performed within 72 hours to decrease the risk of future bleeding episodes. The TIPS procedure is performed by an interventional radiologist who uses angiography to guide placement of a stent that shunts some blood away from the liver (portal vein to the hepatic vein to the inferior vena cava) and reduces pressure in the portal vein (Fig. 28.5).[10] The anatomic location of a TIPS is depicted in Fig. 28.6. Postprocedural care should include observation for overt (cannulation site) or covert (intrahepatic site) bleeding, hepatic or portal vein laceration (resulting in rapid loss of blood volume), and inadvertent puncture of surrounding organs. Other complications include liver failure, bacteremia, and stent stenosis.[21] In addition to angiography, there is an option for surgical portosystemic shunts.[22] The portosystemic shunt operative procedures are depicted in Fig. 28.7.

Nursing Management

The patient care management plan for a patient experiencing acute GI hemorrhage incorporates a variety of patient problems (Box 28.2). The nurse plays a role in gastrointestinal intubation, maintaining surveillance for complications, and educating the patient and family.

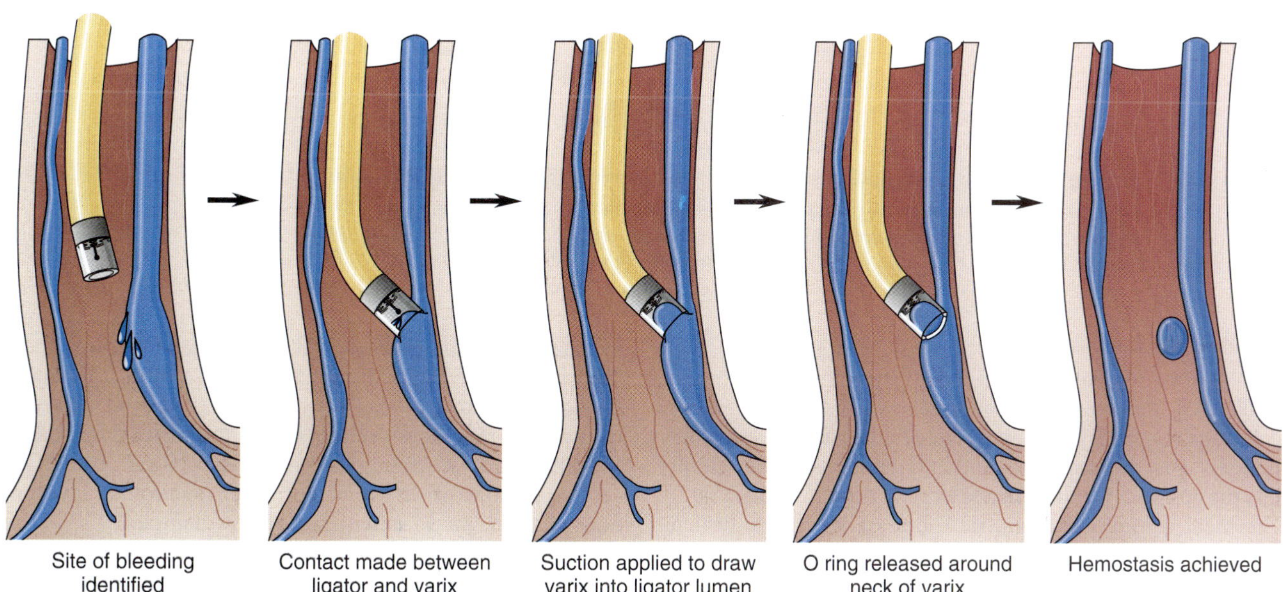

FIG. 28.4 Endoscopic Variceal Ligation. (From Copstead LC, Banasik JL, eds. *Pathophysiology*. 6th ed. Elsevier; 2019.)

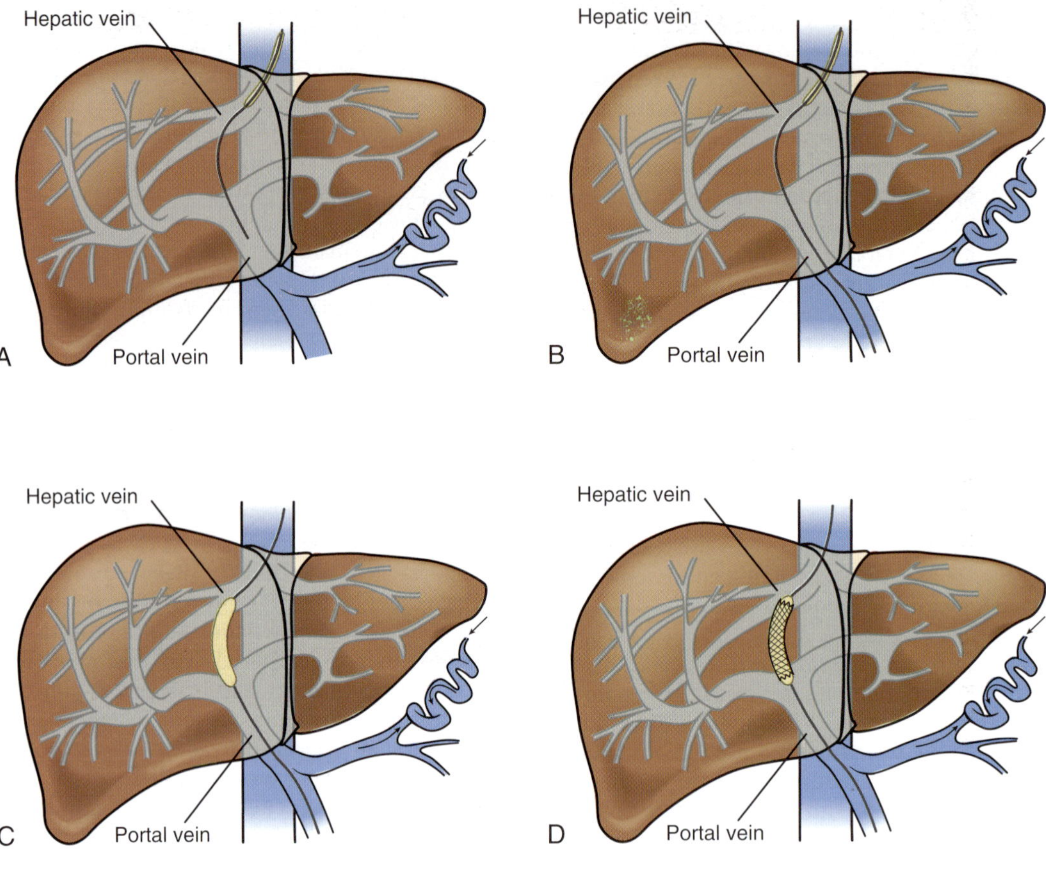

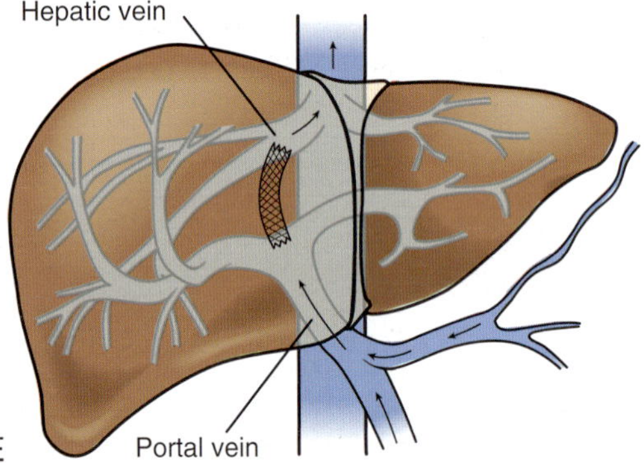

FIG. 28.5 Transjugular Intrahepatic Portosystemic Shunt (TIPS) Procedure. (A) Needle directed through liver parenchyma to portal vein. (B) Needle and guidewire passed down to midportal vein. (C) Balloon dilation. (D) Deployment of stent in liver parenchyma. (E) Intrahepatic shunt from portal to hepatic vein. (From Urden LD, Stacy KM, Lough ME. *Priorities in Critical Care Nursing*. 9th ed. Elsevier; 2023.)

Gastrointestinal Intubation

If gastrointestinal intubation is part of the therapeutic management of GI bleeding, the nurse places and manages the gastrointestinal tube. Nasogastric (NG) tubes are inserted in the nares, through the oropharynx, past the esophagus, and into the stomach. The length of time the nasogastric tube remains in place depends on its use.

The most common nasogastric tubes are the single-lumen Levin tube and the double-lumen Salem sump. Levin tubes are primarily used for feeding. Feeding tubes are discussed in Chapter 6. The Salem sump has one lumen that is used for suction and drainage and another that allows air to enter the patient's stomach and prevents the tube from adhering to the gastric wall and damaging the mucosa. The Salem sump removes remove fluid regurgitated into the stomach, prevents accumulation of swallowed air, may partially decompress the bowel, and reduces the patient's risk for aspiration. It may also be used for collecting specimens and assessing the presence of blood. The NG tube can be placed to gravity, low intermittent suction, or low continuous suction, and in rare instances, it is clamped.

Patient care management focuses on preventing complications common to this therapy, such as ulceration and necrosis of the nares, esophageal reflux, esophagitis, esophageal erosion and stricture, gastric erosion, and dry mouth and parotitis from mouth breathing.

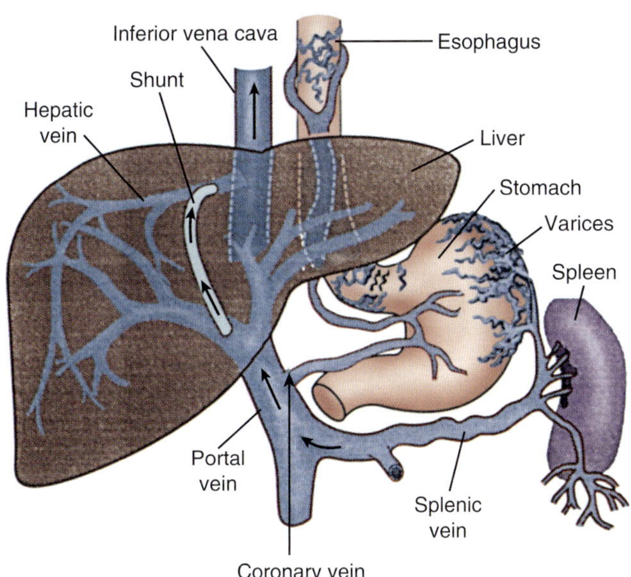

FIG. 28.6 Anatomic Location of Transjugular Intrahepatic Portosystemic Shunt (TIPS). (From Vargas HE, Gerber D, Abu-Elmagd K. Management of portal hypertension-related bleeding. *Surg Clin North Am.* 1999;79(1):1–22. https://doi.10.1016/s0039-6109(0570004-9)

Maintain Surveillance for Complications

All critically ill patients should be considered at risk for GI hemorrhage. Patients at risk also should be assessed for the presence of bright red or coffee ground emesis; bloody nasogastric aspirate; and bright red, black, or dark red stools. Any signs of bleeding should be promptly reported to the provider for immediate medical management.

After an endoscopic procedure, the patient should be continuously observed for signs of gastric perforation. Although a rare complication, gastric perforation constitutes a surgical emergency. Signs and symptoms include sudden, severe, generalized abdominal pain with significant rebound tenderness and rigidity. Perforation should be suspected when fever, leukocytosis, and tachycardia persist despite adequate volume replacement.

Educate the Patient and Family

Early in the hospital stay, the patient and family should be taught about acute GI hemorrhage and its causes and treatments. Closer to discharge, teaching should focus on the interventions necessary for preventing the recurrence of the precipitating disorder and steps to take if another bleed should occur. If the patient abuses alcohol, the patient should be encouraged to stop drinking and be referred to an alcohol cessation program. The patient and family education plan is summarized in Box 28.3.

Interprofessional collaborative management of the patient with acute GI hemorrhage is outlined in Box 28.4.

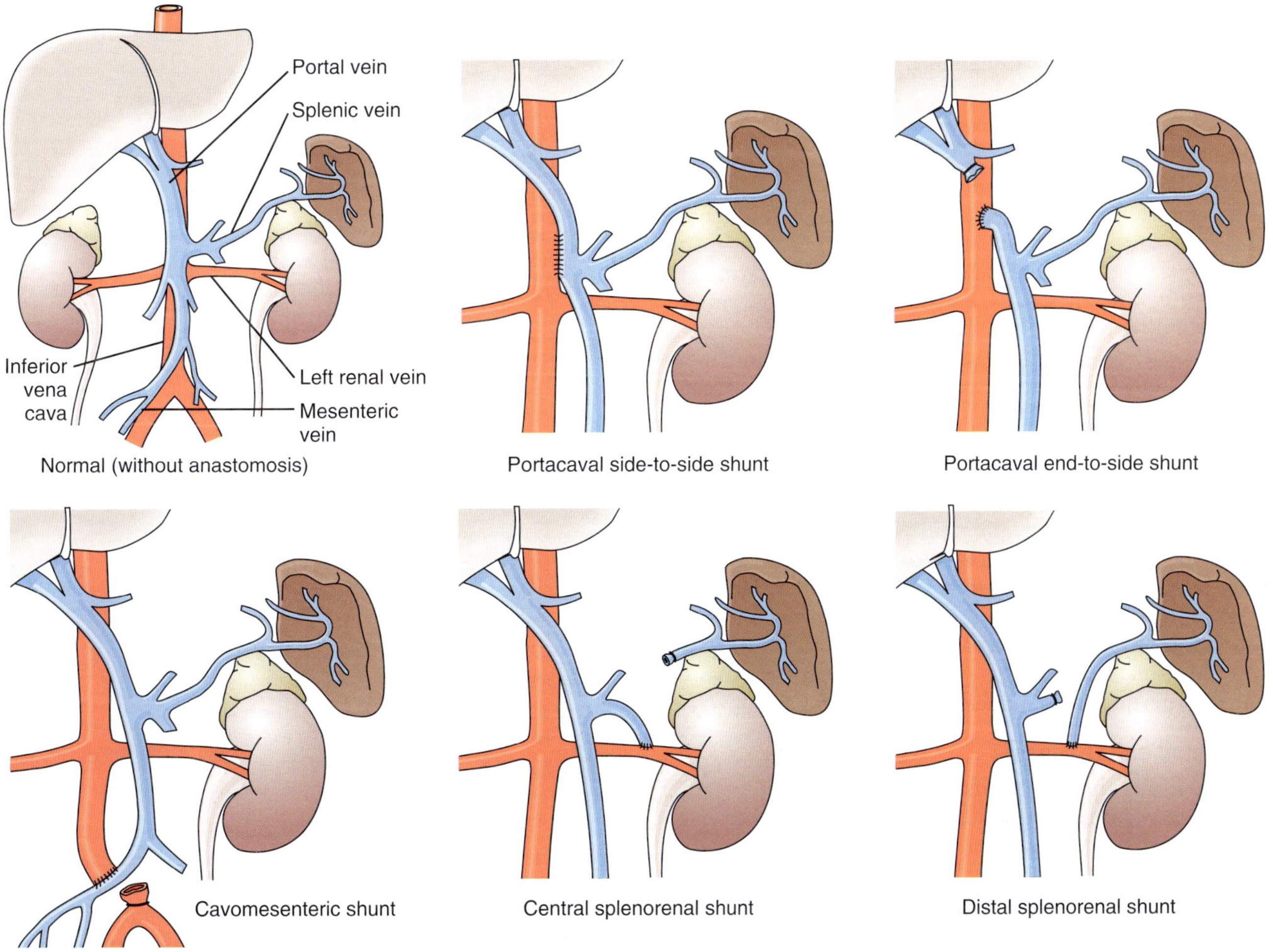

FIG. 28.7 Portosystemic Shunt Operative Procedures. (From Copstead LC, Banasik J, eds. *Pathophysiology.* 6th ed. Elsevier; 2019.)

ACUTE PANCREATITIS

Description and Etiology

Acute pancreatitis is a complex gastrointestinal disease that is characterized by enlargement of the pancreas and enhancement of pancreatic parenchyma with peripancreatic fat inflammation that may involve surrounding tissues, organ systems, or both. The clinical course can range from a mild, self-limiting disease to a systemic process characterized by organ failure, sepsis, and death. Estimated incidence of acute pancreatitis is 110 to 140 per 100,000 people.[23] Reported mortality rates for severe acute pancreatitis are as high as 30%.[24]

Acute pancreatitis is divided into two subtypes: interstitial edematous pancreatitis and necrotizing pancreatitis. Severity classifications are based on local and systemic complications and presence and duration of organ failure (Box 28.5). Interstitial edematous pancreatitis may be classified as mild or moderately severe, while necrotizing pancreatitis is classified as either moderately severe or severe.[23] Approximately 80% of patients with acute pancreatitis have mild or moderately severe pancreatitis. The remaining 20% of patients develop severe pancreatitis.

The most common causes of acute pancreatitis are gallstones and alcohol use.[23] Together, they account for approximately 80% of cases.[23] Less common causes are quite diverse and include hypertriglyceridemia, hypercalcemia, various toxins, ischemia, infections, and the use of certain medications. In 20% of patients with acute pancreatitis, no etiologic factor can be determined.[1,23] The causes of acute pancreatitis are listed in Box 28.6. Key concepts related to acute pancreatitis are summarized in Fig. 28.8.

Pathophysiology

Injury to the acinar cells within the pancreas or other pathophysiologic triggers (e.g., edema, ischemia, infection) lead to intracellular and extracellular activation of enzymes causing premature release of trypsin and other digestive enzymes.[1,23] The digestive enzymes cause autodigestion of the pancreatic cells and tissues resulting in inflammation and vascular damage. Other local effects include fat necrosis and peripancreatic fluid collections, which may become infected and develop into pseudocysts on the pancreas.[23] If injury to the pancreatic cells is mild and without necrosis, edematous pancreatitis develops. If injury to the pancreatic cells is severe, the patient may develop necrotizing pancreatitis. Cellular destruction in pancreatic injury results in the release of toxic enzymes and inflammatory mediators into the systemic circulation and causes injury to vessels and other organs distant from the pancreas. Systemic complications may include vasodilation, hypotension, coagulation abnormalities, systemic inflammatory response syndrome, respiratory distress syndrome, peritonitis, renal failure, sepsis, and shock.[1]

Assessment and Diagnosis

When obtaining the patient history, it is important to gather information regarding previous pancreatitis episodes, family history, and preceding events known to cause pancreatitis including trauma, insect bites, gallstones, alcohol use, and infections (Box 28.6). An accurate list of home medications can be used to determine if the patient is on any medications that have been associated with pancreatitis.[23]

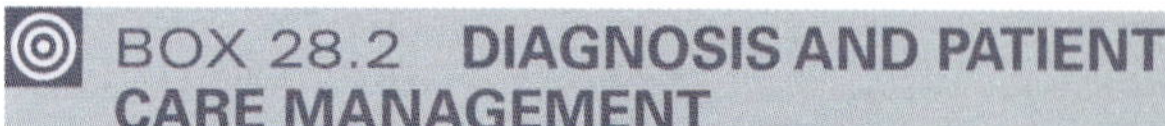

BOX 28.2 DIAGNOSIS AND PATIENT CARE MANAGEMENT

Acute Gastrointestinal Hemorrhage

- Hypovolemia due to absolute loss
- Impaired Cardiac Output due to alterations in preload
- Risk for Aspiration
- Impaired Nutritional Intake due to lack of exogenous nutrients and increased metabolic demand
- Powerlessness due to lack of control over current situation or disease progression
- Impaired Family Coping critically ill family member
- Lack of Knowledge of Treatment Regime due to lack of previous exposure to information (see Patient and Family Education Plan, Box 28.3)

Patient Care Management Plans are located in Appendix A.

BOX 28.3 PATIENT AND FAMILY EDUCATION PLAN

Acute Gastrointestinal Hemorrhage

Before discharge, the patient should be able to teach back the following topics:

- Gastrointestinal hemorrhage
- Specific cause
- Precipitating factor modification
- Interventions to reduce further bleeding episodes
- Importance of taking medications
- Lifestyle changes
- Stress management
- Diet modifications
- Alcohol cessation
- Smoking cessation

BOX 28.4 Teamwork and Collaboration

Interprofessional Collaborative Practice: Acute Gastrointestinal Hemorrhage

- Initiate fluid resuscitation to achieve hemodynamic stability.
  - Crystalloids
  - Colloids
  - Blood and blood products
- Determine the cause of bleeding.
- Control bleeding.
  - Octreotide
  - Endoscopic interventions
  - Transjugular intrahepatic portosystemic shunt
  - Surgery (last resort)
- Provide comfort and emotional support.
- Maintain surveillance for complications.
  - Hypovolemic shock
  - Gastric perforation

The results of a focused physical assessment usually reveal hypoactive bowel sounds and abdominal tenderness, guarding, distention, and tympany. Findings that previously were used to indicate possible pancreatic hemorrhage include Grey-Turner sign (gray-blue discoloration of the flanks) and Cullen sign (discoloration of the umbilical region); however, these signs are not

BOX 28.5 Severity Classifications of Acute Pancreatitis

Mild Severity
- No organ failure
- No local or systemic complications
- Subtypes: Interstitial edematous pancreatitis

Moderate Severity
- Transient organ failure, resolves within 48 hours
- Local or systemic complications without persistent organ failure
- Subtypes: Interstitial edematous pancreatitis, necrotizing pancreatitis

Severe Severity
- Persistent organ failure, lasts for greater than 48 hours
- One or more organs fail
- Subtypes: Necrotizing pancreatitis

BOX 28.6 Causes of Acute Pancreatitis

- Biliary disease (stones, sludge, common bile duct obstruction)
- Alcohol
- Hypertriglyceridemia
- Toxins (ethyl alcohol, methyl alcohol, scorpion, venom, parathion)
- Medications (thiazides, immunosuppressive agents, antiinflammatory drugs)
- Hypercalcemia (hyperparathyroidism)
- Tumors (periampullary, pancreatic head mass, cystic lesions)
- Infections (bacterial, viral, parasitic)
- Trauma (iatrogenic: abdominal, surgical, endoscopic)
- Sphincter of Oddi dysfunction
- Autoimmune diseases
- Ampullary stenosis

Pancreatic strictures
- Pancreatic divisum
- Idiopathic cause

Acute Pancreatitis

Clinical and diagnostic assessments	Signs	Nursing interventions

• History and risk factors
  • Gallstones
  • Alcohol use
  • Insect bites
  • Previous ERCP
• Obtain vital signs
  • Tachycardic
  • Hypotensive
• Clinical assessment
  • Acute onset epigastric or midabdominal pain
  • Nausea and/or vomiting
  • Abdominal distention
  • Diaphoresis
• Laboratory studies
  • Obtain CBC, CMP, lipid panel, amylase, lipase
• Diagnostic procedures
  • Ultrasound, CT, MRI
	• Increased amylase
	• Increased lipase
	• Altered electrolytes
		• Administer fluids as ordered
		• Correct electrolytes as ordered
		• Administer analgesics as ordered
		• Promote nutrition

FIG. 28.8 Summary of Key Concepts Related to "Acute Pancreatitis." *CBC*, Complete blood count; *CMP*, complete metabolic panel; *CT*, computed tomography; *ERCP*, endoscopic retrograde cholangiopancreatography; *MRI*, magnetic resonance imaging.

sensitive or specific and are best used as a sign of abdominal pathology or retroperitoneal bleeding.[25] A palpable abdominal mass may indicate the presence of a pseudocyst or abscess.

The clinical manifestations of acute pancreatitis range from mild to severe and often mimic the manifestations of other disorders (Box 28.7). The patient usually presents with acute onset of abdominal pain in the epigastric or midabdominal area that may radiate to the back.[1] The pain is often described as constant and worse after eating, drinking, or lying supine.[23] Pain ranges from mild and tolerable to severe and incapacitating. Nausea, vomiting, and a low-grade fever are common.[23] Other clinical findings may include diaphoresis, weakness, tachypnea, hypotension, tachycardia,[1] abdominal distention, and decreased bowel sounds.[23] Depending on the extent of fluid loss and hemorrhage, the patient may exhibit signs of hypovolemic shock.[1]

Laboratory tests and findings in acute pancreatitis are summarized in Table 28.2. For patients with recurrent acute pancreatitis with no cause identified, consider genetic testing.

The diagnosis of acute pancreatitis requires two of these three features: (1) abdominal pain that is characteristic of acute pancreatitis; (2) serum lipase or serum amylase values that are at least three times the upper normal value; and (3) evidence of acute pancreatitis on ultrasonography, contrast-enhanced computed tomography, or magnetic resonance imaging (MRI).[1]

Medical Management

The identification and treatment of the causes of pancreatitis are essential to prevent recurrence and may guide treatment decisions. Potential interventions based on cause include medication changes or adjustments, alcohol cessation counseling, and cholecystectomy.[23] The medical management for acute pancreatitis focuses on appropriate fluid resuscitation, nutrition, and identification and management of local and systemic complications.

Fluid Resuscitation

Because pancreatitis is often associated with massive fluid shifts, intravenous crystalloids are administered immediately to ensure tissue perfusion and maintain hemodynamic stability. Electrolytes are monitored closely, and abnormalities such as hypocalcemia, hypokalemia, and hypomagnesemia are corrected. If hyperglycemia develops, exogenous insulin may be required.[26] Current guidelines do not recommend a specific type of fluid for resuscitation; however, there is evidence that lactated Ringer solution may be superior to 0.9% sodium chloride solution due to the antiinflammatory effects of the lactate.[26,27] Fluids should be administered at 5 to 10 mL/kg/h[28] until resuscitation goals are met (e.g., heart rate and blood pressure within acceptable range, fluid responsiveness, increased urine output).[23]

Nutrition Support

The philosophies regarding nutrition support have shifted over time. Detailed information on nutrition is discussed in Chapter 6. Previously, conventional nutrition management was to place the patient on a nothing by mouth (NPO) regimen and institute intravenous hydration. The rationale was to rest the inflamed pancreas and prevent enzyme release. This is no longer the standard of practice.[29] Current guidelines recommend starting oral intake within 24 hours, once abdominal pain is decreasing and inflammatory markers are improving, to protect the gut-mucosal barrier and reduce the incidence of bacterial translocation. Patients who are unable to take oral intake should be started on enteral nutrition, either via the nasogastric or nasoenteric (duodenal or jejunal) route. Enteral nutrition is preferred over total parenteral nutrition.[26] Evidence has shown that enteral nutrition is safe, cost effective, and associated with fewer septic and metabolic complications than parenteral nutrition. Parenteral nutrition is only indicated if the patient is unable to tolerate enteral nutrition.[30] In the past, nasogastric suction was also recommended, but this intervention has not been shown to be beneficial and should be instituted only if the patient has persistent vomiting, obstruction, or gastric distention.

Complications

Local complications include the development of infected pancreatic necrosis and pancreatic pseudocyst.

The necrotic areas of the pancreas can lead to development of a widespread pancreatic infection (infected pancreatic necrosis), which significantly increases the risk of death.[24] Prophylactic antibiotics may not reduce mortality in patients suspected to have necrotizing pancreatitis. Intravenous antibiotics should not be used prophylactically,[26] but if sepsis, abscess, or biliary calculi are evident, they are indicated.[31] When the patient develops infected pancreatic necrosis, surgical intervention is necessary. The procedure of choice is a minimally invasive necrosectomy, which entails careful debridement of the necrotic tissue in and around the pancreas.[24] This procedure is ideally performed after the necrotic area has been clearly demarcated, or "walled-off," typically 4 weeks after the onset of pancreatitis.[24]

A pancreatic pseudocyst is a collection of pancreatic fluid enclosed by a nonepithelialized wall. Cyst formation may result from liquefaction of a pancreatic fluid collection or from direct obstruction in the main pancreatic duct. A pancreatic pseudocyst may (1) resolve spontaneously; (2) rupture, resulting in peritonitis; (3) erode a major blood vessel, resulting in hemorrhage; (4) become infected, resulting in abscess; or (5) invade surrounding structures, resulting in obstruction. Treatment involves drainage of the pseudocyst surgically, endoscopically, or percutaneously.[28]

Acute pancreatitis also affects every organ system (Box 28.8), and recognition and treatment of systemic complications are crucial to management of the patient.

BOX 28.7 Clinical Manifestations of Acute Pancreatitis

- Pain
- Location: left upper quadrant or midepigastrium radiating to the back
- Onset: sudden
- Quality: severe, deep, continuous
- Aggravating factors: food and alcohol
- Nausea and vomiting
- Flushing and diaphoresis
- Low-grade fever
- Abdominal distention
- Abdominal tenderness and guarding
- Abdominal tympany
- Hypoactive or absent bowel sounds
- Jaundice
- Palpable abdominal mass
- Basilar crackles
- Tachypnea
- Tachycardia
- Hypotension

TABLE 28.2 Laboratory Tests and Findings in Acute Pancreatitis

Laboratory Study	Finding in Pancreatitis
Serum amylase	Elevated
Urine amylase	Elevated
Serum lipase	Elevated
Serum triglycerides	Elevated
Cross-reactive protein	Elevated
Glucose	Elevated
Calcium	Decreased[a]
Magnesium	Decreased
Potassium	Decreased
White blood cell count	Elevated
Bilirubin	May be elevated
Liver enzymes	May be elevated
Prothrombin time	Prolonged
Arterial blood gases	Hypoxemia, metabolic acidosis

[a]Hypercalcemia is a cause of pancreatitis and calcium may remain elevated with hyperparathyroidism, thyrotoxicosis, or malignancy.

Nursing Management

The patient care management plan for a patient with acute pancreatitis incorporates a variety of patient problems (Box 28.9). The nurse plays a significant role in providing comfort and emotional support, maintaining surveillance for complications, and educating the patient and family.

Provide Comfort and Emotional Support

Pain management is a priority in acute pancreatitis. Administration of around-the-clock analgesics to achieve pain relief is essential. Morphine, fentanyl, and hydromorphone are the commonly used opioids for pain control. Nonpharmacologic management techniques to assist with pain control include relaxation techniques and laying in the knee-chest position. Pain and pain management are discussed in detail in Chapter 7.

Maintain Surveillance for Complications

The patient is routinely monitored for signs of local or systemic complications (Box 28.8). Intensive monitoring of each of the organ systems is imperative because organ failure is a major indicator of the severity of the disease. Intraabdominal pressure monitoring is initiated if intraabdominal hypertension is suspected. The patient is closely monitored for signs and symptoms of pancreatic infection, which include increased abdominal pain and tenderness, fever, and increased white blood cell count (Box 28.10).[32]

Educate the Patient and Family

Early in the patient's hospital stay, the patient and family should be taught about acute pancreatitis and its causes and treatment. Closer to discharge, teaching should focus on the interventions necessary for preventing recurrence. If sustained, permanent damage to the pancreas has occurred, the patient will require teaching specific to diet modification. Diabetes education may also be necessary. If the patient abuses alcohol, the patient should be encouraged to stop drinking and be referred to an alcohol cessation program. The patient and family education plan is summarized in Box 28.11.

BOX 28.8 Systemic Complications of Acute Pancreatitis

Respiratory
- Early hypoxemia
- Pleural effusion
- Atelectasis
- Pulmonary infiltration
- Acute respiratory distress syndrome
- Mediastinal abscess

Cardiovascular
- Hypotension and shock
- Pericardial effusion
- ST-T changes

Renal
- Acute kidney injury
- Oliguria
- Renal artery or vein thrombosis

Hematologic
- Disseminated intravascular coagulation
- Thrombocytosis
- Hyperfibrinogenemia

Endocrine
- Hypocalcemia
- Hypertriglyceridemia
- Hyperglycemia

Neurologic
- Fat emboli
- Psychosis
- Encephalopathy and coma

Ophthalmic
- Purtscher retinopathy (sudden blindness)

Dermatologic
- Subcutaneous fat necrosis

Gastrointestinal or Hepatic
- Intraabdominal hypertension/abdominal compartment syndrome (>20 mm Hg)
- Hepatic dysfunction
- Obstructive jaundice
- Stress ulceration
- Erosive gastritis
- Paralytic ileus
- Duodenal obstruction
- Bowel infarction
- Massive intraperitoneal bleed
- Perforation
  - Stomach
  - Duodenum
  - Small bowel
  - Colon

mm Hg, Millimeters of mercury.

BOX 28.9 DIAGNOSIS AND PATIENT CARE MANAGEMENT

Acute Pancreatitis

- Acute Pain due to transmission and perception of cutaneous, visceral, muscular, or ischemia impulses
- Hypovolemia due to relative fluid loss
- Impaired Cardiac Output due to alterations in preload
- Impaired Breathing due to decreased lung expansion
- Impaired Nutritional Intake due to lack of exogenous nutrients or increased metabolic demand
- Anxiety due to threat to biologic, psychological, or social integrity
- Impaired Family Coping due to critically ill family member
- Lack of Knowledge of Treatment Regime due to lack of previous exposure to information (see Patient and Family Education Plan, Box 28.11)

Patient Care Management Plans are located in Appendix A.

BOX 28.10 Signs and Symptoms of Pancreatic Infection

- Persistent abdominal pain
- Abdominal tenderness
- Prolonged fever
- Abdominal distention
- Palpable abdominal mass
- Nausea and vomiting
- Increased white blood cell count
- Persistent elevation of serum amylase
- Hyperbilirubinemia
- Elevated alkaline phosphatase level
- Positive culture and Gram stain

BOX 28.11 PATIENT AND FAMILY EDUCATION PLAN

Acute Pancreatitis

Before discharge, the patient should be able to teach back the following:
- Pancreatitis
- Specific cause
- Precipitating factor modification
- Interventions to reduce further episodes
- Importance of taking medications
- Lifestyle changes
- Diet modification
- Stress management
- Alcohol cessation
- Diabetes management, if needed

BOX 28.12 Teamwork and Collaboration

Interprofessional Collaborative Practice: Acute Pancreatitis

- Ensure adequate circulating volume.
- Provide nutrition support.
- Correct metabolic alterations.
- Minimize pancreatic stimulation.
- Provide comfort and emotional support.
- Maintain surveillance for complications.
  - Infected pancreatic necrosis
  - Pancreatic pseudocyst
  - Pancreatic abscess
  - Acute respiratory distress syndrome
  - Acute kidney injury
  - Intraabdominal compartment syndrome (>20 mm Hg)
  - Multiple organ dysfunction syndrome

Interprofessional collaborative management of the patient with pancreatitis is outlined in Box 28.12.

ACUTE LIVER FAILURE

Description and Etiology

Acute liver failure (ALF) is a cluster of diseases characterized by severe and sudden liver cell dysfunction, coagulopathy with increased international normalized ratio and prothrombin time, and hepatic encephalopathy.[33] In ALF, patients are usually healthy before the onset of symptoms. Patients rapidly progress from liver injury to liver failure. Types of ALF are categorized as hyperacute and subacute to distinguish differences in onset, laboratory results, and outcomes. Hyperacute ALF includes acetaminophen overdose and ischemia. The disease progresses over 2 to 4 days, and by day 7, the patient has expired, recovered, or received a liver transplant. The subacute types of ALF progress over 2 weeks or more.[33] Hepatic encephalopathy is present within 26 weeks of the liver injury.[33]

In countries where patients have access to organ transplantation, the mortality rate is approximately 30%. The primary cause of ALF in these countries is intentional or unintentional acetaminophen overdose. Other causes include other drug-induced liver injuries, viral hepatitis, autoimmune hepatitis, Wilson's diseases, and pregnancy-related ALF.[33] More causes of ALF are listed in Box 28.13.

Most patients with preexisting cirrhosis do not meet the diagnostic criteria for ALF; instead, patients with preexisting cirrhosis have characteristics associated with chronic liver failure or acute-on-chronic liver failure. Chronic liver failure is briefly discussed as an indication for liver transplantation in Chapter 35. Key concepts related to acute liver failure are summarized in Fig. 28.9.

Pathophysiology

ALF is a result of widespread necrosis and apoptosis of the hepatocytes. It results in numerous derangements, including impaired bilirubin conjugation, decreased production of clotting factors, depressed glucose synthesis, and decreased lactate clearance. This results in jaundice, coagulopathies, hypoglycemia, and metabolic acidosis. Other effects of ALF include increased risk of infection and altered carbohydrate, protein, and glucose metabolism. Hypoalbuminemia, fluid and electrolyte imbalances, and acute portal hypertension contribute to the development of ascites. Hepatic encephalopathy is believed to result from failure of the liver to detoxify various substances in the bloodstream, and it may be worsened by metabolic and electrolyte imbalances.[1]

BOX 28.13 Causes of Acute Liver Failure

Infections
- Hepatitis A, B, C, D, E, non-A, non-B, non-C
- Herpes simplex virus (types 1 and 2)
- Epstein-Barr virus
- Varicella zoster
- Dengue fever virus
- Rift Valley fever virus

Medications or Toxins
- Industrial substances (chlorinated hydrocarbons, phosphorus)
- Amanita phalloides (mushrooms)
- Aflatoxin (a toxic metabolite of fungus)
- Medications (isoniazid, rifampin, halothane, methyldopa, tetracycline, valproic acid, monoamine oxidase inhibitors, phenytoin, nicotinic acid, tricyclic antidepressants, isoflurane, ketoconazole, trimethoprim-sulfamethoxazole, sulfasalazine, pyrimethamine, octreotide)
- Acetaminophen toxicity
- Cocaine

Hypoperfusion
- Venous obstructions
- Budd-Chiari syndrome
- Veno-occlusive disease
- Ischemia

Metabolic Disorders
- Wilson disease
- Tyrosinemia
- Heat stroke
- Galactosemia

Surgery
- Jejunoileal bypass
- Partial hepatectomy
- Liver transplantation failure

Other Causes
- Reye syndrome
- Acute fatty liver of pregnancy
- Massive malignant infiltration
- Autoimmune hepatitis

Assessment and Diagnosis

A thorough medication and health history is imperative to determine a possible cause. Reviewing ingestion of medications (e.g., weight loss drugs and acetaminophen), toxins, and herbal and nonherbal supplements over the last 6 months can provide information regarding a drug-related etiology. Virus history (e.g., hepatitis), exposure to environmental toxins, and

Acute Liver Failure

Clinical and diagnostic assessments	Signs	Nursing interventions
• History and risk factors • Acetaminophen use • Viral or autoimmune hepatitis • Herbal and non-herbal supplements • Ingested or environmental toxins • Obtain vital signs • Tachycardic • Hypotensive • Clinical assessment • Jaundice • Fatigue • Nausea and/or vomiting • Abdominal distention • Pruritus • Headache • Laboratory studies • Obtain CBC, CMP, coagulation studies, viral studies, autoimmune studies • Diagnostic procedures • Ultrasound, CT	• Hypoglycemia • Prolonged prothrombin time • Decreased plasmin • Decreased plasminogen • Increased fibrin • Low platelets • Increased serum bilirubin • Increased aspartate aminotransferase • Increased alkaline phosphatase • Increased serum ammonia • Metabolic acidosis • Respiratory alkalosis • Hypoalbuminemia • Electrolyte imbalances • Asterixis	• Administer crystalloids, blood, and blood products as ordered • Monitor and manage bleeding if present • Correct electrolytes as ordered • Administer medications as ordered (e.g., lactulose) • Perform renal replacement therapy as ordered • Prepare for transplantation if anticipated

FIG. 28.9 Summary of Key Concepts Related to "Acute Liver Failure." *CBC*, Complete blood count; *CMP*, complete metabolic panel; *CT*, computed tomography.

BOX 28.14 Staging of Hepatic Encephalopathy

I	Euphoria or depression, mild confusion, slurred speech, disordered sleep rhythm; slight asterixis and normal EEG
II	Lethargy, moderate confusion; marked asterixis and abnormal EEG
III	Marked confusion, incoherent speech, sleeping but arousable; asterixis present and abnormal EEG
IV	Coma; initially responsive to noxious stimuli, later unresponsive; asterixis absent and abnormal EEG

EEG, Electroencephalogram.

additional vascular causes such as thrombosis, ischemia, Budd-Chiari syndrome (blocked venous outflow from small hepatic veins to inferior vena cava from thrombosis), and metabolic disorders such as Reye syndrome (acute, often fatal liver disease), Wilson disease (disease of defective copper metabolism that damages liver and brain), galactosemia (rare disease in infants in which they cannot metabolize galactose, resulting in hepatocellular damage), and fructose intolerance should be considered.[33]

Initial signs and symptoms of ALF may include fatigue, lethargy, nausea, vomiting, pruritis, abdominal distention, and headache. As the condition progresses, the patient may demonstrate hyperventilation, jaundice, mental status changes, palmar erythema, spider nevi, bruises, and edema. The patient should be evaluated for the presence of asterixis, or "liver flap," which is best described as the inability to voluntarily sustain a fixed position of the extremities. Asterixis is best recognized by downward flapping of the hands when the patient extends the arms and dorsiflexes the wrists. Hepatic encephalopathy is assessed by using a grading system that stages the encephalopathy according to the patient's clinical manifestations (Box 28.14).[34]

Patients may present with extrahepatic organ failure.

Laboratory Studies

Factors I (fibrinogen), II (prothrombin), V, VII, IX, and X are produced exclusively by the liver. Prothrombin time may be the most useful of these in the evaluation of acute ALF, because levels may be 40 to 80 seconds above control values. Test results show decreased levels of plasmin and plasminogen and increased levels of fibrin and fibrin-split products. Platelet counts may be less than 100,000/mm^3.[34]

Diagnostic laboratory findings include prolonged prothrombin times; elevated levels of serum bilirubin, aspartate aminotransferase, alkaline phosphatase, and serum ammonia; and decreased levels of serum albumin.[34] Arterial blood gases reveal respiratory alkalosis, metabolic acidosis, or both. Hypoglycemia, hypokalemia, and hyponatremia also may be present.[34] Other laboratory tests include ammonia measurement. Continue serial monitoring of laboratory values through the critical illness. Some diagnostic procedures include a liver biopsy, abdominal ultrasound, and computed tomography to assess vasculature of the liver.

Medical Management

Determining the cause of ALF is important because some aspects of treatment are determined based on the cause. Laboratory tests to determine cause include viral tests, such as hepatitis screen, herpes simplex, varicella-zoster, cytomegalovirus, Epstein-Barr, and paravirus. An autoimmune hepatitis screen may also be done to determine the cause, and this screen includes antinuclear antibodies, anti-smooth muscle antibodies, anti-soluble liver antigen, globulin profile, and anti-neutrophil cytoplasmic antibodies.

Because liver transplantation is one of the few definitive treatments for ALF, the patient should be transferred to a critical care unit and strongly considered for referral to a major medical center where transplantation services are available.[35] Information on liver transplant is discussed in Chapter 35.

Initial treatment in ALF includes stopping hepatotoxic medications, ensuring adequate fluid volume using crystalloids, and initiating N-acetyl cysteine in acetaminophen overdoses.[35] Additional treatment includes management of ammonia levels with lactulose. Lactulose, a synthetic ketoanalogue of lactose, splits into lactic acid and acetic acid in the intestine. It may be given orally, through a nasogastric tube, or as a retention enema to decrease production of nitrogenous wastes in the large intestine. The result is the creation of an acidic environment that results in ammonia being drawn out of the portal circulation. Lactulose has a laxative effect.[36]

Complications

Bleeding, metabolic disturbances, infections, cerebral edema, and acute kidney injury are several of the complications that must be managed. Patients are at risk for bleeding due to their coagulopathies. Bleeding is best controlled through prevention. If an invasive procedure (e.g., central line placement, intracranial pressure [ICP] monitor) will be performed or the patient develops active bleeding, vitamin K, fresh frozen plasma (to maintain a prothrombin time), and platelet transfusions may be necessary. Maintaining the patient's hemodynamic status is important while managing any bleeding. Patients are at risk for metabolic disturbances as the liver is an important regulator of glucose, acid–base balance, and electrolyte balance along with the pancreas and kidneys. Metabolic disturbances such as hypoglycemia, metabolic acidosis, hypokalemia, and hyponatremia should be monitored and treated appropriately.[34] Patients at high risk for an infection may need prophylactic antibiotic administration initiated.[35] Encephalopathic patients may develop cerebral edema. To prevent cerebral edema, consider early initiation of continuous renal replacement therapy (CRRT) and keeping serum sodium at a high normal level (145–155 mEq/L). Allowing spontaneous hyperventilation and hypothermia may also prevent cerebral edema. For patients who are known to have cerebral edema, treatment with mannitol is recommended. Other interventions to control ICP include hypertonic saline boluses, increased CRRT removal rates, and use of a vasopressor to maintain the cerebral perfusion pressure greater than 60 mm Hg.[33] Deeper sedation, minimizing stimulation when possible, elevating the head of the bed to 30 degrees, and providing therapeutic plasma exchange may also be beneficial.[33] AKI develops in a vast majority of patients with ALF, and CRRT provides renal support. The multiple complications of ALF need to be recognized, prevented if possible, and managed as appropriate.

Nursing Management

The patient management plan for a patient with ALF incorporates a variety of patient problems (Box 28.15). The nurse plays a significant role in maintaining surveillance for complications and educating the patient and family.

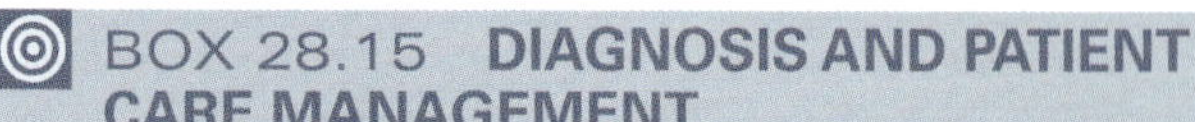

BOX 28.15 DIAGNOSIS AND PATIENT CARE MANAGEMENT

Acute Liver Failure

- Impaired Breathing due to decreased lung expansion
- Impaired Gas Exchange due to ventilation–perfusion mismatching or intrapulmonary shunting
- Impaired Cardiac Output due to alterations in preload
- Impaired Cardiac Output due to alterations in heart rate or rhythm
- Decreased Intracranial Adaptive Capacity due to failure of normal compensatory mechanisms
- Risk for Infection
- Impaired Nutritional Intake due to lack of exogenous nutrients or increased metabolic demand
- Disturbed Body Image due to actual change in body structure, function, or appearance
- Impaired Family Coping due to critically ill family member
- Lack of Knowledge of Treatment Regime due to lack of previous exposure to information (see Patient and Family Education Plan, Box 28.16)

Patient Care Management Plans are located in Appendix A.

BOX 28.16 PATIENT AND FAMILY EDUCATION PLAN

Acute Liver Failure

Before discharge, the patient should be able to teach back the following topics:

- Specific cause
- Precipitating factor modification
- Interventions to reduce further episodes
- Importance of taking medications
- Lifestyle changes
- Diet modification
- Alcohol cessation
- Transplant-specific education as appropriate

BOX 28.17 Teamwork and Collaboration

Interprofessional Collaborative Practice: Acute Liver Failure

Bleeding, metabolic disturbances, infections, and cerebral edema are several of the complications that must be managed.

- Control bleeding.
- Correct metabolic alterations.
- Prevent infection.
- Prevent and treat cerebral edema.
- Comanage acute kidney injury if present.
- Decrease ammonia levels.
- Prepare patient for liver transplantation, if necessary.
- Protect patient from injury.
- Provide comfort and emotional support.

Maintain Surveillance for Complications

As the neurologic condition worsens, respiratory depression and arrest can occur quickly. Continuous pulse oximetry monitoring and arterial blood gas analysis are helpful in assessing adequacy of respiratory efforts. A thorough neurologic assessment should

CASE STUDY 28.1 Patient With Gastrointestinal Issues

Brief Patient History

Mrs. S is a 70-year-old person with a long history of chronic back pain. Mrs. S has been taking nonsteroidal antiinflammatory drugs for several years. Mrs. S was recently started on warfarin for atrial fibrillation.

Clinical Assessment

Mrs. S is admitted to the critical care unit because of vomiting bright red blood. Mrs. S is pale and diaphoretic and complains of epigastric pain.

Diagnostic Procedures

Vital signs include the following: blood pressure of 70/40 mm Hg, heart rate of 130 beats/min (sinus tachycardia), respiratory rate of 30 breaths/min, and temperature of 101.3°F. Her urine output is 15 mL/h, hemoglobin level is 9 g/dL, and international normalized ratio (INR) is 5.3.

Medical Diagnosis

Mrs. S is diagnosed with upper gastrointestinal bleeding.

Questions

1. What major outcomes do you expect to achieve for this patient?
2. What problems or risks must be managed to achieve these outcomes?
3. What interventions could be initiated to monitor, prevent, manage, or eliminate the problems and risks identified?
4. What interventions could be initiated to promote optimal functioning, safety, and well-being of the patient?
5. What technology can be used to monitor this patient and prevent complications?
6. What other interprofessional team members are needed to assist with the management of this patient?
7. What possible learning needs would you anticipate for this patient?
8. What cultural and age-related factors might have a bearing on the patient's plan of care?

be performed at least every 1 to 2 hours,[33] with changes reported immediately.

Educate the Patient and Family

Early in the patient's hospital stay, the patient and family should be taught about ALF and its causes and treatment. Closer to discharge, teaching should focus on the interventions necessary for preventing the recurrence of the precipitating cause. If the patient is considered a candidate for liver transplantation, the patient and family will need specific information regarding the procedure and care (Chapter 35). The patient and family education plan is summarized in Box 28.16.

Interprofessional collaborative management of the patient with ALF is outlined in Box 28.17.

OTHER GASTROINTESTINAL DISORDERS

In the critical care unit, there are several other gastrointestinal disorders that may need to be treated. A summary of these disorders, their common causes, abnormal laboratory findings, confirmatory diagnostic procedures, and therapeutic management is listed in Table 28.3.

PHARMACOLOGY

Many pharmacologic agents are used in the care of patients with GI disorders. Table 28.4 reviews the various agents and any special considerations necessary for administering them.

ADDITIONAL RESOURCES

See Box 28.19 for Internet resources pertaining to gastrointestinal disorders and therapeutic management.

KEY POINTS

Acute Gastrointestinal Hemorrhage

- Acute GI hemorrhage is caused by an external erosion to or internal pressure of the blood vessels leading to vessel rupture and releasing of blood from the broken vessel.
- Medical management focuses on prevention, hemodynamic stability, and control of bleeding.
- Nursing management includes gastrointestinal intubation, surveillance for complications, and patient and family education.

Acute Pancreatitis

- Acute pancreatitis is a complex gastrointestinal disease that is characterized by enlargement of the pancreas and enhancement of pancreatic parenchyma with peripancreatic fat inflammation that may involve surrounding tissues, organ systems, or both.
- Medical management focuses on fluid resuscitation, nutrition support, and control of systemic and local complications.
- Nursing management include providing comfort and emotional support, maintaining surveillance for complications, and educating the patient and family.

Acute Liver Failure

- Acute liver failure is a result of widespread necrosis and apoptosis of the hepatocytes.
- Medical management focuses on control of complications such as bleeding, metabolic disturbances, infections, cerebral edema, and acute kidney injury.
- Nursing management includes maintaining surveillance for complications and educating the patient and family.

Other Gastrointestinal Disorders

- Several other gastrointestinal disorders may need to be treated in the critical care unit, such as small or large bowel obstruction, paralytic ileus, acute mesenteric ischemia, toxic megacolon, abdominal compartment syndrome, acute ascending cholangitis, peritonitis, and perforations.

Pharmacology

- Antacids, histamine-2 antagonists, gastric mucosal agents, gastric proton pump inhibitors, vasopressin, and somatostatin are agents used in the care of patients with GI disorders.

Visit the Evolve site at http://evolve.elsevier.com/Urden/CriticalCareNursing for additional study materials.

TABLE 28.3 Other Gastrointestinal Disorders and Their Therapeutic Management

Disorder	Common Causes	Abnormal Laboratory Findings and Confirmatory Diagnostics	Therapeutic Management
Small bowel obstruction[37]	Mechanical intrinsic luminal obstruction or extrinsic compression: *Adhesions* *Hernias* *Neoplasms*	Low serum bicarbonate levels Low arterial blood pH High lactic acid level Leukocytosis Increased serum amylase Altered coagulation profile Plain abdominal radiograph Ultrasound CT scan MRI Endoscopy	Intravenous crystalloids (balanced isotonic crystalloids, balanced dextrose-saline solutions) with supplemental potassium, antiemetics, bowel rest, nasogastric suction, monitoring of urine output Nonoperative management for up to 72 hours (bowel decompression and nothing by mouth), manual reduction of hernia Surgery: Exploratory laparotomy, lysis of adhesions
Large bowel obstruction,[37] including colonic volvulus[38]	*Mechanical intrinsic luminal obstruction or extrinsic compression:* *Neoplasms* *Volvulus* *Diverticular disease* *Impaired motility*	Low serum bicarbonate levels Low arterial blood pH High lactic acid level Leukocytosis Increased serum amylase Altered coagulation profile Plain abdominal radiograph Ultrasound CT scan MRI Lower endoscopy	Sigmoid volvulus colonoscopy Stents for palliation Endoscopic detorsion procedure Surgery: Resection, sigmoid colectomy
Paralytic ileus,[39] including prolonged postoperative ileus	*Transient interruption of gut motor activity:* *Tactile stimulation during surgery* *Uremia* *Peritonitis* *Hemorrhage* *Retroperitoneal trauma* *Sympathetic overstimulation* *Psychotropic medications* *Gastric autonomic neuropathy* *Opioids* *Anesthetics*	Plain abdominal radiograph in upright posture shows dilated loops of bowel with multiple fluid levels CT scan	*Postoperative ileus often resolves in 24–48 hours* *No fluids and food by mouth until bowel sounds return* *Intravenous crystalloids (normal saline or lactated Ringer solutions)* *Correcting electrolyte imbalances (hypokalemia)* *Rule out mechanical obstruction and pseudo-obstruction* *Prevention:* *Minimally invasive surgical procedures* *Minimal handling of bowel* *Considerations:* *Benefits/risks of NG tube placement and insert if appropriate* *Postoperative chewing gum and early oral feeding* *Gut motility agents* *Multimodal analgesic protocols* *Infusion of antibiotics*
Acute mesenteric ischemia[40]	*Blockage or nonocclusive narrowing of the superior mesenteric artery or vein:* *Thrombosis from preexisting chronic atherosclerotic disease* *Emboli* *Vasculitis* *Aortic dissection* *Mycotic aneurysm* *Mesenteric venous thrombosis* *Hypercoagulability due to inherited disease*	Laboratory results are not definitive but can assist in corroborating suspicion: *Elevated lactate* *Elevated D Dimer* *Leukocytosis* CT with angiography (bowel loop dilation, pneumatosis intestinalis, thrombus identification, free intraperitoneal fluid)	Fluid resuscitation with crystalloid and blood products Supplemental oxygen as needed Broad spectrum antibiotic therapy for up to 4 days Surgery: Emergency laparotomy

TABLE 28.3 Other Gastrointestinal Disorders and Their Therapeutic Management—cont'd

Disorder	Common Causes	Abnormal Laboratory Findings and Confirmatory Diagnostics	Therapeutic Management
Toxic megacolon[41]	*Dilation of the colon:* *Inflammatory bowel diseases* *Septicemia* *Intestinal infections*	Any three of the following: *Fever greater than 38.6°C* *Tachycardia greater than 120 beats/min* *Leukocytosis greater than 10.5 x 10^9/L* *Anemia* *Electrolyte disorders* *Hypovolemia* *Altered mental status* Plain abdominal radiograph (colonic dilation of more than 6 cm)	Reduce inflammation Prevent free perforation *Monitor for signs of impending perforation: abdominal distention, rebound tenderness hemodynamic instability requires immediate surgical intervention* Bowel rest Nasogastric decompression Use of rectal tube Improve motility of the colon: *Enteral feeding* *Use maneuvers to decrease abdominal distention by permitting redistribution or passing of colon gas* *Encourage walking or knee/elbow maneuver in the prone position* Medications: *Gut motility agents* *Empiric antibiotics* *Glucocorticoids* *Infliximab or cyclosporine for patient's refractory to 3 days of intravenous glucocorticoid therapy* For *Clostridioides difficile*[a]–related toxic megacolon: *Discontinue inciting antibiotics* *No steroids due to infectious etiology* Surgery is indicated in patients with colonic perforation, necrosis, or full-thickness ischemia, intraabdominal hypertension or abdominal compartment syndrome, clinical signs of peritonitis, worsening abdominal exam.
Abdominal compartment syndrome[42]	*New organ dysfunction from sustained intraabdominal pressure of 20 mmHg:* *Abdominal surgery* *Abdominal infection* *Intestinal obstruction* *Fluid overload* *Pancreatitis*	Decreased urine output Decreased cardiac output Decreased SV Decreased SVR Decreased oxygen delivery Increased pulmonary artery pressures Increased CVP Hypoxemia Increased airway pressures Decreased ventilatory compliance Increased bladder pressure	Nasogastric tube for decompression Rectal tube for colonic decompression Drainage of abdominal fluid/percutaneous drainage of abscesses Surgical decompression: Laparotomy (temporary closure with vacs, meshes, zippers)
Acute ascending cholangitis[43]	Infection of the biliary tree: *Choledocholithiasis* *Pancreatic cancer* *Primary sclerosing cholangitis* *Stricture of the hepatic ducts* *Biliary stent obstruction*	*Suspected diagnosis—One item in A and one item in B or C* *Certain diagnosis—One item in A, B, C* *A. Systemic inflammation* *Chills* *Fever greater than 38.6°C* *Leukocytes <4 or >10 G/L* *CRP ≥ 10 mg/L* *B. Cholestasis* *Icterus/jaundice* *Abnormal liver function test* *Total bilirubin >1.9 mg/dL* *AST, ALT, ALP and γ-glutamyl transferase >1.5x upper limit of the normal range* *C. Imagery* *Bile duct dilation* *Imagery providing proof of etiology*	Fluid resuscitation Antibiotics Biliary drainage via ERCP and biliary drain Biliary drainage through drain placed in interventional radiology

Continued

TABLE 28.3 Other Gastrointestinal Disorders and Their Therapeutic Management—cont'd

Disorder	Common Causes	Abnormal Laboratory Findings and Confirmatory Diagnostics	Therapeutic Management
Peritonitis[44–46]	*The peritoneum becomes inflamed:* *Bacterial translocation (spontaneous bacterial peritonitis, tuberculous peritonitis* *Peritoneal dialysis catheter leaks* *Appendicitis* *Cholecystitis* *Gastrointestinal perforation*	Positive cultures from peritoneal fluid Abdominal pain Tenderness of abdomen Bloating or fullness Fever	Prophylactic antibiotics Antibiotics for treatment Analgesics IV fluids Vasopressors if needed Surgery to remove infected tissue (e.g., appendicitis)
Gastrointestinal perforation[45] and postoperative anastomotic leaks	A tear, leak, or hole in the gastromucosal area from: Ingestion of sharp objects or caustic substances Medical conditions (e.g., tumors, ulcers) Surgical and/or procedural equipment (e.g., endoscopes, stents, catheters) Incomplete sealing of a surgical connection	Bleeding (depending on location) Collapsed lumen in the digestive tract Nausea Persistent severe pain Distention Chills Fever Increased WBCs Hypotension Altered heart rate	Conservative treatment includes bowel rest and antibiotics. Placement of an NG tube is appropriate in most situations. For upper GI perforations, patient should be admitted for observation. Patient should be kept NPO, receiving IV fluids and broad-spectrum antibiotics. Endoscopy-related (iatrogenic) perforations may be treated by endoscopic closure clips and sutures when feasible. Obtain surgical consultation regardless of success of endoscopic closure.

[a]Prevention of *Clostridioides difficile* is reviewed in Box 28.18.

C, Celsius; *cm*, centimeter; *CT*, computed tomography; *CVP*, central venous pressure; *dL*, deciliter; *ERCP*, endoscopic retrograde cholangiopancreatography; *g*, grams; *IV*, intravenous; *L*, liter; *mg*, milligrams; *mm Hg*, millimeters of mercury; *MRI*, magnetic resonance imaging; *NG*, nasogastric; *pH*, power of hydrogen; *SV*, stroke volume; *SVR*, systemic vascular resistance.

BOX 28.18 Safety

Quality

Prevention of *Clostridioides difficile* Transmission

Clostridioides difficile is a common cause of infectious diarrhea. *C. difficile* is an anaerobic gram-positive bacillus that is spore forming and toxin producing. The spore can live for long periods of time in harsh environments, contributing to the ongoing perseverance in hospitals and health care facilities. Transmission occurs through the fecal-oral route. The clinical manifestations of *C. difficile* range from mild diarrhea to pseudomembranous colitis with toxic megacolon. Major risk factors for *C. difficile* infection include exposure to antibiotics, extended hospitalization, proton pump inhibitors, and advanced age.

Prevention of transmission is crucial to reducing disease outbreaks in health care settings. Interventions are primarily focused on the use of barrier precautions and disinfection. When caring for a patient with *C. difficile* infection:

1. Place the patient in contact precautions.
2. Place the patient in private room if available or cohort patients if private room not available.
3. Use dedicated patient care items and equipment if possible.
4. Ensure disinfection of all shared equipment and the environment.
5. Perform meticulous hand hygiene. Using soap and water prior to the use of alcohol-based hand rubs is recommended.

From Kociolek LK, Gerding DN, Carrico R, et al. Strategies to prevent *Clostridioides difficile* infections in acute-care hospitals: 2022 Update. *Infect Control Hosp Epidemiol* 2023;44(4):527–549. https://doi.10.1017/ice.2023.18

BOX 28.19 Internet Resources

Gastrointestinal Disorders and Therapeutic Management

- Society of Gastroenterology Nurses and Associates, Inc.: https://www.sgna.org
- American Gastroenterological Association: https://www.gastro.org
- American College of Gastroenterology: https://gi.org
- American Society for Gastrointestinal Endoscopy: https://www.asge.org
- International Foundation for Functional Gastrointestinal Disorders: https://www.iffgd.org
- The National Pancreas Foundation: https://pancreasfoundation.org
- American Pancreatic Association: https://www.american-pancreatic-association.org/
- American Liver Foundation: https://www.liverfoundation.org
- American Association for the Study of Liver Diseases: https://www.aasld.org
- Alcoholics Anonymous: https://www.aa.org
- American Society for Parenteral and Enteral Nutrition: https://www.nutritioncare.org

TABLE 28.4 PHARMACOLOGIC MANAGEMENT

Gastrointestinal Disorders

Medication	Dosage	Actions	Special Considerations
Antacids	Variable depending on commercial product used	Used to buffer stomach acid and raise gastric pH	Can cause diarrhea or constipation Electrolyte disturbances if used for an extended period of time
Histamine-2 (H_2) Antagonists			
Cimetidine (Tagamet)	300 mg q6h IV or PO for gastrointestinal ulcers	Used to reduce volume and concentration of gastric secretions	Rare side effects include CNS toxicity (confusion or delirium) and thrombocytopenia
Famotidine (Pepcid)	40 mg daily PO or 20 mg q12h IV for gastrointestinal ulcers		Dosage adjustments recommended for patients with moderate (creatinine clearance <50 mL/min) renal insufficiency Separate PO administration of antacids and cimetidine
Gastric Mucosal Agents			
Sucralfate (Carafate)	1 g NG or PO, given four times a day at least 1 hour before meals and at bedtime	Forms an ulcer-adherent complex with proteinaceous exudates Covers ulcer and protects against acid, pepsin, and bile salts	Requires an acid medium for activation Separate PO administration of antacids and sucralfate May cause severe constipation Delayed absorption effects may influence bioavailability of certain medications
Gastric Proton Pump Inhibitors			
Omeprazole (Prilosec)	20–40 mg daily PO Can be up to 40 mg PO q12h for stress prophylaxis	Inhibits gastric acid secretion by the gastric parietal cells	May increase levels of warfarin May be administered concomitantly with antacids Associated with higher incidence of *Clostridioides difficile* infection
Lansoprazole (Prevacid)	15–30 mg q24h PO 30 mg over 30 min q24h IV		
Esomeprazole (Nexium)	40 mg q24h PO Can be up to 40 mg PO q12h for stress prophylaxis 20–40 mg q24h IV		
Pantoprazole (Protonix)	20–80 mg q24h PO, may be q12h for pathologic hypersecretory syndromes (e.g., Zollinger-Ellison) 40 mg q24h IV, may be up to 80 mg q12h for pathologic hypersecretory syndromes (e.g., Zollinger-Ellison)		
Vasopressin			
(Pitressin Synthetic)	0.2–0.8 units/min IV infusion	Contracts vascular smooth muscle to decrease splanchnic blood flow, reducing portal pressure	Side effects include coronary, mesenteric, and peripheral vasoconstriction
Somatostatin			
Octreotide (Sandostatin)	75–200 mcg SubQ q8h Bolus dose of 50 mcg IV (may repeat once within hour), followed by IV infusion of 50 mcg/h, usually 2–5 days	Decreases splanchnic blood flow, reducing portal pressure	Can cause diarrhea or constipation, abdominal pain, nausea May cause hyperglycemia or hypoglycemia

CNS, Central nervous system; *h*, hour; *IV*, intravenous; *mcg*, microgram; *mg*, milligram; *min*, minute; *NG*, nasogastric; *pH*, power of hydrogen; *PO*, by mouth; *q*, every; *SubQ*, subcutaneous.

REFERENCES

1. Spain SR. Alterations of digestive function. In: Rogers J, ed. *McCance & Huether's Pathophysiology: The Biologic Basis for Disease in Adults and Children*. 9th ed. Philadelphia, PA: Elsevier; 2023:1318–1348.
2. Mackenzie PD, Rogers M, Gallagher M, Rockall T. Management of massive gastrointestinal haemorrhage. *Surg*. 2019;37(10):565–575. https://doi.org/10.1016/j.mpsur.2019.07.013.
3. Nable JV, Graham AC. Gastrointestinal bleeding. *Emerg Med Clin North Am*. 2016;34(2):309–325. https://doi.org/10.1016/j.emc.2015.12.001.
4. Bardou M, Quenot JP, Barkun A. Stress-related mucosal disease in the critically ill patient. *Nat Rev Gastroenterol Hepatol*. 2015;12(5):98–107. https://doi.org/10.1038/nrgastro.2014.235.
5. Quenot JP, Dargent A, Barkun A. Prophylaxis for stress related gastrointestinal bleeding in the ICU: should we adjust to each patient's individual risk? *Anaesth Crit Care Pain Med*. 2019;38(2):99–101. https://doi.org/10.1016/j.accpm.2019.01.012.
6. Tulassay Z, Herszenyi L. Gastric mucosal defense and cytoprotection. *Best Pract Res Clin Gastroenterol*. 2010;24(2):99–108. https://doi.org/10.1016/j.bpg.2010.02.006.
7. Drini M. Peptic ulcer disease and non-steroidal anti-inflammatory drugs. *Aust Prescr*. 2017;40(3):91–93. https://doi.org/10.18773/austprescr.2017.037.
8. Narayanan M, Reddy KM, Marsicano E. Peptic ulcer disease and *Helicobacter pylori* infection. *Mo Med*. 2018;115(3):219–224.
9. McConaghy JR, Decker A, Nair S. Peptic ulcer disease and H. pylori infection: common questions and answers. *Am Fam Physician*. 2023;107(2):165–172.
10. Jothimani D, Rela M, Kamath PS. Liver cirrhosis and portal hypertension: how to deal with esophageal varices? *Med Clin North Am*. 2023;107(3):491–504. https://doi.org/10.1016/j.mcna.2023.01.002.
11. Kovacs TOG, Jensen DM. Varices: esophageal, gastric, and rectal. *Clin Liver Dis*. 2019;23(4):625–642. https://doi.org/10.1016/j.cld.2019.07.005.
12. Wilkins T, Wheeler B, Carpenter M. Upper gastrointestinal bleeding in adults: evaluation and management. *Am Fam Physician*. 2020;101(5):294–300.
13. Sengupta N, Feuerstein JD, Jairath V, et al. Management of patients with acute lower gastrointestinal bleeding: an updated ACG guideline. *Am J Gastroenterol*. 2023;118(2):208–231. https://doi.org/10.14309/ajg.0000000000002130.
14. Stanley AJ, Laine L. Management of acute upper gastrointestinal bleeding. *BMJ*. 2019;364:l536. https://doi.org/10.1136/bmj.l536.
15. Barbateskovic M, Marker S, Granholm A, et al. Stress ulcer prophylaxis with proton pump inhibitors or histamin-2 receptor antagonists in adult intensive care patients: a systematic review with meta-analysis and trial sequential analysis. *Intensive Care Med*. 2019;45(2):143–158. https://doi.org/10.1007/s00134-019-05526-z.
16. Barkun AN, Almadi M, Kuipers EJ, et al. Management of nonvariceal upper gastrointestinal bleeding: guideline recommendations from the International Consensus Group. *Ann Intern Med*. 2019;171(11):805–822. https://doi.org/10.7326/M19-1795.
17. Karakonstantis S, Tzagkarakis E, Kalemaki D, Lydakis C, Paspatis G. Nasogastric aspiration/lavage in patients with gastrointestinal bleeding: a review of the evidence. *Expert Rev Gastroenterol Hepatol*. 2018;12(1):63–72. https://doi.org/10.1080/17474124.2018.1398646.
18. Lau LHS, Sung JJY. Treatment of upper gastrointestinal bleeding in 2020: new techniques and outcomes. *Dig Endosc*. 2021;33(1):83–94. https://doi.org/10.1111/den.13674.
19. Laine L, Barkun AN, Saltzman JR, Martel M, Leontiadis GI. ACG clinical guideline: upper gastrointestinal and ulcer bleeding. *Am J Gastroenterol*. 2021;116(5):899–917. https://doi.org/10.14309/ajg.0000000000001245.
20. McGraw JR, Kiefer RM, Shah A, et al. Outcomes of transarterial embolization for acute nonvariceal upper gastrointestinal bleeding: correlation with periprocedural endoscopy. *J Vasc Interv Radiol*. 2023;34(6):1062–1069. https://doi.org/10.1016/j.jvir.2023.01.026.
21. Patel RK, Chandel K, Tripathy TP, Mukund A. Complications of transjugular intrahepatic portosystemic shunt (TIPS) in the era of the stent graft – what the interventionists need to know? *Eur J Radiol*. 2021;144:109986. https://doi.org/10.1016/j.ejrad.2021.109986.
22. Brand M, Prodehl L, Ede CJ. Surgical portosystemic shunts versus transjugular intrahepatic portosystemic shunt for variceal haemorrhage in people with cirrhosis. *Cochrane Database Syst Rev*. 2018;10(10):CD001023. https://doi.org/10.1002/14651858.CD001023.pub3.
23. Mederos MA, Reber HA, Girgis MD. Acute pancreatitis: a review. *JAMA*. 2021;325(4):382–390. https://doi.org/10.1001/jama.2020.20317.
24. Trikudanathan G, Wolbrink DRJ, van Santvoort HC, Mallery S, Freeman M, Besselink MG. Current concepts in severe acute and necrotizing pancreatitis: an evidence-based approach. *Gastroenterology*. 2019;156(7):1994–2007.e3. https://doi.org/10.1053/j.gastro.2019.01.269.
25. Wright WF. Cullen sign and grey turner sign revisited [published correction appears in *J Am Osteopath Assoc* 2016;116(8):501]. *J Am Osteopath Assoc*. 2016;116(6):398–401. https://doi.org/10.7556/jaoa.2016.081.
26. Hammad AY, Ditillo M, Castanon L. Pancreatitis. *Surg Clin N Am*. 2018;98(5):895–913. https://doi.org/10.1016/j.suc.2018.06.001.
27. Crockett SD, Wani S, Gardner TB, Falck-Ytter Y, Barkun AN, American Gastroenterological Association Institute Clinical Guidelines Committee. American Gastroenterological Association Institute guideline on initial management of acute pancreatitis. *Gastroenterology*. 2018;154(4):1096–1101. https://doi.org/10.1053/j.gastro.2018.01.032.
28. de-Madaria E, Herrera-Marante I, González-Camacho V, et al. Fluid resuscitation with lactated Ringer's solution vs normal saline in acute pancreatitis: a triple-bind, randomized, controlled trial. *United European Gastroenterol J*. 2018;6(1):63–71. https://doi.org/10.1177/2050640617707864.
29. Waller A, Long B, Koyfman A, Gottlieb M. Acute pancreatitis: updates for emergency clinicians. *J Emerg Med*. 2018;55(6):769–779. https://doi.org/10.1016/j.jemermed.2018.08.009.
30. Goodchild G, Chouhan M, Johnson GJ. Practical guide to the management of acute pancreatitis. *Frontline Gastroentoerol*. 2019;10(3):292–299. https://doi.org/10.1136/flgastro-2018-101102.
31. Thomasset SC, Carter CR. Acute pancreatitis. *Surg*. 2016;34(6):292–300. https://doi.org/10.1016/j.mpsur.2016.03.008.
32. Kovacs TO, Jensen DM. Gastrointestinal hemorrhage. In: Goldman L, Schafer A, eds. *Goldman-Cecil Medicine*. 26th ed. Philadelphia, PA: Elsevier; 2020.
33. Tujios S, Stravitz RT, Lee WM. Management of acute liver failure: update 2022. *Semin Liver Dis*. 2022;42(3):362–378. https://doi.org/10.1055/s-0042-1755274.
34. Maher SZ, Schreibman IR. The clinical spectrum and manifestations of acute liver failure. *Clin Liver Dis*. 2018;22(2):361–374. https://doi.org/10.1016/j.cld.2018.01.012.
35. Arshad MA, Murphy N, Bangash MN. Acute liver failure. *Clin Med*. 2020;20(5):505–508. https://doi.org/10.7861/clinmed.2020-0.
36. Khan R, Koppe S. Modern management of acute liver failure. *Gastroenterol Clin North Am*. 2018;47(2):313–326. https://doi.org/10.1016/j.gtc.2018.01.005.
37. Catena F, De Simone B, Coccolini F, Di Saverio S, Sartelli M, Ansaloni L. Bowel obstruction: a narrative review for all physicians. *World J Emerg Surg*. 2019;14:20. https://doi.org/10.1186/s13017-019-0240-7.
38. Alavi K, Poylin V, Davids JS, et al. The American Society of Colon and Rectal Surgeons clinical practice guidelines for the management of colonic volvulus and acute colonic pseudo-obstruction. *Dis Colon Rectum*. 2021;64(9):1046–1057. https://doi.org/10.1097/DCR.0000000000002159.
39. Weledji EP. Perspectives on paralytic ileus. *Acute Med Surg*. 2020;7(1):e573. https://doi.org/10.1002/ams2.573.
40. Yu H, Kirkpatrick IDC. An update on acute mesenteric ischemia. *Can Assoc Radiol J*. 2023;74(1):160–171. https://doi.org/10.1177/08465371221094280.
41. Desai J, Elnaggar M, Hanfy AA, Doshi R. Toxic megacolon: background, pathophysiology, management challenges and solutions [published correction appears in *Clin Exp Gastroenterol*. 2021 Jul 19;14:309-310]. *Clin Exp Gastroenterol*. 2020;13:203–210. https://doi.org/10.2147/CEG.S200760.
42. De Waele JJ. Intra-abdominal hypertension and abdominal compartment syndrome. *Curr Opin Crit Care*. 2022;28(6):695–701. https://doi.org/10.1097/MCC.0000000000000991.

43. An Z, Braseth AL, Sahar N. Acute cholangitis: causes, diagnosis, and management. *Gastroenterol Clin North Am.* 2021;50(2):403–414. https://doi.org/10.1016/j.gtc.2021.02.005.
44. Facciorusso A, Antonino M, Orsitto E, Sacco R. Primary and secondary prophylaxis of spontaneous bacterial peritonitis: current state of the art. *Expert Rev Gastroenterol Hepatol.* 2019;13(8):751–759. https://doi.org/10.1080/17474124.2019.1644167.
45. Lee JH, Kedia P, Stavropoulos SN, Carr-Locke D. AGA clinical practice update on endoscopic management of perforations in gastrointestinal tract: expert review. *Clin Gastroenterol Hepatol.* 2021;19(11):2252–2261.e2. https://doi.org/10.1016/j.cgh.2021.06.045.
46. Peritonitis. National Kidney Foundation. 2023. Accessed October 10, 2023. https://www.kidney.org/atoz/content/peritonitis.

29 Endocrine Anatomy and Physiology

Mary E. Lough and Kathleen M. Stacy

http://evolve.elsevier.com/Urden/CriticalCareNursing

Maintaining dynamic equilibrium among the human body's various cells, tissues, organs, and systems is highly complex and specialized. Two systems regulate these critical relationships: the nervous and endocrine systems. The nervous system communicates by nerve impulses that control skeletal, smooth, and cardiac muscle tissue (see Chapter 20). The endocrine system controls and communicates by distributing potent hormones throughout the body. Fig. 29.1 lists the endocrine glands and their hormones, target tissues, and actions. When stimulated, the endocrine glands secrete hormones into surrounding body fluids. These hormones travel to specific target tissues via the circulation, exerting a pronounced effect. Receptors found on or within these specialized target tissue cells are equipped with molecules that recognize the hormone and bind it to the cell, producing a specific response.

PANCREAS

Anatomy

The pancreas is a long, triangular organ. It is clinically described as consisting of a *head, neck, body*, and *tail*. The head of the organ lies in the C-shaped curvature of the duodenum, and the tail extends behind and below the stomach toward the spleen. The pancreas is approximately 15 cm (6 inches) long and 4 cm (1.5 inches) wide.

Blood Supply

The pancreas receives arterial blood supply from many sources. The head of the pancreas gets its blood supply from both pancreaticoduodenal arteries: the superior pancreaticoduodenal artery, which is a branch of the common hepatic artery (which comes from the celiac trunk), and the inferior pancreaticoduodenal artery, which stems from the superior mesenteric artery. These two blood supplies anastomose. The pancreas's neck, body, and tail receive their blood supply from multiple branches of the splenic artery (another branch of the celiac trunk). Venous drainage occurs through the veins that correspond to the arteries and that ultimately empty into the portal vein. The pancreas has two primary functions: digestive and hormonal.

Exocrine Cells

The pancreatic acini are clusters of specialized exocrine cells within the pancreas that produce and secrete digestive enzymes. Most pancreatic tissue is devoted to producing exocrine digestive enzymes secreted into the pancreatic duct. The duct is 3 mm wide and traverses the length of the pancreas (see Fig. 29.1). The pancreatic duct joins with the common bile duct to allow transport of bile from the liver and gallbladder to the duodenum at the greater duodenal papilla. Because this is the exit for both organs, it presents a danger of a gallstone lodging at the duodenal papilla and blocking the outflow of exocrine pancreatic enzymes. Pancreas exocrine anatomy and pancreatic digestive juices (exocrine) are discussed in more detail in Chapter 26.

Endocrine Cells

The pancreas contains specialized endocrine cells that secrete hormones directly into the bloodstream. The endocrine tissue composes less than 5% of the total volume of the pancreas. The function of the endocrine hormones is the focus of the following discussion.

Physiology

In the pancreas, clusters of cells called *pancreatic islets* (also known as the islets of Langerhans) are composed of distinct cell types: alpha, beta, delta, and PP cells that help regulate blood glucose (Fig. 29.2):

- Alpha cells secrete glucagon and make up about 20% of each islet
- Beta cells secrete insulin and make up about 75% of each islet
- Delta cells secrete somatostatin and make up about 4% of each islet
- PP cells secrete pancreatic polypeptide hormone and make up only 1% of each islet

Most cells that make up the pancreatic islets are glucagon-secreting alpha cells and insulin-secreting beta cells.[1] Glucagon, insulin, somatostatin, and polypeptide hormones are released into the surrounding capillaries to empty into the portal vein, where they are distributed to target cells in the liver. The hormones then travel into general circulation to reach other target cells.

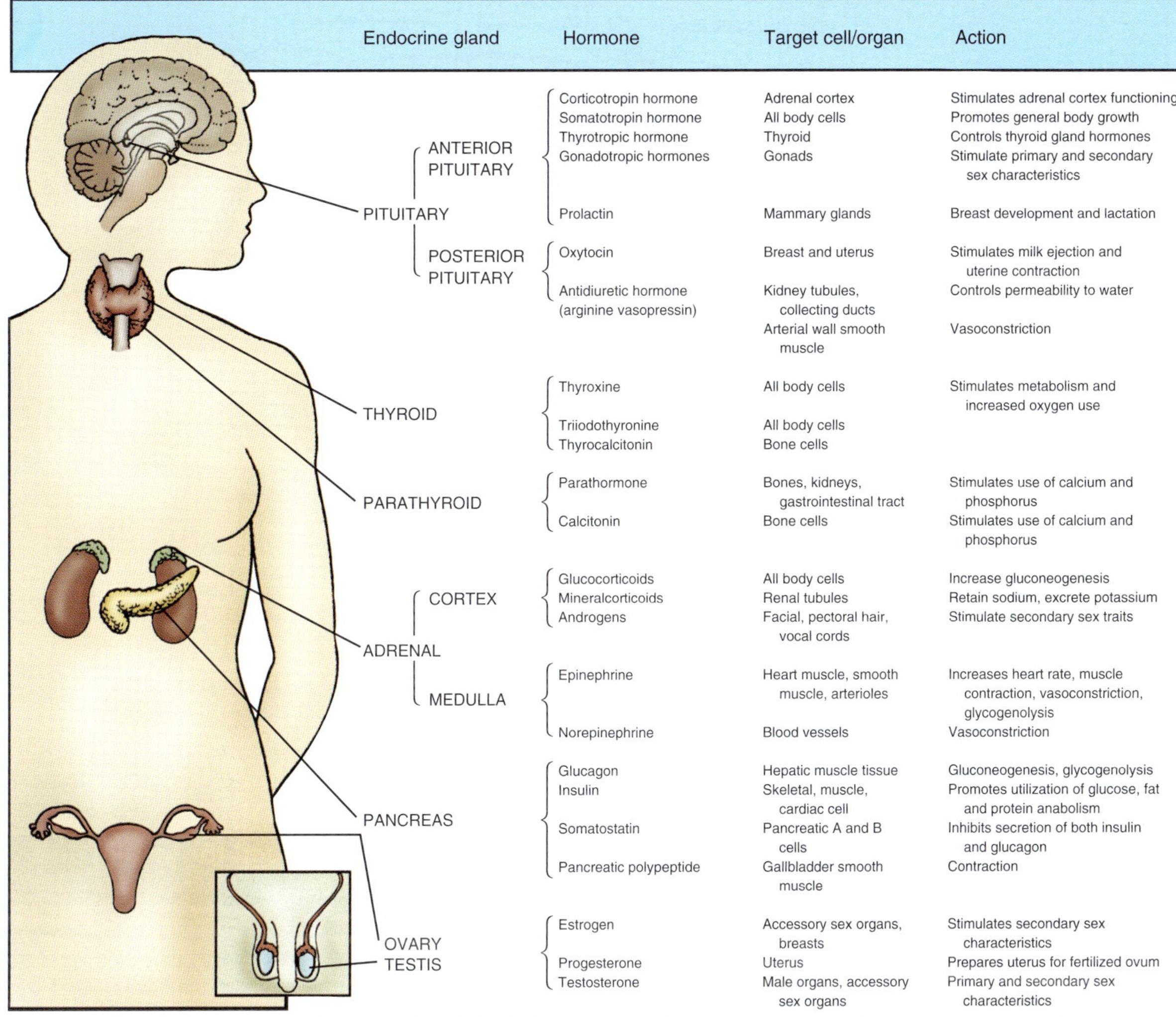

FIG. 29.1 Location of Endocrine Glands With the Hormones They Produce, Target Cells or Organs, and Hormonal Actions.

Insulin

Insulin is a potent anabolic hormone produced by the beta cells of the pancreas. Elevated levels of blood glucose stimulate insulin production. Insulin is the only hormone produced in the body that directly lowers blood glucose levels. Insulin is responsible for storing carbohydrate, protein, and fat nutrients. Insulin also augments potassium transport into the cells, decreases the mobilization of fats, and stimulates protein synthesis (Table 29.1). Box 29.1 defines the terms commonly used when discussing glucose and insulin balance. The main stimulant for insulin secretion is an elevation of serum glucose. The greater the increase in blood glucose, the more insulin the normal pancreas produces. Other hormones inhibit the release of insulin (Table 29.2).

Blood Glucose

Blood glucose is reported in millimoles per liter, the International System of Units (SI) unit of measurement used worldwide. In the United States, blood glucose is measured in milligrams per deciliter. The normal blood glucose range is 70 to 100 mg/dL (3.9 to 5.6 mmol/L). To convert mmol/L of glucose to mg/dL, multiply the mmol/L value by 18. To convert mg/dL of glucose to mmol/L, divide the mg/dL value by 18.

In patients who have symptoms of diabetes, pancreatic beta cell destruction has already occurred. With a diagnosis of type 1 diabetes, all the beta cells are nonfunctional. In type 2 diabetes, about half of the beta cells are already destroyed by the time the patient exhibits signs and symptoms of diabetes.[2] The destruction of the beta cells disrupts the homeostatic ability to regulate blood glucose.[3]

Carbohydrate metabolism. Glucose is admitted to the skeletal, cardiac, and adipose cells for energy in the presence of insulin facilitated by the glucose transporter 4 (GLUT4), as described subsequently. The movement of glucose from the circulation into the intracellular compartment reduces the glucose concentration in the bloodstream and helps preserve the osmolality of the blood. Simultaneously, glucose is available to the cell as its primary energy source. Excess glucose in the form of glycogen is stored in the hepatic and muscle cells for use as fuel later. In skeletal muscle, 90% of the glucose in the cell is converted to glycogen for longer-term storage. Glycogen release protects against the effects of hypoglycemia.[4] However, with a diagnosis of diabetes, glycogen may be too abundant after a meal (postprandial hyperglycemia) and insufficient in hypoglycemic states.[4] Current research suggests that both beta and alpha cells are dysregulated in diabetes.[4]

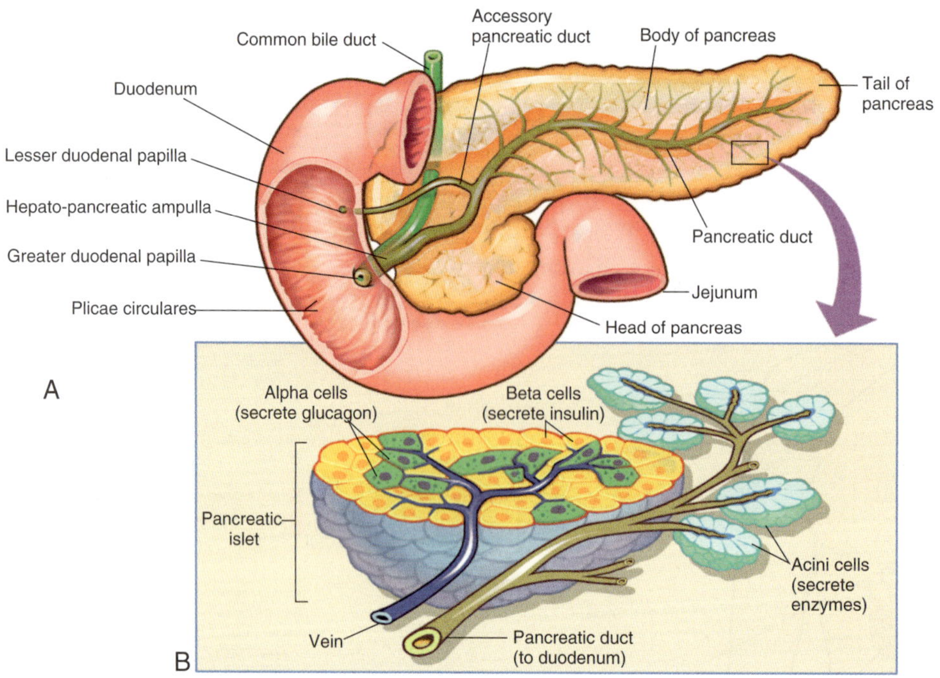

FIG. 29.2 Structures of the Pancreas and Islets of Langerhans. (A) Anatomic structure of the pancreas showing the pancreatic duct and connection to the duodenum. (B) A pancreatic islet with alpha and beta cells (endocrine); nearby are ancini (exocrine) cells. (From Patton K, Bell F, Thompson T, Williamson P. *Anatomy and Physiology*. 11th ed. Elsevier; 2022.)

TABLE 29.1 Pancreatic Endocrine Cells: Target Tissue and Physiologic Response

Cell	Hormone	Stimulant Release Factor	Target Tissue	Physiologic Response
Alpha	Glucagon	↓ Glucose	Hepatocyte	↑ Glucose in bloodstream
		Exercise	Myocyte	↑ Gluconeogenesis
		↑ Amino acids		↑ Glycogenolysis
		SNS stimulation		↑ Fat mobilization
				↑ Protein mobilization
Beta	Insulin	Glucose	Skeletal cells	↓ Blood glucose
			Muscle cells	↓ Fat mobilization
			Cardiac cells	↑ Fat storage
				↓ Protein mobilization
				↑ Protein synthesis
				↑ Glucogenesis
Delta	Somatostatin	Hyperglycemia	Alpha cells	↓ Blood glucose
			Beta cells	↓ Glycogen secretion
				↓ Insulin secretion
PP	Pancreatic polypeptide	Acute hypoglycemia	Gallbladder	↑ Gallbladder contraction
			Smooth muscle	↓ Pancreatic enzyme

SNS, Sympathetic nervous system.

Fat metabolism. Adequate, effective insulin levels are essential for the normal metabolism of lipids. Type 2 diabetes is strongly associated with dyslipidemias and an increased risk of atherogenic cardiovascular disease. The overproduction of large, triglyceride-rich, very-low-density lipoproteins and decreased levels of high-density lipoproteins characterize type 2 diabetes.[5] Carbohydrate and fat metabolism disorders are also associated with metabolic syndrome, a precursor to diabetes and cardiovascular disease.

BOX 29.1 Terms Used for Insulin and Glucose Imbalance

- **Anabolism:** Constructive phase of metabolism in which the body converts simple substances into more complex compounds in the presence of energy
- **Catabolism:** Destructive phase of metabolism in which the body breaks down complex substances to form simpler substances in the presence of energy
- **Gluconeogenesis:** Formation of glucose from noncarbohydrate nutrients (e.g., fats, protein), which occurs in the liver
- **Glycogen:** Storage form of glucose in the liver and muscles
- **Glycogenesis:** Formation of glycogen from glucose and adenosine triphosphate after a meal when both are plentiful
- **Glycogenolysis:** Conversion of glycogen stored in the liver and muscles into usable glucose
- **Osmolality:** Measurement of the number of particles in a solution or the concentration of a solution

Protein metabolism. Insulin and the GLUTs (discussed later in the chapter) facilitate the transfer of glucose across the cell wall. By having glucose (carbohydrate) available as the body's fuel source, protein is spared from use as energy. Protein is then available for critical protein synthesis and amino acid transport into the cells. Protein metabolism also benefits from an adequate insulin supply. The body uses protein for energy sources only in acute hyperglycemia of diabetic ketoacidosis or starvation.

Glucagon

Glucagon, synthesized by alpha cells in the pancreas, has the opposite effect of insulin. Glucagon is released during

TABLE 29.2 **Insulin Release and Inhibition**

Insulin Release (Major Stimulus: High Blood Glucose)	Insulin Inhibition (Major Inhibitor: Low Blood Glucose)
Hormones	
Glucagon	Somatostatin
Corticotropic hormone	Norepinephrine
Thyrotropin	Epinephrine
Somatotropin	
Glucocorticoids	
Incretins	
Medications	
Beta-adrenergic stimulators	Beta-adrenergic blocking agents
Sulfonylurea	Diazoxide
Theophylline	Phenytoin
Acetylcholine	Thiazide or sulfonamide diuretics

hypoglycemia to induce hepatic glucose output.[4] Because glucagon counterregulates insulin levels and raises blood glucose levels, it is a potent *gluconeogenic hormone.* Through *gluconeogenesis*, glucagon can form glucose from noncarbohydrate sources such as fat and protein when required. Glucagon release from the pancreas is stimulated by low blood glucose levels, starvation, exercise, or sympathetic nervous system (SNS) stimulation.[6] Glucagon release protects the brain from the consequences of hypoglycemia.[6]

Glucagon stimulates the release of glycogen stores from liver and muscle cells to meet short-term energy requirements. Through a process called *glycogenolysis*, the glycogen stored in the liver is converted into a glucose form that can be used by the cells.[6]

For long-term energy needs, glucagon stimulates glucose release through the more complex process of gluconeogenesis. In gluconeogenesis, fat and protein nutrients are rapidly broken down into end products that are then changed into glucose.[6]

The insulin-to-glucagon ratio maintains a normal blood glucose level in the healthy body (Box 29.2). When the blood glucose level is high, insulin is released, and glucagon is inhibited. When blood glucose levels are low, glucagon rather than insulin is released to raise the blood glucose level. The brain has a minimal supply of glucose, and glucagon release is essential to protect the brain from the effects of hypoglycemia.

Somatostatin

Somatostatin is a hormone that is produced in the pancreatic delta cells. Somatostatin decreases glucagon secretion; in high quantities, it decreases insulin release (see Table 29.1). Hyperglycemia stimulates the activity of the delta cells. It is theorized that insulin release enables somatostatin to control beta-cell activity. Somatostatin may be involved in regulating the postprandial influx of glucose into cells.

Pancreatic Polypeptide

The PP cells within the pancreatic islets synthesize pancreatic polypeptide hormone.[1] This hormone is released after a meal and remains elevated for several hours, suggesting a role in digestion. Pancreatic polypeptide hormone influences gastrointestinal (GI) motility and gallbladder function.

BOX 29.2 **Insulin-to-Glucagon Ratio: Effects on Carbohydrate, Fat, and Protein Metabolism**

Balanced Insulin and Glucagon	Decreased Insulin and Increased Glucagon
↑ Use of glucose by cells	↓ Use of glucose by cells
↑ Movement of potassium intracellularly	↓ Movement of potassium intracellularly
↑ Carbohydrate metabolism	↑ Blood glucose
↓ Gluconeogenesis	↑ Gluconeogenesis
↑ Glycogen storage	↓ Glycogen storage
↓ Glycogenolysis	↑ Glycogenolysis
↓ Lipolysis	↑ Lipolysis
↓ Fat mobilization	↑ Fat mobilization
↑ Fat storage	↓ Fat stores
↓ Protein mobilization	↑ Hepatic metabolism fats
↑ Protein synthesis	↑ Ketogenesis
	↑ Mobilization of protein
	↑ Proteolysis
	↑ Lipoprotein

Glucose Regulatory Pathways Outside of the Pancreas

The physiology of glucose metabolism has traditionally focused exclusively on the pancreas. With increases in knowledge, glucose metabolism physiology has expanded to include three other critical cellular physiologic pathways: (1) GLUTs in multiple organs, (2) incretin proteins from the GI system, and (3) sodium glucose cotransporter 2 (SGLT2) cells in the kidney tubules.

Glucose Transporters

Human cells take up glucose using facultative glucose transport proteins known as *GLUTs*. These proteins specialize in tissue distribution and function, as described in Table 29.3. GLUT transporter cells are encoded by sodium glucose cotransporter 2 (*SLC2*) genes.[7] At the cellular level, glucose crosses the cell plasma membrane through aqueous pores formed by GLUT transporters. Fourteen GLUTs have been identified.[7] The GLUT number indicates the order in which the molecular sequence and GLUT tissue locations were identified.[7] GLUTs 1 to 5 have been studied in detail.[7]

GLUT1 and GLUT3. The central nervous system (CNS) is freely permeable to glucose transported by GLUT1 and GLUT3. The CNS does not rely on insulin to transport glucose across the neural cell membrane. The brain and other CNS cells require a constant source of glucose because they retain minimal glucose and glycogen stores.

GLUT2. The GLUT2 proteins are associated with glucose sensing and facilitate the rapid entry of glucose into specialized cells. GLUT2 proteins are dispersed in many different tissues, including pancreatic beta cells, hepatoportal vein cells, and the proximal convoluted tubule in the kidney, facilitating glucose resorption back to the bloodstream from the ultrafiltrate.[7,8] In a high-glucose meal, GLUT2 proteins in the intestine may translocate to the apical cell surface to increase glucose absorption from the gut to the bloodstream.[7]

GLUT4. GLUT4 proteins are insulin responsive and insulin dependent because they have a pivotal role in how glucose moves from the bloodstream into muscle and adipose tissue cells.[9,10] After a meal, the levels of sugars and amino acids in the bloodstream rise. This increase signals pancreatic beta cells to release insulin into the bloodstream. As the insulin circulates

TABLE 29.3 Glucose Transporter Functions

Glucose Transporter (GLUT)	Anatomic Locations	Function
GLUT1	Erythrocytes, endothelial cells of the brain Transport across the blood-brain-barrier	Basal glucose uptake
GLUT2	Pancreatic beta cells, liver, kidney, small intestine	High-capacity glucose transporter Can transport fructose
GLUT3	Brain cells, nerve cells (axons and dendrites)	Transports glucose into the brain and neural tissue
GLUT4	Striated muscle and adipose tissue	Insulin-regulated transport in muscle and fat
GLUT5	Intestine, kidney, testis	Transports fructose
GLUT6	Spleen, leukocytes, brain	
GLUT7	Small intestine, colon, testis	Transports fructose
GLUT8	Testis, brain, muscle, adipocytes	Fuel supply of mature spermatozoa
GLUT9	Liver, kidney	
GLUT10	Liver, pancreas	Muscle-specific fructose transporter
GLUT11	Heart, muscle	
GLUT12	Heart, prostate, mammary gland	
GLUT13	Brain	

in the vascular system, it activates an insulin receptor on the plasma membrane of cells, primarily peripheral muscle and adipose cells. This receptor initiates signaling cascades inside the cell to activate GLUT4, which resides in intracellular vesicles (storage areas within the cell) until needed. GLUT4 travels from intracellular storage sites to the plasma membrane in response to the signal from the insulin receptor.[10,11] At the cell surface, GLUT4 facilitates the passive transport of glucose along a concentration gradient into striated muscle and fat cells. This process increases glucose transport into fat cells by 20- to 30-fold in healthy individuals.[9] Glucose transport into skeletal muscle accounts for 85% to 90% of postprandial glucose removal from the bloodstream.[9] In the baseline state (between meals with normal blood glucose), only 4% to 10% of GLUT4 is on the cell surface, whereas 90% is within the cell storage sites.[9] Within 10 to 15 minutes of insulin stimulation of muscle cells, GLUT4 levels at the cell surface double as rapid translocation from the interior to the cell surface occurs. Between meals, the liver normally provides sufficient glucose output to maintain constant circulating blood glucose levels within the normal range.

GLUT5. Fructose absorption is the target for GLUT5 proteins found on the apical membrane of intestinal cells. GLUT5 is of interest because of the high levels of fructose in many modern processed foods and the link between high-fructose foods and obesity.[12]

Incretins in the Gastrointestinal System

Incretins are hormones released from the GI tract after a meal and increase insulin production from the pancreatic beta cells.[13] Two incretins are of particular clinical importance:

- Glucagon-like peptide 1 (GLP-1)
- Glucose-dependent insulinotropic polypeptide (GIP)

The physiology of the incretins has been used to develop new medicines that reduce postprandial blood glucose levels in type 2 diabetes. In normal physiology, more insulin is released after oral glucose ingestion than in response to the same amount of intravenous glucose because of the release of the gut incretins.[13–15] The increase in insulin secretion caused by stimulation from the incretins may make up 70% of the insulin response, depending on the size of the meal.[14,15] This incretin effect is impaired in patients with type 2 diabetes.[14,15] The physiologic effects of GIP and GLP-1 are listed in Table 29.4.

Glucose-dependent insulinotropic polypeptide. GIP is an incretin and is described as a "gut hormone" that is synthesized and predominantly released from the K cells of the duodenum and proximal jejunum.[13,16] GIP acts directly on pancreatic beta cells to increase insulin secretion.[16]

Glucagon-like peptide 1. GLP-1 is an incretin described as a "gut hormone."[16] GLP-1 is synthesized and released from the enteroendocrine L cells of the ileum and colon.[14,16] When blood glucose levels are elevated, GLP-1 stimulates insulin release from the pancreas and inhibits glucagon release from the liver. GLP-1 exerts other beneficial effects, including decreased gastric emptying and satiety (feeling of being full) after a meal. When blood glucose levels are within normal range, GLP-1 inhibits somatostatin release from the pancreatic delta cells and glucagon from the liver.[16,17] The GLP-1 physiologic pathway has been used to develop medications to lower blood glucose. These medications are GLP-1 agonists (GLP-1a) that mimic incretin functions to increase insulin secretion and decrease glucagon release, as described in Chapter 31.

Dipeptidyl peptidase-4. GLP-1 has a short half-life of less than 2 minutes because it is rapidly broken down by the enzyme dipeptidyl peptidase-4 (DPP-4). This physiologic pathway has been used to develop a class of medications known as *Gliptins* to inhibit the DPP-4 enzyme and slow the inactivation of endogenous GLP-1 to reduce postprandial glucose elevation after a meal. Gliptins are DPP-4 inhibitors (DPPI-4i) and have been shown to reduce cardiovascular adverse events.[17]

Sodium Glucose Cotransporter 2 in the Kidneys

The kidney has a further mechanism to maintain a stable blood glucose level. The glomeruli filter about 180 grams of glucose daily, and in the healthy kidney, most are reabsorbed back in the proximal convoluted tubule.

SGL-2. Glucose reabsorption occurs in the proximal convoluted tubule through a dual mechanism: passively via GLUT2 (see earlier description) and actively via SGLT2. Six SGLTs have been identified. SGLT2 is physiologically important in the kidney. Understanding this physiologic pathway has allowed the development of SGLT2 inhibitor medications that increase glucose excretion in the urine. These medications help lower blood glucose in type 2 diabetes and reduce cardiovascular adverse events.[17]

PITUITARY GLAND AND HYPOTHALAMUS

The hypothalamus is linked to the pituitary gland in two distinct ways: (1) a vascular network connects the anterior portion of the pituitary with the hypothalamus, and (2) a separate pathway of nerve fibers connects the posterior pituitary with the hypothalamus. Understanding the proximity of the hypothalamus and the pituitary gland to each other is necessary to appreciate the correlation that exists between these organs.

TABLE 29.4 **Effect of Incretins on Metabolism**

Target Organs and Tissues	GIP	GLP-1
Pancreas	Stimulates insulin synthesis and release from pancreatic beta cells after a meal when blood glucose is elevated Maintains beta cell mass and function Decreases beta cell death (apoptosis) Increases GLUT2 expression in the pancreas	Stimulates insulin synthesis and release from pancreatic beta cells after a meal when blood glucose is elevated Maintains beta cell mass and function Decreases beta cell death (apoptosis) Increases GLUT2 expression in the pancreas Increases somatostatin release from pancreatic delta cells Decreases glucagon release from the pancreas
Liver		Decreases release of glucose from the liver
GI system		Delays gastric emptying
CNS		Decreases appetite and sense of satiety after a meal
Muscle		Increases glucose uptake in muscle
Adipose tissue		Increases glucose uptake and free fatty acid synthesis to triglycerides
Bone	Increases bone formation Decreases bone resorption	Increases bone formation Decreases bone resorption

CNS, Central nervous system; *GI*, gastrointestinal; *GIP*, glucose-dependent insulinotropic polypeptide; *GLP-1*, glucagon-like peptide 1; *GLUT2*, glucose transporter 2.

Anatomy

Hypothalamus

The hypothalamus lies in the base of the brain, superior to the pituitary gland. It is composed of specialized nervous tissue responsible for the integrated functioning of the nervous and endocrine systems, called *neuroendocrine control*.[18] The hypothalamus weighs approximately 4 g and forms the walls and lower portion of the brain's third ventricle. The area that makes up the floor of the third ventricle thickens in the center and elongates and is called the *pituitary stalk*.

Pituitary Stalk

The pituitary gland is suspended from this funnel-shaped portion that may be described as the *infundibular stalk* or the pituitary stalk, as illustrated in Fig. 29.3. The pituitary stalk contains a rich vascular supply and a network of communicating neurons that travel from the hypothalamus to the pituitary.[18] The vascular network and neural pathways transport chemical and neural signals and maintain constant communication between the nervous system and the endocrine system.

Pituitary Gland

The pituitary gland is also called the *hypophysis*. It is attached below the hypothalamus and is recessed in the base of the cranial cavity in a hollow depression of the sphenoid bone known as the *sella turcica*.[19] Secured in such a protected environment, the pituitary is one of the most inaccessible endocrine glands in humans. However, because of this location, the pituitary gland is susceptible to injury from surgical and accidental trauma to the face and head.[19] The pituitary is composed of the anterior and posterior lobes (see Fig. 29.3). Each component within the pituitary has its own origin, morphology, and function.[20]

Anterior pituitary. The anterior lobe of the pituitary, also called the *adenohypophysis*, is the largest portion of the gland. It communicates with the hypothalamus through a vascular network comprising the *superior hypophysial artery*, a capillary network, and the *anterior hypophysial vein* (see Fig. 29.3).[18] The glandular tissue of the anterior pituitary produces several hormones, including adrenocorticotropic hormone (ACTH), thyroid-stimulating hormone (TSH), follicle-stimulating hormone, luteinizing hormone, growth hormone, and prolactin.[20] Information about all the hormones, their target tissues, and their actions is found in Fig. 29.1.

Posterior pituitary. The posterior lobe of the pituitary gland is also known as the *neurohypophysis*. It retains continuity with the hypothalamus through neural fibers running through the infundibular stalk (Fig. 29.3). The neurohypophysis has no glandular properties but functions as an extension of the hypothalamus. It collects, stores, and later releases hormones produced in the hypothalamus. Oxytocin and antidiuretic hormone (ADH) are manufactured in the hypothalamus and stored in the posterior pituitary.[20] The *inferior hypophysial artery* provides blood supply to the posterior pituitary.

Physiology

The hypothalamus gland is known as the "master gland" because of its influence over all areas of body functioning. The hypothalamus controls pituitary gland action and response by secreting *release-inhibiting factors*. These factors control the release or inhibition of hormones. Thyrotropin-releasing hormone (TRH) is an example of a release-inhibiting factor.[20] Virtually every function necessary to maintaining the human body in a state of dynamic equilibrium is regulated in this manner. ADH is one of the most important hormones to understand in caring for a critically ill patient.

Antidiuretic Hormone

ADH, also known as *arginine vasopressin*, is an important hormone responsible for regulating fluid balance within the body.[21,22] ADH acts through specialized vasopressin receptors (V receptors) in specific target tissue:

- V_1 receptors in arterial walls
- V_2 receptors in kidney collecting ducts
- V_3 receptors in pituitary tissue

Function. ADH has two functions: (1) through the V_1 receptors, it constricts smooth muscles within the arterial wall, and (2) through the V_2 receptors, it regulates fluid balance by altering the permeability of the kidney tubule to water.[22] ADH also contributes to controlling the sodium level in the extracellular fluid by controlling plasma osmolality. The sodium ion concentration in the plasma largely determines plasma osmolality. Osmoreceptors in the hypothalamus are sensitive to changes in the circulating plasma osmolality.[22]

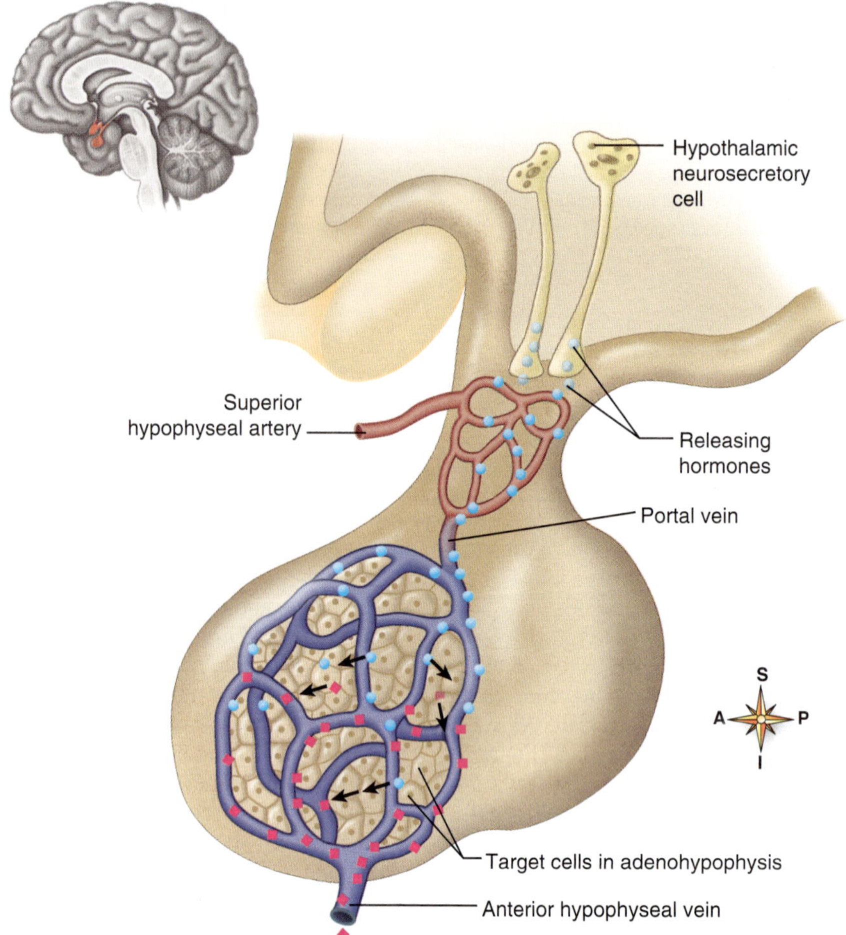

FIG. 29.3 Hypophyseal Portal System. Neurons in the hypothalamus secrete releasing hormones into vessels that carry the releasing hormones directly to the vessels of the adenohypophysis, thus bypassing the typical systemic circulatory route. (From Patton K, Bell F, Thompson T, Williamson P. *Anatomy and Physiology*. 11th ed. Elsevier; 2022.)

Disorders of water metabolism are divided into *hyperosmolar* and *hypoosmolar* states.[22] Hyperosmolar disorders have a deficit of body water relative to body solutes. Hypoosmolar disorders have an excess of body water relative to total body solutes. Different but complementary systems regulate sodium and water metabolism within the body. Sodium metabolism is predominately regulated by the renin-angiotensin-aldosterone system (RAAS), and water metabolism is primarily controlled by arginine vasopressin (AVP) hormone, also known as antidiuretic hormone (ADH).

Hypoosmolar and hyperosmolar states. A low sodium level is associated with a low serum osmolality (hypoosmolar state). When sodium levels rise, plasma osmolality increases (hyperosmolar state). ADH is then released to stimulate water resorption at the nephron to maintain sodium balance. This process decreases water loss from the body and subsequently concentrates and reduces urine volume. Fluid conserved in this manner is returned to the circulating plasma, where it dilutes the plasma concentration (osmolality), as shown in Fig. 29.4.

The release of ADH increases with hypovolemia.[22] Plasma osmotic pressure and circulating blood volume regulate the release of ADH. Stretch receptors in the left atrium are sensitive to volume changes in the plasma that may be caused by vomiting, diarrhea, or blood loss. Bleeding sufficient to lower the blood pressure or emesis sufficient to reduce fluid volume stimulates the release of ADH. Other factors influencing ADH secretion are pain, stress, malignant disease, surgical intervention, alcohol, and some medications. Table 29.5 lists additional factors that affect ADH levels.

THYROID GLAND

Anatomy

The thyroid gland weighs 15 to 25 g in an adult.[23] The size of the adult gland varies according to the availability of dietary iodine in different geographic regions. The gland partially encases the trachea, is wrapped around the second to fourth tracheal rings anteriorly and laterally, and is located posteriorly at the level of the sixth and seventh cervical vertebrae. The thyroid gland lies inferior to the thyroid cartilage and the articulating surface of the cricoid cartilage. This bow-tie-shaped gland has two lateral lobes that are partially covered by the sternohyoid and sternothyroid muscles. The thyroid isthmus, the band of narrow thyroid tissue that connects the lateral lobes, lies directly inferior to the cricoid cartilage, as shown in Fig. 29.5.

Surrounding Nerves

Two vital nerves associated with speech and swallowing pass close to the thyroid gland. The recurrent laryngeal nerve and

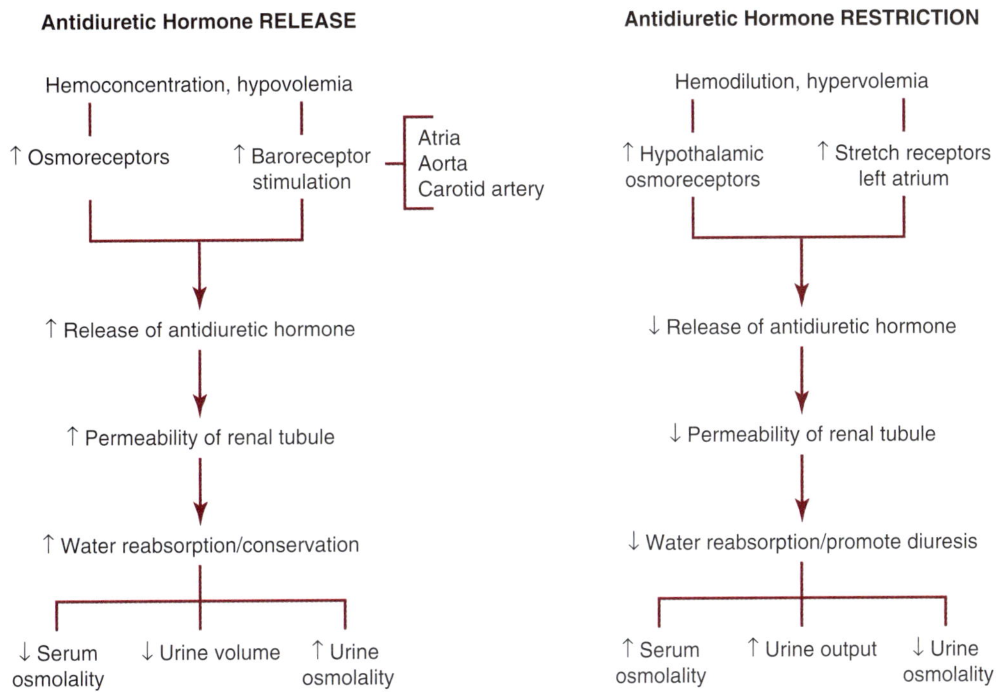

FIG. 29.4 Physiology of the Release and Restriction of Antidiuretic Hormone.

TABLE 29.5 Antidiuretic Hormone Functions

Antidiuretic Hormone Stimulation	Antidiuretic Hormone Restriction
Increased serum osmolality	Decreased serum osmolality
Emesis	Hypervolemia
Hypovolemia	Water intoxication
Hemorrhage	Cold
Pain	Congenital defect
	Carbon dioxide inhalation
Hypothalamic-Pituitary System Damage	
Accidental trauma	Accidental trauma
Surgical trauma	Surgical trauma
Pathologic trauma	Pathologic trauma
Stress: Physical and emotional	
Acute infections	
Malignancies	
Nonmalignant pulmonary disorders	
Stimulated pulmonary baroreceptors	
Nocturnal sleep	
Medications	
Nicotine	Phenytoin
Barbiturates	Chlorpromazine
Oxytocin	Reserpine
Glucocorticoids	Norepinephrine
Anesthetics	Ethanol
Acetaminophen	Opioids
Amitriptyline	Lithium
Carbamazepine	Demeclocycline
Cyclophosphamide	Tolazamide
Chlorpropamide	
Potassium-depleting diuretics	
Vincristine	
Isoproterenol	

superior laryngeal nerve are branches of the vagus nerve. The considerable anatomic variety in the location of these nerves increases the risk of injury during surgical procedures such as thyroidectomy.[23] The functional units of the thyroid gland are spherical cells called *follicles*. Follicles are filled with the protein thyroglobulin.[24]

Blood Supply

The thyroid gland has a rich blood supply from the superior and inferior thyroid arteries. The superior thyroid artery is the first branch of the external carotid artery.[23] Venous drainage is from the superior, middle, and inferior thyroid veins. Lymphatic drainage follows the route of the thyroid veins.[23]

Parathyroid Glands

The parathyroid glands (usually four) are intimately associated with the posterior surface of the thyroid gland. The parathyroid glands derive their name from their anatomic proximity to the thyroid, although they have a different function. The parathyroid glands maintain calcium homeostasis.

Physiology

The functioning of the thyroid gland depends on many factors that respond to a delicate hormonal interplay. The hypothalamus, anterior pituitary, dietary intake of iodine, and circulating protein bodies in the blood all affect thyroid gland function.

Thyroid-Stimulating Hormone

The anterior lobe of the pituitary gland secretes TSH, also known as *thyrotropin*. TSH then stimulates the thyroid gland to produce thyroid hormones.

Iodine and Iodide

In the United States, dietary ingestion of iodine ranges from 200 to 500 mcg per person/day. Iodine is added to table salt to

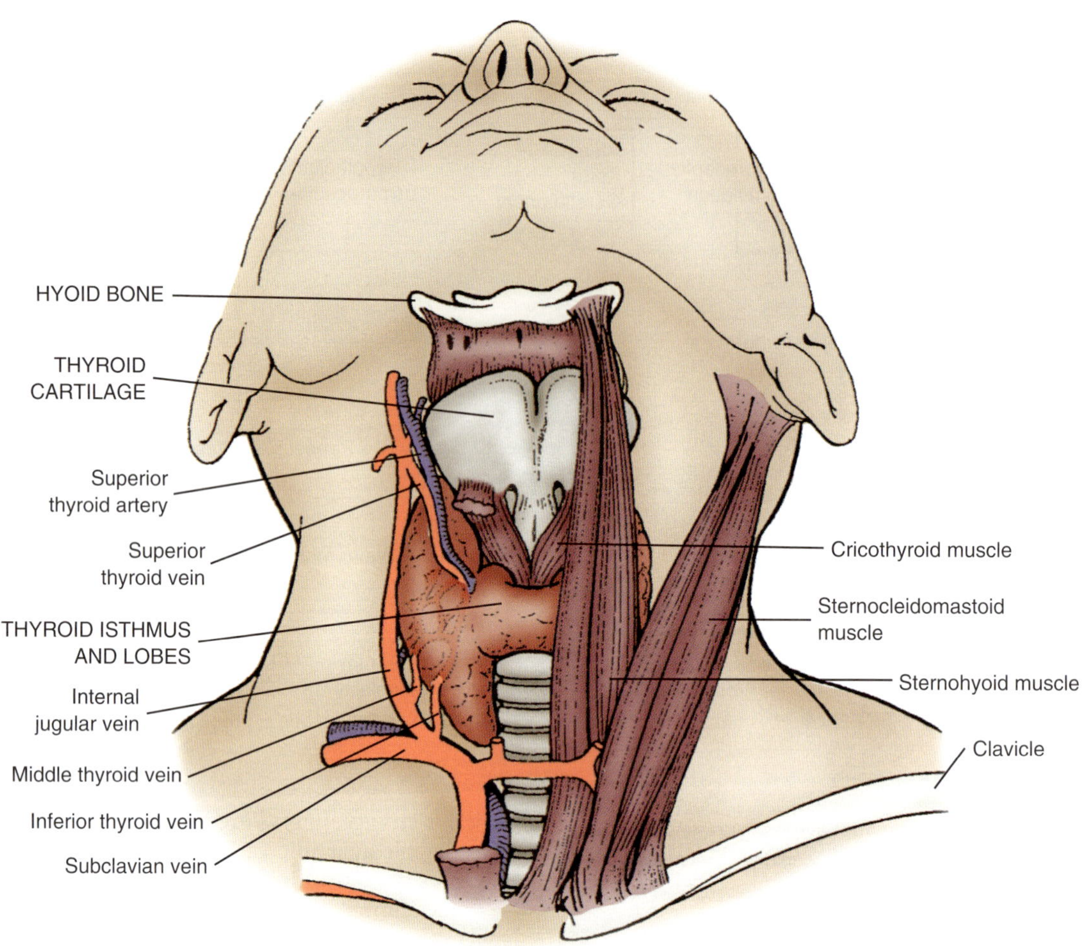

FIG. 29.5 Gross Anatomy of the Human Thyroid.

ensure adequate amounts in the population. Dietary iodine is absorbed and concentrated in the thyroid follicles through a complex process. The iodine is oxidized to iodide by the enzyme thyroid peroxidase. The amino acid tyrosine binds the iodide to thyroglobulin through active transport, eventually yielding triiodothyronine (T_3) and thyroxine (T_4). Most T_3 and T_4 are circulated in the bloodstream bound to proteins. Free thyroid hormone that is not protein bound activates thyroid responses throughout the body and is described as free T_3 and free T_4.

Thyroglobulin

Thyroglobulin is a crucial precursor in the biosynthesis of thyroid hormone. Thyroglobulin is stored in the thyroid follicles until needed. TSH release stimulates thyroglobulin secretion into the bloodstream.[24]

Triiodothyronine and Thyroxine

TSH prompts the thyroid cells to produce thyroid hormones (T_3 and T_4) in the presence of iodine in the thyroid follicles. In the normal thyroid gland, 90% of the thyroid hormone that is produced is in the form of T_4, and 10% is T_3. These hormones are named according to the number of iodine atoms in their structure; T_3 has three iodine atoms, and T_4 has four iodine atoms.[24]

Most T_4 is subsequently converted into the more biologically active T_3. Most T_3 in the bloodstream results from converting T_4 to T_3 in the peripheral tissues, liver, and kidneys. T_3 acts more rapidly on target tissues compared with T_4, and it is more actively potent. Both thyroid hormones affect the rate at which oxygen is used in the body and thus affect all metabolic processes.

Calcitonin

The thyroid gland produces a third hormone, thyrocalcitonin, also called *calcitonin.* This hormone is produced by the parafollicular cells, or C cells, that are scattered among the thyroid follicular cells. Calcitonin acts in concert with parathyroid hormone to maintain normal calcium blood levels. Calcitonin lowers calcium levels in the blood through urinary excretion and promotes calcium absorption in bone. In contrast, parathyroid hormone limits urinary loss and stimulates bones to release calcium. Throughout the remainder of this discussion, thyroid hormone refers collectively to T_3 and T_4, not calcitonin.

Hypothalamic-Pituitary-Thyroid Axis Feedback Loop

The hypothalamic-pituitary-thyroid axis regulates the mechanism for the synthesis and secretion of thyroid hormone.[25] The production and secretion of thyroid hormone are regulated by a feedback mechanism that limits the amount of hormone circulating to the cellular need at that time, as illustrated in Fig. 29.6.

In response to decreased circulating levels of T_3 and T_4, the hypothalamus releases TRH. TRH activates TSH in the anterior pituitary, and TSH stimulates the thyroid gland to manufacture and release the thyroid hormones T_3 and T_4 in the presence of iodine.[25] When serum blood levels of T_3 and T_4 become high,

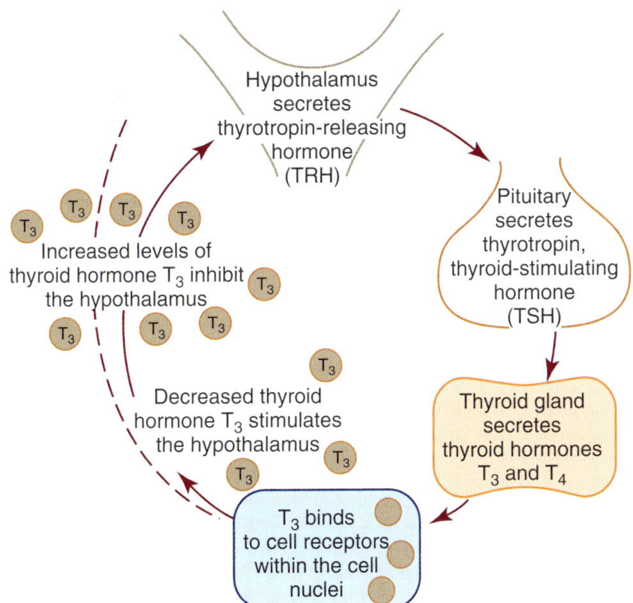

FIG. 29.6 Hypothalamus-Pituitary-Thyroid Axis Feedback Loop.

the pituitary inhibits the production of additional TSH. When levels of T_3 and T_4 become too low, the pituitary is stimulated to secrete additional TSH.

T_4 prompts the activation of beta-adrenergic receptors in widespread areas of the body. These receptors trigger an SNS response and release norepinephrine at sympathetic nerve endings. The effect is stimulation of the cardiac, nervous, and smooth muscle tissue, as well as an increase in metabolism and thermogenesis (increased body heat). Box 29.3 lists the major actions of thyroid hormones in more detail.

BOX 29.3 Thyroid Hormone Functions

- Interact with growth hormone
- Maturation of the skeletal system
- Development of central nervous system
- Stimulate carbohydrate metabolism
- Increase rate of glucose absorption from the gastrointestinal tract
- Increase the rate of glucose use by the cells
- Accelerate the rate of fat metabolism
- Increase cholesterol degradation in the liver
- Decrease serum cholesterol levels
- Increase protein anabolism and catabolism
- Mobilize protein and release amino acids into circulation
- Increase energy from protein nutrients through gluconeogenesis
- Increase demand for vitamins
- Increase oxygen consumption and use
- Increase basal metabolic rate
- Have marked chronotropic and inotropic effects on the heart
- Increase cardiac output
- Stimulate contractility and excitability of myocardium
- Increase blood volume
- Expand respiratory rate and depth necessary for normal hypoxic and hypercapnic drive
- Promote sympathetic overactivity
- Boost erythropoiesis
- Increase metabolism and clearance of various hormones and pharmacologic agents
- Stimulate bone resorption

ADRENAL GLAND

Anatomy

The adrenal glands, also called *suprarenal glands*, are small, yellowish, bilateral, pyramidal, or semilunar-shaped organs located at the superior pole of the kidney. As a neighbor to the kidney, they are retroperitoneal and embedded in the fat pad of the kidney. The normal adrenal gland is 3 to 4 cm in its longest axis and weighs approximately 5 g in adults (Fig. 29.7). Functionally and histologically, two glands exist within the suprarenal gland: (1) the outer cortex and (2) the inner medulla. Both regions secrete hormones integral to the body's response to stress.

Adrenal Cortex

The adrenal cortex is the thicker outer region, making up 85% of the gland. The cortex is composed of three different layers of cells, each with a specific endocrine function: (1) zona glomerulosa, (2) zona fasciculata, and (3) zona reticularis. The cortex secretes cortisol, regulates fluid homeostasis through aldosterone, and secretes androgens.

Adrenal Medulla

The inner region is called the *adrenal medulla*. The inner medulla is a part of the SNS, and it resembles a cluster of neurons more than an endocrine gland. The adrenal medulla contains clusters of specialized chromaffin cells, which are modified preganglionic sympathetic neurons.[26] Different sets of chromaffin cells contain chromaffin granules specific for epinephrine or norepinephrine. The granules for each catecholamine appear in different sets of cells within the adrenal medulla. A chromaffin cell usually contains granules only for one catecholamine or the other.

The SNS stimulates the adrenal medulla by preganglionic bundles of sympathetic nerve fibers that originate in the spinal cord.[26] The role of the chromaffin cells is to secrete the catecholamines epinephrine and norepinephrine. Under physiologic stress, these hormones produce a widespread excitatory effect described as a "surge of adrenaline" or the "fight-or-flight response."[26]

Adrenal Blood Supply

The rich arterial blood supply comes to the adrenal gland from three sources (see Fig. 29.7): (1) the superior suprarenal artery is a branch of the inferior phrenic artery, (2) the middle suprarenal artery branches directly off of the aorta, and (3) the inferior suprarenal artery branches off the renal artery. Venous drainage is usually achieved through a single vein from each adrenal gland. The vein from the right adrenal gland drains into the inferior vena cava, and the left adrenal gland empties into the left renal vein.

Physiology

Hypothalamic-Pituitary-Adrenal Axis

The hypothalamic-pituitary-adrenal (HPA) axis controls vital physiologic stress responses in health and illness.[27] The hypothalamus secretes corticotropin-releasing hormone (CRH), which stimulates the anterior pituitary to release adrenocorticotrophic hormone (ACTH) to stimulate the adrenal cortex to release cortisol into the bloodstream. This process is a feedback loop, so cortisol in the bloodstream will lower ACTH release

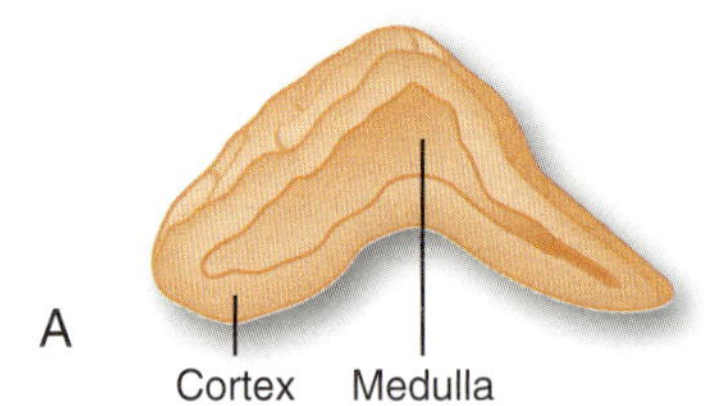

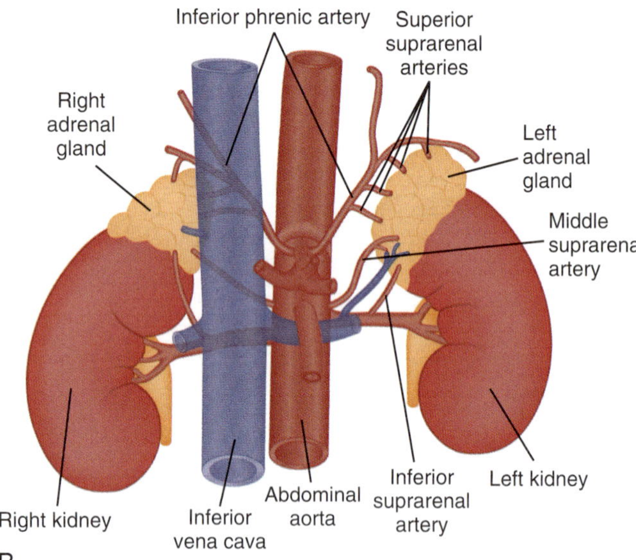

FIG. 29.7 Adrenal Gland. (A) Cross-section of the adrenal gland showing the outer cortex and inner medulla. (B) Anatomic relationship of the adrenal glands to the kidneys.

from the anterior pituitary gland. Under stress-free conditions, cortisol is secreted in a diurnal pattern, and levels are highest in the early morning and lowest in the late evening.[28] Critical illness disrupts normal HPA adrenal physiology with resultant loss of the diurnal pattern.[29]

Adrenal Hormones

The adrenal cortex and the adrenal medulla secrete essential and very different hormones. Each part of the gland is functionally independent.

Adrenal cortex. The adrenal cortex (outer layer) secretes three different classes of hormones, all of which are lipid-based steroid hormones: (1) glucocorticoid, (2) corticosteroid, and (3) mineralocorticoid. The glucocorticoid hormone cortisol is secreted from the zona fasciculata and zona reticularis cells. Cortisol is released in response to physiologic stress caused by infection, trauma, and the fasting state.[27] In hypoglycemia, the release of cortisol triggers other cells in the body to produce energy from fats and amino acids (proteins) to ensure the brain receives a steady supply of glucose. Pharmacologic doses (high doses) of glucocorticoids are used to depress the inflammatory response and inhibit the immune system.

Pharmacologic corticosteroids are administered to prevent rejection of newly transplanted solid organs (see Chapter 35). Corticosteroids are also used to treat inflammatory disorders and are administered when the adrenal gland is cortisol deficient.

The principal mineralocorticoid hormone, aldosterone, is secreted from the zona glomerulosa cells. Secretion of aldosterone is the final step in the RAAS. Aldosterone is secreted in response to intravascular hypovolemia, and its target of action is the distal tubules of the kidneys to retain more sodium and water in the bloodstream. In a healthy person, aldosterone contributes to the body's equilibrium of water and potassium. Fig. 13.18 illustrates the neurohormonal role of the RAAS in heart failure. In patients with heart failure, medications to block aldosterone's effect on the kidneys are often prescribed. The most frequently used medication is spironolactone (Aldactone) (see Neurohormonal Compensatory Mechanisms in Heart Failure in Chapter 13).

Adrenal medulla. The adrenal medulla (inner region) secretes two important catecholamines: epinephrine, also known as *adrenaline*, and norepinephrine, also known as *noradrenaline*. The adrenal medulla acts as a functional extension of the SNS. With stimulation of the SNS, the chromaffin cells in the adrenal medulla are stimulated to secrete predominantly epinephrine and some norepinephrine into the bloodstream. This results in an epinephrine surge described as the fight-or-flight response. In the critical care unit, intravenous infusions of epinephrine and norepinephrine are used in shock states to raise blood pressure. The pharmacologic effects of these catecholamines are described in Table 14.19.

KEY POINTS

Pancreas

- The pancreas is a long, triangular organ approximately 15 cm long and 4 cm wide. It is situated in the C-shaped curvature of the duodenum and extends behind and below the stomach toward the spleen.
- Insulin is released by the beta cells of the pancreas. An elevated blood glucose level is the stimulus for insulin secretion from the pancreas. The higher the blood glucose, the more insulin the normal pancreas produces.
- Glucagon is synthesized from the alpha cells in the pancreas. Its effect is the opposite of the effect of insulin. Glucagon release is stimulated by hypoglycemia, and it stimulates glucose output from the liver.
- In addition to insulin, human cells take up glucose through facultative glucose transport proteins known as GLUTs.
- Incretins are hormones released from the GI tract after a meal that increase insulin production from the pancreatic beta cells.

Pituitary

- The pituitary gland is attached below the hypothalamus and recessed in the base of the skull in a hollow depression known as the *sella turcica.*
- The anterior pituitary gland secretes ACTH, TSH, and other hormones.
- The posterior pituitary gland secretes AVP, also known as antidiuretic hormone (ADH).
- Sodium and water metabolism are regulated by two complementary systems within the body: sodium metabolism by the RAAS and water metabolism by arginine vasopressin (ADH).

Thyroid

- The thyroid gland has a "bow-tie" shape. It is wrapped around the trachea anteriorly and laterally at the sixth and seventh cervical vertebrae level. The thyroid isthmus, the band of narrow thyroid tissue that connects the lateral lobes, lies directly below the cricoid cartilage.

- The thyroid hormones are T_4 and T_3. Most T_4 is converted to the more potent and biologically active T_3 in the peripheral tissues, liver, and kidneys.
- The thyroid gland produces a third hormone, thyrocalcitonin (calcitonin), which acts with parathyroid hormone to maintain normal calcium blood levels.

Adrenal

- The adrenal glands are small, pyramid-shaped organs located at the superior pole of the kidneys.
- The adrenal gland contains a cortex and medulla, representing two functionally different endocrine zones. The adrenal cortex secretes cortisol and aldosterone. The adrenal medulla secretes epinephrine and norepinephrine.

Visit the Evolve site at http://evolve.elsevier.com/Urden/CriticalCareNursing for additional study materials.

REFERENCES

1. Atkinson MA, Campbell-Thompson M, Kusmartseva I, Kaestner KH. Organisation of the human pancreas in health and in diabetes. *Diabetologia*. 2020;63(10):1966–1973. https://doi.org/10.1007/s00125-020-05203-7.
2. Russo GT, Giorda CB, Cercone S, et al. Beta cell stress in a 4-year follow-up of patients with type 2 diabetes: A longitudinal analysis of the BetaDecline Study. *Diabetes Metab Res Rev*. 2018;34(6):e3016. https://doi.org/10.1002/dmrr.3016.
3. Christensen AA, Gannon M. The beta cell in type 2 diabetes. *Curr Diab Rep*. 2019;19(9):81. https://doi.org/10.1007/s11892-019-1196-4.
4. Campbell JE, Newgard CB. Mechanisms controlling pancreatic islet cell function in insulin secretion. *Nat Rev Mol Cell Biol*. 2021;22(2):142–158. https://doi.org/10.1038/s41580-020-00317-7.
5. Hudish LI, Reusch JE, Sussel L. β Cell dysfunction during progression of metabolic syndrome to type 2 diabetes. *J Clin Invest*. 2019;129(10):4001–4008. https://doi.org/10.1172/JCI129188.
6. Wewer Albrechtsen NJ, Holst JJ, Cherrington AD, et al. 100 years of glucagon and 100 more. *Diabetologia*. 2023;66(8):1378–1394. https://doi.org/10.1007/s00125-023-05947-y.
7. Berger C, Zdzieblo D. Glucose transporters in pancreatic islets. *Pflugers Arch*. 2020;472(9):1249–1272. https://doi.org/10.1007/s00424-020-02383-4.
8. Sun B, Chen H, Xue J, Li P, Fu X. The role of GLUT2 in glucose metabolism in multiple organs and tissues. *Mol Biol Rep*. 2023;50(8):6963–6974. https://doi.org/10.1007/s11033-023-08535-w.
9. Klip A, McGraw TE, James DE. Thirty sweet years of GLUT4. *J Biol Chem*. 2019;294(30):11369–11381. https://doi.org/10.1074/jbc.REV119.008351.
10. van Gerwen J, Shun-Shion AS, Fazakerley DJ. Insulin signalling and GLUT4 trafficking in insulin resistance. *Biochem Soc Trans*. 2023;51(3):1057–1069. https://doi.org/10.1042/BST20221066.
11. Bryant NJ, Gould GW. Insulin stimulated GLUT4 translocation - size is not everything!. *Curr Opin Cell Biol*. 2020;65:28–34. https://doi.org/10.1016/j.ceb.2020.02.006.
12. Hernández-Díazcouder A, Romero-Nava R, Carbó R, et al. High fructose intake and adipogenesis. *Int J Mol Sci*. 2019;20(11):2787. https://doi.org/10.3390/ijms20112787.
13. Pais R, Gribble FM, Reimann F. Stimulation of incretin secreting cells. *Ther Adv Endocrinol Metab*. 2016;7(1):24. https://doi.org/10.1177/2042018815618177.
14. Nauck MA, Meier JJ. Incretin hormones: Their role in health and disease. *Diabetes Obes Metab*. 2018;20(Suppl 1):5–21. https://doi.org/10.1111/dom.13129.
15. Drucker DJ, Holst JJ. The expanding incretin universe: from basic biology to clinical translation. *Diabetologia*. 2023;66(10):1765–1779. https://doi.org/10.1007/s00125-023-05906-7.
16. Müller TD, Finan B, Bloom SR, et al. Glucagon-like peptide 1 (GLP-1). *Mol Metab*. 2019;30:72–130. https://doi.org/10.1016/j.molmet.2019.09.010.
17. Elharram CS, Moura M, Abrahamowicz, et al. Novel glucose lowering agents are associated with a lower risk of cardiovascular and adverse events in type 2 diabetes: A population based analysis. *Int J Cardiol*. 2020;310:147–154. https://doi.org/10.1016/j.ijcard.2020.03.025.
18. Clasadonte J, Prevot V. The special relationship: Glia-neuron interactions in the neuroendocrine hypothalamus. *Nat Rev Endocrinol*. 2018;14(1):25–44. https://doi.org/10.1038/nrendo.2017.124.
19. Iskra T, Stachera B, Możdżeń K, et al. Morphology of the sella turcica: A meta-analysis based on the results of 18,364 patients. *Brain Sci*. 2023;13(8):1208. https://doi.org/10.3390/brainsci13081208.
20. Musumeci G, Castorina S, Castrogiovanni P, et al. A journey through the pituitary gland: Development, structure and function, with emphasis on embryo-foetal and later development. *Acta Histochem*. 2015;117(4–5):355. https://doi.org/10.1016/j.acthis.2015.02.008.
21. Kleindienst A, Hannon MJ, Buchfelder M, Verbalis JG. Hyponatremia in neurotrauma: the role of vasopressin. *J Neurotrauma*. 2015;33(7):615. https://doi.org/10.1089/neu.2015.3981.
22. Knepper MA, Kwon TH, Nielsen S. Molecular physiology of water balance. *N Engl J Med*. 2015;372(14):1349. https://doi:10.1056/NEJMra1404726.
23. Mohebati A, Shaha AR. Anatomy of thyroid and parathyroid glands and neurovascular relations. *Clin Anat*. 2012;25(1):19. https://doi.org/10.1002/ca.21220.
24. Coscia F, Taler-Verčič A, Chang VT, et al. The structure of human thyroglobulin. *Nature*. 2020;578(7796):627–630. https://doi.org/10.1038/s41586-020-1995-4.
25. Feldt-Rasmussen U, Effraimidis G, Klose M. The hypothalamus-pituitary-thyroid (HPT)-axis and its role in physiology and pathophysiology of other hypothalamus-pituitary functions. *Mol Cell Endocrinol*. 2021;525:111173. https://doi.org/10.1016/j.mce.2021.111173.
26. Carbone E, Borges R, Eiden LE, et al. Chromaffin cells of the adrenal medulla: Physiology, pharmacology, and disease. *Compr Physiol*. 2019;9(4):1443–1502. https://doi.org/10.1002/cphy.c190003.
27. Russell G, Lightman S. The human stress response. *Nat Rev Endocrinol*. 2019;15:525–534. https://doi.org/10.1038/s41574-019-0228-0.
28. Oster H, Challet E, Ott V, et al. The functional and clinical significance of the 24-hour rhythm of circulating glucocorticoids. *Endocr Rev*. 2017;38(1):3–45. https://doi.org/10.1210/er.2015-1080.
29. Van den Berghe G. Adrenal function/dysfunction in critically ill patients: a concise narrative review of recent novel insights. *J Anesth*. 2021;35(6):903–910. https://doi.org/10.1007/s00540-021-02977-x.

30

Endocrine Clinical Assessment and Diagnostic Procedures

Mary E. Lough and Kathleen M. Stacy

http://evolve.elsevier.com/Urden/CriticalCareNursing

Assessing a patient with endocrine dysfunction is a systematic process that incorporates history taking and physical examination. Most of the endocrine glands are deeply encased in the human body. Although the placement of the glands provides security for the glandular functions, their inaccessibility limits clinical examination. Nevertheless, the endocrine glands may be assessed indirectly. The critical care nurse who understands the metabolic actions of the hormones produced by endocrine glands assesses the physiology of a gland by monitoring the target tissue of the gland, as listed in Fig. 29.1 in Chapter 29. This chapter describes clinical and diagnostic evaluation of the pancreas, the posterior pituitary, and the thyroid gland.

HISTORY

The patient's initial presentation determines the history's rapidity and direction. For a patient in acute distress, the history is curtailed to only a few questions about the patient's chief complaint and precipitating events. For a patient without obvious distress, the endocrine history focuses on four areas: (1) current health status, (2) description of the current illness, (3) medical history and general endocrine status, and (4) family history.

PANCREAS

The endocrine function of the pancreas involves the production and secretion of hormones that play crucial roles in regulating blood sugar levels and various metabolic processes within the body. The key hormones produced by the endocrine cells of the pancreas are insulin, glucagon, somatostatin, and pancreatic polypeptide. These hormones are secreted by specific cell types within the pancreas, primarily found in clusters called islets of Langerhans.

History

Taking a thorough patient history for pancreatic disorders is crucial for accurate diagnosis and appropriate management. A comprehensive history includes gathering information about the patient's symptoms, medical history, family history, lifestyle, and relevant exposures. Taking a thorough patient history for a patient with diabetes is crucial for understanding their condition, management, and potential complications. Data collection for the identification of diabetes complications is outlined in Box 30.1.

Focused Physical Assessment

The focused physical assessment provides information about pancreatic functioning. Clinical manifestations of abnormal glucose metabolism include hyperglycemia, which is the initial assessment priority for a patient with pancreatic dysfunction. Patients with hyperglycemia may be prediabetic, hyperglycemic associated with severe critical illness, or ultimately diagnosed with type 1 or type 2 diabetes.[1] Each of these conditions has specific identifying features. More information on the specific pathophysiology and management of each condition is provided in Chapter 31.

Hyperglycemia

Because severe hyperglycemia affects various body systems, all systems are assessed. The patient may complain of blurred vision, headache, weakness, fatigue, drowsiness, anorexia, nausea, and abdominal pain. On inspection, the patient has flushed skin, polyuria, polydipsia, vomiting, and evidence of dehydration. Progressive deterioration in the level of consciousness, from alert to lethargic or comatose, is observed as the hyperglycemia exacerbates. If ketoacidosis occurs, the patient's breathing becomes deep and rapid (Kussmaul respirations), and the breath may have a fruity odor. Auscultation of the abdomen may reveal hypoactive bowel sounds. Palpation elicits abdominal tenderness. Percussion may reveal diminished deep tendon reflexes. The patient's fluid volume status is assessed as hyperglycemia results in osmotic diuresis. Signs of dehydration include tachycardia, orthostatic hypotension, and poor skin turgor. The critical laboratory tests that assist in assessment are discussed next.

Laboratory Studies

Pertinent laboratory tests for endocrine pancreatic function measure short-term and long-term blood glucose levels, which can identify and diagnose diabetes (Table 30.1).

Blood Glucose

A blood test assesses the fasting plasma glucose (FPG) level after the patient has not eaten for 8 hours (see Table 30.1).[1] A normal FPG level is between 70 and 100 mg/dL.[1] An FPG level between 100 and 125 mg/dL identifies prediabetes.[1] Individuals with prediabetes are at increased risk for complications of diabetes, such as coronary heart disease and stroke. An FPG level of 126 mg/dL (7 mmol/L) or higher is diagnostic of diabetes (see Table 30.1).[1] After a meal, the concentration of glucose increases in the bloodstream. Normal postprandial blood glucose levels are expected to be less than 180 mg/dL (10 mmol/L).[1]

All critically ill patients must have their blood glucose levels monitored frequently while in the hospital. Clinical practice guidelines from the American Association of Clinical Endocrinologists and the American Diabetes Association recommend

BOX 30.1 DATA COLLECTION

Complications of Diabetes

Current Health Status

- The body may be unable to adjust to increased insulin needs resulting from sudden physiologic changes such as infection, injury, or surgery. The patient is assessed for a severe infection, surgical wound, or traumatic injury.
- Recent or current signs and symptoms
- Unexplained changes in weight, thirst, hunger
- Headache, blurred vision
- Long-standing, unhealed infection
- Vaginitis, pruritus
- Leg pain, numbness
- Unexplained change in urinary patterns (e.g., daytime and nighttime, frequency, volume)
- Energy or stamina changes
- Endurance level
- Weakness
- Unexplained, excessive fatigue
- Behavior or mental changes (also ask a family member or significant other for input)
- Memory loss
- Orientation

Assessment of Current Illness: Onset, Characteristics, and Course

- Chronic illness: Physiologic or psychological stress may increase endogenous glucose
- Recent treatments that could be a source of exogenous glucose
- Hyperalimentation
- Peritoneal dialysis
- Hemodialysis
- Medications, including prescription and over-the-counter preparations: Pharmacologic agents may alter pancreatic function by increasing or decreasing the release of endocrine hormones. Medications also may interfere with hormonal action at the receptor site on the target cell.

Medical History: Questions

- Have you had prior pancreatic surgery?
- Have you ever been told that any of the following applied to you?
    - Too much sugar in the urine
    - Too much sugar in the blood
    - Will probably develop too much sugar later in life
- If you answered yes to any of these questions, what treatment, if any, was prescribed?
- Are you currently following such a treatment?

Family History: Questions

- Has a family member ever been diagnosed with diabetes or "sugar in the blood"?
- If so, how was the condition treated?

instituting insulin therapy when a critically ill patient's blood glucose level is greater than 180 mg/dL.[2] A target blood glucose range of 140 to 180 mg/dL is recommended.[2] During administration of a continuous insulin infusion, point-of-care blood glucose testing is performed hourly or according to hospital protocol to achieve and maintain the blood glucose within the target range.[3,4]

Hypoglycemia is defined as a blood glucose level less than 70 mg/dL (3.9 mmol/L).[1] A complication of intensive glucose control is that hypoglycemic episodes may occur more frequently in the hospital and with self-management of glucose levels in diabetes.[2–4]

TABLE 30.1 Blood Glucose Levels

Patient Status	Fasting BG (mg/dL)	Fasting BG (mmol/L)
Hypoglycemia	<70	<3.9
Normal	70–100	>3.9–5.6
Prediabetes	100–125	5.6–6.9
Diabetes	≥126	≥7.0
Diabetes (random test, nonfasting, with symptoms)	≥200	≥11.1

BG, Blood glucose.
Data from American Diabetes Association. Classification and diagnosis of diabetes: standards of medical care in diabetes—2020. *Diabetes Care*. 2020;43(suppl 1): S14–31.

Urine Glucose

Testing the urine for glucose is not recommended for patients with diabetes because too much variation exists in the threshold for glucose when diabetes-related kidney damage has occurred. Urine glucose measurements are affected by variations in fluid intake, reflect an average glucose level, not a specific point in time, and are altered by some medications. Urine glucose testing also does not offer any help in the identification of hypoglycemia. For all these reasons, urine glucose testing should never be used.

Glycated Hemoglobin

Blood testing of glucose is helpful for the daily management of diabetes. However, a different blood test is used to achieve an objective measure of blood glucose over an extended period. The glycated hemoglobin (HbA_{1c}), or A1c, provides information about the average amount of glucose that has been present in the patient's bloodstream over the previous 3 months.[5] During the 120-day lifespan of red blood cells (erythrocytes), the hemoglobin within each cell binds to the available blood glucose through a process known as glycosylation. Typically, 4% to 6% of hemoglobin contains the glucose group A_{1c}. The A1c is less than 5.7% in a person without diabetes.[6] The A1c value in a person with prediabetes is between 5.7% and 6.4%.[6] An acceptable target A_{1c} of less than 7% is appropriate for diabetic patients.[5] The A1c value correlates with specific blood glucose levels, as shown in Table 30.2.[5] The American Diabetes Association recommends using the A1c value both during the initial assessment of diabetes mellitus and for follow-up to monitor treatment effectiveness.[5]

Blood Ketones

Ketone bodies are a byproduct of rapid fat breakdown. Ketone blood levels rise in acute illness, in fasting states, and with sustained elevation of blood glucose in type 1 diabetes in the absence of insulin. In diabetic ketoacidosis, fat breakdown (*lipolysis*) occurs so rapidly that fat metabolism is incomplete, and the ketone bodies (acetone, beta-hydroxybutyric acid, and acetoacetic acid) accumulate in the blood (ketonemia). They are excreted in the urine (ketonuria). A fruity, sweet-smelling odor on the exhaled breath may detect elevated levels of ketones (ketonemia). This distinctive breath odor derives from

TABLE 30.2 Correlation Between Hemoglobin A1c and Plasma Glucose Level

Hemoglobin A1c (%)	Mean Plasma Glucose Level (mg/dL)	Mean Plasma Glucose Level (mmol/L)
5	97 (76–120)	5.4 (4.2–6.7)
6	126 (100–152)	7.0 (5.5–8.5)
7	154 (123–185)	8.6 (6.8–10.3)
8	183 (147–217)	10.2 (8.1–12.1)
9	212 (170–249)	11.8 (9.4–13.9)
10	240 (193–282)	13.4 (10.7–15.7)
11	269 (217–314)	14.9 (12.0–17.5)
12	298 (240–347)	(13.3–19.3)

HbA1c, Glycosylated hemoglobin. The numbers in parentheses represent the 95% confidence intervals (CI) for these values.

From Nathan DM, Kuenen J, Borg R, Zheng H, Schoenfeld D, Heine RJ; for the A1c-Derived Average Glucose (ADAG) Study Group. Translating the A1C assay into estimated average glucose values [published correction appears in *Diabetes Care*. 2009 Jan;32(1):207]. *Diabetes Care*. 2008;31(8):1473–1478. https://doi.org/10.2337/dc08-0545.

eliminating acetone as part of the compensatory response to maintain a normal pH. It is recommended that all patients with diabetes perform self-testing or have their blood tested for the presence of ketones during any alteration in level of consciousness or acute illness accompanied by an elevated blood glucose level. Urine testing for ketones is no longer recommended.[7] Self-test meters to measure blood ketones from a fingerstick are now available.[8,9]

PITUITARY GLAND

The pituitary gland, recessed in the base of the skull, is not accessible for physical assessment. Therefore, the systemic effects of a normally functioning pituitary are used to identify dysfunction. One essential hormone formed in the hypothalamus but secreted through the posterior pituitary gland is antidiuretic hormone (ADH), also known as arginine vasopressin (AVP) or simply vasopressin. ADH is released from the posterior pituitary in response to hypovolemia, changes in plasma osmolality, hypoxia, and acidosis. ADH actions are both antidiuretic and vasoconstrictive.

History

Assessing the history of a patient with potential pituitary issues involves gathering information about their medical, family, and lifestyle history. The patient should be asked about their current symptoms, including headaches, vision changes, hormonal imbalances (e.g., excessive thirst, frequent urination, changes in menstrual cycle), fatigue, and changes in weight. It is also important to explore any preexisting medical conditions such as diabetes, hypertension, thyroid disorders, or other endocrine conditions and determine if the patient has a history of head trauma, radiation exposure to the head or neck, or brain surgery. Inquire about any medications or supplements the patient is currently taking, as some medications can affect the pituitary gland or hormone levels. Investigate if the patient has a family history of endocrine disorders, brain tumors, genetic conditions, or any hereditary factors related to pituitary or hormonal abnormalities. A thorough history, combined with appropriate physical examination and diagnostic tests, is crucial for an accurate assessment of pituitary function and the identification of any related conditions or disorders.

Focused Physical Assessment

ADH controls the amount of fluid lost and retained within the body. Acute posterior pituitary or hypothalamus dysfunction may result in insufficient or excessive ADH production. The clinical signs of posterior pituitary dysfunction often manifest as fluid volume deficit (insufficient ADH production) or fluid volume excess (excessive ADH production).

Hydration Status

One method to determine the effectiveness of ADH production is to conduct a hydration assessment. This assessment includes observations of skin integrity, skin turgor, and buccal membrane moisture. Moist, shiny buccal membranes indicate satisfactory fluid balance. Skin turgor that is resilient and returns to its original position in less than 3 seconds after being pinched or lifted shows adequate skin elasticity. The skin over the forehead is the most reliable for testing tissue turgor because this area of skin is less affected by aging.[9] The skin in the groin and axilla is slightly moist to touch in a well-hydrated patient. In older patients, these typical assessment findings may be absent. Other indicators that the patient's hydration status is adequate for metabolic demands include a balanced intake and output and the absence of thirst. However, the lack of thirst is an unreliable indicator of dehydration in patients with decreased thirst mechanisms, such as older and critically ill patients. The absence of abrupt changes in mental status may also indicate normal hydration. Other indicators of normal hydration include the absence of edema, stable weight, and urine specific gravity within the normal range (1.005 to 1.030).

Vital Signs

Changes in heart rate, blood pressure, and central venous pressure (when available) are helpful to determine fluid volume status. Blood pressure and pulse are monitored frequently. Decreased blood pressure with an increased pulse is characteristic of hypovolemia, whereas elevated blood pressure and a rapid, bounding pulse may indicate hypervolemia. Orthostatic hypotension, which occurs when intravascular fluid volume decreases, is identified by a drop in systolic blood pressure of 20 mm Hg or a drop in diastolic blood pressure of 10 mm Hg when the patient changes position from lying to standing.[10,11]

Weight Changes and Intake and Output

Daily weight changes coincide with fluid retention and fluid loss. Sudden weight changes can result from a change in fluid balance; 1 L of fluid lost or retained equals approximately 2.2 lb, or 1 kg, of weight gained or lost. To use weight as a valid determinant of fluid balance, all extraneous variables must be eliminated; this means the same scale is used at the same time each day. Precise measurement and notation of intake and output are used as criteria for fluid replacement therapy.

Laboratory Studies

No single diagnostic test identifies dysfunction of the posterior pituitary gland. A diagnosis usually is made through the patient's clinical presentation and history. Although serum measurement of ADH is available, it is rarely obtained in critically ill patients.

Serum Antidiuretic Hormone Level

The normal serum ADH reference range is approximately 1 to 5 picograms/mL (pg/mL), although this range may vary according to the clinical laboratory doing the test. Before ADH measurement, all medications that may alter the release of ADH are withheld for a minimum of 8 hours. Common medications that affect ADH levels include morphine sulfate, lithium carbonate, chlorothiazide, carbamazepine, oxytocin, and selective serotonin reuptake inhibitors. Nicotine, alcohol, positive-pressure and negative-pressure ventilation, and emotional stress also influence ADH.

Serum ADH levels are compared with blood and urine osmolality to differentiate the syndrome of inappropriate antidiuretic hormone (SIADH) from central diabetes insipidus (DI).[12] Increased ADH levels in the bloodstream compared with low serum osmolality and elevated urine osmolality confirm the diagnosis of SIADH.[12] Reduced levels of serum ADH in a patient with high serum osmolality, hypernatremia, and reduced urine concentration indicate central DI. Typically, this diagnosis is based on urine output, serum sodium, and serum osmolality rather than serum ADH level.[12] Chapter 31 provides more information about SIADH and DI.

Serum and Urine Osmolality

Values for serum osmolality in the bloodstream range from 275 to 295 mOsm/kg H_2O; there are variations in this range based on the clinical laboratory standard values. Osmolality measurements determine the concentration of dissolved particles in a solution. In a healthy person, a change in the concentration of solutes triggers a chain of events to maintain adequate serum dilution. The most accurate measures of the body's fluid balance are obtained when urine and blood samples are collected simultaneously.

Increased serum osmolality stimulates the release of ADH, which reduces the amount of water lost through the kidney. Body fluid is retained at the kidney tubules and collecting ducts to dilute the particle concentration in the bloodstream. According to one clinical guideline, the hypothalamic vasopressin (ADH) osmoreceptors are maximally inhibited at levels less than 280 mOsm/kg H_2O to eliminate water via the kidney. In contrast, at levels greater than 290 mOsm/kg H_2O, the sensation of thirst and ADH osmoreceptors are maximally stimulated to conserve water.[12] This narrow clinical range is often disrupted in pituitary disease and critical illness.

Decreased serum osmolality inhibits the release of ADH. The kidney tubules increase their permeability and fluid is eliminated from the body in an attempt to regain the normal concentration of particles in the bloodstream. Urine osmolality in a person with normal kidneys depends on fluid intake. With high fluid intake, particle dilution is low but increases if fluids are restricted. Therefore, the expected range for urine osmolality ranges from 50 to 1400 mOsm/kg.

Antidiuretic Hormone Test

The ADH test differentiates neurogenic DI (central) from nephrogenic (kidney) DI or primary polydipsia. In DI, the patient is producing large volumes of dilute urine (see Chapter 31). The patient is challenged with 0.05 to 1.0 mL of intranasally administered ADH in the form of desmopressin (1-deamino-8-D-arginine vasopressin, commonly abbreviated as DDAVP). An intravenous line is inserted before ADH administration, and urine volume and osmolality are measured every 30 minutes for 2 hours before and after the ADH challenge. In central DI (nonfunctional or poorly functional posterior pituitary), the kidney responds to the exogenous ADH by resorbing water at the kidney tubule, making the urine more concentrated.

In nephrogenic DI, the kidney does not respond to the exogenous ADH, and urine osmolality remains unchanged (large volumes of dilute urine). This test is not performed in the critical care unit because of the unstable hemodynamic and volume status of critically ill patients. A different diagnostic test for DI diagnosis is the water deprivation test, which, for the same reasons, is not used in critical care.[13]

Copeptin

At the same time as ADH is released from the posterior pituitary, other biochemical biomarkers are coreleased. These include neurophysin 2 and the C-terminal part of the precursor pre-provasopressin (CTproAVP), more generally known as copeptin.[14–16] This has clinical benefits because copeptin plasma levels reliably relate to ADH levels in healthy and critically ill patients.[14,15] Because measuring ADH directly is technically challenging due to its instability and short half-life in the bloodstream, copeptin is often used as a more practical and reliable alternative to indirectly assess ADH levels.[14–16] For these reasons, copeptin has the potential to be clinically useful in the diagnosis of both nephrogenic DI and partial central DI.[15]

Diagnostic Procedures

In addition to laboratory tests, radiographic examination, computed tomography (CT), and magnetic resonance imaging (MRI) are used to diagnose structural lesions such as cranial bone fractures, tumors, or blood clots in the pituitary region.[17,18] Although these procedures do not diagnose DI or SIADH, they help uncover the likely underlying cause.

Computed Tomography

CT of the base of the skull identifies pituitary tumors, blood clots, cysts, nodules, or other soft tissue masses. This rapid procedure causes no discomfort except requiring the patient to lie perfectly still. CT studies can be performed with or without radiopaque contrast medium. The contrast dye is given intravenously to highlight the hypothalamus, infundibular stalk, and pituitary gland. This dye may cause allergic reactions in iodine-sensitive individuals, and the patient must be asked about iodine allergy before the test. The size and shape of the sella turcica and the position of the hypothalamus, infundibular stalk, and pituitary are identified.[11]

Magnetic Resonance Imaging

MRI enables the radiologist to visualize internal organs and cellular characteristics of specific tissues. MRI uses a magnetic field rather than radiation to produce high-resolution, cross-sectional images. The soft brain tissue and surrounding cerebrospinal fluid make the brain especially suited to assessment with MRI.[18]

THYROID GLAND

The thyroid gland plays a crucial role in the endocrine system, producing hormones that are essential for regulating various bodily functions. Dysfunction of the thyroid gland can result in either overproduction (hyperthyroidism) or underproduction (hypothyroidism) of thyroid hormones.

BOX 30.2 DATA COLLECTION

Hyperthyroidism and Hypothyroidism

- The patient is the best source for the following information. If the patient cannot respond, the following questions can be directed to family, friends, a significant other, or persons involved in the patient's admission to the critical care unit.
- Have you ever been diagnosed with overactive thyroid, increased metabolism, or hyperthyroidism? What about underactive thyroid, slowed metabolism, or hypothyroidism?
- Have you ever been treated for hyperthyroidism or hypothyroidism?
- Have you ever had an operation for thyroid disease?
- Have you ever received radioactive iodine for thyroid disease?
- Are you taking any medicine for thyroid disease? If so, what is the name of the medication, and what is the prescribed dose and frequency?
- When did you first notice the constant restlessness or extreme fatigue?
- Has your weight been the same or changed over the past year?
- Has your appetite changed over the past 6 months?
- Have you lost weight even though your appetite has increased (which may indicate hyperthyroidism)?
- Have you gained or stayed at the same weight even though you have not felt like eating over the past 6 months (which may indicate hypothyroidism)?
- Do you always feel warm (which may indicate hyperthyroidism)?
- Do you open windows in the house even in the winter months?
- Do you wear lightweight clothing even when others wear layers of heavier clothing?
- Do you always feel cold (which may indicate hypothyroidism)?
- Do you wear multiple layers of clothing despite warm weather or the use of a heater or furnace?
- Do you use several blankets and keep windows closed even in warm weather?
- Do you complain about never being able to "warm up"?
- Have you developed any of the following over the past 6 months to 1 year?

Hypothyroidism Indicators	Hyperthyroidism Indicators
Loss of coarse, dry scalp hair and the outer edge of the eyebrow	Hair thinning
	Swelling (face, eyes, legs)
Sleepiness, lethargy, depression	Insomnia, nervousness, anxiety
Weight gain despite decreased appetite	Weight loss despite increased appetite
Severe constipation	Diarrhea
Muscle and joint pain (hands, wrists, feet)	Muscle weakness or wasting; tremors
	Warm, moist skin
Dry, itchy skin	Heat intolerance, sweating
Increased sensitivity to cold	Tachycardia, atrial fibrillation
	Menstruation changes; impaired fertility
Bradycardia	
Menstruation changes; impaired fertility	

History

The history of any patient in a critical care unit should be as detailed as possible. Information regarding the clinical manifestations of hypothyroidism or hyperthyroidism must be obtained from the patient, family, or others with knowledge of the health history. Sample questions pertinent to the detection of thyroid disease are provided in Box 30.2.

Focused Physical Assessment

The thyroid is palpated for tenderness, nodules, and enlargement and is auscultated for bruits. The normal-size thyroid gland is usually neither visible nor palpable in the anterior neck. Palpation may be done from an anterior or posterior approach. Auscultation of the thyroid is accomplished by using the bell portion of the stethoscope to identify a bruit or blowing noise from the circulation through the thyroid gland. The presence of a bruit indicates enlargement of the thyroid, as evidenced by increased blood flow through the glandular tissue.

Laboratory Studies

Controversy exists about routine measurement of thyroid function in adults without clinical symptoms. The U.S. Preventive Services Task Force 2015 review found the research evidence insufficient to recommend routine screening for thyroid disease in asymptomatic adults.[19] However, thyroid hormone blood test screening is recommended for adults 60 years old and older and individuals with symptoms of thyroid dysfunction (hypofunction or hyperfunction).[19] There are no recommendations about thyroid hormone screening for critically ill patients.

Thyroid hormone blood tests measure circulating thyroid hormone levels and assess the integrity of the hormonal negative feedback response within the hypothalamic-pituitary-thyroid axis. Laboratory diagnosis is based on the measurement of thyroid-stimulating hormone (TSH) or the simultaneous measurement of TSH and free thyroxine (FT_4).[20]

Normally, an inverse linear relationship exists between TSH and FT_4.[21] When the hypothalamic-pituitary-thyroid axis is normal, TSH production is inhibited by the presence of free thyroid hormone in the bloodstream (FT_4), and the TSH value is normal.

- Hypothyroidism: High TSH and low FT_4
- Hyperthyroidism: Low TSH, high FT_4, and an increased FT_3-to-FT_4 ratio

Thyroid-Stimulating Hormone

Clinical laboratory analysis of TSH has become more sensitive, allowing more accurate measurement of low thyroid hormone levels. Thyroid hormone reference ranges in adults are listed in Table 30.3.[22] Because serum values vary slightly between laboratory methods, it is imperative to know the normal reference values used by the hospital clinical laboratory.

The serum level of TSH increases as a person ages, which may signal declining thyroid function, as greater stimulation of the thyroid gland by TSH is required.[20] In contrast, T_4 levels fall slightly with advanced age.[20] The average TSH level by age, from a study of 1200 persons (600 males, 600 females), is shown below[20]:

- TSH 0.4–4.3 milliunits/L between 20 to 59 years
- TSH 0.4–5.8 milliunits/L between 60 to 79 years
- TSH 0.4–6.7 milliunits/L older than 80 years

Thyroid Tests in Critically Ill Patients

The incidence of thyroid disease in hospitalized patients is low, estimated at 1% and 2% of all inpatients. In critically ill patients, TSH measurement is usually the first thyroid-related laboratory

TABLE 30.3 Thyroid Hormone Blood Tests

Name of Test	Abbreviation	Reference Value (SI)	Reference Value[a]
Thyroid-stimulating hormone (thyrotropin)	TSH	0.4–4.5 milliunits/L	
Total serum thyroxine	TT_4	581–154 nmol/L	4.0–12.0 mcg/dL
Free thyroxine	FT_4	9–23 pmol/L	0.7–1.8 ng/dL
Total serum triiodothyronine	TT_3	1.2–2.7 nmol/L	100–200 ng/dL
Free triiodothyronine	FT_3	3.2–9.2 pmol/L	208–596 pg/dL
Thyroglobulin[b]	Tg	3.0–40 mcg/L	

[a]Some tests are reported with more than one reference value because clinical laboratories use various reference ranges depending on the specifics of the clinical test.
[b]Thyroglobulin (Tg) reference values should be determined locally because serum thyroglobulin concentrations are influenced by local iodide intake.
SI, International units.
Reference values from Demers LM. Thyroid disease: pathophysiology and diagnosis. *Clin Lab Med.* 2004;24(1):19.

TABLE 30.4 Medications That Influence Diagnostic Thyroid Levels

Increase	Decrease
FT_3	
Increase	*Decrease*
Methadone	Anabolic steroid
Estrogens	Androgens
Progestins	Salicylates
Amiodarone	Phenytoin
	Lithium
	Reserpine
	Propranolol
	Sulfonamides
	Propylthiouracil
	Methylthiouracil
FT_4	
Increase	*Decrease*
Oral contraceptives	Phenytoin
Heparin	Steroids
Aspirin	Diphenylhydantoin
Furosemide	Chlorpromazine
Clofibrate	Lithium
Phenylbutazone	Sulfonylurea
Some NSAIDs	Sulfonamides
Propranolol	Reserpine
Corticosteroids	Chlordiazepoxide
Amiodarone	
TSH	
Increase TSH	*Decrease TSH and TSH Response to TRH*
Metoclopramide	Glucocorticoids
Iodides	Dopamine
Lithium	Heparin
Potassium iodide	Aspirin
Morphine sulfate	Carbamazepine
TBG	
Increase	*Decrease*
Opiates	Androgen therapy
Oral contraceptives	Asparaginase
Estrogens	
Clofibrate	
5-FU	
Perphenazine	

5-FU, 5-Fluorouracil; *FT_3*, free triiodothyronine; *FT_4*, free thyroxine; *NSAIDs*, nonsteroidal antiinflammatory drugs; *TBG*, thyroxine-binding globulin; *TRH*, thyrotropin-releasing hormone; *TSH*, thyroid-stimulating hormone.

test obtained. Most experts recommend obtaining both TSH and FT_4 hormone levels.[23]

Medications and thyroid testing. Additional measurement difficulties involve concomitant use of certain medications that interfere with thyroid function and lower serum levels.[24]

TSH secretion is affected by several medications routinely administered in critical care units. Glucocorticoids in large doses may lower the serum level of FT_3 and inhibit TSH secretion.[22] Dopamine infusions at greater than 1 mcg/kg per minute directly block TSH release.[24] Amiodarone, an antidysrhythmic medication, is an iodine-rich compound structurally similar to T_3 and T_4.[25] At usual doses, amiodarone can increase the daily iodine amount by 50 to 100 times.[25]

Several medications increase the serum level of FT_4 by displacing protein-bound T_4.[24] Medications that displace protein-bound T_4 cause an increase in serum FT_4 levels.[24] Salicylates (aspirin), furosemide (Lasix), and unfractionated and low-molecular-weight heparins raise FT_4 serum levels by this mechanism.[24] A complete list of medications that alter thyroid hormone serum levels is provided in Table 30.4. It is unclear whether it is necessary to adjust the pharmacologic management of critically ill patients in response to these medication-laboratory interactions.

Diagnostic Procedures

Diagnostic procedures often begin with ultrasonography to visualize a thyroid nodule or tumor.[26] A nuclear medicine scan using an oral iodine radioactive isotope may be requested to diagnose hypothyroidism.[27] The thyroid-scanning procedure may also detect the presence of ectopic thyroid tissue, thyroid carcinomas, and the amount of viable thyroid glandular tissue after therapeutic irradiation.

ADRENAL GLAND

Admission to the critical care unit with a primary adrenal disorder is rare. The term *primary* indicates that the principal problem lies within the adrenal gland. Secondary adrenal dysfunction is caused by dysfunction in another gland or by a clinical condition such as sepsis.

The adrenal gland is two glands in one, as described in Chapter 29, which may make the history and presentation complex. The adrenal cortex (outer layer) secretes two classes of hormones; if deficient or released in excess, they may cause clinical symptoms. Two hormones relevant to the care of critically ill patients are (1) the glucocorticoid hormone cortisol and (2) the mineralocorticoid hormone aldosterone. Cortisol is secreted in response to physiologic stress due to infection, trauma, and hypoglycemia. Aldosterone is secreted in response to intravascular hypovolemia. Aldosterone release is the final step in the renin-angiotensin-aldosterone system (RAAS) pathway.

The adrenal medulla (inner layer) also secretes two hormones that cause clinical symptoms if they are deficient or released in excess: epinephrine and norepinephrine. Epinephrine, also known as *adrenaline*, and norepinephrine, also known as *noradrenaline*, are both secreted from the adrenal gland medulla in response to stress.

History

A detailed history may help identify conditions or medications affecting adrenal gland function. Primary endocrine disorders are rare, but a history of uncontrolled hypertension despite three or more oral medications may indicate whether endocrine-related hypertension should be investigated. The medication history may help determine whether the patient takes glucocorticoid tablets, and the patient or family should be asked about using steroid creams for dermatologic conditions and steroid-based inhalers for chronic obstructive lung disease.

Focused Physical Assessment

The physical examination is related to the effects of adrenal dysfunction, and the signs depend on the hormone involved and whether the problem is related to excess or deficiency. This situation means that the signs and symptoms are very diverse. A systematic assessment of all signs and symptoms is essential because adrenal disease is often missed or misdiagnosed.

Adrenal Cortex

Primary cushing syndrome. The excess release of the glucocorticoid hormone cortisol causes Cushing syndrome.[28–30] Excess cortisol produces the classic signs and symptoms listed in Box 30.3. Primary Cushing disease is rare, but if a patient is not taking exogenous steroids, it becomes a diagnosis of exclusion when the relevant constellation of signs and symptoms is present.[29,30] The first step is to obtain a serum adrenocorticotropic hormone (ACTH) level in a patient with overt signs of Cushing syndrome. A serum ACTH level of less than 2.2 pmol/L (10 pg/mL) is considered diagnostic.[30] Imaging of the pituitary gland to search for a tumor or other injury is performed after the low ACTH value has confirmed Cushing syndrome as the cause of the condition.[30]

Secondary cushing syndrome. Symptoms identical to the symptoms of primary Cushing syndrome (see Box 30.3) occur in patients with the secondary form who are on long-term glucocorticoid therapy with pharmacologic doses, such as transplant recipients who take steroids to prevent solid-organ rejection, patients with chronic obstructive lung disease, or patients with chronic inflammatory conditions. When patients are admitted to the critical care unit, it is crucial to ascertain whether they are steroid dependent to avoid the harmful effects of abrupt steroid withdrawal.[30]

BOX 30.3 Causes of Cushing Syndrome

Primary Cushing Syndrome

- Cushing syndrome is divided into adrenocorticotropin-dependent and adrenocorticotropin-independent types. Adrenocorticotropin is also known as adrenocorticotropic hormone (ACTH) or corticotropin.

ACTH-Dependent Cushing Syndrome

- Most cases (80%) result from a pituitary adenoma that causes the pituitary gland to produce excess ACTH. Excess secretion of ACTH stimulates the adrenal cortex to release excess amounts of cortisol into the bloodstream, circumventing the normal inhibitory feedback loop.
- The other 20% of cases are caused by ectopic ACTH secretion from small cell cancers of the lung, metastases, and endocrine tumors.

ACTH-Independent Cushing Syndrome

- Cases are usually caused by a unilateral adrenal tumor: adrenal adenoma (60%) or adrenal carcinoma (40%).

Secondary or Iatrogenic Cushing Syndrome

- The patient takes pharmacologic doses of glucocorticoids, which may be prescribed to prevent rejection after solid-organ transplantation or to treat chronic inflammatory conditions.

Clinical Signs and Symptoms of Cushing Syndrome

- Emotional lability (can range from depression to psychosis)
- Hyperglycemia and poorly controlled type 2 diabetes
- Obesity or weight gain in the abdomen
- Rounded face
- Acne
- Thin skin, bruises easily, poor wound healing
- Hypertension
- Hirsutism (excess hair growth)
- Dorsocervical fat pad ("buffalo hump")
- Decreased libido
- Fatigue, weakness

Primary Aldosteronism

In patients with primary aldosteronism, the adrenal cortex secretes excess mineralocorticoid (aldosterone) unrelated to the RAAS.[31] In other words, the aldosterone secretion is untethered from the normal RAAS feedback loop (see Fig. 13.19 in Chapter 13). Primary aldosteronism occurs in up to 10% of individuals with medication-resistant hypertension and up to 20% in groups with hypertension and hypokalemia.[31] This rare condition may cause the patient to present emergently with severe hypertension and a critically low serum potassium levels (hypokalemia), which can be lethal if not identified and effectively treated. The diagnostic laboratory test recommended for high-risk individuals is an aldosterone-to-renin ratio.[31] A CT scan of the adrenal-kidney structures is obtained to visualize tumors secreting excess aldosterone.[31,32] An invasive diagnostic test is an adrenal venous sampling of cortisol and aldosterone levels obtained by an interventional radiologist to determine whether the condition affects one or both adrenal glands.[31,33] Surgical removal of an aldosterone-secreting tumor may be required.

Adrenal Insufficiency

Adrenal insufficiency is a rare disorder of the adrenal cortex that involves the hyposecretion of glucocorticoids (cortisol), sometimes occurring with the hyposecretion of mineralocorticoids (aldosterone). It is also known as Addison disease after Thomas Addison, who first described the condition.[34,35] Physiologically, adrenal insufficiency may be the inverse of conditions with excess hormone secretion. The laboratory diagnosis involves simultaneous measurements of the serum ACTH level with a cortisol serum level.[35] A low (or normal) serum cortisol in the presence of an elevated ACTH is diagnostic.[35] A serum cortisol value below 100 nmol/L in the early morning is also considered diagnostic.[35]

Adrenal Crisis

An adrenal crisis, also called an Addisonian crisis, is a life-threatening condition in which the adrenal gland is almost nonfunctional, usually because of the destruction of adrenal tissue.[35] The patient presents acutely with critical hypotension, an elevated serum potassium level (hyperkalemia), a low serum sodium level (hyponatremia), and hypoglycemia.

Critical Illness–Related Corticosteroid Insufficiency

The adrenal gland is designed to respond to acute physiologic stress by increasing stress hormones via the hypothalamic-pituitary-adrenal axis. Early in critical illness, a rise in cortisol levels can be documented. However, over time, the adrenal glands often cannot secrete adequate amounts of stress hormones, especially when critical illness is prolonged.[36] This is described as critical illness–related corticosteroid insufficiency (CIRCI).[36] Research into the causes of CIRCI is ongoing.[36]

Adrenal Medulla

Pheochromocytoma. Pheochromocytomas are rare tumors that arise from the catecholamine-producing chromaffin cells of the adrenal medulla.[37] Most produce norepinephrine, but some produce both norepinephrine and epinephrine. These tumors produce a far greater quantity of catecholamines than normal adrenal medullary tissue. The concentrations of catecholamines can be so high within the tumor that it has been likened to a volcano that is ready to erupt. When vast amounts of norepinephrine or epinephrine are released into the bloodstream, it creates a catecholamine storm and a hypertensive crisis that can be life-threatening. The body responds to the catecholamine surge as if to a severe fight-or-flight threat by hypertension, tachycardia, increased respiratory rate, and hyperglycemia. The patient may describe symptoms of headache, dizziness, palpitations, chest pain, anxiety, nervousness, and fatigue (Box 30.4).[37] Because the body perceives the catecholamine onslaught as a signal to be ready to escape a threatening situation, it slows down the gastrointestinal tract, and constipation is another symptom. Patients at greatest risk are admitted to a critical care unit or who undergo surgery and experience a hypertensive crisis during anesthesia.[37]

The recommended laboratory diagnosis of pheochromocytoma is by measurement of plasma and urine fractionated metanephrines.[37,38] Catecholamines are metabolized into metanephrines. Pheochromocytoma-secreted catecholamine levels fluctuate, making blood levels variable, but catecholamine metabolism into metanephrines is constant, which is why this test is preferred.[37] The patient should be supine and resting for 30 minutes before the metanephrine blood level is drawn.[37,38] A 24-hour urine collection of excreted catecholamines may be obtained.[37] Finally, genetic testing of the patient and immediate relatives may be requested.

BOX 30.4 Pheochromocytoma: Signs and Symptoms[a]

Signs	Symptoms
• Hypertension	• Headaches
• Tachycardia	• Dizziness or faintness
• Tachypnea	• Palpitations, chest pain
• Pallor or flushing	• Anxiety and nervousness
• Hyperglycemia or poorly controlled type 2 diabetes	• Excessive sweating
• Decreased gastrointestinal motility	• Weakness, fatigue
	• Weight loss
	• Constipation

[a]Not all patients have all signs and symptoms.

Diagnostic Procedures

CT is the most widely used test to image the adrenal glands. It visualizes the adrenal glands to detect tumors, enlargement, or abnormalities. An MRI may also be performed to provide detailed images of the adrenal glands for evaluation of tumors or other abnormalities. Percutaneous adrenal biopsy is rarely performed in all cases and is unlikely to be performed in critically ill patients. In some cases, this procedure may be performed to examine tissue samples for abnormalities or cancer.

KEY POINTS

- Assessment of a patient with endocrine dysfunction is a systematic process incorporating the medical and family history, physical examination, and laboratory test results.

Pancreas

- Normal fasting blood glucose is between 70 and 100 mg/dL. A fasting blood glucose between 110 and 126 mg/dL identifies prediabetes. A blood glucose level greater than 126 mg/dL is diagnostic of diabetes. Hyperglycemia is a common finding in critically ill patients.

Pituitary

- The normal range of serum ADH is 1 to 5 pg/mL. All medications that may alter ADH release are withheld for at least 8 hours before ADH measurement.
- Serum osmolality ranges from 275 to 295 mOsm/kg H_2O. Urine osmolality ranges from 50 to 1400 mOsm/kg.
- Serum ADH levels are compared with blood and urine osmolality to differentiate SIADH from central DI.

Thyroid

- High TSH and low FT_4 values identify hypothyroidism.
- Low TSH and high FT_4 values identify hyperthyroidism.

Adrenal

- The adrenal gland is designed to respond to acute physiologic stress.
- In prolonged critical illness and septic shock, the adrenal gland may not secrete enough cortisol.
- Other rare adrenal conditions that require specific diagnostic tests include Cushing syndrome, primary aldosteronism, adrenal insufficiency, and pheochromocytoma.

Visit the Evolve site at http://evolve.elsevier.com/Urden/CriticalCareNursing for additional study materials.

REFERENCES

1. ElSayed NA, Aleppo G, Aroda VR, et al. 2. Classification and diagnosis of diabetes: Standards of care in diabetes-2023 [published correction appears in Diabetes Care. 2023 Feb 01] [published correction appears in Diabetes Care. 2023 Sep 1;46(9):1715]. *Diabetes Care*. 2023;46(Suppl 1):S19–S40. https://doi.org/10.2337/dc23-S002.
2. Moghissi ES, Korytkowski MT, DiNardo M, et al. American Association of Clinical Endocrinologists and American Diabetes Association consensus statement on inpatient glycemic control. *Diabetes Care*. 2009;32(6):1119–1131. https://doi.org/10.2337/dc09-9029.
3. Jacobi J, Bircher N, Krinsley J, et al. Guidelines for the use of an insulin infusion for the management of hyperglycemia in critically ill patients. *Crit Care Med*. 2012;40(12):3251–3276. https://doi.org/10.1097/CCM.0b013e3182653269.
4. Pollock F, Funk DC. Acute diabetes management: adult patients with hyperglycemic crises and hypoglycemia. *AACN Adv Crit Care*. 2013;24(3):314–324. https://doi.org/10.1097/NCI.0b013e31829b7d38.
5. ElSayed NA, Aleppo G, Aroda VR, et al. 6. Glycemic targets: standards of care in diabetes-2023. *Diabetes Care*. 2023;46(Suppl 1):S97–S110. https://doi.org/10.2337/dc23-S006.
6. Diabetes Basics. Centers for Disease Control and Prevention (CDC). Reviewed October 25, 2022. https://www.cdc.gov/diabetes/basics/index.html. Accessed September 20, 2023.
7. Brooke J, Stiell M, Ojo O. Evaluation of the accuracy of capillary hydroxybutyrate measurement compared with other measurements in the diagnosis of diabetic ketoacidosis: a systematic review. *Int J Environ Res Public Health*. 2016;13(9):837. https://doi.org/10.3390/ijerph13090837.
8. Guimont MC, Desjobert H, Fonfrède M, et al. Multicentric evaluation of eight glucose and four ketone blood meters. *Clin Biochem*. 2015;48(18):1310–1316. https://doi.org/10.1016/j.clinbiochem.2015.07.032.
9. Morley JE. Dehydration, hypernatremia, and hyponatremia. *Clin Geriatr Med*. 2015;31(3):389–399. https://doi.org/10.1016/j.cger.2015.04.007.
10. Jones PK, Shaw BH, Raj SR. Orthostatic hypotension: managing a difficult problem. *Expert Rev Cardiovasc Ther*. 2015;13(11):1263–1276. https://doi.org/10.1586/14779072.2015.1095090.
11. Dani M, Dirksen A, Taraborrelli P, et al. Orthostatic hypotension in older people: considerations, diagnosis and management. *Clin Med (Lond)*. 2021;21(3):e275–e282. https://doi.org/10.7861/clinmed.2020-1044.
12. Lamas C, del Pozo C, Villabona C. Neuroendocrinology Group of the SEEN. Clinical guidelines for management of diabetes insipidus and syndrome of inappropriate antidiuretic hormone secretion after pituitary surgery. *Endocrinol Nutr*. 2014;61(4):e15–e24. https://doi.org/10.1016/j.endonu.2014.01.005.
13. Christ-Crain M, Winzeler B, Refardt J. Diagnosis and management of diabetes insipidus for the internist: an update. *J Intern Med*. 2021;290(1):73–87. https://doi.org/10.1111/joim.1326.
14. Jalleh R, Torpy DJ. The emerging role of copeptin. *Clin Biochem Rev*. 2021;42(1):17–25. https://doi.org/10.33176/AACB-20-00001.
15. Koch A, Yagmur E, Hoss A, et al. Clinical relevance of copeptin plasma levels as a biomarker of disease severity and mortality in critically ill patients. *J Clin Lab Anal*. 2018;32(9):e22614. https://doi.org/10.1002/jcla.22614.
16. Refardt J, Winzeler B, Christ-Crain M. Copeptin and its role in the diagnosis of diabetes insipidus and the syndrome of inappropriate antidiuresis. *Clin Endocrinol (Oxf)*. 2019;91(1):22–32. https://doi.org/10.1111/cen.13991.
17. Kobalka PJ, Huntoon K, Becker AP. Neuropathology of pituitary adenomas and sellar lesions. *Neurosurgery*. 2021;88(5):900–918. https://doi.org/10.1093/neuros/nyaa548.
18. Nunes RH, Abello AL, Zanation AM, et al. Imaging in endoscopic cranial skull base and pituitary surgery. *Otolaryngol Clin North Am*. 2016;49(1):33–62. https://doi.org/10.1016/j.otc.2015.09.003.
19. LeFevre ML, U.S. Preventive Services Task Force. Screening for thyroid dysfunction: U.S. Preventive Services Task Force recommendation statement. *Ann Intern Med*. 2015;162(9):641–650. https://doi.org/10.7326/M15-0483.
20. Fontes R, Coeli CR, Aguiar F, Vaisman M. Reference interval of thyroid stimulating hormone and free thyroxine in a reference population over 60 years old and in very old subjects (over 80 years): comparison to young subjects. *Thyroid Res*. 2013;6(1):13. https://doi.org/10.1186/1756-6614-6-13.
21. Razvi S, Bhana S, Mrabeti S. Challenges in interpreting thyroid stimulating hormone results in the diagnosis of thyroid dysfunction. *J Thyroid Res*. 2019;2019:4106816. https://doi.org/10.1155/2019/4106816.
22. Demers LM. Thyroid disease: pathophysiology and diagnosis. *Clin Lab Med*. 2004;24(1):19–28. https://doi.org/10.1016/j.cll.2004.01.002.
23. Merchant NB, Mirza FS. Interpretation of thyroid function tests in hospitalized patients. *Hosp Clin Med*. 2015;4(2):243.
24. Soh SB, Aw TC. Laboratory testing in thyroid conditions – pitfalls and clinical utility. *Ann Lab Med*. 2019;39(1):3–14. https://doi.org/10.3343/alm.2019.39.1.3.
25. Trohman RG, Sharma PS, McAninch EA, Bianco AC. Amiodarone and thyroid physiology, pathophysiology, diagnosis and management. *Trends Cardiovasc Med*. 2019;29(5):285–295. https://doi.org/10.1016/j.tcm.2018.09.005.
26. Kapral N, Khot R. Thyroid anatomy and ultrasound evaluation. *Tech Vasc Interv Radiol*. 2022;25(2):100818. https://doi.org/10.1016/j.tvir.2022.100818.
27. Hoang JK, Sosa JA, Nguyen XV, et al. Imaging thyroid disease. *Radiol Clin North Am*. 2015;53:145. https://doi.org/10.1016/j.rcl.2014.09.002.
28. Savas M, Mehta S, Agrawal N, van Rossum EFC, Feelders RA. Approach to the patient: diagnosis of cushing syndrome. *J Clin Endocrinol Metab*. 2022;107(11):3162–3174. https://doi.org/10.1210/clinem/dgac492.
29. Fleseriu M, Auchus R, Bancos I, et al. Consensus on diagnosis and management of Cushing's disease: a guideline update. *Lancet Diabetes Endocrinol*. 2021;9(12):847–875. https://doi.org/10.1016/S2213-8587(21)00235-7.
30. Balomenaki M, Margaritopoulos D, Vassiliadi DA, Tsagarakis S. Diagnostic workup of Cushing's syndrome. *J Neuroendocrinol*. 2022;34(8):e13111. https://doi.org/10.1111/jne.13111.
31. Funder JW, Carey RM, Mantero F, et al. The management of primary aldosteronism: case detection, diagnosis, and treatment: an Endocrine Society Clinical Practice Guideline. *J Clin Endocrinol Metab*. 2016;101(5):1889–1916. https://doi.org/10.1210/jc.2015-4061.
32. Navin PJ, Moynagh MR. Optimal and novel imaging of the adrenal glands. *Curr Opin Endocrinol Diabetes Obes*. 2022;29(3):253–262. https://doi.org/10.1097/MED.0000000000000730.
33. Rossi GP. Update in adrenal venous sampling for primary aldosteronism. *Curr Opin Endocrinol Diabetes Obes*. 2018;25(3):160–171. https://doi.org/10.1097/MED.0000000000000407.
34. Bornstein SR, Allolio B, Arlt W, et al. Diagnosis and treatment of primary adrenal insufficiency: an endocrine society clinical practice guideline. *J Clin Endocrinol Metab*. 2016;101(2):364–389. https://doi.org/10.1210/jc.2015-1710.
35. Betterle C, Presotto F, Furmaniak J. Epidemiology, pathogenesis, and diagnosis of Addison's disease in adults. *J Endocrinol Invest*. 2019;42(12):1407–1433. https://doi.org/10.1007/s40618-019-01079-6.
36. Van den Berghe G. Adrenal function/dysfunction in critically ill patients: a concise narrative review of recent novel insights. *J Anesth*. 2021;35(6):903–910. https://doi.org/10.1007/s00540-021-02977-x.
37. Thomas RM, Ruel E, Shantavasinkul PC, Corsino L. Endocrine hypertension: an overview on the current etiopathogenesis and management options. *World J Hypertens*. 2015;5(2):14–27. https://doi.org/10.5494/wjh.v5.i2.14.
38. Därr R, Kuhn M, Bode C, et al. Accuracy of recommended sampling and assay methods for the determination of plasma-free and urinary fractionated metanephrines in the diagnosis of pheochromocytoma and paraganglioma: a systematic review. *Endocrine*. 2017;56(3):495–503. https://doi.org/10.1007/s12020-017-1300-y.

31

Endocrine Disorders and Therapeutic Management

Mary E. Lough

http://evolve.elsevier.com/Urden/CriticalCareNursing

The endocrine system is almost invisible when it functions well, but it causes widespread disruption when an organ is suppressed, overstimulated, or under physiologic stress. A wide spectrum of possible disorders can result; some are rare, and others are frequently encountered in the critical care unit. This chapter focuses on the neuroendocrine stress associated with critical illness and on disorders of three major endocrine glands: pancreas, posterior pituitary gland, and thyroid gland.

ACUTE NEUROENDOCRINE RESPONSE TO CRITICAL ILLNESS

Major neurologic and endocrine changes occur when an individual is confronted with physiologic stress caused by any critical illness, sepsis, trauma, major surgery, or underlying cardiovascular disease.[1] The normal "fight or flight" response that is initiated in times of physiologic or psychological stress is exacerbated in critical illness through activation of the neuroendocrine system, specifically the hypothalamic-pituitary-adrenal (HPA) axis.[1,2] All endocrine organs are affected by acute critical illness, as shown in Table 31.1.

The fight or flight acute response to physiologic threat is a rapid discharge of the catecholamines *norepinephrine* and *epinephrine* into the bloodstream. Norepinephrine is released from the nerve endings of the sympathetic nervous system. Epinephrine is released from the adrenal glands. These physiologic responses are initiated by the HPA axis.

Hypothalamic-Pituitary-Adrenal Axis in Critical Illness

The pituitary gland has two parts (anterior and posterior) that function under control of the hypothalamus (see Figs. 29.1 and 29.3 in Chapter 29). The *posterior pituitary gland* releases arginine vasopressin (AVP) also known as *vasopressin*, as a component of the physiologic stress response. This hormone is an antidiuretic with a powerful vasoconstrictive effect on blood vessels. The synergistic combination of vasopressin and epinephrine released from the adrenal glands quickly raises blood pressure (BP).

The *anterior pituitary gland* produces several hormones, including *corticotropin* (also called adrenocorticotropic hormone), which stimulates release of *cortisol* from the adrenal cortex. Cortisol release is an important protective response to stress. Increased cortisol levels alter carbohydrate, fat, and protein metabolism so that energy is immediately and selectively available to vital organs. This also contributes to the hyperglycemia observed in critical illness.

The *adrenal gland* produces cortisol from the cortex and epinephrine from the medulla, contributing to the physiologic stress response (see Fig. 29.7 in Chapter 29). Initially, in response to critical illness, cortisol levels rise. However, when the illness is sustained, the adrenal glands may not be able to produce adequate amounts of stress hormones over the long term.[3] This condition is known as *critical illness–related corticosteroid insufficiency* (CIRCI).[2–4]

Hyperglycemia and Hypoglycemia in Critical Illness

Many factors contribute to hyperglycemia in critical illness, including release of glucagon, cortisol, and epinephrine. In response to physiologic stress, *glucagon* is released by the pancreatic alpha cells and stimulates the liver to pour glucose into the bloodstream. In healthy individuals, blood insulin levels control glucagon release. When blood glucose levels are less than 80 mg/dL, the stimulus to release insulin from the pancreatic beta cells is suppressed and the alpha cells are stimulated to release glucagon.

Physiologic Stress and Glucagon Release

The physiologic purpose of glucagon is to prevent hypoglycemia by stimulating the liver to release additional glucose into the bloodstream. However, in diabetes and during critical illness, the normal feedback loop is disrupted. Circulating glucagon can be increased five times the normal value, unrelated to insulin levels, causing hyperglycemia in critical illness.[5] Physiologic stress stimulates release of cortisol and epinephrine from the adrenal glands. These counterregulatory hormones further stimulate glucagon and subsequent release of glucose from the liver.[5]

Under normal physiologic conditions, hyperglycemia and insulin secretion inhibit glucagon release. However, in the acute phase of critical illness, normal physiology is disrupted, and insulin secretion is decreased.[5] This causes a relative insulin deficiency compared with physiologic need. Later in the course of the illness, peripheral tissues may become *insulin resistant*, meaning the tissues are unable to use the available insulin to transport glucose inside the cells.[5]

Physiologic Stress and GLUT Activation

There is a second physiologic system to transport glucose into cells using facilitative *glucose transporters* (GLUTs) (see Table 29.3 in Chapter 29). The normal physiologic stimulus for insulin release from the pancreas is an increase in blood glucose after a meal or hyperglycemia. GLUT2 receptors are located on the surface of the beta cells and transport circulating glucose inside

TABLE 31.1 Endocrine Responses to Stress

Gland or Organ	Hormone	Response or Physical Examination
Adrenal cortex	Cortisol	↑ Insulin resistance → ↑ glycogenolysis → ↑ glucose circulation
		↑ Hepatic gluconeogenesis → ↑ glucose available
		↑ Lipolysis
		↑ Protein catabolism
		↑ Sodium → ↑ water retention to maintain plasma osmolality by movement of extravascular fluid into the intravascular space
		↓ Connective tissue fibroblasts → poor wound healing
	Glucocorticoid	↓ Histamine release → suppression of immune system
		↓ Lymphocytes, monocytes, eosinophils, basophils
		↑ Polymorphonuclear leukocytes → ↑ infection risk
		↑ Glucose
		↓ Gastric acid secretion
	Mineralocorticoids	↑ Aldosterone → ↓ sodium excretion → ↓ water excretion → ↑ intravascular volume
		↑ Potassium excretion → hypokalemia
		↑ Hydrogen ion excretion → metabolic acidosis
Adrenal medulla	Epinephrine	↑ Endorphins → ↓ pain
	Norepinephrine, epinephrine	↑ Metabolic rate to accommodate stress response
		↑ Live glycogenolysis → ↑ glucose
		↑ Insulin (cells are insulin resistant)
		↑ Cardiac contractility
		↑ Cardiac output
		↑ Dilation of coronary arteries
		↑ Blood pressure
		↑ Heart rate
		↑ Bronchodilation → ↑ respirations
		↑ Perfusion to heart, brain, lungs, liver, and muscle
		↓ Perfusion to periphery of body
		↓ Peristalsis
	Norepinephrine	↑ Peripheral vasoconstriction
		↑ Blood pressure
		↑ Sodium retention
		↑ Potassium excretion
Pituitary	All hormones	↑ Endogenous opioids → ↓ pain
Anterior pituitary	Corticotropin	↑ Aldosterone → ↓ sodium excretion → ↓ water excretion → ↑ intravascular volume
		↑ Cortisol → ↑ blood volume
	Growth hormones	↑ Protein anabolism of amino acids to protein
		↑ Lipolysis → ↑ gluconeogenesis
Posterior pituitary	Antidiuretic hormone	↑ Vasoconstriction
		↑ Water retention → restoration of circulating blood volume
		↓ Urine output
		↑ Hypo-osmolality
Pancreas	Insulin	↑ Insulin resistance → hyperglycemia
	Glucagon	↑ Glycolysis (directly opposes action of insulin)
		↑ Glucose for fuel
		↑ Glycogenolysis
		↑ Gluconeogenesis
		↑ Lipolysis
Thyroid	Thyroxine	↓ Routine metabolic demands during stress
Gonads	Sex hormones	Energy and oxygen supply diverted to brain, heart, muscles, and liver

↑, Increased; →, causes; ↓, decreased.

the cell, stimulating insulin release from the beta cell. However, GLUT2 receptor actions do not depend on insulin. The insulin-independent GLUTs (GLUT1, GLUT2, and GLUT3) are active during physiologic stress but may be unable to keep up with the massive increase in glucose production by the liver.[6]

Proactively managing glucagon release in critical illness is not yet feasible and this remains a future goal.[7] Hyperglycemia management is focused on a continuous infusion of insulin to maintain blood glucose levels within a safe range to reduce morbidity and mortality.[5]

Hyperglycemia Management Challenges in Critical Illness

Normal fasting blood glucose levels are between 70 and 100 mg/dL in a healthy person. Critically ill patients frequently have much higher blood glucose levels, and several retrospective analyses have reported that hyperglycemic patients have a higher mortality rate than patients with normal blood glucose values.[5]

The optimal blood glucose range during critical illness remains under debate, although for patient safety, many critical care units have adopted guidelines developed by professional societies.[8] It has taken over 20 years to achieve broad agreement on the management goals for glycemic control. There have been many challenges, such as the difficulty posed by low target levels and efforts to achieve tight glucose control with intensive insulin as described below.

In 2001, a landmark prospective, randomized study appeared to show a significant reduction in morbidity and mortality among critically ill surgical patients whose blood glucose concentration was maintained between 80 and 110 mg/dL with a continuous insulin infusion compared with similar surgical patients whose blood glucose was treated only if it was greater than 180 mg/dL.[9] This initial study was greeted with tremendous enthusiasm, and many critical care units adopted stringent glucose control standards to reduce hyperglycemia-associated morbidity and mortality. However, reproducibility of such tight glucose control in the clinical setting—outside of a research trial—was impossible to achieve, as shown by the results of follow-up clinical studies.[10] The most impactful trial was the NICE-SUGAR trial.[11] This was a prospective randomized trial of 6014 critically ill patients that compared continuous insulin infusion to achieve tight glucose control (target 81 to 108 mg/dL) with a conventional glucose control range (target below 180 mg/dL). In the tight glucose control group, 6.8% had episodes of severe hypoglycemia (less than 40 mg/dL); in the conventional control group, only 0.5% experienced severe hypoglycemia.[11] There was a 2.6% higher risk of death in the intensive glucose control group (27.5% died) compared with the conventional control group (24.9% died).[11] More recent studies have confirmed that lower glucose targets, compared with liberal glucose target ranges, do not improve length of stay in the critical care unit, nor improve patient mortality.[10,12]

Clinical Guidelines for Blood Glucose Management in Critical Illness

As a result of the NICE-SUGAR study just described, clinical practice guidelines were developed by the *American Association of Clinical Endocrinologists* and the *American Diabetes Association* (ADA) that recommend the use of continuous insulin infusions to maintain blood glucose in critical care patients between 140 and 180 mg/dL, with hourly monitoring of blood glucose.[13,14] The range of 140 to 180 mg/dL was selected to minimize the risk of hypoglycemia while avoiding extreme hyperglycemia.[13] More recently, glycemic management guidelines relevant to critical illness were published by the *Society of Critical Care Medicine* (SCCM). The 2024 guideline recommends initiating glycemic control for persistent hyperglycemia at a blood glucose equal or greater than (≥) 180 mg/dL (milligrams per deciliter) or ≥10 mmol/L (millimoles per liter).[8] Guidelines are helpful because stress hyperglycemia (≥180 mg/dL) occurs in almost one-third of critically ill patients[5] and because persistent hyperglycemia is associated with harm.[8]

Glucose Variability

Glucose variability is a relatively new metric that is being examined to determine how variability affects mortality and other outcomes during critical illness.[15] Glucose variability can be calculated in several different ways during critical illness. A consensus around a measurement standard for glucose variability has not been reached, although there are suggestions in the literature based on either designated time periods, or fluctuations between high and low blood glucose values.[16] Some proposed metrics are:

- Time spent outside target range.
- Time spent in hyperglycemia.
- Time spent in hypoglycemia.
- Maximum glucose value minus minimum glucose value.

Insulin Management in Critically Ill Patients

As a result of the research that has highlighted the deleterious effects of hyperglycemia in critically ill patients, most hospitals have developed an institution-specific glucose-insulin algorithm to lower blood glucose into the targeted range. The vigilance of the critical care nurse is pivotal to the success of any intervention to lower blood glucose using a continuous insulin infusion. The most recent SCCM glycemic control guidelines recommend initiating a continuous intravenous (IV) infusion for a blood glucose ≥180 mg/dL (≥10 mm/L) and titrating to a target range of 140 to 200 mg/dL (7.8–11.1 mmol/L).[8] The 2024 guidelines specifically recommend against using lower blood glucose target ranges for most adult critically ill patients to reduce the risk of hypoglycemia.[8]

Frequency of Blood Glucose Monitoring

Monitoring the blood glucose with a point-of-care glucometer is the basis of targeted glucose control. As part of the comprehensive initial assessment, blood sugar is measured by a standard laboratory sample or by a fingerstick capillary blood sample. While the glucose is elevated, and during periods of glycemic instability, blood sample measurements are obtained hourly to allow titration of the insulin drip to achieve a blood glucose within the target range.[8] More frequent blood glucose monitoring is associated with lower rates of hypoglycemia in clinical trials.[8]

Several different blood-sampling methods are available. A capillary fingerstick is perhaps the easiest initial option, although the fingers can become noticeably marked if there are numerous sticks over several days. Trauma to the fingers is also exacerbated if peripheral perfusion is diminished. If a central venous catheter or an arterial line with an attached blood conservation system is in place, this can be a highly efficient system for sampling, because there is no blood wastage. If a blood conservation setup is not attached, use of the venous or arterial catheter for access is unacceptable because of the quantity of "waste" blood that would be discarded.

Point-of-Care Testing for Blood Glucose in Critical Illness

Point-of-care testing with a handheld glucometer is frequently used to allow hourly rapid assessment of the blood glucose and titration of a continuous glucose infusion. The U.S. Food and Drug Administration (FDA) requires that blood glucose testing devices used in the hospital meet standards specific for *Blood Glucose Monitoring Test Systems (BGMS) for Prescription Point-of-Care (POC) Use*.[17] For added safety, it is important to verify very high blood glucose values (hyperglycemia) and very low blood glucose values (hypoglycemia) with a blood sample sent to the clinical laboratory for plasma glucose verification.

Continuous Insulin Infusion

Hospitals use insulin infusion protocols for management of stress-induced hyperglycemia.[13] These protocols are generally implemented and managed by the critical care nurse.[8,14] Effective glucose protocols gauge the insulin infusion rate based on two parameters:

- The current blood glucose value
- The rate of change in the blood glucose level since the last hourly measurement

Protocols vary by hospital, but the underlying concepts are similar and should be based on national guidelines.

The following three examples illustrate blood glucose management strategies that may be used:

- Patient A receives 5 units of continuous IV regular insulin per hour and has a blood glucose measurement of 110 mg/dL, but 1 hour ago it was 190 mg/dL. The insulin rate must be decreased to avoid acute hypoglycemia.
- Patient B receives 5 units of continuous IV regular insulin per hour and has a blood glucose measurement of 150 mg/dL, but 1 hour ago it was 152 mg/dL. In this situation, no change is made in the insulin infusion rate.
- Patient C receives 5 units of continuous IV regular insulin per hour and has a blood glucose measurement of 240 mg/dL, and 1 hour ago it was 193 mg/dL. The insulin rate must be increased to move the patient's blood sugar more rapidly toward the targeted glucose range (i.e., 140 to 200 mg/dL, although this range will vary per individual hospital protocol).

The important point to emphasize is that the *rate of change* of blood glucose is as important as the *most recent* blood glucose measurement. Each of the patients described in the examples may have the same insulin infusion rate but will have different responses depending on their catabolic state. Individualization of the insulin infusion among patients with different diagnoses can be achieved safely as long as the rate of change in response to insulin is considered.

A patient's insulin requirement often fluctuates over the course of an illness. This fluctuation occurs in response to changes in the clinical condition such as development of an infection, caloric alterations caused by stopping or starting enteral or parenteral nutrition, administration of therapeutic steroids, or because the person is less catabolic. A method to allow for corrective incremental changes (up or down) to adapt to the reality of clinical developments and maintain the glucose within the target range is essential. Some protocols alter only the infusion rate, whereas others incorporate bolus insulin doses if the glucose concentration is greater than a preestablished threshold (e.g., 180 mg/dL or 10 mmol/L). Typically, after the blood glucose level has remained within the target range for a number of hours (varies according to the hospital protocol), the time interval between measurements for blood glucose monitoring may be extended to every 2 hours.

Glucose Closed Loop Systems

The algorithms vary by setting, and increasingly computerized algorithms and closed-loop systems are being trialed to increase accuracy, reduce hypoglycemia, and provide real-time blood glucose control during critical illness.[18–21]

Glycemic Instability Protocol Guidelines

The 2024 glycemic management guidelines recommend the following be included in critical care protocols for adults during critical illness:[8]

- Initiate a continuous insulin infusion at ≥180 mg/dL (≥10 mm/L).
- Target a blood glucose range between 140 and 200 mg/dL (7.8–11.1 mmol/L).
- Use a continuous insulin infusion to manage glycemic instability.
- Monitor blood glucose at least hourly when using a continuous insulin infusion.
- Do not use intermittent subcutaneous insulin to manage acute glycemic instability.
- Include computerized decision support within the protocol.
- Computer integration with the electronic health record (EHR) is desirable.

Transition From Continuous Insulin Infusion to Subcutaneous Insulin

The transition from a continuous insulin infusion to intermittent insulin coverage must be handled with care to avoid large fluctuations in blood glucose levels. The ADA recommends administration of subcutaneous basal insulin 2 hours before the IV infusion is discontinued.[13] The intent is to minimize rebound hyperglycemia.[13]

Before the conversion, the regular insulin infusion should be at a stable and preferably low rate, and the patient's blood glucose level should be maintained consistently within the target range. The transition from IV to subcutaneous insulin administration depends on numerous factors, including whether the patient is able to eat a consistent amount of dietary carbohydrate. Therefore, the number of units of insulin transitioned from IV to subcutaneous can range from 50% to 80% of the prior 6 to 8 hours total depending on individual patient needs and the specifics of the transition protocol.[8,13,14,22]

Clinicians use various methods to calculate the quantity of insulin to prescribe during the transition from IV to subcutaneous insulin to maintain stable blood glucose levels. Fig. 31.1 depicts hypothetical examples of how a combination of basal and bolus insulin regimens (prandial insulin) can work in clinical practice. The application of one calculation method is described for a 67-year-old patient, Alice Smith, who is recovering from critical illness and has recently been weaned from mechanical ventilation and extubated.

1. Ms. Smith is in stable condition on a regular insulin drip at 1 unit/h. She is ready to be transitioned to subcutaneous insulin and will be taking food and liquids by mouth. Her total insulin requirement over the previous 24 hours was 32 units. Ms. Smith will now require basal coverage (provided by subcutaneous intermediate or long-acting insulin) and prandial coverage for mealtimes (provided by short-acting or ultra-short-acting subcutaneous insulin).
2. The 30 units of insulin infused during the previous 24 hours is Ms. Smith's required daily insulin dose. To transition to subcutaneous insulin, a proportion of this amount (i.e., 75% to 80%) will be divided between basal and prandial components.[14] In this situation, 75% of the 32 units is 24 units. Half of this amount (12 units) will be administered subcutaneously as intermediate or long-acting insulin; the other half will be administered as short-acting insulin to coincide with meals (i.e., 4 units with each of three meals).
3. The options for insulin administration for Ms. Smith are as follows:
   - *Basal insulin:* 12 units of long-acting insulin once daily *or* 6 units twice daily of intermediate-acting insulin administered subcutaneously.

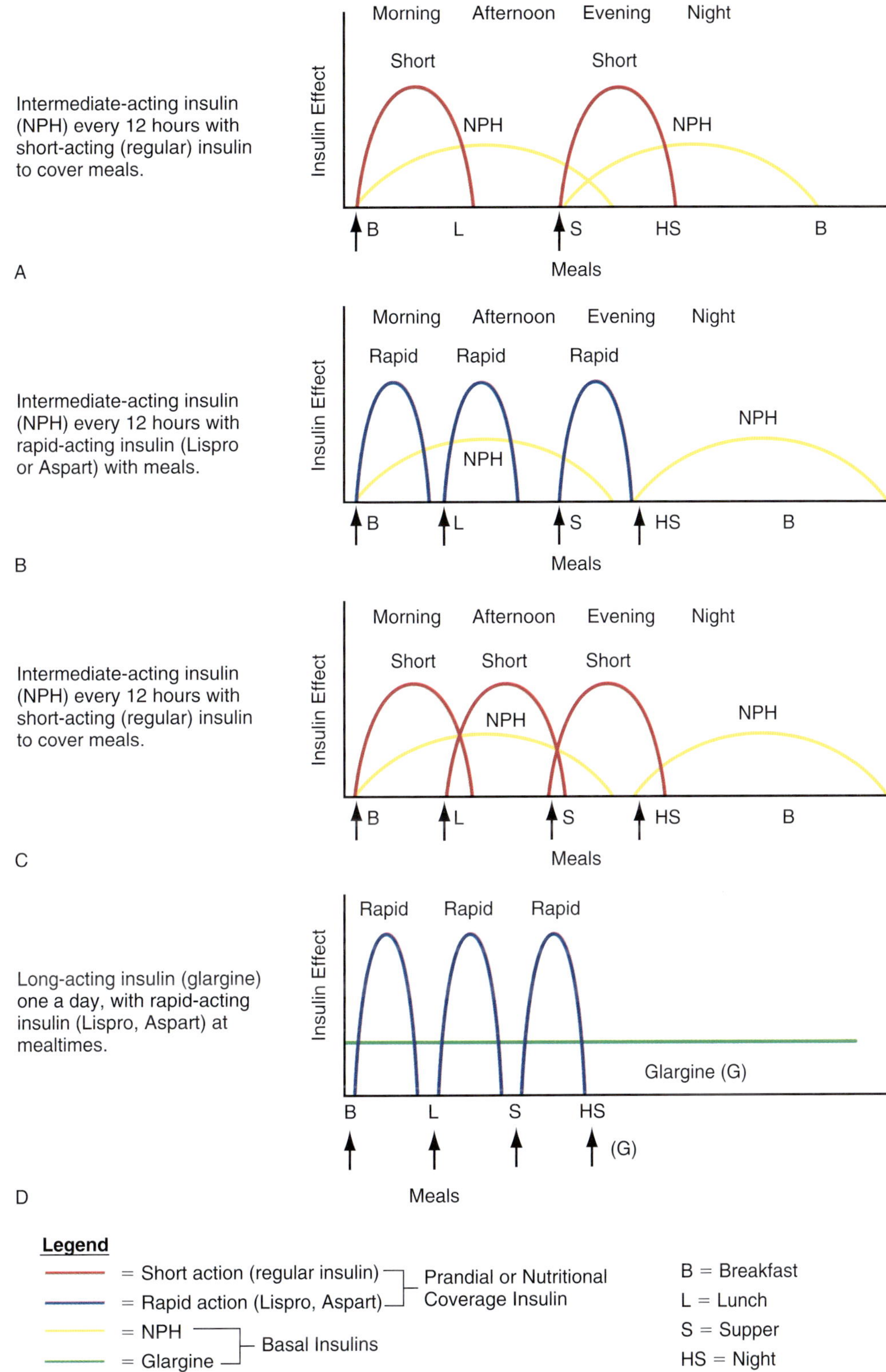

FIG. 31.1 Basal and Nutritional Bolus Insulin Combinations.

- *Prandial insulin:* 4 units of regular insulin given subcutaneously before each meal (short-acting) *or* 4 units of ultra–short-acting insulin given subcutaneously with each meal while verifying current blood glucose level.

Many types of insulin are available for use. These include ultra–short acting, short-acting, intermediate-acting, long-acting, and combination insulin replacement options as listed in Table 31.2. After the transition to subcutaneous insulin is completed, blood glucose is monitored frequently to maintain blood glucose within the target range and detect hyperglycemia or hypoglycemia.[22,23]

Corrective Insulin Coverage

A patient may be prescribed supplemental or corrective doses of insulin in addition to the basal/prandial insulin

TABLE 31.2 PHARMACOLOGIC MANAGEMENT

Insulin[a]

Insulin	Route[b]	Action	Onset/Peak/Duration	Special Considerations
Ultra–Short-Acting Insulins				
Aspart (NovoLog)	Subcutaneous	Insulin replacement, rapid onset	5–15 min/30–90 min/<5 h	Insulin analog almost *immediately* absorbed; must be taken with food Insulin appearance should be clear Must be used in combination with intermediate-acting or long-acting basal insulin regimen; see Fig. 31.1
Lispro (Humalog)	Subcutaneous	Insulin replacement, rapid onset	5–15 min/30–90 min/<5 h	Insulin analog; almost *immediately* absorbed; must be taken with food Shorter duration of action than regular insulin; should be used with basal longer acting insulin; see Fig. 31.1
Glulisine (Apidra)	Subcutaneous	Insulin replacement, rapid onset	5–15 min/30–90 min/<5 h	Insulin analog
Short-Acting Insulin				
Regular	IV or Subcutaneous	Insulin replacement therapy	IV: <15 min Subcutaneous: 30–60 min/ 2–3 h/5–8 h	Only type of insulin suitable for IV continuous infusion or IV bolus administration
Intermediate-Acting Basal Insulin				
NPH	Subcutaneous	Insulin replacement, intermediate action	2–4 h/4–10 h/10–16 h	NPH is not recommended for subcutaneous basal insulin because it has a peak with a less predictable time course than the long-acting insulin analogs
Long-Acting Basal Insulins				
Glargine (Lantus)	Subcutaneous	Long-acting basal insulin analog	2–4 h until steady state/no peak Concentration relatively constant over 20–24 h	Synthetic insulin (analog); differs from human insulin by three amino acids, slow release over 24 h; no peak Decrease dosage by 20% if switching from NPH to glargine Must not be diluted or mixed with other insulins; see Fig. 31.1
Detemir (Levemir)	Subcutaneous	Long-acting basal insulin analog	3–8 h until steady state/no peak/5–23 h	
Combination (Premixed) Insulins				
Various	Subcutaneous	Rapid plus intermediate or long-acting insulin combination	Varies according to combination used	Many combinations exist; examples (long-acting component/short-acting component) include 70/30 regular (70% NPH with 30% regular), NovoLog mix 70/30 (70% aspart-protamine suspension with 30% aspart), and Humalog mix 75/25 (75% lispro-protamine suspension with 25% lispro)

[a]Dosages are individualized according to patient's age and size.
[b]Only regular insulin is suitable for IV use.
IV, Intravenous; *NPH*, neutral protamine Hagedorn.

combination.[13] The use of the trio of basal, prandial, and corrective insulin is designed to eliminate the use of the traditional sliding scale as a solo intervention. Criticisms of the solo corrective (sliding scale) method are that the dosages are rarely reevaluated or adjusted once established, that the scales treat hyperglycemia only after it has occurred. The disadvantage of sliding scales is that they are not proactive in the manner of the basal/bolus/corrective insulin method. Emphatically, the ADA does not recommend solo use of the *corrective scale* previously known as the *sliding scale* to control blood glucose.[13,24]

Supplemental Corrective Insulin

There is a role for corrective coverage in addition to supplemental and prandial insulin. A supplemental correction scale can be used to cover any episodes of hyperglycemia above the target range. The corrective insulin amount can be added to the scheduled insulin administration, depending on when the hypoglycemia is discovered.

After the transition to subcutaneous insulin, it is important to recheck the blood glucose level. The insulin dosage is adjusted based on the patient's *insulin sensitivity,* or stated another way, according to how much insulin is needed to metabolize each 15 g of carbohydrate intake. Patients who are *insulin resistant* require more insulin than patients who are *insulin sensitive.*[25,26]

Hypoglycemia Management

It is important to have a protocol for the management of hypoglycemia.[13] The major drawback to continuous insulin protocols is the risk of hypoglycemia. Whenever hypoglycemia is detected, it is important to *stop* any continuous infusion of insulin.

Hypoglycemia can have different level of severity.[13,27,28]

- **Level 1 Hypoglycemia**: A blood glucose between 54 mg/dL and 70 mg/dL (3.0 and 3.9 mmol/L) describes hypoglycemia.[28] Administration of carbohydrate is indicated to prevent further decline in the blood glucose.[28]
- **Level 2 Hypoglycemia**: A severely low blood glucose less than 54 mg/dL (3.0 mmol/L).[28] Even if there are no obvious signs or symptoms, a severely low blood glucose increases the risk of brain injury, cognitive dysfunction, and death.[28] Urgently administer carbohydrate.
- **Level 3 Hypoglycemia**: A severely low glucose that is associated with mental and physical signs of hypoglycemia.[28] This is a life-threatening event and administration of glucagon may be required.[28]

Following documented hypoglycemia, the blood glucose concentration is monitored frequently; for example, check every 15 minutes until the blood glucose level has increased to >70 mg/dL (>3.9 mmol/L) depending on individual hospital protocols.

Nursing Management

Nursing management of a patient experiencing stress hyperglycemia in critical illness covers a variety of patient problems (Box 31.1). Nursing actions are to monitor blood glucose levels and insulin effectiveness, monitor hyperglycemic side effects of vasopressor therapy, prevent hypoglycemia, make sure nutrition is appropriate, and provide education to the patient's family and supportive others (Box 31.2).

Monitor Blood Glucose and Insulin Effectiveness

The critical care nurse is responsible for the hourly monitoring of blood glucose and titration of the insulin infusion according to the hospital's protocol while the patient is hyperglycemic. The use of standardized protocols makes a systematic approach to the control of blood glucose possible.[8,29,30]

Hypoglycemia Prevention

The 2024 glycemic guidelines do not provide specific recommendations for treating severe hypoglycemia beyond recognition that these episodes be prevented. Instead, the focus is on establishment of safe glycemic ranges and protocols that decrease the risk of hypoglycemia when using a continuous insulin infusion.[8] Additionally, hospitals should have decision support and algorithmic protocols available to advise clinicians about when and how to reverse severe hypoglycemia (≤40 mg/dL; ≤2.2 mmol/L).[8]

One recommendation for the rapid reversal of severe hypoglycemia (≤40 mg/dL) from earlier critical care guidelines is administration of IV dextrose ($D_{50}W$).[31] It is essential to be familiar with the protocols available in each critical care setting.[8]

Monitor Hyperglycemic Side Effects of Vasopressor Therapy

Vasopressors used as continuous infusions to counteract hypotension also raise blood glucose. Epinephrine and norepinephrine stimulate gluconeogenesis (creation of new glucose), increase liver glycogenolysis (glucose production), increase lipolysis (fat breakdown), suppress insulin secretion, and increase peripheral insulin resistance.[30] All these actions elevate blood glucose.

BOX 31.1 DIAGNOSIS AND PATIENT CARE MANAGEMENT

Physiologic Stress of Critical Illness

- Hypovolemia due to relative loss
- Impaired Nutritional Intake due to lack of exogenous nutrients and increased metabolic demand
- Impaired Peripheral Tissue Perfusion due to decreased blood flow
- Risk for Infection
- Delirium due to sensory overload, sensory deprivation, and sleep pattern disturbance
- Patient Care Management plans are located in Appendix A.

BOX 31.2 PATIENT AND FAMILY EDUCATION PLAN

Physiologic Stress of Critical Illness

- Even if the patient is unresponsive because of the underlying critical illness or because of sedation and analgesic medications, brief explanations of procedures are quietly and simply given before interventions.
- During the period of acute illness, questions are answered and information is provided to the family and significant others.
- After recovery, additional information is provided to the patient concerning the illness.

Provide Nutrition

Whenever an insulin infusion is initiated to lower blood glucose, enteral nutritional support should be considered.[13,24,32] Critical illness is associated with significant catabolism of skeletal muscle. The catabolic response to inflammation is much more significant than fasting in a healthy individual because of inflammation, immobility, and the endocrine stress response.[24,31] Enteral nutrition via feeding tube is preferred to IV total parenteral nutrition. Enteral nutrition is associated with better outcomes in critical illness.[24] Enteral nutritional formulas have higher carbohydrate content than total parenteral nutrition, making it easier to manage fluctuations in blood glucose. If enteral nutrition is stopped or slowed, it is vital that the insulin infusion rate is also decreased to avoid hypoglycemia.

Educate the Patient and Family

While the patient is acutely ill, most of the educational interventions are directed to the family at the bedside. Numerous explications are required to describe the IV medications, nutritional needs, purpose of insulin, role of corticosteroids (if applicable), ongoing nursing care, prevention of complications, and management of the underlying disease process. Educational topics to discuss are listed in Box 31.2.

Collaborative Management

Standardized protocols designed to manage the complications of critical illness result in lower morbidity and mortality for patients.[8] Optimally, all disciplines concerned with the endocrine status of the patient will have participated in the hospital's guidelines related to targeted glucose control. Guidelines for blood glucose monitoring in critical illness are described in Box 31.3.

BOX 31.3 Evidence-Based Practice

Hyperglycemia Management in Critical Illness

A summary is provided of evidence and evidence-based recommendations for controlling hyperglycemic symptoms related to physiologic stress of critical illness.

Strong Evidence to Support

- Initiate insulin therapy for persistent hyperglycemia greater than 200 mg/dL.
- Once a continuous insulin infusion is initiated, maintain target blood glucose level between 140 and 200 mg/dL.
- Perform frequent blood glucose monitoring to avoid hypoglycemia defined as blood glucose level less than 70 mg/dL; severe hypoglycemia is less than 40 mg/dL.
- For patients who are eating, maintain preprandial blood glucose below 130 mg/dL; maintain 2-h postprandial blood glucose below 180 mg/dL.
- A multidisciplinary team approach to implement institutional guidelines, protocols, and standardized order sets results in fewer hypoglycemic and hyperglycemic events.

Data from American Diabetes Association Professional Practice Committee. 16. Diabetes care in the hospital: standards of care in diabetes—2024. *Diabetes Care.* 2024;47(Suppl 1):S295–S306. https://doi.org/10.2337/dc24-S016
Honarmand K, Sirimaturos M, Hirshberg EL, et al. Society of Critical Care Medicine guidelines on glycemic control for critically ill children and adults 2024. *Crit Care Med.* 2024;52(4):e161–e181. https://doi.org/10.1097/CCM.0000000000006174
Jacobi J, Bircher N, Krinsley J, et al. Guidelines for the use of an insulin infusion for the management of hyperglycemia in critically ill patients. *Crit Care Med.* 2012;40(12):3251–3276. https://doi.org/10.1097/CCM.0b013e3182653269
Moghissi ES, Korytkowski MT, DiNardo M, et al. American Association of Clinical Endocrinologists and American Diabetes Association consensus statement on inpatient glycemic control. *Diabetes Care.* 2009;32(6):1119–1131. https://doi.org/10.2337/dc09-9029

DIABETES MELLITUS

Diabetes mellitus is a progressive endocrinopathy with multiple manifestations that, without treatment, result in severe hyperglycemia.[33] Only type 1 and type 2 diabetes are discussed in this chapter.

- Type 1 diabetes describes a condition with an absolute loss of insulin that results from autoimmune destruction of the insulin-producing beta cells in the pancreas, so that exogenous insulin administration is required for life.[33]
- Type 2 diabetes describes an insulin deficiency that results from an ongoing nonautoimmune condition that causes pancreatic beta cells to progressively produce less insulin.[33] Insulin resistance and metabolic syndrome often accompany type 2 diabetes.[33] Type 2 diabetes can be managed by medications and alterations in lifestyle as long as the pancreas is producing some insulin.

Diabetes Mellitus Diagnosis

Diabetes mellitus is officially diagnosed by a blood test value known as a *glycated hemoglobin* A1c (A_{1c}).[33] Current guidelines recommend that an A_{1c} be measured on admission to the hospital. The A_{1c} values are:

- Normal $A_{1c} \leq 5.6\%$
- Prediabetes between 5.7% and 6.4%
- Diabetes $\geq 6.5\%$

In the hospital, a fasting plasma glucose (FPG) may also be obtained. The benchmarks for a normal blood glucose value have been progressively lowered as more knowledge has been gained about the benefits of maintaining the plasma glucose level as close to normal as possible.

Fasting Plasma Glucose

Fasting blood glucose values are more likely to be obtained in the critical care unit. The values classified by the ADA are as follows:[33]

- FPG level <100 mg/dL (<5.6 mmol/L) represents a normal fasting glucose.
- FPG level between 100 and 125 mg/dL (5.6 and 6.9 mmol/L) suggests prediabetes.
- FPG level greater than 126 mg/dL (>7 mmol/L) suggests diabetes.

The fasting blood glucose is not a diagnostic test for diabetes. The A_{1c} is used for diagnosis.

The health benefits and importance of maintaining blood glucose at levels as close to normal as possible have been conclusively demonstrated in patients with type 1 and type 2 diabetes. The *Diabetes Control and Complications Trial* (DCCT) demonstrated the powerful benefit of insulin therapy to control type 1 diabetes.[34,35] The *United Kingdom Prospective Diabetes Study* (UKPDS) of type 2 diabetes, and the more recent prospective global DISCOVER study of type 2 diabetes, have demonstrated that lifestyle changes and medications that result in consistently normal glucose levels can reduce microvascular diabetes-related complications and decrease mortality.[36]

Glycated Hemoglobin A_{1c}

For individuals with diabetes, maintenance of blood glucose within a tight normal range is fundamental to avoid the development of microvascular and neuropathic secondary conditions. Although the plasma glucose value produces a snapshot of the blood glucose concentration at a single point in time, the *glycated hemoglobin* A_{1c} measures the percentage of glucose the red blood cells have absorbed from the plasma over the previous 3-month period. The optimal target for patients with diabetes is an A_{1c} value less than 5.7%.[33]

The ADA identifies individuals with an A_{1c} value between 5.7% and 6.4% as being prediabetic or at high risk for developing diabetes and cardiovascular disease.[33]

Type 1 Diabetes

Type 1 diabetes mellitus accounts for between 5% and 10% of all patients with diabetes.[33] Type 1 diabetes is an autoimmune disease that causes progressive destruction of the beta cells of the islets of Langerhans in the pancreas. *Islet autoantibodies* that falsely identify self as a foreign invader to be destroyed can now be identified by laboratory analysis. One or more of these autoantibodies is present in most patients with type 1 diabetes.[33] Over time, the islet autoantibodies render the pancreatic beta cells incapable of secreting insulin and regulating intracellular glucose. The presence of islet autoantibodies with other symptoms is used to confirm a diagnosis of type 1 diabetes.[37] This is especially helpful when symptoms of type 1 diabetes occur in an adult of any age.[37]

In type 1 diabetes, the rate of beta cell destruction is highly variable.[33] It occurs rapidly in some patients and more slowly in others. Some patients, particularly children and adolescents, have ketoacidosis as the first manifestation of their disease.[33]

Genetic predisposition and unknown environmental factors are also believed to play an important role. Patients with type 1 diabetes are prone to development of other autoimmune disorders such as Graves' disease (hyperthyroidism), Hashimoto thyroiditis, Addison disease, autoimmune hepatitis, myasthenia gravis, and pernicious anemia.

Management of Type 1 Diabetes

Patients with type 1 diabetes must receive IV or subcutaneous insulin therapy. Treatment with exogenous insulin replacement restores normal entry of glucose into the cells. The range of insulin replacement options is expanding, and it is essential that critical care nurses be knowledgeable about the different classes of insulin (see Table 31.2).

Insulins are classified according to their duration of action:

- Long acting (basal) (detemir, degludec, glargine)
- Intermediate acting (basal) human NPH insulin (Neutral Protamine Hagedorn)
- Short acting (regular human insulin)
- Rapid acting (aspart, Glulisine, lispro)

There are also several premixed combinations available. Without insulin, the rapid breakdown of noncarbohydrate substrate, particularly fat, leads to ketonemia, ketonuria, and diabetic ketoacidosis (DKA), a life-threatening complication associated with type 1 diabetes (see later discussion).

- Outside the hospital, type 1 diabetes is generally managed with a daily insulin replacement plan that uses a combination of subcutaneous insulin types via a continuous pump with automated insulin delivery.[34,37]
- Basal insulin (30% to 50% is basal)
- Mealtime prandial insulin (approximately 50% to 70% is prandial)
- Corrective insulin

Total daily insulin dose varies among individuals due to differences in age, weight, and carbohydrate intake, with a range of 0.4 to 1.0 units/kilogram/day in a stable situation.[34]

Many hospitals have protocols that permit patients with type 1 diabetes who normally self-manage their insulin replacement with a continuous pump, to continue this regimen under supervision in the hospital.[28,37] Obviously in critical illness self-management is not an option.

Additionally, some patients with type 1 diabetes take oral antihyperglycemic medications, and because these medications also lower blood glucose, hypoglycemia remains a concern.[37]

Type 2 Diabetes

Type 2 diabetes accounts for 90% to 95% of diabetes.[33] Type 2 diabetes is identified by inadequate insulin secretion and insulin resistance with a relative, versus absolute, insulin deficiency. Skeletal muscles become resistant and do not uptake glucose, a mechanism normally facilitated by GLUT4.[38] Risk of developing type 2 diabetes increases with age, obesity, and not being physically active.[33] Often in obese adults the excess adipose tissue is concentrated in the abdominal area. The onset of hyperglycemia occurs gradually, and many people are unaware that they have diabetes. Initially, type 2 diabetes is managed by oral medications (noninsulin therapies) because the pancreatic beta cells remain functional. As progressive beta cell dysfunction occurs, and if insufficient insulin is produced by the beta cells, a basal long-acting insulin may be added to oral noninsulin medications.[39]

Insulin Resistance

Insulin resistance occurs in type 2 diabetes. This is a complex metabolic situation in which organ and tissue cells deny entry to insulin and glucose.[38] This creates the clinical paradox in which elevated serum insulin levels and hyperglycemia are present at the same time. Insulin resistance has a strong association with obesity.[38]

Lifestyle Management for Type 2 Diabetes

For most patients with type 2 diabetes, a program comprising weight reduction, increased physical exercise, and a change in diet pattern are the essential preventative steps.[40] Crash diets are discouraged, and a gradual program of weight loss is recommended. Pharmacotherapy to assist with weight loss can be considered. An exercise program tailored to the individual including brisk walking for 150 minutes per week is often recommended.[33,40]

Type 2 diabetes increases risk of contracting a wide range of cardiovascular and kidney complications that increase morbidity and mortality.[41] In addition to taking medications to control blood glucose, some patients may need medications to lower their BP, lower cholesterol and triglyceride levels, treat coronary artery disease, or manage symptoms of heart failure.[41]

Pharmacologic Management of Type 2 Diabetes

If lifestyle changes are unsuccessful in reversing the pattern of prediabetes or type 2 diabetes, oral noninsulin antihyperglycemic medications are prescribed as recommended by the ADA (Table 31.3 and Box 31.4). These medications are not oral forms of insulin, but they are highly effective at lowering blood glucose by other mechanisms.[34] There are multiple classes of medications to manage type 2 diabetes as described in the next sections and in Table 31.4.

Metformin

Metformin is first-line therapy for patients with type 2 diabetes. Metformin is an *insulin sensitizer*. This oral medication increases insulin sensitivity in the liver, increasing the ability of insulin to suppress hepatic glucose production. Metformin also increases insulin sensitivity at the peripheral cellular level for fat and muscle to increase glucose uptake. Metformin may be used as monotherapy or be combined with other oral medications that lower blood glucose or combined with basal insulin as described in the next sections and in Table 31.3.

In type 2 diabetes, metformin can delay the transition from prediabetes to diabetes.[33,42] This was shown in the *Diabetes Prevention Program Outcomes Study* (DPPOS) where prediabetic participants received metformin and intensive lifestyle management that resulted in fewer eye and kidney complications.[33,43] Gastrointestinal side effects are common with metformin, and this can negatively impact adherence.[43,44] However, higher adherence to taking metformin is associated with a lower risk of progression from prediabetes to diabetes.[43]

Metformin is associated with a rare risk of metabolic acidosis and for this reason is often stopped before a procedure with radiocontrast, especially in patients with a reduced glomerular filtration rate (GFR). Metformin is contraindicated for patients with kidney dysfunction with a low GFR calculated at less than 30 mL/min/1.73 m^2.[45]

Sodium-Glucose Cotransporter-2 Inhibitors

The *sodium-glucose cotransporter-2 inhibitors* (SGLT2i) benefit patients with both type 2 diabetes, cardiovascular disease, and kidney disease[34,44,45] (see Table 31.3). These oral medications, also known as *gliflozins*, inhibit the reabsorption of glucose in

TABLE 31.3 PHARMACOLOGIC MANAGEMENT

Type 2 Diabetes

Medications for Type 2 Diabetes	Lower A_{1c}	Cardiovascular Disease	Cost	Route
Metformin	Yes		Low	Oral
Sulfonylureas	Yes		Low	Oral
Thiazolidinediones	Yes	Avoid in HF	Low	Oral
DPP-4 inhibitors	Yes	Avoid in HF	High	Oral
SGLT2 inhibitors	Yes	Added benefit	High	Oral
GLP-1 RA	Yes	Added benefit	High	Subcutaneous
Insulin	Yes		Low	Subcutaneous

HF, Heart failure.

Data from American Diabetes Association Professional Practice Committee. 9. Pharmacologic approaches to glycemic treatment: standards of care in diabetes—2024. *Diabetes Care.* 2024;47(Suppl 1):S158–S178. https://doi.org/10.2337/dc24-S009

Davies MJ, Aroda VR, Collins BS, et al. Management of hyperglycaemia in type 2 diabetes, 2022. A consensus report by the American Diabetes Association (ADA) and the European Association for the Study of Diabetes (EASD). *Diabetologia.* 2022;65(12):1925–1966. https://doi.org/10.1007/s00125-022-05787-2

BOX 31.4 Oral Antihyperglycemic Medication Classes and Actions

Medications That Sensitize the Body to Insulin (Insulin Sensitizers)

- Biguanides
- Thiazolidinediones

Medications That Stimulate the Pancreas to Make More Insulin (Insulin Secretagogues)

- Sulfonylureas
- Glinides

Medications That Delay Carbohydrate Absorption From Small Intestine

- Alpha-glucosidase inhibitors

Medications That Augment Gut Incretin Hormone Effects

- Incretin mimetics
- Incretin enhancers

Medications That Increase Excretion of Glucose in the Urine

- Sodium-glucose cotransporter2 (SGLT2) inhibitors

the nephron by inhibiting the action of the renal transporter SGLT2.[44] This results in more glucose being excreted in the urine, and blood glucose is reduced as a result. SGLT2i lowers A_{1c} by approximately 0.5% to 1%.[34,44]

The SGLT2i (canagliflozin, dapagliflozin, ertugliflozin, empagliflozin) are used in combination with other antihyperglycemic medications and are recommended by the American Heart Association (AHA) as a component of management in heart failure with reduced ejection fraction (HFrEF) because studies have shown SGLT2i use reduces hospitalizations.[46] The ADA recommends SGLT2i for management of type 2 diabetes.[34] Not unexpectedly, these newer agents are more expensive than older medications.[44] Potential side effects include urinary tract infection related to the increased glucose excreted in the urine.

In 2023 the FDA approved an oral once-daily combination medication (sotagliflozin) that inhibits both SGLT2 in the kidney and SGLT1 in the gastrointestinal system.[41] The primary FDA approved indication is to reduce hospitalization in heart failure.

- The SGLT2i mechanism of action is to increase kidney excretion of glucose in the urine.[41]
- The SGLT1i mechanism of action is to inhibit absorption of glucose into the bloodstream from the intestine.[41]

Glucagon-Like Peptide-1 Receptor Agonists

Glucagon-like peptide-1 receptor agonists (GLP-1 RA) are known as *incretin mimetics* because they augment activity of GLP-1. These medications (albiglutide, exenatide, dulaglutide, liraglutide, lixisenatide, semaglutide) increase insulin secretion from the pancreatic beta cells, lower glucagon levels, and delay gastric emptying. These medications are FDA approved for treatment of type 2 diabetes and in some cases to treat obesity.[44]

As often occurs, these newer medications are more expensive compared with older medications, which is a financial obstacle for many patients.[44] The medications in this class are mostly administered by subcutaneous injection and, depending on the medication, the injection is twice a day, once a day, or once a week using a single or multidose injection pen. GLP-1 RA medications are not a replacement for insulin. In 2023 the FDA approved semaglutide in an oral form.

A GLP-1 RA may be combined with a SGLTi to simultaneously treat type 2 diabetes and to lower the risk of cardiovascular disease and kidney disease.[47] This combination is possible because these drug classes have different mechanisms of action and different adverse risk profiles.[47]

Dipeptidyl Peptidase-4 Receptor Inhibitors

Dipeptidyl peptidase-4 (DPP-4) inhibitors are a class of oral antihyperglycemic medications known as *incretin enhancers* (sitagliptin, vildagliptin, saxagliptin, linagliptin). These medications slow down the degradation of the GLP-1 hormone by the enzyme DPP-4, prolonging the glucose-lowering activity of GLP-1 (see Table 31.3). These agents have the advantage that they rarely cause hypoglycemia.[44]

DPP-4 inhibitors act on the gastric *incretin* hormones. The main therapeutic target is the incretin hormone GLP-1, which is secreted from the gastric mucosa in response to food ingestion. GLP-1 stimulates the pancreatic beta cells to produce insulin. These are more expensive than older medications.[44] See Table 29.4 in Chapter 29 for a description of the physiologic effects of incretin hormones.

TABLE 31.4 PHARMACOLOGIC MANAGEMENT

Medications for Type 2 Diabetes

Medication[a]	Dosage	Action	Onset/Peak/ Duration	Special Considerations
Metformin				
Metformin (Glucophage)[b]	*Initial dosage:* 500 mg bid or 850 mg in morning; *maximum dosage:* 2550 mg tid	Reduces glucose output from liver Increases insulin action by decreasing peripheral insulin resistance	1–3 h/24 h/24–48 h	Temporarily withhold for up to 48 hours post-procedure if patient has received contrast radiography Adverse effects: lactic acidosis (rare); GI upset Contraindicated in male patients with S.Creat of 1.5 mg/dL or greater and female patients with S.Creat of 1.4 mg/dL or greater
Sulfonylureas				
Glipizide (Glucotrol)	*Initial dosage:* immediate-release tablet 5 mg once/day; *maximum dosage:* 40 mg bid	Stimulates insulin release	1 h/1–3 h/12–24 h	Administer with breakfast or after first main meal Also available in extended-release formulation (Glucotrol XL); do not cut, crush, or chew Extended release: *initial dosage:* 5 mg, once daily; *maximum dosage:* 20 mg/day Adjust dosage if creatinine clearance <50 mL/min
Glyburide (DiaBeta; Micronase)	*Initial dosage*: 2.5 mg once/day; *maintenance dosage*: 1.5–20 mg/day	Stimulates insulin release	1 h/4 h/18–24 h	Administer with breakfast or first main meal
Glimepiride (Amaryl)	*Initial dosage:* 1–2 mg once/day; *maximum dosage:* 8 mg once/day	Stimulates insulin release	Duration 24 h	Administer with breakfast or first main meal of day Initial dosage is lower in patients with kidney dysfunction (1 mg once/day)
Meglitinides				
Nateglinide (Starlix)	*Initial dosage*: 120 mg tid; *maximum dosage*: 120 mg tid	Stimulates insulin release	Peak <1 h	Administer 15–30 min before meals Cut dosage in half (i.e., 60 mg tid) for frail older patients and patients near their A_{1c} target
Repaglinide (Prandin)	*Initial dosage*: 1–2 mg tid; *maximum dosage*: 16 mg/day	Stimulates insulin release		Administer 15–30 min before meals Cut dosage in half (i.e., 0.5 mg tid) for frail older patients
Thiazolidinediones				
Pioglitazone (Actos)	*Initial dosage:* 15–30 mg bid; *maximum dosage:* 45 mg once/daily	Increases peripheral insulin sensitivity	Peak 2–3 h	Associated with weight gain, edema, heart failure, bone fractures; extreme caution if used for patients with heart failure; avoid if possible
Rosiglitazone (Avandia)	*Initial dosage:* 4 mg once/day or 2 mg bid; *maximum dosage:* 8 mg once/day or 4 mg bid	Increases peripheral insulin sensitivity		Associated with weight gain, edema, heart failure, LDL cholesterol increase, bone fractures; extreme caution in patients with heart failure; avoid if possible FDA warnings on cardiovascular safety
DPP-4 Receptor Inhibitors				
Sitagliptin	100 mg oral once/day	Inhibits DPP-4 hormone activity		Pancreatitis has occurred
Saxagliptin	2.5–5 mg oral once/day	Prolongs survival of endogenously released incretin hormones		Reduce dosage for sitagliptin and saxagliptin with kidney dysfunction
Linagliptin	5 mg oral once/day			No dosage adjustment for kidney dysfunction needed with linagliptin
SGLT2 Inhibitors				
Dapagliflozin	*Initial dosage:* 5 mg oral once/day; *maximum dosage:* 10 mg once/day	Increases glucose excretion by blocking SGLT2 glucose uptake in nephron		Kidney: Decrease dosage per GFR for various SGLT2 inhibitors

Continued

TABLE 31.4 PHARMACOLOGIC MANAGEMENT—cont'd

Medications for Type 2 Diabetes

Medication[a]	Dosage	Action	Onset/Peak/ Duration	Special Considerations
Canagliflozin	*Initial dosage*: 100 mg/day oral; *maximum dosage*: 300 mg/day	Same as above		Caution with liver failure for some SGLT2s FDA advisory of increased risk of DKA, UTI, AKI, genital yeast infections, Fournier's gangrene in the genital area
Empagliflozin	*Initial dosage*: 10 mg oral in a.m.; *maximum dosage*: 25 mg/day	Same as above		
Ertugliflozin	*Initial dosage*: 5 mg oral in a.m.; *maximum dosage*: 15 mg/day	Same as above		
GLP-1 Receptor Agonists				
Exenatide (Byetta)	*Initial dosage (immediate release)*: 5 mg subcutaneous injection bid; after 1 month may increase to 10 mg bid	Activates GLP-1 receptors in pancreatic beta cells		Avoid if creatinine clearance <30 mL/min
Exenatide extended release (Bydureon)	Extended release: 2 mg once/week			GI side effects (nausea, vomiting diarrhea) Pancreatitis has occurred
Liraglutide (Victoza)	*Initial dosage:* 0.6 mg subcutaneous injection once/day (regardless of meals) for 7 days, then increase to 1.2 mg once/day; may increase to 1.8 mg/day if needed; *maximum dosage:* 1.8 mg/day	Same as above		Pancreatitis has occurred
Alpha-Glucosidase Inhibitors				
Acarbose (Precose)	*Initial dosage*: 25 mg oral tid; *maximum dosage*: 100 mg tid	Delays carbohydrate digestion by blocking absorption of complete carbohydrates in small intestine	Peak 2–3 h	Administer with first bite of each meal GI side effects (flatulence, abdominal pain, diarrhea) Not recommended with severe kidney dysfunction
Miglitol (Glyset)	*Initial dosage*: 25 mg oral tid; *maximum dosage*: 100 mg tid		Peak 2–3 h	Administer with first bite of each meal

[a]Combination medications are too numerous to include in this table.

[b]FDA is alerting patients and health care professionals of a recall of several brands of ER metformin that contain high levels of NDMA. This alert does not affect immediate-release (IR) metformin, which is most often prescribed (https://www.fda.gov/drugs/drug-safety-and-availability/fda-updates-and-press-announcements-ndma-metformin).

AKI, Acute kidney injury; *bid*, twice daily; *DKA*, diabetic ketoacidosis; *DPP-4*, dipeptidyl peptidase-4; *ER*, extended release; *FDA*, U.S. Food and Drug Administration; *GFR*, glomerular filtration rate; *GI*, gastrointestinal; *GLP-1*, glucagon-like peptide-1; *IR*, immediate release; *LDL*, low-density lipoprotein; *NDMA*, N-nitrosodimethylamine; *S.Creat*, serum creatine; *SGLT2*, sodium-glucose cotransporter 2; *tid*, three times daily; *UTI*, urinary tract infection.

Thiazolidinediones

The *thiazolidinediones* (TZD), also known as *glitazones* (pioglitazone and rosiglitazone), are oral medications that belong to a class of medications called *peroxisome proliferator activated receptor gamma modulators*. These medications increase the sensitivity of muscle, fat, and liver cells to insulin. For this reason, thiazolidinediones are known as *insulin sensitizers*. Side effects such as fluid retention and edema limit use of thiazolidinediones. These medications should be avoided in patients with heart failure.[44] Bone loss is also a side effect.[44]

Sulfonylureas

The *sulfonylureas* (glyburide, glipizide, glimepiride, gliclazide) are oral medications that stimulate secretion of insulin from the pancreatic beta cells (see Table 31.3). They are in a category known as *insulin secretagogues*. Sulfonylureas reduce the A_{1c} by 1 to 2 percentage points and have a long duration of action. Sulfonylureas are recommended if cost is a concern.[34,44] Side effects include increased risk of hypoglycemia and weight gain.

The *meglitinides* (repaglinide and nateglinide) also increase insulin secretion (see Table 31.4) and may be prescribed in place of sulfonylureas.[34]

Alpha-Glucosidase Inhibitors

Alpha-glucosidase inhibitors (acarbose, miglitol) are used to reduce postprandial hyperglycemia in type 2 diabetes.[48] Alpha-glucosidase is an enzyme that splits complex carbohydrates into simple sugars in the gastrointestinal tract. These oral medications are taken at the beginning of a meal to inhibit enzyme action and delay gastric absorption of carbohydrates (e.g., bread, corn, pasta, beans) into the bloodstream. These medications lower A_{1c} by approximately 0.5% to 1.5% in persons with type 2 diabetes.[48]

Insulin in Type 2 Diabetes

In some situations, patients with type 2 diabetes will have insulin added to their medication regimen.[34] Patients with an A_{1c} above 10% who are taking two oral antihyperglycemic medications, including metformin, may not benefit from adding a third oral antihyperglycemic medication.[34] Another option is to add a long-acting basal insulin added to the regimen.[44] The addition of subcutaneous insulin requires more intensive blood glucose monitoring and additional education.

Polypharmacy in Diabetes

The availability of varied pharmacologic approaches to reduce blood glucose and manage type 2 diabetes can reduce many long-term complications related to hyperglycemia. Often patients may be taking two or three medications for diabetes (see Table 31.3) and taking additional medications for cardiovascular disease prevention and other health conditions.[39,41,44] One of the unintended consequences of having so many medications to manage type 2 diabetes is *polypharmacy* and risk of medication interactions and hypoglycemia; this is recognized as a particular problem for older adults.

HYPERGLYCEMIC EMERGENCIES

The two hyperglycemic emergencies associated with diabetes are *diabetic ketoacidosis* (DKA) and hyperglycemic hyperosmolar state (HHS).[49,50] In the United States, DKA and HHS account for 168,000 hospital admissions and 207,000 visits to the emergency department each year.[51] In both conditions, treatment focuses on administration of insulin, rehydration, and correction of electrolyte and acid–base imbalances.[49–52] Management of hyperglycemic emergencies is shown in a management algorithm in Fig. 31.2. Hyperglycemia emergencies include both DKA and HHS, but because there are significant differences between DKA and HHS, these conditions are discussed separately in this chapter.

Diabetic Ketoacidosis

DKA is a life-threatening complication of diabetes mellitus. Individuals with type 1 diabetes who are newly diagnosed or already dependent on insulin must be rapidly assessed and treated as listed in the Summary of Key Concepts Related to DKA (Fig. 31.3). The classic diagnostic criteria for DKA include the following criteria.[50]

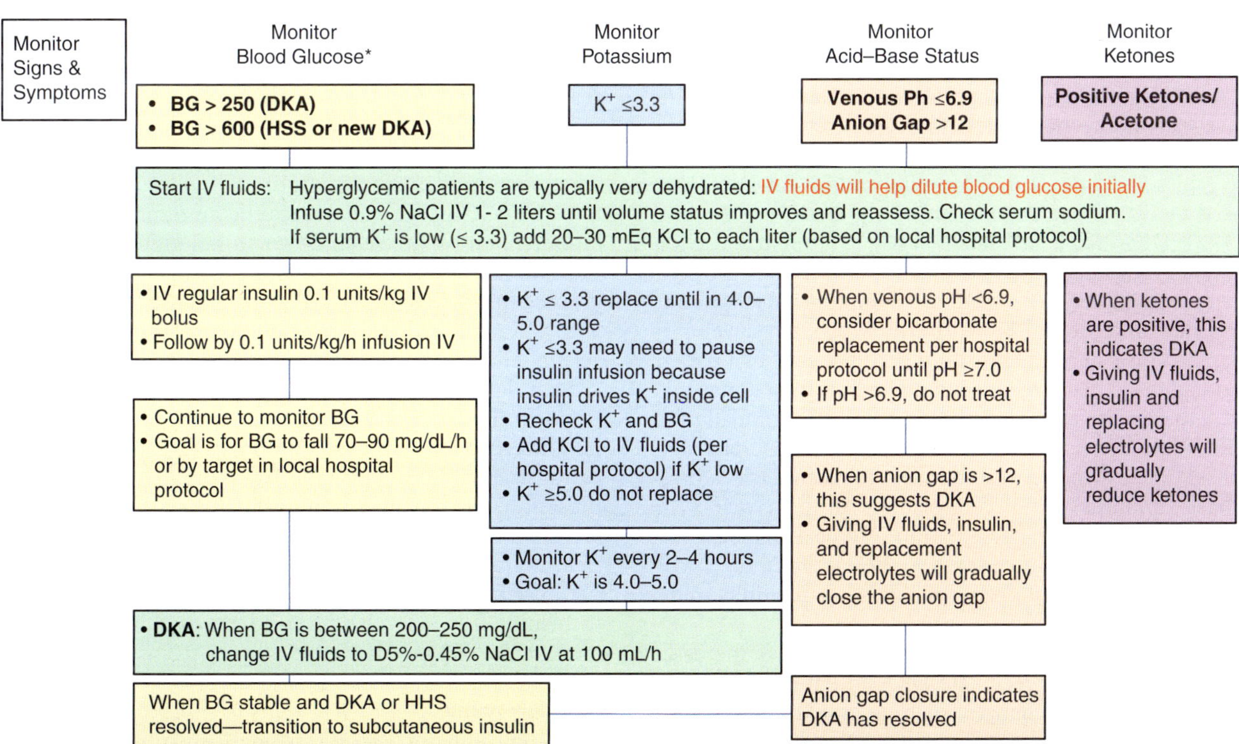

FIG. 31.2 Protocol for Management of Hyperglycemic Emergencies: Diabetic Ketoacidosis and Hyperglycemic Hyperosmolar State. *BG*, Blood glucose; *DKA*, diabetic ketoacidosis; *HHS*, hyperglycemic hyperosmolar state; *IV*, intravenous; *K+*, potassium; *KCl*, potassium chloride; *NaCl*, sodium chloride; *pH*, a measure of the degree to which a solution is acidic or alkaline. *Different hospital protocols may use other blood glucose target values to identify and resolve DKA and HHS. (Data from Kitabchi AE, Umpierrez GE, Miles JM, Fisher JN. Hyperglycemic crises in adult patients with diabetes. *Diabetes Care*. 2009;32(7):1335–1343. https://doi.org/10.2337/dc09-9032. Umpierrez G, Korytkowski M. Diabetic emergencies – ketoacidosis, hyperglycaemic hyperosmolar state and hypoglycaemia. *Nat Rev Endocrinol*. 2016;12(4):222–232. https://doi.org/10.1038/nrendo.2016.15. Mustafa OG, Haq M, Dashora U, Castro E, Dhatariya KK, Joint British Diabetes Societies (JBDS) for Inpatient Care Group. Management of hyperosmolar hyperglycaemic state (HHS) in adults: an updated guideline from the Joint British Diabetes Societies (JBDS) for Inpatient Care Group. *Diabet Med*. 2023;40(3):e15005. https://doi.org/10.1111/dme.15005)

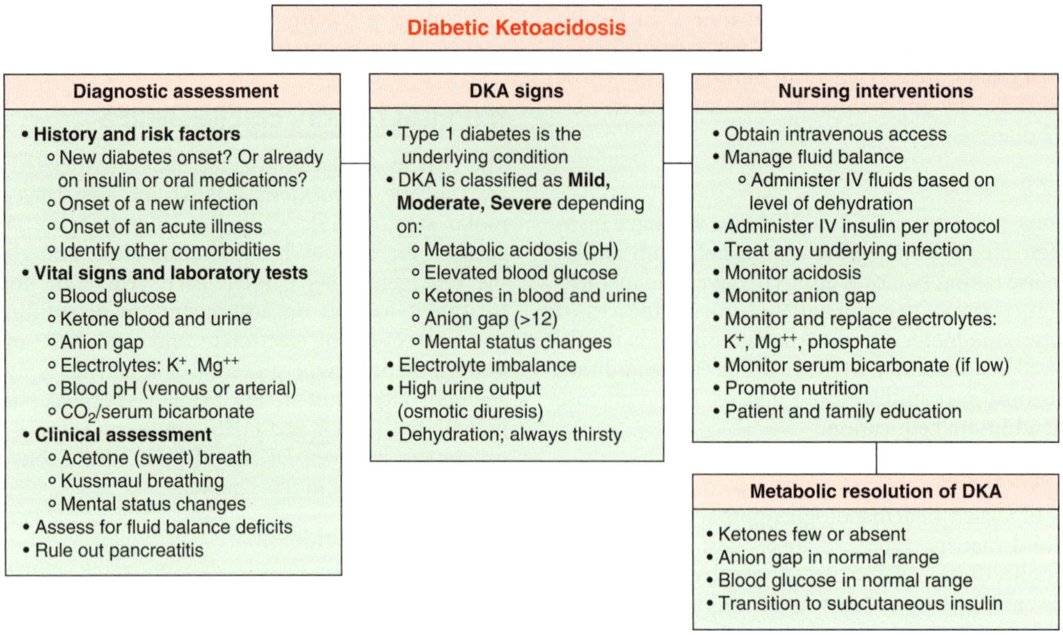

Diabetic Ketoacidosis

Diagnostic assessment

- **History and risk factors**
  - New diabetes onset? Or already on insulin or oral medications?
  - Onset of a new infection
  - Onset of an acute illness
  - Identify other comorbidities
- **Vital signs and laboratory tests**
  - Blood glucose
  - Ketone blood and urine
  - Anion gap
  - Electrolytes: K^+, Mg^{++}
  - Blood pH (venous or arterial)
  - CO_2/serum bicarbonate
- **Clinical assessment**
  - Acetone (sweet) breath
  - Kussmaul breathing
  - Mental status changes
- Assess for fluid balance deficits
- Rule out pancreatitis

DKA signs

- Type 1 diabetes is the underlying condition
- DKA is classified as **Mild, Moderate, Severe** depending on:
  - Metabolic acidosis (pH)
  - Elevated blood glucose
  - Ketones in blood and urine
  - Anion gap (>12)
  - Mental status changes
- Electrolyte imbalance
- High urine output (osmotic diuresis)
- Dehydration; always thirsty

Nursing interventions

- Obtain intravenous access
- Manage fluid balance
  - Administer IV fluids based on level of dehydration
- Administer IV insulin per protocol
- Treat any underlying infection
- Monitor acidosis
- Monitor anion gap
- Monitor and replace electrolytes: K^+, Mg^{++}, phosphate
- Monitor serum bicarbonate (if low)
- Promote nutrition
- Patient and family education

Metabolic resolution of DKA

- Ketones few or absent
- Anion gap in normal range
- Blood glucose in normal range
- Transition to subcutaneous insulin

FIG. 31.3 Summary of Key Concepts Related to Diabetic Ketoacidosis. *CO_2*, carbon dioxide; *DKA*, diabetic ketoacidosis; *IV*, intravenous; *K^+*, potassium; *Mg^{++}*, magnesium; *pH*, a measure of the degree to which a solution is acidic or alkaline.

- Blood glucose greater than 250 mg/dL
- Acidosis with pH less than 7.3
- Serum bicarbonate less than 18 mEq/L
- Moderate or severe ketonemia or ketonuria

DKA is categorized as mild, moderate, or severe depending on the severity of the metabolic acidosis (assessed by blood pH, bicarbonate, ketones) and by the presence of altered mental status (Tables 31.5 and 31.6).[50] Hospitalizations for DKA have increased by 30% since 2010.[53] Before the discovery of insulin in 1921, DKA had a 90% fatality rate.[49] With current treatments, DKA mortality is well below 1%.[53] Infection is the most frequent precipitating cause of DKA.[53] Symptoms of fatigue and polyuria may precede full-blown DKA, which can develop in less than 24 hours in a patient with type 1 diabetes. In a patient with undiagnosed diabetes, it is unknown how long it may take for DKA to develop as the pancreatic beta cells gradually fail. Hospital admission is generally required for DKA related to new-onset type 1 diabetes, and about 5% of recent DKA admissions (last 3 months) are in young adults 18 to 25 years.[49] In adults, DKA is the initial presentation of type 1 diabetes 15% to 20% of the time and in children in 30% to 40 % of cases.[49] DKA accounts for 50% of deaths of children and adults under 24 years of age.[49]

Changes in the type of insulin, change in dosage, or increased metabolic demand can precipitate DKA in patients with type 1 diabetes.[50] Life cycle changes, such as growth spurts in an adolescent, require an increase in insulin intake, as do surgery, infection, and trauma.

Ketoacidosis also occurs with acute pancreatitis. In addition to elevated glucose and acidosis, serum amylase and lipase are abnormally high, which helps to establish pancreatitis as a separate diagnosis from type 1 diabetes. Other nondiabetic causes of ketoacidosis are starvation ketosis and alcoholic ketoacidosis. These cases are distinguished from classic DKA by clinical history and usually by a plasma glucose less than 200 mg/dL.[50]

Insulin Deficiency

Insulin is the metabolic key to the transfer of glucose from the bloodstream into the cell, where it can be used immediately for energy or stored for use later. Without insulin, glucose remains in the bloodstream, and cells are deprived of their energy source. A complex pathophysiologic chain of events follows. The release of glucagon from the liver is stimulated when insulin is ineffective in providing the cells with glucose for energy. Glucagon increases the amount of glucose in the bloodstream by breaking down stored glucose (glycogenolysis). Noncarbohydrates (fat and protein) are converted into glucose (gluconeogenesis). Plasma glucose levels for a patient with DKA typically are greater than 250 mg/dL.[49] Elevated serum glucose levels alone do not define DKA; the other crucial determining factor is the presence of ketoacidosis as listed in Table 31.5.[50] In addition to the low pH (less than 7.3), there is an increased anion gap (greater than 12), indicating metabolic acidosis.[49] Approximately 10% of patients present to the hospital with mild DKA with a plasma glucose less than 250 mg/dL.[50,53] This presentation is known as *euglycemic ketoacidosis* and it can occur in patients taking antihyperglycemic medications (SGLT2i or GLP-1 RA) in addition to insulin.[54] It may also be misdiagnosed because the blood glucose is <250 mg/dL.[54]

Hyperglycemia

Hyperglycemia increases serum osmolality, and the blood becomes hyperosmolar. Cellular dehydration occurs as the hyperosmolar extracellular fluid draws the more dilute intracellular and interstitial fluid into the vascular space to attempt to achieve a normal serum osmolality. Dehydration stimulates catecholamine production to provide emergency support. Catecholamine output stimulates further glycogenolysis, lipolysis, and gluconeogenesis, pouring glucose into the bloodstream.

TABLE 31.5 Diagnostic Criteria for Diabetic Ketoacidosis (DKA) and Hyperglycemic Hyperosmolar State (HHS)

	DKA			HHS
	Mild BG >250 mg/dL (13.9 mmol/L)	**Moderate BG >250 mg/dL (13.9 mmol/L)**	**Severe BG >250 mg/dL (13.9 mmol/L)**	**Plasma Glucose >600 mg/dL**
Arterial pH	7.25–7.30	7.00 to <7.24	<7.00	>7.30
Serum bicarbonate (mEq/L)	15–18	10 to <15	<10	>18
Urine ketone[a]	Positive	Positive	Positive	Negative, or small positive
Serum ketone[a]	Positive	Positive	Positive	Small
Urine or blood beta-hydroxybutyrate (mmol/L)	>3	>3	>3	<3
Effective serum osmolality[b]	Variable	Variable	Variable	>320 mOsm/kg
Anion gap[c]	>10	>12	>12	Variable
Mental status	Alert	Alert/drowsy	Stupor/coma	Stupor/coma

[a]Nitroprusside reaction method.
[b]Effective serum osmolality: 2[measured Na^+ (mEq/L)]+glucose (mg/dL)18.
[c]Anion gap: (Na^+) – (Cl^-+ HCO_3^-) (mEq/L).
Data from Kitabchi AE, Umpierrez GE, Miles JM, et al. Hyperglycemic crises in adult patients with diabetes: a consensus statement from the American Diabetes Association. *Diabetes Care.* 2009;32(7):1335–1343. Umpierrez G, Korytkowski M. Diabetic emergencies—ketoacidosis, hyperglycaemic hyperosmolar state and hypoglycaemia. *Nat Rev Endocrinol.* 2016;12:222–232. Dhatariya KK, Vellanki P. Treatment of diabetic ketoacidosis (DKA)/hyperglycemic hyperosmolar state (HHS): novel advances in the management of hyperglycemic crises (UK versus USA). *Curr Diab Rep.* 2017;17(5):33.

TABLE 31.6 Comparison of Diabetic Ketoacidosis and Hyperglycemic Hyperosmolar State

Characteristics and Laboratory Tests	DKA	HHS
Characteristics		
Cause	Insufficient exogenous glucose for glucose needs	Insufficient exogenous/endogenous insulin for glucose needs
Onset	Sudden (hours)	Slow, insidious (days, weeks)
Precipitating factors	Noncompliance with type 1 diabetes therapy, illness, surgery, decreased activity	Recent acute illness in older patient; therapeutic procedures
Mortality (%)	9–14	10–50
Patients affected	Patients with type 1 diabetes	Patients with type 2 diabetes
Clinical manifestations	Dry mouth, polydipsia, polyuria, polyphagia, dehydration, dry skin, hypotension, weakness	Mental confusion, tachycardia, changes in level of consciousness
	Ketoacidosis, air hunger, acetone breath odor, respirations deep and rapid, nausea, vomiting	No ketosis, no breath odor, respirations rapid and shallow, usually mild nausea/vomiting
Laboratory Tests		
Glucose (mg/dL)	300–800	600–2000
Ketones	Strongly positive	Normal or mildly elevated
pH	<7.3	Normal[a]
Osmolality (mOsm/L)	<350	>350
Sodium	Normal or low	Normal or elevated
Potassium (K^+)	Normal, low, or elevated (total body K^+ depleted)	Low, normal, or elevated
Bicarbonate	<15 mEq/L	Normal
Phosphorus	Low, normal, or elevated (may decrease after insulin therapy)	Low, normal, or elevated (may decrease after insulin therapy)
Urine acetone	Strong	Absent or mild

[a]Exception: In severe HHS, lactic acidosis may develop as a result of dehydration and severe tissue hypoperfusion and ischemia.
DKA, Diabetic ketoacidosis; *HHS*, hyperglycemic hyperosmolar state.

Fluid Volume Deficit

Polyuria (excessive urination) and *glycosuria* (sugar in the urine) occur as a result of the osmotic particle load that occurs with DKA. The excess glucose, filtered at the glomeruli, cannot be reabsorbed at the kidney tubule and spills into the urine. This solute exerts its own osmotic pull in the renal tubules, and less water is returned to circulation through the collecting ducts. As a result, large volumes of water, along with sodium, potassium, and phosphorus, are excreted in the urine, causing a fluid volume deficit. The serum sodium concentration may be decreased because of the movement of water from the intracellular to the extracellular (vascular) space.[53]

Ketoacidosis

In a healthy individual, the presence of insulin in the bloodstream suppresses the manufacture of ketones. In insulin deficiency states, fat is rapidly converted into glucose (gluconeogenesis). *Ketoacidosis* occurs when free fatty acids are metabolized into ketones. Three ketones produced in DKA are:

- 3-beta-hydroxybutyrate
- Acetoacetate
- Acetone

During normal metabolism, the ratio of beta-hydroxybutyrate to acetoacetate is 1:1, with acetone present in only small amounts. In DKA, because of lack of insulin, the quantities of all three ketone bodies increase substantially, and the ratio of beta-hydroxybutyrate to acetoacetate can increase to 10:1. In DKA, the main ketone in the blood is 3-beta-hydroxybutyrate, and the main ketone in the urine is its breakdown product, acetoacetate. Acetone does not cause acidosis and is safely excreted in the lungs, causing the characteristic fruity odor on the exhaled breath.

Ketones are measurable in the bloodstream (ketonemia). Blood tests that measure the quantity of 3-beta-hydroxybutyric acid—the predominant ketone body in the blood—are considered the most useful.[50,54–56] Because ketones are excreted by the kidneys, they are also measurable in the urine (ketonuria). When the blood and urine become clear of ketones, DKA is resolved.

Ketone blood tests are preferred for diagnosis and monitoring of DKA. To test for presence of ketones in blood, direct measurement of 3-beta-hydroxybutyrate is used (see Table 31.5). Point-of-care monitors to test blood ketones exist, and research and development is underway to add a continuous ketone monitoring feature to continuous glucose monitors currently on the market.[57]

Acid–Base Balance

The acid–base balance varies depending on the severity of DKA. A patient with mild DKA typically has a pH between 7.25 and 7.30. In severe DKA, the pH can drop below 7.00 (see Table 31.5).[50] Acid ketones dissociate and yield hydrogen ions, which accumulate and precipitate the fall in serum pH. The level of serum bicarbonate also decreases, consistent with a diagnosis of metabolic acidosis. Breathing becomes deep and rapid (Kussmaul respirations) to release carbonic acid in the form of carbon dioxide (CO_2). Acetone is exhaled, giving the breath its characteristic fruity odor.

Focused Physical Assessment in DKA

The assessment is focused on determining the severity of the hyperglycemia and acidosis and identifying comorbidities or other causes such as infection.

Clinical Manifestations

DKA often has a predictable clinical presentation. It is usually preceded by patient complaints of malaise, headache, polyuria (excessive urination), polydipsia (excessive thirst), and polyphagia (excessive hunger). Nausea, vomiting, extreme fatigue, dehydration, and weight loss follow. Central nervous system (CNS) depression, with changes in the level of consciousness, can lead quickly to coma.[50]

A patient with DKA may be stuporous or unresponsive, depending on the degree of fluid-balance disturbance. Physical examination reveals evidence of dehydration, including flushed dry skin, dry buccal membranes, and skin turgor that takes longer than 3 seconds to return to its original position after the skin has been lifted. Tachycardia and hypotension may signal profound fluid losses. Kussmaul respirations are present, and the fruity odor of acetone may be detected.

Laboratory Studies

Considering the complexity and potential seriousness of DKA, the laboratory diagnosis is straightforward. When the patient has established type 1 diabetes, the presence of hyperglycemia, ketones, and acidosis on a venous blood gas provides rapid diagnostic confirmation of DKA.[55] Many patients have ketone-testing point-of-care devices at home. Other clues may be gleaned from the venous blood chemistry panel. CO_2, if measured, is low in the presence of uncompensated metabolic acidosis, and the anion gap is elevated. Serum sodium may be low as a result of the movement of water from the intracellular space into the extracellular space (vascular and tissues).[50] The serum potassium level is often normal; a low serum potassium level in DKA suggests that a significant potassium deficiency may be present.[50]

Medical Management

Diagnosis of DKA is based on the combination of presenting symptoms, patient history, medical history (type 1 diabetes), precipitating factors (if known), and results of serum glucose and urine ketone testing. After diagnosis, DKA requires aggressive clinical management to prevent progressive decompensation. The goals of treatment are to reverse dehydration, replace insulin, reverse ketoacidosis, and replenish electrolytes.

Reversing Dehydration

A patient with DKA is dehydrated and may have lost 5% to 10% of body weight in fluids. Aggressive IV fluid replacement is provided to rehydrate the intracellular and extracellular compartments and prevent circulatory collapse (see Fig. 31.2).[50,53] Assessment of hydration is an important first step in the treatment of DKA.

IV isotonic normal saline (0.9% sodium chloride [NaCl]) is infused to replenish the vascular deficit and to reverse hypotension. For a severely dehydrated patient, 1 L of normal saline is infused immediately. Laboratory assessment of serum osmolality and the serum sodium concentration can help guide subsequent interventions. If the serum osmolality is elevated and serum sodium is high (hypernatremia), infusions of hypotonic NaCl (0.45) follow the initial saline replacement. The replacement infusion typically includes 20 to 30 mEq of potassium per liter to restore the intracellular potassium debt, provided that kidney function is normal (see Fig. 31.2). In patients without normally functioning kidneys and in patients with cardiopulmonary disease, careful attention must be paid to the volume of fluid replacement to avoid fluid overload.[53]

After the serum glucose level decreases to 200 mg/dL, the infusing solution is changed to a 50/50 mix of hypotonic saline and 5% dextrose (D_5W). Dextrose is added to replenish depleted cellular glucose as the circulating serum glucose decreases to 200 mg/dL.[50] Dextrose infusion also prevents unexpected hypoglycemia when the insulin infusion is continued, but the patient cannot take in sufficient carbohydrate from an oral diet.

Insulin Administration

In moderate to severe DKA, an initial IV bolus of regular insulin at 0.1 unit for each kg of body weight may be administered. Subsequently, a continuous infusion of regular insulin at 0.1 unit/kg/h is infused simultaneously with IV fluid replacement (see Fig. 31.2).[50] In a 70-kg adult, the infusion would be 7 units of insulin per hour. If the blood glucose concentration does not fall by 50 to 70 mg/dL during the first hour of treatment, the glucose measurement should be rechecked. When the blood glucose level is decreasing as expected, the insulin infusion is increased each hour until a steady blood glucose decline of between 50 and 70 mg/dL per hour is achieved.[50] It is important to emphasize that different hospitals' protocols may list other target requirements for decline of hourly blood glucose in DKA/HHS: For example, a decrease of 25 to 75 mg/dL per hour[51] or a decline of up to 100 mg/dL per hour (5 mmol/L)[52] could also be the target reduction depending on the hospital protocol.[51,52]

Frequent assessment of the patient's blood glucose concentration is mandatory in moderate to severe DKA. Initially, blood glucose tests are performed hourly. The frequency decreases to every 2 to 4 hours as the patient's blood glucose level stabilizes and approaches normal. After the BG level has decreased to between 200 and 250 mg/dL, the acidosis has been corrected, and rehydration has been achieved, the insulin infusion rate may be decreased by half to 0.05 unit/kg/hour.[49] This usually represents 3 to 6 units per hour in an adult receiving a continuous IV insulin infusion. It is important to verify that the serum potassium concentration is not lower than 3.3 mEq/L and to replace potassium per local hospital protocol before administering the initial insulin bolus.[50]

Reversing Ketoacidosis

Replacement of fluid volume and insulin interrupts the ketotic cycle and reverses the metabolic acidosis. In the presence of insulin, glucose enters the cells, and the body ceases to convert fats into glucose.

Adequate hydration and insulin replacement usually correct acidosis, and this treatment is sufficient for many patients with DKA. As shown in Fig. 31.2, replacement of bicarbonate is no longer routine except for a severely acidotic patient with a serum pH value lower than 7.0.[50] An indwelling arterial line provides access for hourly sampling of arterial blood gases to evaluate pH, bicarbonate, and other laboratory values in a patient with severe DKA.

Hyperglycemia usually resolves before ketoacidemia does.[50] Patients with type 1 diabetes and DKA may require 6 to 9 L of IV fluid replacement. Volume resuscitation occurs over 24 to 36 hours, with most IV crystalloid administered in the first 8 to 12 hours.[50,52] Patients with a new diagnosis of type 1 diabetes take longer to clear urine ketones and require more insulin to achieve normal glycemic control. This is because the blood glucose is typically very elevated on the initial admission.

Replenishing Electrolytes

Low serum potassium (hypokalemia) occurs as insulin promotes the return of potassium into the cell and metabolic acidosis is reversed. The potassium level must be 3.3 mEq or greater before administering insulin. The potassium level must be checked frequently, as insulin drives potassium into the cells and the serum potassium can drop precipitously. Potassium chloride is administered as soon as the serum potassium falls below normal. Frequent verification of the serum potassium concentration is required for a patient with DKA receiving fluid resuscitation and insulin therapy.

The serum phosphate level is sometimes low (hypophosphatemia) in DKA. Insulin treatment may make this more obvious as phosphate is returned to the interior of the cell. If the serum phosphate level is less than 1 mg/dL, phosphate replacement is recommended.[50]

Nursing Management

Nursing management of a patient with DKA incorporates a variety of patient problems (Box 31.5). The goals of nursing

BOX 31.5 DIAGNOSIS AND PATIENT CARE MANAGEMENT

Diabetic Ketoacidosis

- Risk for Infection
- Hypovolemia due to absolute loss
- Anxiety due to threat to biological, psychological, or social integrity
- Disturbed Body Image due to functional dependence on life-sustaining technology
- Powerlessness due to lack of control over current situation or disease progression
- Lack of Knowledge of Treatment Regime due to lack of previous exposure to information (see Box 31.9, Patient and Family Education Plan for Diabetic Ketoacidosis)

Patient Care Management plans are located in Appendix A.

management are to administer prescribed fluids, insulin, and electrolytes; monitor response to therapy; maintain surveillance for complications; and provide patient education.

Administering Fluids, Insulin, and Electrolytes

Rapid IV fluid replacement requires the use of a volumetric pump. To ensure effective absorption, insulin is administered IV to patients who are severely dehydrated or have poor peripheral perfusion. Patients with DKA are kept on NPO status (nothing by mouth) until hyperglycemia is under control. The critical care nurse is responsible for monitoring the rate of plasma glucose decline in response to insulin. The goal is to achieve a fall in glucose levels of approximately 50 to 70 mg/dL each hour.[50] The coordination involved in monitoring blood glucose, potassium, and often blood gases on an hourly basis is considerable.

When the blood glucose level falls to, or below, 200 mg/dL, a D_5W with 0.45% NaCl solution is infused to prevent hypoglycemia.[50] At this time, it is likely that the insulin dose per hour will also be decreased. The infusion of regular insulin is not discontinued. The goal is to maintain the blood glucose level between 140 and 200 mg/dL until the ketoacidosis subsides, as identified by absence of ketones, until closure of the anion gap and return to a normal venous pH.[50]

Insulin is given subcutaneously after glucose levels, dehydration, hypotension, and acid–base balance return to baseline, when the patient is in stable condition, and taking an adequate oral diet.

Monitoring Response to Therapy

Accurate intake and output (I&O) measurements must be maintained to monitor reversal of dehydration. Hourly urine output is an indicator of kidney function and provides information to prevent overhydration or insufficient hydration. Vital signs, especially heart rate (HR), hemodynamic values, and BP, are continuously monitored to assess response to fluid replacement. Evidence that fluid replacement is effective includes decreased HR, normal BP, and normalizing blood glucose levels. Box 31.6 lists the standard features to be included in an assessment of hydration status. More invasive hemodynamic monitoring, such as a pulmonary artery catheter, is rarely needed. Further evidence of hydration improvement includes a change from a previously weak and rapid pulse to one that is strong and full and a change from hypotension to a gradual elevation of systolic BP. Respirations are assessed frequently for changes in rate, depth, and presence of the fruity acetone odor.

BOX 31.6 Hydration Assessment

- Hourly intake
- Blood pressure changes
- Orthostatic hypotension
- Pulse pressure
- Pulse rate, character, rhythm
- Neck vein filling
- Skin turgor
- Skin moisture
- Body weight
- Central venous pressure
- Hourly output
- Complaints of thirst

Blood glucose is measured each hour in the initial period. Sometimes potassium is measured just as frequently. The serum osmolality and serum sodium concentration are evaluated, and blood urea nitrogen (BUN) and creatinine levels are assessed for possible kidney impairment related to decreased organ perfusion. The purpose of these frequent assessments is to determine that the patient's clinical status is improving.

Transition to Subcutaneous Insulin

When the clinical laboratory indicators are stable and the patient is awake and alert, the transition to subcutaneous insulin and an oral diet can be made. Hyperglycemia is a risk if the subcutaneous insulin dosage is inadequate to maintain a normal blood glucose. In this situation, the anion gap may open up again. Hypoglycemia is also a risk during the transition period. For example, in anticipation of discontinuing the insulin and IV dextrose infusion, a patient receives a subcutaneous dose of insulin and is expected to eat a meal. However, if the patient is then unable to eat an adequate amount, hypoglycemia results from the administration of subcutaneous insulin without adequate carbohydrate.

Surveillance for Complications

A patient with DKA can experience various complications, including fluid volume overload, hypoglycemia, hypokalemia or hyperkalemia, hyponatremia, cerebral edema, and infection.

Fluid Volume Overload

Fluid overload from rapid volume infusion is a serious complication that can occur in a patient with a compromised cardiopulmonary system or kidneys. Neck vein engorgement, dyspnea without exertion, and pulmonary crackles on auscultation signal circulatory overload. Reduction in the rate and volume of infusion, elevation of the head of the bed, and provision of oxygen may be required to manage increased intravascular volume. Hourly urine measurement is mandatory to assess kidney function and adequacy of fluid replacement.

Hypoglycemia

Hypoglycemia is defined as a serum glucose level lower than 70 mg/dL.[50] Most acute care hospitals have specific procedures for management of hypoglycemia (Box 31.7). For example, if hypoglycemia is detected by fingerstick point-of-care testing at the bedside, a blood sample is sent to the laboratory for verification; the physician is notified immediately; and replacement glucose is given IV or orally, depending on the patient's clinical condition, diagnosis, and level of consciousness.

Unexpected behavior changes or decreased level of consciousness, diaphoresis, and tremors are physical warning signs that the patient has become hypoglycemic. These symptoms are especially important to recognize if the frequency of blood glucose testing has lengthened to 2- to 4-hour intervals. Up to 30% of individuals who have type 1 diabetes have impaired awareness of their low blood glucose, greatly increasing their risk of severe hypoglycemia (see Box 31.7). The physical symptoms associated with hypoglycemia and hyperglycemia are listed in Box 31.8.

Hypokalemia and Hyperkalemia

Hypokalemia can occur within the first hours of rehydration and insulin treatment. Continuous cardiac monitoring is required because hypokalemia can cause ventricular dysrhythmias.

Hyperkalemia occurs with acidosis or with overaggressive administration of potassium replacement in patients with kidney disease. Severe hyperkalemia is demonstrated on the cardiac monitor by a large, peaked T wave; flattened P wave; and widened QRS complex (see Fig. 12.81 in Chapter 12). Ventricular fibrillation can follow.

Hyponatremia

Elimination of sodium from the body results from the osmotic diuresis and is compounded by the vomiting and diarrhea that can occur during DKA. Clinical manifestations of hyponatremia include abdominal cramping, postural hypotension, and unexpected behavioral changes. NaCl is infused as the initial IV solution. Maintenance of the saline infusion depends on clinical manifestations of sodium imbalance and serum laboratory values.

Level of Consciousness

Cerebral edema is rare in adults but occurs in 1% of children with DKA with a mortality rate between 20% and 40%.[49] Changes in the patient's neurologic status may be insidious. Alterations in level of consciousness, pupil reaction, and motor function may be the result of fluctuating glucose levels and cerebral fluid shifts. Confusion and sudden complaints of headache are ominous signs that may signal cerebral edema. These observations require immediate action to prevent neurologic damage. Neurologic assessments are performed every hour or as needed during the acute phase of hyperglycemia and rehydration. Assessment of level of consciousness serves as the index of the patient's cerebral response to rehydration therapy.

Skin Care

Skin care takes on new dimensions for patients with DKA. Dehydration, hypovolemia, and hypophosphatemia interfere with oxygen delivery at the cell site and contribute to inadequate perfusion and tissue breakdown. Patients must be repositioned frequently to relieve capillary pressure and promote adequate perfusion to body tissues. A typical patient with type 1 diabetes is of normal weight or underweight. Bony prominences must be assessed for tissue breakdown, and the patient's body weight must be repositioned every 1 to 2 hours. Irritation of skin from adhesive tape, shearing force, and detergents should be avoided. Maintenance of skin integrity prevents unwanted portals of entry for microorganisms.

Oral Care

Care of the mouth, including toothbrushing and use of lip balm, helps keep lips supple and prevents cracking. Prepared sponge sticks or moist gauze pads can be used to moisten oral

BOX 31.7 Hypoglycemia Management

Hypoglycemia Prevention and Management

- Definition: Blood glucose level below 70 mg/dL (3.9 mmol/L)
- The American Diabetes Association recommends 70 mg/dL plasma blood glucose as the alert threshold for hypoglycemia. Most patients with diabetes do not have symptoms with this blood glucose, and this value provides some time to raise the blood glucose and avoid clinical symptoms.
- Bedside point-of-care (POC) glucometers results vary in accuracy. A POC blood glucose less than 70 mg/dL must be double checked by sending a blood sample to the clinical laboratory *stat* to measure the plasma blood glucose.
- Continuous glucose monitoring (CGM) is not yet approved for use within the hospital setting but algorithmic protocols for type 1 patients can be developed for use in the hospital.

Hypoglycemia Prevention in the Hospital

- Close monitoring of blood glucose for all hospitalized patients who receive insulin is vital. Use 70 mg/dL as the threshold and do not wait for clinical symptoms to adjust the insulin infusion or administer glucose.
- Approximately 10% of patients with a diagnosis of diabetes, that are admitted to a critical care unit experience at least one hypoglycemic episode (below 70 mg/dL).

Hypoglycemia Prevention for Diabetes Type 1 and Type 2

- Blood glucose testing to detect hypoglycemia is vital, because many patients with diabetes do not experience symptoms. This is called *hypoglycemia unawareness.* In patients with diabetes who experience frequent episodes of hypoglycemia, the autonomic nervous system becomes less responsive. This is known as *hypoglycemia-associated autonomic failure.*
- Patient education before hospital discharge is essential to teach patients how blood glucose monitoring and dietary interventions are used to prevent hypoglycemia.
- For patients with type 1 diabetes, who will receive several insulin injections daily, continuous glucose monitoring (CGM) is recommended over self-monitoring with a fingerstick when discharged from the hospital to closely monitor blood glucose in real time. CGM is preferably started in the hospital prior to discharge.
- Long-acting basal insulin over NPH is recommended to reduce the risk of hypoglycemia.
- Insulin pumps with algorithim software may also reduce the risk of hypoglycemia.

Clinical Signs and Symptoms of Acute Hypoglycemia

- Sedated and intubated patients may not have signs and symptoms
- Confusion
- Neurologic changes
- Seizures
- Death

Hypoglycemia Management

- Stop insulin infusion (if infusing).
- Administer 25 grams of hypertonic dextrose (D_{50}) IV immediately.
- If blood glucose is dangerously low (below 40 mg/dL), some hospital protocols recommend 50 grams D_{50} IV.
- Repeat blood glucose value in 15 minutes, and ongoing until blood glucose is greater than 70 mg/dL.
- Evaluate insulin regimen.
- Evaluate IV dextrose and carbohydrate nutrition regimen.
- If the patient can safely swallow, provide 25 grams carbohydrate orally and recheck blood glucose.
- Hold subcutaneous insulin. Recheck blood glucose level if subcutaneous insulin has been recently administered and continue to check blood glucose level based on the duration of action of the subcutaneous insulin previously administered.

D50, 50% Dextrose; *IV,* intravenous; *POC,* point-of-care.

Data from Seaquist ER, Anderson J, Childs B, et al. Hypoglycemia and diabetes: a report of a workgroup of the American Diabetes Association and The Endocrine Society. *Diabetes Care.* 2013;36:1384–1395.
McCall AL, Lieb DC, Gianchandani R, et al. Management of individuals with diabetes at high risk for hypoglycemia: an Endocrine Society clinical practice guideline. *J Clin Endocrinol Metab.* 2023;108(3):529–562. https://doi.org/10.1210/clinem/dgac596
American Diabetes Association Professional Practice Committee. 2. Diagnosis and classification of diabetes: standards of care in diabetes—2024. *Diabetes Care.* 2024;47(Suppl 1):S20–S42. https://doi.org/10.2337/dc24-S002.

membranes of unconscious patients. Swabbing the mouth moistens the tissue and displaces the bacteria that collect when saliva, which has a bacteriostatic action, is curtailed by dehydration. Conscious patients must be provided the means to self-remove oral bacteria by toothbrushing and frequent oral rinsing.

Infection Prevention

Strict sterile technique is used to maintain all IV systems. All venipuncture sites are checked every 4 hours for signs of inflammation, phlebitis, or infiltration. Strict surgical asepsis is used for all invasive procedures. Sterile technique is used if urinary catheterization is necessary to obtain urine samples for testing. Urinary catheter care is provided every 8 hours.

Educate the Patient and Family

It is important to be aware of the knowledge level and adherence history of patients with previously diagnosed diabetes to formulate an appropriate teaching plan. Learning objectives include a discussion of target glucose levels, definition of hyperglycemia and its causes, harmful effects, symptoms, and how to manage insulin and diet when one is unwell and unable to eat. Additional objectives include a definition of DKA and its causes, symptoms, and harmful consequences. The patient and family are also expected to learn the principles of diabetes management. Universal precautions must be emphasized for all family caregivers. The patient and family must also learn the warning signs of DKA to report to a health care practitioner. Knowledge-based, independent self-management of blood glucose level and avoidance of diabetes-related complications are the ultimate goals of education of the patient, family, or other support persons using the teach-back method (Box 31.9).

Collaborative Management

In all aspects of patient care management, health care professionals work as a team with the major collaborative goal of providing the best possible outcome for each patient. Current guidelines related to collaborative management of patients with DKA are listed in Box 31.10.

Hyperglycemic Hyperosmolar State

HHS is a potentially lethal complication of type 2 diabetes. The hallmarks of HHS are extremely high levels of plasma glucose

BOX 31.8 Clinical Manifestations of Hypoglycemia and Hyperglycemia

Hypoglycemia	Hyperglycemia
Restlessness	Excessive thirst
Apprehension	Excessive urination
Irritability	Hunger
Trembling	Weakness
Weakness	Listlessness
Diaphoresis	Mental fatigue
Pallor	Flushed, dry skin
Paresthesia	Itching
Headache	Headache
Hunger	Nausea
Difficulty thinking	Vomiting
Loss of coordination	Abdominal cramps
Difficulty walking	Dehydration
Difficulty talking	Weak, rapid pulse
Visual disturbances	Postural hypotension
Blurred vision	Hypotension
Double vision	Acetone breath odor
Tachycardia	Kussmaul respirations
Shallow respirations	Rapid breathing
Hypertension	Changes in level of consciousness
Changes in level of consciousness	Stupor
Seizures	Coma
Coma	

BOX 31.9 PATIENT AND FAMILY EDUCATION PLAN

Diabetic Ketoacidosis

Acute Phase

- Explain rationale for critical care unit admission.
- Reduce anxiety associated with critical care unit.

Predischarge

Before discharge, the patient should be able to teach back the following topics:

- Target glucose levels
- Signs and symptoms of diabetic ketoacidosis
- Self-care monitoring of blood glucose level
- Self-care monitoring of blood ketones
- Insulin regimen
- Sick-day management
- Signs and symptoms to report to a health care practitioner

with resultant elevation in serum osmolality causing osmotic diuresis. Ketosis is absent or mild. Inability to replace fluids lost through diuresis leads to profound dehydration and changes in level of consciousness. Hospitalizations for HHS account for only 1% of diabetes-related hospital admissions.[49] The HHS mortality rate is between 5% and 16%.[49] Because patients with HHS have type 2 diabetes as an underlying disorder, they are generally older adults with cardiovascular and other comorbidities and must be rapidly assessed and treated as listed in the Summary of Key Concepts Related to HHS (Fig. 31.4).

The diagnostic criteria for HHS are as follows and as shown in Table 31.5.[50,52]

BOX 31.10 Evidence-Based Practice

Diabetic Ketoacidosis

A summary is provided of evidence and evidence-based recommendations for controlling symptoms related to diabetic ketoacidosis.

Strong Evidence to Support

Regular insulin by continuous infusion is recommended.
Replace serum potassium if level is lower than 3.3 mEq/L.
Replace serum phosphate if level is lower than 1.0 mg/dL.

Very Little Evidence to Support

No support for use of routine bicarbonate to correct low serum pH; use may be considered if pH is below 7.0.

Data from Kitabchi AE, Umpierrez GE, Miles JM, et al. Hyperglycemic crises in adult patients with diabetes: a consensus statement from the American Diabetes Association. *Diabetes Care.* 2009;32(7):1335–1343.
Umpierrez G, Korytkowski M. Diabetic emergencies—ketoacidosis, hyperglycaemic hyperosmolar state and hypoglycaemia. *Nat Rev Endocrinol.* 2016;12:222–232.
Dhatariya KK, Vellanki P. Treatment of diabetic ketoacidosis (DKA)/hyperglycemic hyperosmolar state (HHS): novel advances in the management of hyperglycemic crises (UK versus USA). *Curr Diab Rep.* 2017;17(5):33.

- Blood glucose >600 mg/dL (>30 mmol/L)
- No significant acidosis, pH >7.3
- Serum bicarbonate >18 mEq/L
- Serum osmolality >320 mOsm/kg
- Absent or mild ketonuria, ≤3.0 mmol/L

Most patients with this level of metabolic disruption experience visual changes, mental status changes, and potentially hypovolemic shock.

HHS occurs when the pancreas produces an insufficient amount of insulin for the high levels of glucose that flood the bloodstream. Older adults with type 2 diabetes and cardiovascular conditions are at highest risk. Infection is the usual trigger for development of HHS; the most common infections are pneumonia and urinary tract infections.[49] Other precipitating causes of HHS include stroke, myocardial infarction, trauma, major surgery, and the physiologic stress of critical illness.

Differences Between Hyperglycemic Hyperosmolar State and Diabetic Ketoacidosis

Clinically, HHS is distinguished from DKA by the presence of extremely elevated serum glucose, more profound dehydration, and minimal or absent ketosis (see Tables 31.5 and 31.6). Another major difference is that protein and fats are not used to create new supplies of glucose in HHS as they are in DKA; as a result, the ketotic cycle is never started or does not occur until the blood glucose level is extremely elevated.

Pathophysiology of HHS

HHS represents a deficit of insulin and an excess of glucagon. Reduced insulin levels prevent the movement of glucose into the cells, allowing glucose to accumulate in the plasma. The decreased insulin triggers glucagon release from the liver, and hepatic glucose is poured into the circulation. As the number of glucose particles increases in the blood, serum hyperosmolality increases. To decrease the serum osmolality, fluid is drawn from the intracellular compartment (inside the cells) into the vascular bed. Profound intracellular volume depletion occurs if the patient's thirst sensation is absent or decreased. HHS may evolve over days or weeks.[50]

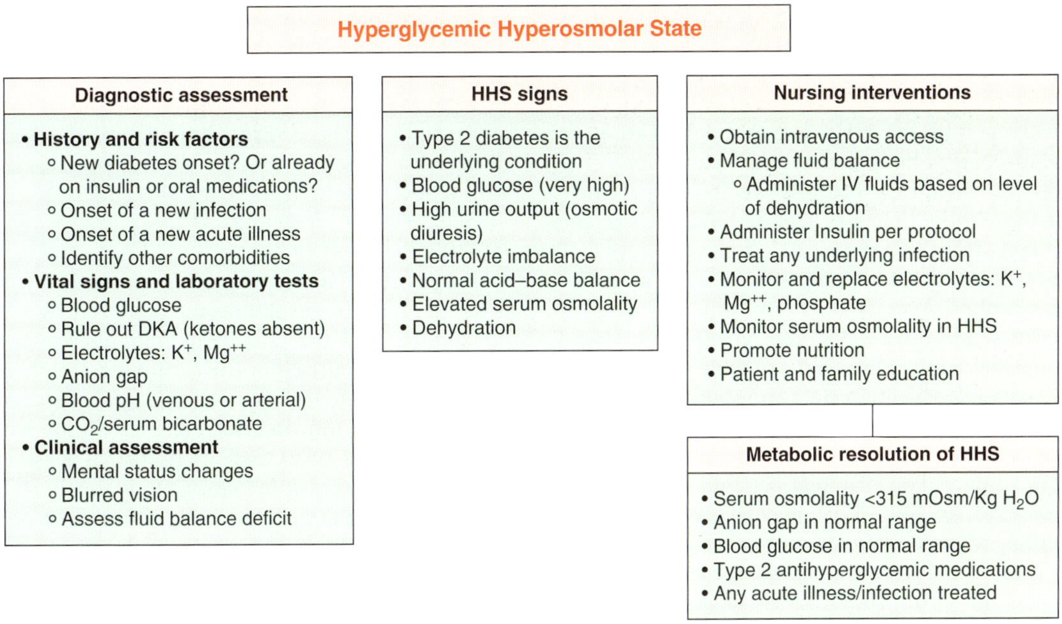

Hyperglycemic Hyperosmolar State

Diagnostic assessment

- **History and risk factors**
  - New diabetes onset? Or already on insulin or oral medications?
  - Onset of a new infection
  - Onset of a new acute illness
  - Identify other comorbidities
- **Vital signs and laboratory tests**
  - Blood glucose
  - Rule out DKA (ketones absent)
  - Electrolytes: K^+, Mg^{++}
  - Anion gap
  - Blood pH (venous or arterial)
  - CO_2/serum bicarbonate
- **Clinical assessment**
  - Mental status changes
  - Blurred vision
  - Assess fluid balance deficit

HHS signs

- Type 2 diabetes is the underlying condition
- Blood glucose (very high)
- High urine output (osmotic diuresis)
- Electrolyte imbalance
- Normal acid–base balance
- Elevated serum osmolality
- Dehydration

Nursing interventions

- Obtain intravenous access
- Manage fluid balance
  - Administer IV fluids based on level of dehydration
- Administer Insulin per protocol
- Treat any underlying infection
- Monitor and replace electrolytes: K^+, Mg^{++}, phosphate
- Monitor serum osmolality in HHS
- Promote nutrition
- Patient and family education

Metabolic resolution of HHS

- Serum osmolality <315 mOsm/Kg H_2O
- Anion gap in normal range
- Blood glucose in normal range
- Type 2 antihyperglycemic medications
- Any acute illness/infection treated

FIG. 31.4 Summary of Key Concepts Related to Hyperglycemic Hyperosmolar State (HHS). *CO_2*, carbon dioxide; *DKA*, diabetic ketoacidosis; *HHS*, hyperglycemic hyperosmolar state; *IV*, intravenous; *K^+*, potassium; *Mg^{++}*, magnesium; *mOsmol/Kg H_2O*, milliosmoles per kilogram water; *pH*, a measure of the degree to which a solution is acidic or alkaline.

Hemoconcentration persists despite removal of large amounts of glucose in the urine (glycosuria). The glomerular filtration and elimination of glucose by the kidney tubules is ineffective in reducing the serum glucose level sufficiently to maintain normal glucose levels. The hyperosmolality and reduced blood volume stimulate release of arginine vasopressin hormone to increase the tubular resorption of water. However, AVP is not powerful enough to overcome the osmotic pull exerted by the glucose load. Excessive fluid volume is lost at the kidney tubule, with simultaneous loss of potassium, sodium, and phosphate in the urine. This chain of events and osmotic diuresis results in progressively worsening hypovolemia.

Hypovolemia reduces perfusion to the kidney, and oliguria develops. Although this process conserves water and preserves the blood volume, it prevents further glucose loss, and hyperosmolality increases. Ketosis is absent or mild in HHS.[50,52]

The sympathetic nervous system reacts to the body's stress response to try to restore homeostasis. Epinephrine, a potent stimulus for gluconeogenesis, is released and additional glucose is added to the bloodstream. Unless the glycemic diuresis cycle is broken with aggressive fluid replacement and insulin administration, intracellular dehydration negatively affects fluid and oxygen transport to the brain cells. Neurologic dysfunction and coma may result. Hemoconcentration increases the blood viscosity, which may result in clot formation; thromboemboli; and cerebral, cardiac, and pleural infarcts.

Focused Physical Assessment in HHS

HHS has a slow, subtle onset and typically develops over several days. Initially, the symptoms may be nonspecific and may be ignored or attributed to the patient's concurrent disease processes. History reveals malaise, blurred vision, polyuria, polydipsia (depending on the patient's thirst sensation), weight loss, and increasing weakness. Progressive dehydration follows and leads to mental confusion, convulsions, and eventually coma, especially in older patients.

The physical examination may reveal a profound fluid deficit. Signs of severe dehydration include longitudinal wrinkles in the tongue, decreased salivation, and increases in heart rate and rapid respirations (Kussmaul air hunger does not occur). In older patients, assessment of clinical signs of dehydration is challenging. Neurologic status is affected as the serum glucose increases. Without intervention, changes in level of conscious occur leading to coma.

Laboratory Studies in HHS

Laboratory studies are used to establish a definitive diagnosis of HHS. Blood glucose levels are strikingly elevated (>600 mg/dL; >30 mmol/L). Serum osmolality is greater than 320 mOsm/kg. Acidosis is absent (arterial pH greater than 7.3), and the serum bicarbonate concentration is greater than 18 mEq/L. Ketonuria is absent or mild.[50,52] The patient may have an elevated hematocrit and depleted potassium and phosphorus levels.

Insulin replacement is prescribed according to the blood glucose result. Some electrolytes also can be tested at the bedside (potassium, sodium, ionized calcium), but usually an arterial line is required for frequent blood sample access. If point-of-care testing is unavailable, traditional serial laboratory tests keep the critical care team apprised of the fluctuating serum electrolyte levels and provide the basis for electrolyte replacement. Intracellular potassium and phosphate levels usually are depleted as a result of prior osmotic diuresis.[50,52]

Elevated BUN and creatinine levels may indicate kidney impairment from severe volume depletion. Metabolic acidosis usually is absent at lower glucose levels. Acidosis may also result from starvation ketosis or from an increase in lactic acid production caused by poor tissue perfusion.

Medical Management of HHS

The goals of medical management are rapid rehydration, insulin replacement, and correction of electrolyte abnormalities, specifically potassium replacement. The underlying stimulus of HHS must be discovered and treated. The same basic principles used to treat DKA are used for patients with HHS.

Rapid Rehydration

The primary intervention for HHS is rapid rehydration to restore the intravascular volume and reduce osmolality.[52] The fluid deficit may be 150 mL/kg of body weight. The average adult (70 kg) can lose more than 7 to 10 L of fluid. Physiologic saline solution (0.9%) is infused at about 1 L/hour, especially for a patient in hypovolemic shock as long as there is not a cardiovascular contraindication. Several liters of volume replacement may be required to achieve a BP and central venous pressure (CVP) within normal range. Infusion volumes are adjusted according to the patient's hydration state and sodium level.[50,52]

Serum sodium concentration is the parameter that is monitored to determine whether to change from isotonic (0.9%) to hypotonic (0.45%) saline. For example, patients with sodium levels equal to or less than 140 mEq/L may be given 0.9% normal saline solution, whereas patients with levels greater than 140 mEq/L are given 0.45% saline solution (see Fig. 31.2).[50] It is difficult to assess the serum sodium level in the presence of hemoconcentration.

Another recommendation is to calculate a *corrected sodium value*. This involves adding 1.6 mEq to the sodium laboratory value for each 100 mg/dL plasma glucose above normal.[50] Sodium input should not exceed the amount required to replace the losses. Careful monitoring of the serum sodium level is recommended to avoid a sodium–water imbalance and hemolysis as the hemoconcentration is reduced.

Insulin Administration

Volume resuscitation lowers the serum glucose level and improves symptoms even without insulin administration. However, insulin replacement is recommended in the treatment of HHS because acidosis can develop if insulin is withheld and because insulin facilitates the cellular use of glucose.

Methods to lower the blood glucose level vary in HHS. One method is to administer an IV bolus of regular insulin (0.15 unit/kg of body weight) initially, followed by a continuous insulin drip. Regular insulin, infusing at an initial rate calculated as 0.1 unit/kg hourly (e.g., 7 units/h for a person weighing 70 kg), should lower the plasma glucose concentration by 50 to 70 mg/dL during the first hour of treatment. If the measured glucose level does not decrease by this amount, the insulin infusion rate may be doubled until the blood glucose is declining at a rate of 50 to 70 mg/dL each hour[50] or as listed in the local hospital protocol.

Insulin Resistance

Type 2 diabetes in manifested not only by hyperglycemia but also by insulin resistance. HHS often develops secondary to an illness such as pneumonia or sepsis. In HHS, circulating counterregulatory hormones, also known as *stress hormones* (cortisol, glucagon, epinephrine), increase blood glucose. Some patients with HHS may require high doses of insulin initially to overcome the hyperglycemia and insulin resistance. Hourly serial monitoring of the blood glucose level permits safe glycemic management and avoids the most common complication, which is hypoglycemia caused by overzealous insulin administration.[50]

Depending on the HHS presentation, guidelines recommend administering adequate IV fluid initially to rehydrate both intracellular and extracellular spaces, as insulin may cause rapid volume and potassium shifts.[52] Thus, it is important to monitor fluid status and ensure that blood glucose does not fall too rapidly when infusing insulin.[52]

After the patient has recovered from the hyperglycemic crisis and insulin has been discontinued, oral medications designed to decrease insulin resistance are individualized to the patient with type 2 diabetes (see Tables 31.3 and 31.4).

Electrolyte Replacement

Increasing the circulating levels of insulin with therapeutic doses of IV insulin promotes the rapid return of potassium and phosphorus into the cell. Serial laboratory tests keep the critical care team apprised of the serum electrolyte levels and provide the basis for electrolyte replacement. Potassium typically is added to the IV infusion (see Fig. 31.2). If the serum potassium concentration is lower than 3.3 mEq/L, it is essential to replenish the serum potassium before giving insulin.[50] Most hospitals have potassium replacement algorithms that are used to treat hypokalemia. Serum phosphate levels are carefully monitored, and phosphate is replaced if the level is lower than 1.0 mg/dL.[50]

Nursing Management

Nursing management of a patient with HHS incorporates a variety of patient problems (Box 31.11). Nursing management goals are similar to the goals outlined for DKA. The critical care nurse administers prescribed fluids, insulin, and electrolytes; monitors the response to therapy; maintains surveillance for complications; and provides patient education.

Administering Fluids, Insulin, and Electrolytes

Rigorous fluid replacement and continuous IV insulin replacement must be controlled with an electronic volumetric pump. Accurate I&O measurements are maintained to monitor fluid balance including the total of all fluids administered minus hourly losses, such as urine output and emesis. If the patient is alert, the fluid and electrolytes are replenished orally and via a peripheral IV line.

If the patient manifests signs of hypovolemic shock, hemodynamic monitoring may include use of an arterial line, although this is not routine. Most critical care units have developed protocols or guidelines to ensure that patients in hyperglycemic crisis are managed safely (see Fig. 31.2). The major responsibility for delivery of insulin, hourly monitoring of blood glucose, and infusion of appropriate crystalloid solutions lies with the critical care nurse (Box 31.12). Many hospitals mandate a double-check procedure for medications such as insulin that have the potential to cause harm if incorrectly administered.

BOX 31.11 DIAGNOSIS AND PATIENT CARE MANAGEMENT

Hyperglycemic Hyperosmolar State

- Risk for Infection
- Hypovolemia due to absolute loss
- Anxiety due to threat to biological, psychological, or social integrity
- Powerlessness due to lack of control over current situation or disease progression
- Lack of Knowledge of Treatment Regime due to previous lack of exposure to information (see Box 31.13, Patient and Family Education Plan for Hyperglycemic Hyperosmolar State)

Patient Care Management plans are located in Appendix A.

BOX 31.12 Hyperglycemia Prevention and Management

Hyperglycemia Definition: Blood glucose above 180 mg/dL

- Two serial blood glucose values above 180 mg/dL are evidence of hyperglycemia in critical care.
- Blood glucose target in critical care is between 140 and 200 mg/dL.

Hyperglycemia Prevention

- In a patient with hyperglycemia without a preexisting history of diabetes, the likely causes are hyperglycemia associated with critical illness or undiagnosed prediabetes.
- **Type 1 diabetes**: A preexisting diagnosis of type 1 diabetes means the patient can never be without insulin coverage. IV or subcutaneous insulin must always be provided and blood glucose checked frequently.
- **Type 2 diabetes**: A preexisting diagnosis of type 2 diabetes means the patient will have an elevated blood glucose when oral medications are stopped. Some patients with type 2 diabetes also have subcutaneous insulin. Hyperglycemia is prevented by use of subcutaneous or IV insulin.
- Use normal saline in IV infusions.
- Monitor blood glucose per hospital protocol.

Hyperglycemia: Clinical Signs and Symptoms

- Hyperglycemia with a history of type 1 diabetes is generally caused by lack of insulin leading to DKA. Symptoms associated with alteration in level of consciousness range from confusion to coma, with dehydration and ketoacidosis.
- Hyperglycemia with a history of type 2 diabetes is often associated with infection leading to HHS, which may take days to weeks to develop. HHS is associated with alteration in level of consciousness and extreme dehydration. Acidosis can develop in HHS when blood glucose levels are extremely high.

Hyperglycemia Management

- Identify the reason for the hyperglycemia (critical illness stress induced, DKA, HHS). Management varies according to the cause. It is essential to also treat the underlying medical/surgical cause of admission to critical care.
- Administer IV insulin according to hospital protocol, with hourly monitoring of blood glucose during the acute phase of hyperglycemia.
- Rehydrate according to hospital protocol and laboratory values.
- Replenish electrolytes according to hospital protocol and laboratory values.

DKA, Diabetic ketoacidosis; *HHS*, hyperglycemic, hyperosmolar syndrome; *IV*, intravenous.

Data from Honarmand K, Sirimaturos M, Hirshberg EL, et al. Society of Critical Care Medicine guidelines on glycemic control for critically ill children and adults 2024. *Crit Care Med.* 2024;52(4):e161–e181. https://doi.org/10.1097/CCM.0000000000006174
Jacobi J, Bircher N, Krinsley J, et al. Guidelines for the use of an insulin infusion for the management of hyperglycemia in critically ill patients. *Crit Care Med.* 2012;40(12):3251–3276. https://doi.org/10.1097/CCM.0b013e3182653269
Kitabchi AE, Umpierrez GE, Miles JM, Fisher JN. Hyperglycemic crises in adult patients with diabetes. *Diabetes Care.* 2009;32(7):1335–1343. https://doi.org/10.2337/dc09-9032
American Diabetes Association Professional Practice Committee. 2. Diagnosis and classification of diabetes: standards of care in diabetes—2024. *Diabetes Care.* 2024;47(Suppl 1):S20–S42. https://doi.org/10.2337/dc24-S002

Monitoring Response to Therapy

BP and HR are monitored to evaluate the degree of dehydration, the effectiveness of hydration therapy, and the patient's fluid tolerance. Because patients with HHS have underlying type 2 diabetes and, if older, are also likely to have preexisting illnesses such as heart failure and kidney failure, it is important to monitor for symptoms of circulatory overload.[52] Symptoms to anticipate include tachycardia, bounding pulse, dyspnea, tachypnea, lung crackles, and engorged neck veins. The astute critical care nurse is aware of the clinical manifestations of fluid overload and observes for potential complications when rehydrating a patient with HHS and diseases involving the heart, lungs, or kidneys.

The serum glucose level should decrease by 50 to 70 mg/dL each hour with insulin administration.[50] This decrease is monitored by hourly blood glucose determinations. Based on the result, the critical care nurse can alter the infusion of insulin according to the local hospital protocol (see Fig. 31.2).

Surveillance for Complications

The potential complications of HHS are similar to the complications described for DKA and include hypoglycemia, hypokalemia or hyperkalemia, and infection. A patient with HHS is at risk for other complications specific to associated disease entities. A history of cardiovascular, pulmonary, or kidney disease, whether known or latent, places the patient with HHS at high risk for complications.[52]

Educate the Patient and Family

As the patient's condition improves and the patient demonstrates readiness to learn, education about type 2 diabetes and avoiding a recurrence of HHS becomes a priority (Box 31.13). Most teaching occurs after the patient has left the critical care unit. Teaching topics include a description of type 2 diabetes and how it relates to HHS, dietary restrictions, exercise requirements, medication protocols, home testing of blood glucose, signs and symptoms of hyperglycemia and hypoglycemia, foot care, and lifestyle modifications.

Collaborative Management

Because HHS is an acute condition superimposed on the chronic health problem of type 2 diabetes, many health professionals provide care and work collaboratively to restore homeostasis for each patient (Box 31.14).[44]

PITUITARY GLAND DISORDERS

Two neuroendocrine disorders of the pituitary gland are discussed in this chapter: diabetes insipidus (DI) and *syndrome of inappropriate antidiuresis* (SIAD) secretion. Both are caused by disruptions in the release of a hormone that helps regulate water balance in the body. This hormone is abbreviated as AVP (*arginine vasopressin*) and is also known as *antidiuretic hormone* (ADH).

DI and SIAD are clinical opposites.

- DI: inadequate or no AVP released from the posterior pituitary—leads to hemoconcentration and dilute urine
- SIAD: excess AVP is released from the posterior pituitary—leads to hemodilution and concentrated urine

These can be long-term chronic conditions, where a patient is admitted to hospital with an unrelated condition, or these may be seen in critical care as acute complications of other disorders.[58] The focus in this chapter is on the acute presentation and management in critical care.

Diabetes Insipidus

DI is recognized clinically by the vast quantities of very dilute urine that is produced in susceptible patients. In a critically ill patient, the extreme diuresis is most likely to be caused by a lack of AVP.[58] Any patient who has sustained a head trauma or had resection of a pituitary tumor has an increased risk of developing DI if AVP is not released from the pituitary gland. It is essential to assess, recognize, and manage this complication quickly as shown in the Summary of Key Concepts Related to DI (Fig. 31.5). Normally, AVP is produced in the hypothalamus and stored in the posterior pituitary gland (see Chapter 29). Physiologically, AVP is released primarily in response to even small elevations in serum osmolality and secondarily in reaction to hypovolemia or hypotension. DI can manifest for several reasons secondary to pathology of the hypothalamus or the pituitary.[58–60]

- The hypothalamus produces insufficient AVP.
- The posterior pituitary fails to release AVP.
- The kidney nephron is resistant (unresponsive) to AVP.

Etiology

DI is divided into two types according to the cause[58,59] (Box 31.15).

- Central DI—AVP Deficiency
- Nephrogenic DI—AVP Resistance

Only central DI is encountered with any frequency in the critical care unit.

BOX 31.13 PATIENT AND FAMILY EDUCATION PLAN

Hyperglycemic Hyperosmolar State

Acute Phase

- Explain rationale for critical care unit admission.

Predischarge

Before discharge, the patient should be able to teach back the following topics:

- Causes of hyperglycemic hyperosmotic state
- Self-care for diabetes
- Signs and symptoms to report to health care practitioner

Central Diabetes Insipidus—AVP Deficiency

In central DI, there is an absolute or relative deficiency of AVP. The inability to synthesize or secrete an adequate amount of AVP results in insufficient water being reabsorbed back to the bloodstream by the kidney tubule, and this causes both dilute urine, and a rise in sodium levels in the bloodstream.[58,60] DI may be summereized as:

- Serum hypernatremia and a high serum osmolality[58,60]
- Dilute urine, with a low urine osmolality[58,60]

BOX 31.14 Evidence-Based Practice

Hyperglycemic Hyperosmolar State

A summary is provided of evidence and evidence-based recommendations for controlling symptoms related to hyperglycemic hyperosmolar state.

Strong Evidence to Support

Regular insulin by continuous infusion is recommended to normalize blood glucose.

Replace serum potassium if the level is less than 3.3 mEq/L.

Replace serum phosphate if the level is less than 1 mg/dL.

A multidisciplinary team approach reduces length of stay and improves clinical outcomes.

Close follow-up after discharge is recommended to maintain glycated hemoglobin (A_{1c}) at less than within a normal range to prevent diabetes-related complications.

Weak Evidence to Support

Use of a sliding insulin scale alone is not best practice because it is associated with both hyperglycemia and hypoglycemia in hospitalized patients.

Data from Kitabchi AE, Umpierrez GE, Miles JM, et al. Hyperglycemic crises in adult patients with diabetes: a consensus statement from the American Diabetes Association. *Diabetes Care.* 2009;32(7):1335–1343.
Umpierrez G, Korytkowski M. Diabetic emergencies—ketoacidosis, hyperglycaemic hyperosmolar state and hypoglycaemia. *Nat Rev Endocrinol.* 2016;12:222–232.
Dhatariya KK, Vellanki P. Treatment of diabetic ketoacidosis (DKA)/hyperglycemic hyperosmolar state (HHS): novel advances in the management of hyperglycemic crises (UK versus USA). *Curr Diab Rep.* 2017;17(5):33.

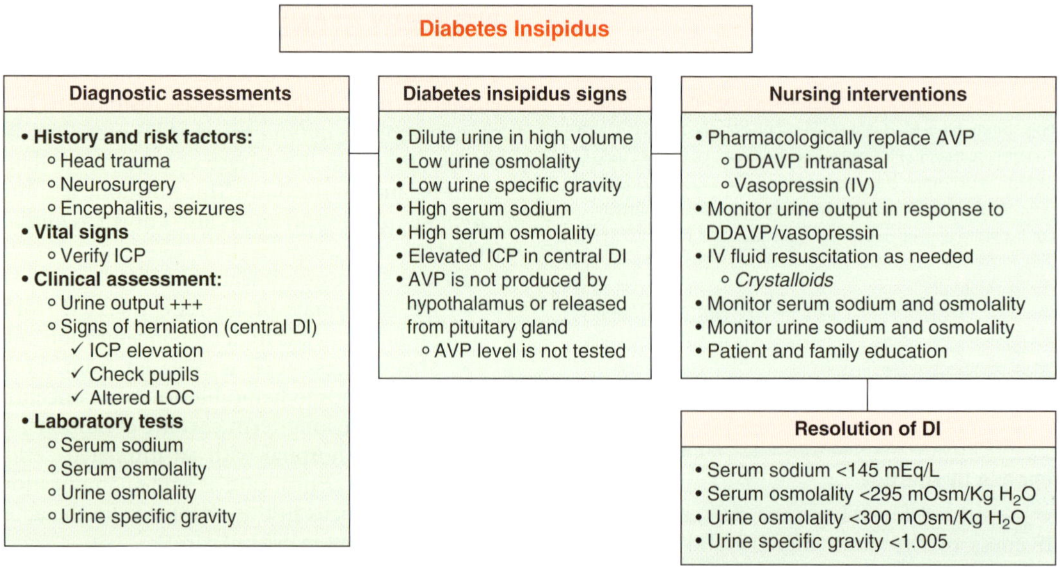

Diabetes Insipidus

Diagnostic assessments

- **History and risk factors:**
  - Head trauma
  - Neurosurgery
  - Encephalitis, seizures
- **Vital signs**
  - Verify ICP
- **Clinical assessment:**
  - Urine output +++
  - Signs of herniation (central DI)
    - ✓ ICP elevation
    - ✓ Check pupils
    - ✓ Altered LOC
- **Laboratory tests**
  - Serum sodium
  - Serum osmolality
  - Urine osmolality
  - Urine specific gravity

Diabetes insipidus signs

- Dilute urine in high volume
- Low urine osmolality
- Low urine specific gravity
- High serum sodium
- High serum osmolality
- Elevated ICP in central DI
- AVP is not produced by hypothalamus or released from pituitary gland
  - AVP level is not tested

Nursing interventions

- Pharmacologically replace AVP
  - DDAVP intranasal
  - Vasopressin (IV)
- Monitor urine output in response to DDAVP/vasopressin
- IV fluid resuscitation as needed
  - *Crystalloids*
- Monitor serum sodium and osmolality
- Monitor urine sodium and osmolality
- Patient and family education

Resolution of DI

- Serum sodium <145 mEq/L
- Serum osmolality <295 mOsm/Kg H_2O
- Urine osmolality <300 mOsm/Kg H_2O
- Urine specific gravity <1.005

FIG. 31.5 Summary of Key Concepts Related to Diabetes Insipidus. *AVP*, Arginine vasopressin; *DDAVP*, desmopressin acetate (synthetic analog of vasopressin); *DI*, diabetes insipidus; *ICP*, intracranial pressure; *IV*, intravenous; *LOC*, level of consciousness; *mOsmol/Kg H_2O*, milliosmoles per kilogram water; < less than; ✓, evaluate/assess.

BOX 31.15 Causes of Diabetes Insipidus

Central Diabetes Insipidus

Primary Diabetes Insipidus (Rare in Critical Care)

- Arginine vasopressin (AVP) deficiency caused by hypothalamic-hypophyseal malformation
- Congenital defect
- Idiopathic

Secondary Diabetes Insipidus (Most Common in Critical Care)

- AVP deficiency caused by damage to hypothalamic–hypophyseal system
- Trauma
- Infection
- Surgery
- Primary neoplasms
- Metastatic malignancies

Nephrogenic Diabetes Insipidus

- Inability of kidney tubules to respond to circulating AVP
- Decrease or absence of AVP receptors
- Cellular damage to nephron, especially loop of Henle
- Kidney damage (e.g., hydronephrosis, pyelonephritis, polycystic kidney)
- Untoward response to medication therapy (e.g., lithium carbonate, demeclocycline)

Dipsogenic Diabetes Insipidus

- Rare form of water intoxication
- Compulsive water drinking

In critical care, the most likely acute cause of central DI is neurosurgery, traumatic head injury, tumors, increased intracranial pressure (ICP), brain death, and infections such as encephalitis or meningitis.

DI is seen with brain death 50% of the time[60] and with traumatic brain injury in 20% to 30% of cases.[60] In patients undergoing surgery on the pituitary gland, transient DI occurs in approximately in 20% to 30% of cases. Permanent DI occurs in 2% to 10% of cases.[61] The degree of hormone replacement required after surgery depends on the quantity of pituitary tissue that has been surgically or endoscopically removed.

Nephrogenic Diabetes Insipidus—AVP Resistance

Nephrogenic DI is most often acquired by exposure to medications or other conditions. It occurs when the vasopressin V_2 receptors on the kidney tubule become nonresponsive to the action of AVP.[59,60]

Pathophysiology of AVP Deficiency and Resistance

The purpose of AVP is to maintain normal serum osmolality, water balance, and circulating blood volume. Normally, AVP binds to the V_2 receptors on the kidney collecting tubules, facilitating insertion of water channels, known as *aquaporins*, along the luminal surface. Even small increases in plasma osmolality are sufficient to stimulate AVP release. Although there are several types of DI, this discussion focuses on central DI, the condition encountered in the critical care unit after neurosurgery or head injury.

In DI, as free water is eliminated, the urine osmolality and specific gravity decrease causing dilute urine. At the same time, in the bloodstream, the serum sodium concentration and serum osmolality increase. Normally, an increase in the serum osmolality to greater than 290 mOsm/kg H_2O (290 mmol/L) triggers synthesis and release of AVP. If the thirst mechanism is intact, thirst sensors are activated in the hypothalamus, causing an acute sensation of thirst that leads the person to drink lots of fluids.[58] In central DI, when insufficient or no AVP is released, the kidney collecting tubules are incapable of concentrating urine and retaining water.

As extracellular dehydration ensues, hypotension and hypovolemic shock can occur. If the patient is alert, extreme thirst will lead the patient to replace lost fluids by drinking lots of water. This excessive intake of water reduces the serum osmolality to a more normal level and prevents dehydration. In a patient with decreased level of consciousness, the polyuria if untreated leads to severe hypernatremia, dehydration, decreased cerebral perfusion, seizures, loss of consciousness, and death.

Focused Physical Assessment in AVP Deficiency

The clinical diagnosis is based on the clinical increase in dilute urine output occurring in the absence of diuretics, a fluid challenge, or hyperglycemia. Central DI is anticipated in conditions in which the underlying disease process is likely to disrupt pituitary function.[60] Central DI that occurs because of increasing ICP is life threatening, and it is imperative that the underlying condition causing ICP elevation be recognized and treated.

Laboratory Studies

The diagnostic tests used to establish the presence of DI and evaluate the body's ability to balance fluid and electrolytes are not specific to the endocrine system. The specific tests are serum sodium, serum osmolality, and urine osmolality (Table 31.7). The combination of an obvious clinical picture of high volumes of hypotonic urine (>3 L of urine output/24 hours) in the presence of these laboratory criteria is sufficient to diagnose central DI.[60]

- Serum sodium level greater than 145 mEq/L
- Serum osmolality greater than 295 mOsm/kg H_2O (greater than 295 mmol/L)
- Urine osmolality less than 300 mOsm/kg H_2O (less than 300 mmol/L)
- Urine specific gravity less than 1.005

Serum Sodium

The serum sodium normal value is 140 mEq/L (range is 135 to 145 mEq/L).

In central DI, the serum sodium level can rise precipitously because of the loss of free water. This hypernatremia is usually associated with serum hyperosmolality.

Serum Osmolality

Serum osmolality has a normal range of 275 to 295 mOsm/kg H_2O.

Severe DI can increase serum osmolality to greater than 320 mOsm/kg H_2O.

Urine Osmolality

Urine osmolality is less than 300 mOsm/kg H_2O (300 mmol/L) in patients with central DI.[61]

For greatest accuracy, the urine sample should be collected and tested simultaneously with the blood sample. This test is rarely performed in the critical care unit and is not accurate once diuretics have been administered.

Antidiuretic Hormone Measurement

Measurement of the baseline serum AVP level is an additional but challenging diagnostic step that is not typically performed in critical care because the clinical circumstances

TABLE 31.7 Laboratory Values for Patients With Diabetes Insipidus and Syndrome of Inappropriate Antidiuretic Hormone

Value	Normal	DI	SIAD
Serum AVP	1–5 pg/mL	Decreased in central DI	Elevated
Serum osmolality (mOsm/L)	275–295	>295	<270
Serum sodium (mEq/L)	135–145	>145	<120
Urine osmolality (mOsm/L)	300–1400	<300	Increased
Urine specific gravity	1.005–1.030	<1.005	>1.030
Urine output	1.0–1.5 L/day	1.0–1.5 L/hour	Below normal

AVP, Arginine vasopressin; *DI,* diabetes insipidus; *pg/mL,* picogram per milliliter; *SIAD,* syndrome of inappropriate antidiuresis.

(e.g., head injury with increased ICP) make further testing unnecessary. Normal AVP levels range from 1 to 5 pg/mL (picograms/mL). With normal hydration, the normal morning fasting serum level is less than 4 pg/mL. When serum AVP levels are severely depressed (less than 0.5 pg/mL), the osmolality in the urine falls (dilute urine) to less than 100 mOsm/kg H_2O and urine output dramatically increases to 800 to 1000 mL/hour.[62]

Copeptin

Copeptin is coreleased with AVP from the posterior pituitary gland and is stable in plasma, facilitating reliable measurements.[58] After pituitary surgery, copeptin levels below 2.6 pmol/L have a specificity of 100% for a diagnosis of DI.[58]

Medical Management

Immediate management of DI requires an aggressive approach. Treatment goals include restoration of circulating fluid volume, pharmacologic AVP replacement, and treatment of the underlying condition.[58,60]

Volume Restoration

Fluid replacement is provided in the initial phase of treatment to prevent circulatory collapse. Patients who are able to drink oral fluids are given voluminous amounts of fluid orally to balance output. For patients who are unable to take sufficient fluids orally, hypotonic IV solutions are infused and carefully monitored to restore the hemodynamic balance.

Medications

Central DI requires immediate pharmacologic management. Table 31.8 presents the medications most frequently prescribed to treat central DI and replace AVP.

Medications Used for Central Diabetes Insipidus

Patients with central DI who are unable to synthesize AVP require replacement with vasopressin or an AVP analog. The most prescribed medication is the synthetic analog *desmopressin* (DDAVP).[58,63] DDAVP can be given intravenously, subcutaneously, orally, or as a nasal spray with dosage titrated according to the patient's antidiuretic response. Close monitoring of urine output is advised.

To avoid a medication error, it is important to be aware that DDAVP is also used to manage other conditions, including hemorrhage caused by platelet disorders, and that the dose ranges for these conditions are different. Other medications to treat central DI are available (see Table 31.8) but are rarely used in critical care. DDAVP is used only for central DI. It has no therapeutic value in nephrogenic DI.

Medications Used for Nephrogenic Diabetes Insipidus

Nephrogenic DI is not typically encountered in critical care unless the patient is admitted with this condition in addition to an unrelated primary diagnosis. The mainstay of therapy for nephrogenic DI is to stop any medications that are inducing the AVP resistance. Nephrogenic DI is treated with thiazide diuretics.[58]

Nursing Management

Nursing management of a patient with DI incorporates a variety of patient problems (Box 31.16). Nursing management is directed toward administration of prescribed fluids and medications, evaluation of response to therapy, surveillance for complications, and provision of patient and family education.

Administration of Fluids

Rapid IV fluid replacement requires the use of a volumetric pump. Initially, a hypotonic IV solution is used to replace fluids lost and reduce the serum hyperosmolality. With any signs of cardiovascular impairment, fluid intake is restricted until urine specific gravity is less than 1.015 and a normal urine output is resumed.

Critical assessment and management of fluid status are the most important initial concerns for patients with DI. Monitoring of heart rate, blood pressure, and central filling pressures provide indications of response to fluid volume replacement. Condition of buccal membranes, skin turgor, daily weight and intake and output measurements, presence of thirst, and temperature provide a basic assessment list that is vital for the patient who is unable to regulate fluid needs and losses. Placement of a urinary catheter may be indicated to monitor the urinary output accurately. Simultaneous urine and blood specimens for determination of osmolality, serum sodium, and serum potassium are obtained, and the results are discussed with the critical care team as necessary.

Administration of Medications

DDAVP by nasal administration is the usual AVP replacement in critical care. The urine output is recorded hourly to evaluate the response to the medication.

Surveillance for Complications

The most dangerous potential complication of AVP replacement is hypertension and vasospasm of cardiac, cerebral, or mesenteric arterial vessels in response to AVP replacement. In most cases, DDAVP is selected for AVP replacement to minimize this risk. A less serious complication of DI is constipation caused by fluid loss; it is treated with dietary fiber, stool softeners, or both.

Patient and Family Education

Educating the patient and the family about the disease process and how it affects thirst, urination, and fluid balance encourages

TABLE 31.8 PHARMACOLOGIC MANAGEMENT

Diabetes Insipidus

Medication	Dosage	Actions	Special Considerations
Central Diabetes Insipidus			
DDAVP (available as IV injection, as nasal spray, rhinal tube)	Nasal: 10–40 mcg single dose or in divided doses Parenteral[a]: 2–4 mcg twice daily	Central DI Antidiuretic Increases water resorption in nephron Prevents and controls polydipsia, polyuria	Few side effects Observe for nasal congestion, upper respiratory infection, allergic rhinitis Monitor intake and output, urine osmolality, serum sodium level
Vasopressin (Pitressin)	IV, IM, subcutaneous Topical: nasal mucosa	Central DI antidiuretic Promotes resorption of water at kidney tubule Decreases urine output Increases urine osmolality Diagnostic aid Increases gastrointestinal peristalsis	Monitor fluid volume often, especially in older patients Assess cardiac status May precipitate angina, hypertension, or myocardial infarction if increased dosage is given to patient with cardiac history Parenteral extravasation can cause skin necrosis
Lypressin (Diapid)	Intranasal: 1–2 sprays (7–14 mcg) in each nostril 4 times daily	Central DI Synthetic AVP Increases resorption of sodium and water in nephron	Proper instillation is important for absorption and action Patient sits upright while holding bottle upright for administration Repeat sprays (>2–3) are ineffective and wasteful; if dosage is increased to 2–3 sprays, shorten time between dosing Cough, chest tightness, shortness of breath
Nephrogenic Diabetes Insipidus			
Thiazide diuretics	Varies according to diuretic chosen, patient's size, and age	Nephrogenic DI Leads to mild fluid depletion Increases resorption of water and sodium in proximal nephron; less fluid travels to distal nephron, excreting less water	Varies according to diuretic chosen
Dipsogenic Diabetes Insipidus			
Anticompulsive disorder medications, anxiolytics, psychopharmacologic agents	Dosage varies	Dipsogenic DI	Varies according to medication chosen

[a]IV or subcutaneous administration.
AVP, Arginine vasopressin; *DDAVP*, desmopressin acetate; *DI*, diabetes insipidus; *IM*, intramuscular; *IV*, intravenous.

BOX 31.16 DIAGNOSIS AND PATIENT CARE MANAGEMENT

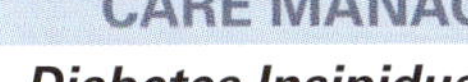

Diabetes Insipidus

- Impaired Cardiac Output due to alterations in preload
- Hypovolemia due to absolute loss
- Lack of Knowledge of Treatment Regime due to lack of previous exposure to information (see Box 31.17, Patient and Family Education Plan for Diabetes Insipidus)

Patient Care Management plans are located in Appendix A.

patients to participate in their care and reduces the feelings of hopelessness (Box 31.17). For most critical care patients, central DI is a temporary condition that resolves as the underlying medical condition (e.g., brain injury) improves. Patients who are discharged with DI are taught, along with their families, the signs and symptoms of dehydration and overhydration and procedures for accurate daily weight and urine specific gravity measurements. Printed information pertaining to medication actions, side effects, dosages, and timetable is provided along with an outline of factors that must be reported to the physician.

BOX 31.17 PATIENT AND FAMILY EDUCATION PLAN

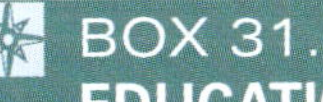

Diabetes Insipidus

Acute Phase

- Explain rationale for critical care unit admission.

Predischarge

Before discharge, the patient should be able to teach back the following topics:

- Patient-specific cause of diabetes insipidus
- Measurement of fluid intake and output
- Urine specific gravity
- Causes of diabetes insipidus
- Disease process of diabetes insipidus
- Nutritional information to prevent constipation and diarrhea
- Medications: Explain purpose, side effects, dosage, and how often to use
- Signs and symptoms to report to health care professional

Collaborative Management

Central DI is a life-threatening condition. The collaborative assessment and clinical skills of all health care professionals and use of a clear plan of care are essential to achieve optimal outcomes for each patient.

Syndrome of Inappropriate Antidiuresis

The opposing syndrome to DI is SIAD, which manifests as a dilutional hyponatremia and highly concentrated urine.[62,64] A patient with SIAD has an excess of AVP hormone secreted into the bloodstream; the excess is more than the amount needed to maintain normal blood volume and serum osmolality. It is essential to assess, recognize, and manage this complication quickly as listed in the Summery of Key Concepts Related to SIAD (Fig. 31.6). In SIAD, excessive water is resorbed back into the bloodstream at the kidney tubule, leading to:

- Dilutional serum hyponatremia and a low serum osmolality[62,64]
- Highly concentrated urine, and a high urine osmolality[62,64]

Etiology

Numerous causes of SIAD have been observed in patients who are critically ill (Box 31.18). Central nervous system injury, tumors, and diseases that interfere with the normal functioning of the hypothalamic-pituitary system can cause SIAD. This is often associated with malignancies that involve the lung, brain, head and neck, gastrointestinal system, gynecologic system, and hematologic system.[64]

Pathophysiology

AVP is a powerful, complex polypeptide compound. When released into the circulation by the posterior pituitary gland, AVP regulates water and electrolyte balance in the body. In SIAD, profound fluid and electrolyte disturbances result from the unsolicited, continuous release of the hormone into the bloodstream. Excessive AVP stimulates the kidney tubules to retain fluid regardless of need. This results in severe overhydration.

Excessive AVP dramatically alters the sodium balance in the extracellular vascular compartment. The overhydration causes a *dilutional hyponatremia* and reduces the sodium concentration to critically low levels. In a healthy adult, hyponatremia inhibits the release of AVP. However, in SIAD, increased levels of circulating AVP are unrelated to the serum sodium concentration. Aldosterone production from the adrenal glands is also suppressed. Serum hypo-osmolality leads to a shift of fluid from the extracellular fluid space into the intracellular fluid compartment (inside the cells) in an attempt to equalize osmotic pressure.

Because minimal sodium is present in this fluid, edema usually does not occur. Without AVP and aldosterone, water is retained (dilutional hyponatremia), and urine output is diminished. The urine has an increased osmolality from the decreased water excretion. Urinary concentration is also elevated by excess sodium in the urine. It is believed that, despite the serum hyponatremia, high levels of AVP promote sodium loss through the kidneys into the urine.

Focused Physical Assessment of SIAD

The clinical manifestations of SIAD secretion relate to the excess fluids in the extracellular compartment and the proportionate dilution of the circulating sodium. Edema usually is not present, although slight weight gain may occur from the expanded extracellular fluid volume. Early clinical manifestations of dilutional hyponatremia include lethargy, anorexia, nausea, and vomiting. If the hyponatremia is chronic, symptoms may not be as noticeable.[65] In contrast, with acute hyponatremia severe neurologic symptoms occur when serum sodium concentration decreases below 125 mEq/L. Symptoms of severe hyponatremia include inability to concentrate, mental confusion, apprehension, seizures, decreased level of consciousness, coma, and death.[65]

Laboratory Values

Patients with SIAD present with very dilute serum, hyponatremia, and concentrated urine. Laboratory values confirm this

Syndrome of Inappropriate Antidiuresis (SIAD)

Diagnostic assessments

- **History and risk factors**
  - Malignancies
  - Head injury
  - Medications
- **Vital signs**
  - BP, HR, RR,
- **Clinical assessment**
  - Mental status changes
  - Seizures
  - Coma
- **Laboratory tests**
  - Serum sodium
  - Serum osmolality
  - Urine osmolality

SIAD signs

- Dilutional hyponatremia
  - Low serum sodium
  - Low serum osmolality
- Low urine output
  - High urine sodium
  - High urine osmolality
- Excess AVP produced
  - AVP level is not tested

Nursing interventions

- Correct fluid and sodium balance
- Restrict fluid intake
- Pharmacologic aquadiuresis
  - Vaptans (IV or PO)
  - Do restrict fluid if on vaptans
- Replace sodium slowly, do not raise more than 10 mEq/L in 24 hours
  - 3% hypertonic sodium (IV) slowly
  - 0.9% crystalloid (IV)
- Monitor serum sodium & osmolality
- Monitor urine sodium & osmolality
- Patient and family education

Resolution of SIAD

- Serum sodium within normal limits
- Resolution of underlying condition that triggered excess ADH production

FIG. 31.6 Summary of Key Concepts Related to Inappropriate Antidiuresis. *AVP*, Arginine vasopressin; *BP*, blood pressure; *HR*, heart rate; *LOC*, level of consciousness; *mEq/L*, milliequivalents per liter; *RR*, respiratory rate; *SIAD*, syndrome of inappropriate antidiuresis.

BOX 31.18 Causes of Syndrome of Inappropriate Antidiuresis (SIAD)

Malignancy Associated With SIAD
- Bronchogenic small cell carcinoma
- Pancreatic adenocarcinoma
- Duodenal, bladder, ureter, and prostatic carcinomas
- Lymphosarcoma, Ewing sarcoma
- Acute leukemia, Hodgkin disease
- Cerebral neoplasm, thymoma

Neurological Diseases Associated With Increased Production/Release of Arginine Vasopressin (AVP)
- Head injury
- Brain abscess
- Hydrocephalus
- Pituitary adenoma
- Subdural hematoma
- Subarachnoid hemorrhage
- Cerebral atrophy
- Guillain-Barré syndrome

Neurogenic Stimuli Capable of Increasing Arginine Vasopressin (AVP)
- Decreased glomerular filtration rate
- Physical or emotional stress
- Pain
- Fear
- Trauma
- Surgery
- Myocardial infarction
- Acute infection
- Hypotension
- Hemorrhage
- Hypovolemia

Pulmonary Diseases Associated With Increased Arginine Vasopressin (AVP)
- Pulmonary tuberculosis
- Viral and bacterial pneumonia
- Empyema
- Lung abscess
- Chronic obstructive lung disease
- Status asthmaticus
- Cystic fibrosis

Endocrine Disturbances Associated With Increased Arginine Vasopressin (AVP)
- Myxedema
- Hypothyroidism
- Hypopituitarism
- Adrenal insufficiency—Addison disease

Medications That Mimic, Increase, Release or Potentiate Increased Arginine Vasopressin (AVP)
- Hypoglycemics
- Insulin
- Tolbutamide
- Chlorpropamide
- Potassium-depleting thiazide diuretics
- Tricyclic antidepressants
- Imipramine
- Amitriptyline
- Phenothiazine
- Fluphenazine
- Thioridazine
- Thioxanthenes
- Thiothixene
- Chlorprothixene
- Chemotherapeutic agents
- Vincristine
- Cyclophosphamide
- Opiates
- Carbamazepine
- Clofibrate
- Acetaminophen
- Nicotine
- Oxytocin
- Vasopressin
- Anesthetics

clinical picture. In SIAD, there is decreased serum osmolality with increased urine osmolality.[65]

- Serum osmolality is low in SIAD (<275 mOsm/kg H_2O)[65]
- Urine osmolality is high in SIAD (>100 mOsm/kg H_2O)[65]

In SIAD the serum sodium is low from dilution, which can cause increasingly severe neurologic symptoms. The urine sodium is elevated congruent with the concentrated urine output of SIAD.[65]

- Serum sodium is low in SIAD (<125 mEq/L)[65]
- Urine sodium is high in SIAD (>30 mEq/L)[65]

Use of diuretics negates the reliability of the urine sodium and urine osmolality levels.[65]

See Table 31.7 for the typical laboratory values associated with SIAD and with DI. Measurement of serum AVP levels is not recommended to diagnosis SIAD in critical care.[65]

Copeptin

Measurement of copeptin as a biomarker for AVP is a focus of research in patients with SIAD.[65,66] Multiple SIAD subsets have been identified with different plasma patterns and concentrations of AVP and copeptin. This may lead to more precise diagnosis and better outcomes in the future.[66]

Medical Management

In the critical care unit, SIAD often occurs as a secondary disease. Ideally, recognition and treatment of the primary disease will reduce the production of AVP. If the patient is receiving any of the medications suspected to cause SIAD, stopping that medication may return AVP levels to normal. Some medications that alter AVP levels are listed in Box 31.18.

The goals of medical management are to restore fluid and sodium balance. Yet research from the *International Hyponatremia Registry*[67] suggests that correction of serum sodium can be difficult to achieve and is not always successful.[67] Also, there are potentially many different causes of SIAD, and SIAD must be differentiated from other causes of hyponatremia.[65] The heterogeneity of SIAD and hyponatremia can make the choice of optimal treatments challenging, although research demonstrates that patients have worse outcomes without treatment.[64] In the next sections the current recommended treatments are presented.

Fluid Restriction

Fluid restriction is a cornerstone of the treatment plan for SIAD.[62] Fluids are generally restricted to 500 to 1000 mL/day.[62]

Sodium Replacement

Patients with severe hyponatremia of less than 120 mEq/L (mmol/L) serum sodium experience severe neurologic symptoms, including seizures. Too-rapid serum sodium correction must be avoided to reduce the risk of *osmotic demyelination syndrome*, which occurs in the white matter of the brain. This is also known as *central pontine myelinolysis* (CPM), although demyelination effects are not limited to the pons or the brainstem. Severe neurologic damage or death can result. The demyelination complication can be avoided by increasing the serum sodium slowly. Guidelines recommend no more than 10 to 12 mEq/L increase in 24 hours and no more than 18 mEq/L rise in 48 hours.[62,68] Caution is advised is the serum sodium is very low (<120 mEq/L). A minimum sodium replacement of 4 to 6 mEq/L per 24 hours is recommended.[68] Serum sodium levels must be evaluated at least every 4 hours during the acute phase of sodium replacement.

In SIAD, a slow infusion of 3% saline (hypertonic saline) may be used to replenish the serum sodium without adding extra volume.[65,68] Hypertonic saline solution (3% or greater) can be dangerous if administered too quickly, as described earlier. Calculation of the quantity of sodium that will be administered each hour and over 24 hours is advised.[64]

Pharmacologic Management

Medications are prescribed when water restriction is ineffective in correcting the SIAD. One pharmacologic option is to increase the action of AVP on the V_2 kidney tubule receptors so that more water is excreted.[62] One class of medications (described next) are the vaptans.

Vasopressin Receptor Antagonists—Vaptans

Vasopressin receptor antagonists are used to treat hyponatremia such as SIAD.[69] Medications in this class are also called *vaptans*. Conivaptan (Vaprisol) is approved for use only in hospitalized patients. These medications excrete water while conserving sodium, known as *aquadiuresis*. There is an initial 20-mg IV loading dose over 30 minutes, followed by a 20-mg/day continuous infusion for up to 4 days.[70] If the sodium correction is inadequate, the infusion dose can be increased to 40 mg/day.[70] Conivaptan is a nonselective vasopressin receptor antagonist, which means that it blocks V_1 receptors in the vasculature and V_2 receptors in the kidney. The patient must be observed carefully to avoid hypotension (caused by V_1 receptor blockade). Hypovolemia is a contraindication. Tolvaptan (Samsca) is an oral medication in the same class. This medication may be initiated in the hospital, where serum sodium levels can be monitored to avoid a too-rapid increase in serum sodium after aquadiuresis.[70]

European guidelines for treatment of hyponatremia do not include vaptans for management of SIAD.[65,69,71] This highlights different ways in which SIAD is managed in different countries and the necessity of patient assessment and clinical judgment when using these medications.

Nursing Management

Nursing management of a patient with SIAD addresses a variety of patient problems (Box 31.19). Nursing management is directed toward restriction of fluids, surveillance for complications, and provision of patient education.

BOX 31.19 DIAGNOSIS AND PATIENT CARE MANAGEMENT

Syndrome of Inappropriate Antidiuresis (SIAD)

- Hypervolemia due to increased secretion of antidiuretic hormone
- Anxiety due to threat to biological, psychological, or social integrity
- Lack of Knowledge of Treatment Regime due to lack of previous exposure to information (see Box 31.20, Patient and Family Education Plan for Diabetes Insipidus)

Patient Care Management plans are located in Appendix A.

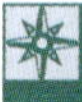

BOX 31.20 PATIENT AND FAMILY EDUCATION PLAN

Syndrome of Inappropriate Antidiuresis (SIAD)

Acute Phase

- Explain reasons for admission to the critical care unit.
- Explain reasons for neurologic changes associated with inappropriate antidiuresis (SIAD) due to increased arginine vasopressin (AVP) secretion.

Predischarge

Before discharge, the patient should be able to teach back the following topics:

- Patient-specific cause of SIAD
- How to measure intake and output
- How to measure urine specific gravity (if indicated)
- Signs and symptoms to report to health care professional

Restriction of Fluids

Thorough, astute nursing assessments are required for care of a patient with SIAD while an attempt is made to correct the fluid and sodium imbalance; the systemic effects of hyponatremia occur rapidly and can be lethal. Fluids are restricted to between 500 and 1000 mL/day. Accurate measurement of I&O is required. Frequent assessment of the patient's hydration status is accomplished with serial measurements of urine output, serum sodium levels, and serum osmolality. Frequent mouth care (moistening of the buccal membrane) may give comfort during the period of fluid restriction. The patient is weighed daily to gauge fluid retention or loss. Weight gain signifies continual fluid retention, whereas weight loss indicates loss of body fluid.

Educate the Patient and Family

Rapidly occurring changes in the patient's neurologic status may worry visiting family members. Sensitivity to the family's fears can be shown by words that express empathy and by providing time for the patient and family to ask questions and express their concerns. Patient and family education about SIAD, its effect on water balance, and the reasons for fluid restrictions should be done using the teach-back method (Box 31.20).

Collaborative Management

SIAD is a complex condition that requires clinical judgment and a team approach to manage the fluid and electrolyte disruption.[64] Effective clinical management requires the skills of many health care professionals working as a team with goals that are clearly communicated to all team members.

PATIENT-CENTERED CRITICAL CARE

Music for Patients in the Critical Care Unit

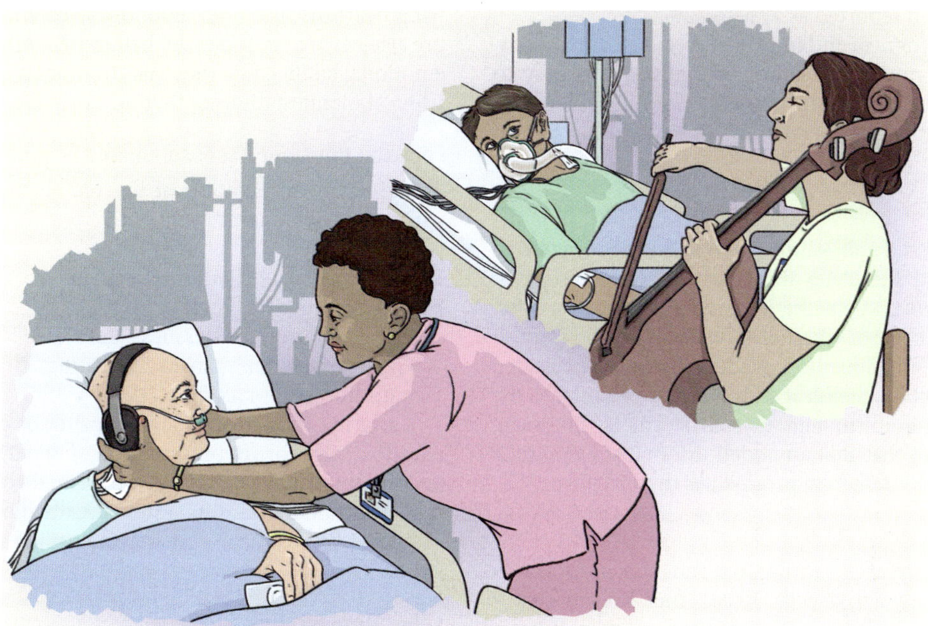

Music can be incorporated into the critical care environment in a number of different ways. Patients can be provided with noise-cancelling earphones that cover the entire ear, or they can use smaller earbuds that insert into the external ear. The earphones or earbuds can be Bluetooth/wireless or wired and attached to a smartphone with a music playlist.

Music is a helpful distractor during painful procedures and has been used as an adjunct to opiates and other pain-relieving medications in critical care. Music may also be used as an adjunct to anxiolytics to decrease feelings of anxiety. The selected music must be something the patient would normally enjoy listening to. Family members can often provide a playlist of favorite music. For patients who like to listen to music, this is a wonderful way to find some respite from the beeping of alarms in the critical care unit.

THYROID GLAND DISORDERS

There are two emergency thyroid disorders. *Thyroid storm* is caused by an excess of thyroid hormone and is an exacerbation of hyperthyroidism. The clinical opposite is *myxedema coma*, which is caused by insufficient thyroid hormone and is an exacerbation of hypothyroidism. Both hyperthyroidism and hypothyroidism are generally nonemergency conditions that are treated outside the hospital and are not discussed in this chapter. This section discusses recognition and management of the two thyroid emergency disorders that are rare but are occasionally seen in the critical care unit.

Thyroid Storm

Thyroid storm always occurs as a complication of preexisting hyperthyroidism.[72] Hyperthyroidism, also called *thyrotoxicosis*, occurs when the thyroid gland produces thyroid hormone in excess of the body's need.[72] The primary cause of hyperthyroidism is *Graves' disease*, an autoimmune condition that affects 2% of women and 0.5% of men globally.[73] Graves' disease is caused by circulating immunoglobulin G antibodies that attack the thyroid-stimulating hormone (TSH) receptor cells on the gland, causing release of thyroid hormone unrelated to the normal physiologic feedback mechanisms. A different cause is the antidysrhythmic medication amiodarone, which can create a painless thyroiditis in 5% to 10% of patients.[72] Conditions associated with hyperthyroidism are described in Box 31.21. The hypothalamic-pituitary-thyroid axis feedback loop is illustrated in Fig. 29.6 in Chapter 29.

BOX 31.21 Conditions Associated With Hyperthyroidism

- Excessive pituitary production of thyroid-stimulating hormone
- Excessive ingestion of thyroid hormone
- Graves' disease
- Toxic adenoma
- Toxic multinodular goiter
- Thyroiditis
- Painless thyroiditis, including amiodarone-induced, lymphocytic, and postpartum variations

Thyroid storm, also called *thyroid crisis*, is a rare and life-threatening exacerbation of hyperthyroidism.[74] The pathophysiology underlying the transition from hyperthyroidism to thyroid storm is not fully understood, as thyroid hormone levels are not necessarily different from patients with hyperthyroidism. Activation of the sympathetic nervous system and enhanced sensitivity to the effects of thyroid hormone are apparent. Stopping antithyroid medications and major stressors such as infection, surgery, trauma, pregnancy, or critical illness can precipitate thyroid storm in any patient with preexisting hyperthyroidism.

In a study of patients with thyroid storm admitted to critical care, *amiodarone-induced thyrotoxicosis* was the most frequently cited cause, followed by Graves' disease.[74] Mortality after thyroid storm in critical care has been reported as 17% to 22%.[73–75]

It is essential to recognize and manage thyroid storm quickly, as if the signs and symptoms are not recognized it is easy to misdiagnose. The key diagnostic and management elements are listed in the Summary of Key Concepts Related to Thyroid Storm (Fig. 31.7).

Etiology

In thyroid storm, excessive endogenous thyroid hormone increases metabolic activity and stimulates the beta-adrenergic receptors, resulting in a heightened sympathetic nervous system response. There is hyperactivity of cardiac tissue, nervous tissue, and smooth muscle tissue, and tremendous heat production with an elevated temperature. The exact biochemical stimulus that precipitates the transition of hyperthyroidism into thyroid storm is unknown, although it is apparent that that an added external stressor such as surgery, pregnancy, or infection precipitates thyroid storm.[74,75]

Pathophysiology

Thyroid hormone increases cellular oxygen consumption in almost all metabolically active cells. Excess metabolism generates heat and critically high fever. Cellular oxygen demands are dramatically increased with increased cardiac output to meet tissue demands. The oxygen demands in the hypermetabolic state are so great that the cardiac system cannot compensate adequately. Hypertension and tachycardia follow.

Gastrointestinal peristalsis increases, resulting in diarrhea, nausea, and vomiting. These symptoms all lead to dehydration and compound the problem of malnutrition and weight loss. Muscular weakness occurs and is compounded by the excessive protein breakdown. Metabolic acidosis is a potential problem.

Hypersensitivity to the increased adrenergic-binding sites potentiates the cardiovascular and nervous system responses to the hypermetabolic state. Atrial fibrillation is a common dysrhythmia in patients with hyperthyroidism, and tachydysrhythmias should be anticipated in thyroid storm, especially in patients with underlying heart disease.[72,74,75] Pulmonary edema and acute heart failure also can occur. Increased beta-adrenergic activity manifests as emotional lability, fine muscular tremors, agitation, and delirium. Clinical manifestations of thyroid storm are listed in Box 31.22.

Focused Physical Assessment and Diagnosis

The clinical presentation of thyroid storm is characterized by various organ systems:

1. Thermoregulation: fever
2. Heart: atrial fibrillation, supraventricular tachycardia, acute heart failure
3. CNS: agitation, restlessness, delirium
4. Gastrointestinal: nausea, vomiting, diarrhea, unexplained jaundice, stupor, coma

Early manifestations may be insidious or missed, creating a paradoxically abrupt presentation of apparently unrelated signs and symptoms. Use of a preestablished thyroid storm scoring system is one method to systematically diagnose thyroid storm (Table 31.9).[72] A score greater than 45 is indicative of thyroid storm.[72]

Laboratory Studies

Laboratory findings are used to confirm the suspicion raised by the clinical signs. The TSH value is extremely low, and thyroid hormones (triiodothyronine [T_3] and thyroxine [T_4]) are high compared with normal values[73] (see Table 30.3 in Chapter 30 for normal reference values). These results, in combination with the clinical picture, provide the diagnosis.

No laboratory test is available to differentiate thyroid storm from its predecessor, thyrotoxicosis, for which the laboratory values may be similar.[72,75] Thyroid storm is identified by a combination of the patient's medical history and exacerbation of clinical manifestations.

Thyroid Storm

Diagnostic assessment

- **History and risk factors**
  - **HYPER**thyroidism history
    - ✓ Graves disease, goiter
  - Thermoregulatory
    - ✓ High temperature
  - Cardiovascular
    - ✓ Tachycardia, dysrhythmias, hypertension
  - Neurologic
    - ✓ Agitation, delirium
  - Gastrointestinal
    - ✓ Nausea, vomiting, diarrhea
    - ✓ Weight loss
  - New infection that may have precipitated thyroid storm/crisis
- **Vital signs:** BP, HR, RR, temperature
- **Clinical assessment**
  - Mental status changes
  - Seizures (rare)
- **Laboratory tests**
  - TSH
  - T_3 & T_4
  - Metabolic panel

Thyroid storm signs

- Hyperthyroidism is the underlying condition
- Hypermetabolic state
- Agitation, anxiety
- High temperature
- Tachycardia and dysrhythmias
- Hypertension
- Rapid respiratory rate
- Thyroid storm score >45
- Low TSH
- Elevated free T_4

Nursing interventions

- Reduce temperature
- Normalize BP and HR
- Administer beta blockers
- Administer antithyroid medications
  - Propylthiouracil
  - Methimazole
  - Iodine (if deficient)
- Patient and family education

Resolution of thyroid storm

- At baseline metabolic rate with normal temperature, BP and HR
- Taking antithyroid medications

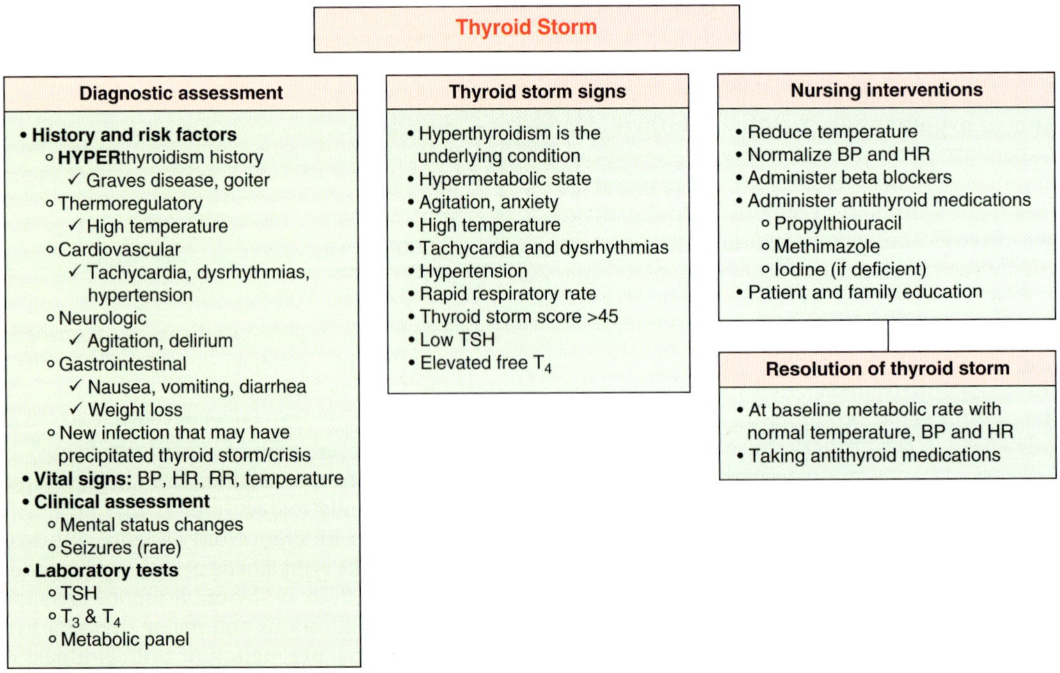

FIG. 31.7 Summary of Key Concepts Related to Thyroid Storm. *BP,* Blood pressure; *HR,* heart rate; *RR,* respiratory rate; *TSH,* Thyroid stimulating hormone; > greater than; ✓, evaluate/assess.

BOX 31.22 Clinical Manifestations of Thyroid Storm

Cardiovascular Signs and Symptoms

Activation of Beta-Adrenergic (B_1) Receptors in Heart

- Tachycardia
- Systolic murmur
- Increased stroke volume
- Increased cardiac output
- Increased systolic blood pressure (BP)
- Decreased diastolic BP
- Extra systoles
- Paroxysmal atrial tachycardia
- Premature ventricular contraction
- Palpitations
- Chest pain
- Increased cardiac contractility
- Acute heart failure
- Pulmonary edema
- Cardiogenic shock

Central Nervous System Signs and Symptoms

Resulting From Increased Catecholamine Response

- Hyperkinesis
- Nervousness
- Muscle weakness
- Confusion
- Convulsions
- Heat intolerance
- Fine tremor
- Emotional lability
- Frank psychosis
- Apathy
- Stupor
- Diaphoresis

Gastrointestinal Signs and Symptoms

- Nausea
- Vomiting
- Diarrhea
- Liver enlargement
- Abdominal pain
- Weight loss
- Increased appetite

Integumentary Signs and Symptoms

- Pruritus
- Hyperpigmentation of skin
- Fine, straight hair
- Alopecia

Thermoregulatory Signs and Symptoms

- Hyperthermia
- Heat dissipation
- Diaphoresis

Serum and Urine Signs

- Hypercalcemia
- Hyperglycemia
- Hypoalbuminemia
- Hypoprothrombinemia
- Hypocholesterolemia
- Creatinuria

TABLE 31.9 Thyroid Storm Diagnostic Criteria

Criteria	Points
Thermoregulatory Dysfunction	
Temperature (°F)	
99.0–99.9	5
100.0–100.9	10
101.0–101.9	15
102.0–102.9	20
103.0–103.9	25
≥104.0	30
Cardiovascular	
Tachycardia (beats/min)	
100–109	5
110–119	10
120–129	15
130–139	20
≥140	25
Atrial fibrillation	
Absent	0
Present	10
Acute heart failure	
Absent	0
Mild	5
Moderate	10
Severe	20
Gastrointestinal-Hepatic Dysfunction	
Manifestation	
Absent	0
Moderate (diarrhea, abdominal pain, nausea/vomiting)	10
Severe (jaundice)	20
Central Nervous System Disturbance	
Manifestation	
Absent	0
Mild (agitation)	10
Moderate (delirium, psychosis, extreme lethargy)	20
Severe (seizure, coma)	30
Precipitant History	
Status	
Positive	0
Negative	10
Scores Totaled	
>45 Thyroid storm	
25–44 Impending storm	
<25 Storm unlikely	

Modified from Burch HB, Wartofsky L. Life-threatening thyrotoxicosis: thyroid storm. *Endocrinol Metal Clin North Am.* 1993;22:263. Bahn RS, Cooper D, Garber J, et al. Hyperthyroidism and other causes of thyrotoxicosis: management guidelines of the American Thyroid Association and American Association of Clinical Endocrinologists. *Endocr Pract.* 2011;17(3):456.

Medical Management

The goal of acute medical management of thyroid storm is to reduce the clinical effects of thyroid hormone as rapidly as possible. This includes preventing cardiac decompensation, reducing hyperthermia, and fluid administration to reverse dehydration caused by fever or gastrointestinal losses. In severe cases, surgical partial thyroidectomy, or *therapeutic plasmapheresis* (plasma exchange) is used to rapidly reduce circulating thyroid hormone levels.[72–75]

Prevent Cardiovascular Collapse

The body's heightened sensitivity to the increased adrenergic and catecholamine receptors must be suppressed. Atrial dysrhythmias need to be controlled, and progression of heart failure must be halted. Beta-blockers are the mainstay of therapy for cardiac protection.[72]

Reduce Hyperthermia

Reduction in body temperature is achieved by use of a cooling blanket and the antipyretic agent acetaminophen.[75] Salicylates (aspirin) are contraindicated because they inhibit protein binding of T_3 to T_4, increasing the level of free, metabolically active thyroid hormone.[75]

Fluid Replacement

Vigorous fluid replacement must be instituted to treat or prevent dehydration. Antibiotic therapy may be warranted in the presence of systemic infection. Dehydration is treated with large volumes of glucose and isotonic sodium solutions to replace circulating fluid and sodium losses from hypermetabolism.

Pharmacologic Management of Thyroid Storm

Pharmacologic treatment is essential in treatment of thyroid storm.[72] A multimodal medication approach is recommended, with monitoring in a critical care unit during the acute phase.[72] Beta-blockers are administered to decrease the peripheral cellular sensitivity to catecholamines, and antithyroid medications are administered to block the synthesis and release of thyroid hormone into the circulation and to inhibit peripheral conversion of T_4 to T_3. Medications used to treat thyroid storm are listed in Table 31.10.

Medications That Block Catecholamine Effect

Beta-adrenergic blocking agents are used to decrease the catecholamine effects of excessive thyroid hormone (see Table 31.10). Beta-blockers have no effect on thyroid hormone but reduce the exaggerated myocardial stimulation and slow the atrioventricular conduction rate. Therapeutic doses vary from patient to patient, but higher doses are typically required for effective control of symptoms. Options include propranolol (oral) or esmolol, a short-acting IV beta-blocker.[72] Nondihydropyridine calcium channel blockers (verapamil, diltiazem) may be used to lower HR in patients who cannot take beta-blockers.[72] However, beta-blockers always represent first-line emergency treatment.[72]

Medications That Block Thyroid Synthesis

The synthesis of new thyroid hormone is blocked by the administration of antithyroid medications. Two agents are frequently used: propylthiouracil (PTU) and methimazole (see Table 31.10).[72–74] These medications are administered by mouth or via a feeding tube. PTU is especially therapeutic because it blocks thyroid synthesis and blocks conversion of T_4 to T_3. Methimazole has a slower rate of action but is more potent than PTU. Both medications act within 1 to 2 hours after absorption from the gastrointestinal tract. These medications have no effect on previously released thyroid hormone.

TABLE 31.10 PHARMACOLOGIC MANAGEMENT

Thyroid Storm

Medication	Dosage	Actions	Special Considerations
Antithyroid Medications			
Propylthiouracil	Loading dose: 500–1000 mg Maintenance dosage: 250 mg every 4 h	Blocks new thyroid hormone synthesis Blocks conversion of T_3 to T_4	May cause rash, nausea, vomiting, agranulocytosis, skin hyperpigmentation Administer with meals to reduce GI effects
Methimazole	60–80 mg/day	Blocks new thyroid hormone synthesis	Monitor signs listed for propylthiouracil. May cause rash, agranulocytosis
Iodine (saturated solution of potassium iodide)	5 drops (0.25 mL or 250 mg) orally every 6 h	Blocks new hormone synthesis	Do not start until 1 h after antithyroid medications have been administered
Hydrocortisone	Loading dose: 300 mg IV Maintenance dosage: 100 mg every 8 h	May block conversion of T_4 to T_3	Prophylaxis against adrenal insufficiency Dexamethasone is an alternative medication
Beta-Blockers			
Propranolol	10–40 mg every 3–4 hours	Beta-adrenergic blockade	Monitor HR and BP response to beta-blockade
Atenolol	25–100 mg, every 12 h or 1–2 times/d	Beta-adrenergic blockade	B_1 receptor selective
Metoprolol	25–50 mg every 8 h or 2–3 times /d	Beta-adrenergic blockade	B_1 receptor selective
Esmolol	50–100 mcg/kg/min IV pump	Beta-adrenergic blockade	Monitor HR and BP response to beta-blockade in critical care unit

BP, Blood pressure; *GI*, gastrointestinal; *HR*, heart rate; *IV*, intravenous/intravenously; T_3, triiodothyronine; T_4, thyroxine.

Based on data from Ross DS, Burch HB, Cooper DS, et al. 2016 American Thyroid Association guidelines for diagnosis and management of hyperthyroidism and other causes of thyrotoxicosis. *Thyroid.* 2016;26(10):1343–1421.

BOX 31.23 DIAGNOSIS AND PATIENT CARE MANAGEMENT

Thyroid Storm

- Hyperthermia due to increased metabolic rate
- Impaired Nutritional Intake due to lack of exogenous nutrients and increased metabolic demand
- Impaired Cardiac Output due to alterations in heart rate or rhythm
- Anxiety due to threat to biological, psychological, and social integrity
- Impaired Sleep due to fragmented sleep
- Lack of Knowledge of Treatment Regime due to lack of previous exposure to information (see Box 31.24, Patient and Family Education Plan: Thyroid Storm)

Patient Care Management plans are located in Appendix A.

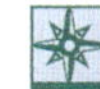

BOX 31.24 PATIENT AND FAMILY EDUCATION PLAN

Thyroid Storm

Acute Phase

- Explain reasons for critical care unit admission.
- Explain reasons for extreme hypermetabolism.

Predischarge

Before discharge, the patient should be able to teach back the following topics:

- Patient-specific cause of thyroid storm
- Medications: purpose, dosage, how often to use, and side effects
- Signs and symptoms to report to health care professional

Medications That Block Release of Thyroid Hormone

Administration of inorganic iodine blocks the release of any preformed thyroxine that is already in the thyroid gland but not yet released.[72] It is essential that iodine therapy not be administered until adequate inhibition of new hormone synthesis has occurred, as described in Table 31.10.[72] The iodide preparations are rapid acting and have a short duration. They are given approximately 1 hour after administration of the antithyroid medications (described in the previous section) to prevent the iodide from being used for thyroid hormone production and possible worsening of the clinical state.

Adrenal Insufficiency and Thyroid Storm

Some patients with thyroid storm have concomitant adrenal insufficiency and may be prescribed hydrocortisone or dexamethasone during the initial stages of thyroid storm management. See Table 31.10 for a list of medications and their nursing implications for a patient with thyroid storm.

Nursing Management

Nursing management of a patient with thyroid storm incorporates a variety of patient problems (Box 31.23). Nursing management is directed toward safe administration and monitoring of the effects of prescribed medications, normalizing body temperature, rehydration with correction of other metabolic derangements, and patient education.

Medication Administration

The timely and ordered sequence of medication administration is essential in the management of thyroid storm (see previous sections on pharmacologic management). The patient in thyroid storm is agitated, anxious, and unable to rest and benefits from a calm environment. The effects of the antithyroid medications, iodides, and beta-adrenergic blocking agents gradually decrease the neurologic symptoms related to catecholamine sensitivity. HR should decrease with beta-blockade.

The patient and family need to be reassured that this extreme agitation is the result of the disease process and that the medications will help control the nonstop fidgeting and tremors. Frequent reassurance and clear, simple explanations of the patient's condition help decrease the fear brought on by the onset of thyroid storm.

Normalize Body Temperature

In thyroid storm, the patient has hyperthermia related to a hypermetabolic state, as evidenced by a critically high body temperature; diaphoresis; hot, flushed skin; intolerance to heat; tachycardia; and tachypnea. Temperature is assessed frequently until normal body temperature is attained. Nursing measures to provide comfort while the patient is intolerant to heat include a room with a cool environment and a fan to circulate air and comfortable, nonrestrictive bedclothes. A tepid sponge bath helps to reduce heat by evaporation, and cold-pack applications to the groin and axilla increase heat loss at major blood vessels. If antipyretic medications are required, acetaminophen is the agent of choice and salicylates are avoided.[75]

Rehydration and Correction of Metabolic Derangements

Hyperthermia, tachypnea, diaphoresis, vomiting, and diarrhea predispose the patient to a fluid volume deficit. Fluids and electrolytes are as vigorously replaced as the decompensated cardiovascular system can tolerate. Glucose solutions are given to replace glycogen stores, which are depleted. Insulin is administered to treat the hyperglycemia that results from mobilization of nutrients and glucocorticoids. Hyponatremia from active loss (e.g., vomiting) is monitored by means of laboratory serum values. Hyponatremia can be prevented or treated with isotonic IV fluid replacement. Additional nursing measures focus on frequent hydration assessments (see Box 31.6).

Educate the Patient and Family

During the critical events surrounding the thyroid storm, the patient and family are given information according to their emotional state and cognitive level of understanding. The cause of the high fever, anxiety, and cardiac dysrhythmias is explained in understandable terms (Box 31.24). The patient and family often are relieved to know that the agitation and nervousness result from circulating hormones that may be decreased by taking daily medications.

Side effects of the specific medication therapy are taught before discharge. Patients treated with beta-blockers are taught to report signs of bradycardia, unexplained fatigue, and orthostatic hypotension, among other untoward effects. Patients discharged with antithyroid medications are alerted to the potential side effect of agranulocytosis (see Table 31.10). Symptoms of *agranulocytosis* include sudden cough, fever, rash, and inflammation. For management of elevated temperature, patients are instructed to use acetaminophen rather than salicylates, because salicylates increase the amount of free thyroid hormone in circulation.

Collaborative Management

Management of patients with thyroid storm is derived from the 2016 guidelines issued by the American Thyroid Association and American Association of Clinical Endocrinologists.[72] A patient with thyroid storm requires interventions by many health care professionals, with clearly communicated goals to facilitate rapid recovery.

Myxedema Coma

A severe deficiency of thyroid hormone produces hypothyroidism.[76] There is a spectrum of hypothyroidism, as defined by laboratory tests and clinical symptoms, that ranges from mild to severe. Mild hypothyroidism has subtle symptoms and is treated in the outpatient setting. *Myxedema coma* is an extreme exacerbation of hypothyroidism. It is associated with respiratory depression, cardiogenic shock, hypothermia, and coma and is often fatal.[77] Mortality is reported to be between 30% and 50%.[77,78]

Myxedema is differentiated from hypothyroidism by the depressive effect on all organ systems but specifically the CNS leading to decreased level of conscious, stupor or coma.[79]

It is essential to recognize myxedema coma because this is a reversible condition if detected early and managed appropriately as listed in the Summary of Key Concepts Related to Myxedema Coma (Fig. 31.8).

Etiology

Myxedema coma is a rare condition, and a high index of suspicion is required to correctly recognize the signs and symptoms in the early stages. A person may be admitted with myxedema coma after a prolonged period of unrecognized or poorly controlled hypothyroidism. The precipitating event is generally a severe infection, trauma, or acute illness, such as a stroke or acute myocardial infarction. More women are affected than men.[80]

These features have been proposed as hallmarks of myxedema coma: precipitating illness, altered mental status, hypothermia, bradycardia, and abnormal thyroid blood levels, specifically increased TSH and low free T_4.[77] See Table 30.3 in Chapter 30 for normal values of TSH and free (unbound) FT_3, and FT_4. The TSH level may be higher than 30 mU/L in myxedema coma.[77]

Hypothyroidism affects all body cells and organs and slows the metabolic rate in every system. Hypothyroidism can be caused by damage to the thyroid gland (primary) or can be secondary to pituitary or hypothalamic dysfunction.

Pathophysiology

The effects of hypothyroidism are widespread and varied. When the basal metabolic rate of oxygen consumption is reduced, cells are unable to maintain the processes necessary to sustain life. Without thyroid hormone, protein synthesis is severely curtailed and amino acid production and repair of tissues are halted. Metabolism of carbohydrate and fat is incomplete and gluconeogenesis cannot supply additional sources of glucose. Lipolysis is ineffective and cholesterol collects in the bloodstream. Hypothermia occurs. All systems are affected.

Skin

The composition of the skin changes as deposits of *hyaluronic acid* (a gel-like substance capable of holding large amounts of fluid) accumulate in the interstitial spaces, giving rise to a full appearance of face, hands, and feet. The skin has an overall yellowish appearance resulting from increased carotene deposits from reduced carotene conversion to vitamin A. The nails and hair are thin and brittle. Absence of thyroid hormone also leads to decreased or absent sweat production. The hyaluronic acid deposits are evident in heart muscle; skeletal muscles; and muscles of the tongue, pharynx, and proximal esophagus. These striated muscular changes of the tongue, pharynx, and esophagus contribute to the hoarse, husky voice. A lack of facial expression is notable in patients with hypothyroidism.

Cardiopulmonary System

Interstitial edema impairs cardiac myocytes, resulting in low cardiac output. Serous fluid accumulation in the pericardial sac can cause cardiac tamponade. A decreased sensitivity to

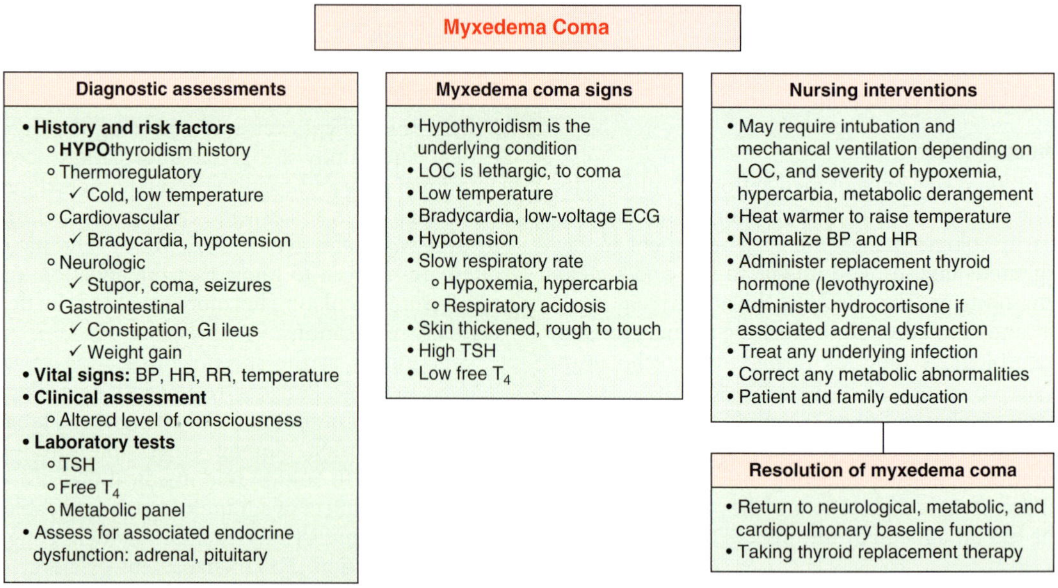

Myxedema Coma

Diagnostic assessments

- **History and risk factors**
  - **HYPO**thyroidism history
  - Thermoregulatory
    - ✓ Cold, low temperature
  - Cardiovascular
    - ✓ Bradycardia, hypotension
  - Neurologic
    - ✓ Stupor, coma, seizures
  - Gastrointestinal
    - ✓ Constipation, GI ileus
    - ✓ Weight gain
- **Vital signs:** BP, HR, RR, temperature
- **Clinical assessment**
  - Altered level of consciousness
- **Laboratory tests**
  - TSH
  - Free T_4
  - Metabolic panel
- Assess for associated endocrine dysfunction: adrenal, pituitary

Myxedema coma signs

- Hypothyroidism is the underlying condition
- LOC is lethargic, to coma
- Low temperature
- Bradycardia, low-voltage ECG
- Hypotension
- Slow respiratory rate
  - Hypoxemia, hypercarbia
  - Respiratory acidosis
- Skin thickened, rough to touch
- High TSH
- Low free T_4

Nursing interventions

- May require intubation and mechanical ventilation depending on LOC, and severity of hypoxemia, hypercarbia, metabolic derangement
- Heat warmer to raise temperature
- Normalize BP and HR
- Administer replacement thyroid hormone (levothyroxine)
- Administer hydrocortisone if associated adrenal dysfunction
- Treat any underlying infection
- Correct any metabolic abnormalities
- Patient and family education

Resolution of myxedema coma

- Return to neurological, metabolic, and cardiopulmonary baseline function
- Taking thyroid replacement therapy

FIG. 31.8 Summary of Key Concepts Related to Myxedema Coma. *BP*, Blood pressure; *ECG*, Electrocardiogram; *GI*, gastrointestinal; *HR*, heart rate; *LOC*, level of consciousness; *RR*, respiratory rate; *TSH:* thyroid stimulating hormone; > greater than; ✓, evaluate/assess.

catecholamines is present even though serum catecholamine levels are elevated. Resting HR and stroke volume are reduced. The force of myocardial contraction is weakened. There is a decrease in systolic BP and an increase in diastolic BP, causing a narrowed pulse pressure. Electrocardiogram (ECG) typically reveals low-voltage QRS complexes and low-voltage, flattened, or inverted T waves and a prolonged Q–T interval.

Pulmonary System

Pleural effusions and muscular changes affect gas exchange. The basal rate of oxygen consumption decreases, with a resulting insensitivity to CO_2. Hypoventilation increases the CO_2 serum content, which increases cerebral hypoxia. Hypoxic and hypercapnic ventilatory drives are severely impaired. Respiratory acidosis can occur. Pleural effusion, reduced vital capacity, and shallow respirations occur with any exertion. Respiratory muscle weakness, sleep apnea, and upper airway obstruction may be present. Respiratory failure and requirement for mechanical ventilation is often the reason for admission to the critical care unit.

Kidneys and Fluid and Electrolyte Balance

Blood flow to the kidneys is reduced, and the glomerular filtration rate, urine specific gravity, and urine osmolality are decreased. Elimination of medications by the kidneys is severely slowed in hypothyroidism.

Nutrition and Elimination

Decreased gastric motility or ileus is an expected complication for a patient with severe hypothyroidism. Food utilization and nutrient mobilization decrease with insufficient thyroid hormone. Intestinal hypomotility occurs, and serum cholesterol increases. Abdominal distention decreased intestinal peristalsis, and eventual paralytic ileus lead to extreme constipation. These findings make the provision of enteral nutrition a challenge.

Thermoregulation

Heat production decreases because of insufficient energy to maintain the base metabolic rate within the cells and hypothermia occurs. The ability to maintain body heat is further restricted by hypoglycemia.

Anemia

Anemia is present in many patients with hypothyroidism.[76] Symptoms of fatigue and depression are associated. Erythropoiesis (red blood cell production) is impaired. Coagulation abnormalities may coexist.[79]

Focused Physical Assessment and Diagnosis

The diagnosis of myxedema coma is based on the clinical manifestations of end-stage hypothyroidism. Severe hyperthyroidism (thyroid storm) and severe hypothyroidism (myxedema) are compared in Box 31.25.

Clinical Presentation

The diagnosis of end-stage hypothyroidism is based on the clinical presentation. Increasing signs of somnolence, depression, and diminished mental acuity signal diminished cellular function. Interstitial edema collects in almost all tissues. Organs become infiltrated with the mucoid-rich mucopolysaccharides, compromising organ function. Patients present with cardiovascular collapse, hypothermia, decreased kidney function, fluid excess, hypoventilation, and severe metabolic disorders.[79,80]

BOX 31.25 Clinical Manifestations of Hyperthyroidism Compared With Hypothyroidism

Hyperthyroidism (Thyrotoxicosis, Thyroid Storm)	Hypothyroidism (Myxedema, Myxedema Coma)
Elevated T_4, T_3	Decreased T_4, T_3
Decreased TSH	Elevated TSH
Hypercalcemia	Hyponatremia
Hyperglycemia	Hypoglycemia
Metabolic acidosis	Respiratory acidosis, metabolic acidosis
Tachycardia, palpitations, atrial fibrillation	Hypercholesterolemia
Angina	Anemia
ST segment wave changes	Bradycardia
Shortened Q–T interval	Peripheral vasoconstriction
Hypertension	Flattened, inverted T waves
AV block, acute heart failure	Prolonged Q–T and P–R intervals
Hypovolemia	Decreased stroke volume, decreased cardiac output
Shortness of breath, tachypnea	Enlarged heart, pericardial effusion
Hypermetabolism	Increased total body fluid with decreased effective arterial blood volume
Polyphagia	Hypoventilation, possible CO_2 retention
Weight loss	Depressed metabolism
Nausea, vomiting, increased peristalsis	Decreased lipolysis, increased cholesterol
Tremor	Weight gain
Extreme restlessness, insomnia, uneasiness, anxiety	Constipation
Emotional instability, despondency	Seizures
Diaphoresis	Slowness, depression
Heat intolerance	Impaired short-term memory
Increased DTRs	Slow, deliberate speech
Muscle weakness or muscle wasting	Thickened tongue
Oligomenorrhea	Coarse, dry, scaly, edematous skin
	Hypothermia
	Delirium (myxedema madness)
	Lethargy → stupor → coma (myxedema coma)
	Diminished DTRs
	Paresthesia of hands
	Menorrhagia

AV, Atrioventricular; *CO_2*, carbon dioxide; *DTRs*, deep tendon reflexes; *T_3*, triiodothyronine; *T_4*, thyroxine; *TSH*, thyroid-stimulating hormone.

Weight gain is attributed to the collection of mucopolysaccharides in the interstitium, the increase in fluid retention, and the decrease in metabolism. Paresthesias of hands and feet are caused by hyaluronic acid accumulation in the synovial sacs, which leads to compression of nerves and carpal tunnel syndrome. Compression of nerves interferes with the simplest hand grasp and the ability to raise one's hands. Reflexes contract briskly but take extended seconds to relax.

Hypothermia is a very distressing symptom. Most cases of myxedema are diagnosed in the winter months. A myxedematous patient has hypotension, decreased cardiac output, and often bradycardia, all related to a decrease in beta-adrenergic stimulation. Symptoms of depression and decreased mental acuity occur as hypothyroidism progresses.

Laboratory Studies

Thyroid hormone blood tests confirm the clinical picture of myxedema coma. TSH is the first test to order if hypothyroidism is suspected. Typically, patients with myxedema have primary hypothyroidism with a high TSH level and a low T_4 level.[80] If the TSH level is normal or low, other nonthyroidal causes of coma must be investigated. TSH is released by the pituitary gland; see Table 30.3 in Chapter 30 for normal reference values. Endocrine studies to evaluate pituitary function and adrenal function should also be undertaken.[80]

Medical Management

The patient's primary admitting diagnosis may mask an underlying hypothyroidism. However, clinical manifestations can trigger the alert clinician to suspect a hypofunctioning thyroid. The primary disease condition and the myxedema coma must be treated immediately to improve the patient's chances for recovery. Myxedema coma often necessitates ventilator support, correction of fluid and electrolyte imbalance, correction of other multisystem abnormalities, corticosteroid supplementation, and thyroid hormone replacement.[78,80]

Pharmacologic Management of Myxedema Coma

Thyroid hormone replacement including type and dosage to treat end-stage hypothyroidism (myxedema coma) is challenging, as dosages often are individualized for each patient.[80] One method is to replete T_4 levels with an initial dose of levothyroxine (100 to 100 mcg administered IV) to saturate the previously empty T_4 binding sites, followed by daily administration of 50 mcg of levothyroxine.[80] If coexisting adrenal compromise is present, patients may first be administered corticosteroids.[80]

Nursing Management

Nursing management of a patient with myxedema coma involves management of a variety of patient problems (Box 31.26). Nursing actions are directed toward management of the precipitating disease and on the severe effect of hypothyroidism on multiple organ systems.

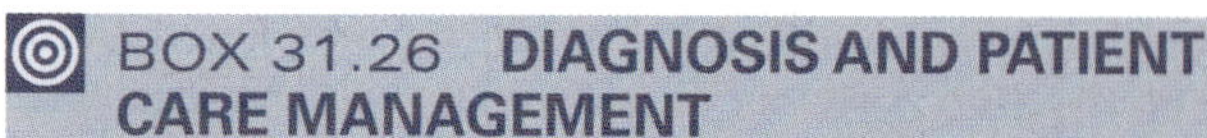

BOX 31.26 DIAGNOSIS AND PATIENT CARE MANAGEMENT

Myxedema Coma

- Hypothermia due to decreased metabolic rate
- Impaired Breathing due to respiratory muscle fatigue or metabolic factors
- Activity Intolerance due to prolonged immobility or deconditioning
- Lack of Knowledge of Treatment Regime due to lack of previous exposure to information (see Box 31.27, Patient and Family Education Plan for Myxedema Coma)

Patient Care Management plans are located in Appendix A.

Pulmonary Care

A patient with myxedema coma who is admitted to the critical care unit may require intubation and mechanical ventilatory support. Individuals who are not intubated are monitored for development of respiratory failure. Arterial blood gas measurements are evaluated to monitor for CO_2 retention and respiratory acidosis.

Cardiac Concerns

Dysrhythmias are common in patients with myxedema and can quickly be identified by continuous ECG monitoring. Expected signs associated with myxedema coma on the ECG include low QRS voltage, flattened or inverted T waves, and prolonged Q–T and P–R intervals.

Thermoregulation

Hypothermia gradually improves as the patient is treated with thyroid hormone. Several warm blankets comfortably wrapped around a patient with mild hypothermia may be sufficient to help raise the body temperature to normal. Active warming devices are also used. Continuous assessments are important to avoid too-rapid heating and vasodilation. Electronic devices that can measure accurately at the extreme lower range of body temperatures are used.

Thyroid Replacement Therapy

Older patients and patients with a cardiac history receive IV thyroid hormone replacement with due precautions. Thyroxine can precipitate angina and dysrhythmias. Improvements in the patient's cardiopulmonary and neurologic status, together with changes in T_4 and TSH laboratory values, are used to gauge the success of thyroid hormone replacement therapy.

Skin Care

Patients with myxedema coma have rough, dry skin. Measures are taken to avoid skin breakdown related to decreased circulation and widespread edema. An emollient for skin hydration follows nonsoap baths. Frequent repositioning minimizes pressure over bony prominences.

Elimination

Constipation is managed on a daily basis to avoid impaction. Use of fiber-enriched enteral nutrition may be helpful in an alert patient. Fluids are encouraged as the hypovolemia is corrected and BP stabilizes. Increased fiber is preferable to use of enemas.

Patient and Family Education

Patients with myxedema coma have decreased comprehension and mental acuity. All instructions, procedures, and activities are explained slowly and provided in written form. The patient and family members may experience myriad emotions with one constant—fear of the unknown. Before any teaching, the nurse evaluates the family's ability to accept the patient's slowed thinking and slowed response time.

All instructions given to the patient or family are given orally and in writing. A written copy of all schedules is given as a reference for home care before discharge. The nurse discusses the medication schedule and the frequency of the medication doses with the patient and family. Side effects of each medication are described. The patient and family need to know the side effects of medications including over-the-counter medications so that they can manage the medications at home. Also, the nurse discusses which signs and symptoms to report to the health care provider (Box 31.27).

Collaborative Management

There are limited guidelines that discuss acute collaborative care management of patients with hypothyroidism and myxedema coma.[76] Early recognition of symptoms and a willingness to

BOX 31.27 PATIENT AND FAMILY EDUCATION PLAN

Myxedema Coma

Acute Phase

- Explain reasons for critical care unit admission.
- Explain reasons for extreme hypometabolism.

Predischarge

Before discharge, the patient should be able to teach back the following topics:

- Patient-specific cause of hypothyroidism and myxedema coma
- Medications: purpose, dosage, how often to use, and side effects
- Signs and symptoms to report to health care professional

request laboratory tests to confirm the diagnosis allow therapy to be instituted as early as possible.

ADRENAL GLAND DISORDERS

The adrenal gland is complex. The adrenal gland is composed of a cortex and a medulla, which each produce different hormones, and multiple adrenal hormonal actions affect other systems within the body. Disease states may be related to either oversecretion or undersecretion of specific hormones. Because the adrenal glands are interconnected with the rest of the endocrine system, it is not uncommon to test for some of the conditions described in the next sections when investigating etiology of pituitary, thyroid, or CNS disorders.

Oversecretion of Adrenal Hormones

Primary Cushing Syndrome

Primary Cushing syndrome is rare. It occurs because of either an excess of adrenocorticotropic hormone (ACTH) from the pituitary gland (pituitary adenoma), another ectopic source (small cell or kidney carcinoma), or from an adenoma within the adrenal cortex that produces excess cortisol.[81] Cortisol levels are normalized by surgical resection. Endocrine diagnostic tests include ACTH and cortisol levels. Additional management is individualized depending on the initial cause.[82]

Secondary Cushing Syndrome

Secondary Cushing syndrome is a cluster of signs and symptoms that occur after taking high-dose corticosteroids for an extended time. In response to exogenous corticosteroids, the adrenal glands stop production of intrinsic hormones. Patients who have been taking steroids before their admission to the hospital need their dosage increased during illness to avoid hypoadrenalism.

Primary Aldosteronism

Primary aldosteronism occurs when the adrenal cortex produces excessive amounts of the mineralocorticoid aldosterone, causing the adrenal glands to lose potassium and conserve sodium.[83–85] The elevated sodium causes fluid retention. Hypertension, hypernatremia, and hypokalemia occur in primary aldosteronism. Presentation in critical care may be for a hypertensive emergency or stroke. Diagnostic tests include blood levels of aldosterone and renin and an imaging study of the adrenal glands.[83–85]

BOX 31.28 Internet Resources

Endocrine Disorders

- American Association of Clinical Endocrinology (AACE): *https://www.aace.com/*
- The Endocrine Society: *https://www.endocrine.org/*
- American Diabetes Association: https://www.diabetes.org/diabetes
- American Thyroid Association Guidelines: *https://www.thyroid.org/professionals/ata-professional-guidelines/*
- Cushing's Support and Research Foundation: https://csrf.net/
- NIH Cushing's: https://www.ninds.nih.gov/disorders/all-disorders/cushings-syndrome-information-page
- National Cancer Institute (NCI), Neuroendocrine tumors, Pheochromocytomas: https://www.cancer.gov/pediatric-adult-rare-tumor/rare-tumors/rare-endocrine-tumor/pheochromocytoma

Pheochromocytoma

Pheochromocytoma tumors originate in the chromaffin cells of the adrenal medulla. These specialized cells produce either norepinephrine and epinephrine, and a pheochromocytoma will dramatically increase the catechol output, leading to a *catecholamine storm* with sustained hypertension that can cause a stroke and end-organ damage.[86] The recommended laboratory diagnosis of pheochromocytoma is to measure plasma and urine fractionated metanephrines, collect 24-hour urinary output for catecholamine measurement, and obtain adrenal imaging studies. Surgical or laparoscopic resection of the tumor provides definitive relief although follow-up is recommended in case of reoccurrence.[87]

Undersecretion of Adrenal Hormones

Addison Disease

Primary adrenal insufficiency, also known as *Addison disease*, describes an intrinsic failure of the adrenal gland to produce normal endogenous corticosteroid hormones (cortisol) and mineralocorticosteroid hormones (aldosterone).[88]

Specific adrenal diagnostic tests include:

- ACTH level
- Cortisol level
- Corticotrophin stimulation test

Adrenal crisis, also known as an Addisonian crisis, although rare, may require admission to a critical care unit and be associated with other endocrine disorders.[89–91] Adrenal crisis is life threatening and can present with hypotension, hyponatremia, hyperkalemia, hypoglycemia, and hypercalcemia.[88] Treatment is focused on replenishing the glucocorticosteroid and mineralocorticosteroid hormones.

Endocrine disorders are often unique because signs and symptoms for the same disorder can vary greatly between patients, and sometimes multiple conditions are present. When the diagnosis or prognosis is unclear, this makes nursing management both challenging and complex and requires a high degree of skill and knowledge.

ADDITIONAL RESOURCES

See Box 31.28 for Internet resources pertaining to endocrine disorders and therapeutic management.

CASE STUDY 31.1 Patient With an Endocrine Disorder

Brief Patient History

Ms. S is a 72-year-old woman with a history of hypertension treated with an angiotensin-converting enzyme inhibitor and thiazide diuretics. She has a past 100-pack/year history of tobacco abuse but quit smoking 2 years ago. She lives independently in a senior apartment. She was brought to the hospital by friends because of a fall. Ms. S states that she has a severe headache but cannot recall whether she hit her head during the fall. She is also having difficulty recalling recent events.

Clinical Assessment

Ms. S is admitted to the critical care unit from the emergency department because of nonspecific electrocardiogram (ECG) changes suggestive of inferior wall ischemia and electrolyte abnormalities. She is awake, alert, and oriented to person, time, and place; she is unable to recall the events leading to her hospitalization. She states that her headache is severe and feels like someone is hitting her head with a hammer. Her skin is warm and dry. Her gait is visibly unsteady.

Diagnostic Procedures

Ms. S's vital signs include blood pressure of 180/92 mm Hg, heart rate of 100 beats/min (sinus rhythm), respiratory rate of 24 breaths/min, and temperature of 98.8°F.

Ms. S reports that her headache is a 10 on the pain rating scale. Laboratory findings include sodium level of 116 mmol/L, potassium level of 3.3 mmol/L, chloride level of 88 mmol/L, carbon dioxide level of 22 mEq/L, magnesium level of 1.8 mg/dL, urinary sodium level of 30 mmol/L, and urine osmolality value of 118 mOsm/L. The test result for troponin I on admission is negative. ECG testing shows a normal sinus rhythm; T wave inversion in leads II, III, and AVF; and a change from prior ECG findings suggestive of inferior wall ischemia. Chest radiography identifies a mass in the right upper lobe that strongly suggests a neoplasm.

Medical Diagnosis

Ms. S is diagnosed with syndrome of inappropriate antidiuresis (SIAD).

Questions

1. What major outcomes do you expect to achieve for this patient?
2. What problems or risks must be managed to achieve these outcomes?
3. What interventions must be initiated to monitor, prevent, manage, or eliminate the problems and risks identified?
4. What interventions should be initiated to promote optimal functioning, safety, and well-being of the patient?
5. What technology can be used to monitor this patient and prevent complications?
6. What other interprofessional team members are needed to assist with the management of this patient?
7. What possible learning needs do you anticipate for this patient?
8. What cultural and age-related factors may have a bearing on the patient's plan of care?

KEY POINTS

Stress of Critical Illness

- The endocrine system is complex, and assessment relies heavily on laboratory tests for confirmation of disease processes. To fully participate in the care of patients with these complex conditions, the critical care nurse must be aware of the intricacies of the endocrine system.
- Physiologic stress associated with critical illness causes increased secretion of stress hormones by the HPA pathway, resulting in secretion of cortisol, stimulation of the sympathetic nervous system, and release of norepinephrine and epinephrine to mobilize glucose. If critical illness is prolonged beyond 7 to 10 days, profound suppression of pituitary, thyroid, and adrenal gland function may occur.

Pancreas: Diabetic Ketoacidosis and Hyperglycemic Hyperosmolar State

- Diagnostic criteria for DKA include blood glucose concentration greater than 250 mg/dL, arterial pH value less than 7.3, serum bicarbonate level less than 18 mEq/L, and moderate or severe ketonemia or ketonuria.
- Diagnostic criteria for HHS include blood glucose concentration greater than 600 mg/dL, arterial pH value higher than 7.3, serum bicarbonate level greater than 18 mEq/L, serum osmolality greater than 320 mOsm/kg H_2O (320 mmol/kg H_2O), and absent or mild ketonuria.

Pituitary: Diabetes Insipidus and Syndrome of Inappropriate Antidiuresis (SIAD)

- Central DI occurs when AVP (vasopressin), also known as antidiuretic hormone (ADH), is insufficient or is not released from the posterior pituitary gland. The excretion of large quantities of hypotonic urine disrupts serum and urinary laboratory values: serum sodium greater than 145 mEq/L, serum osmolality greater than 295 mOsm/kg H_2O (>295 mmol/L), urine osmolality less than 200 mOsm/kg H_2O (<200 mmol/L), and urine specific gravity less than 1.005.
- SIAD occurs when excess AVP (vasopressin), also call ADP, is released from the posterior pituitary gland. This stimulates the kidney tubules to retain water, resulting in fluid overload and hyponatremia manifested by these alterations in serum and urinary laboratory values: decreased serum osmolality (<275 mOsm/kg H_2O) with increased urine osmolality (> 100 mOsm/kg H_2O), low serum sodium (<125 mEq/L), and elevated urinary sodium (>30 mEq/L).

Thyroid: Thyroid Storm and Myxedema Coma

- Thyroid storm is identified by clinical signs such as high fever, tachycardia, hypertension, and tremor as evidence of the rapid metabolic rate. Laboratory values resemble values seen in hyperthyroidism: low TSH and high T_4 levels.
- Myxedema coma is characterized by a precipitating illness, hypothermia, hypoventilation, bradycardia, decreased mental acuity, high TSH, and low T_4 levels.

Adrenal

- Excess secretion of adrenal hormones can produce several different life-threatening conditions: primary Cushing syndrome, primary aldosteronism, a pheochromocytoma tumor may release a catecholamine surge resulting in hypertension.
- Insufficient secretion of adrenal hormones can produce primary adrenal insufficiency, also known as Addison disease.

Visit the Evolve site at http://evolve.elsevier.com/Urden/CriticalCareNursing for additional study materials.

REFERENCES

1. Russell G, Lightman S. The human stress response. *Nat Rev Endocrinol.* 2019;15(9):525–534. https://doi.org/10.1038/s41574-019-0228-0.
2. Fowler C, Raoof N, Pastores SM. Sepsis and adrenal insufficiency. *J Intensive Care Med.* 2023;38(11):987–996. https://doi.org/10.1177/08850666231183396.
3. Téblick A, Peeters B, Langouche L, Van den Berghe G. Adrenal function and dysfunction in critically ill patients. *Nat Rev Endocrinol.* 2019;15(7):417–427. https://doi.org/10.1038/s41574-019-0185-7.
4. Annane D, Pastores SM, Arlt W, et al. Critical illness-related corticosteroid insufficiency (CIRCI): a narrative review from a multispecialty task force of the Society of Critical Care Medicine (SCCM) and the European Society of Intensive Care Medicine (ESICM). *Intensive Care Med.* 2017;43(12):1781–1792. https://doi.org/10.1007/s00134-017-4914-x.
5. Harp JB, Yancopoulos GD, Gromada J. Glucagon orchestrates stress-induced hyperglycaemia. *Diabetes Obes Metab.* 2016;18(7):648–653. https://doi.org/10.1111/dom.12668.
6. Navale AM, Paranjape AN. Glucose transporters: physiological and pathological roles. *Biophys Rev.* 2016;8(1):5–9. https://doi.org/10.1007/s12551-015-0186-2.
7. Wewer Albrechtsen NJ, Holst JJ, Cherrington AD, et al. 100 years of glucagon and 100 more. *Diabetologia.* 2023;66(8):1378–1394. https://doi.org/10.1007/s00125-023-05947-y.
8. Honarmand K, Sirimaturos M, Hirshberg EL, et al. Society of critical care medicine guidelines on glycemic control for critically ill children and adults 2024. *Crit Care Med.* 2024. https://doi.org/10.1097/CCM.0000000000006174. Published online January 19.
9. van den Berghe G, Wouters P, Weekers F, et al. Intensive insulin therapy in critically ill patients. *N Engl J Med.* 2001;345(19):1359–1367. https://doi.org/10.1056/NEJMoa011300.
10. Gunst J, Debaveye Y, Güiza F, et al. Tight blood-glucose control without early parenteral nutrition in the ICU. *N Engl J Med.* 2023;389(13):1180–1190. https://doi.org/10.1056/NEJMoa2304855.
11. NICE-SUGAR Study Investigators, Finfer S, Chittock DR, et al. Intensive versus conventional glucose control in critically ill patients. *N Engl J Med.* 2009;360(13):1283–1297. https://doi.org/10.1056/NEJMoa0810625.
12. Poole AP, Finnis ME, Anstey J, et al. The effect of a liberal approach to glucose control in critically ill patients with type 2 diabetes: a multicenter, parallel-group, open-label randomized clinical trial. *Am J Respir Crit Care Med.* 2022;206(7):874–882. https://doi.org/10.1164/rccm.202202-0329OC.
13. American Diabetes Association Professional Practice Committee. 16. Diabetes care in the hospital: standards of care in diabetes—2024. *Diabetes Care.* 2024;47(Suppl 1):S295–S306. https://doi.org/10.2337/dc24-S016.
14. Moghissi ES, Korytkowski MT, DiNardo M, et al. American Association of Clinical Endocrinologists and American Diabetes Association consensus statement on inpatient glycemic control. *Diabetes Care.* 2009;32(6):1119–1131. https://doi.org/10.2337/dc09-9029.
15. Kulkarni H, Bihari S, Prakash S, et al. Independent association of glucose variability with hospital mortality in adult intensive care patients: results from the Australia and New Zealand Intensive Care Society Centre for Outcome and Resource Evaluation Binational Registry. *Crit Care Explor.* 2019;1(8):e0025. https://doi.org/10.1097/CCE.0000000000000025.
16. Umpierrez GE, P Kovatchev B. Glycemic variability: how to measure and its clinical implication for type 2 diabetes. *Am J Med Sci.* 2018;356(6):518–527. https://doi.org/10.1016/j.amjms.2018.09.010.
17. Klonoff DC, Umpierrez GE, Rice MJ. A milestone in point of care capillary blood glucose monitoring of critically ill hospitalized patients. *J Diabetes Sci Technol.* 2018;12(6):1095–1100. https://doi.org/10.1177/1932296818801607.
18. Davis GM, Faulds E, Walker T, et al. Remote continuous glucose monitoring with a computerized insulin infusion protocol for critically ill patients in a COVID-19 medical ICU: proof of concept. *Diabetes Care.* 2021;44(4):1055–1058. https://doi.org/10.2337/dc20-2085.
19. Salinas PD, Mendez CE. Glucose management technologies for the critically ill. *J Diabetes Sci Technol.* 2019;13(4):682–690. https://doi.org/10.1177/1932296818822838.
20. Spanakis EK, Cook CB, Kulasa K, et al. A consensus statement for continuous glucose monitoring metrics for inpatient clinical trials. *J Diabetes Sci Technol.* 2023;17(6):1527–1552. https://doi.org/10.1177/19322968231191104.
21. Lalani B, Gosselin K, Penno R, Puryear B, Rilo H, Lalani A. A retrospective cohort analysis of two computerized insulin infusion protocols. *J Diabetes Sci Technol.* 2023;17(3):635–641. https://doi.org/10.1177/19322968231163584.
22. Gerhardt JM, Dine SA, Foster DR, et al. Development of a pharmacist-managed protocol for the transition from intravenous to subcutaneous insulin in critically ill adults. *Am J Health Syst Pharm.* 2022;79(suppl 3):S86–S93. https://doi.org/10.1093/ajhp/zxac141.
23. Alshaya AI, DeGrado JR, Lupi KE, Szumita PM. Safety and efficacy of transitioning from intravenous to subcutaneous insulin in critically ill patients. *Int J Clin Pharm.* 2022;44(1):146–152. https://doi.org/10.1007/s11096-021-01325-z.
24. Lambell KJ, Tatucu-Babet OA, Chapple LA, Gantner D, Ridley EJ. Nutrition therapy in critical illness: a review of the literature for clinicians. *Crit Care.* 2020;24(1):35. https://doi.org/10.1186/s13054-020-2739-4.
25. Ibrahim SMH, Shahat EA, Amer LA, Aljohani AK. The impact of using carbohydrate counting on managing diabetic patients: a review. *Cureus.* 2023;15(11):e48998. https://doi.org/10.7759/cureus.48998.
26. Mastrototaro L, Roden M. Insulin resistance and insulin sensitizing agents. *Metabolism.* 2021;125:154892. https://doi.org/10.1016/j.metabol.2021.154892.
27. Agiostratidou G, Anhalt H, Ball D, et al. Standardizing clinically meaningful outcome measures beyond HbA1c for type 1 diabetes: a consensus report of the American Association of Clinical Endocrinologists, the American Association of Diabetes Educators, the American Diabetes Association, the Endocrine Society, JDRF International, The Leona M. and Harry B. Helmsley Charitable Trust, the Pediatric Endocrine Society, and the T1D Exchange. *Diabetes Care.* 2017;40(12):1622–1630. https://doi.org/10.2337/dc17-1624.
28. McCall AL, Lieb DC, Gianchandani R, et al. Management of individuals with diabetes at high risk for hypoglycemia: an Endocrine Society clinical practice guideline. *J Clin Endocrinol Metab.* 2023;108(3):529–562. https://doi.org/10.1210/clinem/dgac596.
29. Kwan TN, Marhoon N, Young M, Holmes N, Bellomo R. Insulin therapy associated relative hypoglycemia during critical illness. *J Crit Care.* 2022;70:154018. https://doi.org/10.1016/j.jcrc.2022.154018.
30. Ware LR, Gilmore JF, Szumita PM. Practical approach to clinical controversies in glycemic control for hospitalized surgical patients. *Nutr Clin Pract.* 2022;37(3):521–535. https://doi.org/10.1002/ncp.10858.
31. Jacobi J, Bircher N, Krinsley J, et al. Guidelines for the use of an insulin infusion for the management of hyperglycemia in critically ill patients. *Crit Care Med.* 2012;40(12):3251–3276. https://doi.org/10.1097/CCM.0b013e3182653269.
32. Wischmeyer PE, Bear DE, Berger MM, et al. Personalized nutrition therapy in critical care: 10 expert recommendations. *Crit Care.* 2023;27(1):261. https://doi.org/10.1186/s13054-023-04539-x.
33. American Diabetes Association Professional Practice Committee. 2. Diagnosis and classification of diabetes: standards of care in diabetes—2024. *Diabetes Care.* 2024;47(Suppl 1):S20–S42. https://doi.org/10.2337/dc24-S002.
34. American Diabetes Association Professional Practice Committee. 9. Pharmacologic approaches to glycemic treatment: standards of care in diabetes—2024. *Diabetes Care.* 2024;47(Suppl 1):S158–S178. https://doi.org/10.2337/dc24-S009.
35. Nathan DM. Realising the long-term promise of insulin therapy: the DCCT/EDIC study. *Diabetologia.* 2021;64(5):1049–1058. https://doi.org/10.1007/s00125-021-05397-4.
36. Arnold SV, Khunti K, Tang F, et al. Incidence rates and predictors of microvascular and macrovascular complications in patients with type 2 diabetes: results from the longitudinal global discover study. *Am Heart J.* 2022;243:232–239. https://doi.org/10.1016/j.ahj.2021.10.181.
37. Holt RIG, DeVries JH, Hess-Fischl A, et al. The management of type 1 diabetes in adults. A consensus report by the American Diabetes Association (ADA) and the European Association for the Study of Diabetes (EASD). *Diabetes Care.* 2021;44(11):2589–2625. https://doi.org/10.2337/dci21-0043.

38. Petersen MC, Shulman GI. Mechanisms of insulin action and insulin resistance. *Physiol Rev*. 2018;98(4):2133–2223. https://doi.org/10.1152/physrev.00063.2017.
39. Samson SL, Vellanki P, Blonde L, et al. American association of clinical Endocrinology consensus statement: comprehensive type 2 diabetes management algorithm – 2023 update. *Endocr Pract*. 2023;29(5):305–340. https://doi.org/10.1016/j.eprac.2023.02.001.
40. American Diabetes Association Professional Practice Committee. 8. Obesity and weight management for the prevention and treatment of type 2 diabetes: standards of care in diabetes—2024. *Diabetes Care*. 2024;47(Suppl 1):S145–S157. https://doi.org/10.2337/dc24-S008.
41. American Diabetes Association Professional Practice Committee. 10. Cardiovascular disease and risk management: standards of care in diabetes—2024. *Diabetes Care*. 2024;47(Suppl 1):S179–S218. https://doi.org/10.2337/dc24-S010.
42. American Diabetes Association Professional Practice Committee. 3. Prevention or delay of diabetes and associated comorbidities: standards of care in diabetes—2024. *Diabetes Care*. 2024;47(Suppl 1):S43–S51. https://doi.org/10.2337/dc24-S003.
43. Walker EA, Gonzalez JS, Tripputi MT, et al. Long-term metformin adherence in the diabetes prevention program outcomes study. *BMJ Open Diabetes Res Care*. 2020;8(1):e001537. https://doi.org/10.1136/bmjdrc-2020-001537.
44. Davies MJ, Aroda VR, Collins BS, et al. Management of hyperglycaemia in type 2 diabetes, 2022. A consensus report by the American Diabetes Association (ADA) and the European Association for the Study of Diabetes (EASD). *Diabetologia*. 2022;65(12):1925–1966. https://doi.org/10.1007/s00125-022-05787-2.
45. American Diabetes Association Professional Practice Committee. 11. Chronic kidney disease and risk management: standards of care in diabetes—2024. *Diabetes Care*. 2024;47(Suppl 1):S219–S230. https://doi.org/10.2337/dc24-S011.
46. Heidenreich PA, Bozkurt B, Aguilar D, et al. 2022 AHA/ACC/HFSA guideline for the management of heart failure: a report of the American College of Cardiology/American Heart Association Joint Committee on Clinical Practice Guidelines. *Circulation*. 2022;145(18). https://doi.org/10.1161/CIR.0000000000001063.
47. Jha KK, Adhikari R, Tasdighi E, Osuji N, Rajan T, Blaha MJ. Transitioning to GLP-1 RAs and SGLT2 inhibitors as the first choice for managing cardiometabolic risk in type 2 diabetes. *Curr Atheroscler Rep*. 2022;24(12):925–937. https://doi.org/10.1007/s11883-022-01066-y.
48. Alssema M, Ruijgrok C, Blaak EE, et al. Effects of alpha-glucosidase-inhibiting drugs on acute postprandial glucose and insulin responses: a systematic review and meta-analysis. *Nutr Diabetes*. 2021;11(1):11. https://doi.org/10.1038/s41387-021-00152-5.
49. Fayfman M, Pasquel FJ, Umpierrez GE. Management of hyperglycemic crises: diabetic ketoacidosis and hyperglycemic hyperosmolar state. *Med Clin North Am*. 2017;101(3):587–606. https://doi.org/10.1016/j.mcna.2016.12.011.
50. Kitabchi AE, Umpierrez GE, Miles JM, Fisher JN. Hyperglycemic crises in adult patients with diabetes. *Diabetes Care*. 2009;32(7):1335–1343. https://doi.org/10.2337/dc09-9032.
51. Firestone RL, Parker PL, Pandya KA, Wilson MD, Duby JJ. Moderate-intensity insulin therapy is associated with reduced length of stay in critically ill patients with diabetic ketoacidosis and hyperosmolar hyperglycemic state. *Crit Care Med*. 2019;47(5):700–705. https://doi.org/10.1097/CCM.0000000000003709.
52. Mustafa OG, Haq M, Dashora U, Castro E, Dhatariya KK, Joint British Diabetes Societies (JBDS) for Inpatient Care Group. Management of hyperosmolar hyperglycaemic state (HHS) in adults: an updated guideline from the Joint British Diabetes Societies (JBDS) for Inpatient Care Group. *Diabet Med*. 2023;40(3):e15005. https://doi.org/10.1111/dme.15005.
53. Long B, Willis GC, Lentz S, Koyfman A, Gottlieb M. Evaluation and management of the critically ill adult with diabetic ketoacidosis. *J Emerg Med*. 2020;59(3):371–383. https://doi.org/10.1016/j.jemermed.2020.06.059.
54. Long B, Lentz S, Koyfman A, Gottlieb M. Euglycemic diabetic ketoacidosis: etiologies, evaluation, and management. *Am J Emerg Med*. 2021;44:157–160. https://doi.org/10.1016/j.ajem.2021.02.015.
55. Dhatariya KK, Glaser NS, Codner E, Umpierrez GE. Diabetic ketoacidosis. *Nat Rev Dis Primers*. 2020;6(1):40. https://doi.org/10.1038/s41572-020-0165-1.
56. Umpierrez G, Korytkowski M. Diabetic emergencies – ketoacidosis, hyperglycaemic hyperosmolar state and hypoglycaemia. *Nat Rev Endocrinol*. 2016;12(4):222–232. https://doi.org/10.1038/nrendo.2016.15.
57. Virdi N, Poon Y, Abaniel R, Bergenstal RM. Prevalence, cost, and burden of diabetic ketoacidosis. *Diabetes Technol Ther*. 2023;25(S3):S75–S84. https://doi.org/10.1089/dia.2023.0149.
58. Angelousi A, Alexandraki KI, Mytareli C, Grossman AB, Kaltsas G. New developments and concepts in the diagnosis and management of diabetes insipidus (AVP-deficiency and resistance). *J Neuroendocrinol*. 2023;35(1):e13233. https://doi.org/10.1111/jne.13233.
59. Arima H, Cheetham T, Christ-Crain M, et al. Changing the name of diabetes insipidus: a position statement of the Working Group for Renaming Diabetes Insipidus. *J Clin Endocrinol Metab*. 2022;108(1):1–3. https://doi.org/10.1210/clinem/dgac547.
60. Harrois A, Anstey JR. Diabetes insipidus and syndrome of inappropriate antidiuretic hormone in critically ill patients. *Crit Care Clin*. 2019;35(2):187–200. https://doi.org/10.1016/j.ccc.2018.11.001.
61. Bockenhauer D, Bichet DG. Pathophysiology, diagnosis and management of nephrogenic diabetes insipidus. *Nat Rev Nephrol*. 2015;11(10):576–588. https://doi.org/10.1038/nrneph.2015.89.
62. Verbalis JG. Disorders of water metabolism: diabetes insipidus and the syndrome of inappropriate antidiuretic hormone secretion. *Handb Clin Neurol*. 2014;124:37–52. https://doi.org/10.1016/B978-0-444-59602-4.00003-4.
63. Atila C, Loughrey PB, Garrahy A, et al. Central diabetes insipidus from a patient's perspective: management, psychological co-morbidities, and renaming of the condition: results from an international web-based survey. *Lancet Diabetes Endocrinol*. 2022;10(10):700–709. https://doi.org/10.1016/S2213-8587(22)00219-4.
64. Warren AM, Grossmann M, Christ-Crain M, Russell N. Syndrome of inappropriate antidiuresis: from pathophysiology to management. *Endocr Rev*. 2023;44(5):819–861. https://doi.org/10.1210/endrev/bnad010.
65. Martin-Grace J, Tomkins M, O'Reilly MW, Thompson CJ, Sherlock M. Approach to the patient: hyponatremia and the Syndrome of Inappropriate Antidiuresis (SIAD). *J Clin Endocrinol Metab*. 2022;107(8):2362–2376. https://doi.org/10.1210/clinem/dgac245.
66. Fenske W, Sandner B, Christ-Crain M. A copeptin-based classification of the osmoregulatory defects in the syndrome of inappropriate antidiuresis. *Best Pract Res Clin Endocrinol Metab*. 2016;30(2):219–233. https://doi.org/10.1016/j.beem.2016.02.013.
67. Verbalis JG, Greenberg A, Burst V, et al. Diagnosing and treating the syndrome of inappropriate antidiuretic hormone secretion. *Am J Med*. 2016;129(5):537.e9–537.e23. https://doi.org/10.1016/j.amjmed.2015.11.005.
68. Sterns RH, Rondon-Berrios H, Adrogué HJ, et al. Treatment guidelines for hyponatremia: stay the course. *Clin J Am Soc Nephrol*. 2023. https://doi.org/10.2215/CJN.0000000000000244. Published online June 28.
69. Krisanapan P, Tangpanithandee S, Thongprayoon C, et al. Safety and efficacy of vaptans in the treatment of hyponatremia from syndrome of inappropriate antidiuretic hormone secretion (SIADH): a systematic review and meta-analysis. *J Clin Med*. 2023;12(17):5483. https://doi.org/10.3390/jcm12175483.
70. Verbalis JG, Goldsmith SR, Greenberg A, et al. Diagnosis, evaluation, and treatment of hyponatremia: expert panel recommendations. *Am J Med*. 2013;126(10 Suppl 1):S1–42. https://doi.org/10.1016/j.amjmed.2013.07.006.
71. Hoorn EJ, Zietse R. Diagnosis and treatment of hyponatremia: compilation of the guidelines. *J Am Soc Nephrol*. 2017;28(5):1340–1349. https://doi.org/10.1681/ASN.2016101139.
72. Ross DS, Burch HB, Cooper DS, et al. 2016 American Thyroid Association guidelines for diagnosis and management of hyperthyroidism and other causes of thyrotoxicosis. *Thyroid*. 2016;26(10):1343–1421. https://doi.org/10.1089/thy.2016.0229.
73. Lee SY, Pearce EN. Hyperthyroidism: a review. *JAMA*. 2023;330(15):1472–1483. https://doi.org/10.1001/jama.2023.19052.

74. Bourcier S, Coutrot M, Kimmoun A, et al. Thyroid storm in the ICU: a retrospective multicenter study. *Crit Care Med.* 2020;48(1):83–90. https://doi.org/10.1097/CCM.0000000000004078.
75. Chiha M, Samarasinghe S, Kabaker AS. Thyroid storm: an updated review. *J Intensive Care Med.* 2015;30(3):131–140. https://doi.org/10.1177/0885066613498053.
76. Garber JR, Cobin RH, Gharib H, et al. Clinical practice guidelines for hypothyroidism in adults: cosponsored by the American Association of Clinical Endocrinologists and the American Thyroid Association. *Endocr Pract.* 2012;18(6):988–1028. https://doi.org/10.4158/EP12280.GL.
77. Chiong YV, Bammerlin E, Mariash CN. Development of an objective tool for the diagnosis of myxedema coma. *Transl Res.* 2015;166(3):233–243. https://doi.org/10.1016/j.trsl.2015.01.003.
78. Bourcier S, Coutrot M, Ferré A, et al. Critically ill severe hypothyroidism: a retrospective multicenter cohort study. *Ann Intensive Care.* 2023;13(1):15. https://doi.org/10.1186/s13613-023-01112-1.
79. Popoveniuc G, Chandra T, Sud A, et al. A diagnostic scoring system for myxedema coma. *Endocr Pract.* 2014;20(8):808–817. https://doi.org/10.4158/EP13460. OR.
80. Bridwell RE, Willis GC, Gottlieb M, Koyfman A, Long B. Decompensated hypothyroidism: a review for the emergency clinician. *Am J Emerg Med.* 2021;39:207–212. https://doi.org/10.1016/j.ajem.2020.09.062.
81. Fassnacht M, Tsagarakis S, Terzolo M, et al. European Society of Endocrinology clinical practice guidelines on the management of adrenal incidentalomas, in collaboration with the European Network for the Study of Adrenal Tumors. *Eur J Endocrinol.* 2023;189(1):G1–G42. https://doi.org/10.1093/ejendo/lvad066.
82. Nieman LK, Biller BMK, Findling JW, et al. Treatment of Cushing's syndrome: an Endocrine Society clinical practice guideline. *J Clin Endocrinol Metab.* 2015;100(8):2807–2831. https://doi.org/10.1210/jc.2015-1818.
83. Funder JW, Carey RM, Mantero F, et al. The management of primary aldosteronism: case detection, diagnosis, and treatment: an Endocrine Society clinical practice guideline. *J Clin Endocrinol Metab.* 2016;101(5):1889–1916. https://doi.org/10.1210/jc.2015-4061.
84. Turcu AF, Yang J, Vaidya A. Primary aldosteronism – a multidimensional syndrome. *Nat Rev Endocrinol.* 2022;18(11):665–682. https://doi.org/10.1038/s41574-022-00730-2.
85. Vaidya A, Carey RM. Evolution of the primary aldosteronism syndrome: updating the approach. *J Clin Endocrinol Metab.* 2020;105(12):3771–3783. https://doi.org/10.1210/clinem/dgaa606.
86. Lenders JWM, Duh QY, Eisenhofer G, et al. Pheochromocytoma and paraganglioma: an Endocrine Society clinical practice guideline. *J Clin Endocrinol Metab.* 2014;99(6):1915–1942. https://doi.org/10.1210/jc.2014-1498.
87. Schreiner F, Beuschlein F. Disease monitoring of patients with pheochromocytoma or paraganglioma by biomarkers and imaging studies. *Best Pract Res Clin Endocrinol Metab.* 2020;34(2):101347. https://doi.org/10.1016/j.beem.2019.101347.
88. Bornstein SR, Allolio B, Arlt W, et al. Diagnosis and treatment of primary adrenal insufficiency: an Endocrine Society clinical practice guideline. *J Clin Endocrinol Metab.* 2016;101(2):364–389. https://doi.org/10.1210/jc.2015-1710.
89. Carsote M, Nistor C. Addison's disease: diagnosis and management strategies. *Int J Gen Med.* 2023;16:2187–2210. https://doi.org/10.2147/IJGM.S390793.
90. Mortimer B, Naganur VD, Satouris P, Greenfield JR, Torpy DJ, Rushworth RL. Acute illness in patients with concomitant Addison's disease and type 1 diabetes mellitus: increased incidence of hypoglycaemia and adrenal crises. *Clin Endocrinol (Oxf).* 2020;93(2):104–110. https://doi.org/10.1111/cen.14219.
91. Martin-Grace J, Dineen R, Sherlock M, Thompson CJ. Adrenal insufficiency: physiology, clinical presentation and diagnostic challenges. *Clin Chim Acta.* 2020;505:78–91. https://doi.org/10.1016/j.cca.2020.01.029.

32

Trauma

Eugene E. Mondor

http://evolve.elsevier.com/Urden/CriticalCareNursing

Trauma is the leading cause of death worldwide for all individuals aged 1 to 45 years.[1] Each year, injury costs the United States hundreds of billions of dollars. In 2019, it was estimated that both medical and work loss cost of injuries, including injury attributable to violence, was $4.2 trillion.[2] It is one of the most demanding health care issues in the United States today. Still, the effect of trauma on an individual's physical injury, psychological adjustment, lost time from work, disability, and costs to society remains largely underappreciated.

Trauma occurs in many forms. Motor vehicle collisions (MVCs) are the leading cause of death from injury worldwide, with more than 1.35 million deaths reported annually.[3] Injuries by firearms and stabbings are being reported with increasing frequency by trauma centers nationwide. Falls, sports-related injuries, work-related mishaps, and intentional self-harm produce physical injury. Coexisting illicit drug use and alcohol abuse are much more commonly encountered by trauma teams. Prehospital, emergency department (ED), and critical care professionals must actively participate in public education and injury prevention.

MECHANISM OF INJURY

Trauma occurs when an external force of energy impacts the body and causes structural or physiologic alterations or *injury*. External forces can be radiation, electrical, thermal, chemical, or mechanical forms of energy. Trauma that occurs from high-velocity impact (mechanical energy) is most common. Mechanical energy can produce blunt or penetrating traumatic injuries. Understanding the mechanism of injury helps health care practitioners predict potential injuries and anticipate the associated care that may be required.

Blunt Trauma

Blunt trauma is often seen with MVCs, falls, contact sports, or blunt-force injuries (e.g., trauma caused by a baseball bat). Blunt injury occurs because of the forces sustained during a rapid change in velocity (deceleration). To estimate the amount of force sustained in an MVC, multiply the person's weight by the miles per hour (speed) the vehicle was traveling. For example, a driver weighing 130 pounds traveling in a vehicle 60 miles/h that hits a brick wall would sustain 7800 pounds of force within milliseconds. As the body stops suddenly, tissues and internal organs continue to move forward. This sudden change in velocity can cause significant external and internal injury. Blunt injury may be difficult to diagnose, as injuries are not always obvious or readily apparent.

Penetrating Trauma

Penetrating injuries—those that puncture the body and damage internal structures—occur with gunshot wounds, stabbings, or other impalements. Damage is created along the path of penetration. Penetrating injuries can be misleading because the appearance of the external wound may not accurately reflect the extent of internal injury. For instance, bullets can create internal cavitation several times larger than the bullet's diameter. Several factors determine the extent of damage sustained due to penetrating trauma. For example, different weapons cause different types of injuries. The severity of a gunshot wound depends on the type of gun, ammunition used, and the distance and angle from which the gun was fired. Pellets from a shotgun blast expand on impact and cause multiple injuries to internal structures. Handgun bullets usually damage what is directly in the bullet's path. Inside the body, the bullet can ricochet off bone and create further damage. With penetrating stab wounds, factors determining the extent of injury include the type and length of object used and the insertion angle. Stab wounds typically produce less serious injury (but not always), as most stabbings are characteristically a low-velocity injury. Specific information that must be elicited about the mechanism of injury is summarized in Box 32.1.

PHASES OF TRAUMA CARE

Care of trauma victims during wartime has enhanced knowledge about trauma, triage, and the importance of rapid transport of injured individuals to medical facilities. Military experience has demonstrated that decreasing the time from injury to definitive care can save more lives. Care of critically injured individuals due to war has provided insight and knowledge that has helped improve civilian trauma care.

BOX 32.1 History of Mechanism of Injury

Blunt Trauma

- Motor vehicle crash extrication time
- Ejection
- Steering wheel deformation
- Location in automobile (passenger, driver, front seat, back seat)
- Restraint status (lap belt, shoulder harness, or combination; unrestrained)
- Speed of motor vehicles, the direction of impact
- Occupants (number and morbidity status)
- Height of fall

Penetrating Trauma

- Weapon used (handgun, shotgun, rifle, knife)
- Caliber of weapon
- Number of shots fired
- Position of victim and assailant when the injury occurred

BOX 32.2 Informatics

Trauma Registry

A trauma registry is a centralized database or system that collects, organizes, and analyzes information about traumatic injuries and their treatments. These data are primarily utilized for research, quality improvement, and policy development in trauma care and injury prevention. Trauma registries are commonly used in hospitals, trauma centers, and health care organizations to track and manage trauma patients' information. In the context of a trauma registry, informatics refers to the application of information technology and data management principles to gather, store, process, and retrieve data related to traumatic injuries. It involves using technology to effectively capture and analyze data for various purposes, including monitoring patient outcomes, identifying trends, and improving the overall quality of trauma care.

Here are some key aspects of trauma registries and informatics:

- Data Collection:
  - Trauma registries collect a wide range of data related to traumatic injuries, such as patient demographics, injury mechanisms, clinical assessments, interventions, outcomes, and follow-up information.
  - These data can be gathered from electronic health records, medical charts, diagnostic reports, and other sources.
- Data Standardization:
  - To ensure consistent and accurate data collection, trauma registries often use standardized data definitions and coding systems, such as the Abbreviated Injury Scale (AIS) or International Classification of Diseases (ICD) codes.
  - Standardization facilitates meaningful comparisons and analyses across different institutions and regions.
- Data Entry:
  - Health care professionals input data into the trauma registry.
  - This activity may involve manual data entry or integration with electronic health record systems for automated data capture.
- Data Analysis:
  - Informatics techniques are applied to the collected data to derive insights, trends, and patterns. Statistical analyses and data visualization tools help health care providers and researchers understand the epidemiology of traumatic injuries, treatment effectiveness, and patient outcomes.
- Quality Improvement:
  - Trauma registries play a crucial role in quality improvement initiatives by identifying areas where trauma care can be enhanced.
  - Regular analysis of registry data can reveal opportunities to streamline processes, reduce complications, and improve patient outcomes.
- Research and Education:
  - The data stored in trauma registries can be used for research purposes to advance knowledge in trauma care.
  - Additionally, registries provide a valuable resource for the training and education of health care professionals involved in trauma management.
- Policy Development:
  - Governments, health care organizations, and public health agencies can use trauma registry data to develop evidence-based policies and interventions to reduce the incidence of traumatic injuries and improve patient care.
- Collaboration and Benchmarking:
  - Trauma centers and hospitals can benchmark their performance against regional, national, or international standards using aggregated data from trauma registries.
  - This activity facilitates a collaborative approach to improving trauma care across different health care facilities.

In summary, trauma registries and informatics are integral to advancing the field of trauma care by providing a systematic way to collect, analyze, and leverage data for research, quality improvement, and policy development. These tools contribute to better patient outcomes and enhance trauma care practices.

Historically, studies reported and statistics demonstrated that deaths resulting from trauma occurred in a trimodal distribution.[4] Development of the Advanced Trauma Life Support (ATLS) guidelines by the American College of Surgeons has enhanced the assessment skills of prehospital care practitioners, expedited transport of critically injured patients, identified the importance of designated trauma care centers, created evidence-based protocols for injured patients, and focused on injury prevention, all which have affected the timing of death after trauma. The development of trauma registries has also contributed to this effort (Box 32.2). With the improvements in trauma resuscitation just described, most deaths occur in a bimodal distribution (Fig. 32.1).[5]

The first peak of trauma deaths occurs within 48 hours after initial injury, and the second peak occurs days to weeks after injury. In the first peak, death often occurs on the scene or very soon after admission to the hospital, usually due to severe traumatic brain injury (TBI) or hemorrhage. During the second peak, death frequently occurs in the critical care unit (CCU) because of complications from the initial injury, such as infection or multiple-organ dysfunction syndrome (MODS). Trauma patients who develop MODS have mortality estimated to be as high as 30%.[6]

The *golden hour* of trauma resuscitation is often viewed as a critical time frame in which the injured patient will die unless definitive care is delivered. However, the golden hour should not be considered a time frame but rather a "window of opportunity" for all trauma care practitioners. Components of the golden hour incorporate activation of emergency medical services, stabilization and transport, triage, initial resuscitation, early surgical consultation, and provision of critical care. The primary goal for a critically injured trauma patient is to minimize the time from injury to definitive care. There is no evidence to suggest that survival rates dramatically decrease in trauma patients after 60 minutes.

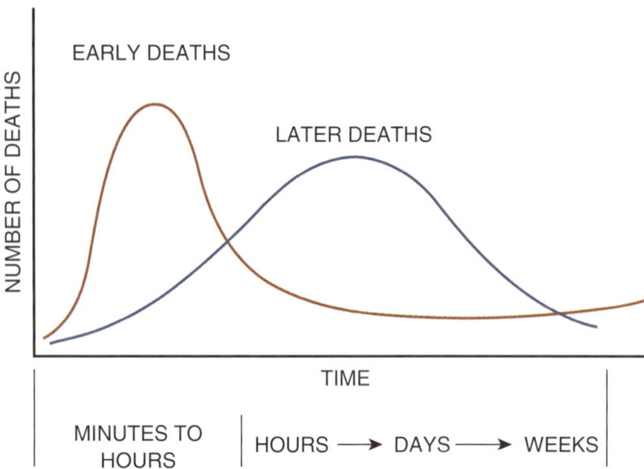

FIG. 32.1 Bimodal Distribution of Trauma Deaths.

Significant advances have been made in managing patients with traumatic injuries in the prehospital, emergency department, and critical care settings. Nursing management of a patient with traumatic injury begins the moment a call for help is received and continues until the patient's death or return to the community. Patients with multiple traumatic injuries are frequently admitted to CCUs, requiring complex nursing care. The care of a trauma patient is viewed on a continuum that includes numerous phases and locations: prehospital care, ED, damage control resuscitation, critical care, intermediate care, and rehabilitation.

Prehospital Care

The goal of prehospital care is the immediate identification of life-threatening injuries and transport (ground or air) to the closest appropriate medical facility. Airway maintenance, recognition and control of external bleeding and shock, and patient immobilization are essential priorities. Initiation of a peripheral intravenous (IV) line, splinting of fractures, and pain management are also vital components. Prehospital personnel should communicate information needed for triage before arrival at the hospital. Advanced planning for multiple-injured patients by trauma teams is essential.

Emergency Department

The ATLS guidelines assist health care practitioners with the essential actions for rapid assessment, immediate identification of life-threatening injuries, and initial resuscitation of trauma patients in the ED.[7] These guiding principles delineate a systematic approach to the initial assessment and care of a trauma patient that includes a rapid primary survey, resuscitation of vital organ systems, a more detailed secondary survey, and initiation of the most appropriate care. Initially developed for physicians, these guidelines have been adopted worldwide by prehospital care practitioners and trauma teams, including emergency and critical care nurses, and provides the framework for the ABCDEs of trauma care.

Primary Survey

On arrival of the trauma patient in the ED, the primary survey is initiated. This initial assessment aims to identify and treat any life-threatening injuries that, if left untreated, could potentially cause the patient's death.

The five steps in the ATLS primary survey are commonly referred to as the *ABCDEs* of trauma resuscitation (Table 32.1):

- **A**irway patency with cervical spine protection
- **B**reathing and ventilation
- **C**irculation with hemorrhage control
- **D**isability: Neurologic status
- **E**xposure or environmental control

Although many trauma centers use this approach, there is ever-present awareness that many trauma patients die from bleeding. Consequently, many trauma facilities have informally adopted the military's *C-ABCDE* approach, where the additional "C" stands for catastrophic hemorrhage.[8] This slight modification to the *ABCDE* approach of ATLS is intended to emphasize the importance of the immediate assessment, identification, and implementation of measures to control hemorrhage in a trauma patient without becoming overly preoccupied with other primary survey components.

Airway. The patient's airway is assessed for patency and possible airway obstruction. Trauma patients are at risk for ineffective airway clearance, especially in the presence of altered consciousness, effects of drugs and alcohol, and maxillofacial or thoracic injuries. Foreign bodies, blood clots, or broken teeth can cause airway obstruction. Airway patency is assessed by inspecting the oropharynx for foreign body obstruction and listening for air movement at the nose and mouth. If the patient can verbally communicate, the airway is likely patent. Patients with a Glasgow Coma Scale (GCS) score of 8 or less or who cannot protect their airway often require placement of a definitive airway.[9] Airway placement must incorporate cervical spine immobilization. The patient's head and neck should not be rotated, hyperflexed, or hyperextended. The cervical spine must be immobilized at all times in all trauma patients until a cervical spinal cord injury (SCI) has been ruled out.

Breathing. The patient is assessed for signs of visible chest movement. An open, clear airway does not always ensure adequate ventilation and gas exchange. Assessment includes visual inspection of chest wall integrity and respiratory rate, depth, and symmetry. Auscultation is performed to assess the presence or absence of breath sounds. Decreased or absent breath sounds or alteration in chest wall integrity may necessitate chest tube placement. Supplemental oxygen is administered to some injured patients. However, it may not be required in the spontaneously breathing trauma patient who is awake, alert, talking, and has a peripheral capillary oxygen saturation (SpO_2) greater than 92%.[10] Endotracheal intubation may be required for patients with a compromised airway caused by mechanical factors, who are unconscious, or who have ventilatory problems. Needle or surgical cricothyroidotomy may be necessary when severe maxillofacial trauma exists, and endotracheal intubation is not an option.[11]

Circulation. The next step is to assess for a palpable pulse and any evidence of external or internal bleeding and, if possible, obtain a baseline measurement of the patient's vital signs. Rapid evaluation of circulatory status includes assessment of level of consciousness (LOC), skin color, and pulse. The LOC provides data on cerebral perfusion. Facial color that is ashen or gray and extremities that are pale or slightly mottled may be ominous

TABLE 32.1 **Primary Survey of Trauma Patient**

Survey Component	Trauma Team Assessment	Immediate Care
A—Airway	Immediately assess the patient's ability to speak Look Are there obvious signs of airway trauma, tachypnea, or accessory muscle use? Listen Can you hear the patient breathing? Feel For air exchange through the mouth Palpate for tracheal deviation	Immobilize spine Nondefinitive airway management Oropharyngeal (unconscious patient) Nasopharyngeal (conscious patient) When in doubt, secure the airway Endotracheal intubation Emergency cricothyrotomy
B—Breathing	Is the patient breathing? Look Is the patient's chest rising and falling? Respiratory rate, rhythm, symmetry Is there any evidence of thoracic trauma? Listen Quickly auscultate air entry Is there air entry in all lobes? Palpate Chest wall integrity	Administer supplemental oxygen For life-threatening conditions (e.g., tension pneumothorax), immediate needle decompression, then chest tube insertion Full-support mechanical ventilation (as required)
C—Circulation	Assess pulse quality and rate Assess for life-threatening conditions (e.g., uncontrolled bleeding, shock) Examine and feel the patient's skin Warm and dry Cool, pale, and clammy	Signs and symptoms of poor tissue perfusion Initiate IV access Administer 1 L of isotonic IV fluid, then reassess hemodynamic status If no pulse, begin CPR
D—Disability	Neurologic assessment GCS score Pupils: Size and reactivity? Is the patient moving all four limbs to command? Any evidence of posturing?	Consider early neurosurgical consultation Consider an early CT scan
E—Exposure	All clothing removed to inspect all body regions Any lacerations, abrasions, or bruises? Stab wounds: Entrance? Gunshot wounds: Entrance? Exit?	Prevent hypothermia Warm blankets Warm IV fluids Increase room temperature

CPR, Cardiopulmonary resuscitation; *CT*, computed tomography; *GCS*, Glasgow Coma Scale; *IV*, intravenous.

signs of hypovolemia and shock. Central pulses (i.e., carotid artery, femoral) are assessed bilaterally for rate, regularity, and quality. Cardiopulmonary resuscitation (CPR) must be initiated immediately if a pulse is absent.

All trauma patients are considered to be in shock. Trauma patients may or may not exhibit significant deterioration in hemodynamic stability. Trauma teams know that vital signs can initially remain stable even in the face of bleeding. Measurement and trending of systolic and diastolic blood pressure, mean arterial pressure (MAP), and SpO_2 readings are more important than individual values. Hypotension in trauma should be attributed to hypovolemia until proven otherwise.[12] External exsanguination is identified and controlled by direct manual pressure on the wound. Internal hemorrhage in trauma requires urgent surgical consultation and transport to interventional radiology for diagnostic imaging or the operating room (OR) for immediate surgery.

Disability. A rapid neurologic assessment is performed. The patient's baseline LOC, pupil size, and reaction are assessed and documented during this vital step. The *AVPU* method can be used to quickly describe the patient's LOC:

- A: Alert
- V: Responds to verbal stimuli
- P: Responds to painful stimuli
- U: Unresponsive

The GCS score can also be used (see Table 21.1).

Exposure. In the final step of the primary survey, all the patient's clothing is removed to facilitate a thorough examination of all body surfaces for the presence of injury. The patient is turned (logrolled) while full spinal precautions are maintained. The spine is carefully palpated for obvious deformity. The occipital lobe, neck, back, buttocks, and extremities are quickly examined for wounds, impaled objects, and bleeding. Immediately after inspection, the patient must be protected from hypothermia. This step can be accomplished through warm blankets, increasing room temperature, and warm IV fluids.

Secondary Survey

The secondary survey begins when the primary survey is completed, after potentially life-threatening injuries have been identified and resuscitation initiated. In reality, primary and secondary surveys may occur almost simultaneously. However, the secondary survey is a more detailed, in-depth physical examination of the trauma patient. A head-to-toe approach is used to examine each body region thoroughly during the secondary survey.

During the secondary survey, the nurse ensures the completion of all necessary procedures, such as an electrocardiogram, radiographic studies (cervical spine, chest, and pelvis), insertion of gastric and urinary catheters, and blood tests. Throughout this survey, the nurse continuously monitors the patient's vital signs (heart rate, blood pressure, MAP, and SpO_2) and response to resuscitation interventions. Emotional support to the patient and family is imperative.

Patient history is also an essential aspect of the secondary survey. The patient's pertinent history can be assessed by use of the mnemonic *AMPLE:*

A: **A**llergies
M: **M**edications (including prescription and nonprescription drugs)
P: **P**ast medical illnesses/**p**regnancy
L: **L**ast meal
E: **E**vents/**e**nvironment related to the injury

Head injury, shock, or the use of drugs and alcohol may preclude obtaining information from the patient. Prehospital care practitioners (paramedics, emergency medical technicians), family members, or sometimes bystanders can be excellent sources of information.

Hemorrhagic shock. Hypovolemic shock resulting from hemorrhage is the most common type of shock in trauma patients.[13] The traditional signs and symptoms of hemorrhagic hypovolemic shock may not appear until approximately 30% to 40% of circulating blood volume is lost.[7] Hemorrhage in trauma must be identified and treated rapidly. To manage this situation two large-bore (14-gauge to 16-gauge) peripheral IV catheters are inserted to administer fluids. If unable to use peripheral IV catheters, an intraosseous device or central venous catheter may be inserted. Initial blood samples to be drawn from trauma patients are identified in Box 32.3. The ideal IV fluid for trauma resuscitation has not been established. Current ATLS guidelines suggest an initial infusion of 1 L of 0.9% normal saline or lactated Ringer solution.[7] Both crystalloid solutions are physiologically isotonic, provide volume to the volume-depleted patient, and are often readily available. For more information about hypovolemic shock see Chapter 33.

When IV fluid is administered, trauma patients may be categorized as *responders, transient responders*, or *nonresponders.*[14] *Responders* are patients whose hemodynamics steadily improve with IV fluid administration. *Transient responders* may exhibit temporary stabilization of vital signs, followed by a decline in patient condition. *Nonresponders* are the most problematic. These patients do not respond to IV fluid, which often indicates that internal bleeding may be present. Overaggressive volume resuscitation with IV fluids must be avoided to prevent unnecessary complications such as pulmonary edema or exacerbation of hemorrhage.

Damage control resuscitation. Damage control resuscitation is an evidence-based strategy employed in trauma centers worldwide to control and assist in stabilizing the trauma patient in hemorrhagic shock.[15] Components of damage control resuscitation include permissive hypotension, massive transfusion protocols, and damage control surgery.[11] Damage control resuscitation begins in the field and continues through the ED, OR, and CCU.

Permissive hypotension. Most trauma practitioners employ permissive hypotension. Permissive hypotension involves low-volume IV fluid resuscitation.[7] The goal is to maintain the blood pressure low enough to prevent the worsening of hemorrhage but high enough to maintain perfusion of vital organs, including the brain. Under any circumstances, it is not considered a substitute for surgical control of bleeding in the hemorrhaging trauma patient.

In adult trauma patients, some authors suggest targeting a systolic blood pressure (SBP) of 70 to 90 mm Hg and MAP of 50 mm Hg,[16] but these targets have not been universally adopted. Individualized assessment of each trauma patient is mandatory. Aggressively infusing IV fluid into a trauma patient may dilute clotting factors, disrupt any formed clots, and exacerbate bleeding. Permissive hypotension is contraindicated in TBI and pregnancy.

Massive transfusion protocols. Given the current emphasis on using blood products over crystalloids and correcting trauma-induced coagulopathy, many trauma centers have developed *massive transfusion protocols* (MTP). While a small percentage of trauma patients require an MTP, having a defined protocol serves as a system-based strategy to facilitate the early, timely release of blood products in what can often be a chaotic situation. The MTP outlines the ratio of packed red blood cells, fresh frozen plasma, platelets, and cryoprecipitate to be administered. This situation is referred to as *hemostatic resuscitation*, where blood components are administered in a ratio that resembles whole blood.[13,17] The optimal ratio of blood components to be administered to bleeding trauma patients is a major focus in trauma research.

Tranexamic acid is an antifibrinolytic agent used to stop bleeding in trauma patients. It is given IV as a loading dose and subsequent IV infusion over 1 hour. *Thromboelastography*, or *TEG*, is a newer technique whereby real-time point-of-care testing of the coagulation profile can be done at the bedside of the trauma patient.[18] Based on the patient's coagulation profile, *TEG* helps identify the most critical blood component required of the trauma patient when the sample is drawn and the results obtained.

Damage control surgery. Trauma is sometimes referred to as a "surgical disease" because the nature and extent of injuries usually require operative management. Damage control surgery is a well-established concept in trauma care. Damage control surgery is a strategy of providing essential surgical interventions to control hemorrhage and limit contamination.[19] The goal is to optimize the physiology of the actively bleeding patient, not complete definitive repair. Permissive hypotension and massive transfusion protocols are often employed simultaneously during damage control surgery. Reconstruction and formal closure of wounds are usually not completed until after resuscitation and stabilization of the patient in the CCU have occurred.

BOX 32.3 Recommended Initial Blood Samples in Trauma Patients

- Complete blood cell (CBC) count
- Electrolyte profile (Na^+, K^+, Cl^-, carbon dioxide, glucose, blood urea nitrogen, creatinine)
- Coagulation parameters: prothrombin time, partial thromboplastin time
- Type and screen (ABO compatibility)
- Amylase
- Toxicology screens
- Liver function studies
- Pregnancy test (for women of childbearing age)
- Lactate

BOX 32.4 Transfer Report Using SBAR Method

S: Situation	Age Sex Mechanism of injury/injuries sustained Admission diagnosis/chief complaint; any loss of consciousness (duration) and current Glasgow Coma Scale score Diagnostic tests and procedures completed Current issues, including any physical assessment abnormalities requiring acute interventions
B: Background	Significant medical and surgical history Home medications
A: Assessments	Current assessment findings, including vital signs, level of consciousness, established airway, and mechanical ventilation settings Medications administered (opiates, sedatives, antibiotics, antifibrinolytics) Diagnostic test results (e.g., completed radiographs, CT scan, angiography) Laboratory results (including implementation of massive transfusion protocol) Family members present and assessment of their current knowledge of the situation, extent of injuries, and treatment plan
R: Recommendations	Identification of any immediate treatment required Description of resuscitation plan, including blood products, diagnostic imaging, possible surgery

Critical Care Phase

Transfer Report

Critically injured trauma patients are frequently admitted to the CCU as direct transfers from the ED, diagnostic imaging, or OR. The critical care team must be aware of all resuscitation strategies that have been initiated up until admission to the CCU. Upon transfer the information needed from prehospital, ED, or OR personnel can be summarized using the **SBAR** communication tool: **S**ituation, **B**ackground, **A**ssessment, and **R**ecommendations (Box 32.4). This information is ideally obtained before the patient's admission to the CCU to ensure the availability of needed personnel, equipment, and supplies. However, this may not always be possible. Table 32.2 summarizes the effects of prehospital, ED, and OR resuscitation measures that can affect the initial management of the trauma patient in the CCU.

Repeat Primary and Secondary Survey

Immediately after the patient arrives in the CCU, the nurse repeats the primary and secondary surveys per ATLS guidelines. Priority nursing care during the critical care phase includes ongoing, repeated physical assessments, monitoring laboratory and diagnostic test results, and observing trends in the patient's response to treatment. The nurse is aware that the second peak of the bimodal distribution of trauma deaths occurs most often in the critical care setting due to complications including prolonged shock states, acute respiratory distress syndrome (ARDS), sepsis, and MODS. Ongoing nursing assessments are imperative for early detection and treatment of complications.

TABLE 32.2 Effects of Trauma Resuscitation

Aspect of Injury or Resuscitation	Effect on Critical Care Management
Prolonged extrication time	Loss of perfusion to vital organs Severity of shock state
Respiratory or cardiac arrest	Loss of perfusion to the brain (anoxic injury), kidneys, and other vital organs
Time on backboard	Potentiates risk of skin breakdown and pressure injuries to the occipital lobe, scapulae, sacrum, coccyx, and heels
Number of units of blood; whether any were not fully crossmatched; packed cells vs. whole blood used	Potentiates risk of acute respiratory distress syndrome (ARDS) and multiple organ dysfunction syndrome (MODS)
Prolonged transportation to a definitive trauma facility	Worsening of patient condition during transport (e.g., hypotension, ongoing bleeding, acid–base imbalance, oxygenation, or ventilation issues) New-onset bleeding or rebleeding decreases perfusion to vital organs

TABLE 32.3 Factors Predisposing Trauma Patients to Impaired Oxygenation

Factor	Impairment
Impaired ventilation	Injury to airway structures, loss of central nervous system regulation of breathing, impaired level of consciousness
Impaired pulmonary gas diffusion	Pneumothorax, hemothorax Aspiration of gastric contents Shifts to the left of oxyhemoglobin dissociation curve (can result from infusion of large volumes of banked blood, hypocarbia or alkalosis, or hypothermia)
Decreased oxygen supply	Reduced hemoglobin (from hemorrhage) Reduced cardiac output (cardiovascular injury, decreased preload from hemorrhage)

Prevention of Hypoxemia

One of the most essential nursing roles is the ongoing assessment of oxygen delivery (supply) and oxygen demand (consumption). Oxygen delivery must be optimized to prevent further system damage. The trauma patient is at high risk for impaired oxygenation due to various factors (Table 32.3). Risk factors must be promptly identified and treated to prevent life-threatening sequelae. Prevention and treatment of hypoxemia depend on accurate assessment of the adequacy of pulmonary gas exchange (arterial blood gas), oxygen supply (fraction of inspired oxygen), and oxygen consumption (assessment of LOC, tissue perfusion, capillary refill, urinary output).

Prevention of Acidosis, Hypothermia, and Coagulopathy

Acidosis (pH less than 7.2), hypothermia (temperature less than 35°C), and clinical coagulopathy are often present in trauma patients. This combination of factors is known as the *lethal triad of death*.[16] For example, hypothermia induced by an open visceral cavity in conjunction with a massive blood transfusion can lead to coagulopathy and continued bleeding, which results in shock and metabolic acidosis. The triad of hypothermia, coagulopathy, and acidosis creates a self-propagating cycle that can eventually lead to an irreversible physiologic insult.

Most recently, trauma teams are becoming increasingly aware of the need to monitor calcium levels during trauma resuscitation. Low calcium levels in trauma patients result from hemodilution from overaggressive IV fluid resuscitation and citrate-containing blood products.[15] As a result, hypocalcemic patients are predisposed to arrhythmias and alterations in coagulation. Calcium levels less than 0.9 mmol/L have been associated with increased mortality rates in trauma patients.[20] The addition of hypocalcemia to the lethal triad has been termed by some as the *diamond of death*.[21] The goal is to continue resuscitation and assist in correcting hypothermia, coagulopathy, acidosis, and hypocalcemia. Rewarming techniques are described in Table 32.4.

Endpoints in Trauma Resuscitation

During resuscitation, all attempts are made to improve cellular oxygenation. Resuscitation aims to ensure adequate tissue perfusion with fluid, oxygen, and nutrients to support cellular function. No single resuscitation endpoint is sufficient. Resuscitation endpoints (variables or parameters) must be viewed across the continuum of trauma resuscitation.

During resuscitation from traumatic hemorrhagic shock, normalization of standard clinical parameters such as blood pressure, heart rate, and urine output is inadequate.[22] Resuscitation endpoints must include physiological, hematologic, and metabolic parameters. Base deficit and lactic acid (lactate) have been well studied in trauma and used to help assess the adequacy of cellular oxygenation and predict the risk of bleeding[23] and 72-hour mortality after injury.[24] Optimal resuscitation endpoints in different types of trauma are ongoing research areas in trauma care.

Frequent and thorough assessments of all body systems are the cornerstone of medical and nursing management of critically injured trauma patients in critical care. These actions can detect subtle changes in patient condition and facilitate the implementation of timely therapeutic interventions to prevent complications often associated with trauma. The nurse must be knowledgeable about specific organ injuries and their associated sequelae. This chapter focuses on the nursing management of adult patients with traumatic injuries in the critical care setting.

SOCIAL DETERMINANTS OF HEALTH

Health Disparities Associated With Trauma

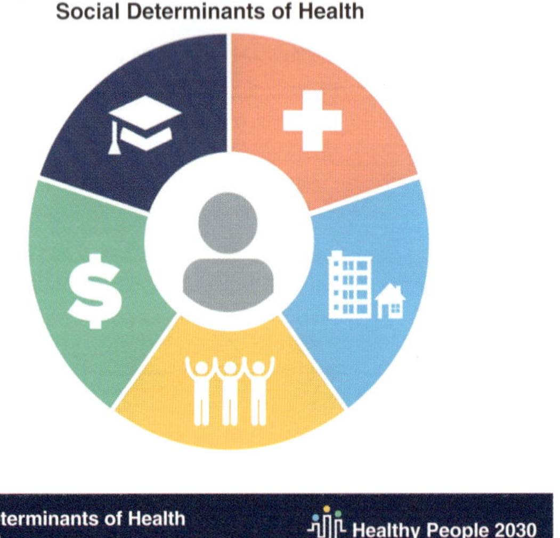

Social disparities can significantly impact a person's exposure to trauma and their ability to recover from it. Individuals from marginalized communities, such as low-income families and communities of color, may be more likely to experience trauma due to increased exposure to violence, crime, and environmental stressors.[1]

Moreover, these individuals may also encounter barriers to accessing adequate resources for recovery, such as quality health care, therapy, and support groups. Language barriers, lack of insurance or finances, and stigma surrounding mental health can all contribute to disparities in trauma recovery.

Social inequality can directly affect an individual's physiological response to trauma. Chronic stress and trauma can lead to an increased risk of health problems, such as cardiovascular disease and obesity, particularly for those who do not have access to resources that promote healthy coping mechanisms.

In conclusion, social disparities and trauma are intimately linked, with those experiencing social inequities being more susceptible to trauma and experiencing more barriers to recovery. Bridging these gaps in resources and support is critical for addressing the impact of trauma on marginalized communities.

Strategies to improve these disparities include the development of:

Improve access to trauma care services, including emergency medical services (EMS), trauma centers, and rehabilitation facilities.

Enhance cultural competence among health care providers to improve communication and understanding between patients and health care professionals.

Improve health literacy among trauma patients by providing clear and understandable information about their condition, treatment options, and posttrauma care.

Implement community outreach programs to raise awareness about trauma prevention, early recognition of trauma symptoms, and appropriate response during emergencies.

Increase diversity among health care providers to better reflect the communities they serve.

Implement trauma-informed care principles throughout the health care system. This approach recognizes the impact of trauma on patients' lives and emphasizes safety, trustworthiness, collaboration, and empowerment in health care interactions.

Reference:

1. Bradley AS, Adeleke IO, Estime SR. Healthcare disparities in trauma: Why they exist and what we can do. *Curr Opin Anaesthesiol.* 2022;35(2):150–153. https://doi.org/10.1097/ACO.0000000000001094.

Illustration from Healthy People 2030, U.S. Department of Health and Human Services, Office of Disease Prevention and Health Promotion. Retrieved August 23, 2023, from https://health.gov/healthypeople/objectives-and-data/social-determinants-health.

TABLE 32.4 Interventions for Rewarming Trauma Patients

Intervention	External Rewarming Procedures	Internal Rewarming Procedures
Passive (Protect patient from heat loss, patient will increase body temperature)	Remove all wet, bloody clothing and linen. Cover the patient with blankets. Expose only those body parts being examined. Avoid bathing the patient until normothermia is achieved. Maintain a warm temperature in the resuscitation room.	
Active (Delivery of heat to the trauma patient, either externally or internally)	Use heating blankets, forced warm air, or pads.	Administer warm, humidified oxygen. Administer warm IV fluids. Administer warm blood products. Perform thoracic, peritoneal, or bladder lavage with warm solutions. Extracorporeal rewarming Intravascular catheters

IV, Intravenous.

SPECIFIC TRAUMA INJURIES

Traumatic Brain Injuries

More than 69 million TBIs occur worldwide each year.[25] In the United States, almost 3 million TBIs are estimated to occur annually.[26] In 2021, approximately 69,000 Americans died and 223,000 were hospitalized with TBI.[27] More than 5 million Americans live with some form of long-term disability due to TBI. TBI can be caused by both blunt and penetrating trauma. The leading causes of TBI include MVCs, violence (suicide and firearm injuries), and falls.[26] Adults 65 years old and older with a TBI that requires hospitalization have the highest percentage of TBI-related mortality.[28] It is estimated that TBI costs the USA approximately 400 billion dollars annually.[29]

Degree of Traumatic Brain Injury

Mild brain injury. Mild TBI is described as a GCS score of 13 to 15 with a loss of consciousness that lasts up to 15 minutes. Patients with mild injury are seen in the ED and often discharged home with a family member who is instructed to evaluate the patient routinely and to bring the patient back to the hospital if any further neurological symptoms appear.

Moderate brain injury. Moderate TBI is described as a GCS score of 9 to 12 with a loss of consciousness for up to 6 hours. Patients with this type of TBI are usually hospitalized. They are at high risk for deterioration from increasing cerebral edema and intracranial pressure (ICP), and serial neurologic assessments are essential. Hemodynamic and ICP monitoring and ventilatory support are usually not required for these patients unless other bodily injuries make them necessary. A computed tomography (CT) scan is obtained on admission. Repeat CT scans are indicated if the patient's neurologic status deteriorates.

Severe brain injury. Patients with a GCS score of 8 or less after resuscitation or patients who deteriorate to that level within 48 hours of admission have a severe TBI.[30] Loss of consciousness may be 6 hours or longer. These patients are admitted to the CCU for continuous neurologic assessment, hemodynamic monitoring, mechanical ventilation, and management of complex care issues. Serial CT scans may be performed to rule out evidence of ongoing bleeding or mass lesions that can be surgically corrected.

Etiology

Injuries of the skull and brain are described by the mechanism of injury, location of injury in the brain, and anatomic changes or losses that occur. Some of the most common abnormalities seen in neurologic trauma are described here.

Skull fracture. Skull fractures are common, but they do not by themselves cause neurologic deficits. Skull fractures can be classified as open (dura mater is torn) or closed (dura mater is not torn), or they can be classified as fractures of the vault or fractures of the base. Common vault fractures occur in the frontal and parietal regions. Basilar skull fractures are usually not visible on conventional skull radiographs; a CT scan is typically required. Assessment findings may include cerebrospinal fluid (CSF) leakage—described as rhinorrhea (from the nose) or otorrhea (from the ear), Battle sign (ecchymosis overlying the mastoid process behind the ear), "raccoon eyes" (subconjunctival and periorbital ecchymosis), or palsy of the seventh cranial nerve.

The significance of a skull fracture is that it identifies a patient with a higher probability of having or developing an intracranial hematoma. A significant amount of force is required to fracture the skull. This external force is evident in Fig. 32.2A, which shows a CT scan of a depressed skull fracture with brain tissue injury. In the same patient, the fragmentation of bone in the skull fracture is even more apparent in the bone window scan shown in Fig. 32.2B. Bone window views help identify bone tumors, and in trauma patients with TBI, a bone window scan provides an enhanced view of cranial abnormalities.

Open skull fractures require surgical intervention to remove bony fragments and close the dura mater. Major complications of basilar skull fractures are cranial nerve injury and CSF leakage. A CSF leak may result in a fistula, which increases the possibility of bacterial contamination and subsequent meningitis.

Concussion. A concussion is a brain injury accompanied by a brief loss of neurologic function, in particular, loss of consciousness. When loss of consciousness occurs, it may last for a few seconds to an hour. Neurologic dysfunctions include confusion, disorientation, and sometimes a period of anterograde or retrograde amnesia.[31] Other clinical manifestations after a concussion are headache, dizziness, nausea, irritability, inability to concentrate, impaired memory, and fatigue. The diagnosis of concussion is based primarily on patient history.

Contusion. Contusion, or "bruising" of the brain, is frequently associated with acceleration–deceleration injuries, which result in bleeding into the superficial parenchyma. Frontal or temporal lobe contusions are most common and can be seen in a *coup–contrecoup mechanism of injury* (Fig. 32.3A). Coup injury affects the cerebral tissue directly under the point of impact. Contrecoup injury occurs in a line directly opposite the point of impact (Fig. 32.3B). The brain contusions caused by the coup and contrecoup impact are visible on a CT scan (Fig. 32.3C).

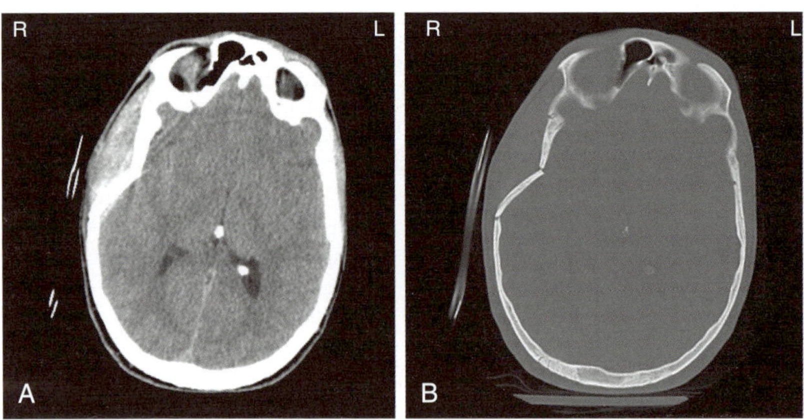

FIG. 32.2 (A) Computed tomography scan of depressed skull fracture shows both brain tissue injury and bone injury. (B) Bone window scan of the same depressed skull fracture more clearly shows the displaced fragments of bone.

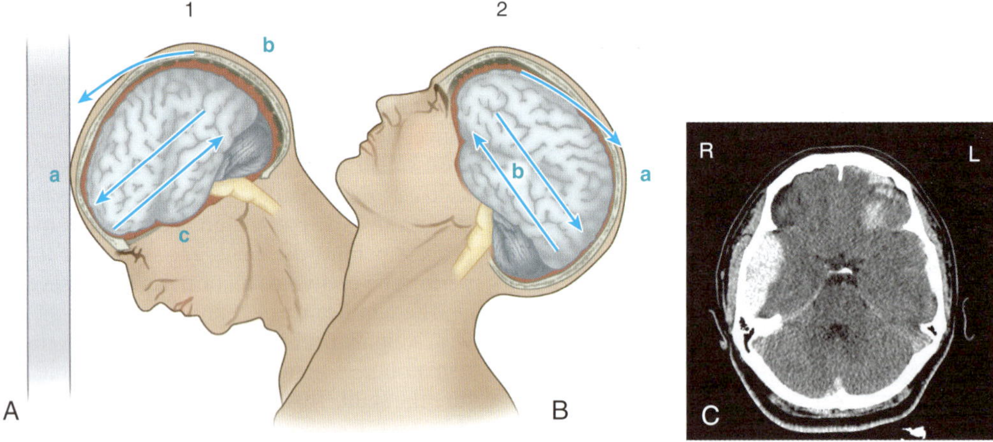

FIG. 32.3 Coup and Contrecoup Head Injury After Blunt Trauma. (A) Coup injury: impact against an object, showing the site of impact and *(a)* direct trauma to the brain, *(b)* shearing of subdural veins, and *(c)* trauma to the base of the brain. (B) Contrecoup injury: impact within the skull, showing *(a)* the site of impact from the brain hitting the opposite side of the skull and *(b)* shearing forces throughout the brain. These injuries occur in one continuous motion; the head strikes the wall (coup) and then rebounds (contrecoup). (C) Computed tomography (CT) scan of a coup and contrecoup head injury. The primary injury is located in the right parietal region, with the contrecoup injury in the left frontal/temporal area. Note that a CT scan is always shown as if the reader is looking at the patient from the foot of the bed, so that right (R) and left (L) are reversed.

Clinical manifestations of a contusion are related to the location of the injury, the degree of contusion, and the presence of associated lesions. Contusions can be small, in which localized areas of dysfunction result in a focal neurologic deficit. Larger contusions can evolve over 2 to 3 days after injury due to further edema and hemorrhage. For this reason, a repeat CT scan in the first 24 hours is often required. A large contusion can produce a mass effect that can cause a significant increase in ICP. Contusions may lead to the development of intracerebral hematomas.

Contusions of the tips of the temporal lobe are common and of particular concern. Because the inner aspects of the temporal lobe surround the opening in the tentorium (where the midbrain enters the cerebrum), edema in this area can cause a rapid deterioration in LOC and can lead to herniation. Because of the particular location of this injury, deterioration can occur with little or no warning.

Diagnosis of contusion is made by CT scan. If contusions are small, focal, or multiple, they are treated medically with serial neurologic assessments. Larger contusions that produce considerable mass effect may require surgical intervention to reduce edema and elevations in ICP. The nurse must pay specific attention to neurologic assessment findings and look for subtle changes in pupillary signs, vital signs, or neurologic signs (e.g., weakness, speech problems), which may indicate a potential worsening of the patient's condition. The outcome of cerebral contusion is highly variable.

Cerebral hematoma. Extravasation of blood creates a space-occupying lesion within the cranial vault that can lead to increased ICP. Three types of hematomas are discussed here and illustrated in Fig. 32.4. The first two, epidural hematoma (EDH) and subdural hematoma (SDH), are extraparenchymal (outside of brain tissue) and produce injury by pressure and displacement of intracranial contents. The third type is intraparenchymal, occurring within the brain tissue. Traumatic intracerebral hemorrhage (ICH) directly damages neural tissue and can produce further injury due to pressure and displacement of intracranial contents.

Epidural hematoma. EDH is a collection of blood between the inner skull and the outermost layer of the dura mater (see Fig. 32.4A). EDH occurs due to trauma to the skull and meninges, as seen in the CT scan in Fig. 32.5A. On a CT scan, brain tissue appears dark gray, and any collection of blood appears light gray. EDHs are most often associated with skull fractures and middle meningeal artery lacerations (two-thirds of patients) or skull fractures with venous bleeding.[7] A blow to the head that causes a linear skull fracture on the lateral surface of the head may tear the middle meningeal artery. As the artery bleeds, it pulls the dura mater away from the skull, creating a pouch that expands into the intracranial space.

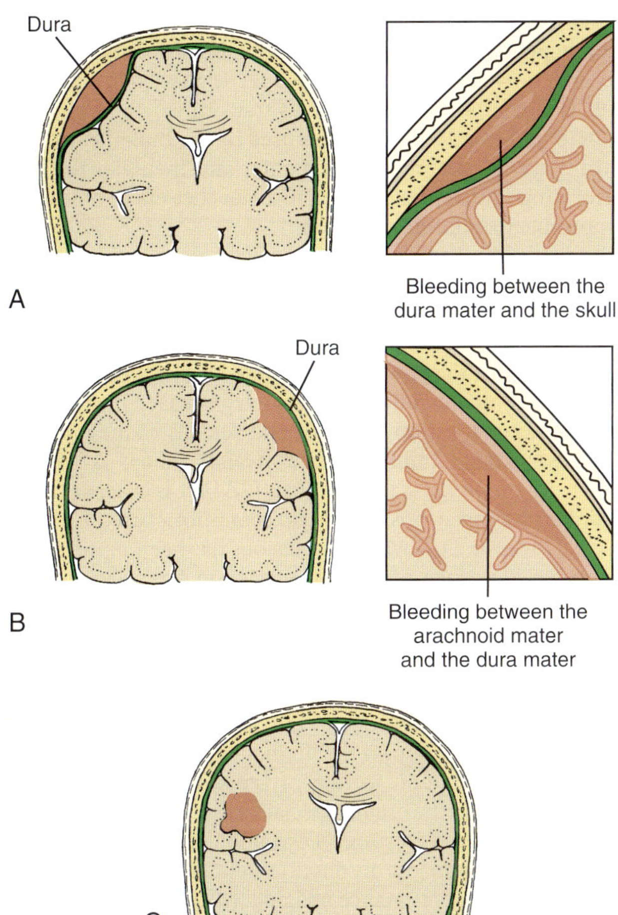

FIG. 32.4 Intracranial Hematomas. (A) Epidural hematoma. (B) Subdural hematoma. (C) Intracerebral hematoma.

The incidence of EDH is relatively low. EDH can occur due to low-impact injuries (e.g., falls) or high-impact injuries such as MVCs. The classic clinical manifestations of EDH include a brief loss of consciousness followed by a period of lucidity. Rapid deterioration in the LOC should be anticipated because arterial bleeding into the epidural space can occur quickly. The patient may complain of a severe, localized headache and may be sleepy. A dilated and fixed pupil on the same side as the impact area is a hallmark of EDH.[31] Diagnosis is based on clinical symptoms and evidence of blood collection in the epidural space on a CT scan. Treatment of EDH requires urgent surgical intervention to remove the blood and to cauterize the bleeding vessels.

Subdural hematoma. SDH, the accumulation of blood between the dura mater and underlying arachnoid membrane, accounts for approximately 30% of severe head injuries.[7] It is most often related to a rupture in the bridging veins between the cerebral cortex and the dura mater (Fig. 32.4B).[31] Acceleration–deceleration and rotational forces are major causes of SDH, which often is associated with cerebral contusions and ICH. Three types of SDH—acute, subacute, and chronic—are based on the time frame from injury and clinical symptoms.

Acute subdural hematoma. Acute SDHs are hematomas that occur after a severe blow to the head. They primarily occur within 72 hours of the initial injury.[32] The severity of the injury determines the clinical presentation of acute SDH to the underlying brain tissue at the time of impact and the rate (speed) at which blood accumulates in the subdural space. The patient often presents with a decreased LOC; in other situations, the patient has a lucid period before deterioration. Careful observation for deterioration in the LOC or lateralizing signs such as inequality of pupils or motor movements is essential. Rapid surgical intervention (e.g., craniectomy, craniotomy, or burr hole evacuation) can reduce mortality.

Subacute subdural hematoma. Subacute SDHs are hematomas that develop 4 days to 3 weeks after trauma.[32] An SDH occurs within the meninges in the subdural space. SDH is diagnosed by alterations in neurologic symptoms and by CT scan (Fig. 32.5B).

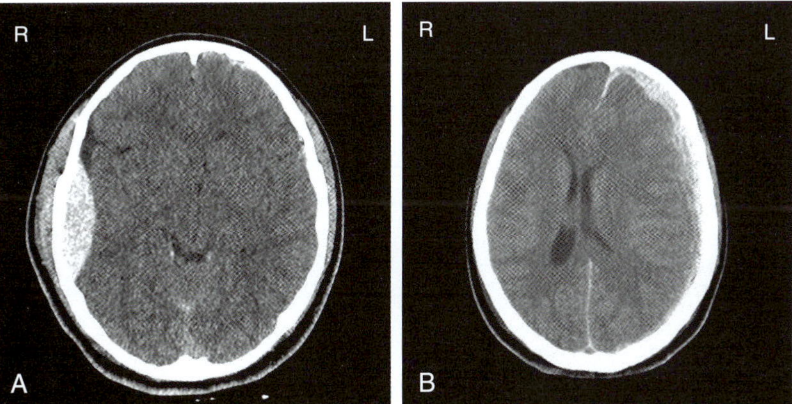

FIG. 32.5 Intracranial Hematomas—Computed Tomography (CT) Scans. (A) CT scan of an epidural hematoma in the right temporal/parietal area. (B) CT scan of a subdural hematoma in the left frontal/temporal area. Note that a CT scan is always shown as if the reader is looking at the patient from the foot of the bed so that right (R) and left (L) are reversed.

In subacute subdural bleeding, the hematoma's expansion occurs slower than that observed in acute SDH and less than an epidural bleed. Clinical deterioration of a patient with a subacute SDH is also usually slower than deterioration with an acute SDH, but treatment by surgical intervention, when appropriate, is the same.

Chronic subdural hematoma. Chronic SDH is diagnosed when symptoms appear 21 days or more after injury. Most patients with chronic SDH are late middle age or older. Individuals at risk for chronic SDH include patients with coordination or balance disturbances and those receiving anticoagulation therapy. Clinical manifestations of chronic SDH are deceptive. The patient may report symptoms such as lethargy, absent-mindedness, headache, vomiting, stiff neck, and photophobia. They may also show signs of transient ischemic attack, seizures, pupillary changes, or hemiparesis. Because a history of trauma is often not significant enough to be recalled, chronic SDH seldom is seen as an initial diagnosis. CT evaluation confirms the diagnosis.

If surgical intervention is required, evacuation of chronic SDH may be accomplished by craniotomy, burr holes, or catheter drainage. The outcome after chronic SDH evacuation varies. The return of neurologic status often depends on the degree of neurologic dysfunction before the intervention occurred. Because this condition is most common in older or debilitated patients, recovery may be slow.

Intracerebral hemorrhage and hematoma. ICH results when bleeding occurs deep within cerebral tissue. Traumatic causes of ICH include depressed skull fractures, penetrating injuries (bullet, knife), or sudden acceleration–deceleration motion. The ICH can act as a rapidly expanding space-occupying lesion; late ICH into the necrotic center of a contused area also is possible (Fig. 32.4C). Sudden clinical deterioration of a patient, 6 to 10 days after trauma, may result from ICH.

Medical management of ICH may include nonsurgical or surgical approaches. Hemorrhages that are minimal or localized and do not cause significant neurologic or other problems are treated without surgery. Control of blood pressure, reversal of anticoagulation, and neuroprotective strategies are the mainstays of treatment.[33] If significant problems with neurologic status occur as a result of the ICH producing a mass effect, neurosurgical intervention is required. The outcome of a patient with an ICH depends on the size and location of the hemorrhage, mass effect, and degree of displacement of other intracranial structures.

Penetrating brain injury. Missile injuries are caused by objects that penetrate the skull to produce significant focal damage but little acceleration–deceleration or rotational injury. The injury may be depressed, penetrating, or perforating (Fig. 32.6). Penetrating brain injuries are the most lethal form of TBI, with mortality rates of up to 90%.[34]

Depressed injuries are caused by skull fractures with bone penetration into cerebral tissue. Penetrating injury is caused by a missile entering the cranial cavity but not exiting. A low-velocity penetrating injury (knife) may involve only focal damage and no loss of consciousness. A high-velocity projectile (bullet) can produce shock waves transmitted throughout the brain in addition to the injury caused by the bullet. Perforating injuries are missile injuries that enter and then exit the brain. Perforating injuries have much less ricochet effect but are still responsible for significant injury.

The risk of infection and cerebral abscesses is a major concern in missile injuries. If fragments of the missile are embedded within the brain, surgery may be required. Careful consideration of the location and risk of increasing neurologic deficit is weighed against the risk of abscess, infection, or permanent disability. The outcome after missile injury is based on the degree of penetration, location of injury, and velocity of the missile.

Diffuse axonal injury. *Diffuse axonal injury* (DAI), also known as *traumatic axonal injury (TAI)*,[35] is a term used to describe prolonged posttraumatic coma not caused by a mass lesion. However, DAI with mass lesions has been reported. DAI covers a wide range of brain dysfunction typically caused by acceleration–deceleration and rotational forces. DAI occurs due to damage to the axons or disruption of the axonal transmission of neural impulses.

The pathophysiology of DAI is related to the stretching, shearing, and tearing of axons due to the brain's movement inside the skull at the time of impact. While not as widespread as initially thought, stretching and tearing of axons result in microscopic lesions throughout the brain, especially deep within cerebral tissue and the base of the cerebrum.[36] Disruption of axonal transmission of impulses results in loss of consciousness. DAI may not be visible on CT or magnetic resonance imaging (MRI) unless surrounding tissue areas are significantly injured, causing small hemorrhages.

DAI can be classified as mild, moderate, or severe based on the extent of lesions. A patient with mild DAI may be in a coma for 24 hours and exhibit periods of decorticate (abnormal flexion) and decerebrate (abnormal extension) posturing. Patients

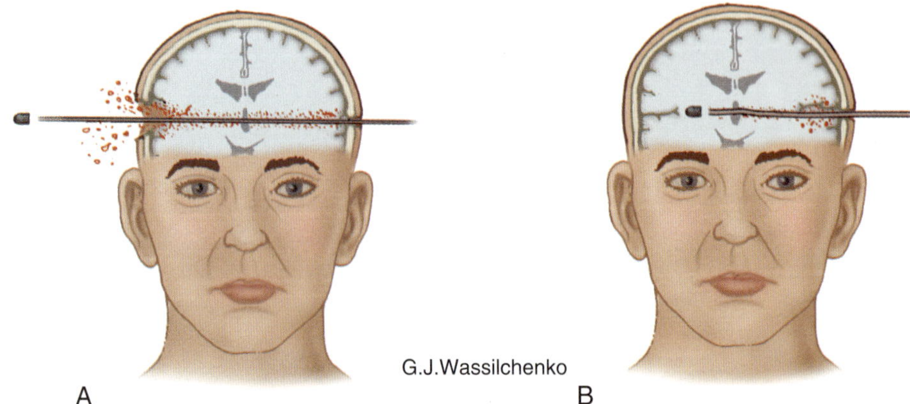

FIG. 32.6 Bullet Wound of the Head. A bullet wound or other penetrating missile injury causes an open (compound) skull fracture and damage to brain tissue. Shock wave effects are transmitted throughout the brain. (A) Perforating injury. (B) Penetrating injury.

with moderate DAI may be in a coma for longer than 24 hours and have flexion and extension posturing episodes. Severe DAI usually manifests as a prolonged, deep coma with periods of hypertension, hyperthermia, and excessive diaphoresis.[37] Treatment of DAI includes support of vital functions. The outcome after severe DAI is often poor because of the extensive physiologic destruction of cerebral pathways.

Pathophysiology

The pathophysiology of TBI can be divided into two main categories: primary brain injury and secondary brain injury. The nurse must understand these two distinct phases of TBI because critical care interventions are often directed at limiting the effects of and reducing morbidity and mortality from primary but, more importantly, secondary brain injury.

Primary injury. Primary TBI occurs at the moment of impact due to mechanical forces to the head. Primary injuries include those injuries that directly damage the brain parenchyma. Examples of primary TBIs include contusion, laceration, shearing injuries, and hemorrhage. Hemorrhage may significantly compress structures within the cranial vault. Primary injury may be mild, with little or no neurologic damage, or severe, with significant brain and tissue damage. The extent of and recovery from injury are often related to whether the primary injury was localized (limited to a specific area) or diffuse (widespread) throughout the brain. Immediately after brain injury, a cascade of neural and vascular processes is activated.

Secondary injury. Secondary injury is the biochemical and cellular response to the initial trauma that can exacerbate the primary injury and cause additional damage and impairment in brain recovery. Secondary injury can be caused by ischemia, hypotension, hypercapnia, cerebral edema, seizures, or metabolic derangements.[31] Hypoxia and hypotension, the best-known culprits for secondary injury,[38] typically are the result of extracranial trauma. A self-perpetuating cycle develops that may cause worsening of the primary injury due to uncontrolled secondary factors.

Cerebral edema. Cerebral edema occurs as a result of the changes in the cellular environment caused by contusion, loss of autoregulation, and increased permeability of the blood-brain barrier. As the pressure inside the cranial vault increases (in an attempt to perfuse the brain), cerebral perfusion decreases, further compromising brain function. Cerebral edema can be localized around the contusion or diffuse due to hypotension or hypoxia. The combined effects of increasing pressure and decreasing perfusion precipitate a downward spiral of events. The extent of cerebral edema can sometimes be minimized by managing aspects of secondary injury, such as oxygenation, ventilation, and perfusion.

Hypotension. Significant hypotension will not adequately perfuse neural tissue. Hypotension is rarely observed in patients with TBI on admission to the hospital unless terminal medullary failure has occurred. If a trauma patient is unconscious and hypotensive, a detailed chest, abdomen, and pelvis assessment must be performed to rule out internal injuries and bleeding.

However, hypertension in a trauma patient with severe TBI is common. With the loss of autoregulation, blood pressure increases, resulting in increased intracranial blood volume and elevating ICP. Hypertension, observed most frequently after initial TBI, is the body's attempt to perfuse the brain when cerebral circulation is compromised.[39]

Ischemia. Tissue ischemia occurs in areas of poor cerebral perfusion due to primary injury, edema, hypotension, or hypoxia. The cells in ischemic areas become edematous. Extreme vasodilation of the cerebral vasculature occurs in TBI in an attempt to supply oxygen and nutrients to the cerebral tissue. This sudden increase in blood volume increases intracranial volume and raises ICP.

Hypercapnia. Hypercapnia is a potent vasodilator of cerebral vessels. Most often caused by hypoventilation in an unconscious patient, hypercapnia results in cerebral vasodilation, increased cerebral blood flow (volume) and increased ICP. These three variables all contribute to worsening TBI.

Assessment and Diagnosis

Neurologic assessment is the most crucial tool for evaluating a patient with a severe TBI because it can provide information about the severity of the injury, offer prognostic information, and dictate the speed with which further evaluation and treatment must proceed. The cornerstone of neurologic assessment is the GCS score, although assessment of the GCS score is not a complete neurologic examination. Pupillary and motor strength assessments must be incorporated into early and ongoing assessments. After specific injuries are identified, a more thorough, focused neurologic assessment, such as examining the cranial nerves, is warranted. To assist with the initial assessment, TBIs are divided into three descriptive categories—mild, moderate, or severe—based on the patient's GCS score and duration of the unconscious state.

Degree of traumatic brain injury

Mild brain injury. Mild TBI is described as a GCS score of 13 to 15 with a loss of consciousness that lasts up to 15 minutes. Patients with mild injury are seen in the ED and often discharged home with a family member who is instructed to evaluate the patient routinely and to bring the patient back to the hospital if any further neurological symptoms appear.

Moderate brain injury. Moderate TBI is described as a GCS score of 9 to 12 with a loss of consciousness for up to 6 hours. Patients with this type of TBI are usually hospitalized. They are at high risk for deterioration from increasing cerebral edema and ICP, and serial neurologic assessments are essential. Hemodynamic and ICP monitoring and ventilatory support are usually not required for these patients unless other bodily injuries make them necessary. A CT scan is obtained on admission. Repeat CT scans are indicated if the patient's neurologic status deteriorates.

Severe brain injury. Patients with a GCS score of 8 or less after resuscitation or patients who deteriorate to that level within 48 hours of admission have a severe TBI.[30] Loss of consciousness may be 6 hours or longer. These patients are admitted to the CCU for continuous neurologic assessment, hemodynamic monitoring, mechanical ventilation, and management of complex care issues. Serial CT scans may be performed to rule out evidence of ongoing bleeding or mass lesions that can be surgically corrected.

Assessment. As in all traumatic injuries, evaluating a critically injured patient with TBI follows the *ABCDE* approach of ATLS. Immediate assessments of airway, breathing, and circulation (ABCs) are the first steps in patient assessment. Patients with moderate to severe TBI may require endotracheal intubation with mechanical ventilation to reduce the risk of hypoxia and hypercapnia. After stabilization of the ABCs, a thorough neurologic assessment is performed.

LOC, motor movements, pupillary response, respiratory function, and vital signs all are part of a complete neurologic assessment of a patient with TBI. LOC is a patient's degree of responsiveness and awareness.[7] Consciousness is assessed by obtaining the patient's response to verbal and painful stimuli. Determination of orientation to person, place, and time assesses mental alertness. Pupils are assessed for size, shape, equality, and reactivity. Asymmetry must be reported immediately. Pupils are also assessed for constriction to a light source (parasympathetic innervation) or dilation (sympathetic innervation). Because parasympathetic fibers are present in the brainstem, pupils that react slowly to light may indicate a brainstem injury. A "blown" pupil is a term used to describe a fixed and dilated pupil that can be caused by compression of the third cranial nerve or transtentorial herniation (see Figs. 21.5 and 22.14). Bilateral fixed pupils can indicate midbrain involvement and poor neurologic outcome.

Neurologic assessments are continuous throughout the patient's stay in the CCU as part of ongoing assessments to detect subtle changes in the patient's condition. Serial assessments include changes in LOC, GCS score, pupils, and hemodynamic status. In these situations, careful clinical observation of trends in the patient's condition is essential. Medications such as analgesics, sedatives, and muscle relaxants may mask neurologic signs in a patient with a severe head injury. When sedation of the patient is required, newer shorter-acting sedatives with a short half-life are used. For example, IV propofol can be turned off, and a neurologic examination can be performed within minutes.

Diagnostic procedures. The cornerstone of diagnostic procedures for evaluating TBI is the CT scan.[7,38] CT is a rapid, noninvasive procedure that can provide invaluable information about the presence of mass lesions (including hemorrhage) and cerebral edema. Serial CT scans may be obtained over several days to assess areas of contusion and ischemia and to detect delayed hematomas. It is important that the patient be continuously observed and monitored during the CT scan and while being transported to and from the scanner. Transporting the patient, moving the patient from the bed to the CT table, and positioning the head flat during the CT scan are all stressful events and can cause severe increases in ICP and decreases in *cerebral perfusion pressure* (CPP).

Medical Management

Surgical management. If a lesion identified on a CT scan is causing a shift of intracranial contents or increasing ICP, surgical intervention is necessary. A craniotomy is performed to remove the EDH, SDH, or large ICH. Patients may also undergo a *decompressive craniectomy* specifically for elevated ICP. This procedure involves the removal of the overlying bone flap to allow the underlying brain tissue to expand and swell. This surgical strategy has demonstrated some benefits but remains controversial.[40]

Nonsurgical management. Nonsurgical management includes management of ICP, maintenance of acceptable CPP, ensuring adequate oxygenation, and prevention and treatment of complications such as pneumonia or infection. The decision of when to initiate ICP monitoring is critical. ICP monitoring may be required for patients with a GCS score of less than 8 and abnormal findings on a head CT scan.[29] Various methods to monitor brain tissue oxygenation may also be used (see Fig. 21.20).

Nursing Management

The management care plan for a patient with a TBI incorporates a variety of patient problems (Box 32.5). Nursing interventions focus on recognizing and reducing increased ICP, limiting or

BOX 32.5 DIAGNOSIS AND PATIENT CARE MANAGEMENT

Traumatic Brain Injury

- Ineffective Tissue Perfusion due to alterations in cerebral blood flow
- Decreased Intracranial Adaptive Capacity due to failure of normal intracranial compensatory mechanisms
- Impaired Verbal Communication due to cerebral speech center injury
- Impaired Breathing due to neuromuscular impairment
- Impaired Gas Exchange
- Risk for Aspiration
- Impaired Nutritional Intake due to lack of exogenous nutrients and increased metabolic demand
- Risk for Infection
- Powerlessness related to lack of control over current situation
- Lack of Knowledge of Treatment Regime due to lack of previous exposure to information

Patient Care Management plans are located in Appendix A.

preventing secondary brain injury, and stabilizing vital signs. Ongoing neurologic assessments are the foundation of care for patients with TBI. Assessments are the primary mechanism for determining the improvement or worsening of the patient's condition. If a secondary injury is to be prevented, all events that increase ICP, reduce MAP, and reduce CPP must be responded to immediately. Initial management of severe TBI frequently occurs in the CCU. All aspects of care, including hemodynamic management, control of ICP, IV fluid therapy, pulmonary care, acid–base balance, maintenance of body temperature, and control of the environment, can affect the outcome after TBI.[41]

Hemodynamic management. In patients with TBI, changes in cardiovascular function and circulating catecholamines may contribute to hemodynamic instability. Heart rate and blood pressure are continually monitored. Although no specific hemodynamic parameters have been universally agreed upon, the Brain Trauma Foundation (BTF) TBI guidelines currently recommend SBP be maintained greater than 100 mm Hg for patients aged 50 to 69 years and greater than 110 mm Hg for patients 15 to 49 years and those over age 70.[42] Isotonic IV fluids (e.g., 0.9% normal saline) and vasopressors may be required if target SBP is not achieved. Arterial blood pressure should be continually monitored because hypotension in a patient with TBI is unusual and may indicate coexisting or undiagnosed injuries.

ICP management. Ongoing monitoring of ICP may be necessary, and in some patients with TBI, insertion of an external ventricular drain may be required. When an external ventricular drain is in situ, best practice evidence suggests keeping ICP less than 22 mm Hg[42,43] (normal ICP is 0 to 15 mm Hg) and maintaining CPP at between 60 to 70 mm Hg[43] to facilitate optimal patient outcomes. Aggressive attempts to maintain CPP greater than 70 mm Hg have not been supported in the literature and should be avoided secondary to increasing risk of cardiac or respiratory problems.[44]

When ICP is too high, administering IV mannitol or hypertonic saline may be necessary. Mannitol (an osmotic diuretic) and hypertonic saline (sterile salt solution) pull fluid from the brain parenchyma and decrease ICP. Mannitol and hypertonic saline are given as intermittent IV boluses. Whether mannitol or hypertonic saline is given to patients with TBI, careful monitoring of the patient's serum sodium and serum osmolality is required.

Pulmonary management. In severe TBI, the patient is often intubated, mechanically ventilated, and placed on a full support mode of mechanical ventilation. No consensus exists for mechanical ventilation in TBI. Still, the best evidence suggests that lung-protective ventilation with tidal volumes of 6 to 8 mL/kg and the lowest amount of positive end-expiratory pressure (PEEP) that prevents hypoxemia is safe.[45] Of utmost importance is ensuring that the TBI patient is not hypoxemic.

Capnography (monitoring of exhaled carbon dioxide levels) is suggested to monitor for hypercapnia. Arterial blood gases (ABGs) are frequently obtained, with particular attention to the arterial partial pressure of carbon dioxide ($PaCO_2$). Most facilities caring for patients with TBI aim to keep the $PaCO_2$ level low to normal at 35 to 45 mm Hg,[46] as increases in $PaCO_2$ would potentially increase cerebral blood flow and worsen ICP. When $PaCO_2$ levels increase, the tidal or minute volume must be increased on the ventilator. Although pulmonary care must be instituted, endotracheal suctioning can elevate ICP.

Temperature management. Cerebral oxygen consumption is increased during periods of increased body temperature. As a result, the goal is to achieve normothermia (36°C to 37°C). Monitoring the patient's temperature, using antipyretics and cooling blankets, and early identification and work-up for infection are essential. A tremendous catecholamine surge after TBI has been associated with infectious complications and potentially preventable mortality.[47] The use of beta-blockers to suppress this catecholamine surge in patients with TBI has been shown to decrease mortality.[47]

In the early postinjury phase, the patient's environment must be controlled. Stimuli that produce pain, agitation, or discomfort can increase ICP. Nursing interventions should not be clustered, and care should be evenly distributed throughout the shift. Explanations can be provided to patients in a calm, soft-spoken manner. Families and significant others are informed about the importance of maintaining a quiet environment. Analgesics and sedatives should be administered as ordered by the practitioner and as required by the patient; they should not be routinely used as first-line agents when ICP increases. Patients should be provided with several rest periods during hospitalization.

New strategies. Newer strategies have demonstrated promise in treating patients with traumatic brain injury. IV ketamine boluses have been correlated with ICP reductions and CPP increases.[48] Several biomarkers are being investigated, including calcium protein B (S100b), neuron-specific enolase (NSE), and glial fibrillary acidic protein (GFAP).[49] In the not-too-distant future, biomarkers may assist clinical assessment and diagnostic imaging in helping predict the severity and outcome of TBI. Animal therapy and its impact on cognitive scores of hospitalized patients with severe TBI has had some effect on patients.[50] Without question, much more research is required.

Spinal Cord Injuries

Approximately 18,000 new SCIs occur in the United States annually.[51] Since the 1970s, the median age at injury has increased from 28 years to the current median age of 43 years.[51] Over 80% of SCI patients are male, and 90% are attributable to traumatic injury.[52] The diagnosis of SCI begins with a detailed history of events surrounding the incident, precise evaluation of sensory and motor function, and radiographic studies of the spine.

Etiology

The most frequent cause of SCI is MVCs (38%), followed by falls (30%), violence (14.6%), and sporting activities (9%).[53] Hyperflexion, hyperextension, rotation, and axial loading are four distinct forces by which the spinal cord can be injured. The spinal cord may also be injured by penetrating trauma.

Hyperflexion. Hyperflexion injury is often seen in the cervical area, especially at C5 to C6, because this is the most mobile portion of the cervical spine. This type of injury is often caused by sudden deceleration motion, as in head-on collisions. The damage occurs from cord compression due to fracture fragments or dislocation of the vertebral bodies. Instability of the spinal column occurs because of rupture or tearing of the posterior muscles and ligaments.

Hyperextension. Hyperextension injuries involve the backward and downward motion of the head. With this injury, often seen in rear-end MVCs, the spinal cord is stretched and distorted. Neurologic deficits associated with this injury are usually caused by contusion and ischemia of the cord without significant bony involvement. *Whiplash* is a mild form of hyperextension injury.

Rotational. Rotational injuries often occur in conjunction with a flexion or extension injury. This injury may occur in the cervical, thoracic, or lumbar sections of the cord. Severe rotation of the neck or body results in tearing of the posterior ligaments and displacement (rotation) of the spinal column.

Compression (axial loading). Compression injury (axial loading) occurs from a vertical force along the spinal cord. This injury is commonly seen in a fall from a height where the person lands on the feet or buttocks. Compression injuries may cause *burst fractures* of the vertebral body, often sending bony fragments into the spinal canal or spinal cord (Fig. 32.7).

Penetrating injuries. Penetrating injury to the spinal cord can be caused by a bullet, knife, or any other object that penetrates the cord. These injuries often cause permanent damage by anatomically transecting the spinal cord.

Pathophysiology

SCIs result from a mechanical force that disrupts neurologic tissue, vascular supply, or both. Similar to the pathophysiology of TBI, injury to the spinal cord occurs through both primary and secondary injury mechanisms (Box 32.6). Primary injury is the neurologic and vascular damage that occurs at the moment of impact, possibly caused by blunt or penetrating injury. Secondary injury, which occurs within minutes of injury, refers to the complex biochemical processes affecting cellular function that arise from hemorrhage, inflammation, edema, ischemia, cytokine release, and vascular injury.[54]

This cascade of events immediately after SCI may lead to spinal cord ischemia and loss of neurologic function. Additionally, electrolyte and biochemical changes, the accumulation of glutamate (the most prevalent neurotransmitter in our brains), and disruption of the blood–spinal cord barrier promote cellular death.[55] These secondary pathophysiologic events result in direct and indirect damage to the spinal cord by allowing an influx of calcium ions into neurons.[56] This extends the level of injury and functional deficit and potentially worsens long-term outcomes. Knowledge of the pathophysiology of secondary processes has led to the development of newer therapies that target cellular changes contributing to injury. Despite ongoing research efforts at repairing primary SCI, minimizing damage by reducing secondary injury has shown the most promise.

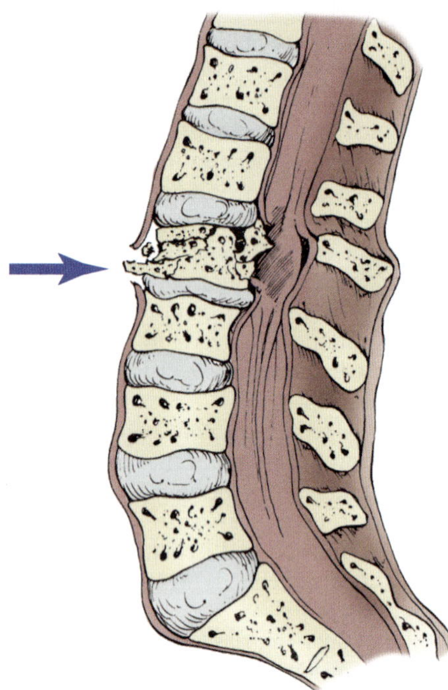

FIG. 32.7 Spinal Cord Compression Burst Fracture. Compression injuries cause burst fractures of the vertebral body (see arrow), often sending bony fragments into the spinal canal or spinal cord. Mechanisms of injury include hyperflexion, hyperextension, rotation, axial loading (vertical compression), and missile or penetrating injuries.

BOX 32.6 Primary and Secondary Mechanisms of Acute Spinal Cord Injury

Primary Injury Mechanisms
- Impact and persistent compression (most common)
- Impact and transient compression
- Distraction (two adjacent vertebrae pulled apart; spinal cord stretches)
- Laceration/transection
- Missile injuries, dislocations, sharp bony fragments

Secondary Injury Mechanisms

Acute Phase
- Hemodynamic effects (e.g., bradycardia, hypotension, hypoxemia, shock, and hemorrhage)
- Vascular damage (e.g., decreased peripheral resistance, decreased cardiac output, increased—then decreased—levels of circulating catecholamines)
- Ion imbalance
- Accumulation of neurotransmitters (increased intracellular glutamate)
- Free radical formation
- Influx of calcium
- Inflammation, edema, inflammatory cytokines
- Necrotic cell death

Subacute Phase
- Demyelination of surviving axons
- Apoptosis
- Glial scar formation around the injury
- Matrix remodeling

Chronic Phase
- Maturation of glial scar formation

Adapted from Alizadeh A, Dyck SM, Karimi-Abdolrezaee S. Traumatic spinal cord injury: An overview of pathophysiology, models and acute injury mechanisms. *Front Neurol.* 2019;10:282. https://doi.org/10.3389/fneur.2019.00282.

Spinal shock. As discussed earlier, hypovolemic shock in trauma occurs in response to a deficit of fluid volume, often related to bleeding. *Spinal shock* is a condition that occurs shortly after traumatic injury to the spinal cord. Spinal shock is a complete loss of all muscle tone and normal reflex activity below the level of injury,[7] including loss of rectal tone. In other words, spinal shock is a "concussion" of the spinal cord. Patients with spinal shock may appear completely without function below the area of injury, although not all of the area may be destroyed. On average, it may occur 30 to 60 minutes after injury and lasts 4 to 12 weeks or longer.[57]

Neurogenic shock. Neurogenic shock results from injury to the descending sympathetic pathways in the spinal cord. This injury results in loss of vasomotor tone and sympathetic innervation to the heart. Patients with SCI at T6 or above may have profound neurogenic shock due to interruption of the sympathetic nervous system and loss of vasoconstrictor response below the level of the injury. Hypotension, bradycardia, and peripheral vasodilation are hallmark signs and symptoms of neurogenic shock. Blood pressure support may be required with IV fluids and vasopressors, such as norepinephrine (Levophed). The duration of this shock state can persist for up to 6 weeks after injury.[58] Neurogenic shock is discussed further in Chapter 33.

The mechanism of injury often assists trauma teams in distinguishing between these three types of shock. In hypovolemic shock, the patient is often tachycardic. In neurogenic shock, the patient is generally bradycardic. In spinal shock, priapism may be present.

Functional injury of the spinal cord. Functional injury of the spinal cord refers to the degree of disruption of normal spinal cord function. This injury depends on what specific sensory and motor structures within the cord are damaged. SCIs are classified as complete or incomplete. The most frequent diagnosis at discharge has been incomplete tetraplegia (47.6%), followed by complete paraplegia (19.9%) and incomplete paraplegia (19.6%).[59] SCI cannot be classified until spinal shock has resolved.

Complete injury. Complete SCI results in a total loss of sensory and motor function below the level of injury. Regardless of the mechanism of injury, the result is a complete dissection of the spinal cord and its neurochemical pathways, resulting in one of two conditions: tetraplegia or paraplegia.

Tetraplegia. With tetraplegia, the injury occurs between the C1 and T1 levels. Residual muscle function depends on the specific cervical segments involved. The potential functional status resulting from different neurologic levels of injury is described in Table 32.5.

Paraplegia. With paraplegia, the injury occurs in the thoracolumbar region (T2 to L1). Patients with injuries in this area may have full or limited use of their arms, and all require a wheelchair. In rare circumstances, a few patients may have limited ability to ambulate short distances with crutches, braces, or other orthotic devices. Thoracic, L1, and L2 injuries produce paraplegia with variable innervation to intercostal and abdominal muscles.

Incomplete injury. Incomplete SCI results in a mixed loss of voluntary motor activity and sensation below the level of the lesion. Incomplete SCI exists if any function remains below

TABLE 32.5 Quadriplegia Functional Status

Neurologic Level (Vertebrae) of Complete Injury	Functional Ability
C1–C4	Requires electric wheelchair with breath, head, or shoulder controls
C5	Needs electric wheelchair with hand control and/or manual wheelchair with rim projections; may require adaptive devices to assist with ADLs
C6	Independent in manual wheelchair on level surface; may need hand controls; adaptive devices may be needed for ADLs
C7	Requires manual wheelchair on most surfaces
C8–T1	May need adaptive devices

ADL, Activities of daily living.

TABLE 32.6 Muscle Strength Scale

5=	Active movement against maximal resistance
4=	Active movement through ROM against resistance
3=	Active movement through ROM against gravity
2=	Active movement through ROM with gravity eliminated
1=	Flicker or trace of contraction
0=	No contraction; total paralysis

ROM, Range of motion.

the level of injury. Incomplete injuries can result in various syndromes, which are classified according to the degree of motor and sensory loss below the level of injury. Some of the more common incomplete injury syndromes are described here.

Brown-séquard syndrome. Brown-Séquard syndrome is associated with damage to only one side of the cord due to penetrating trauma or crush injury. This injury produces a loss of voluntary motor movement on the same side as the injury (hemiparaplegia), with coexisting loss of pain, temperature, and sensation on the opposite side (hemianesthesia).[60] Functionally, the side with the best motor control has little or no sensation, whereas the side with sensation has little or no motor control.

Central cord syndrome. Associated with cervical hyperextension–hyperflexion injury and damage to the central region of the spinal cord, central cord syndrome is the most common type of incomplete SCI. This injury produces loss of motor and sensory function more pronounced in the upper extremities than in the lower extremities.[7] Various degrees of sensory impairment (pain, temperature) and bowel and bladder dysfunction may exist.

Anterior cord syndrome. Anterior cord syndrome occurs due to direct anterior spinal cord compression (occlusion) of the anterior spinal artery or hyperflexion of the cervical spine.[60] Injury occurs to the anterior gray horn cells (motor), spinothalamic tracts (pain), anterior spinothalamic tract (light touch), and corticospinal tracts (temperature).[61] The result is a loss of motor function and loss of the sensations of pain and temperature below the level of injury. However, below the level of injury, position sense and sensations of pressure and vibration remain intact.

Posterior cord syndrome. Posterior cord syndrome is most often associated with blockage of the posterior spinal artery from a tumor. In trauma with extreme cervical hyperextension injury, the posterior column may be damaged. This results in the loss of position sense, pressure, and vibration below the level of injury. Motor function and sensation of pain and temperature often remain intact. These patients may be unable to ambulate because the loss of position sense impairs spontaneous movement. This type of SCI is extremely rare.

Assessment and Diagnosis

Screening the trauma patient for SCI is an integral part of the assessment for all trauma teams. However, the initial neurologic examination may not accurately indicate eventual motor and sensory loss. The first assessment focuses on the rapid and accurate identification of present, absent, or impaired functioning of the motor, sensory, and reflex systems that coordinate and regulate vital functions. Once the patient has been stabilized, a more detailed motor and sensory examination, which includes an assessment of all 32 spinal nerves for evidence of dysfunction, can be performed.

Dermatomes. Carefully mapped pathways for the sensory portion of the spinal nerves, called *dermatomes*, can assist in localizing the functional (sensory) level of injury. The American Spinal Injury Association (ASIA) suggests that motor function and strength may be graded on a six-point scale (Table 32.6). The initial evaluation must be performed correctly, and findings must be thoroughly documented so that subsequent serial assessments can rapidly identify deterioration. ASIA has developed a form that outlines the necessary assessments for the initial and ongoing classification of SCIs (Fig. 32.8). Ongoing spinal cord assessments must be documented during the critical care phase.

Assessment. Attention to the ABCs of the ATLS approach is imperative in a patient with known or suspected SCI on admission to the CCU, similar to patients with TBI and all other trauma patients. Ensuring a patent airway is of primary concern. Breathing patterns and gas exchange are assessed after the airway has been evaluated and secured. The level of SCI often dictates the degree of altered breathing patterns that exist (Table 32.7). Because injuries above the C3 level result in paralysis of the diaphragm, patients with these injuries require intubation and mechanical ventilation.

Diagnosis. Radiographic evaluations identify the severity of damage to the spinal cord. Initial evaluation on admission to the ED or CCU should include anteroposterior and lateral radiograph views of all areas of the spinal cord. In many medical centers, CT scan has replaced plain radiography as the principal modality for cervical spine assessment after trauma. A CT scan of all seven cervical vertebrae and the top of T1 must be obtained to rule out cervicothoracic injury. Flexion and extension views can identify subtle ligament injuries. MRI may also be used for definitive diagnosis of SCI. The Canadian C-Spine Rule (CCR) and the National Emergency X-Radiography Utilization Study (NEXUS) are two widely accepted criteria used to help rule out cervical SCI in trauma patients.[62]

Medical Management

After the initial assessment of the trauma patient has occurred and a diagnosis of SCI is confirmed, the medical and nursing plan of care is determined. The primary goal is to preserve the remaining neurologic function with surgical or nonsurgical interventions.

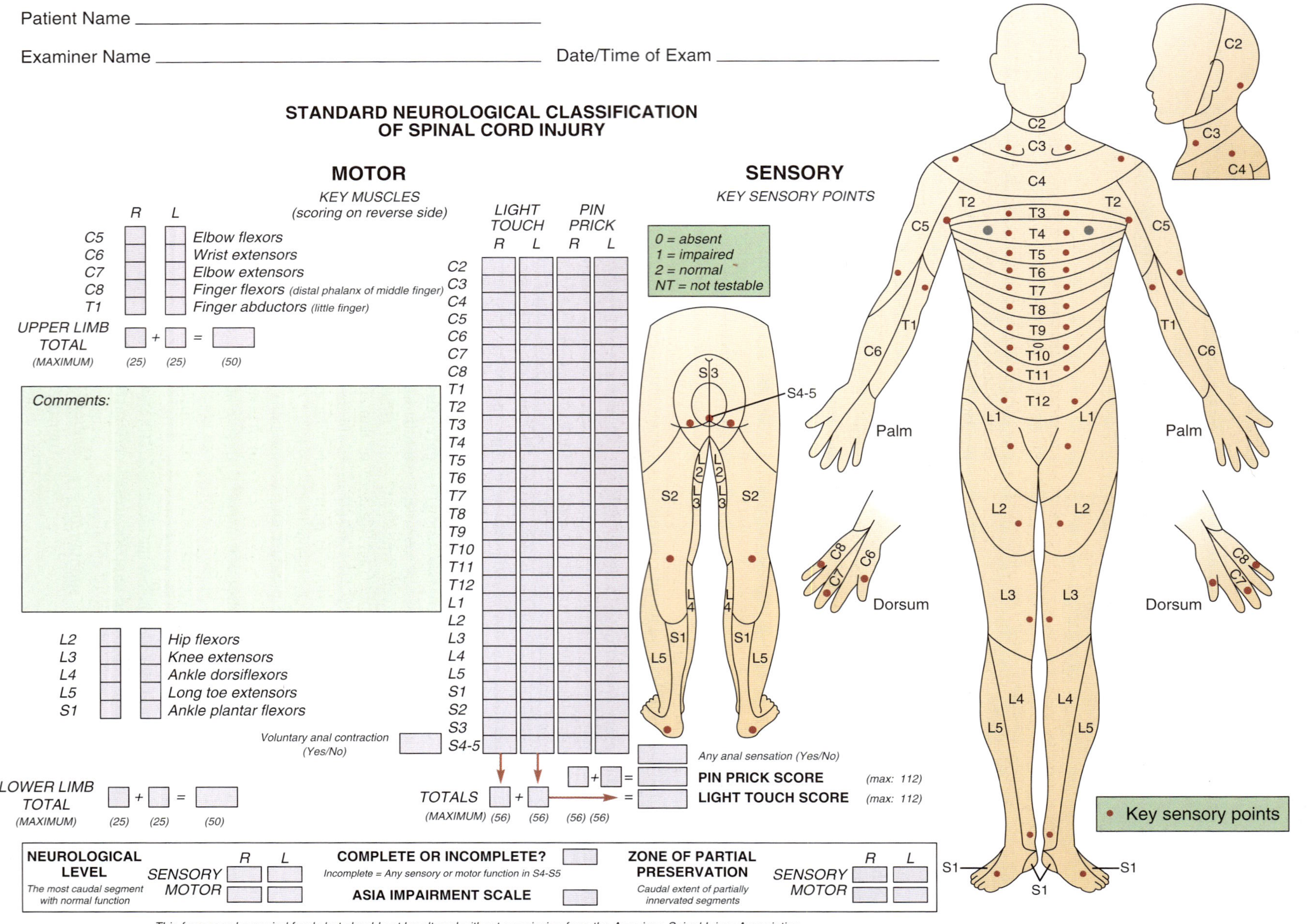

Patient Name ______________________

Examiner Name ______________________ Date/Time of Exam ______________________

STANDARD NEUROLOGICAL CLASSIFICATION OF SPINAL CORD INJURY

MOTOR

KEY MUSCLES (scoring on reverse side)

	R	L	
C5			Elbow flexors
C6			Wrist extensors
C7			Elbow extensors
C8			Finger flexors (distal phalanx of middle finger)
T1			Finger abductors (little finger)

UPPER LIMB TOTAL (MAXIMUM) ☐ (25) + ☐ (25) = ☐ (50)

Comments:

	R	L	
L2			Hip flexors
L3			Knee extensors
L4			Ankle dorsiflexors
L5			Long toe extensors
S1			Ankle plantar flexors

Voluntary anal contraction (Yes/No) ☐

LOWER LIMB TOTAL (MAXIMUM) ☐ (25) + ☐ (25) = ☐ (50)

SENSORY

KEY SENSORY POINTS

	LIGHT TOUCH R	LIGHT TOUCH L	PIN PRICK R	PIN PRICK L
C2				
C3				
C4				
C5				
C6				
C7				
C8				
T1				
T2				
T3				
T4				
T5				
T6				
T7				
T8				
T9				
T10				
T11				
T12				
L1				
L2				
L3				
L4				
L5				
S1				
S2				
S3				
S4-5				
TOTALS (MAXIMUM)	(56)	(56)	(56)	(56)

0 = absent
1 = impaired
2 = normal
NT = not testable

Any anal sensation (Yes/No) ☐

☐ + ☐ = ☐ **PIN PRICK SCORE** (max: 112)

☐ + ☐ = ☐ **LIGHT TOUCH SCORE** (max: 112)

NEUROLOGICAL LEVEL The most caudal segment with normal function		R	L
	SENSORY	☐	☐
	MOTOR	☐	☐

COMPLETE OR INCOMPLETE? ☐
Incomplete = Any sensory or motor function in S4-S5

ASIA IMPAIRMENT SCALE ☐

ZONE OF PARTIAL PRESERVATION Caudal extent of partially innervated segments		R	L
	SENSORY	☐	☐
	MOTOR	☐	☐

This form may be copied freely but should not be altered without permission from the American Spinal Injury Association.

FIG. 32.8 American Spinal Injury Association Classification of Spinal Cord Injuries. *SCI*, Spinal cord injury.

MUSCLE GRADING

0 total paralysis

1 palpable or visible contraction

2 active movement, full range of motion, gravity eliminated

3 active movement, full range of motion, against gravity

4 active movement, full range of motion, against gravity and provides some resistance

5 active movement, full range of motion, against gravity and provides normal resistance

5* muscle able to exert, in examiner's judgment, sufficient resistance to be considered normal if identifiable inhibiting factors were not present

NT not testable. Patient unable to reliably exert effort or muscle unavailable for testing due to factors such as immobilization, pain on effort or contracture.

ASIA IMPAIRMENT SCALE

☐ **A = Complete**: No motor or sensory function is preserved in the sacral segments S4-S5.

☐ **B = Incomplete:** Sensory but not motor function is preserved below the neurological level and includes the sacral segments S4-S5.

☐ **C = Incomplete:** Motor function is preserved below the neurological level, and more than half of key muscles below the neurological level have a muscle grade less than 3.

☐ **D = Incomplete:** Motor function is preserved below the neurological level, and at least half of key muscles below the neurological level have a muscle grade of 3 or more.

☐ **E = Normal:** Motor and sensory function are normal.

CLINICAL SYNDROMES (OPTIONAL)

☐ Central Cord
☐ Brown-Sequard
☐ Anterior Cord
☐ Conus Medullaris
☐ Cauda Equina

STEPS IN CLASSIFICATION

The following order is recommended in determining the classification of individuals with SCI.

1. Determine sensory levels for right and left sides.
2. Determine motor levels for right and left sides.
   Note: in regions where there is no myotome to test, the motor level is presumed to be the same as the sensory level.
3. Determine the single neurological level.
   This is the lowest segment where motor and sensory function is normal on both sides, and is the most cephalad of the sensory and motor levels determined in steps 1 and 2.
4. Determine whether the injury is Complete or Incomplete (sacral sparing).
   If voluntary anal contraction = **No** *AND all S4-5 sensory scores =* **0** *AND any anal sensation =* **No**, *then injury is COMPLETE. Otherwise injury is incomplete.*
5. Determine ASIA Impairment Scale (AIS) Grade:

Is injury Complete? If **YES**, AIS=A Record ZPP
(For ZPP record lowest dermatome or myotome on each side with some (non-zero score) preservation)

NO ↓

Is injury motor incomplete? If **NO**, AIS=B
(Yes=voluntary anal contraction OR motor function more than three levels below the motor level on a given side.)

YES ↓

Are at least half of the key muscles below the (single) neurological level graded 3 or better?

NO ↓ AIS=C

YES ↓ AIS=D

If sensation and motor function is normal in all segments, AIS=E
Note: AIS E is used in follow up testing when an individual with a documented SCI has recovered normal function. If at initial testing no deficits are found, the individual is neurologically intact; the ASIA Impairment Scale does not apply.

FIG. 32.8, cont'd

TABLE 32.7 Effects of Spinal Cord Injury on Ventilatory Functions

Neurologic Level (Vertebrae) of Complete Injury	Respiratory Function	Comment
C1–C2	Paralysis of diaphragm	Ventilator dependent
C3–C5	Various degrees of diaphragm paralysis	Some diaphragm control; may need ventilatory support; weaning depends on preinjury pulmonary status
C6–T11	Various degrees of impaired intercostal muscles and abdominal muscles	Compromised respiratory function; reduced inspiratory ability; paradoxical breathing patterns; ineffective cough, sneeze

Initial spine stabilization. Stabilization of the spinal cord is mandatory to prevent further injury, and spinal precautions are maintained until otherwise ordered. This action includes stabilization of the head and neck with manual (handheld) traction during the initial assessment, including intubation and establishment of ventilatory support. A hard collar, spine boards, bed rest, and logrolling maneuvers are widely used nationwide, although there is limited evidence to indicate true clinical benefit.[63] However, until cervical and spinal radiographs have been completed, reviewed, and cleared, or definitive stabilization has been achieved, it is unlikely that pre- and in-hospital immobilization protocols will change anytime in the near future. The assessment and authorization to remove the cervical collar, known as *clearance of the cervical spine*, is challenging in a patient with SCI in the CCU. Clearance of the cervical spine is made difficult by alteration in mentation due to coexisting injury, alcohol or illicit substance use, analgesia, and sedation; intubation and mechanical ventilation; surgical procedures; and a focus on other more distracting injuries. The Eastern Association of Surgeons in Trauma developed guidelines for cervical spine clearance (Table 32.8).

Venous thromboembolism prophylaxis. As with any immobilized patient, venous thromboembolism (VTE) risk is high. However, detection of VTE, especially in the lower limbs, is difficult because pain and tenderness are not evident to a patient with SCI. Prevention of VTE is imperative and may include a combination of therapies such as low-dose heparin, low-molecular-weight heparin, pneumatic sequential compression devices, and embolic hose.[69]

Surgical management. Unstable injuries include disrupted ligaments, tendons, and a vertebral column that cannot maintain normal alignment. Identifying and immobilizing unstable injuries are particularly important for a patient with an incomplete neurologic deficit. Without adequate stabilization, movement and dislocation of the unstable vertebral column may cause a complete neurologic deficit. Surgical intervention decompresses the cord (relief of pressure on spinal nerves) and realigns and stabilizes the spine. Various surgical procedures may be performed to achieve decompression and stabilization after SCI. Unfortunately, there is no evidence to suggest that earlier surgical intervention enhances long-term outcomes.[64]

TABLE 32.8 Evidence-Based Practice Guidelines for Cervical Spine Clearance

Trauma Patient Population	Recommendation
Awake, asymptomatic Not intoxicated, neurologically normal exam, no complaints of neck pain or tenderness, full range of motion of cervical spine, no distracting injuries	Neck is palpated in all directions for tenderness or pain. If physical examination is negative for pain or tenderness, CT of cervical spine is not required. Cervical collar may be removed.
Awake, symptomatic All other trauma patients with suspected cervical injury must be radiologically evaluated, including patients with neck pain or tenderness, whether alert or with altered mental status/neurologic deficit, or distracting injury	Obtain high-quality CT scan Consultation with neurosurgery, spine service If CT is positive for injury, options: 1. Continue c-spine precautions until patient asymptomatic. 2. Discontinue c-spine precautions after normal flexion-extension radiographs. 3. Discontinue c-spine precautions after normal MRI. 4. Discontinue c-spine precautions at discretion of the practitioner.
Obtunded	Obtain high-quality CT scan If CT is negative for injury, options: Options: 1. Discontinue c-spine precautions after flexion-extension views under fluoroscopy. 2. Discontinue c-spine precautions after normal MRI. 3. Discontinue c-spine precautions at the discretion of the physician.

CT, Computed tomography; *MRI*, magnetic resonance imaging.
Adapted from Hadley MN, Walters BC. Introduction to the guidelines for the management of acute cervical spine and spinal cord injuries. *Neurosurgery*. 2013;72(Suppl 2):5–16. https://doi.org/10.1227/NEU.0b013e3182773549.

Laminectomy. In this procedure, the lamina (which forms the posterior portion of the spinal canal) is removed to allow decompression and removal of bony fragments or material from the canal.

Spinal fusion. This technique involves surgical fusion of two to six vertebral bodies to stabilize and prevent motion. An anterior or posterior surgical approach may accomplish this procedure. Fusion is accomplished using bone chips taken from the iliac crest, bone bank, or artificial bone substitute and using wires, pins, or rods.

Other spinal cord surgical options. Pedicle screw fixation has become one treatment option for thoracic and lumbar fracture fixation.[65] This procedure helps stabilize fractured thoracic and lumbar segments of the spinal column. Vertebral plates and bone grafting may also be used.

Nonsurgical management. If the injury to the spinal cord is stable, nonsurgical management is the treatment of choice. Nonsurgical management for cervical and thoracolumbar injuries is discussed in this section.

Cervical injury. Management of cervical injuries involves immobilizing the fracture and realigning any dislocation. This process is accomplished through skeletal traction that consists of the use of two-point tongs, which are inserted into the skull

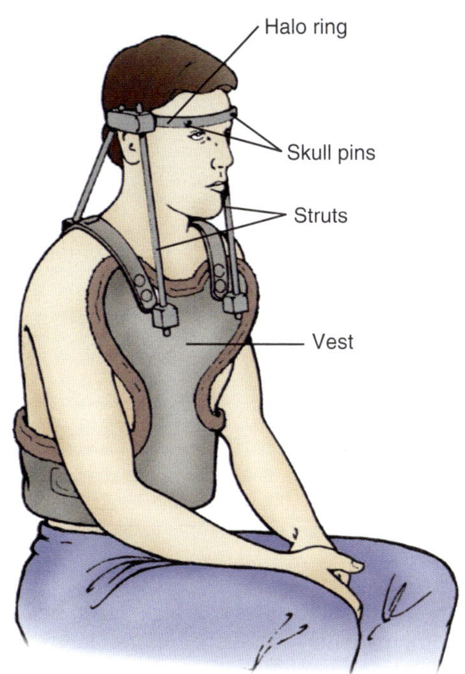

FIG. 32.9 Halo Vest. The halo traction device immobilizes the cervical spine, which allows the patient to ambulate and participate in self-care.

through shallow burr holes and are connected to weights. Several types of cervical tongs are used. Gardner-Wells and Crutchfield tongs are the most common. These tongs can be applied by experienced personnel using a local anesthetic at the bedside. Weights are applied gradually, with frequent neurologic and radiographic evaluations, until the fracture is reduced (realigned).

After the procedure, the patient must be immobilized on a kinetic therapy bed or a regular bed. The kinetic therapy bed is advantageous for cervical immobilization because it maintains alignment of the spinal column while providing a constant turning motion to reduce pulmonary complications and the incidence of skin breakdown. The use of cervical skeletal traction on a regular bed is also acceptable. However, it is more challenging to provide adequate care to the pulmonary and integumentary systems because of the extensive degree of immobility.

Halo traction braces may be used for some patients with cervical spine injuries. The halo vest consists of a metal ring secured to the skull with two occipital and two temporal screws. The metal ring is attached to steel bars that anchor to the plastic vest to provide cervical immobilization (Fig. 32.9). The halo traction brace immobilizes the cervical spine but allows the patient to ambulate and participate in self-care.

Thoracolumbar injury. Nonsurgical management of a patient with a thoracolumbar injury is undertaken in the absence of a neurologic injury. Traditionally, this approach frequently involved immobilization. Current best practice recommends adequate pain relief and early mobilization within the comfort and safety of the patient.[66] A short period of bed rest may be required initially after injury, but maintaining a balance between activity and rest is essential. If necessary, a brace may be ordered to help decrease patient discomfort and encourage mobility. Coordination between the patient, nursing, and physiotherapy is integral to the nonoperative management of thoracolumbar injury.

BOX 32.7 DIAGNOSIS AND PATIENT CARE MANAGEMENT

Spinal Cord Injury

- Impaired Gas Exchange due to alveolar hypoventilation
- Impaired Breathing due to decreased lung expansion
- Impaired Breathing due to musculoskeletal fatigue or neuromuscular impairment
- Impaired Cardiac Output due to sympathetic blockade
- Autonomic Dysreflexia due to excessive autonomic response to noxious stimuli
- Activity Intolerance due to prolonged immobility or deconditioning
- Disturbed Body Image due to actual change in body structure, function, or appearance
- Lack of Knowledge of Treatment Regime due to lack of previous exposure to information

Patient Care Management plans are located in Appendix A.

Nursing Management

The patient care management plan for the patient with SCI incorporates a variety of patient diagnoses (Box 32.7). Nursing actions during the critical care phase optimize hemodynamic stability and prevent life-threatening complications while maximizing the function of all organ systems. Nursing interventions aim to prevent secondary damage to the spinal cord and manage the complications of the neurologic deficit. Because almost all body systems are affected by SCI, nursing management must include interventions that promote the optimal functioning of each system. Moreover, patients with SCIs have complex psychosocial needs that require significant emotional support from the health care team.

Neurologic care. Assessment, monitoring, and trending of the patient's GCS score and sensory and motor function are essential aspects of nursing the SCI patient in critical care. The use of methylprednisolone as a neuroprotective agent in SCI is controversial.[67] There is no consensus on the efficacy of this medication or any other medication in enhancing recovery of cord function after injury. Current best practice guidelines suggest not administering corticosteroids in traumatic SCI.[7,56]

Cardiovascular care. Maintaining hemodynamic stability and ensuring adequate tissue perfusion is necessary to promote injured spinal cord tissue recovery. Hypotension (SBP less than 90 mm Hg) should be avoided or corrected immediately after acute SCI. Alteration in tissue perfusion because of hypotension may require the administration of IV fluids. After the fluid volume status has been optimized, inotropic or vasopressor support (or both) may be implemented if SBP or MAP remains low. An accurate assessment of fluid volume status is required because pulmonary edema is a threat to patients with SCI. It is widely accepted as best practice to maintain the MAP greater than 85 to 90 mm Hg for the first 5 to 7 days post-SCI.[68] This treatment helps facilitate optimal perfusion to the injured spinal cord and helps facilitate functional recovery.

Dysrhythmias. A patient with SCI is at high risk for or may exhibit alterations in cardiovascular stability, including dysrhythmias. The risk for cardiovascular instability is profound in patients with SCI at the C3 to C5 levels, although alterations in cardiovascular function occur with most injuries above T6. Symptomatic bradyarrhythmias may be treated with an inotropic medication such as isoproterenol or anticholinergic medication such as atropine. Both medications increase heart rate but also increase myocardial oxygen consumption. For persistent low heart rates that produce symptoms, another option may be a temporary transcutaneous or transvenous pacemaker.

Pulmonary care. Pulmonary complications are the most common cause of mortality in patients with SCI.[69] Initial and ongoing nursing assessments of respiratory status are vital for identifying actual or potential impairment in ventilation. Evaluations include assessment of respiratory rate and rhythm, observation of symmetry of chest expansion and use of accessory muscles, inspection of quantity and character of secretions, and auscultation of breath sounds. Serial ABG values provide information on the adequacy of gas exchange.

Ventilatory support. Intubation and mechanical ventilation are frequently required in acute SCI. Neuromuscular blocking agent *succinylcholine* (suxamethonium) should not be administered to patients with SCI as this medication may aggravate existing injury due to fasciculation during induction and produce hyperkalemic cardiac arrest. Patients with lesions at C3 to C5 may eventually be able to be weaned from the ventilator. Some patients with C3 injuries may require mechanical ventilation only at night. Weaning can be complex because of the physiological demands placed on the diaphragm and the psychological effects of fear of the inability to breathe. Various weaning methods are available, and a well-coordinated approach by the nurse, practitioner, respiratory therapist, and patient is essential. Weaning difficulties are common, and reintubation, including tracheostomy tube insertion, is sometimes required.

Airway clearance. Ineffective airway clearance and impaired gas exchange are problems for a patient with SCI due to hypoventilation (paralysis of respiratory muscles), increased bronchial secretions, and atelectasis secondary to decreased cough. Nursing interventions are directed at improving and maintaining adequate gas exchange.

Frequent suctioning of the airway is required. Caution must be used with vigorous suctioning because stimulation of the vagus nerve (which runs alongside the trachea) can cause profound bradycardia. Hyperoxygenation with 100% oxygen before suctioning is recommended.

Repositioning may facilitate the removal of secretions. Kinetic therapy beds, which can rotate up to 60 degrees on each side, may provide continual postural drainage and mobilization of secretions. A cough assistance technique can further aid in mobilizing secretions in the presence of an ineffective cough (Fig. 32.10). This procedure is similar to abdominal thrusts (formerly known as the Heimlich maneuver). Exact hand placement may vary, and assessing which hand placement works best for the patient is important. Cough assist machines are also commercially available.

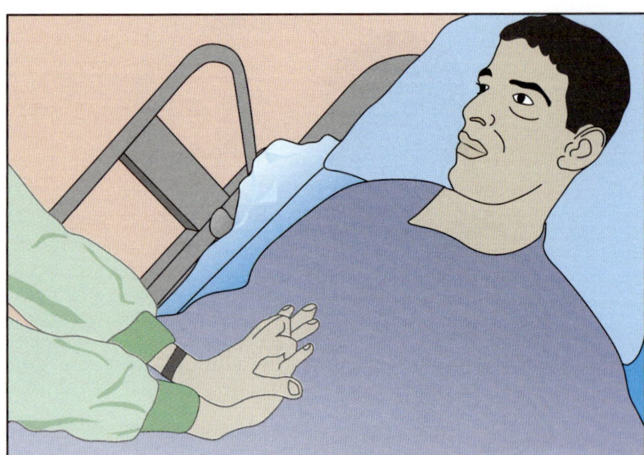

FIG. 32.10 Cough Assistance. One hand or both hands are placed over the upper diaphragm. After the patient inhales, pressure is directed inward and upward as the patient attempts to cough.

Gastrointestinal and genitourinary care. Immediately after SCI injury, bowel and bladder tone are flaccid. Innervation between the brain and the defecation center in the sacral cord has been disrupted.

Bowel issues. Abdominal distention, constipation, and fecal impaction are problems often encountered in SCI patients in early recovery. In the critical care phase, a bowel program may be initiated to prevent fecal impaction and encourage normal, regular bowel function. The patient should not go longer than 2 to 3 days without a bowel movement. Laxatives and stool softeners may be needed, especially if the patient receives opiates. Aspects of a successful bowel program include consistent timing of evacuation, proper positioning, physical activity, appropriate fluid intake, a high-fiber diet, and reflex stimulation for patients with upper motor neuron injuries.[70] The SCI patient and caregivers are essential in planning and modifying the plan based on experiences. Bowel retraining is a major focus of the intermediate care and rehabilitation phase of treatment.

Bladder issues. The degree of bladder and urinary sphincter dysfunction depends on the location and completeness of the injury. A urinary drainage catheter is inserted on admission, but it should be removed 3 to 4 days later or as soon as possible, at which time the patient is placed on an intermittent catheterization schedule of every 4 to 6 hours. It is not unusual for male patients with an upper motor neuron injury to experience a reflexogenic erection when catheterized. An overdistended bladder in a patient with an injury at T6 or above may trigger autonomic dysreflexia.

Autonomic dysreflexia. Autonomic dysreflexia is a life-threatening complication that occurs most commonly in the first year after SCI. This condition is caused by a massive sympathetic response to a noxious stimulus (e.g., full bladder, fecal impaction) that results in severe hypertension, bradycardia, facial flushing, pounding headache, nausea, blurred vision, and anxiety.[71] Immediate intervention is needed to prevent cerebral hemorrhage and seizures. Treatment is aimed at alleviating the noxious stimuli. Suggestions for treatment of autonomic dysreflexia are provided in Box 32.8.

Integumentary and musculoskeletal care. Patients with SCI are at extremely high risk for pressure injuries because of the lack of motor control and sensation. Prevention is the best treatment. Diligent assessments, meticulous skin care, and frequent position changes are required. Any evidence of skin breakdown or pressure injury development should be assessed, documented, and reported immediately to the most appropriate health care practitioner. Specialty surfaces or low-air-loss beds may be necessary to prevent pressure injury in patients with SCI.

Prevention of contractures. Immobilized patients are at high risk for contractures. Muscle fibers shorten and produce a contracture when a muscle is denervated, as in the case of SCI. Irreversible contractures may result in skin breakdown, inability to perform activities of daily living, poor wheelchair posture, and inability to use adaptive devices. Physical and occupational

BOX 32.8 Autonomic Dysreflexia

- If the patient is supine, immediately sit the patient upright.
- Begin frequent vital sign monitoring, including blood pressure every 5 minutes.
- Loosen tight clothing and constrictive devices.
- Immediately begin assessment for an underlying cause.
- If an indwelling urinary catheter is not placed, catheterize the patient.
- If an indwelling catheter is present, immediately:
  - Check the system for kinks, obstructions to flow, and correct placement.
  - Irrigate the bladder with a small sterile amount of fluid using strict aseptic technique.
  - If not draining, remove the catheter and replace immediately using aseptic technique.
- Perform a digital examination to check for the presence of stool; if present, gently remove it.
- If systolic blood pressure is greater than 150 mm Hg, consider a rapid-onset, short-duration antihypertensive agent.
- Do not hesitate to call for immediate medical assistance.
- Search for other possible causes (e.g., infected or ingrown toenail, pressure injury).

therapy personnel should be consulted early in the patient's hospitalization. Range-of-motion exercises are initiated as soon as the spine has been stabilized. Footdrop devices should be applied on admission to prevent contractures and skin breakdown of the heels. Hand splints should be used for individuals with quadriplegia. Hand and foot splints should be removed every 2 hours, and the extremities should be examined for evidence of skin breakdown.

Pin care. Care management of a patient in skull traction or halo vest includes inspection of pins and traction for security, correct positioning, and maintenance of skin integrity. Traction bars of the halo vest must never be used to lift or reposition the patient, and the wrench that comes with the halo jacket must be immediately available at all times in case of cardiac arrest.

Temperature management. Another consequence of sympathetic nervous system dysfunction is loss of thermoregulation *(poikilothermy)*, in which the external environment regulates body temperature. Heat or cold for therapeutic or comfort measures may be required but must be used cautiously. Profound changes in body temperature must be avoided. Before anti-pyretics are given for hyperthermia, a cooling blanket is typically used. Hypothermia can produce bradyarrhythmias and sinus arrest and may impair wound healing.

Maximizing psychosocial adaptation. Nursing management of the patient with SCI must include dedicated emotional support. In the CCU, the patient, family, and significant others often experience anxiety, grief, denial, anger, frustration, and hopelessness because of the nature of the injury, profound and immediate changes required in lifestyle, and long-term neurologic deficits that may remain unknown.

Appropriate nursing interventions include promoting support systems, often involving family and friends, and using coping mechanisms and adaptive skills. Simple, accurate, and consistent information may help alleviate some fear and anxiety. Feelings of powerlessness may be reduced by including the patient and family in patient care and decision making. Further psychosocial support can be provided by social workers, occupational therapists, psychologists, and members of the clergy.

Maxillofacial Injuries

The face represents a direct link to self and to expression by playing a significant role in personal identity, appearance, and communication. Vital functions that depend on facial integrity include mastication, deglutination, respiration, and perception of the environment by vision, hearing, speech, and olfaction. Consequently, maxillofacial trauma can produce long-term adverse effects with varying degrees of sensory, emotional, and psychosocial consequences.

Etiology

Maxillofacial injury can occur from blunt or penetrating trauma. Blunt trauma for this injury is exemplified by the unbelted driver or passenger thrown into the dashboard or windshield. Associated injuries may include concussion, skull fracture, SCI, and fractures of other bones. Bullet wounds to the face can be life-threatening injuries because of bleeding and airway obstruction.

Pathophysiology

The facial skeleton is an energy-absorbing shield to protect the brain, eyes, spinal cord, and pharynx. Maxillofacial trauma can result in soft tissue injury ranging from abrasions to destruction of most of the face with accompanying maxillofacial skeletal fractures. Nasal bones, the zygoma, and the mandibular condyle are the most susceptible to fracture.

Maxillofacial skeletal injuries. Fractures of the maxilla are diagnosed according to the *Le Fort classification*. Le Fort fractures are classified into three broad categories, depending on the level of the fracture (Fig. 32.11). The most common, Le Fort I, consists of horizontal fractures, including the nasal floor, septum, and teeth.[72] The entire palate moves separately from the lower maxilla (floating palate). Le Fort II fractures are an extension of a Le Fort I fracture and resemble a pyramidal fracture. They involve the midface: orbit, hard palate, and nasal bones (floating maxilla).[73] In a Le Fort III fracture, this transverse fracture involves both zygomas and the nose, nasal bridge, and upper part of the maxilla,[38] resulting in complete craniofacial disruption (floating face). Often associated with severe skull and brain injuries, CSF frequently leaks with Le Fort II and III fractures because there is usually communication between the cranial base and the cribriform plate. A combination of Le Fort fractures is often observed in patients with multisystem trauma.

Assessment and Diagnosis

Major or minor facial deformities should not distract the trauma team from the standardized ABCDE approach of ATLS primary and secondary surveys.

Assessment. During the secondary survey, a comprehensive examination of facial structures is part of the detailed head-to-toe assessment. Assessment of the face involves careful inspection and palpation of the orbit and soft tissues. A small abrasion or contusion of the face may seem unremarkable. However, the effect on the underlying structures might have disrupted facial bone integrity, the parotid gland, or the facial nerve. The mouth is inspected for traumatic tooth dislodgment, recognizing that some teeth may intrude into the underlying alveolar bone. The ear canal is inspected for occult lacerations of the tympanic membrane.

Maxillofacial trauma often is associated with TBI and traumatic SCI. An altered LOC in the presence of maxillofacial fractures strongly suggests neurotrauma. Fractures involving the

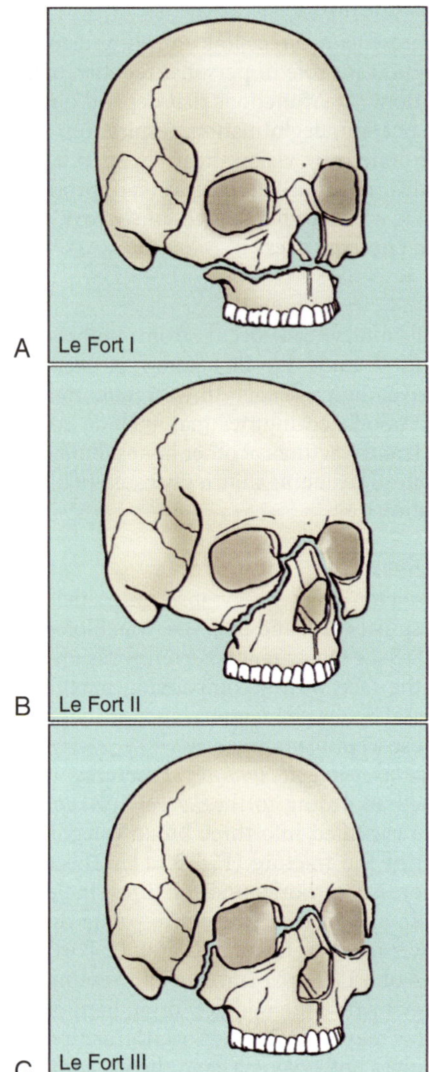

FIG. 32.11 Le Fort Classification. Fractures of the maxillae are diagnosed according to the Le Fort classification, which consists of three broad categories based on the level of the fracture. (A) Le Fort I. (B) Le Fort II. (C) Le Fort III.

skull and tearing of the dura mater may enable bacteria from the nose or oral cavity to enter the CSF, placing the patient at risk for meningitis. Nasal and auditory canals must be inspected for discharge. The presence of rhinorrhea or otorrhea should be immediately reported to the practitioner, and a sample should be tested for glucose to help confirm the drainage is CSF.

Diagnosis. CT scan determines the location and displacement of fractures.[74] MRI is also valuable in assessing associated head, neck, and vascular structures for injury and extent of trauma.

Medical Management

Le Fort I and II fracture treatment may include closed reduction and intermaxillary fixation. In contrast, all Le Fort III fractures require open reduction and intermaxillary fixation with wires, plates, and screws. Life-threatening complications associated with maxillofacial trauma include airway obstruction and head and cervical spine injuries.

Patients with maxillofacial trauma are at high risk for ineffective airway clearance. The tongue, hemorrhage, foreign objects,

BOX 32.9 DIAGNOSIS AND PATIENT CARE MANAGEMENT

Maxillofacial Trauma

- Risk for Aspiration
- Risk for Infection
- Impaired Swallowing due to neuromuscular impairment, fatigue
- Acute Pain due to transmission and perception of cutaneous, visceral, muscular, or ischemic impulses
- Disturbed Body Image due to actual change in body structure, function, or appearance
- Impaired Nutritional Intake due to lack of exogenous nutrients and increased metabolic demand
- Lack of Knowledge of Treatment Regime due to lack of previous exposure to information

Patient Care Management plans are located in Appendix A.

broken teeth, vomit, bone fragments, or edema can obstruct the airway. The "look, listen, and feel" methods (see Table 32.1) should be used to assess airway obstruction. An artificial airway may be required. An oral endotracheal tube may be used unless there is a laryngeal fracture. Nasotracheal or nasogastric intubation is contraindicated in unstable facial fractures (e.g., fracture of the cribriform plate), as the tube could inadvertently be placed through the fractured base of the skull and into the brain. In severe maxillofacial trauma, a surgical airway (tracheostomy) may be the best choice for patients with hypopharynx swelling or hemorrhage.

Profuse bleeding through the nares may occur with nasal, maxillary, or cranial base fractures. As a result, patients with maxillofacial trauma are at risk for fluid volume deficit related to hemorrhage due to bleeding from ethmoid or maxillary sinuses. Control of bleeding with nasal packing, ligation, or arterial embolization may be required. IV fluids are administered to correct deficient fluid volume status.

Nursing Management

The management plan for the patient with maxillofacial trauma incorporates a variety of patient problems (Box 32.9). Nursing interventions are aimed at maintaining and protecting the cervical spine and airway. A reverse Trendelenburg position is necessary if cervical spines are not cleared. Once the cervical spine is cleared, the head of the bed is elevated 30 degrees to reduce the risk of aspiration. Serial GCS assessments, IV fluids, mechanical ventilation, and blood products are essential aspects of care.[75] Patients may have an oral endotracheal tube or a tracheostomy. Proper orogastric tube functioning must be ensured. If vomiting occurs, the patient is immediately placed in a side-lying or forward position and oral or nasal suctioning is used. Antiemetics may be administered. If the mandible has been wired postoperatively, wire cutters must always be available at the bedside, especially for the nonintubated patient. Although seldom necessary, cutting the wires prevents aspiration in case of vomiting or gaining immediate access to the oral cavity for airway protection. Complications may include CSF leaks and epistaxis.[75]

Thoracic Injuries

Thoracic injuries involve trauma to the chest wall, lungs, heart, great vessels, and esophagus. Second only to head injury or SCI, thoracic injuries account for 25% of trauma deaths.[76]

Etiology

Blunt thoracic trauma to the chest is most often caused by MVCs or falls. Various types of blunt trauma are associated with specific injury patterns. In penetrating thoracic injury, the object involved determines the degree of damage to underlying structures. Low-velocity weapons (e.g., .22-caliber gun, knife) usually damage only what is in the direct path of the weapon. Stab wounds involving the anterior chest wall between the midclavicular lines, the angle of Louis, and the epigastric region are of particular concern because of the heart's and great vessels' proximity. High-velocity weapons can cause considerable thoracic injury because of greater kinetic energy.

Chest Wall Injuries

Rib fractures. Fractures of the ribs can be minimal and cause minor discomfort or be severe and life threatening, mainly when multiple ribs are fractured, the patient is an older adult, or when preexisting cardiopulmonary disease is present.

Pathophysiology. Because arteries and veins are protected by the scapula, clavicle, humerus, and muscles, fractures of the first and second ribs are frequently associated with a high degree of force applied to the thorax. As a result, neurovascular injuries of the brachial plexus or great vessels may occur. Fractures to the middle ribs may be associated with lung injury, including pulmonary contusion and pneumothorax. Fractures to the lower ribs (7th to 12th) may be associated with abdominal trauma, such as spleen and liver injuries.

Assessment and diagnosis. Localized pain that increases with respiration or that is elicited by rib compression may indicate rib fractures. The pain associated with rib fractures can be aggravated by chest wall movement. The patient often splints fractured ribs, takes shallow breaths, and may refuse to cough. These actions can result in atelectasis and pneumonia. A definitive diagnosis of rib fractures can be made with a chest radiograph or CT scan.

Management. Interventions include pain control to improve chest expansion and facilitate gas exchange and early mobilization. The primary goal of pain management in patients with rib fractures is patient comfort and prevention of pneumonia. Pain management interventions are multimodal, tailored to the individual patient and the patient's response to therapy. Nonsteroidal antiinflammatory medications, intercostal nerve blocks, thoracic epidural analgesia, and opiates may be considered.[77] External splints are not recommended because they may limit chest wall expansion and worsen existing atelectasis. Surgical plating of fractured ribs has not yet gained widespread acceptance. This procedure is most often reserved for those patients with severe chest wall deformity, accompanied by pain and problems with oxygenation and ventilation, that, without this newer surgical intervention, would possibly require many months of hospitalization.[78]

Flail chest. A flail chest, caused by blunt trauma, disrupts the continuity of chest wall structures. Typically, a flail segment occurs when two or more ribs are fractured in two or more places and are no longer attached to the thoracic cage, producing a free-floating segment of the chest wall.[79] A flail chest is a clinical diagnosis wherein the so-called flail segment (or floating segment) moves paradoxically compared with the rest of the chest wall (Fig. 32.12).

Pathophysiology. During inspiration, the intact portion of the chest wall expands while the injured part is sucked in. During expiration, the chest wall moves in, and the flail segment moves out. Although the flail segment increases the work of breathing, the leading cause of hypoxemia is often underlying pulmonary contusions.[80] The physiologic effects of impaired chest wall motion of a flail chest include decreased tidal volume and vital capacity and impaired cough that lead to hypoventilation and atelectasis.

Assessment and diagnosis. Diagnosis is made by clinical inspection of the thorax, which reveals paradoxical chest movement. Palpation of the chest may indicate crepitus and tenderness near fractured ribs. A chest radiograph shows multiple rib fractures. ABGs may demonstrate evidence of hypoxemia, but this does not aid in the diagnosis.

Management. Interventions focus on ensuring adequate oxygenation and analgesia to improve ventilation. Priorities include multimodal pain relief strategies, repeated assessments of airway patency and breathing (rate, rhythm depth), and in some situations, intubation and mechanical ventilation may be required. Surgical stabilization of severe flail chest has successfully repaired severe deformity and reduced pain in some patient situations.[81]

Lung Injuries

Pulmonary contusion. A pulmonary contusion is a bruise of the lung. Pulmonary contusion is often associated with blunt trauma and other chest injuries, such as rib fractures and flail chest. Pulmonary contusions can occur unilaterally or bilaterally.

Pathophysiology. A contusion manifests initially as a hemorrhage followed by alveolar and interstitial edema. Alveoli can rupture, and hematomas and atelectasis can develop. Capillary damage and edema directly affect lung function, negatively affecting gas exchange across the alveolar–capillary membrane. As inflammation and edema increase, lung compliance may decrease, resistance may increase, and decreased pulmonary blood flow may decrease.[77] These processes cause a ventilation–perfusion mismatch that results in progressive hypoxemia and poor ventilation.

Assessment and diagnosis. Clinical manifestations of pulmonary contusion may take 24 to 72 hours after injury to develop.[82] Inspection of the chest wall may reveal ecchymosis at the site of impact. Diminished breath sounds and coarse crackles may be auscultated over the contused lung. The patient may have a cough and blood-tinged sputum. Abnormal lung function can manifest as arterial hypoxemia. Diagnosis is made primarily by the mechanism of injury and imaging studies consistent with pulmonary infiltrates corresponding to the area of external chest impact that manifest within 24 to 72 hours of injury. Pulmonary contusions may worsen over the next few days after injury and slowly resolve in about 7 days unless complications from infection or ARDS occur.

Management. Aggressive respiratory care is the cornerstone for nonintubated patients with pulmonary contusion. Interventions include deep-breathing exercises, incentive spirometry, early mobilization, or noninvasive positive pressure ventilation. Adequate pain control is achieved with nonsteroidal antiinflammatory medications, opiates, intercostal nerve blocks, or thoracic epidural analgesia. Removal of airway secretions is essential to avoid infection and to improve ventilation. Patients with unilateral contusions are placed with the injured side up and the uninjured side down ("good lung down"). This positioning helps correct any existing ventilation–perfusion mismatch. Patients with severe pulmonary contusions may continue to exhibit signs of decompensation, such as respiratory

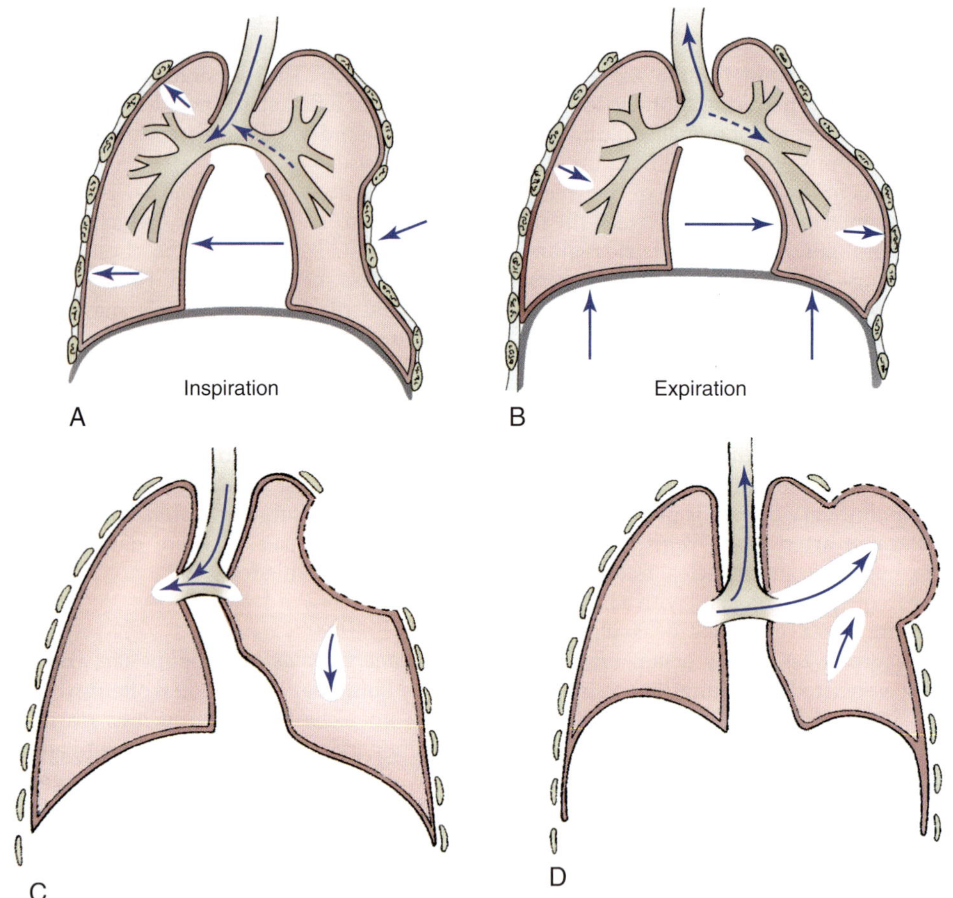

FIG. 32.12 Flail Chest. (A) Normal inspiration. (B) Normal expiration. (C) The area of the lung underlying the unstable chest wall sucks in on inspiration. (D) The same area expands outwards on expiration. During inspiration, notice movement of the mediastinum toward the opposite lung.

acidosis and increased work of breathing, despite aggressive nursing management. Endotracheal intubation and mechanical ventilation with PEEP may be required. Complications resulting from pulmonary contusions include pneumonia, hemothorax, pneumothorax, lung abscesses, pulmonary embolism, and ARDS.[82]

Pneumothoraces. Pleural damage is common in trauma. These conditions include *pneumothorax* (air in the pleural space), *hemothorax* (blood in the pleural space), or *hemopneumothorax* (air and blood in the pleural space). Pneumothoraces may be managed with chest tubes, analgesia, or surgical consultation, depending on the size of the pneumothorax, the hemodynamic stability of the patient, and the effects on oxygenation and ventilation. *Open pneumothorax, tension pneumothorax*, and *massive hemothorax*, three additional potentially life-threatening respiratory problems in trauma, warrant special consideration.

Open pneumothorax. An open pneumothorax ("sucking chest wound") is caused by penetrating trauma.

Pathophysiology. Large open thoracic wounds (greater than two-thirds the diameter of the trachea) allow communication between the atmosphere and the intrathoracic cavity.[7] As air moves in and out of the hole in the chest, a sucking sound can be heard on inspiration. Respiratory mechanics become impaired.

Assessment and diagnosis. Shortness of breath, tachycardia, and hypotension may be observed. *Subcutaneous emphysema* indicates that air is trapped in the tissues beneath the skin. This condition may be palpated around the wound as *crepitus*, a crackling sensation the examiner feels when lightly palpating the affected area.

Management. Initial management of an open pneumothorax is accomplished by promptly inserting a chest tube. If a chest tube is not immediately available, covering the wound at end-expiration with a sterile occlusive dressing taped securely on three sides and large enough to overlap the edges of the wound should be used.[7] As the patient breathes in, the dressing gets sucked in to occlude the wound and prevent air from entering the thoracic cavity. On expiration, the dressing moves outward, permitting the patient to exhale. Commercially available nonocclusive chest seals, such as the Sentinel® and Russell®, are used by many prehospital personnel. Surgical intervention is often required to close the wound.

Tension pneumothorax. A tension pneumothorax is caused by an injury that perforates the chest wall or pleural space.

Pathophysiology. During inspiration, air flows into the pleural space and becomes trapped. As the pressure in the pleural space increases, the lung on the injured side collapses and causes the mediastinum to shift to the opposite (uninjured) side (Fig. 32.13). As pressure builds, the shift exerts pressure on the heart and thoracic aorta, resulting in decreased venous return and cardiac output. Oxygenation and ventilation are affected because the collapsed lung does not participate in gas exchange.

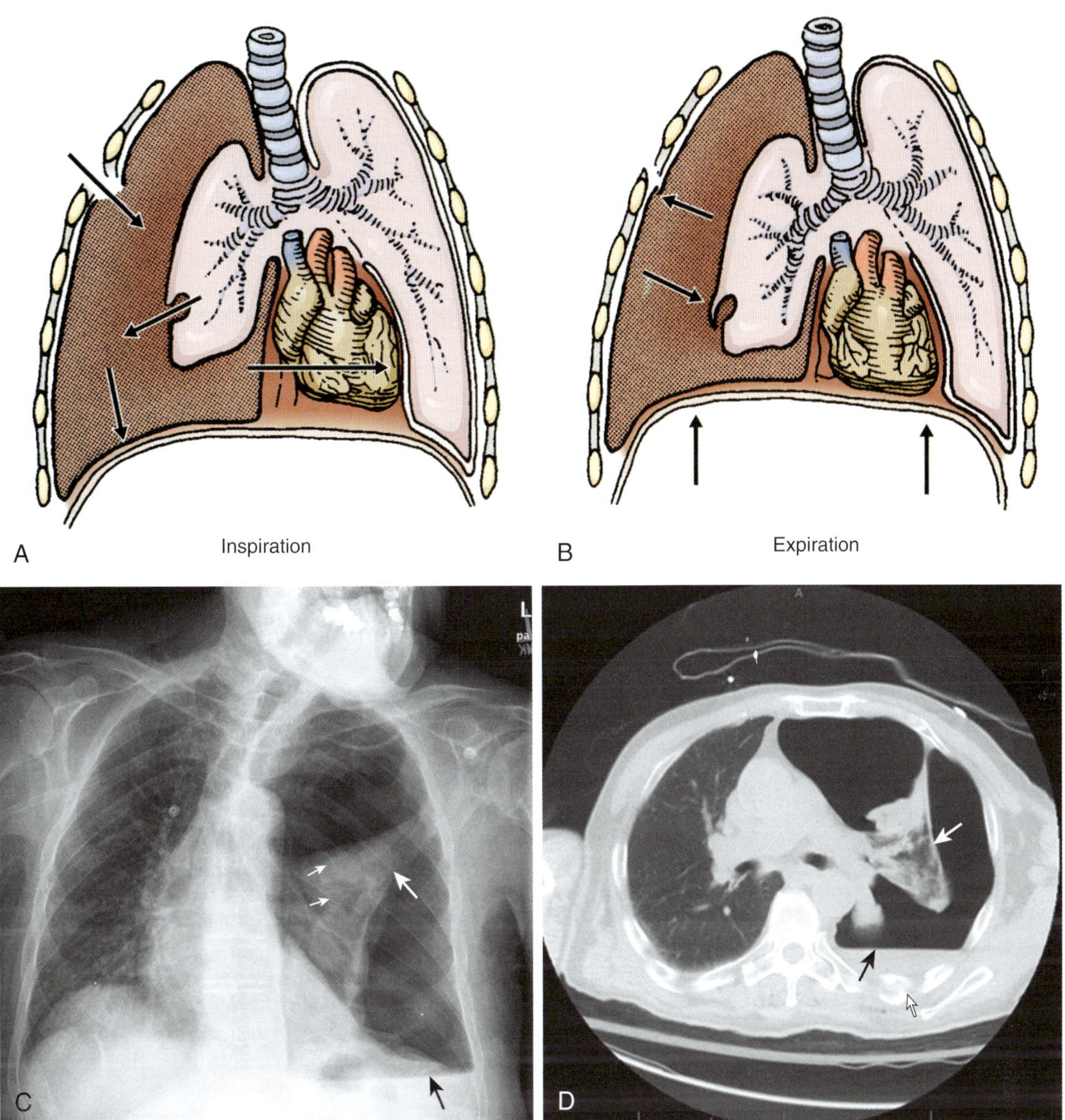

FIG. 32.13 Traumatic Tension Pneumothorax. (A and B) Pathophysiology of a tension pneumothorax. During inspiration, air enters the pleural space through a one-way valve either from the outside or from the lung itself. On expiration, the injury/valve closes and traps increasing amounts of air in the pleural space. Eventually, the mediastinum shifts and cardiac filling and ultimately cardiac output are compromised. (C) This elderly patient sustained a tension hemopneumothorax after slipping and falling on ice. The left hemithorax is very dark (radiolucent) because of total collapse of the left lung (large white arrow). Note the dramatic shift of the mediastinum to the right, indicative of tension. Multiple posterior rib fractures are present but are difficult to appreciate on this film (small white arrows). The air-fluid level (black arrow) indicates the presence of air in the pleural cavity in addition to fluid (blood). (D) A computed tomography scan of the same patient again demonstrates the findings seen on the conventional radiograph. (From Roberts, JR, ed. *Roberts and Hedges' Clinical Procedures in Emergency Medicine and Acute Care.* 7th ed. Elsevier; 2019.)

Assessment and diagnosis. Clinical manifestations of a tension pneumothorax include shortness of breath, tachycardia, hypotension, and sudden chest pain extending to the back, neck, or shoulders. On the injured side, breath sounds may be decreased or absent. Percussion of the chest reveals a hyperresonant sound over the affected side. Tracheal deviation (a late sign of tension pneumothorax) can be observed as the trachea shifts away from the injured side. Diagnosis is made by immediate clinical assessment. An Extended Focused Assessment with Sonography for Trauma (E-FAST) exam can help detect the presence of air in the pleural space (Box 32.10).

Management. When a tension pneumothorax is suspected in any trauma patient, there is no time for a chest radiograph because this potentially lethal condition must be treated immediately. Needle decompression is the immediate treatment of choice. Current ATLS guidelines suggest inserting a 5-cm to 8-cm needle at the fifth intercostal space, slightly anterior to the midaxillary line.[7] In contrast, the most recent Trauma Nursing Care Course (TNCC) guidelines advocate for a

BOX 32.10 FAST and E-FAST Exams

FAST (Focused Assessment with Sonography for Trauma) and E-FAST (Extended Focused Assessment with Sonography for Trauma) are both rapid bedside ultrasound techniques used to assess trauma patients for potential internal injuries,[1] particularly in blunt trauma—the main difference between the two lies in the scope and areas they cover during the ultrasound examination. The exam is typically performed by emergency medical personnel, including emergency practitioners and trauma surgeons, at the patient's bedside.[1]

The FAST exam is a rapid ultrasound examination designed to evaluate four specific areas in the abdomen and chest to identify the presence of free fluid, which could indicate internal bleeding. These four areas are:

- Right Upper Quadrant (RUQ): Assessing the space around the liver and right kidney.
- Left Upper Quadrant (LUQ): Evaluating the space around the spleen and left kidney.
- Suprapubic Area: Examining the pelvic region for fluid.

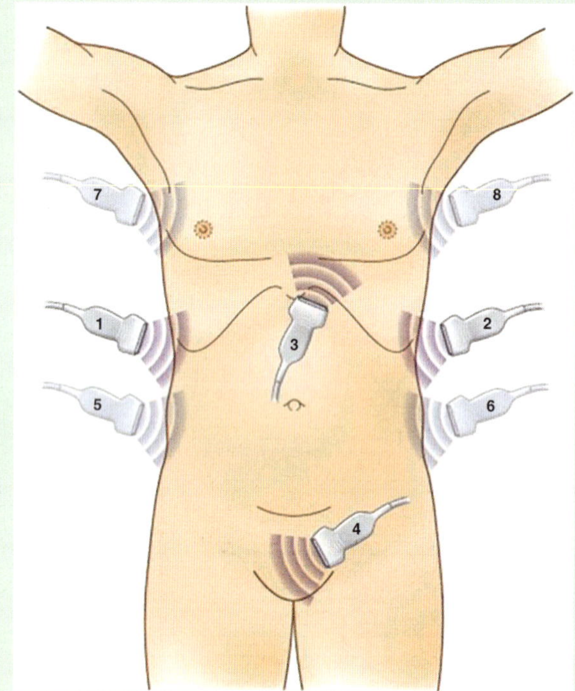

From Curtis K, Ramsden C, Shaban, R, et al. eds. *Emergency and Trauma Care for Nursing and Paramedics.* 3rd ed. Elsevier Australia; 2019.

- Pericardial Space: Checking for fluid around the heart.

The E-FAST extension of the FAST exam includes additional assessment areas. In addition to the four areas covered by FAST, E-FAST also examines the thoracic (chest) cavity. This information can help detect injuries to the lungs or other thoracic structures. The additional areas assessed in E-FAST are:

- Thoracic (Chest) Cavity: Assessing the pleural spaces on both sides of the chest for the presence of fluid or air.

Both techniques provide rapid and valuable information about potential internal injuries in trauma patients, aiding in quick decision making and appropriate patient management.[1]

Placement of ultrasound probes during FAST and extended FAST technique. 1, Right hypochondrium (Morison's pouch). 2, Left hypochondrium. 3, Pericardium. 4, Pelvis (retrovesical space). 5, Right renal fossa. 6, Left renal fossa. 7, Right chest base. 8, Left chest base.

The FAST and E-FAST exams are valuable tools for quickly assessing trauma patients for potential internal injuries. However, like any medical diagnostic technique, it has its limitations, including:

- The quality can vary based on the skill and experience of the operator performing the ultrasound. Proper technique, positioning, and interpretation of ultrasound images require training and expertise. Inexperienced operators might miss subtle findings or misinterpret images, leading to false negatives or positives.
- Ultrasound has limitations in terms of the structures it can visualize. It focuses on detecting fluid collections, which can indicate injury but might not directly visualize specific injuries to solid organs or other structures within the thorax or abdomen.
- The exam might not detect small amounts of fluid or minor injuries, especially in low-velocity trauma or injuries that don't cause significant fluid accumulation.
- The effectiveness can be impacted by obesity, bowel gas, subcutaneous emphysema, and patient positioning. These factors can affect the clarity of ultrasound images and make it more challenging to interpret findings accurately.
- As with any diagnostic test, false positives (indicating an injury that isn't present) and false negatives (missing an actual injury) are possible. Some injuries might not produce significant fluid accumulation initially, leading to false negatives. On the other hand, the presence of fluid might not always indicate trauma-related bleeding, resulting in false positives.

The FAST and E-FAST exams are just one part of the overall assessment of a trauma patient. It should be used with other clinical findings, patient history, and additional diagnostic tests to provide a comprehensive evaluation.[1]

Reference:

1. Savoia P, Jayanthi SK, Chammas MC. Focused assessment with sonography for trauma (FAST). *J Med Ultrasound.* 2023;31(2):101–106. https://doi.org/10.4103/jmu.jmu_12_23.

large-bore (14-gauge) needle inserted over the second rib midclavicular line (on the affected side) and using the fifth intercostal space as an alternative option.[83] A needle at least 8 cm long will penetrate the pleural space and relieve the tension pneumothorax approximately 90% of the time.[84] This procedure allows the release of air from the pleural space. A hissing sound is heard as the tension pneumothorax is converted to a simple pneumothorax. A chest tube is immediately inserted after needle decompression.

Massive hemothorax. Blunt or penetrating thoracic trauma can cause bleeding into the pleural space, resulting in a hemothorax (Fig. 32.14).

Pathophysiology. A massive hemothorax results from accumulating more than 1500 mL of blood in the thoracic cavity.[85] The source of bleeding may be the intercostal or internal mammary arteries, lungs, heart, or great vessels. Lacerations to the lung parenchyma are low-pressure bleeds and typically stop bleeding spontaneously. Arterial bleeding from hilar vessels usually requires immediate surgical intervention. Increasing blood loss into the pleural space causes decreased venous return and cardiac output.

Assessment and diagnosis. Assessment findings for patients with massive hemothorax reveal diminished or absent breath sounds over the affected lung and collapsed neck veins (hypovolemia) or distended neck veins (coexisting tension pneumothorax).[79] Massive hemothorax is diagnosed based on hypotension associated with the absence of breath sounds or dullness to percussion on one side of the chest. Hypovolemic

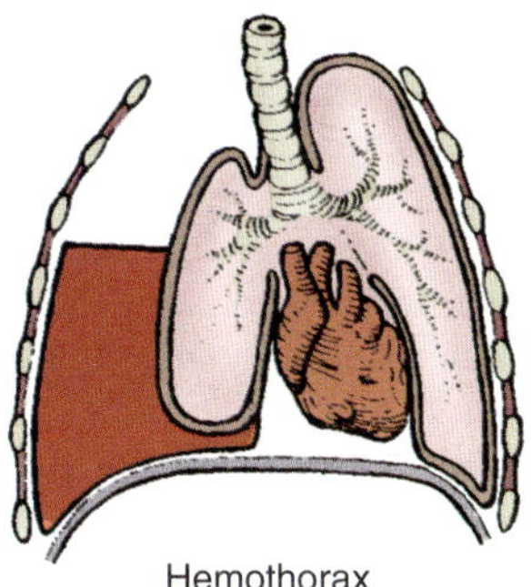

FIG. 32.14 Blunt or penetrating thoracic trauma can cause bleeding into the pleural space to form a hemothorax.

shock may be present. An E-FAST exam can help detect the presence of blood in the pleural space (Box 32.10).

Management. This potentially life-threatening condition must be treated immediately. Resuscitation with IV fluids is initiated to treat hypovolemic shock. A chest tube is placed on the affected side to allow drainage of blood. An MTP may be required. Emergency thoracotomy may be necessary for patients who require persistent blood transfusions or who have significant bleeding (greater than 20 mL/kg, or 200 mL/h for 2 to 4 hours, or more than 1500 mL on initial tube insertion) or when there are accompanying injuries to major cardiovascular structures.[7]

Heart and Vascular Injuries

Heart and vascular injuries can result from either blunt or penetrating trauma. The most common causes of blunt cardiac trauma include high-speed MVCs, direct blows to the chest, and falls. Because of its mobility and its location between the sternum and thoracic vertebrae, the heart is particularly susceptible to blunt traumatic injury. Sudden acceleration (from contact with a steering wheel) can cause the heart to be thrown against the sternum (Fig. 32.15). Sudden deceleration can cause the heart to be thrown against the thoracic vertebrae by a direct blow to the chest, such as blows caused by a baseball, animal kick, or fall.

Penetrating cardiac trauma can occur from mechanical injuries from gunshot wounds, stabbings, or other impalements. The chest wall offers little protection to the heart from penetrating trauma. The most common site of injury is the right ventricle because of its anterior position in the mediastinum. Pre- and in-hospital mortality rates from penetrating cardiac trauma are reported to be between 5% and 76%.[86] Most deaths occur minutes after injury due to exsanguination, tamponade, or shock. Trauma teams must be aware of three potentially lethal cardiac and vascular injuries: blunt cardiac injury (BCI), cardiac tamponade, and blunt traumatic aortic injury (BTAI).

Blunt cardiac injury. BCI covers a broad spectrum of possible cardiac issues in trauma patients, including myocardial contusion, septal valve rupture, and coronary artery dissection. The chambers most often injured are the right atrium and right ventricle because of their anterior position in the chest.

Pathophysiology. The most common form of BCI is a myocardial contusion, which is injury to the heart muscle itself. The impact can cause direct damage to the myocardium, disrupting the cardiac muscle fibers and potentially impairing cardiac contractility. Myocardial contusions can range from mild to severe, with varying levels of functional impairment.

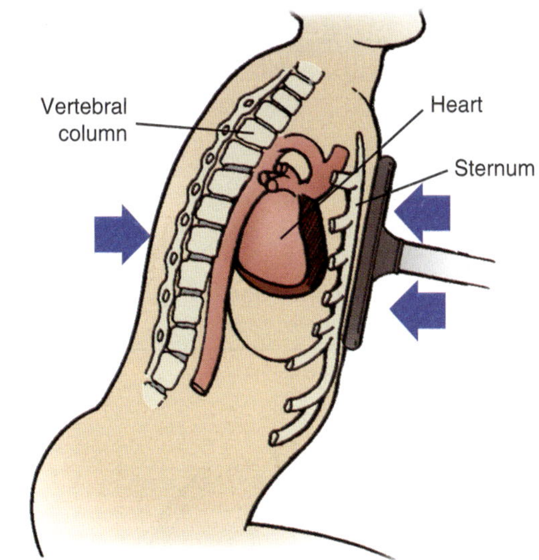

FIG. 32.15 Blunt Cardiac Trauma. Sudden acceleration (e.g., from contact with the steering wheel) can cause the heart to be thrown against the sternum.

BCI can disrupt the normal electrical conduction pathways of the heart, leading to dysrhythmias. The impact can cause conduction disturbances, such as heart block or bundle branch blocks, as well as atrial or ventricular arrhythmias. Arrhythmias can further compromise cardiac output and oxygen delivery to the body. Severe BCI can lead to damage to the heart's valves and other structural components. The force of impact can cause valve leaflet tears, rupture of chordae tendineae, or even damage to the papillary muscles. This can result in valvular insufficiency or stenosis, affecting cardiac function.

Assessment and diagnosis. Few clinical signs and symptoms are specific to BCI. Evidence of external chest trauma, such as steering wheel imprint or sternal fractures, should raise suspicion for BCI. However, the presence of a sternal fracture does not predict the incidence of BCI. The patient may complain of chest pain like anginal pain, but the pain is not relieved with nitroglycerin. Chest discomfort is usually caused by associated injuries, including fractured ribs. Unexplained tachycardia or the presence of a new bundle branch block should increase awareness for BCI.

Guidelines for screening BCI from the Eastern Association of Surgeons in Trauma are listed in Box 32.11. The patient should have a chest radiograph and be monitored for new onset of dysrhythmias. A 12-lead electrocardiogram may reveal dysrhythmias, ST segment changes, or bundle branch block.[79] Cardiac biomarkers, such as troponin, are of little diagnostic help for BCI. Unexplained shock and hypotension heighten suspicion for BCI. In symptomatic patients, echocardiography may reveal possible wall motion abnormalities, pericardial fluid, or valve tearing or rupture.[87]

Management. Medical management is aimed at preventing and treating complications. This approach includes hemodynamic monitoring in a CCU and possible administration of antidysrhythmic medications. A "watch and see" approach is advised for hemodynamically stable patients. Surgical consultation may be required for the unstable patient for ruptured valves and pericardial fluid accumulation.

Cardiac tamponade. Cardiac tamponade is the progressive accumulation of blood in the pericardial sac (Fig. 32.16). In

BOX 32.11 EAST Guidelines for Screening of Blunt Cardiac Injury

- Obtain an admission electrocardiogram (ECG) for all patients in whom there is suspected blunt cardiac injury (BCI).
- If ECG is abnormal, the patient should be admitted for continuous ECG monitoring for 24 to 48 hours.
- If the patient is hemodynamically unstable, an echocardiogram may be performed.
- Cardiac biomarkers such as cardiac troponin T values do not help predict which patients will have BCI-related complications.

EAST, Eastern Association for the Surgery of Trauma.

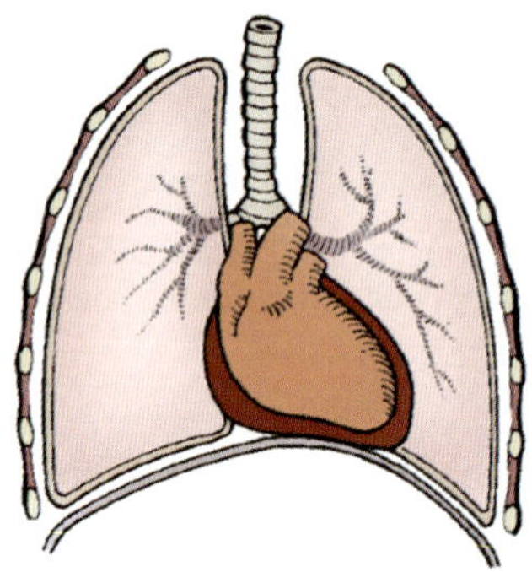

FIG. 32.16 Cardiac tamponade is the progressive accumulation of blood in the pericardial sac.

traumatic injury, cardiac tamponade can occur as a result of either blunt or penetrating origins.

Pathophysiology. After an injury, blood accumulation increases intracardiac pressure and compresses the atria and ventricles. The amount of blood needed to cause changes in patient hemodynamics depends on the amount of blood in the pericardial sac and the speed with which the fluid has accumulated.[88] As intracardiac pressure continues to increase, this leads to decreased venous return, preload, and cardiac output. Myocardial hypoxia, heart failure, and cardiogenic shock may occur.

Assessment and diagnosis. Classic assessment findings associated with cardiac tamponade include elevated central venous pressure (with neck vein distention), muffled heart sounds, and hypotension. These signs are known as *Beck's triad.* These signs are present in only 10% to 58% of traumatic cardiac tamponade.[89] Focused assessment with sonography for trauma (FAST) in the ED is rapid and highly accurate, and it may be used to identify cardiac tamponade in the trauma patient quickly.

Management. While preparing for immediate pericardiocentesis, first-line actions include administering oxygen, monitoring vital signs, and administering IV fluids to increase cardiac output. Ultrasound-guided pericardiocentesis involves fluid aspiration from the pericardial sac using a large-bore needle. This procedure helps restore normal transmural pressure and improve the patient's hemodynamic status.[90] The inherent risk in this procedure is potential laceration of the coronary artery when a blind insertion is used. Longer-term definitive treatment may involve a pericardiotomy, percutaneous catheter drainage, or pericardial window.[90]

Blunt traumatic aortic injury. BTAI is one of the most lethal thoracic injuries and the second most common cause of death in blunt trauma. Of patients with BTAI, 85% die before reaching the hospital.[91] Associated injuries include a first or second rib fracture, high sternal fracture, left clavicular fracture at the level of the sternal margin, and massive hemothorax.

Pathophysiology. BTAI should be suspected in all trauma patients with a rapid deceleration or acceleration mechanism of injury. The thoracic aorta is relatively mobile and may tear at fixed anatomic points within the thorax. Approximately 75% of BTAI patients will rupture at the aortic isthmus (the most mobile and weakest portion of the aorta), but other areas may be injured.[92] A complete rupture of the aorta causes death by hemorrhage. The aorta, a relatively rigid structure, can be subjected to extreme stretching and shearing forces during these events. The initial mechanical impact can cause a tear or rupture of the intimal layer of the aortic wall. This can create a communication between the true lumen (inner channel of the aorta) and the false lumen (a new channel created within the layers of the aortic wall). Blood can flow into the false lumen, causing the layers of the aortic wall to separate and form an aortic dissection. The dissection can extend along the length of the aorta and compromise blood flow to vital organs. As blood enters the false lumen and dissects along the aortic wall, it can accumulate within the layers of the wall, forming an intramural hematoma. This further weakens the aortic wall and can lead to rupture.

In severe cases, the mechanical stress and weakened aortic wall can lead to rupture.

Rupture of the aorta results in massive internal hemorrhage, leading to life-threatening hypovolemic shock. The rupture can occur into the pericardial space (hemopericardium) or into the thoracic cavity (hemothorax), further compromising cardiac and respiratory function. BTAI can also affect the aortic valve, causing valve dysfunction due to the displacement of the aortic root or direct damage to the valve leaflets. This can lead to aortic regurgitation (backward flow of blood) and further compromise cardiac output.

Assessment and diagnosis. Blood pressure is measured in both arms because a tear in the aortic arch may create a pressure gradient resulting in blood pressure changes between the upper extremities. Patients may also present asymptomatic. Additional clinical assessment findings include a pulse deficit at any site, unexplained hypotension, sternal pain, precordial systolic murmur, hoarseness, dyspnea, and lower extremity sensory deficits.[79]

An initial upright chest radiograph is obtained after spine radiographs have been completed and the spine is cleared. Radiographic findings suggesting aortic injury include widened mediastinum, abnormal shape of the aorta, and deviation of the left main stem bronchus.[91] Contrast-enhanced CT (time permitting) and transesophageal echocardiography (TEE) are the gold standard for diagnosis.[92]

Management. Blood pressure management is the primary goal to minimize injury during the resuscitation phase for a patient with blunt traumatic aortic injury. Minimizing stress on the vessel is achieved by maintaining the heart rate less than 100 beats/min, ideally using a beta-blocker. The aim is to keep SBP less than 100 mm Hg and MAP 60 to 70 mm Hg by using beta-blockers such as esmolol or labetalol.[93] If beta-blockers are contraindicated, calcium channel blockers may be used. IV nitroglycerin or sodium nitroprusside may be added as adjuncts when initial blood pressure and MAP goals are unmet.[7] Early surgical consultation and urgent endovascular repair should be anticipated. The most common operative procedure for blunt aortic injury is endoluminal stent grafts.[93]

Postoperative care is also directed toward stabilizing blood pressure to minimize vessel stress while maintaining tissue perfusion, which is accomplished using medications described earlier. Careful assessment for stroke and postoperative paraplegia is needed because of the degree of injury to the aorta. Paraplegia is closely related to the degree of aortic injury affecting spinal perfusion and duration of intraoperative aortic cross-clamping time. The patient is monitored for hemorrhage, bowel ischemia (e.g., tube feeding intolerance, lactic acidosis), infection, and respiratory failure postoperatively. Acute kidney injury (AKI), which may manifest as low urine output and rising serum creatinine, may occur because blood flow to the mesentery and kidney may have been compromised due to the injury or surgery.

Abdominal Injuries

Abdominal injuries are frequently associated with multisystem trauma. Abdominal injuries are the third leading cause of death in trauma. Injuries to the abdomen may be the result of blunt or penetrating events.

Pathophysiology

Blunt abdominal injuries occur most often from MVCs, assaults, and falls. Blunt abdominal trauma can produce injuries to the liver, spleen, and diaphragm. Deceleration and direct forces can produce retroperitoneal hematomas. Penetrating abdominal trauma is primarily caused by stabbings, gunshot wounds, or other impalements. Commonly injured organs from stab wounds are the colon, liver, spleen, and diaphragm. Gunshot wounds to the abdomen usually are more serious than stab wounds. A bullet can travel in erratic paths and ricochet off bone inside the abdomen. Death from penetrating injuries depends on the extent of damage to major vascular structures and resultant intraabdominal hemorrhage.

Assessment and Diagnosis

Initial assessment of the trauma patient, whether in the ED or CCU, follows the primary and secondary survey techniques outlined by ATLS guidelines.[7] The initial physical assessment of the abdomen may be nonspecific or unreliable, given possible coexisting influences of alcohol, illicit drugs, analgesics, or an altered LOC.

Assessment. A distended abdomen may indicate blood, fluid, or gas accumulation from a perforated organ or a ruptured blood vessel. Purplish discoloration of the flanks or umbilicus (Cullen sign) may signify blood in the abdominal wall. Ecchymosis in the flank area (Grey-Turner sign) may indicate retroperitoneal bleeding or a pancreatic injury. A hematoma in the flank area suggests kidney injury.

Auscultation may reveal normal or absent bowel sounds. The abdomen is assessed for rebound tenderness and rigidity, indicative of peritoneal inflammation. Referred pain to the left shoulder (Kehr sign) may indicate a ruptured spleen or irritation of the diaphragm from bile or other material in the peritoneum. The locations of entry and exit sites associated with penetrating trauma are identified and documented. Physical examination of the abdomen alone is unreliable in a patient suspected to have abdominal trauma.

Diagnosis. Insertion of a nasogastric or orogastric tube serves as a valuable diagnostic and therapeutic aid. These tubes can decompress the stomach, and drainage can be checked for blood. Laboratory test results may be nonspecific for patients with abdominal trauma. Because of hemoconcentration, hemoglobin and hematocrit results may not reflect actual values. Serial measurements help diagnose abdominal injuries. An increasing lactate level is highly suggestive of mesenteric hypoperfusion and shock.[94]

Diagnostic imaging may occur during the ATLS secondary survey. Diagnostic peritoneal lavage, an invasive technique in which a small catheter is inserted into the abdominal cavity, and the abdomen is assessed for the presence of blood, is rarely performed. A bedside ultrasound, CT scan, and FAST exam have primarily replaced diagnostic peritoneal lavage as a superior diagnostic tool in abdominal trauma. Although FAST has good sensitivity and specificity, it is not intended to replace the CT scan.[95] CT is the mainstay of diagnostic evaluation in a hemodynamically stable patient with abdominal trauma. Abdominal CT provides information about specific organ injuries, pelvic injuries, and retroperitoneal hemorrhage. Hemodynamically unstable patients with a positive FAST examination generally undergo damage control surgery to achieve hemostasis.

Management

Medical and nursing management vary according to specific organ injuries. Liver, spleen, and bowel injuries, seen most frequently in patients with multisystem trauma, are discussed here.

Liver injuries. The liver is a commonly injured abdominal organ in trauma and is a significant cause of hemorrhage after injury. Abdominal CT is the most reliable diagnostic tool to identify and assess the severity of injury to the liver.[7] The severity of liver injuries is graded to provide a mechanism for determining the amount of trauma sustained, the care needed, and possible outcomes (Table 32.9). Nonsurgical management is considered the standard of care for hemodynamically stable patients with blunt liver injury.[96]

Nonsurgical management. Care of trauma patients with severe liver injuries can be challenging. Serial serum hematocrit

TABLE 32.9 Liver Injury Scale

Grade[a]	Injury	Criteria
I	Hematoma	Subcapsular, <10% surface area
	Laceration	Capsular tear, <1 cm parenchymal depth
II	Hematoma	Subcapsular, 10%–50% surface area; intraparenchymal <10 cm in diameter
	Laceration	1–3 cm parenchymal depth, <10 cm long
III	Hematoma	Subcapsular, >50% surface area or expanding; ruptured subcapsular or parenchymal hematoma; intraparenchymal hematoma >10 cm or expanding
	Laceration	>3 cm parenchymal depth
IV	Laceration	Parenchymal disruption involving 25%–75% of hepatic lobe
	Bleeding	Active bleeding beyond liver and into the peritoneum
V	Laceration	Parenchymal disruption involving >75% of hepatic lobe
	Vascular	Juxtahepatic venous injuries (retrohepatic vena cava, central major hepatic veins)

[a]Advance one grade for multiple injuries up to grade III.

and hemoglobin levels and vital signs are monitored over several days. Hemodynamic instability can result from hemorrhage and hypovolemic shock, leading to fluid volume deficit, impaired cardiac output, and decreased tissue perfusion. An MTP may be implemented to restore blood volume and correct coagulopathies.

Surgical management. Continued hemodynamic instability (e.g., hypotension, decreased cardiac output) despite aggressive medical intervention may indicate ongoing hemorrhage, in which case an exploratory laparotomy may be required to identify and correct the source of bleeding. Resection of devitalized tissue is necessary for massive injuries. Hemorrhage is common with liver injuries, and ligation of hepatic arteries or veins may be required. Damage-control surgery involves ligating bleeding vessels and packing the liver in traumatic liver injury. Drains may be placed intraoperatively to prevent hematoma development. The patient's postoperative course may be complicated by coagulopathy, acidosis, hypothermia, and hypocalcemia. Jaundice may occur as a sign of liver dysfunction, but it may also be caused by the reabsorption of hematomas or the breakdown of transfused red blood cells.

Spleen injuries. The spleen is also a commonly injured organ in abdominal trauma and, like the liver, can be a source of life-threatening hemorrhage. Splenic injuries, like liver injuries, are graded to determine the amount of trauma sustained, the care required, and possible outcomes (Table 32.10). Hemodynamically stable patients may be monitored in the CCU, trending serial hematocrit and hemoglobin values and vital signs. The current trend favors nonsurgical management. Embolization therapy is a possible option in all grades of spleen injury to help decrease blood loss from the spleen. Patients with splenic injury who exhibit hemodynamic instability and progressive deterioration may require immediate surgical intervention with laparotomy.[97]

TABLE 32.10 Spleen Injury Scale

Grade[a]	Injury	Criteria
I	Hematoma	Subcapsular, <10% surface area
	Laceration	Capsular tear <1 cm, parenchymal depth
II	Hematoma	Subcapsular 10%–50% surface area; intraparenchymal <5 cm in diameter
	Laceration	1–3 cm parenchymal depth
III	Hematoma	Subcapsular >50% surface area; ruptured subcapsular or intraparenchymal hematoma; intraparenchymal hematoma ≥5 cm or expanding
	Laceration	>3 cm parenchymal depth
IV	Bleeding	Any vascular injury in presence of injury to spleen or active bleeding *within* spleen capsule
	Laceration	Parenchymal laceration involving segmental or hilar vessels producing major devascularization (>25% of spleen)
V	Bleeding	Any vascular injury in presence of injury to spleen or active bleeding *beyond* spleen capsule into peritoneum Completely shattered spleen
	Vascular	Hilar vascular injury that devascularizes spleen

[a]Advance one grade for multiple injuries up to grade III.

Modified from Kozar RA, Crandall M, Shanmuganathan K, et al; AAST Patient Assessment Committee. Organ injury scaling 2018 update: spleen, liver, and kidney. *J Trauma Acute Care Surg.* 2018;85(6):1119–1122. https://doi.org/10.1097/TA.0000000000002058.

Traditional postoperative care is provided after a splenectomy. The spleen plays a significant role in preventing infection against different organisms, including *Streptococcus, Neisseria*, and *Haemophilus*.[98] Patients who have had a splenectomy are at risk for developing postsplenectomy sepsis with streptococcal pneumonia. These patients require the polyvalent pneumococcal vaccine (Pneumovax) 14 days postoperatively to help promote immunity against pneumococcal bacteria.[99] Patients should also receive *Haemophilus influenzae* type B and meningococcal vaccines within 2 weeks of splenectomy.[99] Complications after splenic trauma include wound infection, sepsis, subdiaphragmatic abscess, and fistulas of the colon, pancreas, and stomach.

Complications. Two major life-threatening conditions after abdominal trauma are missed hollow viscus injuries and abdominal compartment syndrome. It is crucial that the patient be monitored closely after an abdomen injury for immediate recognition and prevention of complications. Signs and symptoms are often subtle and nonspecific, so synthesis of physical assessment findings, diagnostic imaging tests, and laboratory results are essential for the early detection of abdominal complications.

Missed hollow viscus injuries. The term *hollow viscus* refers to the hollow organs in the abdomen, such as the stomach, small intestine, and large intestine. While relatively uncommon, hollow viscus injuries can result from penetrating (17%) or blunt (1%) trauma.[100] Diagnosing a hollow viscus injury is challenging because these injuries may not be readily identifiable during the primary or secondary assessments or may not appear on an initial CT scan or ultrasound. A delay in the time to diagnosis contributes to complications. Regardless of the mechanism of injury, intestinal contents (e.g., bile, stool, enzymes, bacteria) can leak into the peritoneum and cause numerous complications, including septic shock. Surgical resection and repair are almost always required.

The patient's postoperative course is usually affected by the degree of septic shock the patient is experiencing as a result of leakage of intestinal contents from perforated structures within the abdominal cavity. Important interventions include monitoring vital signs, administering analgesia and antibiotics, trending hemoglobin and hematocrit values, and observing all fluid exiting from all gastrointestinal tubes and drains. If frank blood is observed exiting from any tube or drain, the health care practitioner is notified immediately. Enteral nutrition is generally not initiated until the bowel has had time to heal and only after consultation and approval by the surgeon. The patient is observed for signs of worsening hemodynamic instability and abscess or fistula formation.

Abdominal compartment syndrome. Abdominal compartment syndrome is end-organ dysfunction caused by intra-abdominal hypertension (IAH). Increased pressure can be caused by bleeding, ileus, mesenteric edema, or a noncompliant abdominal wall. Increased pressure within the abdominal cavity can impinge on diaphragmatic excursion and affect ventilation. Clinical manifestations of abdominal compartment syndrome include decreased cardiac output, decreased tidal volume, increased peak pulmonary pressure, decreased urine output, and hypoxia.[101]

Intraabdominal pressure monitoring. Intraabdominal pressure (IAP) can be measured through various commercially available devices or a simple pressurized tubing setup. In both instances, the urinary bladder acts as a transducer to estimate the degree of IAP after injecting 25 mL of sterile saline. IAH is defined as an IAP greater than or equal to 12 mm Hg (normal IAP is 5 to 7 mm Hg).[102] IAH may be graded as follows:

- IAH grade I (12 to 15 mm Hg)
- IAH grade II (16 to 20 mm Hg)
- IAH grade III (21 to 25 mm Hg)
- IAH grade IV (greater than 25 mm Hg)[102]

The abdominal perfusion pressure (APP) is calculated as MAP – IAP. The APP should be maintained within 50 to 60 mm Hg to ensure adequate blood supply to the gut.

Surgical management. Surgical decompression of the abdomen may be required for abdominal pressures greater than 20 to 25 mm Hg accompanied by a taut, tense abdomen and signs of organ dysfunction such as deteriorating heart, lung, and kidney status. After surgical decompression is completed and the pressure is relieved, the patient may return to the CCU with an "open abdomen." For example, the abdomen may be temporarily closed with biological mesh or sutured closed. Negative pressure wound therapy (NPWT) is currently the preferred strategy.[103] After 4 to 7 days, fascial and skin closure may be possible. In the days or weeks following the surgery, depending on its size, the open abdomen may also be allowed to heal with synthetic mesh or by secondary intention and eventual skin grafting.[104]

Genitourinary Injuries

Trauma to the genitourinary tract seldom occurs as an isolated injury. A genitourinary injury must be suspected in any patient with pelvic fracture; blunt trauma to the lower chest or flank; contusions, hematoma, or tenderness over the flank, lower abdomen, or perineum; genital swelling or discoloration; blood at the urethral meatus; hematuria after Foley catheter placement; or difficulty with micturition.[7] Similar to all other traumatic injuries, genitourinary injuries can result from blunt or penetrating trauma.

Pathophysiology

The pathophysiology of genitourinary injuries can vary based on the specific organ involved and the mechanism of injury. The kidneys are vulnerable to trauma due to their location and proximity to the ribs and spine. Damage to the kidneys can result in renal contusions (bruising), lacerations (tears), or even ruptures. Trauma to the bladder can lead to rupture of the bladder. Bladder rupture can lead to urine leaking into the peritoneal cavity, causing peritonitis, an inflammation of the abdominal lining. Bladder injuries are further subdivided into extraperitoneal ruptures (60%), intraperitoneal ruptures (30%), or combined injuries (10%).[105] Urethral injuries can result from pelvic fractures, straddle injuries (falling onto a hard object between the legs), or catheterization procedures. Incomplete or complete disruption of the urethra can lead to difficulty in passing urine and blood in the urine. Ureteral injuries are less common but can occur due to trauma. If the ureter is damaged, urine can leak into the surrounding tissues, leading to urinoma (accumulation of urine) and potential infection. Testicular injuries can result from direct trauma, causing testicular rupture or hematoma. Scrotal injuries can also lead to hematocele (blood collection in the scrotum).

Assessment and Diagnosis

Assessment. Evaluation of genitourinary trauma begins after the ATLS primary survey has been completed. Specific assessment findings may heighten suspicion of genitourinary trauma. A conscious patient may complain of flank pain or colic pain. Rebound tenderness can be elicited if intraperitoneal extravasation of urine has occurred. Inspection may reveal blood at the urethral meatus. Bluish discoloration of the flanks may indicate retroperitoneal bleeding, whereas perineal discoloration may indicate a pelvic fracture and possible bladder or urethral injury. Hematuria is a common assessment finding with genitourinary trauma. However, the absence of gross or microscopic hematuria does not exclude a urinary tract injury.[106]

Kidney and bladder injuries. Injury to the kidney may be reflected by flank ecchymosis and fracture of inferior ribs or spinous processes. Gross or microscopic hematuria may be present; however, the degree of blood in the urine does not reflect the true extent of kidney damage. Gross hematuria can exist with minor injuries and sometimes clears within a few hours. Injury to the bladder may present with lower abdominal bruising, distention, and pain. The patient may be unable to void.

Diagnosis

The CT scan is considered the first-line diagnostic test to help evaluate the genitourinary system for evidence of blunt traumatic injury. Contrast-enhanced CT can help identify the presence of upper and lower urinary tract for trauma. CT is the most accurate modality available for diagnosing kidney injury because it can assess the extent of parenchymal laceration, urine extravasation, surrounding hemorrhage, and the presence of vascular injury. Penetrating kidney trauma may require a renal angiogram, which can also be used to embolize bleeding vessels. Sonography for testicular injury and MRI scans may also be used in genitourinary trauma.

Management

Medical and nursing management vary according to specific organ injuries. After admission to the CCU, assessment of the patient is done according to ATLS guidelines. Consultation with a urologist may be necessary. Primary interventions for genitourinary trauma include assessing hemorrhage, maintaining fluid and electrolyte balance, and maintaining patency of drains and tubes. Measurement of urinary output includes drainage from the urinary catheter, nephrostomy, or suprapubic tubes. Urinary output should be at least 0.5 mL/kg/h.[7] Urine output is measured hourly until bloody drainage and clots have cleared. Gentle irrigation of drainage tubes may be required to clear clots and maintain patency. Monitoring the patient's hemoglobin, potassium, creatinine, and urea is essential. Kidney and bladder injuries are further discussed here

Kidney trauma. Kidney injuries are graded I through V to assist trauma teams in determining the extent of the injury. Grade I, the most frequently occurring kidney injury, reflects small contusion and hematoma, while grade V identifies avulsion injury, devascularization, and active bleeding.[107]

Contusions and minor lacerations usually are treated medically with observation in hemodynamically stable patients. Operative interventions may be required in patients with kidney injuries who are hemodynamically unstable with a devascularized segment or are actively hemorrhaging. Angiographic embolization is used when possible. Postoperative and post-injury complications following kidney trauma include hemorrhage, infection, infarction, extravasation, calcification, and AKI.

Bladder trauma. Many bladder injuries result from blunt trauma,[108] although penetrating mechanisms can also induce injury. Similarly, bladder injuries can be classified from grade I (mild injury with small hematoma) through grade V (lethal laceration that may extend into the neck of the bladder).[109] The type of injury depends on the location and strength of blunt force and the volume of urine in the bladder at the time of injury. Extraperitoneal rupture of the bladder may be managed conservatively with catheterization and antibiotics for 7 to 10 days. Unresolved extravasation from intraperitoneal rupture requires surgical intervention. The ideal treatment for bladder injury is unknown.

Musculoskeletal Injuries

Fractures of the arms, hands, wrists, legs, and feet are common in trauma. Although painful, orthopedic fractures are often not life threatening. However, when injured, the pelvis poses potentially life-threatening consequences for a trauma patient.

Pelvic Fractures

The pelvis is a ring-shaped structure composed of the hip bones (ilium, ischium, pubis), sacrum, and coccyx. The pelvis protects the lower urinary tract, major blood vessels, and nerves of the lower extremities. Pelvic trauma can result in urologic and neurologic dysfunction and severe, life-threatening hemorrhage.

Etiology. Blunt trauma to the pelvis can be caused by MVCs, falls, or a crush injury. Pelvic fractures constitute a spectrum of complexity ranging from a single nondisplaced fracture to a life-threatening condition in which multiple fractures and crush injuries are associated with significant internal injuries and hemorrhage. There is no universally agreed-on classification system for pelvic fractures. Pelvic fractures may be *stable* (intact pelvic ring) or *unstable* (nonintact pelvic ring). Pelvic fractures may be open (continuity with vagina, rectum, or external body surface) or closed. The Young-Burgess system is most frequently used by trauma teams and classifies pelvic fractures based on forces applied to the pelvic ring.[110]

Pathophysiology. When the pelvic ring is disrupted, the radius increases, increasing blood volume capacity. Pelvic injuries may be associated with damage to underlying arterial and venous vessels. There is also loss of the tamponade effect of the pelvis with severe disruption of the pelvic ring, contributing to further bleeding. Because the pelvic area is a highly vascular compartment, it can sequester a large volume of blood. The mortality rate from pelvic trauma ranges from 8% to 16%.[111] Death within 24 hours of injury is most often caused by hemorrhagic shock.

Anteroposterior compression pelvic injury. When force is applied in the anteroposterior direction, the pelvic diameter widens. In this case, the injury can be completely ligamentous, manifesting as an open sacroiliac joint or open pubic symphysis. This type of compression injury is commonly associated with vascular injury. There are three types of anteroposterior compression pelvic fractures, classified according to severity of injury:

- *Type I anteroposterior injury* includes disruption of the pubic symphysis with less than 2.5 cm of diastasis and insignificant posterior pelvic involvement.
- *Type II anteroposterior injury* includes disruption of the pubic symphysis of more than 2.5 cm with tearing of associated ligaments.
- *Type III anteroposterior injury* is a complete disruption of the pubic symphysis, posterior ligament complexes, and hemipelvic involvement. This type of injury is known as the unstable "open book" pelvic fracture.

Lateral compression pelvic injury. Lateral compression forces produce a shortening of the pelvic diameter and typically do not involve ligamentous injury. The pelvic volume is reduced in this type of injury, so hemorrhage is not as common, but localized bleeding may occur. Lateral compression fractures are classified according to the severity of the injury as follows:

- *Type I lateral compression injury* includes posterior sacroiliac joint compression without ligament disruption or an oblique pubic ramus fracture. This type of fracture is considered stable.
- *Type II lateral compression injury* includes rupture of the posterior sacroiliac ligament or internal rotation of the hemipelvis with a crush injury of the sacrum and an oblique pubic ramus fracture.
- *Type III lateral compression injury* includes the findings of type II lateral compression injury with additional evidence of anteroposterior compression to the contralateral hemipelvis. This type of fracture is considered unstable.

Vertical shear. A vertical shear pelvic injury occurs when force is applied in a perpendicular plane across the anterior and posterior aspects of the ring. Complete disruption of the hemipelvis associated with major hemipelvic displacement and instability occurs. This type of injury typically occurs in people who fall from a great height and land on one extremity. This injury is the most severe type of pelvic fracture, the most unstable, and often associated with significant visceral damage.[112]

Combined pelvic injuries. Combined pelvic injuries are a combination of injury types that do not fit into any single category. Most combined pelvic fracture injuries are unstable.

Assessment and diagnosis

Assessment. Signs of pelvic fracture include swelling, tenderness, and bruising around the pubis, iliac bones, hips, or sacrum. Perianal ecchymosis (scrotum or vulva) may be present, indicating extravasation of urine or blood. Pain or crepitus on palpation, or "rocking" of the iliac crests, suggests a fractured pelvis, but this is inconclusive.[113] Lower extremity rotation or leg shortening is also suspicious for a pelvic injury. Other possible assessment findings are lower limb paresis, swollen testicles, and vaginal, rectal, or urethral bleeding, which may or may not be accompanied by hematuria. Patients with a suspected pelvic injury should have a rectal examination to assess for SCI (reduced or absent rectal tone) or occult rectal bleeding.

Diagnosis. The diagnosis of pelvic fracture is made by an anteroposterior pelvic radiograph (with the patient in the supine position) or a CT scan of the pelvis. Additional radiographs may be required for definitive treatment, but obtaining additional films depends on the patient's hemodynamic stability.

Management. Pelvic fractures are serious injuries that require prompt and specialized medical treatment. The approach to treating pelvic fractures depends on the severity of the fracture, the stability of the pelvic ring, the presence of associated injuries, and the overall status of the patient. Initial assessment of a trauma patient with a pelvic fracture on admission to the

CCU proceeds according to ATLS guidelines. Before the patient is moved, the practitioner should have classified the pelvic fracture as *stable* or *unstable*. A stable pelvic injury implies no further pathologic displacement of the pelvis can occur with turning or moving. An unstable pelvic fracture means further pathologic displacement of the pelvis can occur with turning or moving.

IV fluid resuscitation and hemorrhage control are the mainstays of pelvic fracture management. Massive blood loss contributes to alterations in tissue perfusion. On admission, the patient may exhibit hemodynamic instability with abnormal coagulation factors. Interventions include IV fluids and blood products, with the recognition that a MTP may be required.

Interventional radiology management. The priority in trauma management of pelvic fractures is to prevent or control life-threatening hemorrhage. For unstable polytrauma patients with ongoing hemorrhage and pelvic instability, pelvic angiography with embolization is one option.[114] Additionally, patients with evidence of arterial extravasation on pelvic CT scans may require angiography and embolization independent of hemodynamic status.

Surgical management. *Damage control orthopedics*—nondefinitive surgical repair of the orthopedic injury—is another option. This time-limited approach may involve exploratory laparotomy, pelvic packing, or the application of a pelvic external fixator. Once the patient has stabilized, and generally after several days, definitive management of pelvic fractures may be done with internal screws, nails, or plates to create stability, prevent or correct deformity, and facilitate early mobilization.

Nursing management of external fixation devices aims to ensure patient comfort, prevent hospital-acquired pressure injury (HAPI), and prevent infection. Most institutions have protocols for pin site care of the external fixator device.

Nonsurgical management. Hemodynamically stable patients with stable pelvic fractures may be treated conservatively with ongoing monitoring of vital signs and collaboration with surgeons for physical therapy and progressive mobility. Essential nursing care includes neurovascular assessment of the lower extremities. Neurologic injury secondary to a pelvic fracture may be transient and temporary. Any sudden change in sensation or movement requires prompt notification of the practitioner.

Temporary pelvic binders may be applied initially at the scene to help reduce the pelvic ring size and limit the extent of bleeding.[115] Application of pelvic binders may also be accomplished by wrapping the pelvis with a bed sheet or commercially available binder between the greater trochanter and the iliac crests. The advantages of this technique are that it is quick, does not involve specialized training, allows continued access to the patient during trauma resuscitation, and does not require specialized equipment. Although pelvic binders may limit hemorrhage, improvement in mortality remains unclear.

Open pelvic fractures may necessitate complex, time-consuming, and sometimes painful dressing changes. Pain management strategies are essential for these patients. Patients with pelvic fractures may have a prolonged critical care course with various degrees of complications. A patient with a pelvic fracture often has other associated injuries, complicating recovery and rehabilitation after injury. The patient is at high risk for several postinjury problems, including pain, urogenital injuries, development of VTE, ARDS, wound infection, and sepsis.

COMPLICATIONS OF TRAUMA

As a result of vast improvements in prehospital and ED care of trauma patients, many more patients are surviving their initial multisystem injuries, transport to the hospital, and damage control operative procedures. Within the CCU, after resuscitation, stabilization, and damage control or definitive surgery, this is often a period of significant vulnerability for trauma patients. Ongoing nursing assessments are imperative for detecting complications associated with traumatic injuries early. Complications increase critical care and hospital length of stay, increase costs, and are associated with increased morbidity and mortality. Some of the most important complications in the care of critically injured patients in the critical care, intermediate care, and rehabilitation phases are identified in this section.

Pain

Pain may come from many sources, including surgery, procedures, and injuries. Relief of pain is a significant component in the care of trauma patients. Several different pain management strategies may be used with the trauma patient, including continuous IV infusions, thoracic and lumbar epidural infusions, intercostal nerve blocks, and nonsteroidal antiinflammatory medications.[116] Pain relief measures are individualized for each patient based on injuries, contraindications, allergies, and patient, practitioner, and institutional preferences or protocols. Multimodal pain management approaches in the trauma patient may be required (see Pain Management in Chapter 7).

Venous Thromboembolism

VTE, including deep vein thrombosis (DVT) and pulmonary emboli, is a significant cause of morbidity and mortality in trauma patients with multiple injuries. Patients with major trauma are at very high risk for VTE. Factors that form the basis of VTE pathophysiology are exacerbated in trauma, including direct endothelial injury due to the trauma, hypercoagulopathy from trauma-induced coagulopathy, and blood stasis from immobility. VTE may develop into a life-threatening acute pulmonary embolism (PE) (see Figs. 18.7 and 18.8). More information on PE is available in Chapter 18.

Trauma patients are at the greatest risk for developing VTE early in their hospitalization. Prevention is key. Routine thromboprophylaxis for a high-risk trauma patient includes using low-molecular-weight heparin (starting as soon as it is considered safe) and mechanical prophylaxis, such as pneumatic sequential compression devices. Strategies must be individualized for each patient. Early mobilization, ensuring the comfort and safety of the patient, and considering known injuries can also help prevent the development of VTE.

Acute Compartment Syndrome

Compartment syndrome is a condition in which increased pressure within a limited space compromises circulation, resulting in ischemia and necrosis of tissues within that space.[117] Among patients at high risk for developing compartment syndrome are patients with upper and lower extremity trauma, including fractures, vascular ruptures, massive tissue and crush injuries, or venous obstruction.

Clinical manifestations of compartment syndrome include obvious swelling and tightness of a limb, paresthesia, and extreme pain on passive stretch in the affected extremity.[7] Diminished pulses and decreased capillary refill do not reliably identify compartment syndrome because they may be intact until after irreversible damage has occurred. Elevated intracompartmental pressures confirm the diagnosis. Treatment can consist of simple interventions such as removing an occlusive dressing, bivalving (cutting) a cast, or more complex interventions, including surgical decompressive fasciotomy.

Acute Respiratory Distress Syndrome

Posttraumatic respiratory failure is often related to fractured ribs, pneumonia, or ARDS. ARDS can be caused by direct or indirect lung injury (see Acute Respiratory Distress Syndrome in Chapter 18). Direct injuries in trauma patients, including aspiration, inhalation, and pulmonary contusion, or indirect injuries, including sepsis and massive transfusion, can all contribute to ARDS. When ARDS in trauma occurs, it generally develops 24 to 72 hours after the initial injury. Intubation, mechanical ventilation, low tidal-volume ventilation, and use of PEEP are the mainstays of ARDS treatment.[118] In severe cases of ARDS, and when spinal radiographs have been cleared, and it is safe to do so, the trauma patient may need to be placed in the prone position to help facilitate oxygenation.

Hypermetabolism

Within 24 to 48 hours after traumatic injury, it was previously thought a predictable hypermetabolic response occurred after traumatic injury. Recent research has questioned whether or not such a response occurs.[119] Without question, stress hypermetabolism occurs in some patients after a major injury and is characterized by increased metabolic rate and oxygen consumption. Energy requirements increase to promote immune function and tissue repair. The goal of early nutrition is to maintain host defenses by supporting this hypermetabolism and preserving lean body mass.

Nutritional Support

Nutrition support is an essential component in the care of critically ill trauma patients. Most nutrition experts advocate beginning enteral nutrition as early as possible. Unless otherwise ordered, current guidelines recommend enteral feedings be initiated within 24 to 48 hours for all trauma patients.[120] Enteral feeding sites include the gastric route and any site beyond the pylorus of the stomach, including the duodenum and jejunum. Diminished or absent bowel sounds are not a contraindication to initiating tube feeds. Small bowel function and the ability to absorb nutrients remain intact despite gastroparesis and absent bowel sounds. Patients at risk for pulmonary aspiration due to gastric retention or gastroesophageal reflux should receive enteral feedings into the duodenum or jejunum. If enteral feeding is unsuccessful, parenteral nutrition should be initiated. See Chapter 6 for additional information on nutrition management.

Acute Kidney Injury

Assessment and ongoing monitoring of kidney function are critical to the trauma patient's survival. AKI is not entirely uncommon after traumatic injury. The cause of posttraumatic AKI is complex and may involve various factors besides the initial injury (Box 32.12).

Prevention of kidney failure is the best treatment, and it begins with ensuring sufficient IV fluid volume to maintain adequate renal perfusion. Serial assessments of blood urea nitrogen and creatinine levels are commonly used to evaluate kidney function. Progressive deterioration in kidney function requires prompt diagnosis and treatment (see Acute Kidney Injury in Chapter 25).

BOX 32.12 Etiologic Factors in Posttraumatic Acute Kidney Injury (AKI)

Patient Specific

- Preexisting kidney disease
- Hypertension
- Heart failure
- Diabetes
- Chronic kidney disease
- Chronic liver disease

Trauma Specific

- Prolonged shock states
- Profound acidosis
- Systemic inflammatory response syndrome or reperfusion injury
- Abdominal compartment syndrome
- Muscle ischemia; myoglobinuria
- Microemboli
- Nephrotoxic medications
- Radiocontrast dye

Rhabdomyolysis and Myoglobinuria

Patients with muscle trauma and crush injuries are susceptible to rhabdomyolysis and, if left untreated, can develop AKI. Prolonged immobility and crush injuries can compromise blood flow. Decreased arterial blood flow results in insufficient oxygen transport and ischemia. This situation initiates a cascade of cellular events, including depletion of adenosine triphosphate (ATP) and failure of ATP pumps, which leads to the necrosis of skeletal muscle cells.[121]

As cells die, intracellular contents, particularly potassium and myoglobin, are released. Myoglobin, a muscular pigment, is a large molecule lodged in the glomerulus resulting in myoglobinuria (myoglobin in the urine). Circulating myoglobin can lead to the development of AKI by several mechanisms: volume depletion, renal vasoconstriction, decreased renal perfusion, proximal tubule cytotoxicity, cast formation with tubular obstruction, accumulation of iron, and direct toxic effects of myoglobin in the kidney tubules.[122]

Rhabdomyolysis should be suspected in all patients who experience immobility or crush injuries in which blood flow to the muscle is interrupted for a prolonged time. Dark tea-colored urine suggests myoglobinuria. Testing for myoglobin in the urine can be done but may take some time. The most rapid screening test is a serum creatine kinase (CK) level. Increased creatine kinase levels are associated with muscle damage and renal failure. Urine output is monitored hourly, and trends in serial creatine kinase levels should be monitored frequently.

When rhabdomyolysis is diagnosed, treatment is aimed at preventing permanent kidney failure. Prevention of kidney dysfunction is paramount through the aggressive administration of IV fluids. IV fluids increase renal blood flow and decrease the concentration of nephrotoxic pigments. Alkalinization of the urine and administration of diuretics have been studied, but their roles in the prevention or management of rhabdomyolysis are not firmly established. Nursing management is directed toward maintaining urinary output, achieving fluid and electrolyte balance, monitoring CK levels, and optimizing hemodynamics to prevent deterioration in kidney function.

Fat Embolism Syndrome

Fat embolism syndrome can occur as a complication of orthopedic trauma. The clinical onset of fat embolism syndrome is as early as 12 hours after initial injury but generally within 72 hours.[123] Fat embolism syndrome appears to develop due to fat droplets that leak from fractured bone with embolization of the fat droplets to the lungs. These droplets are broken down into free fatty acids that are toxic to the pulmonary microvascular membranes. Pulmonary fat emboli alter pulmonary hemodynamics and pulmonary vascular permeability. The lung becomes highly edematous and hemorrhagic. This situation may lead to the development of ARDS.

Signs and symptoms may be subtle and nonspecific. The patient may become restless and slightly confused. Hypoxemia, neurologic impairment, and a petechial rash are classic signs and symptoms but may not always be present.[124] The patient may or may not exhibit tachypnea with some degree of respiratory distress. Hypoxia is a common finding. A chest radiograph may reveal patchy infiltrates; a CT scan is often performed to rule out pulmonary embolism. Diagnosis is clinical and based on patient history, usually involving orthopedic injury. Nursing care is supportive.

Transfusion-Related Acute Lung Injury

A patient receiving multiple blood products, particularly red blood cells, must be monitored for *transfusion-related acute lung injury* (TRALI). Signs of TRALI are similar to signs of ARDS, although there is a time-based relationship between the new onset of respiratory distress and the transfusion of blood products.[125] TRALI may occur 6 hours after a transfusion, as evidenced by fever, hypoxemia, and hypotension. Bilateral infiltrates may appear on the chest x-ray, often described as a "white out" in clinical practice. Treatment is supportive, including lung-protective strategies (low tidal-volume ventilation and PEEP) and, if possible, avoidance of subsequent transfusions.

Infection

Infection is a major source of mortality and morbidity in CCUs. Trauma patients are at risk for infection because of contaminated wounds, intubation and mechanical ventilation, invasive catheters, host susceptibility (including preexisting medical conditions), adverse effects of trauma on the immune system, and the critical care environment. Nursing management must include interventions to decrease and eliminate the patient's risk of infection. Standard interventions for the prevention of ventilator-associated pneumonia (VAP), catheter-associated urinary tract infection (CAUTI), and central line bloodstream infection (CLABSI) apply to trauma patients. Strict aseptic technique is required for all invasive procedures, catheter care, and dressing changes. Prompt removal of unnecessary lines, tubes, and drains, and hand hygiene are paramount to supporting optimal patient outcomes.

Wound Management

Wound contamination poses a significant infection risk for trauma patients, especially with injuries resulting from deep or penetrating trauma. Exogenous bacteria (from the external environment) can enter through open wounds. Exogenous bacteria can be dirt, grass, or debris inoculated into the wound at the time of injury or microorganisms introduced by personnel during wound care. Endogenous bacteria (from the internal environment) can be released due to gastrointestinal or genitourinary perforation.

Meticulous wound care is essential. Wound care goals include removing dead and devitalized tissue, allowing for wound drainage, and promoting wound epithelialization and contraction. Wound healing is accomplished through interventions that promote tissue perfusion, including administering oxygen and IV fluids and ensuring adequate nutritional support.

Sepsis

Traumatic injury initiates both inflammatory and immunological reactions within the body related to the severity of trauma. However, it is not always clear who is most at risk for sepsis posttraumatic injury. One recent study identified that risk factors for sepsis post injury were strongly correlated with age, spinal and chest injuries, presence of shock, packed red blood cells, and positive blood alcohol levels at admission.[126] The same authors also reported that trauma patients with sepsis had an increased length of stay and required more days of mechanical ventilation, IV vasopressors, and renal replacement therapy.[126]

Possible sources of sepsis in adult trauma patients are contaminated wounds, invasive catheters, and severe damage to internal organs and structures. The source of the septic nidus must be promptly investigated. Gram stain and cultures of blood, urine, sputum, invasive catheters, and wounds are obtained. Broad-spectrum antibiotic therapy is often initiated before receiving definitive positive culture results. It is based on the patient's current condition, nature of traumatic injury, hemodynamic stability severity, and infection probability.

Missed Injury

Once the trauma patient's condition has stabilized, nursing assessment of a patient with multiple injuries may reveal missed injuries. Missed injuries have a reported incidence of approximately 0.6% to 39%.[127] Primarily orthopedic, missed injuries may cause morbidity and mortality. Several factors in critical care contribute to missed injuries. Patient factors include individuals with head injuries and a GCS score of 8 or less, intoxicated at admission, higher ISSs, and patients receiving analgesia and sedation. Clinician factors may include lack of experience, error in radiologic interpretation, failure to engage other services, or responsibility for several trauma patients with multiple competing demands.

In the CCU, a missed injury may be suspected if the patient fails to respond appropriately to medical or surgical intervention. Hypotension and a falling hematocrit level despite fluid administration may indicate new-onset or continued bleeding. Changes in the character of drainage from wounds or catheters may represent biliary or duodenal injuries. The practitioner must be notified immediately because potential complications of hemorrhage and infection may be life threatening. In the intermediate care unit and rehabilitation facility, small bone fractures and sprains may manifest as the patient begins to mobilize. Nurses and other health care team members play vital roles in identifying missed injuries, particularly when patients regain consciousness and begin to increase their activity.

Multiple Organ Dysfunction Syndrome

Trauma patients are at high risk for MODS, a clinical syndrome characterized by reversible impairment of two or more organ systems during infection or after shock or traumatic injury.[128] It has been estimated that up to 61% of late trauma deaths in ICU are related to MODS.[129] It has been suggested that the development of MODS post trauma may be associated with aging, immunosuppression, and infection.[130]

MODS often appears after admission to the critical are unit and is believed to have a multifactorial etiology. Trauma patients may experience MODS at two different times post injury. Within a few days after ICU admission, the proinflammatory response releases immune mediators into the bloodstream. This situation is known as the *first hit* of MODS.[128] The *second hit*, which may occur later during hospitalization, is thought to occur as a result of infection or surgical interventions.[128] In both situations, the patient often remains in the CCU for prolonged periods. Treatment is supportive, and priorities include controlling or eliminating the source of inflammation, maintaining oxygen delivery, minimizing oxygen consumption, and meeting nutritional and metabolic support for individual organs (see Chapter 33 for an in-depth discussion of MODS).

SPECIAL CONSIDERATIONS IN TRAUMA

Intimate Partner Violence and Trauma

Intimate partner violence (IPV), previously referred to as domestic violence, constitutes a major public health issue in North America. It has been reported that approximately 1 in 3 women and 1 in 4 men endure some type of IPV (spouse, previous spouse, or partner) during their lifetime.[131] IPV takes many forms, including physical violence, sexual violence, and stalking. More than 61 million women and 53 million men have endured some form of psychological aggression by their partners at some point in their life.[131] IPV is a leading cause of injury and death to women.

IPV can occur in all age groups and cultures and in heterosexual and same-sex relationships. Trauma care centers and EDs are seeing increased numbers of individuals affected by IPV. In particular, the incidence of IPV occurs more frequently in low- and middle-income countries.[132]

Injuries reported as a result of IPV include head injuries, lacerations, gastrointestinal bleeding, and sexually transmitted diseases. Posttraumatic stress disorder is also frequently observed in women who are the victims of IPV. Major risk factors for IPV in women are having a current partner with alcohol issues and mental illness.[133]

Many health care facilities and EDs routinely screen patients for IPV. Ensure that patients are provided privacy, make sure that they feel safe, and offer appropriate medical and social service assistance. Key interventions for victims of IPV are listed in Box 32.13.

BOX 32.13 Key Interventions With Victims of Intimate Partner Violence

When intimate partner violence (IPV) is suspected or confirmed, health care practitioners can assist victims in many ways:

Communication
- Discuss intimate partner violence with patients privately.
- Patients should be fully clothed.
- Respect confidentiality.
- Listen attentively and nonjudgmentally.
- Believe and validate the patient's experiences.

Assess the Patient
- Assess for possible injury or risk of immediate or future harm.

Provide Information
- Let the patient know that IPV is a common problem.
- Let the patient know that the IPV is not their fault.

Follow-up
- Assist the patient with making a "safety" plan.
- Provide information/contact numbers on community resources.
- Offer information about local shelters to the patient in a way that is safe for the patient to take with them. This information could be a printed card for a purse or wallet or entering a shelter phone number into the patient's cell phone using a code name.
- The situation may need to involve a social worker or social services.
- Notify law enforcement agencies when child abuse is suspected.
- Respect the patient's right to make decisions.

Adapted from Dicola, D, Spaar, E. Intimate partner violence. *Am Fam Physician.* 2016;94(8):646–651.

Alcohol and Substance Abuse and Trauma

Both alcohol and substance abuse have been implicated in traumatic injury. In 2020, more than 11,654 people died in alcohol-related MVCs, approximately 30% of all trauma deaths.[134] Alcohol can alter consciousness, affect behavior, and impair judgment and concentration. Alcohol screening is now a routine component of care in many trauma hospitals. A strong correlation exists between IPV, alcohol use, substance abuse, and violence-related injuries.[135]

Any substance can be abused, including alcohol, prescription medications, and illegal drugs such as cocaine, heroin, and crystal methamphetamine. In 2018, 12.6 million Americans reported driving under the influence of marijuana or other illicit substances.[136] Substance abuse embodies the potential to impair judgment and enhance impulsivity. Emergency and critical care teams screen trauma patients on admission for the presence of alcohol and illicit substances by obtaining blood and urine samples. The Alcohol Use Disorders Identification Test (Table 32.11) is an inexpensive, rapid test validated in trauma centers and can be used to screen for problem drinking.

Trauma in Pregnancy

Physical trauma affects 1 in 12 pregnant women.[137] MVCs are the primary mechanism for most traumatic injuries in pregnancy; falls and IPV are also leading contributors.[138] In the United States, trauma is the leading cause of maternal death from a nonobstetrical origin. Approximately 20% of all maternal deaths in the United States are related to trauma.[139]

The physiological changes of pregnancy require special consideration by trauma teams. A hyperdynamic, hypervolemic state occurs due to pregnancy, with increases in heart rate, cardiac output, and stroke volume. Hormonal changes in pregnancy enhance edema of upper airways and increase oxygen consumption, tidal volume, and minute ventilation, creating a chronically compensated respiratory alkalosis. The pregnant trauma patient is less tolerant of hypoxemia. The E-FAST is less sensitive to detecting hemorrhage due to more fluid within the abdomen. An increase in plasma volume creates the "physiological anemia" of pregnancy.

The admission of a pregnant trauma patient to the ED or CCU necessitates the ABC approach of ATLS, where the focus

TABLE 32.11 AUDIT Alcohol Screening Questionnaire

Question	Score[a]
How often do you have a drink containing alcohol?	Never Monthly or less 2–4 times per month 2–3 times per week 4 or more times per week
How many standard drinks containing alcohol do you have on a typical day when drinking?	1 or 2 3 or 4 5 or 6 7–9 10 or more
How often do you have 6 or more drinks on one occasion? During the past year, how often have you found that you were not able to stop drinking once you had started? During the past year, how often have you failed to do what was normally expected of you because of drinking? During the past year, how often have you needed a drink in the morning to get yourself going after a heavy drinking session? During the past year, how often have you had a feeling of guilt or remorse after drinking? During the past year, have you been unable to remember what happened the night before because you had been drinking?	Never Less than monthly Monthly Weekly Daily or almost daily
Have you or someone else been injured as a result of your drinking? Has a relative or friend or doctor, or other health worker been concerned about your drinking or suggested you cut down?	No Yes, but not in the past year Yes, during the past year

[a]Scores for each question range from 0 to 4, with the first response for each question (never) scoring 0, the second (less than monthly) scoring 1, the third (monthly) scoring 2, the fourth (weekly) scoring 3, and the fifth response (daily or almost daily) scoring 4. For the last two questions, which only have three responses, the scoring is 0, 2, and 4. A score of 8 to 14 is associated with harmful or hazardous drinking, and a score of 15 or more by is likely to indicate alcohol dependence. See https://auditscreen.org for more information.
AUDIT, Alcohol Use Disorders Identification Test.

of trauma teams is on the resuscitation and stabilization of the mother initially. Both mom and fetus are evaluated during the secondary survey. The mom's health is the priority in the resuscitation of the pregnant trauma patient.

Modification of Standard Protocols

Some crucial modifications as a result of the pregnancy are required by trauma teams. The patient is always placed in a left lateral decubitus position. This position will relieve compression of the aorta, improve venous return, and increase cardiac output by 30% for mom and fetus.[140] Supplemental oxygen is required. Intubation, if required, should occur early, generally with a smaller endotracheal tube. The most experienced practitioner should intubate, and alternative airway adjuncts should be immediately available. The target oxygen saturation is greater than 94%. IV fluid resuscitation, vasopressors and inotropes, massive transfusion protocol, tranexamic acid, and damage-control surgery are all part of the resuscitation of the critically injured pregnant patient. Diagnostic imaging, including bedside ultrasound, radiographs, CT, and MRI, should be undertaken as necessary, understanding that the fetus is most vulnerable during the first trimester. Signs and symptoms of hypovolemia and hemorrhagic shock may initially go unnoticed until the patient is in significant distress, so always suspect that the patient is in shock until proven otherwise.

BOX 32.14 Factors That Predispose Older Adults to Motor Vehicle Crashes

- Alterations in visual and auditory acuity
- Deterioration in strength and slower reaction times
- Decrease of cerebral skills
- Reduction of motor skills
- Exacerbation of acute or chronic medical conditions
- Medications that may interfere with safe driving

Placental Abruption

Placental abruption is the most frequently observed complication for the pregnant patient with a traumatic injury.[139] Premature labor and uterine rupture can also occur as consequences of trauma. Strategies for managing pregnant trauma patients must be individualized and consider current injuries, hemodynamic stability, ongoing bleeding, gestational age, and any known complications encountered during the pregnancy. Specific assessment and management issues for the obstetric patient are discussed in Chapter 37.

Trauma and the Older Adult

Older adults are predisposed to traumatic injuries because of the inevitable consequences of aging. The ability to react to or avoid environmental hazards is impaired because of age-related deterioration of the senses and changes in motor strength, postural stability, balance, and coordination.

Etiology

Older adults are most at risk for falls. Factors that predispose older people to falls are summarized in Box 32.14. Because falls are often caused by an underlying medical condition (syncope, dysrhythmias, hypotension), management of an older adult who has experienced a fall must include an evaluation of events and conditions immediately preceding the traumatic injury.

The involvement of older adults in MVCs is a consequence of the increasing age of the general population and the growing number of older drivers and occupants of motor vehicles. In 2020, 7500 older adults were killed, and more than 200,000 older adult patients were triaged in EDs in the United States.[141] Factors that predispose older adults to MVCs are summarized in Box 32.15.

Limited Physiologic Reserve

The concept of *limited physiologic reserve* in an older adult trauma patient highlights the critical difference between the average younger trauma patient with normal physiologic reserve and the older patient with underlying physiologic derangements.[142] Age-related changes in virtually every organ system may not produce evidence of organ dysfunction in the resting state. At the same time, the ability of organs to augment function in response to traumatic stress may be significantly compromised.

BOX 32.15 Risk Factors for Falls in Older Adults

Acute Illness
- Cerebrovascular accidents
- Dysrhythmias
- Syncope
- Diabetes

Cognitive Impairment
- Dementia

Neuromuscular Disorders
- Arthritis
- Lower extremity weakness
- Essential tremor
- Unstable gait

Medications
- Analgesics
- Antidepressants
- Antihypertensives
- Benzodiazepines
- Diuretics
- Phenothiazines

Assessment and Diagnosis

On admission to the adult ICU, older adult trauma patients are assessed using the principles of ATLS. A comprehensive older adult trauma assessment should include a complete medical and medication history and cognitive and frailty assessments. A low threshold exists for a CT scan of the head, especially when patients are receiving anticoagulation therapy for preexisting conditions. When a head injury is suspected or confirmed, systemic anticoagulation must be corrected as soon as possible after admission. Traumatic injury combined with a prolonged international normalized ration (INR) dramatically increases the risk of significant hemorrhage.

Challenges posed by older trauma patients in EDs and CCUs include accurately identifying the injury and recognizing altered physiology due to aging. Frailty, polypharmacy, cognitive decline, and refusal of treatment pose additional difficulties. TBI, chest trauma, and fractures of the pelvis, hip, and extremities are injuries frequently observed in the geriatric trauma population.[143]

Modification of Standard Protocols

Clinicians increasingly recognize that trauma protocols must be individualized for older trauma patients. As an example, fluid resuscitation is an integral part of trauma resuscitation. Older adult patients on long-term diuretic therapy may require additional volume and enhanced potassium supplementation due to chronic volume and potassium depletion. At the same time, these patients may be less likely to tolerate aggressive fluid resuscitation because of preexisting cardiac or pulmonary issues. Small IV fluid boluses, clearing cervical spines quickly, ensuring adequate pain control, early mobilization, and the importance of family in the care of the older trauma patient cannot be underestimated.

Outcomes

It is widely recognized that the best outcomes for this patient population are achieved through early, appropriate, aggressive trauma care, with admission to a trauma center with resources and protocols to provide excellent care to injured adults regardless of age. In one recent study, more than one-half of trauma patients greater than 70 years of age survived their initial injuries, emphasizing the importance that patients should not be excluded from trauma care based on age alone.[144] Trauma in older adults, however, is associated with longer critical care stays, an increased number of life-threatening complications, and higher mortality rates, even when the injuries are less severe.[145] Possible explanations include preexisting medical conditions, limited physiologic reserve, and decreased ability to compensate for severe injury.

Discharge Planning

Older patients who survive traumatic injuries often face changes in functional status after injury. Relatively minor trauma can be the event that changes an older person's lifestyle from one of relative independence to one that requires prolonged rehabilitation or skilled nursing care. Early advanced care planning in the CCU involving patients and families is paramount. Discharge planning and rehabilitation may also begin in the critical care or intermediate care unit (see Chapter 39 for an in-depth discussion regarding the older adult).

Mass Casualty Events

With increasing frequency, emergency and critical care staff respond to mass casualty incidents (MCI) or events (MCE). While some confusion exists between these two terms in the literature, it is understood that these situations produce more casualties than prehospital, hospital, and other facilities can adequately address and often exceeds available resources.

Causes of MCEs can range from naturally occurring events (e.g., hurricane, tornado, flood, earthquake, or wildfire), accidental (e.g., multiple car pile-ups on the freeway), or intentional (e.g., explosive device) circumstances. Injuries may include blunt and penetrating injuries, gunshot wounds, stabbings, burns, and orthopedic injuries. Every MCE is unique and can place the health care system under considerable pressure and health care workers under much stress.

Mass Shootings

More recently, mass shootings have appeared with increasing frequency in the United States. The Federal Bureau of Investigation (FBI) reported 50 active shooter incidents in 25 states in 2022, and over 100 people were killed.[146] This was a 66% increase in mass shootings since 2018. Mass shooter events necessitate principles of disaster triage. Shock, hemorrhage, blood loss, and facial, vascular, and orthopedic injuries are common. Psychological issues may or may not be readily or immediately apparent amongst patients and families at the time of the event, but the long-lasting effects of such catastrophic events cannot be ignored.

Triage

Triage plays an essential role in MCE. Two currently used methods for triaging a large number of casualties include START (Simple Triage and Rapid Assessment) and SALT (Sort-Assess-Lifesaving Interventions-Treatment and/or Transport).[7] In brief, using the START model, patients are briefly assessed for injury, color coded (indicating the level of care required), and sent to the most appropriate area (e.g., diagnostic imaging, OR, ICU, or unit). A secondary triage is often undertaken after initial categorization to ensure patients have been accurately triaged, to reevaluate patient condition, and to ensure disposition (transfer) of the patient to the most appropriate point in the health care system. During an MCE, the focus is doing the greatest good for the greatest number of individuals.

Disaster Planning

Simulation of large-scale disaster planning for designated prehospital care practitioners, trauma centers, and community hospitals is frequently practiced annually across the country. Disasters can

PATIENT-CENTERED CRITICAL CARE

The Older Adult in Critical Care

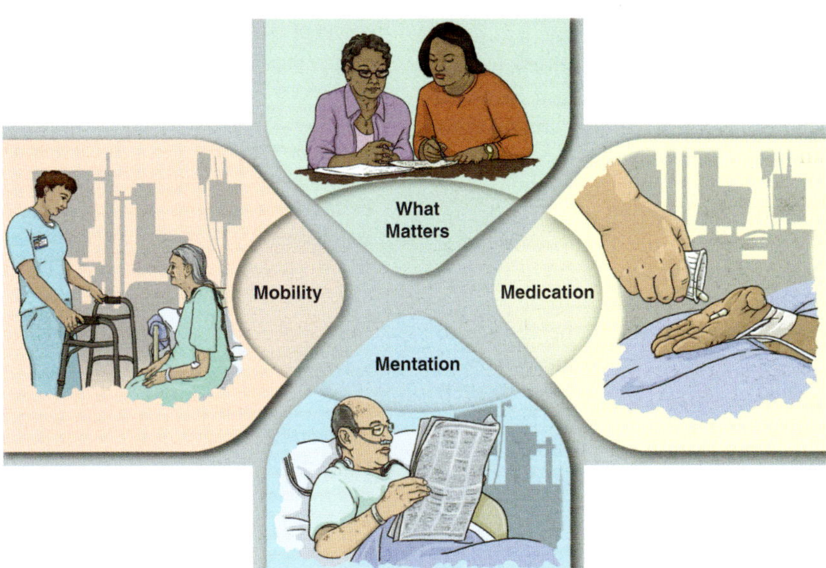

There are ways to adapt the critical care unit to be more hospitable to the needs of older adults. Examples include having large clocks to display time, large calendars to display the day of the week and date, and whiteboards to identify names of primary caregivers.

Geriatricians recommend that older adults undergo a comprehensive cognitive assessment before major elective surgeries. This evaluation is needed because prior cognitive impairment is a decisive risk factor for developing delirium with permanent cognitive decline. To combat the risk of delirium, some hospitals use a program called the *Hospital Elder Life Program*, which includes steps to prevent delirium. This program is based on the research of Dr. Sharon Inouye. The components are similar to those advocated for all patients in critical care: encourage periods of at least 4 to 6 hours of uninterrupted rest at night (if possible), encourage sleep without the use of benzodiazepines or similar medications, ensure the patient has eyeglasses or hearing aids, and promote early mobility as soon as possible.

The Institute for Healthcare Improvement (IHI) advocates for age-friendly health systems and has published a framework using 4Ms to care for older adults.

The four components are:

- What Matters
  - Know and align care with each older adult's specific health outcome goals and care preferences, including but not limited to end-of-life care and across care settings.
- Medication
  - If necessary, use age-friendly medication that does not interfere with What Matters, Mobility, or Mentation.
- Mentation
  - Prevent, identify, treat, and manage dementia, depression, and delirium.
- Mobility
  - Ensure that older adults move safely every day to maintain function and do What Matters.

The 4Ms constitute a core framework for caring for older adults in critical care and across all settings.

More information is available at http://www.ihi.org/Engage/Initiatives/Age-Friendly-Health-Systems/Documents/IHIAgeFriendlyHealthSystems_GuidetoUsing4MsCare.pdf.

occur anywhere at any time. CCUs must ensure proper education and staff preparation, including disaster simulation, the ability to practice triage, and become familiar with emergency preparedness protocols.[147] Challenges often identified when mass casualties occur at one time involve communication, transportation, and security.[148] Significant physiological and psychological stress on prehospital and hospital care practitioners due to MCEs cannot be underestimated. Debriefings after such events and psychological counseling are frequently required.

Meeting Needs of Family Members and Significant Others

The effect of traumatic injury can be devastating for patients, family members, and significant others. Trauma can precipitate a crisis within the family. The family often faces an unexpected situation for which the members have had little time to prepare. Family members may exhibit physical and sociocultural reactions and a combination of emotional responses, including anger, fear, powerlessness, confusion, and mistrust. Recovery from traumatic injury can be long and frustrating for families. During this time, the family may exhaust social and financial support systems. It is crucial to recognize, assess, and address the effect of stressors on families of trauma patients.

Family Presence During Trauma Resuscitation

A trend has evolved to move away from a paternalistic model of care to one that incorporates family into all aspects of trauma care. Although it is common for family members to be present during CPR, one question is whether they should be allowed to stay and observe trauma teams during resuscitation events.[149] Although many family members wish to remain close to their loved ones during hospitalization, should family be permitted to witness aggressive trauma interventions in a busy ED or CCU? Much more conversation and research is needed about this very important question.

Family Participation in Care

Although it may be challenging, family members should be encouraged, to the extent that they are able and wish to do so, to participate in patient care while maintaining the comfort and safety of the patient. For example, bathing, brushing teeth, combing hair, and reading to the patient are excellent strategies to involve families in caring for the injured patient.

Trauma Support Groups

Another valuable intervention is to bring families of trauma patients together in support groups. Support of family members caring for trauma patients post discharge is essential. There is increasing awareness that caregivers of trauma patients experience physical and emotional challenges for several months post discharge.[150] Trauma family support groups can offer sharing of experiences, coping strategies, expression of emotions, mutual support, and education about hospital and community resources and services.

ADDITIONAL RESOURCES

See Box 32.16 for Internet resources pertaining to trauma.

BOX 32.16 Internet Resources

Trauma

- American College of Surgeons: Trauma Quality Improvement Program (TQIP), https://www.facs.org/quality-programs/trauma/quality/trauma-quality-improvement-program/
- Centers for Disease Control and Prevention (CDC): Injury Prevention & Control, https://www.cdc.gov/injury/index.html
- Eastern Association for the Surgery of Trauma (EAST), https://www.east.org/
- Emergency Nurses Association (ENA), https://www.ena.org/
- ENA: Trauma Nursing Core Course (TNCC), https://www.ena.org/education/tncc
- Society of Trauma Nurses: https://www.traumanurses.org/

CASE STUDY 32.1 Patient With Trauma

Brief Patient History

Mr. G is a 25-year-old male. He was a pedestrian crossing the street in a marked crosswalk when he was hit by a pickup truck traveling approximately 40 miles/h (64 km/h). He was ejected onto the side of the road. There is visible external damage to the front passenger panel of the truck. On arrival, emergency medical services personnel determined the patient was awake, restless, and agitated, not following commands. His respiratory rate was 22 breaths/min, and his breathing was shallow and unlabored. His oxygen saturation on pulse oximetry (SpO_2) was 87%. There was blood oozing from the right side of his head and an obvious deformity to his right leg. He was placed in a hard collar, immobilized, and given oxygen via a 15-L nonrebreather mask. He was immediately transported to the hospital.

Clinical Assessment

Mr. G is admitted to the emergency department. The advanced trauma life support (ATLS) primary survey is completed, and these assessment findings are identified:

- Airway: moaning incomprehensibly
- Breathing: 26 breaths/min, shallow; obvious right-sided deformity (flail chest)
- Circulation: pale, cool; palpable carotid and femoral pulses
- Disability: Glasgow Coma Scale (GCS) score 12 (motor, 5; verbal, 3; eyes, 4); moving all four limbs but not to command
- Exposure: right scalp laceration; several abrasions; lacerations over face, back, and legs

Diagnostic Procedures

Admission radiographs identify fractured right ribs 3 through 8, a fractured right femur. Computed tomography (CT) scan shows a small subdural hematoma (SDH) and liver laceration.

Medical Diagnosis

Mr. G is diagnosed with SDH (secondary to trauma), flail chest, fractured ribs, fractured right femur, and grade III liver laceration.

Admission to Critical Care Unit (CCU)

On admission to the adult CCU after the CT scan, reassessment of the patient is done with these assessment findings: heart rate, 142 beats/min (sinus tachycardia); respiratory rate, 30 breaths/min, short, shallow, and labored; blood pressure, 85/46 mm Hg (MAP 59 mmHg); SpO_2, 86%; temperature, 96.3 °F (35.7°C); Glasgow Coma Scale score 8. The patient has an altered level of consciousness, does not respond to voice, and only reacts very briefly to a peripheral painful stimulus.

Questions

1. What major outcomes do you expect to achieve for this patient?
2. What problems or risks must be managed to achieve these outcomes?
3. What interventions could be initiated to monitor, prevent, manage, or eliminate the problems and risks identified?
4. What interventions could be initiated to promote optimal functioning, safety, and well-being of the patient?
5. What technology can be used to monitor this patient and prevent complications?
6. What other interprofessional team members are needed to assist with the management of this patient?
7. What possible learning needs would you anticipate for this patient?
8. What cultural and age-related factors might have a bearing on the patient's plan of care?

KEY POINTS

- Trauma is costly in terms of disability, health care dollars, and lives lost.
- Traumatic injuries most frequently involve high-velocity impact and may be caused by blunt or penetrating mechanisms.

Phases of Trauma Care

- Assessment of the trauma patient is performed systematically, using the principles of the Advanced Trauma Life Support (ATLS) program.
- The initial ATLS primary survey focuses on airway, breathing, circulation, disability, and exposure.
- The more detailed secondary survey is an in-depth, head-to-toe physical assessment.
- Resuscitation of the trauma patient involves hemostasis to control hemorrhage, goal-directed volume support to restore cellular oxygenation, maintenance of normothermia, and prevention and correction of acidosis, coagulopathy, and hypocalcemia.
- Assessment and reassessment of the trauma patient in the CCU is essential.

Specific Trauma Injuries

- In critical care, managing severe TBIs and SCIs focuses on preventing secondary injury by maintaining oxygen delivery to the brain and spinal cord and avoiding complications of prolonged bed rest and immobility.
- Airway compromise is a primary care focus for a patient with maxillofacial injuries.
- Chest wall and pulmonary injuries require multimodal pain management approaches and frequent reassessment of oxygenation and ventilation status.
- Pneumothoraces are often treated with the insertion of chest tubes.
- BCI is associated with an increased risk of dysrhythmias.
- Abdominal trauma often has nonspecific signs and symptoms; maintaining increased awareness of abdominal complications is critically important.
- Liver and spleen injuries are associated with an increased risk of bleeding.
- Kidney and bladder injuries are often managed medically.
- Pelvic fractures may result in tremendous blood loss, and the nurse must remain alert for signs of hemorrhagic shock.
- Complications of trauma may include VTE, infection, sepsis, missed injury, and multiple organ dysfunction syndrome (MODS).

Visit the Evolve site at http://evolve.elsevier.com/Urden/CriticalCareNursing for additional study materials.

REFERENCES

1. Centers for Disease Control and Prevention. WISQARS Leading Causes of Death Visualization Tool; 2024. https://wisqars.cdc.gov/lcd/?o=LCD&y1=2022&y2=2022&ct=10&cc=ALL&g=00&s=0&r=0&ry=2&e=0&ar=lcd1age&at=groups&ag=lcd1age&a1=0&a2=199. Accessed December 9, 2024.
2. Peterson C, Miller GF, Barnett SB, et al. Economic cost of injury – United States, 2019. *MMWR Morb Mortal Wkly Rep*. 2021;70:1655–1659.
3. World Health Organization. Road Traffic Injuries Fact Sheet; 2022. https://www.who.int/news-room/fact-sheets/detail/road-traffic-injuries. Accessed December 9, 2024.
4. Rauf R, von Matthey F, Croenlein M, et al. Changes in the temporal distribution of in-hospital mortality in severely injured patients - an analysis of the Trauma Register. *PLoS One*. 2019;14(2):e0212095. https://doi.org/10.1371/journal.pone.0212095.
5. Bardes JM, Inaba K, Schellenberg M, et al. The contemporary timing of trauma deaths. *J Trauma Acute Care Surg*. 2018;84(6):893–899. https://doi.org/10.1097/TA.0000000000001882.
6. Cole E, Gillespie S, Vulliamy P, et al. Multiple organ dysfunction after trauma. *Br J Surg*. 2020;107(4):402–412. https://doi.org/10.1002/bjs.11361.
7. American College of Surgeons. *Advanced Trauma Life Support*. 10th ed. Chicago: American College of Surgeons; 2018.
8. Ferrada P, Callcut RA, Skarupa, et al. Circulation first – the time has come to question the sequencing of care in the ABCs of trauma; an American Association for the Surgery of trauma multicenter trial. *World J Emerg Surg*. 2018;13:8. https://doi.org/10.1186/s13017-018-0168-3.
9. Powers-Jarvis RS. Initial assessment. In: *Trauma Nursing Core Course Provider Manual*. 8th ed. Burlington: Emergency Nurses Association; 2020.
10. Eskesen TG, Baekgaard JS, Steinmetz J, et al. Initial use of supplementary oxygen for trauma patients: a systematic review. *BMJ Open*. 2018;8:e020880. https://doi.org/10.1136/bmjopen-2017-020880.
11. Milici JJ. Shock. In: *Trauma Nursing Core Course Provider Manual*. 8th ed. Burlington: Emergency Nurses Association; 2020.
12. Ntourakis D, Liasis L. Damage control resuscitation in patients with major trauma: prospects and challenges. *J Emerg Crit Care Med*. 2020;4:34. https://doi.org/10.21037/jeccm-20-24.
13. Fecher A, Stimpson A, Ferrigno L, et al. The pathophysiology and management of hemorrhagic shock in the polytrauma patient. *J Clin Med*. 2021;10:4793. https://doi.org/10.3390/jcm10204793.
14. Vishwanathan K, Chhajwani S, Gupta A, et al. Evaluation and management of haemorrhagic shock in polytrauma: clinical practice guidelines. *J Clin Orthop Trauma*. 2021;13:106–115. https://doi.org/10.1016/j.jcot.2020.12.003.
15. Iyengar KP, Venkatesan AS, Jain VK, et al. Risks in the management of polytrauma patients: clinical insights. *Orthop Res Rev*. 2023;15:27–38. https://doi.org/10.2147/ORR.S340532.
16. Ntourakis D, Liasis L. Damage control resuscitation in patients with major trauma: prospects and challenges. *J Emerg Crit Care Med*. 2020;4:34. https://doi.org/10.21037/jeccm-20-24.
17. Dauer E, Goldberg A. What's new in trauma resuscitation? *Adv Surg*. 2019:221–233. https://doi.org/10.1016/j.yasu.2019.04.010.
18. Lee C, Rasmussen TE, Pape HC, et al. The polytrauma patient: current concepts and evolving care. *OTA Int*. 2021;4(2S):e108. https://doi.org/10.1097/OI9.0000000000000108.
19. Leibner E, Andreae M, Galvagno SM, et al. Damage control resuscitation. *Clin Exp Emerg Med*. 2020;7(1):5–13. https://doi.org/10.15441/ceem.19.089.
20. Vargas M, Garcia A, Caicedo Y, et al. Damage control in the intensive care unit: what should the intensive care physician know and do? *Colomb Med*. 2021;52(2):e4174810. https://doi.org/10.25100/cm.v52i2.4810.
21. Wray JP, Bridwell RE, Schauer SG, et al. The diamond of death: hypocalcemia in trauma and resuscitation. *Am J Emerg Med*. 2021;41:104–109. https://doi.org/10.1016/j.ajem.2020.12.065.
22. Belaunzaran M, Raslan S, Ali A, et al. Utilization and efficacy of resuscitation endpoints in trauma and burn patients: a review article. *Am Surg*. 2022;88(1):10–19. https://doi.org/10.1177/00031348211060424.
23. Arboleda NS, Diaz AR, Zuniga AJ, et al. Shock index, lactate and base deficit as bleeding predictors in trauma patients from a complex emergency department: a prospective cohort study. *Panamerican J Trauma, Crit Care Emerg Surg*. 2023;12(1):42–46. https://doi.org/10.5005/jp-journals-10030-1416.
24. Qi J, Bao L, Yang P, et al. Comparison of base excess, lactate and pH predicting 72-h mortality of multiple trauma. *BMC Emerg Med*. 2021;21:80. https://doi.org/10.1186/s12873-021-00465-9.
25. Wiles MD, Braganza M, Edwards H, et al. Management of traumatic brain injury in the non-neurosurgical intensive care unit: a narrative review of current evidence. *Anaesthesia*. 2023;73:510–520. https://doi.org/10.1111/anae.15898.
26. Niziolek G, Sandsmark DK, Pascual JL. Neurotrauma. *urrO Pin Crit Care*. 2022;28:715–724. https://doi.org/10.1097/MCC.00000000026.0001005.

27. Centers for Disease Control and Prevention. *Traumatic Brain Injury and Concussion*; 2023. https://www.cdc.gov/traumaticbraininjury/index.html.
28. Maas AIR, Menon DK, Manley GT, et al. Traumatic brain injury: progress and challenges in prevention, clinical care, and research. *Lancet Neurol*. 2022;21:1004–1060. https://doi.org/10.1016/S1474-4422(22)00309-X.
29. Dietvorst S, Depreitere B, Meyfroidt G. Beyond intracranial pressure: monitoring cerebral perfusion and autoregulation in severe traumatic brain injury. *Curr Opin Crit Care*. 2023;29:85–88. https://doi.org/10.1097/MCC.0000000000001026.
30. Ismail N. Severe traumatic brain injury. *Mediterranean JEM*. 2020;28:33–42. http://www.mjemonline.com/index.php/mjem/article/view/96.
31. Manthey DE, Tsuruoka S, Alson RL. Head trauma and traumatic brain injury. In: Alson RL, Han K, Campbell JE, eds. *International Trauma Life Support for Emergency Care Providers*. 9th ed. Hoboken, NJ: Pearson Education; 2020.
32. Kang HG, Cho KY, Lee RS, et al. Delayed operation of acute subdural hematoma in subacute stage by trephine drainage using urokinase. *Korean J Neurotrauma*. 2019;15(2):103–109. https://doi.org/10.13004/kjnt.2019.15.e32.
33. Tenny S, Thorell W. Intracranial hemorrhage. In: *StatPearls*. NCBI Bookshelf version. StatPearls Publishing; 2023. https://www.ncbi.nlm.nih.gov/books/NBK470242/. Accessed August 23, 2023.
34. D'Agostino R, Kursinskis A, Parikh P, et al. Management of penetrating traumatic brain injury: operative versus non-operative intervention. *J Surg Res*. 2021;257:101–106. https://doi.org/10.1016/j.jss.2020.07.046.
35. Bruggeman GF, Haitsma IK, Dirven CMF, et al. Traumatic axonal injury (TAI): definitions, pathophysiology and imaging-a narrative review. *Acta Neurochir*. 2021;163:31–44. https://doi.org/10.1007/s00701-020-04594-1.
36. Kearns C. Diffuse Axonal Injury; 2023. https://radiopaedia.org/articles/diffuse-axonal-injury. Accessed December 9, 2024.
37. Zheng RZ, Lei ZQ, Yang RZ, et al. Identification and management of paroxysmal sympathetic hyperactivity after traumatic brain injury. *Front Neurol*. 2020;11:81. https://doi.org/10.3389/fneur.2020.00081.
38. Campbell MR. Head trauma. In: *Trauma Nursing Core Course Provider Manual*. 8th ed. Burlington, MA: Emergency Nurses Association; 2020.
39. Krishnamoorthy V, Chaikittisilpa N, Kiatchai T, et al. Hypertension after severe traumatic brain injury: friend of foe? *J Neurosurg Anesth*. 2017;29(4):382–387. https://doi.org/10.1097/ANA.0000000000000370.
40. Vrettou CS, Mentzelopoulos SD. Second- and third-tier therapies for severe traumatic brain injury. *J Clin Med*. 2022;11:4790. https://doi.org/10.3390/jcm11164790.
41. Wiles MD. Management of traumatic brain injury: a narrative review of current evidence. *Anaesthesia*. 2022;77(Supp 1):102–112. https://doi.org/10.1111/anae.15608.
42. Carney N, Totten AM, O'Reilly C, et al. Guidelines for the management of severe traumatic brain injury, fourth edition. *Neurosurgery*. 2016;80(1):6–15. https://doi.org/10.1227/NEU.0000000000001432.
43. Wittenberg C. Recognizing and managing traumatic brain injury. *Nurs Crit Care*. 2018;13(1):20–27. https://doi.org/10.1097/01.CCN.0000527221.34428.02.
44. Musick S, Alberico A. Neurologic assessment of the neurocritical care patient. *Front Neurol*. 2021;12:588989. https://doi.org/10.3389/fneur.2021.588989.
45. Meyfroidt G, Bouzat P, Casaer M, et al. Management of moderate to severe traumatic brain injury: an update for the intensivist. *Inten Care Med*. 2022;48:649–666. https://doi.org/10.1007/s00134-022-06702-4.
46. Godoy DA, Murillo-Cabezas F, Suarez JI, et al. "THE MANTLE" bundle for minimizing cerebral hypoxia in severe traumatic brain injury. *Crit Care*. 2023;27:13. https://doi.org/10.1186/s13054-022-04242-3.
47. Schroeppel TJ, Sharpe JP, Shahan CP, et al. Beta-adrenergic blockade for attenuation of catecholamine surge after traumatic brain injury: a randomized pilot trial. *Trauma Surg Acute Care Open*. 2019;18;4(1):e000307. https://doi.org/10.1136/tsaco-2019-000307.
48. Dengler BA, Karam O, Barthol CA, et al. Ketamine boluses are associated with a reduction in intracranial pressure and an increase in cerebral perfusion pressure: a retrospective observational study of patients with severe traumatic brain injury. *Crit Care Res Pract*. 2022:3834165. https://doi.org/10.1155/2022/3834165.
49. Posti JP, Raj R, Luoto TM. How do we identify the crashing traumatic brain injury patient – the neurosurgeon's view. *Opin Crit Care*. 2020;27(2):87–94. https://doi.org/10.1097/MCC.0000000000000799.
50. Horton L, Griffen M, Chang L, et al. Efficacy of animal-assisted therapy in treatment of patients with traumatic brain injury: a randomized trial. *J Trauma Nurs*. 2023;30(2):68–74. https://doi.org/10.1097/JTN.0000000000000705.
51. National Spinal Cord Injury Statistical Center. Traumatic Spinal Care Injury Demographics at a Glance; 2024. https://sites.uab.edu/nscisc/files/2024/06/Traumatic_SCI_Infographic_Demographics_2024.pdf. Accessed December 9, 2024.
52. American Association of Neurological Surgeons. Spinal Cord Injury; 2023. https://www.aans.org/en/Patients/Neurosurgical-Conditions-and-Treatments/Spinal-Cord-Injury. Accessed December 9, 2024.
53. Morano JM, Morano MJ, Wagner NE, et al. Management of acute traumatic brain injury and acute spinal cord injury. *Int Anesth Clin*. 2021;59(2):17–24. https://doi.org/10.1097/AIA.0000000000000314.
54. Hills TE. Caring for patients with a traumatic spinal cord injury. *Nursing*. 2020;50(12):30–40. https://doi.org/10.1097/01.NURSE.0000721724.96678.5a.
55. Quadri SA, Farooqui M, Ikram A, et al. Recent update on basic mechanisms of spinal cord injury. *Neurosurg Rev*. 2020;43:425–441. https://doi.org/10.1007/s10143-018-1008-3.
56. Taylor EC, Fitzpatrick CE, Thompson SE, et al. Acute traumatic spinal cord injury. *Adv Emerg Nurs J*. 2022;44(4):272–280. https://doi.org/10.1097/TME.0000000000000428.
57. Volski A, Ackerman DJ. Neurogenic shock. In: Stawicki SP, Swaroop M, eds. *Clinical Management of Shock – the Science and Art of Physiological Restoration*; 2020. https://doi.org/10.5772/intechopen.89915.
58. Sacino A, Rosenblatt K. Early management of acute spinal cord injury-Part 1: initial injury to surgery. *J Neuroanaesth Crit Care*. 2019;6(3):213–221. https://doi.org/10.1055/s-0039-1694688.
59. SCI-Info Pages. Spinal Cord Injury Facts and Statistics; 2023. https://www.sci-info-pages.com/spinal-cord-injury-facts-and-statistics/. Accessed December 9, 2024.
60. Clarkson AW. Spinal trauma. In: *Trauma Nursing Core Course Provider Manual*. 8th ed. Burlington, MA: Emergency Nurses Association; 2020.
61. Pearl NA, Dubensky L. Anterior cord syndrome. In: *StatPearls*. NCBI Bookshelf version. StatPearls Publishing; 2023. https://www.ncbi.nlm.nih.gov/books/NBK559117. Accessed August 23, 2023.
62. Vazirizadeh-Mahabadi M, Yarahmadi M. Canadian C-spine rule versus NEXUS in screening of clinically important traumatic cervical spine injuries; a systematic review and meta-analysis. *Arch Acad Emerg Med*. 2023;11(1):e5. https://doi.org/10.22037/aaem.v11i1.1833.
63. Maschmann C, Jeppesen E, Rubin MA, et al. New clinical guidelines on the spinal stabilisation of adult trauma patients – consensus and evidence based. *Scand J Trauma Resusc Emerg Med*. 2019;27:77. https://doi.org/10.1186/s13049-019-0655-x.
64. Lee BJ, Jeong JH. Early decompression in acute spinal cord injury: review and update. *J Korean Neurosurg*. 2023;66(1):6–11. https://doi.org/10.3340/jkns.2022.0107.
65. Tabarestani TQ, Lewis NE, Kelly-Hedrick M, et al. Surgical considerations to improve recovery in acute spinal cord injury. *Neurospine*. 2022;19(3):689–702. https://doi.org/10.14245/ns.2244616.308.
66. American College of Surgeons. Best Practice Guidelines: Spine Injury; 2022. https://www.facs.org/media/k45gikqv/spine_injury_guidelines.pdf. Accessed December 9, 2024.
67. Peev N, Zileli M, Sharif S, et al. Indications for nonsurgical treatment of thoracolumbar spine fractures: WFNS spine committee recommendations. *Neurospine*. 2021;18(4):713–724. https://doi.org/10.14245/ns.2142390.195.
68. Lee YS, Kim KT, Kwon BK. Hemodynamic management of acute spinal cord injury: a literature review. *Neurospine*. 2021;18(1):7–14. https://doi.org/10.14245/ns.2040144.072.
69. Wang TY, Park C, Zhang H, et al. Management of acute traumatic spinal cord injury: a review of the literature. *Front Surg*. 2021;8:698736. https://doi.org/10.3389/fsurg.2021.698736.

70. Rodriguez GM, Gater DR. Neurogenic bowel and management after spinal cord injury: a narrative review. *J Pers Med.* 2022;12:1141. https://doi.org/10.3390/jpm12071141.
71. Balik V, Sulla I. Autonomic dysreflexia following spinal cord injury. *AJNS.* 2022;17:165–172. https://doi.org/10.1055/s-0042-1751080.
72. Van Wicklin SA. Le fort maxillary fractures. *Plastic Aesth Nursing.* 2022;42(2):56–67. https://doi.org/10.1097/PSN.0000000000000441.
73. Shah V. Le Fort Fracture Classification; 2023. https://radiopaedia.org/articles/le-fort-fracture-classification?case_id=le-fort-type-1-fracture&lang=us. Accessed December 9, 2024.
74. Rosello EG, Granado AMQ, Garcia MA, et al. Facial fractures: classification and highlights for a useful report. *Insights Imaging.* 2020;11:49. https://doi.org/10.1186/s13244-020-00847-w.
75. Pswarayi R, Burns C. Le fort III fractures: an approach to resuscitation and management. *Ann Med Surg.* 2022;81:104513. https://doi.org/10.1016/j.amsu.2022.104513.
76. Tran J, Haussner W, Shah K. Traumatic pneumothorax: a review of current diagnostic practices and evolving management. *J Emerg Med.* 2021;61(5):517–528. https://doi.org/10.1016/j.jemermed.2021.07.006.
77. Beloy V, Dull M. Blunt chest wall trauma: rib fractures and associated injuries. *JAAPA.* 2022;35(11):25–31. https://doi.org/10.1097/01.JAA.0000885136.91189.83.
78. Lodhia JV, Eyre L, Smith M, et al. Management of thoracic trauma. *Anaesthesia.* 2022;78:225–235. https://doi.org/10.1111/anae.15934.
79. Bauza GM, Peitzman AB. Thoracic trauma. In: Alson RL, Han K, Campbell JE, eds. *International Trauma Life Support for Emergency Care Providers.* 9th ed. Hoboken, NJ: Pearson Education; 2020.
80. Yapanto AM. Flail chest: a literature review. *J Eduvest-J Universal Studies.* 2022;2(4):660–672. https://doi.org/10.59188/eduvest.v2i4.428.
81. Yahn CA, McNally AP, Deivert K, et al. Outcomes of trauma patients with flail chest and surgical rib stabilization. *Am Surg.* 2022;88(4):810–812. https://doi.org/10.1177/00031348211056260.
82. Rendeki S, Molnar TF. Pulmonary contusion. *J Thorac Dis.* 2019;11(Suppl 2):S141–S151. https://doi.org/10.21037/jtd.2018.11.53.
83. Casey RM. Thoracic and neck trauma. In: *Trauma Nursing Core Course Provider Manual.* 8th ed. Burlington, MA: Emergency Nurses Association; 2020.
84. Azizi N, Avest E, Hoek AE, et al. Optimal anatomical location for needle chest decompression for tension pneumothorax: a multicentre prospective cohort study. *Injury.* 2021;52:213–218. https://doi.org/10.1016/j.injury.2020.10.068.
85. Kim M, Moore JE. Chest trauma; Current recommendations for rib fractures, pneumothorax, and other injuries. *Curr Anesth Rep.* 2020;10:61–68. https://doi.org/10.1007/s40140-020-00374-w.
86. Dumani S, Ibrahimi A, Likaj E, et al. Cardiac trauma. Management strategies short panoramic view. *Albanian J Trauma Emerg Surg.* 2023;7(1):1189–1195. https://doi.org/10.32391/ajtes.v7i1.318.
87. Sixta S, Kozar R. Management of the severely injured trauma patient. In: Roberts PR, Todd SR, eds. *Comprehensive Critical Care: Adult.* 2nd ed. Mount Prospect, IL: Society of Critical Care Medicine; 2017.
88. Stashko E, Meer JM. Cardiac tamponade. In: *StatPearls.* NCBI Bookshelf version. StatPearls Publishing; 2023. https://www.ncbi.nlm.nih.gov/books/NBK431090/#article-18905.s2. Accessed August 23, 2023.
89. Gupta B, Singh Y, Bagaria D, et al. Comprehensive management of the patient with traumatic cardiac injury. *Anesth Anal.* 2023;136(5):877–893. https://doi.org/10.1213/ANE.0000000000006380.
90. Adler Y, Ristic AD, Imazio M, et al. Cardiac tamponade. *Nat Rev Dis Primers.* 2023;9(1):36. https://doi.org/10.1038/s41572-023-00446-1.
91. Dahal R, Acharya Y, Tyroch AH, et al. Blunt thoracic aortic injury and contemporary management strategy. *Angiology.* 2022;73(6):497–507. https://doi.org/10.1177/00033197211052131.
92. Mazzaccaro D, Righini P, Fancoli F, et al. Blunt thoracic aortic injury. *J Clin Med.* 2023;12:2903. https://doi.org/10.3390/jcm12082903.
93. Scalea TM, Feliciano DV, DuBose JJ, et al. Blunt thoracic aortic injury: endovascular repair is now the standard. *J Am Coll Surg.* 2019;228(4):605–610. https://doi.org/10.1016/j.jamcollsurg.2018.12.022.
94. Morales C, Ascuntar J, Londono JM, et al. Lactate clearance: prognostic mortality marker in trauma patients. *Colom J Anesth.* 2019;47(1):41–48. https://doi.org/10.1097/CJ9.0000000000000084.
95. Savoia P, Jayanthi SK, Chammas MC. Focused assessment with sonography for trauma (FAST). *J Med Ultrasound.* 2023;31(2):101–106. https://doi.org/10.4103/jmu.jmu_12_23.
96. Hetherington A, Cardosa FS, Lester ELW, et al. Liver trauma in the intensive care unit. *Curr Opin Crit Care.* 2022;8(2):184–189. https://doi.org/10.1097/MCC.0000000000000928.
97. Larsen JW, Thorsen K, Soreide K. Splenic injury from blunt trauma. *Br J Surg.* 2023;110(9):1035–1038. https://doi.org/10.1093/bjs/znad060.
98. Coccolini F, Montori G, Catena F, et al. Splenic trauma: WSES classification and guidelines for adult and pediatric patients. *World J Emerg Surg.* 2017;12:40. https://doi.org/10.1186/s13017-017-0151-4.
99. Luu S, Spelman D, Woolley IJ. Post-splenectomy sepsis: preventative strategies, challenges and solutions. *Infect Drug Resist.* 2019;12:2839–2851. https://doi.org/10.2147/IDR.S179902.
100. Smyth L, Bendinelli C, Lee N, et al. WSES guidelines on blunt and penetrating bowel injury: diagnosis, investigations, and treatment. *World J Emerg Surg.* 2022;17:13. https://doi.org/10.1186/s13017-022-00418-y.
101. Ghosh L, Gantioque R, Sotelo C. Abdominal compartment syndrome in adult trauma patients. *J Nurse Pract.* 2021;17(8):932–934. https://doi.org/10.1016/j.nurpra.2021.05.014.
102. Rajasurya V, Surani S. Abdominal compartment syndrome: often overlooked conditions in medical intensive care units. *World J Gastroenterol.* 2020;21;26(3):266–278. https://doi.org/10.3748/wjg.v26.i3.266.
103. Einav S, Zimmerman FS, Tankel J, et al. Management of the patient with the open abdomen. *Curr Opin Crit Care.* 2021;27(6):726–732. https://doi.org/10.1097/MCC.0000000000000879.
104. De Laet I, Malbrain MLNG, De Waele JJ. A clinician's guide to management of intra-abdominal hypertension and abdominal compartment syndrome in critically ill patients. *Crit Care.* 2020;24(1):97. https://doi.org/10.1186/s13054-020-2782-1.
105. Kang L, Geube A. Bladder trauma. In: *StatPearls.* NCBI Bookshelf version. StatPearls Publishing; 2023. https://www.ncbi.nlm.nih.gov/books/NBK557875/#article-18359.s2. Accessed August 23, 2023.
106. Coccolini F, Moore EE, Kluger Y, et al. Kidney and uro-trauma: WSES-AAST guidelines. *World J Emer Surg.* 2019;14:54. https://doi.org/10.1186/s13017-019-0274-x.
107. American Association for the Surgery of Trauma. Injury Scoring Scale: A Resource for Trauma Care Professionals; 2019. https://www.aast.org/resources-detail/injury-scoring-scale#kidney. Accessed December 9, 2024.
108. Gutierrez JO, Vasquez-Lopez S, Betancur-Marquez CM, et al. Blunt bladder trauma: laparoscopic repair. *Urol Case Rep.* 2022;40:101947. https://doi.org/10.1016/j.eucr.2021.101947.
109. Mahat Y, Leong JY, Chung PH. A contemporary review of adult bladder trauma. *J Inj Violence Res.* 2019;11(2):101–106. https://doi.org/10.5249/jivr.v11i2.1069.
110. Coleman JR, Moore EE, Vintimilla DR, et al. Association between young-burgess pelvic ring injury classification and concomitant injuries requiring urgent intervention. *J Clin Orthop Trauma.* 2020;11(6):1099–1103. https://doi.org/10.1016/j.jcot.2020.08.009.
111. Cheung J, Wong CKK, Yang MLC, et al. Young–Burgess classification: inter-observer and inter-method agreement between pelvic radiograph and computed tomography in emergency polytrauma management. *Hong Kong J Emerg Med.* 2021;28(3):143–151. https://doi.org/10.1177/1024907919857008.
112. Knipe H. Young and Burgess Classification of Pelvic Ring Fractures; 2023. https://radiopaedia.org/articles/young-and-burgess-classification-of-pelvic-ring-fractures. Accessed December 9, 2024.
113. Mejia D, Parra MW, Ordonez CA, et al. Hemodynamically unstable pelvic fracture: a damage control surgical algorithm that fits your reality. *Colomb Med (Cali).* 2020;51(4):e4214510. https://doi.org/10.25100/cm.v51i4.4510.
114. Mostafa AMHAM, Kyriacou H, Chimutengwende-Gordon M, et al. An overview of the key principles and guidelines in the management of pelvic fractures. *J Perioper Pract.* 2021;31(9):341–348. https://doi.org/10.1177/1750458920947358.
115. Braithwaite S, Seitz SR. Extremity trauma. In: Alson RL, Han K, Campbell JE, eds. *International Trauma Life Support for Emergency Providers.* 9th ed. Hoboken, NJ: Pearson Education; 2020.

116. Gessner DM, Horn JL, Lowenberg DW. Pain management in the orthopaedic trauma patient: non-opioid solutions. *Injury*. 2020;51(Suppl 2):S28–S36. https://doi.org/10.1016/j.injury.2019.04.008.
117. Mortensen SJ, Orman S, Serino J, et al. Factors associated with development of traumatic acute compartment syndrome: a systematic review and meta-analysis. *Arch Bone Joint Surg*. 2021;9(3):263–271. https://doi.org/10.22038/abjs.2020.46684.2284.
118. Banavasi H, Nguyen P, Osman H, et al. Management of ARDS-What works and what does not. *Am J Med Sci*. 2021;362(1):13–23. https://doi.org/10.1016/j.amjms.2020.12.019.
119. Byerly S, Vasileiou G, Qian S, et al. Early hypermetabolism is uncommon in trauma intensive care unit patients. *J Parenter Enteral Nutr*. 2022;46(4):771–781. https://doi.org/10.1002/jpen.1945.
120. Li PF, Wang YL, Fang YL, et al. Effect of early enteral nutrition on outcomes of trauma patients requiring intensive care. *Chin J Traumatol*. 2020;23:163–167. https://doi.org/10.1016/j.cjtee.2020.04.006.
121. Kodadek L, Carmichael IISP, Seshadri A, et al. Rhabdomyolysis: an American association for the surgery of trauma critical care committee clinical consensus document. *Traum Surg Acute Care Open*. 2022;7:e000836. https://doi.org/10.1136/tsaco-2021-000836.
122. Subashri M, Sujit S, Thirumalvalavan K, et al. Rhabdomyolysis-associated acute kidney injury. *Indian J Nephrol*. 2023;33(2):114–118. https://doi.org/10.4103/ijn.ijn_247_21.
123. Rothberg DL, Makarewich CA. Fat Embolism and fat embolism syndrome. *J Am Acad Orthop Surg*. 2019;27(8):e346–e355. https://doi.org/10.5435/JAAOS-D-17-00571.
124. Luff D, Hewson DW. Fat embolism syndrome. *BJA Educ*. 2021;21(9):322–328. https://doi.org/10.1016/j.bjae.2021.04.003.
125. Van Wonderen SF, Klanderman RB, Vlaar APJ. Understanding transfusion-related acute lung injury (TRALI) and its complex pathophysiology. *Blood Trans*. 2022;20:443–445. https://doi.org/10.2450/2022.0232-22.
126. Eriksson J, Lindstrom AC, Hellgren E, et al. Postinjury sepsis-Associations with risk factors, impact on clinical course, and mortality: a retrospective observational study. *Crit Care Explor*. 2021;3(8):e0495. https://doi.org/10.1097/CCE.0000000000000495.
127. Al Babtain I, Almalki Y, Asiri D, et al. Prevalence of missed injuries in multiple trauma patients at a level-1 trauma center in Saudi Arabia. *Cureus*. 2023;15(2):e34805. https://doi.org/10.7759/cureus.34805.
128. Asim M, Amin F, El-Menyar A. Multiple organ dysfunction syndrome: contemporary insights on the clinicopathological spectrum. *Qatar Med J*. 2020;2020(1):22. https://doi.org/10.5339/qmj.2020.22.
129. Ting RS, Lewis DP, Yang KX, et al. Incidence of multiple organ failure in adult polytrauma patients: a systematic review and meta-analysis. *J Trauma Acute Care Surg*. 2023;94(5):725–734. https://doi.org/10.1097/TA.0000000000003923.
130. Cole E, Gillespie S, Vulliamy P, et al. Multiple organ dysfunction after trauma. *BJS*. 2020;107:402–412. https://doi.org/10.1002/bjs.11361.
131. Centers for Disease Control and Prevention. Intimate Partner Violence Prevention; 2024. https://www.cdc.gov/intimate-partner-violence/about/index.html. Accessed December 9, 2024.
132. Ghoshal R, Douard AC, Sikder S, et al. Risk and protective factors for IPV in low- and middle-income countries: a systematic review. *J Aggress, Maltreat Trauma*. 2023;32(4):505–522. https://doi.org/10.1080/10926771.2022.2154185.
133. Normandin PA. Special populations: the interpersonal-violence trauma patient. In: *Trauma Nursing Core Course Provider Manual*. 8th ed. Burlington, MA: Emergency Nurses Association; 2020.
134. Centers for Disease Control and Prevention. Impaired Driving; 2024. https://www.cdc.gov/impaired-driving/facts/?CDC_AAref_Val=https://www.cdc.gov/transportationsafety/impaired_driving/impaired-drv_factsheet.html. Accessed December 9, 2024.
135. Miller E, McCaw B. Intimate partner violence. *N Engl J Med*. 2019;380:850–857. https://doi.org/10.1056/NEJMra1807166.
136. Centers for Disease Control and Prevention. Drug-Impaired Driving in the United States; 2020. https://www.cdc.gov/impaired-driving/media/pdfs/Drug-Impaired-Driving-Summary-Sheet-LD-508.pdf. Accessed December 9, 2024.
137. Wilkerson RG, Yuan S, Windsor TA. Trauma in pregnancy: a comprehensive overview. *Trauma Rep*. 2020;21(3):1–11.
138. Tibbott J, Di Carlofelice M, Menon R, et al. Trauma and pregnancy. *Obstet Gynecol*. 2021;23:258–264. https://doi.org/10.1111/tog.12769.
139. Downing J, Sjeklocha L. Trauma in pregnancy. *Emerg Med Clin N Am*. 2023;41:233–245. https://doi.org/10.1016/j.emc.2022.12.001.
140. Bradley WJ. Trauma in pregnancy. In: Alson RL, Han K, Campbell JE, eds. *International Trauma Life Support for Emergency Care Providers*. 9th ed. Hoboken, NJ: Pearson Education; 2020.
141. Centers for Disease Control and Prevention. Older Adult Drivers. https://www.cdc.gov/transportationsafety/older_adult_drivers/index.html; 2022.
142. Clare D, Zink KL. Geriatric trauma. *Emerg Med Clin North Am*. 2021;39(2):257–271. https://doi.org/10.1016/j.emc.2021.01.002.
143. Ferrah N, Dipnall J, Gabbe B, et al. Injury profiles and clinical management of older patients with major trauma. *Austral J Ageing*. 2022;41:116–125. https://doi.org/10.1111/ajag.13000.
144. Van Wessem KJP, Leenen LPH. Geriatric polytrauma patients should not be excluded from aggressive injury treatment based on age alone. *Eur J Trauma Emerg Surg*. 2022;48:357–365. https://doi.org/10.1007/s00068-020-01567-y.
145. Lin PC, Wu NC, Su HC, et al. Comprehensive comparison between geriatric and nongeriatric patients with trauma. *Medicine (Baltimore)*. 2022;101(7):e28913. https://doi.org/10.1097/MD.0000000000028913.
146. Federal Bureau of Investigation. Active Shooter Incidents in the United States in 2022; 2023. https://www.fbi.gov/file-repository/active-shooter-incidents-in-the-us-2022-042623.pdf/view. Accessed December 9, 2024.
147. Gallagher JJ, Adamski J. Mass casualties and disaster implications for the critical care team. *AACN Adv Crit Care*. 2021;32(1):76–88. https://doi.org/10.4037/aacnacc2021235.
148. DeNolf RL, Kahwaji CI. EMS mass casualty management. In: *StatPearls*. NCBI Bookshelf version. StatPearls Publishing; 2022. https://www.ncbi.nlm.nih.gov/books/NBK482373/. Accessed August 24, 2023.
149. Afzali Rubin M, Svensson TL, Herling SF, et al. Family presence during resuscitation. *Cochrane Database Syst Rev*. 2023;9;5(5):CD013619. https://doi.org/10.1002/14651858.CD013619.pub2.
150. Tabata-Kelly M, Ruan M, Dey T, et al. Postdischarge caregiver burden among family caregivers of older trauma patients. *JAMA Surg*. Published online July 05, 2023. https://doi.org/10.1001/jamasurg.2023.2500.

Sepsis, Shock, and Multiple Organ Dysfunction Syndrome

Kathrine Anne Winnie and Kimberly Sanchez

http://evolve.elsevier.com/Urden/CriticalCareNursings

Sepsis, shock, and multiple organ dysfunction syndrome (MODS) are life-threatening emergencies, requiring immediate medical management and nursing intervention. This chapter presents an overview of sepsis and the general shock response, or shock syndrome. Information is also provided regarding the pathogenesis and clinical management of MODS.

SEPSIS

Description and Etiology

Sepsis is a life-threatening clinical syndrome caused by an infection and dysregulated physiologic systemic response; the body's response to infection injures its own tissues and organs.[1] It is characterized by perfusion abnormalities with organ dysfunction. Both the international consensus and the Centers for Medicare & Medicaid Services (CMS) criteria for sepsis are used in clinical practice (Table 33.1).[2,3]

Sepsis is caused by a wide variety of microorganisms, including gram-negative and gram-positive aerobes, anaerobes, fungi, and viruses. Among all ages, the most common causes of sepsis were diarrheal diseases and lower respiratory infection sepsis.[4] Anyone may be at risk for sepsis as everyone may be affected by an infection, but the most susceptible are neonates, older adults, pregnant or recently pregnant women, hospitalized patients, patients in critical care units, immunocompromised people, and people with chronic conditions.[4]

Pathophysiology

Sepsis is a complex systemic response that is initiated when a microorganism enters the body and stimulates the inflammatory and immune response.[5]

In a host–pathogen interaction, the body's natural response is to identify the microorganism, mobilize immune defenses to eliminate the microorganism, and activate clotting mechanisms to keep the infection localized.[5] This entire process is extremely complex and usually regulated internally by the body to keep it a localized response.[5]

The body's ability to regulate and limit the extent of damage by the microorganism and the body's tolerance of subsequent damage from future microorganism exposure is variable among individuals.[5] For this reason, the dysregulated response seen with sepsis is not clearly understood.[5] What is known is that the dysregulated response is an overactivation of the body's natural inflammatory and immune response that leads to leaking mediators into circulation via vascular or lymphatic vessels, resulting in the systemic activation or suppression of several pathways (e.g., metabolic, neural, hormonal, coagulation).[5] The body's initial, natural response compromises the organ initially affected by the microorganism (e.g., lungs with the SARS-CoV-2 virus) and this dysregulated response compromises distant organs as leaked mediators circulate.[5] The extent of distant organ compromise is variable among individuals and not well understood.[5]

Hallmarks of sepsis are increased vascular permeability and activated coagulation pathways.[5] The gap junctions in endothelial cells widen, increasing permeability and loss of intravascular volume to the interstitium.[5] These fluid shifts result in edema and intravascular hypovolemia.[5] Tissue factor is released from endothelial cells and the release of tissue factor initiates the coagulation cascade, producing widespread microvascular thrombi.[5] These macro- and microvascular changes directly affect the heart, resulting in systolic and diastolic dysfunction, and lead to distant organ hypoperfusion.[5] The other neural and hormonal pathways that are activated also affect vascular tone and responsiveness to catecholamines, further contributing to decreased blood flow to distant organs.[5] Blood flow to distant organs may also be influenced by variable microvasculature flow, whether it be absent, sluggish, or increased, all of which result in blood shunting to or from an organ and leads to tissue hypoxia.[5] Tissue hypoxia is one reason for an elevated lactate.[5] In the absence of tissue hypoperfusion and hypoxia, elevated lactate levels may develop from mitochondrial dysfunction, leading to an inadequate production of adenosine triphosphate (ATP) for cellular metabolism.[5] The systemic effects of the dysregulated response affects multiple organs and their physiological function and may lead to life-threatening consequences.[5]

Assessment and Diagnosis

Screening, early identification, and appropriate management of sepsis improve outcomes.[1] Effective management of sepsis depends on timely recognition.[1] Screening for sepsis is variable among organizations but some screening measures include systemic inflammatory response syndrome (SIRS) criteria (Table 33.1), sequential organ failure assessment (SOFA) criteria (Table 33.1), vital signs, signs and symptoms of an infection, or early warning scores.[1] The screening process may be manual or automated,[1] leveraging informatics (Box 33.1).

Common findings, indicative of sepsis, from a focused physical assessment include tachypneic respiratory pattern,[6] increased rate of heart sounds,[7] decreased intensity of S2 heart sounds,[7] bounding or thready pulse,[8] and skin temperature warmer cooler than usual to touch.[9] The clinical manifestations may be nondescript signs and symptoms of an infection, including a cough, shortness of breath, nasal congestion, stiff neck, fever, chills, sweats, burning or pain

TABLE 33.1 Criteria for Sepsis

Variables	International Consensus Criteria for Sepsis[2]	Centers for Medicare & Medicaid Services Criteria for Sepsis[3]
Infection	Confirmed	Suspected Two or more SIRS criteria: • Temperature >38°C or <36°C • Heart rate >90 beats/min • Respiratory rate >20 breaths/min • Leukocyte count over 12,000 mm^3 or under 4000 mm^3 or immature band/neutrophil ratio exceeds 10%
Organ Dysfunction	Two or more SOFA criteria: • PaO_2/FiO_2 ratio mmHg <400 • Mechanical ventilation • Platelet <150 $x10^3$/µL • Bilirubin ≥1.2 mg/dL • MAP <70 • On dopamine • On dobutamine • On epinephrine • On norepinephrine • GCS <15 • Creatinine ≥1.2 mg/dL • UO <500 mL	One or more variable of organ dysfunction: • Acute respiratory failure evidenced by a new need for invasive or non-invasive mechanical ventilation • Platelet <100 $x10^3$/microliter • INR >1.5 or aPTT >60 sec • Bilirubin >2 mg/dL • SBP <90 mmHg • MAP <65 mmHg • Creatinine >2.0 mg/dL • Lactate >2 mmol/L (18.0 mg/dL) • Physician documentation indicating >40 mmHg decrease in SBP is related to infection and not another cause

aPTT, Activated partial thromboplastin time; *C*, Celsius; *dL*, deciliter; *FiO_2*, fraction of inspired oxygen; *GCS*, Glasgow Coma Scale; *INR*, international normalized ratio; *MAP*, mean arterial pressure; *mg*, milligram; *min*, minute; *mL*, milliliter; *mm*, millimeters; *mmHg*, millimeter of mercury; *mmol*, millimole; *PaO_2*, arterial oxygen pressure; *sec*, second; *SBP*, systolic blood pressure; *SIRS*, systemic inflammatory response syndrome; *SOFA*, sequential organ failure assessment; *UO*, urine output.

BOX 33.1 Informatics

Information Technology and Early Identification of Sepsis

Early detection and diagnosis of sepsis is crucial for improving patient outcomes and reducing the risk of complications. Information technology plays a significant role in enhancing the early detection and diagnosis of sepsis.[a] Informatics contributes to this process via several different mechanisms:

- Data Integration: Informatics allows for integrating various sources of patient data, including electronic health records (EHRs), vital signs monitors, laboratory results, and more. By consolidating these data, a comprehensive view of a patient's condition is obtained, making it easier to identify signs of sepsis.
- Real-Time Monitoring: Informatics solutions can continuously monitor patient data in real time. Algorithms can be designed to detect abnormal patterns or trends that might indicate the onset of sepsis. For instance, if a patient's heart rate, respiratory rate, and temperature suddenly spike, an informatics system could trigger an alert for health care practitioners to investigate further.
- Machine Learning and Predictive Analytics: Machine learning algorithms can analyze large datasets to recognize subtle patterns that might not be apparent to human clinicians. These algorithms can predict the likelihood of sepsis development based on patient characteristics, allowing health care practitioners to intervene early.
- Clinical Decision Support Systems: Clinical decision support systems can analyze a patient's medical history, vital signs, laboratory results, and other clinical data to identify patterns consistent with sepsis. They can alert health care providers when specific criteria are met, helping to detect sepsis early and initiate appropriate interventions.

Incorporating informatics into sepsis detection and diagnosis processes can enhance the speed, accuracy, and consistency of identifying patients at risk or with early signs of sepsis. However, it's important to remember that information technology is supportive and should not replace clinical judgment. Health care practitioners should always exercise critical thinking and make informed decisions based on a combination of clinical expertise and informatics-driven insights.[A]

Reference

A Amland RC, Hahn-Cover KE. Clinical decision support for early recognition of sepsis. *Am J Med Qual.* 2019;34(5):494–501. https://doi.org/10.1177/1062860619873225.

with urination, unusual discharge from an orifice, erythema or swelling in an area, or malaise.[10] Additionally, abnormal vital signs, decreased urine output, altered mental status, or altered hemodynamic measures may also provide an indication of sepsis. Hemodynamic measures are discussed in detail in Chapter 12.

Laboratory tests for diagnosis of sepsis may include lactate,[1] arterial blood gas, complete blood count with differential, complete metabolic panel, and coagulation studies. Microbiology specimen types may depend on the suspected location of the infection[11] but often include blood cultures in adults with suspected sepsis.[1] The diagnosis of sepsis depends on criteria used (Table 33.1).[2,3]

Medical Management

Treatment of a patient with sepsis requires a multifaceted approach, and early treatment is critical for optimal patient outcomes.[1] This approach includes identifying and treating the infection, supporting the cardiovascular system and enhancing tissue perfusion with hemodynamic management, as well as maintaining oxygenation and ventilation. Dysfunction of the individual organ systems must be prevented.

Hour-1 Bundle: Initial Resuscitation

The hour-1 bundle is intended to minimize the time to treatment and promote immediate intervention.[12] The hour-1 bundle lists interventions that should be implemented within the first hour after recognition of sepsis (Box 33.2).[12]

Treatment of the Infection

The infection should be treated with antimicrobials. Patients with sepsis and a high risk for having multidrug-resistant (MDR) microorganisms should have both a gram-negative and gram-positive antimicrobial administered.[1] If the patient with sepsis is not at high risk for having an MDR microorganism, two gram-negative agents should be administered.[1] Patients with sepsis and a high risk for a fungal infection should have an antifungal agent administered, but those with a low risk of fungal infection should not have empiric antifungal therapy.[1] Once susceptibilities are available, antimicrobials should be evaluated.[1] Discontinuation of antimicrobials should be based on daily clinical evaluation and procalcitonin levels, with shorter durations of therapy being recommended over longer durations.[1]

BOX 33.2 Evidence-Based Practice

Surviving Sepsis Campaign Hour-1 Bundle[1,12]

- Measure lactate level
  - Remeasure lactate if initial lactate is elevated (>2 mmol/L)
- Obtain blood cultures before administering antibiotics (if can be done with <45-minute delay in antibiotic administration)
- Administer broad-spectrum antibiotics
- Start rapid administration of 30 mL/kg crystalloid for hypotension or lactate level ≥4 mmol/L
- Infuse vasopressors if hypotensive during or after fluid resuscitation to maintain MAP ≥65 mm Hg

kg, Kilogram; *L*, liter; *mL*, milliliter; *mm Hg*, millimeter of mercury; *mmol*, millimole;.

Patients with suspected sepsis have antimicrobials started as part of the hour-1 bundle but need to have continuous evaluation of likely infectious or noninfectious causes.[1] If a noninfectious cause is identified, empiric antimicrobials should be discontinued.[1]

Hemodynamic Management

A patient with sepsis with signs of hypoperfusion requires immediate volume resuscitation. Balanced crystalloids should be used instead of normal saline[1] to augment intravascular volume in the fluid-responsive patient. If large volumes of crystalloids are administered, albumin may be considered for administration.[1] Fluid responsiveness and lactate trends should guide fluid resuscitation.[1] See Chapter 12 for information on fluid volume responsiveness.

Maintenance of Oxygenation and Ventilation

Optimization of oxygenation and ventilation are often needed for patients with sepsis. If hypoxemia is present in patients with sepsis, high-flow nasal oxygen is preferred over noninvasive ventilation.[1] Should invasive ventilation be needed, low tidal volume ventilation strategies (6 mL/kg), plateau pressures less than 30 cm H_2O, and higher positive end-expiratory pressures are preferred.[1] Prone positioning

Shock Syndrome

Clinical and diagnostic assessments

- History and risk factors
  - Hypovolemic
    - GI hemorrhage from ulcerations or varices
    - Trauma/burns
  - Cardiogenic
    - MI
    - Arrythmias
    - Valvular dysfunction
  - Obstructive
  - Distributive
    - Infection
    - Allergen
    - Brain or spinal cord injury, anesthesia, or neuropathies
- Obtain vital signs
  - Hypoperfusion (e.g., decreased BP, decreased CO, changes in HR)
- Clinical assessment
  - Any signs of global tissue hypoperfusion
- Laboratory studies
  - Obtain serum lactate, arterial blood gas, mixed venous oxygen saturation, CBC, CMP, coagulation studies, amylase, lipase
- Diagnostic procedures
  - Assist with endoscopy, angiography, ultrasound, ECG, ECHO

Signs

- Hypotension
- Tachycardia
- Decreased cardiac index
- Tachypnea
- Altered mental status
- Decreased urine output or incontinence or retention
- Skin temperature and color changes

Nursing interventions

- Administer crystalloids, blood, and blood products as ordered
- Monitor fluid responsiveness
- Administer medications as ordered (e.g., vasopressors)
- Titrate vasopressors to target BP goals as ordered
- Maintain large-bore IVs
- Trend laboratory studies
- Manage treatment of causative factors
- Perform organ supportive therapies (MCS, RRT) as ordered

FIG. 33.1 Summary of Key Concepts Related to "Shock Syndrome." *BP*, Blood pressure; *CO*, cardiac output; *GI*, gastrointestinal; *HR*, heart rate; *MI*, myocardial infarction; *CBC*, complete blood count; *CMP*, complete metabolic panel; *ECG*, electrocardiogram; *ECHO*, echocardiogram; *MCS*, mechanical circulatory support; *RRT*, renal replacement therapy.

PATIENT-CENTERED CRITICAL CARE

Open Visiting and Family Areas in Critical Care

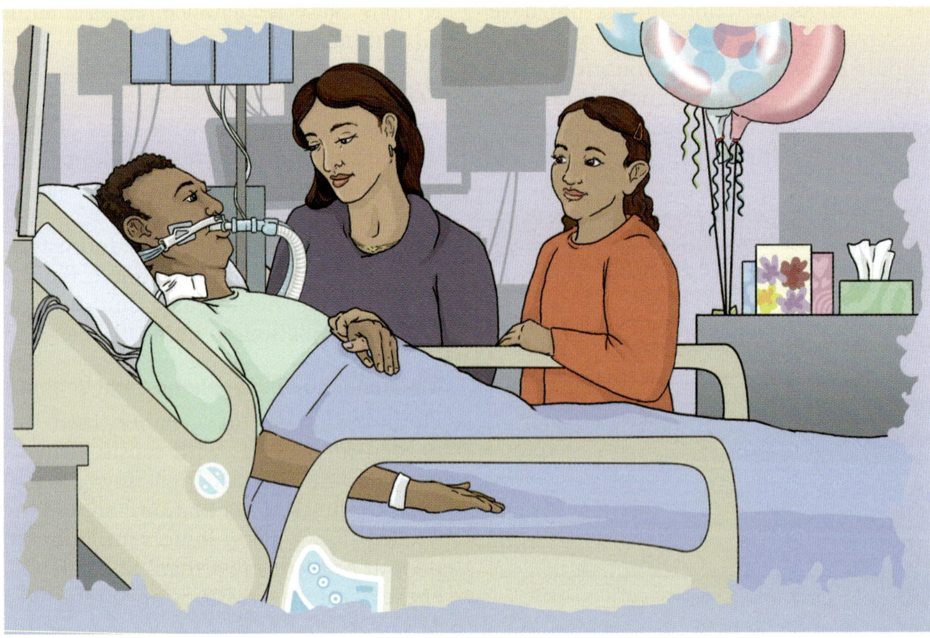

The modern critical care unit is designed to keep in mind the needs of critically ill patients and their families. In newly constructed hospitals, an area of critical care patient rooms is specifically designated for the family. This may include a seating area during the day that transitions to a bed for one family member to sleep overnight, and there may be a small closet for family belongings. Some settings have shower facilities for families. There is not a standard model, but the concept is to include the patient's family to decrease their anxiety. Of course, older hospitals can also be family friendly, but most were not designed to accommodate family members.

A critical care nurse working in a patient-centered critical care unit with an "open visiting" policy may find family members at the bedside at any time of day or night. The family-focused model has been the norm in pediatric hospitals for decades but is becoming more common in adult critical care. Communication with the family about the workflow and about what is happening to the patient is essential, especially in the first few days. In general, the number of family members who can be in the room is limited to 2 at one time. The exception is for end-of-life care, in which there may be many more family members in attendance.

The purpose of the patient-centered model is to decrease the family's stress about the experience of having a loved one in the critical care unit. The health care team is encouraged to consider close significant others/family members as part of the patient's team rather than using the traditional term "visitors."

may also be needed.[1] See Chapter 19 for further management of respiratory disorders.

Prevention of Complications

Patients with sepsis may have several complications that should be mitigated if possible. Patients at risk for gastrointestinal bleeding should have stress ulcer prophylaxis administered (see Chapter 28).[1] Pharmacologic venous thromboembolism (VTE) prophylaxis, with low-molecular-weight heparin, and mechanical VTE prophylaxis is recommended, unless contraindicated.[1] Blood glucose should be managed with insulin if the glucose level is ≥180 mg/dL, with a target glucose range of 144 to 180 mg/dL.[1] Fluid volume status should be optimal with consideration of renal replacement therapies, as needed (see Chapter 25).[1] Malnutrition should be prevented by initiating enteral nutrition within 72 hours, if possible (see Chapter 6).[1]

SHOCK SYNDROME

Description and Etiology

Shock is an acute, widespread syndrome of acute circulatory failure characterized by impaired tissue perfusion that results in cellular, metabolic, and hemodynamic alterations.[13] Ineffective tissue perfusion occurs when an imbalance develops between cellular oxygen supply and cellular oxygen demand.[13] This imbalance can occur for a variety of reasons and eventually results in cellular dysfunction and death.

Shock can be classified as hypovolemic, cardiogenic, obstructive, or distributive depending on the pathological cause.[13] *Hypovolemic shock*, the most commonly occurring shock, results from absolute or relative loss of circulating or intravascular volume.[13] Absolute loss includes loss of whole blood, plasma, or other bodily fluids. Relative loss includes vasodilation, increased capillary membrane permeability, and decreased colloidal osmotic pressure. Conditions that lead to hypovolemic shock are hemorrhage, burns, severe dehydration, and severe vomiting or diarrhea.[13] *Cardiogenic shock* results from the impaired ability of the heart to pump.[13] Conditions that lead to cardiogenic shock include myocardial ischemia or infarction, cardiac arrhythmias, and heart valve dysfunction.[13] *Obstructive shock* is caused by a blockage of circulating blood flow, affecting preload and afterload.[13] Conditions that can lead to obstructive shock are tension pneumothorax, pulmonary embolus, cardiac tamponade, and heart valve stenosis.[13] *Distributive shock* results from maldistribution of circulating blood and can be further classified as septic, anaphylactic, or neurogenic.[13] Septic shock is hypotension from sepsis that is not resolved despite adequate fluid resuscitation.[2] Anaphylactic shock is the result of a severe, systemic hypersensitivity reaction to an allergen.[13] Neurogenic shock is the result of the loss of sympathetic tone from brain or spinal cord injury, spinal anesthesia, or neuropathies.[13]

The shock syndrome is a pathway involving a variety of pathological processes that may be categorized into four stages: initial, compensatory, progressive, and refractory.[13] Progression through each stage varies with the patient's prior condition, duration of initiating event, response to therapy, and correction of the underlying cause.

Key concepts related to shock syndrome are summarized in Fig. 33.1.

Pathophysiology

During the *initial stage*, the body works to maintain homeostasis, regulating blood pressure, heart rate, and respirations.[13] Hemodynamic changes are subtle. Clinical signs are present (e.g., pale appearance, anxious).[13]

During the *compensatory stage*, mechanisms are mediated by the sympathetic nervous system and consist of neural, hormonal, and chemical responses that maintain blood pressure and respond to the oxygen supply and demand imbalance.[13] Epinephrine increases heart rate and contractility to improve nutrient and oxygen delivery, and norepinephrine enhances arterial and venous constriction, shunting blood to the vital organs for better perfusion.[13] Low blood flow to the kidneys triggers the renin-angiotensin-aldosterone-system response, with the release of aldosterone from the adrenal glands signaling the kidneys to reabsorb sodium and water leading to an increase in blood pressure.[13] Activation of renin eventually results in the production of angiotensin II, which causes vasoconstriction to also increase blood pressure.[13] Baroceptors detect a change in blood pressure and the response is peripheral vasoconstriction.[13]

During the *progressive stage*, the patient may need organ support.[13] When the cause of shock is not or cannot be addressed, the compensatory mechanisms begin failing to meet the tissue metabolic needs and the shock cycle is perpetuated.[13] Blood pressure and cardiac output decrease.[13] As tissue perfusion becomes ineffective and tissue is damaged from ongoing hypoxia, the cells switch from aerobic to anaerobic metabolism to produce energy.[13] Anaerobic metabolism produces small amounts of energy but a large amount of lactic acid, producing lactic acidemia.[13] Inflammatory mediators cause vasodilation and a decrease in preload.[13] Multiple organ systems fail.[13]

During the *refractory stage*, there is impaired vasoconstriction from hypoxia and lactic acidemia and impaired vascular response to catecholamine, resulting in pathologic vasodilation.[14] Additionally, there is a reduced amount of endogenous vasoactive hormones and excess amounts of vasodilatory nitric oxide, further contributing to the extensive vasodilation.[14] In this stage, the patient becomes unresponsive to treatment and death is expected in more than 50% of the cases.[14] As the individual organ systems die, MODS (discussed later) occurs and death is the final outcome.

Assessment and Diagnosis

Clinical manifestations vary according to the underlying cause of shock, the stage of the shock, and the patient's response to shock. Clinical manifestations for shock are compared in Table 33.2. Vital signs, hemodynamic measures, laboratory studies, and diagnostic procedures help in the diagnosis of shock. Hemodynamic measures, such as cardiac index, central venous pressure, pulmonary artery occlusion pressure, systemic vascular resistance, and fluid responsiveness, are discussed in detail in Chapter 12. Laboratory studies may include global indicators of systemic perfusion, such as serum lactate, arterial blood gas, and mixed venous oxygen saturation levels. Other laboratory studies may include complete blood count, comprehensive metabolic panel, coagulation studies, amylase, and lipase. Diagnostic procedures may include electrocardiogram, echocardiogram, heart catheterization, angiography, endoscopy (for bleeding), and ultrasound. Diagnosis for anaphylaxis, in particular, is reviewed in Box 33.3. A patient with evidence of global tissue hypoperfusion is considered to be in a shock state.[13]

Medical Management

The medical management of shock includes the improvement and preservation of circulating blood volume and tissue perfusion, the identification and treatment of the underlying cause, and prevention and treatment of organ failure.

Hemodynamic Stability

The initial treatment priority is the restoration of adequate circulating blood volume. For patients with obstructive shock, restoration of circulating blood volume is best accomplished by immediately addressing the obstruction through etiology-specific interventions (e.g., pericardiocentesis for cardiac tamponade).[18] In the other types of shock, circulating blood volume is increased through the administration of crystalloids, blood, and blood products.[16] The volume of crystalloids can range from 10 to 30 mL/kg and should be administered as quickly as possible to restore circulating blood volume.[1,15,19,21] Blood and blood product administration should be based on the patient's need for replacement and should follow a restrictive transfusion strategy.[1,16,22] Fluid responsiveness, lactate trends, and capillary refill should guide fluid resuscitation.[1] See Chapter 12 for information on fluid volume responsiveness.

Pharmacologic agents, including vasoconstrictors, vasodilators, inotropes, and antidysrhythmics, may also be used to promote hemodynamic stability in nonobstructive shock states and those agents are listed in Box 33.4. Vasoconstrictor agents are used to increase afterload by increasing the systemic vascular resistance (SVR) and improving the patient's

TABLE 33.2 Clinical Manifestations for Shock

Type of Shock	Cardiovascular Manifestations	Pulmonary Manifestations	Neurologic Manifestations	Kidney Manifestations	GI Manifestations	Other Alterations
Hypovolemic Shock[15,16]	Hypotension Tachycardia Decreased cardiac index Decreased preload Decreased right atrial pressure Increased systemic vascular resistance Decreased pulmonary artery occlusion pressure Weak, thready pulse Narrow pulse pressure Delayed capillary refill	Tachypnea	Altered mental status	Decreased urine output	Loose stool if blood present in GI tract	Cool skin Mottling, pale, or cyanotic skin
Cardiogenic Shock[17]	Hypotension Tachycardia Decreased cardiac index Increased preload Increased right atrial pressure Variable systemic vascular resistance Increased pulmonary artery occlusion pressure Weak, thready pulse Narrow pulse pressure Chest pain Diminished heart sounds Dysrhythmias	Tachypnea Crackles Pulmonary edema Hypoxemia	Altered mental status	Decreased urine output	---------	Cool, pale, moist skin Peripheral edema
Obstructive Shock[18]	Hypotension Tachycardia Decreased cardiac index Preload, right atrial pressure varies based on location of obstruction Pulsus paradoxus Chest pain	Tachypnea Air hunger	Altered mental status	Decreased urine output	Abdominal pain	Cool, pale, diaphoretic skin
Distributive Shock						
Septic Shock	Hypotension Tachycardia Increased cardiac index (early) and decreased cardiac index (late) Decreased preload (early) and increased preload (late) Decreased right atrial pressure Decreased systemic vascular resistance Decreased pulmonary artery occlusion pressure Full, bounding pulse Wide pulse pressure	Increased respiratory rate (early) or decreased respiratory rate (late) Crackles Decreased HCO_3^- Decreased PaO_2 Decreased $PaCO_2$ (early) or increased $PaCO_2$ (late)	Altered mental status	Decreased urine output	---------	Pink, warm, flushed skin Increased or decreased temperature

TABLE 33.2 **Clinical Manifestations for Shock—cont'd**

Type of Shock	Cardiovascular Manifestations	Pulmonary Manifestations	Neurologic Manifestations	Kidney Manifestations	GI Manifestations	Other Alterations
Anaphylactic Shock	Hypotension Tachycardia Bradycardia Decreased cardiac index Decreased preload Decreased right atrial pressure Decreased systemic vascular resistance Decreased pulmonary artery occlusion pressure Chest pain	Angioedema Stridor Wheezing Hoarseness Dyspnea Rhinitis Chest tightness Cough	Altered mental status Dizziness Headache Sense of impending doom Syncope or near syncope	Incontinence	Dysphagia Nausea Vomiting Diarrhea Cramping abdominal pain	Pruritus Erythema Urticaria Sense of warmth
Neurogenic Shock[19,20]	Hypotension Bradycardia Decreased cardiac index Decreased preload Decreased systemic vascular resistance	Respiratory rate dysregulation	Impaired thermoregulation Dizziness Syncope or near syncope	Incontinence or retention	---------	Pink, warm, flushed skin

GI, Gastrointestinal.

BOX 33.3 **Clinical Criteria for Diagnosing Anaphylaxis[21]**

Anaphylaxis is highly likely when one of the following two criteria is fulfilled:

1. Acute onset of an illness (minutes to several hours) with involvement of the skin or mucosal tissue or both (e.g., generalized hives; pruritus or flushing; swollen lips, tongue, and uvula) *and at least one of the following:*
   a. Respiratory compromise (e.g., dyspnea, wheeze [bronchospasm], stridor, reduced peak expiratory flow, hypoxemia)
   b. Reduced blood pressure or associated symptoms of end-organ dysfunction (e.g., collapse, syncope, incontinence)
   c. Persistent gastrointestinal symptoms (e.g., crampy abdominal pain, vomiting, diarrhea), especially after food allergens
2. Acute onset hypotension[a] or bronchospasm or laryngeal involvement that occur rapidly after exposure *to a likely allergen for that patient* (minutes to several hours), even in the absence of skin findings

[a] Adults: Systolic blood pressure of <90 mm Hg or >30% decrease for the person's baseline

blood pressure level. Vasodilator agents are used to decrease preload or afterload, or both, by decreasing venous return and SVR. Positive inotropic agents are used to increase contractility. Antidysrhythmic agents are used to influence heart rate. Initially, vasoconstrictors should help reach and maintain a mean arterial pressure (MAP) of 65 mmHg.[1,17] In patients with neurogenic shock, though, the goal MAP is 85 to 90 mmHg to improve spinal cord perfusion.[19] In septic and neurogenic shock, norepinephrine should be the first-line pharmacologic agent.[1,19] In septic shock, norepinephrine is followed by vasopressin, then epinephrine.[1] Inotropic

BOX 33.4 **Pharmacologic Agents Used in the Treatment of Shock**

Vasoconstrictors
- Epinephrine (Adrenalin)
- Norepinephrine (Levophed)
- Alpha-range dopamine (Intropin)
- Phenylephrine (Neo-Synephrine)
- Vasopressin (Pitressin)

Vasodilators
- Nitroprusside (Nipride, Nitropress)
- Nitroglycerin (Nitrol, Tridil)
- Hydralazine (Apresoline)
- Labetalol (Normodyne, Trandate)

Inotropes
- Dopamine (Intropin)
- Dobutamine (Dobutrex)
- Epinephrine (Adrenalin)
- Norepinephrine (Levophed)
- Milrinone (Primacor)

Antidysrhythmics
- Amiodarone (Cordarone)
- Adenosine (Adenocard)
- Procainamide (Pronestyl)
- Labetalol (Normodyne, Trandate)
- Verapamil (Calan, Isoptin)
- Esmolol (Brevibloc)
- Diltiazem (Cardizem)
- Lidocaine (Xylocaine)

agents, such as dobutamine, may also be needed in addition to norepinephrine to augment cardiac function.[1,17] In cardiogenic shock, vasopressin is preferred as the first-line pharmacologic agent as it has less pulmonary vasoconstriction when compared to norepinephrine.[17] In anaphylactic shock, epinephrine is the first-line pharmacologic agent as it promotes bronchodilation, vasoconstriction, increases myocardial contractility, and inhibits further release of biochemical mediators.[21] For patients with ongoing requirements for vasoconstrictors, it is recommended to use intravenous corticosteroids to attempt to accelerate the resolution of the shock syndrome.[1]

To enhance evaluation of treatment goals, invasive blood pressure and hemodynamic monitoring is recommended. These monitoring mechanisms are discussed in Chapter 12.

Promote Oxygenation and Ventilation

In addition to achieving hemodynamic stability, medical management should focus on promoting tissue perfusion. Adequate tissue perfusion depends on an adequate supply of oxygen being transported to the tissues and the cell's ability to use it. In critical care, oxygen supply should focus on achieving an oxygen saturation greater than 92%. If invasive ventilation is needed, low tidal volume ventilation strategies (6 mL/kg) pressures are preferred.[1,17] Oxygen consumption at the cellular level may be impacted by acidemia. In the presence of acute kidney injury and severe metabolic acidosis (pH ≤7.2), it is recommended to use sodium bicarbonate therapy.[1]

Identify and Treat Underlying Cause

Identification and treatment of the underlying cause is occurring simultaneously while ensuring hemodynamic stability and promoting oxygenation and ventilation in order to prevent further physiological insult. For hypovolemic shock, the source of absolute or relative volume loss should be identified and stopped. For cardiogenic shock, heart failure may need pharmacologic or mechanical circulatory management, myocardial ischemia or infarction may need revascularization, cardiac arrhythmias may need pharmacologic management, and heart valve dysfunction may need surgical intervention. For septic shock, prompt identification of the infection and source control interventions are recommended as soon as medically possible.[1] For anaphylactic shock, the offending allergen must be identified and removed.

Prevent Complications

Treatment should focus on preventing and treating organ failure to reduce mortality. Fluid volume status should be optimal with consideration of renal replacement therapies, as needed (see Chapter 25).[1,17] Cardiac function should be optimized with consideration of mechanical circulatory support devices as they have been shown to improve survival when utilized early.[17]

MULTIPLE ORGAN DYSFUNCTION SYNDROME

Description and Etiology

MODS is one of the most common syndromes in critical care in which two or more organ systems have acute and potentially reversible dysfunction.[23]

Three scoring systems are currently used to determine the severity of MODS: SOFA, logistic organ dysfunction score, and multiple organ dysfunction score. All three scoring systems include a measure of the cardiovascular system (heart rate, mean arterial pressure, central venous pressure), respiratory system (PaO_2/FiO_2 ratio), hematological system (platelets, white blood cell count), central nervous system (Glasgow coma scale), renal system (blood urea nitrogen, creatinine, urine output), and hepatic system (bilirubin, prothrombin time).[23] In addition to these scoring systems, matrix metalloproteinases, an inflammatory mediator, may be a potential biomarker to assess the severity of organ injury, with an increased level indicating an increased innate immune cell response.[23] MODS can be classified as primary, if organ dysfunction was a direct consequence of an initial insult, or secondary, if the involved organs were not directly affected by the initial insult.[24] Primary MODS results from a well-defined insult in which organ dysfunction occurs early and is directly attributed to the insult itself. Direct insults initially cause localized inflammatory responses.[24] Secondary MODS is a consequence of widespread sustained systemic inflammation that results in dysfunction of organs not involved in the initial insult.[24]

MODS is common in critical care, with an incidence up to 50%.[23] Mortality associated with MODS ranges from 44% to over 76% and is influenced by the number of involved organ systems and the severity of dysfunction.[23] Mortality risk increases in the presence of cardiovascular and neurological dysfunction.[23] Mortality is 100% in cases with seven organs in failure.[23] The most common cause of MODS is the dysregulated inflammatory and immune response of sepsis.[23] Noninfectious causes also contribute to MODS and include trauma, burns, surgery, shock, tissue ischemia, or necrosis.[23]

Pathophysiology

Because sepsis is the most common cause of MODS, the pathophysiological process is similar to sepsis, resulting in an altered regulation of the patient's inflammatory and immune response. Dysregulation of the inflammatory and immune response leads to widespread damage to vascular endothelium and organs.[23] A simplified pathophysiology of organ failure, inclusive of sepsis pathophysiology, is depicted in Fig. 33.2. A more detailed pathophysiology of MODS, inclusive of primary and secondary MODS, is depicted in Fig. 33.3.

Assessment and Diagnosis

MODS is a systemic syndrome with organ-specific manifestations. The clinical manifestations of cardiovascular, pulmonary, neurologic, kidney, gastrointestinal (including gallbladder, liver), endocrine, and hematologic alterations seen in MODS are outlined in Box 33.5. The clinical manifestations of and diagnostic criteria for organ-specific failure are discussed in detail throughout this book:

- Heart failure, along with other cardiovascular disorders, is discussed in detail in Chapter 13.
- Acute lung failure and acute respiratory distress syndrome, along with other pulmonary disorders, is discussed in detail in Chapter 18

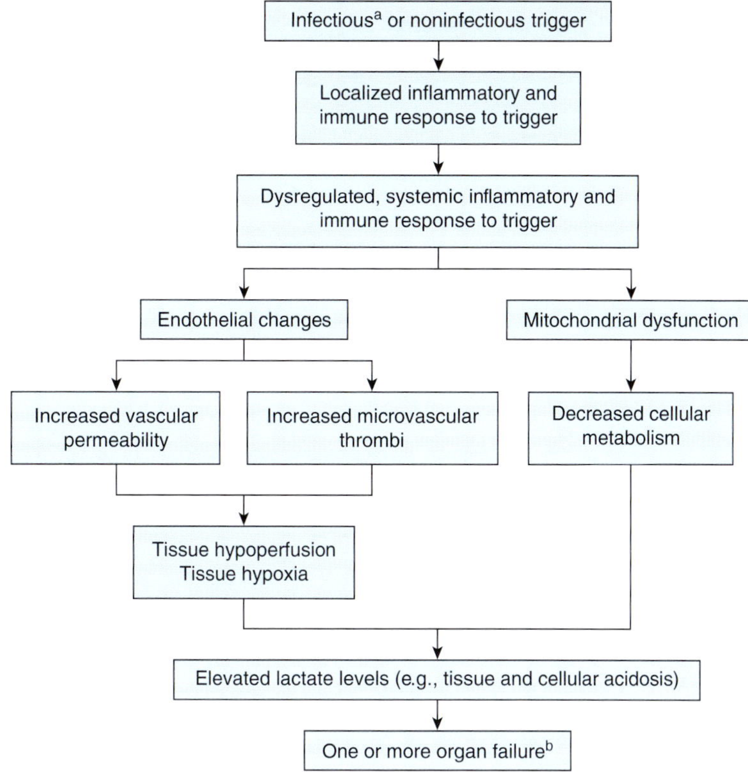

FIG. 33.2 Simplified Pathophysiology of Organ Failure. [a]Infectious is the most common cause of multiple organs dysfunction syndrome. [b]Multiple organ dysfunction syndrome is two or more organ system with dysfunction.

- Neurologic disorders are discussed in detail in Chapter 22.
- Acute kidney injury, along with other kidney disorders, is discussed in detail in Chapter 25.
- Gastrointestinal disorders, acute pancreatitis, and acute liver failure are discussed in detail in Chapter 28.
- Endocrine disorders are discussed in detail in Chapter 31.
- Disseminated intravascular coagulation, along with other hematologic disorders, is discussed in detail in Chapter 36.

Medical Management

There is no specific treatment for MODS; rather support of the failing organs is the priority in critical care.[23] A patient with MODS requires interprofessional collaboration in clinical management similar to sepsis (treatment of the infection, hemodynamic management, oxygenation and ventilation maintenance), as sepsis is the most common cause of MODS. Supporting the organ is the focus of medical management. *Cardiovascular support* may be provided using mechanical circulatory support devices, including intraaortic balloon pumps (IABPs), temporary or permanent ventricular assist devices (VADs), and extracorporeal membrane oxygenation (ECMO). These therapies are discussed in detail in Chapter 14. *Pulmonary support* may be provided using noninvasive or invasive mechanical ventilation and positioning therapy. These therapies are discussed in detail in Chapter 19. *Neurologic support* may include interventions to regulate body temperature, ventilation status, metabolic demand, blood pressure, seizures, and intracranial pressures. These interventions are discussed in detail in Chapter 22. *Kidney support* may be provided with renal replacement therapies, including continuous renal replacement therapy or intermittent hemodialysis. These therapies are discussed in detail in Chapter 25. *Gastrointestinal support* includes interventions to increase perfusion and resume enteral feeding when clinically appropriate. Nutrition is discussed in detail in Chapter 6. *Endocrine support* may include interventions to regulate blood glucose. These interventions are discussed in detail in Chapter 31. *Hematologic support* may include plasma exchange[23] or blood and blood product replacement.

NURSING MANAGEMENT

The patient care management for the patient with sepsis, shock, or MODS is a complex and challenging responsibility. It requires an in-depth understanding of the pathophysiology of the disease, prevention strategies, evaluation of intake and output, assessment of organ perfusion, promotion of nutrition, and providing comfort and emotional support. Patient and family education is also a component of nursing management.

Patient Care Management Plans

The patient care management plan for a patient with sepsis (Box 33.6), hypovolemic shock (Box 33.7), cardiogenic shock

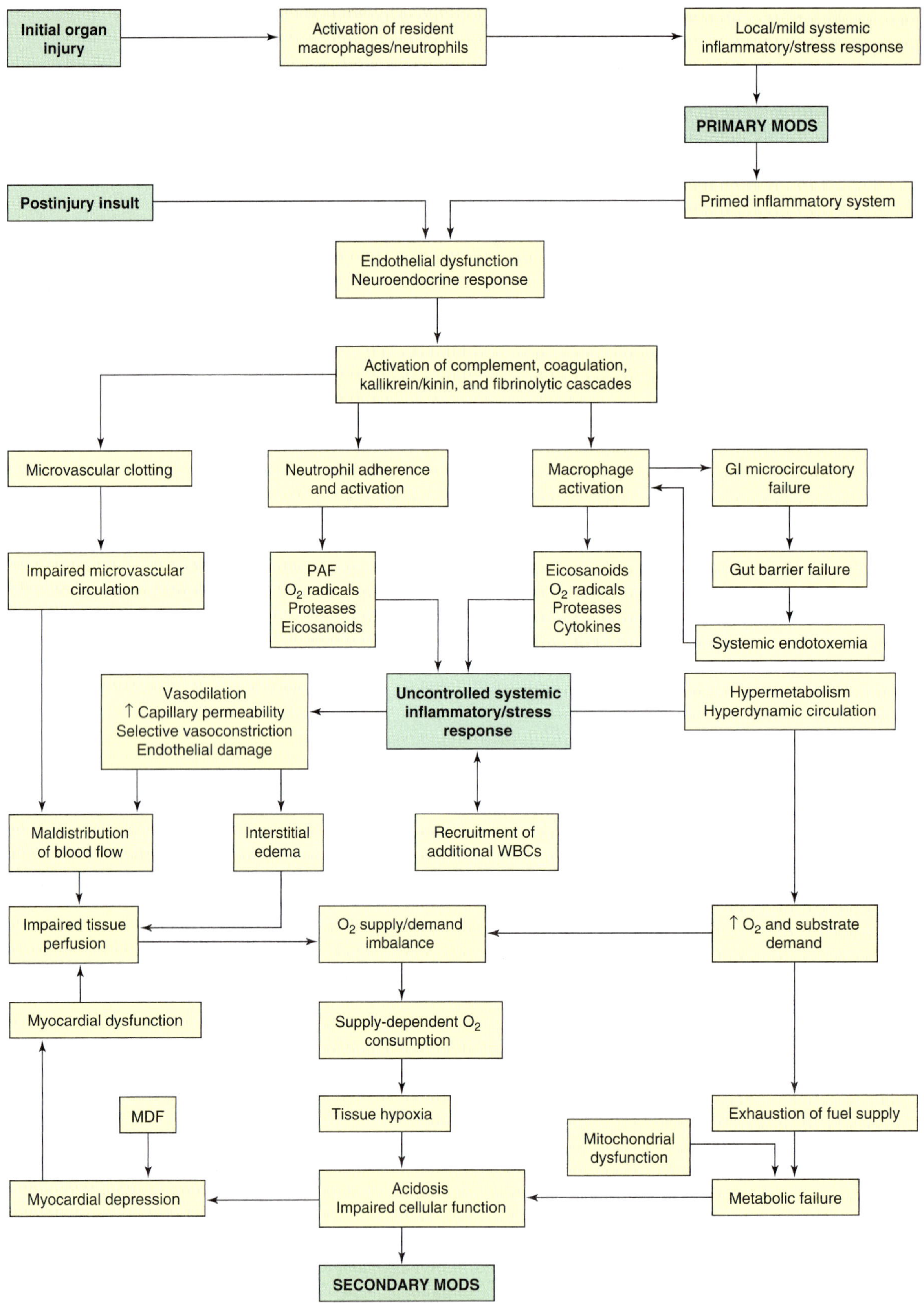

FIG. 33.3 Pathophysiology of Multiple Organ Dysfunction Syndrome. *GI*, Gastrointestinal; *MDF*, myocardial depressant factor; *MODS*, multiple organ dysfunction syndrome; *O_2*, oxygen; *PAF*, platelet-activating factor; *WBCs*, white blood cells. (From Rogers J. *McCance & Huether's Pathophysiology: The Biologic Basis for Disease in Adults and Children*. 9th ed. Elsevier; 2023.)

BOX 33.5 Clinical Manifestations of Organ Dysfunction

Cardiovascular

Hyperdynamic
- Decreased pulmonary artery occlusion pressure
- Decreased systemic vascular resistance
- Decreased right atrial pressure
- Decreased left ventricular stroke work index
- Increased oxygen consumption
- Increased cardiac output, cardiac index, and heart rate

Hypodynamic
- Increased systemic vascular resistance
- Increased right atrial pressure
- Increased left ventricular stroke work index
- Decreased oxygen delivery and consumption
- Decreased cardiac output and cardiac index

Pulmonary
- Dyspnea
- Patchy infiltrates
- Refractory hypoxemia
- Respiratory acidosis
- Abnormal O_2 indices
- Pulmonary hypertension

Neurologic
- Lethargy
- Altered level of consciousness
- Fever
- Increased intracranial pressure
- Encephalopathy

Kidney
- Increased serum creatinine and blood urea nitrogen
- Decreased glomerular filtration rate
- Oliguria, anuria, or polyuria
- Abnormal urinary indices
- Altered electrolytes
- Edema or other signs of fluid volume overload

Gastrointestinal
- Abdominal distention and ascites
- Intolerance to enteral feedings
- Paralytic ileus
- Upper or lower gastrointestinal bleeding
- Diarrhea
- Ischemic colitis
- Mucosal ulceration
- Decreased bowel sounds
- Bacterial overgrowth in stool
- Acute mesenteric ischemia
- Increased intraabdominal pressures
- Malabsorption

Gallbladder
- Right upper quadrant tenderness or pain
- Abdominal distention
- Unexplained fever
- Decreased bowel sounds

Liver
- Jaundice
- Hepatomegaly
- Increased serum bilirubin
- Increased liver enzymes
- Increased serum ammonia
- Decreased serum transferrin
- Abnormal coagulation studies
- Asterixis

Endocrine and Nutrition
- Decreased lean body mass
- Muscle wasting
- Severe weight loss
- Negative nitrogen balance
- Hyper- or hypoglycemia
- Hypertriglyceridemia
- Increased serum lactate
- Decreased serum albumin, serum transferrin, prealbumin, and retinol-binding protein
- Increased amylase and lipase

Hematologic
- Thrombocytopenia
- Disseminated intravascular coagulation
- Infection
- Decreased lymphocyte count
- Anergy

BOX 33.6 DIAGNOSIS AND PATIENT CARE MANAGEMENT

Sepsis

- Hypovolemia due to relative loss
- Ineffective Tissue Perfusion due to microvascular changes
- Stress Overload due to critical illness and critical care unit environment
- Anxiety due to threat to biologic, psychological, or social integrity
- Impaired Family Coping due to a critically ill family member
- Lack of Knowledge of Treatment Regime due to lack of previous exposure to information (see Patient and Family Education Plan, Box 33.13)

Patient Care Management plans are located in Appendix A.

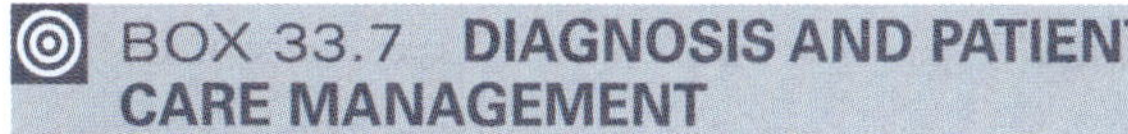

BOX 33.7 DIAGNOSIS AND PATIENT CARE MANAGEMENT

Hypovolemic Shock

- Hypovolemia due to absolute loss
- Hypovolemia due to relative loss
- Impaired Cardiac Output due to alterations in preload
- Risk for Infection
- Anxiety due to threat to biologic, psychological, or social integrity
- Impaired Family Coping due to a critically ill family member
- Lack of Knowledge of Treatment Regime due to lack of previous exposure to information (see Patient and Family Education Plan, Box 33.13)

Patient Care Management plans are located in Appendix A.

 BOX 33.8 **DIAGNOSIS AND PATIENT CARE MANAGEMENT**

Cardiogenic Shock

- Impaired Cardiac Output due to alterations in contractility
- Impaired Cardiac Output due to alterations in heart rate or rhythm
- Impaired Nutritional Intake due to lack of exogenous nutrients and increased metabolic demand
- Risk for Infection
- Impaired Family Coping due to a critically ill family member
- Lack of Knowledge of Treatment Regime due to lack of previous exposure to information (see Patient and Family Education Plan, Box 33.13)

Patient Care Management plans are located in Appendix A.

 BOX 33.9 **DIAGNOSIS AND PATIENT CARE MANAGEMENT**

Neurogenic Shock

- Hypovolemia due to relative loss
- Impaired Cardiac Output due to sympathetic blockade
- Hypothermia due to exposure to cold environment, trauma, or damage to the hypothalamus
- Risk for Infection
- Anxiety due to threat to biologic, psychological, or social integrity
- Impaired Family Coping due to a critically ill family member
- Lack of Knowledge of Treatment Regime due to lack of previous exposure to information (see Patient and Family Education Plan, Box 33.13)

Patient Care Management plans are located in Appendix A.

 BOX 33.10 **DIAGNOSIS AND PATIENT CARE MANAGEMENT**

Anaphylactic Shock

- Hypovolemia due to relative loss
- Impaired Cardiac Output due to alterations in preload
- Impaired Cardiac Output due to alterations in afterload
- Impaired Breathing due to decreased lung expansion
- Impaired Gas Exchange due to ventilation-perfusion mismatching or intrapulmonary shunting
- Risk for Infection
- Impaired Adaptation due to situational crisis and personal vulnerability
- Impaired Family Coping due to a critically ill family member
- Lack of Knowledge of Treatment Regime due to lack of previous exposure to information (see Patient and Family Education Plan, Box 33.13)

Patient Care Management plans are located in Appendix A.

 BOX 33.11 **DIAGNOSIS AND PATIENT CARE MANAGEMENT**

Septic Shock

- Hypovolemia due to relative loss
- Impaired Cardiac Output due to alterations in preload
- Impaired Cardiac Output due to alterations in afterload
- Impaired Cardiac Output due to alterations in contractility
- Impaired Gas Exchange due to ventilation-perfusion mismatching or intrapulmonary shunting
- Impaired Nutritional Intake due to lack of exogenous nutrients and increased metabolic demand
- Risk for Infection
- Anxiety due to threat to biologic, psychological, or social integrity
- Impaired Family Coping due to a critically ill family member
- Lack of Knowledge of Treatment Regime due to lack of previous exposure to information (see Patient and Family Education Plan, Box 33.13)

Patient Care Management plans are located in Appendix A.

(Box 33.8), neurogenic shock (Box 33.9), anaphylactic shock (Box 33.10), septic shock (Box 33.11), and MODS (Box 33.12) may include numerous patient problems, depending on the progression of the process.

Prevent and Monitor for Complications

Prevention of sepsis, shock, and MODS is one of the primary responsibilities of the nurse in the critical care unit. Prevention includes identification of patients at risk and reduction of their risk factors, including monitoring neurologic status and limiting exposure to microorganisms and allergens. Early identification and treatment result in decreased mortality.

Preventing Infection

Handwashing, aseptic technique, and an understanding of evidence-based interventions to reduce nosocomial infection in critically ill patients are essential components of preventive nursing care.

Patients are assessed closely for inflammation and infection. Subtle expressions of infection warrant investigation. Nursing measures include strict adherence to standards of practice to prevent infection. Practices related to infection control with invasive hemodynamic monitoring, urinary catheters, endotracheal tubes, intracranial pressure monitoring devices, total parenteral nutrition, and wound care must be stringent to prevent further infection.

Monitoring Intake and Output

As the nurse is administering large-volume, rapid administration of crystalloids, blood, and blood products, it is important to assess intake and output to aid in determining fluid balance, in addition to other clinical assessment of fluid volume overload or deficit. A patient in hypovolemic shock requires continuous evaluation of intravascular volume. Accurate monitoring of intake and output and daily weights are essential components of preventive nursing care.

Assessing Organ Perfusion

A head-to-toe assessment, informed by invasive and noninvasive monitoring, may provide information about organ perfusion to supplement the laboratory studies and diagnostic procedures. Assessment of cardiopulmonary status provides information on oxygen supply and demand. Nursing may enhance oxygen delivery through administration of supplemental oxygen and managing invasive or noninvasive delivery devices (e.g., mechanical ventilator). Nursing may limit myocardial oxygen demand through the administration of pharmacologic agents or through limiting duration of activity, while still engaging in some activity to prevent muscle atrophy. Assessment of neurologic status is important to note

BOX 33.12 DIAGNOSIS AND PATIENT CARE MANAGEMENT

Multiple Organ Dysfunction Syndrome

- Decreased Cardiac Output due to alterations in preload
- Decreased Cardiac Output due to alterations in afterload
- Decreased Cardiac Output due to alterations in contractility
- Impaired Gas Exchange due to ventilation-perfusion mismatching or intrapulmonary shunting
- Imbalanced Nutrition: Less Than Body Requirements due to lack of exogenous nutrients and increased metabolic demand
- Risk for Infection
- Acute Pain due to transmission and perception of cutaneous, visceral, muscular, or ischemic impulses
- Acute Confusion due to sensory overload, sensory deprivation, and sleep pattern disturbance
- Anxiety due to threat to biologic, psychological, or social integrity
- Compromised Family Coping due to a critically ill family member
- Lack of Knowledge of Treatment Regime due to lack of previous exposure to information (see Patient and Family Education Plan, Box 33.13)

Patient Care Management plans are located in Appendix A.

changes in mental status and motor response. Assessment of kidney function through intake and output monitoring may provide information on ensuing kidney injury. Bowel function or dysfunction (e.g., nausea, vomiting, diarrhea) is indicative of perfusion and should be assessed regularly for signs of delayed gastric emptying, obstruction, or ischemia. A full body assessment is warranted considering the systemic impact of sepsis, shock, and MODS.

Promote Nutrition

The nurse should collaborate with the dietician and provider to promote nutrition. Detailed information on nutrition support in critical illness is discussed in Chapter 6.

Provide Comfort and Emotional Support

The psychosocial needs of the patient and family dealing with sepsis, shock, and MODS are extremely important. These needs are based on situational, familial, and patient-centered variables. Nursing interventions for the psychosocial stress of critical illness include providing information on patient status, explaining procedures and routines, supporting the family, encouraging the expression of feelings, facilitating problem solving and shared decision making, offering open and individualized visitation schedules, involving the family in the patient's care, and promoting a calm and quiet environment. Patients and families should be given the option of open or individualized visitation, including presence during invasive procedures and resuscitation, as this helps decrease anxiety, improves well-being, and improves communication.[25]

Educate the Patient and Family

Patient education should focus on the pathophysiological process of sepsis, shock, or MODS. Additionally, patient-specific risk factors (e.g., allergens) and prevention strategies should be reviewed. Education about how to recognize and respond to signs and symptoms of a recurrence is essential to prevent a future life-threatening event. Short-term and long-term therapies are also important for the continued management of sepsis, shock, and MODS. The patient and family education plan is summarized in Box 33.13.

Interprofessional collaborative management of a patient with sepsis, shock, or MODS is outlined in Box 33.14.

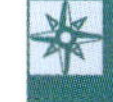

BOX 33.13 PATIENT AND FAMILY EDUCATION PLAN

Sepsis, Shock, or Multiple Organ Dysfunction Syndrome

Before discharge, the patient should be able to teach back the following topics:

- Pathophysiology of sepsis, shock, or multiple organ dysfunction syndrome as a life-threatening systemic syndrome
- Specific risk factors and prevention strategies
- Strategies to promote tissue perfusion
- Emphasize the importance of nutrition.
- Describe sign and symptoms that warrant follow-up with health care professionals.
- Explain need for ongoing follow-up with health care professional.
- Explain purpose of long-term therapies as appropriate (e.g., medications, mechanical circulatory support, dialysis, mechanical ventilation, transplantation).
- Describe complications associated with sepsis, shock, or multiple organ dysfunction syndrome.

BOX 33.14 Teamwork and Collaboration

Interprofessional Collaborative Practice: Sepsis, Shock, or Multiple Organ Dysfunction Syndrome

- Identify underlying cause of and treat accordingly:
  - Administer antimicrobials.
  - Remove infected tissue.
  - Correct lactic acidosis.
- Hemodynamic management:
  - Administer fluids (crystalloids, colloids, blood, and other blood products).
  - Administer vasoactive medications.
  - Administer positive inotropic medications.
  - Ensure adequate organ and extremity perfusion.
- Maintain oxygenation and ventilation:
  - Establish a patent airway.
  - Administer oxygen, as needed
  - Initiate mechanical ventilation.
  - Ensure sufficient hemoglobin and hematocrit.
  - Decrease oxygen demand
- Treat individual organ dysfunction:
  - Gastrointestinal
  - Hepatobiliary
  - Pulmonary
  - Renal
  - Cardiovascular
  - Coagulation system
- Initiate nutrition support therapy.
- Prevent and maintain surveillance for complications.
- Assess response to therapy.
- Provide comfort and emotional support.

ADDITIONAL RESOURCES

Refer to Box 33.15 for Internet resources related to sepsis, shock, and MODS.

BOX 33.15 Internet Resources

Sepsis, Shock, and Multiple Organ Dysfunction Syndrome

- American Society for Parenteral and Enteral Nutrition (ASPEN): https://www.nutritioncare.org/
- International Sepsis Forum (ISF): https://internationalsepsisforum.com/
- Sepsis Alliance (SA): https://www.sepsis.org/
- Surviving Sepsis Campaign: https://www.sccm.org/SurvivingSepsisCampaign/Home
- Shock Society: https://www.shocksociety.org/
- Society for Cardiovascular Angiography & Interventions (SCAI) Shock Resource Center: https://scai.org/clinical-practice/quality-improvement/scai-shock-resource-center
- American Spinal Injury Association (ASIA): https://asia-spinalinjury.org/
- The Food Allergy Research & Education (FARE): https://www.foodallergy.org/
- Anaphylaxis UK: https://www.anaphylaxis.org.uk/

CASE STUDY 33.1 Patient With Systemic Inflammatory Response Syndrome

Brief Patient History

Mr. Z is a 38-year-old construction worker who sustained a liver laceration after falling from a roof. Mr. Z required an exploratory laparotomy for splenectomy and repair of the liver laceration 4 days earlier. Mr. Z's medical history reveals no chronic health problems.

Clinical Assessment

Mr. Z is admitted to the critical care unit from the telemetry unit with acute respiratory insufficiency and hypotension. He is using his accessory muscles to breathe. His abdomen is distended, and there are no bowel sounds. Small amounts of dark green drainage are visible in the nasogastric tube. There is no sign of redness or drainage around the surgical wound.

Diagnostic Procedures

Vital signs are as follows: blood pressure of 78/55 mm Hg, heart rate of 142 beats/min (sinus tachycardia), respiratory rate of 35 breaths/min, temperature of 103.1° F, and urine output of 20 mL over the past 8 hours. Arterial blood gas values on a 100% nonrebreather mask are as follows: pH of 7.22, arterial partial pressure of oxygen of 54 mm Hg, arterial partial pressure of carbon dioxide of 69 mm Hg, bicarbonate level of 18 mEq/L, and oxygen saturation of 88%. The chest radiograph reveals infiltrates in the right lower lobe. Laboratory data reveal a hemoglobin level of 9.8 g/dL, hematocrit of 29%, and white blood cell count of 18,000 mm^3.

Medical Diagnosis

Mr. Z is diagnosed with sepsis.

Questions

1. What major outcomes do you expect to achieve for this patient?
2. What problems or risks must be managed to achieve these outcomes?
3. What interventions could be initiated to monitor, prevent, manage, or eliminate the problems and risks identified?
4. What interventions could be initiated to promote optimal functioning, safety, and well-being of the patient?
5. What technology can be used to monitor this patient and prevent complications?
6. What other interprofessional team members are needed to assist with the management of this patient?
7. What possible learning needs would you anticipate for this patient?
8. What cultural and age-related factors might have a bearing on the patient's plan of care?

KEY POINTS

Sepsis

- Sepsis is a life-threatening clinical syndrome caused by an infection and dysregulated physiologic systemic response; the body's response to infection injures its own tissues and organs.
- Hallmarks of sepsis are increased vascular permeability and activated coagulation pathways.
- Treatment of a patient with sepsis requires a multifaceted approach and includes identifying and treating the infection, supporting the cardiovascular system and enhancing tissue perfusion with hemodynamic management, as well as maintaining oxygenation and ventilation. Dysfunction of the individual organ systems must be prevented.

Shock Syndrome

- Shock is an acute, widespread syndrome of acute circulatory failure characterized by impaired tissue perfusion that results in cellular, metabolic, and hemodynamic alterations.
- A patient with evidence of global tissue hypoperfusion is considered to be in a shock state.
- The medical management of shock includes the improvement and preservation of circulating blood volume and tissue perfusion, the identification and treatment of the underlying cause, and prevention and treatment of organ failure.

Multiple Organ Dysfunction Syndrome

- Multiple organ dysfunction syndrome (MODS) is one of the most common syndromes in critical care in which two or more organ systems have acute and potentially reversible dysfunction.
- MODS is a systemic syndrome with organ-specific manifestations and the manifestations of cardiovascular, pulmonary, neurologic, kidney, gastrointestinal (including gallbladder, liver), endocrine, and hematologic alterations should be evaluated when assessing and diagnosing MODS.
- There is no specific treatment for MODS; rather support of the failing organs is the priority in critical care.

Nursing Management

- The patient care management for the patient with sepsis, shock, or MODS requires an in-depth understanding of the pathophysiology of the disease, prevention strategies, evaluation of intake and output, assessment of organ perfusion, promotion of nutrition, comfort, and emotional support, and education of the patient and family.

Visit the Evolve site at http://evolve.elsevier.com/Urden/CriticalCareNursing for additional study materials.

REFERENCES

1. Evans L, Rhodes A, Alhazzani W, et al. Surviving Sepsis Campaign: International guidelines for management of sepsis and septic shock 2021. *Crit Care Med.* 2021;49(11):e1063–e1143. https://doi.org/10.1097/CCM.0000000000005337.
2. Singer M, Deutschman CS, Seymour CW, et al. The third international consensus definitions for sepsis and septic shock (Sepsis-3). *JAMA.* 2016;315(8):801–810. https://doi.org/10.1001/jama.2016.0287.

3. Centers for Medicare & Medicaid Services. Specifications manual for national hospital inpatient quality measures: discharges 01-01-24 (1Q24) through 06-30-24 (2Q24); 2023. From https://qualitynet.cms.gov/inpatient/specifications-manuals#tab1. Accessed October 11, 2023.
4. World Health Organization. Sepsis; 2023. From https://www.who.int/news-room/fact-sheets/detail/sepsis. Accessed October 11, 2023.
5. Arina P, Singer M. Pathophysiology of sepsis. *Curr Opin Anaesthesiol.* 2021;34(2):77–84. https://doi.org/10.1097/ACO.0000000000000963.
6. Ball JW, Dains JE, Flynn JA, Solomon BS, Stewart RW. Chapter 14. Chest and lungs. In: Ball JW, Dains JE, Flynn JA, Solomon BS, Stewart RW, eds. *Seidel's Guide to Physical Examination.* 10th ed. Philadelphia, PA: Elsevier; 2023:290–325.
7. Ball JW, Dains JE, Flynn JA, Solomon BS, Stewart RW. Chapter 15. Heart. In: Ball JW, Dains JE, Flynn JA, Solomon BS, Stewart RW, eds. *Seidel's Guide to Physical Examination.* 10th ed. Philadelphia, PA: Elsevier; 2023:326–363.
8. Ball JW, Dains JE, Flynn JA, Solomon BS, Stewart RW. Chapter 16. Blood vessels. In: Ball JW, Dains JE, Flynn JA, Solomon BS, Stewart RW, eds. *Seidel's Guide to Physical Examination.* 10th ed. Philadelphia, PA: Elsevier; 2023:364–382.
9. Ball JW, Dains JE, Flynn JA, Solomon BS, Stewart RW. Chapter 9. Skin, hair, and nails. In: Ball JW, Dains JE, Flynn JA, Solomon BS, Stewart RW, eds. *Seidel's Guide to Physical Examination.* 10th ed. Philadelphia, PA: Elsevier; 2023:133–188.
10. Centers for Disease Control and Prevention. Know the signs and symptoms of infection; 2023. From https://www.cdc.gov/cancer/preventinfections/symptoms.htm. Accessed October 11, 2023.
11. Miller JM, Binnicker MJ, Campbell S, et al. A guide to utilization of the microbiology laboratory for diagnosis of infectious diseases: 2018 update by the Infectious Diseases Society of America and the American Society for Microbiology. *Clin Infect Dis.* 2018;67(6):e1–e94. https://doi.org/10.1093/cid/ciy381.
12. Surviving Sepsis Campaign. Adult patients; 2019. From https://www.sccm.org/SurvivingSepsisCampaign/Guidelines/Adult-Patients. Accessed October 12, 2023.
13. Blumlein D, Griffiths I. Shock: aetiology, pathophysiology and management. *Br J Nurs.* 2022;31(8):422–428. https://doi.org/10.12968/bjon.2022.31.8.422.
14. Jentzer JC, Vallabhajosyula S, Khanna AK, Chawla LS, Busse LW, Kashani KB. Management of refractory vasodilatory shock. *Chest.* 2018;154(2):416–426. https://doi.org/10.1016/j.chest.2017.12.021.
15. Cannon JW. Hemorrhagic shock. *N Engl J Med.* 2018;378(4):370–379. https://doi.org/10.1056/NEJMra1705649.
16. Hill B, Mitchell A. Hypovolaemic shock. *Br J Nurs.* 2020;29(10):557–560. https://doi.org/10.12968/bjon.2020.29.10.557.
17. Vahdatpour C, Collins D, Goldberg S. Cardiogenic shock. *J Am Heart Assoc.* 2019;8(8):e011991. https://doi.org/10.1161/JAHA.119.011991.
18. Zotzmann V, Rottmann FA, Muller-Pelzer K, Bode C, Wengenmayer T, Staudacher DL. Obstructive shock, from diagnosis to treatment. *Rev Cardiovasc Med.* 2022;23(7):248. https://doi.org/10.31083/j.rcm2307248.
19. Stein DM, Knight 4th WA. Emergency neurological life support: Traumatic spine injury. *Neurocrit Care.* 2017;27(Suppl 1):170–180. https://doi.org/10.1007/s12028-017-0462-z.
20. Mojtahedzadeh M, Taghvaye-Masoumi H, Najafi A, Dianatkhah M, Sharifnia H, Shahrokhi M. Management of hypotension and bradycardia caused by spinal cord injury. The usefulness of midodrine and methylxanthines. *Iran J Pharm Res.* 2019;18(4):2131–2135. https://doi.org/10.22037/ijpr.2019.1100824.
21. Cardona V, Ansotegui IJ, Ebisawa M, et al. World allergy organization anaphylaxis guidance 2020. *World Allergy Organ J.* 2020;13(10):100472. https://doi.org/10.1016/j.waojou.2020.100472.
22. Cable CA, Razavi SA, Roback JD, Murphy DJ. RBC transfusion strategies in the ICU: a concise review. *Crit Care Med.* 2019;47(11):1637–1644. https://doi.org/10.1097/CCM.0000000000003985.
23. Gourd NM, Nikitas N. Multiple organ dysfunction syndrome. *J Intensive Care Med.* 2020;35(12):1564–1575. https://doi.org/10.1177/0885066619871452.
24. Selzer MC, Cheek DJ, Rogers JL. Chapter 48. Shock, multiple organ dysfunction syndrome, and burns in adults. In: McCance RJ, ed. *Huether's Pathophysiology: The Biologic Basis for Disease in Adults and Children.* 9th ed. Philadelphia, PA: Elsevier; 2023:1557–1590.
25. Dragoi L, Munshi L, Herridge M. Visitation policies in the ICU and the importance of family presence at the bedside. *Intensive Care Med.* 2022;48(12):1790–1792. https://doi.org/10.1007/s00134-022-06848-1.

34

Burns

Jennifer Seigel, Robyn Myers, and Carrie Wilson

http://evolve.elsevier.com/Urden/CriticalCareNursing

Burn incidence has decreased worldwide but remains a common injury.[1] Approximately 486,000 burn injuries require medical treatment annually.[2] Burn injuries requiring hospitalization total approximately 40,000 per year, and 60% of these patients are admitted to one of the 128 specialized burn centers in the United States.[2]

Severely burn-injured patients have significant risk of morbidity and mortality[3] and face lengthy hospitalizations, although these have decreased. The decreases in morbidity, mortality, and lengthy hospitalizations for patients with burns are attributed to fire and burn prevention education, advancements in surgical-critical care management, management of patients in specialized burn centers, regulation of consumer products, and implementation of occupational safety standards. Many programs and organizations are dedicated to the prevention of burn injury. Societal changes including decreased smoking and alcohol abuse, changes in home cooking practices, and reduced industrial employment also have contributed to the decline in burn incidence. However, despite a decline in overall burn incidence, because of an increase in child maltreatment, burn injury as a result of physical abuse remains a differential diagnosis in patients with burns.[4] Great advances have been made in the care of patients with burns. With improvements in fluid resuscitation, better critical care management, and the trend toward early excision and grafting, mortality rates have decreased. Focusing management on early eschar excision and grafting leads to earlier resolution of the inflammatory response, decreased infection rates, improved mortality, better functional outcome, and reduced lengths of hospital stay.[5]

To provide comprehensive, holistic care to patients with burns, close collaboration is required among members of the interprofessional team. The burn team comprises nurses, physicians, physical therapists, occupational therapists, recreational therapists, nutritionists, psychologists, social workers, family members, and spiritual support staff members. The patient's response to a major burn injury is dramatic and involves multisystem alterations. Knowledge of local and systemic changes associated with patient needs is essential in providing care, which places extraordinary demands on a nurse in a burn practice, who must be both a specialist and a broad-based generalist. The purpose of this chapter is to provide a basic understanding of the complexities of burn care and the patient's response to burn injury.

ANATOMY AND FUNCTIONS OF THE SKIN

The skin is the largest organ of the human body, ranging from 0.2 m^2 in a newborn to more than 2 m^2 in an adult. The integumentary system consists of three layers: (1) epidermis, (2) dermis, and (3) hypodermis (Fig. 34.1).

Epidermis

The epidermis is composed of dead, cornified cells that act as a tough protective barrier against the environment. It serves as a barrier to bacteria and moisture loss.[6] From the surface inward, the five epidermal layers are: (1) stratum corneum, (2) stratum lucidum, (3) stratum granulosum, (4) stratum spinosum, and (5) stratum germinativum. The deepest layer of the epidermis contains fibronectin, which adheres the epidermis to the basement membrane. The epidermis regenerates every 2 to 3 weeks.

Dermis

The second, thicker layer, the dermis, is 1 to 2 mm thick and lies below the epidermis and regenerates continuously. The dermis is composed of two layers: (1) the more superficial, papillary layer next to the stratum germinativum and (2) the deeper, reticular layer. The dermis, composed primarily of connective tissue and collagenous fiber bundles made from fibroblasts, provides nutrition support to the epidermis.

The dermis contains blood vessels; sweat and sebaceous glands; hair follicles; nerves to the skin and capillaries that nourish the avascular epidermis; and sensory fibers that detect pain, touch, and temperature. Mast cells in the connective tissue perform the functions of secretion, phagocytosis, and production of fibroblasts.

Hypodermis

The hypodermis is beneath the dermis and contains fat, smooth muscle, and areolar tissues. The hypodermis is composed of adipose lobules along with some skin appendages like the hair follicles, sensory neurons, and blood vessels and acts as a heat insulator, shock absorber, and nutrition depot.[6]

The skin provides functions crucial to human survival, including maintenance of body temperature; a barrier to evaporative water loss; metabolic activity (vitamin D production); immunologic protection by preventing microbes from entering the body; protection against the environment through the sensations of touch, pressure, and pain; and overall cosmetic appearance.

PATHOPHYSIOLOGY AND ETIOLOGY OF BURN INJURY

A burn injury results in tissue loss or damage.[7] Injury to tissue can be caused by exposure to thermal, electrical, chemical, or

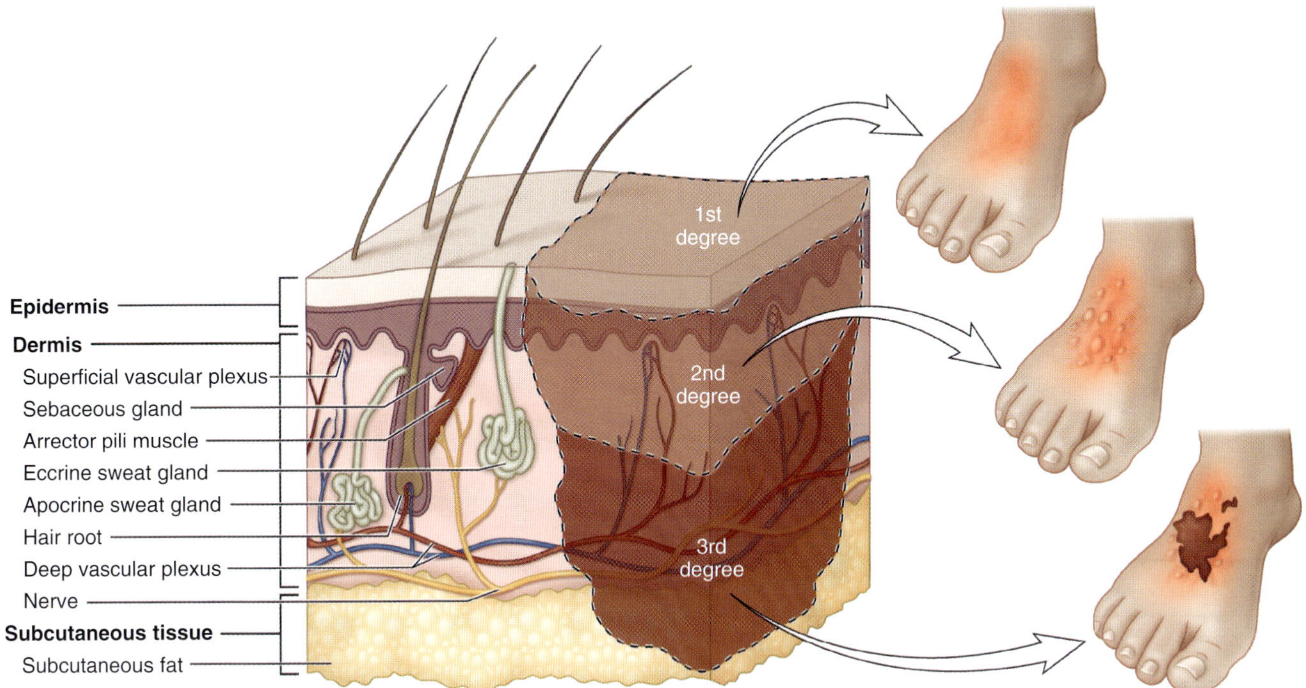

FIG. 34.1 Anatomy of the Skin. (From Dains JE. Integumentary system. In: Thompson JM, McFarland GK, Hirsch JE, et al., eds. *Mosby's Clinical Nursing*. 5th ed. Mosby; 2002.)

radiation sources.[7] The temperature or causticity of the burning agent and duration of tissue contact with the source determine the extent of tissue injury.[8] Tissue damage can occur at various temperatures, usually between 40° C (104° F) and 44° C (111.2° F). The burn wound itself is responsible for the local and systemic effects seen in the patient with burns. Tissue damage is caused by enzyme malfunction and denaturation of proteins. Prolonged exposure or higher temperatures can lead to cell necrosis and a process known as *protein coagulation*. The areas extending outward from this central area of injury sustain various degrees of damage and are identified by zones of injury.[3,7]

Zones of Injury

Three concentric zones are present in burn injury: (1) zone of coagulation, (2) zone of stasis, and (3) zone of hyperemia[3] (Fig. 34.2). The zone of coagulation, or central zone, is the site of most severe damage, and the peripheral zone is the site of least severe damage. The zone of coagulation is usually the site of greatest heat transfer, leading to irreversible skin death.[3] This area is surrounded by the zone of stasis, which is characterized by impaired circulation that can lead to cessation of blood flow caused by a pronounced inflammatory reaction. This area is potentially salvageable;[3] however, local or systemic factors can convert it into a full-thickness injury. Some factors that can lead to deeper wound conversion are toxic mediators of the inflammatory process, infection, inappropriate volume resuscitation, malnutrition, chronic illness, or the local wound care provided. It may take 48 to 72 hours to determine the full extent of injury in this area. The outermost area, the zone of hyperemia, has vasodilation and increased blood flow but minimal cell involvement.[3] Early spontaneous recovery can occur in this area.[3,7]

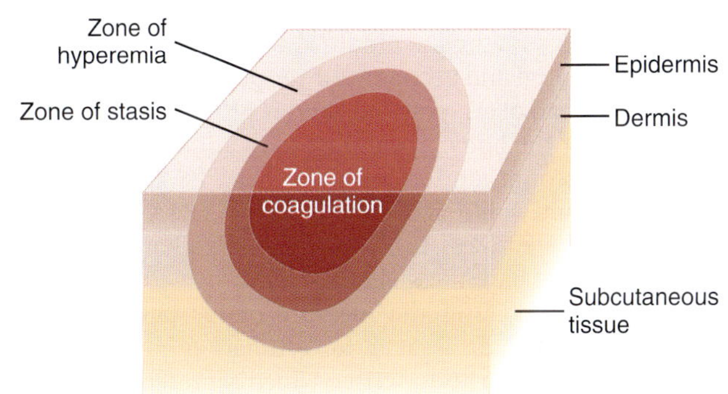

FIG. 34.2 Zones of Burn Injury.

CLASSIFICATION OF BURN INJURY

Burns are classified primarily according to the size and depth of injury. However, the type and location of the burn and the patient's age and medical history are also significant considerations. Recognition of the magnitude of burn injury, which is based on the above-mentioned factors, is crucial in the overall plan of care and in decisions concerning patient management and appropriate referral to a burn center (Box 34.1).[2] The patient's age, burn size, and inhalation injury are the cardinal determinants of survival. A significant decrease in inpatient mortality was seen among patients with extensive burns. Extensive burns can lead to hypermetabolic, hypercatabolic state leaving patients immunocompromised with an increased risk of infection, sepsis, and multisystem organ failure.[8] Adults with >40% total burn surface area (TBSA) burned and children with >60% TBSA burned are at high risk for morbidity and mortality.

BOX 34.1 Burn Center Referral

Patients with the following burn injuries are best treated in a certified burn center:

- Partial-thickness burns of 10% or more of total body surface area
- Full-thickness (third-degree) burns in any age group
- Burns of face, hands, feet, genitalia, perineum, or major joints that may result in cosmetic or functional disability
- Electrical burns, including lightning injury
- Inhalation injuries
- Chemical burns
- Burns in patients with preexisting medical disorders (e.g., diabetes mellitus, symptomatic cardiopulmonary disease) that could complicate management, prolong recovery, or affect mortality
- Burn injuries with concomitant trauma (e.g., fractures) in which the burn injury poses the greatest risk of morbidity or mortality may be stabilized initially in a trauma center before transfer to a burn center
- Burns in children in hospitals without qualified personnel or equipment for the care of children
- Burn injuries in patients who will require special social, emotional, or long-term rehabilitative intervention

Size of Injury

Several different methods can be used to estimate the size of the burn area. A quick and easy method is the *rule of nines* (or *Berkow formula*), which often is used in the prehospital setting for initial triage of a patient with burns (Fig. 34.3). In this method, the adult body is divided into different surface areas of 9% per area. This method is modified for assessing infants and very small children and accounts for proportionate growth. For example, the head of a 1-year-old child is proportionately larger than the rest of the body, in contrast to in adults, so the child's head would account for 19% of his or her TBSA, whereas the head of an adult would account for 7% of TBSA. Designated burn centers have access to *Berkow formula* charts, but local hospitals may not have these charts.

Another method uses the measure of the palmar surface of the victim's hand as a gauge for estimating burn area. The palmar surface (fingertip to wrist), which represents 1% of the TBSA, also can be useful in making burn estimates in the prehospital setting or for estimating the percentage of involvement in small and scattered areas of burn.[7]

In the hospital setting, the Lund and Browder method (Fig. 34.4) is the most accurate and accepted method for determining the percentage of burn. Surface area measurements are assigned to each body part in terms of the age of the patient. This method is highly recommended for use with children younger than 10 years because it corrects for smaller surface areas of the lower extremities. It is also recommended for adult burn victims because of its accuracy.

Depth of Burn Injury

Because the management of burn wounds is closely tied to the correct assessment of wound severity, some newer strategies other than observation are being investigated. Some of these techniques have taken into account the presence of denatured collagen, wound edema, and altered blood flow. One such technique is noncontact laser Doppler imaging, which can give a color perfusion map of the burn wound.[9] Other techniques of assessing the burn depth include use of current optical techniques to complement clinical examination, but these optical

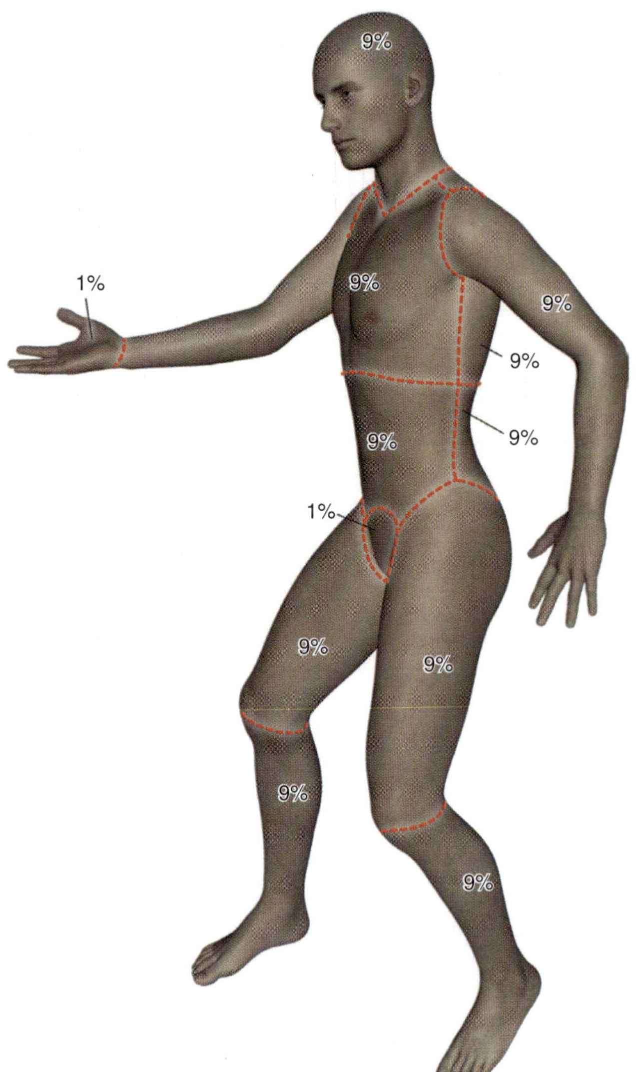

FIG. 34.3 Estimation of Adult Burn Injury. Rule of Nines: Anterior and posterior view. (From Walls RM, Hockberger R, Gausche-Hill M, Erickson TB, Wilcox SR, eds. *Rosen's Emergency Medicine Concepts and Clinical Practice*. 10th ed. Elsevier; 2023.)

techniques are based on the premise that functioning blood vessels are retained in viable tissue.[9] Clinical examination is approximately 75% accurate in assessing burn wound depth, but current optical techniques (e.g., three-dimensional photography, B-mode harmonic ultrasound technology, color-coded tissue elastography, hyperspectral imaging, fluorescent dye indocyanine green [ICG], laser speckle contrast imaging [LSI], and ultrasound Doppler imaging) have both advantages and disadvantages.[9] Use of harmonic ultrasound technology would be useful in assessing burn wound depth and looking at blood flow dynamics, whereas in a noncontact and noninvasive setting, LSI would be more advantageous in assessing tissue vascularization.[9] Research with these techniques is ongoing, but they are limited in their clinical usefulness currently. Future imaging platforms may change burn wound care from time of initial assessment all the way through the healing period.

Traditionally, burn depth has been classified in degrees of injury based on the amount of injured epidermis, dermis, or both: first-degree, second-degree, third-degree, or fourth-degree burns. However, these terms are not descriptive of the

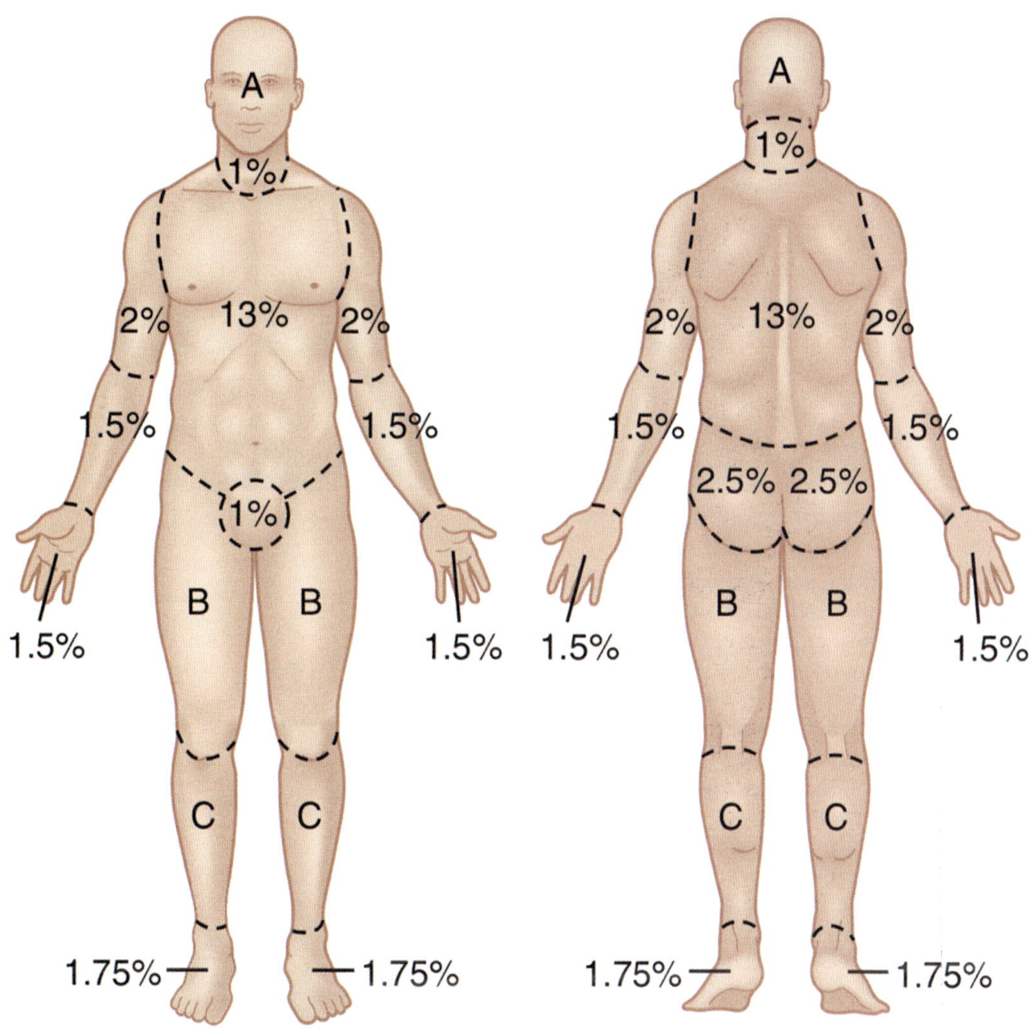

Relative percentages of areas affected by growth

Age	Half of head (A)	Half of one thigh (B)	Half of one leg (C)
Infant	9.5	2.75	2.5
1 yr	8.5	3.25	2.5
5 yr	6.5	4	2.75
10 yr	5.5	4.25	3
15 yr	4.5	4.25	3.25
Adult	3.5	4.75	3.5

FIG. 34.4 Lund and Browder Burn Estimate Chart and Diagram. (From Walls RM, Hockberger R, Gausche-Hill M, Erickson TB, Wilcox SR, eds. *Rosen's Emergency Medicine Concepts and Clinical Practice*. 10th ed. Elsevier; 2023.)

burn surface. The depth of the burn is defined by how much of the skin's two layers are destroyed by the heat source.[5,7] Burns are classified as superficial, partial-thickness, or full-thickness burns. These descriptions are based on the surface appearance of the wound. Superficial burns include first-degree burns and are limited to the epidermis.

Partial-Thickness Burns

Partial-thickness burns include various stages of second-degree burns.[7,10] Some authorities further separate partial-thickness burns as superficial or deep-dermal partial-thickness burns.

A superficial (first-degree) burn involves only the first two or three of the five layers of the epidermis. Erythema and mild

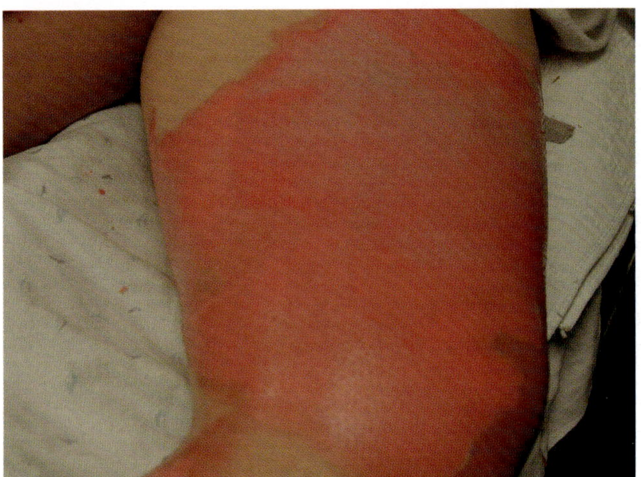

FIG. 34.5 Partial-Thickness Burn to Left Thigh.

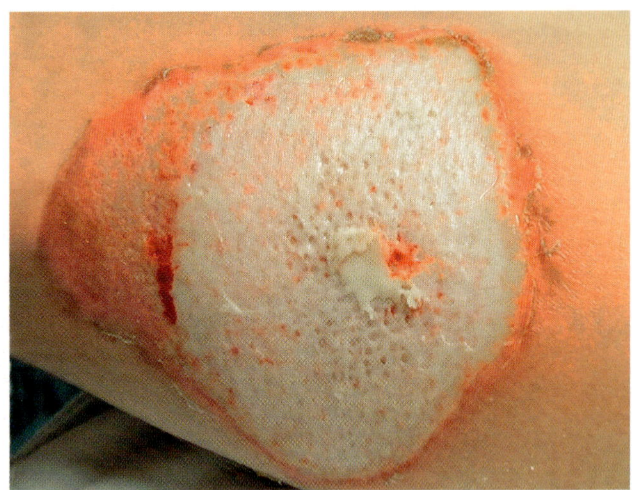

FIG. 34.6 Deep-Dermal Partial-Thickness Burn to Thigh.

discomfort characterize superficial partial-thickness wounds. Pain, the chief symptom, usually resolves in 48 to 72 hours. Common examples of these burn injuries are sunburns and minor steam burns such as may occur while cooking. These wounds usually heal in 2 to 7 days and do not require medical intervention aside from pain relief, management of pruritus (itching), and oral fluids. Swelling can be a common complication that may require intervention. Superficial burns are not included in the calculation of percent burn.

A partial-thickness (second-degree) burn involves all the epidermis and part of the underlying dermis.[7] These burns usually are caused by brief contact with flames, hot liquid, or exposure to dilute chemicals (Fig. 34.5). A light to bright red or mottled appearance characterizes superficial second-degree burns. These wounds may appear wet and weeping, may contain bullae, and are extremely painful and sensitive to air currents. These burns blanch painfully.[7] The microvessels that perfuse this area are injured, and permeability is increased, resulting in leakage of large amounts of plasma into the interstitium. This fluid lifts off the thin, damaged epidermis, causing blister formation. Despite the loss of the entire basal layer of the epidermis, a burn of this depth heals in 7 to 21 days. Minimal scarring can be expected. Mid-dermal partial-thickness wounds commonly take 4 to 6 weeks to heal.

Deep-dermal partial-thickness (second-degree) burns involve the entire epidermal layer and deeper layers of the dermis.[7] These burns often result from contact with hot liquids or solids or with intense radiant energy. A deep-dermal partial-thickness burn usually is not characterized by blister formation. Only a modest plasma surface leakage occurs because of severe impairment in blood supply. The wound surface usually is red with patchy white areas that blanch with pressure. The appearance of the deep-dermal wound changes over time. Dermal necrosis and surface coagulated protein turn the wound from white to yellow (Fig. 34.6). These wounds have a prolonged healing time. They can heal spontaneously as the epidermal elements germinate and migrate until the epidermal surface is restored, or they may require a skin substitute or surgical excision and grafting for wound closure. This process of healing by epithelialization can take up to 6 weeks. Left untreated, these wounds can heal primarily with unstable epithelium, late hypertrophic scarring, and marked contracture formation.[7,10] Partial-thickness injuries can become full-thickness injuries if they become infected, if blood supply is diminished, or if further trauma occurs to the site. The treatment of choice is surgical excision and skin grafting.

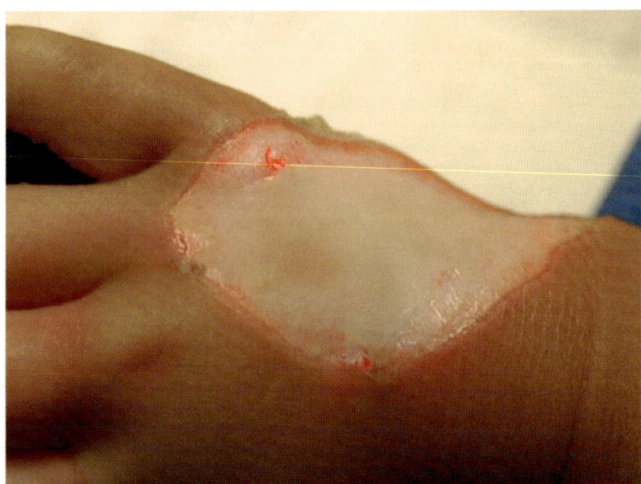

FIG. 34.7 Full-Thickness Burn to Back of Hand.

Full-Thickness Burns

A full-thickness (third-degree) burn involves destruction of all the layers of the skin down to and including the subcutaneous fat (Fig. 34.7).[7,10] Full-thickness burns include third-degree burns.[7,10] Fourth-degree burns extend through all skin layers and extend into muscle, tendon, and bone. The subcutaneous tissue is composed of adipose tissue, includes the hair follicles and sweat glands, and is poorly vascularized. A full-thickness burn appears pale white or charred, red or brown, and leathery. The surface of the burn may be dry, and if the skin is broken, fat may be exposed. Full-thickness burns usually are painless and insensitive to palpation. Because all the epithelial elements are destroyed, the wound does not heal by epithelialization. Wound closure of small full-thickness burns (less than 4 cm^2 area) can be achieved with healing by contraction. All other full-thickness wounds require skin grafting for closure. Extensive full-thickness wounds leave the patient extremely susceptible to infections, fluid and electrolyte imbalances, alterations in thermoregulation, and metabolic disturbances.

The exact depth of many burn wounds cannot be clearly defined on the first inspection, and many burn wounds may contain superficial, mid-dermal, and deep-dermal wounds. A major difficulty is distinguishing deep-dermal partial-thickness from full-thickness injury. It is important to identify the depth of injury for appropriate treatment. Deep-dermal partial-thickness wounds that do not heal within a relatively short time are treated with wound excision and grafting. Burn wounds can evolve over time, and they require frequent reassessment. Special consideration must always be given to very young patients and older patients because of their thin dermal layer. Older adults may also have reduced sensation and blood supply, causing them to be more susceptible to a full-thickness injury. Time of burn injury can lead to higher mortality. Burn injuries in these two age groups may be more severe than they initially appear.

The TBSA of the burn is calculated at the same time that assessment for wound depth occurs. This calculation provides the basis for determining the amount of fluid required for treatment. All burn wound surface area percentages except for superficial burns are used to calculate the patient's fluid requirements.

Types of Injury

Thermal Burns

The most common type of burn is a thermal burn caused by steam, scalds, contact with heat, or fire. Each year nearly 10,000 children experience severe disability as a result of thermal injury.[5] Toddlers are most often affected by scald burns, and mortality is highest in the 0- to 2-year age group because of their incompletely developed immune and organ systems.[5] Contact with hot foods (burns) are also common.[10] The length of time the hot object is in contact with the skin determines the depth of injury. Children have thinner skin and will sustain a deeper burn at any temperature.[5] Non–food-related thermal burns can occur from fireworks, irons, curling irons, campfires, and fire pits in young children.

Burns associated with the use of lighters, lighter fluid, fire, firecrackers, and gasoline are seen in adolescents. Electrical burns are most likely to occur where there is exposure to live electrical wires from high-voltage lines, appliances, lightning, or faulty wiring.[10] Contact and flame burns tend to be deep-dermal or full-thickness injuries.

Electrical Burns

Electrical and lightning injuries result in 1000 deaths per year in the United States.[11] Electrical injuries account for 4% of patient admissions to burn centers.[2] Low-voltage (alternating) current (60 to 1000 V) or high-voltage (alternating or direct) current (greater than 1000 V) can cause electrical burns.[11] Children have the highest incidence of electrical injury. These accidents occur as a result of insertion of an object into an outlet or by biting or sucking on an electrical cord. These burns can lead to tissue destruction and contracture formation.[10] Electrical burns occur most often in the home; in adults, electrical injuries occur most often in the workplace.[11] Common situations that may increase the risk for electrical injuries include occupational exposure and accidents involving household current.

Chemical Burns

Acid and alkali agents cause chemical burns. Alkali burns commonly result in more severe injuries compared with acid burns. Acid and alkali agents are found in many household and industrial substances such as liquid concrete. Chemical burns most commonly occur in the domestic setting as a result of nonintentional exposure to household chemicals in children younger than 10 years of age and are preventable.[12] Chemical burns occur most often as a result of deliberate harm in children older than 10 years of age.[12] The concentration of the chemical agent and the duration of exposure are the key factors that determine the extent and depth of damage. Progression of injury from chemical burns to their complete depth may be delayed, and the full extent of the injury may not be apparent until 48 hours after injury. Time must not be wasted in looking for a specific neutralizing agent, because the injury is related directly to the concentration of the chemical and the duration of the exposure, and the heat of neutralization can extend the injury.

Radiation Burns

Burns associated with radiation exposure are uncommon. Radiation burns usually are localized and indicate high radiation doses to the affected area. Radiation burns may appear identical to thermal burns.[13] The major difference is the time between exposure and clinical manifestation; it can be days to weeks, depending on the level of the radiation dose. Radiation injury can occur with exposure to industrial equipment such as accelerators and cyclotrons and to equipment used for medical treatment.

Location of Injury

Location of injury can be a determining factor in differentiating the level of care required. According to triage criteria from the American College of Surgeons, burns on the face, hands, feet, genitalia, major joints, and perineum are best treated in a burn center. These burns involve functional areas of the body and often require specialized intervention (Fig. 34.8). Injuries to these areas can result in significant long-term morbidity from impaired function and altered appearance.

Patient Age and History

Patient age and history are significant determinants of survival. Patients considered most at risk are children younger than 2 years and adults older than 60 years. Inhalation injury, electrical burns, and all burns complicated by trauma and fractures (considered major injuries) significantly increase the risk for death. Obtaining the patient's medical history is important, especially

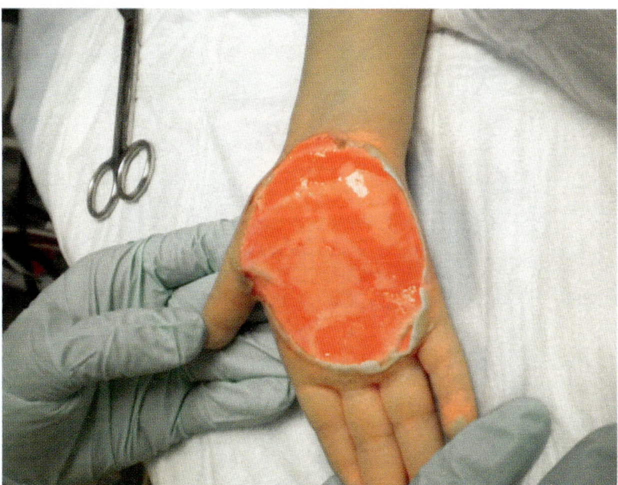

FIG. 34.8 Partial-Thickness Contact Burn to Palm.

a history related to cardiac, pulmonary, or kidney dysfunction; diabetes; and central nervous system disorders. It is essential to obtain a thorough history, especially for nonverbal patients. Attention should be paid to the description of the burn event to rule out nonaccidental trauma (Fig. 34.9). Social services such as child protective services and the police should be consulted if abuse or neglect is suspected.

Child Abuse

The most recent statistics show 3.9 million referrals were made for child maltreatment, and of those, 16.7% of cases are investigated and substantiated for abuse.[4] There were a nationally estimated 588,229 victims of child abuse and neglect.[4] According to this report, 1820 children died as a result of abuse and neglect.[4]

Child abuse or maltreatment should be a differential diagnosis when caring for children with burn injury, because about 18% of children who are maltreated sustain physical abuse.[4] Burns account for approximately 5.8% to 8.8% of all abuse cases annually.[14] Most often, burns in children are accidental but are related to failure of the caregiver or parent to provide adequate supervision. However, the developmental age and size of the child are of key importance in ruling out accidental and nonaccidental burn injuries. The patterns of burns—that is, inflicted burns consistent with immersion or dunking or contact—can be diagnostic of child abuse regardless of history.[14] A delay in seeking treatment or isolated scald or contact burns to the hands, feet, genitalia, or buttocks without a clearly defined mechanism should prompt further investigation for nonaccidental trauma.[10]

INITIAL EMERGENCY BURN MANAGEMENT

The goals of acute care of a patient with thermal injuries are to save life, minimize disability, and prepare the patient for definitive care. The burn injury may involve multiple organ systems, and the approach to the injured patient should be expeditious and methodical in identifying problems and establishing priorities of care.

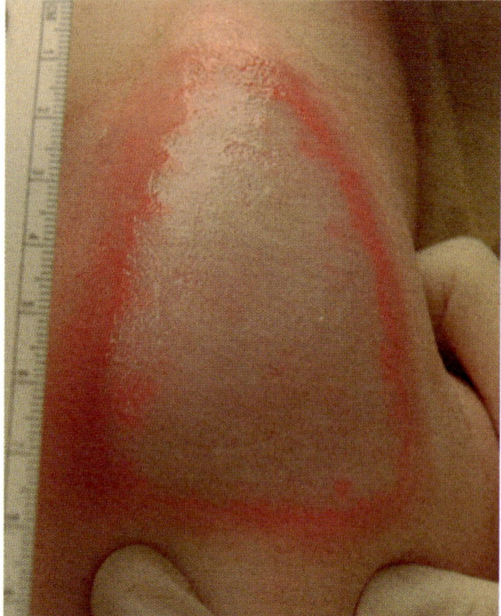

FIG. 34.9 Partial-Thickness Iron Burn to Right Buttock from Nonaccidental Trauma.

The resuscitation phase begins immediately after the burn insult has occurred; therefore, the nurse is concerned with patient management at the scene until admission to an appropriate medical facility. As with any major trauma, the first hour after injury is crucial; however, the first 24 to 36 hours after injury also are important in management of patients with burns. Management during this period has a major effect on the patient's survival and ultimate rehabilitation.

Obtaining a history regarding the nature of the injury is important in management of a patient with burns. Explosion of a water heater, propane gas, or grain elevator and other types of explosions often throw the patient some distance and may result in concomitant orthopedic, neurologic, and internal trauma. If the burns are chemical, it is valuable to know the specific agents involved. It also helps to know what substance was burned or inhaled and how long the patient was exposed to smoke or superheated air. A detailed patient history should include the mechanism of injury, patient's age, location and size of burn, type and amount of fluid already administered, known allergies, status of tetanus immunization, and significant medical history.

All rings, watches, and jewelry are removed from injured limbs to avoid a tourniquet effect when edema occurs as a result of fluid shifts and fluid resuscitation.

Airway Management

The first priority of emergency burn care is to secure and protect the airway. If there is any possibility of underlying cervical instability, cervical precautions must be initiated. In patients with facial burns, exposure to fire in an enclosed space, or both, inhalation injury should be suspected. Carbon monoxide poisoning is associated with high mortality rates. Carboxyhemoglobin (HbCO) levels are obtained, and oxygen therapy is initiated. Patients with HbCO level elevated greater than 10% and arterial partial pressure of oxygen (PaO_2)/fraction of inspired oxygen (FiO_2) ratio less than 200 have a high probability of needing respiratory support.[6] All patients with major burns or suspected inhalation injury are initially administered 100% oxygen. The nurse should continue to observe the patient for clinical manifestations of impaired oxygenation such as tachypnea, agitation, anxiety, and upper airway obstruction (e.g., hoarseness, stridor, wheezing). Early intubation may be lifesaving in a patient who has an inhalation injury, because it may be impossible to perform this procedure later, when edema has obstructed the larynx. The need for frequent blood sampling and the benefit of continuous blood pressure monitoring may necessitate placement of an arterial line.

Respiratory Management

Circumferential, full-thickness burns to the chest wall can lead to restriction of chest wall expansion and decreased compliance. Decreased compliance requires higher ventilatory pressures to provide the patient with adequate tidal volumes. In a patient who has not undergone intubation, clinical manifestations of chest wall restriction include rapid, shallow respirations; poor chest wall excursion; and severe agitation. Arterial blood gas analysis reveals a decrease in oxygen tension and an increasing arterial partial pressure of carbon dioxide ($PaCO_2$) level. Patients receiving mechanical ventilation have increasing peak airway pressure values.

Escharotomies (burn eschar incisions) may be needed immediately to increase compliance and for improved ventilation.[6] These incisions usually are made bilaterally along the anterior axillary lines and are connected by a transverse incision at the costal margin (Fig. 34.10).

Circulatory Management

The extent and depth of the burn are assessed. The extent of TBSA of the burn is calculated for estimation of fluid resuscitation requirements (Table 34.1); the Parkland formula is the most widely used method of calculation.[6] Burn shock is caused by loss of fluid from the vascular compartment into the area of injury resulting in hypovolemia. The larger the percentage of burn area, the greater is the potential for development of shock. Lactated Ringer solution is infused through a large-bore cannula in a peripheral vein.[6] Lactated Ringer solution, an isotonic crystalloid, is the resuscitation fluid used most often. Given in large amounts, it can restore cardiac output to normal in most patients. It is preferred over normal saline because it most closely matches extracellular fluid. Because isotonic salt solutions generate no difference in osmotic pressure between plasma and the interstitial space, the entire extracellular space must be expanded to replace intravascular losses. Diuretics should not be given during the resuscitative phase of burn care.

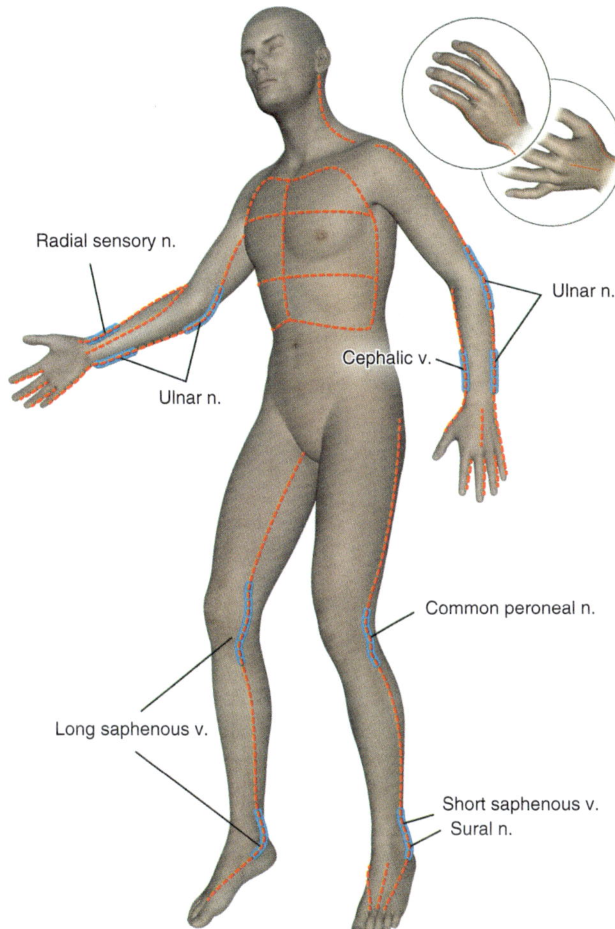

FIG. 34.10 Location of Escharotomy Incisions. (From Walls RM, Hockberger R, Gausche-Hill M, Erickson TB, Wilcox SR, eds. *Rosen's Emergency Medicine Concepts and Clinical Practice.* 10th ed. Elsevier; 2023.)

According to the Parkland formula (see Table 34.1), 50% of the calculated amount of fluid is administered to the patient in the first 8 hours after injury, 25% is given in the second 8 hours, and 25% is given in the third 8 hours. Calculated fluid requirements are guidelines. Fluid resuscitation is a dynamic process. The rate of fluid administration is adjusted according to the individual's response, which is determined by monitoring urine output, heart rate, blood pressure, and level of consciousness. Meticulous attention to the patient's intake and output is imperative to ensure that he or she is appropriately resuscitated. Underresuscitation may result in inadequate cardiac output, leading to inadequate organ perfusion and the potential for wound conversion from a partial-thickness to full-thickness injury.[6] Overresuscitation may lead to moderate to severe pulmonary edema, to excessive wound edema causing a decrease in perfusion of unburned tissue in the distal portions of the extremities, or to edema inhibiting perfusion of the zone of stasis resulting in wound conversion. Fluid requirements may be much higher than estimated by using the Parkland formula. The recommendations for these situations are included later in this chapter. For pediatric patients, dextrose-containing intravenous fluid is added at a maintenance rate along with Parkland resuscitation fluid. Pediatric patients need continuous dextrose infusions for vital organs.

Continuous monitoring with electrocardiograms (ECGs) should be used in patients with serious thermal burn injury and in the presence of electrical burns, inhalation injury, or associated traumatic injury. ECG lead placement may present a challenge with extensive burns, and nontraditional locations on nonburned skin should be selected instead.

TABLE 34.1 Formulas for Fluid Replacement or Resuscitation in First 24 Hours

Fluid and Dose Rate	ABA Consensus	Parkland	Modified Brooke	Brooke	Hypertonic
Electrolyte solution	Ringer lactate	Ringer lactate	Ringer lactate	Ringer lactate	Hypertonic lactated saline (sodium, 250 mEq/L)
Dose: mL/kg/% burned[a]	2–4 50% of fluid over first 8 hr; 50% of fluid over next 16 hr	4	2	1.5	Rate based on urine output of 30–50 mL/h

Examples using ABA consensus formula: An 85-kg patient with 35% TBSA burn

2 mL × 85 kg × 35% = 5950 mL in first 24 h	3 mL × 85 kg × 35% = 8925 mL in first 24 h	4 mL × 85 kg × 35% = 11,900 mL in first 24 h
2975 mL in first 8 h = 372 mL/h	4462 mL in first 8 h = 558 mL/h	5950 mL in first 8 h = 744 mL/h
2975 mL in next 16 h = 186 mL/h	4462 mL in next 16 h = 279 mL/h	5950 mL in next 16 h = 372 mL/h

ABA, American Burn Association; *TBSA*, total body surface area.
[a]Adjust these rates to maintain urine output >30 mL/h in adults or 1 mL/kg/h in children.

Pathophysiology of Burn Shock

Burn injuries greater than 20% of TBSA can result in burn shock.[6] *Shock* is defined as inadequate cellular perfusion. Significant burn injury results in hypovolemic shock and tissue trauma. Both cause the production and release of several local and systemic mediators. Burn shock can occur even when hypovolemia is corrected.

The first component of burn shock is hypovolemic shock. At the cellular level, the burning agent produces dilation of the capillaries and small vessels, increasing the capillary permeability. Plasma seeps out into the surrounding tissue, producing blisters and edema. The type, duration, and intensity of the burn all affect the amount and extent of fluid loss. This progressive fluid loss in extensive burns results in significant intravascular fluid volume deficit. Edema occurs locally in the burn wound and systemically in unburned tissues. Edema formation is unique to thermal injury.

Burn edema has been attributed to several factors. Barrier property changes of the capillary wall occur by direct injury and indirect mediator-modulated changes. Increases in permeability of protein and water occur, resulting in edema. In most forms of shock, capillary pressure decreases as a result of arteriolar vasoconstriction. However, an increase in capillary pressure has been found in burned tissue in the first minutes to hours after burn injury, causing capillary leak for the first 24 hours. Coupled with this increase in capillary pressure is a negative interstitial hydrostatic pressure that occurs in the dermis layer of burned skin after thermal injury. This negative interstitial hydrostatic pressure represents an edema-generating mechanism that occurs for approximately 2 hours after injury. Plasma colloid osmotic pressure is decreased as a result of protein leakage into the extravascular space. Plasma is then further diluted with fluid resuscitation. The osmotic pressure is decreased, and further fluid extravasation can occur.

In addition to leaking capillaries, local and systemic mediators cause edema and the cardiovascular problems seen in patients with burns. These mediators include histamine, prostaglandins, kinins, and oxygen radicals, and they increase arteriolar vasodilation. Manipulation of these mediators to stop the cascade of burn edema and burn shock is being researched.

The intravascular fluid changes combined with the action of inflammatory mediators and vasoconstriction mediators result in hemodynamic consequences in patients with burns. The hemodynamic alterations include decreased myocardial contractility and cardiac output despite adequate volume resuscitation, increased systemic vascular resistance, and increased pulmonary vascular resistance. Increased pulmonary vascular resistance can lead to pulmonary edema. Large but judicious volumes of resuscitation fluids are required to maintain the vascular volume during the first few hours after a large burn injury to provide optimal resuscitation. Early and full fluid resuscitation can prevent the complications of acute kidney injury (AKI), cardiovascular collapse, and death from shock. However, overresuscitation increases edema formation, which can further impair tissue oxygen diffusion. The nurse must assess the patient's fluid status and response to resuscitation to obtain the optimal response.

Kidney Management

If fluid resuscitation is inadequate, AKI may occur. In the emergency department, an indwelling urinary catheter should be placed for burns greater than 20% of TBSA to monitor urine output and the effectiveness of fluid resuscitation.[6] A catheter may be necessary if the burn extends into the perineal area because of the presence or development of edema. Urinary catheters with temperature probes should be used whenever possible. The nurse measures urine output hourly. Adequate urine output for adults is 0.5 to 1 mL/kg/h, or 30 to 50 mL/h; in children, it is 1 to 2 mL/kg/h.[6]

Gastrointestinal System Management

Patients with burns of greater than 20% of TBSA are prone to gastric dilation as a result of paralytic ileus. Nasogastric or orogastric tubes are placed in these patients to prevent abdominal distention, emesis, and potential aspiration. This decrease in gastrointestinal (GI) function is caused by the effects of hypovolemia and the neurologic and endocrine response to injury. GI activity usually returns in 24 to 48 hours. Prophylaxis with histamine blockers or sucralfate is initiated because patients with burns are prone to ileus. These acute ulcerations of the duodenum are caused by sloughing of the gastric mucosa resulting from loss of plasma volume after severe burns. Enteral nutrition has been shown to be protective of gastric mucosal integrity and to improve intestinal flow, gastric motility, and intestinal blood flow in patients with burns.[15] Enteral nutrition should be started as soon as possible. Patients with severe burns can be safely fed in the duodenum or jejunum within 6 hours of burn injury.[15] Enteral feeds should be promptly initiated for patients with burns via nasoduodenal or nasojejunal tube.

Extremity Pulse Assessment

Edema formation may cause neurovascular compromise to the extremities; frequent assessments are necessary to evaluate pulses, skin color, capillary refill, and sensation. Arterial circulation is at greatest risk with circumferential burns. If not corrected, reduced arterial flow causes ischemia and necrosis. The Doppler flow probe is one of the best ways to evaluate arterial pulses. An escharotomy may be required to restore arterial circulation and to allow for further swelling. The escharotomy can be performed at the bedside with a sterile field and scalpel. Care must be taken to avoid major nerves, vessels, and tendons. The incision extends through the length of the eschar, over joints, and down to the subcutaneous fat. The incision is placed laterally or medially on the extremity. If a single incision does not restore circulation, bilateral incisions are required (see Fig. 34.8). If escharotomy is required before the patient is transferred to a burn center, consultation with the receiving physician is advised.

Laboratory Assessment

Initial laboratory studies include complete blood count, electrolytes, blood urea nitrogen (BUN), creatinine, urinalysis, glucose, and blood screening. Special situations such as inhalation injury warrant arterial blood gas measurements, HbCO level determination, cultures, alcohol and drug screens, and cyanide levels. A baseline assessment of nutrition status, including albumin and prealbumin, is helpful in monitoring future nutrition needs. Also, creatinine kinase, urinalysis, and urine myoglobin are good indicators of rhabdomyolysis seen in the setting of electrical burn injuries.[6] An ECG is obtained for all patients with electrical burns or preexisting heart disease. Serum lactate is also another good inflammatory marker indicating burn severity.[6]

Wound Care

In the emergent phase, topical antimicrobial therapy is not a priority. However, the wounds must be covered with clean, dry dressings or sheets. All restrictive jewelry or clothing should be removed. Every attempt must be made to keep the patient warm because of the high risk of hypothermia. The administration of tetanus prophylaxis is recommended for all burns covering more than 10% of the TBSA and for patients with an unknown immunization history.

Burn Center Referral

After initial treatment and stabilization at an emergency department, referral to a burn center is considered (see Box 34.1). A burn center must be able to deliver all therapy required including rehabilitation and must perform personnel training and burn research. Patients meeting the criteria for referral need the expertise of an interprofessional team. Referring hospitals must always contact the burn center in their region.[16] Providers in the field should cover the burns with clean, dry cloths until arrival at the burn center. Early communication between the initial provider and the burn center is encouraged.[16]

Special Management Considerations

Inhalation Injury

Inhalation injury can occur in the presence or absence of cutaneous injury. Inhalation injuries are strongly associated with burns sustained in a closed or confined space, and they are associated with increased mortality.[6] Inhalation injury can occur in three basic forms, alone or in combination: carbon monoxide poisoning, direct heat injury, and chemical damage. The three types of inhalation injury are carbon monoxide poisoning, upper airway injury, and lower airway injury.

Immediate lifesaving measures in patients with burns include management of the airway. The patient with burns may exhibit few or no signs of airway distress; however, thermal injury to the airway must be anticipated if facial burns, singed eyebrows and nasal hair, carbon deposits in the oropharynx, and carbonaceous sputum are present or if the history suggests confinement in a burning environment. Any of these findings indicates acute inhalation injury and requires immediate and definitive care. To prevent the necessity of tracheostomy or cricothyrotomy, the use of early intubation and respiratory support must be considered before tracheal edema occurs. Inhalation injury increases the patient's risk of developing pneumonia and acute respiratory distress syndrome (ARDS).[6] Management of ARDS necessitates mechanical ventilatory support and, in extreme cases, high-frequency oscillatory ventilation or extracorporeal membrane oxygenation. The occurrence of inhalation injury with cutaneous burns increases the fluid requirements during resuscitation to a higher level than would be predicted by the cutaneous burn alone.

Carbon monoxide poisoning. Carbon monoxide poisoning is the leading cause of death in persons found dead at the scene of a fire who have few or no cutaneous thermal injuries. Carbon monoxide is a colorless, odorless, and tasteless gas. Inhalation of carbon monoxide, a byproduct of the incomplete combustion of carbon, results in its bonding to available hemoglobin, producing HbCO, which effectively decreases oxygen saturation of hemoglobin. The affinity of hemoglobin molecules for carbon monoxide is approximately 200 to 250 times greater than that for oxygen.[15] HbCO binds poorly with oxygen, reducing the oxygen-carrying capacity of blood and causing hypoxemia. The shortage of oxygen at the tissue level is worsened by a shift to the left of the oxyhemoglobin dissociation curve, reflecting the fact that the oxygen in the hemoglobin is not readily given up to the cells.

Measurement of arterial oxygen saturation is of limited value, because oxygen saturation may be quite high despite dangerously low levels of oxygen content. Because the pulse oximeter cannot distinguish between oxyhemoglobin and HbCO, it is an unreliable predictor of tissue oxygenation during the initial stages of carbon monoxide poisoning.[15] Arterial blood gases and oxygen saturation are used to accurately assess the hemoglobin oxygen saturation level. A serum HbCO level should be obtained at presentation. Normal HbCO levels are less than 2%. HbCO levels of 40% to 60% often produce unresponsiveness; levels of 15% to 40% may result in various degrees of central nervous system dysfunction. Levels of 10% to 15%, which can be found in cigarette smokers, rarely produce serious symptoms but may cause a headache.

The major clinical manifestations of severe carbon monoxide poisoning are related to the central nervous system and the heart. Symptoms associated with carbon monoxide poisoning include headache, dizziness, nausea, vomiting, dyspnea, and confusion.[15] In severe cases, carbon monoxide poisoning may lead to myocardial ischemia, cardiac dysfunction, and central nervous system complications caused by reduced oxygen delivery and the already compromised circulatory system. Early signs of carbon monoxide poisoning may include tachycardia, tachypnea, confusion, and lightheadedness. As the carbon monoxide level rises, patients exhibit a decreased level of responsiveness, which may progress to unresponsiveness and respiratory failure.

The treatment of choice for carbon monoxide poisoning is high-flow oxygen administered at 100% through a tight-fitting nonrebreathing mask or endotracheal intubation. The half-life of carbon monoxide in the body is 5 hours at room air (21% oxygen), 2 hours at 40% oxygen, and 40 to 60 minutes at 100% oxygen.[15] The half-life of carbon monoxide is 30 minutes in a hyperbaric oxygen chamber at three times atmospheric pressure. The use of hyperbaric oxygen in the care of patients with burns is controversial, because wheezing and airway debris is a contraindication to hyperbaric chamber use.[17] Because of the rapid removal of carbon monoxide with the administration of 100% oxygen, the time required to transport a patient who has received oxygen in the field should always be considered to prevent possible underestimation of inhalation injury.

Upper airway injury. Burns of the upper respiratory tract include burns involving the pharynx, larynx, glottis, trachea, and larger bronchi. Injuries are caused by direct heat or by chemical inflammation and necrosis. Respiratory injury is most often confined to the upper airway. The heat exchange capability is so efficient that most heat absorption and damage occur in the pharynx and larynx above the vocal cords.

Heat damage may be severe enough to cause upper airway obstruction at any time, beginning from the moment of injury through the resuscitation period. Caution is needed for patients with severe hypovolemia, because supraglottic edema may be delayed until fluid resuscitation is underway and third spacing occurs.[17] Patients must be monitored for hoarseness, stridor, audible airflow turbulence, and the production of carbonaceous sputum. Maximal edema occurs 24 hours after injury with upper airway injuries, and these patients should be observed in the critical care unit for a minimum of 24 hours.

The prediction of an upper airway obstruction is based on consideration of several variables: extent of injury to the face and neck, presence of blisters on or redness of the posterior pharynx, signs of singed nasal hair, increased HbCO levels, increased rate and decreased depth of breathing, hoarseness and stridor (which indicates a significant decrease in the diameter of the airway), increased amount of sputum, and circumstances of the burn event (whether it occurred in an enclosed space or involved superheated gases or steam).[17] Steam has a heat-carrying capacity many times that of dry air, and it is capable of overwhelming the extremely efficient heat-dissipating capabilities of the upper airway.

Intubation is recommended whenever airway patency is questionable, rather than delaying intubation until airway obstruction is so severe that intubation becomes a challenge. After the airway is secure, priority is given to minimizing airway edema, maintaining pulmonary hygiene, and treating bronchospasm. Elevating the head of the bed to 30 degrees or higher decreases airway edema. Therapeutic deep breathing and coughing, early mobility, suctioning, and bronchodilators assist in mobilizing and removing secretions. Fiberoptic bronchoscopy may be required to remove secretions in some patients. Mechanical ventilatory support is necessary when respiratory fatigue or failure occurs. Precautions to prevent ventilator-associated pneumonia should be implemented to avoid secondary infection.

Lower airway injury. Heated air rarely causes lower airway injury. If it does, it usually is associated with a higher mortality rate. Lower airway injuries are typically caused by chemical damage to mucosal surfaces. Tracheobronchitis with severe spasm and wheezing may occur in the first minutes to hours after injury. The onset of symptoms is unpredictable after smoke inhalation, and patients at risk must be closely monitored for at least 24 to 48 hours after injury.

Historically, the most accurate method of documenting lower airway injury is the ventilation-perfusion lung scan; however, the study is cumbersome and rarely used. Prolonged retention or symmetry of washout of the radioisotope indicates pulmonary parenchymal injury on the side of the retained emissions. Plain chest radiography and computed tomography (CT) scan are faster and more readily available and can also evaluate lower airway injury.[17]

Patients with inhalation injuries are at risk for developing pneumonia and ARDS. Ventilator management strategies for hypoxia and ARDS in patients with burns can be challenging. Lung protective ventilation with low tidal volumes, higher levels of positive end-expiratory pressure, and permissive hypercarbia have shown optimal outcomes and minimized ventilator-induced lung injury.[17] Nebulized heparin has been shown to increase clearance of airway debris and improve patient outcomes.[18] Treatment of lower airway injury is largely symptomatic. As with upper airway injury management, aggressive pulmonary hygiene, removal of secretions, ventilatory support, and careful fluid resuscitation so as to avoid exacerbating pulmonary edema and ARDS are indicated when caring for patients with burns and lower airway inhalation injuries.

Nonthermal Burns

Chemical burns. Chemical burns can be caused by a variety of products. Acids, alkalis, and organic and inorganic compounds cause chemical burns. The acid or base quality determines the injurious nature of a product. The injury is caused by the pH of the product or by the concentration of the product. In the past, irrigation with neutralizing solutions was recommended to limit the extent and depth of chemical burns. This practice is no longer advocated, because neutralizing agents may cause reactions that are exothermic (produce heat), increasing the extent and depth of the burn. It also is possible that the neutralizing agent is neither immediately known nor available. Instead, large amounts of water should be used to flush the area. Clothing and shoes should be removed if they have been in contact with the chemical. Alkali burns of the eyes require continuous irrigation for many hours after the injury. Removal of contact lenses is necessary before irrigation. Litmus paper may be used to assess for neutrality or if further irrigation is needed.[6]

Treatments for chemical burns vary. Phenol burns are first diluted, and then the skin is wiped quickly with polyethylene glycol or vegetable oil to decrease the severity of the burn. Areas exposed to hydrofluoric acid must be copiously irrigated with water; the burned area then can be treated with 2.5% calcium gluconate gel. The patient may need calcium gluconate supplements because the fluoride ion precipitates serum calcium, causing hypocalcemia. White phosphorus can ignite if kept dry, and these wounds must be covered with a moist dressing. After a tar or asphalt injury, the removal of tar or asphalt is best accomplished with the use of petroleum-containing distillates. The solution can be placed directly on the wound and gently wiped off. Routine debridement of loose skin should be initiated after tar removal.

Electrical burns. In electrical burns, the type and voltage of the circuit, resistance, pathway of transmission through the body, and duration of contact are considered in determining the amount of damage sustained. In these situations, the rescuer also may be injured if he or she becomes part of the electrical circuit. The rescuer must disconnect the electrical source to break the circuit or must know how to avoid becoming part of the circuit. The use of appropriately insulated equipment that diverts the circuit elsewhere is essential. Extreme caution must be used in the rescue of victims.

Electricity always travels toward the ground. The body conducts electrical current as a whole, as opposed to the earlier belief that it traveled most quickly through the nerves and circulatory system. Electrical burns are caused by the thermal conversion of electricity into heat within the tissues, which can cause the skin to only be minimally affected; however, there may be extensive damage to the underlying tissues.[6]

The electrical burn process can result in a profound alteration in acid–base balance and rhabdomyolysis, resulting in myoglobinuria, which poses a serious threat to kidney function. Myoglobin is a normal constituent of muscle. With extensive muscle destruction, it is released into the circulatory system and filtered by the kidneys. It can be highly toxic and can lead to AKI. Fluid resuscitation for a patient with an electrical burn does not correlate with the Parkland formula, and the fluid is adjusted according to the patient's urine output. If myoglobin is present in the urine, a urine output of at least 1 mL/kg/h must be established until the urine is clear of all myoglobin pigment.[19]

If hemoglobinuria is identified, the clinician should assume that the patient has myoglobinuria and acidosis. Sodium bicarbonate may be administered to bring the pH level into the normal range, to correct a documented acidosis, or to alkalize urine to promote myoglobin excretion. Diuretics such as mannitol also may be administered to increase renal blood flow and glomerular filtration rate to facilitate myoglobin clearance.[19] Sodium bicarbonate infusions and diuretic therapy are called *forced alkaline diuresis*. A baseline ECG and myocardial biomarker levels should be obtained while the patient is in the emergency department. The following criteria are used for monitoring the cardiac status of patients with burns:

- A history of loss of consciousness or cardiac arrest
- Documentation of cardiac dysrhythmia at the scene of the accident or in the emergency department
- Abnormal ECG findings on admission
- TBSA burns of greater than 20%
- Very young age or advanced age
- Prior history of heart disease

Other patients with burns may be admitted to nonmonitored settings and observed closely. Cardiac dysrhythmias must be treated promptly, and a protocol to rule out myocardial infarction must be followed.

BURN NURSING MANAGEMENT

The clinical course of a burn injury has three phases: (1) resuscitative, (2) acute care, and (3) rehabilitative. Each phase has a unique set of actual and potential problems. The resuscitative phase begins with initial hemodynamic response to the injury and lasts until capillary integrity is restored and the repletion of plasma volume by fluid replacement occurs. Spontaneous diuresis demonstrates that capillaries have regained their integrity. The acute phase begins with the onset of diuresis of fluid mobilized from the interstitial space and ends with the closure of the burn wound. The major focus of the acute phase is wound healing, wound closure, and prevention of infection. The rehabilitative phase begins when the patient is admitted to the hospital, with correction of functional deficits and scar management being major considerations. The rehabilitative phase may last months to years, depending on the severity of injury. Psychosocial support of the patient and the family should continue in this phase.

Resuscitation Phase

Life-threatening airway and breathing problems, cardiopulmonary instability, and hypovolemia characterize the resuscitation phase, or shock phase. Burn injury affects the structure and function of almost every organ.[20] The magnitude of this pathophysiologic response is proportional to the extent of cutaneous injury. The goal of the resuscitation phase is to maintain vital organ function and perfusion. Emergent interventions for inhalation injury, airway management, and hypovolemia are concurrently addressed.

Oxygenation Alterations

Early diagnosis of inhalation injury is essential to minimize complications and to decrease the mortality rate. Three oxygenation complications are associated with smoke inhalation during the resuscitation phase: (1) carbon monoxide poisoning, (2) upper airway obstruction, and (3) chemical pneumonitis. Evaluation of a patient for inhalation injury includes physical assessment (e.g., singed facial hairs, mucosal burns of nose or mouth, carbonaceous sputum), arterial blood gas analysis, HbCO levels, chest radiography, flexible fiberoptic bronchoscopy, ventilation-perfusion lung scan, and pulmonary function tests.[17] Critical care nursing management includes the following:

- Assess breath sounds and the rate and quality of respirations.
- Administer oxygen, as prescribed.
- Monitor HbCO levels.
- Elevate the head of the bed and implement ventilator-associated pneumonia precautions.
- Assess and assist with pulmonary secretion suctioning.
- Observe for signs of airway obstruction (e.g., increased respiratory rate and heart rate, increased work of breathing, use of accessory muscles, stridor, wheezing, hoarseness, and crackles).
- Prepare for endotracheal intubation and mechanical ventilation.
- Maintain accurate and timely documentation.

Impaired gas exchange. The most common pulmonary burn complication is carbon monoxide poisoning. High-flow oxygen should be administered at 100% through a nonrebreathing mask or endotracheal intubation until the HbCO level is less than 10% to 15%.

Chemical pneumonitis is caused by inhalation of the byproducts of combustion of substances such as cotton, aldehydes, oxides of sulfur, and nitrogen. Burning polyvinyl chloride yields at least 75 potentially toxic compounds, including hydrochloric acid and carbon monoxide. Within days after a burn, ARDS commonly develops in patients with chemical pneumonitis. The primary clinical manifestation of ARDS is hypoxemia that is refractory to oxygen therapy. Early signs include increased pH, decreased $PaCO_2$, and increased respiratory rate. Ventilatory support with the use of positive end-expiratory pressure is the treatment of choice.

Ineffective airway clearance. Laryngeal swelling and upper airway obstruction may occur at any time during the first 24 hours after a burn injury. Endotracheal intubation must be accomplished early, because this simple procedure can become extremely difficult in the presence of laryngeal edema.[15] Enough time is usually available to intervene after obtaining the history and transporting the patient to the primary hospital. Consequent edema may not manifest for up to 48 hours after the burn incident. A patient who has not initially undergone intubation must be carefully monitored during this critical period. When prolonged ventilatory failure is expected as a result of severe inhalation, a tracheostomy is performed.

Extubation is done only after ensuring pulmonary edema has resolved and if the patient can meet extubation criteria: level of consciousness assessed as *awake*, intact cough and gag reflexes, inspiratory effort greater than −25 cm H_2O in adults, vital capacity of 10 mL/kg, and decreased volume and tenacity of sputum.[17] Resolution of airway edema can be assessed by deflating the endotracheal cuff and observing the patient's ability to breathe around the endotracheal tube.

Although uncommon, laryngospasm must be addressed. Laryngospasm usually is brought on by airway irritation from inhalation of noxious agents.

Fluid Resuscitation

Current resuscitation protocols emphasize fluid delivery rates based on the extent of burn injury and the patient's weight. The patient's weight measured in kilograms must be obtained on admission to the hospital. The extent of the burn is calculated by using one of the methods previously described. Several formulas are available to guide fluid resuscitation and should be used to assist in the management of fluid replacement (see

Table 34.1). The formulas differ primarily in terms of administration, volume, and sodium content. The actual amount of fluid given to any patient must be based on that individual's response. The goal of fluid resuscitation is to maintain end organ perfusion and avoid fluid overload.[21]

The type of fluid used in resuscitation and at what point a switch should be made to a colloid solution are controversial topics. No clear-cut guidelines for resuscitation exist. The administration of crystalloid fluid (e.g., lactated Ringer solution) for the first 24 to 36 hours after the burn is the most common practice.[22] Lactated Ringer solution is the crystalloid solution of choice because of its physiologic similarity to the composition of extracellular fluid. The addition of lactated Ringer solution with 5% dextrose should be considered as maintenance fluid, especially in the first 24 hours. Assessment for secondary injuries that would affect the choice of fluid should be performed. Ideally, the capillary leak seals approximately 24 hours after the injury, making it possible to give colloid without leakage of protein into the interstitium. Colloid deficits can be considered for replacement in the next 24 hours with albumin. Colloid replacement can increase circulating volume and decrease fluid needs.[21] In addition to colloid, maintenance fluids are given to replace evaporative losses, and the amount is adjusted according to the patient's serum electrolyte levels, urine output, weight, volume status, and clinical assessment.

Deficient fluid volume. Physiologic effects of the burn complicate the tissue damage that occurs after the burn insult. Coagulation factors are affected, protein is denatured, and cellular content is ionized. These factors, coupled with dilation of capillaries and small vessels, lead to increased capillary permeability and fluid shifts from the intravascular space to the interstitial space. The lymphatic system, which normally carries away the increased interstitial fluid, may be damaged or overloaded and unable to function to its normal capacity.

In addition to the protein and electrolyte shift, an increased insensible water loss occurs. In a healthy adult, this loss is estimated to be 35 to 50 mL/h. Insensible water loss in a patient with burns may be 300 to 3000 mL/day. This increase may be related to temperature elevation, tracheostomy, and the size of the burn.

Burn shock is proportional to the extent and depth of injury. The loss of plasma begins almost immediately after the injury and reaches its peak within the first 48 hours. Desired clinical responses to fluid resuscitation include urinary output of 0.5 to 1 mL/kg per hour, heart rate less than 120 beats/min, blood pressure in the normal to high range, mean arterial pressure greater or equal to 65 mm Hg, normal lactate, clear lung sounds, clear sensorium, and absence of intestinal events such as nausea and paralytic ileus.[23] Heart rate, blood pressure, and central venous pressure values are not always accurate or reliable predictors of successful fluid resuscitation.

Electrolytes should be monitored frequently during resuscitation. Hyperkalemia can occur during this phase because of (1) the release of potassium from damaged cells; (2) metabolic acidosis; and (3) impaired kidney function caused by hemoglobinuria, myoglobinuria, or decreased renal perfusion. The patient must be assessed for clinical manifestations of hyperkalemia. Treatment includes correction of acidosis. During the resuscitation phase, using cation-exchange resins or intravenously administered insulin and hypertonic dextrose to transport potassium back into the cell is not recommended because of the unpredictable nature of fluid shifts that occur.

Hypokalemia can occur during the resuscitation phase because of the massive loss of fluids and electrolytes through the burn wounds or because of hemodilution. During the acute phase, it may be related to hemodilution; inadequate replacement; loss associated with diuresis, diarrhea, vomiting, nasogastric drainage, and long hydrotherapy sessions; or the shift of potassium from the intravascular space to the cell after the acidosis has been corrected. Nursing interventions include treating nausea and vomiting, limiting immersive hydrotherapy sessions to less than 30 minutes, preventing fluid volume excess, and judicious replacement of potassium.

Hyponatremia is common during the resuscitation phase because of the loss of sodium through the burn wound, the shift of fluid into the interstitial space, vomiting, nasogastric drainage, diarrhea, and the use of hypotonic salt solutions during the early phase of resuscitation. During this phase, it may be necessary to monitor serum sodium levels every 4 to 8 hours. Hyponatremia also may occur during the acute phase because of hemodilution and loss through the wound, lengthy hydrotherapy sessions, and excessive diuresis resulting from the fluid shift back into the intravascular space. Interventions are followed for treating nausea and vomiting, hydrotherapy sessions are limited, and intravenous replacement of sodium is considered. During diuresis, which occurs during the acute phase, restricting free water intake usually is the only required intervention to increase the serum sodium level.

Tissue Perfusion

Ineffective kidney tissue perfusion. Urinalysis to determine the myoglobin level may be performed soon after burn injury. Myoglobinuria can be detected grossly by the dark, port-wine color of the urine. Myoglobin is extremely toxic to the kidneys and can cause massive tubular destruction. It is best treated with rapid fluid administration and forced diuresis with diuretics such as mannitol, an osmotic diuretic.[19] The goal is an hourly urine output that is at least double the general recommendations to flush the kidney tubules. All other diuretics are avoided because they would deplete the already compromised intravascular volume. Sodium bicarbonate is sometimes given intravenously to alkalinize the urine and assist in the elimination of heme pigments.[19]

Maintaining and monitoring the renal system is vital in management of patients with burns. Impairment of the renal system may be related to hemoglobinuria, myoglobinuria, hypoperfusion, and hypovolemia. Urinary output must be monitored every hour for the first 48 to 72 hours, and specific gravity values can be used to determine the adequacy of hydration status and renal competency. The urine glucose concentration is monitored, as are urine sodium, creatinine, and BUN levels. Use of an indwelling urinary catheter is appropriate for the first 48 to 72 hours. Because of the tremendous risk of infection related to indwelling catheters, they are removed as soon as possible. However, leaving the catheter in place may be necessary if perineal burns are involved. Oliguria may be associated with AKI but is usually related to inadequate fluid resuscitation in patients with burns. More commonly, AKI occurs early during resuscitation or late secondary to sepsis.[18] Other signs of kidney failure include increasing creatinine, BUN, phosphorus, and potassium levels; excessive fluid-weight gain; excessive edema; elevated blood pressure; lethargy; and confusion.

The presence of glucose in the urine causes osmotic diuresis. In this clinical situation, urine output is an unreliable estimate of volume status. Because of the increased loss of fluid through the kidneys, glucosuria may suggest the need for additional fluid beyond the original estimates.

Ineffective cerebral tissue perfusion. The patient's neurologic status is assessed frequently during the first few days. Changes may be related to an associated head injury that occurred at the time of burn injury, hypoperfusion related to hypovolemia, hypoxemia associated with inadequate ventilation, carbon monoxide poisoning, or electrolyte imbalances. Patients with electrical burns or major thermal burns may have peripheral neurologic injuries, which may not become evident for several days after the injury. The neurologic assessment includes use of the Glasgow Coma Scale. It is not unusual for the patient to be agitated, restless, and extremely anxious during the resuscitation phase of burn injury as a result of hypovolemia, pain, and fear of disfigurement or death. However, the possibility of neurologic involvement must not be overlooked. Maintaining an adequate mean arterial pressure is essential to ensure adequate cerebral perfusion pressure.

Ineffective peripheral tissue perfusion. Ineffective peripheral tissue perfusion results from third spacing of fluid during the resuscitation phase, which restricts blood flow to extremities.[21] As hypovolemia ensues, vasoconstriction increases, which can be potentiated by the loss of body temperature. Peripheral tissue perfusion must be monitored carefully in all patients with burns. Burned as well as unburned areas are carefully assessed for warmth, color, and peripheral pulses. Capillary refill time should be less than 2 seconds in unburned areas. Any clinical manifestation of diminished systemic tissue perfusion must be reported immediately. Nursing actions are taken to minimize any compromise of peripheral circulation. Close monitoring of appropriate fluid resuscitation and careful positioning of the patient are necessary to prevent compromised blood flow. Crossed legs, dependent positions, and pillows under the patient's knees should be avoided. Specialty mattresses and beds may be helpful to prevent secondary skin breakdown and assist with positioning and pulmonary hygiene. The limbs should be elevated above the heart to decrease peripheral edema and enhance venous return. Assisted range-of-motion exercises can help decrease edema.

Monitoring the peripheral circulation is crucial in a patient with circumferential, full-thickness burns on the extremities. The resulting edema may severely compromise the venous system and then the arterial system. Neurovascular integrity of extremities with circumferential burns must be assessed every hour for the first 24 to 48 hours using the six *Ps*: *pulselessness, pallor, pain, paresthesia, paralysis*, and *poikilothermy*. Careful, ongoing assessment is necessary, especially for patients who are intubated and may be unable to communicate pain or paresthesia. The use of a Doppler flowmeter may be necessary. Loss of pulses is a late sign of compromised vascular flow. If any changes are observed, the provider must be notified immediately. Numbness and paresthesia may occur only 30 minutes before loss of pulses. Irreversible nerve ischemia resulting in loss of function may begin after 12 to 24 hours. An escharotomy may become necessary to allow the underlying tissue to expand. In deeper wounds, a fasciotomy, which involves incision into the fascia, may be necessary.

Ineffective gastrointestinal tissue perfusion. Paralytic ileus is a common GI complication that can occur during resuscitation or when sepsis develops, because blood flow can decrease up to 60%. An abdominal examination should be performed every 2 hours during the initial phase and every 4 hours thereafter. If clinical manifestations of a paralytic ileus occur, oral intake is withheld, and a nasogastric tube may be inserted and placed on low suction. Paralytic ileus can be related to hypokalemia, the sympathetic response to severe trauma, or decreased tissue perfusion related to hypovolemia. In large burns (>60% TBSA) or circumferential abdominal burns, the abdominal examination should include careful evaluation for abdominal compartment syndrome.

A stress ulcer may develop as a result of decreased tissue perfusion to the GI tract, a change in the quantity or quality of mucus (which has a pH of 1), or an increase in gastric acid secretion resulting from the stress response. Gastric acid should be maintained above a pH of 5 through the administration of antacids, histamine blockers, or proton-pump inhibitors to prevent the development of these ulcers. The patient should be carefully monitored for GI bleeding. All stools and gastric content should be monitored for blood. The patient should be observed for epigastric discomfort or fullness, decreased blood pressure, or increased pulse.

Other Considerations in the Resuscitation Phase

Hypothermia. Maintenance of thermoregulation is a nursing challenge. A patient with extensive burn injury is at high risk for hypothermia. Hypothermia is especially problematic during initial treatment, during hydrotherapy, during dressing changes, and immediately after surgery. Heat is lost through open burn wounds by means of evaporation and radiation. The patient's core temperature should be maintained between 37.6° C (99.6° F) and 38.3° C (101° F).

Risk for infection. Preventing infection in patients with burns is challenging and involves complex decision-making. Considerable debate has been ongoing about the infection control precautions to use with patients with burns. The burn wound is the most common source of infection in the patient with burns. The loss of the protective mechanism of the skin and contamination from the patient's own bacterial flora can lead to bloodstream infections. Diagnosis of burn sepsis is based on evaluation of both clinical examination and laboratory findings. Some centers advocate routine wound surveillance cultures and wound biopsy to identify infection early. Frequent wound inspection is needed to assess for changes in appearance such as an increase in exudate, odor, or color to minimize the risk of bacteremia. Patients should not be treated with antibiotics prophylactically; rather, treatment should be based on clinical examination and laboratory findings.[23]

Cross-contamination by direct contact is a significant source of infection and a subsequent cause of sepsis. Effective handwashing technique cannot be overemphasized. Nurses must wash their hands and change gloves when moving from area to area on the same patient. For example, after changing the chest dressing, which may be contaminated with sputum from the tracheostomy, hands must be washed and gloves changed before the nurse moves to the legs. Gowns, gloves, and masks should be worn whenever contact with body fluids occurs. These garments also must be changed and hands washed before caring for a different patient. Maintaining patient-specific dressings and topical agents is recommended. Equipment such as thermometers, intravenous pumps, and stethoscopes should be designated for each patient or, when shared, should be cleaned with appropriate bactericidal cleansers between patients.

Whichever precautions are used, everyone coming in contact with the patient, including the patient's family and visitors, must be knowledgeable about the standard for infection control. These precautions should be strictly followed by all.

Invasive monitoring. The decision to use invasive monitoring techniques requires careful consideration of the potential risk factors, and how the collected data will influence the course of treatment. Invasive monitoring should be considered if treatment seems ineffective or if complicating factors such as severe respiratory involvement, major life-threatening injuries, head injuries, or pneumothorax occur. Patients with preexisting medical conditions such as chronic obstructive pulmonary disease, acute heart failure, and kidney failure also may require invasive monitoring.

Invasive monitoring includes direct measurement of central venous pressure, pulmonary artery pressure, arterial pressure, core temperature, cardiac output, systemic vascular resistance, and pulmonary vascular resistance. The use of an arterial line is considered if serial and frequent arterial blood gas values are required for respiratory management or for hemodynamic instability requiring the titration of vasoactive medications. Central venous catheters can be helpful in the early stages of fluid resuscitation to deliver the massive volume of fluids required. The provider selects the catheter insertion site based on burn location and the purpose of the catheter. It is preferable not to insert catheters through burned skin. It may be appropriate to use a multilumen catheter that can serve as a route for fluid resuscitation, maintenance fluids, antibiotic therapy, and vasoactive medications. The risks involved include the increased chance of infection, potential for pneumothorax, and difficulty with insertion if hypovolemia is present.

Pulmonary artery catheters are placed only when necessary for optimal care. They may be essential to the survival of a septic patient despite the risks involved. Pulmonary artery catheters can provide data about pulmonary artery occlusion pressure, cardiac output, stroke volume, systemic vascular resistance and pulmonary vascular resistance, core temperature, and mixed venous oxygen saturation levels.

Centrally placed intravascular catheters require meticulous care. Strict guidelines should be established and monitored. Catheters are inserted under sterile conditions, and the dressings are changed under the same conditions. Because infection is such a major concern, all invasive catheters should be removed as early as possible.

Laboratory assessment. Laboratory assessment is another important aspect of burn care. Because of the invasive nature of drawing blood, it is done only if absolutely indicated. Consideration should be given to the age of the patient, the size of the burn, the time since injury, and any underlying disease process. White blood cell counts usually are monitored for elevation, a sign of sepsis. However, it is not unusual for the white blood cell count to fall to less than 5000/mm^3 within 48 hours after injury. The value may decrease even more, 1500/mm^3 to 2000/mm^3, with the use of silver sulfadiazine (SSD). Hemoglobin and hematocrit data can be useful in the resuscitative phase to guide fluid administration. If surgical debridement is required, monitoring blood counts in the postoperative period is important. Serum chemistry information is helpful for ongoing assessment of kidney function and electrolyte balance. The myriad tests available should be used appropriately and as indicated by individual patient needs.

Acute Care Phase

The acute care phase of burn management begins after resuscitation and lasts until complete wound closure is achieved. The early postresuscitation phase is a period of transition from the shock phase to the hypermetabolic phase. Major cardiopulmonary and wound changes occur that substantially alter the manner of patient care from that given during resuscitation. Cardiopulmonary stability is optimal during this period because wound inflammation and infection have not developed. Hypermetabolic changes can be complicated with the onset of wound infection and sepsis. Early wound excision and skin grafting procedures, local wound care, nutrition support, and infection control characterize this phase.

Nurses play a major role in promoting the healing process. As skilled clinicians of the burn team, nurses provide wound care, hydrotherapy, debridement, preoperative and postoperative management, and pain management.

Physiologic Attempts to Restore Skin Integrity

Immediately after injury, the body responds by initiating a series of physiologic changes to restore skin integrity. These physiologic changes include the inflammatory phase, proliferative phase, and maturation phase.

Inflammatory phase. The inflammatory phase begins immediately after injury. A wound disrupts the blood vessels and results in bleeding, which induces the wound healing process.[24] Vascular changes and cellular activity characterize this period. Changes in the severed vessels occur in an attempt to wall off the wound from the external environment. Platelets, activated as a result of vessel wall injury, aggregate; blood coagulation is initiated; and in larger vessels, smooth muscle tissue contraction occurs, resulting in a reduction in the diameter of the vessel lumen. These brief but important compensatory mechanisms protect the patient from excessive blood loss and increased exposure to bacterial contamination. As vasodilation occurs, blood supply to the wound site increases and is observed as erythema and exudates. Granulocytes invade the wound within 24 hours and initiate the phagocytosis of necrotic tissue and bacteria. Fibroblasts migrate to the wound and multiply, producing a bed of collagen.

Proliferative phase. The proliferative phase of healing occurs approximately 4 to 20 days after injury. Formation of granulation tissue is key in this phase. The key cell in this phase of healing, the fibroblast, rapidly synthesizes collagen. Collagen synthesis provides the needed strength for a healing wound. Epithelial cells migrate across the wound bed and multiply to a great extent. After these cells contact each other, the wound is covered. This process is known as *epithelialization*. The wound contraction process occurs when specialized fibroblasts known as *myofibroblasts* pull down the wound edges in an effort to close the wound.

Maturation phase. The maturation phase, or remodeling phase, of healing occurs approximately 21 days after injury. During this period, the wound develops tensile strength and the collagen becomes increasingly more organized. Both the quantity and quality of the new collagen determines the strength and integrity of the wound. Scar remodeling may continue for 2 years after the injury. Regardless of how well the collagen realigns itself, the tissue of the wound will never regain the degree of strength or intactness inherent in uninjured tissue.

Impaired Tissue Integrity

Management of the burn wound is the top priority after the resuscitation phase. The depth of the burn wound is the principal determinant of wound management. Expedient closure of the wounds decreases the potential for many complications such as fluid and electrolyte imbalances, loss of proteins and nitrogen, and infection. The major goal of burn wound care is wound closure. Initial debridement is done by removal of blisters and loose skin. The assessment of wound depth by the clinician guides the treatment based on whether the wound will close in a reasonable time with dressings or will require surgical debridement. The assessment of wound depth can be a difficult challenge. There are many alternative dressing regimens for wound closure that are temporary, semipermanent, or permanent. The following objectives must be met for optimal wound closure: control of infection through meticulous cleansing and debridement, promotion of epithelialization, and preparation of the wound for grafting and closure. Other goals are reduction of scarring and contracture formation and providing patient comfort with appropriate psychological support and pharmacologic intervention.

Factors affecting healing of the burn wound. Sources of contamination include the patient's endogenous flora found on the skin, the upper respiratory tract, and the GI tract. Exogenous flora found in the patient care setting include bacteria carried by staff members and present in the environment. Patient-specific factors that predispose the patient to infection include age, diabetes, steroid therapy, extreme obesity, severe malnutrition, and infections in remote sites. Because wound healing and clinical infection are inflammatory responses, it is essential to differentiate between normal wound inflammation in the presence of colonization of microorganisms and that of invading organisms. In diagnosing infection, the importance of microbiologic results must be evaluated in conjunction with clinical findings such as excessive erythema, edema, pain, and purulence. Multidrug-resistant pathogens are increasing; therefore, the appropriate diagnosis and choice of antimicrobial treatment should be guided by the intensity of colonization with these organisms as indicated by cultures from various sites. Clinical findings in conjunction with burn wound biopsy or culture results determine the diagnosis of wound infection. A burn wound infection can delay healing and increase scarring, and invasive infection can result in death of the patient. Other factors that affect wound healing are tissue hypoxia from low blood flow to the burn wound, presence of eschar that requires debridement, exudate on the wound that can be harmful to the granulating wound or consume oxygen in the wound, and trauma to the wound from daily dressing changes or lack of protection from the outside environment.

Wound cleansing. A variety of equally appropriate methods can be used to cleanse burn wounds. At some centers, a mild antimicrobial cleansing agent may be used such as hypochlorous acid. Wounds are gently cleaned with a gauze dressing or washcloth and patted dry before application of topical agents. Hydrotherapy facilitates the removal of debris and loose eschar; however, the prevalence of immersion hydrotherapy has been decreasing. Frequent cleansing and inspection of the wound and unburned skin are performed to assess for signs of healing and local infection. Wound care exposure is limited as much as feasible to prevent hypothermia and decrease exposure to bacteria. Measures to reduce pain and hypothermia are used. Premedication with analgesics, opiates, and sedatives are used for comfort during wound cleaning.

Wound care. Although many options for burn wound care are available, the basic principle of maintaining a moist wound environment while preventing wound infection is the standard of care. Benefits include preventing wound desiccation, optimal function of local wound growth factors and proteolytic enzymes to remove dead tissue, increased epithelialization and collagen synthesis, and decreased wound fluid loss. The most common regimen for burn wound care involves the application of a topical antimicrobial agent, followed by a primary nonstick dressing. An outer layer is applied to provide increased absorption, compression, and occlusion. Some clinicians use the method of covering the wound with a thin layer of gauze or nonstick dressing that can be impregnated with a petroleum product, with or without a topical antimicrobial. This method is useful for less severe wounds when the amount of drainage has decreased and wound closure has almost been achieved. Lastly, a popular method for wound care is using silver-impregnated dressings. These dressings are more costly, but they reduce the dressing change frequency.

Topical antibiotic therapy. Burn injuries destroy the function of the skin's protective mechanism, including the function of sebaceous glands. Sebaceous glands normally secrete sebum, which contains fatty acids, including oleic acid. In addition to lubricating the skin, sebum is believed to help destroy some microorganisms, such as streptococci and some strains of staphylococci. Serum is lost from damaged capillaries, providing a rich nutrition medium for bacterial colonization. Topical antibiotic agents are used to control this colonization. Burn infection continues to be a concern during treatment, and topical use of antimicrobial agents plays an important role in the control of burn wound infection. Effective antibacterial agents should control colonization so that specimens for wound biopsy reveal fewer than 10^5 microorganisms per gram of tissue. With more than 10^5 microorganisms per gram of tissue, control of wound sepsis with topical antibiotics is questionable, and oral or intravenous therapy may then be considered. The topical antibiotics selected must meet several criteria: side effects must be minimal, resistant strains must not develop with use, application must be easy and rapid, and use must be relatively economical. The most commonly used topical antibiotics are SSD (Silvadene cream), mafenide acetate cream (Sulfamylon), bacitracin ointment, and silver impregnated into the primary dressing (Table 34.2). With multidrug-resistant pathogens increasing, deciding on the appropriate topical treatment is important. Studies show that multidrug-resistant organisms showed more resistance to topical antimicrobial treatments than non–multidrug-resistant organisms.[24]

SSD is a broad-spectrum antimicrobial agent with bactericidal action against many gram-negative and gram-positive bacteria associated with burn wound infection. SSD is indicated for use with partial-thickness and full-thickness wounds. It is a white cream that is applied once or twice daily to the burn wound. Moisture provided by the wound exudate may give the SSD cream layer a yellow-gray pseudo eschar. A common side effect of SSD is leukopenia resulting from bone marrow suppression, which may develop 24 to 72 hours after application. Rebound to normal leukocyte levels follows onset within 2 to 3 days, and it is not necessary to discontinue SSD use.

Mafenide acetate cream penetrates through burn eschar and is bacteriostatic against many gram-negative and gram-positive organisms. However, the most recent research shows a decrease in effectiveness against these organisms likely due to heavy use in burn care that can produce resistant organisms.[24] Its use is limited because the application is uncomfortable for the patient, it creates a burning sensation, and it is rapidly absorbed, requiring

TABLE 34.2 PHARMACOLOGIC MANAGEMENT

Topical Antimicrobial Agents

Agent	Advantages	Disadvantages	Implications
SSD	Painless application Broad spectrum Easy application Rare sensitivities	May produce transient leukopenia by bone marrow suppression Minimal eschar penetration Some gram-negative resistance	Monitor WBC count Observe wounds for tunneling and subeschar infection Monitor culture reports
Mafenide acetate cream	Broad spectrum (especially *Pseudomonas* coverage) Easy application Penetrates eschar	Painful application Rare acid–base imbalance Frequent sensitivities	Provide adequate analgesia Monitor arterial blood gases Observe for hyperventilation Observe for rashes
Bacitracin	Painless application Nonirritating Transparent Nontoxic	No eschar penetration No gram-negative or fungal coverage	
Pure silver	Painless application Broad spectrum, including fungus and resistant organisms Rare sensitivity Less frequent dressing changes	Can be more costly	Ensure knowledge of proper application Observe for signs of silver sensitivities

SSD, Silver sulfadiazine; *WBC*, white blood cell.

dressing changes two or three times daily. It is used routinely for coverage of small wounds involving anatomic areas that contain cartilage such as the ears and nose. Metabolic acidosis can result from the use of mafenide acetate. The patient must be observed closely for hyperventilation (see Table 34.2).

Bacitracin ointment is a topical agent applied to superficial burns and facial burns. Bacitracin is effective against gram-positive organisms such as *Staphylococcus aureus* and Streptococci.[24] Most gram-negative organisms and yeast are resistant. Bacitracin is applied to the wound one or two times daily and covered with a nonstick dressing. The ease of use, cost, and accessibility make it a common treatment in burn wounds. A yeast rash is commonly associated with repeated bacitracin usage. Triple antibiotic ointment (TAO) is a combination of bacitracin zinc, polymyxin B sulfate, and neomycin sulfate. This broad-spectrum coverage has activity against both gram-positive and gram-negative organisms.

Although SSD is still the standard of care in many parts of the world, advances in technology have led to newer silver dressings. Silver has long been used for the treatment of wounds because of its broad-spectrum bacteriostatic properties against gram-negative and gram-positive bacteria. Silver has minimal side effects and minimal bacterial resistance. The wound moisture activates the silver and releases it into the wound. An advantage of silver dressings is that the dressing does not need to be changed daily because of the sustained release of silver.[25] These dressings are a popular choice by patients and providers because they decrease dressing change frequency.

Wound debridement. Eschar is the nonviable tissue that forms after a burn injury. This tissue has no blood supply, and polymorphonuclear leukocytes, antibodies, and systemic antibodies cannot reach these areas. Eschar provides an excellent medium for bacterial growth, and it is vital that loose eschar is debrided as necessary. Debridement facilitates wound healing by removing contaminated tissue of foreign bodies and bacteria, controlling the inflammation, and removing the devitalized tissue, preparing the wound bed for grafting or biological dressing application.[26] The three types of debridement are mechanical, enzymatic, and surgical.

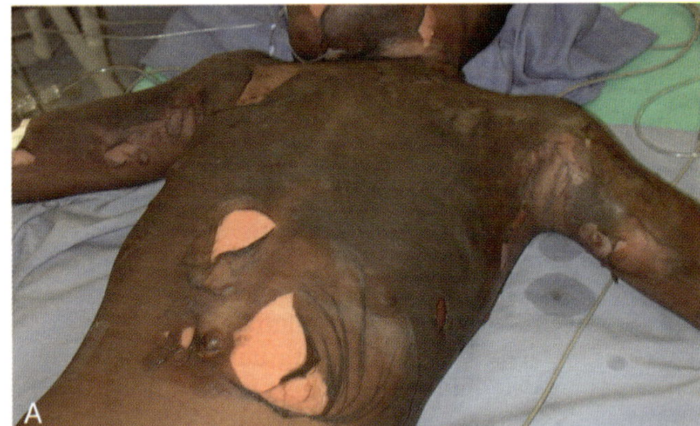

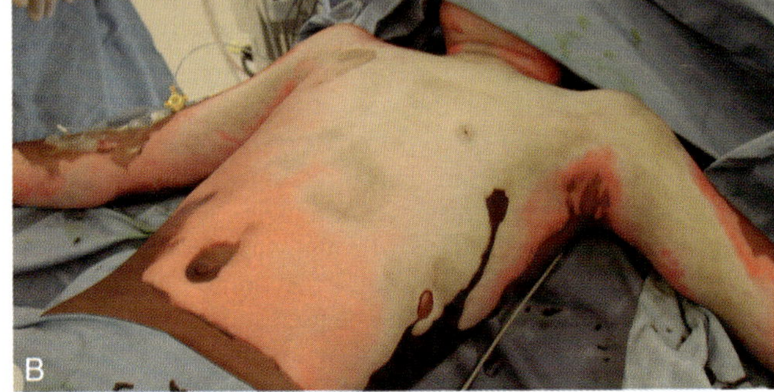

FIG. 34.11 Anterior Trunk and Bilateral Arm Burn. (A) Before mechanical debridement. (B) After mechanical debridement.

Mechanical Debridement. Mechanical debridement includes rough debridement, wet-to-dry debridement, and sharp debridement with the use of scissors and forceps or curette (Fig. 34.11).[27] Wet-to-dry or wet-to-wet dressing to further debride the wound bed is less popular because of the related pain and tissue trauma.

Enzymatic Debridement. Enzymatic debridement involves the topical application of proteolytic substances to the wound bed such as SANTYL. These agents are useful in softening eschar and dissolving devitalized tissue while sparing healthy tissue. They promote the separation of eschar, which can lead to earlier wound closure.

The gold standard of debridement remains surgical debridement, which is performed by a surgeon.[26] The goal of debridement is to remove nonviable tissue down to bleeding viable tissue with an electric dermatome or surgical knife. Surgical excision is performed to mechanically remove necrotic tissue from the burn wound; it may be performed by tangential excision or fascial excision. Tangential excision involves sequentially excising the eschar down to bleeding, viable tissue and then placing a split-thickness skin graft over the wound. Fascial excision is used when the wounds are deep and the fat does not appear viable.

Skin substitutes. To assist in wound closure, many temporary and permanent skin substitute dressings have gained popularity in the United States. Temporary substitutes are designed for placement on partial-thickness or clean, excised wounds. Permanent substitutes provide a permanent skin replacement.

Skin substitutes must possess properties that mimic the native epidermis and dermis. They are made from various synthetic materials such as nylon, polyurethane, or solid silicone polymers. Skin barrier substitutes must possess several properties to accomplish their desired effect as a temporary wound covering to protect the granulating tissue and to preserve a clean, viable wound surface for future autografting (Box 34.2). The most important property of these materials is adherence so that the skin substitute can simulate the function of the skin. Adherence must be uniform to prevent fluid accumulation beneath the surface of the substitute, which can lead to bacterial proliferation.

For application of skin substitutes, the wound must be clean and ideally should have a bacterial count of fewer than 10^5 microorganisms per gram of tissue. The burn wound must be free from eschar, and hemostasis must exist.

BOX 34.2 Ideal Properties of Skin Substitutes

- Adherence
- Decreased pain
- Easy application and removal
- Intact bacterial barrier
- Shelf storage capability
- Inexpensive in relation to alternatives
- Nonantigenic
- Similar to normal skin in transport of water vapor
- Elastic and durable
- Hemostatic
- Decreased protein and electrolyte loss
- Enhanced natural healing processes

Definitive Burn Wound Closure

The primary goal of burn wound management is wound closure during the acute phase. Early excision and grafting of full-thickness (third-degree) burns is the standard in burn centers.[27] Some deep-dermal partial-thickness burns that have a prolonged healing time may also benefit from excision and grafting. Early excision should be undertaken to improve functional and cosmetic results, decrease infection risk, decrease in-hospital time, and reduce the cost of burn care. Surgical debridement may begin 3 to 5 days after the burn insult, as soon as hemodynamic stability has been achieved. Some physicians operate within 24 hours of admission if the patient is hemodynamically stable. To minimize contraction, burn wounds over joint surfaces should be excised and grafted as soon as possible. In patients with massive burns, excision procedures are commonly staged, requiring the patient to return to the operating room every 2 to 3 days until all wounds have been excised. Table 34.3 summarizes advantages and disadvantages of different graft types.

Autograft. An autograft is a skin graft harvested from a healthy, uninjured donor site on the patient with burns and then placed over the patient's burn wound to provide permanent coverage of the wound. Autografts are the only grafts that provide permanent wound coverage. Preferred sites for obtaining these grafts are the thighs, back, and abdomen; however, grafts can be harvested from almost anywhere on the body. Autografting with the patient's own skin from a donor site is the preferred choice for wound closure. However, with large TBSA burns, availability of donor sites can be problematic. When an autograft is unavailable, many alternative methods are used to achieve this goal. Skin substitutes can be used until the patient's own skin is available for harvesting. Previously used and healed donor sites can be used again on later return visits to the operating room.

Sheets of the patient's epidermis and a partial layer of the dermis are harvested with use of a dermatome. These grafts are referred to as *split-thickness skin grafts* and can be applied to the wound bed as a sheet or in meshed form (Fig. 34.12). The size of the mesh is based on the areas requiring grafting and the availability of donor skin. This meshing prevents serum

TABLE 34.3 Types of Grafts

Graft	Use	Advantages	Disadvantages
Autograft	Provides permanent coverage of burn wounds Used in sheets or meshed form	Permanent coverage Nonantigenic Least expensive Meshing allows small amount of tissue to cover large area	Lack of available donor sites, which may delay wound coverage Donor sites are painful partial-thickness wounds Must be done in surgical suite
Homograft (allograft)	Temporary wound coverage	Can be placed at bedside or in operating room Allows for vascularization over deep wound Provides better control over bacterial growth than xenograft	Possibility of disease transmission Antigenic; body rejects in approximately 2 weeks Not readily available to all burn centers Expensive Requires rigorous quality controls

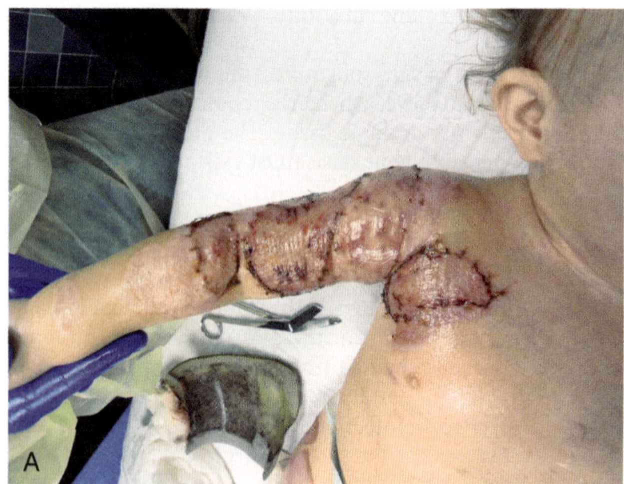

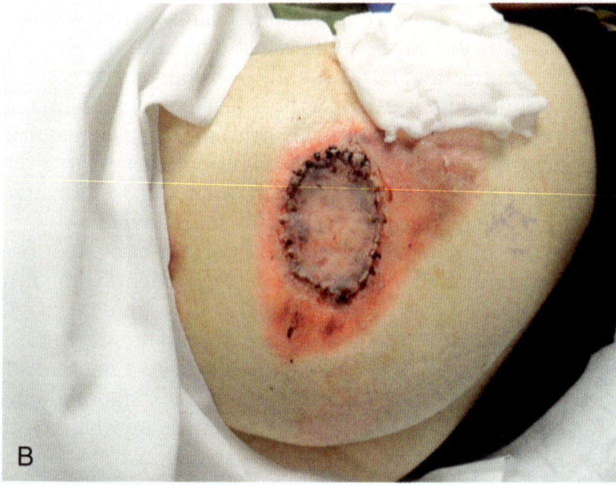

FIG. 34.12 (A) Split-thickness skin graft. (B) Sheet graft to left buttock.

accumulation under the graft and permits coverage of a surface area larger than its original surface. Sheet grafts are placed on the face, neck, lower portions of the arms, and hands when possible. Mesh grafts can cover more area but may not produce the cosmetic appearance desired; therefore, they are usually placed on areas covered by clothing.

Grafts can be secured with sutures, fibrin glue, or staples.[27] The choice of dressing that is placed over the graft varies widely based on physician and institution preference. One choice is fine mesh gauze impregnated with an emollient. It is placed over the graft, covered with a heavy gauze dressing, and secured to the patient with or without a splint, depending on the anatomic area of the graft. A vacuum-assisted closure (VAC) device provides a safe and effective method for securing split-thickness skin grafts, and it is associated with improved graft survival.[27] VAC therapy can be used to secure the graft in place. The VAC is removed on postoperative day 3 to 5 for assessment of adherence and graft survival. Nurses, in collaboration with the interprofessional team, provide proper positioning, splinting, and pain management in the postoperative period. Great care must be taken not to disturb the graft. Care of the donor site is equally important, because it represents a wound similar to that of a partial-thickness injury. Donor sites can be covered with many different types of dressings depending on surgeon and institution preference.

Biosynthetic skin substitutes. The common purpose of skin substitutes is to replicate the properties of normal skin.[27] Skin substitutes include homografts (allografts) and heterografts (xenografts). Homograft skin can be obtained from living donors or deceased donors (cadaver skin). With advances in cryopreservation, a homograft harvested from cadaver skin can be frozen and stored in a tissue bank. Because it is possible to transmit disease through the application of a homograft, tissue banks must adhere to strict guidelines. Before application, homograft skin is tested for various transmissible diseases, including human immunodeficiency virus and hepatitis B surface antigens. Homograft skin can be applied as a biological dressing for debridement at the bedside or as temporary wound coverage on excised burn wounds. Vascular ingrowth occurs, and the homograft seals the wound and protects it from bacterial invasion; however, it is rejected approximately 2 weeks after its application. Disadvantages include the homograft antigenicity, lack of accessibility, difficulties with storage and quality control, expense of procurement, and possibility of disease transmission from the donor. Homografts are harvested during the first 4 hours after death, and they are taken from the abdomen, thighs, and back. Homografts usually are available only in centers in which the rigorous processing procedure can be achieved. These centers usually have skin and tissue bank facilities. Procurement of the allograft is much the same as for any other donated organ.

A xenograft (heterograft) is a graft transferred between two different species to provide temporary wound coverage. The most common and widely accepted xenograft is pigskin (porcine skin). Pigskin is available in frozen and shelf forms. The pigskin is packaged in a variety of ways and in various sizes. It can be meshed or nonmeshed. Pigskin can be used for temporary coverage of burn wounds and donor sites. After the pigskin is in place, it may be dressed with antibacterial-impregnated dressings or other forms of dressings. Pigskin usually is removed or dissolves because of lack of blood supply in 5 to 7 days (see Table 34.3).

Synthetic skin. The lack of available donor sites for major burn injury often delays wound closure. In an effort to minimize infection and to promote healing, many attempts have been made to develop skin substitutes that seal the wound in a functional and cosmetically acceptable fashion. A dermal substitute has become very popular, with its ultrathin layer of epidermal autograft used successfully. The dermal substitute is intended to be placed on freshly excised, full-thickness burns, and the outer silicone membrane is replaced with an ultrathin epithelial autograft 2 to 3 weeks later. A technique that involves the growth and subsequent graft placement of cultured epithelial autograft (CEA) has also become an adjunct to the treatment of burn wounds. A complex process that allows for separation of keratinocytes is performed. The CEA is grown over 2 to 3 weeks to achieve a graft size of 25 cm^2. This represents an expansion of 50 to 70 times the original specimen. These confluent sheets of cultured epithelial cells are attached to a gauze backing and placed on the wound. Published results reveal that graft acceptance is unpredictable, because the CEA lacks dermis. Even when grafts take initially, graft loss can occur later. Compared with other methods, the CEA also is more fragile, and the technique is costly. This therapy is being recommended as an adjunct for traditional split-thickness skin grafts, and it continues to be investigated and combined with newer dermal skin substitutes.

Other Considerations in the Acute Phase

Imbalanced nutrition: less than body requirements. The basal metabolic rate of a patient with burns may be elevated 40% to 100% above the normal rate, depending on the amount of TBSA involved. The metabolic rate is influenced by the amount of protein and albumin lost through the wounds; the catabolic response associated with stress, injuries, fluid loss, fever, infection, and immobility; sex; and height and weight of the patient before the injury. A 10% loss of total body mass leads to immune dysfunction; 20% leads to decreased wound healing; 30% leads to severe infections; a 40% loss leads to death. Severely burned, catabolic patients can lose 25% of total body mass after acute severe burn injury.

The goal in nutrition management of a patient with burns is to provide adequate calories to enhance wound healing. To achieve this goal, nutrition support and a reduction of energy demand are imperative. Every effort should be made to reduce the release of catecholamines, which increase metabolic rate. Pain, fear, anxiety, and cold stimulate release of catecholamine stores. Appropriate interventions for each of these stimuli must be performed. Examples of nonpharmacologic interventions include early excision and burn wound closure; elevation of the environmental temperature to thermal neutrality (31.5° C ± 0.7° C); and high-carbohydrate, high-protein feeds.

Because of the increased nutrition needs of patients with large-surface-area burns, oral feedings are usually inadequate, and supplemental enteral feedings are necessary. After burn injury, intestinal mucosal damage and increased bacterial translocation occur, resulting in decreased absorption of nutrients. Therefore, nutritional support should ideally be initiated within 24 hours of injury via an enteral route.[28] Enteral feedings may be gastric or postpyloric; both are widely used. Caloric requirements are calculated on the basis of the size of the burn; the age, height, and weight of the patient; and stress factors. The daily protein requirement may increase to two to four times the normal 0.8 g/kg of body weight. Carbohydrates and fat are used for energy and to spare proteins required for wound healing. Daily caloric intake can be 2 to 20 times higher than normal. Vitamins and minerals usually are given in doses higher than normal. Serum albumin, prealbumin, iron, zinc, calcium, phosphate, and potassium values are monitored, and supplements are given as needed. Initiating early enteral feedings has shown to alleviate malnutrition and stress reaction, strengthen immunity, and promote gastrointestinal mobility, thereby promoting wound healing.

Pain management. Burn injuries are very painful. Pain management must be addressed early and frequently reassessed. Pain is an individualized and subjective phenomenon, and it has physiologic and psychological components. Pain results from the acute burn injury and occurs throughout the phases of healing. Injury interacts with the sensory neural fibers by impacting the heat-induced vascular tissue damage and inflammatory mediators.[28] The heat-induced vascular damage induces hypoxia in the nerves. The inflammatory mediators directly impact the nerves.[28] Background pain is related to the physiologic changes associated with the burn injury and includes the damage or exposure of the nerve endings within partial-thickness burns and donor sites. Range of motion of the affected limbs and routine activities contribute to background pain. Breakthrough pain is described as episodes of pain more severe than background pain; breakthrough pain is not relieved by routine pain medications. Procedural pain includes pain caused by interventions such as daily wound care, arterial punctures, physical and occupational therapy, and the use of splints.

Initially after burn injury, opioids are administered intravenously in small doses and titrated to effect. The constant background pain may be addressed with the use of a patient-controlled analgesia device. After hemodynamic stability has occurred and GI function has returned, oral opioids can be useful. Intramuscular or subcutaneous injections must not be administered, because absorption by these routes is unpredictable. Additional premedication and analgesics are necessary during therapeutic procedures. Acetaminophen and nonsteroidal antiinflammatory drugs can be useful in patients who are not at risk for bleeding. Anxiolytics and antidepressants also should be considered and used appropriately. The nurse must be flexible with dosing and should assess the effectiveness of medication. The nurse should assure the patient that pain control issues will be continually addressed.

Pain continues even after healing; some patients describe the itching, tingling, and paresthesia as being as uncomfortable as the initial injury. Paresthesia are abnormal neurologic sensations of numbness, tingling, or burning that can last 1 year or longer after injury. Inadequate pain management is an issue in many burn units because of the fear of opioid side effects and opioid addiction and the lack of pain evaluation or treatment protocols.

Loss of control, forced dependence, loneliness, and separation from home and family can contribute to anxiety, which heightens the patient's perception of pain. The patient's fears abound in thoughts of disfigurement and loss of love, function, and job. The psychological experience or subjective component may be related to past experiences, anxiety, and altered coping mechanisms. Attention to the psychological component of the patient's pain may lead to useful strategies that decrease perceived pain. If possible, past experiences with pain, hospitalization, and successful coping strategies should be explored. Pain is a psychological and physical experience that accumulates over time and becomes part of the individual's deepest psychology.

Nonpharmacologic techniques such as imagery, hypnosis, virtual reality, and distraction can be effective in reducing anxiety and the pain experience.[29] Giving the patient some control over pain management also can reduce anxiety and the perception of pain. The perception of pain often is increased in a patient who is anxious and lacks control of the situation.

Treatment strategies need to be individualized. Failure to adequately treat pain can increase burn hypermetabolism, result in loss of confidence between the burn team and patient, and lead to the development of psychiatric disorders. The nurse must assess and discuss on a regular basis the patient's psychological status and avoid using psychotropic medication for analgesia and opioids for anxiety and depression. See Chapter 7 for more information on pain and pain management.

Rehabilitation Phase

The rehabilitation phase is one of recuperation and healing physically and emotionally. This phase can last several years. Psychological rehabilitation is equal in importance to physical rehabilitation in patients with burns. The patient may require extensive reconstructive surgery. Psychologically, the patient focuses on attaining specific personal goals related to achieving as much preburn function as possible. A person's preburn level of physical and emotional functioning can greatly affect the course of recovery. Minor and major accomplishments must be praised. This phase is characterized by scar management techniques and by physical and occupational therapies.

The burn team and the patient prepare for the transition to the outside world. Group therapy is a valuable tool used at many burn centers. Patients, family members, and health care providers express ideas and feelings. Patients with burns often establish priorities and make realistic decisions about their lives. Staff intervention during this phase is primarily of a supportive nature.

Impaired Physical Mobility

Tremendous advances have been made in the physical care of patients with burns. As more patients with larger and deeper burns survive, the challenge to maintain their optimal mobility and cosmetic appearance has been met with increased success. Despite advances in other areas of burn care, contractures still develop after a burn injury. A contracture is the shortening of a scar over a joint surface and is the primary cause of functional deficits in patients with burns (Fig. 34.13).[30] Around 40% to 55% of burn patients experience joint scar contractures at discharge.[30] Contractures develop as a result of various factors including the extent, depth, location, and configuration of the burn; the position of comfort the patient most frequently assumes; the relative underlying muscle strength; and the patient's motivation and compliance. The affected body parts should be positioned to prevent long-term deformity. Frequent change of position also is important and may need to be performed as often as every hour. Although contracture prevention is the goal, many patients with burns will develop self-limiting contractures despite aggressive prevention measures and good care. Early identification of high-risk patients is a useful endeavor.[30]

Splints can be used to prevent or correct contracture or to immobilize joints after grafting. If splints are used, they must be checked daily for proper fit and effectiveness. Splints that are used to immobilize body parts after grafting must be left on at all times except to assess the graft site for pressure points during every shift. Splints may also be used in the rehabilitation phase to correct severe contracture. Serial casting has also been shown to be effective in correcting scar contractures when traditional methods have failed or are not feasible.[30] Orthosis can be a faster way to correct contracture compared to massage and compression. Active exercise is encouraged and is preferred, although active-assisted or gentle-passive exercises also may be an important part of the rehabilitation program. Active exercise maintains muscle mass, aids in restoring protein structures within the muscle tissue, aids in venous and lymphatic return, and reduces the risk of pulmonary embolus and deep vein thrombosis. The patient's tolerance must be carefully evaluated. The number of repetitions of an exercise is proportional to the degree of anticipated contracture and the patient's tolerance. Anticipation of the patient's pain also must be carefully considered. Before range-of-motion exercises and activities of daily living are performed, the need for pain medication must be assessed. The nursing management plans for a patient with burn injuries are summarized in Box 34.3 and Box 34.4.

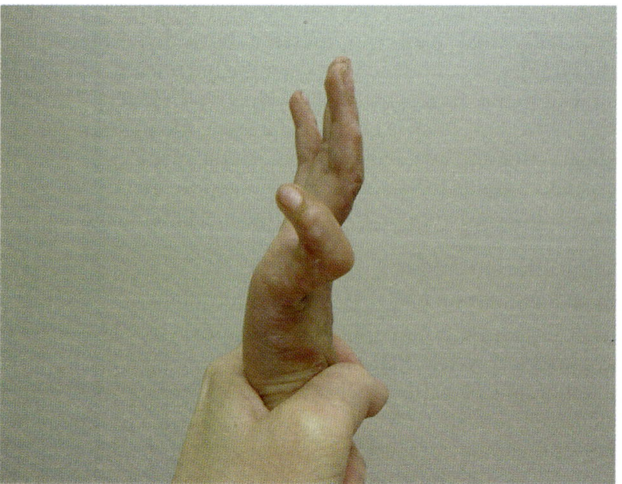

FIG. 34.13 Severe Contracture to Bilateral Lower Extremities.

Scar Management

The goal of scar management is to minimize scarring, making the skin flat, elastic, and close to the original color. A person's skin response to a burn injury can be barely noticeable, such as slight color change, or can lead to cosmetic disfigurement and dysfunction. It is important to inform the patient that the tissue may not return to the preburn texture or appearance despite good efforts. Excess collagen deposit results in a pathologic

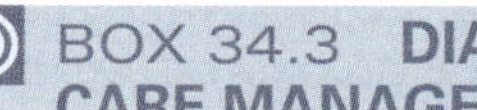

BOX 34.3 DIAGNOSIS AND PATIENT CARE MANAGEMENT

Resuscitative and Acute Phase in Burn Injury

- Acute Pain due to transmission and perception of cutaneous, visceral, muscular, or ischemic impulses
- Impaired Gas Exchange due to ventilation-perfusion mismatching or intrapulmonary shunting
- Impaired Airway Clearance due to excessive secretions or abnormal viscosity of mucus
- Hypovolemia due to relative loss
- Risk for Infection
- Disturbed Body Image due to actual change in body structure, function, or appearance
- Powerlessness due to lack of control over current situation or disease progression
- Impaired Nutritional Intake due to lack of exogenous nutrients and increased metabolic demand
- Anxiety due to threat to biological, psychological, or social integrity
- Lack of Knowledge of Treatment Regime due to lack of previous exposure to information

Patient Care Management plans are located in Appendix A.

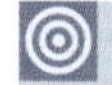

BOX 34.4 DIAGNOSIS AND PATIENT CARE MANAGEMENT

Rehabilitative Phase in Burn Injury

- Activity Intolerance due to prolonged immobility or deconditioning
- Disturbed Body Image due to actual change in body structure, function, or appearance
- Impaired Adaptation due to situational crisis and personal vulnerability
- Lack of Knowledge of Treatment Regime due to lack of previous exposure to information

Patient Care Management plans are located in Appendix A.

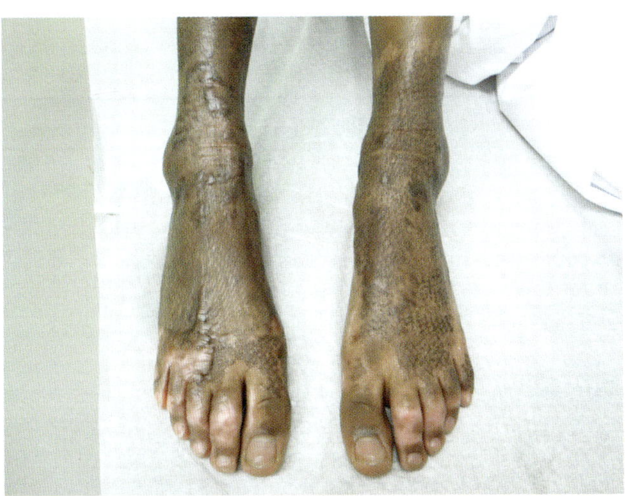

FIG. 34.14 Healed Split-Thickness Skin Graft to Bilateral Feet.

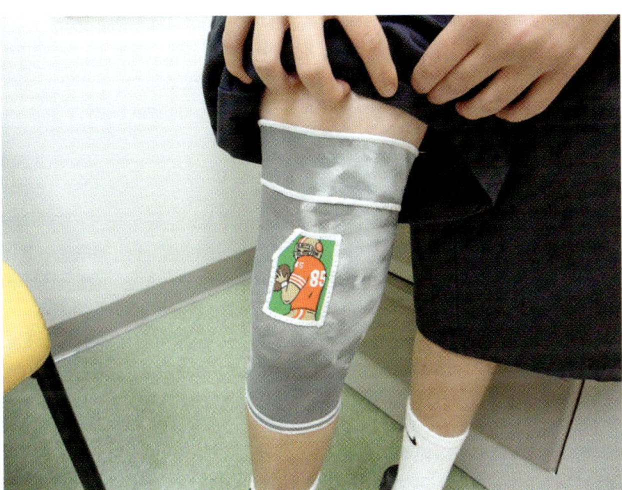

FIG. 34.15 Compression Garment to Right Leg.

hypertrophic scar that is thick and can be painful and itchy.[31] The highest risk for scar tissue development is associated with deep partial-thickness and full-thickness burns because of their depth and increased risk of infection. Areas of the skin that required skin grafting also have a visible scar (Fig. 34.14). Scar maturation occurs 6 months to 2 years from the time of the injury. One method to reduce scar formation is timely application of uniform pressure. Custom-made elastic pressure garments are worn for 6 months to 1 year, if needed (Fig. 34.15). These garments reduce scar blood flow and may provide force that helps developing collagen to organize. Although compression therapy is one of the main methods of prophylaxis and treatment of burn scars, its mechanism is not totally understood.

Additional approaches to reduce scarring are scar massage, high-SPF sun protection, silicone gel sheeting, laser therapy, and steroid treatment. Scar massage works by stretching the scar and providing moisture and is most helpful in preventing contractures. Sun protection over the healed burn may decrease the long-term pigment change to the injured area. Silicone gel sheets are used alone over the scar or in conjunction with compression to soften the scar by maintaining scar hydration and tension reduction. Injectable steroids are used for treatment of hypertrophic scars; however, they have some side effects that may make them undesirable. Corticosteroid injections inhibit fibroblast growth and enhance collagen breakdown, leading to a flatter and softer scar. If less-invasive techniques have been unsuccessful for troublesome scars that cause pain or inhibit full range of motion, surgical excision may be recommended.

Itching

Pruritus is common in the maturing burn wound and commonly replaces burn pain. Itching can be extremely uncomfortable for the patient and should be continually assessed. Research has shown that burn pruritus can continue for years after the healed burn injury and has negative long-term effects for the patient.[32] A mild, non–alcohol-based skin cream or lotion is applied every 4 hours and as needed to healed areas to lubricate the skin until natural lubrication occurs. Patients can be relieved of discomfort by the administration of an antipruritic agent such as diphenhydramine and by the application of moisturizing creams. Further research needs to be done on how to standardize itching assessment and treatment.

Age Considerations

Children are vulnerable to burn injury and account for almost one-fourth (24%) of all burn injuries.[33] Children carry the burden of the injury for the remainder of their lifetime; however, there are limited data available that examine the long-term effects. The majority of pediatric burn injuries are a result of a scald or contact with hot food. Other common causes are fireworks, campfires, irons, and house fires. Unfortunately, some burn injuries are also a result of child abuse. The larger BSA–to–body-mass ratio and thinner skin of a child predisposes the child to hyperthermia, and fluid losses are proportionately higher in children and require close monitoring. The Lund and Browder method (Fig. 34.4) can be used to more precisely calculate the BSA based on age. In addition, children have a smaller airway diameter, making a lower threshold for intubation. A burn injury is a stressful and traumatic event for the child and the loved ones. Some evidence shows that a parent's response to stress influences how the child reacts.[33] It is important to address the child's pain and anxiety appropriate to their age. Many burn centers have a Child Life Specialist who is trained in distraction techniques and comfort measures. National prevention and education efforts have been useful to decrease burn injuries in children.

Burn care of an older adult presents its own unique challenges, especially with the growing number of aging people in society. There is not a consensus on what age defines *older adult;* however, we do know that with increasing age, complications and risk for mortality increase. Even a small burn can lead to poor outcomes.[34] Older adults have preexisting conditions, lower immune function, a thinning of the skin, decreased sensation, and sometimes mental alteration. All of these contribute to worsened outcomes. Age is not always an ideal predictor of the outcome; it is related more to the person's frailty, aging progression, and functionality.[8]

Interprofessional Collaborative Care

An interprofessional collaborative approach to burn treatment is an integral part of providing quality care. This approach involves considering all aspects of the patient's care when treatment decisions are made. The burn team should work together to address all needs of the patient and the family. The team should meet frequently to review patient care and maximize patient and family support. The interprofessional team includes, but is not limited to, nurses and physicians and individuals from social work, nutrition, physical and occupational therapy, respiratory therapy, psychology, pain service, child life services, and utilization review.

Outpatient Burn Care

Outpatient burn care can be considered for patients with minor burns. Patients with larger burns can be transitioned to outpatient care when ready. It is cost-effective and removes the potential for a wound infection by endemic, drug-resistant microorganisms within the hospital environment. The hospital environment also changes many self-care routines such as diet, family contact, hygiene, and coping mechanisms. However, patients considered for outpatient burn care must be screened carefully. Nursing evaluation of the patient and the family includes consideration of motivation, willingness to participate in care, ability to understand and perform the necessary procedures, potential aversions to wound care or dressing changes, and reliability of transportation. The transition to outpatient care must also include consideration of physical and occupational therapy needs and involve exercises designed to accelerate return to activities of daily living such as work, school, or both. Home health nurses are helpful in monitoring patients.

Support of the Patient With Burns

Burn injuries are physically and psychologically traumatic and life altering for the patient. The family of the patient with burns is also affected, and their needs should be remembered during the healing process. Guilt is often associated with burn injuries, especially when the victim is a child. It is important for care providers to support the patient with burns physically and psychologically. Health care providers heal and support the patient throughout the hospital stay but often forget that the patient's biggest challenges may still lie ahead after hospitalization.

Many resources are available to help patients with burns cope after they are home, and these resources should be provided by the hospital team during the inpatient stay. Research has shown that many patients have difficulty returning to work. Work capacity may be assessed by a coordinator during the rehabilitation process. Programs are available to help with issues including social and school reentry, support for sexual considerations, and dealing with scars.

Stressors of Burn Nursing

Burn units can be stimulating yet stressful workplaces in that they offer fast-paced, high-technology atmosphere. The physical environment can be a difficult one for a variety of reasons. The amount of equipment necessary to maintain the patient can be overwhelming and can limit the workspace dramatically. The temperature of the room usually is kept at approximately 85° F and can become much warmer, depending on the amount of equipment in the room. The various odors in the room may be very unpleasant. Noise levels within a unit also are distressing. It can be overwhelming for clinicians to work in a demanding burn unit environment where they are repeatedly exposed to stressful events.[35] A recent study showed that burn nurses are at higher risk of anxiety, depression, and burnout; however, more research is needed in this area.[35] While burn nurses do well with supporting the patient and family, they still need to do self-care for themselves. The decision to specialize in burn nursing requires careful consideration.

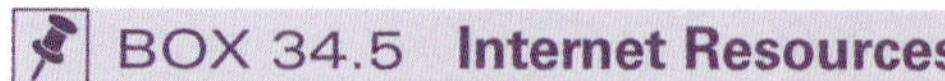
BOX 34.5 Internet Resources

Burns

- American Burn Association: http://www.ameriburn.org

ADDITIONAL RESOURCES

Internet resources related to this chapter are located in Box 34.5.

CASE STUDY 34.1 Patient With Burns

Brief Patient History

Ms. J is a 40-year-old victim of a motor vehicle crash. She was found conscious at the scene and pulled out of a burning car to safety by a passerby. The paramedics at the scene reported her as awake but disoriented and anxious. She is otherwise healthy and is the mother of a 5-year-old child, who was also rescued at the scene with no injuries.

Clinical Assessment

Ms. J is sent from the emergency department to the trauma unit. She is intubated and sedated on arrival. She has partial-thickness burns covering her face, including her nose, lips, and neck. She has areas of partial-thickness and full-thickness burns to both her hands and to her chest and left leg. Her breath sounds are auscultated as present bilaterally, but she is wheezing, and her sputum has a dark carbon appearance. She has a triple-lumen catheter in her right femoral vein with good blood return to all ports.

Diagnostic Procedures

Ms. J has a carboxyhemoglobin level of 3.4% and arterial blood gas values as follows: pH of 7.27, arterial partial pressure of carbon dioxide of 29 mm Hg, arterial partial pressure of oxygen of 313 mm Hg, bicarbonate of 14 mEq/L (mmol/L), and oxygen saturation of 88% on 100% fraction of inspired oxygen. Her serum cyanide level is 45 mmol/L. The chest radiograph obtained on arrival in the emergency department was normal. Blood pressure is 85/50 mm Hg, heart rate is 136 beats/min (sinus tachycardia), respiratory rate is 14 breaths/min, and temperature is 96.3° F.

Medical Diagnosis

Ms. J is diagnosed with burns covering 40% of total body surface area, inhalation injury, and cyanide toxicity.

Questions

1. What major outcomes do you expect to achieve for this patient?
2. What problems or risks must be managed to achieve these outcomes?
3. What interventions could be initiated to monitor, prevent, manage, or eliminate the problems and risks identified?
4. What interventions could be initiated to promote optimal functioning, safety, and well-being of the patient?
5. What technology can be used to monitor this patient and prevent complications?
6. What other interprofessional team members are needed to assist with the management of this patient?
7. What possible learning needs do you anticipate for this patient?
8. What cultural and age-related factors may have a bearing on the patient's plan of care?

KEY POINTS

- Burn care is highly complex, and decisions regarding appropriate management of burn injuries are best managed by certified burn centers, where the most accurate burn size estimates can be made.
- Burn size, type of injury, location of the burn, and the patient's age and history all are determinants of survival.
- Size and depth of burns are divided into four main categories: (1) superficial (first-degree) burns, which are injuries to epidermis; (2) partial-thickness (second-degree) burns, which involve the epidermis and dermis of the skin, and can be superficial or deep-dermal partial-thickness burns; and (3) full-thickness (third-degree) burns, which involve destruction of skin layers from the epidermis down to and including the subcutaneous tissue.
- Accurate fluid resuscitation of a patient with burns for more severe burn injuries (greater than 10% of TBSA) is crucial to prevent AKI that may result in acute kidney failure, cardiovascular collapse, and death from burn shock. The Parkland formula is a guide for determining resuscitation fluid (e.g., lactated Ringer) volume.
- Careful assessment of intake and output of the patient with burns is critical to achieve the optimal patient response to fluid resuscitation.
- After the resuscitative phase of patients with burns, the acute care phase of wound healing, wound closure, and prevention of infection begins. This hypermetabolic phase can be complicated by wound infection and sepsis.
- The gold standard of burn wound care includes the application of a topical antimicrobial agent followed by a gauze dressing to absorb excess drainage, with an outer layer to provided increased absorption, compression, and occlusion. Silver dressings have shown positive results in the prevention of bacterial growth without silver toxicity.
- The rehabilitative phase of care of the patient with burns starts from admission of the patient and may last years, depending on future surgical procedures, therapy needs, contracture prevention, and psychological or emotional needs of the patient.
- All the interprofessional needs of patients with burns must be addressed for these patients to be able to perform in and feel accepted back into society.

Visit the Evolve site at http://evolve.elsevier.com/UrdenCCN for additional study materials

REFERENCES

1. Smolle C, Cambiaso-Daniel J, Forbes AA, et al. Recent trends in burn epidemiology worldwide: a systematic review. *Burns*. 2017;43:249–257. https://doi.org/10.1016/j.burns.2016.08.013.
2. American Burn Association. Burn incidence fact sheet. https://ameriburn.org/who-we-are/media/burn-incidence-fact-sheet/. Accessed September 14, 2023.
3. Kaddoura I, Abu-Sittah G, Ibrahim A, Karamanoukian R, Papazian N. Burn injury: review of pathophysiology and therapeutic modalities in major burns. *Ann Burns Fire Disasters*. 2017;30(2):95–102.
4. Child Maltreatment 2021. U.S. Department of Health & Human Services, Administration for Children and Families, Administration on Children, Youth and Families, Children's Bureau. https://www.acf.hhs.gov/cb/data-research/child-maltreatment. Accessed September 14, 2023.
5. Palmieri TL. Pediatric burn resuscitation. *Crit Care Clin*. 2016;32(4):547–559. https://doi.org/10.1016/j.ccc.2016.06.004.
6. Cartotto R, Burmeister DM, Kubasiak JC. Burn shock and resuscitation: review and state of the science. *J Burn Care Res*. 2022;43(3):567–585. https://doi.org/10.1093/jbcr/irac025.
7. Douglas HE, Dunne JA, Rawlins JM. Management of burns. *Surgery*. 2017;35(9):511–518. https://doi.org/10.1016/j.mpsur.2017.06.007.
8. Strassle PD, Williams FN, Napravnik S, et al. Improved survival of patients with extensive burns: Trends in patient characteristics and mortality among burn patients in a tertiary care burn facility, 2004–2013. *J Burn Care Res*. 2022;38(3):187–193. https://doi.org/10.1097/BCR.0000000000000456.
9. Sen CK, Ghatak S, Gnyawali SC, Roy S, Gordillo GM. Cutaneous imaging technologies in acute burn and chronic wound care. *Plast Reconstr Surg*. 2016;138(3S):119S–128S. https://doi.org/10.1097/PRS.0000000000002654.
10. Shah AR, Liao LF. Pediatric burn care: unique considerations in management. *Clin Plast Surg*. 2017;44(3):603–610. https://doi.org/10.1016/j.cps.2017.02.017.
11. Zemaitis MR, Foris LA, Lopez RA, Huecker MR. Electrical injuries. In: *StatPearls*. Treasure Island, FL: StatPearls; 2023.
12. D'Cruz R, Pang TCY, Harvey JG, Holland AJA. Chemical burns in children: aetiology and prevention. *Burns*. 2015;41(4):764–769. https://doi.org/10.1016/j.burns.2014.10.020.
13. Hundeshagen G, Milner SM. Chapter 41. Radiation injuries and vesicant burns. In: Herndon D, ed. *Total Burn Care*. 5th ed. Philadelphia, PA: Elsevier; 2017:414–421.
14. Hodgman EI, Pastorek RA, Saeman MR, et al. The Parkland Burn Center experience with 297 cases of child abuse from 1974 to 2010. *Burns*. 2016;42(5):1121–1127. https://doi.org/10.1016/j.burns.2016.02.013.
15. Rose JJ, Wang L, Xu Q, et al. Carbon monoxide poisoning: pathogenesis, management, and future directions of therapy. *Am J Respir Crit Care Med*. 2017;195(5):596–606.
16. Chambers SB, Garland K, Dai C, DeLyzer T. Adherence of burn outpatient clinic referrals to ABA criteria in a tertiary center: creating unnecessary referrals? *J Burn Care Res*. 2021;42(6):1275–1279. https://doi.org/10.1093/jbcr/irab117.
17. Sheridan RL. Fire-related inhalation injury. *N Engl J Med*. 2016;375(5):464–469.
18. Nielson CB, Duethman NC, Howard JM, Moncure M, Wood JG. Burns: pathophysiology of systemic complications and current management. *J Burn Care Res*. 2017;38(1):e469–e481. https://doi.org/10.1097/BCR.0000000000000355.
19. Gibran N. Chapter 15. Electrical injuries. In: Greenhalgh DG, ed. *Burn Care for General Surgeons and General Practitioners*. Switzerland: Springer International Publishing; 2016:193–200.
20. Kraft R, Herndon DN, Finnerty CC, Shahrokhi S. Jeschke. Occurrence of multiorgan dysfunction in pediatric burn patients: incidence and clinical outcome. *Ann Surg*. 2014;259(2):381–387. https://doi.org/10.1097/SLA.0b013e31828c4d04.
21. Gillenwater J, Garner W. Acute fluid management of large burns: pathophysiology, monitoring, and resuscitation. *Clin Plast Surg*. 2017;44(3):495–503. https://doi.org/10.1016/j.cps.2017.02.008.
22. Guilabert G, Usua G, Martin N, Abarca L, Barret JP, Colomina MJ. Fluid resuscitation management in patients with burns: update. *Br J Anaesth*. 2016;117(3):284–296. https://doi.org/10.1093/bja/aew266.
23. Lopez ON, Cambiaso-Daniel J, Branski LK, Norbury WB, Herndon DN. Predicting and managing sepsis in burn patients: current perspectives. *Ther Clin Risk Manag*. 2017;13:1107–1117. https://doi.org/10.2147/TCRM.S119938.
24. Nethery W, Warner P, Burkee P, Dwyer A, Zembrodt J, Fowler L. Efficacy of topical antimicrobial agents against bacterial isolates from burn wounds. *J Burn Care Res*. 2020;41(4):739–742. https://doi.org/10.1093/jbcr/iraa048.

25. Nherera LM, Trueman P, Roberts CD, Berg L. A systematic review and meta-analysis of clinical outcomes associated with nanocrystalline silver use compared to alternative silver delivery systems in the management of superficial and deep partial thickness burns. *Burns*. 2017;43(5):939–948. https://doi.org/10.1016/j.burns.2017.01.004.
26. Harats M, Kornhaber RA, Trodler G, Shoham Y, Haik J. 515 enzymatic debridement for burns: off label experience. *J Burn Care Res*. 2018;39(1):S230. https://doi.org/10.1093/jbcr/iry006.437.
27. Leon-Villapalos J, Dziewulski P. *Skin Autografting*. UpToDate; 2022. https://www.uptodate.com/contents/skin-autografting. Accessed September 14, 2023.
28. Clark A, Imran J, Madni T, Wolf SE. Nutrition and metabolism in burn patients. *Burns Trauma*. 2017;5:11. https://doi.org/10.1186/s41038-017-0076-x.
29. Wardhan R, Fahy BG. Regional anesthesia and acute pain management for adult patients with burns. *J Burn Care Res*. 2023;44(4):791–799. https://doi.org/10.1093/jbcr/irad069.
30. Schetzsle S, Lin WWC, Purushothaman P, Ding J, Kwan P, Tredget EE. Serial casting as an effective method for burn scar contracture rehabilitation: A case series. *J Burn Care Res*. 2023;44(5):1062–1072. https://doi.org/10.1093/jbcr/irad078.
31. Tredget EE, Shupp JW, Schneider JC. Scar management following burn injury. *J Burn Care Res*. 2017;38(3):146–147. https://doi.org/10.1097/BCR.0000000000000548.
32. Nedelec B, Carrougher GJ. Pain and pruritus post burn injury. *J Burn Care Res*. 2017;38(3):142–145. https://doi.org/10.1097/BCR.0000000000000534.
33. Brown EA, De Young A, Kimble R, Kenardy J. Review of a parent's influence on pediatric procedural distress and recovery. *Clin Child Fam Psychol Rev*. 2018;21(2):224–245. https://doi.org/10.1007/s10567-017-0252-3.
34. Tomtschik J, Sweitzer K, Cook C, O'Shea A, Bell D. Racial, ethnic, and socioeconomic disparities in burn care access: a single-center retrospective study. *J Burn Care Res*. 2023:irad109. https://doi.org/10.1093/jbcr/irad109.
35. Cox CA, Krout K, Navabi P, Markiewitz ND, McColl M, Caffre J. 9 Prevalence of burnout syndrome in burn center clinical staff. *J Burn Care Res*. 2018;39(S1):S9. https://doi.org/10.1093/jbcr/iry006.013.

35

Organ Donation and Transplantation

Schawnté P. Williams-Taylor, Teresa J. Shafer, Gabriela Oro, Tara Jean Redwantz, Melissa Voltz, Ellen Arce, and Roy Lee

http://evolve.elsevier.com/Urden/CriticalCareNursing

Organ transplantation provides the only opportunity for patients with end-stage organ disease to have an enhanced quality of life and an extended survival. Organ transplantation is accepted as often the only treatment option for some end-stage organ disease. Success rates in patients treated, as well as increases in organ donation, have improved as the field of organ donation and transplantation has evolved.[1] Such evolution has come as a result of increased cultural acceptance of brain death, donation, and transplantation; legal and political efforts to facilitate organ donation; improved procurement and allocation processes; advances in organ preservation, organ recovery, surgical techniques in transplantation, immunology, and immunosuppression; and management of infectious diseases.[2]

ORGAN DONATION

In the United States, more than 103,000 people are waiting for a lifesaving organ transplant (Fig. 35.1).[3] In 2022, the *Organ Procurement Transplant Network* (OPTN) reported 21,372 donors, of which 14,905 were deceased donors and 6467 were living donors. The categories of organ donors are described in Table 35.1. In total, 46,325 transplants were performed in 2022. This number is encouraging, although insufficient, as one patient is added to a transplant waiting list every 10 minutes.[3] It is also vital to ensure that that all members of society have equitable access to organ donation and transplantation.[4] Ongoing collaboration between organ procurement organizations; transplant centers; and critical care nurses, physicians, and other health care workers is necessary to have a significant effect in saving lives through organ, tissue and eye donation, and transplantation.

Role of the Critical Care Nurse in Organ Donation

The critical care nurse is an essential member of the team in the donation process, linking the hospital to the *organ procurement organization* (OPO), physicians, and families of potential donors. The Centers for Medicare and Medicaid Services (CMS) guidelines, The Joint Commission standards, and hospital policies require that patients meeting criteria for imminent death and cardiac death be referred to an OPO in a timely manner.[5] Once the notification has been made, nurses must follow the established donation policies for their hospital in accordance with federal guidelines and state laws. Hospitals will already have worked with their federally designated OPO to develop their hospital policy to ensure that it meets these regulations and laws.

Continued hemodynamic support is necessary during the process of declaration of brain death. Patients progressing to brain death undergo many physiologic changes that can compromise the viability of organs for transplantation. Ensuring that oxygenation and perfusion of the organs is maintained along with electrolyte and acid–base balance preserves the opportunity for donation.

Collaboration between the nurse and the OPO staff is necessary to protect the rights of the patient, who may already have made the decision to donate by indicating his or her decision on a donor registry. After declaration of death, the family is informed that the patient has died. OPO staff will already have checked the donor registry to determine whether the individual is a donor and, if so, will inform the family of such and what and how the donation will proceed. If the patient has not made the first-person decision to be a donor, the OPO staff will have a donation conversation with the family to inform of what can be donated. The family can then make the decision about donation.

Because organ donation and transplantation are now mainstream, families often talk about donation well in advance of brain death declaration because they anticipate the direction in which the patient's condition is proceeding. Exactly when donation is discussed varies, and the nurse should be flexible and attentive to the family's informational needs, ensuring first and foremost that the experts, the OPO staff, are there to guide the information-giving process.

During the interval after pronouncement of death and until donation authorization is obtained either by checking the donor registry or by receiving authorization from the family, medical management of the potential donor is continued by the medical and nursing staff, as required by state law and the *Uniform Anatomical Gift Act*. After authorization for donation, the OPO assumes the care of the donor, providing direction for medical management. The goal of medical management of the patient shifts toward optimal preservation of organ function so that the organs are suitable for transplant.

After death of the patient, nurses and OPO staff together advocate for their patient by ensuring the patient's donation decision is honored or, if the patient had not made such a decision during his or her lifetime, upholding the family's right to be offered the opportunity to donate organs and tissues.[6] Once authorization (formerly known as *consent*) is obtained, the OPO coordinator and nurse collaborate on management of the donor according to established donor management protocols. Such protocols include managing fluid and electrolyte imbalances secondary to brain death. Patients commonly have a low circulating volume or high serum sodium levels, as hypertonic sodium may have been administered to prevent brain herniation. The donor management phase corrects deficits in the

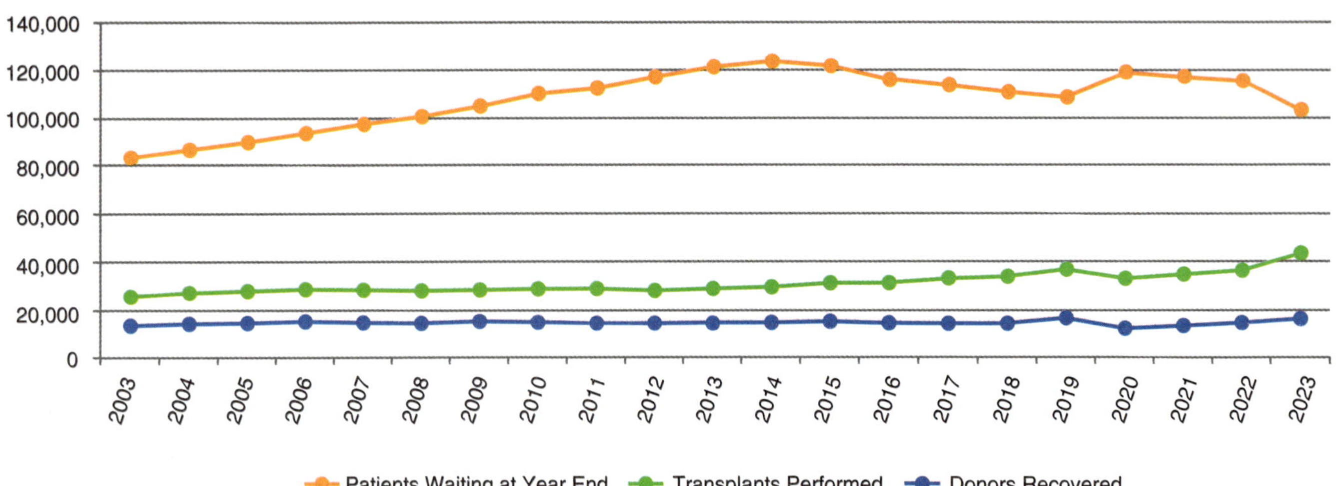

FIG. 35.1 Growth in U.S. Transplant Waiting List Outpaces Growth in Deceased Organ Donors. (2020 data are through October 25, 2020.). ((From Department of Health and Human Services. Organ Procurement Transplant Network. Statistics. http://optn.transplant.hrsa.gov/.) Accessed October 25, 2020.)

TABLE 35.1 Categories of Organ Donors

Brain-dead donor	Donor declared dead by neurologic criteria for brain death.
Donation after cardiac death	Donor declared dead by circulatory criteria for death.
Living related donor	Living family member related by blood who donates a kidney, portion of the liver, pancreas, intestine, or lung to another family member.
Living, unrelated donor (directed/nondirected)	Living individual not related to a patient requiring a transplant who donates a kidney, portion of the liver, pancreas, intestine, or lung to another individual. The donor may be anonymous or altruistic.
Living donor, paired donation	Allocated paired kidney exchange or paired exchange involves two pairs of living kidney donors and transplant candidates who do not have matching blood types. The two candidates "trade" donors so that each candidate receives a kidney from a donor with compatible blood type.

From United Network for Organ Sharing (UNOS) https://unos.org and the Oran Procurement and Transplant Network (OPTN) https://optn.transplant.hrsa.gov. Accessed October 25, 2023.

patient's physiologic status to provide optimal organ function before surgical recovery and preservation. Compassionate nursing care encompasses skilled donor management and continued support of the family.[6]

The critical care nurse monitors and records vital signs, intake and output, and oxygenation status; obtains specimens for laboratory tests; and assists with central line insertions and multiple diagnostic assessments such as chest radiograph, bronchoscopy, electrocardiogram (ECG), or echocardiogram to evaluate organ function. The donor management phase of the donation process starts after brain death and continues until the patient is taken to the operating room and organs are recovered.

Educational initiatives to increase the attitudes and knowledge of health care professionals can impact outcomes in organ donation and transplantation.[7] It is important that nurses are knowledgeable about the organ donation process. Nurses must assess their own beliefs that pertain to organ donation because the attitude of the nurse and care given to the family can affect the outcome of the donation.

Organ Procurement Organization as Part of the Health Care Team

Organ procurement organizations in partnership with hospitals must develop effective donation programs as required by federal regulations. Building an effective donation program requires collaboration and commitment from nurses, physicians, respiratory therapists, social workers, pastoral care, and the OPO.

The U.S. federal government has made clear the responsibility placed on hospitals to actively engage and work through the donation process with OPOs, identifying and making referrals to the OPO while the OPO is managing the donor assessment, obtaining authorization, donor management and optimization of end organ function, allocating organs, and facilitating the recovery process. It is also important for the health care team to be knowledgeable of the donation pathways and to notify the OPO in a timely manner.

Nurses and other members of the health care team are key in providing care and support to families. In preparing for the donation conversation with potential donor families it is important that huddles occur to plan for meeting with the family.[8]

A retrospective observational study showed increased authorization rates by implementing a standardized effective request process. Key elements of the standardized effective request process include:

- Timely referral to the OPO
- Development of a huddle
- Declaration of death by neurological criteria in a brain-dead patient, or in death by circulatory criteria
- A donation conversation does not occur until the family has made a decision to proceed to comfort care
- Enactment of the agreed-upon plan established in the huddle[9]

National Donation and Transplantation Laws

Organ transplantation is the only medical and surgical therapy that is regulated entirely by law. From donation to

TABLE 35.2 National Organ Donation and Transplantation Laws

Laws	Type	First Enacted
Uniform Anatomical Gift Act (UAGA)	State law	1968; revised in 1987 and 2006
National Organ Transplant Act (NOTA)	Federal law	1984
Uniform Determination of Death Act (UDDA)	State laws	1980
Hospital conditions of participation—organ donation; Centers for Medicare and Medicaid Services (CMS)	Federal regulation	1998
Medical examiner laws preventing or restricting ability of medical examiner or coroner to deny organ donation	State laws	Year varies by state
Omnibus Budget Reconciliation Act (OBRA)	Federal law	1986

transplantation, the federal government, and to some extent state governments, monitor the administrative and financial aspects of this process. These regulations ensure that organs are shared on a fair and equitable basis. In addition, the responsibilities and functions of health care professionals are sanctioned and safeguarded by these laws so that their responsibilities may be discharged with assurance and protection medically, legally, and ethically. The major laws are listed in Table 35.2.

Uniform Anatomical Gift Act

The Uniform Anatomical Gift Act of 1968 established the legal framework for organ and tissue donation and donor designation, as well as the priority of legal next-of-kin for authorization in the absence of donor designation. It required that the physician pronouncing or certifying death may not in any way participate in the procedures for removing or transplanting anatomic gifts. It also protects health care professionals from liability associated with donation. The act was later amended to require hospitals to establish agreements with an OPO to coordinate recovery. It prohibits the sale or purchase of organs or tissues. This act clarifies who can provide authorization for donation in the absence of known donor wishes.[10]

Uniform Determination of Death Act

The Uniform Determination of Death Act of 1981 states that an individual is dead who has sustained either:

- Irreversible cessation of circulatory and respiratory functions
- Irreversible cessation of all functions of the entire brain, including the brainstem

A determination of death must be made in accordance with accepted medical standards. Most states have adopted similarly worded Determination of Death Acts in their state statutes.

National Organ Transplant Act

The National Organ Transplant Act of 1984 mandated the establishment of the national OPTN. The *United Network for Organ Sharing* (UNOS) administers the national contract to operate the OPTN and houses the database that contains the list of waiting recipients nationwide and by which all donor and recipient matches are determined. This act also made it illegal to buy or sell organs and tissues.

Omnibus Budget Reconciliation Act

The Omnibus Budget Reconciliation Act requires OPOs to coordinate the recovery and transplantation process at local levels and requires hospitals to be affiliated with a federally mandated OPO. There is only one designated OPO per service area. This act gave families the right to know about organ and tissue donation by mandating that all hospitals participating in the CMS reimbursement program institute a "required request" policy to ensure that families of potential donors are made aware of the option of organ or tissue donation and their option to decline. Hospitals must have a signed agreement with an OPO, tissue bank, and eye bank.[5]

Medical Examiner/Coroner State Laws

Before 1994, thousands of lives were lost because of medical examiner and coroners (ME/C) denial of medically suitable organs for transplantation. There were only three states with laws that addressed the issue of ME/C prevention of potential organ donors from donating medically suitable transplantable organs. In 1992 it was estimated that 1223 (11.4% of ME/C cases) organs were denied recovery for waiting patients by ME/Cs.[11] Since that time, ME/C laws require or encourage the release of organs for transplantation. In some states, medical examiners or justices of the peace cannot deny organ donation under any circumstances. In other states, they cannot deny organ donation unless the ME/C is physically present at the donation surgery viewing the organ(s). In situations such as these, the ME/C may request a biopsy while in surgery. These state laws were passed to provide protection for recipients waiting at centers so that every possible organ that can be recovered is being recovered to save a life (see Table 35.2). Since 1994, after numerous publications and intense focus from multiple parties to address the problem.[12,13] this has saved the lives of thousands of patients waiting. The number of organs lost should be "zero"; with continued work, eventually all states will have these laws, resulting in even more lives saved.

Overview of the Donation Process

The CMS requires hospitals to notify their respective OPOs of all deaths, including patients meeting imminent death criteria and cardiac death, to increase the potential for organ, tissue, and eye donation. The types of organ donor referrals made to the OPO are listed in Table 35.3. All patients meeting imminent death criteria must be referred within the agreed-on time (usually within 1 hour) of meeting criteria. All cardiac deaths must be referred, regardless of age, medical condition, or cause of death.[5] The nurse or hospital designee makes the initial call to the OPO to provide demographic information, admitting diagnosis, and current neurologic status of the patient. Most OPOs have either in-house staff or on-call coordinators who respond to the initial referral call from the hospital. On site, the OPO coordinator communicates with the bedside nurse and physicians involved in the care of the patient to obtain information about the patient's present hospital course, the past medical history, and the plan of care.

Determining medical suitability is solely the responsibility of the OPO. Speaking to the family about donation is also the responsibility of the OPO, unless designated requestors at the hospital have been trained to do so.[5]

TABLE 35.3 Types of Referrals to the Organ Procurement Organization

ORGAN REFERRAL		TISSUE REFERRAL
Brain Death	**Donation After Circulatory Determination of Death**	**Cardiac Arrest**
Irreversible, nonsurvivable brain injury. Patient currently maintained on a ventilator. Tests performed to confirm brain death (e.g., clinical examination, apnea test). First-person authorization/authorizing agent gives authorization for donation. Patient is maintained in critical care unit while donation evaluation and work-up is completed. To operating room for organ recovery. Organ donors may also donate tissue and corneas.	Irreversible, nonsurvivable brain injury. Patient currently maintained on a ventilator. Any ventilator-dependent patient where plans are to forego life-sustaining treatment. Patient has not progressed to brain death. Family decides to withdraw life-sustaining therapies. Family authorizes donation. Patient is extubated, circulatory arrest within 60–90 min, rapid recovery of organs in operating room. Organ donors may also donate tissue and corneas.	Patient may or may not have sustained a brain injury. Patient not currently on a ventilator. No cardiac or respiratory activity. First-person authorization/authorizing agent gives authorization for donation. May donate tissue and corneas (e.g., bone, heart valves, skin).

Types of Referrals

Two types of referrals are discussed:

- Brain dead: Death by neurological criteria
- Cardiac death: Death by circulatory criteria

Death by Neurological Criteria

Imminent death referral criteria for patients with severe acute brain injury include:

- Mechanical ventilation dependent
- In a critical care unit or emergency department
- Clinical findings consistent with a low Glasgow Coma Score, typically 5 or less
- Physicians are evaluating a diagnosis of brain death or have ordered that life-sustaining therapies be withdrawn, pursuant to the family's decision[8]

Patients meeting the imminent death referral criteria may be or become brain dead (discussed later in chapter), resulting in *donation after brain death* (DBD), also known as death by neurological criteria.

Patients declared dead by neurologic criteria constitute only 1% of total deaths in the United States.

Cardiac Death

Cardiac death referrals provide the opportunity for patients to be tissue and eye donors (discussed later in chapter) after cardiac asystole. Because of the relatively rare occurrence of brain death or withdrawal of treatment, many more deceased patients could have the opportunity to donate tissue and eyes. Transplantable tissues include bone, skin, fascia, cartilage, tendons, ligaments, saphenous veins, heart valves, eyes, and corneas.

The decision to withdraw life-sustaining therapies, whether because of an advance directive or surrogate decision making, must always be separated from the organ donation decision. When a patient from whom treatment is being withdrawn has also executed a legal document or gift (as a document or gift or on a donor registry), that legal document must be honored, regardless of the mode of death, whether brain death or cardiac circulatory death. To accomplish both compassionate end-of-life care and the patient's goal of donation, the withdrawal of life-sustaining therapies and family support need to be carefully coordinated.

Donor Evaluation

Once the initial call is made to the OPO, an organ coordinator will contact the critical care nurse and request specific information regarding the patient's age; sex; race; neurologic, ventilatory, and hemodynamic status; as well as the hospital's plan of care. On site, the OPO coordinator will assess the patient and review the medical records, history of the current hospitalization, and major procedures to obtain information on surgeries, therapies, current medications, past medical history, laboratory values specific to each organ, pulmonary status, systemic infection, diagnostic reports, and hemodynamic status.[14] The time between brain death declaration and organ procurement is often marked by significant hemodynamic instability. During this time, optimal medical management is crucial to ensure posttransplant graft survival.

If the patient is not brain dead or there are no plans to withdraw or decelerate support, the OPO coordinator collaborates with the critical care nurse on a follow-up plan for ongoing evaluation. The OPO continues to follow the patient until the patient meets neurologic criteria for brain death, death is declared, or there is a plan to withdraw life-sustaining therapies. Many patients referred to the OPO do not become donors because they do not meet brain death criteria or there are no plans to withdraw life-sustaining therapies, as the patient's status may improve.

Brain Death

Brain death is the irreversible cessation of all brain functions including the brainstem. The clinical diagnosis of brain death is based on guidelines established by the American Academy of Neurology. The practice of brain death declaration varies based on hospital policy and state legislation. Neurologists, neurosurgeons, intensivists, and anesthesiologists usually perform the brain death evaluation. Before establishing brain death, certain conditions must be confirmed, including the cause and the irreversibility of coma and confounding factors such as the following:

- Absence of severe hypothermia, defined as a core temperature of 32°C or less
- Absence of hypotension, defined as a systolic blood pressure of 90 mm Hg or less
- Absence of evidence of illicit drug abuse, defined by a careful history, calculation of clearance, and, if needed, a normal drug screen
- Absence of recent or current administration of neuromuscular-blocking medications, defined by the presence of four twitches with maximal ulnar nerve stimulation by a train-of-four peripheral nerve stimulation, as shown in Fig. 20.17 in Chapter 20.

- Absence of electrolyte, acid–base, or endocrine dysfunction, as defined by severe acidosis and marked deviation from normal values.

Clinical Examination for Brain Death

The bedside clinical examination has three components:
1. Absence of cerebral motor reflexes
2. Absence of brainstem reflexes
3. Absence of respiratory drive

Cerebral Motor Responses

Cerebral motor responses to pain in all extremities are absent in brain death. These motor responses can be stimulated by the application of pressure to the nail beds or supraorbital ridge. Some motor responses may occur spontaneously during apnea testing because of the presence of hypoxia or hypotension and are considered spinal cord reflexes. These may also be elicited in the presence of respiratory acidosis and can include spontaneous flexion and muscle stretch reflexes in the arms and legs that can resemble grasping movements. It is important to determine whether the patient has been given any neuromuscular blocking medications that may induce pharmacologic motor weakness.

Brainstem Reflexes

Brainstem reflexes that are tested include pupillary signs, ocular movements, facial sensory and motor responses, and pharyngeal and tracheal reflexes.

Pupillary Reflexes

Pupillary signs are evaluated by absence of the light reflex, which is consistent with brain death. Most often, the pupils are round, oval, or irregularly shaped, although dilated pupils may remain even after brain death has occurred. This dilation may exist if the sympathetic cervical pathways to the pupillary dilator muscle are intact. Medications do not normally alter pupil response, although the application of topical medications or severe trauma to the eye may affect pupil reactivity.[15]

Oculocephalic Reflex

Ocular movements are lost with brain death. The oculocephalic reflex, also described as *doll's eyes*, involves fast turning of the head to both sides. In brain death, this should not generate any eye movements. Neck movements should be avoided in patients with a traumatic brain injury or cervical spine injury.

Oculovestibular Reflex

Because the oculovestibular reflex is tested using ice water or normal saline, it is sometimes called *cold calorics*. The head of the bed is elevated 30 degrees, and approximately 50 mL of ice water or normal saline is injected into the ear; no movement of the eye toward the side of the stimulus should be present. It is recommended that the patient be observed for up to 1 minute after each ear irrigation, and 5 minutes should be allowed before testing the opposite ear. Medications that can influence the oculovestibular reflex include sedatives, aminoglycosides, tricyclic antidepressants, anticholinergics, and antiseizure agents.

Corneal and Jaw Reflexes

Facial sensory and motor responses are elicited by testing for corneal and jaw reflexes. Stroking a cotton-tipped swab gently across the cornea tests the corneal reflexes. Grimacing in response to pain can be elicited by applying deep pressure to the nail beds, the supraorbital ridge, or the temporomandibular joint. Severe trauma within these areas could inhibit interpretation of facial brainstem reflexes.[16]

Gag and Cough Reflexes

Pharyngeal and tracheal reflexes are absent in patients with brain death. The gag reflex can be evaluated by stimulating the posterior part of the pharynx with a tongue blade. The cough reflex can be tested with bronchial suctioning.[17]

Apnea Testing

The loss of brainstem function results in the loss of centrally controlled breathing with resultant apnea. The respiratory neurons are controlled by cerebral chemoreceptors that sense changes in the arterial partial pressure of carbon dioxide ($PaCO_2$) and pH of the cerebrospinal fluid that accurately reflect changes in plasma $PaCO_2$.

Guidelines for determination of death recommend achieving $PaCO_2$ levels greater than 60 mm Hg for maximal stimulation of brainstem respiratory centers. Prerequisites and the procedure for apnea testing are outlined in Box 35.1. The prerequisites that should be addressed before the apnea test are to prevent cardiac dysrhythmias, hypotension, and decreased oxygen saturation. If any of these conditions occur during the apnea test, the test should be aborted and additional brain death confirmatory testing should be performed (Box 35.2). In cases where a patient is a carbon dioxide retainer or the clinical examination is unreliable

BOX 35.1 Apnea Test

Prerequisites

- Normothermia
- Systolic blood pressure ≥90 mm Hg
- Euvolemia
- Eucapnia
- Normoxemia

Procedure

- Pulse oximeter is connected to the patient to monitor oxygen saturation.
- Preoxygenate for 10 min with fraction of inspired oxygen of 100%.
- Reduce ventilation frequency to 10 breaths/min and reduce positive end-expiratory pressure to 5 cm H_2O.
- If pulse oximetry oxygen saturation remains >90%, obtain baseline arterial blood gas, including arterial partial pressure of carbon dioxide ($PaCO_2$), pH, bicarbonate, and base excess.
- Disconnect ventilator.
- Place a cannula at the level of the carina and deliver 100% O_2, 6 L/min.
- Observe closely for respiratory movements for 8 to 10 min. Respiration is defined as abdominal or chest excursions that produce adequate tidal volumes.
- Abort if blood pressure remains <90 mm Hg systolic or declining despite increasing vasopressors.
- Abort if oxygen saturation is <80% for 2 min or drops steadily (consider retry with T-piece and continuous positive airway pressure).
- If no breathing drive is observed, measure arterial partial pressure of oxygen, $PaCO_2$, and pH after approximately 8 min.
- If respiratory movements are absent and $PaCO_2$ is ≥60 mm Hg (or 20 mm Hg increase in $PaCO_2$ over a baseline normal $PaCO_2$), the apnea test result is positive (i.e., it supports the clinical diagnosis of brain death).
- If the patient breathes, repeat test a few hours later.

From Wijdicks EFM. The clinical diagnosis of brain death. In: *The Comatose Patient*. Oxford University Press; 2008.

BOX 35.2 Confirmatory Tests in Brain Death

Cerebral Angiography

- Contrast medium under high pressure in both anterior and posterior circulation injections
- No intracerebral filling at the level of the carotid or vertebral artery entry to the skull
- Patent external carotid circulation
- Possible delayed filling of superior longitudinal sinus

Electroencephalography

- Minimum of eight scalp electrodes
- Electrode dependencies should be between 100 and 10,000
- Integrity of entire recording system should be tested
- Electrode distances should be at least 10 cm
- Sensitivity should be increased to at least 2 microvolts for 30 min with inclusion of appropriate calibrations
- High-frequency filter setting should be at 30 Hz, and low-frequency setting should not be below 1 Hz
- There should be no electroencephalographic reactivity to intense somatosensory or audiovisual stimuli

Transcranial Doppler Ultrasonography

- Bilateral insonation
- The probe is placed at the temporal bone above the zygomatic arch or the vertebrobasilar arteries through the suboccipital transcranial window
- The abnormalities should include a lack of diastolic or reverberating flow, small systolic peaks in early systole, and a lack of flow found by the investigator who previously demonstrated normal velocities

Cerebral Scintigraphy (Technetium Tc-99m Exametazime)

- Injection of isotope within 30 min of reconstitution
- Static image of 500,000 counts at several time intervals: immediately, between 30 and 60 min, and at 2 h
- Correct intravenous injection needs to be confirmed with additional liver images demonstrating uptake (optional)

This information is based on the American Academy of Neurology Guidelines. From Wijdicks EFM. The clinical diagnosis of brain death. In: *The Comatose Patient.* Oxford University Press; 2008.

because of head trauma, confirmatory testing is necessary. Confirmatory testing is mandatory in children.

Confirmatory Tests

Additional confirmatory testing for the determination of brain death may include cerebral angiography, electroencephalography, transcranial Doppler, and cerebral scintigraphy, although these diagnostic procedures are not required (see Box 35.2).

Donation After Circulatory Determination of Death

Patients not meeting all necessary criteria for brain death, but who have a nonsurvivable injury when the family and physician have made the decision to withdraw life support, are potential donors after circulatory death determination. Donation after *circulatory determination of death* (DCD) is based on the cessation of circulatory and respiratory functions.[18] Previously, DCD donors were known as non–heart-beating donors, asystolic donors, or donation after cardiac death donors. Patients who do not meet brain death criteria but have a nonsurvivable condition such as a catastrophic neurologic injury, high spinal cord injury, or a medical condition requiring mechanical ventilation are candidates for DCD. Organs are recovered after cardiac asystole and a 3- to 5-minute wait period. Cardiac asystole must occur within 60 to 90 minutes for organ donation to occur. Before the enactment of brain death laws in the 1970s, all organ donors were DCD donors. Interest in DCD has increased because of (1) family interest in organ donation when neurologic criteria for brain death have not been met and (2) the continued national demand for organs.[4,19]

Controlled Donation After Circulatory Determination of Death

DCD donors are classified as *controlled* or *uncontrolled DCD donors*. Controlled DCD occurs when the family has already decided to withdraw life-sustaining support and death is declared at the time of circulatory arrest. In controlled DCD, families, health care providers, and OPO staff are involved in the timing and planning of the time when support will be withdrawn.[17]

Uncontrolled Donation After Circulatory Determination of Death

Uncontrolled DCD describes a situation in which cardiac arrest has occurred and resuscitation efforts are determined to be futile. The uncontrolled DCD process is rapid, as the patient is undergoing cardiopulmonary resuscitation. After authorization from the family, the patient is taken to the operating room for immediate recovery of organs, primarily kidneys.

Uncontrolled DCD is an opportunity to increase the number of organs available for transplantation; however, there is a higher incidence of primary graft nonfunction and delayed graft function.[20]

Outcomes in Donation After Circulatory Death

There has been a paradigm shift in organ preservation methods to utilize machine perfusion devices to improve organ transplantation outcomes. With the use of normothermic regional perfusion, outcomes in donation after circulatory death have shown overall patient and graft survival is favorable in liver, kidney, and lung transplantation.[20]

The normothermic regional perfusion technique allows oxygenated blood to perfuse to the abdomen (abdominal normothermic regional perfusion) and to the chest and abdomen (thoracoabdominal regional perfusion). This also allows more time for surgeons to evaluate the organs while in situ.[21]

Traditionally delayed graft nonfunction in DCD donation is higher when normothermic perfusion is not utilized in comparison to brain dead donors. The use of normothermic regional perfusion has expanded graft utilization and optimized transplantation outcomes for heart, lung, liver, pancreas, and kidneys.[20]

Authorization for Donation

"Presumed consent" is the donation law in some European countries.[22] This is a system in which a person is deemed a donor after death unless they have specifically indicated they do not want to be a donor. This is not the law in the United States. The United States retains a voluntary system, often referred to as *opting-in*.[22] The architecture of U.S. organ donation law, also termed *Gift Law*, is the Uniform Anatomical Gift Act, which is enacted in all 50 states.[23,24] The OPO coordinator is an advocate for the donor/donor family and potential recipients. Many factors are important in working with potential donor families. The nurse and OPO coordinator are important in providing a safe, comfortable environment for families in a position to make decisions about donation. Assessing the needs of the family is crucial to the outcome of the donation conversation. The timing of the conversation is also important; donation does not consist of simply asking the family if they wish to donate. The critical care nurse should inform the family that an expert member of the health care team is available to provide information and answer their questions about donation.[8,9] Research indicates that families who are satisfied with their hospital experience are more predisposed to donate. Receiving timely information is critical to families' satisfaction with their hospital experience.[25,26]

Many myths and misconceptions surround organ donation. Common misconceptions from families surround religious beliefs, cultural milieus, concerns about possible body disfigurement, concerns about the ability to have an open casket funeral, and costs to the family. Another common misperception is that hospital staff will not attempt to save the life of their loved one if they believe the patient could be a donor. These misperceptions must be debunked with the family.[27] Finally, research has shown that the way the donation request is made is an important factor in a family's ultimate decision, regardless of preexisting attitudes. Many families report that donation has helped their healing in the grieving process and say that donation represents something positive in their loss.[28]

Donor Management

The donor management phase includes ongoing collaboration between the OPO coordinator and OPO medical director, critical care nurse, intensivist, respiratory therapist, and transplant professionals to ensure optimal preservation of organ function for organ recovery and transplantation. Standing orders for the care of an organ donor are provided by the OPO. These encompass required testing and screening of donors, as well as parameters for continued medical management of the cadaveric donor, as listed in Box 35.3. The goals of donor management are to maximize oxygenation and provide optimal organ perfusion to maintain the viability of organs for transplantation.

BOX 35.3 Donor Care Protocols

The Organ Procurement Organization (OPO) coordinator should write orders to initiate standard donor care.

1. Transfer care to [Name of OPO].
2. Discontinue all prior orders.
3. Assess blood pressure, heart rate, temperature, urine output, central venous pressure (CVP) (if central venous catheter present), pulmonary artery occlusion pressure (PAOP) (if pulmonary artery [PA] catheter present) every hour.
4. Reorder mechanical ventilator parameters as previously set.
5. Maintain head of bed at 30 to 40 degrees elevation.
6. Continue routine pulmonary suctioning and side-to-side body positioning.
7. Warming blanket to maintain body temperature above 36.5°C.
8. Maintain sequential compression devices.
9. Continue chest tube suction or water seal as previously ordered (if present).
10. Nasogastric (orogastric) tube to low intermittent suction (if present).
11. Intravenous fluid: dextrose 5% in 0.45% saline plus 20 mEq potassium chloride per liter at 75 mL/h.
12. Call OPO coordinator if mean arterial pressure is <70 mm Hg, systolic pressure is >170 mm Hg, heart rate is <60 or >130 beats/min, temperature is <36.5°C or >37.8°C, urine output is <75 or >250 mL/h, or CVP or PAOP is <8 or >18 mm Hg.
13. Medications:
    - Pantoprazole 40 mg intravenously every 24 h, first dose now
    - Artificial tears every 1 h and as needed to prevent corneal drying
    - Albuterol and Atrovent unit dose per aerosol every 4 h
    - Antibiotics previously ordered continued at same dose and frequency
    - Vasoactive medication infusions (dopamine, norepinephrine) at previously ordered concentrations and infusion rates
14. Review all medications previously ordered. Most anticonvulsants, pain medications, laxatives, gastrointestinal motility agents, eye drops, antihypertensives, antinausea agents, subcutaneous heparin, osmotic agents (mannitol), and diuretics are unnecessary during donor care and will be discontinued automatically with order number 2 above. Review any other medications in question with the physician.
15. Send electrolytes, magnesium, ionized calcium, complete blood count, platelets, glucose, blood urea nitrogen, creatinine, phosphorus, arterial blood gas, prothrombin time/international normalized ratio, and partial thromboplastin time STAT and repeat every 4 h.
16. Send blood for type and screen with above blood draw (if not previously done).
17. Fingerstick blood glucose every 2 h; call OPO coordinator if blood glucose <90 or >180 mg/dL.
18. Order electrocardiogram STAT.
19. Order radiography STAT with indication "initial donor evaluation."
20. Add other orders for specific organ evaluation as indicated.
21. The above order set provides a "safety net" of call orders so that the coordinator is alerted to significant changes in donor status. It also prescribes the foundation for ongoing monitoring of physiologic and laboratory variables.

Modified from Powner DJ, O'Connor KJ. Adult clinical donor care. In: LaPointe-Rudow D, Ohler L, Shafer TJ, eds. *A Clinician's Guide to Donation and Transplantation.* Applied Measurement Professionals; 2006.

Donor Management Goals

Donor management goals are preset critical care end points used to increase the number of organs transplanted per donor, as listed in Table 35.4. The Health Resources and Services Administration has advocated for the implementation of donor management goals by OPOs.[29,30]

Patients with critical neurologic impairment present with many clinical challenges: including

- Hypotension
- Diabetes insipidus
- Disseminated intravascular coagulation
- Heart dysrhythmias
- Pulmonary edema
- Metabolic acidosis

There is increasing evidence that control of these pathophysiologic changes by active clinical management increases the number and quality of organs available for transplantation, which ultimately affects the potential recipient.[31,32] Further assessment of the donor by the OPO coordinator includes screening for any transmissible diseases, including serologic tests for infectious diseases such as human immunodeficiency virus (HIV), hepatitis, syphilis, cytomegalovirus (CMV), and Epstein-Barr virus. The OPO coordinator conducts a medical-social history questionnaire with the authorizing person or others who can provide information on the donor's past medical and social history. The questionnaire comprises standard questions about the donor's past behavioral, medical, social, and sexual health. These survey questions are approved by UNOS, by the U.S. Food and Drug Administration, and by other accrediting agencies for organ and tissue donation.

Organ Allocation

The OPTN is responsible for operating the national database, which lists all patients waiting for an organ transplant in the

TABLE 35.4 Donor Management Clinical Parameters

Parameter	Clinical Goal
1. Mean arterial pressure	60–100 mm Hg
2. Central venous pressure	4–10 mm Hg
3. Ejection fraction	>50%
4. Vasopressors	<1 and low dose
5. Arterial blood gas pH	7.3–7.45
6. PaO_2/FiO_2 ratio	>300
7. Serum sodium	135–155 mEq/L
8. Blood glucose	<150 mg/dL
9. Urine output (averaged over 4 h)	0.5–3.0 mL/kg/h over 4 h

FiO_2, Fraction of inspired oxygen; *PaO_2*, arterial partial pressure of oxygen.

United States. The UNOS manages the national list. The OPO coordinator accesses the UNOS computer to generate a donor-specific list of potential recipients from the national list. Potential recipients are matched with the donor based on blood type, height, weight, human leukocyte antigen (HLA), distance from the donor, waiting time on the list, and severity of illness. The national system in place for organ allocation is fair and equitable for patients requiring a transplant. The list does not reference race, sex, or socioeconomic status. Organs are offered electronically to the transplant team of the first person on the list. If the organ is refused for any reason, the transplant hospital of the next patient on the list is contacted. The process continues until a match is made. Once a patient is selected and contacted and all testing is complete, surgery is scheduled, and the transplant takes place.

Organ Recovery

Once all recipients have been identified, the OPO coordinator schedules the operating room time and coordinates arrival of the surgical recovery teams for organ retrieval. The OPO coordinator and critical care nurse coordinate the transport, collaborating with operating room and anesthesiology staff. The nurse ensures the donor is connected to a transport monitor; oxygen and emergency medications must be available. In the operating room, hemodynamic support and continued medical management are coordinated among the OPO staff, anesthesiologist, and recovery surgeons.

Organs are first flushed with preservative solution containing electrolytes and nutrients. The organs are then removed from the donor, examined individually in a sterile basin, and packed in sterile containers for transport. For heart, heart and lung, and lungs, transport is immediate. For pancreas and liver, time to transplant ranges from 6 to 20 hours. For kidneys, approximately 24 hours may elapse before transplantation. Tissue typing is primarily carried out between kidney and pancreas donors and recipients and is less common among heart, heart and lung, and single-lung donors and recipients.

Tissue Donation

Families can save many lives through tissue and eye donation. This donation could affect the lives of 60 to 80 individuals awaiting tissue transplantation. There are approximately 40,000 tissue donors per year, and an estimated 2.5 million Americans receive tissue transplants each year, from sight-saving corneas, heart valves, musculoskeletal tissue as bone grafts and tendons, skin, nerve, and vascular tissue. Patients with cardiac death can donate tissues if deemed medically suitable after further evaluation and screening by tissue organizations working with the OPO. After the authorization process, if tissue recovery is going to be delayed, it is imperative that the body of the donor is cooled. The American Association of Tissue Banks standards require that tissue be recovered within 24 hours of cardiac death, provided that the body has received sufficient cooling. The recovery of tissue is performed in the operating room using sterile technique. Donors may be both organ and tissue donors, with tissue recovery following organ recovery. OPO-trained specialists perform the recovery and bring the necessary supplies required for tissue recovery. Hospital operating room staff are not required for tissue recovery.[33]

Organ Donation Nursing Responsibility

Organ and tissue donation save lives. Critical care nurses are in a unique position to affect the lives of many patients—patients who can give the gift of life and patients awaiting a lifesaving transplant. Nurses collaborate closely with the OPO to honor the decision of patients and their families. Nursing care does not stop when a patient meets the criteria to become an organ donor. Provision of expert nursing care, compassion, and support of families facing end-of-life decisions is part of daily nursing practice.

IMMUNOLOGY OF TRANSPLANTATION

Organ transplantation has become a widely accepted treatment for end-stage heart, lung, liver, kidney, and pancreatic disease. Significant advancements have been achieved in the realms of organ recovery and conservation, surgical methodologies, as well as the prevention, detection, and management of rejection. Ultimately, the long-term success of transplantation depends on the immune system's tolerance for the transplanted organ. Virtually every cell in the human body carries distinctive molecules that enable the immune system to distinguish self from nonself. An intact immune system recognizes and eliminates any foreign biologic material recognized as nonself. Successful organ transplantation requires suppression or downregulation of the immune response. To best understand the principles of immunosuppressive therapy, it is important to have some understanding of the cells of the immune system, the immune response, and the process of organ rejection.

Immune System

Whenever the body is presented with a substance recognized as nonself, a primary immune response is elicited. There are three phases of any primary immune response:

- Recognition of the substance as nonself
- Proliferation of immunocompetent cells
- Action against the foreign substance (effector phase)

During the primary response, immunologic memory is established so that any subsequent encounter with the same substance induces a more rapid and intense immune response. Subsequent encounters are called *secondary immune responses*.

An antigen is a substance that can elicit an immune response. Every cell has antigens on its surface that are determined by a series of a linked family of genes known as the *major histocompatibility complex (MHC)*.[34] When tissue from an individual is transplanted into someone with a different genetic makeup, the antigens present on the transplanted tissue cells are promptly identified as foreign, triggering an immediate rejection response.

The MHC determines the antigens to which the immune system should respond. The human MHC is called the HLA complex because these markers were first discovered on lymphocytes.

HLAs are divided into two classes.[34]

1. Class I antigens consist of HLA-A, HLA-B, and HLA-C loci and are expressed on the plasma membranes of all nucleated cells.
2. Class II antigens consist of HLA-DR, HLA-DQ, and HLA-DP loci and are expressed on activated immune cells.

Because of the potential for millions of different arrangements of these antigens, the chances of finding a donor organ with identical genetic markers as a recipient are almost nil unless the donor and recipient are identical twins.

Cells of the Immune System

The immune system contains a variety of cells responsible for general defense, as well as very specific immune responses. When a particular antigen (foreign protein) appears, the cells of the immune system are stimulated to multiply and mount a response. Immune cells are originally produced in bone marrow as stem cells, and their descendants become specialized lymphocytes or phagocytes (Fig. 35.2).

The divisions of the immune system are described as *innate* or *adaptive* (Fig. 35.3). The innate or natural immune system is always active because its purpose is to immediately identify and destroy foreign (nonself) antigens.

- Innate immunity includes epithelial barriers, phagocytes, mast cells, complement, natural killer (NK) cells, and innate lymphoid cells (see Fig. 35.3).
- The adaptive immune system comprises specialized white cells known as *lymphocytes*.

Activation causes proliferation and differentiation of the specialized lymphocytes in response to a foreign antigen (nonself protein). The adaptive immune system is designed to fight infections and retain memory of the infecting organism. However, the adaptive immune system is also stimulated after organ transplantation (foreign tissue) unless the immune system is suppressed by medications, as described in the section on Immunosuppressive Medications.

Lymphocytes

The two major classes of lymphocytes important to organ transplantation are *B cells* and *T cells*.

- B lymphocytes, known as *humoral immunity*, secrete antibodies that mark an antigen for destruction by macrophages and other parts of the immune system. B cells remain in bone marrow to complete their maturation (see Fig. 35.2).
- T lymphocytes confer *cell-mediated immunity*. T cells migrate to the thymus gland and mature there (see Fig. 35.2). In the thymus, T cells acquire the ability to distinguish self from nonself.

After they have matured, some B and T cells are stored in the lymph nodes, whereas other cells circulate in the blood and lymphatic system.

B Cells: Humoral Immunity

Humoral immunity is mediated by B cells, which are responsible for the production of antibodies or immunoglobulin. When a B cell encounters an antigen to which it is specifically coded to respond, the B cell enlarges, divides, and differentiates into a plasma cell. The plasma cell then produces and secretes antigen-specific antibody. B cells function as antigen-presenting cells.[35] After exposure to an antigen, the immune system retains a memory of that antigen. Subsequent exposure stimulates the B-cell memory cells, resulting in a rapid mobilization of antibody-secreting cells. Antibodies function through multiple mechanisms, with their central role being to label antigens for elimination by immune system cells such as macrophages and other effector cells.[36]

T Cells: Cell-Mediated Immunity

T lymphocytes provide cell-mediated immunity. Approximately 65% to 80% of all lymphocytes are T cells, of which there are three basic types: helper T cells, cytotoxic T cells, and regulatory T cells (Fig. 35.4).

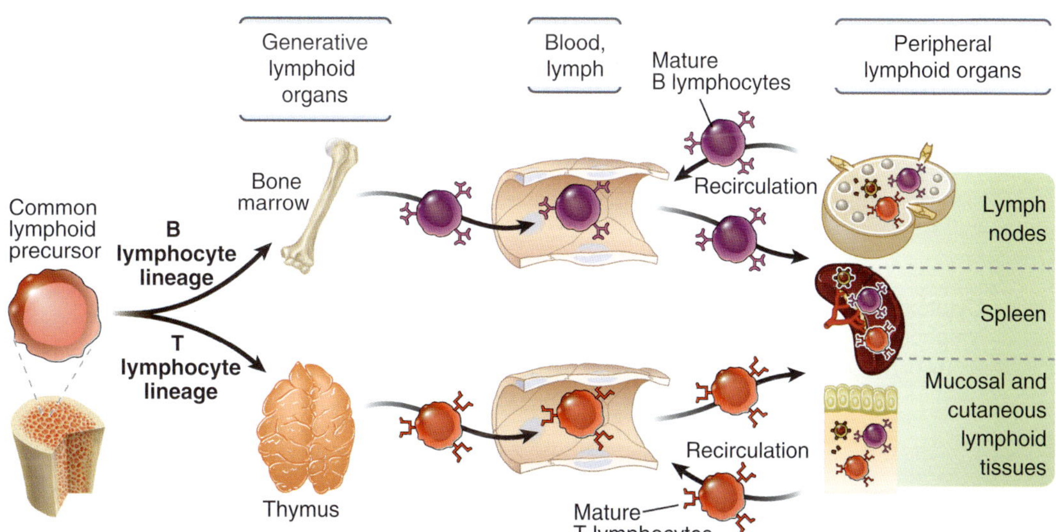

FIG. 35.2 Lymphocyte Development and Distribution. Lymphocytes develop from common lymphoid precursor cells in bone marrow. There are two lineages, B lymphocytes and T lymphocytes, that enter the thymus gland. Mature lymphocytes reside in the peripheral lymphoid organs (lymph nodes, spleen, and mucosal and cutaneous lymphoid tissues) and respond and circulate in lymph and blood as an activation-response to foreign antigens. (From Abbas AK, Lichtman AH, Pillai S. *Basic Immunology: Functions and Disorders of the Immune System*. 7th ed. Elsevier; 2024.)

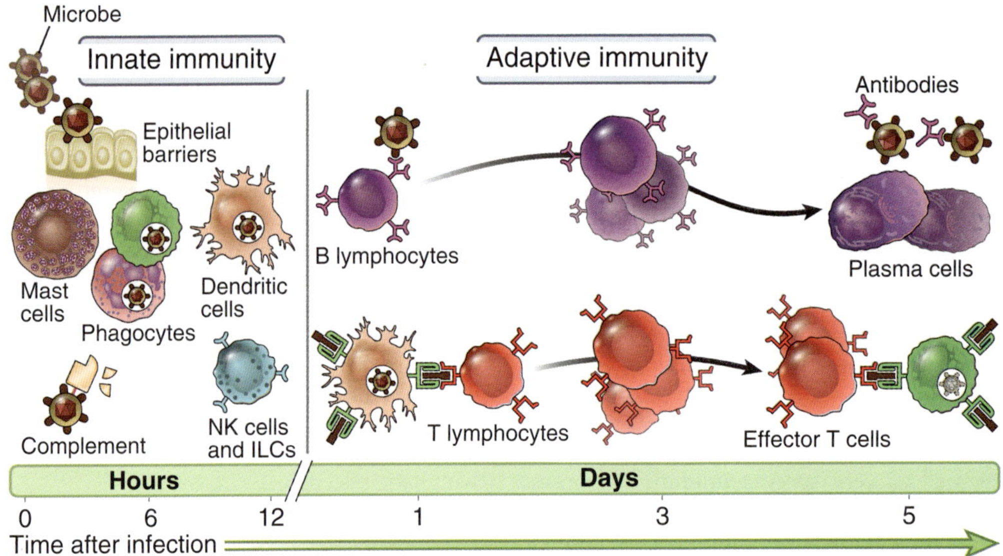

FIG. 35.3 Innate Immunity and Adaptive Immunity. The immune system has several different parts. Innate immunity is the first line of host defense and includes the skin barrier, phagocytic cells, mast cells, complement, and natural killer *(NK)* cells to provide an immediate initial defense against infection. Adaptive immunity, also known as *acquired immunity,* develops more slowly as lymphocytes proliferate and differentiate to provide a more specialized defense against foreign antigens. B lymphocytes produce antibodies from plasma cells. T lymphocytes eradicate infected cells or cells with foreign antigen. *ILC,* Innate lymphoid cells; *NK cells,* natural killer cells. (From Abbas AK, Lichtman AH, Pillai S. *Basic Immunology: Functions and Disorders of the Immune System.* 7th ed. Elsevier; 2024.)

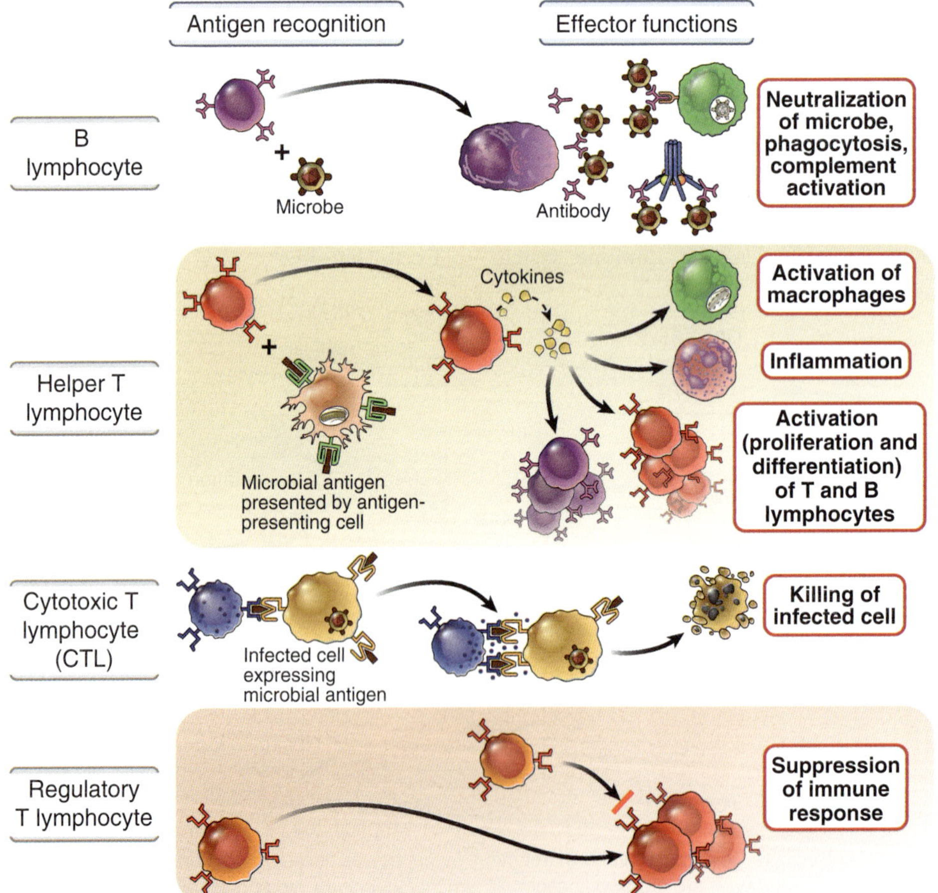

FIG. 35.4 B Lymphocytes and Different Classes of T Lymphocytes and Their Actions. Helper T lymphocytes recognize foreign antigens. Cytotoxic T lymphocytes kill cells with foreign antigen markers. Regulatory T lymphocytes regulate the immune system. (From Abbas AK, Lichtman AH, Pillai S. *Basic Immunology: Functions and Disorders of the Immune System.* 7th ed. Elsevier; 2024.)

Helper T Cells

Helper T lymphocytes upregulate the immune response by stimulating B cells to differentiate into plasma cells and begin antibody production. Helper T cells use chemical mediators to activate cytotoxic T cells and stimulate macrophages and NK cells. Helper T cells are identified by surface glycoproteins known as *CD4* or *T4 markers*. Fig. 35.4 illustrates the helper T cell activation process.

Cytotoxic T Cells

Cytotoxic T lymphocytes are responsible for killing invading foreign cells (see Fig. 35.4). Their primary role is to rid the body of cells that have become infected or have been transformed by cancer and eliminate nonself tissue (organ transplant). Cytotoxic T cells are also called *T8* or *CD8 lymphocytes*, referring to a marker that distinguishes cytotoxic T cells from other T cells. Cytotoxic T cells are activated by macrophages that present the foreign antigen to immature cytotoxic T cells. With the assistance of helper T cells and their release of chemical mediators, the cytotoxic T cells mature and kill foreign cells that carry that specific antigen (see Fig. 35.4).

A third type of T cell is the regulatory T lymphocyte. These cells regulate the immune response and play an important role in keeping the immune response controlled and turning off the response after the antigenic threat is no longer present (see Fig. 35.4). Regulatory T cells regulate tolerance to self-antigens, thereby preventing autoimmune diseases.

Graft Rejection

Rejection of any transplanted organ occurs when the donor and the recipient differ at MHC class I antigens. The transplanted organ may also be described as a *graft*. The recipient's immune system attacks nonself antigens called *alloantigens* and stimulates an *alloreactive response* from recipient T cells that recognize the transplanted tissue as nonself.[37] Graft rejection can occur at different time intervals and has different injury patterns. The three types of rejection patterns are hyperacute rejection, acute rejection, and chronic rejection.

Hyperacute Rejection

Hyperacute rejection is a humoral-mediated response that occurs within hours after transplantation and results in immediate graft failure. Blood type must be matched in organ transplantation to prevent a hyperacute rejection (Fig. 35.5). In blood transfusions only ABO and Rhesus (Rh) groups must match. However, matching numerous polymorphic MCH differences between donor and recipient is much more difficult and is the reason some transplants use closely related donors. In hyperacute rejection, alloantigen (nonself antigen) on the epithelium of the newly transplanted organ is attacked by the circulating antibodies in the recipient's immune system (see Fig. 35.5A). Hyperacute rejection is prevented by testing for the presence of preformed antibodies in the recipient and by selecting donors with compatible blood types. Hyperacute rejection causes complement activation, endothelial damage, inflammation, thrombosis, and graft failure.

Sensitization can be the result of previous blood transfusions, multiple pregnancies, or a previous organ transplant. Short and long-term mechanical circulatory support systems such as extracorporeal membrane oxygenator (ECMO), left ventricular assist devices (LVAD), and total artificial hearts (TAH) may be used as a bridge to eventual heart transplantation. However, these may also lead to further sensitization of potential recipients because of the physical properties of these devices, although this remains controversial.[38–40]

Acute Rejection

Acute rejection tends to occur weeks to months after transplantation but can occur at any time. Recipient cytotoxic T lymphocytes react against alloantigens (nonself antigens) on the epithelium of the transplanted organ, causing cell damage and inflammation (see Fig. 35.5B).

Chronic Rejection

Chronic rejection occurs at varying times after transplantation and progresses for years until it leads to ultimate failure of the transplanted organ. Chronic rejection is the result of both humoral-mediated and cellular-mediated immune responses. Chronic inflammation results in a chronic inflammatory reaction in the transplanted organ vasculature, intimal smooth muscle cell proliferation, diffuse scarring, and occlusion of the organ vasculature, eventually leading to ischemia and necrosis of tissue (see Fig. 35.5C).

IMMUNOSUPPRESSIVE MEDICATIONS

Immunosuppression protocols vary among institutions and according to the type of organ transplanted. The primary goal of immunosuppression is to prevent allograft rejection while minimizing medication-related toxicities. Immunosuppressive regimens can be classified as:

- Maintenance therapy
- Induction therapy
- Rejection treatment

Maintenance Therapy

Maintenance immunosuppression regimens vary widely from organ to organ, and from institution to institution, but typically combine different medications from different classes with differing mechanisms of action. Maintenance regimens aim to provide maintenance immunosuppression throughout the patient's transplanted life to prevent rejection but with the goal of eventually minimizing the intensity of immunosuppression that is both compatible with preventing rejection and minimizing medication-related toxicities. Maintenance regimens combine medications from the following classes of immunosuppressives:

- Calcineurin inhibitor (cyclosporine or tacrolimus)
- Antimetabolite (mycophenolate mofetil or azathioprine)
- Proliferation signal inhibitor (sirolimus or everolimus)
- Corticosteroid (prednisone)

Table 35.5 summarizes the various immunosuppressive medications. Absolute care must be taken to monitor the effectiveness of medication therapy and to minimize unnecessarily high doses, which could predispose patients to greater risks for infection, malignancy, or other toxic effects. Additionally, knowledge of drug interactions will be of paramount importance because many commonly used medications, herbals, and supplements can interact with many of the immunosuppressive medications.

Rejection treatment regimens aim to reverse any acute cellular or antibody-mediated rejection and are discussed later in the chapter.

Corticosteroids

Corticosteroids (methylprednisolone and prednisone) have complex and diverse effects on the immune system. They are used for maintenance therapy and to treat acute rejection and were one of the first immunosuppressive agents used in transplantation. The antiinflammatory actions of steroids provide important protection of the transplanted organ against permanent damage from the body's natural immune response. As maintenance therapy, steroids impair the sensitivity of T cells

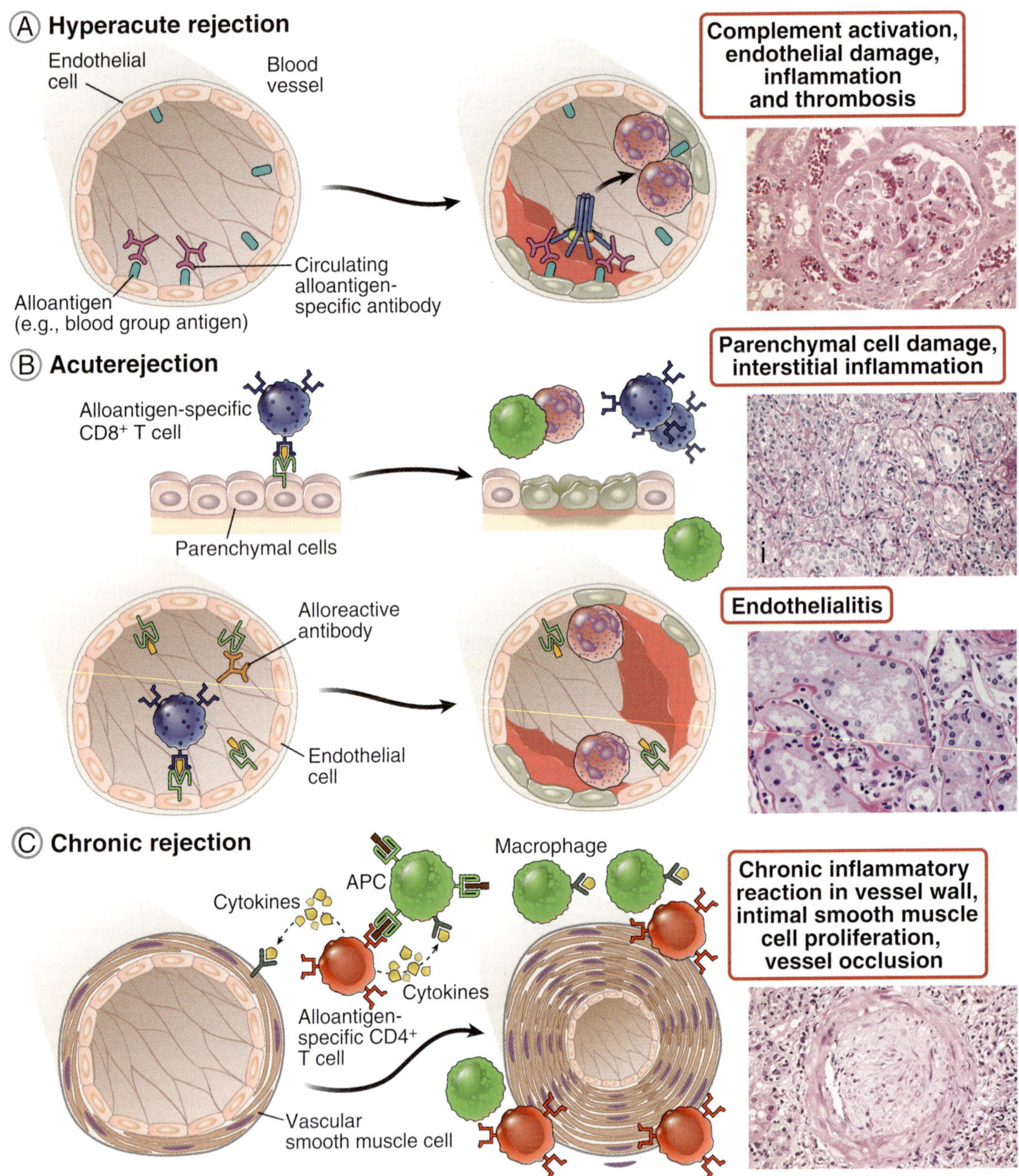

FIG. 35.5 Graft Rejection Mechanisms and Histologic Appearance. (A) Hyperacute rejection. (B) Acute rejection. (C) Chronic rejection. *APC,* Antigen-presenting cell. (From Abbas AK, Lichtman AH, Pillai S. *Basic Immunology: Functions and Disorders of the Immune System*. 7th ed. Elsevier; 2024.)

to antigen, decrease the proliferation of sensitized T cells, and impair the production of cytokines and growth factors.

Long-term steroid therapy is associated with numerous adverse effects and predisposes the patient to an increased risk of infection (see Table 35.5). A primary goal of corticosteroid therapy is to titrate the medication dose to as low a dose as possible. An ideal therapeutic regimen would allow for elimination of the medication altogether. Corticosteroids are associated with psychosis, anxiety, Cushing syndrome, edema, diabetes, insomnia, osteoporosis, glaucoma, cataracts, avascular necrosis of joints, fragile skin that is easily traumatized, poor wound healing, susceptibility to skin cancers, steroid-induced acne, and obesity.

Cyclosporine

Cyclosporine belongs to a class of immunosuppressants called calcineurin inhibitors. The primary mechanism of action is to suppress activation of T cells by binding to cyclophilin to inhibit calcineurin that, in turn, inhibits the production of interleukin-2 (IL-2). Because cyclosporine specifically targets T cells, the patient's immune system is not completely impaired, and some ability to protect the body from infection is preserved.

Several formulations of cyclosporine are available. The older, "nonmodified" version of cyclosporine is characterized by more erratic pharmacokinetics and lower bioavailability. The newer, "modified" formulations are characterized by more predictable pharmacokinetics and higher bioavailability. Because the two formulations are different, they are not considered bioequivalent and, thus, are not interchangeable. Care must be taken when changing between formulations, with close monitoring of drug concentrations in the blood.

When given orally, the medication is typically dosed twice daily. Therapeutic drug monitoring is required in the blood and

SOCIAL DETERMINANTS OF HEALTH

Health Disparities Associated With Medication Adherence

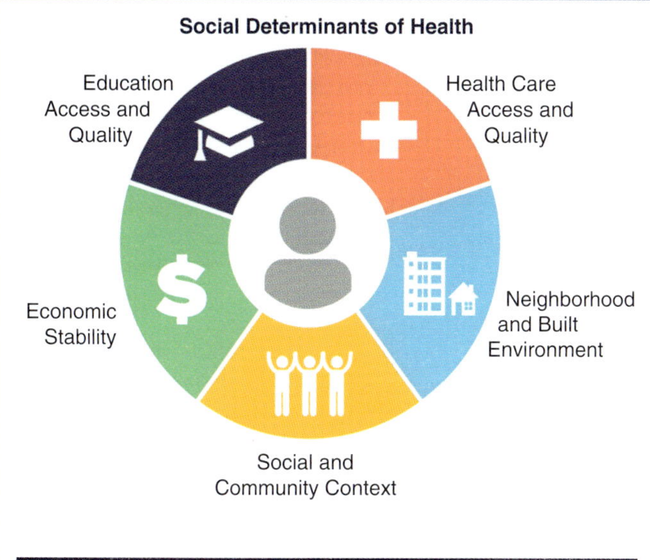

Medication adherence is crucial for managing chronic conditions, preventing disease progression, and improving overall health outcomes. Several social factors can influence medication adherence:

- Socioeconomic Status: Individuals with limited financial resources may struggle to afford prescription medications and health care costs. Even with insurance, high medication costs can be a significant barrier to adherence. Low-income individuals may also face challenges related to transportation to pharmacies and health care appointments.
- Health Insurance Coverage: Comprehensive health insurance covering prescription medications can improve medication adherence. Those without insurance or with inadequate coverage may be more likely to skip doses or delay refills due to the cost.
- Access to Health Care Services: Limited access to health care practitioners, including primary care physicians and specialists, can hinder the prescribing and monitoring of medications. People in rural or underserved areas may have difficulty accessing health care services, impacting medication adherence.
- Education and Health Literacy: Understanding why medications are prescribed, how to take them, and their potential side effects is essential for adherence. Individuals with low health literacy may struggle to comprehend health care instructions, leading to nonadherence.
- Cultural and Language Barriers: Cultural beliefs, language differences, and medication misunderstandings can affect adherence. Health care practitioners must communicate effectively and provide information in a culturally sensitive and language-appropriate manner.
- Social Support: Patients with limited social support may be less likely to adhere to their medication regimens. A robust support system, including family and friends, can positively influence medication adherence.
- Food Insecurity: Some medications require specific dietary considerations, such as taking with or without food. The lack of access to sufficient and nutritious food, can make it challenging for individuals to follow these instructions.
- Transportation: Difficulty in accessing transportation to health care facilities and pharmacies can lead to missed appointments and delayed medication refills, affecting adherence.
- Social Stigma and Discrimination: Stigmatization of certain medical conditions or social groups can lead to reluctance to seek medical care and take prescribed medications.

Strategies to enhance adherence among individuals facing these challenges include providing clear and culturally appropriate education, offering assistance and outreach programs, and expanding telehealth services. By recognizing and addressing factors affecting medication adherence, health care practitioners and systems can improve health outcomes and reduce health care disparities.

Reference:

1. Wilder ME, Kulie P, Jensen C, et al. The impact of social determinants of health on medication adherence: a systematic review and meta-analysis. *J Gen Intern Med.* 2021;36(5):1359–1370. https://doi.org/10.1007/s11606-020-06447-0.

Illustration from Healthy People 2030, U.S. Department of Health and Human Services, Office of Disease Prevention and Health Promotion. Retrieved August 23, 2023, from https://health.gov/healthypeople/objectives-and-data/social-determinants-health.

a 12-hour trough level must periodically be monitored. The therapeutic trough range varies considerably and can depend on several factors, such as the time from transplant and any active infection or malignancies. Generally, however, the goal trough level can range anywhere between 25 and 400 ng/mL. Although peak cyclosporine blood concentrations have been correlated to better match AUCs (area under the curve), they are also much more difficult to accurately monitor.

Side effects of cyclosporine include hypertension, hyperlipidemia, hirsutism, gingival hyperplasia, nephrotoxicity, neurotoxicity (e.g., tremors, seizures), diabetes, electrolyte abnormalities (e.g., hyperkalemia, hypomagnesemia), and thrombotic microangiopathies. Cyclosporine is less commonly used than tacrolimus, a newer and more potent calcineurin inhibitor.

Tacrolimus

Tacrolimus (FK506) is a calcineurin inhibitor with similar activity to cyclosporine in that it also impairs T-cell activation and proliferation by inhibiting the formation of IL-2. However, instead of mediating inhibition of calcineurin via cyclophilin, it mediates this inhibition through a protein called FK binding protein (FKBP).

Tacrolimus comes in many different formulations. When given orally, it is typically given twice daily with the immediate release formulation and once daily with the extended-release formulations. As with cyclosporine, therapeutic drug monitoring is required by monitoring 12- or 24-hour trough blood levels depending on the oral formulation used. The therapeutic trough range varies considerably and can depend on several factors. Generally, however, the goal trough can range anywhere between 4 and 20 ng/mL.

Side effects are similar to cyclosporine. However, tacrolimus is more likely to cause diabetes, nephrotoxicity, and neurotoxicity. Interestingly, tacrolimus can also cause alopecia, unlike cyclosporine.

Studies comparing cyclosporine with tacrolimus as a primary immunosuppressant in kidney and heart transplant recipients have found tacrolimus to be better at preventing acute rejection, with similar overall allograft and patient survival.[41,42] In liver transplants, however, tacrolimus also appears to be superior for survival and graft loss compared with cyclosporine.[43]

TABLE 35.5 PHARMACOLOGIC MANAGEMENT

Organ Transplantation

Medication	Dosage[a]	Action	Special Considerations
Azathioprine	1–3 mg/kg once daily	Converted to thioguanine nucleotide, which is incorporated into replicating DNA and halts replication	May need to adjust dose for severe bone marrow suppression (leukopenia, thrombocytopenia)
Cyclosporine[b], oral solution, and capsules	Therapeutic trough range: 25–400 ng/mL Standard po dosage ranges for specific organs: Liver: 4–12 mg/kg/day[c] Kidney: 6–12 mg/kg/day, tapered to 5–10 mg/kg/day[c] Heart: 4–10 mg/kg/day[c]	Calcineurin inhibitor that blocks IL-2 synthesis	Must perform therapeutic medication concentration monitoring in the blood Monitor for nephrotoxicity, hypertension, neurotoxicity (e.g., tremors, headaches, seizures), diabetes, electrolyte abnormalities (e.g., hyperkalemia, hypomagnesemia), bone marrow suppression
Mycophenolate mofetil (MMF) (CellCept)	1–3 g/day po[c]	Inhibits inosine monophosphate dehydrogenase, which inhibits de novo guanosine nucleotide synthesis; T and B cells require this pathway for proliferation	Monitor for bone marrow suppression and gastrointestinal side effects
Mycophenolate sodium (MPA) (Myfortic)	720–2160 mg/day po[c]	Action same as MMF	Conversions between MMF and mycophenolate sodium should provide equimolar amounts of MPA. • 250 mg MMF = 180 mg MPA
Prednisone	Doses vary by institution and are tapered to some long-term maintenance dose or off (institution specific)	Suppresses inflammatory response	Tapered to as low a dosage as tolerated; dosage is increased with rejection. Side effects can include psychosis, depression, mood changes, moon face, edema, diabetes, anxiety, insomnia, ulcers, sodium retention, osteoporosis, obesity, cataracts, impaired wound healing
Rabbit antithymocyte globulin (Thymoglobulin)	1–1.5 mg/kg/day IV for 1–7 days	Depletes circulating T lymphocytes	Monitor for leukopenia and thrombocytopenia Used as rescue therapy for other transplantation procedures Monitor for infusion-related reactions Premedication with acetaminophen, diphenhydramine, and corticosteroids recommended
Sirolimus (Rapamune)	Loading dose up to 15 mg on day 1, then 2–5 mg/day po adjusted to trough level of 4–15 ng/mL (depending on organ, time from transplant, and center)	Mechanistic target of rapamycin inhibitor; halts progression of cell cycle	Synergistic effects when used with cyclosporine or tacrolimus. Adjust trough goals for cyclosporine or tacrolimus. Monitor for bone marrow suppression, hyperlipidemia, mucositis, edema, pulmonary toxicity, thrombosis, nephrotoxicity, wound healing complications, and proteinuria.
Everolimus (Zortress)	0.75–1 mg po twice daily adjusted to trough level of 3–8 ng/mL	Mechanistic target of rapamycin inhibitor; halts progression of cell cycle	Monitor for bone marrow suppression, hyperlipidemia, mucositis, edema, pulmonary toxicity, thrombosis, nephrotoxicity, wound healing complications, and proteinuria. Synergistic effects when sued with cyclosporine or tacrolimus. Adjust trough goals for cyclosporine or tacrolimus.
Tacrolimus, immediate release (Prograf)	0.075–0.2 mg/kg/day po[c] Therapeutic trough range: 4–20 ng/mL	Calcineurin inhibitor that blocks IL-2 synthesis	Must perform therapeutic medication concentration monitoring in blood. Monitor for nephrotoxicity, hypertension, neurotoxicity (e.g., tremors, headaches, seizures), diabetes, electrolyte abnormalities (e.g., hyperkalemia, hypomagnesemia), bone marrow suppression.

[a]These dosage ranges are general guidelines. Significant variations in dosages occur based on institutional practices, other medications being used in combination, type of transplantation, and patient response to the medications.

[b]Nonmodified cyclosporine preparations (e.g., Sandimmune) are not bioequivalent to modified cyclosporine preparations (e.g., Gengraf and Neoral) and cannot be used interchangeably; Gengraf and Neoral are bioequivalent.

[c]Daily dose is divided and administered 12 hours apart.

g, grams; *IV*, intravenous; *mg*, milligrams; *ng*, nanograms; *po*, per os (oral administration).

Most centers now use tacrolimus as their primary calcineurin inhibitor of choice but may switch to cyclosporine if the patient is exhibiting intolerable tacrolimus-associated toxicity, such as uncontrollable diabetes.

Azathioprine

Azathioprine (Imuran) is a prodrug that is converted into mercaptopurine and, subsequently, a purine analog that is incorporated into DNA and inhibits nucleotide synthesis. This, in turn, inhibits the proliferation of T and B lymphocytes when activated by antigen. Azathioprine is used as a maintenance medication in conjunction with other immunosuppressive medications but never alone. A major adverse effect is myelosuppression, resulting in leukopenia, thrombocytopenia, and anemia. The medication dose can be adjusted or temporarily withheld if leukopenia occurs. The actual minimum acceptable white blood cell count varies with institutional preferences and the type of organ transplanted. Most centers have abandoned the use of azathioprine in favor of mycophenolate mofetil.[44] Other side effects can include nausea, vomiting, hepatotoxicity, and pancreatitis. Therapeutic monitoring of azathioprine blood levels is not required.

Mycophenolate Mofetil

Mycophenolate mofetil (CellCept) is a prodrug that is rapidly hydrolyzed into its active form, mycophenolic acid. Mycophenolic acid is a selective inhibitor of the enzyme inosine monophosphate dehydrogenase (IMPDH), which is crucial for de novo guanine nucleotide synthesis. By blocking this pathway, mycophenolate mofetil effectively inhibits T- and B-lymphocyte proliferation, thereby suppressing cellular-mediated and humoral-mediated rejection.[44]

The use of mycophenolate mofetil in transplant recipients appears to be associated with significant reductions in rejection, mortality, and graft loss as well.[45,46] As such, most centers now use mycophenolate mofetil over azathioprine as their antimetabolite agent of choice.

Mycophenolate mofetil is typically given twice daily. Although therapeutic monitoring is usually not performed, some centers will monitor mycophenolic acid trough levels in the blood. A reason for this variation in practice may have to do with variable outcomes with trough monitoring.

Side effects consist mainly of gastrointestinal symptoms, such as nausea, vomiting, diarrhea, gastritis, and upset stomach. Bone marrow suppression can also be seen, though not to the same extent as with azathioprine. As with azathioprine, some centers adjust mycophenolate mofetil doses based on white blood cell counts and gastrointestinal side effects.

The gastrointestinal side effects of mycophenolate mofetil are sometimes difficult to tolerate for patients and can lead to dose interruptions or omissions. A newer and potentially better tolerated enteric-coated formulation of mycophenolate called *mycophenolate sodium* (Myfortic) is available. This may be helpful for patients who do not tolerate the traditional mycophenolate mofetil formulation. Several studies have shown that mycophenolate sodium is therapeutically similar and has a comparable safety profile. Mycophenolate is typically combined with a calcineurin inhibitor (cyclosporine or tacrolimus).[44]

It should be noted that mycophenolate is associated with an increased risk of congenital malformations and miscarriages, particularly in the first trimester of pregnancy, when used by pregnant women. As such, women of reproductive potential in the United States must be counseled about pregnancy prevention and planning. Alternative agents should be considered for women considering pregnancy.

Sirolimus

Sirolimus (Rapamune), formerly rapamycin, is an immunosuppressive agent that is also a macrolide antibiotic known for its powerful antifungal properties. Cyclosporine and tacrolimus inhibit cytokine production, whereas the mechanism of action of sirolimus is to block the effect of cytokines on the proliferation of lymphoid cells (T and B lymphocytes) by inhibiting a protein (mechanistic target of rapamycin [mTOR]) that is essential for cytokine-driven T-cell proliferation. These medications are known as *proliferation signal inhibitors*, or mammalian target of rapamycin inhibitors (mTORi).[47,48]

Sirolimus inhibits the proliferation of nonlymphoid cells such as endothelial and smooth muscle cells, as well as fibroblasts, which slows the progression of graft vasculopathy in heart transplant recipients. However, the fibroblasts and endothelial cells that are inhibited by sirolimus are also responsible for wound healing, leading to an increase in the incidence of impaired wound healing compared with patients who received other immunosuppressants.[47,49] Many centers delay the introduction of sirolimus into the immunosuppressive regimen until the recipient is several months from transplantation and has had the opportunity to heal any surgical wounds. Another immunosuppressant agent is often substituted for sirolimus for several weeks to months before any scheduled surgical procedure to decrease the risk of delayed wound healing.

Other side effects of this medication include hyperlipidemia, pulmonary toxicity, lymphocele and fluid accumulation, proteinuria, increased serum creatinine, hepatic artery thrombosis, bronchial anastomotic dehiscence, mucositis, and myelosuppression.

Although dosages vary among institutions, a loading dose is often administered before initiating a maintenance dose to achieve trough medication blood concentrations of 5 to 15 ng/mL. Because of its prolonged half-life (approximately 60 hours), sirolimus is administered once daily. Sirolimus has also been shown to have synergistic effects when combined with cyclosporine and tacrolimus, which can result in a lower dose requirement for these medications. Because cyclosporine and tacrolimus can be nephrotoxic, lower doses of these two medications can be advantageous. Sirolimus also specifically interacts with cyclosporine and must be administered 4 hours after the dose of cyclosporine.

Everolimus

Everolimus (Zortress) is an analog of sirolimus with a shorter half-life (approximately 30 hours) and more rapid time to steady state. Similar to sirolimus, everolimus is a proliferation signal inhibitor and works by blocking IL-2 mediated signal transduction in activated lymphocytes. A synergistic effect of everolimus and calcineurin inhibitors such as cyclosporine and tacrolimus allow for lower doses of those medications to be used.

Side effects of sirolimus and everolimus are similar. Everolimus can cause bone marrow suppression, edema, graft thrombosis, hyperglycemia, hyperlipidemia, hypertriglyceridemia, mucositis, nephrotoxicity, pulmonary toxicity, and wound healing complications.[47] In the United States, the Food and Drug Administration (FDA) issued a black box warning for everolimus in de novo heart transplantation because an increased risk of mortality (usually associated with infections) was observed within the first 3 months of transplantation. Therefore, the use of everolimus is not recommended early after heart transplantation. As with sirolimus, therapeutic monitoring is required, and doses are adjusted to achieve trough blood level medication concentrations of 3 to 8 ng/mL.

mTORi may be used in certain heart transplant populations to reverse or slow the progression of kidney injury, cardiac allograft vasculopathy, and malignancies. It may also be somewhat protective from cytomegalovirus (CMV) infections. In lung transplant recipients, mTORi use may be associated with better rejection outcomes versus azathioprine and mycophenolate but appears to be no better at preventing bronchiolitis obliterans syndrome.[50,51]

Belatacept

Belatacept (Nulojix) is a fusion protein that acts as a selective T-cell costimulation blocker by binding to CD80 and CD86 receptors on antigen-presenting cells. This blocks CD28-mediated interaction between antigen-presenting cells and T cells that is needed to activate T lymphocytes.

Belatacept is probably most used in kidney transplants to minimize the use of calcineurin inhibitors because of the development of severe side effects. In the United States, belatacept has a black box warning in liver transplantation and is not recommended in this population because of the increased risk of graft loss and death. Belatacept is only available as an intravenous formulation.

Induction Therapy

Induction regimens aim to provide intense postoperative immunosuppression when the risk of rejection may be the highest. Induction therapy can be divided into depleting (cytolytic) or nondepleting regimens.

- Depleting regimens use agents that cause rapid T-cell destruction. Depleting agents include antithymocyte globulin and alemtuzumab.
- Nondepleting regimens use agents that only prevent T-cell proliferation. Nondepleting agents include basiliximab.

Induction therapy involves the intraoperative or postoperative use of potent immunosuppressive agents for a limited period of time. The purpose of induction is to provide intense immunosuppression early on when the risk of rejection may be at its highest or to induce tolerance to the transplanted graft. Induction therapy may be particularly useful in highly sensitized patients and those who carry preformed HLA antibodies. The use of induction therapy varies from center to center and from organ to organ and partially reflects the ongoing debate regarding the need for and effectiveness of induction therapy. According to the 2021 Annual Report from the *Scientific Registry of Transplant Recipients* (SRTR), induction therapy is administered to approximately 49% of heart,[52] 82% of lung,[53] 91% of kidney,[54] and 31% of liver,[55] transplant recipients.

Antithymocyte Globulin

Antithymocyte globulin (ATG) antibodies are made by injecting human thymocytes into an animal, usually a horse or a rabbit. The animal then produces antibody in response to the foreign human antigen. Antibody to human thymocytes can then be extracted from the serum of the animal. ATG causes rapid depletion of T cells by acting on T-cell surface antigens and inducing complement-mediated cytolysis. ATG also interferes with the normal functioning of B cells, dendritic cells, and natural killer cells. Depending on the protocol of the institution, ATG may be administered as induction therapy or to treat acute rejection.

Antithymocyte antibodies are polyclonal antibodies, and two versions are available in the United States: equine ATG and rabbit ATG. Data from kidney transplants suggest that rabbit ATG may result in a lower incidence of rejection compared with equine ATG because of its greater potency and duration of action.

Infusion-related reactions and serum sickness reactions characterized by fever, chills, myalgia, tachycardia, and hemodynamic instability are common. Premedication with acetaminophen, diphenhydramine, and corticosteroids is highly recommended. Leukopenia and thrombocytopenia are also common and may necessitate dose adjustments.

Because ATG is a cytolytic medication, it has been associated with an increased incidence of malignancy, possibly due to the suppression of cytotoxic T cells that normally play an important role in identifying and eliminating malignant cells. Additionally, ATG may increase the overall risk of infections. For that reason, transplant centers may use ATG only to reverse rejections that are unresponsive to treatment with increased corticosteroids. Duration of action likely is dependent on the cumulative dose but can last for weeks to months.

Interleukin-2 Receptor Antagonists

Basiliximab is currently the only IL-2 receptor antagonist available in the United States. Basiliximab is a chimeric (murine/human) monoclonal antibody directed against the IL-2 receptor found on T lymphocytes. Thus, basiliximab prevents IL-2 mediated activation and proliferation of T lymphocytes. Unlike ATG, basiliximab is not cytolytic and is considered a nondepleting agent. As it is a nondepleting agent, its duration of action is less than ATG's. Based on the package insert, duration may only be approximately 1 month.

Basiliximab is well tolerated, with fewer incidences of infusion-related reactions, leukopenia, thrombocytopenia, and other adverse reactions.

Alemtuzumab

Alemtuzumab is a depleting monoclonal antibody that binds to CD52 that is expressed on both T and B cells. It is a potent immunosuppressive medication that can last for months, if not years, in certain individuals. However, it is no longer commonly used. It was originally approved for the treatment of chronic lymphocytic leukemia.

Rituximab

Rituximab is a monoclonal antibody directed against CD20-positive B cells that is present on almost all B cells except for plasma cells. As it works by activating complement-dependent cytolysis, it can be considered a depleting agent. Few transplant centers use rituximab as an induction agent as it may cause harm in some cases. More commonly, rituximab is used as part of a desensitization regimen or to treat antibody-mediated rejection as part of a multimodal approach.

Acute Rejection Treatment

Although induction and maintenance immunosuppressive therapy has advanced over the decades to decrease allograft rejection and mortality rates, allograft rejection still occurs to varying degrees in all solid organ transplants. When rejection occurs, it can generally be divided into two categories: cellular- and antibody-mediated rejection. Acute cellular rejection is predominantly mediated by T cells, whereas acute antibody-mediated rejection is mediated by B-cells. Depending on the type of acute rejection occurring, different treatment options are available, such as methylprednisolone, antithymocyte globulin, intravenous immune globulin (IVIG), rituximab, bortezomib, carfilzomib, eculizumab, and tocilizumab.

TRANSPLANT CANDIDATE EVALUATION

When an individual has progressed to end-stage organ function and is considered for transplant, each type of organ transplant has specific criteria to determine indications. The specific indications and contraindications are explained for each organ within that section of the chapter. All transplant candidates undergo a comprehensive evaluation with components that are organ specific, although many points of the evaluation are required for all organ transplants. Thus, a comprehensive health evaluation of all body systems and comorbidities is conducted. This involves blood tests and other diagnostic procedures to ensure transplantation is the appropriate medical treatment. All other aspects of the person's physical and mental health are evaluated, including psychiatric and social screenings. After transplant, the recipient must adhere to a rigorous medication regimen, and there may be unexpected complications. The psychiatric evaluation will examine how the person has previously coped with difficult life situations.[56]

In addition to satisfying medical and mental health criteria, patients are psychosocially evaluated for the presence of active social support, current absence of chemical dependence and abstinence in concordance with respective transplant program's selection criteria, and commitment to adhering to a strict lifetime medical regimen and follow-up. This psychosocial evaluation is included to ensure adequate social and emotional support for the recipient during and after the transplant period. Although different transplant centers may have individualized criteria, there are many similarities, including that the final candidacy is typically decided by the entire transplant team.[56–60]

An extensive work-up must be completed to determine eligibility of the recipient for transplant. Each type of transplanted organ has individualized relative and absolute contraindications. Relative contraindications considered for organ transplant include advanced age and preexisting malignancy, excluding hepatic malignancies for liver transplants. Preexisting malignancy, once considered an absolute contraindication because of the potential for recurring cancer or development of secondary cancers resulting from therapeutic immunosuppression, is now considered only a relative contraindication if the potential recipient has been free of malignancy for a specific number of years and if there are no signs of metastasis.[59]

Individuals may not be eligible for transplant based on absolute contraindications, including active infection (delay transplant until treated); significant chronic functional impairment of other vital organs (unless a candidate for multiorgan transplant); active or recent malignancy with exceptions for hepatic malignancy for liver transplant; excessive obesity; evidence of active drug abuse, alcohol abuse, or tobacco use; severe chronic disabling illness (i.e., connective tissue disease, neurologic disease); untreated HIV; severe deconditioning potentiating unlikely survival of major surgery; unwillingness to receive blood products; and active mental illness or psychosocial instability that would limit ability to comply with care needs posttransplant.[57–59,61,62]

Once potential eligibility for transplant has been determined, the patient must undergo extensive testing to determine suitability of organ transplant. A physician specializing in the medical management of the failing organ and an evaluation specific for the type of organ to be transplanted must be completed to determine candidacy. Multiple laboratory tests including blood type, cross-matching, panel reactive antibodies (PRA), HLA phenotype, antibodies for multiple viruses, serology, chemistry profiles, lipid panel, coagulation studies, HIV, hepatitis, and other laboratory tests specific to the organ being transpla nted.[34,58,59,62] Screening also occurs to rule out alcohol abuse, drug abuse, and serum cotinine for tobacco abuse.

Other tests and procedures for transplant work-up entail electrocardiogram; chest radiography; computed tomography (CT) scan; urine culture; bacterial and fungal cultures (if indicated); pulmonary function tests; bone mineral density study; dental evaluation; prostate, rectal, and gynecologic examinations; mammogram; and colonoscopy (if older than 50 years). Based on results, specialty consultations may be required for gastroenterology, infectious disease, endocrine, nutrition, cardiology, nephrology, psychiatry, gynecology, rheumatology, or others.[59] Examples of a pretransplantation history are listed with the transplantation criteria for each solid organ later in this chapter.

In addition to the multiple laboratory blood tests, diagnostic tests, and procedures, the patient may also meet with a transplant social worker, transplant pharmacist, financial counselor, psychiatrist (when indicated), and transplant coordinator. Transplant support groups are encouraged but may be required by some transplant programs. Based on laboratory and test results, the recipient may need to participate in cardiac and/or pulmonary rehabilitation to enable successful transplant outcomes. Once work-up results have been obtained, the patient information is typically presented to a multidisciplinary transplant evaluation committee for determination of eligibility.[58–60]

Evaluation Decision

At the conclusion of the evaluation, one of several outcomes is possible for the patient:

- Transplant candidate
- Not a candidate for transplant
- Deferred and may be a candidate sometime in the future if specific criteria are met

The specific criteria for a future transplant candidate may be of a physical nature or incomplete testing for incidental findings, meaning it is too early in the disease process to list, in which case the patient will be reevaluated at set intervals. The criteria may also be psychosocial. For example, the patient must attend a formal alcohol or drug rehabilitation program or undergo treatment for depression.[56]

Transplant Recipient Listing

After candidacy has been determined and the patent is ready for transplantation, the candidate is entered into the national computer system operated by UNOS. Candidates are listed and receive organs based on the type of organ needed, described in each organ section of the chapter. Distribution of organs is strictly regulated by a regional, state, and national network organized by the UNOS and contracted by the federal government.[56,63] In addition to candidate status, other variables such as age, local organ donation rate, and blood type affect the length of time a candidate will wait for transplant. For example, blood type O organs are compatible with recipients with all blood types. Because these organs can be allocated to non-type O recipients, patients who are blood type O generally spend more time on the waiting list before receiving organs.[52] There is also some regional variability that affects median wait times. This variability is related to population density of the regions and number of transplant centers within each region, which can often compete for the same donors. The wait can be weeks, months, or years and varies by organ, blood group, and location in the country. The waiting period is always challenging because there are so many unknowns. For this reason, candidates and their families are encouraged to join one of the support groups that are hosted at many centers. Organs are a limited resource, and only a fraction of recipients in need receive an organ.[63]

Waiting for Transplant

Next, one of the most difficult phases begins: the waiting period. It is impossible to anticipate when an appropriate organ will become available. The patient may feel that their life is put "on hold." Because of the shortage of donors, it is common for patients in critical care units to die while awaiting transplantation; this is especially true for pediatric recipients. Moreover, knowing that another person must die so that one may live can cause feelings of guilt as the patient hopes for an organ to become available. Patients with end-stage organ failure know that the only alternative to transplantation is death. By understanding the basic psychosocial processes that patients experience while awaiting transplantation, nurses can facilitate health promotion activities.

Pretransplant Support Groups

It is important for the patient and family to receive ongoing psychosocial assessment and to attend pretransplantation support groups, which are available at most transplant centers. Psychosocial aspects must be considered because many individuals wait a substantial length of time for an organ to become available.[63]

Financial Stress 3>

Financial stress can affect psychosocial well-being because the individual is not likely to be medically and/or physically able to maintain employment and potentially insurance benefits.

Financial concerns are a major source of stress in these patients.[63] Many transplant recipients had chronic organ failure before their surgery. They often were disabled for some time and already have experienced financial stressors related to illness. As these patients live longer posttransplant, issues of insurability, continued disability, and the ability to obtain work will have to be addressed.[63] The federal government helps to pay for the immunosuppressant medications for 36 months after kidney transplantation for recipients younger than 65 years. Recipients older than 65 years with Medicare are covered for life. However, the Medicare copayment system is complex, and many transplant recipients have financial concerns about the costs of their immunosuppressive medications.[64] Transplantation offers hope for survival but at considerable expense. Many insurance providers, including Medicare, provide partial reimbursement for transplant procedures. The costs to patients can be staggering.[61,63] Transplant centers must continuously find innovative ways to control rising costs because of decreasing reimbursements, complexity of patient care, and increasing patient loads.

Remaining on the Transplant List

Once listed, specific indications must be followed to remain on the transplant list. Regular follow-up with the transplant center, laboratory tests and procedures specific to the organ needed for transplant, and transplant list status are evaluated at regular intervals. If the recipient's condition changes while listed, prompt follow-up with the transplant center is required. Evaluation and testing may be required to update the individual's listing status. Individuals waiting for transplant are chronically ill with end-stage organ failure. As a result, complications related to organ failure can increase as the wait time lengthens and require medical intervention and, at times, admission to the critical care unit for life-sustaining medical interventions. This medical care at times includes interventions such as ventilation, ventricular assist devices, ECMO,[57] intravenous inotropic medications, treatment of electrolyte imbalances, dialysis, insulin infusions, infections, gastrointestinal procedures, treatment of coagulation disorders, and nutrition support, among others. While listed, patients should remain as active as possible and continue rehabilitation efforts to prevent further physical deterioration and to assist in ensuring successful transplant outcomes.[63]

Vaccinations

Vaccinations tend to be more effective when patients are not immunosuppressed; thus patients should receive vaccines such as herpes zoster; influenza; measles, mumps, and rubella; varicella (based on laboratory results); hepatitis A and B; tetanus; pneumonia; and human papillomavirus before transplant.[65] Specific vaccines for travel or exposure are indicated on an individualized basis and risk factors.

Available Organ

Once an organ becomes available for transplant, the transplant center coordinator will conduct initial assessment for matching and notify the surgeon. The surgeon will obtain information necessary about the donor and recipient to determine whether the organ is a match and viable for transplant. At this time the transplant team coordinates how the organ will be harvested and delivered to the transplant center. While organ surgical procurement is occurring, the recipient is notified and reports to the transplant center. Once the surgical team visualizes the organ to be transplanted and determines definitive viability, the recipient is prepared in an operating room for transplant. With organs such as lungs, on visual assessment the organ is often determined not to be acceptable. This information is communicated to the transplant center and the patient is notified of the outcomes and discharged to continue waiting for an organ. Further sections of this charter discuss organ-specific transplants.

Patient and Family Education

Patient and family education is imperative for successful organ transplantation outcomes and survival. Education should begin during the evaluation phase for transplant listing. Education will continue while the patient is wait listed, after organ transplant, and throughout the patient's life. The multidisciplinary team includes transplant coordinators, physicians, nurse practitioners, physician assistants, social workers, pharmacists, nurses, dietitians, discharge planners, and visiting nurses. Multiple methods are used to provide education, such as handouts, a transplant binder or folder, and educational videos.[63]

Primary caregivers must be a part of the learning experience to ensure understanding of the entire process from selection through posttransplantation. Health care providers educate on the process of being assessed for transplant and the evaluation process. Once listed, patient and family education begin with the requirements for staying active on the transplant wait list. Education related to immediate postoperative recovery will be provided. Also, while awaiting an organ the patient and family will gain a better understanding of the posttransplant process and lifestyle changes required after transplant.[63] Transplant pharmacology, specifically immunosuppressive medication doses, frequencies, indications, side effects, and what to do if a dose is missed, can be introduced before transplant (see Table 35.5). Education regarding posttransplant self-care, follow-up appointment frequency, posttransplant procedures, laboratory tests, indications for when to contact the transplant center, and assessment for signs and symptoms of infection and/or rejection can be initiated pretransplant. Lifestyle changes include limiting exposure to sick contacts, safety precautions, potential dietary restrictions and healthy diet, and other restrictions based on organ-specific recommendations. Patient and family education will continue immediately posttransplant during hospitalization and includes all essential information for discharge.

HEART TRANSPLANTATION

The first human heart transplantation was performed at the University of Cape Town, South Africa in 1967 by Christian Barnard; the patient survived 18 days. In 1968 Shumway et al. performed the first successful heart transplant in the United States at Stanford University. The number of heart transplantation procedures grew dramatically for the first few years and then rapidly declined because of poor results. Over time, technologic and surgical advancements in addition to pharmacologic developments led to significantly increased survival. These advancements included the development of the endomyocardial biopsy to detect allograft rejection, the introduction of T-cell–specific agents such as rabbit antithymocyte globulin, the ability of laboratories to measure specific T cells (rosette counts) in the blood, and the introduction of the immunosuppressive medication cyclosporine (previously described). Over 131,000 adult transplants and over 15,000 pediatric heart transplants that have been performed since 1982 in more than 480 transplant centers. Survival after heart transplant has also improved, with adults averaging over 90% survival at 1 year and 86% survival at 5 years.[66,67]

Indications and Selection

Heart transplantation is indicated for individuals with *stage D heart failure*, or end-stage cardiac disease where symptoms of heart failure can no longer be managed with conventional medical therapy. Additional considerations include no alternate surgical options offering more favorable long-term outcomes and if the individual's short-term prognosis is poor without transplantation. The most common conditions requiring heart transplantation are nonischemic cardiomyopathies of various origins (idiopathic, viral, valvular) accounting for approximately 51% of cases, and ischemic cardiomyopathies accounting for about 32% of cases.[66,67] Other, less common etiologic factors include severe heart failure resulting from chemotherapy, radiation treatment, myocardial tumor, and complex congenital defects. Many centers grade the severity of heart failure by the classification developed by the New York Heart Association (NYHA) (Table 35.6), which is based on the amount of exertion required to cause symptoms. Most patients who need a heart transplant are categorized as NYHA class IV.

In addition to the evaluations for all transplant recipients, specific contraindications to heart transplantation are listed in Box 35.4. Heart transplant recipients range from neonates to older adults, with upper age limits varying among transplant institutions. Advanced age was previously considered an absolute

TABLE 35.6 New York Heart Association Class and Physical Manifestation of Heart Failure

NYHA Class	Physical Manifestation
I	No limitation of physical activity; no dyspnea, fatigue, or palpitations with ordinary activity
II	Slight limitation of physical activity; patients have fatigue, palpitations, and dyspnea with ordinary physical activity but are comfortable at rest
III	Marked limitation of activity; less than ordinary physical activity results in symptoms, but patients are comfortable at rest
IV	Symptoms are present at rest, and any physical exertion exacerbates symptoms

NYHA, New York Heart Association.

BOX 35.4 Heart Transplantation Contraindications

Medical Contraindication

Absolute	Relative
Elevated pulmonary artery pressures	Advanced age (>70 years)
Irreversible severe kidney, liver, or lung disease	Diabetes mellitus with end-organ damage or poor glycemic control
Recent or unresolved pulmonary infarction	Body mass index >35 kg/m ^{2}
Chronic liver dysfunction	Severe cachexia or malnutrition
Active malignancy or recent malignancy with high risk of recurrence	Systemic disease with high probability of recurrence in transplanted heart
Active uncontrolled infection	Kidney dysfunction
Severe symptomatic cerebrovascular disease	Significant peripheral vascular disease that may limit rehabilitation or refractory to revascularization
History of primary central nervous system lymphoma and visceral Kaposi sarcoma	

Psychosocial Contraindications

Absolute	Relative
Inadequate social support system	Inadequate social support system
Illicit substance use	Illicit substance use
Alcohol dependence	Alcohol dependence
Nicotine abuse	Nicotine abuse
Active psychotic symptoms	Active psychotic symptoms
Dementia or severe cognitive-behavioral disabilities	Dementia or severe cognitive-behavioral disabilities

Data from: Mehra MR, Canter CE, Hannan MM, et al. The 2016 International Society for Heart Lung Transplantation listing criteria for heart transplantation: a 10-year update. *J Heart Lung Transplant.* 2016;35(1):1–23.

contraindication to transplantation, but it is now considered a relative contraindication, based on physiologic versus chronological age. Severe liver and kidney dysfunction that is not believed to be reversible by an increase in cardiac output is a contraindication for heart transplantation alone. However, combined organ transplants such as heart and kidney, or heart and liver transplant, can be considered for certain individuals.[68] Diabetes mellitus, as an example, is a relative contraindication if adequately treated and if the patient is exhibiting no sign of end-organ damage such as nephropathy, neuropathy, or retinopathy. Recent pulmonary infarctions increase the risk for postoperative infection and complicates oxygenation and ventilation. Therefore, a recent history of pulmonary infarction often precludes transplantation.

Heart transplant candidates are prioritized based on medical urgency, which is determined by the patient's need for inotropic support with invasive hemodynamic monitoring, mechanical ventilation, or mechanical assist devices such as a left ventricular assist device, ECMO, or an intraaortic balloon pump (IABP).

The heart allocation system has changed as of October 2018. The new allocation score classifies patients who require this degree of assistance as status 1 or 2; all other heart transplantation candidates are listed as status 3 through 6 (Table 35.7). Since the allocation changes, the number of transplants performed has remained stable and continues to slightly increase, with over 4000 heart transplants performed in the United States in 2022.[3]

TABLE 35.7 Classification of Heart Transplant Candidates

Status	Definition
1	VA ECMO
	Nondischargeable, surgically implanted, nonendovascular biventricular support device
	MCSD with life-threatening ventricular arrhythmias
2	Nondischargeable, surgically implanted, nonendovascular LVAD
	IABP
	V-tach/V-fib, mechanical support not required
	MCSD with device malfunction/mechanical failure
	TAH, BiVAD, RVAD, or VAD for single-ventricle patients
	Percutaneous endovascular MCSD
3	Dischargeable LVAD for discretionary 30 days
	Multiple inotropes or single high-dose inotrope with continuous hemodynamic monitoring
	VA ECMO after 7 days; percutaneous endovascular circulatory support device or IABP after 14 days
	Nondischargeable, surgically implanted, nonendovascular LVAD after 14 days
	MCSD with one of the following: device infection, hemolysis, pump thrombosis, right heart failure, mucosal bleeding, or aortic insufficiency
4	Dischargeable LVAD without discretionary 30 days
	Inotropes without hemodynamic monitoring
	Retransplant
	Diagnosis of one of the following: congenital heart disease (CHD), ischemic heart disease with intractable angina, hypertrophic cardiomyopathy, restrictive cardiomyopathy, or amyloidosis
5	On the waitlist for at least one other organ at the same hospital
6	All remaining active candidates

BiVAD, Biventricular assist device; *IABP*, intraaortic balloon pump; *LVAD*, left ventricular assist device; *MCSD*, mechanical circulatory support device; *RVAD*, right ventricular assist device; *TAH*, total artificial heart; *VA ECMO*, veno-arterial extracorporeal membrane oxygenation; *VAD*, ventricular assist device; *V-Fib*, ventricular fibrillation; *V-tach*, ventricular tachycardia.
Data from Organ Procurement and Transplantation Network Policies. Policy 6: allocation of heart and heart-lungs. http://optn.transplant.hrsa.gov/media/1200/optn_policies.pdf. Accessed October 12, 2020.

Heart Transplantation Surgical Procedure

Two surgical approaches for heart transplantation are discussed:

- Biatrial technique
- Bicaval technique

Biatrial Technique

The standard surgical procedure for orthotopic heart transplantation was originally developed by Lower and Shumway in 1960.[69] A standard median sternotomy is used, the great vessels are cannulated, and cardiopulmonary bypass is instituted after anticoagulation and standard hypothermia are achieved. The donor heart is prepared by interconnecting the pulmonary veins to form a single left atrial cuff and by trimming the aorta and pulmonary artery to fit the recipient's anatomy. The entire recipient heart is removed except the posterior walls of the atria that contain the openings of the pulmonary veins and vena cava. Four major anastomoses are performed between the donor heart and the recipient's native atrial remnant and great vessels. In order, they are anastomoses of the right and left atria, the aorta, and the pulmonary artery (Fig. 35.6). The posterior native atrial remnant remains innervated by the parasympathetic and sympathetic nerve fibers from the autonomic nervous system. However, the donor heart is denervated, resulting in a faster resting heart rate of 90 to 100 beats/min. The rate of the transplanted heart is the normal intrinsic rate generated by the donor sinoatrial node located in the right atrium.

Although it was long regarded as the gold standard for heart transplantation, the standard biatrial technique had disadvantages related to the large atrial cavities. The loss of normal atrial anatomy increased the risk of mitral and tricuspid valve regurgitation, atrial septal aneurysm, atrial thrombus formation, and tachydysrhythmias.

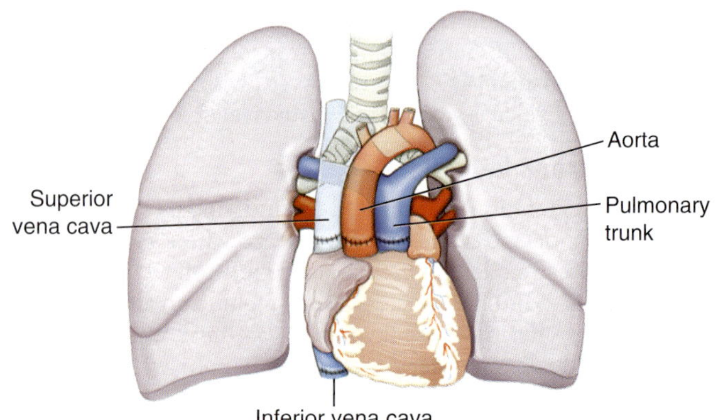

FIG. 35.6 Surgical Procedure for Heart Transplantation.

Bicaval Technique

The bicaval technique was originally reported by Sievers et al. in 1991 and is now the usual method for orthotopic heart transplant.[70] The anastomotic sites of the bicaval technique include the left atrial cuff, which contains the orifices of pulmonary veins; the superior vena cava and inferior vena cava; and the aorta and the main pulmonary artery (see Fig. 35.6). This technique leaves the recipient with more anatomically normal atria. Benefits of the bicaval technique include preserved sinoatrial node function with decreased incidence of atrial dysrhythmias and mitral and tricuspid regurgitation.

Postoperative Medical and Nursing Management

Immediate postoperative management of the heart transplant recipient resembles management of patients undergoing other cardiac surgery procedures. The care management plan components following a heart transplant are listed in Box 35.5.

Low cardiac output often occurs posttransplant because of prolonged ischemic time (time from excision of the donor heart to removal of the aortic cross-clamp after implantation into the recipient), reperfusion injury, and hypothermia. One of the more recent innovations helping extend this limited ischemic time is the *Organ Care System* (OCS™) heart system. This portable warm perfusion system has allowed transplant centers to further extend ischemic time and cross prior prohibitive distances while keeping heart transplants viable.[71]

Dysrhythmias may occur because of myocardial irritation, local ischemia, edema around the atrial suture line, and disruption of the sinoatrial nodal blood supply. An ECG abnormality unique to a biatrial transplanted heart is the presence of a second P wave, which is generated by the native sinoatrial node that has been left in the atrial cuff. Because this impulse does not cross the suture line, it can conduct only through the remnant of the native recipient atria. This impulse is not seen in hearts that are transplanted using the bicaval technique because the native right atrium with the sinoatrial node is removed.

Temporary epicardial pacing or isoproterenol, a powerful beta-adrenergic agonist, are sometimes used in the postoperative period for chronotropic (heart rate) support. The chronotropic and vasodilator properties of isoproterenol effectively sustain the heart rate, increase cardiac output, and decrease pulmonary vascular resistance. Pulmonary vascular resistance may be increased as a result of preexisting left ventricular failure and may be a cause of transient right ventricular dysfunction in the newly transplanted heart. Dopamine and epinephrine are often used for inotropic support in the postoperative period. However, the use of inotropic and chronotropic medications is highly individualized based on institutional preference. Generally, inotropic medications are gradually discontinued over 24 to 48 hours as tolerated by the patient, and the need for isoproterenol decreases as the heart begins to maintain its normal intrinsic rate of approximately 100 beats/min. Temporary pacing is required only occasionally, and less than 10% of transplant recipients require a permanent pacemaker implant.

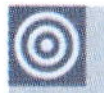

BOX 35.5 DIAGNOSIS AND PATIENT CARE MANAGEMENT

Heart Transplantation

- Risk for Infection
- Impaired Cardiac Output due to alterations in preload
- Impaired Cardiac Output due to alterations in afterload
- Impaired Cardiac Output due to alterations in heart rate or rhythm
- Disturbed Body Image due to actual change in body structure, function, or appearance
- Anxiety due to threat to biological, psychological, or social integrity
- Lack of Knowledge of Treatment Regime due to lack of previous exposure to information

Patient Care Management plans are located in Appendix A.

Cardiac tamponade does not occur with greater frequency in heart transplantation compared with other heart surgeries, but tamponade may be more difficult to detect because of an enlarged pericardial sac secondary to long-standing cardiomyopathy.

Early Postoperative Complications

Primary Graft Dysfunction

Primary graft dysfunction (PGD) stands as the primary factor contributing to early mortality following cardiac transplantation, a condition that can be typically seen within the first 24 hours following transplantation. PGD is characterized by the dysfunction of either a single or both ventricles of the transplanted heart, leading to low blood pressure as a result of inadequate cardiac output, compromising the recipient's circulatory requirements.[72] There is a professional consensus to determine severity of clinical findings in Box 35.6.[72]

Secondary Graft Dysfunction

This is early graft dysfunction that can be attributed to an obvious cause such as hyperacute rejection, pulmonary hypertension, or sepsis. The occurrence of hyperacute rejection in heart transplants is uniformly fatal unless emergency hemodynamic support such as ECMO is initiated until retransplantation can be performed. Signs and symptoms of hyperacute rejection are not subtle. The donor heart becomes cyanotic, and graft failure and hemodynamic collapse occur within minutes. Careful ABO matching and advances in antibody screening have made occurrence of hyperacute rejection rare.

Signs and Symptoms of Rejection

Acute cellular rejection in heart transplant recipients can occur at any time, although it is most likely to occur during the first 3 to 6 months after transplantation. The clinical signs and symptoms of rejection are listed in Box 35.7.

Rejection Surveillance

Diagnosis of heart transplant rejection is determined by fluoroscopic or echocardiography-guided endomyocardial biopsy. A

BOX 35.6 Signs and Symptoms of Heart Transplant Rejection

R	Rub (pericardial friction)
E	Electrocardiogram voltage decreased
J	Jugular venous distention
E	Edema (peripheral, sudden onset)
C	Cardiac dysrhythmias (atrial, bradycardia)
T	Tiredness
I	Intolerance of exercise
O	Onset of low-grade fever
N	New S_3 or S_4 heart sound
E	Enlarged cardiac silhouette
P	Pulmonary crackles, wheezes
I	Increased weight
S	Shortness of breath
O	Onset of hypotension
D	Disturbance in mood
E	Echocardiogram findings (systolic function, left ventricular mass/thickness)

From Cupples SA. Heart transplantation. In: Cupples SA, Ohler L, eds. *Transplantation Nursing Secrets*. Hanley & Belfus; 2003.

BOX 35.7 Indications for Heart-Lung and Lung Transplant

Pulmonary Vascular Disease
- Primary pulmonary hypertension
- Eisenmenger syndrome
- Cardiomyopathy with pulmonary hypertension

Restrictive Lung Disease
- Idiopathic pulmonary fibrosis
- Sarcoidosis
- Asbestosis
- Histiocytosis X
- Bronchiolitis obliterans organizing pneumonia
- Desquamative interstitial pneumonitis

Obstructive Lung Disease
- Emphysema—idiopathic
- Emphysema—alpha-1-antitrypsin deficiency
- Cystic fibrosis
- Bronchiectasis
- Bronchopulmonary dysplasia
- Idiopathic and posttransplant obliterative bronchiolitis
- Lymphangioleiomyomatosis

TABLE 35.8 Cardiac Biopsy Grading

Grade	Nomenclature
0R	No rejection
1R, mild	Interstitial and/or perivascular infiltrate with up to one focus of myocyte damage
2R, moderate	Two or more foci of infiltrate with associated myocyte damage
3R, severe	Diffuse infiltrate with multifocal myocyte damage, ± edema, ± hemorrhage, ± vasculitis

bioptome is percutaneously inserted through the right internal jugular vein and advanced through the right atrium to the right ventricle. The femoral, subclavian, and left internal jugular veins are alternative sites for venous access, although the right internal jugular vein provides the most direct access. *Endomyocardial tissue* is obtained from the interventricular septum. The samples are microscopically evaluated for interstitial and perivascular infiltration. Heart biopsies are graded according to the severity of the interstitial infiltration of lymphocytes. The standardized cardiac biopsy grading scale ranges from mild to severe (Table 35.8).[73]

The frequency of surveillance biopsies varies from center to center. Generally, biopsies are performed more frequently in the first few weeks and months after transplant and are performed less frequently as time goes on. Many centers stop performing routine biopsies after 2 to 5 years and rely instead on clinical assessment to determine the need for biopsy. A major but rare complication of biopsy is ventricular perforation, which can result in cardiac tamponade. Pneumothorax is another potential complication of endomyocardial biopsy and may result from perforation of the visceral pleura during cannulation of the jugular vein; clinical manifestations are a sudden onset of sharp pain in the affected side and dyspnea.

Despite the invasive nature and potential for complications associated with endomyocardial biopsy, this procedure remains the gold standard to confirm suspected rejection in heart transplantation. Alternative methods from noninvasive monitoring with comparable sensitivity and specificity remain elusive, although significant progress has been with the development and application of *gene expression profile* (GEP) testing,[74] and more recently, donor-derived cell-free DNA testing (dd-cf DNA).

The GEP testing measures the genes expressed by activated T cells as a marker of possible rejection.[74] The dd-cf DNA testing is a supplemental noninvasive surveillance monitoring blood test that measures the amount of graft injury and is usually more sensitive to detect antibody mediated rejection.[75] Many heart transplant programs use the test as a trigger for performing endomyocardial biopsy to rule out rejection.

Treatment of acute rejection episodes may require intravenously administered corticosteroids. Recurrence of acute rejection is managed with various pharmacologic agents, depending on the patient's clinical condition and institutional preference. Strategies include augmenting current maintenance immunosuppression or switching to alternatives such as tacrolimus, mycophenolate mofetil, or sirolimus. Other agents used for recurrent rejection include polyclonal antibodies such as antilymphocyte globulin or antithymocyte globulin. Salvage therapy for persistent rejection that has not responded to conventional immunosuppression includes multiple steroid boluses, anti–T-cell antibodies, or total lymphoid irradiation in which low-dose ionizing radiation is used to treat the lymphoid tissue. Transplant centers tend to have specific experiential protocols for treatment of recurrent rejections.

Infection Surveillance

Infection surveillance is a high priority for an immunocompromised patient. It is well known that immunosuppression predisposes the patient to infection by a multitude of opportunistic pathogens that cannot easily be prevented with infection control. Development of infection is encountered most often in the early postoperative period when immunosuppression is maximized. Infection is a leading cause of death during this period (up to 2 years after surgery). Great care must be taken to use aseptic technique for all intravenous line and dressing changes. Centers differ in their protective practices regarding the transplant recipient. Some use reverse isolation, whereas others put transplant recipients in rooms with other patients and simply use standard precautions.

Development of fever is aggressively investigated, with systematic blood, wound, and respiratory tract cultures; chest radiographs; and observation. Because steroids are known to suppress the body's inflammatory reaction, an elevated temperature generally is considered significant when it reaches 38°C (100.4°F). Nurses must be suspicious of any new productive cough, dry cough, change in type of secretions, or change in chest radiograph findings.

CMV is a particular threat to transplant recipients. CMV is a herpesvirus that can produce latent infection that persists and can be reactivated throughout life. In the United States more than half of all adults are infected with CMV.[76] CMV can be transmitted through organ and blood product donation. Transplantation from a CMV-seropositive donor to a CMV-seronegative recipient poses the highest risk to the recipient for acquiring a primary infection. The antiviral agent valganciclovir can inhibit viral replication and ameliorate symptoms and is used in the prophylaxis and treatment of CMV infections.[77] CMV immune globulin can be administered for prevention of primary CMV disease and for treatment of CMV disease.[78]

Patient and Family Education

Thorough, effective, and ongoing education of patients and their family and/or caregivers is vital to successful long-term outcomes after heart transplantation. Patients and caregivers are taught about transplant medications, self-monitoring for signs of infection and rejection, and safety precautions. Prior to discharge, patients are also provided with guidelines for maintaining a heart-healthy diet and increasing physical activity. Patients may be required to check their blood glucose, blood pressure, temperature, and daily weight at home. At first, frequent clinic visits are needed to monitor progress and adjust medications. A schedule is established for routine laboratory tests and clinic visits to ensure long-term success of the transplant.

Long-Term Considerations

Chronic immunosuppression results in significant morbidity. Steroid administration can result in osteoporosis, avascular necrosis of joints, fragile skin, and obesity. Cyclosporine can cause kidney damage, excessive hair growth, gingival hyperplasia, tremor, and hypertension necessitating pharmacologic control. Azathioprine can be hepatotoxic (see Table 35.5). Tacrolimus can cause kidney damage, hypertension necessitating pharmacologic control, excessive hair loss, and tremors.[79] Sirolimus can delay wound healing and cause lower extremity edema, hypertriglyceridemia, hypertension necessitating pharmacologic control, and mouth ulcers.[80] Concomitant use of these immunosuppressants also leaves patients more susceptible to malignancies and late infections.[81]

Initial causes of death include graft failure, infection, and multiorgan failure. Cause of death 3 to 5 years after transplant is most often related to malignancy, cardiac allograft vasculopathy, and kidney failure.[81]

Cardiac Graft Vasculopathy

Cardiac graft vasculopathy, or coronary artery disease in the transplanted heart, is believed to develop as a result of chronic rejection and is a major cause of late morbidity and mortality. It is a diffuse and rapidly progressive type of coronary disease that causes concentric narrowing of the coronary arteries. Since patients are denervated at the time of transplant, these patients rarely complain of angina. Because the lesions are discrete, they are generally not amenable to interventions such as angioplasty or bypass grafting. The pathophysiology is completely different from typical atherosclerotic coronary artery disease, as illustrated in Fig. 35. 7.

Patients with denervated hearts usually cannot feel anginal pain, although reinnervation of transplanted hearts can occur over time. Cardiac graft vasculopathy can cause ischemic injury, heart failure, or sudden death. Graft vasculopathy is diagnosed initially by angiographic screening and later in the course of the disease by silent infarctions observed on the 12-lead ECG. Patients may have the disease and demonstrate no clinical sequelae. Many transplant programs have initiated baseline and annual angiographic studies to look for the development and progression of graft vasculopathy. Proliferation signal inhibitor medications such as sirolimus and everolimus are sometimes used as prophylaxis against graft vasculopathy or to slow its progression. However, the only definitive treatment for advanced graft vasculopathy is retransplantation.

Pregnancy After Heart Transplant

A subset of heart transplant recipients are women of reproductive age who pursue pregnancy posttransplantantion.[82] The Transplant Pregnancy Registry International reports that 91 women experienced 157 pregnancies between 1987 and 2016.[82] According to the report, 69% of women had a live birth with 26% miscarriage rate, making pregnancy successful in almost two-thirds of cases.[82] Most transplant centers recommend close monitoring during pregnancy due to fluid shifts and potential labile immunosuppression levels. The recommendation is to wait at least 1 year from transplant before becoming pregnant.[82] Pregnancy risks include preeclampsia, rejection, and infection.[82]

Long-Term Functional Status

Compared with end-stage heart disease before transplant, heart transplant recipients report improvement in their functional status and health-related quality of life. The median recipient age for heart transplant is 55 years.[81] Some recipients return to work; 22% are employed at 1 year and 33% at 2 years post heart transplant.[83] At 1 to 3 years after transplant, 80% of recipients report no activity limitations.[83]

HEART-LUNG TRANSPLANTATION

Combined heart-lung transplant is recommended for patients who have concomitant end-stage heart failure and end-stage lung disease. The first experimental heart-lung transplants were performed on dogs in the 1940s and then on primates in the 1970s with good success. This success was in part related to improvements in immunosuppressant medications (described earlier in the chapter) that prevented rejection. Reitz et al. performed the first human heart-lung en bloc transplant at Stanford University in 1981 in a 45-year-old woman with end-stage primary pulmonary hypertension, who survived for more than 5 years.[84,85]

Indications and Selection

Heart-lung transplantation is a viable option for patients with end-stage cardiopulmonary failure such as congenital cardiac anomalies with pulmonary hypertension, primary pulmonary hypertension with irreversible right-sided heart failure, primary parenchymal lung disease with severe right-sided heart failure and, less commonly, cystic fibrosis. Although heart-lung transplantation is the most common among multiorgan transplants, relatively few heart-lung transplants are performed.[86] In 2022, there were 51 heart-lung transplants performed in the United States, a mere fraction when compared to other solid organ transplants.[3] According to the International Society for Heart and Lung Transplantation (ISHLT), there are over 184 transplant centers worldwide that perform heart-lung transplants, and in 2016 only 58 heart-lung transplants were performed worldwide, with 18 of these transplants performed in the United States.[3] Box 35.7 lists indications for heart-lung, single-lung, and double-lung transplantation.

Patients with end-stage cardiopulmonary or pulmonary disease who have exhausted conventional medical management with the capacity for full rehabilitation may be considered for

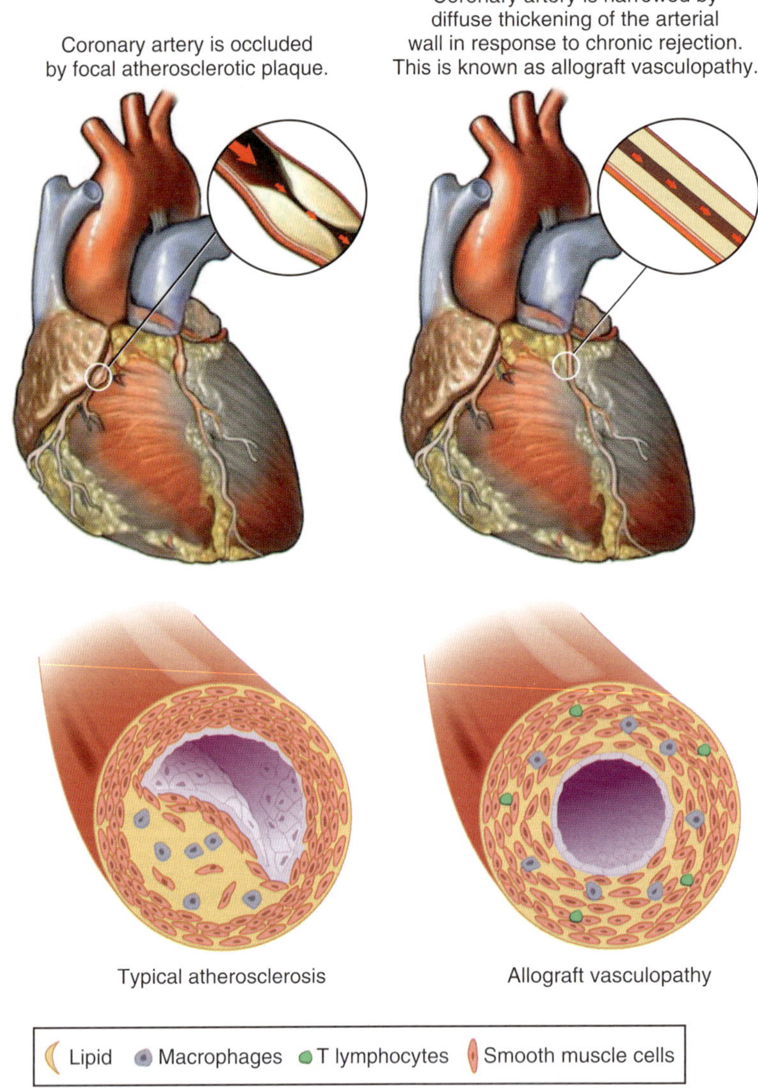

FIG. 35.7 Allograft Vasculopathy Compared With Typical Atherosclerosis.

combined heart-lung transplantation. Potential transplant candidates are those who failed medical management of end-stage organ disease and are terminally ill but must have the strength and stamina to survive the long wait, complex surgery, and rigorous rehabilitation after transplantation. Although there are general standards that all centers adhere to in the candidate selection process, relative contraindications vary by case in most centers. Box 35.8 lists absolute and relative contraindications for heart-lung, single-lung, and double-lung transplantation.

Heart-Lung Transplant Surgical Procedure

Suitable donors are required for the success of a heart-lung transplant. All potential donors are primarily brain dead from an event that leads to donor ventilator dependence to keep potential organs viable. There has been an emergence of case reports of use of DCD for heart-lung "en blocs," utilizing modified lung OCS™ to aid in extending warm perfusion times and bridging longer distances.[87,88] Advancements such as these may aid transplant centers in recovering and utilizing additional otherwise unused organs in the future.

Heart-lung blocs are at risk for pulmonary edema, embolism, infectious processes, and atelectasis. Besides these risks, underlying donor pathology and chest trauma also determine whether donor organs are suitable for placement.

Donor Heart-Lung Procurement Surgery

Lung tissue has a relatively short preservation time, generally 4 to 6 hours, leading to procurement distance limits with its traditional recovery process. Donors must meet brain death criteria and have preserved lung function with no evidence of infection, malignancy, or cardiopulmonary pathology. Donors with a history of smoking may be accepted if they meet the above-mentioned criteria.

To overcome the shortage of donor lungs, suboptimal lungs are occasionally accepted. Lungs that have experienced trauma, aspiration, or infection may have deteriorated pulmonary function. Interventions such as fluid management, toileting of airways by bronchoscopy, modification of ventilatory parameters, and preconditioning through ex vivo lung perfusion are sometimes performed to optimize donor lungs for transplantation.[89] Although most donors are younger than 55 years, older donors may be accepted if they meet all other criteria. Lung fields must be clear on radiologic findings with arterial oxygenation greater than 100 mm Hg on 40% inspired oxygen. A 100% oxygen

BOX 35.8 Contraindications for Heart-Lung and Lung Transplant

Absolute Contraindications

- Malignancy in the last 5 y; lung transplantation for localized bronchoalveolar cell carcinoma is considered on a case-by-case basis
- Ductal carcinoma of the breast is considered on a case-by-case basis
- Untreatable advanced dysfunction of another major organ system
- Coronary artery disease with significant impairment of left ventricular function; heart-lung transplantation may be considered
- *Burkholderia cepacia* genomovar I, III, VI
- Noncurable chronic extrapulmonary infection
- Significant chest wall/spinal deformity
- Mantle radiation
- Documented nonadherence to follow-through with medical therapy or office follow-up, or both
- Untreatable psychological condition associated with inability to comply with medical therapy
- Absence of consistent or reliable social support system
- Active substance addiction

Relative Contraindications

- Age older than 65 y for single-lung transplant
- Age older than 60 y for bilateral lung transplant
- Corticosteroid >20 mg/day
- Critical or unstable clinical condition
- Severely limited functional status with poor rehabilitation potential
- Colonization with highly resistant or highly virulent bacteria, fungi, or mycobacteria
- Obesity, defined as body mass index exceeding 30 kg/m^2
- Symptomatic osteoporosis
- Mechanical ventilation
- Coronary artery disease with percutaneous intervention with no cardiac dysfunction

Other medical conditions that have not resulted in end-stage organ damage such as diabetes mellitus, systemic hypertension, peptic ulcer disease, or gastroesophageal reflux should be optimally treated before transplant.

challenge must show an arterial partial pressure of oxygen greater than 300 mm Hg.[90,91]

The donor and potential recipients are matched for ABO compatibility and organ size. Chest circumference, wall dimensions, and height-adjusted and weight-adjusted lung volumes are assessed. A donor with slightly smaller lungs than the recipient helps prevent postoperative compression atelectasis. Finally, inspection of the donor organs during procurement is essential for assessing lesions and trauma, which may affect transplant outcomes.[90,91]

During procurement, a sternotomy is made to inspect the heart and lungs. Once it is determined that the organs are suitable, the heart and lungs are mobilized. Prostaglandins are administered into the pulmonary artery.[92] The donor heart is then flushed with cold cardioplegia solution while the donor lungs are flushed with cold modified Collins solution, Perfadex®, or University of Wisconsin solution.[93] Once the heart and lungs are perfused, they are removed and placed in cold electrolyte solution for transport using sterile technique.[94]

Recipient Heart-Lung Transplant Surgery

Cardiopulmonary bypass is used for the recipient operation. The phrenic nerves and bronchial artery circulation are preserved and maintained to prevent bleeding complications in the postoperative period. The heart-lung en bloc is placed with the tracheal anastomosis performed first, followed by the atrial anastomosis and then the aortic anastomosis. The donor trachea is kept short because of limited vascular blood supply in the area (Fig. 35.8)

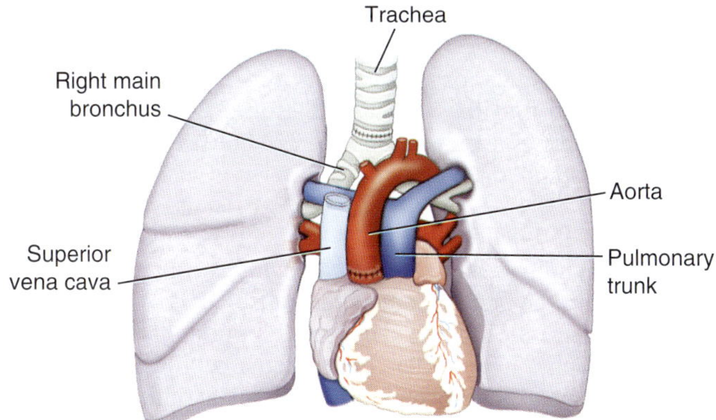

FIG. 35.8 Heart-Lung Transplant En Bloc Surgical Procedure. Incisions in trachea and aorta are shown. The heart is attached to a remnant atrial cuff, which contains the openings of the superior and inferior vena cava and pulmonary veins (not shown).

Postoperative Nursing and Medical Management after Heart-Lung Transplant

The heart-lung transplant recipient is admitted to the critical care unit immediately after surgery and monitored for general hemodynamic stability, oxygenation, bleeding, ischemia-reperfusion injury, acute rejection, infection, deep vein thrombosis, pulmonary emboli, and multiorgan function.

Mechanical Ventilation

Ventilator settings are determined partially by the underlying disease process and patient progression. Regular suctioning of secretions is crucial to maintain airway clearance. Extubation is performed after satisfactory gas exchange and lung mechanics are accomplished, and most patients are extubated within 24 to 48 hours. Evaluation for graft dysfunction, reperfusion injury, gas trapping, and phrenic nerve injury is ongoing. Early mobilization following extubation is essential for effective pulmonary hygiene and may help prevent reintubation. Bronchoscopy is used to assess for potential complications such as stenosis, dehiscence, infection, and rejection and to assess the anastomosis.

Fluids

Care must be maintained when managing fluids in the early postoperative period. The lungs are extremely sensitive to volume overload. Pulmonary artery occlusion pressure and daily weight may be used to determine volume status and the need for diuretics. Overdiuresis results in hypotension and prerenal azotemia. Most patients are maintained on low-dose dopamine for the first 24 to 48 hours for inotropic support and kidney vasodilation. Epinephrine may also be used for inotropic support. Prostaglandin E_1 and nitroprusside provide pulmonary and systemic vasodilation. Nitric oxide, a potent vasodilator, is useful in decreasing pulmonary artery pressures and improving oxygenation.[93]

Pleural Drainage

Pleural drainage must be observed and documented, and careful attention should be paid to signs of active bleeding from the mediastinal and pleural chest tubes. Frank blood of more than 100 mL per hour over 3 hours should be a concern in patients with normal coagulation. Exploratory surgery of the chest may be required to find the source of bleeding. When chest tube drainage produces less than 200 mL in 24 hours without a noted air leak, chest tubes can be removed.

Ischemia-Reperfusion Injury

Reperfusion injury, also called *primary graft dysfunction*, usually occurs within the first 72 hours after transplantation and is typified by nonspecific alveolar damage with pulmonary infiltrates on radiography, hypoxemia, lung edema with poor pulmonary compliance, and normal or low left atrial filling pressures. Severe cases require ventilation, moderate levels of positive end-expiratory pressure and fraction of inspired oxygen, pharmacologic therapy, and perhaps nitric oxide or ECMO.[93]

Rejection Surveillance

Acute cellular rejection is a significant risk factor in development of chronic rejection, which is associated with poor outcomes; thus early diagnosis and treatment of rejection is essential.

Clinical manifestations of rejection in the heart-lung or lung transplant recipient can include shortness of breath, cough, fever, fatigue, wheezes, crackles, and decrease in lung function noted on pulmonary function tests. However, the potential signs of rejection are also potential signs of pulmonary infection. Patients with a decline in lung function on pulmonary function tests with a decrease in forced expiratory volume in 1 second greater than 10% and a decrease in forced vital capacity greater than 10% should be further evaluated for rejection. Desaturation may also occur with exercise oximetry.

Rejection of the lungs is diagnosed by transbronchial biopsy. Rejection of the heart has been traditionally diagnosed by endomyocardial biopsy of the heart, but advances in heart rejection detection and management have been changing because of the availability of gene expression profile and donor-derived cell free DNA testing in single-organ transplants.[74,75] It is important to mention that some patients are asymptomatic when rejection is present; thus many transplant centers perform surveillance bronchoscopies at specific intervals within the first year after heart-lung or lung transplant for early diagnosis and treatment of a rejection episode.[95] Heart biopsy is not recommended after 4 to 6 months posttransplant and is performed only with symptoms of heart failure or left ventricular or biventricular dysfunction on echocardiography.

Pulmonary function testing should be used as an adjunct to clinical evaluation and biopsy, not solely to diagnose acute lung rejection.[95] Spirometry has been shown to have a sensitivity of greater than 60% for detecting infection or rejection grade A2 and higher, but it cannot differentiate between the two. The ability to detect rejection diminishes further in single-lung transplants because of the effect of native lung dysfunction hindering the results.[95] Some patients with marked decreased in lung function without underlying infection and biopsy-proven rejections may be treated empirically with high doses of steroids, normally methylprednisolone 10 mg/kg intravenously daily for 3 consecutive days. Severe grades of rejection may also warrant the use of rabbit antithymocyte globulin. Table 35.9 depicts pulmonary grading of lung rejection.[95]

Humoral rejection is mediated by antibody and complement.[95] Antibody-mediated rejection can occur immediately after transplantation (hyperacute) or months later. Clinical manifestations are similar to the symptoms of acute cellular rejection. Antibodies are either preformed antibodies or represent antidonor antibodies that develop after transplantation.[96] Blood testing for donor-specific antibodies (DSA) provides a method for determining whether a recipient has built antibodies specific to the donor after transplant. Treatment for antibody-mediated rejection warrants high-dose steroids, plasmapheresis, immunoglobulin, and rituximab (Rituxan). Intractable rejection can be treated with monoclonal or polyclonal antibodies, total lymphoid irradiation, or methotrexate.

Infection

Infectious complications are one of the most common causes of morbidity and mortality after heart-lung transplantation. Direct exposure to microbes, denervation of the graft with impaired cough reflex, impaired lymphatic drainage, infections

TABLE 35.9 Pathologic Grading of Lung Rejection

Category	Grade	Meaning	Appearance
A: Acute rejection	0	None	Normal lung parenchyma
	1	Minimal	Inconspicuous small mononuclear perivascular infiltrates
	2	Mild	More frequent, more obvious perivascular infiltrates; eosinophils may be present
	3	Moderate	Dense perivascular infiltrates; extension into interstitial space; can involve endothelialitis, eosinophils, and neutrophils
	4	Severe	Diffuse perivascular, interstitial, and air-space infiltrates with lung injury; neutrophils may be present
B: Airway inflammation	0	None	No evidence of bronchiolar inflammation
	1 R	Low grade	Infrequent, scattered, or single-layer mononuclear cells in bronchiolar submucosa
	2 R	High grade	Larger infiltrates of larger and activated lymphocytes in bronchiolar submucosa; can involve eosinophils and plasmacytoid cells
	X	Ungradable	No bronchiolar tissue available
C: Chronic airway rejection—obliterative bronchiolitis	0	Absent	If present, describes intraluminal airway obliteration with fibrous connective tissue
	1	Present	
D: Chronic vascular rejection—accelerated graft vascular sclerosis		Not graded	Fibrointimal thickening of arteries and poor cellular hyaline sclerosis of veins; usually requires open lung biopsy for diagnosis

Modified from Martinu T, Chen DF, Palmer SM. Acute rejection and humoral sensitization in lung transplant recipients. *Proc Am Thorac Soc.* 2009;6(1):54.

transferred from the donor, infection from the native lung in single-lung transplants, and immunosuppression all contribute to infection risk.[97] Evidence of infection after heart-lung transplantation can be found in blood cultures, sputum, and urine and while performing a bronchoscopy with bronchoalveolar lavage. Samples of fluid from bronchial lavage are cultured for presence of bacteria or fungi and tested for viruses.

Antimicrobial prophylaxis for *Pneumocystis jirovecii* with sulfamethoxazole and trimethoprim is used in most centers because of successful prevention of this bacterial infection with additional antimicrobial effects against *Toxoplasma gondii* and *Nocardia* species. There are many other bacterial colonizers and infections seen after heart-lung transplantation and lung transplantation but no widely used prophylaxis.[97]

Candida and *Aspergillus* infections are the most common fungal infections in transplant patients. Prophylactic antifungal medications are used by many centers, but there are no clear data regarding optimal treatment or duration.

CMV is the most common viral infection in transplant recipients (described earlier in chapter). CMV may occur within the first few months after transplantation and can also occur later on. Universal prophylaxis and preemptive therapy are the main measures taken to prevent occurrence. CMV infection occurs in 25% to 50% of heart transplant recipients but is highest in lung transplant recipients, with a reported incidence of 54% to 92% in recipients not taking prophylactic antiviral medications.[97–99] Intravenous ganciclovir followed by oral valganciclovir (Valcyte) are the primary prophylactic antiviral medications to prevent CMV infection.[97] Longer-term survival is decreased in recipients who receive a lung from a CMV-positive donor.[100]

Other common viruses after transplant include respiratory syncytial virus, influenza, adenovirus, human metapneumovirus, and parainfluenza. These are not treated prophylactically but as they occur. Nevertheless, viral infections still pose a threat to recipient health and may lead to allograft injury over time.

Immunosuppression

Immunosuppressive therapy begins with the induction phase, perioperatively and immediately after transplantation, followed by maintenance therapy that continues for the life of the allograft. As noted earlier in this chapter, induction medication regimens are different from maintenance medications, and their use varies by transplant center. Maintenance immunosuppression is the key to prevention of acute and chronic rejections throughout the life of the graft. Most centers use a three-medication regimen consisting of a calcineurin inhibitor, antimetabolite, and corticosteroid (see previous section, Immunosuppressive Medications).

Patient and Family Education

To improve outcomes, patient and family education should begin during the evaluation process and continue after transplant. A significant factor that affects a patient's outcome posttransplant is the patient's ability to self-manage an extensive medication regimen and follow complex instructions. Effective education is an essential component in management of post–heart-lung transplant patients.[101] Patients and their family and/or primary caregivers must be part of the learning experience to ensure understanding of the entire process from selection through posttransplantation. Posttransplant patient education should include medication education, emphasis on medication adherence, self-monitoring for signs and symptoms of complications, and tips for maintaining a healthy lifestyle, including fundamental lifestyle changes, keeping up with medical appointments, healthy diet, exercising, and protection from the sun.[102]

Long-Term Considerations

Chronic rejection can affect either or both the heart and lungs in combined heart-lung transplant patients. Chronic rejection of the heart manifests as coronary allograft vasculopathy as described earlier in this chapter. Chronic rejection of the lungs is often referred to as *chronic allograft dysfunction* (CLAD) and can manifest as either an obstructive or a restrictive phenotype. Bronchiolitis obliterans syndrome (BOS) is the hallmark of CLAD and is the primary cause of morbidity and mortality after heart-lung transplantation. Restrictive allograft syndrome (RAS) is characterized by fibrotic changes predominantly concentrated in upper lobes and restrictive pulmonary function tests. RAS, although less common than BOS, is associated with poorer outcomes.

Bronchiolitis Obliterans Syndrome

Bronchiolitis obliterans syndrome is graded by spirometry and defined as an irreversible decline in forced expiratory volume in 1 second (FEV_1) with measurements taken 3 weeks apart, after excluding other causes of allograft dysfunction.[102] Caused by dense fibrotic scar tissue affecting the small airways, clinical manifestations of chronic rejection include progressive dyspnea, cough, negative sputum cultures, and worsening airflow obstruction without obvious cause. By 5 years after lung transplant, more than 50% of survivors have BOS symptoms.[102]

Factors such as acute cellular rejection and lymphocytic bronchiolitis are known to be associated with BOS. Nonimmune mechanisms such as PGD, infections, airway ischemia, and gastroesophageal reflux may also trigger an inflammatory-immune response leading to BOS.[102] Therefore the balancing act with immunosuppression dosage to prevent rejection and infection is a careful art. Investigation of patient gastrointestinal complaints should be done promptly to avoid aspiration risk leading to allograft damage. Currently, there is no cure for chronic rejection. Research is ongoing to discover interventions to slow the process and eliminate BOS. Table 35.10 depicts the BOS classification system.[102]

TABLE 35.10 Bronchiolitis Obliterans Syndrome Classification System

BOS Stage	Description
0	FEV_1 >90% of baseline and $FEF_{25\%-75\%}$ >75% of baseline (No BOS)
0-p[a]	FEV_1 81%–90% of baseline and/or $FEF_{25\%-75\%}$ ≤75% of baseline (Potential BOS)
1	FEV_1 66%–80% of baseline (Mild BOS)
2	FEV_1 51%–65% of baseline (Moderate BOS)
3	FEV_1 ≤50% of baseline (Severe BOS)

[a]0-p=Potential BOS.

BOS, Bronchiolitis obliterans syndrome; *$FEF_{25\%-75\%}$*, forced expiratory flow, midexpiratory phase; *FEV_1*, forced expiratory volume in 1 second.

Modified from Ahmad S, Shlobin OA, Nathan SD. Pulmonary complications of lung transplantation. *Chest.* 2011;139(2):402.

Comorbidities

Numerous morbidities develop over time in transplant patients, including hypertension and hyperlipidemia from calcineurin inhibitor medications, diabetes mellitus from corticosteroids and calcineurin inhibitors, kidney disease from calcineurin inhibitors, cancers such as skin cancer, and posttransplant lymphoproliferative disease from immunosuppressive agents.

Although the success rate for heart-lung transplantation is not at the level of other organ transplants, heart-lung transplantation remains a viable option for patients with cardiopulmonary end-stage disease.

Survival after heart-lung transplant has made steady improvement with a median survival of 5.8 years.[103] For heart-lung transplant recipients who received their transplant between 2004 and 2014, this represents 63% 1-year survival, 45% 3-year survival, and 32% 10-year survival.[103]

SINGLE-LUNG AND DOUBLE-LUNG TRANSPLANTATION

Lung transplantation is a viable option for patients with end-stage pulmonary disease without end-stage cardiac disease. Chronic obstructive pulmonary disease (32%), interstitial lung diseases (24%), cystic fibrosis (16%), and alpha-antitrypsin deficiency (5%) are the main diseases warranting a lung transplant.[104] Lung transplantation is considered when life expectancy is no more than 36 months despite maximum medical management with disease symptoms classified as NYHA class III or IV.

Suitable donor lungs are a scarce resource, and single-lung transplantation can provide benefit to two recipients from one donor. Consequently, single-lung versus double-lung transplant surgery is thoughtfully considered during patient evaluation. Some advantages of a single-lung transplant include shorter waitlist time, decreased need for cardiopulmonary bypass and intubation time, and it typically warrants a shorter hospitalization. Single lung transplants are suitable in certain conditions such as pulmonary fibrosis and emphysema. Since conditions such as cystic fibrosis can infect both lungs, only double-lung transplants are warranted for this disease. However, improved quality of life and success rates of double-lung transplants have made double-lung transplantation the preferred method of surgery for those in need of a lung transplant regardless of the illness.

COVID-19 and Lung Transplant

Shortly after the declaration of the COVID-19 pandemic, lung transplant was utilized as a lifesaving measure in a limited number of patients who suffered from irreparable lung injury from COVID-19.[105] Since then, hundreds of lung transplants for COVID-19 have been performed. Many critically ill COVID-19 patients are difficult to manage, requiring high levels of sedation, paralytics and ECMO due to acute respiratory distress syndrome.[106] Earlier in the pandemic lung transplants were offered to those who had persistent lung failure and remained critically ill for several weeks or months.[107] As time into the pandemic went on, physicians became more experienced with use of ECMO in COVID-19 patients and functional and pulmonary improvement without transplant was observed.[106] The timing of lung transplant in COVID-19 patients remains highly challenging, and delayed recovery from the viral infection must be thoughtfully considered against complications of prolonged critical illness. However, with the availability of vaccines, improved therapeutics, and less virulent variants of the virus, the number of lung transplants due to COVID-19 appears to be declining.

Lung Transplantation Surgical Procedures

The surgical procedure is different depending on whether the surgery is for single-lung, double-lung, or lobar transplant. For patients with end-stage lung disease who are not candidates for a transplant, surgery to reduce lung volume is an option.

Single-Lung Transplant Surgical Procedure

The lung with the worst function is chosen for excision. If both lungs have equal function, the right lung is selected for explantation (lung removal). Implantation (donor lung placement) in the right lung position avoids maneuvering around the heart.

A thoracotomy incision is made anteriorly or posteriorly at the fourth or fifth intercostal space. Alternatively, a sternotomy incision can be used. The lung is collapsed while the blood vessels are tied off. The lung is then removed at the bronchus. Next, the donor lung is placed, and the blood vessels are attached. Finally, the implanted lung is inflated, and the incision is closed.[94] The surgical procedure for single-lung transplantation is illustrated in Fig. 35.9.

Lung hyperinflation is a common complication after single-lung transplantation.[94] Graft compression by the hyperinflated native lung can cause mediastinal shift and respiratory failure. Lobectomy and lung volume reduction surgery (LVRS) are two methods to prevent graft compression leading to decreased ventilation of the allograft. The native lung can also be a source of infections or develop a pneumothorax.

Double-Lung Transplantation Surgical Procedure

Double-lung (bilateral) transplant is the preferred surgical procedure for patients with cystic fibrosis or bronchiectasis given the significance of infections in both lungs, which would remain in the native lung if both lungs were not transplanted. A double-lung transplant can be performed simultaneously (see en bloc Fig. 35.8) or sequentially (Fig. 35.10). Bilateral lung transplant is increasingly selected over single-lung transplant.

Transverse thoracosternotomy, clamshell incision, and median sternotomy are the incisional approaches used in double-lung transplant surgery. The first lung is collapsed, and the blood vessel is tied off and cut at the corresponding bronchi.

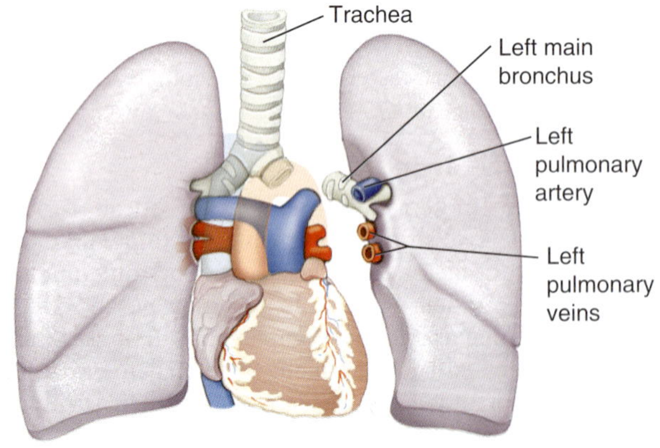

FIG. 35.9 Single-lung transplantation procedure shows where incisions will be for the left main bronchus, left pulmonary artery, and left pulmonary veins.

The new lung is then placed, and the vessels are reattached. The same process is repeated for the second lung to be placed. Patients with pulmonary hypertension may be placed on cardiopulmonary bypass during the surgery to avoid right heart failure.[94] The surgical procedure for a sequential double-lung transplant is shown in Fig. 35.10.

Lung Volume Reduction Surgery

LVRS is an option that may be available to patients with end-stage lung disease with comorbidities. LVRS may be indicated in patients with emphysema who have relative or absolute contraindications to transplant. The technique involves reducing the lung volume by wedge resection of the emphysematous tissue.[94] LVRS may decrease the mismatch between the hyperinflated lungs and the chest cavity. This may lead to elastic recoil and improved expiratory flow.

LVRS should be considered for patients with chronic medical conditions that make them ineligible for transplant, such as active hepatitis B, hepatitis C with biopsy-proven liver disease, HIV infection, and organ system dysfunction. Medical conditions that may be acceptable for LVRS, include limited-stage non–small cell cancer with resection, lack of family support, psychiatric conditions, or a history of poor adherence with treatment.

Living Donor Lobar Lung Transplantation

Living lobar lung transplant was introduced at the University of Southern California in 1993 for patients who were too ill to wait for cadaveric organs. Two donors are required to donate either a right or left lower lobe of their own lung, and the recipient receives bilateral lower lobe transplants.[108,109] Cystic fibrosis is the most frequent diagnosis for living lung transplantation.[108] The risk of complications or death is higher than in cadaveric donor transplants because it involves two healthy living donors, as well as the recipient. The recipient must also meet the requirements for cadaveric lung transplant and be on the waiting list.

Postoperative Nursing and Medical Management After Lung Transplant

Postoperative management for lung transplant recipients is similar to the management of heart-lung transplant recipients. Ventilation, hemodynamic monitoring, fluid management, drainage, immunosuppression, ischemia-reperfusion injury, rejection, and infection are monitored in the same way. Typically, single-lung transplant recipients have an easier time weaning off the ventilator and have shorter hospitalizations. Ventilation issues may warrant bronchoscopy while the patient is still intubated. Airway complications such as partial anastomotic dehiscence and stenosis are common and are diagnosed by bronchoscopy. Airway dehiscence is treated by reoperation or close observation and supportive care, whereas stenosis may require stent placement in the affected airway.

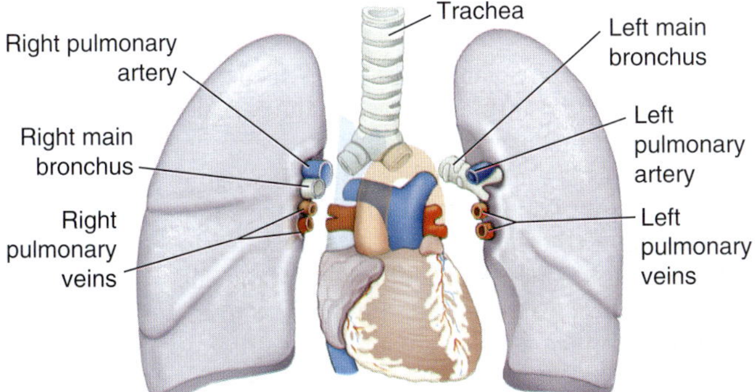

FIG. 35.10 Simultaneous double-lung transplantation procedure in which both lungs are sequentially replaced shows where incisions will occur between the right and left pulmonary veins, right and left pulmonary arteries, and right and left bronchi.

Aggressive postoperative pulmonary hygiene is essential to promote airway clearance because surgical denervation of the lungs diminishes the cough reflex after surgery. Ischemia-reperfusion injury and disrupted pulmonary lymphatics can increase vascular permeability, leading to interstitial edema. Other potential postoperative complications are dysrhythmias, deep vein thrombosis, pulmonary emboli, and pneumothorax, all of which are prevalent in the early postoperative period.

Patient and Family Education

Patient and family and/or caregiver education begins before transplant in the evaluation period and continues throughout the life of the patient. Education includes information regarding infection prevention, signs and symptoms of infection, importance of medication adherence to prevent allograft rejection, lifestyle modifications, dietary recommendations, and follow-up care instructions. It is important that lung transplant patients continue to follow up with their lung transplant center as they will need lifelong specialized care.

Long-Term Considerations

BOS is the histopathologic finding of chronic lung rejection (see Table 35.10). BOS affects 10%, 27%, and 50% of lung transplant recipients at 1, 3, and 5 years.[110] Acute rejection, infectious episodes, cancer, hypertension, diabetes mellitus, kidney dysfunction, gastrointestinal disturbances, and psychosocial issues all are very common short-term and long-term problems after transplantation and need to be addressed regularly. Median survival after primary lung transplant is 6.5 years,[104] although some recipients survive more than 20 years.[111]

LIVER TRANSPLANTATION

Liver transplantation was first attempted in canine models in the 1950s. The outcomes were unsuccessful because of technical complications, infection, and graft failure. Efforts to improve surgical technique continued, and successful liver transplantation in dogs was achieved several years later. Later in 1963 Starzl performed the first human liver transplant, although the patient died intraoperatively. In 1967, Starzl performed the first successful human liver transplant in a patient with malignant hepatoma.[112]

The adjusted patient survival rate after liver transplantation is approximately 90% at 1 year, approximately 85% at 3 years, and approximately 70% at 5 years.[55,113,114] Survival is affected by the pretransplant diagnosis, the donor liver (deceased or living donation), and age.[55,113,114] In 2018 there were 8250 liver transplants performed in the United States.[113]

Indications and Selection

Liver transplantation must be considered for any patient who has irreversible acute or chronic liver disease that is progressive and there is no therapy of established efficacy. Diseases of the liver may be categorized as chronic, vascular, fulminant or subfulminant, inborn errors of metabolism, and hepatic

BOX 35.9 End-Stage Liver Diseases Commonly Treated With Liver Transplantation

Cholestatic Liver Diseases
- Biliary atresia
- Primary sclerosing cholangitis
- Primary biliary cirrhosis

Chronic Hepatocellular Diseases
- Viral hepatitis (types A, B, C, D, E)
- Alcoholic liver disease (Laennec disease)
- Autoimmune hepatitis
- Cryptogenic cirrhosis
- Medication-induced liver disease

Vascular Diseases
- Budd-Chiari syndrome
- Venoocclusive disease

Acute and Subacute Liver Failure
- Viral hepatitis (types A, B, C, D, E)
- Medication-induced liver failure (acetaminophen, isoniazid overdoses)
- Fulminant Wilson disease

Inborn Metabolic Disorders
- Wilson disease
- Alpha-1-antitrypsin deficiency
- Hemochromatosis
- Tyrosinemia
- Glycogen storage disease, types I and II

Primary Hepatic Malignancies
- Hepatocellular carcinoma
- Hemangioendothelioma
- Hepatoblastoma

malignancies. Box 35.9 lists the most common diseases in patients who undergo liver transplantation. In the United States the most common indication for liver transplantation in adults is chronic viral hepatitis C. However, the availability of interferon-free treatment of hepatitis C patients with advanced liver cirrhosis restores liver function and has decreased the number of patients with hepatitis C waiting for a liver transplant in the United States.[55,113,114] Cholestatic disease, biliary atresia, and metabolic disorders are the most common diseases leading to transplantation in pediatric patients.

Candidate selection is an important aspect of transplantation. Given the shortage of available organs, the transplant team must have reasonable assurance of a successful outcome. The timing of transplantation is of utmost importance. The patient must not be so ill as to be unable to survive the surgery yet must be experiencing significant deterioration in their quality of life. Body mass index (BMI) plays a role in posttransplantation survival. Patients who are underweight (BMI less than 20) or morbidly obese (BMI greater than 40) are at greater risk for death after transplantation.[55,113,114] In general, liver transplantation is not to be offered to patients in the following situations:

- Unlikely to survive major surgery
- Would not survive the effects of long-term immunosuppression
- Have a disease that is likely to recur quickly and fatally after transplantation
- Unable or unwilling to comply with long-term medical regimens

BOX 35.10 Contraindications to Liver Transplantation

Absolute Contraindications	Relative Contraindications
Brain death	Physiologic age
Metastatic malignancy	Advanced renal disease
Extrahepatic malignancy	Multiple hepatic malignancies
Active drug abuse or alcohol abuse	Moderate cardiopulmonary disease
Advanced cardiopulmonary disease	Peripheral vascular disease
Acquired immunodeficiency syndrome	Psychosocial behaviors indicating noncompliance with medical regimens
Extrahepatic sepsis	Human immunodeficiency virus infection

The absolute contraindications listed in Box 35.10 fall under these four specific categories. Having one relative contraindication may not rule out transplantation but having several predicts a poor outcome. Chronologic age is less important than physiologic age and liver transplantation in older adults is increasing.[55,113,114] Certain diseases can recur after transplantation, including viral hepatitis, sclerosing cholangitis, and biliary malignancies. In the case of viral hepatitis, serologic indicators of viral replication are monitored closely. Early treatment is indicated. Multicenter protocols are important in evaluating the outcomes of transplants in patients with diseases that recur. The decision to offer liver transplantation to any patient must be based on evaluation criteria, which may vary among institutions. The criteria are modified as advances in technical ability, immunosuppression, and perioperative management develop.

Recipient Liver Transplant Evaluation

A candidate for liver transplantation undergoes a thorough evaluation to determine the cause and severity of the liver disease, to establish the need for transplantation rather than other interventions, and to identify objective indications and contraindications. Evaluation begins with a carefully elicited patient history (Box 35.11). A comprehensive approach includes laboratory, radiographic, and diagnostic testing and multidisciplinary consultations (Box 35.12). Not every patient undergoes every test and consultation. Careful assessment of medical history and a good physical examination directs initial diagnostic testing. For example, a patient with a history of malignancy would undergo extensive testing to rule out metastases, whereas a patient with acute liver failure may have a more abbreviated work-up focused on determining the cause and potential for hepatic recovery.

Initially, the transplant candidate is seen and examined by a hepatologist and transplant surgeon. The patient is evaluated for comorbidities that can potentially negatively impact a good outcome. Any history of drug abuse or alcohol abuse is discussed, and if this is an issue, referral to addictive behavior psychiatry is made for further evaluation. Additionally, the effect of liver disease on the patient's functional level and the availability of social support are reviewed. Physical examination not only serves as a confirmation of advanced liver disease but also as an opportunity to document clinical signs that may affect successful liver transplant, including loss of muscle mass and debility. Discussions regarding recurrent disease after transplantation and possible hepatitis C virus antiviral therapies before or after transplantation are just as important. Surgical evaluation may

BOX 35.11 Pretransplantation History for a Patient With End-Stage Liver Disease

- Risk factors for viral hepatitis: transfusions, intravenous drug abuse, tattoos, other parenteral exposure
- Family history of liver disease
- Associated disorders: hypothyroidism, osteoporosis, infertility, arthritis
- Onset, duration, and description of symptoms and complications: jaundice, lethargy, bleeding disorders, pruritus, confusion, ascites, edema, melenic stools, abdominal pain, bone pain or fractures, chronic diarrhea, gynecomastia (in men), amenorrhea (in women)
- Current and past medical history: hospitalizations, surgeries
- Social history: exposure to alcohol, drug abuse, toxins, tobacco products
- Status of immunizations

identify additional factors that may complicate the transplant operation, including prior abdominal surgery, obesity, and the candidate's general health and ability to undergo a major surgical procedure. During the evaluation, the surgeon educates the patient and family about the spectrum of donor and graft types, the complexity of the proposed surgery, potential complications, rejection rates, and other aspects of liver transplant, including long-term immunosuppression and its side effects.

As with other organs, a multitude of evaluations are completed, and objective criteria are used to place a patient on the waiting list. These data are used in a formula to determine the patient's liver disease score, which is directly associated with risk of death within 3 months. A higher Model for End-Stage Liver Disease (MELD) score indicates a higher degree of illness and risk of death.[115]

Model for End-Stage Liver Disease

The MELD formula is used in all U.S. transplant centers to calculate the risk of 3-month mortality in patients 12 years old or older.[115] The MELD objective criteria include serum total bilirubin, serum creatinine, prothrombin time, international normalized ratio (INR), and whether the patient has undergone hemodialysis at least twice in the past 2 weeks. The MELD score ranges from 6 to 40, with higher numbers indicating more severe illness. In January 2016 serum sodium was added to the MELD score, creating a MELD-Na score. The serum sodium was added because hyponatremia is associated with higher mortality rates.

Waitlist Placement and MELD Score

The current liver allocation policy is to take the "sickest first" to receive a transplant. Patients with acute liver failure are classified as status 1 and are placed at the top of the list.

The "Share 35" policy was approved and implemented on June 18, 2013. Share 35 mandates that deceased donor livers are offered to regional candidates with a MELD score of 35 or greater before local candidates with a MELD score of less than 35. The policy was implemented to reduce geographic disparities in waitlist mortality.

Additionally, requests may be made to the UNOS regional review board to assign a higher than calculated score for a patient with special problems that are not addressed using only objective criteria. Patients who have hepatocellular carcinoma that meet specific tumor criteria are automatically given a MELD score of 22 because the risk of metastasis outside the liver within 3 months is high. Once metastasis occurs, the patient is no longer deemed a transplant candidate. Other exceptions include disorders such as primary sclerosing cholangitis and polycystic liver disease.

The frequency of recalculation of the MELD score is determined by the score itself.[115]

- MELD scores greater than 25 are evaluated every 7 days.
- MELD scores between 19 and 24 are evaluated every 30 days.
- MELD scores between 11 and 18 are evaluated every 90 days.
- MELD scores below 10 are recalculated yearly, barring any exacerbation of the liver disease or patient condition.

Pediatric End-Stage Liver Disease

The Pediatric End-Stage Liver Disease (PELD) formula is used to calculate risk of 3-month mortality for patients younger than

BOX 35.12 Sample Evaluation Before Liver Transplantation

Laboratory Tests
- Liver function profile: transaminases (aspartate transaminase, alanine transaminase, gamma-glutamyltransferase), alkaline phosphatase, bilirubin, albumin, prothrombin time, partial thromboplastin time, clotting factors, cholesterol, triglycerides
- Kidney function profile with electrolytes: blood urea nitrogen, creatinine, sodium, potassium, carbon dioxide, chloride
- Hematology: complete blood count, reticulocytes, erythrocyte sedimentation rate
- Thyroid function: serum triiodothyronine (T_3) radioimmunoassay, serum thyroxine (T_4) radioimmunoassay, thyroid-stimulating hormone, T_4 and T_3 uptake
- Serology studies for hepatic viruses and other infectious diseases: viral hepatitis (A, B, C, D, E), cytomegalovirus, Epstein-Barr virus, herpesvirus 1 and 2, parvovirus, human immunodeficiency virus, rapid plasma reagin
- Blood type and antibody screen
- Immunologic profiles: antinuclear antibody, antimitochondrial antibody, anti–smooth muscle antibody, immunoglobulins (IgA, IgG, IgM)
- Nutrition profiles: vitamin levels (A, D, E, B_{12}, folate), iron studies with ferritin
- Tumor markers: alpha-fetoprotein, carcinoembryonic antigen, prostate-specific antigen
- Miscellaneous: ceruloplasmin, alpha-1-antitrypsin level and phenotype

Urine
- 24-h protein and electrolytes, cultures, creatinine clearance, urinalysis, copper

Stool
- Ova, cysts, parasites, occult blood, 48-h fecal fat, cultures

Gastrointestinal Work-Up
- Endoscopy, colonoscopy, endoscopic retrograde cholangiopancreatography, liver biopsy

Pulmonary Profile
- Arterial blood gases, pulmonary function studies

Radiographic and Diagnostic Tests
- Chest radiograph, ultrasound studies of liver including vascular studies

Optional Tests
- Doppler studies, sinus radiography, computed tomography (abdomen, chest, head), electrocardiography, echocardiography, cardiac stress test, cardiac catheterization, mammography, peripheral vascular studies, carotid ultrasonography, abdominal angiography, percutaneous cholangiography, bone mineral density

12 years.[116] The PELD objective criteria include date of birth, sex, weight, height, serum albumin, serum total bilirubin, prothrombin time, and INR.

Pretransplantation Phase

A patient with end-stage liver disease who is awaiting a transplant can pose many nursing care challenges in the critical care unit. The clinical issues often include:

- Hepatic encephalopathy
- Coagulopathy
- Portal hypertension, ascites, varices
- Severe fluid and electrolyte imbalances
- Heart failure
- Pulmonary failure
- Kidney failure (hepatorenal syndrome)

Hepatic Encephalopathy

Frequent mental status assessments are important in determining the patient's continued candidacy for transplantation. Hepatic encephalopathy may improve with the administration of antibiotics and laxatives, or the patient may proceed to grade IV coma. Later stages of hepatic encephalopathy may be clinically indistinguishable from cerebral hemorrhage. Diagnostic studies may be needed to evaluate the possibility of an intracranial bleed. Some centers use intracranial pressure monitoring catheters with these patients. The head of the bed is maintained at 30 to 45 degrees to avoid even slight increases in intracranial pressure (ICP). Protection of the airway is especially important in an encephalopathic patient who is not intubated. In these circumstances, if hematemesis or vomiting occurs, intubation and use of paralytic agents may be necessary to protect the patient's airway.

Nutritional Support

Patients who have chronic liver disease are malnourished because of poor dietary intake and impaired digestion, absorption, and metabolism of nutrients. They require supplements of the fat-soluble vitamins (A, D, E, and K). Recommended dietary intake for patients with chronic liver disease includes 35 to 40 kcal/kg/day and 1.2 to 1.5 g/kg/day of protein using ideal body weight for patients with ascites and actual body weight for patients without ascites.

Portal Hypertension

Consequences of portal hypertension must be corrected. Gastrointestinal hemorrhage from varices may respond to administration of propranolol or may require procedures such as banding and sclerotherapy. Portal hypertension may be reduced by a *transjugular intrahepatic portosystemic shunt* (TIPS) performed by an interventional radiologist. Rarely, the patient may need to undergo surgical intervention with a vascular shunt created between the portacaval system and the mesangial, splenic, or renal vascular system. However, surgically created vascular shunts are usually not considered in patients who are transplant candidates. Patients with massive ascites usually have total body fluid overload but are intravascularly contracted and require sodium restriction and administration of colloidal fluids, such as albumin with diuretics. Careful documentation of fluid intake and output, daily weight determinations, and frequent measurement of vital signs are needed to monitor fluid status. Ascites can interfere with lung expansion and can compromise oxygenation. Patients with large, distended abdomens also find adequate oral nutrition difficult. Use of diuretics to control ascites is common but can compromise kidney function or worsen hepatorenal syndrome. Paracentesis (removal of ascites) may be required for intractable ascites. However, frequent large-volume paracentesis procedures can contribute to kidney and heart compromise related to fluid volume shifts.

Spontaneous Bacterial Peritonitis

Spontaneous bacterial peritonitis (SBP) can manifest in a patient with end-stage liver disease by an acute decline in liver and kidney function accompanied by fever, abdominal pain, and hepatic encephalopathy. SBP is commonly caused by translocation of bacteria from the intestinal lumen. SBP is diagnosed when the paracentesis fluid shows increased white blood cells, with or without a positive culture. Patients are treated aggressively with antibiotics and are temporarily deferred from transplantation during treatment for and recovery from bacterial peritonitis.

Determining Donor Liver Suitability

The two criteria necessary for matching a donor liver to a recipient are blood type and body size. HLA tissue typing is not used in the matching of donor livers because it has not been shown to significantly affect patient outcomes. Donors are carefully screened for infectious diseases and metastatic carcinomas because these can be transmitted to the recipient. The transplant center is notified by the regional OPO that a liver is available. If the organ is accepted, a member of the transplant team contacts the patient.

In very urgent situations, the donor blood type (e.g., type O) may be incompatible with the recipient blood type (e.g., type A). Despite this ABO incompatibility, liver transplants can occur in urgent situations and can be successful. There may be some early postoperative complications, such as mild hemolysis, higher incidence of acute cellular rejection, and increased postoperative hepatic vascular and biliary complications, but innovative use of immunosuppressive regimens and plasmapheresis have improved graft survival of patients with recipient–donor ABO incompatibility.

Extended-criteria donor (ECD) livers, including livers from DCD donors, livers with a cold ischemia time longer than 12 hours, hepatitis C antibody–positive livers, and livers from donors older than 60 years, are expanding the donor pool and shortening waiting times.[117] The use of ECD livers can lead to complications and worsen outcomes. For example, the use of livers from DCD donors can lead to biliary complications, livers from donors with advanced age or fatty liver can cause delayed graft function, and livers from high-risk donors can increase the rate of infection in the recipient.[118] Despite the shortcomings of ECD livers, many lives are saved.

After a donor liver becomes available, it is necessary to expedite the preoperative preparation of the recipient. The use of newer preservation solutions has allowed for longer cold ischemia time. Cold ischemia is the length of time from when the organ is removed from the donor, flushed, and packed in ice for storage until the time when it is transplanted.

Living Donor Lobe Liver Transplant

Many liver transplant centers in the United States offer living donor liver transplantation (LDLT). In 2020, there were 425 adult liver transplants from living donors.[114] By comparison, in 2020 there were 7979 adult liver transplants from deceased donors.[114] LDLT is more common in pediatric liver transplantation.

LDLT began in 1989 with adult-to-child donations, commonly from a parent to their infant. The left lateral hepatic lobe is resected, leaving the donor with the larger mass of liver remaining. LDLT of the lateral segment of the left lobe of the liver has become highly successful in pediatric transplantation. Adult-to-adult LDLT began in the 1990s. Some transplant centers perform adult-to-adult right lobe and, less frequently, left lobe LDLT.

Living Donor Liver Transplantation Complications

Complications for the donor after partial hepatectomy are graded by the *Clavien Severity System* grades I through IV.[114,119]

- Grade I complications are not life threatening and do not result in permanent disability.
- Grade II complications require medications or transfusion.
- Grade III complications can be potentially life threatening and require invasive therapy, including a return to the operating room.
- Grade IV complications lead to disability or death.

Most LDLT complications are grade I and II and include urinary tract infection, rash, dysrhythmia, wound infection, pulmonary emboli, pleural effusion, postoperative bleeding, bile leak, or biliary stricture.[119] More serious grade III and IV complications that have been reported for the liver donor include pleural effusions requiring chest tubes, bleeding requiring surgery, biliary complications requiring surgery, wound dehiscence, hepatic artery thrombosis, intraabdominal abscess, splenectomy, perforated gastric ulcer, deep vein thrombosis, and death.

Individuals who donate a part of their liver in the United States have a perioperative risk of mortality of 1.7 per 1000 donors.[120] The risk of a catastrophic donor outcome such as acute liver failure or early death is estimated at 2.9 per 1000 donors.[120] Living donors must undergo a rigorous evaluation to determine eligibility to donate. This evaluation includes both physical health and psychosocial assessments. During this evaluation, the mass of the liver is measured, and the volume that can be safely removed is determined. The volume of liver that can safely be removed must be of sufficient mass to be able to support the recipient adequately.

Donor Advocate

Each center that performs living donor procedures must have a donor advocate who is not a member of the transplant team. The donor advocate is involved in all phases of the procedure to ensure donor safety and well-being.

Postoperative Care of the Living Donor

Postoperative care of the living donor is similar to any patient who has undergone a liver resection. Liver regenerates rapidly after LDLT. Full restoration of liver volume appears to occur more slowly in the donor than in the recipient.[120] Critical care nurses play an important role in caring for donors and must be vigilant in assessing for complications and initiating early interventions.

Liver Transplantation Surgical Procedure

Liver transplantation surgery is lengthy and technically difficult, often lasting 4 to 12 hours. The patient is taken to the operating room for anesthesia induction, insertion of large-bore intravenous catheters that allow high-volume fluid infusion, and insertion of a pulmonary artery catheter for hemodynamic monitoring. Continuous renal replacement therapy (CRRT) may be continued or initiated in the operating room. The patient is positioned on the operating room table in such a way as to minimize pressure that could cause ischemia and chronic injury to tissue and peripheral nerves. Liver transplantation surgery can be divided into three stages:

- recipient hepatectomy
- vascular anastomoses with donor liver
- biliary anastomosis

Recipient Hepatectomy

Stage 1 is the longest and most difficult part of the surgery because it involves removal of the native liver. It is further complicated by coagulopathies, adhesions, portal hypertension, and venous collaterals. Before completion of this stage, the patient may be placed on venovenous bypass (Fig. 35.11), although not all patients require this procedure. A centrifugal pump cycles the blood out through iliac and portal vein cannulas and returns it to the central circulation through the axillary or subclavian vein. Advances in surgical techniques, anesthesia, and fluid management have shortened the length of surgery enough to warrant elimination of venovenous bypass in many cases.

Vascular Anastomoses With Donor Liver

Stage 2 comprises the four vascular anastomoses: suprahepatic inferior vena cava, infrahepatic vena cava, hepatic artery, and portal vein. Many variations and adaptations such as vascular

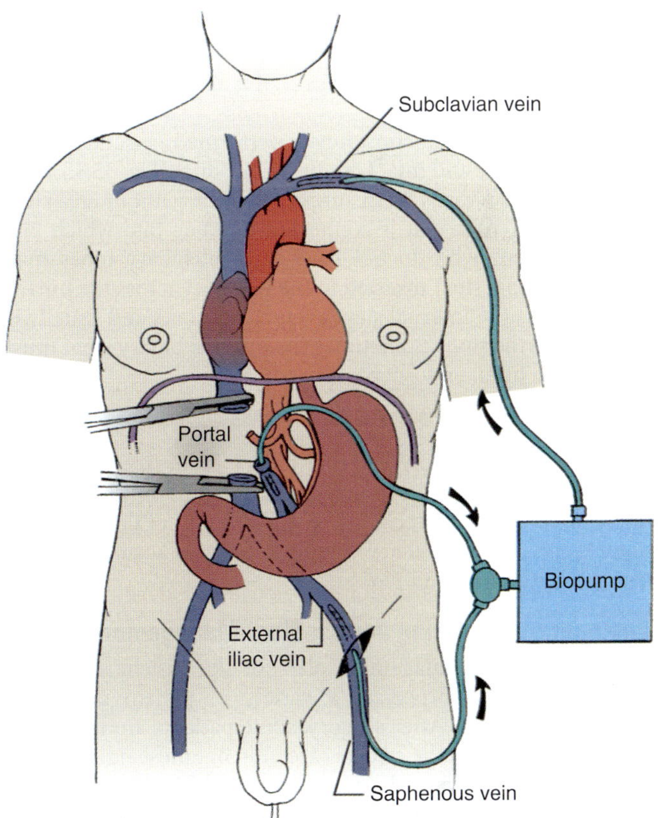

FIG. 35.11 Venovenous Bypass During Removal of Native Liver. The portal and iliac veins are cannulated, and blood is circulated by a centrifugal pump to the subclavian vein.

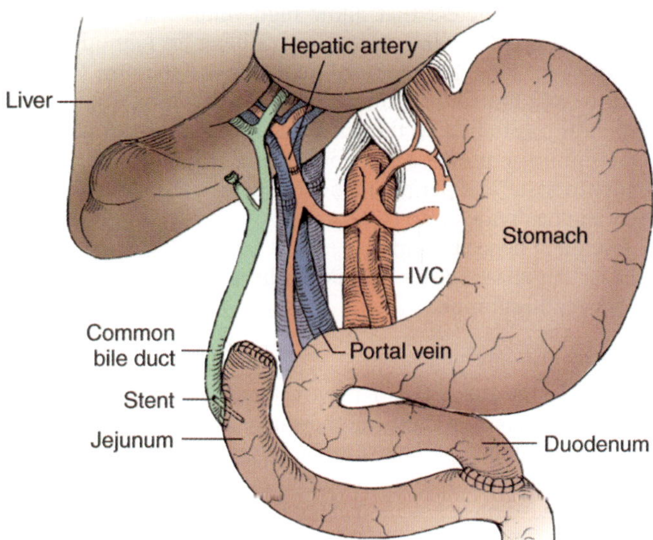

FIG. 35.12 Roux-en-Y Procedure (Choledochojejunostomy) for Liver Transplant. *IVC*, Inferior vena cava.

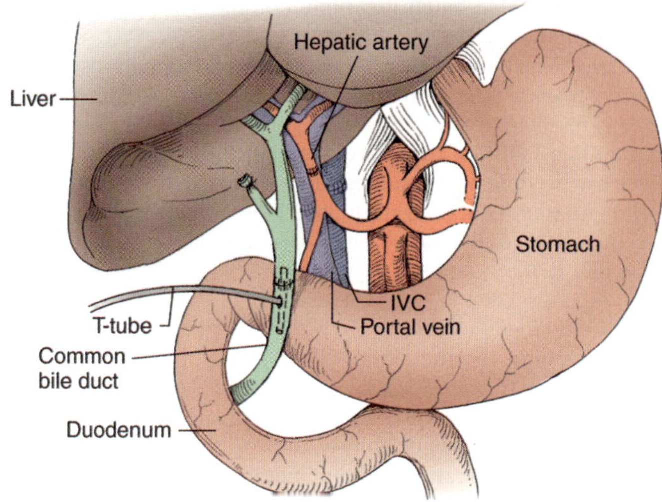

FIG. 35.13 Choledochocholedochostomy Procedure for Liver Transplantation. *IVC*, Inferior vena cava.

patches may be used, depending on the anatomy of the donor and the recipient. If venovenous bypass is used, it is removed after the infrahepatic vena cava anastomosis and before the hepatic artery anastomosis.

Biliary Anastomosis

Stage 3 can be achieved by *choledochojejunostomy* (bile duct to jejunum) or by *choledochocholedochostomy* (bile duct to bile duct).

- Choledochojejunostomy is performed in patients with diseased bile ducts, such as patients with biliary atresia or sclerosing cholangitis (Fig. 35.12). It is also known as a *Roux-en-Y* procedure.
- Choledochocholedochostomy is performed in patients who have a healthy and intact common bile duct (Fig. 35.13).

The patient returns from surgery with or without an external stent or T-tube that is connected to a bag into which bile drains. Patients who do not have external biliary tubes may have an internal stent inserted in the bile duct across the biliary anastomosis. The internal stent eventually moves and usually is passed with the stool. Sometimes the internal biliary stent must be removed by an endoscopic procedure.

Bile Drains

Careful attention to any external biliary drain line is important. If the patient has an external biliary drain, the critical care nurse documents color, character, and amount of drainage and reports any changes. Biliary complications can occur after liver transplantation (Box 35.13).

BOX 35.13 Common Complications After Liver Transplantation

Pulmonary Complications
- Pleural effusion
- Pulmonary edema
- Pneumonia
- Pneumothorax or hemothorax
- Atelectasis
- Paralysis of right diaphragm

Biliary Complications
- Leaks
- Strictures
- Obstruction
- Infection (cholangitis)
- Breakdown of anastomosis

Gastrointestinal Complications
- Bleeding and ulceration
- Gastrointestinal infections (cytomegalovirus, *Candida, Clostridioides difficile*)
- Bowel perforations

Vascular Complications
- Hepatic artery thrombosis
- Portal vein thrombosis
- Vena caval thrombosis
- Peripheral and central line sepsis
- Hepatic vein thrombosis

Postoperative Nursing and Medical Management

The patient care management plan for the patient after liver transplantation incorporates a variety of patient problems, listed in Box 35.14. After surgery, some patients are extubated before they arrive in the critical care unit, but most arrive before reversal of anesthesia and remain intubated for 12 to 24 hours. Immediate goals include:

- Reestablishment of normal body temperature
- Hemodynamic stabilization
- Maintenance of an effective airway

Postoperative hypothermia is common after orthotopic liver transplantation. The critical care nurse must achieve rewarming safely by using methods such as warming blankets, heating lamps, and head covers.

Hemodynamic Stabilization

Hemodynamic stabilization is a particular challenge, because the patient may arrive hypervolemic, euvolemic, or hypovolemic and may be hypertensive or hypotensive. Assessment of total body fluids compared with intravascular fluid status is important.

BOX 35.14 DIAGNOSIS AND PATIENT CARE MANAGEMENT

Liver Transplantation

- Risk for Infection
- Impaired Nutritional Intake due to lack of exogenous nutrients and increased metabolic demand
- Disturbed Body Image due to actual change in body structure, function, or appearance
- Anxiety due to threat to biological, psychological, and social integrity
- Lack of Knowledge of Treatment Regime due to lack of previous exposure to information

Patient Care Management plans are located in Appendix A.

Because of inherent presurgical problems with decreased serum albumin, some centers tend to keep the patient "dry." Hypervolemia often results in third spacing, with resultant ascites and a leaking wound. Accurate measurements of hemodynamic function such as arterial blood pressure, peripheral blood pressure, central venous pressure, pulmonary artery occlusion pressure or wedge pressure, urinary output, patency of drains, and bile totals are assessed frequently to evaluate volume status. Choice of replacement fluids and pharmacologic agents for correction of volume and blood pressure abnormalities is specific to the transplant center. These protocols vary in their use of albumin or fresh frozen plasma and in the use of intravenous dopamine or prostaglandin, as well as other agents and solutions. However, the goals are the same: Optimize tissue perfusion and deliver oxygen to all tissues, especially the newly transplanted graft.

Electrolyte Management

Electrolyte abnormalities can occur after liver transplantation. Disturbances in potassium and magnesium levels are common. High serum levels of electrolytes are usually associated with acute kidney injury; low levels can be related to medication side effects (e.g., diuretic therapy). The presence of hypernatremia or hyponatremia complicates the correction of volume status and fluid replacement. Calcineurin inhibitors can cause hypomagnesemia, which lowers seizure thresholds. Because these medications can also cause seizures, careful monitoring and replacement of magnesium is important.

Pulmonary Management

Ventilatory support of the patient is maintained until the anesthetic agent has been metabolized and cleared by the new liver and the patient awakens. Frequent measurement of arterial blood gas levels, continuous pulse oximetry, and assessment of breath sounds are needed. The patient may require changes in ventilatory settings, suctioning to remove secretions, or administration of pharmacologic agents to correct acid–base imbalances. Pulmonary complications are common, as listed in Box 35.13. While the patient is on ventilatory support, pneumonia can be avoided by maintaining the head of bed elevated at 30 degrees, turning the patient frequently, providing good oral care, and brushing the patient's teeth. After extubation, patients must be encouraged to perform incentive spirometry exercises and to turn, cough, and deep breathe frequently to help prevent atelectasis and pneumonia. Respiratory treatments with bronchodilators, prophylactic antimicrobials, and chest physiotherapy also may be used. Early mobilization and physical therapy are encouraged.

Coagulopathy Management

Management of coagulopathies is important in the early postoperative phase. Characterization and careful measurement of drain lines and drainage from incisions are needed, along with other nursing assessments of blood loss such as identifying signs of hypovolemia, tachypnea, tachycardia, or poor peripheral oxygenation. A sudden increase in abdominal girth, sanguineous incisional drainage or coffee-ground nasogastric output, or black tarry stools are hallmarks of bleeding problems and must be reported immediately. Laboratory monitoring during the first 24 hours after surgery is necessary to assess blood loss and coagulopathies and includes hematocrit, hemoglobin, platelet count, prothrombin time, partial thromboplastin time, fibrinogen, and fibrin split products. Reversal of coagulopathies is done judiciously, with consideration for the potential to thrombose newly anastomosed blood vessels in the liver. Blood products such as platelets, fresh frozen plasma, and specific factors can be given with pharmacologic agents such as vitamin K.

Neurologic Management

Neurologic assessment of the patient is important in the early postoperative phase to determine mental status and graft function. Patients who were encephalopathic preoperatively are usually slower to clear mentally. Nevertheless, with good liver function, the patient should be alert and oriented within 1 to 2 days; the improved mental status reflects a functional new liver. Certain pharmacologic agents, including immunosuppressants, can cause peripheral and central neurologic side effects that may alter neurologic status. Induction therapy may be used to delay the initiation of immunosuppressant medications associated with neurologic and nephrogenic side effects.

Pain Management

The critical care nurse must always be aware of the potential for intracranial bleeds in a patient who has coagulopathies, serum sodium imbalances, and hemodynamic instability. All these conditions can interfere with pain management because the pharmacologic agents used for pain can mask deterioration in mental status. Medications to relieve pain are administered, but other nonpharmacologic nursing interventions also must be used. See Chapter 7 for more detailed information regarding pain management.

Blood Glucose Management

Blood glucose levels after liver transplant can be altered by steroid administration, graft function, calcineurin inhibitors, and preexisting diabetes. Intensive blood glucose control (less than 150 mg/dL) during liver transplantation surgery has been associated with a lower infection rate and lower mortality. Perioperative hyperglycemia was associated with increased risk of liver allograft rejection in a retrospective study.[121] Low serum glucose in the absence of insulin administration can indicate primary nonfunction of the liver allograft.

Kidney Function

Kidney function can be altered by several mechanisms after liver transplantation, including cyclosporine or tacrolimus administration, acute kidney injury, intrinsic kidney disease, and poor liver function. Patients are managed with attention to fluid and electrolyte imbalances; by avoidance of nephrotoxic medications; and occasionally with ultrafiltration, continuous renal replacement therapy, or intermittent hemodialysis. With good liver function, kidney function usually improves. However, certain immunosuppressive agents and antimicrobials can deleteriously affect the kidney. Adjustments in dose or avoidance of use must be balanced with assessment of kidney and liver function. Daily monitoring of cyclosporine or tacrolimus serum levels is vital to determining adequate immunosuppression, and daily serum creatinine levels are necessary to monitor for acute kidney injury. As the patient's condition continues to improve, the frequency of laboratory testing may decrease.

Infection Prevention

Immunosuppressive therapy places the transplant recipient at an increased risk for infection. Infectious complications are common and continue to be the leading cause of death among orthotopic liver transplant recipients. The potential for infection is greatest when patients receive high doses of immunosuppressants. All persons who come into contact with the transplant recipient throughout the hospitalization must practice good handwashing techniques and standard precautions to prevent the transmission of infection. Infections are treated with appropriate antimicrobials specific to the invading organism. Prophylactic therapies are commonly used as well. Removal of central lines, arterial lines, urinary catheters, and drains is accomplished as early as is safe for the patient to avoid line-associated infections.

Nutrition Management

The nasogastric tube is removed when its output is minimal, bowel sounds have returned, and the patient is extubated. Patients who undergo a Roux-en-Y biliary anastomosis keep the nasogastric tube longer because postoperative ileus is more common. If oral nutrition is delayed longer than several days, total parenteral nutrition may be started. Consultation with a dietitian should be sought. Prealbumin levels may be measured to assess nutrition status. Otherwise, nutrition may begin orally or through a feeding tube as soon as the patient is extubated. When bowel function returns, the diet is advanced as tolerated.

Liver Function Tests

Graft function is monitored with the standard laboratory biomarkers serum aspartate aminotransferase (AST), alanine aminotransferase (ALT), alkaline phosphatase, and gamma-glutamyltransferase; serum bilirubin; and prothrombin time. The serum levels of the biomarkers are measured frequently during the first few postoperative days. These levels may continue to rise for a few days before peaking and subsequently falling. As liver function improves, the frequency of laboratory testing decreases.

Liver Graft Nonfunction

A patient with suspected primary nonfunction of a liver graft demonstrates:

- Hemodynamic instability
- Progressive deterioration of kidney function
- Coagulopathies and abnormal serum liver function laboratory tests
- Hypoglycemia
- Mechanical ventilatory dependence
- Inability to awaken from anesthesia

Continued nonfunction of the graft necessitates relisting the patient for another donor liver. Early signs of optimal graft function include improving kidney function, mental alertness, a high to normal serum glucose concentration, and early extubation. The serum ALT, AST, gamma-glutamyltransferase, and alkaline phosphatase levels may peak on the third or fourth day but should subsequently decrease. The serum bilirubin concentration may take 1 week before beginning to decrease, and there may be a mild elevation when the external biliary drainage tube is clamped or after a blood transfusion.

Rejection Surveillance

Acute rejection is a cellular-mediated event and should be suspected if the serum liver enzymes, especially AST and ALT, become elevated compared with previous levels. Elevations in total bilirubin following a rise in AST/ALT can precede any other sign of acute rejection of the liver allograft. Certain infections, such as CMV, can also cause liver function test values to increase, and these are ruled out.

Sometimes the patient also exhibits fever, a decrease in bile output (if a T-tube is still connected to a drainage bag), and a change in the color and viscosity of the bile. At first, the patient may not have any other physical symptoms, but eventually late signs of rejection may occur, including jaundice, malaise, dark urine, and clay-colored stools.

Tests to investigate the likelihood of rejection include:

- Liver function tests (AST/ALT) increase, without other reasons for these elevations.
- Doppler, ultrasound, and angiography to rule out mechanical and vascular complications
- Endoscopic retrograde cholangiopancreatography
- Hepatoiminodiacetic acid scanning
- Transhepatic cholangiography may reveal biliary obstruction or leakage.
- Liver biopsy may be indicated to determine the cause of liver dysfunction if the other tests are inconclusive.

Acute rejection can occur at any time after transplantation, but most commonly it occurs during the first few months and sometimes the first week after surgery. Most liver transplant recipients experience at least one acute rejection episode. Treatment of acute rejection requires increasing immunosuppression. Immunosuppressant protocols vary from center to center and are usually successful at reversing acute rejection.

Chronic rejection is both a humoral and a cellular event and is progressive over time and nonreversible. It results in destruction and loss of bile ducts. It is sometimes treated with plasmapheresis to remove circulating antibodies along with pharmacologic immunotherapies that bind B cells. Chronic rejection in a liver transplant recipient usually requires retransplantation if the patient is still a candidate.

Transfer Out of Critical Care

After the patient is stable and the transplanted liver is functional, central venous catheters and arterial lines are removed. The urinary catheter is removed as soon as the patient is awake enough to be continent. Drain lines are removed as drainage outputs become minimal. As the patient begins to participate in self-care, plans are made for transfer out of the critical care unit to the transplant progressive care nursing where laboratory data and vital signs continue to be routinely monitored. Self-care is promoted. Increasing levels of physical therapy are encouraged, diet is advanced, and much of the nurse's interventions are directed toward teaching the patient and family.

Patient and Family Education

Considerable attention is focused on patient and family education and discharge planning. Discharge booklets are helpful in the education process. It is essential for the patient to learn how to self-administer medications, monitor vital signs, care for the incision and the T-tube (if present), prevent infections, follow safe living practices, and identify problems that must promptly receive medical attention.

Because patients are commonly discharged within 2 weeks after orthotopic liver transplant, it is important for discharge instructions to begin as soon as the patient is mentally alert. Patients discharged early may require home health nurse referrals to assist with follow-up of incision care, intravenous therapies, and other procedures. Education must be provided about rejection surveillance, signs and symptoms of infection, lifestyle changes as needed, long-term medication considerations, and the follow-up visit schedule.

Long-Term Considerations After Liver Transplant

Liver transplant recipients who do not live in the same city in which their surgery was performed usually remain in the immediate area of the transplant center after discharge before returning home. During this period, they may be monitored by a home health nurse and be seen in clinic several times a week by the transplant team. Continued serologic testing is performed to monitor graft function, to determine blood levels of certain immunosuppressive agents, and to identify postoperative complications. Although many of these complications can be managed successfully in the outpatient setting, readmissions do occur. Because rejections, readmissions, grieving for the donor, and pharmacologic side effects can create anxiety for the family and the patient, they are encouraged to attend transplantation support groups if offered by the center. After patients return home, they are encouraged to resume a close relationship with their local primary care physician and gastroenterologist.

With the proliferation in the numbers of liver transplants being performed, it is not unreasonable for recipients to be admitted to a non–tertiary care hospital for management of some long-term posttransplantation complications. Nurses who work for hospitals that do not perform transplants may have the opportunity to care for these patients. Nurses in these settings must also become knowledgeable about the signs and symptoms of rejection, administration of immunosuppressant medications, monitoring of immunosuppressant levels, and medication-to-medication interactions with the immunosuppressants. Every transplant recipient has a coordinator who follows the patient at the transplant center. The transplant coordinator is also available for consultation with community health care providers who have questions about transplant recipients.

Liver transplant recipients need long-term follow-up surveillance for hypertension, kidney failure, obesity, dyslipidemias, biliary and infectious complications, and malignancies. Early intervention affects the quality and length of life. Behavior modifications and therapeutic lifestyle changes should be frequently reinforced to positively affect long-term health. Close management of posttransplant complications and avoidance of rehospitalization is important in reducing costs. Advanced practice nurses who work in transplant centers offer an effective economic model in the delivery of safe patient care.

Future Considerations for Liver Transplantation

A limiting factor in liver transplantation continues to be the shortage of organ donors (see Fig. 35.1). Attention is being focused on ways to increase the number and availability of donor organs. This includes reduced-size organs, split-liver technique (in which one liver is divided and transplanted into two recipients), and living liver donors. Expanded criteria for deceased liver donors include DCD, advanced donor age, steatosis, hepatitis C–positive allografts, human T-cell lymphotropic virus–positive allografts, hepatitis B core antibody–positive allografts, donors with active infections, and high-risk donors. Studies are exploring the roles of xenografts and bioartificial liver devices that can support a patient who is awaiting a homograft. As recipients live longer and healthier lives, pregnancy after transplantation will become more common.[122]

KIDNEY TRANSPLANTATION

The first successful kidney transplantation was performed in 1954 in Boston. Today, it is the treatment of choice for patients with end-stage kidney disease. Kidney transplantation allows the recipient to lead a much less restricted lifestyle and provides a more cost-effective treatment method than long-term dialysis. Advances in the study of the immune system and the development of new immunosuppressant medications have allowed for increased graft survival rates for deceased donor and living donor kidney transplants. Transplant centers use a combination of immunosuppressive medications to prevent rejection to lower the doses of each medication so that the associated side effects can be minimized.

In 2021, the Scientific Registry of Transplant Recipients reported[123]

- 127,671 patients listed awaiting a donor kidney transplant
- 25,488 kidneys transplanted in 2021 in the United States
- 19,518 from deceased donor
- 5970 from living donor

According to national statistics, the total number of kidney transplant recipients alive with a functioning kidney graft is projected to surpass 250,000 within the next 2 years.[123]

Indications and Selection

Many disease processes can lead to end-stage kidney disease. For this reason, potential recipients must undergo numerous laboratory tests and some noninvasive physical testing before they can be approved as candidates (Box 35.15). Because after transplantation the patient's immune system will be purposely and controllably compromised, there are several contraindications to kidney transplantation (Box 35.16). If any of these contraindications are present, the patient's risk is determined to be too high for transplantation and the immunosuppressant regimen that follows. The alternative for such a patient is to decrease or eliminate the risk factors that can be controlled and be reevaluated later. If the candidate is unwilling to eliminate controllable high-risk behaviors, the only alternative for survival is to remain on dialysis.

Kidney Donation

A donor kidney can come from a deceased donor or from a living donor.

Deceased Kidney Donation

Most kidneys transplanted in the United States come from a deceased donor who meets the criteria for brain death or cardiac

BOX 35.15 Evaluation Before Kidney Transplantation

- Chemistry 24-panel test; human leukocyte antigen tissue typing; prothrombin time; partial thromboplastin time; complete blood count with differential; platelet count; human immunodeficiency virus; hepatitis; cytomegalovirus; Epstein-Barr virus; lipid profile; urine for analysis, culture, and sensitivities; 24-h urine for creatinine clearance and protein (if patient still produces urine); dialysate fluid for culture and sensitivity (if patient is undergoing continuous ambulatory peritoneal dialysis)
- Kidney ultrasonography or spiral computed tomography, chest radiography (posteroanterior and lateral views), electrocardiography, stress test and cardiac catheterization (if indicated), weight management (if indicated), colonoscopy (if age >55 y), mammography (for women age >35 y), venography (for patients with diabetes)
- Consultants: psychologist or psychiatrist, urologist, transplantation surgeon or transplantation nephrologist, social worker, dietitian, chaplain, financial counselor

BOX 35.16 Contraindications to Kidney Transplantation

- Malignancy during the past 3 years
- Active infectious process
- Advanced cardiopulmonary disease
- High risk for surgery
- Nonadherence to current medical regimen
- Illicit drug abuse or alcohol abuse
- Other serious contributing disease processes

death (described earlier in the chapter). Donor and recipient are matched by ABO blood type. A simplified description of the current organ allocation criteria is provided.

The priority for a deceased donor kidney is to those candidates who are listed for a combined kidney and a simultaneous second organ (pancreas, heart, or liver) transplant.[124] The second priority is given to candidates who have a perfect HLA match with the donor kidney because this optimizes graft survival. The third priority is by local geographic region.[124] Organ allocation is managed through the OPTN/UNOS registry (described in the beginning of the chapter). Deceased kidney donors are further classified by donor age:[124]

- Standard criteria donor kidneys (normal kidney function, or ≤35 years of age).
- ECD kidneys (donor age ≥60 years or ≥50 years with comorbidities such as hypertension or elevated creatinine).
- DCD donor kidneys[124]

Living Kidney Donation

The first successful kidney transplant was a living donor transplant between identical twins in 1954. In most cases today, the living donor is related to the recipient. Family members are often the most likely to be compatible living kidney donors. However, successful living-donor transplants are also common with a kidney donated from unrelated people such as friends, coworkers, or religious congregation members.

Living Kidney Paired Donation

An innovative option is kidney paired donation.[125,126] A person may want to donate one of his or her kidneys to a family member, but the person's blood type is incompatible with the intended recipient. In this situation, they could participate in a donation exchange with another living donor–recipient pair, as shown in Fig. 35.14A. This could also be a three-way living donor exchange, as shown in Fig. 35.14B. Several other variations have also been used, involving a "chain" of donor-to-recipient transplants.[125–127] Clinical outcomes for cooperative kidney paired donation early graft survival are equivalent to standard living donor donation.[128]

Kidney Transplantation Surgical Procedure

When the kidney to be transplanted is procured from the donor, whether living or deceased, the ureter, renal vein, and renal artery are dissected, leaving as much length as possible. When kidneys are retrieved from a deceased donor, an aortic patch is often taken where the renal artery inserts into the aorta. This minimizes posttransplant renal artery stenosis.[129]

Living Donor Kidney Laparoscopic Nephrectomy

If the donor is living, the procurement is typically by laparoscopic nephrectomy. Open surgical kidney removal is rare today. After the kidney is secured, it is flushed with a cold electrolyte preservative solution until the venous return is clear. This usually requires 100 to 200 mL of solution. The kidney is then transported to the operating room to be transplanted.

Deceased Donor Kidney Transplantation

If the kidney is from a deceased donor, it is flushed with a cold electrolyte preservative solution and simultaneously cooled externally as quickly as possible. It can be transported on a kidney perfusion machine or packed in an iced preservation solution. After the kidney is procured and placed in the hypothermic solution, it can be maintained for 48 to 72 hours before it must be transplanted. Most transplant centers attempt to transplant the organ within 24 hours after procurement to avoid cold ischemic injury and acute kidney injury. At the time of procurement, the kidney is assessed in situ for color, shape, and form. It is palpated to determine firmness, and often a biopsy sample is taken to rule out undiagnosed kidney dysfunction. One concern is the proportion of deceased kidney donors recovered but not transplanted (nonuse rate) was 17.9% in 2011 and has increased to 24.6% in 2021.[54]

Kidney Transplant Recipient Surgery

The patient is anesthetized, and a urinary catheter is placed. A curvilinear incision is made 3 to 4 cm above the symphysis pubis and extended to the iliac crest (Fig. 35.15A). The muscles and fascia are divided and retracted medially to expose the iliac vessels. The kidney is placed in the extraperitoneal space of the right or left iliac fossa. The donor renal artery is anastomosed to the external iliac artery, and the donor renal vein is sutured to the external iliac vein (Fig. 35.15B).[129] The native kidney is not removed.

After the revascularization procedures are completed, the ureteral anastomosis is performed. The most common method used is ureteroneocystostomy. During this procedure, an incision is made in the dome of the recipient's bladder and the donor ureter is tunneled through the recipient's mucosal layer and sutured to the mucosal opening. Tunneling of the ureter prevents urinary reflux into the transplanted kidney,[129] A stent is often placed in the ureter to decrease postoperative risk of stenosis of the ureter. The stent is retrieved 2 to 4 weeks after transplant.[129]

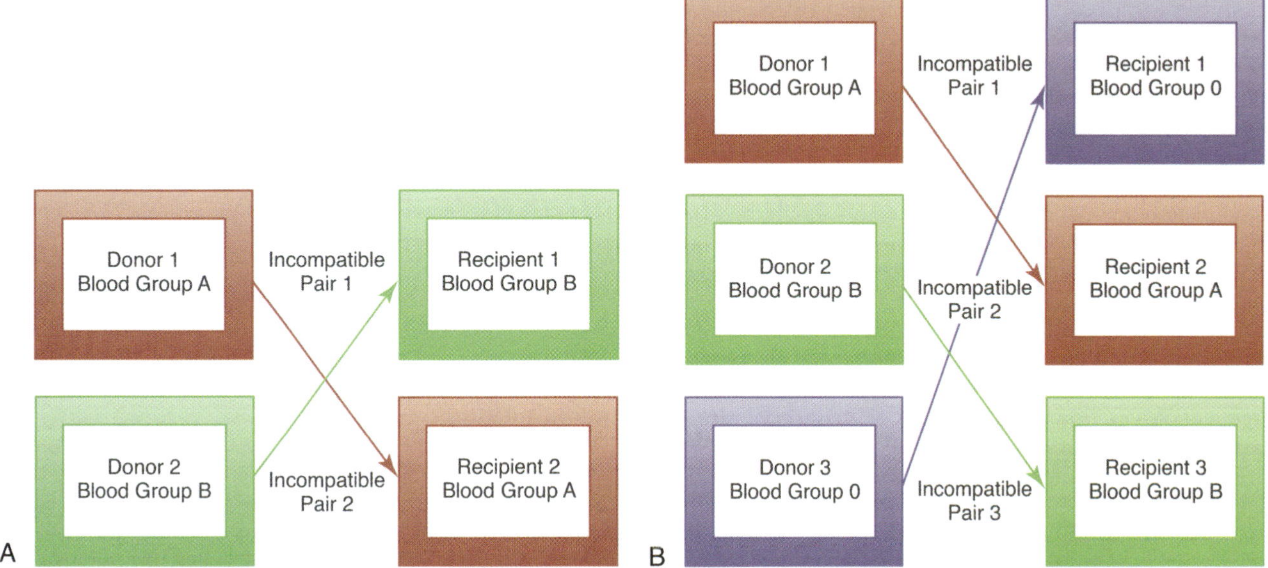

FIG. 35.14 Kidney paired donation is an option for a person who wants to donate a kidney to a family member but does not have a compatible blood type with the intended recipient. With this option, donors can participate in a donation exchange with another living donor–recipient pair (A). There could also be a three-way living donor exchange (B).

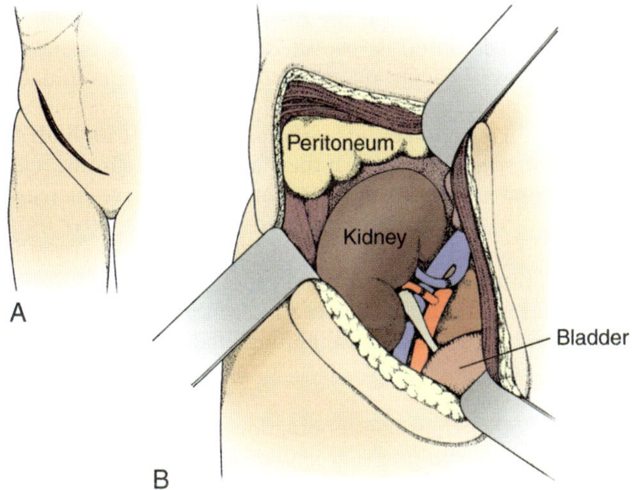

FIG. 35.15 Placement of the Kidney Graft Into the Iliac Fossa. (A) The incision in the right side of the abdomen is used for graft implantation in the right iliac fossa. (B) The iliac vessels are exposed. (Modified from Smith SL. *AACN Tissue and Organ Transplantation: Implications for Professional Nursing Practice*. Mosby; 1990.)

During the surgery, a central venous pressure of 8 to 16 mm Hg is maintained, and a systolic blood pressure at least as high as the patient's baseline value should be maintained to ensure adequate perfusion of the transplanted kidney.

Postoperative Nursing and Medical Management of the Kidney Transplant Recipient

After the transplantation is completed and the patient is stable and ready for leave the recovery room, most transplant centers admit the patient directly to the organ transplantation unit or to the critical care unit. Serious complications can occur in the immediate postoperative period, and a sound knowledge base of medical/surgical nursing, kidney function, anatomy, and immunosuppressive medications is imperative. The patient care management plan for a patient after kidney transplant incorporates a variety of patient problems as listed in Box 35.17.

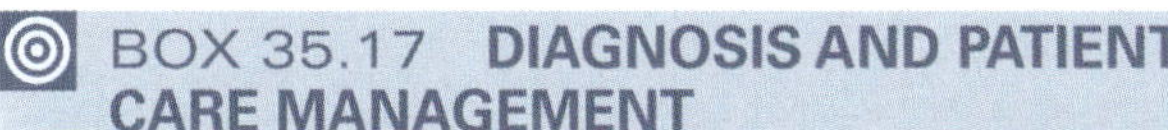

BOX 35.17 DIAGNOSIS AND PATIENT CARE MANAGEMENT

Kidney Transplantation

- Risk for Infection
- Impaired Nutritional Intake due to lack of exogenous nutrients and increased metabolic demand
- Disturbed Body Image due to actual change in body structure, function, or appearance
- Anxiety due to threat to biological, psychological, and social integrity
- Lack of Knowledge of Treatment Regime due to lack of previous exposure to information

Patient Care Management plans are located in Appendix A.

Fluid Status

If the transplanted kidney is producing urine, the patient's fluid status is monitored closely. Adequate hydration is an absolute necessity for continued graft function in the immediate postoperative period. Hypovolemia can lead to compromised blood flow to the kidney, acute kidney injury, and possible graft failure. Urine output volume and color should be monitored at least every 30 minutes. The new kidney will be producing large amounts of urine, and fluid replacement, usually maintained in a 1:1 ratio, must be sustained.

Electrolytes

Electrolyte balance is also of grave concern. Because of the large volumes of urine produced, the potential exists for hypokalemia, hypomagnesemia, and hypocalcemia, leading to possible cardiac compromise. Electrolytes must be monitored at least every 4 to 6 hours and replaced as necessary in the first 24 hours. Assessment of the blood urea nitrogen (BUN) and the creatinine concentration also is necessary every 4 to 6 hours to monitor graft function and determine the need for dialysis within the first 24 to 48 hours. Electrolytes, BUN, and creatine are monitored daily until discharged.

Postoperative Complications

The complete blood count and platelet count should be monitored every 4 to 6 hours. Blood loss during the operation is minimal, usually 500 mL or less. Abrupt decreases or continuously falling counts may indicate hemorrhage at an anastomosis site, which requires a return to the operating room for repair. Even with minimal blood loss during surgery, transfusion of blood products after the surgery can be necessary.

Frequent observation and assessment of the surgical incision is needed to evaluate for drainage and swelling.

Urine output volume and color should be monitored at least every 30 minutes. The bladder anastomosis is fragile, and clots can commonly occlude the catheter. The bladder must remain decompressed for several days to promote proper healing.

If clots occlude the end of the catheter, gentle irrigation or aspiration may be necessary. If the clot cannot be dislodged or aspirated out, it may be necessary to change the catheter. Painful bladder spasms can also occur, and opiates, usually in the form of a belladonna and opium suppository or an oral urinary antispasmodic, may be required to relax the bladder.

Immunosuppression

Initiation of induction immunosuppressant therapy begins at the time of transplantation, usually in the form of a polyclonal antithymocyte/antilymphocyte intravenous compound or an intravenous monoclonal antibody compound. These compounds remove the lymphocytes from the patient's system, preventing rejection and suppressing the immune system until oral medications can be safely administered and blood levels are sufficient to allow discontinuation of the intravenous agent. Because the patient is now immunocompromised, strict aseptic technique is required for all procedures to prevent infection. For specific immunosuppression details, see the earlier section on Immunosuppressive Medications.

Infection Risk

Thorough handwashing, aseptic dressing changes, discontinuation of any unnecessary invasive lines, and limiting the number of visitors are necessary protective measures. Because of the transplant recipient's immunocompromised status, subtle changes in the temperature, white blood cell count, or wound drainage can signal an active infection. Transplant recipients are also susceptible to infection by opportunistic native organisms such as *Candida*, pneumocystis pneumonia, CMV, Epstein-Barr virus, and herpes simplex virus.[130]

Preparation for Discharge Home

The average length of hospital stay after uncomplicated kidney transplantation is 3 to 5 days. During the first few days, the patient must learn the self-care routines essential for graft survival. Medication regimens are complex, and most centers initiate a self-medication program at the patient's bedside as a training tool. Patients and families are taught the signs and symptoms of infection and graft rejection (Box 35.18), the protocols of the transplant clinic, and new dietary limitations.

BOX 35.18 Signs and Symptoms of Kidney Rejection

- Increased tenderness over transplanted kidney site
- Decreased urine output
- Increased serum creatinine levels, greater than patient's baseline level
- Fever
- Rapid weight gain (4–6 lb in a 24-h period)
- Swelling, usually in the hands and feet

Frequent transplant clinic visits to check the functioning of the organ and to adjust the doses of immunosuppressant medications are necessary for the first few months after transplantation.

Patient and Family Education

Adherence to the medical regimen required to maintain a transplanted organ is a major focus of education. Patients are reluctant to take immunosuppressive medications if they are experiencing severe side effects. Decreasing the dosage of the medications can often alleviate these symptoms but may lead to a rejection episode.

Long-Term Considerations

Rejection of the transplanted kidney is an ongoing concern for all kidney transplant recipients. The graft function is monitored closely, and if rejection is suspected, a biopsy is performed. If the biopsy reveals acute rejection, rescue therapy is initiated. This therapy can be in the form of high-dose intravenous steroids for mild rejection or intravenous monoclonal antibody for moderate to severe rejection. If the biopsy reveals chronic rejection, the oral immunosuppressant medications are increased or returned to the higher doses used immediately after transplantation. No two patients' immune systems are exactly alike, and the immunosuppressant medication regimen required to prevent rejection must be tailored to each patient individually. The goal is to create a balance among medications that allows the patient to fight off most infections but avoid rejection of the transplanted organ.

As with other transplant populations, women of childbearing age may become pregnant after kidney transplant. Careful management is required throughout the pregnancy.[131] Live births are reported as 75%, miscarriages occur in 15%, and stillbirths occur in 5%.[131] Risks to the mother include preeclampsia, pregnancy-induced hypertension, gestational diabetes, and rejection.[131]

PANCREAS TRANSPLANTATION

Pancreas transplantation offers the opportunity of normal glucose control without the use of exogenous insulin. Patients with type 1 diabetes mellitus who are dependent on exogenous insulin are at high risk to develop chronic kidney disease.

The first pancreas transplants were performed in 1966, with little success.[132] Advances in immunosuppressive medications, diagnosis of rejection, management of the exocrine secretions, and improved surgical techniques have improved the success rate of pancreas transplantation.

Over 63,000 pancreas transplants have now been performed worldwide but only 8% are pancreas alone.[133] Most pancreas

BOX 35.19 Evaluation Before Pancreas Transplantation

- Blood chemistries, tissue typing, and viral studies similar to those for kidney transplantation candidates
- Complete cardiovascular work-up, including cardiac catheterization
- Complete vascular studies, particularly of the lower extremities, to ensure proper vascularization of graft
- Nerve conduction studies to evaluate for neuropathy
- Urologic and bladder function studies
- Consultations as required for all transplantation candidates

transplants are performed simultaneously with other organs, usually a kidney.[133,134]

In 2021, 963 pancreases were transplanted, and 820 of those were kidney-pancreas transplants.[135] Most recipients had type 1 diabetes, and a smaller number had type 2 diabetes.[135] There is no difference in survival between recipients with type 1 and type 2 diabetes. Pancreas graft survival is at 53% at 5 years and 36% at 10 years for pancreas transplant alone.[136] For simultaneous kidney-pancreas transplant survival is higher, at 73% at 5 years and 56% at 10 years.[136]

Indications and Selection

Patients who are selected for pancreas transplantation must undergo a thorough evaluation similar to that for other solid organ transplants (Box 35.19). The disease processes involved in diabetes mellitus and their effects on all major body systems require that special care be taken to ensure the candidate is in the best possible condition before transplantation. Severe and often life-threatening complications can occur after transplantation if the major body systems have not been fully evaluated beforehand.

Pancreas Transplantation Surgical Procedure

The surgical techniques for pancreas transplantation are diverse, and different programs use different methods. However, the principles are consistent, and all include the following three precepts:

- Provide adequate arterial blood flow to the pancreas and duodenal segment
- Provide adequate venous outflow from the pancreas
- Provide management of the pancreatic exocrine secretions

The cold-ischemia time of the pancreas before implantation should be minimized. The pancreas allografts do not tolerate cold ischemia as well as kidney allografts. Ideally, the pancreas should be revascularized within 24 hours from the time of cross-clamping. The abdomen is entered through a midline incision. The pancreas graft is transplanted into the right iliac fossa, with the head of the pancreas placed downward into the pelvis.[132] Most transplantation centers place both organs on the right side, although some put the pancreas on the right and the kidney on the left. The native pancreas is not removed.

Arterial and Venous Revascularization

Arterial flow to the pancreas graft is provided from the recipient's iliac artery. Venous outflow from the transplanted graft can be via an anastomosis to the portal vein or to the iliac vein.[132] The iliac vein is more commonly used. Graft outcomes

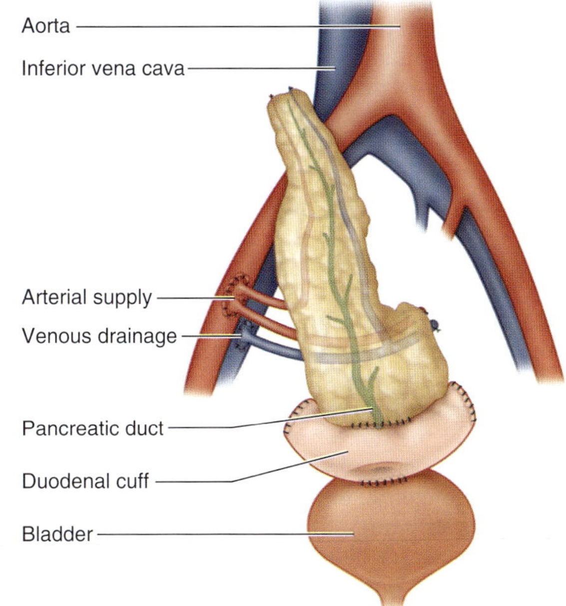

FIG. 35.16 Exocrine Pancreatic Management by Urinary Diversion. (Modified from Smith SL. *AACN Tissue and Organ Transplantation in Pancreas Transplantation: Implications for Professional Nursing Practice*. Mosby; 1990.)

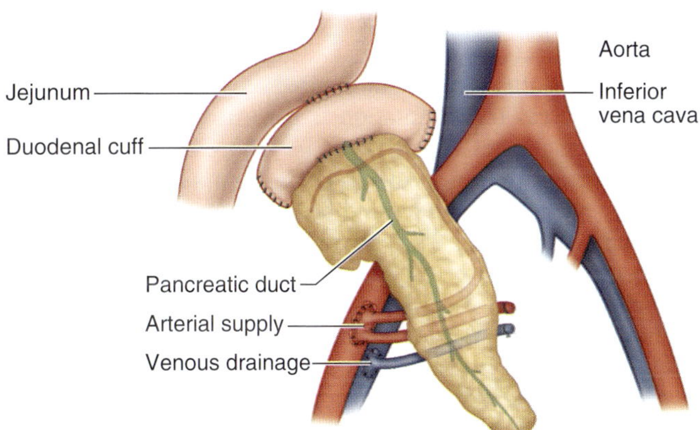

FIG. 35.17 Exocrine Pancreatic Management by Enteric Exocrine Diversion. A segment of the donor duodenum (oversewn duodenal cuff) is transplanted with the pancreas graft.

and survival are similar with both venous anastomosis methods.[132]

Exocrine Drainage

The exocrine drainage of the pancreas is one of the most challenging aspects of the transplantation procedure. The head of the pancreas is positioned to drain downward into either the bladder (Fig. 35.16) or more commonly, the bowel (Fig. 35.17).

Enteric Exocrine Drainage

Enteric drainage is the draining of pancreatic exocrine secretions into the bowel. The pancreas and a segment of the donor duodenum are transplanted onto the recipient's small bowel. All the enzymes drain into the bowel and are excreted with the stool. Exocrine drainage into the duodenum most closely approximates normal physiology. However, complications with the side-to-side anastomosis can cause peritonitis. To decrease this risk, a Roux-en-Y duodenojejunostomy is constructed (see Fig. 35.17).[132] One disadvantage of enteric drainage is that it is impossible to monitor pancreatic enzymes as a direct measure of pancreatic function. Nevertheless, enteric drainage is the more commonly used technique.[132]

Bladder Exocrine Drainage

Bladder drainage is the draining of pancreatic exocrine secretions into the bladder (see Fig. 35.16). A major advantage of this method is that direct monitoring of graft function is possible by measuring urinary amylase. A decrease in urinary amylase precedes irreversible hyperglycemia associated with acute cellular rejection of the transplanted pancreas.[132] The disadvantage of bladder exocrine drainage is that it is associated with genitourinary complications such as recurrent urinary tract infections, prostatitis, urethritis, and hematuria. Other complications include urinary bicarbonate loss and metabolic acidosis.[132] Additional surgery to change the drainage method from bladder to enteric drainage is required in 30% of pancreas transplant recipients within 5 years and in 50% of recipients within 15 years.[132]

Postoperative Nursing and Medical Management

After surgery, the patient is taken to the critical care unit. Although these patients now have a functioning pancreas, they are at high risk for surgical complications because of the long-term effects of diabetes. Oxygenation, hemodynamics, and cardiac status must be monitored closely. If simultaneous kidney-pancreas transplantation is performed, fluid and electrolyte management is indicated, including intravenous fluid replacement; monitoring of intake and output; and measurements of pancreas enzymes and fasting glucose. A nasogastric tube can be placed for 24 to 48 hours after surgery. A continuous insulin drip may be used to prevent hyperglycemia until the new pancreas graft is fully functional. Frequent blood glucose monitoring is essential for patient safety while the continuous insulin infusion is in place.

The same aseptic techniques used for kidney transplant recipients are used for pancreas transplant recipients. An increased potential for urinary catheter occlusion exists for pancreas transplant recipients who have undergone a urinary diversion procedure. The exocrine pancreatic enzymes make the urine more viscous and may irritate the anastomosis site on the bladder, causing an increased risk of bleeding. Continuous bladder irrigation may be necessary to keep the urinary drainage catheter patent. The patient care management plan after a pancreas or pancreas-kidney transplant incorporates a variety of patient problems, as listed in Box 35.20.

Patient and Family Education

Patient and family education is adapted as needed when there is a simultaneous pancreas-kidney transplant. The primary focus is on the importance of taking the immunosuppressive medications, infection prevention, and recognition of symptoms that may indicate rejection. After a successful pancreas transplant exogenous inulin is no longer required because the functional pancreas will produce insulin. However, patients with functional pancreas grafts should continue to monitor glucose at home but some forget to continue this practice as they no longer require insulin. Continued monitoring with frequent clinic visits is required for several months after pancreas transplantation.

Long-Term Considerations

Rejection can be very difficult to detect. Serum amylase levels after pancreas-only transplantation are ineffective in monitoring graft function, and blood glucose levels become elevated only in the late stages of rejection. Urine amylase levels in patients with the urinary diversion are an effective means of monitoring for rejection. If kidney transplantation has been performed simultaneously, an increase in the serum creatinine level is predictive of rejection. Because of the fragility of pancreas tissue, a pancreas biopsy is rarely performed. However, a kidney biopsy specimen may be obtained to determine rejection and treatment options. Treatment of pancreas rejection is the same as for all other types of organ rejection.

ADDITIONAL RESOURCES

See Box 35.21 for Internet resources related to organ donation and transplantation.

BOX 35.20 DIAGNOSIS AND PATIENT MANAGEMENT

Pancreas Transplantation

- Risk for Infection
- Impaired Nutritional Intake due to lack of exogenous nutrients and increased metabolic demand
- Disturbed Body Image related to actual change in body structure, function, or appearance
- Anxiety related to threat to biological, psychological, and social integrity
- Lack of Knowledge of Treatment Regime due to lack of previous exposure to information

Patient Care Management plans are located in Appendix A.

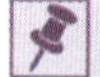

BOX 35.21 Internet Resources

Organ Donation and Transplantation

Donation

- Organ Procurement and Transplantation Network (OPTN): http://optn.transplant.hrsa.gov
- United Network for Organ Sharing (UNOS): https://www.unos.org
- US Government on Organ Donation and Transplantation: http://organdonor.gov

Transplantation

- International Liver Transplantation Society (ILTS): https://ilts.org
- International Pancreas and Islet Transplant Association: https://www.tts.org/
- International Society for Heart and Lung Transplantation (ISHLT): http://www.ishlt.org
- International Transplant Nurses Society (ITNS): http://www.itns.org
- Lung Transplant Foundation: http://www.lungtransplantfoundation.org
- National Kidney Foundation (NKF): https://www.kidney.org
- The Transplantation Society (TTS): https://www.tts.org

CASE STUDY 35.1 Patient With a Transplant

Brief Patient History

Mr. V is a 42-year-old man with chronic viral hepatitis C. He has a Model for End-Stage Liver Disease (MELD) score greater than 25. Mr. V is in acute fulminant liver failure and is on the waiting list to receive a liver transplant. Mr. V was hospitalized 2 weeks ago with ascites, hepatorenal syndrome, and hepatic encephalopathy. He has been treated with diuretics, antibiotics, and laxatives. Before transplantation, he remained in the intermediate care unit and was not intubated. He is now undergoing liver transplantation.

Clinical Assessment

Mr. V is admitted to the critical care unit from the operating room after receiving an orthotopic liver transplant. He is intubated and sedated. Mr. V moves all extremities but does not follow commands. He has a nasogastric tube, pulmonary artery catheter, arterial line, urinary catheter, abdominal drain (draining bright red blood), and external biliary drain in place. Continuous renal replacement therapy is in progress.

Diagnostic Procedures

Baseline vital signs include the following: blood pressure of 100/60 mm Hg, heart rate of 118 beats/min (sinus tachycardia), respiratory rate of 20 breaths/min, temperature of 98.3°F, and oxygen saturation of 98%.

Urine output was 75 mL/h and is now 15 mL/h. Central venous pressure is 14 mm Hg, pulmonary artery pressure is 30/16 mm Hg, pulmonary artery occlusion pressure is 18 mm Hg, and intraabdominal pressure is greater than 25 mm Hg.

His current laboratory values include the following:

- White blood cell count: 3100 cells/mm^3
- Hematocrit: 25.3%
- Hemoglobin: 8.6 g/dL
- Platelet count: 47,000/microliter
- Aspartate aminotransferase: 315 units/L
- Aminotransferase: 230 units/L
- Alkaline phosphatase: 380 units/L
- Gamma-glutamyltransferase: 1040 units/L
- Total bilirubin: 12.5 mg/dL
- Prothrombin time: 21.3 s
- International normalized ratio: 2.5
- Partial thromboplastin time: 69.9 s
- Blood urea nitrogen: 39 mg/dL
- Serum creatinine: 1.4 mg/dL
- Potassium: 3.8 mEq/L (mmol/L)

Medical Diagnosis

Mr. V is diagnosed with intraabdominal hypertension and abdominal compartment syndrome.

Questions

1. What major outcomes do you expect to achieve for this patient?
2. What problems or risks must be managed to achieve these outcomes?
3. What interventions could be initiated to monitor, prevent, manage, or eliminate the problems and risks identified?
4. What interventions could be initiated to promote optimal functioning, safety, and well-being of the patient?
5. What technology can be used to monitor this patient and prevent complications?
6. What other interprofessional team members are needed to assist with the management of this patient?
7. What possible learning needs would you anticipate for this patient?
8. What cultural and age-related factors might have a bearing on the patient's plan of care?

KEY POINTS

Organ Donation

- The fields of organ donation and solid-organ transplantation have made dramatic progress in the past 50 years. This trajectory is expected to continue. As transplantation becomes more widespread, more nurses will encounter patients who have undergone solid-organ transplantation. Even more likely is that critical care nurses will assist with the care of a potential organ donor. Knowledge of the rationales for care is essential to delivering safe and high-quality patient care.
- There are 58 OPOs in the United States, Puerto Rico, Guam, and Bermuda. They are nonprofit corporations that provide organ donation services to a designated regional area.
- There are many more individuals listed for transplants than the number of donor organs available.

The Immune System

- Almost every human cell carries distinctive molecules that allow the immune system to distinguish self from nonself. The immune system contains multiple specialized defenses to identify and eliminate foreign material recognized as nonself. To prevent rejection, organ transplantation requires suppression or downregulation of the immune response.

Immunosuppressive Medications

- The recipient of an organ transplant is required to adhere to a strict regimen of immunosuppressive medications to avoid rejection of the organ by the recipient's own immune system, which recognizes the foreign graft as nonself. The immunosuppressants increase vulnerability to infection. The goal is to create a balance among medications that allows the patient to fight off most infections but avoid rejection of the transplanted organ.

Transplant Candidate Evaluation

- When an individual has progressed to end-stage organ function and is considered for transplant, each type of solid-organ transplant has organ-specific indications and contraindications. In addition, there is a comprehensive health assessment, a psychological assessment, and screening for social support before being listed for transplant.

Heart Transplantation

- A transplanted heart must come from a deceased donor. Immediate postoperative management of the heart transplant recipient is similar to that for patients undergoing other heart surgery procedures.

Lung Transplantation

- Transplanted lungs come from a deceased donor. Lungs have a limited ischemic time of approximately 4 hours, which limits the geographic area for donor procurement. Relatively few lungs are available for donation.

Liver Transplantation

- Liver transplants may come from a deceased donor or from a living donor who donates a section of the liver. Before transplantation, the severity of liver disease and level of placement on the transplantation waiting list is determined by the MELD score for patients older than 12 years. The postoperative course is highly variable. Many liver transplant recipients were encephalopathic before transplantation and may have a complicated course afterward. Other patients who have a lower MELD score and receive a functional liver may recover very quickly and should be alert and oriented within 1 to 2 days.

Kidney Transplantation

- Kidney transplants come from a deceased donor or from a living donor who donates one kidney. Postoperative management of fluid status is vital to ensure that the kidney is functional and to avoid volume overload. The bladder must remain decompressed by a urinary catheter for several days to promote effective healing.

Pancreas Transplantation

- Pancreas transplantation is usually performed in tandem with kidney transplantation because most recipients have type 1 diabetes mellitus that has caused the kidney failure.

Visit the Evolve site at http://evolve.elsevier.com/Urden/CriticalCareNursing for additional study materials.

REFERENCES

1. The history of organ donation and transplantation | UNOS. Accessed November 6, 2023. https://unos.org/transplant/history/
2. Linden PK. History of solid organ transplantation and organ donation. *Crit Care Clin.* 2009;25(1):165–184, ix. https://doi.org/10.1016/j.ccc.2008.12.001.
3. Organ Procurement and Transplantation Network (OPTN). Data - OPTN. ; 2023. https://optn.transplant.hrsa.gov/data/. Accessed September 24, 2023.
4. National Research Council. In: Kizer KW, English RA, Hackmann M, eds. *Realizing the Promise of Equity in the Organ Transplantation System.* National Academies Press; 2022:26364. https://doi.org/10.17226/26364.
5. Federal Register. 1998;63(Issue 119). Published 1998. https://www.govinfo.gov/content/pkg/FR-1998-06-22/html/98-16490.htm. Accessed September 23, 2023.
6. O'Leary GM. Deceased donor organ donation: the critical care nurse's role. *Nurs Crit Care.* 2018;13(4):27–32. https://doi.org/10.1097/01.CCN.0000534920.55430.ba.
7. Araujo CAS, Siqueira MM. The effect of educational initiatives on the attitude and knowledge of health care professionals regarding organ donation and transplantation: an integrative literature review. *Transplant Proc.* 2023;55(1):13–21. https://doi.org/10.1016/j.transproceed.2022.09.037.
8. Wojda TR, Stawicki SP, Yandle KP, et al. Keys to successful organ procurement: an experience-based review of clinical practices at a high-performing health-care organization. *Int J Crit Illn Inj Sci.* 2017;7(2):91–100. https://doi.org/10.4103/IJCIIS.IJCIIS_30_17.
9. Bly JD, Atluri S, Graham-Stephenson A, et al. What is the effect of organ donation authorization rates when utilizing a standardized effective request process? *Crit Care Explor.* 2022;4(1):e0615. https://doi.org/10.1097/CCE.0000000000000615.
10. Revised Uniform Anatomical Gift Act; 2006. National Conference of Commissioners on Uniform State Law. 2006:7–14. July.
11. Shafer T, Schkade LL, Warner HE, et al. Impact of medical examiner/coroner practices on organ recovery in the United States. *JAMA.* 1994;272(20):1607–1613.
12. Shafer TJ, Schkade LL, Siminoff LA, Mahoney TA. Ethical analysis of organ recovery denials by medical examiners, coroners, and justices of the peace. *J Transpl Coord.* 1999;9(4):232–249. https://doi.org/10.7182/prtr.1.9.4.q022hjm60630w514.
13. Shafer TJ, Schkade LL, Evans RW, O'Connor KJ, Reitsma W. Vital role of medical examiners and coroners in organ transplantation. *Am J Transplant.* 2004;4(2):160–168. https://doi.org/10.1046/j.1600-6143.2003.00327.x.
14. Ellis MKM, Sally MB, Malinoski DJ. Management of the potential organ donor. In: Salim A, Brown C, Inaba K, Martin MJ, eds. *Surgical Critical Care Therapy.* Springer International Publishing; 2018:67–75. https://doi.org/10.1007/978-3-319-71712-8_7.
15. Wijdicks EFM. *The Comatose Patient.* Oxford University Press; 2014. https://doi.org/10.1093/med/9780199331215.001.0001.
16. Bernat JL, Capron AM, Bleck TP, et al. The circulatory-respiratory determination of death in organ donation. *Crit Care Med.* 2010;38(3):963–970. https://doi.org/10.1097/CCM.0b013e3181c58916.
17. Institute of Medicine (US) Committee on Non-Heart-Beating Transplantation II. The Scientific and Ethical Basis for Practice and Protocols. Non-heart-beating Organ Transplantation: Practice and Protocols. National Academies Press (US); 2000. http://www.ncbi.nlm.nih.gov/books/NBK225025/. Accessed September 23, 2023.
18. Schroder JN, Patel CB, DeVore AD, et al. Transplantation outcomes with donor hearts after circulatory death. *N Engl J Med.* 2023;388(23):2121–2131. https://doi.org/10.1056/NEJMoa2212438.
19. Bekki Y, Croome KP, Myers B, Sasaki K, Tomiyama K. Normothermic regional perfusion can improve both utilization and outcomes in DCD liver, kidney, and pancreas transplantation. *Transplant Direct.* 2023;9(3):e1450. https://doi.org/10.1097/TXD.0000000000001450.
20. Suberviola B, Mons R, Ballesteros MA, et al. Excellent long-term outcome with lungs obtained from uncontrolled donation after circulatory death. *Am J Transplant.* 2019;19(4):1195–1201. https://doi.org/10.1111/ajt.15237.
21. Hessheimer AJ. In situ normothermic regional perfusion in controlled donation after circulatory determination death: organ utilization, outcomes, and elusiveness of a randomized clinical trial. *Transplantation.* 2023;107(2):311–312. https://doi.org/10.1097/TP.0000000000004281.
22. Vela RJ, Pruszynski J, Mone T, Niles P, Peltz M. Differences in organ donation and transplantation in states within the United States and in European countries: is there a benefit to opting out? *Transplant Proc.* 2021;53(10):2801–2806. https://doi.org/10.1016/j.transproceed.2021.09.029.
23. Glazier AK. Organ donation and the principles of gift law. *Clin J Am Soc Nephrol.* 2018;13(8):1283–1284. https://doi.org/10.2215/CJN.03740318.
24. Glazier A, Mone T. Success of opt-in organ donation policy in the United States. *JAMA.* 2019;322(8):719–720. https://doi.org/10.1001/jama.2019.9187.
25. Dicks SG, Burkolter N, Jackson LC, Northam HL, Boer DP, van Haren FMP. Grief, stress, trauma, and support during the organ donation process. *Transplant Direct.* 2020;6(1):e512. https://doi.org/10.1097/TXD.0000000000000957.
26. Kentish-Barnes N, Siminoff LA, Walker W, et al. A narrative review of family members' experience of organ donation request after brain death in the critical care setting. *Intensive Care Med.* 2019;45(3):331–342. https://doi.org/10.1007/s00134-019-05575-4.
27. Anker AE, Feeley TH. Why families decline donation: the perspective of organ procurement coordinators. *Prog Transplant.* 2010;20(3):239–246. https://doi.org/10.1177/152692481002000307.
28. Stouder DB, Schmid A, Ross SS, Ross LG, Stocks L. Family, friends, and faith: how organ donor families heal. *Prog Transplant.* 2009;19(4):358–361. https://doi.org/10.1177/152692480901900412.
29. Malinoski DJ, Patel MS, Daly MC, Oley-Graybill C, Salim A, UNOS Region 5 DMG workgroup. The impact of meeting donor management goals on the number of organs transplanted per donor: results from the United Network for Organ Sharing Region 5 prospective donor management goals study. *Crit Care Med.* 2012;40(10):2773–2780. https://doi.org/10.1097/CCM.0b013e31825b252a.
30. Malinoski DJ, Patel MS, Ahmed O, et al. The impact of meeting donor management goals on the development of delayed graft function in kidney transplant recipients. *Am J Transplant.* 2013;13(4):993–1000. https://doi.org/10.1111/ajt.12090.

31. Kotloff RM, Blosser S, Fulda GJ, et al. Management of the potential organ donor in the ICU: Society of Critical Care Medicine/American College of Chest Physicians/Association of Organ Procurement Organizations Consensus Statement. *Crit Care Med.* 2015;43(6):1291–1325. https://doi.org/10.1097/CCM.0000000000000958.
32. McKeown DW, Bonser RS, Kellum JA. Management of the heartbeating brain-dead organ donor. *Br J Anaesth.* 2012;108(Suppl 1):i96–107. https://doi.org/10.1093/bja/aer351.
33. American Association of Tissue Banks (AATB). The American Association of Tissue Banks; 2023. https://www.aatb.org/. Accessed September 24, 2023.
34. Nakamura T, Shirouzu T, Nakata K, Yoshimura N, Ushigome H. The role of major histocompatibility complex in organ transplantation- donor specific anti-major histocompatibility complex antibodies analysis goes to the next stage. *Int J Mol Sci.* 2019;20(18):4544. https://doi.org/10.3390/ijms20184544.
35. Stolp J, Turka LA, Wood KJ. B cells with immune-regulating function in transplantation. *Nat Rev Nephrol.* 2014;10(7):389–397. https://doi.org/10.1038/nrneph.2014.80.
36. Karahan GE, Claas FHJ, Heidt S. B cell immunity in solid organ transplantation. *Front Immunol.* 2016;7:686. https://doi.org/10.3389/fimmu.2016.00686.
37. Lakkis FG, Lechler RI. Origin and biology of the allogeneic response. *Cold Spring Harb Perspect Med.* 2013;3(8):a014993. https://doi.org/10.1101/cshperspect.a014993.
38. Chiu P, Schaffer JM, Oyer PE, et al. Influence of durable mechanical circulatory support and allosensitization on mortality after heart transplantation. *J Heart Lung Transplant.* 2016;35(6):731–742. https://doi.org/10.1016/j.healun.2015.12.023.
39. Dardas TF. Impact of mechanical circulatory support on posttransplant outcomes. *Cardiol Clin.* 2018;36(4):551–560. https://doi.org/10.1016/j.ccl.2018.06.009.
40. Goetz RL, Kaleekal TS, Wille KM, et al. HLA sensitization in patients bridged to lung transplantation with extracorporeal membrane oxygenation. *Transplant Direct.* 2023;9(7):e1497. https://doi.org/10.1097/TXD.0000000000001497.
41. Grimm M, Rinaldi M, Yonan NA, et al. Superior prevention of acute rejection by tacrolimus vs. cyclosporine in heart transplant recipients--a large European trial. *Am J Transplant.* 2006;6(6):1387–1397. https://doi.org/10.1111/j.1600-6143.2006.01300.x.
42. Webster AC, Woodroffe RC, Taylor RS, Chapman JR, Craig JC. Tacrolimus versus ciclosporin as primary immunosuppression for kidney transplant recipients: meta-analysis and meta-regression of randomised trial data. *BMJ.* 2005;331(7520):810. https://doi.org/10.1136/bmj.38569.471007.AE.
43. Haddad EM, McAlister VC, Renouf E, Malthaner R, Kjaer MS, Gluud LL. Cyclosporin versus tacrolimus for liver transplanted patients. *Cochrane Database Syst Rev.* 2006;2006(4):CD005161. https://doi.org/10.1002/14651858.CD005161.pub2.
44. Staatz CE, Tett SE. Pharmacology and toxicology of mycophenolate in organ transplant recipients: an update. *Arch Toxicol.* 2014;88(7):1351–1389. https://doi.org/10.1007/s00204-014-1247-1.
45. Kobashigawa J, Miller L, Renlund D, et al. A randomized active-controlled trial of mycophenolate mofetil in heart transplant recipients. Mycophenolate Mofetil Investigators. *Transplantation.* 1998;66(4):507–515. https://doi.org/10.1097/00007890-199808270-00016.
46. Wagner M, Earley AK, Webster AC, Schmid CH, Balk EM, Uhlig K. Mycophenolic acid versus azathioprine as primary immunosuppression for kidney transplant recipients. *Cochrane Database Syst Rev.* 2015;12:CD007746. https://doi.org/10.1002/14651858.CD007746.pub2.
47. Ventura-Aguiar P, Campistol JM, Diekmann F. Safety of mTOR inhibitors in adult solid organ transplantation. *Expert Opin Drug Saf.* 2016;15(3):303–319. https://doi.org/10.1517/14740338.2016.1132698.
48. Zeiser R, Robson SC, Vaikunthanathan T, Dworak M, Burnstock G. Unlocking the potential of purinergic signaling in transplantation. *Am J Transplant.* 2016;16(10):2781–2794. https://doi.org/10.1111/ajt.13801.
49. Katabathina V, Menias CO, Pickhardt P, Lubner M, Prasad SR. Complications of immunosuppressive therapy in solid organ transplantation. *Radiol Clin North Am.* 2016;54(2):303–319. https://doi.org/10.1016/j.rcl.2015.09.009.
50. Glanville AR, Aboyoun C, Klepetko W, et al. Three-year results of an investigator-driven multicenter, international, randomized open-label de novo trial to prevent BOS after lung transplantation. *J Heart Lung Transplant.* 2015;34(1):16–25. https://doi.org/10.1016/j.healun.2014.06.001.
51. Snell GI, Valentine VG, Vitulo P, et al. Everolimus versus azathioprine in maintenance lung transplant recipients: an international, randomized, double-blind clinical trial. *Am J Transplant.* 2006;6(1):169–177. https://doi.org/10.1111/j.1600-6143.2005.01134.x.
52. Colvin MM, Smith JM, Ahn YS, et al. OPTN/SRTR 2021 annual data report: heart. *Am J Transplant.* 2023;23(2):S300–S378. https://doi.org/10.1016/j.ajt.2023.02.008.
53. Valapour M, Lehr CJ, Schladt DP, et al. OPTN/SRTR 2021 annual data report: lung. *Am J Transplant.* 2023;23(2):S379–S442. https://doi.org/10.1016/j.ajt.2023.02.009.
54. Lentine KL, Smith JM, Miller JM, et al. OPTN/SRTR 2021 annual data report: kidney. *Am J Transplant.* 2023;23(2 Suppl 1):S21–S120. https://doi.org/10.1016/j.ajt.2023.02.004.
55. Kwong AJ, Ebel NH, Kim WR, et al. OPTN/SRTR 2021 annual data report: liver. *Am J Transplant.* 2023;23(2):S178–S263. https://doi.org/10.1016/j.ajt.2023.02.006.
56. Lewandowski AN, Skillings JL. Who gets a lung transplant? Assessing the psychosocial decision-making process for transplant listing. *Glob Cardiol Sci Pract.* 2016;2016(3):e201626. https://doi.org/10.21542/gcsp.2016.26.
57. Leard LE, Holm AM, Valapour M, et al. Consensus document for the selection of lung transplant candidates: an update from the International Society for Heart and Lung Transplantation. *J Heart Lung Transplant.* 2021;40(11):1349–1379. https://doi.org/10.1016/j.healun.2021.07.005.
58. Mahmud N. Selection for liver transplantation: indications and evaluation. *Curr Hepatol Rep.* 2020;19(3):203–212. https://doi.org/10.1007/s11901-020-00527-9.
59. Mehra MR, Canter CE, Hannan MM, et al. The 2016 International Society for Heart Lung Transplantation listing criteria for heart transplantation: a 10-year update. *J Heart Lung Transplant.* 2016;35(1):1–23. https://doi.org/10.1016/j.healun.2015.10.023.
60. Volk ML, Biggins SW, Huang MA, Argo CK, Fontana RJ, Anspach RR. Decision making in liver transplant selection committees: a multicenter study. *Ann Intern Med.* 2011;155(8):503–508. https://doi.org/10.7326/0003-4819-155-8-201110180-00006.
61. Flattery MP, Dale C. Solid organ transplantation: the evaluation process. In: Cupples SA, Larret S, McCalmont V, Ohler L, eds. *Core Curriculum for Transplant Nurses.* 2nd ed. Wolters Kluwer; 2017:1–30.
62. Malinis M, Boucher HW, AST Infectious Diseases Community of Practice. Screening of donor and candidate prior to solid organ transplantation-guidelines from the American society of transplantation infectious diseases community of practice. *Clin Transplant.* 2019;33(9):e13548. https://doi.org/10.1111/ctr.13548.
63. Bernardina DK, Phillips DK. Education for transplant patients and caregivers. In: Cupples SA, Larret S, McCalmont V, Ohler L, eds. *Core Curriculum for Transplant Nurses.* 2ed ed. Wolters Kluwer; 2017:50–85.
64. Tanriover B, Stone PW, Mohan S, Cohen DJ, Gaston RS. Future of Medicare immunosuppressive drug coverage for kidney transplant recipients in the United States. *Clin J Am Soc Nephrol.* 2013;8(7):1258–1266. https://doi.org/10.2215/CJN.09440912.
65. Danziger-Isakov L, Kumar D, AST ID Community of Practice. Vaccination of solid organ transplant candidates and recipients: guidelines from the American society of transplantation infectious diseases community of practice. *Clin Transplant.* 2019;33(9):e13563. https://doi.org/10.1111/ctr.13563.
66. Khush KK, Cherikh WS, Chambers DC, et al. International Thoracic Organ Transplant Registry of the International Society for Heart and Lung Transplantation: thirty-sixth adult heart transplantation report - 2019; focus theme: donor and recipient size match. *J Heart Lung Transplant.* 2019;38(10):1056–1066. https://doi.org/10.1016/j.healun.2019.08.004.

67. Khush KK, Hsich E, Potena L, et al. International Thoracic Organ Transplant Registry of the International Society for Heart and Lung Transplantation: thirty-eighth adult heart transplantation report - 2021; focus on recipient characteristics. *J Heart Lung Transplant.* 2021;40(10):1035–1049. https://doi.org/10.1016/j.healun.2021.07.015.
68. Kittleson MM, Sharma K, Brennan DC, et al. Dual-organ transplantation: indications, evaluation, and outcomes for heart-kidney and heart-liver transplantation: a scientific statement from the American Heart Association. *Circulation.* 2023;148(7):622–636. https://doi.org/10.1161/CIR.0000000000001155.
69. Lower RR, Shumway NE. Studies on orthotopic homotransplantation of the canine heart. *Surg Forum.* 1960;11:18–19.
70. Sievers HH, Weyand M, Kraatz EG, Bernhard A. An alternative technique for orthotopic cardiac transplantation, with preservation of the normal anatomy of the right atrium. *Thorac Cardiovasc Surg.* 1991;39(2):70–72. https://doi.org/10.1055/s-2007-1013934.
71. Schroder JN, D'Alessandro D, Esmailian F, et al. Successful utilization of Extended Criteria Donor (ECD) Hearts for Transplantation - Results of the OCS™ heart EXPAND trial to evaluate the effectiveness and safety of the OCS heart system to preserve and assess ECD hearts for transplantation. *J Heart Lung Transplant.* 2019;38(4, Suppl):S42. https://doi.org/10.1016/j.healun.2019.01.088.
72. Kobashigawa J, Zuckermann A, Macdonald P, et al. Report from a consensus conference on primary graft dysfunction after cardiac transplantation. *J Heart Lung Transplant.* 2014;33(4):327–340. https://doi.org/10.1016/j.healun.2014.02.027.
73. Stewart S, Winters GL, Fishbein MC, et al. Revision of the 1990 working formulation for the standardization of nomenclature in the diagnosis of heart rejection. *J Heart Lung Transplant.* 2005;24(11):1710–1720. https://doi.org/10.1016/j.healun.2005.03.019.
74. Pham MX, Teuteberg JJ, Kfoury AG, et al. Gene-expression profiling for rejection surveillance after cardiac transplantation. *N Engl J Med.* 2010;362(20):1890–1900. https://doi.org/10.1056/NEJMoa0912965.
75. Crespo-Leiro M, Zuckermann A, Stypmann J, et al. Increased plasma levels of donor-derived cell-free DNA correlate with rejection in heart transplant recipients: the CARGO II multicenter trial. *J Heart Lung Transplant.* 2015;34(4):S31–S32. https://doi.org/10.1016/j.healun.2015.01.075.
76. Centers for Disease Control and Prevention (CDC). About Cytomegalovirus and Congenital CMV Infection; 2023. https://www.cdc.gov/cmv/overview.html. Accessed September 26, 2023.
77. Eriksson M, Jokinen JJ, Söderlund S, Hämmäinen P, Lommi J, Lemström K. Low-dose valganciclovir prohylaxis is efficacious and safe in cytomegalovirus seropositive heart transplant recipients with anti-thymocyte globulin. *Transpl Infect Dis.* 2018;20(3):e12868. https://doi.org/10.1111/tid.12868.
78. Schulz U, Solidoro P, Müller V, et al. CMV immunoglobulins for the treatment of CMV infections in thoracic transplant recipients. *Transplantation.* 2016;100(Suppl 3):S5–10. https://doi.org/10.1097/TP.0000000000001097.
79. Zuckermann A. 415 Five-year results of a multicenter observational study comparing tacrolimus and cyclosporine in heart transplantation. *J Heart Lung Transplant.* 2011;30(suppl 4):S142. https://doi.org/10.1016/j.healun.2011.01.424.
80. Stallone G, Infante B, Grandaliano G, Gesualdo L. Management of side effects of sirolimus therapy. *Transplantation.* 2009;87(8S):S23–S26. https://doi.org/10.1097/TP.0b013e3181a05b7a.
81. Khush KK, Cherikh WS, Chambers DC, et al. The International Thoracic Organ Transplant Registry of the International Society for Heart and Lung Transplantation: thirty-fifth adult heart transplantation report-2018; focus theme: multiorgan transplantation. *J Heart Lung Transplant.* 2018;37(10):1155–1168. https://doi.org/10.1016/j.healun.2018.07.022.
82. Punnoose LR, Coscia LA, Armenti DP, Constantinescu S, Moritz MJ. Pregnancy outcomes in heart transplant recipients. *J Heart Lung Transplant.* 2020;39(5):473–480. https://doi.org/10.1016/j.healun.2020.02.005.
83. Cramer CL, Marsh K, Krebs ED, et al. Long term employment following heart transplantation in the United States. *J Heart Lung Transplant.* 2023;42(7):880–887. https://doi.org/10.1016/j.healun.2022.12.025.
84. Deuse T, Sista R, Weill D, et al. Review of heart-lung transplantation at Stanford. *Ann Thorac Surg.* 2010;90(1):329–337. https://doi.org/10.1016/j.athoracsur.2010.01.023.
85. Reitz BA. The first successful combined heart-lung transplantation. *J Thorac Cardiovasc Surg.* 2011;141(4):867–869. https://doi.org/10.1016/j.jtcvs.2010.12.014.
86. Shudo Y, Kasinpila P, Lingala B, Kim FY, Woo YJ. Heart-lung transplantation over the past 10 years: an up-to-date concept. *Eur J Cardiothorac Surg.* 2019;55(2):304–308. https://doi.org/10.1093/ejcts/ezy253.
87. Loor G, Warnecke G, Villavicencio M, et al. Results of the OCS lung EXPAND international trial using portable normothermic OCS lung perfusion system (OCS) to recruit and evaluate Extended Criteria Donor (ECD) lungs. *J Heart Lung Transplant.* 2018;37(4 Suppl):S147. https://doi.org/10.1016/j.healun.2018.01.356.
88. Messer S, Page A, Kaul P, et al. Successful combined heart-lung transplant from a Donation after Circulatory Determined Death (DCD) donor. *J Heart Lung Transplant.* 2020;39(4 Suppl):S20–S21. https://doi.org/10.1016/j.healun.2020.01.1149.
89. Divithotawela C, Cypel M, Martinu T, et al. Long-term outcomes of lung transplant with ex vivo lung perfusion. *JAMA Surg.* 2019;154(12):1143–1150. https://doi.org/10.1001/jamasurg.2019.4079.
90. Naik PM, Angel LF. Special issues in the management and selection of the donor for lung transplantation. *Semin Immunopathol.* 2011;33(2):201–210. https://doi.org/10.1007/s00281-011-0256-x.
91. Snell GI, Westall GP. Selection and management of the lung donor. *Clin Chest Med.* 2011;32(2):223–232. https://doi.org/10.1016/j.ccm.2011.02.002.
92. Latchana N, Peck JR, Whitson B, Black SM. Preservation solutions for cardiac and pulmonary donor grafts: a review of the current literature. *J Thorac Dis.* 2014;6(8):1143–1149. https://doi.org/10.3978/j.issn.2072-1439.2014.05.14.
93. Hayanga JA, Lira A, Vlahu T, et al. Procedural volume and survival after lung transplantation in the United States: the need to look beyond volume in the establishment of quality metrics. *Am J Surg.* 2016;211(4):671–676. https://doi.org/10.1016/j.amjsurg.2015.12.010.
94. Boasquevisque CHR, Yildirim E, Waddel TK, Keshavjee S. Surgical techniques: lung transplant and lung volume reduction. *Proc Am Thorac Soc.* 2009;6(1):66–78. https://doi.org/10.1513/pats.200808-083GO.
95. Martinu T, Pavlisko EN, Chen DF, Palmer SM. Acute allograft rejection: cellular and humoral processes. *Clin Chest Med.* 2011;32(2):295–310. https://doi.org/10.1016/j.ccm.2011.02.008.
96. Wallace WD, Li N, Andersen CB, et al. Banff study of pathologic changes in lung allograft biopsy specimens with donor-specific antibodies. *J Heart Lung Transplant.* 2016;35(1):40–48. https://doi.org/10.1016/j.healun.2015.08.021.
97. Nosotti M, Tarsia P, Morlacchi LC. Infections after lung transplantation. *J Thorac Dis.* 2018;10(6):3849–3868. https://doi.org/10.21037/jtd.2018.05.204.
98. Kotton CN. Management of cytomegalovirus infection in solid organ transplantation. *Nat Rev Nephrol.* 2010;6(12):711–721. https://doi.org/10.1038/nrneph.2010.141.
99. Le Page AK, Jager MM, Kotton CN, Simoons-Smit A, Rawlinson WD. International survey of cytomegalovirus management in solid organ transplantation after the publication of consensus guidelines. *Transplantation.* 2013;95(12):1455–1460. https://doi.org/10.1097/TP.0b013e31828ee12e.
100. Kurihara C, Fernandez R, Safaeinili N, et al. Long-term impact of cytomegalovirus serologic status on lung transplantation in the United States. *Ann Thorac Surg.* 2019;107(4):1046–1052. https://doi.org/10.1016/j.athoracsur.2018.10.034.
101. Gerity SL, Silva SG, Reynolds JM, Hoffman B, Oermann MH. Multimedia education reduces anxiety in lung transplant patients. *Prog Transplant.* 2018;28(1):83–86. https://doi.org/10.1177/1526924817746910.
102. Rebafka A, Bennett C, Jones J, Carrier J, Kugler C, Edwards D. Lung transplant recipients' experiences of and attitudes towards self-management: a qualitative systematic review protocol. *JBI Database System Rev Implement Rep.* 2018;16(4):831–837. https://doi.org/10.11124/JBISRIR-2017-003524.

103. Yusen RD, Edwards LB, Dipchand AI, et al. The Registry of the International Society for Heart and Lung Transplantation: thirty-third adult lung and heart-lung transplant report-2016; focus theme: primary diagnostic indications for transplant. *J Heart Lung Transplant.* 2016;35(10):1170–1184. https://doi.org/10.1016/j.healun.2016.09.001.
104. Chambers DC, Cherikh WS, Goldfarb SB, et al. The International Thoracic Organ Transplant Registry of the International Society for Heart and Lung Transplantation: thirty-fifth adult lung and heart-lung transplant report-2018; focus theme: multiorgan transplantation. *J Heart Lung Transplant.* 2018;37(10):1169–1183. https://doi.org/10.1016/j.healun.2018.07.020.
105. Tasoudis P, Lobo LJ, Coakley RD, et al. Outcomes following lung transplant for COVID-19-related complications in the US. *JAMA Surg.* 2023:e233489. https://doi.org/10.1001/jamasurg.2023.3489. Published online August 16.
106. Weder MM, Aslam S, Ison MG. Lung transplantation for COVID-19-related lung disease: clinical experience and call for a global registry. *Transplantation.* 2023;107(1):18–20. https://doi.org/10.1097/TP.0000000000004327.
107. Bermudez CA, Crespo MM. The case for prolonged ECMO for COVID-19 ARDS as a bridge to recovery or lung transplantation. *Transplantation.* 2022;106(4):e198–e199. https://doi.org/10.1097/TP.0000000000004063.
108. Date H. Living-related lung transplantation. *J Thorac Dis.* 2017;9(9):3362–3371. https://doi.org/10.21037/jtd.2017.08.152.
109. Date H. Living-donor lobar lung transplantation. Published online September 11 *J Heart Lung Transplant.* 2023;(23):S1053–2498. https://doi.org/10.1016/j.healun.2023.09.006. 02013-2.
110. Knoop C, Estenne M. Chronic allograft dysfunction. *Clin Chest Med.* 2011;32(2):311–326. https://doi.org/10.1016/j.ccm.2011.02.009.
111. Miggins JJ, Reul RM, Barrett S, et al. Twenty-year survival following lung transplantation. *J Thorac Dis.* 2023;15(6):2997–3012. https://doi.org/10.21037/jtd-22-1414.
112. Starzl TE, Groth CG, Brettschneider L, et al. Orthotopic homotransplantation of the human liver. *Ann Surg.* 1968;168(3):392–415. https://doi.org/10.1097/00000658-196809000-00009.
113. Kwong A, Kim WR, Lake JR, et al. OPTN/SRTR 2018 annual data report: liver. *Am J Transplant.* 2020;20(Suppl s1):193–299. https://doi.org/10.1111/ajt.15674.
114. Kwong AJ, Ebel NH, Kim WR, et al. OPTN/SRTR 2020 annual data report: liver. *Am J Transplant.* 2022;22(Suppl 2):204–309. https://doi.org/10.1111/ajt.16978.
115. Organ Procurement and Transplantation Network - OPTN. MELD calculator - OPTN; 2023. https://optn.transplant.hrsa.gov/data/allocation-calculators/meld-calculator/. Accessed September 24, 2023.
116. Organ Procurement and Transplantation Network - OPTN. PELD calculator - OPTN; 2023. https://optn.transplant.hrsa.gov/data/allocation-calculators/peld-calculator/. Accessed September 24, 2023.
117. Harring TR, O'Mahony CA, Goss JA. extended donors in liver transplantation. *Clin Liver Dis.* 2011;15(4):879–900. https://doi.org/10.1016/j.cld.2011.08.006.
118. deLemos AS, Vagefi PA. Expanding the donor pool in liver transplantation: extended criteria donors. *Clin Liver Dis (Hoboken).* 2013;2(4):156–159. https://doi.org/10.1002/cld.222.
119. Hall EC, Boyarsky BJ, Deshpande NA, et al. Perioperative complications after live-donor hepatectomy. *JAMA Surg.* 2014;149(3):288–291. https://doi.org/10.1001/jamasurg.2013.3835.
120. Muzaale AD, Dagher NN, Montgomery RA, Taranto SE, McBride MA, Segev DL. Estimates of early death, acute liver failure, and long-term mortality among live liver donors. *Gastroenterology.* 2012;142(2):273–280. https://doi.org/10.1053/j.gastro.2011.11.015.
121. Wallia A, Parikh ND, Molitch ME, et al. Posttransplant hyperglycemia is associated with increased risk of liver allograft rejection. *Transplantation.* 2010;89(2):222–226. https://doi.org/10.1097/TP.0b013e3181c3c2ff.
122. Durst JK, Rampersad RM. Pregnancy in women with solid-organ transplants: a review. *Obstet Gynecol Surv.* 2015;70(6):408–418. https://doi.org/10.1097/OGX.0000000000000194.
123. Hart A, Smith JM, Skeans MA, et al. OPTN/SRTR 2018 annual data report: kidney. *Am J Transplant.* 2020;20(Suppl s1):20–130. https://doi.org/10.1111/ajt.15672.
124. Smith JM, Biggins SW, Haselby DG, et al. Kidney, pancreas and liver allocation and distribution in the United States. *Am J Transplant.* 2012;12(12):3191–3212. https://doi.org/10.1111/j.1600--6143.2012.04259.x.
125. Leeser DB, Aull MJ, Afaneh C, et al. Living donor kidney paired donation transplantation: experience as a founding member center of the National Kidney Registry. *Clin Transplant.* 2012;26(3):E213–222. https://doi.org/10.1111/j.1399-0012.2012.01606.x.
126. Leeser DB, Thomas AG, Shaffer AA, et al. Patient and kidney allograft survival with national kidney paired donation. *Clin J Am Soc Nephrol.* 2020;15(2):228–237. https://doi.org/10.2215/CJN.06660619.
127. Melcher ML, Leeser DB, Gritsch HA, et al. Chain transplantation: initial experience of a large multicenter program. *Am J Transplant.* 2012;12(9):2429–2436. https://doi.org/10.1111/j.1600-6143.2012.04156.x.
128. Verbesey J, Thomas AG, Ronin M, et al. Early graft losses in paired kidney exchange: experience from 10 years of the National Kidney Registry. *Am J Transplant.* 2020;20(5):1393–1401. https://doi.org/10.1111/ajt.15778.
129. Lenhan TR, Tan JC. Clinical management of the adult kidney transplant recipient. In: 11th ed. Yu ASL, Chertow GM, Luyckx V, Marsden HA, Skorecki K, Taaleds MW, eds. *Benner and Rector's the Kidney.* Vol 2. Elsevier; 2020:2244–2287.
130. Agrawal A, Ison MG, Danziger-Isakov L. Long-term infectious complications of kidney transplantation. *CJASN.* 2022;17(2):286–295. https://doi.org/10.2215/CJN.15971020.
131. Shah S, Venkatesan RL, Gupta A, et al. Pregnancy outcomes in women with kidney transplant: Metaanalysis and systematic review. *BMC Nephrol.* 2019;20(1):24. https://doi.org/10.1186/s12882-019-1213-5.
132. Dhanireddy KK. Pancreas transplantation. *Gastroenterol Clin North Am.* 2012;41(1):133–142. https://doi.org/10.1016/j.gtc.2011.12.002.
133. Moein M, Papa S, Bahreini A, Saidi R. Pancreas transplant alone in the USA, where do we stand? *World J Surg.* 2023;47(9):2250–2258. https://doi.org/10.1007/s00268-023-07062-w.
134. Jarmi T, Brennan E, Clendenon J, Spaulding AC. Mortality assessment for pancreas transplants in the United States over the decade 2008-2018. *World J Transplant.* 2023;13(4):147–156. https://doi.org/10.5500/wjt.v13.i4.147.
135. Kandaswamy R, Stock PG, Gustafson SK, et al. OPTN/SRTR 2018 annual data report: pancreas. *Am J Transplant.* 2020;20(Suppl s1):131–192. https://doi.org/10.1111/ajt.15673.
136. Gruessner AC, Gruessner RWG. Long-term outcome after pancreas transplantation: a registry analysis. *Curr Opin Organ Transplant.* 2016;21(4):377–385. https://doi.org/10.1097/MOT.0000000000000331.

36

Hematologic and Oncologic Emergencies

Carol Ann Suarez

http://evolve.elsevier.com/Urden/CriticalCareNursing

Understanding the pathology of a disease, the areas of assessment on which to focus, and the usual medical management allows the critical care nurse to more accurately anticipate and plan nursing interventions. This chapter focuses on hematologic and oncologic disorders commonly seen in the critical care environment.

OVERVIEW OF COAGULATION AND FIBRINOLYSIS

Hemostasis, the ability of the body to control bleeding and clotting, is an intricate balancing act between the coagulation mechanism and fibrinolysis. These four major actions are involved in achieving hemostasis: (1) local vasoconstriction to reduce blood flow, (2) platelet aggregation at the injury site and formation of a platelet plug, (3) formation of a fibrin mesh to strengthen the plug, and (4) dissolution of the clot after tissue repair is complete.[1] Disruption of the normal hemostatic balance can result in devastating hemorrhagic or thrombotic conditions.

Coagulation Mechanism

The coagulation mechanism consists of 13 factors that work together through a series of feedback loops to achieve hemostasis (Table 36.1 and Fig. 36.1). Depending on the initial triggering event, the extrinsic or intrinsic coagulation pathway is initiated.[1] The extrinsic pathway begins when vascular injury occurs, resulting in release of tissue factor and activation of coagulation factor VII. The intrinsic pathway is activated when the damaged subendothelium comes into direct contact with circulating blood. In this contact phase, proteins activate additional coagulation factors (XII, XI, IX, and VIII).[1] At this point, the two pathways converge into a common pathway and prothrombin and fibrinogen are converted to their active forms, resulting in clot formation.[2,3]

TABLE 36.1 Coagulation Factors

Factor	Common Name
I	Fibrinogen
II	Prothrombin
III	Tissue factor or thromboplastin
IV	Calcium
V	Proaccelerin
VI	Accelerin
VII	Proconvertin
VIII	Antihemophilic A factor
IX	Christmas factor/antihemophilic B factor
X	Stuart factor
XI	Plasma thromboplastin antecedent
XII	Hageman factor
XIII	Fibrin-stabilizing factor

Clot Formation

Platelets are activated by the arrival of thrombin at the site of injury (Fig. 36.2). Local platelets change shape, become sticky, and begin to aggregate along the vessel wall. Activated platelets undergo degranulation, releasing several factors to assist in clot formation. Serotonin and histamine, two potent vasoconstrictors, help limit blood loss while the clot is forming. The prostaglandin thromboxane A_2 contributes to vasoconstriction and promotes further platelet degranulation. Adenosine diphosphate recruits platelets by increasing adherence and degranulation,[2] and the process continues.

At the convergence of the intrinsic and extrinsic pathways, factor X is converted into its active form, enabling the conversion of prothrombin to thrombin. Thrombin then converts fibrinogen to fibrin. Strands of fibrin form and radiate around the newly formed clot, essentially creating a net in which platelets, red blood cells (RBCs), and white blood cells (WBCs) are trapped. The clot is further secured to the site as platelet actomyosin causes the clot to contract and consolidate.[1]

Regulatory Mechanisms

Under normal conditions, feedback systems prevent the coagulation process from spinning out of control. Prostacyclin I_2, a prostaglandin released from damaged endothelial cells, counteracts the effects of thromboxane A_2, serotonin, and histamine through vasodilation and inhibition of platelet degranulation.[1,2] Another means of regulating clot formation is through inhibition of enzymes necessary for activation of coagulation factors along the intrinsic and extrinsic pathways, preventing the conversion of prothrombin to thrombin. The most important of these regulators is antithrombin III; however, protein C and protein S also play a role in thrombin inhibition.[4]

Fibrinolysis

The process of fibrinolysis promotes dissolution and remolding of the clot to promote repair of the vessel wall and maintain flow through the vessel lumen (Fig. 36.2D). Fibrinolysis begins as soon as the fibrin clot is formed. Circulating plasminogen, a precursor to the powerful enzyme plasmin, binds to fibrin and is trapped within the newly formed clot. The injured epithelial wall releases tissue-type plasminogen activator, which converts plasminogen to its active state, plasmin. The plasmin begins to digest the fibrin, rapidly breaking down the clot.[3] When fibrin

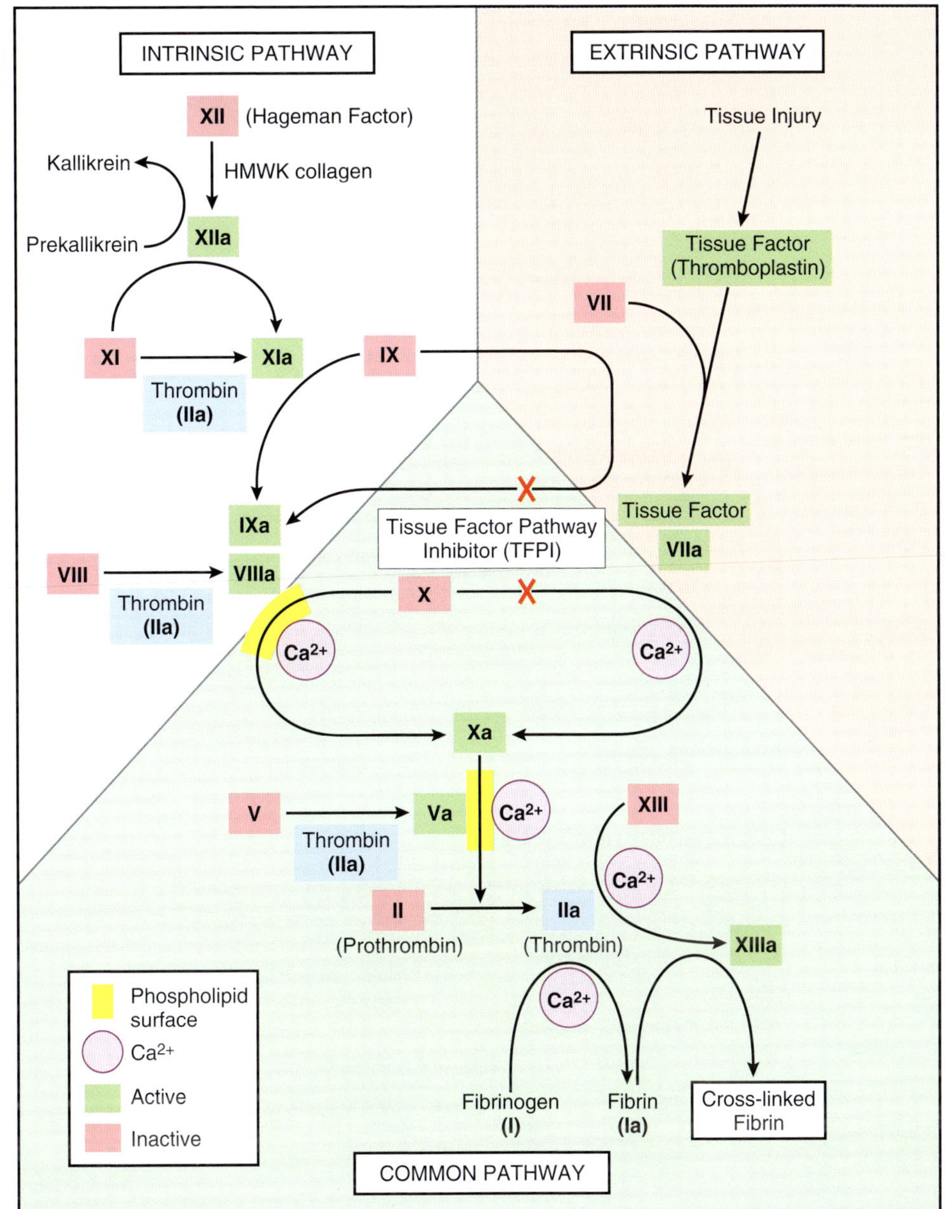

FIG. 36.1 Coagulation Cascade. Factor IX can be activated either by factor XIa or by factor VIIa; in laboratory tests, activation predominantly depends on factor XIa of the intrinsic pathway. Factors in red boxes represent inactive molecules; activated factors are indicated with a lower case "a" and a green box. Note also the multiple points where thrombin (factor IIa; light blue boxes) contributes to coagulation through positive feedback loops. The red "X's" denote points of action of the tissue factor pathway inhibitor, which inhibits the activation of factors X and IX by factor VIIa. *HMWK*, High-molecular-weight kininogen. (From Kumar V, Abbas AK, Aster JC, eds. *Robbins and Cotran Pathologic Basis of Disease*. 8th ed. Saunders; 2010.)

is broken down, the fibrin degradation products released act as anticoagulants.

DISSEMINATED INTRAVASCULAR COAGULATION

Description and Etiology

Disseminated intravascular coagulation (DIC) is a condition characterized by systemic activation of coagulation, potentially leading to thrombotic obstruction of small and midsize vessels, thereby contributing to organ dysfunction.[5] An understanding of the etiologic and pathophysiologic mechanisms of DIC can assist in anticipating occurrence of the syndrome, recognizing its signs and symptoms, and prompting intervention. Also known as *consumptive coagulopathy*, DIC is characterized by bleeding and thrombosis, both of which result from depletion of clotting factors, platelets, and RBCs. If not treated quickly, DIC will progress to multiple organ failure and death.[6]

Etiology

Many clinical events can prompt the development of DIC in a critically ill patient, but the exact underlying trigger may not be identifiable (Box 36.1). DIC is always secondary to an underlying condition, such as severe infection, solid or hematologic malignancies, trauma, or obstetric calamities.[5]

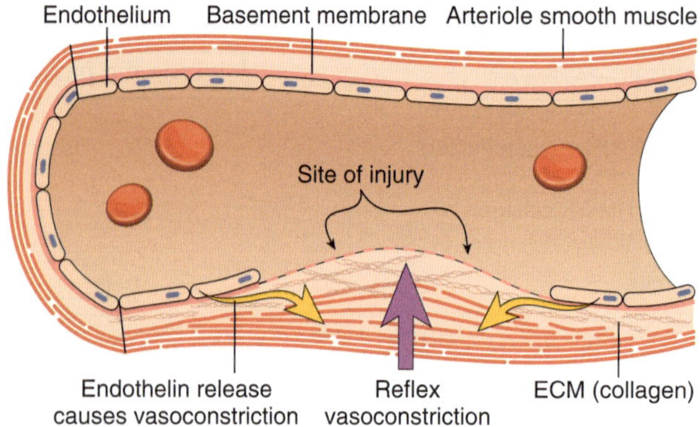

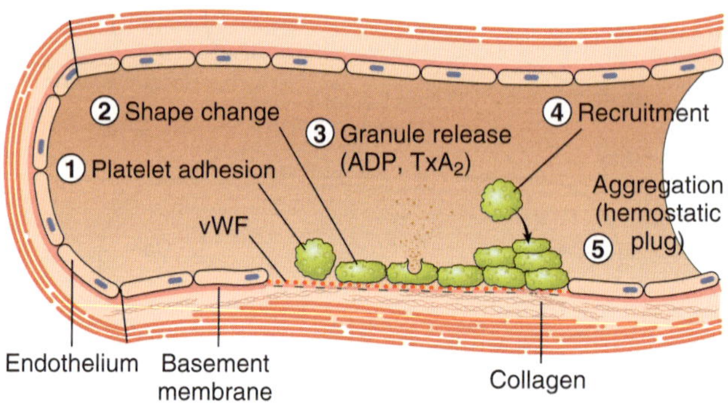

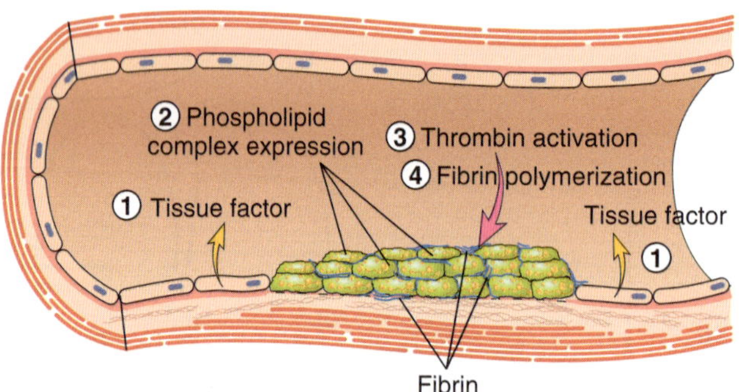

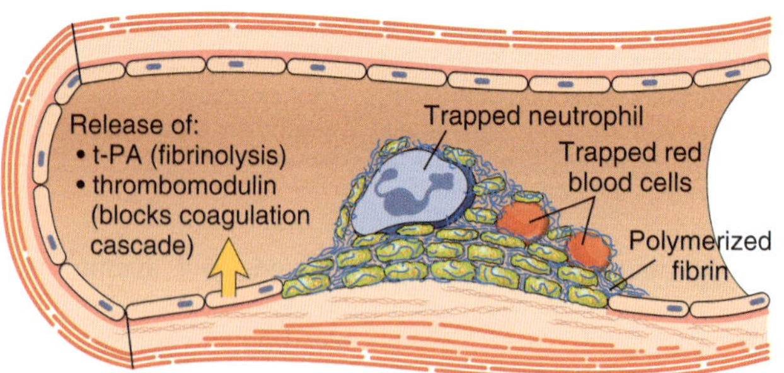

FIG. 36.2 Normal Hemostatic Process. Diagrammatic representation of the normal hemostatic process. (A) After vascular injury, local neurohumoral factors induce a transient vasoconstriction. (B) Platelets adhere to exposed extracellular matrix (ECM) by means of von Willebrand factor (vWF) and are activated, undergoing a shape change and granule release. Released adenosine diphosphate (ADP) and thromboxane A_2 (TxA_2) lead to further platelet aggregation to form the primary hemostatic plug. (C) Local activation of the coagulation cascade (involving tissue factor and platelet phospholipids) results in fibrin polymerization, "cementing" the platelets into a definitive secondary hemostatic plug. (D) Counterregulatory mechanisms, such as release of tissue-type plasminogen activator (t-PA) (fibrinolytic) and thrombomodulin (interfering with the coagulation cascade), limit the hemostatic process to the site of injury. (From Kumar V, Abbas AK, Aster JC, eds. *Robbins and Cotran Pathologic Basis of Disease*. 10th ed. Elsevier; 2021.)

Sepsis, particularly sepsis resulting from gram-negative organisms, can be identified as the cause of DIC in 20% of cases, making it the most common cause of DIC. Endotoxins serve as a trigger for activation of tissue factor and the extrinsic coagulation pathway. Metabolic acidosis and hypoperfusion associated with shock syndromes can result in increased formation of free radicals and damage to tissues. Tissue factor is activated, resulting in DIC. Massive trauma or burns are frequently associated with DIC. Direct tissue damage activates the extrinsic coagulation pathway, and damage to endothelial surfaces activates the intrinsic pathway.[2] Obstetric emergencies, such as abruptio placentae, retained placenta, or incomplete abortion, are also associated with the development of DIC. Tissue factor is concentrated in the placenta, and damage or disruption of this structure can activate coagulation pathways, resulting in coagulopathy.[7]

BOX 36.1 Causes of Disseminated Intravascular Coagulation

Obstetric Complications
- Abruptio placentae
- Placenta previa
- Retained dead fetus
- Septic abortion
- Amniotic fluid embolism
- Toxemia of pregnancy

Infections
- Gram-negative sepsis
- Gram-positive sepsis
- Meningococcemia
- Rocky Mountain spotted fever
- Histoplasmosis
- Aspergillosis
- Malaria

Neoplasms
- Carcinomas of pancreas, prostate, lung, and stomach
- Acute promyelocytic leukemia
- Tumor lysis syndrome
- Chemotherapy

Massive Tissue Injury
- Trauma
- Crush injuries
- Burns
- Extensive surgery
- Heat stroke
- Acute transplant rejection

Miscellaneous
- Acute intravascular hemolysis
- Snakebite
- Giant hemangioma
- Shock
- Heat stroke
- Vasculitis
- Aortic aneurysm
- Liver disease
- Cardiac arrest

Pathophysiology

Regardless of the cause, the common thread in the development of DIC is damage to the endothelium that results in activation of the coagulation mechanism (Fig. 36.3).[1] The extrinsic coagulation pathway plays a major role in the development of DIC. Direct damage to the endothelium results in the release of tissue factor and activation of this pathway. The secondary surge of thrombin formation as a result of activation of the intrinsic coagulation pathway leads to the massive disruption of the delicate balance that is hemostasis. Excessive thrombin formation results in rapid consumption of coagulation factors and depletion of regulatory substances—protein C, protein S, and antithrombin.[4] With no checks and balances, thrombi continue to form along damaged epithelial walls, resulting in occlusion of the vessels. As occlusion reaches a critical level, tissue ischemia ensues, leading to further tissue damage and perpetuating the process. Eventually, end-organ function is affected by the ischemia, and failure is evident.[1]

In response to the formation of clots, the fibrinolytic system is activated. As plasmin breaks down the fibrin clots, fibrin split products are released, and they act as anticoagulants.[2,6] Coupled with depletion of circulating clotting factors, activation of fibrinolysis results in excessive bleeding. The end result is shock and further tissue ischemia that aggravate end-organ dysfunction and failure. Death is imminent if this destructive cycle is not interrupted.[7]

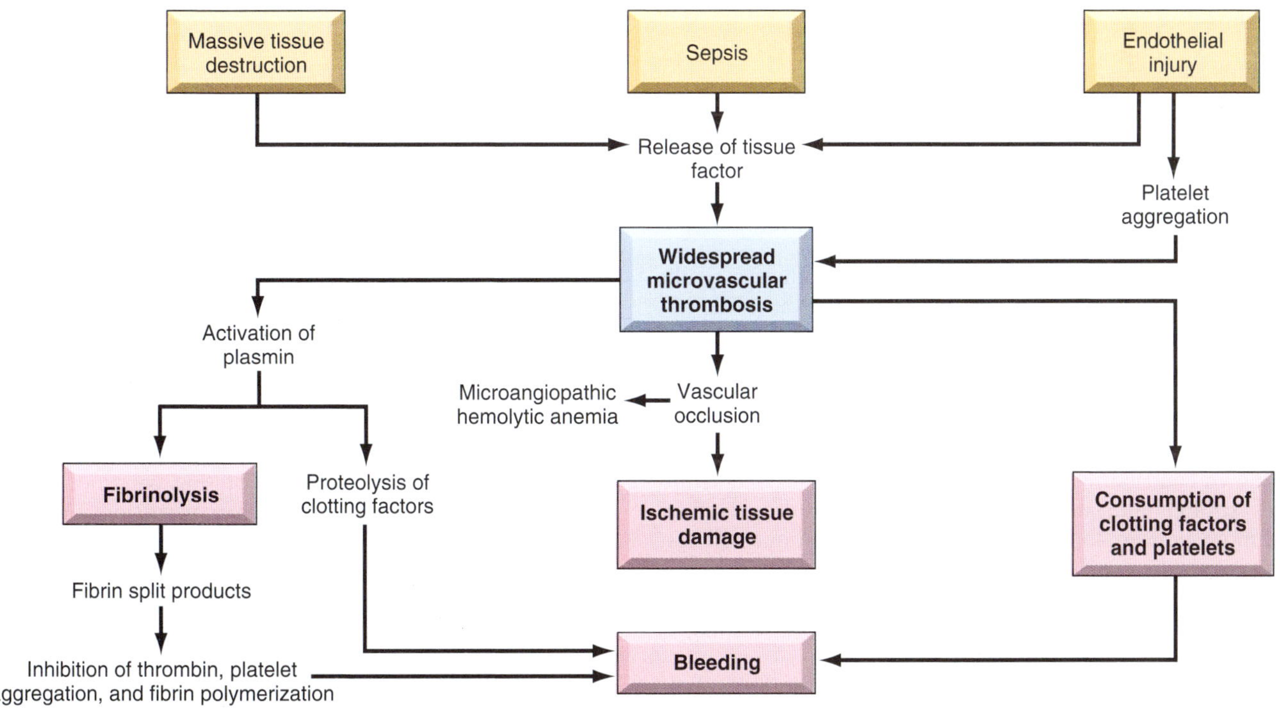

FIG. 36.3 Pathophysiology of Disseminated Intravascular Coagulation. (From Kumar V, Abbas AK, Aster JC, eds. *Robbins and Cotran Pathologic Basis of Disease*. 10th ed. Elsevier; 2021.)

TABLE 36.2 Signs and Symptoms of Disseminated Intravascular Coagulation

System	Signs Related to Hemorrhage	Signs Related to Thrombi
Integumentary	Bleeding from gums, venipunctures, and old surgical sites; epistaxis; ecchymoses	Peripheral cyanosis, gangrene
Cardiopulmonary	Hemoptysis	Dysrhythmias, chest pain, acute myocardial infarction, pulmonary embolus, respiratory failure
Renal	Hematuria	Oliguria, acute kidney injury
Gastrointestinal	Abdominal distention, hemorrhage	Diarrhea, constipation, bowel infarct
Neurologic	Subarachnoid hemorrhage	Altered level of consciousness, ischemic stroke

Assessment and Diagnosis

Favorable outcomes for patients with DIC depend on accurate and timely diagnosis of the condition. Realization of the role underlying pathology plays, recognition of clinical manifestations, and assessment of appropriate laboratory values are key steps in this process.

Assessment

Clinical manifestations are related to the two primary pathophysiologic mechanisms of DIC: the formation of thrombi and bleeding. Thrombi in peripheral capillaries can lead to cyanosis, particularly in the fingers, toes, ears, and nose. In severe, untreated cases, this peripheral ischemia may progress to gangrene.[2,6] As the condition progresses, ischemia worsens, and end organs are affected. The result of this more central ischemia can be respiratory insufficiency and failure, acute kidney injury, bowel infarction, and ischemic stroke. The tissue damage that results perpetuates the anomalies of DIC.[2]

As coagulation factors are depleted, bleeding from intravenous and other puncture sites is observed. Ecchymoses may result from routine interventions such as the use of a manual blood pressure cuff, bathing, or turning. Bloody drainage may also occur from surgical sites, drains, and urinary catheters. With the progression of DIC, the patient is at risk for severe gastrointestinal or subarachnoid hemorrhage.[2,6] Table 36.2 lists common signs and symptoms of DIC.

Diagnosis

Laboratory tests used to diagnose DIC essentially assess the four basic characteristics of this syndrome: (1) increased coagulant activity, (2) increased fibrinolytic activity, (3) impaired regulatory function, and (4) end-organ failure.[2,6]

Continuous activation of the coagulation pathways results in the consumption of coagulation factors. Because of this, prothrombin time, activated partial thromboplastin time, and international normalized ratio values are elevated. Although the platelet count may be within normal ranges, serial examination reveals a declining trend in values. An unexpected drop of at least 50% in the platelet count, particularly in the presence of known contributing factors and associated signs and symptoms, strongly indicates DIC.[1] Fibrinogen levels drop as more and more clots are formed. Thrombus formation in small vessels narrows the vessel lumen, forcing RBCs to squeeze through. The resulting damage and fragmentation of these cells can be seen on microscopic examination of blood samples. Damaged, fragmented RBCs are called *schistocytes*.[2,6]

In response to the excess clotting activity, the fibrinolytic process accelerates, and levels of byproducts increase. This is reflected in markedly elevated levels of fibrin degradation products. Another key laboratory test used to evaluate the degree of clot dissolution and the severity of the coagulopathy is the d-dimer level.[1] d-dimers exclusively indicate clot degradation because, in contrast to fibrin degradation products, which also result from the breakdown of free circulating fibrin, d-dimers result only from dissolution of clots.[2] With progression of the coagulopathy, normal regulatory mechanisms are disrupted, as reflected in decreasing levels of inhibitory factors such as protein C, factor V, and antithrombin III.[2,6,8]

TABLE 36.3 Laboratory Studies in Disseminated Intravascular Coagulation

Test	Value
Prothrombin time (PT)	>12.5 s
Platelets	<50,000/mm^3 or at least 50% drop from baseline
Activated partial thromboplastin time (aPTT)	>40 s
d-dimer	>250 ng/mL
Fibrin degradation products (FDP)	>40 mg/mL
Fibrinogen	<100 mg/dL

Unchecked DIC resulting in occlusion of vessels and tissue ischemia leads to end-organ dysfunction. Common findings in advanced DIC include respiratory failure, indicated by abnormal arterial blood gas (ABG) levels; liver failure, indicated by increasing liver enzymes; and renal impairment, indicated by increasing blood urea nitrogen (BUN) and creatinine levels.[8]

No single laboratory study can confirm the diagnosis of DIC, but several key results are strong indicators of the condition (Table 36.3). The International Society on Thrombosis and Hemostasis emphasizes early detection of DIC through observation of abnormal trends in laboratory values.[9]

Medical Management

The primary intervention in DIC is prevention. Being aware of the conditions that commonly contribute to the development of DIC and treating them vigorously and without delay provide the best defense against this devastating condition.[2,6,8] After DIC is identified, maintaining organ perfusion and slowing consumption of coagulation factors are paramount to achieving a favorable outcome.[1,2]

Multiple organ dysfunction syndrome (MODS) frequently results from DIC and exacerbates the underlying pathology.[7] It is essential to prevent end-organ ischemia and damage by supporting blood pressure and circulating volume. Administration of intravenous fluids and inotropic agents and, if overt hemorrhaging is evident, infusion of packed RBCs are appropriate interventions to replace blood volume and essential, oxygen-carrying RBCs.

In the presence of severe platelet depletion (less than 50,000/mm^3) and severe hemorrhage, platelet transfusions are often indicated.[6,8] However, caution must be used when administering platelets, because antiplatelet antibodies may be formed. These antibodies may become activated during future platelet transfusions and elicit DIC.[2]

Replacement of clotting factors in a patient with DIC is thought by some authorities to perpetuate the coagulopathy; however, there is little scientific evidence to support this theory.[1] Fibrinogen levels less than 100 mg/dL indicate the appropriateness of administering cryoprecipitate. A prolonged prothrombin time indicates the need for fresh-frozen plasma.[2,6,8]

Slowing consumption of coagulation factors by inhibiting the processes involved in clot formation is another strategy used to treat DIC. The use of heparin, particularly low-molecular-weight heparin, to prevent formation of future clots is controversial.[6] It is contraindicated in patients with DIC associated with recent surgery or with gastrointestinal or central nervous system bleeding. However, heparin has been beneficial in obstetric emergencies such as retained placenta or incomplete abortion, severe arterial occlusions, or MODS caused by microemboli.[2,6] Inhibitors such as aminocaproic acid may be used in conjunction with heparin.[2,6]

Thrombin production in DIC surpasses production of antithrombins and other regulatory factors that would normally be present to inactivate thrombin and its subsequent actions. The use of antithrombin III has been approved in the United States. Ongoing research is yielding mixed results in the treatment of DIC.[2]

Nursing Management

The patient care management plan for a patient with DIC incorporates a variety of patient problems (Box 36.2). Assessment and monitoring are the primary weapons in the arsenal against DIC. Knowing the diseases and conditions that are most often associated with DIC and understanding the pathophysiologic mechanisms involved enables appropriate monitoring and intervention should the situation arise. Nursing actions are driven by the specific cause of the DIC, although some common interventions are appropriate for all patients with DIC. The nurse has a significant role in supporting the patient's vital functions, initiating bleeding precautions, providing comfort and emotional support, and maintaining surveillance for complications.

Support Vital Functions

Supporting the patient's vital physiologic functions is critical to the outcome of the patient. The administration of intravenous fluids, blood products, and medications is essential to providing adequate hemodynamic support and ensuring adequate tissue oxygenation to combat DIC and prevent end-organ damage. Blood products may include packed RBCs, fresh frozen plasma, platelet concentrations, and cryoprecipitates. The patient should be closely monitored for any adverse reaction to blood products. Medications may include heparin, antibiotics for infection (depending on the underlying cause), vasoactive agents for hemodynamic support, and analgesics for pain.

Close monitoring of vital signs, hemodynamic parameters, intake and output, and appropriate laboratory values assists in the administration and titration of appropriate agents. Frequent assessments of the patient's neurologic status, kidney function, cardiopulmonary function, and integumentary condition facilitate the early identification of impaired tissue or organ perfusion. Particular parameters to include are mental status and level of consciousness; BUN and creatinine levels; prothrombin time, activated partial thromboplastin time, and international normalized ratio values; urine output; vital signs and hemodynamic values including cardiac rhythm and oxygen saturation; and skin integrity.

Initiate Bleeding Precautions

Awareness of the patient's bleeding potential necessitates adjustments to normal nursing interventions (Box 36.3). Unnecessary venipunctures or arterial punctures that may result in bleeding, bruising, or hematomas are avoided. Blood is drawn from existing arterial or venous lines. The use of manual or automatic blood pressure cuffs is avoided whenever possible. If tracheal or oral suctioning is necessary, the use of low-level suction is recommended. Meticulous skin care is advised, keeping the skin moist and using specialty mattresses and beds as appropriate to prevent breakdown. Gentle care is used when bathing or turning the patient to prevent bruising or hematoma formation. The

BOX 36.2 DIAGNOSIS AND PATIENT CARE MANAGEMENT

Disseminated Intravascular Coagulation

- Hypovolemia due to absolute loss
- Impaired Cardiac Output due to alterations in preload
- Risk for Infection
- Anxiety due to threat to biological, psychological, or social integrity
- Impaired Family Coping due to a critically ill family member

Patient Care Management plans are located in Appendix A.

BOX 36.3 Safety

Bleeding Precautions and Injury Prevention

- Handle the patient gently.
- Use a draw sheet when repositioning the patient in bed.
- Instruct the patient to notify the nurse immediately if bleeding or bruising is noted.
- Protect the patient from trauma.
- Instruct the patient to notify the nurse immediately if any trauma occurs.
- Apply ice to areas of trauma.
- Avoid rectal temperatures, enemas, and suppositories.
- If suppositories are prescribed, lubricate liberally and administer with caution.
- Initiate fall precautions.
- Avoid IM injections and venipunctures.
- Apply firm pressure to any puncture sites for at least 10 min or until site no longer oozes blood.
- If necessary, use a small-gauge needle or IV cannula.
- Observe IV sites every few hours for bleeding.
- Avoid the use of manual or automatic blood pressure cuff.
- When using a cuff for BP, remove cuff immediately after using it.
- Do not leave cuff on the patient.
- Shave the patient with an electric shaver only.
- Use a soft-bristled toothbrush when providing mouth care.
- Test urine and stool for occult blood as ordered.
- Inform patient not to strain or push too hard when have a bowel movement.

BP, Blood pressure; *IM*, intramuscular; *IV*, intravenous

patient is continually assessed for signs of bleeding, petechiae, and ecchymosis.

Provide Comfort and Emotional Support

The development of DIC in an already critically ill patient can be stressful for the patient and his or her family members. It is imperative to provide psychosocial support throughout this crisis. Calm reassurance and uncomplicated explanations of the care the patient is receiving can help allay much of the anxiety experienced. All treatments and interventions are explained before carrying them out, and questions should be answered at a level understandable to the patient and family. The use of an interpreter when English is not the primary language can enhance understanding and help avoid misconceptions. Providing spiritual support as requested may also be of assistance.

Intraprofessional collaborative management of the patient with DIC is outlined in Box 36.4.

THROMBOCYTOPENIA

Description and Etiology

Thrombocytopenia is defined as a platelet count less than $150,000/mm^3$ or a decrease of greater than 50% from the last measurement.[10,11] This disorder is described as mild when the platelet count is between $70,000/mm^3$ and $150,000/mm^3$, moderate when the platelet count is between $20,000/mm^3$ and $70,000/mm^3$, and severe when the platelet count is less $20,000/mm^3$.[10] When the platelet count decreases to less than $50,000/mm^3$, the patient is at severe risk for bleeding.[10,11] Thrombocytopenia occurs in 20% to 45% of critically ill patients.[11]

Etiology

Onset of thrombocytopenia often follows a viral infection, pregnancy, administration of certain medications (e.g., heparin, thiazide diuretics, chemotherapeutic agents), malignancies, splenomegaly, blood transfusions, or alcoholism.[11] Regardless of the precipitating condition, the development of thrombocytopenia occurs via one of these five mechanisms: (1) decreased platelet production, (2) increased platelet destruction, (3) splenic sequestration of platelets, (4) massive consumption of platelets,[11,12] and (5) hemodilution.[12] One form of thrombocytopenia seen in critically ill patients is immune thrombocytopenic purpura (ITP), which may also be referred to as *idiopathic thrombocytopenic purpura*.[11,12]

BOX 36.4 Teamwork and Collaboration

Disseminated Intravascular Coagulation

- Identify and eliminate underlying cause.
- Provide hemodynamic support to prevent end-organ ischemia.
  - Intravenous fluids
  - Assess arterial blood gases
  - Positive inotropic agents
- Administer blood and blood components.
  - Fresh frozen plasma
  - Platelets
  - Cryoprecipitate
  - Antithrombin III
- Administer medications.
  - Heparin
  - Aminocaproic acid
- Initiate bleeding precautions.
- Maintain surveillance for complications.
  - Hypovolemic shock
  - Peripheral ischemia
  - Central ischemia
  - Multiple-organ dysfunction syndrome
- Provide comfort and emotional support.

Pathophysiology

In ITP, lymphocytes produce antibodies that begin to destroy existing platelets. The cause of this autoimmune response is unknown.[13] With insufficient platelets available, the normal coagulation pathways are disrupted. Inadequate hemostasis ensues, and bleeding results. Life-threatening gastrointestinal or intracerebral bleeding can occur.[13,14]

Assessment and Diagnosis

ITP is characterized by the gradual onset of signs and symptoms.[13] The diagnosis of ITP is a diagnosis of exclusion and is primarily based on findings in the patient's history and physical examination. ITP is thought to be present when the patient develops a low platelet count and no other cause can be identified.[14]

Assessment

Petechial hemorrhages, which manifest as small red spots primarily on legs and oral mucosa, are most indicative of a platelet disorder. In contrast, larger hematomas are most commonly associated with coagulation disorders. Bruising unrelated to trauma is another common sign of ITP.[13] The signs and symptoms of ITP are listed in Table 36.4.

Unusual bleeding is a hallmark of ITP. Excessive bleeding from the gums after dental work, spontaneous epistaxis, blood in the urine or stool, and unusually heavy menses in women are typical features of ITP. Rarely, retinal hemorrhage or intracerebral bleeding may be observed.

Diagnosis

A complete blood cell count reveals a severely diminished platelet count, often falling below $30,000/mm^3$, for a patient with ITP.[14] However, the numbers of RBCs and WBCs, the hemoglobin level, results of coagulation studies, and bleeding times are normal.[14]

Medical Management

In most cases, ITP resolves spontaneously, and treatment is unnecessary. In mild cases in which diminished platelet counts

TABLE 36.4 Diagnostic Data for Immune Thrombocytopenic Purpura

System or Study	Signs and Symptoms
Integumentary	Petechial hemorrhage of lower extremities, ecchymoses, gingival bleeding, spontaneous epistaxis
Neurologic	Sudden, severe headache; nausea and vomiting; seizures; focal neurologic deficits; decreased level of consciousness
Renal	Hematuria
Gastrointestinal	Hematemesis, melena, hematochezia
Other	Heavy menses in women, retinal hemorrhage
Laboratory	Decreased platelet count, often <30,000 mm^3

BOX 36.5 DIAGNOSIS AND PATIENT CARE MANAGEMENT

Immune Thrombocytopenic Purpura

- Hypovolemia due to absolute loss
- Powerlessness due to lack of control over current situation and/or disease progression
- Disturbed Body Image due to actual change in body structure, function, or appearance

Patient Care Management plans are located in Appendix A.

result in symptoms, administration of oral corticosteroids is appropriate.[13,14] Platelet counts increase to normal levels within 2 to 6 weeks, and dosages can then be tapered.

In patients exhibiting life-threatening hemorrhage, rapid intervention is necessary. Administration of intravenous immunoglobulin suppresses the platelet-destroying antibody response. This therapy is extremely expensive and is reserved for the most severe manifestations of ITP.[13] High-dose methylprednisolone can be given intravenously and is very effective in treating ITP.[13] Platelet transfusion is recommended after administration of intravenous immunoglobulin or methylprednisolone. When steroid therapy fails to arrest the condition, surgical removal of the spleen is considered.[14]

Nursing Management

The patient care management plan for a patient with ITP incorporates a variety of patient problems (Box 36.5). The nurse has a significant role in supporting the patient's vital functions, initiating bleeding precautions, providing comfort and emotional support, and maintaining surveillance for complications.

Recognizing potential hazards and providing a safe care environment is of utmost importance (see Box 36.3). For example, padding bed rails can protect the patient from bruising. Substituting sponge-tipped oral care devices for firm-bristled toothbrushes can help minimize mucosal trauma and bleeding. The patient is instructed on how to blow the nose gently to avoid instigating epistaxis. When shaving patients, an electric razor is used to reduce the risk of laceration associated with a blade. Venipuncture and intramuscular injections are avoided. In the event venipuncture is required, prolonged pressure on the site may be necessary to arrest bleeding. Careful administration of prescribed medications and monitoring for adverse effects of platelet transfusions and for complicating or contributing factors, such as hemorrhage and infection, are critical to the patient's outcome.

Interprofessional collaborative management of the patient with ITP is outlined in Box 36.6.

BOX 36.6 Teamwork and Collaboration

Immune Thrombocytopenic Purpura

- Administer medications.
  - Glucocorticoids
  - Intravenous immunoglobulin/plasmapheresis
- Prepare patient for splenectomy if unresponsive to medication therapy.
- Administer platelets.
- Initiate bleeding precautions.
- Maintain surveillance for complications.
  - Intracranial or other major hemorrhage
  - Severe blood loss
- Provide comfort and emotional support.

HEPARIN-INDUCED THROMBOCYTOPENIA

Description and Etiology

Another form of thrombocytopenia seen in critical care patients is heparin-induced thrombocytopenia (HIT). There are two distinct types of HIT. The most common form is non–immune-mediated HIT, formally known as *type 1 HIT*.[15] Seen in 30% of patients receiving heparin therapy, this nonautoimmune condition manifests within a few days of initiation of therapy. Platelet depletion is moderate, counts are usually less than 100,000/mm^3, and the condition is transient, often resolving spontaneously. Discontinuation of heparin is not required. The second form is type 2 HIT, or *immune-mediated HIT*,[15] which is less commonly encountered but is more severe.[15,16] This discussion is limited to immune-mediated HIT.

Etiology

Immune-mediated HIT is a response to the administration of heparin therapy. It has been observed in 0.5% to 5% of patients treated with unfractionated heparin and has occurred after exposure to low-molecular-weight heparin, although to a lesser degree.[15] The disorder is characterized by severe thrombocytopenia during heparin therapy. Diagnostically, it is identified by a platelet count less than 50,000/mm^3 or at least a 50% decrease from the baseline platelet count from the initiation of therapy. Onset usually occurs 5 to 10 days from the first exposure to heparin, but the onset can occur within hours of a reexposure to heparin.[15,16] The risk of developing HIT is higher in women, surgical patients, and patients with major trauma.[15] High-risk surgical procedures include cardiac surgery and orthopedic surgery.[15]

Pathophysiology

The thrombocytopenia that occurs with immune-mediated HIT is related to the formation of heparin-antibody complexes. These complexes release a substance known as *platelet factor 4*. Platelet factor 4 attracts heparin molecules, forming immunogenic complexes that adhere to platelet and endothelial surfaces (Fig. 36.4). Activation of platelets stimulates the release of thrombin and the subsequent formation of platelet clumps.[15,16]

Patients with immune-mediated HIT are at greater risk for thrombosis than bleeding. Thrombotic complications develop in 20% to 50% of patients and can occur in both the venous and the arterial system.[15] Vessel occlusion can result in the need for limb amputation, stroke, acute myocardial infarction, and death.[15–17] The resultant formation of fibrin- and platelet-rich thrombi is the primary characteristic of HIT that distinguishes it from other forms of thrombocytopenia and gives rise to its more descriptive name: white clot syndrome.[16]

Assessment and Diagnosis

HIT can be associated with severe consequences. Rapid recognition of risk factors and subsequent development of signs and symptoms is essential in treating this condition.

Assessment

Common signs and symptoms are listed in Table 36.5. The clinical manifestations of HIT are related to the formation of thrombi and subsequent vessel occlusion.[15] Most thrombotic events are venous, although venous and arterial thrombosis can

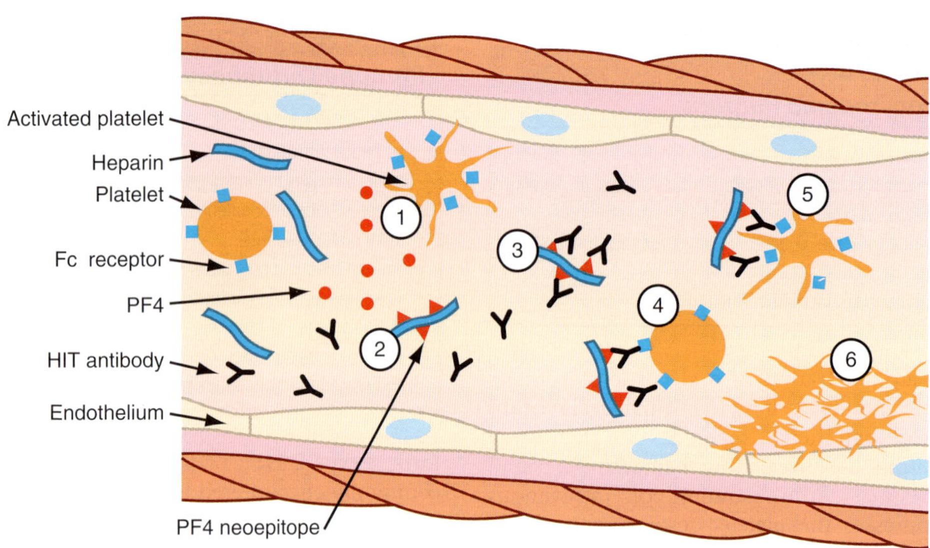

FIG. 36.4 Pathophysiology of Heparin-Induced Thrombocytopenia (HIT). *(1)* Activated platelets release procoagulant proteins from α-granules, including platelet factor 4 (PF4). Administered heparin binds PF4 *(2)*, which undergoes a conformation change and expresses a new antigen (neoepitope). Individuals with HIT produce an immunoglobulin G (IgG) antibody that specifically reacts *(3)* with multiple identical neoepitopes on the heparin-PF4 complex. The reaction forms heparin-PF4-IgG immune complexes. Platelets express FcγRIIa receptors (Fcγ receptor) that react *(4)* with the Fc portion of IgG in immune complexes. Cross-linking of Fc receptors *(5)* results in FcγRIIa-dependent platelet activation. The activated platelets mediate a series of events that lead to further activation of the coagulation cascade, resulting in thrombin generation. Further release of PF4 from newly activated platelets leads to a cycle of continuing platelet activation and *(6)* formation of a primary clot. The reaction can be enhanced by the release of platelet-derived microparticles that are rich in surface phosphatidylserine and increase activation of coagulation and by the binding of heparin-PF4 complexes and HIT-IgG to the vascular endothelium (not shown). (From Rogers J, ed. *McCance & Huether's Pathophysiology: The Biologic Basis for Disease in Adults and Children.* 9th ed. Elsevier; 2023.))

occur. Thrombotic events typically include deep vein thrombosis, pulmonary embolism, limb ischemia thrombosis, thrombotic stroke, and myocardial infarction.[15,18] The presence of blanching and the loss of peripheral pulses, sensation, or motor function in a limb indicate peripheral vascular thrombi. Neurologic signs and symptoms such as confusion, headache, and impaired speech can signal the onset of cerebral artery occlusion and stroke. Acute myocardial infarction may be heralded by dyspnea, chest pain, pallor, and alterations in blood pressure. Thrombi in the pulmonary vasculature may be evidenced by pleuritic pain, rales, and dyspnea.

Diagnosis

The key indicator for identifying HIT is the platelet count. General consensus in the literature considers a platelet count of less than 100,000/mm^3 or a sudden drop of 50% from the patient's baseline after initiation of heparin therapy to strongly indicate HIT.[15–18]

Two types of assays are available to assist in confirming the diagnosis of HIT: activation assays, based on platelet aggregation or the release of granular contents such as serotonin, and assays that identify the HIT antigen. Activation assays are highly sensitive in detecting the presence of HIT. The most common assay used is heparin-induced platelet aggregation. Serotonin release assay is used by a few institutions. The enzyme-linked immunosorbent assay identifies the presence of the HIT antigen.[16,17]

Medical Management

Early identification is critical to managing the effects of immune-mediated HIT. Current guidelines suggest that platelet count monitoring be performed every 2 or 3 days from day 4 to day 14 for high-risk patients.[19] When a decrease in the platelet count is detected, heparin therapy is discontinued immediately, and the patient is tested for the presence of heparin antibodies.[15–19] If the original indication for heparin still exists or new thromboses occur, an alternative form of anticoagulation is usually necessary.[19]

Direct Thrombin Inhibitors

Direct thrombin inhibitors (DTIs) are being used with increasing frequency to treat HIT. DTIs bind directly to the thrombin molecule, inhibiting its action.[18] Argatroban is the only medication approved for use in the United States at the present time (Table 36.6). Warfarin, although commonly used to treat deep vein thrombosis, is not indicated as a sole agent in treating HIT because of its prolonged onset of action. Studies have shown that the use of warfarin without concomitant use of DTIs can significantly increase the incidence of thrombosis in patients with HIT.[18]

Nursing Management

The patient care management plan for a patient with HIT incorporates a variety of patient problems (Box 36.7). The nurse has a significant role in decreasing the incidence of heparin exposure, maintaining surveillance for complications, providing comfort and emotional support, and educating the patient and family. Prevention of HIT is a major nursing focus, because most critically ill patients receive heparin as part of their plan of care and thus are at risk for this disorder. Initial assessment is crucial to identifying patients at risk for HIT. A medical history that includes previous heparin therapy, deep vein thrombosis,

TABLE 36.5 Diagnostic Data for Heparin-Induced Thrombocytopenia

System or Study	Signs and Symptoms
Cardiac	Chest pain, diaphoresis, pallor, alterations in blood pressure, dysrhythmias
Vascular	Arterial: pain, pallor, pulselessness, paresthesia, paralysis Venous: pain, tenderness, unilateral leg swelling, warmth, erythema, palpable cord, pain on passive dorsiflexion of foot, spontaneous maintenance of relaxed foot in abnormal plantar flexion (Homans sign)
Pulmonary	Dyspnea, pleuritic pain, rales, chest pain, chest wall tenderness, back pain, shoulder pain, upper abdominal pain, syncope, hemoptysis, shortness of breath, wheezing
Renal	Thirst, decreased urine output, dizziness, orthostatic hypotension
Gastrointestinal	Abdominal pain, vomiting, bloody diarrhea, abnormal bowel sounds
Neurologic	Confusion, headache, impaired speech patterns, hemiparesis or hemiplegia, vision disturbances, dysarthria, aphasia, ataxia, vertigo, nystagmus, sudden decrease in consciousness
Laboratory	Platelets <50,000/mm^3 or sudden drop of 30%–50% from baseline; positive results for HIPA, SRA, ELISA

ELISA, Enzyme-linked immunosorbent assay; *HIPA*, heparin-induced platelet aggregation; *SRA*, serotonin release assay.

TABLE 36.6 PHARMACOLOGIC MANAGEMENT

Heparin-Induced Thrombocytopenia

Medication	Dosage	Action	Special Considerations
Argatroban	Loading dose: none IV infusion: 2 mcg/kg/min not to exceed 10 mcg/kg/min	Used to inhibit thrombin	Obtain baseline aPTT 2 h after therapy started Monitor aPTT; maintain INR 1.5–3.0 times initial baseline Reduce dosage in patients with known or suspected hepatic impairment

aPTT, Activated partial thromboplastin time; *INR*, international normalized ratio; *IV*, intravenous.

or cardiovascular surgery that involved the use of cardiopulmonary bypass can signal potential problems.

Decrease Incidence of Heparin Exposure

Ensuring that all heparin has been removed from the patient's hemodynamic pressure monitoring system, avoiding the use of heparin-coated catheters, and discontinuing heparin flushes to maintain the patency of other intravenous lines are essential elements of nursing management.

Maintain Surveillance for Complications

Patients with HIT remain at high risk for thrombotic complications for several days or weeks after cessation of heparin. Key nursing actions include vigilant monitoring, early recognition of signs and symptoms, and strategies to prevent deep vein thrombosis. Prompt notification of the physician of any complications that occur is critical to patient outcome.

BOX 36.7 DIAGNOSIS AND PATIENT CARE MANAGEMENT

Heparin-Induced Thrombocytopenia

- Impaired Peripheral Tissue Perfusion due to decreased blood flow
- Ineffective Tissue Perfusion due to decreased myocardial blood flow
- Ineffective Tissue Perfusion due to decreased kidney blood flow
- Ineffective Tissue Perfusion due to decreased gastrointestinal blood flow
- Ineffective Tissue Perfusion due to decreased cerebral blood flow
- Powerlessness due to lack of control over current situation or disease progression
- Lack of Knowledge of Treatment Regime due to lack of previous exposure to information (see Box 36.8, Patient and Family Education Plan for Heparin-Induced Thrombocytopenia)

Patient Care Management plans are located in Appendix A.

BOX 36.8 PATIENT AND FAMILY EDUCATION PLAN

Heparin-Induced Thrombocytopenia

Before discharge, the patient should be able to teach back the following topics:

- Pathophysiology of disease
- Purpose of heparin
- Measures to avoid future exposure to heparin
- Identify different types of heparin (unfractionated and low-molecular-weight forms)
- Encourage the purchase of a medical alert bracelet or similar type of warning device
- Tell any new health care provider about the heparin allergy and previous reaction

Educate the Patient and Family

Early in the patient's hospital stay, the patient and family are taught about HIT, its etiologies, and its treatment (Box 36.8). Education of the patient and family is part of prevention of subsequent episodes in patients sensitized to heparin. Closer to discharge, the patient's education plan focuses on the interventions necessary for preventing the reoccurrence of HIT, including measures to avoid future exposure to heparin. The use of medical alert bracelets and listing heparin allergies in the medical record are necessary to avoid this serious complication in the future.

Interprofessional collaborative management of the patient with HIT is outlined in Box 36.9.

SICKLE CELL ANEMIA

Description and Etiology

Sickle cell anemia (SCA) is a hereditary disease in which RBCs form an abnormal sickle or crescent shape. RBCs carry oxygen to the body and are normally shaped like a disk.[20,21] The sickle-shaped cells have a shortened life span; are unable to carry adequate oxygen to tissues and become trapped in the vasculature because of their shape; and can cause severe pain, increased risk of infection, and life-threatening complications.[20,21]

BOX 36.9 Teamwork and Collaboration

Heparin-Induced Thrombocytopenia

- Stop all heparin exposure.
  - Unfractionated and low-molecular-weight heparin by any route
  - No heparin flushes
  - No heparin-coated vascular access devices
- Begin therapy with an alternative anticoagulant.
  - Argatroban
- Maintain surveillance for complications.
  - Deep vein thrombosis
  - Pulmonary emboli
  - Acute limb ischemia
  - Ischemic stroke
  - Acute myocardial infarction
- Administer antifibrinolytic therapy (as indicated) if thrombosis occurs.
- Prepare patient for surgical embolectomy (as indicated) if thrombosis occurs.
- Provide comfort and emotional support.

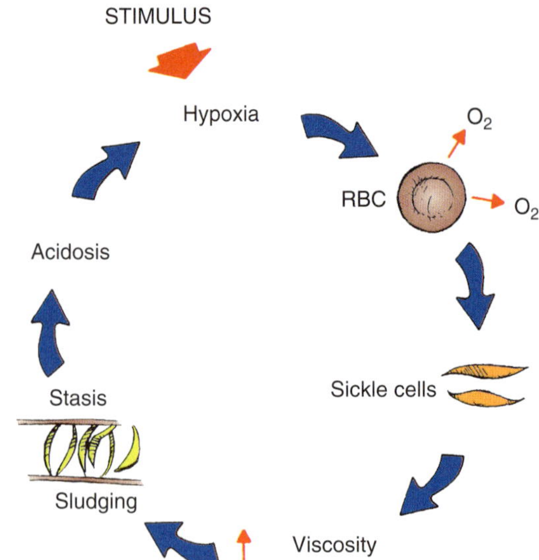

FIG. 36.5 Cycle Causing Vasoocclusive Episodes in Sickle Cell Anemia. *RBC,* Red blood cell. (From Hockenberry M, Coody D. *Pediatric Oncology and Hematology: Perspectives on Care.* Mosby; 1986.)

Etiology

SCA is an autosomal recessive genetic disorder. An individual with normal hemoglobin has two copies of hemoglobin A (HbA) gene. An individual with SCA has two copies of hemoglobin S (HbS) gene. Individuals who have one gene for HbS and one gene for HbA are known as *carriers* of the sickle cell trait (HbAS). When two carriers have a child, there is a 25% chance that the child will have SCA (HbSS), a 50% chance that the child will have sickle cell trait (HbAS), and a 25% chance that the child will have entirely normal hemoglobin (HbAA).[22] This genetic trait is found in people of African, Caribbean, Central American, South American, Saudi Arabian, Indian, and Mediterranean descent.[21] Most patients in the United States are African American.[21] The disease is not prevalent in persons of Asian or Pacific Islander descent.

SCA is usually diagnosed during the first few years of life secondary to manifestation of initial symptoms. Prenatal screening that consists of DNA analysis from fetal cells is now available for at-risk couples.[22] This screening should be offered as part of their prenatal counseling. More than 40 states offer universal neonatal screening for hemoglobinopathies.[22]

Pathophysiology

Sickle cell disease (SCD) is a chronic inflammatory condition that is characterized by hemolysis and vasoocclusion. The cause of SCA is a mutation in the genetic sequence in the beta chain gene of the hemoglobin. This results in a sequence of the replacement of valine with glutamic acid at the N-terminal amino acid position 6 of the protein chain.[20] This substitution leads to the production of HbS.[21]

Normal RBCs contain hemoglobin that are flexible, biconcave disks. When deoxygenated, RBCs containing predominantly HbS distort into a crescent or sickle shape. In this form, the hemoglobin becomes rigid and friable, causing vasoocclusion in the small vessels of the circulatory system.[20] This tends to occur during times of physiologic stress, such as physical overexertion, muscle tissue ischemia, dehydration, infection, or extreme temperatures.[21] Although these conditions have a tendency to exacerbate the condition, most of the sickling events have no identifying cause.[21]

The RBCs become lodged in the vasculature and the microcirculation causing stasis and obstruction of blood flow and damage to the surrounding organs, tissue ischemia, infarction, and, if not corrected, eventually necrosis (Fig. 36.5). In addition, hemolysis of the RBCs occurs, resulting in anemia.[20]

Assessment and Diagnosis

SCA can be associated with severe consequences. Rapid recognition of signs and symptoms is essential in treating this condition.

Assessment

Various clinical manifestations are associated with SCA (Fig. 36.6). The patient may present with a low-grade fever, bone or joint pain, pinpoint pupils, inability to follow commands, photophobia, tachycardia, tachypnea, decreased respiratory excursion, hepatomegaly, nonpalpable spleen, and pretibial ulcers.[23]

Diagnosis

Initial laboratory studies include a complete blood count, a peripheral blood smear, and a quantitative hemoglobin electrophoresis. Sickle cells constitute 5% to 10% of the blood smear. The elevated reticulocyte count (greater than 10%) is characteristically accompanied by the presence of Howell-Jolly bodies. Howell-Jolly bodies are small remnants of nuclear material from hemolyzed erythrocytes reflective of hyposplenia or autoinfarction and target cells (an erythrocyte with a deeply stained core surrounded by a lighter stained margin that resembles a target with a bull's eye). Typically, an elevated WBC count occurs during and after a crisis. Other tests might include an indirect bilirubin level, which will be elevated following hemolysis. The haptoglobin level will be low or absent because it cannot be replaced quickly enough after severe hemolysis. Haptoglobin, a glycoprotein, exists to bind free hemoglobin that is released from hemolyzed erythrocytes.

Medical Management

SCA is an incurable disease; however, treatment options are available for management of symptoms and complications. Bone marrow transplant offers a cure in a limited number of cases.[20]

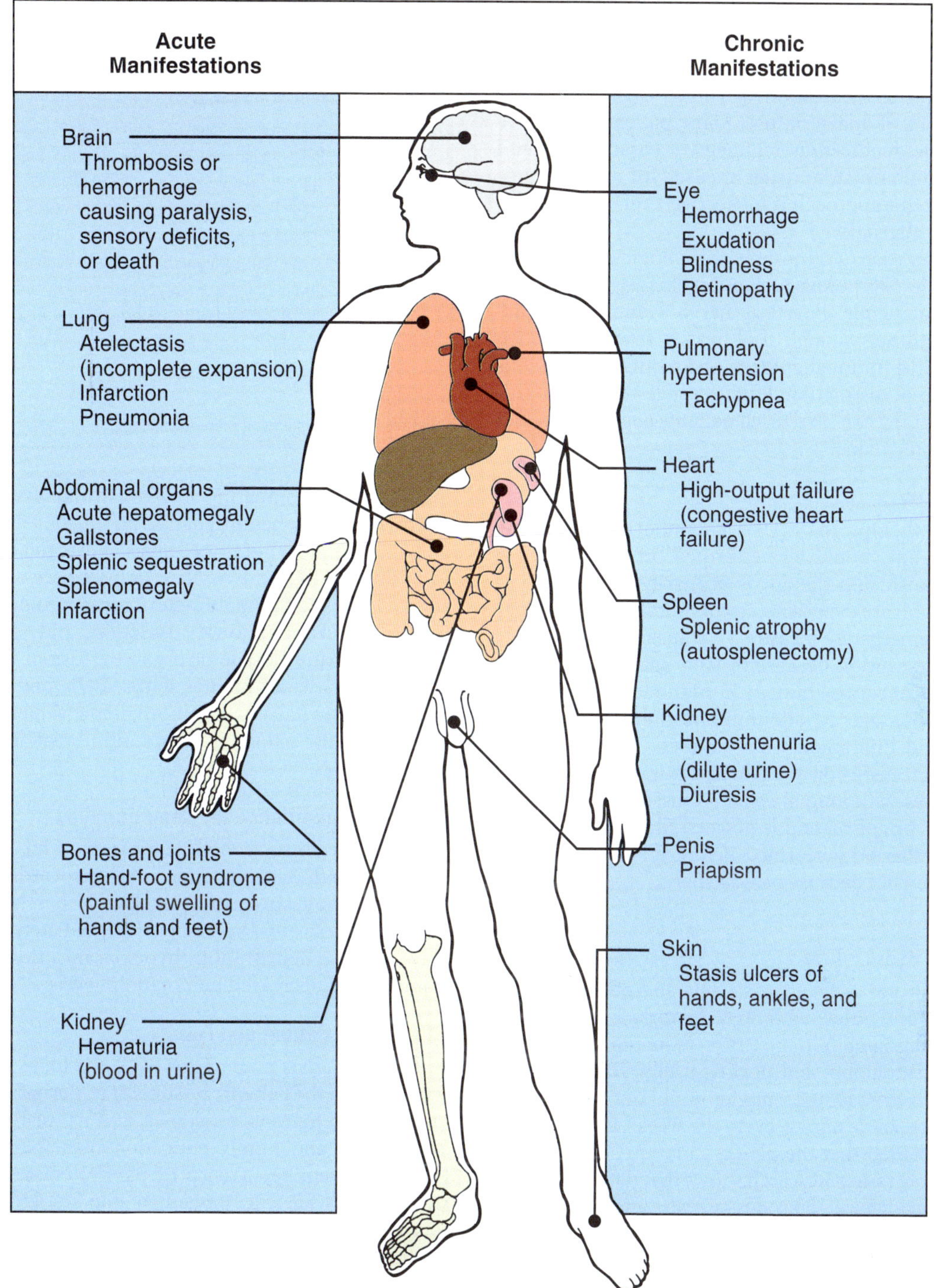

FIG. 36.6 Clinical Manifestations of Sickle Cell Disease. (Rogers J, ed. *McCance & Huether's Pathophysiology: The Biologic Basis for Disease in Adults and Children.* 9th ed. Elsevier, 2023.)

Medical interventions are aimed at preventing infections, managing pain, transfusing RBCs, and administering hydroxyurea. Patients with chronic disease are more effectively managed through a multidisciplinary approach.[20] It is also important to look at other issues that may exacerbate the patient disease process, such as diet, poor housing, inadequate housing, lack of education, poor access to services, and poor lifestyle choices.

Prevent Infection

Both children and adults with SCA are more prone to infection and have a more difficult time fighting off infection.[23] SCA can result in damage to the spleen from constant sickling of the RBCs, and damage to the spleen can prevent the destruction of bacteria in the blood. Prophylactic administration of oral antibiotics starting at age 2 months can decrease the chances of a pneumococcal infection and early death. Vaccinations against pneumococcal infections, meningitis, hepatitis, and influenza are important to prevent future infections.[23]

Pain Management

Pain associated with SCA can be acute or chronic in nature. The most common type of pain associated with SCA is vasoocclusive pain. It is commonly treated with antiinflammatory and opioid or nonopioid analgesics.[23,24] The pain associated with SCA can vary enormously; therefore numerous different approaches may be required. The medication of choice is influenced by the patient's history of analgesia use. Some patients may have extremely intricate medication regimens.[23] Paracetamol and nonsteroidal antiinflammatory drugs are used for mild to moderate pain relief. If this approach is ineffective, oral or parenteral opiates may be an alternative.[23,24]

For patients who wish to try nonpharmacologic pain control, approaches include psychological support, massage, acupuncture, and transcutaneous electrical nerve stimulation. Distraction can be another valuable tool to use. Television, video games, repeating inspirational phrases, and mental calculations can also be a form of distraction. Studies suggested that cognitive behavioral therapy can help teach patients coping strategies for acute and chronic pain.[23]

Transfusion Therapy

RBC transfusion therapy in SCD is an important lifesaving treatment option but should be performed only after careful consideration. Transfusion therapy is primarily used for treatment of patients who are experiencing complications secondary to SCD or as an emergency measure.[24] Transfusion therapy is used with extreme caution because of risks such as iron overload; exposure to hepatitis, human immunodeficiency virus, and other infectious agents; alloimmunization; induction of hyperviscosity; and limitations on resources. The indications for having a blood transfusion or exchange are recurrent painful vasoocclusive crises with long hospital admissions, acute chest syndrome, stroke, priapism, and leg ulcers. Blood transfusions or exchange can also be performed before major operations, such as hip replacement because of avascular necrosis of the hip bone.[23]

Administration of Hydroxyurea

Hydroxyurea is an oral agent that is a safe and effective treatment for children and adults with SCA. It works by increasing the level of fetal hemoglobin in the RBCs, reducing the concentration of sickle hemoglobin and sickling itself.[23] The patient is usually started at a dosage of 15 mg/kg orally once a day. The dosage is increased by 5 mg/kg every 12 weeks until 35 mg/kg is reached, provided that the patient's blood count remains within an acceptable range. Research shows that patients receiving hydroxyurea had fewer episodes of pain and acute chest syndrome and had a decreased need for blood transfusion and hospitalizations compared with patients who received no treatment. Research showed that hydroxyurea can be used as an alternative to regular blood transfusions.[24]

Nursing Management

The patient care management plan for a patient with SCA incorporates a variety of patient problems (Box 36.10). The nurse has a significant role in supporting the patient's vital functions, providing comfort and emotional support, maintaining surveillance for complications, and educating the patient and family.

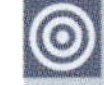

BOX 36.10 DIAGNOSIS AND PATIENT CARE MANAGEMENT

Sickle Cell Anemia

- Acute Pain due to transmission and perception of cutaneous, visceral, muscular, or ischemic impulses
- Impaired Peripheral Tissue Perfusion due to decreased blood flow
- Ineffective Tissue Perfusion due to decreased kidney blood flow
- Ineffective Tissue Perfusion due to decreased gastrointestinal blood flow
- Ineffective Tissue Perfusion due to decreased cerebral blood flow
- Powerlessness due to lack of control over current situation or disease progression
- Lack of Knowledge of Treatment Regime due to lack of previous exposure to information (see Box 36.11, Patient and Family Education for Sickle Cell Anemia)

Patient Care Management plans are located in Appendix A.

Support Vital Functions

The nurse must recognize and support the patient's vital physiologic functions. Administration of intravenous fluids, blood products, and inotropic agents to provide adequate hemodynamic support and tissue oxygenation is essential in preventing or combating end-organ damage. Close monitoring of vital signs, hemodynamic parameters, intake and output, and appropriate laboratory values assists the critical care nurse in administering and titrating appropriate agents.[24] Frequent assessments include parameters for neurologic status, kidney function, cardiopulmonary function, and skin integrity that indicate impaired tissue or organ perfusion. Particular parameters to include are mental status, BUN and creatinine levels, urine output, vital signs, hemodynamic values, cardiac rhythm, ABG and pulse oximetry values, skin breakdown, ecchymoses, or hematomas.[24]

Maintain Surveillance for Complications

The nurse needs to be vigilant for signs of life-threatening complications such as septicemia, acute myocardial infarction, priapism, ischemic stroke, and shock.[20] If there are any significant concerns, these must be reported immediately. Other issues that may arise are dehydration, hypoxia, infection, skin and tissue viability, and decreased hemoglobin levels.

Educate the Patient and Family

Although there is no cure for SCA, the focus of care is prevention. Early in the patient's hospital stay, the patient and family are taught about SCA, its etiologies, and its treatment (Box 36.11). The patient and family education plan focuses on measures to help prevent recurrence of painful episodes. If the patient smokes, they are encouraged to stop smoking and is referred to a *smoking cessation program*. In addition, the importance of continuous medical follow-up is stressed. While research continues to try to find a cure, nurses must continue to be sensitive to the effects of the disease on the patient and the family and the need to be culturally sensitive.[20]

Interprofessional collaborative management of the patient with SCA is outlined in Box 36.12.

TUMOR LYSIS SYNDROME

Description and Etiology

Tumor lysis syndrome (TLS) refers to a variety of metabolic disturbances that may be seen with the treatment of cancer. A potentially lethal complication of various forms of cancer treatment, TLS occurs when large numbers of neoplastic cells are rapidly killed, resulting in the release of large amounts of potassium, phosphate, and uric acid into the systemic circulation. It

BOX 36.11 PATIENT AND FAMILY EDUCATION PLAN

Sickle Cell Anemia

Before discharge, the patient should be able to teach back the following topics:

- Pathophysiology of disease
- Precipitating factor modification
- Importance of taking medications
- Increased risk of infection
- Maintenance of adequate hydration (especially during febrile periods and hot weather)
- Use of pharmacologic and nonpharmacologic methods of pain management
- Avoidance of situations that can precipitate condition such as extreme cold
- Smoking cessation and avoidance of secondhand smoke
- Importance of plenty of rest and relaxation and avoiding exhaustive exercise
- Genetic screening
- Encourage the purchase of a medical alert bracelet or similar type of warning device

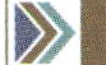

BOX 36.12 Teamwork and Collaboration

Sickle Cell Anemia

- Prevent infection.
  - Prophylactic antibiotics
  - Vaccinations
- Manage pain.
  - Pharmacologic management
  - Nonpharmacologic management
- Administer blood.
- Administer hydroxyurea.
- Maintain surveillance for complications.
  - Septicemia
  - Splenic sequestration
  - Acute kidney injury
  - Acute myocardial infarction
  - Acute limb ischemia
  - Ischemic stroke
  - Anemia
  - Deep vein thrombosis
- Provide comfort and emotional support.

is most commonly seen in patients with lymphoma, leukemia, large bulky tumors, or multiple metastatic conditions who are receiving cytotoxic chemotherapy.[25,26]

Etiology

Although most often associated with the use of chemotherapeutic medications, TLS has also been associated with immunotherapy, monoclonal antibody therapy, radiation therapy, and hormone therapy.[25–27] In rare instances, TLS can occur spontaneously.[25] Certain preexisting conditions can place the patient at higher risk for developing TLS, including dehydration, hypotension, elevated uric acid, splenomegaly, and chronic renal insufficiency.[25,27]

Pathophysiology

The primary mechanism involved in the development of TLS is the destruction of massive numbers of malignant cells by chemotherapy or radiation therapy (Fig. 36.7). Massive destruction of cells releases large amounts of potassium, phosphorus, and nucleic acids, leading to severe metabolic disturbances such as hyperuricemia, hyperkalemia, hyperphosphatemia, and hypocalcemia (Table 36.7). Vomiting, diarrhea, and other insensible fluid losses from fever or tachypnea also contribute to these electrolyte disturbances.[25] Death of patients with TLS is most often caused by complications of acute kidney injury or cardiac arrest.[25–27]

Hyperuricemia

Hyperuricemia occurs 48 to 72 hours after the initiation of anticancer therapy.[25] Tumor cells undergo rapid growth and development, and large amounts of nucleic acids are present within them. When therapy is initiated, tumor cell destruction releases nucleic acids, which are metabolized into uric acid. Metabolic acidosis ensues, resulting in crystallization of the uric acid in the distal tubules of the kidney and leading to obstruction of urine flow. Glomerular filtration rates decrease as the kidneys are unable to clear the increasing amounts of uric acid. Consequently, acute kidney injury eventually occurs.[28] Acute kidney injury is discussed further in Chapter 25.

Hyperuricemia associated with TLS can be potentiated by several other factors, including elevated uric acid levels before the initiation of therapy. Other causes of increased uric acid production are elevated WBC counts; destruction of WBCs; and enlargement of the lymph nodes, spleen, or liver.[25]

Hyperkalemia

Hyperkalemia occurs within 6 to 72 hours after the initiation of chemotherapy. This is the most deleterious of all the manifestations of TLS.[25] In addition to the release of nucleic acids, tumor cell destruction also results in the release of potassium. Renal insufficiency related to hyperuricemia prevents adequate excretion of potassium, and levels rise. The resultant hyperkalemia may have a profound effect on intracellular and extracellular fluid levels.[29] Left untreated, hyperkalemia can have devastating consequences, including cardiac arrest and death.[25]

Hyperphosphatemia and Hypocalcemia

Hyperphosphatemia and hypocalcemia occur 24 to 48 hours after the initiation of therapy.[25] Phosphorus levels also rise as a consequence of tumor cell destruction. Calcium ions then bind with the excess phosphorus, creating calcium phosphate salts and bringing about hypocalcemia. These salts precipitate in the kidney tubules, worsening renal insufficiency. Hypocalcemia causes tetany and cardiac dysrhythmias, which can result in cardiac arrest and death.[28,29]

Assessment and Diagnosis

Detection and recognition of TLS is accomplished through assessment of clinical manifestations, evaluation of laboratory findings, and other diagnostic tests. Table 36.8 summarizes common findings in TLS.[25,27]

Assessment

Clinical manifestations are related to the metabolic disturbances associated with TLS.[27] The patient's history reveals an unexplained weight gain after initiation of chemotherapy or radiation therapy. The weight gain is associated with fluid retention secondary to electrolyte disturbances. Other early signs heralding the onset of TLS include diarrhea, lethargy, muscle

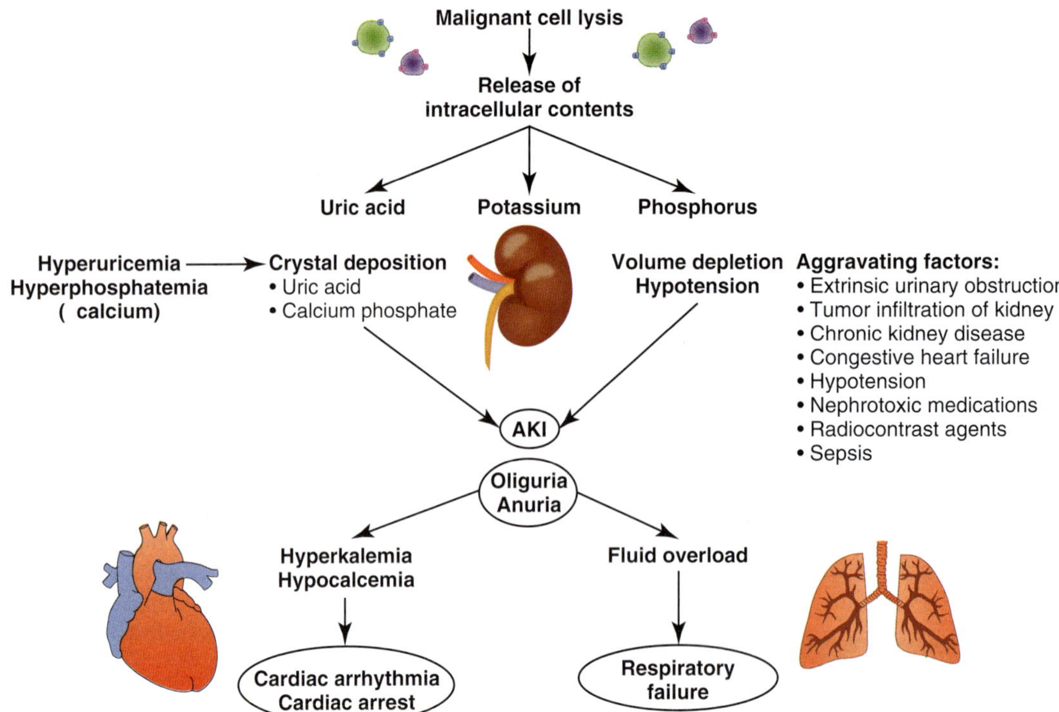

FIG. 36.7 Tumor Lysis Syndrome. Metabolic abnormalities in tumor lysis syndrome and clinical consequences. *AKI*, Acute kidney injury. (From Abu-Alfa AK, Younes A. Tumor lysis syndrome and acute kidney injury: evaluation, prevention and management. *Am J Kidney Dis.* 2010;55[5 Suppl 3]:S1-S13.)

TABLE 36.7 Electrolyte Abnormalities in Tumor Lysis Syndrome

Electrolyte	Pathophysiology	Clinical Consequence	Treatment Options
Potassium	Rapid expulsion of intracellular K^+ into circulation due to cell lysis	Adverse skeletal and cardiac manifestations (e.g., ventricular dysrhythmias, weakness, paresthesias)	Insulin/glucose, sodium bicarbonate, inhaled beta-agonist, K^+-binding resins, dialysis, calcium gluconate
Phosphate	Release of intracellular PO_4^- due to cell lysis May be compounded by renal dysfunction	Muscle cramps, tetany, dysrhythmias, seizures	Dialysis, phosphate binders
Calcium	Precipitation of calcium phosphate complex because of rapid increase in phosphorus concentration	Muscle cramps, tetany, dysrhythmias, seizures, acute kidney injury (acute nephrocalcinosis)	Calcium gluconate (treatment should be reserved for patients with neuromuscular irritability)
Uric acid	Cell lysis leads to increased levels of purine nucleic acids into circulation that are metabolized to uric acid	Renal failure (uric acid nephropathy)	Hydration, dialysis, xanthine oxidase inhibitors, alkalization of urine, urate oxidase

From Davidson MB, Thakkar S, Hix JK, et al. Pathophysiology, clinical consequences, and treatment of tumor lysis syndrome. *Am J Med.* 2004;116(8):546–554.

cramps, nausea, vomiting, paresthesias, and weakness.[26] Physical examination reveals positive Chvostek and Trousseau signs related to hypocalcemia. Hyperactive deep tendon reflexes indicate hyperkalemia and hypocalcemia.[27] Potassium and calcium disturbances result in changes that can be seen on the electrocardiogram, such as peaked or inverted T waves, altered Q–T intervals, widened QRS complexes, and dysrhythmias.[25]

Diagnosis

Laboratory findings demonstrate electrolyte disturbances such as elevated potassium and phosphorus levels and a decreased calcium level. Uric acid levels are increased. Elevated levels of BUN and creatinine and decreased creatinine clearance also indicate TLS. Metabolic acidosis is confirmed by the presence of decreased pH, bicarbonate levels, and arterial partial pressure of carbon dioxide ($PaCO_2$) on ABG measurements.[26]

Medical Management

Medical interventions are aimed at maintaining adequate hydration, treating metabolic imbalances, and preventing life-threatening complications (see Table 36.7).[26,29]

Adequate Hydration

Administration of intravenous fluids may be necessary early in the course of treatment if inadequate hydration exists. The administration of isotonic saline (0.9% normal saline) reduces

TABLE 36.8 Diagnostic Data for Tumor Lysis Syndrome

Diagnostic Parameter	Findings
Clinical	Weight gain, edema, diarrhea, lethargy, muscle cramps, nausea and vomiting, paresthesia, weakness, oliguria, uremia, seizures
Laboratory	↑ Potassium, phosphorus, uric acid, BUN, Cr ↓ Calcium, Cr clearance, pH, bicarbonate, $PaCO_2$
Diagnostic	Positive Chvostek and Trousseau signs, hyperactive deep tendon reflexes, dysrhythmias, ECG changes

BUN, Blood urea nitrogen; *Cr*, creatinine; *ECG*, electrocardiogram; *$PaCO_2$*, arterial partial pressure of carbon dioxide; ↑, increased; ↓, decreased.

serum concentrations of uric acid, phosphate, and potassium.[27] The use of nonthiazide diuretics to maintain adequate urine output may be required. If acute kidney injury occurs, hemodialysis is considered.[27]

Metabolic Imbalances

Electrolytes and ABGs are closely monitored. Dietary restrictions of potassium and phosphorus may be necessary. The goals in treating hyperuricemia are to inhibit uric acid formation and to increase renal clearance.[29] This can be accomplished through the administration of sodium bicarbonate to increase the pH of the urine to greater than 7.0, which increases the solubility of uric acid, preventing subsequent crystallization. Allopurinol administration can also inhibit uric acid formation.[27]

Life-Threatening Complications

If potassium levels rise dangerously, sodium polystyrene sulfonate (Kayexalate) may be given orally, or if the patient is unable to tolerate oral medications because of nausea and vomiting, rectal instillation may be used. If the patient is oliguric, glucose and insulin infusions may be given to facilitate lowering the potassium levels. A 10% solution of calcium gluconate may be administered to stabilize cardiac tissue membranes to prevent life-threatening dysrhythmias.[30] Phosphorus-binding antacids can be used for treating hyperphosphatemia. Stool softeners may be necessary to treat the constipation often associated with the administration of these antacids. Calcium gluconate may be required to replace calcium, but it should be used judiciously.[25]

Nursing Management

The patient care management plan for a patient with TLS incorporates a variety of patient problems (Box 36.13). The nurse has a significant role in monitoring fluid and electrolytes, providing comfort and emotional support, maintaining surveillance for complications, and education of the patient and family.

Monitor Fluid and Electrolytes

Assessment and continued monitoring of the patient is an important role of the critical care nurse when caring for a patient with TLS. Recognizing critical laboratory changes or development of symptoms and notifying the physician in a timely manner are essential. Insertion of a urinary catheter and maintenance of the intravenous line site are necessary to ensure adequate intake and output. Vital signs are monitored frequently, and the patient's weight is monitored daily.

Maintain Surveillance for Complications

Nursing interventions are aimed at preventing complications. Seizure precautions are instituted, especially if calcium levels are disrupted. Insertion of a nasogastric tube is appropriate if nausea or vomiting occurs. Dietary adjustments are necessary, such as potassium and phosphorus restrictions in the presence of elevated serum levels and providing additional fiber to combat the constipation associated with the administration of antacids.[30]

Educate the Patient and Family

Early in the patient's hospital stay, the patient and family are taught about TLS, its etiologies, and its treatment. All treatments and interventions are explained before carrying them out, and questions should be answered at a level understandable to the patient and family. Before discharge, potential risk factors and identification of early signs and symptoms are reviewed.

Interprofessional collaborative management of the patient with TLS is outlined in Box 36.14.

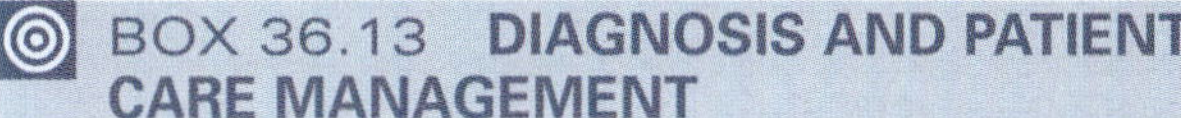

BOX 36.13 DIAGNOSIS AND PATIENT CARE MANAGEMENT

Tumor Lysis Syndrome

- Hypervolemia due to renal dysfunction
- Impaired Cardiac Output due to alterations in contractility
- Anxiety due to threat to biological, psychological, or social integrity
- Impaired Adaptation due to a situational crisis and personal vulnerability

Patient Care Management plans are located in Appendix A.

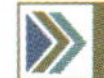

BOX 36.14 Teamwork and Collaboration

Tumor Lysis Syndrome

- Facilitate adequate kidney function.
  - Volume hydration with 0.9% normal saline
  - Nonthiazide diuretics
- Treat hyperkalemia.
  - Kayexalate
  - Glucose and insulin
- Treat hyperuricemia.
  - Sodium bicarbonate
  - Allopurinol
- Treat hyperphosphatemia.
  - Dietary restrictions
  - Phosphorus-binding antacids
- Treat hypocalcemia.
  - Calcium gluconate
- Maintain surveillance for complications.
  - Acute kidney injury
  - Cardiac dysrhythmias
- Provide comfort and emotional support.

SUPPORTING NURSE WELL-BEING

Environmental Wellness

I have worked in the Trauma ICU for almost 5 years and am still excited about my job. The teamwork among my colleagues is stellar, and I feel like I am learning something new every day. Our hospital had just received its second Magnet™ designation, and our unit is recognized as a Beacon unit by AACN. So we have a healthy work environment regarding support for nurses, resources, shared governance, education, and EBP. I volunteered for the Environmental Enhancement Committee when committee assignments came up for this year. Although I knew little about it, I have learned a lot about what we are and can do for our hospital that will be environmentally friendly. Six months ago, I took up composting at home and now have gorgeous roses, giant sunflowers, and tomatoes! We discussed a new initiative at our latest condominium association meeting and are moving forward to create a group to study this and make recommendations. So, I feel like I can make a difference and positive change in our environment!

The above vignette illustrates how one nurse chose to address issues that affect the environment, both inside settings and outside. It also delineates that significant practice changes do not have to be undertaken by one person. It is a cumulative effect that will ultimately make a difference for all of us. Environmental wellness is the recognition of the connectedness between ourselves and the world around us. The natural environment (the air, water, and land that surrounds us) and the environment we create (our homes, workplaces, and communities) significantly impact our health and well-being.[1] It includes having good health by occupying pleasant and stimulating environments that support well-being. Environmental health promotes interaction with nature and creates an enjoyable personal environment (both in and out of the workspace. Ways to foster environmental wellness include:

- Recycling paper, cans, and glass as much as possible
- Using reusable bags and water bottles, coffee cups, and other food containers
- Replace chemical cleaning products with natural alternatives
- Bike, walk, carpool, or use public transportation, if feasible
- Turning off lights, appliances, and electric devices when not in use
- Compost or recycle foods and vegetation per your local regulations
- Replace chemical yard/flower pesticides and products with natural alternatives
- Shop at farmer's markets and roadside fruit and vegetable stands
- Grow your food and share it with others
- Use long-lasting light bulbs and batteries
- Avoid single-use plastic products
- Volunteer for clean-ups and other related environmental activities in the community
- Conserve water
- Advocate for environmentally friendly products and practices in your work and the community
- Plant a tree
- Educate your children and grandchildren about the environment

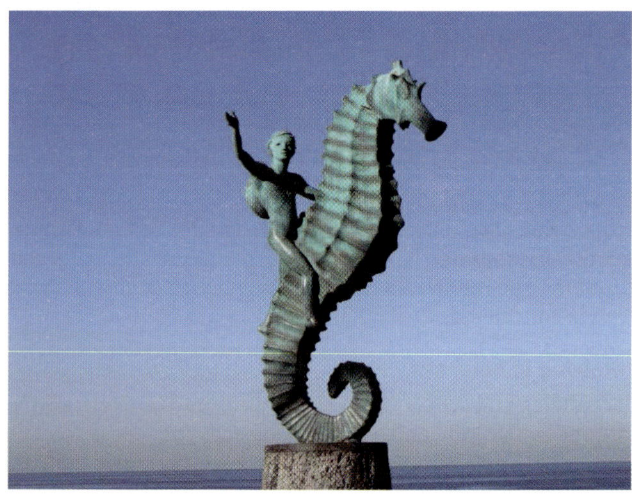

Let us permit nature to have her way. She understands her business better than we do.

Michel de Montaigne

Reference:

1. Environmental Wellness. University of New Hampshire. Accessed 8-5-2023. https://www.unh.edu/health/environmental-wellness.

HOSPITAL-ACQUIRED ANEMIA

Etiology

Hospital-acquired anemia (HAA) is commonly seen in critically ill patients. It results from inflammation, iron deficiency, trauma, surgery, gastrointestinal bleeding, and iatrogenic blood loss from diagnostic testing. Inflammation causes decreased RBC production and increased destruction of RBCs by macrophages.[31] Characteristics of patients most at risk for developing HAA include those with anemia on admission, advanced age, significant comorbidities, diagnoses requiring frequent blood sampling, and interventions that can result in blood loss.[32] Studies have shown that 33% to 75% of transfusions administered in the critical care unit are related to hospital-acquired anemia.[33] For these reasons, research has focused on minimizing iatrogenic blood losses, improving blood salvage techniques, and developing alternatives to traditional blood transfusion therapy.

Blood Conservation Strategies

As more patients and clinicians opt for the limited use of blood products, strategies for conserving blood and preventing unnecessary loss become an important part of the critical care nurse's standard of care. These strategies include minimizing blood loss, managing oxygen delivery and consumption, stimulating the production of RBCs, and understanding transfusion safety and alternative agents.[34,35]

Minimizing Blood Loss

Frequent blood draws in critically ill patients have been associated with the development of anemia. Blood losses correspond to the actual volume of samples and discards when drawing from venous access lines. Critical care nurses can be instrumental in significantly decreasing blood loss in this area. The use of pediatric collection tubes and point-of-care testing are techniques that yield valid diagnostic results but require smaller blood samples. Closed-loop vascular devices that retain the sterility of the potential discard and allow its return to the patient are also being used.[36] Noninvasive monitoring devices such as pulse oximetry and capnography can reduce the need for ABG analysis.

The critical care nurse is vital in preventing and managing hemorrhagic blood loss in critically ill patients. Control of hypertension, which can contribute to significant bleeding, can be accomplished through fluid management and administering antihypertensive and vasodilatory medications as needed. Blood salvage devices can collect shed blood and return it to the patient.[35] Several pharmacologic agents can assist in achieving

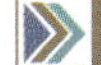

BOX 36.15 Evidence-Based Practice

Red Blood Cell (RBC) Transfusion Thresholds and Storage Guidelines

Recommendation 1:

- For hospitalized adult patients and critically ill patients who are hemodynamically stable: Transfusion is not indicated until the hemoglobin level is 7 g/dL.
- For patients undergoing orthopedic surgery, cardiac surgery, and those with preexisting cardiovascular disease: Transfusion is not indicated until the hemoglobin level is 8 g/dL.
- Due to insufficient evidence these recommendations do not apply to patients with acute coronary syndrome, severe thrombocytopenia, and chronic transfusion-dependent anemia.

Recommendation 2:

- RBC units should be used at any point within their shelf life.
- There is insufficient evidence to support the administration of "fresher blood" to critically ill patients.

Data from Carson JL, Guyatt G, Heddle NM, et al. Clinical practice guidelines from the AABB: Red blood cell transfusion thresholds and storage. *JAMA.* 2016;316(19):2025–2035. https://doi.org/10.1001/jama.2016.9185.

hemostasis and can prevent further blood loss. Desmopressin is a potent vasoconstrictor that also affects clotting factor VIII.[34] Aminocaproic acid (Amicar) inhibits the activation of plasminogen.[34] All these agents and devices work to control bleeding.

Managing Oxygen Delivery and Consumption

Illness-related stress, blood loss from surgery, infection, pain, and anxiety contribute to the higher-than-normal need for oxygen by critically ill patients.[32] Monitoring pulse oximetry is useful in identifying activities and interventions that can contribute to the imbalance between supply and demand. Supplemental oxygen therapy assists in maintaining available oxygen supplies. Promoting a restful environment by modulating nursing care activities and providing pain and sedation control can decrease oxygen demand. It is important to monitor cardiac output and other hemodynamic parameters to manage interventions that optimize oxygen delivery. The administration of fluids and inotropic agents optimizes blood pressure and cardiac output, and vasodilators are used to decrease afterload and improve the efficiency of cardiovascular function.[35]

Encouraging Safer Transfusions and Alternative Agents

Finding ways to decrease the risks associated with blood transfusions and make the blood supply safer for patients is a high priority. Better and more sensitive screening tests, irradiation, and removal of leukocytes are a few of the current methods in use. Plasma expanders manufactured from nonhuman sources are also available. Autologous transfusion, in which the patient donates their blood before a surgical procedure or other anticipated need, has been a common practice for many years. Recombinant DNA technology is being used to develop safe alternatives to blood transfusions. The use of blood from other species is being researched in the quest to provide safe and effective products for use in severe anemia.[34] Current RBC transfusion thresholds and storage guidelines are presented in Box 36.15.

ADDITIONAL RESOURCES

See Box 36.16 for Internet resources pertaining to hematologic disorders and oncologic emergencies.

BOX 36.16 Informatics

Internet Resources Hematologic and Oncologic Emergencies

- American Association of Critical-Care Nurses (AACN): https://www.aacn.org/
- American College of Physicians (ACP): https://www.acponline.org/
- American College of Surgeons: https://www.facs.org/
- American Medical Association (AMA): https://www.ama-assn.org/
- American Society of Clinical Oncology (ASCO): https://www.asco.org/
- American Society of Hematology: https://www.hematology.org/
- British Society for Haematology: https://b-s-h.org.uk/
- Cancer Network: https://www.cancernetwork.com/
- National Heart, Lung, and Blood Institute: https://www.nhlbi.nih.gov/
- Society of Critical Care Medicine (SCCM): https://www.sccm.org/Home

CASE STUDY 36.1 Patient With Hematologic Disorders and Oncologic Emergencies

Brief Patient History

Mr. L, an otherwise healthy, 23-year-old African American man, presents with a week-long history of diarrhea, nausea, and vomiting after attending a barbecue the previous weekend.

Clinical Assessment

Mr. L is admitted to the critical care unit from the emergency department with hypotension, fever, and leukocytosis.

Diagnostic Procedures

Vital signs are as follows: blood pressure of 65/42 mm Hg, heart rate of 145 beats/min (sinus tachycardia), respiratory rate of 35 breaths/min, and temperature of 102.4 °F. His white blood cell count is 25,000/mm^3 with 15% bands, lactate level is 7 mmol/L, prothrombin time is 25 s, and platelet count is 22,000/mm^3. Blood cultures show gram-negative bacilli.

Medical Diagnosis

Mr. L is diagnosed with severe sepsis and disseminated intravascular coagulation.

Questions

1. What major outcomes do you expect to achieve for this patient?
2. What problems or risks must be managed to achieve these outcomes?
3. What interventions could be initiated to monitor, prevent, manage, or eliminate the problems and risks identified?
4. What interventions could be initiated to promote optimal functioning, safety, and well-being of the patient?
5. What technology can be used to monitor this patient and prevent complications?
6. What other interprofessional team members are needed to assist with the management of this patient?
7. What possible learning needs would you anticipate for this patient?
8. What cultural and age-related factors might have a bearing on the patient's plan of care?

KEY POINTS

Coagulation and Fibrinolysis

- Hemostasis is the ability of the body to control bleeding and clotting.
- Four actions are involved in achieving hemostasis: local vasoconstriction to reduce blood flow, platelet aggregation at

the injury site and formation of a platelet plug, formation of a fibrin mesh to strengthen the plug, and dissolution of the clot after tissue repair.

Disseminated Intravascular Coagulation

- DIC is characterized by bleeding and thrombosis, which result from depletion of clotting factors, platelets, and RBCs and, if left untreated, will result in death.
- Medical management focuses on identification of the underlying cause; provision of hemodynamic support to preserve end-organ function; and administration of blood, blood components, and medications to interrupt the process.
- Nursing actions include initiating bleeding precautions, providing comfort and emotional support, and maintaining surveillance for complications (e.g., hypovolemic shock, ischemia, multiple-organ dysfunction syndrome).

Idiopathic Thrombocytopenia Purpura

- Idiopathic thrombocytopenia purpura is caused by an autoimmune response that results in the destruction of existing platelets.
- Medical management focuses on administration of glucocorticoids, immunoglobulin, and platelets.
- Nursing actions include initiating bleeding precautions, providing comfort and emotional support, and maintaining surveillance for complications (e.g., intracranial hemorrhage, severe blood loss).

Heparin-Induced Thrombocytopenia

- There are two forms of heparin-induced thrombocytopenia: type 1 and type 2. Type 1 is more common, milder, and transient. Type 2 is the result of an autoimmune response to the administration of heparin and is more severe than type 1.
- Medical management focuses on discontinuation of all heparin, initiation of anticoagulation with an alternative anticoagulant, and treatment of thrombosis.
- Nursing actions include providing comfort and emotional support and maintaining surveillance for complications (e.g., deep vein thrombosis, pulmonary emboli, limb ischemia, ischemic stroke, acute myocardial infarction).

Sickle Cell Anemia

- SCA is a disease passed down through families in which RBCs form an abnormal sickle or crescent shape.
- Medical management focuses on prevention of infection, management of pain, and administration of RBCs and hydroxyurea.
- Nursing actions include supporting the patient's vital functions, providing comfort and emotional support, maintaining surveillance for complications (e.g., ischemic stroke, acute myocardial infarction, acute limb ischemia, acute kidney injury), and educating the patient and family.

Tumor Lysis Syndrome

- Tumor lysis syndrome occurs when a large number of neoplastic cells are rapidly killed, resulting in the release of large amounts of potassium, phosphate, and uric acid in the systemic circulation.
- Medical management focuses on preservation of kidney function and treatment of electrolyte disorders (hyperkalemia, hyperuricemia, hyperphosphatemia, and hypocalcemia).
- Nursing actions include providing comfort and emotional support and maintaining surveillance for complications (e.g., acute kidney injury, dysrhythmias).

Hospital-Acquired Anemia

- Anemia of critical illness occurs as a result of inflammation, iron deficiency, trauma, surgery, gastrointestinal bleeding, and iatrogenic blood loss from diagnostic testing.
- Blood conservation strategies include minimizing blood loss, managing oxygen delivery and consumption, and stimulating production of RBCs.

Visit the Evolve site at http://evolve.elsevier.com/Urden/CriticalCareNursing for additional study materials.

REFERENCES

1. Turner KC. Structure and function of the hematologic system. In: Rogers J, ed. *McCance & Huether's Pathophysiology: The Biologic Basis for Disease in Adults and Children*. 9th ed. St. Louis: Elsevier; 2023.
2. Levi M. Pathogenesis and diagnosis of disseminated intravascular coagulation. *Int J Lab Hematol*. 2018;40(Suppl 1):15–20. https://doi.org/10.1111/ijlh.12830.
3. Sang Y, Roest M, de Laat B, et al. Interplay between platelets and coagulation. *Blood Rev*. 2021;46:100733. https://doi.org/10.1016/j.blre.2020.100733.
4. Smith L. Disseminated intravascular coagulation. *Semin Oncol Nurs*. 2021;37(2):151135. https://doi.org/10.1016/j.soncn.2021.151135.
5. Popescu NI, Lupu C, Lupu F. Disseminated intravascular coagulation and its immune mechanisms. *Blood*. 2022;139(13):1973–1986. https://doi.org/10.1182/blood.2020007208.
6. Iba T, Levi M, Levy JH. Sepsis-induced coagulopathy and disseminated intravascular coagulation. *Semin Thromb Hemost*. 2020;46(1):89–95. https://doi.org/10.1055/s-0039-1694995.
7. Adelborg K, Larsen JB, Hvas AM. Disseminated intravascular coagulation: epidemiology, biomarkers, and management. *Br J Haematol*. 2021;192(5):803–818. https://doi.org/10.1111/bjh.17172.
8. Levi M, Sivapalaratnam S. Disseminated intravascular coagulation: an update on pathogenesis and diagnosis. *Expert Rev Hematol*. 2018;11(8):663–672. https://doi.org/10.1080/17474086.2018.1500173.
9. Iba T, Levi M, Thachil J, Levy JH. Disseminated intravascular coagulation: the past, present, and future considerations. *Semin Thromb Hemost*. 2022;48(8):978–987. https://doi.org/10.1055/s-0042-1756300.
10. Lee EJ, Lee AI. Thrombocytopenia. *Prim Care*. 2016;43(4):543–557. https://doi.org/10.1016/j.pop.2016.07.008.
11. Thachil J, Warkentin TE. How do we approach thrombocytopenia in critically ill patients? *Br J Haematol*. 2017;177(1):27–38. https://doi.org/10.1111/bjh.14482.
12. Cooper N, Ghanima W. Immune thrombocytopenia. *N Engl J Med*. 2019;381(10):945–955. https://doi.org/10.1056/NEJMcp1810479.
13. Bohn JP, Steurer M. Current and evolving treatment strategies in adult immune thrombocytopenia. *Memo*. 2018;11(3):241–246. https://doi.org/10.1007/s12254-018-0428-7.
14. Neunert C, Terrell DR, Arnold DM, et al. American Society of Hematology 2019 guidelines for immune thrombocytopenia. *Blood Adv*. 2019;3(23):3829–3866. https://doi.org/10.1182/bloodadvances.2019000966.
15. Hogan M, Berger JS. Heparin-induced thrombocytopenia (HIT): review of incidence, diagnosis, and management. *Vasc Med*. 2020;25(2):160–173. https://doi.org/10.1177/1358863X19898253.
16. Gruel Y, De Maistre E, Pouplard C, et al. Diagnosis and management of heparin-induced thrombocytopenia. *Anaesth Crit Care Pain Med*. 2020;39(2):291–310. https://doi.org/10.1016/j.accpm.2020.03.012.
17. Sakr Y. What's new about heparin-induced thrombocytopenia type II. *Intensive Care Med*. 2015;41(10):1824–1827. https://doi.org/10.1007/s00134-015-3811-4.

18. Arepally GM, Padmanabhan A. Heparin-induced thrombocytopenia: a focus on thrombosis. *Arterioscler Thromb Vasc Biol.* 2021;41(1):141–152. https://doi.org/10.1161/ATVBAHA.120.315445.
19. Cuker A, Gowthami M, Arepally BH, et al. American Society of Hematology 2018 guidelines for management of venous thromboembolism: heparin-induced thrombocytopenia. *Blood Adv.* 2018;2(22):3360–3392. https://doi.org/10.1182/bloodadvances.2018024489.
20. Hoppe C, Neumayr L. Sickle cell disease: monitoring, current treatment, and therapeutics under development. *Hematol Oncol Clin North Am.* 2019;33(3):355–371. https://doi.org/10.1016/j.hoc.2019.01.014.
21. Onimoe G, Rotz S. Sickle cell disease: a primary care update. *Cleve Clin J Med.* 2020;87(1):19–27. https://doi.org/10.3949/ccjm.87a.18051.
22. Jorde LB. Genes and genetic diseases. In: Rogers J, ed. *McCance & Huether's Pathophysiology: The Biologic Basis for Disease in Adults and Children.* 9th ed. St. Louis: Elsevier; 2023.
23. Brandow AM, Liem RI. Advances in the diagnosis and treatment of sickle cell disease. *J Hematol Oncol.* 2022;15(1):20. https://doi.org/10.1186/s13045-022-01237-z.
24. Pinto VM, Balocco M, Quintino S, Forni GL. Sickle cell disease: a review for the internist. *Intern Emerg Med.* 2019;14(7):1051–1064. https://doi.org/10.1007/s11739-019-02160-x.
25. Durfee EM. Tumor lysis syndrome. *Crit Care Nurse.* 2022;42(3):19–25. https://doi.org/10.4037/ccn2022795.
26. Delaney E, Nilolai C, Coe K. Metabolic emergencies. In: Brant JM, ed. *Core Curriculum for Oncology Nursing.* 7th ed. St. Louis: Elsevier; 2023.
27. Webster JS, Kaplow R. Tumor lysis syndrome: implications for oncology nursing practice. *Semin Oncol Nurs.* 2021;37(2):151136. https://doi.org/10.1016/j.soncn.2021.151136.
28. Durani U, Hogan WJ. Emergencies in haematology: tumour lysis syndrome. *Br J Haematol.* 2020;188(4):494–500. https://doi.org/10.1111/bjh.16278.
29. Puri I, Sharma D, Gunturu KS, Ahmed AA. Diagnosis and management of tumor lysis syndrome. *J Community Hosp Intern Med Perspect.* 2020;10(3):269–272. https://doi.org/10.1080/20009666.2020.1761185.
30. Williams SM, Killeen AA. Tumor lysis syndrome. *Arch Pathol Lab Med.* 2019;143(3):386–393. https://doi.org/10.5858/arpa.2017-0278-RS.
31. Weiss G, Ganz T, Goodnough LT. Anemia of inflammation. *Blood.* 2019;133(1):40–50. https://doi.org/10.1182/blood-2018-06-856500.
32. Bressman E, Jhang J, McClaskey J, Ginzburg YZ. Tackling the unknowns in understanding and management of hospital acquired anemia. *Blood Rev.* 2021;49:100830. https://doi.org/10.1016/j.blre.2021.100830.
33. Shander A, Javidroozi M, Lobel G. Patient blood management in the intensive care unit. *Transfus Med Rev.* 2017;31(4):264–271. https://doi.org/10.1016/j.tmrv.2017.07.007.
34. Hayden SJ, Albert TJ, Watkins TR, et al. Anemia in critical illness: insights into etiology, consequences, and management. *Am J Respir Crit Care Med.* 2012;185(10):1049–1057. https://doi.org/10.1164/rccm.201110-1915CI.
35. Hudgins K, Carter E. Blood conservation: exploring alternatives to blood transfusions. *Crit Care Nurs Q.* 2019;42(2):187–191. https://doi.org/10.1097/CNQ.0000000000000252.
36. Shander A, Corwin HL. A narrative review on hospital-acquired anemia: keeping blood where it belongs. *Transfus Med Rev.* 2020;34(3):195–199. https://doi.org/10.1016/j.tmrv.2020.03.003.

37

The Obstetric Patient

Kathrine Anne Winnie and Kimberly Sanchez

http://evolve.elsevier.com/Urden/CriticalCareNursing

The most recent statistics show the number of pregnancy-related deaths in the United States is 17.6 deaths per 100,000 live births, a greater than twofold increase in over 30 years.[1] An alarming trend in maternal mortality in the United States is ethnicity-specific pregnancy-related deaths per 100,000 live births, with the highest being among non-Hispanic Native Hawaiian or other Pacific Islander persons (62.8), followed by non-Hispanic Black persons (39.9), non-Hispanic American Indian or Alaskan Native persons (32), non-Hispanic white persons (14.1), non-Hispanic Asian persons (12.8), and Hispanic persons (11.6).[1] Although the reason for the increased risk of a woman dying from pregnancy-related causes is unclear, an increasing number of pregnant women in the United States have chronic health conditions such as hypertension, diabetes, and chronic heart disease.[1] These conditions may put a pregnant woman at higher risk of pregnancy complications. Box 37.1 summarizes the leading causes of death among pregnant women.

This chapter does not focus on every aspect of managing a critically ill obstetric patient. Instead, the focus of this chapter is to provide a synopsis of the more commonly seen conditions or concerns in the realm of critical care obstetrics. Critical care obstetrics encompasses two distinct populations: (1) women who are pregnant and become compromised by injury or critical illness and (2) women with preexisting disorders who become pregnant. The manifestations and management of many critical illnesses are often similar in pregnant and nonpregnant patients, although the change in physiological parameters associated with pregnancy must be considered.

The two priorities for a pregnant critically ill woman are (1) supporting fetal growth and development and (2) optimizing maternal health. Clinical decisions must be made in light of the maternal–fetal risk–benefit ratio, considering teratogens (e.g., radiation) and fetal viability. When developing the plan of care, the parameters of gestational age, fetal weight, parental desires, and maternal–fetal mortality must be considered.

PHYSIOLOGIC ALTERATIONS IN PREGNANCY

During pregnancy, a woman's body undergoes major physiologic changes. These changes are necessary to allow for fetal growth and development and maternal adaptation to pregnancy. The changes are so dramatic that they would probably be considered pathologic in a nonpregnant woman. Pregnancy alters organ systems and changes the patient's physiological response to interventions.

In pregnancy, peripheral vasodilation and an increase in circulating blood volume result in hemodynamic changes (Table 37.1).[2-4] Cardiac output increases beginning in the first weeks of pregnancy and continues to increase.[3] In the later weeks of pregnancy, cardiac output decreases slightly due to a reduced stroke volume from compression of the inferior vena cava and the abdominal aorta by the uterus that is compensated by an elevated heart rate.[3,5] Cardiac output peaks, with a 60% to 80% increase, immediately after delivery.[5]

The pulmonary system undergoes anatomical and physiological changes during pregnancy. Hyperventilation, shortness of breath, and dyspnea are commonly seen in pregnancy. Oxygen consumption increases by approximately 20% throughout pregnancy.[2,4] To meet this need for additional oxygen, ventilatory changes must occur. As the pregnancy progresses, functional residual capacity is reduced as a result of the anatomical changes to the thorax (Fig. 37.1). Respiratory alkalosis is expected in pregnancy due to an increase in tidal volume, which in turn decreases the partial pressure of carbon dioxide (pCO_2).[4]

Venous stasis and an increase in clotting factors result in a hypercoagulable state during pregnancy.[4]

The vasodilatory state in pregnancy increases renal blood flow, glomerular filtration rate, and renal plasma flow.[4]

Anatomical and physiological changes to the gastrointestinal system include reduced lower esophageal sphincter tone and reduced gastric motility, predisposing a pregnant woman to aspiration.[4]

There are several changes in the endocrine system with an altered glucose metabolism, specifically maternal insulin resistance, being the most relevant to managing a critically ill pregnant woman.[4]

These expected physiologic alterations in pregnancy may add a level of complexity to the management of a new critical illness or injury. Alternatively, preexisting disorders may be impacted by these otherwise expected physiological alterations in pregnancy, resulting in needing higher level of care. Understanding the physiologic changes uniquely present

BOX 37.1 Pregnancy-Related Deaths[1]

- Cardiovascular diseases—14.5%
- Infection or sepsis—14.3%
- Hemorrhage—12.1%
- Thrombotic pulmonary or other embolism—10.5%
- Hypertensive disorders of pregnancy—6.3%
- Amniotic fluid embolism—6.1%
- Cerebrovascular accidents—5.8%
- Anesthesia complications—0.2%
- Other noncardiovascular medical conditions—11.1%

during pregnancy allows the clinician to provide comprehensive care to the pregnant woman experiencing critical illness or injury.

As a result of the expected physiologic alterations in pregnancy, special considerations exist for women with preexisting disorders who become pregnant (Table 37.2).[6-17]

DISORDERS RELATED TO PREGNANCY

Preeclampsia and Eclampsia

Description and Etiology

Preeclampsia is a syndrome that affects both the mother and the fetus. Preeclampsia is characterized by gestational hypertension along with one or more predefined new-onset conditions at or after 20 weeks' gestation.[18] Gestational hypertension is defined as systolic blood pressure of 140 mm Hg or greater or diastolic blood pressure of 90 mm Hg or greater, or both, on at least two occasions.[18]

TABLE 37.1 Hemodynamic Changes Associated With Pregnancy[2-4]

Parameter	Pregnancy Normal Value[a]	Change
Mean arterial pressure (mm Hg)	90.3 ± 5.8	No significant change
Central venous pressure (mm Hg)	3.6 ± 2.5	No significant change
Pulmonary artery occlusion pressure (mm Hg)	7.5 ± 1.8	No significant change
Heart rate (beats/min)	83 ± 10	Increase 17%
Cardiac output (L/min)	6.2 ± 1.0	Increase 43%
Systemic vascular resistance (dyn • sec • cm^{-5})	1210 ± 266	Decrease 21%
Colloid oncotic pressure (mm Hg)	18 ± 1.5	Decrease 14%
Plasma volume (mL)	3700 - 4200	Increase 30%–50%

[a]Values may change during labor and delivery

cm, Centimeter; *L*, liter; *min*, minute; *mL*, millilitre; *mm Hg*, milliliters of mercury; *sec*, second.

The new-onset conditions include (a) proteinuria, (b) other maternal organ dysfunction (e.g., neurologic complication such as altered mental status, pulmonary complication such as pulmonary edema, hematologic complication such as thrombocytopenia, kidney complication such as acute kidney injury, liver complication

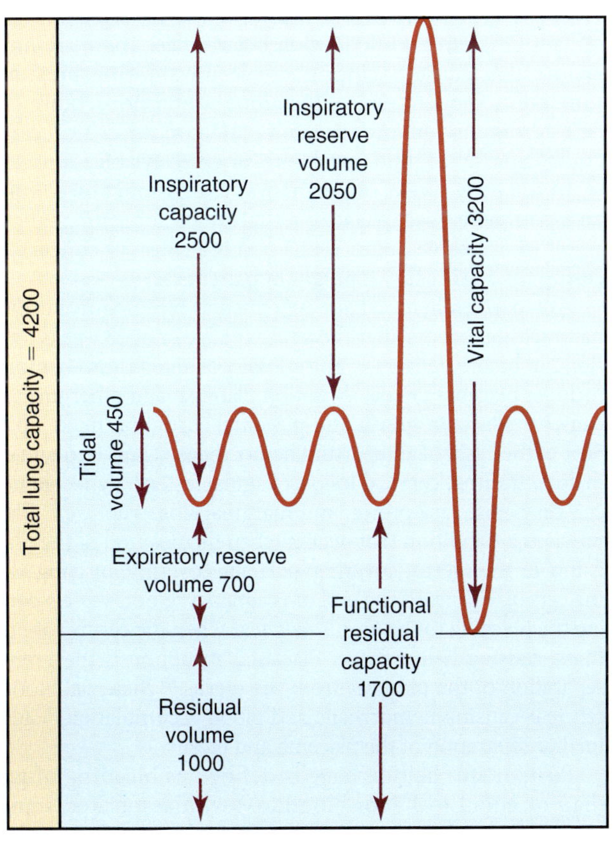

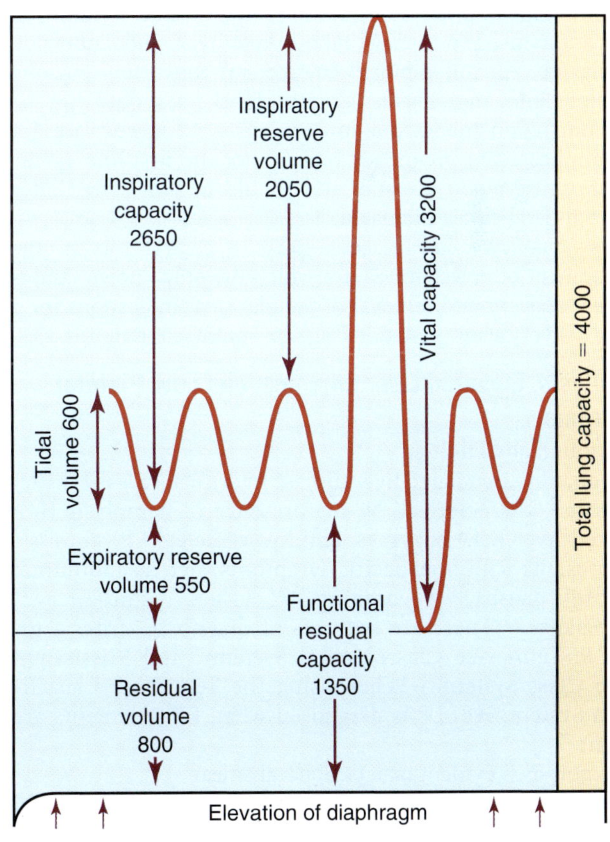

FIG. 37.1 Pulmonary Volumes and Capacities (in milliliters) During Pregnancy. (From Bonica JJ, MacDonald J. *Principles and Practice of Obstetric Analgesia and Anesthesia.* 2nd ed. Williams & Wilkins; 1995.)

with or without right upper quadrant or epigastric pain), and (c) uteroplacental dysfunction (e.g., placental abruption).[18]

The etiology of preeclampsia is unclear with multifactorial risk factors.[19,20] These risk factors include maternal characteristics (e.g., age, body mass index),[19,20] comorbidities (e.g., hypertension, diabetes mellitus, hyperparathyroidism),[19,20] immune factors,[19,20] multifetal pregnancies,[19,20] and maternal infection.[20]

Table 37.3 summarizes eclampsia, its medical management, and associated maternal and fetal considerations.[18,21,22]

Pathophysiology

Preeclampsia develops from poor placental implantation and subsequent maternal vascular dysfunction.[19,20] When the placenta does not implant deeply in the uterus, the spiral arterioles may not remodel into high flow vessels.[19,20] Rather, the inadequate spiral arteriolar remodeling leads to narrow maternal vessels, compromising placental flow and contributing to placental ischemia.[19,20]

As pregnancy continues into the later trimesters, the poorly implanted placenta secretes an increasing amount of antiangiogenic factors.[19,20] These antiangiogenic factors produce systemic endothelial damage, resulting in maternal hypertension and organ injury.[19,20]

Medical Management

Once the diagnosis of preeclampsia is made, medical management focuses on antihypertensive therapy and timed fetal delivery.[18]

Antihypertensive therapy. The target blood pressure for antihypertensive therapy should be a diastolic blood pressure of 85 mm Hg, despite systolic blood pressure value.[18] Common medications used to manage blood pressure include labetalol, hydralazine, and nifedipine.[18]Angiotensin-converting enzyme inhibitors and angiotensin receptor blockers should not be given during pregnancy due to fetotoxicity.[18] Diuretics are not contraindicated in pregnancy but are not the first-line agents for managing blood pressure and should be considered after maternal–fetal risk is evaluated.[18]

Timely delivery. The placenta plays a central role in the development of preeclampsia, for which the only known cure is a timely delivery and removal of the placenta. Indications for a timely delivery at any gestational age are summarized in Box 37.2.

Hemolysis, Elevated Liver Enzymes, and Low Platelet Syndrome

Description and Etiology

A pregnancy-associated liver disease in critical care is HELLP syndrome, characterized by the presence of hemolysis (H), elevated liver (EL) enzymes, and low platelet (LP) counts[23] and presents with nonspecific symptoms such as abdominal pain,[23,24] nausea,[23,24] vomiting,[23,24] visual disturbances,[24] and malaise.[23] There are two sets of diagnostic criteria for HELLP: Tennessee Classification System[25] and Mississippi Triple Class System.[26] When using the Tennessee Classification System, HELLP is diagnosed when four elements are present:[25]

1. hemolysis is evident on a peripheral smear
2. lactate dehydrogenase (LDH) levels are greater than 600 units per liter (or a total bilirubin is greater than 1.2 milligrams per deciliter)
3. aspartate aminotransferase (AST) levels are greater than 70 units per liter
4. platelet counts are less than 100 $x10^9$ per liter

When using the Mississippi Triple Class System, HELLP is diagnosed with the presence of hemolysis, elevated LDH, and elevated AST and divided into three classes based on platelet counts indicative of disease severity.[26] In all classes, there is evidence of hemolysis on a peripheral smear, LDH levels are greater than or equal to 600 units per liter, and AST levels are greater than or equal to 40 units per liter.[26] Class severity is divided based on platelet counts:[26]

Class 1: the platelet levels are less than or equal to 50 $x10^9$ per liter

Class 2: the platelet levels are greater than 50 $x10^9$ per liter and less than or equal to 100 $x10^9$ per liter

Class 3: the platelet levels are greater than 100 $x10^9$ per liter and less than or equal to 150 $x10^9$ per liter

The etiology of HELLP is not fully understood, but some risk factors include multiple deliveries and age over 30 years.[23]

Pathophysiology

In HELLP, obstruction and limited blood flow to the liver damages hepatocytes and results in loss of liver function and possible rupture.[23,27]

Medical Management

Once the diagnosis of HELLP is made, medical management focuses on stabilizing the pregnant woman and planning for a timely delivery once maternal–fetal risk is evaluated.[27]

Hemorrhage

Description and Etiology

Hemorrhage is defined as acute blood loss from a damaged vessel, and it is not an uncommon occurrence. There are multiple factors that cause vaginal tract bleeding during pregnancy.[28] Limited or moderate bleeding alone would not require critical care admission but any pregnant patient in the critical care unit could experience mild, moderate, or excessive bleeding.

In the early weeks of pregnancy, vaginal tract bleeding from an incomplete miscarriage or a ruptured ectopic pregnancy may result in excessive hemorrhage and is a cause of concern when caring for a critically ill pregnant patient.[29,30]

Antepartum hemorrhage is defined as bleeding from the vaginal tract that occurs after the fetus is viable or at 28 weeks of gestation but before delivery.[28] The etiology of antepartum hemorrhage includes placenta previa, abruption placenta, and other unclassified causes.[28] Placenta previa and placental abruption make up about 50% of the cases of antepartum hemorrhage.[28] Less frequent causes include trauma, cervical lesions, vaginal lesions, gynecologic cancer, cervicitis, vasa previa, and marginal sinus rupture.[28] Placenta previa is a condition that occurs when the position of the placenta is low in the uterus, covering, partially covering, or lying close to the cervix.[28] Toward the end of pregnancy, blood vessels connecting the placenta to the uterus may tear when the cervix softens and thins, causing hemorrhage. Placental abruption is the premature separation of the placenta from the uterus.[28] Maternal blood vessels tear causing hemorrhage and blood accumulation, leading to further separation of the placenta and uterus.

Postpartum hemorrhage is defined as bleeding of greater than or equal to 1 L or blood loss with associated signs and symptoms of hypovolemia within 24 hours after vaginal or cesarean delivery.[31] The etiology of postpartum hemorrhage can be summarized following the *four Ts* as a mnemonic: (1) tone, (2) trauma (e.g., genital tract lacerations or uterine

TABLE 37.2 Preexisting Maternal Disorders, Considerations in Pregnancy, and Their Therapeutic Management

Disorder	Description	Considerations During Pregnancy	Therapeutic Management
Cardiac Disorders			
Atrial septal defect (ASD)[6,7]	A passage between the atria allowing blood flow from the left to the right atrium. An ASD is a congenital cardiac anomaly.	Most pregnant women with ASD tolerate pregnancy and delivery without complications. The most common complications seen with ASD among pregnant women are dysrhythmias and heart failure.	Cardiology follow-up and management based on clinical symptoms.
Ventricular septal defect (VSD)[7,8]	A passage between the ventricles allowing blood flow from the left to the right ventricles. A VSD is a congenital cardiac anomaly.	Most women with a VSD have the defect repaired in childhood. The most common complication seen with VSD among pregnant women is preeclampsia and premature labor.	Cardiology follow-up and management based on clinical symptoms.
Eisenmenger syndrome[8]	Complication from other cardiac lesions that cause left-to-right shunting. It is more likely to occur with ASD or VSD.	It is not recommended for women with Eisenmenger syndrome to become pregnant. If a woman with Eisenmenger syndrome does become pregnant, termination of pregnancy is recommended.	Close cardiology follow-up if a woman decides to continue the pregnancy.
Patent ductus arteriosus (PDA)[7]	A passage between the aorta and pulmonary artery allowing blood flow from the aorta to the pulmonary artery. A PDA is a congenital cardiac anomaly.	Most women with a PDA have the defect repaired in childhood. Most pregnant women with a PDA tolerate pregnancy and delivery without complications.	Cardiology follow-up and management based on clinical symptoms.
Tetralogy of Fallot[7]	Defect composed of four heart problems, including VSD, overriding aorta, pulmonary stenosis, and right ventricular hypertrophy. Tetralogy of Fallot is a congenital cardiac anomaly.	Most women with repaired Tetralogy of Fallot tolerate pregnancy and delivery without complications. It is not recommended for women with unoperated Tetralogy of Fallot to become pregnant.	Cardiology follow-up and management based on clinical symptoms.
Coarctation of the aorta[7,9]	Narrowing or constriction of the aorta.	Most pregnant women with coarctation of the aorta tolerate pregnancy and delivery without complications.	Cardiology follow-up and management based on clinical symptoms.
Aortic stenosis[7]	Narrowing of the aortic valve increasing the workload of the left ventricle.	Women with mild to moderate stenosis tolerate pregnancy and delivery without complications. Women with severe stenosis or symptomatic stenosis should consider valve replacement or repair prior to becoming pregnant.	Cardiology follow-up and management based on clinical symptoms.
Mitral stenosis[10]	Narrowing of the mitral valve impeding filling of the left ventricle.	The hemodynamic changes expected in pregnancy are not well tolerated among women with mitral stenosis. The most common complications seen with mitral stenosis among pregnant women are atrial arrhythmias and heart failure.	Close cardiology follow-up.
Marfan syndrome[11]	Autosomal dominant disorder of connective tissue in which serious cardiovascular involvement, usually dissection or rupture of the aorta, may occur.	The most common complication seen with Marfan syndrome among pregnant women is aortic dissection.	Cardiac surgery during pregnancy is recommended.
Respiratory Disorders			
Asthma	The bronchial airways of the lungs become inflamed and constricted, limiting ventilation and oxygenation.	Poorly controlled asthma may lead to maternal–fetal hypoxia. Women who may not be compliant with medical regimens while pregnant for fear of fetal harm should be informed that well-controlled asthma does not appear to affect pregnancy adversely, whereas poorly controlled asthma greatly increases pregnancy risk.[13]	Sufficient fetal oxygenation requires a maternal arterial partial pressure of oxygen (PaO_2) greater than 70 mm Hg, which corresponds to an oxygen saturation of 95%.[12] The most commonly used agents in this category that are safe for use during pregnancy are inhaled steroids, systemic steroids, mast cell stabilizers, methylxanthines, and leukotriene antagonists. Rescue agents, used to provide immediate symptomatic relief, include inhaled beta-agonists and inhaled anticholinergics.[13,14]

Continued

TABLE 37.2 Preexisting Maternal Disorders, Considerations in Pregnancy, and Their Therapeutic Management—cont'd

Disorder	Description	Considerations During Pregnancy	Therapeutic Management
Respiratory Disorders			
Cystic fibrosis (CF)	Autosomal recessive, multisystem disease that affects the exocrine glands and epithelial tissues of the pancreas, sweat glands, and mucous glands of the respiratory, digestive, and reproductive tracts.[15]	It is recommended for women with CF to have a forced expiratory volume (FEV) of 50% or more before becoming pregnant. Women with lower FEVs may still become pregnant but risk more complications.[15]	Increased pulmonologist follow-up.
Pulmonary hypertension[16]	Increase in mean pulmonary arterial pressure (greater or equal to 20 mm Hg at rest)	It is not recommended for women with pulmonary hypertension to become pregnant. If a woman with pulmonary hypertension does become pregnant, termination of pregnancy is recommended.	Close cardiology and pulmonary follow-up if a woman decides to continue the pregnancy.
Hematology Disorders			
Sickle cell disease[17]	Inherited hemoglobinopathy in which the hemoglobin molecule crystalizes and red blood cells change into a sickle shape.	Pregnant women with sickle cell disease experience the following complications: preeclampsia, eclampsia, thromboembolic events, infections, cesarean section delivery, stillbirth, and preterm delivery.	An interprofessional approach, including hematologists, obstetrician, and pain management providers, is needed to manage the care of pregnant women with sickle cell disease.

TABLE 37.3 Summary of Eclampsia

Definition	Management	Maternal and Fetal Considerations
Eclampsia is the occurrence of a seizure in a woman with preeclampsia who has no other cause for seizure.[21,22]	Seizure management:[18] • Magnesium loading dose of 4 g intravenously over 20 minutes, followed by an intravenous infusion of 1 g per hour for 24 hours after last seizure or fetal delivery (whichever is later) Hypertension management: • Labetalol 10–80 mg intravenously, with a max cumulative dose of 300 mg[18] • Hydralazine 5–10 mg intravenously, with a max cumulative dose of 20 mg[18] • Nicardipine intravenous infusion of 3–5 mg per hour[21]	Obtain emergent obstetric consult for • Fetal heart rate monitoring[22] • Possible delivery of fetus[21,22] Place pregnant woman in left lateral decubitus position (improves placental blood flow and reduces aspiration risk)[21]

rupture), (3) tissue (e.g., retained placental tissue), and (4) thrombin (e.g., clotting factor deficiency).[31] *Tone* refers to uterine atony, which is the most common cause of PPH.[31] Overdistention of the uterus, fatigue caused by prolonged labor or rapid forceful labor, and inhibition of contractions by medications constitute major risk factors for atony.[31] Any damage to the genital tract during delivery constitutes *trauma*.[31] Trauma also includes cesarean delivery, uterine rupture, and cervical or vaginal sidewall lacerations.[31] *Tissue* includes retained placenta or failure of complete separation of the placenta, which occurs with placenta accreta.[31] With *thrombin*, coagulation disorders may be preexisting or acquired.[31]

Pathophysiology

External erosion to or internal pressure of the blood vessels lead to vessel rupture and release of blood from the broken vessel. Blood may be retained inside the body or exit the body depending on the location of the hemorrhage, amount of blood lost, and rate of the loss. Circulating blood volume is decreased and, as a result, tissue oxygen demand is not met. Hypoperfusion of organs can lead to ischemia and organ failure.

Medical Management

Rapid recognition and diagnosis of PPH is essential to successful management. Priorities in the medical management of maternal hemorrhage include hemodynamic stability and bleeding control.[27,32] Antepartum hemorrhage control involves timely delivery. PPH control includes management of the *four Ts:* tone, trauma, tissue, and thrombin.

Hemodynamic stability. The initial treatment priority is the restoration of adequate circulating blood volume to treat or prevent shock. This is accomplished with the administration of intravenous infusions of crystalloids, blood, and blood products. The expected physiologic alterations in pregnancy may alter ranges in vital signs and laboratory values, which should be taken into consideration during medical management.[31]

Postpartum hemorrhage control

Uterine atony management. Uterine atony management includes bimanual uterine massage, uterine agent administration, uterine tamponade, and possible hysterectomy.[31,32] A bimanual uterine massage is performed by pressing on the abdominal wall over the fundus with one hand while pushing against the body of the uterus through the vagina with the other hand.[33] Examples of uterotonic agents include oxytocin, methylergonovine, carboprost, and misoprostol.[31,32] These agents should be administered as part of the first-line treatment of PPH from uterine atony.[31] Multiple agents may be used if uterine atony continues.[31] If uterine atony persists, uterine tamponade is recommended.[31,32] Uterine tamponade includes balloon tamponade, gauze packing, or use of uterine compression sutures.[31,32] Lastly, if needed, a hysterectomy may be indicated as a life-saving measure.[32]

Obstetric trauma management. Genital tract lacerations should be sutured[32] and vascular ligation should be considered if a uterine artery laceration is suspected.[31] Hematomas may need to be managed with embolization or an incision and drainage.[31] With uterine rupture, surgical intervention is needed to attempt to reconstruct the uterus.[31]

Tissue management. Retained products of conception should be examined with ultrasonography or with a manual intrauterine examination.[31,32] If retained tissue is identified, manual removal is recommended, followed by mechanical extraction if manual removal of the tissue was unsuccessful.[31,32]

Coagulopathy management. Administering blood and blood component therapy may be needed in managing coagulopathies contributing to PPH.

Amniotic Fluid Embolism

Description and Etiology

Amniotic fluid embolism (AFE) is when amniotic fluid enters the maternal circulation throughout pregnancy, during labor, or in the postpartum period and presents as cardiovascular collapse, respiratory distress, and coagulopathy.[34] It has been described as the *anaphylactic syndrome of pregnancy*.[34] Although rare, AFE is an obstetric emergency.[34]

The etiology of AFE is unknown but multiple risk factors have been identified.[34,35] These risk factors include placental accreta (growth of the placenta into the uterine wall), placental abruption, gestational age, and early delivery.[34,35] There are no specific diagnostic criteria or tests for AFE.[34,35]

Pathophysiology

The pathophysiology of AFE is not completely understood and necessitates further research.[34,36]

Medical Management

Management consists of life-saving measures to maintaining oxygenation and supporting cardiac function.[34] Supportive therapy consists of vasopressors, inotropes, mechanical ventilation, blood component therapy, and timely delivery.[34] Aggressive fluid administration should be limited and if used should be informed by close hemodynamic monitoring.[34,36] Extracorporeal membrane oxygenation should be considered.[34]

Venous Thromboembolism

Description and Etiology

Venous thromboembolism (VTE), which includes deep vein thrombosis (DVT) and pulmonary embolism (PE), is discussed in detail in Chapter 13 and Chapter 18, respectively. The risk of developing a VTE during pregnancy is increased due to expected physiologic changes, including a hypercoagulable state, uterine compression of inferior vena cava and left iliac vein, and venous stasis from hormones.[37,38] Physiologic changes and symptoms associated with pregnancy may obscure the diagnosis of VTE during pregnancy, necessitating a thorough history and physical examination, laboratory work-up, and diagnostic imaging.[37,38] Timely and accurate identification of DVT during pregnancy is important to prevent it from progressing to a PE, with DVTs being more common in the left leg during pregnancy.[37,38]

Medical Management

Medical management of VTE is similar among pregnant and nonpregnant patients.[37,38] Systemic anticoagulation with low-molecular-weight heparin or unfractionated heparin is recommended.[37,38] Because of the risk of adverse effects on the fetus, vitamin K antagonists (e.g., warfarin) and direct oral anticoagulants (e.g., apixaban) are not recommended and should be avoided.[37,38] An inferior vena cava filter may be implanted, and a suprarenal position is preferred to prevent displacement of the filter from uterine compression.[37,38] Systemic thrombolysis, thrombectomies, and extracorporeal membrane oxygenation should be considered after maternal–fetal risk is evaluated.[37,38]

Disseminated Intravascular Coagulation

Description and Etiology

There is no universal definition of disseminated intravascular coagulation (DIC) in pregnancy and traditional risk scoring systems do not account for the expected physiologic alterations in pregnancy.[39] In pregnancy, clotting potential is increased,

BOX 37.2 Indications for a Timely Delivery at Any Gestational Age[30]

- Abnormal neurological features (severe intractable headache or repeated visual scotomata)
- Repeated episodes of severe hypertension despite treatment with three classes of antihypertensive agents
- Pulmonary edema
- Progressive thrombocytopenia
- Transfusion of any blood product
- Abnormal and rising serum creatinine and/or liver enzymes
- Hepatic dysfunction (INR > 2 in absence of disseminated intravascular coagulation or warfarin), hematoma, or rupture
- Abruption with evidence of maternal or fetal compromise
- Nonreassuring fetal status (including death)

BOX 37.3 Maternal and Fetal Conditions Associated With Obstetric Disseminated Intravascular Coagulation

- Placental abruption
- Maternal hemorrhage
- Preeclampsia
- Amniotic fluid embolism
- Acute fatty liver of pregnancy
- Hemolysis, elevated liver enzymes, and low platelets (HELLP) syndrome
- Any retained products of conception
- Septic abortion
- Stillbirth
- Uterine rupture

SOCIAL DETERMINANTS OF HEALTH

Increasing Early and Adequate Prenatal Care

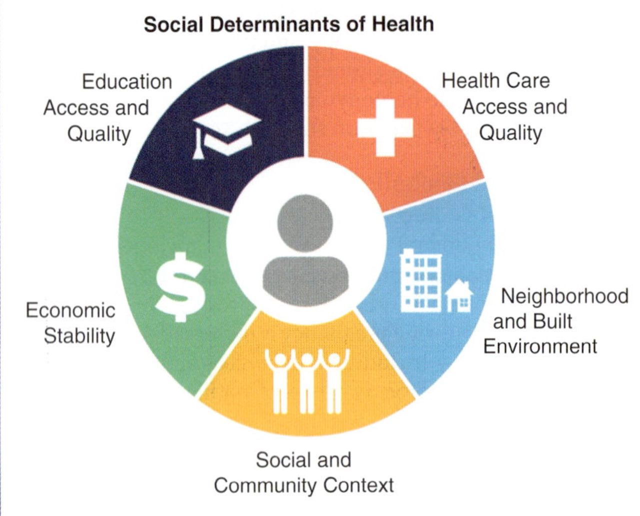

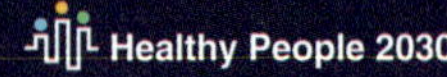

Prenatal care is the care received while pregnant and should begin as soon as a woman is or may be pregnant.[1] Prenatal care is most effective when it starts early and continues throughout pregnancy. Routine prenatal care visits are usually scheduled monthly for up to 28 weeks' gestation, then twice a month for up to 36 weeks' gestation, then weekly until delivery.[1] More frequent prenatal care visits may be warranted if there is a concern for pregnancy-related complications or if a health problem is identified while pregnant.[1] At prenatal care visits, providers obtain a health history, perform a physical exam, check vital signs of the mother and fetus as well as check for indicators of fetal growth, review blood tests, and calculate the delivery date.[1] Consistent prenatal care visits promote communication between the pregnant woman and the interprofessional team and allow for regular monitoring of maternal health and fetal growth. In 2022, almost 75% of pregnant women received early and adequate care, determined by the month prenatal care started and the number of prenatal visits prior to delivery.[2] Delayed and insufficient prenatal care disproportionally affects women living in rural areas and persons from racial and ethnic minorities.[3]

The practices and policies limiting access to early and adequate prenatal care places pregnant women at an increased risk for unhealthy behaviors and adverse outcomes by up to 30%, including prenatal smoking, labor complications, low birth weight, and reduced breastfeeding habits.[3]

Improving payment models for maternity care may mediate the social determinants of health that contribute to delayed and insufficient prenatal care.[3] Efforts should focus on interventions to improve prenatal care but not substitute the need to address underlying inequities in the distribution of resources. Current strategies to promote early and adequate prenatal care are focused on developing local community health programs, utilizing federal supplemental programs, and changing local and federal policies.[3]

References:

1. *Prenatal Care and Tests.* U.S. Department of Health and Human Services; 2021. from. https://www.womenshealth.gov/pregnancy/youre-pregnant-now-what/prenatal-care-and-tests. Accessed March 1, 2024.
2. Increase the Proportion of Pregnant Women Who Receive Early and Adequate Prenatal Care – MICH-08. U.S. Department of Health and Human Services Accessed March 1, 2024 from https://health.gov/healthypeople/objectives-and-data/browse-objectives/pregnancy-and-childbirth/increase-proportion-pregnant-women-who-receive-early-and-adequate-prenatal-care-mich-08.
3. *Healthy women, Healthy Pregnancies, Healthy Futures: Action Plan to Improve Maternal Health in America.* U.S. Department of Health and Human Services; 2020. from. https://aspe.hhs.gov/sites/default/files/private/aspe-files/264076/healthy-women-healthy-pregnancies-healthy-future-action-plan_0.pdf. Accessed March 1, 2024.

Illustration from Healthy People 2030, U.S. Department of Health and Human Services, Office of Disease Prevention and Health Promotion. Retrieved September 8, 2022, from https://health.gov/healthypeople/objectives-and-data/social-determinants-health.

anticoagulation properties are decreased, and fibrinolysis is decreased, promoting blood flow through the placenta and protecting against maternal bleeding during delivery.[39] Some obstetric DIC scoring systems have been developed with varying sensitivity and specificity but additional research and consensus on a definition of DIC in pregnancy is needed.[39]

DIC is a thrombohemorrhagic disorder[39] and is discussed in detail in Chapter 36. Obstetric DIC, particularly, presents with bleeding rather than thrombotic clinical manifestations and develops as a complication of maternal and/or fetal conditions.[39] These conditions are summarized in Box 37.3, with placental abruption being the most common condition leading to obstetric DIC.[39]

Pathophysiology

In obstetrical DIC, the expected increase in coagulation pathway activation in the placenta, needed to prepare for blood loss during delivery, is altered by maternal or fetal conditions (Box 37.3) and results in the procoagulation factors entering the maternal circulation.[39] In the maternal circulation, a fibrinolytic response is activated, limiting the formation of clots and interfering with platelet activation.[39] As a result, the clinical manifestations of hemorrhage are noted in obstetric DIC.[39]

Medical Management

Primary goals of managing obstetric DIC are identification of the underlying condition, removal of the trigger or initiating event, timely delivery, volume replacement, including blood component therapy, and monitoring of laboratory values.[39] Heparin therapy is controversial.[39]

Peripartum Cardiomyopathy

Description and Etiology

Peripartum cardiomyopathy (PPCM) is systolic heart failure marked by left ventricular dysfunction (an ejection fraction less than 45%) in women when no other cause of heart failure is identified.[40,41] PPCM is a potentially life-threatening pregnancy-associated disease that occurs usually in the last month of pregnancy and up to 5 months after delivery.[40–42] The etiology of PPCM is not fully understood but multiple risk factors include black race, multifetal pregnancy, preeclampsia, hypertension, and advanced maternal age.[40,42] PPCM is a diagnosis of exclusion and most women are diagnosed after delivery rather than during the pregnancy.[40] A common complication of PPCM is cardiogenic shock.[41] Symptoms are identical to those of classic heart failure and may be confused with expected symptoms of pregnancy.[40] Heart failure is discussed in detail in Chapter 13.

Pathophysiology

Controversy regarding exact causes of PPCM continues, but recent studies suggest the disease is caused by vascular dysfunction, triggered by maternal hormones.[41] The most recent information has also indicated that many cases of PPCM have genetic underpinnings.[40,41]

Medical Management

Medical management of PPCM is similar to nonpregnant patients, focusing on improving cardiac function.[40] The prognosis of PPCM is positively related to the recovery of ventricular function.[40] Systemic anticoagulation with low-molecular-weight heparin or unfractionated heparin is recommended.[40] Because of the risk of adverse effects on the fetus, vitamin K antagonists (e.g., warfarin) are not recommended and should be avoided.[40] Beta-blockers, except atenolol, are recommended.[40] Loop diuretics, isosorbide dinitrate, and digoxin may be used. Renin-angiotensin-aldosterone system inhibitors, including angiotensin-converting enzyme inhibitors and angiotensin-receptor blockers, are not recommended and should be avoided.[40] In the setting of severe PPCM, intravenous nitroglycerin should be considered and used with caution to avoid hypoperfusion of the placenta.[40] Mechanical circulatory support has been used during pregnancy.[40]

Acute Myocardial Infarction

Description and Etiology

Myocardial infarction is discussed in detail in Chapter 13. A pregnancy-related myocardial infarction (PAMI) can occur throughout pregnancy and up to 12 weeks postpartum.[43] The highest incidence of PAMI occurs in the later weeks of pregnancy and postpartum.[44] The risk of PAMI is increased due to expected physiologic changes, including a hypercoagulable state and an increase in plasma volume.[44] The most common causes of PAMI are spontaneous coronary artery dissection, atherosclerosis, thromboembolism without atherosclerosis, and coronary vasospasm.[43–45] PAMI is identified similar to the nonpregnant population and is diagnosed by ischemic symptoms, elevated cardiac biomarkers, and electrocardiographic changes.[43,44] PAMI most often presents as an ST-elevation myocardial infarction and the anterior wall is the most common location of the myocardial infarction.[43,45]

Medical Management

Medical management of PAMI is similar to nonpregnant patients, focusing on restoring myocardial blood flow and balancing myocardial oxygen supply and demand.[43–45] Nitroglycerin should be used cautiously to avoid hypoperfusion of the placenta.[43,45] Aspirin is recommended, but dual antiplatelet therapy with aspirin and P2Y12 inhibitors should be considered after maternal–fetal risk is evaluated.[43–45] Systemic anticoagulation with low-molecular-weight heparin or unfractionated heparin is recommended.[43–45] Beta-blockers, except atenolol, are recommended.[43,45] Statins and renin-angiotensin-aldosterone system inhibitors, including angiotensin-converting enzyme inhibitors and angiotensin-receptor blockers, are not recommended and should be avoided.[43–45] Coronary angiograms, angioplasty, and bypass surgery all have been successfully used during pregnancy.[43–45]

OTHER DISORDERS WHILE PREGNANT

Trauma

Trauma is the leading nonobstetric cause of death among pregnant women.[46–50] Motor vehicle accidents (MVA) and domestic/intimate partner violence account for most cases of maternal trauma, whereas falls, burns, homicide, suicide, penetrating trauma (e.g., gunshot or stab wounds), and toxic exposure represent the remaining cases of maternal trauma.[47,48] Placental abruption is most commonly seen in maternal trauma cases.[47] Additionally, maternal trauma may result in uterine rupture, premature delivery, and fetal death.[47,48] The most common cause of fetal death in maternal trauma is maternal death.[49] The second leading cause of fetal death is placental abruption.[50]

Improper use of seat belts is a contributing factor to adverse maternal and/or fetal outcomes during MVA.[47–49] Seat belts should be under the abdomen and across pelvis with shoulder straps across the clavicle and between breasts to reduce pressure on uterus.[47]

In the first weeks of pregnancy, the fetus is usually well protected from external trauma because the uterus is located within the pelvis and is protected by bony structures.[49] As a result, direct fetal injury is not usually seen with blunt abdominal trauma.[48] In the middle and later weeks of pregnancy, as the enlarging uterus expands out of the pelvis, maternal abdominal organs are displaced upward and laterally.[49] Some protection is provided to the maternal abdominal organs because the uterus and fetus now occupy much of the abdominal cavity; however, the growing fetus becomes more vulnerable to penetrating trauma.[48]

Initial assessment and management of obstetric trauma are provided in Table 37.4. Additional information related to trauma is discussed in Chapter 32.

Pneumonia

Pneumonia is the leading cause of infection-related death among pregnant women.[51] With the decreased functional residual capacity from the anatomical changes to the thorax (Fig. 37.1), maternal tolerance to respiratory infections is decreased.[51] Pregnancy itself is an independent risk factor for the development of a pneumonia and disorders related to pregnancy increase that risk.

A pneumonia may develop throughout pregnancy, but poorer outcomes are noted if the pneumonia develops in the later weeks of pregnancy.[51] Symptoms of pneumonia may be justified as physiologic changes and symptoms associated with pregnancy, delaying a diagnosis of pneumonia until more severe symptoms of pneumonia develop.[51] When completing diagnostic imaging, protective shielding is recommended. Antimicrobials, except tetracyclines, are recommended in the medical management of pneumonia.[43,45] Data suggest that infants born to mothers whose pregnancies have been complicated by pneumonia are more likely to be born preterm and to have a lower birth weight.[51] Pneumonia is discussed in detail in Chapter 18.

Acute Respiratory Distress Syndrome

Acute respiratory distress syndrome (ARDS) is discussed in detail in Chapter 18. It is important to note that pregnant women may need noninvasive or invasive ventilation if unable to maintain a partial pressure of oxygen greater than 70 mm Hg or an oxygen saturation greater than 95%.[42] Timely delivery is recommended when ARDS develops from obstetric causes, including preeclampsia, placental abruption, and amniotic fluid embolism, among others.[42] When a pregnant woman requires invasive ventilation, it is more like to result in an early delivery because of an increased risk of fetal distress.[42]

TABLE 37.4 Initial Assessment and Management of Obstetric Trauma

Assessment	Management, Rationale, or Purpose
Primary Survey	
Airway	
Signs of Obstruction	
Same as for nonpregnant patient	Remove visible debris with caution because of increased hyperemia of nasal or oral area. Decrease risk of aspiration (because of enlarged uterus and effects of progesterone) by lateral tilt or by inserting NGT or OGT. Emergency cricothyrotomy or tracheotomy, if performed, is done above usual site because of upward displacement of thoracic structures.
Breathing	
Signs of Ineffective Respiration	
Same as for nonpregnant patient with exception of the following: SpO_2 <95 PaO_2 <100 mm Hg $PaCO_2$ >30 mm Hg pH <7.40 Tidal volume <800 mL Labored respirations RR <20 breaths/min or >24 beats/min	100% oxygen by mask because passages tend to be hyperemic and a tendency for breathing through mouth exists. Elevate head of bed, if possible, to decrease pressure on thoracic structures caused by elevated diaphragm. Oral intubation using smaller size (5.5–6.5 Fr) endotracheal tubes to reduce risk of bleeding caused by increased vascularity of area. Gastric decompression with OGT (or small NGT if patient does not tolerate OGT placement) because prone to ileus and gastric reflux. Physiologic monitoring (RR, SpO_2, $ETCO_2$) Obtain ABGs, chest radiograph. Emergent needle decompression or chest tube insertion for hemopneumothorax; may need to reassess entry point because of upward or outward displacement of thorax. The chest tube insertion point is usually between the third and fourth intercostal spaces.
Circulation	
Signs of Ineffective Circulation	
Same as for nonpregnant patient with exception of the following: Systolic blood pressure <110 mm Hg Mean arterial pressure <80 mm Hg Central venous pressure <6 mm Hg Pale, moist, cool skin	Diagnostic peritoneal lavage may be performed; open technique is usually preferred. Assess for possible placental abruption. Normally hypervolemic skin is warm and slightly moist because of progesterone and may mask signs of hypoperfusion. Central venous catheter or large-bore IV access to upper extremity sites because of potential for impeded venous return from lower extremities. Fluid resuscitation. LR solution is recommended because it has the potential to metabolize into bicarbonate through intrinsic body pathways; do not administer blood products through same IV line. With 0.9 NS, can administer blood products through line; may decrease risk of developing maternal alkalosis (compared with LR solution). O-negative blood may be given until type and cross-matching are done. Replace 3 mL per 1 mL of blood lost to compensate for hypervolemia associated with pregnancy. Use caution because of increased risk of pulmonary edema caused by decreased colloidal osmotic pressure. May apply MAST, but *do not* inflate abdominal compartment. Left uterine displacement, manually or with wedge for 30-degree tilt to the side, even if on a backboard, to maximize venous return.
Secondary Survey	
Focused Obstetric History	
Gestational age Single versus multiple pregnancy Number of pregnancies, live births, abortions Name of obstetrician Rh factor Prenatal complications Past vaginal drainage, bleeding, clots Past abdominal pain or uterine contractions	Keep the mother alive. Keep the baby where it is. Perform vaginal examination to determine fetal presentation, status of amniotic membrane, and presence of fetal parts or umbilical cord in vagina. Avoid manipulating cord because of risk of spasms. Emergent delivery; vaginal versus cesarean; live versus perimortem.

TABLE 37.4 Initial Assessment and Management of Obstetric Trauma—cont'd

Assessment	Management, Rationale, or Purpose
Secondary Survey	
Maternal Studies	
Unexpected Diagnostic Study Results	
WBC >18,000/mm³	Insert a urinary Foley catheter with caution because of risk of bleeding caused by increased pelvic vascularity; consider using a smaller size catheter.
RBC <6,500,000/mm³	
Hg <12 g/dL	Consider significance of positive toxicity results. Is the fetus at risk for issues such as drug withdrawal or fetal alcohol syndrome?
Hct <32%	
Platelets <200 x10⁹/L	Hct and Hg values that are below those identified may put the mother and fetus at risk for hypoxia.
Fibrinogen >400 mg/dL	Use caution when performing a rectal examination to assist in determining fetal position or traumatic damage; pelvic vascular congestion contributes to development of hemorrhoids and predisposes the mother to bleeding from this site.
BUN <9 mg/dL	
Creatinine >0.5 mg/dL	
Na⁺ slightly increased	Obtain radiologic studies, as needed; however, implement measures to decrease risk to fetus.
Glucose slightly decreased	Left axis deviation may be seen on 12-lead ECG as a normal variant.
Fetal Studies	
Signs of Fetal Distress	
Fetal heart rate <100–110 or >160 beats/min	Ultrasound to evaluate fetus
Nonreassuring patterns on fetal monitor	Assess fundal height, firmness, contractions every 30 min.
Fundal height not appropriate for gestational age	Fetal monitoring (with pocket Doppler, ultrasonography, or fetal monitor) for a minimum of 4 hours and up to 24 hours as allowed based on interventions provided to mother
Vaginal drainage, bleeding, clots present	
Abdominal pain, uterine firmness, or contractions present	Differentiate uterine pain or contractions from other sources of abdominal pain.
Amniocentesis:	Administer tocolytics, as needed.
Presence of RBCs	L/S ratio and presence of PG to determine fetal lung maturity.
L/S ratio and presence of PG	Kleihauer-Betke result indicates break in the integrity of placental circulation if fetal cells are present.
Kleihauer-Betke test to detect presence of fetal blood in maternal bloodstream	
Tertiary Survey	
Aspect of Care	
Administer "follow-up meds"	Prophylactic measures:
	Choose broad-spectrum antibiotics, nonteratogenic agents.
	Tetanus toxoid does not cross placenta.
	Rh-negative mothers:
	May become Rh immunized within 72 h
	Administer Rh immune globulin (300 mcg/15 mL of fetal blood or 30 mL of whole blood) if possibility of mother having received Rh-positive blood.
	Breach in integrity of the placenta of Rh-positive fetus as evidenced by positive Kleihauer-Betke test result

ABGs, Arterial blood gases; *BUN*, blood urea nitrogen; *CBC*, complete blood count; *ECG*, electrocardiogram; *$ETCO_2$*, end-tidal carbon dioxide; *Hct*, hematocrit; *Hg*, hemoglobin; *IV*, intravenous; *LR*, lactated Ringer; *L/S*, lecithin-to-sphingomyelin ratio; *MAST*, military antishock trousers; *Na⁺*, sodium ion; *NGT*, nasogastric tube; *NS*, normal saline; *OGT*, orogastric tube; *$PaCO_2$*, arterial partial pressure of carbon dioxide; *PaO_2*, arterial partial pressure of oxygen; *PG*, phosphatidylglycerol; *RBC*, red blood cell; *RR*, respiration rate; *SpO_2*, oxygen saturation measured by pulse oximetry; *WBC*, white blood cell.

Cardiac Arrest

The American Heart Association recommends that the standard resuscitation algorithm be followed with a few modifications in maternal cardiac arrest.[52] Specifically, considerations include uterine displacement and preparation for perimortem cesarean delivery. Left lateral uterine displacement through manual manipulation or through the use of a wedge under the woman's hip improves venous return by decreasing uterine compression of the inferior vena cava.[50,52] Perimortem cesarean delivery is indicated in situations incompatible with maternal survival.[52] Delivery should occur with 5 minutes of arrest if initial resuscitation efforts are unsuccessful.[52] The term resuscitative hysterotomy describes a perimortem cesarean delivery performed at or after 20 weeks' gestation and has been shown to improve maternal outcomes.[52]

Although not modifications to the standard resuscitation algorithm, it is important to note current guidelines recommend standard hand position when performing chest compression during maternal cardiac arrest and this is the lower half of the sternum.[52] Additionally, the guidelines recommend intravenous access be obtained above the diaphragm.[52] Lastly, current guidelines reinforce that electrical therapies, such as defibrillation, cardioversion, and pacing, are not contraindicated in pregnancy, but all fetal monitoring devices should be removed.[52]

PHARMACOLOGY

In 2001, the U.S. Food and Drug Administration (FDA) placed medications into risk categories regarding use during pregnancy along with potential effects on the growing fetus.[53] In 2014, the FDA completed major revisions to prescription drug labeling to cover the use of medicines more thoroughly during pregnancy and breastfeeding.[53] They published the *Content and Format of Labeling for Human Prescription Drug and Biological Products: Requirements for Pregnancy and Lactation Labeling*, referred to as the Pregnancy and Lactation Labeling Rule (PLLR).[53] This new ruling went into effect June 30, 2015.[53] The PLLR format assists health care providers in rating the risks and benefits of the medications, which enables providers to provide informed counseling to nursing mothers.[53] The pregnancy letter categories—A, B, C, D, and X—were removed.[53] Box 37.4 presents a comparison of the old prescription medication labeling with the new PLLR labeling.[53] The Females and Males of Reproductive Potential subsection (8.3) is a new labeling that includes pregnancy testing, contraception recommendations, and information about infertility as it relates to the medication.[53]

Physiologic alterations in pregnancy influences pharmacokinetic properties (e.g., absorption, distribution, metabolism, and elimination) of medications.[54] In pregnancy, *absorption* through the gastrointestinal tract is decreased due to reduced gastric motility, but absorption through the intramuscular, subcutaneous, or inhaled routes is increased due to increased blood flow and ventilatory adaptations[54] (Fig. 37.1). With the increase in plasma volume, the volume of *distribution* for medications is altered and may reduce plasma drug concentrations for hydrophilic medications (e.g., antibiotics).[54] Lipophilic medications (e.g., fentanyl), in contrast, may have an increased plasma drug concentration with the placental and maternal hormones displacing medications normally in a protein-bound state.[54] Lastly, both *metabolism* and *elimination* may be increased due to heightened kidney and liver function during pregnancy.[54] Pharmacologic therapies must take into account the pharmacokinetic changes that may occur during pregnancy as a result of the expected physiologic alterations.[54] This may inform loading and maintenance dosing of medications, along with serum concentration measurements of certain prescribed therapies.[54] Ultimately, therapeutic regimens should consider maternal–fetal risk and benefits.[54]

BOX 37.4 Safety

FDA Pregnancy and Lactation Labeling Rule (PLLR)

Prescription Drug Labeling Sections 8.1–8.3: Use in Specific Populations

Former Labeling	New Labeling
8.1 Pregnancy	8.1 Pregnancy—includes Labor and Delivery
8.2 Labor and Delivery	8.2 Lactation—includes Nursing Mothers
8.3 Nursing Mothers	8.3 Females and Males of Reproductive Potential

From U.S. Food & Drug Administration. Pregnancy and Lactation Labeling (Drugs) Final Rule. http://www.fda.gov/Drugs/DevelopmentApprovalProcess/DevelopmentResources/Labeling/ucm093307.htm. Accessed March 1, 2024.

NURSING MANAGEMENT

Maintain Surveillance for Complications

Maternal Monitoring

As with a nonpregnant patient, the critical care nurse should routinely monitor signs of local or system complications. Information from the patient's history, physical assessments findings, vital sign measures, hemodynamic values, and laboratory tests should all be considered and communicated among the interprofessional team. Care of the obstetric patient experiencing critical illness requires collaborative efforts among the patient, the family, obstetrics nurses, perinatal nurses, critical care nurses, critical care physicians, and obstetric physicians. Critical care nursing practices and interprofessional collaborative practices are discussed in Chapter 1.

Fetal Monitoring

Fetal assessment is often performed by a perinatal nurse while collaborating with the critical care nurse in the management of the obstetric patient.[55] Fetal assessment components include auscultation, palpation, electronic fetal monitoring, and ultrasound or Doppler flow studies.[55] Fetal monitoring provides information on fetal oxygenation as well as maternal cardiopulmonary and metabolic function. Fetal monitoring may inform the need for a timely delivery.[55]

ADDITIONAL RESOURCES

See Box 37.5 for Internet resources related to the obstetric patient.

BOX 37.5 Internet Resources

The Obstetric Patient

- Association of Women's Health, Obstetric and Neonatal Nurses. AWHONN. https://www.awhonn.org/
- Centers for Disease Control and Prevention. Reproductive Health, Maternal and Infant Health. https://www.cdc.gov/reproductivehealth/maternalinfanthealth/index.html
- Every Mother Counts (EMC) – Improving Maternal Health. https://everymothercounts.org/
- Health Resources & Service Administration. Maternal and Child Health Bureau. https://mchb.hrsa.gov/
- Maternal Health Task Force, Global Maternal Health News and Resources https://www.mhtf.org/resources/
- World Health Organization – Maternal Health https://www.who.int/health-topics/maternal-health#tab=tab_1
- World Health Organization-Partnership for Maternal, Newborn, and Child Health. https://www.who.int/pmnch/en/

CASE STUDY 37.1 Patient With Obstetric Issues

Brief Patient History

Mrs. S is a 40-year-old black female, gravida 2, para 1. She delivered a preterm baby boy by cesarean delivery this morning. Mrs. S has experienced chills, malaise, and abdominal pain since the operation, and she has been given morphine for pain relief but is still complaining of abdominal pain.

Clinical Assessment

Mrs. S is admitted to the critical care unit with hypotension, tachypnea, and tachycardia. She is lethargic, curled up in bed, and groaning. She does not follow commands or answer questions. No urine output has occurred over the last 4 h, and since placement of a urinary catheter, only 10 mL of dark amber urine has accumulated.

Diagnostic Procedures

Her admission vital signs are as follows: blood pressure of 60/35 mm Hg, heart rate of 145 beats/min (sinus tachycardia), respiratory rate of 30 breaths/min, temperature of 97.5 °F, hemoglobin level of 5 g/dL, and platelet level of 30 x 10^9/L. Ultrasound reveals a large fluid collection in the abdomen.

Medical Diagnosis

Mrs. S is diagnosed with an intraabdominal hemorrhage.

Questions

1. What major outcomes do you expect to achieve for this patient?
2. What problems or risks must be managed to achieve these outcomes?
3. What interventions must be initiated to monitor, prevent, manage, or eliminate the problems and risks identified?
4. What interventions should be initiated to promote optimal functioning, safety, and well-being of the patient?
5. What technology can be used to monitor this patient and prevent complications?
6. What other interprofessional team members are needed to assist with the management this patient?
7. What possible learning needs would you anticipate for this patient?
8. What cultural and age-related factors might have a bearing on the patient's plan of care?

KEY POINTS

- Critical care obstetrics encompasses two distinct populations: (1) women who are pregnant and become compromised by injury or critical illness and (2) women with preexisting disorders who become pregnant.
- The two priorities for a pregnant critically ill woman are (1) supporting fetal growth and development and (2) optimizing maternal health.
- Clinical decisions must be made in light of the maternal–fetal risk–benefit ratio, considering teratogens (e.g., radiation) and fetal viability.
- When developing the plan of care, the parameters of gestational age, fetal weight, parental desires, and maternal–fetal mortality must be considered.

Visit the Evolve site at http://evolve.elsevier.com/Urden/CriticalCareNursing for additional study materials.

REFERENCES

1. Centers for Disease Control and Prevention. Pregnancy mortality surveillance system; 2023. From https://www.cdc.gov/reproductivehealth/maternal-mortality/pregnancy-mortality-surveillance-system.htm. Accessed February 18, 2014.
2. Oxford-Horrey CM, Patel SS. Chapter 1. Basic hemodynamic monitoring in obstetric patients. In: Foley MR, Strong THJ, Garite TH, eds. *Obstetric Intensive Care Manual*. 5th ed. McGraw-Hill Education; 2018.
3. Mulder EG, de Haas S, Mohseni Z, et al. Cardiac output and peripheral vascular resistance during normotensive and hypertensive pregnancy - a systematic review and meta-analysis. *BJOG*. 2022;129(5):696–707. https://doi.org/10.1111/1471-0528.16678.
4. Soma-Pillay P, Nelson-Piercy C, Tolppanen H, Mebazaa A. Physiological changes in pregnancy. *Cardiovasc J Afr*. 2016;27(2):89–94. https://doi.org/10.5830/CVJA-2016-021.
5. Morton A. Physiological changes and cardiovascular investigations in pregnancy. *Heart Lung Circ*. 2021;30(1):e6–e15. https://doi.org/10.1016/j.hlc.2020.10.001.
6. Bredy C, Mongeon FP, Leduc L, Dore A, Khairy P. Pregnancy in adults with repaired/unrepaired atrial septal defect. *J Thorac Dis*. 2018;10(Suppl 24):S2945–S2952. https://doi.org/10.21037/jtd.2017.10.130.
7. American Heart Association. About congenital heart defects; 2023. From https://www.heart.org/en/health-topics/congenital-heart-defects/about-congenital-heart-defects. Accessed March 1, 2024.
8. Harris IS. Management of pregnancy in patients with congenital heart disease. *Prog Cardiovasc Dis*. 2011;53(4):305–311. https://doi.org/10.1016/j.pcad.2010.08.001.
9. Ramlakhan KP, Tobler D, Greutmann M, et al. ROPAC investigators group. Pregnancy outcomes in women with aortic coarctation. *Heart* Oct 29;107(4):290–298. https://doi.org/10.1136/heartjnl-2020-317513.
10. Wichert-Schmitt B, Steckham KE, Pfaller B, et al. Cardiac complications in pregnant women with isolated mitral stenosis and their association with echocardiographic changes during pregnancy. *Am J Cardiol*. 2021;158:81–89. https://doi.org/10.1016/j.amjcard.2021.07.037.
11. Goland S, Elkayam U. Pregnancy and Marfan syndrome. *Ann Cardiothorac Surg*. 2017;6(6):642–653. https://doi.org/10.21037/acs.2017.10.07.
12. Rush B, Martinka P, Kilb B, McDermid RC, Boyd JH, Celi LA. Acute respiratory distress syndrome in pregnant women. *Obstet Gynecol*. 2017;129(3):530–535. https://doi.org/10.1097/AOG.0000000000001907.
13. Murphy VE, Schatz M. Asthma in pregnancy: a hit for two. *Eur Respir Rev*. 2014;23(131):64–68.
14. Briggs G, et al. *Drugs in Pregnancy and Lactation*. 11th ed. Baltimore: Williams & Wilkins; 2017.
15. Planning for a safe pregnancy. Cystic Fibrosis Foundation. From https://www.cff.org/managing-cf/planning-safe-pregnancy. Accessed March 1, 2024.
16. Mei JY, Channick RN, Afshar Y. Pregnancy and pulmonary hypertension: from preconception and risk stratification through pregnancy and postpartum. *Heart Fail Clin*. 2023;19(1):75–87. https://doi.org/10.1016/j.hfc.2022.08.019.
17. Moukalled NM, Bou Fakhredin R, Taher AT. Pregnancy and sickle cell disease: an overview of complications and suggested perinatal care. *Expert Rev Hematol*. 2022;15(12):1055–1061. https://doi.org/10.1080/17474086.2022.2151432.
18. Magee LA, Brown MA, Hall DR, et al. The 2021 International Society for the Study of Hypertension in Pregnancy classification, diagnosis & management recommendations for international practice. *Pregnancy Hypertens*. 2022;27:148–169. https://doi.org/10.1016/j.preghy.2021.09.008.
19. Chappell LC, Cluver CA, Kingdom J, Tong S. Pre-eclampsia. *Lancet*. 2021;398(10297):341–354. https://doi.org/10.1016/S0140-6736(20)32335-7.
20. Rana S, Lemoine E, Granger JP, Karumanchi SA. Preeclampsia: pathophysiology, challenges, and perspectives. [published correction appears in Circ Res. 2020 Jan 3;126(1):e8] *Circ Res*. 2019;124(7):1094–1112. https://doi.org/10.1161/CIRCRESAHA.118.313276.

21. Boushra M, Natesan SM, Koyfman A, Long B. High risk and low prevalence diseases: Eclampsia. *Am J Emerg Med.* 2022;58:223–228. https://doi.org/10.1016/j.ajem.2022.06.004.
22. Yang TJ, Sangal RB, Conlon LW. Eclampsia. *J Educ Teach Emerg Med.* 2021;6(3):S33–S61. https://doi.org/10.21980/J8PS8R.
23. Petca A, Miron BC, Pacu I, et al. HELLP syndrome-holistic insight into pathophysiology. *Medicina (Kaunas).* 2022;58(2):326. https://doi.org/10.3390/medicina58020326.
24. Rimaitis K, Grauslyte L, Zavackiene A, Baliuliene V, Nadisauskiene R, Macas A. Diagnosis of HELLP syndrome: a 10-year survey in a perinatology centre. *Int J Environ Res Public Health.* 2019;16(1):109. https://doi.org/10.3390/ijerph16010109.
25. Sibai BM, Ramadan MK, Usta I, Salama M, Mercer BM, Friedman SA. Maternal morbidity and mortality in 442 pregnancies with hemolysis, elevated liver enzymes, and low platelets (HELLP syndrome). *Am J Obstet Gynecol.* 1993;169(4):1000–1006. https://doi.org/10.1016/0002-9378(93)90043-i.
26. Martin Jr JN, Rinehart BK, May WL, Magann EF, Terrone DA, Blake PG. The spectrum of severe preeclampsia: comparative analysis by HELLP (hemolysis, elevated liver enzyme levels, and low platelet count) syndrome classification. *Am J Obstet Gynecol.* 1999;180(6 Pt 1):1373–1384. https://doi.org/10.1016/s0002-9378(99)70022-0.
27. Griffin KM, Oxford-Horrey C, Bourjeily G. Obstetric disorders and critical illness. *Clin Chest Med.* 2022;43(3):471–488. https://doi.org/10.1016/j.ccm.2022.04.008.
28. Singh R, Aditya V, Agarwal S, Maurya G, Kumari A, Sharma NR. Identifying the risk factors of antepartum haemorrhage and to evaluate the feto maternal outcome in antepartum haemorrhage cases. *Int J Reprod Contracept Obstet Gynecol.* 2021;10(10):3786–3792. https://doi.org/10.18203/2320-1770.ijrcog20213838.
29. Ghosh J, Papadopoulou A, Devall AJ, et al. Methods for managing miscarriage: a network meta-analysis. *Cochrane Database Syst Rev.* 2021;6(6):CD012602. https://doi.org/10.1002/14651858.CD012602.pub2.
30. Tonick S, Conageski C. Ectopic pregnancy. *Obstet Gynecol Clin North Am.* 2022;49(3):537–549. https://doi.org/10.1016/j.ogc.2022.02.018.
31. Committee on Practice Bulletins-Obstetrics. Practice Bulletin No. 183: postpartum hemorrhage. *Obstet Gynecol.* 2017;130(4):e168–e186. https://doi.org/10.1097/AOG.0000000000002351.
32. Bienstock JL, Eke AC, Hueppchen NA. Postpartum hemorrhage. *N Engl J Med.* 2021;384(17):1635–1645. https://doi.org/10.1056/NEJMra151324.
33. Evensen A, Anderson JM, Fontaine P. Postpartum hemorrhage: prevention and treatment. *Am Fam Physician.* 2017;95(7):442–449.
34. Coggins AS, Gomez E, Sheffield JS. Pulmonary embolism and amniotic fluid embolism. *Obstet Gynecol Clin North Am.* 2022;49(3):439–460. https://doi.org/10.1016/j.ogc.2022.02.015.
35. Mazza GR, Youssefzadeh AC, Klar M, et al. Association of pregnancy characteristics and maternal mortality with amniotic fluid embolism. *JAMA Netw Open.* 2022;5(11):e2242842. https://doi.org/10.1001/jamanetworkopen.2022.42842.
36. Guntupalli KK, Hall N, Karnad DR, Bandi V, Belfort M. Critical illness in pregnancy: part I: an approach to a pregnant patient in the ICU and common obstetric disorders. *Chest.* 2015;148(4):1093–1104. https://doi.org/10.1378/chest.14-1998.
37. Lao TT. Pulmonary embolism in pregnancy and the puerperium. *Best Pract Res Clin Obstet Gynaecol.* 2022;85(Pt A):96–106. https://doi.org/10.1016/j.bpobgyn.2022.06.003.
38. Kalaitzopoulos DR, Panagopoulos A, Samant S, et al. Management of venous thromboembolism in pregnancy. *Thromb Res.* 2022;211:106–113. https://doi.org/10.1016/j.thromres.2022.02.002.
39. Erez O, Othman M, Rabinovich A, Leron E, Gotsch F, Thachil J. DIC in pregnancy - pathophysiology, clinical characteristics, diagnostic scores, and treatments. *J Blood Med.* 2022;13:21–44. https://doi.org/10.2147/JBM.S273047.
40. Davis MB, Arany Z, McNamara DM, Goland S, Elkayam U. Peripartum cardiomyopathy: JACC state-of-the-art review. *J Am Coll Cardiol.* 2020;75(2):207–221. https://doi.org/10.1016/j.jacc.2019.11.014.
41. Arany Z. Peripartum cardiomyopathy. *N Engl J Med.* 2024;390(2):154–164. https://doi.org/10.1056/NEJMra2306667.
42. Guntupalli KK, Karnad DR, Bandi V, Hall N, Belfort M. Critical illness in pregnancy: Part II: common medical conditions complicating pregnancy and puerperium. *Chest.* 2015;148(5):1333–1345. https://doi.org/10.1378/chest.14-2365.
43. Kim JA, Kim SY, Virk HUH, et al. Acute myocardial infarction in pregnancy. *Cardiol Rev.* 2024. https://doi.org/10.1097/CRD.0000000000000681. Published online February 27.
44. Merlo AC, Rosa GM, Porto I. Pregnancy-related acute myocardial infarction: a review of the recent literature. *Clin Res Cardiol.* 2022;111(7):723–731. https://doi.org/10.1007/s00392-021-01937-5.
45. Alameh A, Jabri A, Aleyadeh W, et al. Pregnancy-associated myocardial infarction: a review of current practices and guidelines. *Curr Cardiol Rep.* 2021;23(10):142. https://doi.org/10.1007/s11886-021-01579-z.
46. Liggett MR, Amro A, Son M, Schwulst S. Management of the pregnant trauma patient: a systematic literature review. *J Surg Res.* 2023;285:187–196. https://doi.org/10.1016/j.jss.2022.11.075.
47. Patel S, Qabbani A, Sheridan R, DuMont T, Kautza B, Arshad H. Trauma in pregnancy. *Crit Care Nurs Q.* 2023;46(4):398–402. https://doi.org/10.1097/CNQ.0000000000000475.
48. LA Rosa M, Loaiza S, Zambrano MA, Escobar MF. Trauma in pregnancy. *Clin Obstet Gynecol.* 2020;63(2):447–454. https://doi.org/10.1097/GRF.0000000000000531.
49. Greco PS, Day LJ, Pearlman MD. Guidance for evaluation and management of blunt abdominal trauma in pregnancy. *Obstet Gynecol.* 2019;134(6):1343–1357. https://doi.org/10.1097/AOG.0000000000003585.
50. Sakamoto J, Michels C, Eisfelder B, Joshi N. Trauma in pregnancy. *Emerg Med Clin North Am.* 2019;37(2):317–338. https://doi.org/10.1016/j.emc.2019.01.009.
51. Ashby T, Staiano P, Najjar N, Louis M. Bacterial pneumonia infection in pregnancy. *Best Pract Res Clin Obstet Gynaecol.* 2022;85(Pt A):26–33. https://doi.org/10.1016/j.bpobgyn.2022.07.001.
52. Panchal AR, Bartos JA, Cabañas JG, et al. Adult basic and advanced life support writing group. Part 3: adult basic and advanced life support: 2020 American heart association guidelines for cardiopulmonary resuscitation and emergency cardiovascular care. *Circulation.* 2020;142(16_suppl_2):S366–S468. https://doi.org/10.1161/CIR.0000000000000916.
53. United States Food & Drug Administration. Pregnancy and lactation labeling (drugs) final rule; 2021. From http://www.fda.gov/Drugs/DevelopmentApprovalProcess/DevelopmentResources/Labeling/ucm093307.htm. Accessed March 1, 2024.
54. Heavner MS, Cucci MD, Barlow B, et al. Caring for two in the ICU: pharmacologic management of pregnancy-related complications. *Pharmacotherapy.* 2023;43(7):659–674. https://doi.org/10.1002/phar.2837.
55. Cypher RL. A standardized approach to electronic fetal monitoring in critical care obstetrics. *J Perinat Neonatal Nurs.* 2018;32(3):212–221. https://doi.org/10.1097/JPN.0000000000000343.

38

The Pediatric Patient

Cynthia A. Lewis

http://evolve.elsevier.com/Urden/CriticalCareNursing

Developmental and physiologic differences between adults and children older than 1 month are discussed in this chapter. Although children may experience medical conditions similar to those of adults, they are assessed and managed differently. During periods of stress, children may maintain physiologic stability for a period, but they may then decompensate quickly. Children are *not* small adults. Box 38.1 describes the differences between children and adults. Many of the laboratory values, medications, blood product dosages, methods of administration, and other therapeutic modalities for children are different from those used with adults. Heart rate and blood pressure should be within normal range for age (Tables 38.1 and 38.2). Blood pressure measurement is the most important diagnostic tool and should be monitored in children with symptoms of hypertension. This includes children admitted to critical care units.[1]

ADMISSION TO THE CRITICAL CARE UNIT

Regardless of the anticipated outcome, admission to a critical care unit is stressful for families. Critical care nurses who successfully deal with pediatric patients see the child and the family as an integral unit and are perceptive to the entire family's needs.[2] Knowledge of normal growth and development and the ability to assess the child's developmental level are essential for working with children and their parents. Nurses caring for pediatric patients can conceptualize using a developmental perspective as the ideal norm.[2] The developmental stages include the different age groups: infancy (0 to 12 months), toddlers (1 to 3 years), preschoolers (3 to 5 years), school-age children (6 to 12 years), and adolescents (12 to 18 years).

Although some critically ill children may be managed in adult critical care units in certain situations, children need the services of various pediatric subspecialists or pediatric intensivists, and they must be transferred to a tertiary care pediatric critical care unit. This situation is also true for pediatric trauma patients. The risk of death or significant disabilities is significantly lower for children who receive care from health care professionals at a facility that is expert in providing care to pediatric trauma patients.[3] Conditions that may require transfer to a hospital with a pediatric critical care unit include the need for high-frequency ventilation, extracorporeal membrane oxygenation, or cardiac surgery and treatment for some neurologic conditions that require intracranial pressure (ICP) monitoring. Transfer is also considered for children who do not respond to treatment.

CARDIOVASCULAR SYSTEM

Anatomy and Physiology

The cardiac anatomy and physiology of infants and children differ from adults in various aspects. At birth, the heart is more horizontally positioned and becomes more vertically oriented as the child grows. The heart's size relative to the body is larger in infants than in older children and adults. The myocardial wall is relatively thicker in infants, especially the right ventricle due to the higher pulmonary vascular resistance in utero. The tricuspid valve in neonates is closer to the cardiac apex compared to adults. The foramen ovale is present in fetuses; it allows blood flow between the right and left atria, bypassing the nonfunctional fetal lungs. It typically closes soon after birth as pulmonary resistance drops and becomes the fossa ovalis. Another fetal structure connects the pulmonary artery to the descending aorta, allowing blood to bypass the lungs. It typically closes within the first few days of life. Infants and children have a faster heart rate compared to adults. Newborns often have heart rates around 120 to 160 beats per minute (bpm), which gradually decrease with age to reach adult levels. Stroke volume is limited in infants and doesn't significantly change with heart rate. Hence, cardiac output is heavily reliant on heart rate in this age group. The infant heart relies more on calcium for contractility and is more sensitive to changes in calcium levels. Infants and children have a higher metabolic rate, leading to increased oxygen consumption. This makes them more susceptible to rapid decompensation in cases of shock or heart failure.[4]

Congenital Heart Defects

The differences in cardiovascular function between children and adults are related to early physical development and the presence or absence of congenital cardiac disease. Congenital heart defects (CHDs) occur during the embryologic development of the heart, whereas acquired defects occur after birth. Most fetal cardiac development occurs between the fourth and seventh weeks of fetal life. The heart is most susceptible to teratogenic influences at this time.[4] Approximately 90% of CHDs are caused by a genetic predisposition and an adverse response to environmental teratogens during cardiac development. Environmental factors alone account for only approximately 1% of all CHDs. Approximately 5% to 8% of CHDs are associated with genetic anomalies or syndromes.[4] Although more than 35 well-recognized cardiac defects have been documented, the most common is ventricular septal defect.

Some CHDs may be diagnosed with ultrasonography before birth, and some parents decide to undergo delivery at a tertiary

(i.e., decrease in systolic blood pressure by more than 10 mm Hg during inspiration). The treatment is supportive and includes fluids, adequate oxygenation and ventilation, vasopressors, and a possible pericardiocentesis.[5]

Tension pneumothorax. A second type of obstructive shock is caused by a *tension pneumothorax*,[5] which is caused by the entry of air into the pleural space. This is most often seen in a pediatric patient when chest trauma has occurred or when an intubated child on positive-pressure ventilation deteriorates suddenly. The signs and symptoms include diminished breath sounds on the affected side, distended neck veins, tracheal deviation, and a rapidly deteriorating clinical condition of the child that may result in bradycardia, hypotension, and hypoxemia. The treatment is immediate needle decompression over the third rib at the midclavicular line. The decompression should lead to an escape of air. The decompression should be followed by an insertion of a chest tube.

Pulmonary embolism. A third but rare cause of obstructive shock is a *massive pulmonary embolism*,[5] which results from partial or total obstruction of the pulmonary artery. The symptoms include signs of cyanosis, hypotension, and right heart failure. Treatment includes adequate oxygenation and ventilation, and fluid therapy is administered if the patient is poorly perfused. Additional diagnostic tests and medications, such as fibrinolytic agents, may be required.

Ductal-dependent congenital heart lesion. A fourth type of obstructive shock is caused by a *ductal-dependent congenital heart lesion*.[5] Because systemic circulation is supported by the right side of the heart through the ductus arteriosus, these lesions are called *ductal-dependent lesions*. The affected infant shows signs of severe shock, acute heart failure, hypotension, poor perfusion, lethargy, and acidosis. The infant is treated with prostaglandin E_1 to maintain the patency of the ductus arteriosus.

Cardiopulmonary Arrest

The pediatric patient must be assessed for manifestations of respiratory failure and shock because failure to recognize these problems may result in the development of cardiopulmonary failure and respiratory or cardiac arrest. In pediatric patients, respiratory arrest usually precedes cardiac arrest. In an arrest situation, oxygen is administered and an airway is established and maintained (see Assessment and Oxygen Devices in this chapter). In the event of a cardiac arrest, compressions are started and an intravenous or intraosseous line is established.

Intraosseous Access

Intraosseous placement is recommended as an alternative means to deliver intravenous fluids and medications in children of all ages when vascular access is not obtained within 90 seconds or after three attempts. Intraosseous access is often achieved in 30 to 60 seconds and is the preferred route over the endotracheal route for medications. Any medication or fluid that is administered by a peripheral intravenous line may be given by the intraosseous route.[5] The preferred site is the broad, flat portion of the anteromedial surface of the tibia approximately 1 to 2 cm below the tibial tuberosity. Other interventions are based on the cardiac rhythm and the cause of the arrest.

Cardiopulmonary Resuscitation

Pulseless arrest includes the following dysrhythmias: asystole, ventricular fibrillation (VF), pulseless ventricular tachycardia (VT), and pulseless electrical activity (PEA).[5] Treatment of asystole starts with cardiopulmonary resuscitation (CPR; rate of 15 compressions to two breaths with two rescuers), airway maintenance with oxygenation, attachment to a monitor or defibrillator, and obtaining intravenous or intraosseous access. After an advanced airway is in place, chest compressions may continue without pauses for breaths. A child requires 8 to 10 breaths per minute. The next step in the treatment algorithm depends on whether the rhythm is shockable.[5]

Shockable rhythms. The rhythms of VF or VT are shockable. On a manual defibrillator, the initial dose of electricity is 2 J/kg. Immediately after the shock, compressions are resumed for 2 minutes (five cycles). The compressions support the heart while it is in a recovery state, even if a perfusion rhythm has returned.[5] If VT or VF persists, another shock is administered at 4 J/kg, compressions are resumed, and epinephrine is given. The first dose of epinephrine is 0.01 mg/kg (1:10,000 at 0.1 mL/kg) given intravenously or intraosseous; if given endotracheally, the dose is 0.1 mg/kg (1:1000 at 0.1 mL/kg). Subsequent doses may be given every 3 to 5 minutes. Maximum dosage is 1 mg (1 mL). After 2 minutes of CPR, the patient's rhythm should be checked. If the VT or VF rhythm continues, the patient is defibrillated again at 4 J/kg, compressions are resumed immediately, and an antiarrhythmic medication such as amiodarone (5 mg/kg) is given intravenously or intraosseous.[5]

Nonshockable rhythms. If the rhythm is not shockable, as in asystole or PEA, the first action after starting CPR is to give epinephrine at the same dose listed previously. After five cycles or 2 minutes of CPR, the patient's rhythm is checked, and if asystole or PEA persists, CPR and dosing with epinephrine every 3 to 5 minutes are continued. The treatment needs to include reversible causes, which include hypovolemia, hypoxia, hydrogen ion (acidosis), hypoglycemia, hypokalemia or hyperkalemia, hypothermia, tension pneumothorax, tamponade, toxins, and thrombosis (pulmonary or coronary).[5]

Postresuscitation Management

The primary goals of postresuscitation management of a pediatric patient include[5]:

1. Optimization and stabilization of airway, oxygenation, ventilation, and cardiopulmonary function to restore and maintain vital organ perfusion and function, especially the brain
2. Prevention of any secondary organ injury
3. Identification and treatment of the cause of any acute illnesses
4. Initiation of measures to help improve long-term, neurologically intact survival of the child.
5. Minimization of the risk of deterioration of the child during transport to the next level of care

The nurse should assess the patient using a systematic approach. In addition to primary assessments, the approach should include a review of the patient's history, a thorough physical examination, the use of invasive and noninvasive monitoring techniques, and the use of appropriate laboratory testing.[5]

PULMONARY SYSTEM

Anatomy and Physiology

The airway anatomy and physiology of infants and children differ significantly from those of adults. Understanding these differences is crucial, especially in scenarios such as cardiopulmonary resuscitation and anesthesia, where management of the airway is critical. Infants and children have a relatively larger

TABLE 38.3 Clinical Indicators for Infants or Children at Risk for Respiratory Failure

Assessment Area	Physical Findings	Discussion Points
Respiratory rate	Infant: >60 breaths/min Child: >40 breaths/min	Tachypnea usually first sign of distress in an infant; fatigue is a common contributing factor in respiratory failure
	Slow or irregular	Late signs: apnea, gasping, or agonal respirations
Mechanics	Retractions (intercostal, supraclavicular, substernal) Paradoxical movements (chest in and abdomen out) Signs of diaphragm fatigue, respiratory alternans:	
	Grunting	Closing of glottis to create "auto-PEEP" to keep alveoli open at end expiration
	Stridor	Sign of upper airway obstruction
	Wheezing	Sign of lower airway obstruction
Air entry	Changes in pitch rather than volume of breath sounds	Chest expansion sometimes is barely perceptible in a normal, spontaneously breathing infant. Small, thin chest wall causes breath sounds from any area of the lungs to be easily referred throughout the chest, even over fluid or atelectasis. Listen for bilateral breath sounds high in the axillae because these are the two most separated points.
Color or temperature	Central coolness, pallor, or cyanosis	Peripheral changes may be normal in an infant or child
Heart rate	<5 y: <60 or >180 beats/min 5–10 y: <60 or >160 beats/min >10 y: <50 or >140 beats/min	Infants and children have limited ability to increase stroke volume; with hypoxemia, the heart rate increases to improve cardiac output. If bradycardia occurs with cardiorespiratory distress, arrest may be imminent.
Neurologic status	Infant: hypotonia	Sign of hypoxia for infants
	Child: irritability	Early sign of hypoxia, often manifested as a decreased responsiveness to parents or to pain
	Decreased level of consciousness	

PEEP, Positive end-expiratory pressure.
Data from Hazinski MF, ed. *Nursing Care of the Critically Ill Child.* 3rd ed. Elsevier; 2013.

head, which can cause flexion of the neck when lying supine. This can obstruct the airway. Table 38.3 outlines the assessment areas for pediatric patients at risk for respiratory failure.[4]

Upper Airway

The upper airway of the infant and child is different from that of the adult. The epiglottis is located at the level of the cervical spine. It is located at C1 in the newborn, at C3 in the older infant, and at C4 to C5 in the adult.

Epiglottis and tongue. The infant's epiglottis is large and floppy, and because of its high placement, it may press against the pharyngeal soft palate on inspiration. The infant's tongue is large relative to its head size. The tongue fills most of the oral cavity. Because of this anatomy, the infant usually is an obligatory nose breather until 4 to 6 months of age, after which the larynx descends with growth.[2] Oral breathing is a very complex process for an infant, and it never occurs alone. Oronasal breathing is possible, but only 30% to 40% of ventilation may be provided orally. During sleep, oronasal breathing may occur spontaneously and last for about 20 seconds.

Larynx. The larynx of the infant and young child, in contrast to that of the adult, is a funnel-shaped structure, with the narrowest portion at the cricoid ring.[4] The larynx is pliable because the cartilage is less developed, making it easier to collapse on inspiration or expiration. With changes in intrathoracic pressure, collapse may occur even with crying.[4] By age 8 to 10 years, the larynx has grown cylindrical, has assumed the narrowest portion at the glottic opening, and has increased in length, width, and internal diameter. By the age of 12 years, the diameter has grown to 1.8 cm.

Submucosal layer of larynx. The submucosal layer of the larynx is also looser in the infant and young child, and fluid accumulates more easily in that space. Within the airway's relatively rigid confines, any accumulation of fluid encroaches into the airway space. Along with a shorter and narrower airway, any decrease in airway radius leads to an exponential increase in airflow resistance, which increases the work of breathing. Turbulent airflow, as occurs with crying, doubles the already increased airflow resistance.[5] Fig. 38.1 illustrates the changes in airway diameter and airflow resistance with obstruction from edema in an adult and in an infant. An infant or child with an abnormally small jaw and low-set ears should be considered as having a potentially difficult airway to manage, and a consultation with an anesthesiologist is needed if airway management is required.

Lower Airway

Alveolar collapse is more likely in the infant and young child because of the smaller alveolar size. Infants and young children are at greater risk for ventilation–perfusion mismatch and atelectasis without this collateral ventilation. Infants and children have a higher metabolic rate compared with adults, and oxygen consumption per kilogram is higher. Hypoxemia develops more rapidly in the context of respiratory compromise in young children than in adults.[4]

Chest Mechanics

The respiratory structure and mechanics of infants and young children are very different from those of mature adults. In the infant and young child, the chest wall is more compliant because bones are smaller and more cartilaginous. The ribs are

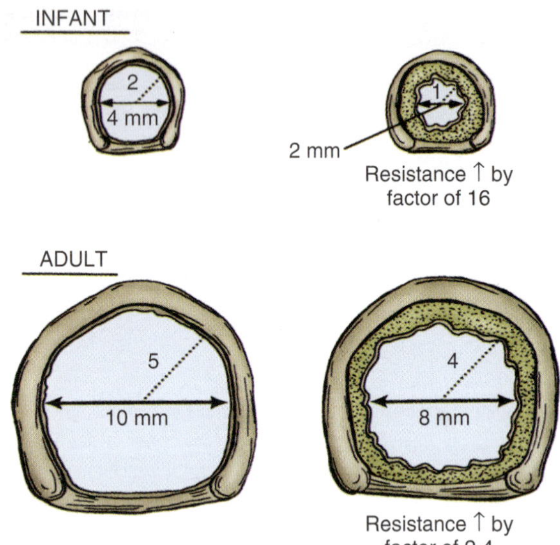

FIG. 38.1 Effects of Edema on Airway Resistance. Effects of edema on airway resistance are shown by proportional increases in airflow resistance with 1 mm of circumferential edema in an infant versus an adult. (From Hazinski MF. Children are different. In: Hazinski MF, ed. *Nursing Care of the Critically Ill Child.* 3rd ed. Elsevier; 2013.)

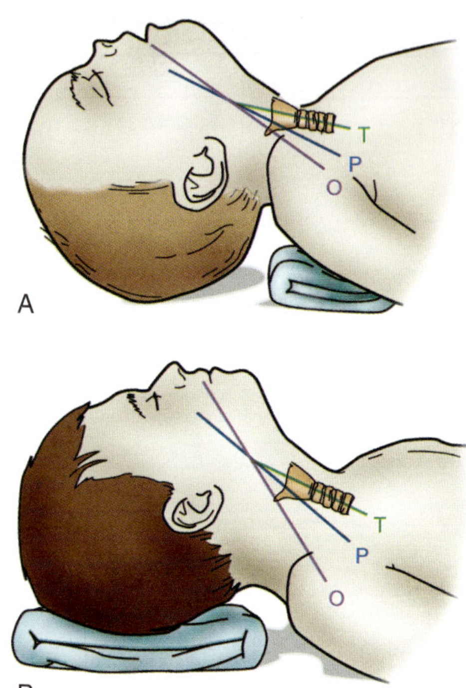

FIG. 38.2 Correct Airway Positioning for Ventilation. Correct airway positioning for ventilation is shown for (A) an infant and (B) a child. Better airflow is provided with straight alignment of the oropharynx *(O)*, pharynx *(P)*, and trachea *(T)*. (From Cote CJ, Todres ID. The pediatric airway. In: Cote CJ, Lerman J, Anderson BJ, eds. *A Practice of Anesthesia for Infants and Children.* 2nd ed. Saunders; 1993:55.)

more horizontally placed, providing less of a bellowing action on inspiration. Accessory muscles are less developed, and the external intercostals do not contribute to pulling the ribs up on inspiration. The diaphragm is the principal muscle for inspiration. The diaphragm is more horizontal in the chest of an infant and tends to pull the lower ribs inward on inspiration.[6]

Because of these mechanics, infants and toddlers depend almost totally on diaphragmatic contraction for lung expansion. Anything that impedes diaphragmatic contractions may result in respiratory compromise. The intercostal muscles are inadequately developed before school age, and they are unlikely to help with effective ventilation if the diaphragm is impaired.[4] With any decrease in lung compliance, as with lung disease, diaphragmatic contractions, which cause decreased intrathoracic pressure, produce intercostal and substernal retractions rather than inflation of the lungs.[6] The greater the chest wall retractions, the more the diaphragm must contract to offset the changes in intrathoracic pressure to generate an adequate tidal volume for the child. The compliant chest wall of the infant or the young child should expand easily outward with positive-pressure ventilation. If the chest wall does not expand bilaterally during positive-pressure ventilation, either the ventilation effort is inadequate or the airway is obstructed.[4]

Oxygenation and Ventilation Delivery Devices

An infant or child usually experiences respiratory failure more often than primary heart failure. In contrast to older adults, who may have underlying cardiovascular disease, infants and children tend to demonstrate bradycardia and apnea in cardiopulmonary failure and not ventricular dysrhythmias.[5] For an infant or child who is conscious and needs supplemental oxygen, the device of comfort must be selected.[4] Minimizing anxiety and fear in the child is paramount to decrease the work of breathing.

Airway Positioning

Knowledge of childhood anatomy is necessary to establish a patent airway. An infant or toddler younger than 2 years of age, because of the large occiput, needs to have a small roll or towel placed under the upper shoulders, with the jaw slightly extended into a "sniffing" position.[5] Optimal positioning of the head should assist in maintenance of a patent airway or help when bag-mask ventilation is required.[5] This head positioning displaces the tongue and lines up the posterior pharynx and tracheal opening for a clear airway. For infants younger than 6 months, correct head positioning still may not prevent the large tongue from falling back into the posterior pharynx. Oral airways must not be used unless the infant is unconscious, because the airway tip may stimulate laryngospasm as a result of the higher placement of the larynx. Side-lying placement, with the neck in a neutral position, should be attempted.[4] The older child needs to have a folded towel placed under the head, with the neck in an extended position to maintain a patent airway.[4] Fig. 38.2 illustrates proper head positioning for the infant and the child. A child who is conscious must be allowed to assume a position of choice for airway maintenance.

Supplemental Oxygen Devices

Many of the oxygen devices used for adults also are used for children. One technique is oxygen "blow-by," which uses oxygen tubing to blow oxygen approximately 2 to 3 inches from the child's face. Because of the unpredictability of the actual oxygen percentage that is delivered, the child should never be left unattended with blow-by as an oxygen delivery method. Oxygen simple face masks may aggravate the child and often are not well tolerated because of the snug fit of the mask to ensure adequate delivery of oxygen.[7] It is imperative that a minimum flow rate is used with the simple face mask to flush out the carbon dioxide that accumulates in the mask.[7] One option in older infants and

TABLE 38.4 Supplemental Oxygen Devices and Oxygen Administration in Infants and Children

Device	Administration	Discussion Points
Nasal cannula	Infant Child	Minute volume, inspiratory/expiratory times, and amount of mouth breathing affects infant FiO_2 by nasal cannula differently from an adult given the same gas flow and O_2 percent Low-flow O_2 devices are inaccurate for FiO_2 delivery; titrate to patient's O_2 saturation readings
O_2 blow-by	10–15 L/min	Better tolerated than O_2 masks Short-term method of O_2 delivery Titrated to child's O_2 saturation Allows child or parent to hold tubing
Simple mask	0.4–0.5 FiO_2	Entrains room air; FiO_2 does not correlate with high flow rates
Nonrebreather mask	0.9–0.95 FiO_2	No entrainment of room air; O_2 flow is determined by child's minute ventilation
Self-inflating resuscitation bag	Infant: <3 mo: 0.25-L bag 3 mo–4 y: 0.5-L bag Child: 5–10 y: 1-L bag >10 y: 1.5-L bag	Do not use bags with leaf-flap outlet valves or with spring-loaded PEEP valves
Flow-inflating resuscitation bag	Spontaneously breathing: Flow rate 3 × minute ventilation Not spontaneously breathing: 8–10 L/min flow rate	Set O_2 flow rate at level necessary to achieve desired level of ventilation
Peak inspiratory pressure	≤20–30 cm H_2O	
Ventilatory mask size	<6 mo old: 0 6 mo–3 y: 1 3–6 y: 2 >6 y: 3	Fit and placement on face same as for adult

FiO_2, Fraction of inspired oxygen; *O_2*, oxygen; *PEEP*, positive end-expiratory pressure.
Data from Hazinski MF, ed. *Nursing Care of the Critically Ill Child.* 3rd ed. Elsevier; 2013.

children is to use a nasal prong or cannula.[6] This method allows the child to talk and eat without a facial obstruction.

The appropriate device for oxygen delivery is determined by the patient's age, size, inspiratory flow rate (tidal volume mL/s), and fraction of inspired oxygen (FiO_2) needed.[8] Oxygen delivery devices may be divided into two different classes: low-flow devices and high-flow devices. Low-flow (variable performance) devices are unable to deliver an oxygen flow rate sufficient enough to supply the patient's inspiratory flow rate. This allows the child to entrain room air with supplemental oxygen on inspiration. The FiO_2 the child receives depends on his or her respiratory rate and tidal volume. High-flow (fixed performance) devices may deliver an oxygen flow rate that meets or exceeds the child's inspiratory flow rate. This allows a higher FiO_2 to be consistently delivered.[8] Nursing care for a child receiving supplemental oxygen delivery should include monitoring and recording the type of oxygen delivery device, the liter flow (L/min), the FiO_2, and the patient's response to the oxygen therapy.

Manual Resuscitation Bag

An adult-sized, self-inflating resuscitation bag may be carefully used on an infant, provided that only the force needed to cause appropriate chest expansion is used.[4] In general, two types of manual resuscitation bags are used: the self-inflating bag and the flow-dependent bag. Self-inflating bags do not require a gas source to provide ventilation, but flow-dependent bags do require a gas flow.[8] Resuscitation bag sizes, along with other supplemental oxygen devices and oxygen administration, are summarized in Table 38.4. Leaf-flap outlet valves should be avoided when a self-inflating bag is used to assist spontaneous ventilation in an infant, because the infant cannot generate enough negative inspiratory pressure to open the valve.[4] Resuscitation bags equipped with spring-loaded, positive end-expiratory pressure (PEEP) valves to provide continuous positive airway pressure (CPAP) must not be used with a spontaneously breathing child for the same reason previously discussed.[4] Flow-inflating bags have no flow valves that require opening on inspiration and therefore may be used to provide supplemental oxygen, PEEP, or CPAP to a spontaneously breathing infant or child.[4] Pressure manometers may be attached to these bags to measure peak inspiratory pressure. Ventilatory masks are measured in the child, as in the adult, from the bridge of the nose to the point before the end of the chin. Using a correctly sized mask for an infant or child is critical for adequate oxygenation and ventilation of the patient.

Endotracheal Intubation

Endotracheal tube (ETT) placement and management is an important intervention to maintain the airway in a pediatric patient with respiratory failure.[5] Preoxygenation of the child before intubation is very important. Bag-mask ventilation is an effective way to assist the child's ventilation. Attempts for intubation should be no longer than approximately 30 seconds per attempt to prevent deterioration in heart rate or the child's appearance. Box 38.2 provides formulas as a guideline for ETT

BOX 38.2 Endotracheal Tube Measurement

Size

- For infants and toddlers: size based on age 1 to 2 y = 3.5 mm
- For children >2 years old: (age in years + 16) ÷ 4
- For any age: compare circumference of the child's little finger with the external diameter size of the ETT
- Cuffed tube: external diameter one-half size smaller than appropriate-sized uncuffed tube

Depth of Insertion

- From teeth to midtrachea: internal diameter of ETT × 3

Cuff Pressure

- Allow for a slight air glottic leak

ETT, Endotracheal tube.
Modified from Hazinski MF. *Nursing Care of the Critically Ill Child*. 3rd ed. Elsevier; 2013.

measurements in pediatric patients. It is important to ensure that pediatric emergency equipment of the correct size is used.

Broselow system. Many facilities use length-based or color-coded resuscitation tapes, such as the Broselow system.[5,9] This tape gives an estimate of the child's body weight based on the crown-to-heel length and may be used to determine the appropriate size of resuscitation equipment and medication dosages for the child. Each color bar on the Broselow tape has specific information regarding equipment sizing and medication doses for the specific weight range of the child when time to treatment is critical.[9] Fig. 38.3 provides an illustration of a Broselow tape.

Confirmation of placement. When correctly placed, the tip of the ETT should be 1 to 2 cm above the carina, no higher than the first rib.[4] After the child is intubated, bilateral breath sounds should be assessed high in the axillae along with bilateral chest expansion. The easy transmission of sounds in the chest of the child may be mistaken for breath sounds in the event of accidental esophageal intubation. Initial confirmation of tube placement after assessment of bilateral breath sounds and adequate chest expansion is made with the use of the colorimetric carbon dioxide (CO_2) detector. This device detects the delivery of CO_2 after six breaths. Additional confirmation of the correct placement of the ETT must be obtained by using a capnography waveform.[5] This is a very reliable indicator of exhaled CO_2 and tracheal tube placement, because a perfusing cardiac rhythm is needed to deliver CO_2 to the lungs. During a cardiac arrest, CO_2 may not be present, and CO_2 may not be detected even if the ETT is in the correct location. Reexpansion of the bulb of the esophageal detector device indicates ETT placement.[10] A chest radiograph is obtained once the ETT is taped in place to confirm proper tube depth and the position.

Securing endotracheal and nasotracheal tubes. A small infant or child has less facial area for tape adherence for securing the tubes. A method with a low incidence of accidental extubation uses two pieces of cloth tape, split halfway down the middle, creating a Y shape (Fig. 38.4). The skin of a child is more fragile than that of an adult. Cloth tape may be irritating to the child's skin. A soft foam dressing (e.g., Mepilex) may be applied to the cheeks, with the securing tape attached to the top of the dressing. Breath sounds should be auscultated before and after taping or retaping of the tubing to ensure that the ETT position has not changed.[4] Commercially manufactured devices to secure ETTs are available, but these may be limited in infant and pediatric sizes. No single method of securing a tube has been identified as superior for minimizing ETT dislodgment.[10]

Endotracheal tube dislodgement. ETT dislodgment may occur more easily in an infant or young child and cause acute deterioration of the patient's condition. The tip of the ETT is pulled upward with neck extension or when the head is turned completely to the side. Conversely, the ETT moves downward with neck flexion. With the trachea of the young child being short, an ETT placed higher or lower may become dislodged or intubate the bronchus. ETT obstruction may occur with high placement, neck flexion, or head rotation, which may cause the bevel of the ETT to press against the tracheal wall, occluding the lumen. Secretions and mucus plugs may more easily occlude the lumen of a small-diameter ETT. Assessment of the tube by the bedside nurse is critical in the evaluation of proper functioning of the child's ETT.

Monitoring of the patient. The nurse and the respiratory therapist must ensure that the child's ETT remains patent and in correct placement to maintain correct oxygenation and ventilation. Causes of acute deterioration in an intubated pediatric patient may be remembered by using the mnemonic *DOPE*:[4]

*D*isplacement of the tube
*O*bstruction of the tube
*P*neumothorax (or other air leak)
*E*quipment failure

Suction equipment and a bag-valve mask need to be readily available for resuscitation if any of these intubation complications occur.

Mechanical Ventilation

Many types of unconventional mechanical ventilation (e.g., high-frequency, oscillation, jet ventilation) are used, but for most infants and children, standard means of positive-pressure ventilation support use volume- or pressure-controlled ventilators. The type of ventilation chosen depends on the child's size, minute ventilation requirements, and lung compliance. Newer ventilators need to have flow and pressure triggers that are sensitive enough to ventilate infants and children. The choice of ventilation mechanisms depends on the respiratory compliance of the child, the ability to breathe spontaneously, and the predicted clinical course of the underlying condition or disease.

Assessment of the child is very important, because the patient may not respond in the expected manner to the current ventilator settings, and a new mode needs to be instituted.[6,11] For the older child, non–continuous-flow, volume-limited ventilation in synchronized intermittent mandatory ventilation mode is used most often. Pressure support ventilation is also used in the child in conjunction with other modes to assist with spontaneous breathing, especially during the weaning process. Currently used ventilators have flow triggering designed for infants. This type of synchronized ventilation mode is used almost exclusively for the ventilation of infants and children. Box 38.3 outlines the characteristics for the ideal pediatric ventilator for the infant and child.[12]

Ventilator–patient asynchrony. Ventilator–patient asynchrony may have several causes. The Hering-Breuer reflex is a vagal reflex in which the child's sensing of positive lung inflation sets off immediate expiration and lung deflation stimulates inspiration. Apnea, or active expiration during the ventilator's inspiratory cycle, also may cause asynchrony. The use of adult

Equipment	GRAY* 3-5 kg	PINK Small Infant 6-7 kg	RED Infant 8-9 kg	PURPLE Toddler 10-11 kg	YELLOW Small Child 12-14 kg	WHITE Child 15-18 kg	BLUE Child 19-23 kg	ORANGE Large Child 24-29 kg	GREEN Adult 30-36 kg
Resuscitation bag		Infant/child	Infant/child	Child	Child	Child	Child	Child	Adult
Oxygen mask (NRB)		Pediatric	Pediatric	Pediatric	Pediatric	Pediatric	Pediatric	Pediatric	Pediatric/ adult
Oral airway (mm)		50	50	60	60	60	70	80	80
Laryngoscope blade (size)		1 Straight	1 Straight	1 Straight	2 Straight	2 Straight	2 Straight or curved	2 Straight or curved	3 Straight or curved
ET tube (mm)†		3.5 Uncuffed 3.0 Cuffed	3.5 Uncuffed 3.0 Cuffed	4.0 Uncuffed 3.5 Cuffed	4.5 Uncuffed 4.0 Cuffed	5.0 Uncuffed 4.5 Cuffed	5.5 Uncuffed 5.0 Cuffed	6.0 Cuffed	6.5 Cuffed
ET tube insertion length (cm)	3 kg 9-9.5 4 kg 9.5-10 5 kg 10-10.5	10.5-11	10.5-11	11-12	13.5	14-15	16.5	17-18	18.5-19.5
Suction catheter (F)		8	8	10	10	10	10	10	10-12
BP cuff	Neonatal #5/infant	Infant/child	Infant/child	Child	Child	Child	Child	Child	Small adult
IV catheter (ga)		22-24	22-24	20-24	18-22	18-22	18-20	18-20	16-20
IO (ga)		18/15	18/15	15	15	15	15	15	15
NG tube (F)		5-8	5-8	8-10	10	10	12-14	14-18	16-18
Urinary catheter (F)	5	8	8	8-10	10	10-12	10-12	12	12
Chest tube (F)		10-12	10-12	16-20	20-24	20-24	24-32	28-32	32-38

FIG. 38.3 Broselow Pediatric Color-Coded Resuscitation Tape. *BP*, Blood pressure; *ET*, endotracheal; *F*, French; *IO*, intraosseous; *IV*, intravenous; *NG*, nasogastric; *NRB*, nonrebreathing. *For Gray column, use Pink or Red equipment sizes if no size is listed. †Per 2010 AHA Guidelines, in the hospital, cuffed or uncuffed tubes may be used. (Adapted from Broselow Pediatric Emergency Tap. Distributed by Armstrong Medical Industries, Lincolnshire, IL. Copyright © 2017 Vital Signs, Inc. All rights reserved.)

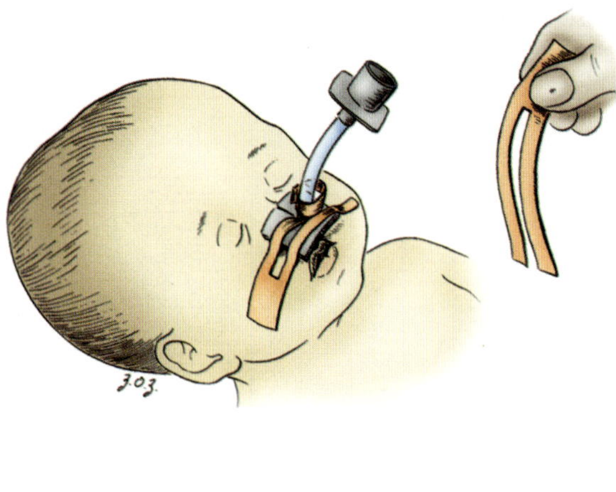

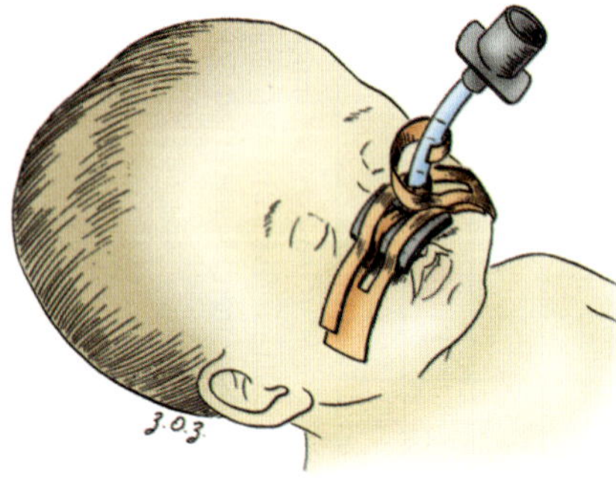

FIG. 38.4 Securing an Endotracheal Tube With Split Taping. (Modified from Kline-Tilford A, Sorce LR, Levin DL, et al. Pulmonary disorders. In: Hazinski MF, ed. *Nursing Care of the Critically Ill Child.* 3rd ed. Elsevier; 2013.)

ventilators not appropriately adapted for an infant or child may cause asynchrony. In a small child, decreased tidal volume and increased respiratory rates occur to cope with respiratory compromise. Adult ventilators may not sense rapidly enough, if at all, any spontaneous respiratory efforts, which leads to increased work of breathing in the child. Asynchrony may lead to poor oxygenation or volutrauma. Significant asynchrony may require sedation, alone or with neuromuscular blockade.

Weaning. Criteria for weaning and extubation are much more extensive for adults than for children, but some guidelines exist for these procedures. Synchronized intermittent mandatory ventilation with pressure support ventilation is used for weaning from positive-pressure ventilation. Pressure support ventilation allows the child to have greater control over breathing, and asynchrony is not a problem. Box 38.4 outlines the indicators for initiating weaning and extubation.[6,10] Supplemental oxygen may be supplied after extubation by a nasal cannula or a ventilation mask. Noninvasive ventilation devices such as nasal or facial CPAP, or heated high flow nasal cannula (HHFNC), may be an option for the patient, but if the child cannot be managed using these options, reintubation may be necessary.

Extubation complications. Postextubation croup may occur in small children. Manifestations arising from airway edema include hoarseness, stridor, or a crowing cough that begins immediately or up to 3 hours after extubation. Initial treatment consists of keeping the child calm. Procedures must be withheld, if possible, and crying must be prevented to avoid increasing airway resistance. Supplemental humidified oxygen should be administered to the child immediately after extubation, and a cool mist should continue to be provided. More severe symptoms may be treated with racemic epinephrine along with intravenous or inhaled steroid therapy. Intubation equipment and personnel qualified to intubate should be available after extubation in case the patient requires reintubation.

BOX 38.3 Characteristics of a Pediatric Ventilator

Specifications

- Volume, pressure, or time cycled; mixed modes of ventilation
- Assist/control, CPAP, PSV, SIMV
- Tidal volume range of 20–450 mL/breath (minute ventilation of 0.4–0.6 L/min)
- Respiratory rate of 1–1000/min (high-frequency ventilation capability is also desirable)
- Variable inspiratory flow of 0.5–40 L/min
- Variable inspiratory/expiratory flow ratios
- Adjustable peak inspiratory pressure of 10–80 cm H_2O
- Adequate humidification
- Provision for PEEP/CPAP

Visual Indicators

- Proximal airway pressure (patent airway)
- Proximal airway temperature (patent airway)
- FiO_2 (high and low)
- Inspiratory/expiratory times
- Flow rate (L/min)
- Tidal volume
- Minute ventilation

Alarms

- High and low pressure
- Apnea
- Loss of PEEP
- Power failure/disconnect
- Loss of air/oxygen
- High temperature
- Failure to cycle
- Output jacks to allow ventilator alarms to be connected to a remote alarm in nursing stations

CPAP, Continuous positive airway pressure; *FiO_2,* fraction of inspired oxygen; *PEEP,* positive end-expiratory pressure; *PSV,* pressure support ventilation; *SIMV,* synchronized intermittent mandatory ventilation.

Modified from Hazinski MF, ed. *Nursing Care of the Critically Ill Child.* 3rd ed. Elsevier; 2013.

BOX 38.4 Evidence-Based Practice

Indicators for Initiating Weaning of a Pediatric Patient

- Achievement of baseline mental status
- Presence of cough and gag reflexes
- Absence of fever
- Spontaneous respiratory effort
- Normal acid–base balance
- Oxyhemoglobin saturation ≥90% or PaO_2 ≥60 mm Hg (in the absence of cyanotic heart disease)
- FiO_2 <0.5
- PEEP <7 cm H_2O
- $PaCO_2$ <50 mm Hg
- Stable hemodynamically
- Stable ventilation support for ≥24 h
- No plans that will require significant sedation or operative procedures in the next 12 h

FiO_2, Fraction of inspired oxygen; *$PaCO_2$,* arterial partial pressure of carbon dioxide; *PaO_2,* arterial partial pressure of oxygen; *PEEP,* positive end-expiratory pressure.

From Hazinski MF, ed. *Nursing Care of the Critically Ill Child.* 3rd ed. Elsevier; 2013:483.

Tracheostomy

The tracheostomy has become an increasingly common procedure in children and can be an elective or an emergency

TABLE 38.5 Guidelines for Intubation Equipment and Tracheostomy Tubes for Pediatrics

	EQUIPMENT CHOICES BASED ON AGE AND WEIGHT							
	3 mo	6 mo	1 y	3 y	6 y	8 y	12 y	16 y
Factors	**6 kg**	**8 kg**	**10 kg**	**15 kg**	**20 kg**	**25 kg**	**40 kg**	**60 kg**
ETT size (mm)	3.0–3.5	3.5–4.0	4.0–4.5	4.5–5.0	5.0–5.5	6.0 c/u	7.0 c	7.0–8.0 c
Laryngoscope blade	0–1 s	0–1 s	1 s	2 s	2 s	2 s/c	3 s/c	3 s/c
Stylet (Fr)	6	6	6	6	14	14	14	14
Suction catheter (Fr)[a]	6–8	8	8	8–10	10	10–12	12–14	12–14
Shiley Tracheostomy								
Shiley size (mm)	0	1	1–12	4	4	4	6	6
Internal diameter (mm ID)	3.4	3.7	3.7–4.1	5	5	5	7	7
Length (cm)	4	4.1	4.1–4.2	4.6	4.6	4.6	6.7	6.7

[a]Catheter size twice the ID size of any tracheal tube.

c/u, Cuffed or uncuffed; *ETT*, endotracheal tube; *Fr*, French sizing; *ID*, internal diameter; *s/c*, straight or curved.

Data from Hazinski MF, ed. *Nursing Care of the Critically Ill Child.* 3rd ed. Elsevier; 2013.

procedure. It also can be combined with mechanical ventilation.[7] Some reasons for having a tracheotomy performed include upper airway obstruction caused by anatomic abnormalities, the anticipated need for prolonged ventilation as children with chronic diseases are living longer, or the need for effective pulmonary hygeine.[13] Children who have had a tracheostomy need to be closely monitored for complications such as hemorrhage, edema, aspiration, accidental decannulation, tube obstruction, and the entrance of free air into the pleural cavity.[7]

Several types of tracheostomy tubes are available for children; the plastic, single-cannula type is the most popular for in-hospital care because it has few complications. Silastic tubes have been recommended for the infant and the child because they are pliable and bend with tracheal movement. Uncuffed tubes usually are preferred for pediatric patients to prevent subglottic stenosis.[14] The diameter of the tracheostomy tube should be carefully selected to avoid any damage to the tracheal wall, to minimize the work of breathing, and to promote translaryngeal airflow, when possible. Occlusion of the tracheostomy tube can be a life-threatening event and is a greater risk to infants and children than adult patients due to the smaller diameter of the tube. Maintaining the patency of the tracheotomy tube is accomplished with suctioning and routine tube changes to prevent the formation of crusting in the tube.[13] Table 38.5 describes tracheostomy tube sizes for infants and children.

Bronchiolitis

Bronchiolitis is an inflammation of the small airways in the lungs, called the bronchioles. It is primarily caused by viral infections, with the respiratory syncytial virus (RSV) being the most common causative agent. However, other viruses, such as parainfluenza, adenovirus, and rhinovirus, can also cause bronchiolitis. Bronchiolitis affects the lower respiratory tract and results in obstruction of the small airways.

Bronchiolitis is one of the diseases that primarily affects very young infants and is the most common disease in infants and children younger than 2 years of age.[15] Although this disease has a relatively low mortality rate (200 to 500 deaths per year), it is the most frequent cause of hospitalization in the infant population.[15] Bronchiolitis is one of the most common diagnoses in children who present in the hospital and critical care units with respiratory failure.[16]

Respiratory Syncytial Virus

RSV causes annual epidemics of acute respiratory illness in children ranging from mild respiratory disease to severe lower respiratory disease including bronchiolitis and pneumonia.[17] The peak incidence for viral bronchiolitis occurs during midwinter and into early spring. RSV is highly contagious and may be spread by close contact through droplets. RSV infection has an overall low mortality rate, but the mortality rate is 37% among infected infants with congenital heart disease. In children younger than 2 years of age, 40% of RSV infections may progress to lower respiratory infections.[15] Recent data suggest that up to 30% of infants are infected with two or more viruses.[6] Patients with cystic fibrosis or bronchopulmonary dysplasia or who are immunocompromised are also at greater risk for more serious disease and for occurrence beyond 1 year of age. Meticulous handwashing by clinical staff is the most important step to prevent hospital-acquired infections in other patients or staff members.[18]

Children who have had a hospital admission for RSV bronchiolitis are three times more likely to also have a diagnosis of lower lung dysfunction at 6 years old and a higher incidence of asthma at 13 years and 18 years old.[19] The chance of recovery from RSV may be excellent; however many children develop recurrent respiratory symptoms post infection. This is thought to be in part from the loss of cilia from the airway epithelial surfaces during the acute illness as the epithelium is replaced with nonciliated tissue.[19]

Pathophysiology

The virus typically enters the respiratory tract through inhalation or direct contact. Once the virus infects the epithelial cells lining the bronchioles, it induces a local inflammatory response. This response brings white blood cells to the infected area, leading to swelling and inflammation of the bronchioles. Infected epithelial cells may die and slough off, contributing to luminal obstruction. The inflammatory process also stimulates mucus production. The accumulation of mucus, combined with cellular debris from the inflammation, can block the small bronchioles.

The disease is characterized by mucosal edema, inflammation, increased mucus production, and sloughing of epithelial cells. Obstruction of the bronchioles occurs, resulting in hypoxemia and hypercapnia.[15] Widespread fine end-inspiratory crackles and an expiratory wheeze are heard on auscultation. This clinical pattern may be seen during the first year of life, with most hospital admissions occurring within the first 6 months of life.[15]

Pathologic pulmonary dynamics involve lung hyperinflation almost two times normal. Obstruction occurs in a patchy distribution with complete obstruction, leading to atelectasis and partial obstruction, which results in hyperinflation. Inspiratory resistance and expiratory resistance are present, along with ventilation–perfusion mismatch, which leads to hypoxemia and some degree of CO_2 retention. The probable mechanism in addition to the ventilation–perfusion mismatch is hypoventilation, which results from a marked increase in the work of breathing in the infant.[6]

Assessment

The first symptoms to appear are symptoms of an upper respiratory tract infection—sneezing and rhinorrhea. In many cases, a family member has had a respiratory illness. After 2 to 3 days, respiratory distress ensues with increased respirations, coughing, nasal flaring, chest retractions, wheezing, irritability, and feeding difficulties. Fever and lung rhonchi may or may not occur. After bronchiolar obstruction has occurred, patients present with increased work of breathing. This may lead to muscle fatigue and respiratory failure if the work of breathing exceeds the capacity of the patient's respiratory muscles. Infants tolerate respiratory loads poorly and are susceptible to fatigue because of the immature pattern of their muscle fibers.[20]

Management

The overall treatment for bronchiolitis is supportive. Oxygen continues to be the primary therapy to decrease the work of breathing and oxygen demands. Depending on the severity of illness, the infant may receive supplemental humidified oxygen by mask, HFNC, or mechanical ventilation.[6,21]

High-flow nasal cannula. HFNC is a frequently used modality for noninvasive respiratory support in the management of acute respiratory distress due to bronchiolitis. This therapy helps to decrease work of breathing by matching flow rates to the inspiratory demand of the child and washing out the carbon dioxide in the nasopharyngeal dead space, which will improve oxygenation by creating a reservoir of oxygen in the nasopharynx. The HFNC device is being used across care settings, including the critical care units, emergency rooms, and some care units to deliver a high gas flow rate of greater than 2 L/min. The starting flow rates are determined on the child's weight and starting flow rates are 2 L/kg/min for <12 kg patient to a maximum of 50 L/kg/min for a patient weighting >50 kg.[22] In addition, there are recommended guidelines for a weight-based approach for delivering HFNC and suggested clinical thresholds for weaning and discontinuing the HFNC when the patient's FiO_2 is <0.40 and there is no severe respiratory distress.[22]

Lack of efficacy of medications. RSV causes airway obstruction, and no medication therapy has demonstrated an ability to rapidly reduce this obstruction. Suctioning of the airways will be required to help alleviate the signs and symptoms of airway obstruction from mucous secretions. The mucus will be thick and initially cause the infant to be suctioned frequently. Inhaled beta-2 agonists, anticholinergic agents, and corticosteroids during the acute or recovery phase have been tried with various degrees of success.[15] The evidence found in the literature shows the use of a clinical pathway for the treatment of bronchiolitis to be effective. A decrease in the use of therapies such as bronchodilators, glucocorticoids, antibiotics, and chest physiotherapy and a decrease in admission rates and length of stay have occurred in association with the use of a bronchiolitis clinical pathway.[15]

RSV prophylaxis. The current recommendation from the American Academy of Pediatrics for the prevention of RSV is administration of the monoclonal antibody palivizumab (Synagis; MedImmune). Clinicians may administer palivizumab prophylactically to selected high-risk infants and children within the first year of life. This prophylaxis is recommended for infants born before 29 weeks, 0 days of gestation. The treatment is not recommended for otherwise healthy infants born after 29 weeks. Within the first year of life, this prophylaxis is recommended for preterm infants with chronic lung disease of prematurity, defined as birth at less than 32 weeks of age, with an oxygen requirement of greater than 21% for at least 28 days at birth.[18] Palivizumab is administered in five monthly doses, 15 mg/kg per dose administered intramuscularly, during the RSV season, usually beginning in November or December.[18] Administration of more than five doses is not recommended within the continental United States. In 2023, a new vaccine was created for the protection against severe RSV disease. The Centers for Disease Control and Prevention, CDC, have taken their strongest position on recommending this new RSV immunization to infants entering or born during the RSV season due to the fact that RSV is the leading cause for infant hospitalization in the United States.[23]

Status Asthmaticus

Asthma is a chronic inflammatory disorder of the airways in which many cells and cellular elements, including mast cells, eosinophils, T lymphocytes, neutrophils, and epithelial cells, play a role.[24] An acute asthma exacerbation is an event of progressive wheezing, cough, chest tightness, shortness of breath, or a combination of all these symptoms. Asthma is identified as the disease with a triad of physiologic processes—airway inflammation, edema, and airway hyperactivity. Inflammation has been recognized as the primary underlying cause in the pathogenesis of this disease.[24]The treatment for asthma is aimed at decreasing and reducing airway inflammation.

Pathophysiology

The universal feature of the inflammatory response in asthma includes the activation and infiltration of the airway by cells. The early phase in the inflammation reaction is caused by a trigger, and this may be different with each child. The immediate response to this trigger is bronchospasm and smooth muscle contraction caused by the mediators from the various inflammatory cells in the airway. If this early phase is not responsive to beta-2 agonists, a late phase will occur approximately 6 to 9 hours after the initial exposure to the trigger.[24] This will lead to increased release of the mediator cells in the airway and produce cellular infiltration, airway edema, mucus secretions, bronchospasm, and smooth muscle contraction. Without treatment, atelectasis and mucus plugging may occur in the child.

SOCIAL DETERMINANTS OF HEALTH

Health Disparities Associated in Children With Asthma

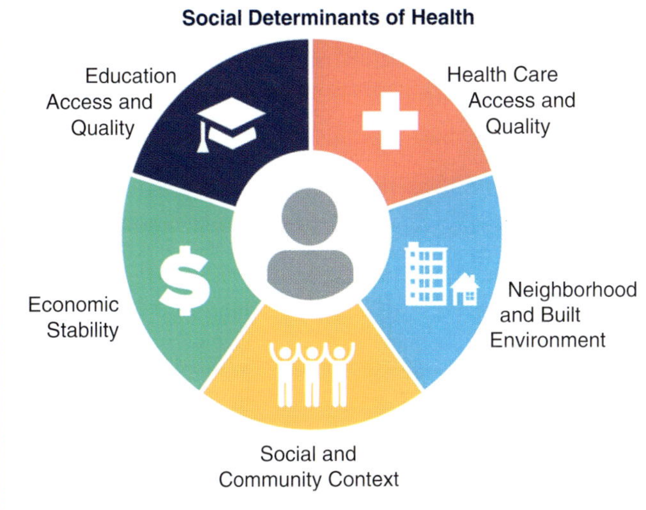

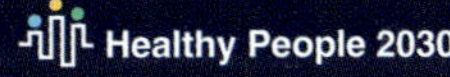

Asthma impacts those with the disease in many ways that may differ by demographic group and can change over time. Among children, asthma is more common for males than females; blacks and American Indian/Alaska Natives have the highest asthma rates compared to other racial and ethnic groups. Children ages 5 to 17 years old have the highest prevalence rates and those less than 5 years of age have the highest asthma attack rates compared to other age groups. Lastly, 2.2 million children missed more than 7.9 million school days in 2018 as the result of their asthma disease.[1] The American Academy of Pediatrics reported that 27.7% of children under the age of 18 years live below the poverty level; of that, 30.7% are White, non-Hispanic; 43.1 % are Black; 41.7% are Hispanic (any race); and 29.3% are Asian, with a single mother.[2]

The American Lung Association launched a *Little Airways, Little Voices* initiative that explores current and future treatments in childhood asthma. According to the reports, asthma disparities and barriers to diagnosis, treatment, and prevention impact children's lives. It also examines the need for new treatment options that reduce asthma symptoms, have fewer asthma symptoms, have fewer side effects, and allow children to participate in more activities.[1]

It is known that outpatient screening for social determinants of health (SDOH) improve patient referral to and use of appropriate resources. Researchers recounted that hospitalization serves as an opportunity for SDOH screening and linkage to; resources. However, providers actually screening for determinants are in the minority. SDOH identified in their study include access to health care and/or insurance; housing, housing conditions, and/or utilities; abuse (physical, psychological, sexual, neglect); language barriers; parent education/literacy; transportation barriers; school and/or school services; food insecurity; income source; and community violence.[3]

Strategies to improve these disparities include the development of:

- SDOH screening in all health care settings: outpatient, primary care, hospitals, schools, emergency departments, and urgent care centers
- Public policies to expand access to care, increase economic stability, improve education, and enhance the physical environment
- Interventions to enhance culturally competent clinical management, expanded adoption of childhood asthma education and outreach programs, and initiation of community-based partnerships
- Adopt existing pediatric asthma guidelines and protocols
- Additional research to identify and test models of care

1. https://www.lung.org/research/trends-in-lung-disease/asthma
2. https://www.childstats.gov/americanchildren/tables/health8a.asp
3. Schwartz B, Herrmann LE, Librizzi J, et al. Screening for social determinants of health in hospitalized children. *Hospital Pediatrics* 2020;10(1):29–36.

Illustration from Healthy People 2030, U.S. Department of Health and Human Services, Office of Disease Prevention and Health Promotion. Retrieved September 8, 2022, from https://health.gov/healthypeople/objectives-and-data/social-determinants-health.

Assessment and Diagnosis

Assessing severe asthma in an infant is different compared with assessment in an older child because of the anatomic and physiologic differences between them. Physiologic changes may progress rapidly to respiratory failure in the infant. Table 38.6 outlines guidelines for classifying the severity of an asthma exacerbation. A moderate asthma episode requires hospitalization with close monitoring. In a severe event, the child may be able to speak only in short phrases or not at all. The position of comfort or degree of agitation should be noted; sitting upright and unable to lie down indicates severe distress.[25] A severe episode requires critical care, with intubation and ventilation equipment readily available.[6]

Management

Standard treatment for a pediatric patient who has asthma includes receiving oxygen, beta-adrenergic therapy, corticosteroids, and anticholinergic medications, as indicated.[6,24] Pharmacologic therapy is based on the concept of reducing airway inflammation. The child and family should be informed of the management approach and plan of care. If properly and effectively treated, pediatric patients who have status asthmaticus may return to their usual state of health, but they will require close follow-up by a pediatrician or pulmonologist.[24]

Beta-adrenergic agonist and anticholinergic medications. Beta-adrenergic agonists are the first-line agents in the treatment of asthma. Beta-agonist medications that are selective for beta-2 receptors on airway smooth muscle (e.g., albuterol, levalbuterol) are preferred to avoid the stimulation of the beta-1 cardiac receptors.[24] These medications are given by nebulization intermittently or continuously. Anticholinergic medications in conjunction with beta-agonists improve pulmonary function in children, especially school-age patients.[24] These medications may decrease bronchomotor tone and secretions. The most commonly administered inhaled anticholinergic is ipratropium bromide. This medication works synergistically with beta-agonists to improve and prolong bronchodilation. Ipratropium bromide should be administered with albuterol in a nebulizer and not given alone.

Corticosteroid medications. Corticosteroids are also an important part of the treatment for airway inflammation. Corticosteroids may be administered orally or parenterally. Both methods are equally efficacious in the treatment of asthma.[24] The peak effect for corticosteroids is virtually the same with either route. Treatment for asthma should not have to be delayed because of a lack of intravenous access in a pediatric patient. The corticosteroid of choice is a glucocorticoid (e.g., prednisone, prednisolone, methylprednisolone).

Intravenous magnesium sulfate. Intravenous magnesium sulfate is administered to pediatric patients as an adjunct therapy,

TABLE 38.6 Guidelines for Assessing Severe Asthma in Infants and Children

	PHYSICAL FINDINGS		
Assessment Area	**Infant**	**Child**	**Discussion Points**
Respiratory rate	Increase of >50% above normal	Can range from normal to >95th percentile for age	Sleeping rates in infants and resting rates in children are good measures of obstruction; awake or activity rates are too variable.
Level of consciousness	Decreased	May be decreased	Assess response to parents and pain.
Accessory muscle use	Retractions in less-than-severe states	Severe intercostal, tracheosternal, and sternocleidomastoid retractions and nasal flaring	In infants, compliant chest wall produces retractions earlier in course. In children, retractions and flaring correlate well with degree of obstruction and with PEF <50% of predicted for age.
Color	Pallor, grayness, or cyanosis	Possible cyanosis	
Dyspnea		Can speak only single words or short phrases; cannot count to 10 in one breath	Infants and children are drowsy or confused.
Quality of cry	Softer and shorter as FEV_1 decreases		
Oxygen saturation	<90% in less-than-severe states	<90% on room air	Infants have greater ventilation–perfusion mismatch. In children, hypoxemia correlates well with degree of obstruction.
Auscultation (breath sounds)	Wheezing; becoming inaudible because of decreased air movement	Same as in infant	Presence and volume of wheezing is the least sensitive predictor of obstruction.
$PaCO_2$	If >50 mm Hg or if rising 5–10 mm Hg/h, consider mechanical ventilation	Can range from <40 mm Hg with respiratory distress to >40 mm Hg as air movement significantly decreases	$PaCO_2$ is best measure of ventilation in infants. Continually rising $PaCO_2$ of >40 mm Hg in a child occurs when PEF is <20% of predicted for age. Hypercapnia develops more readily in young children than adults.
PEF	≥70%		PEF is not needed in cases of severe asthmatic exacerbation. This is used after asthma is under control.
Feeding/sucking ability	Decreased or absent		

FEV1, Forced expiratory volume in 1 second; *$PaCO_2$*, arterial partial pressure of carbon dioxide; *PEF*, peak expiratory flow.
Data from Bolick B, Madden M, Severin P, et al., eds. *Pediatric Acute Care: A Guide For Interprofessional Practice.* 2nd ed. Elsevier, 2021

as it provides smooth muscle relaxation to patients with severe or life-threatening asthma events to decrease inflammation and improve pulmonary function.[25] Magnesium is a physiologic calcium antagonist, which has a direct effect on the calcium uptake in the muscle, causing smooth muscle relaxation.[6] Magnesium sulfate (25 to 75 mg/kg/dose, maximum dose 2000 mg) is administered intravenously, usually over 20 minutes.[26]

Heliox. Critical care management of a child with status asthmaticus involves humidified oxygen to maintain an oxygen saturation of more than 95%, combined with the pharmacologic therapies. Heliox is a mixture of 79% helium and 21% oxygen, which makes this mixture lighter than air. This mixture should be delivered using a Heliox flowmeter.[20] Administration of heliox is effective in decreasing airway resistance and in decreasing the work of breathing. Heliox can be administered via nasal cannula, high flow nasal cannula, nonrebreathing mask, and both invasive and noninvasive ventilation devices.[20] The use of heliox does not appear to have adverse effects, and its administration may improve the status of the child.[20]

Ventilation. The use of noninvasive positive-pressure ventilation by means of nasal prongs or a facemask may avoid the need for intubation. Some indications for considering mechanical ventilation are respiratory muscle fatigue, markedly diminished or absent breath sounds, pulsus paradoxus greater than 20 to 40 mm Hg, deterioration in mental status, and arterial partial pressure of oxygen (PaO_2) less than 70 mm Hg on 100% FiO_2.[24]

SARS-CoV-2

Starting in 2019, this novel virus, COVID-19, rapidly spread throughout the world, resulting in a pandemic. The spectrum of this virus is from asymptomatic infection to severe pneumonia with acute respiratory distress and multiorgan failure with the children requiring critical care support. Underlying conditions are associated with an increased rate of hospitalization and intensive care admissions. Infants less than 1 year have also been associated with increased rates of hospitalization. Having multiple underlying health conditions is also associated with an increased risk of severe disease. In studies of children admitted to intensive care units with COVID-19–related illness, most but not all the children presented with one or more underlying condition. The most common conditions include chronic pulmonary disease, obesity, neurologic and developmental conditions, and cardiovascular conditions.[27,28] Approximately one-third of

TABLE 38.7 **Modified Glasgow Coma Scale for Infants and Children**[a]

	Child	Infant	Score
Eye opening	Spontaneous	Spontaneous	4
	To verbal stimuli	To verbal stimuli	3
	To pain only	To pain only	2
	No response	No response	1
Verbal response	Oriented, appropriate	Coos and babbles	5
	Confused	Irritable cries	4
	Inappropriate words	Cries to pain	3
	Incomprehensible words or nonspecific sounds	Moans to pain	2
	No response	No response	1
Motor response	Obeys command (e.g., child holds up two fingers, wiggles toes, or sticks out tongue)	Moves spontaneously and purposefully	6
	Localizes painful stimulus (e.g., child reaches for hand that is rubbing sternum or pinching trapezius)	Withdraws to touch	5
	Withdraws in response to pain (e.g., child adducts each extremity when medial aspect is pinched)	Withdraws in response to pain	4
	Flexion in response to pain (e.g., decorticate posturing when sternum is rubbed or trapezius muscle pinched)	Decorticate posturing (abnormal flexion) in response to pain	3
	Extension in response to pain (e.g., decerebrate posturing when sternum rubbed or trapezius pinched)	Decerebrate posturing (abnormal extension) in response to pain	2
	No response (flaccid)	No response (flaccid)	1

[a]Modifications in parentheses from Milonovich L, Eichler V. Neurological disorders. In: Hazinski MF, ed. *Nursing Care of the Critically Ill Child.* 3rd ed. Elsevier; 2013:587.
Data from Tasker RC. Head and spinal cord trauma. In Nichols DG, ed. *Rodgers Textbook of Pediatric Intensive Care.* 4th ed. Philadelphia: Lippincott Williams & Wilkins, 2008; originally proposed in Morray JP, et al. Coma scale for use in brain-injured children. *Crit Care Med.* 1984;12:1018.

the children with COVID-19 had severe disease that required an intensive care or stepdown unit for care, required invasive mechanical ventilation, or had an in-hospital death.[28]

Multisystem inflammatory syndrome in children (MIS-C) is a rare but serious condition that is associated with COVID-19.[27] The clinical features of MIS-C may be similar to those of Kawasaki disease, Kawasaki disease shock syndrome, or toxic short syndrome. The clinical presentation is of persistent fever, hypotension, gastrointestinal symptoms, rash, myocarditis, and laboratory findings associated with increased inflammatory markers, but respiratory symptoms may not be present. Treatment has consisted of supportive measures that are directed against the inflammatory process. These measures have included fluid resuscitation, inotropic support, respiratory support, if needed, and in rare cases extracorporeal membranous oxygenation. The antiinflammatory medications have included the use of intravenous gamma globin, IVIG, and steroids. Aspirin has been part of the treatment due to the concern for coronary artery involvement.

NEUROLOGICAL SYSTEM

The nervous system grows rapidly before birth, and growth continues during infancy and childhood. Compared with an adult, an infant or toddler's head size is proportionally larger than the rest of the body. When infants fall, the head usually leads, and a significant head injury may occur.[4]

Anatomy and Physiology

The skull is more flexible because the skull bones are not fused and are separated by spaces called *fontanels*. The anterior fontanel is the junction of the coronal, sagittal, and frontal sutures, whereas the posterior fontanel is the junction of the parietal and occipital bones. By age 3 months, the posterior fontanel is usually closed, and the anterior fontanel is closed by age 20 months. The brain of a young child has a high water content and contains less myelin compared with the brain of an adult. This makes the child's brain more homogeneous and less compartmentalized.[4] Shear hemorrhages and diffuse brain injuries are more common in children than in adults. Spinal cord injuries are less common in children than in adults because the spine of the child is elastic, and the vertebrae are less likely to fracture. However, in children with head injuries or multisystem trauma, spinal cord injuries should always be suspected until ruled out.[4]

Cerebral blood flow and oxygen consumption are increased in childhood in relation to increased metabolic needs. Hyperemia, tissue hypoxia, and acidosis result in cerebral arterial dilation and increased cerebral blood flow. Hyperventilation decreases cerebral blood flow, but severe hypercarbia may result in decreased oxygen consumption and use. Normal cerebral perfusion pressure (CPP) values in children are unknown. It is thought that CPP should be in the range of 40 to 60 mm Hg, but this figure may vary, because perfusion is determined by blood flow and not by blood pressure.[4] CPP must be maintained at a level to maintain blood flow. A patient with a normal CPP does not necessarily have effective cerebral perfusion.

Assessment

Cognitive function cannot be evaluated until the preschool and early childhood years, but level of consciousness, movement, and pupils can be evaluated in pediatric patients. The Glasgow Coma Scale (GCS) is used for older children and has been modified for use in infants and younger children (Table 38.7). Survival and recovery of a patient with a GCS score of 5 to 8 are better for children than for adults.[4] Evaluation of reflexes in children is similar to that in adults, with a couple of exceptions. Although a positive Babinski reflex is an abnormal response in adults, this response is normal in children until age 1 year.[7] In the first few months of life, grasp is reflexive in an infant. With severe neurologic disease or injury, grasp may revert to a reflex as opposed to a purposeful response, and the grasp response may not indicate improvement of the child's neurologic status.

Responsiveness

Responsiveness in a pediatric patient should be evaluated in relation to the child's age, clinical condition, and changes in responsiveness over time. Infants and children should always respond to their parents or caregivers and to a painful stimulus. A decrease in responsiveness is abnormal and should be investigated.[4] If the child is older than 2 years, the ability to follow commands may be assessed by asking him or her to hold up two fingers or wiggle the toes. This action is not accomplished by a reflex action.

Motor Function

When a child is unconscious, the most important component of the GCS to assess is the motor function.[4] The patient's central and peripheral responses to a painful stimulus need to be assessed. A central stimulus is applied to the head and trunk above the nipple line. The peripheral stimulus may be assessed at the medial aspect of each extremity. The patient's best response is the one that is recorded for the GCS score.

Signs of Increased Intracranial Pressure

Signs of increased ICP in pediatric patients include a change in responsiveness, a deterioration in the ability to follow commands, a change in the response to pain, and pupil dilation with light stimulation.[4] The Cushing triad sign of an increased ICP may be observed only during cerebral herniation and should not be used as an early indicator of ICP. If any neurologic deterioration is detected in a pediatric patient, a complete neurologic assessment is required, including the child's vital signs and consultation with the patient's physician.

Seizures

Seizures are brief manifestations of the brain's electrical system that result from cortical neuronal discharge. Regardless of the etiology, the basic mechanism of a seizure is the same. Abnormal electrical discharge may arise from central areas of the brain that may affect consciousness. This activity may be restricted to one area of the cerebral cortex or spread to other portions of the brain. Seizures are the most commonly observed neurologic deficit in children and may occur with various central nervous system conditions. The symptoms depend on the origin of the electrical location in the brain (Box 38.5). At least 8% of the general population will experience one or more seizures in their lifetime, and approximately 1% will develop epilepsy, involving recurring seizures.[29]

Etiology

The incidence of causative factors that are associated with seizures in children is related to the child's age. In infants, the most common factors are related to birth traumas (i.e., anoxia, congenital defects, intracranial bleeds).[29] A febrile seizure is the most common form of childhood seizures, with an occurrence rate of 2% to 5% of all children. In children who are older than 3 years, the most common cause of seizures is idiopathic epilepsy.[29]As children enter adolescence, hormonal and metabolic changes may alter the seizure threshold. A child who is in an unconscious state must be evaluated for a history of seizures because unconsciousness may be the result of a postictal state.

BOX 38.5 Causes of Seizures in Children

Nonrecurrent (Acute)	Recurrent (Chronic)
• Febrile episodes	• Idiopathic epilepsy
• Intracranial infection	• Epilepsy resulting from:
• Intracranial hemorrhage	• Trauma
• Space-occupying lesions (cyst, tumor)	• Hemorrhage
• Acute cerebral edema	• Anoxia
• Anoxia	• Infections
• Toxins	• Toxins
• Drugs	• Degenerative phenomena
• Tetanus	• Congenital defects
• Lead (encephalopathy)	• Parasitic brain disease
• *Shigella, Salmonella*	• Hypoglycemic injury
• Metabolic alterations	• Epilepsy—sensory stimulus
• Hypocalcemia	• Epilepsy—stimulating states
• Hypoglycemia	• Narcolepsy and catalepsy
• Hyponatremia or hypernatremia	• Psychogenic causes
• Hypomagnesemia	• Tetany from hypocalcemia, alkalosis
• Alkalosis	
• Disorders of amino acid metabolism	• Hypoglycemic states
• Deficiency states	• Hyperinsulinism
• Hyperbilirubinemia	• Hypopituitarism
	• Adrenocortical insufficiency
	• Hepatic disorders
	• Uremia
	• Allergy
	• Cardiovascular dysfunction or syncopal episodes
	• Migraine

Modified from Hockenberry M, Wilson D, Rodgers C, eds. *Wong's Essentials of Pediatric Nursing.* 11th ed. Elsevier; 2022.

Nursing Management

Nursing management of seizures includes providing a safe environment for the child, monitoring respiratory status and perfusion, assessing for the cause of the seizure, determining methods to prevent additional seizures, and documenting the seizure activity. Children admitted to the critical care unit may require intubation for respiratory complications of seizures, for the sedative effects of anticonvulsants, or for status epilepticus. Anticonvulsant therapy may be indicated for prolonged or recurrent seizures. The primary therapy for seizure disorders is administration of the appropriate antiepileptic medication or a combination of medications to provide the desired effort without causing undesirable side efforts. Medications that may be used for a child with seizures include phenobarbital, phenytoin (Dilantin), levetiracetam (Keppra), fosphenytoin, and benzodiazepines (lorazepam, diazepam).[29]

Status Epilepticus

Status epilepticus is a medical emergency that requires immediate intervention to prevent possible brain injury or death.[29] This condition is characterized by two or more unprovoked seizures that may be caused by a variety of pathologic processes in the brain.[29] Causes may include high fever, meningitis, encephalitis, metabolic disorders, and abrupt cessation of anticonvulsant medications. Cerebral blood flow, metabolic requirements, and oxygen needs all increase when a seizure occurs. A video electroencephalogram is required to confirm status epilepticus in patients in a deep coma or with pharmacologic paralysis.

Magnetic resonance imaging may be performed to evaluate the brain for any anatomic abnormalities. The goal of treatment is to control the seizures or reduce their frequency and severity, to discover the correct cause of the seizures, or to evaluate the child for possible epilepsy surgery.[29] This will allow the child to live as normal a life as possible. Treatment includes short-term administration of benzodiazepines such as diazepam, lorazepam, or midazolam. The critical care nurse should assess and evaluate the child to ensure that the patient has a patent airway, adequate ventilation effort, adequate oxygenation, and systemic perfusion. Clinical documentation should contain the patient's neurologic assessment, including the seizure manifestation and duration. With rapid treatment of the seizures, it may be possible to prevent neuronal damage, systemic complications, and even death from status epilepticus.[30]

Bacterial Meningitis

Meningitis is an acute inflammation of the meninges, the outer covering of the brain and spinal cord, and cerebrospinal fluid. The pathogens usually come from a distant site and colonize. They enter the bloodstream, producing sepsis, and they invade the meninges.[31] The highest incidence is found among infants younger than age 1 year. Meningococcal meningitis is readily transmitted by droplet infection from nasopharyngeal secretions. The risk of transmission increases with the number of contacts. This may occur most frequently in school-age children or adolescents.[29]

Assessment

The clinical manifestations of bacterial meningitis include fever, chills, headache, vomiting, irritability or lethargy, photophobia, nuchal rigidity, and a positive Kernig (pain with extension of the legs) or Brudzinski sign (flexion of the neck stimulates flexion at the knees and hips).

One of the most dramatic and serious complications usually associated with meningococcal infection is meningococcal sepsis or meningococcemia. When the onset is severe and sudden, it is known as *Waterhouse-Friderichsen syndrome.* This syndrome is characterized by overwhelming septic shock, disseminated intravascular coagulation, massive bilateral adrenal hemorrhage, and purpura.[29] Meningococcemia requires emergency treatment and critical care because of the high mortality rate.[29] The late stages of this disease may produce increased ICP and cardiovascular collapse. Symptoms in infants are less specific and may include lethargy, vomiting, bulging fontanels, hypothermia or hyperthermia, diarrhea, and poor feeding.

Nursing Management

Nursing management must include early recognition and immediate start of therapies to prevent possible disabilities. Initial management includes use of isolation precautions, initiation of antibiotic therapy, maintenance of ventilation and hydration, reduction of increased ICP, management of systemic shock, control of seizures and temperature, and provision of family education and support.[29] Because of the sudden nature of the illness, emotional support of the child and parents is extremely important. Parents frequently feel guilty for not having suspected the seriousness of this disease. They should be kept informed about their child's progress and all procedures and results.[29] The complications of bacterial meningitis may include the development of hearing loss, hydrocephalus, loss of digits or parts of extremities, and possible death. The long-term effect on infants manifests as communicating hydrocephalus; in the older child, the effects are related to the inflammatory process or vasculitis associated with the disease. Hearing impairment is the most common sequela of this disease.[29] Evaluation of the child's hearing for possible hearing loss is needed for at least 6 months after the infection.

TRAUMA

Any experience a child perceives as threatening has long-term consequences for the child's holistic health and qualities as a trauma. If the experience is traumatic, the outcome will depend on the three E's of trauma: the event, the experience of the event, and the effects. Traumatic events can affect an infant or child's development and possibly have repercussions for their lifetime.[32]

Unintentional injury is the leading cause of death in children between ages 1 and 17 years. The number of children in this age range dying of their injuries is higher compared with the total number of pediatric patients dying of the next nine leading causes.[3] Current evidence suggests that most injured children are not being treated in pediatric trauma centers. Approximately 47% of pediatric trauma care occurs in nontrauma centers.[33] The best outcome after pediatric trauma occurs when the clinical team is prepared and knowledgeable about the unique aspects of the injured child.[9] Much of the anxiety of taking care of injured pediatric patients is eliminated by having instruments, equipment, and medication dosages carefully precalculated. One effective practice in many centers is the use of the Broselow tape that is color coded for specific weight groups of infants and children for weight-based equipment sizing and medication dosing (see Fig. 38.3).

Head Trauma

Describe the causes, classification, complications, and management of head trauma in children.

Head trauma in pediatric patients is due to closed head injuries resulting from motor vehicle accidents, bicycle crashes, falls, or child abuse.[34] During infancy and childhood, the head is proportionally larger compared with the rest of the body. As a result, a child may be propelled headfirst in unrestrained crashes, causing acceleration–deceleration injuries when their heads hit objects. Child abuse resulting from blunt trauma to the head or from shaking is the leading cause of head injury among infants and young children.[34]

Traumatic brain injury (TBI) is the leading cause of childhood death and disability in developing nations. In the United States, 435,000 children visit the emergency department each year because of head trauma; of these patients, 37,000 require hospitalization.[35]Morbidity and mortality associated with head trauma are attributed to injury suffered in two distinct phases: the *primary* phase and the *secondary* phase.

Primary Phase

The primary phase of injury occurs at the moment of impact, when the mechanical forces cause direct disruption of the brain parenchyma. Primary injuries may be focal or diffuse in nature. Examples of focal brain injuries include intracranial contusion and extraaxial hemorrhage (epidural, subdural, or subarachnoid hemorrhage). Diffuse brain injury is typically produced by acceleration or deceleration forces that result in shear trauma at the interface of the white and gray matter.[35]

Secondary Phase

The secondary phase of injury comprises sequelae of local and systemic events triggered by the primary injury. The three basic mechanisms leading to secondary brain injury are ischemia, energy failure, and excitotoxicity resulting in cell death.[35] Other factors that may contribute to secondary brain injury include axonal injury and death, cerebral edema, and ICP abnormalities.[35]

Classification of Head Injuries

Head injuries are classified on the basis of the GCS score for the patient: mild injuries with a GCS score of 13 to 15, which may be associated with brief loss of consciousness, disorientation, headache, or vomiting; moderate TBI with a GCS score of 9 to 12; and severe TBI with a GCS score of less than 8. Patients with moderate or severe TBI typically have more significant symptoms compared with symptoms seen with mild TBI and abnormal brain imaging. Children with severe TBI need to be admitted to a critical care unit for aggressive management and treatment of increased ICP.[34] Several studies on children with severe TBI have reported that the ICP remains greater than 20 mm Hg despite initial therapies and protocols to address the ICP. In cases as these, more aggressive interventions maybe indicated,[34] and therapy should be directed to maintain ICP below this level (20 mm Hg).

Management

Treatment goals include measures to ensure adequate cerebral oxygenation and prevention of secondary brain injury. The child's plan of care includes providing optimal ventilation and oxygenation, maintaining a normal arterial partial pressure of carbon dioxide ($PaCO_2$), normothermia, avoiding hyponatremia, normalizing electrolytes, monitoring serum osmolality, maintaining a normal ICP with monitoring and interventions, and maintaining adequate systemic and cerebral perfusion pressures.[34] Complications of head injuries include hemorrhage, infections, cerebral bleeding, cerebral edema, seizures, and brain herniation.

Treatment is based on the clinical signs in the patient. Treatment for epidural hematoma is surgical intervention. Subdural hematomas are more common in children; treatment of a subdural hematoma may also be surgical intervention for large hematomas associated with increased ICP.[4] Children, especially infants, are at risk for seizures after severe head injury. A child admitted to the critical care unit with a TBI must be constantly monitored for cerebral edema and signs of increased ICP. Two other potential complications of head injury—diabetes insipidus and syndrome of inappropriate antidiuretic hormone—are discussed in Chapter 31. Nursing interventions include precise neurologic assessment, which includes use of GCS scores and monitoring for signs of increased ICP. Children who survive severe head injuries often require extended rehabilitation services to improve long-term outcomes. The pediatric rehabilitation team should be involved in the care of the child while the child is in the critical care unit.

Psychological effects. The psychological effect of injury on a child cannot be underestimated. Studies have shown that 60% of injured children have posttraumatic stress disorder symptoms immediately after the injury. Symptoms continue to be experienced 18 months after injury in 38% of children.[9]

Working with the family of a child with a head injury is challenging. Information given to the parents must be accurate and consistent. The parents may be guilt ridden, especially if they feel they could have prevented the injury. Parents are encouraged to interact with the child soothingly and gently, even if the child cannot respond. Reading books, making a video of home activities or family members, and bringing familiar toys or stuffed animals to the child are ways to involve the family in the care of the child.

End-of-life issues. If the child is not expected to survive, the parents should be informed. The child should be evaluated for brain death and possible organ donation. Before the tests begin, the parents are offered the opportunity to spend time with the child. If brain death has been determined, the parents are informed of the test results. Parents may be asked to discontinue the critical care treatment for their child. The priorities for the critical care nurse include providing comfort and dignity for the child and the family.[36] The most important aspects of care for the families at this time are to show a genuinely caring attitude, to extend kindness and understanding, and to be present with them.[36] Parents must always be approached in a sensitive and compassionate manner. The critical care nurse is typically the member of the team who is closest to the family and the best person to help the family members prepare for the death of the child. Special circumstances such as the impending arrival of additional family members may influence the timing of the decision. Parents must be allowed to spend as much time as they desire with the child to see that everything possible has been done for their child.

GASTROINTESTINAL SYSTEM

Anatomy and Physiology

After birth, growth and maintenance of the small intestine require nutritional components and the stimulation that comes from having food in the gut lumen. The intestinal tracts of infants and young children are larger in relation to body weight compared with intestinal tracts of adults. Sodium and water conservation, which occurs in the large intestine, is an immature process in the infant. For the first 2 years of life, gut immunity is lower, and mucosal binding for bacterial toxins is greater. With these differences in immunity, sensitivity, and greater potential for fluid loss, infants and toddlers have greater morbidity and mortality rates associated with enteric infections compared with adults.[4]

Management

Fluid Replacement

The child's fluid requirements involve replacing output and insensible losses and extra fluid for the production of new intracellular and extracellular fluid during growth. Fluid maintenance for a child with normal renal and cardiac status may be calculated using several formulas, but these account only for basal metabolic needs and growth. The amount of fluid given to a pediatric patient must be determined by the child's clinical condition, fluid balance, and insensible water losses.[4] Table 38.8 provides guidelines for normal fluid and electrolyte maintenance for infants and children. Box 38.6 provides adjustments to fluid maintenance based on level of activity or increased metabolic rate associated with disease.

TABLE 38.8 Normal Fluid and Electrolyte Maintenance for Infants and Children

Component	Weight of Infant or Child	Total Amount
Fluids	1–10 kg	100 mL/kg/day (may be increased to 150 mL/kg for caloric requirements)
	11–20 kg	1000 mL + 50 mL/each kg over 10 kg
	>20 kg	1500 mL + 25 mL/each kg over 20 kg *or* 100 mL/100 kcal/day can be used for children of any weight *or* 1500 mL/m^2/day can be used for children >10 g
Sodium		2–4 mEq/kg/day
Potassium		1–2 mEq/kg/day
Hourly fluid maintenance	1–10 kg	4 mL/kg/hour
	11–20 kg	40 mL + 2 mL/kg over 10 kg
	>20 kg	60 mL + 1 mL/kg over 20 kg

Data from Hazinski MF, ed. *Nursing Care of the Critically Ill Child.* 3rd ed. Elsevier; 2013.

BOX 38.6 Adjustments to Fluid Maintenance

- Fever or hypothermia: increases or decreases 0.42 mL/kg for each 1°C greater than or less than 37°C
- Tachypnea: increases 25% to 30%
- Humidified mechanical ventilation: decreases 12%
- Activity of non–critically ill, resting child: increases 10%
- Restless or active child: increases 30%
- Diaphoresis: increases 10% to 25%
- High-humidity environment: decreases 25% to 40%

Modified from Hazinski MF. *Nursing Care of the Critically Ill Child.* 3rd ed. Elsevier; 2013.

Fluid and electrolyte requirements are based on the patient's history, degree of dehydration, and presenting symptoms. Infants and children need more calories per body weight compared with adults for energy expenditure because of growth. Critical illness has a major effect on the nutritional status of a child because children are especially susceptible to malnutrition.

Nutrition

Suboptimal nutritional intake may result in malnutrition and is associated with adverse clinical outcomes, including longer periods of ventilation, higher risk of hospital-acquired infections, longer critical care unit stays, and increased mortality. Nutritional support after the initial nutritional assessment is an essential aspect of care for the child. It is recommended that critically ill children undergo a nutritional assessment within 48 hours of being admitted and be reevaluated at least weekly by a dedicated dietitian.[37] Critical care nurses play an important role in the feeding of critically ill children. Many procedures such as placing an enteral access device (EAD), checking gastric retentions, performing mouth care, and administering enteral or parenteral nutrition are important to the outcomes of the child and within the nursing domain.[37]

Parenteral nutrition. Providing needed calories in the face of fluid restrictions is a significant problem for an infant or child who is critically ill if the intestinal tract is nonfunctional. One method that may provide the necessary nutrition is parenteral nutrition. This form of nutrition is given by the intravenous route, and although it does not provide greater nutrition compared with enteral feedings, it may give sufficient support until enteral feeding is possible.[4] Box 38.7 outlines daily dextrose, lipid, and amino acid amounts; administration rates; and intravenous line concentration limits for an infant or child receiving total parenteral nutrition. The total parenteral nutrition solution should be tailored to account for the unique needs of each patient. Determination of the child's individual nutrient requirements may vary, depending on such factors as age, weight, organ dysfunction, disease state, metabolic condition, body composition, and current medications.[38]

Enteral nutrition. The enteral route is an important route for providing nutrition to a child.[37] Its advantages are convenience, safety, and low cost. The enteral route also is important in maintaining gastrointestinal mucosal integrity and immunologic function.[37]

Formulas. Many different formulas based on age, host factors, and nutritional requirements are available for the infant or child. Amounts for formula feeds are based on needed kilocalories per kilogram per day for the child, the tolerance of the child to the formula, and their clinical condition. For a full-term infant younger than 1 year, cow's milk-based formulas (Enfamil, Similac) or soy-based formulas (Isomil, ProSobee) are most commonly given. Standard dilution for infant formulas is 20 kcal/ounce.[37] Human breast milk is highly recommended for feedings for infants. Feedings designed specifically for children between 1 and 6 years old include infant formulas, pediatric follow-up formulas, pediatric enteral formulas, various homemade and pureed feedings, and commercial adult formulas.[39] Adult formulas may be given to children older than 6 years. Osmolite and Isocal are preferred for their isotonicity and caloric and protein content.

Feeding procedures. Continuous gavage feedings have advantages over bolus feedings. The risk for aspiration is less, particularly for an infant with reflux. In practice, the individual child's tolerance ultimately dictates the method of how the formula is delivered. Feeding pumps are used to control the rate of continuous-drip feeding. The important features of the enteral pump for use with children is the ability to provide low delivery rates (less than 5 mL/h) and to advance in small increments (1 to 5 mL/h).[39]

Feeding tubes. Gastric and duodenal or jejunal feeding tubes, EADs, are used to administer enteral feeds in a critically ill child.[37] Gastric feeding tubes can be placed easily at the bedside by the nurse. The patency and correct placement of a new EAD must be confirmed prior to any feeding or medication administration. Radiographic confirmation remains the current standard for initial tube verification. In situations where the child's EAD location verification is needed and radiologic placement confirmation is not possible, two methods of tube verification are recommended. These nonradiographic methods can be tube length measurement and pH testing.[37] Determining the insertion length of a nasogastric tube in a child has traditionally been the same as that in an adult—naris to ear to xyphoid process. However,

BOX 38.7 Evidence-Based Practice

Total Parenteral Nutrition Administration for Term Infants and Children

	Infants and Children			
Per 24 Hours	**10 kg**	**10–20 kg**	**20 kg**	**Adolescents**
Fluids (mL/kg)	100–125	1000 mL: add 50 mL/kg for each extra kg >10 kg		1500 mL: add 20–25 mL for each extra kg >20 kg
Calories (kcal/kg)	75–90	75–90	>40	30–60
Protein (g/kg)	2–2.5	1.5–2.5	1.5–2.5	1–2
Maximum peripheral: 2 g/kg/day				
Maximum central: 3.5 g/kg/day				
Dextrose (%)	5–30	5–30	5–30	5–30
Maximum peripheral: 10%–12.5%				
Maximum central: 30%				
Fat (g/kg/day)	1–3	1–3	1–3	1–3
	Infants and Children (>2.5 kg and <11 y)			**Children and Adults (>11 y)**
Vitamins (mL/day)	5 mL/day			10 mL/day
MVI-peds (vitamin K = 0.2 mg/5 mL)				
MVI-13 (vitamin K = 0.15 mg/10 mL)				
Heparin[a]	0–0.5 units/mL			0–0.5 units/mL
Levocarnitine[b]	>30 days = 5 mg/kg/day			>30 days = 1–5 mg/kg/day

[a]Recommended for slow infusion rates.

[b]Prematurity or TPN dependent.

MVI, Multiple vitamins for infusion; *PN*, parenteral nutrition; *TPN*, total parenteral nutrition.

Data from Mehta NM, Skillman HE, Irving SY, et al. Guidelines for the provision and assessment of nutrition support therapy in the pediatric critically ill patient: Society of Critical Care Medicine and American Society for Parenteral and Enteral Nutrition. *JPEN J Parenter Enteral Nutr.* 2017;41(5):706–742. https://doi.org/10.1177/0148607117711387.

TABLE 38.9 Guidelines for Gavage Feeding in Infants and Children

Parameters	Age and Size Determinations				
Age	3 mo	6 mo	2 y	5 y	10 y
Tube size	6 Fr	8 Fr	10 Fr	12 Fr	14 Fr

Method	Initial volume and rate	Advancement volume and rate
Bolus	2–5 mL/kg every 3–4 h over 20 min	2–5 mL/kg every other feeding
Continuous	1–2 mL/kg/h; initial volume not to exceed 55 mL/h regardless of child's weight	1–2 mL/kg every 8–12 h

Fr, French sizing.

Data from Konek S, Becker PJ, eds. *Samour and King's Pediatric Nutrition in Clinical Care.* 5th ed. Jones & Bartlett; 2019.

this measurement may not always allow for all the side holes of a feeding tube to be in the stomach. Measuring to a point between the xyphoid and the umbilicus is a safer method. Table 38.9 provides guidelines for gavage feeding tube sizes and feeding rates for infants and children. Nasoduodenal or transpyloric tubes are recommended to reduce the risk of aspiration in the presence of delayed gastric emptying or reflux. These tubes also ensure the delivery of enteral feeds to the main sites of nutrient absorption. Gastric retention, diarrhea, and abdominal distention may limit the use of enteral nutrition. Parenteral nutrition should be considered when it is impossible to obtain enteral access, when enteral nutrition cannot meet the child's nutritional requirements, or when the child has a contraindication to enteral nutrition such as a mechanical obstruction of the gastrointestinal tract.[37]

PAIN MANAGEMENT

Research in the 2000s and 2010s has witnessed remarkable growth in pediatric pain management. Research has proven that infants and children do feel pain, and when they are not treated, morbidity and mortality rates and hyperalgesia are increased. A negative effect on the development of the infant or child may occur. Children experience pain not only from life-threatening diseases but also from injuries, surgeries, burns, and infections. Children in pain frequently receive too little medication or they may receive no medication at all. This is due to a misconception that children do not experience pain the same as adults. Children will express pain in varying ways during different developmental ages. An accurate assessment of the critically ill or injured child's pain is vital for appropriate pain control. [40]

Physiology

Neurotransmitters and peripheral and central neural pathways for pain transmission are developed and are functional before birth, and they continue to mature during the first 2 years of life. After age 2 years, the perception of pain is the same for adults and children, but the psychosocial and behavioral expressions of the responses to pain change with the child's growth and developmental stage.[4] The nerve tracts to the brain are myelinated by 30 weeks of gestation, and the thalamocortical tracts are myelinated by 37 weeks of gestation, indicating that neonates are able to perceive all forms of pain. No perfect guide exists for providing analgesia to a pediatric patient. Children may demonstrate wide variations in the medications needed, the duration and dosing requirements, and the responses to the medications.[4] Each child must be monitored for his or her response to the pain therapy.

The physiologic effects of untreated pain in a child may result in:

- Hyperglycemia from decreased insulin secretion with breakdown of carbohydrate and fat stores
- Metabolic acidosis from increased use of fat
- Increased corticosteroids, growth hormone, and catecholamines
- Increased pulmonary vascular resistance
- Hypoxemia

Assessment

Pain assessment is the key to effective pain management. Many of the factors that influence pain in an adult also influence pain in a child. However, one difference is the influence of parental anxiety and behavior regarding their child's overall experience of pain. Although most pain research has involved procedural pain, it is important to be cognizant of the acute and chronic pain and distress associated with the critical care unit and its repetitive procedures.

The child may not spontaneously express his or her need for pain treatment. Staff members must be vigilant and actively explore a child's level of pain whenever the potential for pain exists. A child's verbal statement of pain is the most reliable indicator in acute pain management. However, this approach may not be possible with a preverbal child, a child who cannot comprehend the request to symbolically identify pain, or a child who has a significantly altered level of consciousness or is intubated. For children up to age 3 years, behavioral scales are used as the primary source for pain assessment, and physiologic parameters are used as secondary sources. One such tool is the Face, Legs, Activity, Crying, and Consolability (FLACC) postoperative pain scale.

For children at least 6 years old, self-reports are the primary assessment tool, with behavioral scales used as secondary sources. For children 3 to 6 years old, self-reports may be used, but with a caveat. Many self-report scales have been tested as effective with this age group, but younger children ages 3 to 4 years may have difficulty using them. Cognitive ability may not be advanced enough, or the child might have regressed in cognitive ability because of the illness. The child's rating may indicate a mood state rather than pain. Within this age group, self-reports and behavioral scales may need to be used together to get a true picture of the child's pain. One of the most valuable clues to pain relief is a change in behavior and vital signs after the administration of pain medication.

Parents often are the primary source of information about how their child exhibits pain. Parents are sensitive to changes in the child's behavior and often want to be involved in efforts for the child's pain relief. Encouraging parents to be involved gives them a sense of control and help. Parents usually know what comfort measures to take with their children when they are in pain. For most children, having the supportive presence of their parents provides the most comfort. (See Chapter 7 for a discussion of pain rating scales.)

Management of Pain

Some general principles are applied to the management of pain in children:

- *Prevention of pain:* If pain can be anticipated, pain should be treated prophylactically.
- *Adequate assessment:* Developmentally appropriate assessment tools are available.
- *Multimodal approach:* Analgesics; physical strategies such as massage, acupuncture, and hot or cold therapies; and behavioral, cognitive, and psychological approaches are available.
- *Parental involvement:* Parents are the best source of information about their child. They should be taught different strategies to help their child cope with the pain.
- *Nonnoxious routes:* The route of administration of analgesia should be as painless as possible.
- *Pain control during procedures:* Inadequate pain control during procedures may create an atmosphere of anxiety and increased pain during subsequent procedures.

Nonsteroidal Antiinflammatory Drugs

Nonsteroidal antiinflammatory drugs (NSAIDs) are effective for the management of mild to moderate pain, and they may be used in combination with opioids. They have superior antiinflammatory properties compared with aspirin or acetaminophen.[4] The drawbacks to NSAIDs are that a ceiling effect exists, and they affect the gastric mucosa, decrease platelet aggregation, and cause peptic ulcer formation and hepatic dysfunction. It is recommended that a histamine-2 receptor blocker be given concurrently for prolonged use of these medications.[26] The use of NSAIDs should be avoided in children with a history of severe renal disease, dehydration, or heart failure.[26] Examples of NSAIDs commonly used are ibuprofen and ketorolac. Ketorolac is the only NSAID that is approved for parenteral use by the U.S. Food and Drug Administration.[41] Use of ketorolac IV should be done judiciously, as there is an increased risk of gastrointestinal ulceration and bleeding.

NSAIDS can be given intravenously or orally and work well in combination with opioids for pain control. NSAIDS provide analgesia for longer durations than opioids with fewer potential side effects and are approved for use in children older than 6 months.[41] Ketorolac, an NSAID, given intravenously, provides excellent analgesic effect and has been shown to lead to shorter hospital stays, less gastrointestinal discomfort, and decreased opioid requirement. However, the use of ketorolac for longer than 72 hours does carry a risk for gastrointestinal and renal damage.[41]

Opioid Analgesics

Opioid analgesics are the most important class of medications for the relief of moderate to severe pain. Administration of opioids requires decisions about the route of administration of the medication, the choice of opioids, and the method of administration. The most commonly used opioids for children are morphine, fentanyl, and hydromorphone. Methadone is an extremely long-acting opioid, but it is not used as commonly for acute pain control. This medication is used for weaning from iatrogenic opioid dependency or for control of chronic pain.[4] Meperidine is not a medication of choice because it decreases cardiac output and causes tachycardia. The medication's metabolite lowers the child's seizure threshold, causing hyperexcitability with multiple dosing. Opioids can be administered by intravenous push, continuous infusion, patient-controlled analgesia, or epidural injection.

Naloxone is an opioid antagonist that is required if the child becomes unresponsive after receiving opioids. The child's respirations will become shallow and less than 8 per minute, and the pupils become pinpoint. The patient will need to be observed for the response to the medication.[26]

Pain medications can be given in different routes other than oral or intravenous. Transdermal fentanyl (Duragesic) is available as a patch for continuous pain control. This medication should not be used for acute pain because of the peak effect taking 12 to 24 hours. The use of anesthetics such as nitrous oxide can be administered by inhalation. This medication provides either partial or complete analgesia for pain procedures that child might have to endure.[42]

Topical Anesthetics

The use of topical analgesic ointments reduces the local pain of procedures such as suturing or venipuncture and reduces the child's anticipated pain and anxiety over the upcoming procedure. The use of these agents has been expanded to include pain reduction for lumbar punctures or bone marrow aspiration. Some ointments take approximately 10 to 60 minutes to be effective. ELA-Max is a topical formulation of 4% lidocaine that is encapsulated by liposomes, which create lipid solubility and allow transdermal medication delivery. ELA-Max provides anesthesia in approximately 30 minutes.[26] LAT (lidocaine, adrenaline, tetracaine) provides skin anesthesia about 15 minutes after application on intact skin. Lidocaine iontophoresis allows active transdermal delivery of lidocaine under the influence of a low-level electric current.

Nonpharmacologic Management

Nonpharmacologic techniques should be used to supplement, not replace, the use of pain medications. Some nonpharmacologic interventions that may be used in children include distraction, relaxation, guided imagery, and cutaneous stimulation. The use of these techniques may decrease the perceived threat of pain, provide a sense of control, enhance the child's comfort, and promote rest or sleep. These nonpharmacologic techniques are safe, noninvasive, and usually inexpensive, and most are independent nursing functions.

Oral sucrose is a valuable analgesic option for neonates undergoing a brief painful procedure. It has a rapid onset of effect and short-lived action thought to be mediated by the release of endogenous brain opioids. Use of sugar has a low risk, and it is simple to administer to the neonate.[43]

Opioid-Related Issues

The number of children admitted to hospital intensive care units for opioid poisoning has nearly doubled over a decade. The curiosity nature of young children makes them vulnerable to harm from accidental medication injections, as opposed to the adolescent patient who is more likely to have intention ingestions for recreational or self-harm purposes. About 43% of opioid-related hospitalizations require admission to an intensive care unit for critical care support.[44]

PSYCHOSOCIAL ISSUES OF THE CHILD AND FAMILY

An unplanned admission of a child to a critical care unit, including children with illnesses or injuries, is a traumatic event for parents and for the child. In a crisis situation, parents may feel overwhelmed and become focused solely on the physiological well-being of their child. If the child is conscious, he or she desperately needs the continual physical presence and emotional support of the parents; however, this is a time when it may be very difficult for the parents to help their child emotionally. Critical care nurses encounter the child and family at a very emotionally vulnerable time. Parents may view nurses and physicians as their lifeline, controlling the needs and the life of their child.[4] A common complaint of families and patients is the lack of accuracy, clarity, and consistency of the information that is presented to them. Family members indicate a willingness and desire that bad news be empathetically communicated.[45] The critical care nurse needs to be knowledgeable about childhood cognitive and emotional development and about family dynamics to assist the child and the family through this health crisis. The next sections address some common issues that hospitalized children and their families face during hospitalization.

The Ill Child's Experience of Critical Illness

The term *family-centered care* defines the focus of care for a child because the nursing care of a child involves not only the child but also the family as a whole. Family-centered care supports the child's family by prioritizing the family members' needs and values and empowering the family unit.[46] Two basic concepts in family-centered care are *enabling* and *empowering*. The critical care staff enable families by creating opportunities and means for family members to be present during examinations and procedures.[36] Empowerment describes the interaction of the staff members with the families in a way that allows the families to maintain control or acquire a sense of control over their lives.

The emotional reactions of the child to hospitalization depend on the type and quantity of stress produced by the illness itself, the hospitalization experience, and the notions that the child has about the situation. The final outcome is influenced by the child's age and level of development. A child in the critical care unit experiences significant stress, and the important question is whether the child's capacity to cope physically or emotionally in an age-appropriate fashion is exceeded.

Three elements that help a child cope successfully with a crisis are: (1) a resilient personality, (2) a supportive family, and (3) an outside support system.[4] The critical care health team members serve as the outside support system, applying the family-centered concept as they reinforce and strengthen the coping efforts of the child and family. A communication tool that places safety as a priority standardizes the summary of clinical rounds and plan of care should be used utilized. This tool can be customized to the PICU and will facilitate an increase in the family and patient's satisfaction.[45] Nurses must take every opportunity to reassure the parents that they are an integral part of their child's care and recovery. When children were asked who or what helped the most while they were in the pediatric critical care unit, they stated their nurses were the most helpful and said then it was their families.[47] This is not a surprising finding considering that critical care nurses function as communicators, translators, and care coordinators within the hospital and are also at the patient's bedside around the clock.[47]

A child who is critically ill needs the physical presence of the parents (or primary caretaker) at the bedside. Young children are most frightened by the separation from their parents. Unrestricted visitation (i.e., 24 h/day) for parents is imperative. The parents are the most reassuring people in the child's eyes and are needed psychologically by the child to believe that he or she will not be abandoned, left to be unsafe, or left in pain and distress. Anxiety and fear are easily heightened when the child recognizes scary words or fills in ambiguities heard with his or her own distorted interpretations. For a child who is very ill and prostrate, anxieties may fester within, unknown to staff members. Every member of the health care team should have an understanding of the five phases of development of logical thought—infancy, toddlerhood, preschool age, school age, and adolescence—to communicate effectively with a child and should understand the basis of a child's perceptions, fears, and misunderstandings.[4]

Parents' Experience of a Child's Critical Illness

When their child is admitted to the critical care unit, parents may experience a staged response similar to the grief process.[4] With a sudden illness or injury, the initial emotions may be shock, disbelief, and denial. These feelings may last for a few hours or a few days. Parents may question the diagnosis or want to prove the providers wrong. The situation may feel unreal, as if it were not happening to them. It may be difficult to grasp the totality of what has happened to their child. They may feel paralyzed and not know what they should do next. The parents may find it difficult to remember and process explanations given to them about what is happening with their child. This is usually a defense against pain. Forgetting may result in some parents feeling that staff members do not explain much to them. Other parents may feel that this is a sign of their own inadequacy. Explanations about their child's condition may have to be given in small increments of information with compassion and repetition. Some parents may appear to be competent and composed during the height of the crisis, but this should not be interpreted as their being less stressed or anxious.

Parents need to be reunited with their child, if this is their wish, as soon as they have been prepared about what to expect. However, parents may be afraid to see their child. Changes in their child's appearance and in the child's emotional reactions will be very upsetting to parents. If the child is conscious and relatively alert, the parents need to be informed that their child may show some form of regressive behavior such as withdrawal or anger, which is to be expected given the stress of the situation and the degree of illness or injury. Parents also may feel frightened about touching or talking to their child, believing that this may harm the child. They must be reassured that they can do this and that if they have any concerns, staff members will be present in the room to help them.

Intense anxiety may make parents question whether their reactions are normal. They wonder how other parents feel or behave. They may be extremely frightened by the intensity of their feelings and may wonder whether they are going to have a breakdown. These feelings are common in a crisis, and parents need to hear that their feelings are understandable. Some parents may behave with hostility toward staff or family members. Some may behave quite rigidly, visiting only briefly or not asking questions in an attempt to maintain composure.

Anger is an emotion that usually takes its toll after the crisis period, usually with longer critical care unit stays. Destructive anger occurs when parents seek justification for their anger by blaming others for their child's condition. They are unreasonably critical of the health care team and may make complaints about the child's care as a manifestation of their anger. Parents may become depressed as they realize the severity of their child's condition. At this time, parents should be given an opportunity to express their feelings and participate in activities such as bathing the child.

The critical care nurse can assist the parents by clarifying information and by helping them support their child.[48] During crises, communication with the parents must be frequent and clear. Key elements to effective communication include communication at frequent, predictable intervals; use of consistent, understandable terminology; provision of opportunities for parents to ask questions and express opinions; and assistance of support personnel.[4] The primary focus in decision making should be the interests of the child.[45]

Critical care nurses who provide direct care to the child and parents have the greatest degree of contact with the family. In addition to the nurse's role in psychological assessment and intervention, other support staff members should be available to assist the family. The creation of an ethical working environment in the critical care unit is a necessary precondition for addressing ethical issues raised by specific parent situations.[45] Clinical nurse specialists assess parental worries and concerns and, based on the assessment, help the parents make plans to address their concerns.[49] Social workers provide the family with support and advocacy during their time of crisis. Many critical care units also have access to child life specialists, chaplains, discharge planners, and ethicists to assist in providing psychosocial support to the families. Concern for the psychosocial and developmental well-being of pediatric patients and their families is the primary focus of the child life specialist.[46]

An important role of the critical care nurse is to mobilize and introduce the families to the support staff available in their institutions for their support. This case study discusses some of these concepts.

ADDITIONAL RESOURCES

See Box 38.8 for Internet resources related to the care of pediatric patients.

BOX 38.8 Internet Resources

The Pediatric Patient

- American Association of Critical-Care Nurses (AACN) https://www.aacn.org/
- American Academy of Pediatrics (AAP) https://www.aap.org/en-us/Pages/Default.aspx
- Cystic Fibrosis Foundation (CFF) https://www.cff.org/
- National Association of Neonatal Nurses (NANN) http://nann.org/
- Society of Pediatric Nurses (SPN) http://www.pedsnurses.org/

CASE STUDY 38.1 The Pediatric Patient

Brief Patient History

A 2-month-old infant of a single non–English-speaking mother is admitted directly to the critical care unit with a history of vomiting and diarrhea over the past 24 hours. The mother reports that the infant was irritable yesterday but is more lethargic today. The infant has had three wet diapers over the past 24 hours, and the urine appears dark. The infant does not tolerate any formula or Pedialyte orally.

Focused Physical Assessment

Physical assessment reveals the following: weight, 7 kg (weight 1 week prior, 7.6 kg); temperature, 38.5°C; pulse, 180 beats/min; respiratory rate, 46 to 50 breaths/min; blood pressure, 60/43 mm Hg; and pulse oximetry, 93%. The infant's lips and mucous membranes are dry and tacky. Her fontanel is sunken. Extremities are cool and mottled, nail beds are dusky, and capillary refill is 4 seconds. Pulses are rapid and weak centrally and peripherally. The infant is lethargic.

Diagnostic Procedures

The infant is placed on oxygen and intravenous access is attained. A point-of-care glucose test reveals blood sugar of 50 mg/dL.

Medical Diagnosis

The infant is diagnosed with hypovolemic, hypotensive shock and hypoglycemia.

Questions

1. What major outcomes do you expect to achieve for this patient?
2. What problems or risks must be managed to achieve these outcomes?
3. What interventions could be initiated to monitor, prevent, manage, or eliminate the problems and risks identified?
4. What interventions could be initiated to promote optimal functioning, safety, and well-being of the patient?
5. What technology can be used to monitor this patient and prevent complications?
6. What other interprofessional team members are needed to assist with the management of this patient?
7. What possible learning needs would you anticipate for this patient?
8. What cultural and age-related factors might have a bearing on the patient's plan of care?

KEY POINTS

- Children are physically, physiologically, and emotionally immature, and they are different from adults.
- Complete respiratory failure may develop rapidly in a child when respiratory distress is present.
- In infants and children, most cardiac arrests result from progressive respiratory failure, shock, or both.
- Bradycardia is an ominous sign in a seriously ill or injured child.
- Hypotension is typically only a late sign of hypotensive shock in children.
- Head injury is a primary insult to a child. Patient outcomes are compromised if secondary insults such as hypotension or hypoxemia occur.
- Most children in the critical care unit experience pain and anxiety, and they should be treated accordingly.
- The concept of family-centered care recognizes that the family is the one constant in a child's life.

Visit the Evolve site at http://evolve.elsevier.com/Urden/CriticalCareNursing for additional study materials.

REFERENCES

1. Hockenberry M. Children, their families and the nurse. In: Hockenberry M, Wilson D, Rodgers C, eds. *Wong's Essentials of Pediatric Nursing*. 11th ed. St Louis: Elsevier; 2022.
2. Mullen J, Pate MF. Caring for critically ill children and their families. In: Slota M, ed. *AACN Core Curriculum for Pediatric High Acuity, Progressive, and Critical Care Nursing*. 3rd ed. New York: Springer; 2019.
3. Blayney F, Young C. Multisystem issues. In: Slota M, ed. *AACN Core Curriculum for Pediatric High Acuity, Progressive, and Critical Care Nursing*. 3rd ed. New York: Springer; 2019.
4. Hazinski MF. Children are different. In: Hazinski MF, ed. *Nursing Care of the Critically Ill Child*. 3rd ed. St. Louis: Elsevier; 2013.
5. American Heart Association. *Pediatric Advanced Life Support*. Dallas: American Heart Association; 2020.
6. Flasch E, Brueck N, Lynn J, Henningfeld J. Pulmonary system. In: Slota M, ed. *AACN Core Curriculum for Pediatric High Acuity, Progressive, and Critical Care Nursing*. 3rd ed. New York: Springer; 2019.
7. Napolitano N, Berlinski A, Walsh BK, et al. AARC Clinical practice guideline: management of pediatric patients with oxygen in the acute care setting. *Respir Care*. 2021;66(7):1214–1223. https://doi.org/10.4187/respcare.09006.
8. Slota M. Bioinstrumentation: Principles and techniques. In: Hazinski MF, ed. *Nursing Care of the Critically Ill Child*. 3rd ed. St. Louis: Elsevier; 2013.
9. Waibel E. Traumatic injuries. In: Bolick B, Madden M, Severin P, et al., eds. *Pediatric Acute Care: A Guide for Interprofessional Practice*. 2nd ed. St. Louis: Elsevier; 2021.
10. Kline-Tilford A, Levin DL, Source L, et al. Pulmonary disorders. In: Hazinski MF, ed. *Nursing Care of the Critically Ill Child*. 3rd ed. St. Louis: Elsevier; 2013.
11. Kneyber MCJ, de Luca D, Calderini E, et al. Recommendations for mechanical ventilation of critically ill children from the Paediatric Mechanical Ventilation Consensus Conference (PEMVECC). *Intensive Care Med*. 2017;43(12):1764–1780. https://doi.org/10.1007/s00134-017-4920-z.
12. Kuch B. Respiratory monitoring and support. In: Hazinski MF, ed. *Nursing Care of the Critically Ill Child*. 3rd ed. St. Louis: Elsevier; 2013.
13. Anderson C, Herring R. Pediatric nursing interventions and skills. In: Hockenberry M, Wilson D, Rodgers C, eds. *Wong's Essentials of Pediatric Nursing*. 11th ed. St Louis: Elsevier; 2022.
14. Baum R. Mechanical ventilation. In: Kliegman R, St Geme JW, eds. *Nelson's Textbook of Pediatrics*. 21st ed. Philadelphia: Elsevier; 2020.
15. Zentz SE. Care of infants and children with bronchiolitis: a systematic review. *J Pediatr Nurs*. 2011;26(6):519–529. https://doi.org/10.1016/j.pedn.2010.07.008.
16. Dalziel SR, Haskell L, O'Brien S, et al. Bronchiolitis. *Lancet*. 2022;400(10349):392–406. https://doi.org/10.1016/S0140-6736(22)01016-9.
17. American Academy of Pediatric Updated Guidance: Use of Palivizumab Prophylaxis to Prevent Hospitalizations From Severe Respiratory Syncytial Virus Infection During The 2022-2023 Season. Updated November 11, 2022. Accessed October 21, 2023. https://www.aap.org/en/pages/2019-novel-coronavirus-covid-19-infections/clinical-guidance/interim-guidance-for-use-of-palivizumab-prophylaxis-to-prevent-hospitalization/.
18. American Academy of Pediatrics. Updated Guidance: Use of Palivizumab Prophylaxis to Prevent Hospitalization From Severe Respiratory Syncytial Virus Infection During the 2022-2023 RSV Season. Update November 17, 2022. Accessed October 21, 2023. https://www.aap.org/en/pages/2019-novel-coronavirus-covid-19-infections/clinical-guidance/interim-guidance-for-use-of-palivizumab-prophylaxis-to-prevent-hospitalization/.
19. Cunningham S, Williams T. Bronchiolitis. In: Bush A, Deterding R, Li AM, et al., eds. *Kendig's and Willmott's Disorders of the Respiratory Tract in Children*. 10th ed. Philadelphia: Elsevier; 2024.
20. Pitts, T. Thinking Outside Intubation: The Pros and Cons of Heliox Therapy. American Association for Respiratory Care Newsroom. Published December 22, 2022. Accessed November 18, 2024. https://www.aarc.org/news/thinking-outside-intubation-the-pros-and-cons-of-heliox-therapy/.

21. Kline-Tilford A, Kane J. Ventilation support. In: Bolick B, Madden M, Severin P, et al., eds. *Pediatric Acute Care: A Guide for Interprofessional Practice*. 2nd ed. St. Louis: Elsevier; 2021.
22. Richards-Belle A, Davis P, Drikite L, et al. FIRST-line support for assistance in breathing in children (FIRST-ABC): A master protocol of two randomised trials to evaluate the non-inferiority of high-flow nasal cannula (HFNC) versus continuous positive airway pressure (CPAP) for non-invasive respiratory support in paediatric critical care. *BMJ Open*. 2020;10(8):e038002. https://doi.org/10.1136/bmjopen-2020-038002.
23. Centers for Disease Control and Prevention. *RSV Immunization Guidance for Infants and Young Children*. Updated August 30, 2024. Assessed November 18, 2024. https://www.https://www.cdc.gov/rsv/hcp/vaccine-clinical-guidance/infants-young-children.html.
24. Cloutier MM, Teach SJ, Lemanske Jr RF, Blake KV. The 2020 focused updates to the NIH asthma management guidelines: key points for pediatricians. *Pediatrics*. 2021;147(6):e2021050286. https://doi.org/10.1542/peds.2021-050286.
25. Bryant R. Long term respiratory dysfunction: asthma. In: Hockenberry M, Wilson D, Rodgers C, eds. *Wong's Essentials of Pediatric Nursing*. 11th ed. St Louis: Elsevier; 2022.
26. Lexi-Comp Online Formulary. Accessed on March 4th, 2023. http://online.lexi.com/lco/action/doc/retrieve/docid/pdh-f/128905?searchUrl5%2Flco%2Faction%2Fsearch%3Fq%3DMagnesium%2520Sulfate%26t%3Dname%26va%3Dmagnesium%2520sulfate
27. Nikolopoulou GB, Maltezou HC. COVID-19 in children: where do we stand? *Arch Med Res*. 2022;53(1):1–8. https://doi.org/10.1016/j.arcmed.2021.07.002.
28. Yasuhara J, Kuno T, Takagi H, Sumitomo N. Clinical characteristics of COVID-19 in children: a systematic review. *Pediatr Pulmonol*. 2020;55(10):2565–2575. https://doi.org/10.1002/ppul.24991.
29. Hockenberry M. The child with cerebral dysfunction. In: Hockenberry M, Wilson D, Rodgers C, eds. *Wong's Essentials of Pediatric Nursing*. 11th ed. St Louis: Elsevier; 2022.
30. Smith G, Wagner JL, Edwards JC. Epilepsy update, Part 1: Refining our understanding of a complex disease. *Am J Nurs*. 2015;115(5):40–49. https://doi.org/10.1097/01.NAJ.0000465030.89975.e8.
31. Vernon-Levett P. Neurologic system. In: Slota M, ed. *AACN Core Curriculum for Pediatric High Acuity, Progressive, and Critical Care Nursing*. 3rd ed. New York: Springer; 2019.
32. Ochoa C, Chokshi N, Upperman JS, et al. Prior studies comparing outcomes from trauma care at children's hospitals versus adult hospitals. *J Trauma*. 2007;63(6 Suppl):S87–S95. https://doi.org/10.1097/TA.0b013e31815acc0f.
33. McDowell BM, Pasek TA, Perlick C, Kostie K. Trauma-informed care: pediatric intensive care nurses at the root of children's safety and trust. *Crit Care Nurse*. 2022;42(6):66–72. https://doi.org/10.4037/ccn2022215.
34. Blayney F, et al. Multiple trauma. In: Slota M, ed. *AACN Core Curriculum for Pediatric High Acuity, Progressive, and Critical Care Nursing*. 3rd ed. New York: Springer; 2019.
35. O'Brien N, Lovett M. Traumatic brain injury. In: Bolick B, Madden M, Severin P, et al., eds. *Pediatric Acute Care: A Guide for Interprofessional Practice*. 2nd ed. St. Louis: Elsevier; 2021.
36. Hesselgrove J, Santucci G. Impact of chronic illness, disability, or end of life care of the child and family. In: Hockenberry M, Wilson D, Rodgers C, eds. *Wong's Essentials of Pediatric Nursing*. 11th ed. St Louis: Elsevier; 2022.
37. Mehta NM, Skillman HE, Irving SY, et al. Guidelines for the provision and assessment of nutrition support therapy in the pediatric critically ill patient: Society of Critical Care Medicine and American Society for Parenteral and Enteral Nutrition. *JPEN J Parenter Enteral Nutr*. 2017;41(5):706–742. https://doi.org/10.1177/0148607117711387.
38. Ratz N. Parental nutrition. In: Bolick B, Madden M, Severin P, et al., eds. *Pediatric Acute Care: A Guide for Interprofessional Practice*. 2nd ed. St. Louis: Elsevier; 2021.
39. Cohen A, Ruffin A. Enteral nutrition. In: Konek S, Becker PJ, eds. *Samour and King's Pediatric Nutrition in Clinical Care*. 5th ed. Burlington, MA: Jones & Bartlett; 2019.
40. Mullen J, Pate MJ. Caring for critically ill children and their families. In: Slota M, ed. *AACN Core Curriculum for Pediatric High Acuity, Progressive, and Critical Care Nursing*. 3rd ed. New York: Springer; 2019.
41. Coit C, Shannon E. Approaches to pediatric musculoskeletal pain: opioids and so much more. *Orthop Nurs*. 2019;38(2):138–147. https://doi.org/10.1097/NOR.0000000000000523.
42. Hellsten M. Pain assessment and management in children. In: Hockenberry M, Wilson D, Rodgers C, eds. *Wong's Essentials of Pediatric Nursing*. 11th ed. St Louis: Elsevier; 2022.
43. Pasek TA, Huber JM. Hospitalized infants who hurt: a sweet solution with oral sucrose. *Crit Care Nurse*. 2012;32(1):61–69. https://doi.org/10.4037/ccn2012912.
44. Kane JM, Colvin JD, Bartlett AH, Hall M. Opioid-related critical care resource use in US children's hospitals [published correction appears in Pediatrics. 2018 Jun;141(6). *Pediatrics*. 2018;141(4):e20173335. https://doi.org/10.1542/peds.2017-3335.
45. Perkin R. Ethical issues in pediatric critical care. In: Hazinski MF, ed. *Nursing Care of the Critically Ill Child*. 3rd ed. St. Louis: Elsevier; 2013.
46. Pike M, Banderas C. Child life: developmental considerations. In: Bolick B, Madden M, Severin P, et al., eds. *Pediatric Acute Care: A Guide for Interprofessional Practice*. 2nd ed. St. Louis: Elsevier; 2021.
47. Hallman ML, Bellury LM. Communication in pediatric critical care units: a review of the literature. *Crit Care Nurse*. 2020;40(2):e1–e15. https://doi.org/10.4037/ccn2020751.
48. Pietsch J, Chung D. Care of the child with burns. In: Hazinski MF, ed. *Nursing Care of the Critically Ill Child*. 3rd ed. St. Louis: Elsevier; 2013.
49. McNelis AM, Buelow J, Myers J, Johnson EA. Concerns and needs of children with epilepsy and their parents. *Clin Nurse Spec*. 2007;21(4):195–202. https://doi.org/10.1097/01.NUR.0000280488.33884.1d.

39

The Older Adult Patient

Fiona Winterbottom and Misty Jenkins

CRITICAL CARE AND THE OLDER ADULT

Future Trends in Older Adult Aging

Trends in older adult admissions to intensive care units (ICUs) are shifting due to worldwide demographic changes.[1] Sixteen percent of the population, or one in seven Americans, is over 65 years old. That number is expected to increase to 21% by 2040. Number of adults greater than 85 years old is predicted to double from 6.6 million in 2019 to 14.4 million by 2040, representing a 118% increase in individuals over the age of 85. [2]

Implications for Health Care Delivery

Older adults will account for almost a quarter of the total population, requiring transformation of societal structure, health care redesign, creative reimbursement models, and innovative training.[1] Another factor to consider regarding aging demographics is the increase in racial and ethnic minorities, which is predicted to increase to 34% by 2040. The largest growing minorities include Hispanics at 160%, followed by Asian Americans at 102% and African Americans at 80%.[2]

Community living statistics will also be important in future health care delivery planning. More than half of individuals over 65 years of age currently live with a spouse or partner, with 70% of older men and 48% of older women being married, and 27% of older adults living alone. The number of people living in nursing homes is approximately 1% in those aged 65 to 75, 2% in adults 75 to 84, and 8% for those over 85. [2]

Older Adults in the Future Requiring Critical Care

Nearly 1 in 10 adults 65 or older live below the poverty line with another 4% (2.6 million) living in near poverty. This number is higher in African Americans, Hispanics, and older women. Notably, the percentage of older adults who completed high school increased from 28% in 1970 to 89% in 2020.[2] These statistics are important when considering the types of patients who will require care in the ICU and for postacute care needed for older adult survivors.

As adults age, reserve capacity decreases, compounded by geriatric syndromes that include delirium, sensory deficit, reduced cognition, functional decline, frailty, and multimorbidity leading to decreased physical independence and increased mortality.[3] Many older adults have at least one chronic condition, with many having multimorbidity, frailty, dementia, and disability making them vulnerable to adverse outcomes. Depression is a common problem among older adults, but clinical depression is not a normal part of aging. See SDOH Depression in the Older Adult box.

Older Adults With Greater Chronicity and Morbidity

A Medicare-linked health and retirement survey reviewed older adults admitted to ICUs between 1998 and 2015. The survey showed increases in ICU admissions of older adults with preexisting disability from 15.5% to 24%, frailty from 36.6% to 45%, and multimorbidity from 54% to 71%, respectively. Interestingly, rates of dementia did not change significantly in the survey.[3] Understanding demographic trends is imperative to support the growing prevalence and preexisting frailty of critically ill older adults, their families, and to provide training to interprofessional health care staff.

Older adults currently account for 20% of ICU admissions, indicating a need to incorporate geriatric-focused interventions and principles into ICU care. Older adult issues can be considered as predisposing, precipitating, or perpetuating.[1] Predisposing factors include frailty and vulnerability to adverse outcomes. Precipitating factors are acute and trigger serious decline. Perpetuating factors are conditions that prolong illness and impede recovery.[1]

Transition to Future Models of Care to Address Changing Needs

Due to the increasing number of older adults being admitted to ICU there is an urgent need to develop optimal models of care to support this growing population. Proposed models of care include geriatric ICUs, dedicated geriatric beds, geriatric assessment by a geriatrician, or geriatric assessment without a geriatrician.[4] Other adaptive approaches incorporate geriatric best practices such as checklists, care bundles of care, and targeted education programs into existing care delivery systems.[4]

Geriatric-focused interdisciplinary team models include geriatricians, critical care physicians, cardiologists, pharmacists, nurses, geriatric advanced practice nurses (APNs, both Clinical Nurse Specialists [CNSs] and Nurse Practitioners), physical therapists, respiratory therapists, speech therapists, occupational therapists, and social workers. These comprehensive teams can provide prompt assessment, team management, medication review, early mobility, sleep optimization, social assessment, goals of care alignment, and support for patients and families.

Established Evidence-Based Eldercare Models

Models such as the *Acute Care for Elders* (ACE) program and *Nurses Improving Care for Healthsystem Elders* (NICHE) promote evidence-based practices for interdisciplinary patient-centered care of older adults to support physical, cognitive, and mental health function to prevent hospital-acquired geriatric

SOCIAL DETERMINANTS OF HEALTH

Depression in the Older Adult

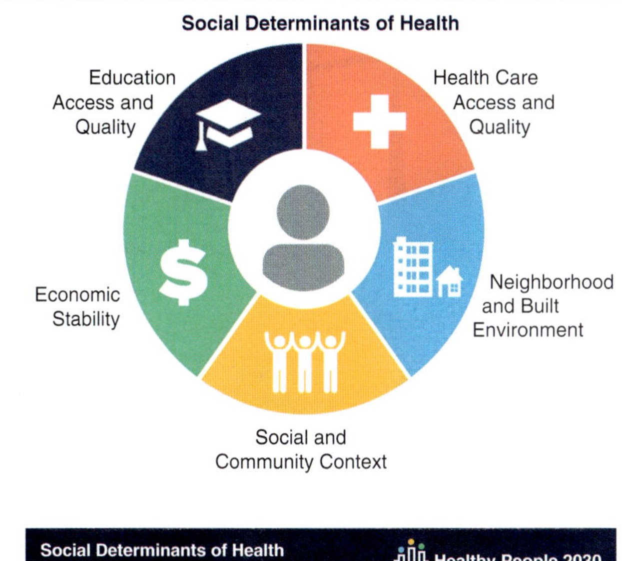

Feeling down every once in a while is a normal part of life, but if these feelings last a few weeks or months, one may have depression. Depression is a serious mood disorder. It can affect the way one feels, acts, and thinks. Depression is a common problem among older adults, but clinical depression is not a normal part of aging. In fact, studies show that most older adults feel satisfied with their lives, despite having more illnesses or physical problems than younger people. However, if one has experienced depression as a younger person, it might be more likely to have depression as an older adult.[1]

Estimates for depression in the older adult are as follows: 1%–5% for those living in the general community; 11.5% for those who are hospitalized; and 13% for those who require home health. It is characterized by feelings of sadness, anxiety, and/or apathy that last at least 2 weeks. It is different from the normal feelings that one has of sadness or grief after the death of a loved one. About 80% of older adults have at least one chronic health condition.[1]

There are many things that can be risk factors for depression. Changes in the brain can affect mood and result in depression. Others may experience depression after a major life event, like a loved one's death or major health event, or their own medical diagnoses. Addition causes of depression include caregiver stress, elder abuse, stroke, cancer, decreased activity/exercise, social isolation, alcoholism, drug addiction, financial issues, chronic pain, and decreased functional activity.[1] It is important that the older adult be assessed for depression in the various health care settings in which they are provided care. There are many assessment tools and toolkits that can be used and community referrals to assist them in their wellness journeys back to mental health wellness.

The following are some symptoms of depression found in older adults:[1]

- Apathy, or a sense of not caring about anything
- Persistent sadness
- Irritability
- Fatigue and low energy
- Feelings of guilt and worthlessness
- A sense of hopelessness
- Less of interest in activities once enjoyed
- Trouble concentrating and other cognitive changes
- Insomnia or oversleeping
- Overeating or a decrease in appetite
- Slower speech or movement
- Digestive problems that persist
- Physical pains that do not get better with treatment
- Recurring thoughts of death

Reference:

1. https://www.nia.nih.gov/health/depression-and-older-adults

Illustration from Healthy People 2030, U.S. Department of Health and Human Services, Office of Disease Prevention and Health Promotion. Retrieved September 8, 2022, from https://health.gov/healthypeople/objectives-and-data/social-determinants-health.

syndromes such as pressure injury, incontinence, falls, functional decline, and delirium.[4]

Immobility

Older adult patients are at risk of many complications of immobility, with those requiring mechanical ventilation for extended periods at the highest rate of mortality.[5] See Box 39.1.

Modifiable factors to reduce critical illness impairment and improve outcomes include (1) decreasing duration of mechanical ventilation, (2) prevention of immobility, (3) identification of delirium, (4) reduction in sleep disruption, and (5) family involvement in care.[6] Functional status before ICU admission is a strong predictor of the ability to recover, and disability after and from critical illness varies irrespective of age.

BOX 39.1 Complications of Immobility in the Older Adult

- Aspiration pneumonia
- Falls
- Deep vein thrombosis
- Loss of independence
- Pulmonary emboli
- Deconditioning
- Pressure injuries
- Bowel paralysis
- Pain
- Increased length of stay

Frailty

Frailty is described as reduced ability to adapt to health stressors based on factors in addition to chronological age.[7] Frailty can be classified as phenotypic or multidimensional. Phenotypic focuses on physical criteria such as weight loss, physical activity, and muscle strength. Multidimensional approaches identify frailty by examining a range of issues such as signs, symptoms, disabilities, and disease processes that would increase the risk of adverse outcomes.

Systematic reviews have identified frailty as a predictor of:

- in-hospital mortality
- increased length of stay
- discharge to a nursing home

Frailty assessment. Frailty assessment tools such as the *Katz Index of Independence in Activities of Daily Living, Barthel Index*, and *Frailty Index* are validated instruments to measure functional status in older adults.[7] Frailty assessments are a way to identify individuals at risk of poor outcomes and support

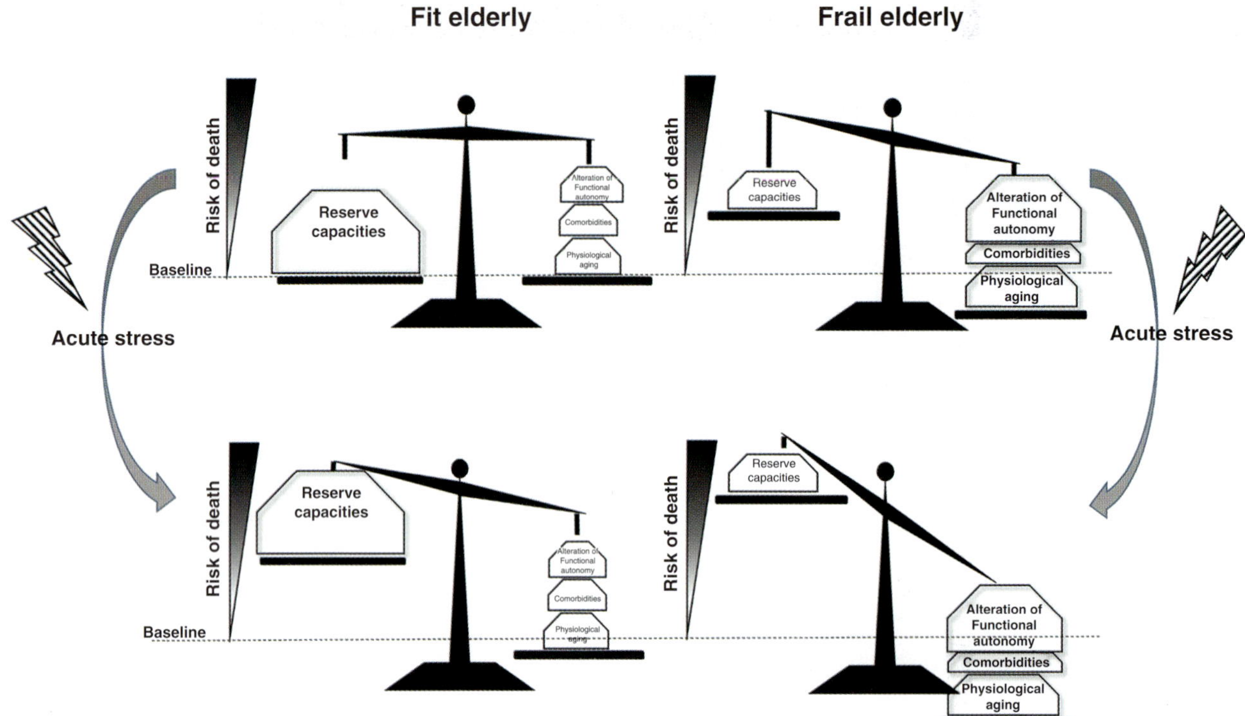

FIG. 39.1 Effect of Acute Stress on Fit and Frail Older Adults. Physiologic aging, comorbidities, and functional dependency are the main components of frailty syndrome, leading to decrease in reserve capacities. At baseline, impact of frailty on survival is slight, but its weight dramatically grows in case of acute stress (all medical events leading to critical care unit admission) and increase the risk of death comparatively to older adults. (Guidet B, Vallet H, Boddaert J, et al. Caring for the critically ill patients over 80: a narrative review. *Ann Intensive Care.* 2018; 8(1):114. doi: 10.1186/s 13613-018-0458-7)

complex patients by personalizing care. Fig. 39.1 illustrates the effect of stress on fit and frail older adults.

The Clinical Frailty Scale, (CFS), *Hospital Frailty Risk Score* (HFRS), *Frailty Index* (FI), and *Tilburg Frailty Indicator* are frailty tools available for prognostication short- and long-term outcomes.[8] The *CFS* is the most widely used instrument for ICU studies and is validated in people aged 65 and older. The choice of frailty measure used will depend greatly on the clinical setting and purpose for frailty assessment, such as to guide interventions, resource planning, prognostication, and even clinical research.[8]

Family and Caregiver Discharge Assessment and Preparation

Thorough discharge planning assessment and caregiver preparation may result in improved outcomes for patients, families, and health care systems. Unpaid caregivers such as family and friends provide approximately 34 billion hours of care and $470 billion in care labor.[9] Caregivers are often unprepared and receive little advice or education on medication management or clinical care before patients are discharged from the hospital.[9] Involving families in caregiving at admission can optimize understanding and planning for discharge.

Several instruments exist to assist with family caregiving assessment and education needs including novel tools that utilize artificial intelligence (AI) and machine learning.[10] Technology is advancing at a rapid rate and can support many aspects of health care. The therapeutic goal of most elderly patients should be to improve or maintain functional independence and alleviate pain.

Conversations with patients and caregivers should include expected outcome, patient values, and understanding that age is associated with an increased risk of iatrogenic complications.[11]

The American Thoracic Society recommends five goals to aid communication between clinician and families, including (1) establishing a trusting relationship; (2) providing emotional support; (3) understanding diagnosis, prognosis, and treatment options; (4) viewing the patient as a person; and (5) creating conditions for meaningful and difficult discussions.[5]

See Box 39.2, Informatics: Wearables and the Older Adult. It describes the role of technology in facilitating safety of the older adult by utilizing various types of technology.

AGE-RELATED CHANGES OF THE CARDIOVASCULAR SYSTEM

The greatest risk factor for cardiovascular disease in older adults is age. Cardiac and arterial system changes result in reduced cardiovascular function and reserve, leaving an older adult at increased risk for:[1,12,13]

- cardiac decompensation
- atherosclerosis
- hypertension
- myocardial infarction
- stroke

Pathological alterations of aging include increased arterial stiffness resulting in hypertrophy and altered left ventricular (LV) function.[1,12,13]

Dysrhythmias

Dysrhythmias increase with age, such as atrial fibrillation, paroxysmal supraventricular tachycardia, and premature

BOX 39.2 Informatics

Wearables and the Older Adult

Informatics and wearables play a significant role in enhancing the quality of life and well-being of older adults. As the global population ages, there is an increasing interest in utilizing technology to address this demographic group's unique challenges and needs. Here's how informatics and wearables are being used for older adults:

1. Health Monitoring: Wearable devices such as smartwatches, fitness trackers, and health monitors can continuously track various health parameters such as heart rate, blood pressure, sleep patterns, and physical activity. These devices provide valuable data to users and health care professionals, enabling early detection of potential health issues and timely intervention.
2. Fall Detection and Prevention: Falls are a major concern for older adults, often leading to serious injuries. Wearables equipped with accelerometers and gyroscope sensors can detect sudden movements and changes in posture that might indicate a fall. These devices can automatically send alerts to caregivers or emergency services, ensuring quick assistance.
3. Medication Management: Wearables and mobile apps can help older adults manage their medications by sending reminders to take pills or providing information about the correct dosage and timing. Some platforms also allow caregivers to remotely monitor medication adherence and receive notifications if doses are missed.
4. Cognitive Health: Cognitive decline is an issue among older adults. Cognitive training apps and games available on tablets and smartphones can help improve memory, attention, and problem-solving skills. These apps can be tailored to the individual's cognitive abilities and progress.
5. Social Engagement: Isolation and loneliness are prevalent concerns for older adults. Wearables and communication apps enable them to stay connected with friends and family through video calls, messaging, and social media. Some devices also offer features like location sharing for safety purposes.
6. Chronic Disease Management: Informatics solutions can assist in managing chronic conditions like diabetes and hypertension. Wearables can track relevant parameters, such as blood sugar levels or blood pressure, and send alerts or recommendations based on the collected data.
7. Remote Monitoring: Informatics technologies allow health care providers to remotely monitor older adults with chronic illnesses. Vital signs, symptoms, and other relevant data can be collected through wearables and transmitted to health care professionals for assessment and intervention, reducing the need for frequent in-person visits.
8. Personalized Health Insights: Data collected from wearables can be analyzed to provide personalized health insights and recommendations. This information can guide older adults towards healthier lifestyle choices and adopting habits supporting their overall well-being.
9. User-Friendly Interfaces: Designing user interfaces that are intuitive and easy to navigate is crucial for older adults who might not be as familiar with technology. Large fonts, simple icons, and voice commands can make wearables and informatics platforms more accessible to this demographic.

It is important to consider ethical and privacy concerns when implementing informatics and wearables for older adults. Data security, informed consent, and the option to control what information is shared should be central to the design and deployment of these technologies.

In summary, informatics and wearables offer numerous opportunities to enhance the lives of older adults by promoting health, safety, social engagement, and overall well-being. As technology advances, there is great potential to develop even more tailored solutions that cater to the unique needs of this demographic.

ventricular contraction, and can be predictive of future cardiac morbidity and mortality. Increased incidence of atrial fibrillation in the older adult is thought to be related to structural remodeling, decreasing compliance and increasing loading of blood vessels and electrical changes that generally require rate control and anticoagulation.[12,13]

Myocardial Infarction

Myocardial infarction (MI) incidence increases with age due to decreasing cardiovascular reserves and age-related myocardial and vascular stiffening, chronotropic incompetence, and other physiological changes of age.[12] Non–ST-segment elevation MIs (N-STEMI) or type 2 MIs are more common in older adults and are generally a result of supply/demand mismatch, whereas type 1 MIs are usually due to plaque erosion or rupture. Type 2 MIs most frequently occur with situations where oxygen demand and supply are mismatched, such as tachyarrhythmias, bradyarrhythmia, hypertension, anemia, and shock.

Therapeutic decisions must be carefully weighed in older adults with multimorbidity given complex cardiac regimen, elevated risks of bleeding, and exacerbation of other concomitant active conditions.[12]

Heart Failure

Heart failure (HF) is a common indicator of end-stage cardiovascular conditions such as coronary artery disease, chronic valvular heart disease, and persistent atrial fibrillation that may be related to chronic inflammation in the setting of diabetes mellitus (DM), hypertension, obesity, and chronic kidney disease (CKD).[12] Valvular heart disease can be acute due to valve lesions from endocarditis, chordal or papillary muscle rupture, aortic dissection, myocardial ischemia, prosthetic valve dysfunction, or iatrogenic injury where patients become acutely decompensated due to LV dysfunction or volume overload. Algorithms and clinical practice guidelines for diagnosis and treatment and management of valvular heart disease in older adults are the same as those for younger adults.[12] Health care is so dependent in all aspects upon technology to deliver care and support to patients and that application continues to grow. Refer to Informatics Box 39.3 for recommended actions to take after a cyberattack.

Polyvascular Disease

Inflammation has emerged as an important risk marker of systemic atherosclerosis and may play a role in progression of polyvascular disease leading to increased risk for cardiovascular events.[14] Many cardiovascular risk factors including advanced age, smoking, and diabetes are shared between peripheral artery disease (PAD), coronary artery disease (CAD), and other atherosclerotic diseases, though there may be different patterns of risk factors in different beds.[14]

Endothelial dysfunction, frailty, and immobility contribute to reduced vasodilation reserve, a prothrombotic environment, and decreased anticoagulant properties leading to increased risk of deep vein thrombosis, venous ulcers, arterial-ischemic ulcers, foot ulcers, and vasculitis.[15] The American Heart Association/American College of Cardiology recommend ankle-brachial index (ABI) screening in adults over 65 years as prevalence of PAD almost doubles over each additional decade of life starting

BOX 39.3 Informatics

After a Cyberattack

Preserving patient safety after a cyberattack is of utmost importance in health care organizations. Cyberattacks can disrupt critical systems, compromise patient data, and jeopardize patient care. To ensure patient safety in the aftermath of a cyberattack, these steps should be considered:

- Activate an Incident Response Plan (IRP):
  - Outline the roles and responsibilities of staff during a cyberattack.
  - Activate the plan immediately to ensure a coordinated response.
- Initiate Containment and Isolation:
  - Isolate affected systems from the network to prevent the spread of the attack.
  - Disconnect compromised devices and systems until they are adequately secured.
- Assess Impact:
  - Determine the extent of the breach and assess potential risks to patient safety.
  - Identify critical systems, medical devices, and patient records that might have been compromised.
- Communicate:
  - Maintain open communication with staff, patients, and relevant stakeholders.
  - Inform patients about the breach and its potential impact on their data and care.
- Preserve Patient Care Continuity:
  - Implement manual processes if necessary to ensure uninterrupted patient care.
  - Rely on paper records or alternate systems if electronic systems are compromised.
- Initiate Data Recovery and System Restoration:
  - Work with IT and cybersecurity experts to recover lost or compromised data and restore systems to normal functionality.
  - Ensure that data recovery processes are secure and do not introduce additional vulnerabilities.
- Complete Cybersecurity Upgrades:
  - Strengthen cybersecurity measures to prevent future attacks, including updating software, implementing multifactor authentication, and enhancing network monitoring and intrusion detection systems.
- Ensure Medical Device Safety:
  - If medical devices are compromised, consult with device manufacturers to assess potential risks to patient safety.
  - Isolate affected devices, update firmware if necessary, and ensure their safe operation before reintegrating them into patient care.
- Provide Staff Training:
  - Train staff members on cybersecurity best practices and how to recognize potential threats.
- Regulatory and Legal Compliance:
  - Comply with relevant data breach reporting requirements and notify appropriate regulatory bodies.
  - Ensure that legal obligations are met while managing the aftermath of the attack.
- Continuous Monitoring and Improvement:
  - Establish a continuous monitoring process to detect and respond to future threats.
  - Regularly review and update cybersecurity protocols to adapt to evolving risks.
- Collaboration and Information Sharing:
  - Collaborate with other health care organizations and cybersecurity experts to share information and best practices for mitigating and recovering from cyberattacks. A collective effort can help enhance overall patient safety.

The goal is to protect patient safety while addressing a cyberattack's immediate and long-term impacts. By following a well-prepared incident response plan and prioritizing patient care, health care organizations can effectively navigate the challenges posed by cyber threats. Patient safety should never be compromised due to a cyberattack.

Additional information can be found in the following resource: The Joint Commission, Preserving patient safety after a cyberattack. *Sentinel Event Alert.* 2023;(67):1–7. https://www.jointcommission.org/-/media/tjc/newsletters/sea-67-cybersecurity-7-26-23-final.

at age 40.[14] Risk assessment and prevention of complications for cardiovascular patients can improve longevity and quality of life in older adults.

Hypertension

In the United States, hypertension prevalence among adults is approximately 45% with blood pressure control worsening for older adults despite growing evidence of reductions in stroke and HF in patients older than 80 years.[16] Prevalence of hypertension increases from 27% in patients younger than 60 years to 74% in adults older than 80 years.[17] The longitudinal Framingham Heart Study demonstrated that 90% of the participants with normal blood pressure at age 55 years ultimately developed hypertension.[17]

Medication Management

Older adults with stable ischemic heart disease and hypertension should be prescribed a beta-blocker, calcium channel blocker, angiotensin-converting enzyme inhibitor (ACEI), or an angiotensin II receptor blocker (ARB) with the addition of other medications such as thiazide diuretics and mineralocorticoid receptor agonists for tighter control.[18]

Baroreceptor reflex response. Baroreflex-mediated tachycardia response to depressor agents is also attenuated in older adults. Orthostatic hypotension results from alteration in distribution of blood volume and position change, resulting in a reduction in cardiac output (CO) and blood pressure (BP). The baroreceptor reflex response also mediates changes in peripheral resistance and force of myocardial contraction, offsetting the drop in BP. Prevalence of orthostatic hypotension is greater in older patients; therefore, a judicious number of antihypertensive medications is recommended.[18]

Pathophysiology of hypertension. Pathophysiology of hypertension in the older adult includes mechanical hemodynamic variations, arterial stiffness with decreased capacitance and recoil, neurohormonal changes with decline in the renin-angiotensin-aldosterone system, autonomic dysregulation, and renal dysfunction. Systolic BP (SBP) increases with age, whereas diastolic BP (DBP) initially increases and then decreases due to central arterial stiffness leading to a widened pulse pressure.[17]

Increased left ventricle wall stiffness and reduced relaxation from increased interstitial connective tissue, myocyte hypertrophy, and changes in calcium channels in the sarcoplasmic reticulum may result in decreased cardiac reserve, sensitivity to changes in volume status, and resultant congestive HF and pulmonary edema.[17]

Preventative strategies. While preventative strategies and advanced therapies have greatly improved life expectancy, the associated economic cost has contributed to increased financial and societal burdens.[12,13] While many older adults with multimorbidity may not be eligible for advanced therapies, such as transplant and mechanical circulatory support, the majority of patients currently treated with transcatheter valve therapy are octogenarians with multiple comorbidities.[13]

Cardiac Medication Considerations in Older Adults

Treatment with medication should be considered when nonpharmacologic interventions such as diet, exercise, smoking cessation, stress reduction, and avoidance of excessive alcohol intake are unsuccessful.[17] Hypertension therapy should target an SBP less than 130 mm Hg for adults greater than 65 years of age.[16] Improved cardiovascular outcomes have been seen in older adults with use of thiazide diuretics, ACEIs, angiotensin II receptor blockers, and calcium channel blockers.[17,18] Arrythmias should be managed with focus on hemodynamic stability. Ventricular rate may be controlled with beta blockade, calcium channel blockers, or amiodarone to allow for increased left ventricle filling time and improved stroke volume.[5] See Table 39.1 for Cardiac Medication Considerations in Older Adults.

Goals of atrial fibrillation management should include decreasing volume overload and treating acute infection as well as considering the risk of cardioembolic stroke and bleeding complications associated with anticoagulation.[17] Anticoagulation therapy can also be complicated by polypharmacy, simultaneous use of antiplatelet medications, uncontrolled hypertension, and poorly controlled anticoagulation therapy; therefore, close attention to medication reconciliation and contraindications is needed. See Table 39.2 for Age-Related Changes in Pharmacokinetics.

TABLE 39.1 Cardiac Medication Considerations in Older Adults

Medication	Clinical Considerations
Thiazide Diuretics	
Hydrochlorothiazide Chlorthalidone Bendrofluazide	Recommended for initial hypertensive therapy ↓ Peripheral vascular resistance ↓ Intravascular volume ↓ BP Generally well tolerated in older adults ↓ Cardiovascular, cerebrovascular, renal adverse outcomes May exacerbate arrhythmias, hyperuricemia, glucose intolerance, dyslipidemia
Nonthiazide Diuretics	
Indapamide—sulfonamide diuretic	Increase blood glucose Do not increase uric acid Can cause potassium-independent prolongation of Q–T interval
Furosemide—loop diuretic	Increase blood glucose May cause headaches, fever, anemia May cause electrolyte disturbances
Mineralocorticoid Antagonists	
Spironolactone/eplerenone	Useful in hypertension when combined with other agents Cause potassium retention Not associated with adverse metabolic effects
Beta-Blockers	
Metoprolol	Indicated for older adult patients with: Hypertension, CAD, HF Certain arrhythmias Migraine headaches Senile tremor
Calcium Antagonists	
Phenylalkylamines—verapamil	Variable effects on heart muscle, sinus node function, atrioventricular conduction, peripheral arteries, coronary circulation
Benzothiazepines—diltiazem	Effective in older adult patients with hypertension due to increasing arterial stiffness, decreased vascular angina and supraventricular arrhythmias, compliance, diastolic dysfunction
Dihydropyridines—nicardipine	Should be avoided in patients with HF
ACEIs	
Captopril (Capoten) Enalapril (Vasotec) Lisinopril (Prinivil, Zestril)	Block conversion of angiotensin I to angiotensin II in tissue and plasma Lower peripheral vascular resistance and BP without reflex stimulation of heart rate and contractility Reduce morbidity and mortality in patients with HF, reduced systolic function, post-MI Retard progression of diabetic renal disease and hypertensive nephrosclerosis
Angiotensin Receptor Blockers	
Losartan (Cozaar) Valsartan (Diovan)	Selectively block AT1 receptor subtype to: Reduce BP Protect kidneys Reduce mortality and morbidity in HF patients Considered first line and as an alternative to ACEIs in older adult hypertensive patients with diabetes mellitus, hypertension, and HF who cannot tolerate ACEIs

TABLE 39.1 Cardiac Medication Considerations in Older Adults—cont'd

Medication	Clinical Considerations
Direct Renin Inhibitors	
Aliskiren	Effective for BP lowering without dose-related increases in adverse events in older adult patients May be used in combination therapy
Nonspecific Vasodilators	
Hydralazine Minoxidil	Fourth-line antihypertensive because of unfavorable side effects Tachycardia Fluid accumulation and atrial arrhythmias (minoxidil) when used as part of combination regimens Centrally acting agents (e.g., clonidine) are not first-line treatments in older adults because of sedation and/or bradycardia Abrupt discontinuation leads to increased BP and heart rate, which may aggravate ischemia and/or HF These agents should not be considered in noncompliant patients but may be used as part of a combination regimen if needed after several other agents are deployed
Centrally Acting Agents	
Clonidine	Not first-line treatments in older adults because of sedation and/or bradycardia Abrupt discontinuation leads to increased BP and HR

ACEIs, Angiotensin-converting enzyme inhibitors; *BP*, blood pressure; *CAD*, coronary artery disease; *HF*, heart failure; *MI*, myocardial infarction.
Adapted from Aronow WS, Fleg JL, Pepine CJ, et al. ACCF/AHA 2011 expert consensus document on hypertension in the elderly: a report of the American College of Cardiology Foundation task force on clinical expert consensus documents. *J Am Coll Cardiol.* 2011;57:2037.

TABLE 39.2 Age-Related Changes in Pharmacokinetics

Pharmacokinetic Parameter	Definition	Age-Related Changes
Absorption	Medication moves from site of administration to bloodstream; affected by mode of administration	Decreased absorptive surface area of small intestine and gastrointestinal motility Decreased splanchnic blood flow Increased gastric acid pH Changes in body skin/fat
Distribution	Medication is delivered from bloodstream to target tissues; affected by blood flow	Decreased lean body mass and total body water Increased total body fat Decreased serum albumin/plasma proteins Decreased red blood cells
Metabolism	Metabolic breakdown of a medication that renders it active or inactive; affected by mode of administration	Decreased liver mass Decreased medication metabolism Decreased total liver blood flow
Excretion	Removal of medication through an eliminating organ, often the kidney; some medications are excreted in bile or feces, in saliva, or through the lungs	Decreased renal blood flow/glomerular filtration rate Decreased distal renal tubular secretory function

Adapted from Rodrigues DA, Herdeiro MT, Figueiras A, Coutinho P, & Roque F. (2020). Elderly and polypharmacy: physiological and cognitive changes. In *Frailty in elder adults - understanding and managing complexity.* IntechOpen. https://www.intechopen.com/chapters/71815.

Goals of care related to cardiac arrest should be considered in older adults as survival rates diminish with age. Overall rates of return of spontaneous circulation (ROSC) and immediate survival of cardiopulmonary arrest for older adults' ranges from 11% to 30% with 1-year survival rates of 50% to 60%.

For those who experience out-of-hospital arrest, survival rates after cardiac arrest and CPR are even lower. Advanced care planning can help patients and families align goals of care with beneficial or unwanted interventions.[12]

AGE-RELATED CHANGES OF THE RESPIRATORY SYSTEM

Many age-related changes affect the pulmonary system, including (1) alterations in compliance of the chest wall, (2) strength of respiratory muscles, (3) connective tissue changes in the lung parenchyma leading to (4) reduced elasticity, (5) dysfunctional mucociliary transport resulting in, (6) difficulty with secretion clearance, (7) reduction in alveoli number, and (8) size affecting the alveolar-arterial (A-a) gradient and ventilation-perfusion

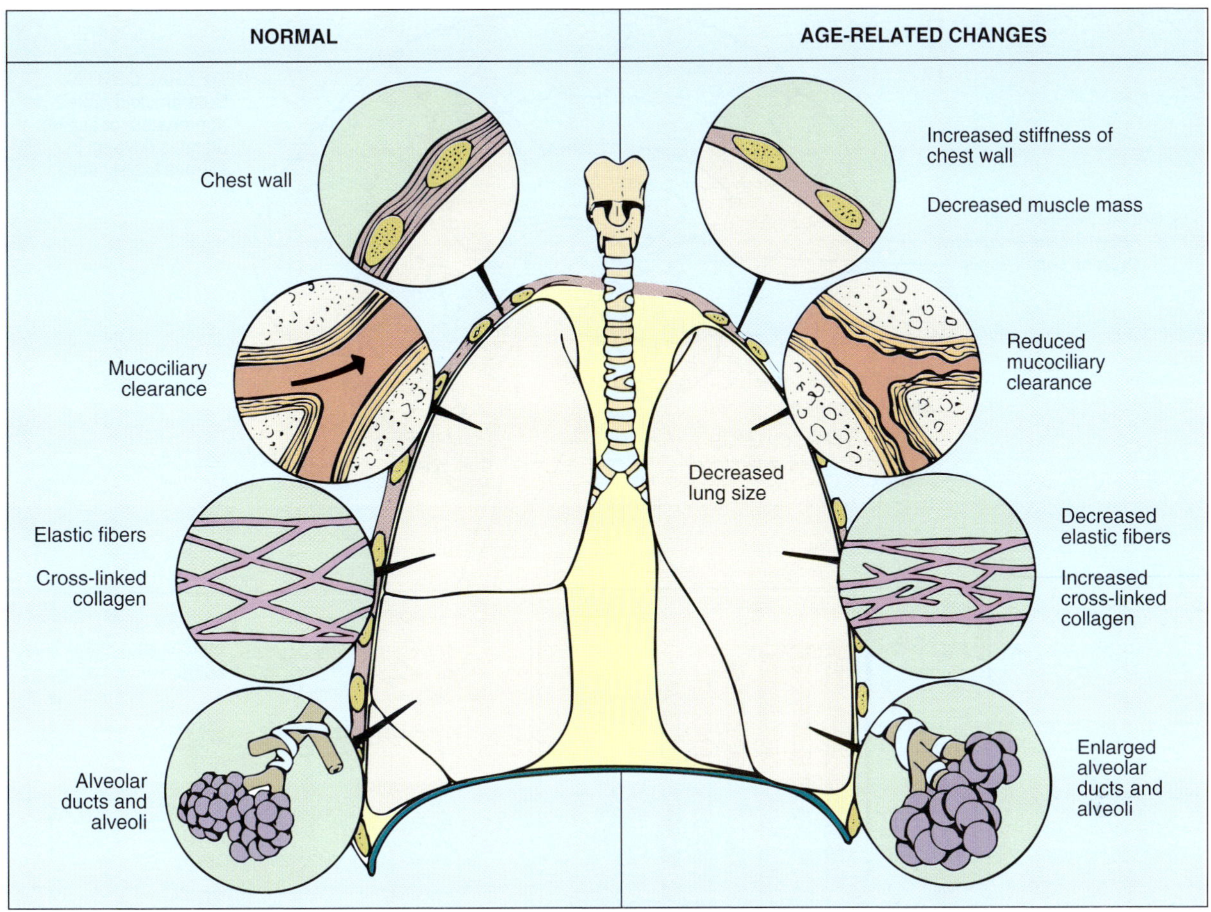

FIG. 39.2 Age-Related Changes in the Respiratory System. With advancing age, the compliance of the chest wall and lung tissue changes. There is also a reduced clearance of mucus by the cilia that line the pulmonary tree and an enlargement of the alveolar ducts and alveoli.

mismatch.[5] See Fig. 39.2 for age-related changes in the respiratory system.

Thorax Changes

The aging thorax has a greater anterior-posterior diameter than that in younger adults, and there is some degree of dorsal kyphosis due to osteoporosis. Rib mobility declines due to contractures of intercostal muscles and calcification of costal cartilage, decrease in chest wall compliance, shape of thorax, and changes in chest wall mechanics leading to deterioration in respiratory function.

During aging, skeletal muscle progressively atrophies, and its energy metabolism decreases. Respiratory muscle performance is impaired by geometric modifications of the rib cage, decreased chest wall compliance, and increases in functional residual capacity (FRC) resulting from decreased elastic recoil of the lung.

Chest Wall Compliance and Pulmonary Function Studies

Changes in chest wall compliance result in a greater contribution of breathing from the diaphragm and abdominal muscles and a lesser contribution from thoracic muscles, leading to increases in residual volume and decrease in vital capacity. There is an age-associated decrease in effectiveness of cough reflex and decrease in ciliary responsiveness and motion that predisposes older adult patients to aspiration and hospital-acquired infections.[5]

Pulmonary function studies may be the best way to assess respiratory impairment in older adults. Dynamic lung volumes and flow rates depend on resistance of airways and chest wall compliance and are limited by collapse of small airways during forced expiration. Breathing exercises generate lung volumes of forced vital capacity, which is an untimed lung volume, and 1-second forced expiratory volume, which is a timed lung volume. These spirometry tests can assist in assessing restrictive respiratory patterns. Reduced timed lung volume is exhibited in chronic obstructive pulmonary disease (COPD), asthma, bronchiectasis, and cystic fibrosis.

Other conditions that display reductions in timed and untimed lung volumes include kyphosis, scoliosis, myasthenia gravis, diaphragmatic paralysis, pleural effusions or fibrosis, and pulmonary hypertension. The application of conventional quality control standards to objective assessment of pulmonary function in older patients may prove difficult because of mood alterations, fatigability, lack of cooperation, or cognitive impairment.[5]

Acute Respiratory Failure

The incidence of acute respiratory failure increases with each decade of life resulting in a greater number of older adults being admitted to ICU for respiratory failure. Critically ill older adults are at increased risk for acute lung failure with chronic illness, major organ dysfunction, and decreased pulmonary reserve

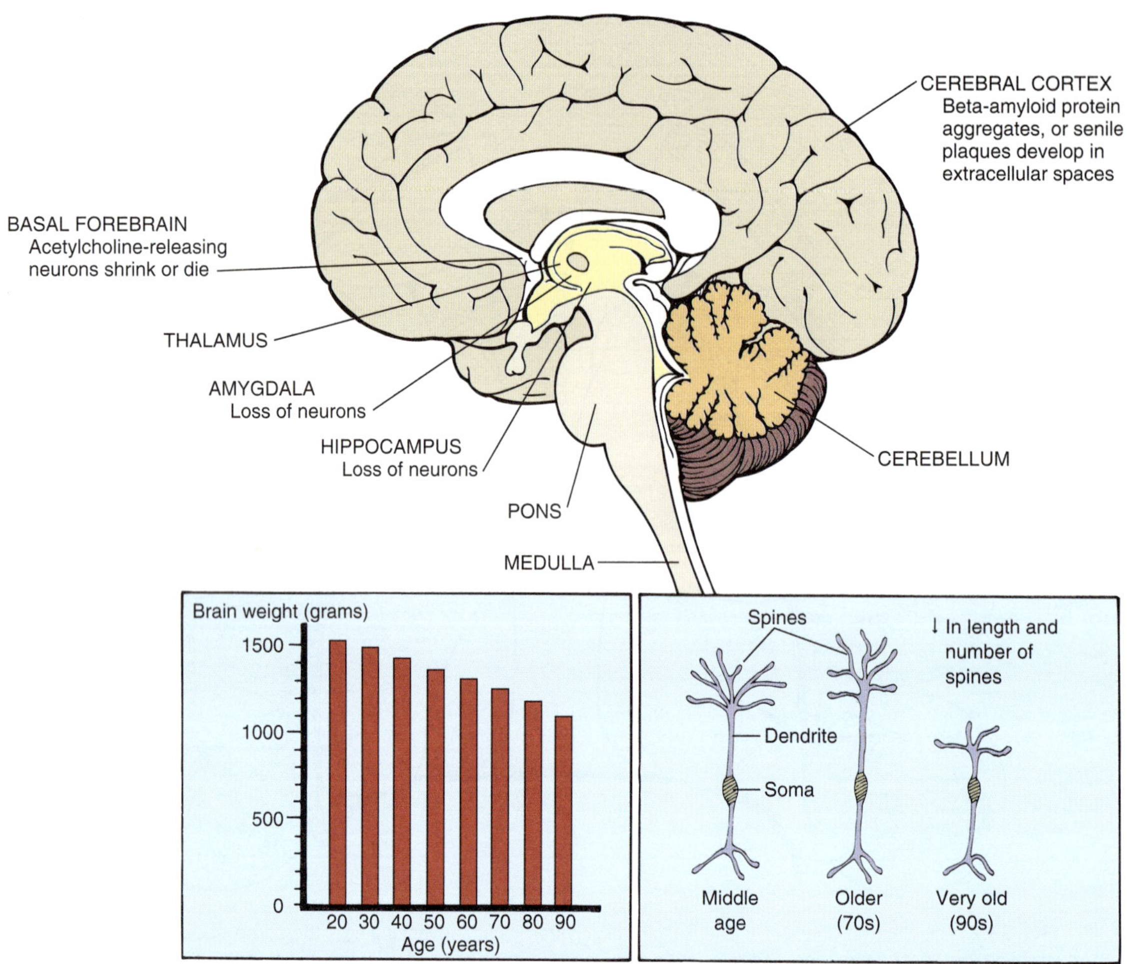

FIG. 39.3 Age-Related Changes in the Brain. (From Selkoe DJ. Aging brain, aging mind. *Sci Am.* 1992;267:134.)

contributing to the incidence of acute lung failure. Reduction in T-cell function, decline in mucociliary clearance, decrease in swallowing ability, and loss of cough reflex can increase the frequency and severity of pneumonia in older adults

Pneumonia

The clinical presentation of pneumonia in older adults may be atypical and include a nonproductive cough, delirium, anorexia, falls, and dizziness. *Noninvasive ventilation* (NIV) is highly effective for respiratory support during COPD exacerbations. Absolute contraindications for NIV include respiratory arrest, inability to maintain one's own airway, loss of airway reflexes, upper airway obstruction, copious secretions, emesis, and patient refusal.

Pulmonary Embolism

Older adults have a higher occurrence of pulmonary embolism as a result of predisposing conditions such as malignancy, postoperative states, and immobility where treatment with systemic anticoagulation places an older adult at a greater risk for adverse events.[5]

NEUROCOGNITIVE AGE-RELATED CHANGES

Loss of cognitive function has become one of the greatest threats of aging, with forecasts indicating that the population of Americans with either Alzheimer dementia or mild cognitive impairment will increase from 6.08 million in 2017 to 15 million in 2060.[2] See Fig. 39.3 for changes in the older adult brain.

Delirium in the Older Adult

Critically ill older adults are especially susceptible to acute brain dysfunction, which is commonly referred to as delirium in the ICU.[19] Older adults in the ICU with neurologic pathology such as traumatic brain injury, stroke, or postoperative cardiac or neurosurgical intervention are at risk for delirium.[5] The diagnostic and statistical manual of mental disorders (DSM-5) defines delirium as attention disturbance that develops rapidly without another preexisting, established, or evolving neurocognitive disorder.

Delirium Subtypes

Delirium has three subtypes: (1) hypoactive, lack of awareness and decreased motor activity; (2) hyperactive, combative, or agitated; and (3) mixed, a combination of both subtypes. The older adult is more likely to have hypoactive delirium with only 30% of delirium being recognized.[20] Morbidity and mortality rates from delirium can be similar to those from MI if left untreated.[20]

TABLE 39.3 Neurocognitive Age-Related Changes and Impairment

Age-Related Change	Resultant Impairment
Loss of gray and white matter volume and integrity	Impaired oxygen delivery
Decreased cerebral blood flow	Slowed metabolism
Increased blood-brain barrier permeability	Altered function of neurotransmitter, e.g., acetycholine, dopamine, serotonin, glutamate, that then negatively affects cognition, motor function, and regulation of sleep-wake cycles

Pathology and Impact of Delirium

The brain loses grey and white matter volume and integrity, cerebral blood flow, and increases blood-brain barrier permeability with aging. The result is impaired oxygen delivery, slowed metabolism, and altered function of neurotransmitters such as acetylcholine, dopamine, serotonin, and glutamate that impact cognition, motor function, and regulation of sleep-wake cycles.[5] See Table 39.3 for neurocognitive age-related changes and resultant impairment.

Orthostatic Hypotension

Endothelial dysfunction induces increases in endothelin-1 and decreasing bioavailability of nitric oxide influencing arterial dilation as well as other neurohormonal mechanisms affecting the renin-angiotensin-aldosterone system.[17] Orthostatic hypotension occurs in older adults as a result of decreased baroreflex sensitivity resulting in increased falls and cerebrovascular effects. Medications such as beta-blockers and diuretics may compound the possibility of developing orthostatic hypotension in those with cardiovascular disease as their ability to compensate is limited.[17]

Cerebral Blood Flow

Cerebral blood flow decreases with age and influences changes in blood pressure, barometric response to positional change, and cerebrovascular disease including ischemic and hemorrhagic strokes and vascular dementia.[17] Advancing age is also a risk factor for cerebral microbleeds, which is associated with decline in cognitive function and inability to perform activities of daily living and increased frailty.[6]

AGE-RELATED CHANGES OF RENAL SYSTEM

Aging Kidney

Aging is associated with various and complex abnormalities of hormones and systems that are important in water homeostasis and risk factors for CKD.[21] The *aging kidney* atrophies and has reduced function characterized by reduced renal mass, renal blood flow, glomerular sclerosis, tubular atrophy, fibrointimal hyperplasia, mesangial cell expansion, and impaired renal tubular capacity.[22]

BOX 39.4 Key Risks for Dehydration in the Older Adult

Reduced Thirst Sensation: Aging diminishes the ability to sense thirst, leading to lower fluid intake even when the body needs water.
Decreased Renal Function: The kidneys' ability to concentrate urine and conserve water declines with age, resulting in higher fluid loss.
Chronic Illnesses: Conditions such as diabetes, heart disease, or kidney disease can increase the risk of dehydration due to medication effects or fluid imbalances.
Medications: Diuretics, laxatives, and certain antihypertensive drugs can promote fluid loss, raising dehydration risk.
Cognitive Impairments: Dementia or other cognitive issues may lead to forgetting or neglecting to drink fluids.
Medications: Diuretics, laxatives, and certain antihypertensive drugs can promote fluid loss, raising dehydration risk.
Cognitive Impairments: Dementia or other cognitive issues may lead to forgetting or neglecting to drink fluids.
Mobility Challenges: Limited mobility or physical frailty may make it harder to access fluids or seek help when thirsty.
Reduced Fluid Reserves: Older adults have less total body water than younger individuals, making them more vulnerable to the effects of fluid loss.
Heat Sensitivity: Older adults are less efficient at regulating body temperature, increasing the risk of dehydration in hot environments.
Social and Psychological Factors: Isolation, depression, or financial constraints may limit access to fluids or awareness of hydration needs.

Decrease in Functional Nephrons

Mitochondrial energy production is reduced, disturbing active transport by kidney tubules, glucose reabsorption, and increased urine protein.[22] The number of functional nephrons and functional reserve decreases with age, contributing to reduced glomerular filtration rate (GFR) and creatinine clearance ratio.[22] After age 40, the GFR declines by about 8 mL/min/1.73 m^2 per decade. Renal blood flow declines by about 10% per decade and is approximately 300 mL/min at age 90 compared with 600 mL/min at age 40.[21]

Dehydration and Hypertension

Reduction in functional nephrons impairs sodium retention, dilution of urine, excretion of water, and renal tubular sensitivity/renal responsiveness to vasopressin, predisposing older adults to dehydration.[22] Box 39.4 outlines key risks for dehydration in the older adult. Hypertension stresses vessel walls, leading to thickening, and reduction in elasticity of the tunica intima and contributing to endothelial injury and decreased renal blood flow.[22] The renin-angiotensin-aldosterone system may be reduced in older adults by 30% to 50% compared with the younger population because of development of atheromatous plaques that limit vessel elasticity.[22]

Impact of Diabetes Mellitus and Heart Failure on the Older Adult

Twenty to thirty percent of older adults have DM and are at risk of developing diabetic nephropathy, including glomerular and microvascular injury, caused by excess blood glucose toxicity, leading to microinfarcts and decreased functional nephrons.[22] HF accounts for up to 20% of hospital admissions in patients older than 65 years of age in part due to hemodynamic changes of inadequate cardiac response to elevation of pulmonary and systemic venous pressures and decompensated renal function changes frequently, increasing risk of mortality.[22]

Cardiorenal Syndrome

Cardiorenal syndrome (CRS) type 1 is the term used to characterize the association between abrupt worsening of cardiac function and renal dysfunction. This phenomenon may be due to low renal perfusion, low CO, hypovolemia, venous congestion, renal intrinsic disease, or caused by drugs used in the treatment of HF, such as ACEIs and angiotensin-receptor blockers.[22]

Chronic Kidney Disease

CKD is defined as a GFR less than 60 mL/min/1.73 m^2 or by the presence of kidney damage for 3 or more months.[23] Main causes of *CKD* are diabetes, hypertension, or glomerulonephritis. Complications include anemia bone disease and increased risk of cardiovascular disease and cancer. People with CKD have diminished quality of life (QOL) and often poorer socioeconomic circumstances as CKD progresses.[23]

Acute Kidney Injury

Acute kidney injury (AKI) is commonly seen in the critical care unit and carries a mortality rate upwards of *50%*.[23] AKI occurs in 7% to 18% of hospital admissions and 57% of ICU admissions.[24] AKI is defined as an increase in serum creatinine (SCr) greater than or equal to 0.3 mg/dL in 48 hours or an increase up to 1.5 times the SCr baseline within 7 days or a urine output <0.5 mL/kg/h for more than 6 hours.[24]

AKI is characterized by acute damage to the kidney that results in alteration in acid-base balance, electrolyte abnormalities, and increase of nitrogen products.[23] Comorbidities that contribute to increased risk of AKI include hypertension, DM, heart disease, and CKD. Because medical procedures can induce AKI due to the lower drug excretion capacity of these patients and cause iatrogenic AKI, the use of contrasts and nephrotoxic drugs should be carefully considered.[23]

Renal Replacement Therapy

One therapy for critically ill patients with severe AKI is renal replacement therapy (RRT). Five to fifteen percent of critically ill patients developing AKI requiring RRT with rates of AKI-related mortality increasing substantially over the last 2 decades.[25] Studies have looked at RRT initiation timing because no clear guidelines exist. Most studies to date have found no significant benefit to initiation of early RRT.

Early RRT may also increase additional risk of invasive procedures and care expense.[26] These findings would indicate that the important decision to initiate dialysis treatment in older adults could be delayed until goals of care interventions are aligned with patients and surrogate decision makers.

AKI and ICU-acquired weakness (ICU-AW). Vigilance and attention to risk factors by the critical care nurse may prevent clinical deterioration to a point of AKI.[26] A more recent phenomenon is AKI and ICU-AW, which may have an incidence of up to 80%. ICU-AW is defined as muscle weakness and wasting resulting from critical illness. Muscle wasting occurs rapidly during critical illness with up to 30% of muscle mass lost in the first 10 days after ICU admission. ICU-AW is associated with increased mortality, hospital readmission, long-term functional impairment, and lower quality of life.[25] Risk factors include preexisting comorbidity, high severity of illness, sepsis, acute respiratory failure, prolonged immobilization, hyperglycemia, advanced age, RRT, corticosteroids, sedatives, or paralytics.

Approximately 40% of patients with end-stage renal disease in the United States are older than 65 years of age. Critical care nurses who are knowledgeable in the trajectory of renal disease can recognize signs of deterioration and alert interprofessional teams to patient conditions, which may prevent or reduce renal injury. Aging is associated with an increase in various disorders.

Water Balance Syndromes

Water balance syndromes are often seen in older hospitalized patients and carry an increased risk of death. The kidneys play a major role in regulation of body water with dehydration representing decline in total body water.[21] Dehydration can result from hyperglycemia and can be seen simultaneously with hypo- and hypernatremia. Dysnatremia is a cause or surrogate marker of underlying diseases. Hypernatremia appears to increase the risk of death more than hyponatremia.[27]

Risk factors for hypernatremia include increased water loss and decreased water intake. Etiologies for increased water loss include osmotic diuresis (diuretic-induced free water loss, glycosuria), uncompensated diabetes insipidus, age-associated impaired concentrating capacity, resistance to vasopressin action (age-related and acquired, e.g., drugs), renal tubular disease, osmotic diarrhea, insensible fluid losses with excessive sweating, or tachypnea.[21]

Causes for decreased water intake include impaired thirst perception, which is blunted in older adults and impaired cognition or physical impairments to enabling access to fluids that lead to dehydration, hypernatremia, and hyperosmolarity.[21,27] Many older adult patients are unable to communicate their needs effectively and are especially susceptible to abnormalities of their electrolyte and body water homeostasis.

Increased water loss from urination via diuretics and poorly controlled or undiagnosed diabetes may cause dehydration in older adults. Other causes of dehydration include diabetes insipidus, excessive sweating, and insensible fluid loss, especially in older adults with fever and in those with an increased respiratory effort, diarrhea, and vomiting.[21]

Polypharmacy can also affect water balance in older adults. Nonsteroidal antiinflammatory agents commonly lead to sodium retention. Diuretics can promote sodium loss and impair the diluting capacity and concentrating capacity of the kidney.[21]

Syndrome of inappropriate antidiuretic hormone secretion (SIADH) can be induced by several drugs, including psychotropics (antidepressants, selective serotonin reuptake inhibitors [SSRIs]), phenothiazines, antineoplastic agents (vincristine, cyclophosphamide), carbamazepine, chlorpropamide, clofibrate, and opioids.[21] Symptoms of dehydration in adults include thirst, confusion, dizziness, and fatigue. Delirium, dementia, and cognitive dysfunction are common causes of dehydration in older adults, leading to agitation, hallucinations, and anxiety.

Hyponatremia is the most common electrolyte disorder seen in clinical practice. Risk factors for hyponatremia fall into three categories: (1) increased free water intake, (2) decreased ability to excrete water, and (3) sodium depletion.[21] Causes for a reduced ability to excrete water in older adults include decreased renal diluting capacity; increased vasopressin secretion and/or action related to idiopathic, drug-induced, inflammatory pulmonary disease; or malignancy with SIADH and CNS disease.

In the older adult population, SIADH is a common cause of hyponatremia.[21] Hyponatremia in older adults is associated with neurocognitive decline, gait instability, falls, osteoporosis, bone loss, incidence of bone fractures, hospital readmission rates, need for long-term care, and mortality.[21]

Hypervolemic hyponatremia can be seen in patients with acute HF, cirrhosis, or renal impairment; it can be exercise induced with ingestion of excess water during exercise and weight gain. Beer potomania, caused by ingestion of large volumes of beer, can lead to retention of water and dilutional hyponatremia.[21] These patients consume low amounts of sodium and have long-term depletion of sodium stores.[21]

DIABETES IN OLDER ADULTS

Diabetes is underdiagnosed and can be found in at least 25% of older adults, with prevalence continuing to increase rapidly over coming decades with higher risks for geriatric syndromes.[28] Diabetes results in higher mortality, reduced functional status, increased risk for institutionalization, and elevated risk for acute and chronic microvascular and cardiovascular complications requiring frequent screening and follow-up.[28] Age-related changes such as insulin resistance and diminished pancreatic islet function add to the risk for developing type 2 diabetes in older adults.

Diabetic Care Management

Recommendations for diabetic management reflect the three major classes of older adults: (1) Healthy (few coexisting chronic illnesses, intact cognitive and functional status); (2) older adults with complex/intermediate medical conditions (multiple coexisting chronic illnesses) or activities of daily living (ADL) impairments or mild-to-moderate cognitive impairment); and (3) older adults with a very complex/poor health (end-stage chronic illnesses or moderate-to-severe cognitive impairment or more than two ADL impairments). [28]

Older adults, particularly adults with diabetes, are more likely to require hospitalization than younger adults. Critically ill hospitalized patients should be evaluated with a personalized plan based on disease and therapeutic goals where less strict targets may be appropriate for patients with multiple comorbidities and reduced life expectancy. Geriatric syndromes are more likely to occur in older adults with diabetes, such as cognitive dysfunction, frailty, functional impairment, and falls due to peripheral neuropathy, vision and hearing difficulty, and gait/balance problems.[28]

For older adult patients who require insulin, it is important to remember that insulin therapy requires good visual and motor coordination, which may be challenging for some older adults. Several tools exist for older adults with diabetes such as those for prognostication, health literacy, self-management, and numeracy that can help with shared decision-making, therapeutic interventions, and goal alignment.[28]

AGE-RELATED CHANGES OF THE GASTROINTESTINAL SYSTEM AND NUTRITION

Aging Gastrointestinal Physiology Impact

Aging physiology predisposes older adults to impaired energy regulation, metabolism derangements, and malnutrition.[29] Older adults are at risk of malnutrition syndromes, which include protein-energy malnutrition, starvation, sarcopenia, and cachexia.[29] Hospitalized, malnourished older adult patients are at a higher risk for morbidity and mortality than healthy older adults.[29] Poor nutrition is linked to inferior outcomes in critically ill older adults as stress-related catabolism and proinflammatory cytokines result in deterioration of nutritional status, increasing length of stay, risk of infection, and poor prognosis.[30]

Sarcopenia represents a state involving muscle mass loss with its associated functional decline with causes due to nutritional deficiencies, impaired response of skeletal muscle to nutrients, and endocrine dysregulation.[29] Hormonal imbalances lead to muscle catabolism and decreases in insulin, estrogen, and testosterone.[31]

Nutritional Screening Tools

Various risk-screening tools exist such as nutritional assessments recommended by the European Society for Clinical Nutrition and Metabolism (ESPEN), Nutritional Risk Screening 2002 (NRS-2002), Nutritional Risk in the Critically ill (NUTRIC), and the Geriatric Nutritional Risk Index (GNRI). GNRI is simple, designed for older adults, and requires minimal participation by patients, making it useful for ICU.[30] Nutritional and swallow screening are needed in all older adult hospitalized patients to identify those at higher nutritional and aspiration risk.

Feeding Goals

Feeding goals should be achieved within 48 hours in older adult ICU patients with oral or enteral nutrition via gastric feeding as the first-line choice. Small bowel feeding can be attempted in those at high risk for aspiration or those who can have an enteral feeding tube placed in the small bowel. Obstacles that promote cessation of feeding must be identified and minimized daily to reduce risks and negative outcomes of malnutrition.

AGE-RELATED CHANGES OF THE LIVER

Change in Liver Physiology and Liver Dysfunctions

Physiologic changes in the senescent liver include a decrease in reduced liver weight, volume, blood flow, and number of hepatocytes, as well as the loss of metabolic function. Age reduces detoxification in the liver and can have significant effect on pharmacokinetics and medication uptake in the older adult. Etiologies of hepatic dysfunction include viral diseases, autoimmune diseases, alcoholic liver diseases, and nonalcoholic steatohepatitis (NASH).[31]

Nonalcoholic fatty liver disease (NAFLD) and NASH affect 30% and 5% of the American population, respectively.[32] NAFLD rates are increasing in parallel to rates of obesity and diabetes, with cirrhosis being the third leading cause of death in these patients.

Treatment for Liver Conditions

Although there have been many advances in therapeutic interventions for hepatic diseases, there is currently no standard therapy to treat liver cirrhosis, but lifestyle modifications can be made to alter liver disease trajectory.[32] Hepatic encephalopathy is characterized by disturbance of consciousness, which can also be hazardous to older adult patients who have increased risk of falls, aspiration, and other accidental injury.

The treatment for hepatic encephalopathy is to increase bowel activity that may induce diarrhea and result in dehydration. Lactulose and rifaximin may be used as a therapeutic option for treatment of hepatic encephalopathy in older adult patients.

Hepatic Encephalopathy

A major decompensating event that causes hepatic encephalopathy or brain dysfunction due to underlying liver disease and portal hypertension can lead to coma. Hepatic encephalopathy is a treatable disease that predisposes patients to chronic malnutrition, nutritional deficiency, thiamine deficiency, cognitive impairment, and alcohol neurotoxicity and can cause alcoholic cerebellar degeneration. It is treatable with nutritional intravenous therapy (see below).

The American Academy of Neurology recommends also screening for other reversible causes of cirrhosis or liver failure, such as vitamin B12 deficiency and perhaps homocysteine levels; this reflects the function of three vitamin B elements including folate vitamin B12 and B6 tests for syphilis human immunodeficiency virus and Lyme disease should also be considered in patient it will have cognitive impairment. Awareness of cirrhosis and hepatic encephalopathy in patients with liver disease will help to increase surveillance and interventions.[33]

TABLE 39.4 Complications and Management of Liver Cirrhosis in Older Adults

Complications	Management (General)	Considerations Should Be Given in Older Adult Patients
Ascites	Sodium restrictions	Electrolyte abnormalities
	Antimineral corticoid	Changes in circulation dynamics
	Furosemide	Body weight
	Torsemide	Pulse and blood pressure
	Albumin infusion	Verification of blood biochemistry and urinalysis
Hepatic encephalopathy	Optimization of bowel movement	Diarrhea
	Laxatives	Frequent diarrhea that causes electrolyte abnormalities
	Branched-chain amino acids	Skin troubles from frequent defecation
	Synthetic disaccharide lactulose	Dehydration
	Rifaximin	Cardiac stress and fluctuation of electrolytes
	Intravenous drip infusion of Fischer solution	
Gastrointestinal bleeding/varices	Nonselective beta-blockers	Arrhythmia
	Endoscopic therapy	Fluctuation of blood pressure
		Heart failure
		Aspiration pneumonia
Sarcopenia	Risk of fall-related injury	Nutritional monitoring (serum markers including the albumin, cholesterol level)
		Muscle volume
		Administration of branched-chain amino acid preparations
Skin symptoms	Skin moisturizers	Likely to have dry skin
	Bile salts	Frequently suffer from wound infections and persistent skin inflammation
	Rifampicin	Nalfurafine hydrochloride
	Antihistamines	
Hepatocellular carcinoma	Use of phase contrast for the diagnosis	Renal function
	Surgical therapy	Cardiac function
	Transarterial chemotherapy	Bone marrow function
	Needle guided local therapy	History of cerebral bleeding
	Molecular-targeted therapies	Hypertension
		Renal function
Cirrhotic cardiomyopathy		Cardiac function
Spontaneous bacterial peritonitis		Sarcopenia
Hepatorenal syndrome		Further clinical trials and information from retrospective studies are necessary
Acute and chronic kidney injury		
Hyponatremia		

From Brennan-Cook J, Turner RL. Promoting skin care for older adults. *Home Healthc Now.* 2019;37(1):10–16.

Complications of Liver Failure

Strategies to differentiate between hepatic encephalopathy and other disease processes include risk factors, time course, cognitive testing, and brain imaging.[31] Another complication of liver failure is *ascites,* which refers to fluid collection in the abdomen, and is a poor prognostic indicator in liver disease.[13] Ascites can cause organ compression and edema that leads to difficulty in walking and falls in older adults.

Gastrointestinal bleeding is also a complication that occurs due to gastroesophageal varices, portal hypertension, gastropathy, and intestinopathy, while also increasing risk of mortality in older adults. Hepatocellular carcinoma, bacterial infections, renal impairment, cardiopulmonary dysfunction, spontaneous bacterial peritonitis, acute and chronic kidney injury, cirrhotic cardiomyopathy, hepatorenal syndrome, and hyponatremia are all complications of liver disease and present increasing challenges with advancing age.[31] See Table 39.4 for Complications and Management of Liver Cirrhosis in Older Adults.

AGE-RELATED CHANGES IN THE IMMUNE SYSTEM

Infections in older adults are the leading cause of morbidity and mortality and are generally more complicated than infections in younger individuals.[34] Adults older than 65 years of age are three to five times more likely to die of an infection than younger adults and are more susceptible to hospital-acquired infections due to immunosenescence, or age-related changes in the immune system.[34]

Immunosenescence combined with comorbidities and geriatric syndromes influence outcomes of older adults with infectious diseases. As the aging population increases, there will be increasing costs and ethical issues associated with invasive ICU interventions.[34]

Risk of Sepsis and Sepsis Shock in the Older Adult

Mechanical ventilation and renal replacement therapy will be a concern as the rate of pneumonia, urinary tract infections, and bacteremia lead to increased risk of sepsis and septic shock.[34] Approximately 60% of hospitalized older adult patients with sepsis present with nonspecific symptoms, including altered mental status, anorexia, and generalized weakness; therefore, it is imperative that clinicians are aware of this atypical presentation so that early recognition, early resuscitation, early antibiotics, and early source control can be initiated.[34,35]

Chronic Critical Illness Condition

There is also a subset of patients who progress to a state of chronic critical illness appearing to be in a persistent inflammatory response state with a dysregulated immune system response.[36] These patients display weakness, inability to perform basic activities of daily living, recurrent infections, decreased wound healing, and a prolonged catabolic state.[36] Critical care nurses need to be aware that these patients are at increased risk of nosocomial infections and hospital acquired conditions.

AGE-RELATED CHANGES IN THE SKIN AND INTEGUMENTARY SYSTEM

The skin is the largest organ that protects the body from pathogens, chemicals, and physical injury through a variety of biological functions using skin microbiota, inflammatory processes, and adaptive immunity.[37] The skin's primary function is thermoregulation, protection from mechanical stress, and safety from microbes that becomes less elastic, drier, and more wrinkled with age.[37] Skin layers include the epidermis, dermis, and hypodermis, which change with age, becoming less elastic and drier with less ability to regenerate and heal wounds.[37]

Diminished wound healing is particularly important in the critical care environment, where increased opportunity to develop pressure injuries and infections exists. Hospital-acquired pressure injury in ICU has prevalence rates between 12% and 24.5% and attributed costs of $26.8 billion annually.[38,39]

Frequent cleansing with alkaline soap increases surface pH, removes the lipid film layers, worsens skin dryness, and decreases skin barrier function and medications such as diuretics, laxatives, antilipemics, and antiandrogens that can exacerbate xerosis, leading to itching, scratching, inflammation, and infections.[40] Critically ill patients are at high risk for the development of pressure injuries due to the severity of their condition, immobility, and medications such as vasopressors. Patients receiving norepinephrine are three times more likely to develop a pressure injury.[39]

Comprehensive risk assessment, appropriate support surface selection, and pressure relief using slow gradual turns or small micro-shifts are recommended for patients with hemodynamic instability to allow reperfusion to areas of compromised tissue oxygenation.[39]

Skin tears are a significant problem for older adult critical care unit patients with friable skin. A skin tear is a wound caused by shear, friction, and/or blunt force resulting in separation of skin layers.[41] A skin tear can be partial thickness, where there is separation of the epidermis from the dermis, or full thickness, where there is separation of both the epidermis and dermis from underlying structures.[41]

Evidence suggests that skin tears may occur more frequently than pressure injuries.[41] In the past few years there has been an increased focus and research into skin tears. The International Skin Tear Advisory Panel developed a classification system and best practice recommendations to assess and treat skin tears based on degree of severity.[41] See Table 39.5 for Age-Related Changes That May Affect Skin Integrity.

AGE-RELATED CHANGES IN THE MUSCULOSKELETAL SYSTEM

Falls can be particularly damaging to older adults; 25% of older Americans experience falls with injury that result in cognitive and physical dysfunction and loss of independence.[42] The critical care unit and acute care settings are particularly dangerous for older adults with cognitive impairment because they have increased risk of falling compared with older adults without cognitive impairment. Vascular dementia, Lewy body dementia, Alzheimer dementia, Parkinson disease, and other neurodegenerative and movement disorders predispose older adults to falls.[42] See Box 39.5 for factors associated with an increased risk of falling.

Hospitalized older adults should undergo a complete fall assessment that includes attention to intrinsic, behavioral, environmental, social, and economic components.[42] Bone density is also an independent predictor of poor survival in ICU elderly

TABLE 39.5 Age-Related Changes That May Affect Skin Integrity

Body System	Age-Related Changes	Effects on Skin
Cardiac	Decreased blood flow Fragile capillaries	Delayed wound healing Increased bruising
Neurologic	Decreased sensation Decreased memory Increased confusion Decreased vision	Increased risk of physical injury (burns) May not sense skin breakdown May forget to care for skin Risk for falls and skin damage May not visualize skin breakdown
Musculoskeletal	Decreased mobility	Increased risk for skin breakdown and pressure injuries May have difficulty reaching areas for good skin care
Genitourinary	Increased incontinence Increased moisture Dehydration	Risk for skin breakdown and increased irritation Risk for infection Dry scaly skin
Gastrointestinal	Increased incontinence and diarrhea episodes Decreased appetite Decreased intake/malnutrition Decreased chewing ability with less dentition	Risk for skin irritation and breakdown Delayed wound healing
Immune	Decreased immunity Decreased ability to regulate temperature	Risk for skin infection Increased risk for skin cancer

Data from Brennan-Cook J, Turner RL. Promoting skin care for older adults. *Home Healthc Now*. 2019;37(1):10–16.

BOX 39.5 Safety

Factors Associated With an Increased Risk of Falling

Biological/Intrinsic

Impaired Mobility

- Balance deficit
- Gait deficit
- Muscle weakness
- Advanced age
- Chronic illness/disability
- Cognitive impairment
- Stroke
- Parkinson disease
- Diabetes
- Arthritis
- Heart disease
- Incontinence
- Foot disorders
- Visual impairment
- Acute illness

Behavioral

- History of falls
- Fear of falling
- Polypharmacy
- Use of:
  1. Antipsychotics
  2. Sedatives/hypnotics
  3. Antidepressants
  4. Excessive alcohol
  5. Risk-taking behaviors
- Lack of exercise
- Inappropriate footwear/clothing
- Inappropriate assistive devices use
- Poor nutrition or hydration
- Lack of sleep

Social and Economic

- Low income
- Lower level of education
- Illiteracy/language barriers
- Poor living conditions
- Living alone
- Lack of support networks and social interaction
- Lack of transportation
- Cultural/ethnicity

Environmental

- Poor building design and/or maintenance
- Inadequate building codes
- Stairs
- Home hazards
- Lack of:
  1. Handrails
  2. Curb ramps
  3. Rest areas
  4. Grab bars
  5. Good lighting or sharp contrasts
- Slippery or uneven surfaces
- Obstacles and tripping hazards

Source: Public Health Agency of Canada. (2014). *Seniors falls in Canada, a second report*. https://www.canada.ca/en/public-health/services/publications/healthy-living/seniors-falls-canada-second-report.html. Cheung C. (2017). Older adults, falls, and skin integrity. *Adv Skin Wound Care*. 2017;30(1):40–46.

adults.[43] While bone density scans are not routine in ICUs, computed tomography (CT) scans are commonplace and can provide a simple prognostication tool.[43]

Osteoblast and osteoclast activity reduces calcium absorption into bone, causing osteoporosis, bone demineralization, and decreased bone mass that increases risk of falls. Osteoporosis results in delicate bones that are at risk for fractures and may result in mortality and decrease QOL for older adults. Medication review is needed for all older adults, specifically to consider the drug-drug, drug-disease, and drug-age interactions that lead to perturbations in balance, equilibrium, and hypotension.

The use of four or more medications increases an older adult's risk of falling with strongest links with use of benzodiazepines, SSRIs, tricyclic antidepressants, neuroleptics, and anticonvulsants.[42] Many older adults will survive their ICU hospitalization but then have a long journey of recovery with up to 65% of survivors experiencing loss of muscle mass, polyneuropathy, and sarcopenia and not achieve functional recovery within 6 months of the critical illness.

Long-term recovery after critical illness in older adults is a multifaceted process that encompasses physical, cognitive, and psychological challenges. Older adults often experience prolonged physical impairments, such as muscle weakness and reduced mobility, due to extended bed rest and the catabolic effects of critical illness.[44] Comprehensive recovery requires interdisciplinary care, including physical therapy, cognitive rehabilitation, nutritional support, and mental health interventions, tailored to address the unique vulnerabilities of this population and promote the best possible quality of life.

Fig. 39.4 illustrates and summarizes physiologic changes that occur in all systems of the older adult.

Box 39.6 lists Internet resources related to the older adult that enhance content in this chapter.

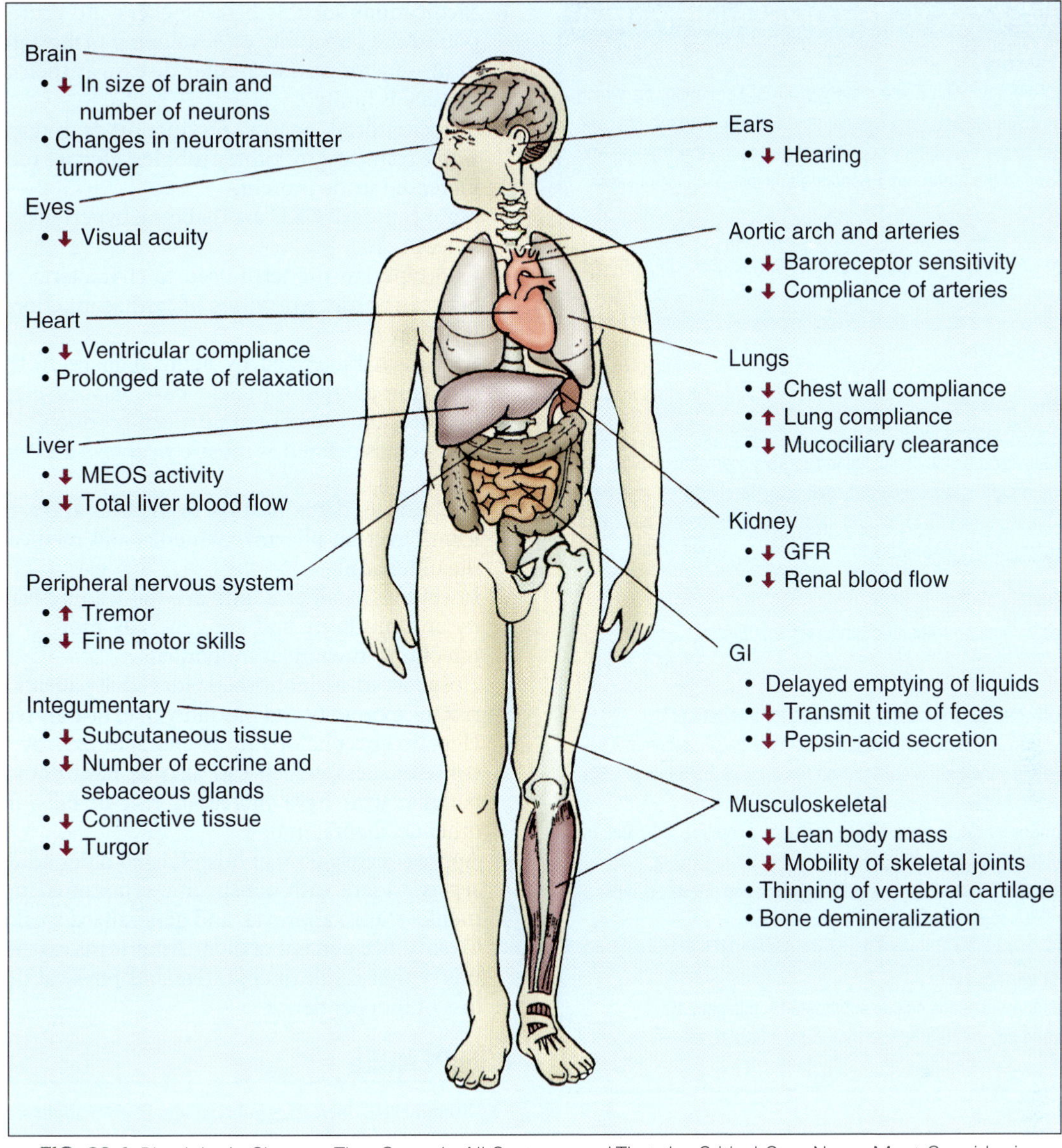

FIG. 39.4 Physiologic Changes That Occur in All Systems and That the Critical Care Nurse Must Consider in Caring for an Older Adult Patient in the Critical Care Unit. *GFR*, Glomerular filtration rate; *GI*, gastrointestinal; *MEOS*, microsomal enzyme oxidative system.

BOX 39.6 Internet Resources

The Older Adult Patient

- Advocacy Centre for the Elderly http://www.advocacycentreelderly.org/
- American Board of Internal Medicine https://abimfoundation.org/what-we-do/choosing-wisely
- American Board of Internal Medicine https://abimfoundation.org/what-we-do/health-equity-inclusion/commitment-to-act-for-health-equity
- Advocacy Services for Elderly help@americorp.gov
- American Geriatrics Society https://www.americangeriatrics.org/
- Geriatric Nursing Society https://geriatricscareonline.org/
- Healthy Aging, National Aging Council: https://www.nia.nih.gov/health/what-do-we-know-about-healthy-aging
- National Council on Aging: https://www.nia.nih.gov/about/naca
- NIA Alzheimer's Disease: https://www.nia.nih.gov/about/nia-and-national-plan-address-alzheimers-disease
- Wound, Ostomy, and Continence Nursing Society https://www.wocn.org/

KEY POINTS

- Many older adults have at least one chronic condition, with many having multimorbidity, frailty, dementia, and disability, making them vulnerable to adverse outcomes.
- Older adults will account for almost a quarter of the total population, requiring transformation of societal structure, health care redesign, creative reimbursement models, and innovative training.
- Older adults currently account for 20% of ICU admissions, indicating a need to incorporate geriatric-focused interventions and principles into ICU care.
- Older adult patients are at risk of many complications of immobility, with those requiring mechanical ventilation for extended periods at the highest rate of mortality.
- Frailty assessments are a way to identify individuals at risk of poor outcomes and support complex patients by personalizing care.

CASE STUDY 39.1 The Older Adult Patient

Brief Patient History

Mr. S is a 70-year-old man who has a history of atrial fibrillation, for which he takes warfarin, hypertension, and chronic obstructive pulmonary disease and who presented to the emergency department at 3 a.m. after tripping and falling while walking to the bathroom. He reported no loss of consciousness.

Focused Clinical Assessment

Mr. S is admitted to the critical care unit from the emergency department. Nursing assessment findings include drowsiness, confusion, and mild left hemiparesis. He also has a raised area of ecchymosis on his right forehead and complains of a headache.

Diagnostic Procedures

The patient's admission laboratory test results are unremarkable except for an international normalized ratio of 4. Computed tomography scan of the head without contrast shows a right-sided subdural hematoma. Baseline vital signs are as follows: blood pressure of 170/65 mm Hg, heart rate of 80 beats/min (atrial fibrillation), respiratory rate of 20 breaths/min, and temperature of 98.4 °F.

Medical Diagnosis

Mr. S is diagnosed with acute traumatic subdural hematoma.

Questions

1. What major outcomes do you expect to achieve for this patient?
2. What problems or risks must be managed to achieve these outcomes?
3. What interventions must be initiated to monitor, prevent, manage, or eliminate the problems and risks identified?
4. What interventions could be initiated to promote optimized functioning, safety, and well-being of the patient?
5. What technology can be used to monitor this patient and prevent complications?
6. What other interprofessional team members are needed to assist with the management of this patient?
7. What possible learning needs do you anticipate for this patient?
8. What cultural and age-related factors may have a bearing on the patient's plan of care?

- Therapeutic goal of most elderly patients should be to improve or maintain functional independence and alleviate pain.
- Dysrhythmias such as atrial fibrillation, paroxysmal supraventricular tachycardia, and premature ventricular contraction increase with age and can be predictive of future cardiac morbidity and mortality.
- HF is a common indicator of end-stage cardiovascular conditions such as coronary artery disease, chronic valvular heart disease, and persistent atrial fibrillation that may be related to chronic inflammation in the setting of DM, hypertension, obesity, and CKD.
- The clinical presentation of pneumonia in older adults may be atypical and include a nonproductive cough, delirium, anorexia, falls, and dizziness.
- The incidence of acute respiratory failure increases with each decade of life resulting in a greater number of older adults being admitted to ICU for respiratory failure.
- Critically ill older adults are especially susceptible to acute brain dysfunction, which is commonly referred to as delirium in the ICU.
- The brain loses grey and white matter volume and integrity and cerebral blood flow and increases blood-brain barrier permeability with aging.
- Medications such as beta-blockers and diuretics may compound the possibility of developing orthostatic hypotension in those with cardiovascular disease as their ability to compensate is limited.
- Mitochondrial energy production is reduced, disturbing active transport by kidney tubules, glucose reabsorption, and increased urine protein.
- Main causes of CKD are diabetes, hypertension, or glomerulonephritis.
- CRS type 1 is the term used to characterize the association between abrupt worsening of cardiac function and renal dysfunction.
- AKI is characterized by acute damage to the kidney that results in alteration in acid-base balance, electrolyte abnormalities, and increase of nitrogen products.
- ICU-AW is defined as muscle weakness and wasting resulting from critical illness.
- Age reduces detoxification in the liver and can have a significant effect on pharmacokinetics and medication uptake in the older adult.
- Infections in older adults are the leading cause of morbidity and mortality and are generally more complicated than infections in younger individuals.
- Hospitalized, malnourished older adult patients are at increased risk for morbidity and mortality than healthy older adults.
- Hepatic encephalopathy is characterized by disturbance of consciousness, which can also be hazardous to older adult patients who have increased risk of falls, aspiration, and other accidental injury.
- Approximately 60% of hospitalized older adult patients with sepsis present with nonspecific symptoms, including altered mental status, anorexia, and generalized weakness.
- Twenty-five percent of older Americans experience falls with injury that result in cognitive and physical dysfunction and loss of independence.

REFERENCES

1. Brummel NE. Increasing vulnerability in older adults with critical illness: implications for clinical care and research. *Chest*. 2022;161(6):1436–1437. https://doi.org/10.1016/j.chest.2022.02.014.
2. Living TA for C. *2020 Profile of Older Americans*. US Department of Health and Human Services. Published online 2021.
3. Cobert J, Jeon SY, Boscardin J, et al. Trends in geriatric conditions among older adults admitted to US ICUs between 1998 and 2015. *Chest*. 2022;161(6):1555–1565. https://doi.org/10.1016/j.chest.2021.12.658.
4. Wissanji T, Forget MF, Muscedere J, Beaudin D, Coveney R, Wang HT. Models of care in geriatric intensive care—a scoping review on the optimal structure of care for critically ill older adults admitted in an ICU. *Crit Care Explor*. 2022;4(4):e0661. https://doi.org/10.1097/CCE.0000000000000661.
5. Brunker LB, Boncyk CS, Rengel KF, Hughes CG. Elderly patients and management in intensive care units (ICU): clinical challenges. *Clin Interv Aging*. 2023;18. https://doi.org/10.2147/CIA.S365968.
6. Devlin JW, Skrobik Y, Gélinas C, et al. Clinical practice guidelines for the prevention and management of pain, agitation/sedation, delirium, immobility, and sleep disruption in adult patients in the ICU. *Crit Care Med*. 2018;46(9):E825–E873. https://doi.org/10.1097/CCM.0000000000003299.
7. Boreskie KF, Hay JL, Boreskie PE, Arora RC, Duhamel TA. Frailty-aware care: giving value to frailty assessment across different healthcare settings. *BMC Geriatr*. 2022;22(1). https://doi.org/10.1186/s12877-021-02722-9.
8. Chong E, Ho E, Baldevarona-Llego J, et al. Frailty in hospitalized older adults: comparing different frailty measures in predicting short- and long-term patient outcomes. *J Am Med Dir Assoc*. 2018;19(5):450–457.e3. https://doi.org/10.1016/j.jamda.2017.10.006.

9. Fields B, Carbery M, Schulz R, Rodakowski J, Terhorst L, Still C. Evaluation of face validity and acceptability of the care partner hospital assessment tool. *Innov Aging.* 2023;7(2). https://doi.org/10.1093/geroni/igad011.
10. Wunderlich P, Wiegräbe F, Dörksen H. Digital case manager—a data-driven tool to support family caregivers with initial guidance. *Int J Environ Res Public Health.* 2023;20(2). https://doi.org/10.3390/ijerph20021215.
11. Guidet B, Vallet H, Boddaert J, et al. Caring for the critically ill patients over 80: a narrative review. *Ann Intensive Care.* 2018;8(1). https://doi.org/10.1186/s13613-018-0458-7.
12. Damluji AA, Forman DE, Van Diepen S, et al. Older adults in the cardiac intensive care unit: factoring geriatric syndromes in the management, prognosis, and process of care: a scientific statement from the American Heart Association. *Circulation.* 2020;141(2). https://doi.org/10.1161/CIR.0000000000000741.
13. Goyal P, Kwak MJ, Al Malouf C, et al. Geriatric cardiology: coming of age. *JACC: Advances.* 2022;1(3). https://doi.org/10.1016/j.jacadv.2022.100070.
14. Aday AW, Matsushita K. Epidemiology of peripheral artery disease and polyvascular Disease. *Circ Res.* 2021;128(12):1818–1832. https://doi.org/10.1161/CIRCRESAHA.121.318535.
15. Mayrovitz HN, Wong S, Mancuso C. Venous, arterial, and neuropathic leg ulcers with emphasis on the geriatric population. *Cureus.* 2023;15(4):1–11. https://doi.org/10.7759/cureus.38123.
16. Chiu N, Chiu L, Aggarwal R, Raber I, Bhatt DL, Mukamal KJ. Trends in blood pressure treatment intensification in older adults with hypertension in the United States, 2008 to 2018. *Hypertension.* 2023;80(3):553–562. https://doi.org/10.1161/HYPERTENSIONAHA.122.19882.
17. Oliveros E, Patel H, Kyung S, et al. Hypertension in older adults: assessment, management, and challenges. *Clin Cardiol.* 2020;43(2). https://doi.org/10.1002/clc.23303.
18. Whelton PK, Carey RM, Aronow WS, et al. 2017 ACC/AHA/AAPA/ABC/ACPM/AGS/APhA/ASH/ASPC/NMA/PCNA Guideline for the Prevention, Detection, Evaluation, and Management of High Blood Pressure in Adults: A Report of the American College of Cardiology/American Heart Association Task Force on Clinical Practice Guidelines. *Hypertension.* 2018;71(6):e13-e115.
19. Stollings JL, Kotfis K, Chanques G, Pun BT, Pandharipande PP, Ely EW. Delirium in critical illness: clinical manifestations, outcomes, and management. *Intensive Care Med.* 2021;47(10):1089–1103. https://doi.org/10.1007/s00134-021-06503-1.
20. Heppner HJ, Haitham H. Intensive care of geriatric patients—a thin line between under- and overtreatment. *Wiener Medizinische Wochenschrift.* 2022;172(5–6). https://doi.org/10.1007/s10354-021-00902-1.
21. Koch CA, Fulop T. Clinical aspects of changes in water and sodium homeostasis in the elderly. *Rev Endocr Metab Disord.* 2017;18(1):49–66. https://doi.org/10.1007/s11154-017-9420-5.
22. Yokota LG, Sampaio BM, Rocha EP, Balbi AL, Prado IRS, Ponce D. Acute kidney injury in elderly patients: narrative review on incidence, risk factors, and mortality. *Int J Nephrol Renovasc Dis.* 2018;11:217–224. https://doi.org/10.2147/IJNRD.S170203.
23. Webster AC, Nagler EV, Morton RL, Masson P. Chronic kidney disease. *The Lancet.* 2017;389(10075):1238–1252. https://doi.org/10.1016/S0140-6736(16)32064-5.
24. Schaubroeck HAI, Vargas D, Vandenberghe W, Hoste EAJ. Impact of AKI care bundles on kidney and patient outcomes in hospitalized patients: a systematic review and meta-analysis. *BMC Nephrol.* 2021;22(1). https://doi.org/10.1186/s12882-021-02534-4.
25. Teixeira JP, Mayer KP, Griffin BR, et al. Intensive care unit–acquired weakness in patients with acute kidney injury: a contemporary review. *American Journal of Kidney Diseases.* 2023;81(3):336–351. https://doi.org/10.1053/j.ajkd.2022.08.028.
26. Chaudhuri D, Herritt B, Heyland D, et al. Early renal replacement therapy versus standard care in the ICU: a ystematic review, meta-analysis, and cost analysis. *J Intensive Care Med.* 2019;34(4):323–329. https://doi.org/10.1177/0885066617698635.
27. Grangeon-Chapon C, Dodoi M, Esnault VLM, Favre G. Osmotic stress and mortality in elderly patients with kidney failure: a retrospective study. *Clin Interv Aging.* 2019;14:225–229. https://doi.org/10.2147/CIA.S158987.
28. Older adults: standards of medical care in diabetes-2021. *Diabetes Care.* 2021;44::S168–S168. https://doi.org/10.2337/dc21-s012.
29. Lugli AK, de Watteville A, Hollinger A, Goetz N, Heidegger C. Review medical nutrition therapy in critically Ill patients treated on intensive and intermediate care units: a literature review. *J Clin Med.* 2019;8(9). https://doi.org/10.3390/jcm8091395.
30. Peng JC, Zhu YW, Xing SP, Li W, Gao Y, Gong WW. Association of geriatric nutritional risk index with all-cause hospital mortality among elderly patients in intensive care unit. *Front Nutr.* 2023;10. https://doi.org/10.3389/fnut.2023.1117054.
31. Kamimura K, Sakamaki A, Kamimura H, et al. Considerations of elderly factors to manage the complication of liver cirrhosis in elderly patients. *World J Gastroenterol.* 2019;25(15):1817–1827. https://doi.org/10.3748/wjg.v25.i15.1817.
32. Rinella ME. Nonalcoholic fatty liver disease a systematic review. *JAMA.* 2015;313(22):2263–2273. https://doi.org/10.1001/jama.2015.5370.
33. Bajaj JS, Gentili A, Wade JB, Godschalk M. Specific challenges in geriatric cirrhosis and hepatic encephalopathy. *Clinical Gastroenterology and Hepatology.* 2022;20(8). https://doi.org/10.1016/j.cgh.2022.04.035.
34. Esme M, Topeli A, Yavuz BB, Akova M. Infections in the elderly critically-ill patients. *Front Med (Lausanne).* 2019;6. https://doi.org/10.3389/fmed.2019.00118.
35. Evans L, Rhodes A, Alhazzani W, et al. Surviving sepsis campaign: international guidelines for management of sepsis and septic shock 2021. *Intensive Care Med.* 2021;47(11):1181–1247. https://doi.org/10.1007/s00134-021-06506-y.
36. Nomellini V, Kaplan LJ, Sims CA, Caldwell CC. Chronic critical illness and persistent inflammation: what can we learn from the elderly, injured, septic, and malnourished? *Shock.* 2018;49(1):4–14. https://doi.org/10.1097/SHK.0000000000000939.
37. Khalid KA, Nawi AFM, Zulkifli N, Barkat MA, Hadi H. Aging and wound healing of the skin: a review of clinical and pathophysiological hallmarks. *Life.* 2022;12(12). https://doi.org/10.3390/life12122142.
38. Cox J, Edsberg LE, Koloms K, VanGilder CA. Pressure injuries in critical care patients in US hospitals: results of the International Pressure Ulcer Prevalence Survey. *Journal of Wound, Ostomy and Continence Nursing.* 2022;49(1):21–28. https://doi.org/10.1097/WON.0000000000000834.
39. Cox J, Schallom M, Jung C. Identifying risk factors for pressure injury in adult critical care patients. *AmerJ Crit Car.* 2020;29(3):204–213. https://doi.org/10.4037/ajcc2020243.
40. Brennan-Cook J, Turner RL. Promoting skin care for older adults. *Home Healthc Now.* 2019;37(1). https://doi.org/10.1097/NHH.0000000000000722.
41. Campbell KE, Baronoski S, Gloeckner M, et al. Skin tears: prediction, prevention, assessment and management. *Nurs Prescribing.* 2018;16(12). https://doi.org/10.12968/npre.2018.16.12.600. http://www.skintears.org/.
42. Cheung C. *Older Adults, Falls, and Skin Integrity C M E 1 AMA PRA Category 1 Credit TM ANCC 1.0 Contact Hours CLINICAL SCENARIO C L I N I C A L M A N A G E M E N T Extra.* Vol 30.; 2017. http://cme.lww.com
43. Schulze-Hagen MF, Roderburg C, Wirtz TH, et al. Decreased bone mineral density is a predictor of poor survival in critically ill patients. *J Clin Med.* 2021;10(16). https://doi.org/10.3390/jcm10163741.
44. Kaushik R, Ferrante LE. Long-term recovery after critical illness in older adults. *Curr Opin Crit Care.* 2022;28(5):572–580. https://doi.org/10.1097/MCC.0000000000000981.

A APPENDIX

Patient Care Management Plans

Kathleen M. Stacy

PATIENT CARE MANAGEMENT PLAN

Activity Intolerance

Activity Intolerance Due to Cardiopulmonary Dysfunction

Signs and Symptoms

- Chest pain with activity
- Electrocardiogram (ECG) changes with activity
- Heart rate is >15 beats/min above baseline with activity for patients on beta-blockers or calcium channel blockers
- Heart rate remains elevated above baseline 5 min after activity
- Breathlessness with activity
- SpO_2 <92% with activity
- Postural hypotension when moving from supine to upright position
- Patient reports fatigue with activity

Outcomes

- Heart rate is <20 beats/min above baseline with activity and is <10 beats/min above baseline with activity for patients on beta-blockers or calcium channel blockers.
- Heart rate returns to baseline 5 min after activity.
- Chest pain with activity is absent.
- Patient reports tolerance to activity.

Interventions and Rationale

1. Encourage active or passive range-of-motion exercises while the patient is in bed **to keep joints flexible and muscles stretched.**
2. Teach the patient to refrain from holding breath while performing exercises and **to avoid Valsalva maneuver.**
3. Encourage performance of muscle-toning exercises at least three times daily **because a toned muscle uses less oxygen when performing work than an untoned muscle.**
4. Progress ambulation **to increase tolerance to activity.**
5. Teach the patient to take pulse **to determine activity tolerance:** Take pulse for a full minute before exercise and then for 10 s and multiply by 6 at exercise peak.
6. Collaborate with the practitioner regarding administration of fluids to ensure that the patient is hydrated to 24-hour fluid requirements per body surface area **to increase preload and increase stroke volume and cardiac output.**

Activity Intolerance Due to Prolonged Immobility or Deconditioning

Signs and Symptoms

- Decrease in systolic blood pressure is >20 mm Hg.
- Increase in heart rate is >20 beats/min with postural change.
- Syncope occurs with postural change.
- Patient reports lightheadedness with postural change.

Outcomes

- Decrease in systolic blood pressure is <10 mm Hg.
- Increase in heart rate is <10 beats/min with postural change.
- Syncope or lightheadedness is absent with postural change.
- Hypoxemia is absent.
- Patient reports tolerance to activity.

Interventions and Rationale

1. Collaborate with the practitioner regarding the patient's activity level and the need for physical therapy **to ensure the patient's safety.**
2. Collaborate with the physical therapist to develop a progressive activity plan for the patient **to return to prior level of function.**

For Patient on Bed Rest

1. Instruct the patient how to perform straight-leg raises, dorsiflexion or plantar flexion, and quadriceps-setting and gluteal-setting exercises **to increase muscular and vascular tone.**
2. Reposition the patient incrementally **to avoid syncope:**
   a. Head of bed to 45 degrees and hold until symptom-free
   b. Head of bed to 90 degrees and hold until symptom-free
   c. Dangle until symptom-free
   d. Stand until symptom-free and ambulate

For Patient on Mechanical Ventilation

1. Collaborate with the practitioner, respiratory care practitioner, and physical therapist regarding the patient's eligibility for early progressive mobility **to ensure patient is ready and able to participate.**
2. Initiate early progressive mobility program when the patient is ready **to limit the effects of prolonged immobility.**
   a. Elevate the head of the bed.
   b. Turn patient every 2 hours.
   c. Perform passive range of motion at least three times a day.
   d. Progress patient to active range of motion when ready.
   e. Place bed in chair position to position patient in upright/leg-down position.
   f. Initiate bed mobility activities such as sitting on the edge of the bed (dangling).
   g. Initiate transfer training.
   h. Implement pregait activities such as standing at the side of the bed and marching in place.
   i. Progress patient to ambulation.
3. Monitor the patient's response to activity and discontinue activity if patient shows signs of intolerance **to ensure patient safety:**
   a. Hypoxemia
   b. Hypotension
   c. Dysrhythmias or ECG changes

PATIENT CARE MANAGEMENT PLAN

Acute Pain

Acute Pain Due to Transmission and Perception of Cutaneous, Visceral, Muscular, or Ischemic Impulses

Signs and Symptoms

Subjective

- Patient verbalizes presence of pain.
- Patient rates pain on a scale of 1 to 10 using a visual analog scale.

Objective

- Increase in blood pressure, heart rate, and respiratory rate
- Pupillary dilation
- Diaphoresis, pallor
- Skeletal muscle reactions (e.g., grimacing, clenching fists, writhing, pacing, guarding, or splinting of affected part)
- Apprehension, fearful appearance
- May not exhibit any physiologic change

Outcomes

- Patient verbalizes that pain is reduced to a tolerable level or is totally relieved.
- Patient's pain rating is lower on a scale of 1 to 10.
- Blood pressure, heart rate, and respiratory rate return to baseline 5 min after intravenous (IV) administration of an opioid analgesic or 20 min after intramuscular administration of an opioid analgesic.

Interventions and Rationale

1. Modify variables that heighten the patient's experience of pain.
    a. Explain to the patient that frequent, detailed, and seemingly repetitive assessments will be conducted to allow the nurse to better understand the patient's pain experience, not because the existence of pain is in question.
    b. Explain the factors responsible for pain production in the individual. Estimate the expected duration of the pain if possible.
    c. Explain diagnostic and therapeutic procedures to the patient in relation to sensations the patient should expect to feel.
    d. Reduce the patient's fear of addiction by explaining the difference between drug tolerance and drug dependence. **Drug tolerance is a physiologic phenomenon in which a medication begins to lose effectiveness after repeated doses; drug dependence is a psychological phenomenon in which opioids are used regularly for emotional, not medical, reasons.**
    e. Instruct the patient to ask for pain medication when pain is beginning and not to wait until it is intolerable.
    f. Explain that the practitioner will be consulted if pain relief is inadequate with the present medication.
    g. Instruct the patient in the importance of adequate rest, especially when it reduces pain **to maintain strength and coping abilities and to reduce stress.**
2. Collaborate with the practitioner regarding pharmacologic interventions.
    a. For postoperative or posttraumatic cutaneous, muscular, or visceral pain, perform the following:
        (1). Medicate with an opioid analgesic to break the pain cycles as long as level of consciousness and vital signs are stable.
        (2). Check the patient's previous response to similar dosage and opioids.
        (3). Establish optimal analgesic dose that brings optimal pain relief.
        (4). Offer pain medication at prescribed regular intervals rather than making the patient ask for it **to maintain more steady blood levels.**
        (5). Consider waking the patient to avoid loss of opiate blood levels during sleep.
        (6). If administering medication on as-needed (PRN) basis, give it when the patient's pain is just beginning, rather than at its peak.
            (a). Advise the patient to intercept pain, not endure it, or several hours and higher doses of opioid analgesics may be necessary to relieve pain, leading to a cycle of undermedication and pain alternating with overmedication and drug toxicity.
        (7). Perform rehabilitation exercises (turn, deep breathe, leg exercises, ambulate) shortly before peak of drug effect **because this will be the optimal time for the patient to increase activity with the least risk of increasing pain.**
        (8). When making the transition from one drug to another or from intramuscular or IV to oral medication, use an equianalgesic chart. **Equianalgesic means approximately the same pain relief. The patient's response should be closely monitored to determine whether the right analgesic choice was made.**
        (9). To assess effectiveness of pain medication, do the following:
            (a). Reevaluate pain 15 to 30 min after IV and 30 to 60 min after oral medication administration; observe the patient's behavior, and ask the patient to rate pain on a scale of 1 to 10.
            (b). Collaborate with the practitioner to add or delete other medications that potentiate the action of analgesics, such as antiemetics, hypnotics, sedatives, or muscle relaxants.
            (c). Observe for indicators of undertreatment: report of pain not relieved; observed restlessness, sleeplessness, irritability, and anorexia; decreased activity level.
            (d). Observe for indicators of overtreatment: hypotension or bradycardia; respiratory rate <10/min; excessive sedation.
        (10). Evaluate the patient's level of sedation and respiratory rate at regular intervals **to avoid oversedation.**
            (a). Respirations should be counted for a full minute and qualified according to rhythm and depth of chest excursion.
            (b). Consider the use of capnography (end-tidal carbon dioxide monitoring) as an early indicator of hypoventilation and oversedation.
        (11). If patient-controlled analgesia (PCA) is used, perform the following:
            (a). Instruct the patient on what the drug is, the dose, and how often it can be self-administered by pushing the button to activate the PCA machine. For example, "When you have pain, instead of asking the nurse to bring medication, push the button that activates the machine and a small dose of the pain medicine will be injected into your IV line. You can keep your pain under control by administering additional medicine as soon as your pain begins to return or increases. Push the button before undertaking a painful activity, such as ambulation. Try to balance your pain relief against sleepiness, and don't activate the machine if you start to feel sleepy. If your pain medicine seems to stop working despite pushing the button several times, call the nurse to check your IV. If you are not receiving adequate pain relief, the nurse will call your doctor."
            (b). Monitor vital signs, especially blood pressure and respiratory rate, every hour for the first 4 hours, and assess postural heart rate and blood pressure before initial ambulation.
            (c). Monitor respiratory rate every 2 hours while the patient is on PCA.
            (d). If the patient's respiratory rate decreases to <10 breaths/min or if patient is overly sedated, anticipate administration of naloxone.

Continued

PATIENT CARE MANAGEMENT PLAN

Acute Pain—cont'd

(12). If epidural opioid analgesia is used, do the following:
- (a). Keep the patient's head elevated 30 to 45 degrees after injection **to prevent respiratory depressant effects.**
- (b). Observe closely for respiratory depression for 24 hours after injection. Monitor respiratory rate every 15 min for 1 hour, every 30 min for 7 hours, and every hour for the remaining 16 hours.
- (c). Assess for adequate cough reflex.
- (d). Avoid use of other central nervous system depressants, such as sedatives.
- (e). Observe for reports of pruritus, nausea, and vomiting.
- (f). Anticipate administration of naloxone for respiratory depression (and smaller doses of naloxone for pruritus).
- (g). Assess for and treat urinary retention.
- (h). Assess epidural catheter site for local infection. Keep the catheter taped securely **to prevent catheter migration.**

For peripheral vascular ischemic pain (hypothetic vascular occlusion of leg), do the following:

(13). Correctly identify and differentiate ischemic pain from other types of pain. (NOTE: Ischemic pain is usually a burning, aching pain made worse by exercise and lessened or relieved by rest. Eventually, the pain occurs at rest. Coldness and pallor of the extremity may be noted, especially if the limb is elevated above the heart level. Rubor and mottling of the skin may be evident from prolonged tissue anoxia and inability of damaged vessels to constrict. Eventually, cyanosis and gangrenous tissue will be evident. Chronic ischemia leads to visible changes in the limb, such as flaking skin, brittle nails and hair, leg ulcers, and cellulitis.)

(14). Administer pain medications and evaluate their effectiveness as previously described. The pain of ischemia is chronic and continuous and can make the patient irritable and depressed.

(15). Treat the cause of the ischemic pain and institute measures to increase circulation to the affected part.

3. Initiate nonpharmacologic interventions.
   - a. Treat contributing factors.
   - b. Apply comfort measures.
     - (1). Use relaxation techniques, such as back rubs, massage, warm baths, music, and aromatherapy.
       - (a). Use blankets and pillows to support the painful part and reduce muscle tension.
       - (b). Encourage slow, rhythmic breathing.
     - (2). Encourage progressive muscle relaxation techniques.
       - (a). Instruct the patient to inhale and tense (tighten) specific muscle groups and then relax the muscles as exhalation occurs.
       - (b). Suggest an order for performing the tension and relaxation cycle (e.g., start with facial muscles and move down body, ending with toes).
     - (3). Encourage guided imagery.
       - (a). Ask the patient to recall an experienced image that is very pleasurable and relaxing and involves at least two senses.
       - (b). Have the patient begin with rhythmic breathing and progressive relaxation and then travel mentally to the scene.
       - (c). Have the patient slowly experience the scene (e.g., how it looks, sounds, smells, feels).
       - (d). Ask the patient to practice this imagery in private.
       - (e). Instruct the patient to end the imagery by counting to three and saying, "Now I'm relaxed." If the person does not end the imagery and falls asleep, the purpose of the technique is defeated.

PATIENT CARE MANAGEMENT PLAN

Anxiety

Anxiety Due to Threat to Biologic, Psychological, or Social Integrity

Signs and Symptoms

Subjective

- Verbalizes increased muscle tension
- Expresses frequent sensation of tingling in hands and feet
- Relates continuous feeling of apprehension
- Expresses preoccupation with a sense of impending doom
- Reports difficulty falling asleep
- Repeatedly expresses concerns about changes in health status and outcome of illness

Objective

- Psychomotor agitation (fidgeting, jitteriness, restlessness)
- Tightened, wrinkled brow
- Strained (worried) facial expression
- Hypervigilance (scans environment)
- Startles easily
- Distractibility
- Sweaty palms
- Fragmented sleep patterns
- Tachycardia
- Tachypnea

Outcomes

- Patient effectively uses learned relaxation strategies.
- Patient demonstrates significant decrease in psychomotor agitation.
- Patient verbalizes reduction in tingling sensations in hands and feet.
- Patient is able to focus on the tasks at hand.
- Patient expresses positive, future-based plans to family and staff.
- Patient's heart rate and rhythm remain within limits commensurate with physiologic status.

Interventions and Rationale

1. Instruct the patient in the following simple, effective relaxation strategies:
   a. If not contraindicated for cardiovascular reasons, tense and relax all muscles progressively from toes to head. Progressive toe-to-head relaxation releases the muscular tension that may be a stress-related effect resulting from the threat or change in the patient's health status and outcome of illness.
   b. Perform slow deep-breathing exercises. Deep-breathing exercises provide slow, rhythmic, controlled breathing patterns that relax the patient and distract them from the effects of their illness and hospitalization.
   c. Focus on a single object or person in the environment. Focusing on a single object or person helps the patient dismiss myriad disorienting stimuli from their visual-perceptual field, which can have a dizzying, distorted effect. A clear sensorium allows them to feel more in control of their environment.
   d. Listen to soothing music or relaxation tapes with eyes closed. Music or words expressed in soft, low tones tend to produce soothing, relaxing effects that counteract or inhibit escalating anxiety and provide respites from the patient's situational crisis. Closed eyes eliminate distracting visual stimuli and promote a more restful environment.
2. Actively listen to and accept the patient's concerns regarding the threats from their illness, outcome, and hospitalization. **Active listening and unconditional acceptance validate the patient as a worthwhile individual and assure them that their concerns, no matter how great, will be addressed. Knowledge that they have an avenue for ventilation will assuage anxiety.**
3. Help the patient distinguish between realistic concerns and exaggerated fears through clear, simple explanations. *Sample statements:* "Your lab results show that you're doing okay right now." "The shortness of breath you're experiencing is not unusual." "The pain you described is expected, and this medication will relieve it." **A patient who is informed about their progress and is reassured about expected symptoms and management of care will be better equipped to maintain a more realistic perspective of their illness and its outcome. Anxiety emanating from imagined or exaggerated fears will likely be assuaged or averted.**
4. Provide simple clarification of environmental events and stimuli that are not related to the patient's illness and care. *Sample statements:* "That loud noise is coming from a machine that is helping another patient." "The visitor behind the curtain is crying because they had an upsetting day." "That gurney is here to take another patient to x-ray." **Clarification of events and stimuli that are unrelated to the patient helps to disengage from the extant anxiety-provoking situations, avoiding further anxiety and apprehension.**
5. Assist the patient in focusing on building on prior coping strategies to deal with the effects of their illness and care. *Sample statements:* "What methods have helped you get through difficult times in the past?" "How can we help you use those methods now?" (See the patient management plan for Impaired Adaptation for interventions that assist patients to use coping strategies effectively.) **Use of previously successful coping strategies in conjunction with newly learned techniques arms the patient with an arsenal of weapons against anxiety, providing them with greater control over the situational crisis and decreased feelings of doom and despair.**
6. Give the patient permission to deny or suppress the effects of their illness and hospitalization with which they cannot cope or control. *Sample statements:* "It's perfectly okay to ignore things you can't handle right now." "How can we help ease your mind during this time?" "What are some things or tasks that may help distract you?" **Adaptive denial can be helpful in reducing feelings of anxiety in patients with a life-threatening illness.**

PATIENT CARE MANAGEMENT PLAN

Autonomic Dysreflexia

Autonomic Dysreflexia Due to Excessive Autonomic Response to Noxious Stimuli

Signs and Symptoms

- Paroxysmal hypertension (sudden increase in both systolic and diastolic blood pressure [BP] >20 mm Hg above patient's normal BP); for many patients with spinal cord injury, normal BP may be 90/60 mm Hg
- Pounding headache
- Bradycardia (may be a relative slowing, so the heart rate may still appear within the normal range)
- Profuse sweating (above the level of the injury) especially in the face, neck, and shoulders
- Pilomotor erection (goose bumps) above the level of the injury
- Cardiac dysrhythmias (atrial fibrillation, premature ventricular contractions, and atrioventricular conduction abnormalities)
- Flushing of the skin (above the level of the injury) especially in the face, neck, and shoulders
- Blurred vision
- Appearance of spots in the visual fields
- Nasal congestion
- Feelings of apprehension or anxiety

Outcomes

- BP returns to patient's baseline level.
- Heart rate and rhythm return to patient's baseline level.
- Headache is absent.
- Sweating, flushing, and piloerection above level of injury are absent.
- Visual disturbances and nasal congestion are absent.
- Feelings of apprehension or anxiety are absent.

Interventions and Rationale

1. Place the patient on a cardiac monitor and assess for bradycardia or other dysrhythmias. Disturbances of cardiac rate and rhythm can occur because of autonomic dysfunction associated with dysreflexia.
2. Check the patient's BP every 3 to 5 min, as BP may fluctuate very quickly.
3. Sit the patient upright and lower their legs if possible to decrease venous return and BP.
4. Loosen any clothing or constrictive devices to decrease venous return and BP.
5. Investigate for and remove the instigating cause of dysreflexia:
   a. Bladder
      (1). If an indwelling catheter is not in place, catheterize the patient immediately.
         (a). Before inserting the catheter, instill 2% lidocaine jelly into the urethra and wait 2 min, if possible.
         (b). Drain 500 mL of urine and recheck BP.
         (c). If BP is still elevated, drain another 500 mL of urine.
         (d). If BP declines after the bladder is empty, serial BPs must be monitored closely because the bladder can go into severe contractions, causing hypertension to recur.
      (2). If an indwelling catheter is in place, check the catheter and tubing for kinks, folds, constrictions, or obstructions and for correct placement. If a problem is found, correct it immediately.
      (3). If the catheter is plugged, irrigate it gently with no more than 10 to 15 mL of sterile normal saline solution at body temperature.
      (4). If unable to irrigate the catheter, remove it and prepare to reinsert a new catheter. Proceed with its lubrication, drainage, and observation as outlined above.
      (5). Avoid manually compressing or tapping on the bladder.
   b. Bowel: If systolic BP is >150 mm Hg, proceed to Step 6 before checking for a fecal impaction.
      (6). With a gloved hand, instill a topical anesthetic agent (2% lidocaine jelly) generously into the rectum **to decrease flow of impulses from bowel.**
      (7). Wait 2 minutes, if possible, **for sensation in area to decrease.**
      (8). With a gloved hand, insert a lubricated finger into the rectum and check for the presence of stool.
      (9). If stool is felt, gently remove, if possible.
   c. Skin
      (1). Loosen clothing or bed linens as indicated.
      (2). Inspect skin for pimples, boils, pressure ulcers, and ingrown toenails, and treat as indicated.
6. If symptoms of dysreflexia do not subside, collaborate with the practitioner regarding the administration of antihypertensive medications (e.g., nifedipine [immediate-release form], nitrates [sodium nitroprusside, isosorbide dinitrate, or nitroglycerin ointment], hydralazine, mecamylamine, diazoxide, phenoxybenzamine, captopril, prazosin).
   a. Administer medications and monitor their effectiveness.
   b. Assess BP and heart rate.
7. Instruct the patient about causes, symptoms, treatment, and prevention of dysreflexia.
8. Encourage the patient to carry a medical bracelet or informational card to present to medical personnel in the event dysreflexia may be developing.

PATIENT CARE MANAGEMENT PLAN

Decreased Intracranial Adaptive Capacity

Decreased Intracranial Adaptive Capacity Due to Failure of Normal Intracranial Compensatory Mechanisms

Signs and Symptoms

- Intracranial pressure (ICP) >15 mm Hg, sustained for 15 to 30 min
- Headache
- Vomiting, with or without nausea
- Seizures
- Decrease in Glasgow Coma Scale score of 2 or more points from baseline
- Alteration in level of consciousness, ranging from restlessness to coma
- Change in orientation: disoriented to time, place, or person, or all three
- Difficulty or inability to follow simple commands
- Increasing systolic blood pressure of more than 20 mm Hg with widening pulse pressure
- Bradycardia
- Irregular respiratory pattern (e.g., Cheyne-Stokes, central neurogenic hyperventilation, ataxic, apneustic)
- Change in response to painful stimuli (e.g., purposeful to inappropriate or absent response)
- Signs of impending brain herniation:
- Hemiparesis or hemiplegia
- Hemisensory changes
- Unequal pupil size (1 mm or more difference)
- Failure of pupil to react to light
- Disconjugate gaze and inability to move one eye beyond midline if third, fourth, or sixth cranial nerves involved
- Loss of oculocephalic or oculovestibular reflexes
- Possible decorticate or decerebrate posturing

Outcomes

- ICP is <15 mm Hg.
- Cerebral perfusion pressure is >60 mm Hg.
- Clinical signs of increased ICP are absent.

Interventions and Rationale

1. Maintain adequate cerebral perfusion pressure.
   a. Collaborate with the practitioner regarding administration of volume expanders, vasopressors, or antihypertensives **to maintain the patient's blood pressure within normal range.**
   b. Implement measures to reduce ICP.
      (1). Elevate head of bed 30 to 45 degrees **to facilitate venous return.**
      (2). Maintain head and neck in neutral (avoid flexion, extension, or lateral rotation) **to enhance venous drainage from the head.**
      (3). Avoid extreme hip flexion.
      (4). Collaborate with the practitioner regarding administration of steroids, osmotic agents, and diuretics and need for drainage of cerebrospinal fluid if a ventriculostomy is in place.
      (5). Assist the patient to turn and move self in bed (instruct the patient to exhale while turning or pushing up in bed) **to avoid isometric contractions and Valsalva maneuver.**
2. Maintain patent airway and adequate ventilation and supply oxygen **to prevent hypoxemia and hypercarbia.**
3. Monitor arterial blood gas values and maintain arterial partial pressure of oxygen (PaO_2) >80 mm Hg, arterial partial pressure of carbon dioxide ($PaCO_2$) >35 mm Hg, and pH at 7.35 to 7.45 **to prevent cerebral vasodilation.**
4. Avoid suctioning beyond 10 sec at a time; hyperoxygenate and hyperventilate before and after suctioning **to avoid hypoxemia.**
5. Plan patient care activities and interventions around the patient's ICP response. Avoid unnecessary additional disturbances and allow the patient up to 1 hour of rest between activities as frequently as possible. **Studies have shown the direct correlation between patient care activities and increases in ICP.**
6. Maintain normothermia with external cooling or heating measures as necessary. Wrap hands, feet, and male genitalia in soft towels before cooling measures **to prevent shivering and frostbite.**
7. Collaborate with the practitioner to control seizures with prophylactic and PRN anticonvulsants. **Seizures can greatly increase the cerebral metabolic rate.**
8. Collaborate with the practitioner regarding administration of sedatives, barbiturates, or paralyzing agents **to reduce cerebral metabolic rate.**
9. Counsel family members to maintain a calm atmosphere and avoid disturbing topics of conversation (e.g., patient condition, pain, prognosis, family crisis, financial difficulties).
10. If signs of impending brain herniation are present, implement the following:
    a. Notify the practitioner at once.
    b. Ensure that head of bed is elevated 45 degrees and that the patient's head is in a neutral plane.
    c. Administer a mainline intravenous infusion slowly to the keep-open rate.
    d. Drain cerebrospinal fluid as ordered if a ventriculostomy is in place.
    e. Prepare to administer osmotic agents and/or diuretics.
    f. Prepare the patient for an emergency computed tomography head scan and/or emergency surgery.

PATIENT CARE MANAGEMENT PLAN

Delirium

Delirium Due to Sensory Overload, Sensory Deprivation, and Sleep Pattern Disturbance

Signs and Symptoms

Early Symptoms

- Sudden onset of global cognitive function impairment (hours to days)
- Restlessness, agitation, and combative behavior
- Drowsiness (can lead to loss of consciousness)
- Slurring of speech, inappropriate statements or "word salad," mumbling, or inappropriate gestures
- Short attention span (needs questions repeated); inability to learn new material
- Disordered sleep/wake cycle
- Disorientation to person, time, place, and situation
- Difficulty in separating dreams from reality (may experience bizarre dreams or nightmares)
- Anger at staff for continued questions about their orientation

Later Symptoms

- Symptoms that tend to fluctuate throughout the day and night
- Continuations of early symptoms, which may be more frequent or of longer duration
- Illusions
- Hallucinations
- Extreme agitation (e. g., attempts to climb out of bed, pull out catheters, rip off dressings)
- Calling out in loud voice, swearing, or attempting to bite or hit people who approach patient

Outcomes

- Absence of or diminished confusion
- Absence of or diminished sensory overload
- Absence of or diminished sensory deprivation
- Absence of or diminished sleep pattern disturbance

Interventions and Rationale

1. Determine and document the patient's dominant spoken language, their literacy level, and the languages in which they are literate. **Sometimes people are not literate in their spoken language, or, less commonly, they are literate only in their second language.**
2. Determine and document the patient's premorbid degree of orientation, cognitive capabilities, and any sensory/perceptual deficits.

For Sensory Overload

1. Initiate each nurse-patient encounter by calling the patient by name and identifying yourself by name. This fosters reality orientation and assists the patient in filtering irrelevant or impersonal conversation.
2. Assess the patient's immediate physical environment from their viewpoint, and explain equipment, its sounds, and its therapeutic purpose. Demonstrate audible and visual alarms and explain possible alarm conditions. This decreases alienation of the patient from the technologic environment and reduces the inherent sense of fear and urgency accompanying alarm conditions.
3. Provide preparatory sensory information by explaining procedures in relation to the sensations the patient will experience, including duration of sensations. Preparatory sensory information enhances learning and lessens anticipatory anxiety.
4. Limit noise levels. Audible alarms cannot and must not be silenced, and many critical but noisy activities must take place in the critical care unit. However, it has been shown that noise levels produced by clinical personnel exceed levels designated as acceptable and are often greater than levels generated by technologic devices.
    a. Keep staff conversations soft enough that they are inaudible to the patient whenever possible.
    b. Assume that everything said at or around a patient's bedside is intended for that patient's awareness and that it will be interpreted as pertaining to them. **As in the discussion that follows, conversations about the patient but not to them foster depersonalization and delusions of reference.**
    c. Enforce nighttime noise limits.
2. Readjust alarm limits on physiologic monitoring devices as the patient's condition changes (improves or deteriorates) **to lessen unnecessary alarm states.**
3. Consider use of headphones and digital music player with the patient's favorite music and/or subliminal or classical music. **This can effectively filter out assaultive noise of the critical care environment and supplant it with familiar, soothing sounds and rhythms.**
4. Modify lighting. **Day and night cycles need to be simulated with environmental lighting.**
    a. Never turn on overhead fluorescent lights abruptly without warning the patient, assisting the patient out of the supine position, and shielding their eyes with gauze or a face cloth. **Continuous bright lighting sustains anxiety and promotes circadian rhythm desynchronization.**
5. Shield patients from viewing urgent and emergent events in the critical care unit. Resuscitation efforts, albeit difficult to conceal, engender fear in the patient and a sense of instability and vulnerability (e. g., "I'm next").
    a. When such an event occurs, elicit the patient's cognitive and emotional reaction; thoughts, impressions, and feelings need to be shared, and misconceptions need to be clarified.
6. Ensure patients' privacy, modesty, and dignity. Physical exposure and nudity, although they seemingly pale in importance compared with priorities such as physiologic assessment and stabilization, are primal indignities for all individuals.
    a. Keep the patient minimally exposed. When it becomes necessary to expose the patient, verbally apologize for this necessity. **To be naked is to feel vulnerable; to be vulnerable is to feel fearful.**

For Sensory Deprivation

1. Provide reality orientation in four spheres (personal, place, time, and situation) at more frequent intervals than when testing.
    a. Convey this information in the context of routine conversation. *Sample statements:* "Mr. Clark, this is Tuesday morning and you're in University Hospital. Your heart surgery was yesterday morning, and you're doing well. My name is Joe, and I'm your nurse today." **The patient is made to feel patronized by repetitions such as, "Do you know where you are?" Given the effects of general anesthesia, opioid analgesics, sedatives, and sleep, it is expected that some degree of disorientation will exist normally.**
2. Ensure the patient's visual access to a calendar.
3. Apprise the patient of daily news events and the weather.
4. Touch patients for the express purpose of communicating caring. Hold their hands, stroke their brows, and rub the skin on an aspect of the arms. **Touch is the universal language of caring. In the setting of critical care, in which there is considerable physical body manipulation, it is useful and important to contrast assaultive touch with comforting touch. Touch can be used as a technique for distraction from painful stimuli when used in conjunction with uncomfortable procedures.** (See later discussion of the use of touch in management of the patient experiencing hallucinations.)

PATIENT CARE MANAGEMENT PLAN

Delirium—cont'd

5. Foster liberal visitation by family members and significant others. Encourage significant others to touch the patient as consistent with their individual comfort level and cultural norms.
6. Structure and identify opportunities for the patient to exercise decision-making skills, however small. **Although not so designated, patients with sensory alterations also experience a type of cognitive deprivation.**
7. Assist patients to find meaning in their experiences. **Patients need to find meaning and to identify their roles in the experience of critical illness and critical care.**
   a. Explain the therapeutic purpose of all they are asked to do for themselves and all that is done with them and for them.
   b. Avoid statements such as, "Will you turn to that side for me?" or "I need you to swallow this medication." **These statements implicitly convey that the maneuver has some value for the nurses instead of the patients.**
   c. Similarly, use "thank you" judiciously. **This simple salutation, when used indiscriminately, suggests something was done to benefit the nurses, not the patients.**

For Hallucinations

1. Approach the patient with a calm, matter-of-fact demeanor. The goal of this interaction is for the nurse to demonstrate external control. This helps decrease the anxiety and fear that generally accompany hallucinations and allows the patient to feel safe. Anxiety is transferable.
2. Address the patient by name. This is a useful presentation of reality because self-identity is the last sphere of orientation to vanish.
3. In responding to the patient's description of the hallucination, do not deny, argue, or attempt to disprove the existence of the perceived event. Statements such as, "There are no voices coming from that air vent," or "Look, I'm brushing my hand across the wall, and there are no bugs," confuse the patient further because the hallucination, although frightening, is their perceived reality.
4. Express to the patient that your experiences are dissimilar and acknowledge how frightening theirs must be. *Sample statements:* "I don't hear (or see) what you do, but I know how frightening such an experience must be to you. I'm Joe, your nurse, and I'm going to stay with you until the voices (or visions) go away." Validating the patient's feelings demonstrates acceptance and sensitivity to the experience and promotes trust.
5. Remain with any patient who is experiencing a hallucination. Feelings of fear and anxiety often accelerate when a patient is left alone. They need someone to represent a nonthreatening reality.
6. Do not explore the content of the hallucination with the patient by asking about its nature or character. The nurse is the patient's link with reality. Pursuit of a detailed description of a hallucination may signify to the patient that the nurse accepts their sensory distortion as factual. This may further confuse the patient and distance them more from reality.
   a. Ascertain that the voices are not telling the patient to harm themself by asking simply and concretely, "What are the voices saying?" **The nurse can help bridge the gap between the patient's misperception and reality by addressing the feelings (e. g., fear, anxiety) and/or meanings (e. g., danger, death) engendered by the hallucination.**
   b. Determine how the misperception affects the patient emotionally, acknowledge those feelings, and use a calm, controlled, matter-of-fact approach to provide the trust and comfort the patient needs to tolerate this frightening experience. **In other words, the nurse should deal with the intent more than the content of the hallucination. The resultant decrease in anxiety will enable the patient to focus more accurately on their immediate environment.**
7. Talk concretely with the patient about things that are really happening. *Sample statements:* "How does your chest incision feel this afternoon, Mr. Clark?" "Your sister Kate was here to see you, but you were sleeping. She went down to the cafeteria and will be back." "Your secretions are a little easier for you to cough up today." **Interpretation of reality-based stimuli by the nurse encourages the patient to focus on actual circumstances and discourages a preoccupation with sensory misperceptions.**
8. Distract the patient by changing the topic. **This tactic is useful in situations of escalating anxiety and confusion or when all else fails. Topics need to consist of basic themes that are universally understood and culturally congruent such as music, food, or weather, or topics of special interest to the patient such as hobbies, crafts, or sports.**
   a. Avoid topics that evoke strong emotions such as politics, religion, or sexuality. This is especially true in regard to a patient with reality distortions; sometimes hallucinations and delusions are expressions of repressed conflicts associated with religious, sexual, or aggressive issues. Pursuit of such subjects could increase confusion and anxiety.
9. Avoid the use of touch as an intervention strategy for any patient who demonstrates escalating anxiety or paranoid, suspicious, or mistrustful thoughts. **Although touch can be useful in the management of patients with sensory alterations, for patients experiencing hallucinations (as well as delusions and illusions), touch can be readily misinterpreted as aggression or pain, and it can provide the basis for a tactile illusion.**
10. For auditory hallucinations:
    a. *Patient behaviors:* Head cocked as if listening to an unseen presence; lips moving.
    b. *Therapeutic nurse responses:* "Mr. Clark, you appear to be listening to something." If the patient acknowledges voices: "I don't hear any voices, but I know this is troubling you. The voices will go away. Nothing is going to harm you. I'm Joe, your nurse, and I'll be here with you."
    c. *Nontherapeutic nurse responses:* "Tell me about your conversations with these voices." "To whom do these voices belong—anyone you know?"
11. For visual hallucinations:
    a. *Patient behaviors:* Staring into space as if focused on an unseen object; startled movements and anxious facial expression.
    b. *Therapeutic nurse responses:* "Mr. Clark, something seems to be troubling you. Tell me what it is." If the patient states he visualizes people, images, or the devil in his environment and implies a sense of danger, respond, "There are only nurses and doctors here, Mr. Clark. I know this must be upsetting, but these images will go away. We're here with you in the hospital. Nothing will happen to you."
    c. *Nontherapeutic nurse responses:* "Describe the people you see. What are they wearing?" "What does the devil mean in your life? What about God?"

For Delusions

1. Explain all unseen noises, voices, and activity simply and clearly. **They readily feed a delusional system.** Sample statements: "That is Dr. Smith. He's come to see you and other patients here in the hospital." "The voices and activity you hear are from the bedside of the patient behind this curtain. He's being helped by one of the nurses."
2. Avoid the "negative challenge" of the patient's delusions (e. g., "Nobody here stole your belongings" or "Doctors and nurses do not harm people"). Similarly, avoid defending the referents of the patient's belief: "Nurses are good," or "Doctors mean well." **A delusion is a belief, albeit false, that cannot be changed with logic. To attempt this change is to challenge the patient's belief system and escalate their anxiety, further blurring the boundaries between reality and the patient's internally based "logic."**

Continued

PATIENT CARE MANAGEMENT PLAN

Delirium—cont'd

3. For a patient with persecutory delusions who refuses food, fluids, or medications because of a belief that they have been poisoned or the medications are tainted, permit the refusal unless it is a life-threatening event. Try again in 20 minutes; allow the patient to choose an alternative selection of food or to read the label on the unit's medication. **Coercion, show of force, or engagement in complicated, logical justifications will heighten the patient's suspiciousness and possibly reinforce the delusional belief. When the patient feels more in control, they need not rely on the "paradoxical" quality of the delusion to equip them with a false sense of power. Their power instead is derived from making reality-based decisions.**
4. Staff members should be particularly careful not to engage in unnecessary laughter or whispering within view of a delusional patient. **The delusional patient is hypervigilant, scanning the environment for evidence to corroborate or confirm their belief that staff members are colluding against them; laughter and whispers easily suggest this belief, this delusion of reference. This rationale also pertains to the patient experiencing hallucinations and/or illusions.**
5. Observe the principles detailed in the third intervention in the For Hallucinations section.

For Illusions

1. Interpret a reality-based stimulus for the patient in a calm, matter-of-fact manner. Seen and unseen noises, voices, activity, and people can provide the stimulus for a sensory misinterpretation, an illusion.
2. Minimize stimulation in the patient's immediate environment. Interventions detailed previously under "For Sensory Overload" are especially relevant here.
3. Address the feeling and meaning associated with the experience, not the content of the sensory misinterpretation.
   a. *Patient behaviors:* Eyes darting, startled movements, frightened facial expression. "I know who you are. You're the devil come to take me to hell."
   b. *Therapeutic nurse responses:* "I'm Joe, your nurse. I know this experience is troubling for you. You're in the hospital, and no one here will harm you."
   c. Nontherapeutic nurse responses: "There are no such things as devils and angels." "Do you think the devil would be dressed in white?" **The first nontherapeutic nurse response carries a parental tone (e. g., "You know better than that."), infantilizing the patient and adding to their feelings of powerlessness over the environment. The second nontherapeutic response reflects obvious logic, which is not in the patient's sensory domain; it cannot be processed and only adds to their confused state.**
4. Observe the principles detailed in the fifth intervention of the "For Hallucinations" section.

PATIENT CARE MANAGEMENT PLAN

Disturbed Body Image

Disturbed Body Image Due to Actual Change in Body Structure, Function, or Appearance

Signs and Symptoms

- Actual change in appearance, structure, or function
- Avoidance of looking at body part
- Avoidance of touching body part
- Hiding or overexposing body part (intentional or unintentional)
- Trauma to nonfunctioning part
- Change in ability to estimate spatial relationship of body to environment
- Verbalization of the following:
    - Fear of rejection or reaction by others
    - Negative feeling about body
    - Preoccupation with change or loss
- Refusal to participate in or to accept responsibility for self-care of altered body part
- Personalization of part or loss with a name
- Depersonalization of part or loss by use of impersonal pronouns
- Refusal to verify actual change

Outcomes

- Patient verbalizes the specific meaning of the change to them.
- Patient requests appropriate information about self-care.
- Patient completes personal hygiene and grooming daily with or without help.
- Patient interacts freely with family or other visitors.
- Patient participates in the discussions and conferences related to planning their medical and patient management in the critical care unit and transfer from the unit.
- Patient talks with trained visitors (support group representatives) at least twice about their loss.

Interventions and Rationale

1. Evaluate the patient's mental, physical, and emotional state; recognize assets, strengths, response to illness, coping mechanisms, past experience with stress, and support system.
2. Appraise the response of the family and significant others. **Body image is derived from the "reflected appraisals" of family and significant others.**
3. Determine the patient's goals and readiness for learning.
4. Provide the necessary information to help the patient and family adapt to the change. Clarify misconceptions about future limitations.
5. Permit and encourage the patient to express the significance of the loss or change; note nonverbal behavior responses.
6. Allow and encourage the patient's expression of anxiety. **Anxiety is the most predominant emotional response to a body image disturbance.**
7. Recognize and accept the use of denial as an adaptive defense mechanism when used early and temporarily.
8. Recognize maladaptive denial as that which interferes with the patient's progress and/or alienates support systems. Use confrontation.
9. Provide an opportunity for the patient to discuss sexual concerns.
10. Touch the affected body part **to provide the patient with sensory information about altered body structure and/or function.**
11. Encourage and provide movement of the altered body part **to establish kinesthetic feedback. This enables the patient to know their body as it now exists.**
12. Prepare the patient to look at the body part. Call the body part by its anatomic name (e.g., stump, stoma, limb) as opposed to "it." **The use of impersonal pronouns increases a sense of fantasy and depersonalization of the body part.**
13. Allow the patient to experience excellence in some aspect of physical functioning—walking, turning, deep breathing, healing, self-care—and point out progress and accomplishment. **This helps to balance the patient's sense of dysfunction with function.**
14. Avoid false reassurance. Acknowledge the difficulty of incorporating the altered body part or function into one's body image. **This evidences the nurse's sensitivity and promotes trust.**
15. Talk with the patient about their life, generativity, and accomplishments. **Patients with disturbances in body image frequently see themselves in a distortedly "narrow" sense. Encouraging a wider focus of themselves and their life reduces this distortion.**
16. Help the patient explore realistic alternatives.
17. Recognize that incorporating a body change into one's body image takes time. Avoid setting unrealistic expectations and **inadvertently reinforcing a low self-esteem.**
18. Suggest the use of additional resources such as trained visitors who have mastered situations similar to those of the patient.
    a. Refer the patient to a psychiatric nurse, psychologist, or psychiatrist if needed.

Disturbed Body Image Due to Functional Dependence on Life-Sustaining Technology

Signs and Symptoms

- Actual change in function requiring permanent or temporary replacement
- Refusal to verify actual loss
- Verbalization of the following: feelings of helplessness, hopelessness, powerlessness, fear of failure to wean from technology

Outcomes

- Patient verifies actual change in function.
- Patient does not refuse or fight technologic intervention.
- Patient verbalizes acceptance of expected change in lifestyle.

Interventions and Rationale

1. Evaluate the patient's response to the technologic intervention.
2. Assess responses of the family and significant others. **Body image is derived from the "reflected appraisals" of family and significant others.**
3. Provide information needed by the patient and family.
4. Promote trust, security, comfort, and privacy.
5. Recognize anxiety. Allow and encourage its expression. **Anxiety is the most predominant emotion accompanying body image alterations.** Implement a patient management plan for anxiety due to threat to biological, psychological, or social integrity.
6. Assist the patient to recognize their own functioning and performance in the face of technology. For example, assist the patient to distinguish spontaneous breaths from mechanically delivered breaths. **The activity will assist in weaning the patient from the ventilator when feasible. To establish realistic, accurate body boundaries, a patient needs to help separate themself from the technology that is supporting their functioning. Any participation or function on the part of the patient during periods of dependency is helpful in preventing and/or resolving an alteration in body image.**
7. Plan for discontinuation of the treatment (e.g., weaning from a ventilator). Explain the procedure that will be followed and be present during its initiation.
8. Plan for transfer from the critical care environment.
9. Document care, ensuring an up-to-date management plan is available to all involved caregivers.

PATIENT CARE MANAGEMENT PLAN

Hyperthermia

Hyperthermia Due to Increased Metabolic Rate

Signs and Symptoms

- Increased body temperature above normal range
- Seizures
- Flushed skin
- Increased respiratory rate
- Tachycardia
- Skin warm to touch
- Diaphoresis

Outcomes

- Temperature is within normal range.
- Respiratory rate and heart rate are within patient's baseline range.
- Skin is warm and dry.

Interventions and Rationale

1. Monitor temperature every 15 min to 1 hour until within normal range and stable, then every 4 hours to maintain close **surveillance for temperature fluctuations and evaluate effectiveness of interventions.**
   a. Use temperature taken from the pulmonary artery catheter or bladder catheter if available **because these methods closely reflect core body temperature.**
   b. Use tympanic membrane temperature if core body temperature devices are unavailable.
   c. Use rectal temperature if none of the aforementioned methods are available.
2. Collaborate with the practitioner regarding administration of antithyroid medications **to block the synthesis and release of thyroid hormone.**
3. Collaborate with the practitioner regarding the use of a cooling blanket **to facilitate heat loss by conduction.**
   a. Wrap hands, feet, and male genitalia to protect them from maceration during cooling and decrease chance of shivering.
   b. Avoid rapidly cooling the patient and overcooling the patient because this initiates the heat-conserving response (i.e., shivering).
4. Place ice packs in patient's groin and axilla **to facilitate heat loss by conduction.**
5. Maintain the patient on bed rest **to decrease the effects of activity on the patient's metabolic rate.**
6. Provide tepid sponge baths **to facilitate heat loss by evaporation.**
7. Decrease the patient's room temperature **to facilitate radiant heat loss.**
8. Place a fan near the patient to circulate cool air **to facilitate heat loss by convection.**
9. Provide the patient with a nonrestrictive gown and lightweight bed coverings **to allow heat to escape from the patient's trunk.**
10. Collaborate with the practitioner and the respiratory care practitioner regarding administration of oxygen to maintain oxygen saturation >90% **because the patient has increased oxygen consumption resulting from an increased metabolic rate.**
11. Collaborate with the practitioner regarding use of antipyretic medications **to facilitate patient comfort.**
12. Collaborate with the practitioner regarding the use of intravenous (IV) and oral fluids **to maintain adequate hydration of the patient.**

PATIENT CARE MANAGEMENT PLAN

Hypervolemia

Hypervolemia Due to Increased Secretion of Antidiuretic Hormone (ADH)

Signs and Symptoms

- Headache
- Decreased sensorium
- Weight gain over short period
- Intake greater than output
- Increased pulmonary artery occlusion pressure
- Increased right atrial pressure
- Urine output is <30 mL/h.
- Serum sodium is <120 mEq/L.
- Serum osmolality is <275 mOsm/kg.
- Urine osmolality greater than serum osmolality
- Urine sodium is >200 mEq/L.
- Urine specific gravity is >1.03.

Outcomes

- Weight returns to baseline.
- Urine output is >30 mL/h.
- Serum sodium is 135 to 145 mEq/L.
- Urine specific gravity is 1.005 to 1030.

Interventions and Rationale

1. Monitor cardiac rhythm continuously for dysrhythmias **caused by electrolyte imbalance.**
2. Restrict the patient's fluids to 500 mL less than output per day **to decrease fluid retention.**
3. Provide the patient chilled beverages high in sodium content such as tomato juice or broth **to increase sodium intake.**
4. Collaborate with the practitioner regarding administration of demeclocycline, lithium, or opioid agonists **to inhibit renal response to ADH.**
5. Collaborate with the practitioner regarding administration of hypertonic saline and furosemide **for rapid correction of severe sodium deficit and diuresis of free water.**
   a. Administer hypertonic saline at a rate of 1 to 2 mL/kg/h until the patient's serum sodium is increased no greater than 1 to 2 mEq/L/h.
6. Weigh the patient daily (at same time, in same amount of clothing, and preferably with same scale) **to ensure accuracy of readings.**
7. Provide frequent mouth care to prevent breakdown of oral mucous membranes.
8. Initiate seizure precautions because the patient is at high risk as a result of hyponatremia.
   a. Pad the side rails of the bed to protect the patient from injury.
   b. Remove any objects from the immediate environment that could injure the patient in the event of a seizure.
   c. Keep an appropriate-size oral airway at bedside to assist with airway management after the seizure.
9. Collaborate with the practitioner regarding the administration of medications to prevent constipation **caused by decreased fluid intake and immobility.**
10. Maintain surveillance for symptoms of hyponatremia (e.g., headache, abdominal cramps, weakness) and congestive heart failure (e.g., dyspnea, rales, increased central venous pressure, and pulmonary artery occlusion pressure).

Hypervolemia Due to Renal Dysfunction

Signs and Symptoms

- Weight gain that occurs during a 24- to 48-hour period
- Dependent pitting edema
- Ascites in severe cases
- Fluid crackles on lung auscultation
- Exertional dyspnea
- Oliguria or anuria
- Hypertension
- Engorged neck veins
- Decrease in urinary osmolality as renal failure progresses
- Right atrial pressure is >8 mm Hg
- Pulmonary artery occlusion pressure is >12 mm Hg

Outcomes

- Weight returns to baseline.
- Edema or ascites is absent or reduced to baseline.
- Lungs are clear to auscultation.
- Exertional dyspnea is absent.
- Blood pressure returns to baseline.
- Heart rate returns to baseline.
- Neck veins are flat.
- Mucous membranes are moist.

Interventions and Rationale

1. Promote skin integrity of edematous areas by frequent repositioning and elevation of areas where possible. Avoid massaging pressure points or reddened areas of skin **because this results in further tissue trauma.**
2. Plan patient care to provide rest periods **so as not to heighten exertional dyspnea.**
3. Weigh the patient daily at same time, in same amount of clothing, and preferably with same scale.
4. Instruct the patient about the correlation between fluid intake and weight gain, using commonly understood fluid measurements; for example, ingesting 4 cups (1000 mL) of fluid results in an approximate 2-lb weight gain in the anuric patient.

PATIENT CARE MANAGEMENT PLAN

Hypothermia

Hypothermia Due to Decreased Metabolic Rate

Signs and Symptoms

- Reduction in body temperature below normal range
- Shivering
- Pallor
- Piloerection
- Hypertension
- Skin cool to touch
- Tachycardia
- Decreased capillary refill

Outcomes

- Temperature is within normal range.
- Heart rate is within patient's baseline range.
- Skin is warm and dry.
- Capillary refill is normal.

Interventions and Rationale

1. Monitor temperature every 15 min to 1 hour until within normal range and stable and then every 4 hours **to maintain close surveillance for temperature fluctuations and to evaluate effectiveness of interventions.**
   a. Use temperature taken from pulmonary artery catheter or bladder catheter if available **because these methods closely reflect core body temperature.**
   b. Use tympanic membrane temperature **if core body temperature devices are unavailable.**
   c. Use rectal temperature if none of the aforementioned methods are available.
2. Collaborate with the practitioner regarding administration of thyroid medications **to replace lacking thyroid hormone.**
3. Collaborate with the practitioner regarding the use of a fluid-filled heating blanket **to facilitate rewarming by conduction.**
4. Initiate forced air–warming therapy **to facilitate convective heat gain.**
5. Provide the patient with warm blankets **to facilitate heat transfer to the patient.**
6. Increase the patient's room temperature **to decrease radiant heat loss.**
7. Replace wet patient gown and bed linen promptly **to decrease evaporative heat loss.**
8. Warm intravenous fluids and blood products **to facilitate rewarming by conduction.**

Hypothermia Due to Exposure to Cold Environment, Trauma, or Damage to the Hypothalamus

Signs and Symptoms

- Core body temperature <35°C (95°F)
- Skin cold to touch
- Slurred speech, incoordination
- At temperatures <33°C (91.4°F):
  - Cardiac dysrhythmias (atrial fibrillation, bradycardia)
  - Cyanosis
  - Respiratory alkalosis
- At temperatures <32°C (89.6°F):
  - Shivering replaced by muscle rigidity
  - Hypotension
  - Dilated pupils
- At temperatures <28°C to 29°C (82.4°F to 84.2°F):
  - Absent deep tendon reflexes
  - Three to four breaths/min to apnea
  - Ventricular fibrillation possible
- At temperatures <26°C to 27°C (78.8°F to 80.6°F):
  - Coma
  - Flaccid muscles
  - Fixed, dilated pupils
  - Ventricular fibrillation to cardiac standstill
  - Apnea

Outcomes

- Core body temperature is >35°C (95°F).
- Patient is alert and oriented.
- Cardiac dysrhythmias are absent.
- Acid–base balance is normal.
- Pupils are normoreactive.

Interventions and Rationale

1. Monitor the patient's core body temperature continuously.
2. Collaborate with the practitioner regarding the need for intubation and mechanical ventilation.
   a. Heated air or oxygen can be added **to help rewarm the body core.**
   b. Do not hyperventilate a patient with hypothermia **because carbon dioxide production is low, and this action may induce severe alkalosis and precipitate ventricular fibrillation.**
3. Maintain cardiopulmonary resuscitation and advanced cardiac life support until core body temperature is at least 29.5°C (85.1°F) before determining that the patient cannot be resuscitated. **Electrical defibrillation is usually successful in terminating ventricular fibrillation if the temperature is >28 °C (82.4 °F).**
4. Administer cardiac resuscitation drugs sparingly because as the body warms, peripheral vasodilation occurs. Drugs that remain in the periphery are suddenly released, leading to a bolus effect that may cause fatal dysrhythmias.
5. Monitor arterial blood gas values to direct further therapy and ensure that pH, arterial partial pressure of oxygen (PaO_2), and arterial partial pressure of carbon dioxide ($PaCO_2$) are corrected for temperature.
6. Rewarm the patient rapidly because the pathophysiologic changes associated with chronic hypothermia have not had time to evolve.
   a. Institute rapid, active rewarming by immersion in warm water (38°C to 43°C) (100.4°F to 109.4°F).
   b. Apply thermal blanket at 36.6°C to 37.7°C (97.9°F to 99.9°F). Some researchers suggest rewarming only the torso or trunk first, leaving the extremities exposed to room temperature. **This is done to prevent early peripheral vasodilation with abrupt redistribution of intravascular volume. This also prevents colder blood trapped in the extremities from returning to the body core before the heart is rewarmed.**
   c. Perform rapid core rewarming with heated (37°C to 43°C [98.6°F to 109.4°F]) intravenous infusion, hemodialysis, peritoneal dialysis, and colonic or gastric irrigation fluids.
7. Monitor peripheral circulation because gangrene of the fingers and toes is a common complication of accidental hypothermia.

PATIENT CARE MANAGEMENT PLAN

Hypovolemia

Hypovolemia Due to Absolute Loss

Signs and Symptoms

- Cardiac output is <4 L/min
- Cardiac index is <2.2 L/min
- Pulmonary artery occlusion pressure is <6 mm Hg
- Right atrial pressure is <2 mm Hg
- Tachycardia
- Narrowed pulse pressure
- Systolic blood pressure is <100 mm Hg
- Urinary output is <30 mL/h
- Pale, cool, moist skin
- Apprehensiveness

Outcomes

- Cardiac output is >4 L/min, and cardiac index is >2.2 L/min.
- Pulmonary artery occlusion pressure is >6 mm Hg or returns to baseline level.
- Right atrial pressure is >2 mm Hg or returns to baseline level.
- Heart rate is normal or returns to baseline level.
- Systolic blood pressure is >90 mm Hg.
- Urinary output is >30 mL/h.

Interventions and Rationale

1. Secure the airway and administer oxygen to maintain oxygen saturation >92%.
2. Place the patient in the supine position with the legs elevated **to increase preload.** For the patient with a head injury, consider using the low-Fowler position with legs elevated.
3. For fluid repletion, use the 3:1 rule, replacing three parts of fluid for every unit of blood lost.
4. Administer crystalloid solutions using the fluid challenge technique: Infuse precise boluses of fluid (usually 5 to 20 mL/min) over 10-min periods; monitor hemodynamic pressures serially **to determine successful challenging.** If the pulmonary artery occlusion pressure elevates >7 mm Hg above the beginning level, the infusion should be stopped. If the pulmonary artery occlusion pressure rises only to 3 mm Hg above baseline or falls, another fluid challenge should be administered.
5. Replete fluids first before considering use of vasopressors **because vasopressors increase myocardial oxygen consumption out of proportion to the reestablishment of coronary perfusion in the early phases of treatment.**
6. When blood replacement is indicated, replace it with fresh-packed red blood cells and fresh-frozen plasma **to keep clotting factors intact.**
7. Move or reposition the patient minimally *to decrease or limit tissue oxygen demands.*
8. Evaluate the patient's anxiety level, and intervene through patient education or sedation **to decrease tissue oxygen demands.**
9. Maintain surveillance for signs and symptoms of fluid overload.

Hypovolemia Due to Decreased Secretion of Antidiuretic Hormone (ADH)

Signs and Symptoms

- Confusion and lethargy
- Decreased skin turgor
- Thirst
- Weight loss over short period
- Decreased pulmonary artery occlusion pressure
- Decreased right atrial pressure
- Urinary output is >6 L/day
- Serum sodium is >148 mEq/L
- Serum osmolality is >295 mOsm/kg
- Urine osmolality is <100 mOsm/kg
- Urine specific gravity is <1.005

Outcomes

- Weight returns to baseline.
- Urinary output is >30 mL/h and <200 mL/h.
- Serum osmolality is 280 to 295 mOsm/kg.
- Urine specific gravity is 1.010 to 1.030.

Interventions and Rationale

1. Record intake and output every hour, noting color and clarity of urine **because color and clarity are an indication of urine concentration.**
2. Monitor cardiac rhythm continuously for dysrhythmias **caused by electrolyte imbalance.**
3. Collaborate with the practitioner regarding administration of vasopressin or desmopressin **to replace ADH.**
   a. Monitor the patient for adverse effects of medications (e.g., headache, chest pain, abdominal pain) **caused by vasoconstriction.**
   b. Report adverse effects to the practitioner immediately.
4. Collaborate with the practitioner regarding intravenous fluid and electrolyte replacement therapy **to restore fluid balance, correct dehydration, and maintain electrolyte balance.**
   a. Administer hypotonic saline **to replace free water deficit.**
5. Provide oral fluids low in sodium such as water, coffee, tea, or orange juice **to decrease sodium intake.**
6. Weigh the patient daily at same time, in same amount of clothing, and preferably with same scale **to ensure accuracy of readings.**
7. Reposition the patient every 2 hours **to prevent skin integrity issues caused by dehydration.**
8. Provide mouth care every 4 hours **to prevent breakdown of oral mucous membranes.**
9. Collaborate with the practitioner regarding administration of medications to prevent constipation **caused by dehydration.**
10. Maintain surveillance for symptoms of hypernatremia (muscle twitching, irritability, seizures), hypovolemic shock (hypotension, tachycardia, decreased central venous pressure and pulmonary artery occlusion pressure), and deep vein thrombosis (calf pain, tenderness, swelling).

Hypovolemia Due to Relative Loss

Signs and Symptoms

- Pulmonary artery occlusion pressure <6 mm Hg
- Right atrial pressure <2 mm Hg
- Tachycardia
- Narrowed pulse pressure
- Systolic blood pressure <100 mm Hg
- Urinary output <30 mL/h
- Increased hematocrit level

Outcomes

- Pulmonary artery occlusion pressure is >6 mm Hg or returns to baseline level.
- Right atrial pressure is >2 mm Hg or returns to baseline level.
- Systolic blood pressure is >90 mm Hg.
- Urinary output is >30 mL/h.
- Hematocrit level is normal.

Interventions and Rationale

1. Collaborate with the practitioner regarding administration of intravenous fluid replacements (usually normal saline solution or lactated Ringer solution) at a rate sufficient to maintain urinary output >30 mL/h. Colloid solutions are avoided in the initial phases (but can be used later) because of the possibility of increased edema formation **as a result of increased capillary permeability.**

PATIENT CARE MANAGEMENT PLAN

Impaired Adaptation

Impaired Adaptation Due to Situational Crisis and Personal Vulnerability

Signs and Symptoms

- Verbalization of inability to cope. *Sample statements:* "I can't take this anymore." "I don't know how to deal with this."
- Ineffective problem solving (problem lumping). *Sample statements:* "I have to eliminate salt from my diet. They tell me I can no longer mow the lawn. This hospitalization is costing a mint. What about my kids' future? Who's going to change the oil in the car? This is an incredible amount of time away from work."
- Ineffective use of coping mechanisms
- Projection: blames others for illness or pain
- Displacement: directs anger and/or aggression toward family
  - *Sample statements:* "Get out of here. Leave me alone."
- Cursing, shouting, or demanding attention; striking out or throwing objects
- Denial: of severity of illness and need for treatment
- Noncompliance. *Examples:* activity restriction; refusal to allow treatment or to take medications
- Suicidal thoughts (verbalizes desire to end life)
- Self-directed aggression. *Examples:* disconnects or attempts to disconnect life-sustaining equipment; deliberately tries to harm self
- Failure to progress from dependent to more independent state (refusal or resistance to care for self)

Outcomes

- Patient verbalizes beginning ability to cope with illness, pain, and hospitalization. *Sample statements:* "I'm trying to do the best I can." "I want to help myself get better."
- Patient demonstrates effective problem solving (lists and prioritizes problems from most to least urgent).
- Patient uses effective behavioral strategies to manage the stress of illness and care.
- Patient demonstrates interest or involvement in illness or environment. *Examples:* Patient does the following:
  - Requests medications when anticipating pain
  - Questions course of treatment, progress, and prognosis
  - Asks for clarification of environmental stimuli and events
  - Seeks out supportive individuals in their environment
  - Uses coping mechanisms and strategies more effectively to manage situational crisis
  - Demonstrates significant reduction in impulsive, angry, or aggressive outbursts (projection, shouting, cursing) directed toward family
  - Verbalizes future-based plans with cessation of self-directed aggressive acts and suicidal thoughts
  - Willingly complies with treatment regimen
  - Begins to participate in self-care

Interventions and Rationale

1. Actively listen and respond to the patient's verbal and behavioral expressions. Active listening signifies unconditional respect and acceptance for the patient as a worthwhile individual. It builds trust and rapport, guides the nurse toward problem areas, encourages the patient to express concerns, and promotes compliance.
2. Offer effective coping strategies to help the patient better tolerate the stressors related to their illness and care. Give permission to vent feelings in a safe setting. Sample statements: "I don't blame you for feeling angry or frustrated." "Others who are ill like you have expressed similar feelings." "I will listen to anything you want to share with me." "We don't have to talk; I'd like to sit here with you." "It's perfectly okay to cry." Individuals who are provided with opportunities to express their feelings will be better able to release pent-up emotions and derive a greater sense of relief and comfort. They are less likely to resort to overly impulsive, aggressive acts, which may harm self or others.
3. Inform the family of the patient's need to displace anger occasionally but that you will be working with the patient to help them release their feelings in a more constructive, effective way. Family members who are well informed are better equipped to cope with their loved one's emotional anguish and outbursts. They are less likely to waste energy on feelings of guilt, fear, anger, or despair and can use their strength to help the patient in more constructive ways. The knowledge that their loved one is being cared for emotionally as well as physically provides family members with a greater sense of comfort and understanding. They will feel nurtured and respected by the nurse's attempt to include them in the process.
4. With the patient, list and number problems from the most to least urgent. Assist the patient in finding immediate solutions for the most urgent problems, postpone finding solutions for problems that can wait, delegate some problems to family members, and help the patient to acknowledge problems that are beyond their control. Listing and numbering problems in an organized fashion help to break them down into more manageable "pieces" so that the patient is better able to identify solutions for problems that are solvable and to suppress problems that are less relevant or not amenable to interventions.
5. Identify individuals in the patient's environment who best help them cope and identify those who do not. Validate your observations with the patient. Sample statements: "I notice you seemed more relaxed during your daughter's visit." "After the chaplain left, you were able to sleep a bit longer than usual; would you like to see them more often?" "Your grandson was a bit upset today; I'll be glad to talk to him if you like." Supportive persons can invoke a calming effect on the patient's physiologic and psychological states. Conversely, well-meaning but nonsupportive individuals can have a deleterious effect on the patient's ability to cope and must be carefully screened and counseled by the nurse.
6. Teach the patient effective cognitive strategies to help them better manage the stress of critical illness and care. Help the patient construct pleasant thoughts, situations, or images that can simultaneously inhibit unpleasant realities. Examples: a day at the beach, a walk in the park, drinking a glass of wine, or being with a loved one. Pleasant thoughts and images constructed during critical illness and care tend to inhibit or reduce the intensity of the unpleasant, stressful effects of the experience.
7. Assist the patient in using coping mechanisms more effectively so that the patient can better manage their situational crisis.
   a. Suppression of problems beyond their control
   b. Compensation for illness and its effects; focusing on their strengths, interests, family, and spiritual beliefs
   c. Adaptive displacement of anger, fear, or frustration through healthy, verbal expressions to staff. **Effective use of coping mechanisms helps to assuage the patient's painful feelings in a safe setting. The patient is strengthened and need not resort to the use of more ineffective defenses to eliminate anxiety.**
8. Initiate a suicidal assessment if the patient verbalizes the desire to die, states that life is not worth living, or exhibits self-directed aggression. *Sample statement:* "We know that this is a bad time for you. You're saying repeatedly that you want to die. Are you planning to harm yourself?" If the response is "yes," remain with the patient, alert staff members, and provide for psychiatric consultation as soon as possible. Continue to express concern to the patient and protect them from harm. **Suicidal thoughts as a result of ineffective coping or exhaustion of coping devices are a common occurrence**

PATIENT CARE MANAGEMENT PLAN

Impaired Adaptation—cont'd

in critically ill patients. If the mood state is distressing enough, a patient may seek relief by attempting a self-destructive act. Although the patient may not imminently have the energy to succeed in their attempt, voicing a specific plan signifies a depressed mood state and depletion of coping strategies. Immediate intervention is needed because the attempt may be successful when the patient's energy is restored.

9. Encourage the patient to participate in self-care activities and treatment regimens in accordance with their level of progress. Offer praise for their efforts toward self-care. **Patients who take an active role in their own treatment and progress are less apt to feel like helpless or powerless victims. This greater sense of control over their illness and environment will guide them more swiftly toward becoming as independent as possible.**

PATIENT CARE MANAGEMENT PLAN

Impaired Airway Clearance

Impaired Airway Clearance Due to Excessive Secretions or Abnormal Viscosity of Mucus

Signs and Symptoms

- Abnormal breath sounds (displaced normal sounds, adventitious sounds, diminished or absent sounds)
- Ineffective cough with or without sputum
- Tachypnea, dyspnea
- Verbal reports of inability to clear airway

Outcomes

- Cough produces thin mucus.
- Lungs are clear to auscultation.
- Respiratory rate, depth, and rhythm return to baseline.

Interventions and Rationale

1. Assess sputum for color, consistency, and amount.
2. Assess for clinical manifestations of pneumonia.
3. Provide for maximal thoracic expansion by repositioning, deep breathing, splinting, and pain management **to avoid hypoventilation and atelectasis.** If hypoventilation is present, implement the patient management plan for Impaired Breathing Due to Decreased Lung Expansion.
4. Maintain adequate hydration by administering oral and intravenous fluids (as ordered) **to thin secretions and facilitate airway clearance.**
5. Provide humidification to airways by an oxygen delivery device or artificial airway **to thin secretions and facilitate airway clearance.**
6. Administer bland aerosol every 4 hours **to facilitate expectoration of sputum.**
7. Collaborate with the practitioner regarding administration of the following:
   a. Bronchodilators to treat or prevent bronchospasms and facilitate expectoration of mucus
   b. Mucolytics and expectorants to enhance mobilization and removal of secretions
   c. Antibiotics to treat infection
8. Assist with directed coughing exercises **to facilitate expectoration of secretions.** If the patient is unable to perform cascade cough, consider using huff cough (patients with hyperactive airways), end-expiratory cough (patient with secretions in the distal airway), or augmented cough (patient with weakened abdominal muscles).
   a. Cascade cough—instruct the patient to do the following:
      (1). Take a deep breath, and hold it for 1 to 3 s.
      (2). Cough out forcefully several times until all air is exhaled.
      (3). Inhale slowly through the nose.
      (4). Repeat once.
      (5). Rest, and then repeat as necessary.
   b. Huff cough—instruct the patient to do the following:
      (1). Take a deep breath, and hold it for 1 to 3 s.
      (2). Say the word "huff" while coughing out several times until air is exhaled.
      (3). Inhale slowly through the nose.
      (4). Repeat as necessary.
   c. End-expiratory cough—instruct the patient to do the following:
      (1). Take a deep breath, and hold it for 1 to 3 s.
      (2). Exhale slowly.
      (3). At the end of exhalation, cough once.
      (4). Inhale slowly through the nose.
      (5). Repeat as necessary, or follow with cascade cough.
   d. Augmented cough—instruct the patient to do the following:
      (1). Take a deep breath, and hold it for 1 to 3 s.
      (2). Perform one or more of the following maneuvers to increase intraabdominal pressure:
         (a). Tighten knees and buttocks.
         (b). Bend forward at the waist.
         (c). Place a hand flat on the upper abdomen just under the xiphoid process and press in and up abruptly during coughing.
         (d). Keep hands on the chest wall and press inward with each cough.
      (3). Inhale slowly through the nose.
      (4). Rest and repeat as necessary.
9. Suction the patient as necessary **to assist with secretion removal.**
10. Reposition the patient at least every 2 hours or use kinetic therapy **to mobilize and prevent stasis of secretions.**
11. Allow rest periods between coughing sessions, suctioning, or any other demanding activities **to promote energy conservation.**

PATIENT CARE MANAGEMENT PLAN

Impaired Breathing

Impaired Breathing Due to Decreased Lung Expansion

Signs and Symptoms

- Abnormal respiratory patterns (hypoventilation, hyperventilation, tachypnea, bradypnea, obstructive breathing)
- Arterial blood gas (ABG) values (increased arterial partial pressure of carbon dioxide [$PaCO_2$], decreased pH)
- Unequal chest movement
- Shortness of breath, dyspnea

Outcomes

- Respiratory rate, rhythm, and depth return to baseline.
- Minimal or absent use of accessory muscles
- Chest expands symmetrically.
- ABG values return to baseline.

Interventions and Rationale

1. Treat pain, if present, **to prevent hypoventilation and atelectasis.** Implement the patient management plan for Acute Pain Due to Transmission and Perception of Cutaneous, Visceral, Muscular, or Ischemic Impulses.
2. Position the patient in high-Fowler or semi-Fowler position **to promote diaphragmatic descent and maximal inhalation.**
3. Assist with deep-breathing exercises and incentive spirometry with sustained maximal inspiration 5 to 10 times/h **to help reinflate collapsed portions of the lung.**
   a. Deep breathing—instruct the patient to do the following:
      (1). Sit up straight or lean forward slightly while sitting on edge of bed or chair (if possible).
      (2). Take in a slow, deep breath.
      (3). Pause slightly or hold breath for at least 3 s.
      (4). Exhale slowly.
      (5). Rest and repeat.
   b. Incentive spirometry—instruct the patient to do the following:
      (1). Exhale normally.
      (2). Place lips around the mouthpiece and close mouth tightly around it.
      (3). Inhale slowly and as deeply as possible, noting the maximal volume of air inspired.
      (4). Hold maximal inhalation for 3 s.
      (5). Take the mouthpiece out of mouth and slowly exhale.
      (6). Rest and repeat.
4. Assist the practitioner with intubation and initiation of mechanical ventilation as indicated.

Impaired Breathing Due to Musculoskeletal Fatigue or Neuromuscular Impairment

Signs and Symptoms

- Unequal chest movement
- Shortness of breath, dyspnea
- Use of accessory muscles
- Tachypnea
- Thoracoabdominal asynchrony
- Abnormal ABG values (increased $PaCO_2$, decreased pH)
- Nasal flaring
- Assumption of three-point position

Outcomes

- Respiratory rate, rhythm, and depth return to baseline.
- Use of accessory muscles is minimal or absent.
- Chest expands symmetrically.
- ABG values return to baseline.

Interventions and Rationale

1. Prevent unnecessary exertion to limit drain on the patient's ventilatory reserve.
2. Instruct the patient in energy-saving techniques to conserve the patient's ventilatory reserve.

Assist with pursed-lip and diaphragmatic breathing techniques to facilitate diaphragmatic descent and improved ventilation.
   a. Diaphragmatic breathing—instruct the patient to do the following:
      (1). Sit in the upright position.
      (2). Place one hand on the abdomen just above the waist and the other on the upper chest.
      (3). Breathe in through the nose and feel the lower hand push out; the upper hand should not move.
      (4). Breathe out through pursed lips, and feel the lower hand move in.

4. Position the patient in the high-Fowler or semi-Fowler position **to promote diaphragmatic descent and maximal inhalation.**
5. Assist the practitioner with intubation and initiation of mechanical ventilation as indicated.

Impaired Breathing Due to Respiratory Muscle Fatigue or Metabolic Factors

Signs and Symptoms

- Dyspnea and apprehension
- Increased metabolic rate
- Increased restlessness
- Increased use of accessory muscles
- Decreased tidal volume
- Increased heart rate
- Abnormal ABG values (decreased arterial partial pressure of oxygen [PaO_2], increased arterial partial pressure of carbon dioxide [$PaCO_2$], decreased pH, decreased arterial oxygen saturation [SaO_2])
- Decreased cooperation

Outcomes

- Metabolic rate and heart rate are within the patient's baseline.
- Patient experiences eupnea.
- ABG values are within the patient's baseline.

Interventions and Rationale

1. Collaborate with the practitioner regarding application of pressure support to the ventilator to assist the patient in overcoming the work of breathing imposed by the ventilator and endotracheal tube.
2. Carefully snip excess length from the proximal end of the endotracheal tube to decrease dead space and decrease the work of breathing.
3. Collaborate with the practitioner and dietitian to ensure that at least 50% of the diet's nonprotein caloric source is in the form of fat rather than carbohydrates to prevent excess carbon dioxide production.
4. Collaborate with the practitioner and respiratory care practitioner regarding the best method of weaning for individual patients because each situation is different and various weaning options are available.
   a. Consider initiating a daily spontaneous awakening trial ("sedation vacation") and spontaneous breathing trial.
   b. Monitor the patient for signs of weaning intolerance.
5. Collaborate with the practitioner and physical therapist regarding a progressive ambulation and conditioning plan **to promote overall muscle conditioning and respiratory muscle functioning.** Implement the patient management plan for Activity Intolerance Due to Prolonged Immobility or Deconditioning.

Continued

PATIENT CARE MANAGEMENT PLAN

Impaired Breathing—cont'd

6. Determine the most effective means of communication for the patient **to promote independence and reduce anxiety.**
7. Develop a daily schedule and post it in the patient's room to coordinate care and facilitate the patient's involvement in the plan.
8. Treat pain, if present, **to prevent respiratory splinting and hypoventilation.** Implement the patient management plan for Acute Pain Due to Transmission and Perception of Cutaneous, Visceral, Muscular, or Ischemic Impulses.
9. Ensure that the patient receives at least 2- to 4-hour intervals of uninterrupted sleep in a quiet, dark room. Collaborate with the practitioner and respiratory care practitioner regarding use of full ventilatory support at night **to provide respiratory muscle rest.**
10. Place the patient in the semi-Fowler position or in a chair at the bedside **for best use of ventilatory muscles and to facilitate diaphragmatic descent.**
11. Explain the weaning procedure to the patient before the trial **so that the patient will understand what to expect and how to participate.**
12. Monitor the patient during the weaning trial for evidence of respiratory muscle fatigue **to avoid overtiring the patient.**
13. Collaborate with the practitioner and occupational therapist to provide diversional activities during the weaning trial **to reduce the patient's anxiety.**
14. Collaborate with the practitioner and respiratory care practitioner regarding removal of the ventilator and artificial airway **after the patient has been successfully weaned.**

PATIENT CARE MANAGEMENT PLAN

Impaired Cardiac Output

Impaired Cardiac Output Due to Alterations in Preload

Signs and Symptoms

- Cardiac output is <4.0 L/min
- Cardiac index is <2.5 L/min/m^2
- Heart rate is >100 beats/min
- Urine output is <30 mL/h or 0.5 mL/kg/h
- Decreased mentation, restlessness, agitation, confusion
- Diminished peripheral pulses
- Blue, gray, or dark purple tint to tongue and sublingual area
- Systolic blood pressure <90 mm Hg
- Subjective complaints of fatigue

Reduced Preload

- Right atrial pressure is <2 mm Hg
- Pulmonary artery occlusion pressure is <6 mm Hg

Excessive Preload

- Right atrial pressure is >8 mm Hg
- Pulmonary artery occlusion pressure is >12 mm Hg

Outcomes

- Cardiac output is 4 to 8 L/min.
- Cardiac index is 2.5 to 4 L/min/m^2.
- Right atrial pressure is 2 to 8 mm Hg.
- Pulmonary artery occlusion pressure is 6 to 12 mm Hg.

Interventions and Rationale

1. Collaborate with the practitioner regarding administration of oxygen to maintain peripheral oxygen saturation (SpO_2) >92% **to prevent tissue hypoxia.**
2. Maintain surveillance for signs of decreased tissue perfusion and acidosis **to facilitate early identification and treatment of complications.**
3. Monitor fluid balance and daily weights to facilitate regulation of the patient's fluid balance.

For Reduced Preload Resulting from Volume Loss

1. Collaborate with the practitioner regarding administration of crystalloids, colloids, blood, and blood products **to increase circulating volume.**
2. Limit blood sampling, observe intravenous lines for accidental disconnection, apply direct pressure to bleeding sites, and maintain normal body temperature **to minimize fluid loss.**
3. Position the patient with legs elevated, trunk flat, and head and shoulders above the chest **to enhance venous return.**
4. Encourage oral fluids (as appropriate), administer free water with tube feedings, and replace fluids that are lost through wound or tube drainage **to promote adequate fluid intake.**
5. Maintain surveillance for signs of fluid volume excess and adverse effects of blood and blood product administration **to facilitate early identification and treatment of complications.**

For Reduced Preload Resulting From Venous Dilation

1. Collaborate with the practitioner regarding administration of vasoconstrictors **to increase venous return.**
2. Maintain surveillance for adverse effects of vasoconstrictor therapy **to facilitate early identification and treatment of complications.**
3. If the patient is hyperthermic, administer tepid bath, hypothermia blanket, or ice bags to the axilla and groin **to decrease temperature and promote vasoconstriction.**

For Excessive Preload Resulting From Volume Overload

1. Collaborate with the practitioner regarding administration of the following:
   a. Diuretics to remove excessive fluid
   b. Vasodilators to decrease venous return
   c. Inotropes to increase myocardial contractility
2. Restrict fluid intake and double-concentrate intravenous drips **to minimize fluid intake.**
3. Position the patient in the semi-Fowler or high-Fowler position **to reduce venous return.**
4. Maintain surveillance for signs of fluid volume deficit and adverse effects of diuretic, vasodilator, and inotropic therapies **to facilitate early identification and treatment of complications.**

For Excessive Preload Resulting From Venous Constriction

1. Collaborate with the practitioner regarding administration of vasodilators **to promote venous dilation.**
2. Maintain surveillance for adverse effects of vasodilator therapy **to facilitate early identification and treatment of complications.**
3. If the patient is hypothermic, wrap them in warm blankets or administer a hyperthermia blanket **to increase temperature and promote vasodilation.**

Impaired Cardiac Output Due to Alterations in Afterload

Signs and Symptoms

- Cardiac output is <4 L/min.
- Cardiac index is <2.5 L/min/m^2.
- Heart rate is >100 beats/min.
- Urine output is <30 mL/h.
- Decreased mentation, restlessness, agitation, confusion
- Diminished peripheral pulses
- Blue, gray, or dark purple tint to tongue and sublingual area
- Systolic blood pressure is <90 mm Hg.
- Subjective complaints of fatigue

Reduced Afterload

- Pulmonary vascular resistance is <100 dyn · sec · cm^{-5}.
- Systemic vascular resistance is <800 dyn · sec · cm^{-5}.

Excessive Afterload

- Pulmonary vascular resistance is >250 dyn · sec · cm^{-5}.
- Systemic vascular resistance is >1200 dyn · sec · cm^{-5}.

Outcomes

- Cardiac output is 4 to 8 L/min.
- Cardiac index is 2.5 to 4 L/min/m^2.
- Pulmonary vascular resistance is 80 to 250 dyn · sec · cm^{-5}.
- Systemic vascular resistance is 800 to 1200 dyn · sec · cm^{-5}.

Interventions and Rationale

1. Collaborate with the practitioner regarding administration of oxygen to maintain SpO_2 >92% **to prevent tissue hypoxia.**
2. Maintain surveillance for signs of decreased tissue perfusion and acidosis **to facilitate early identification and treatment of complications.**

For Reduced Afterload

1. Collaborate with the practitioner regarding administration of vasoconstrictors **to promote arterial vasoconstriction and prevent relative**

Continued

PATIENT CARE MANAGEMENT PLAN

Impaired Cardiac Output—cont'd

hypovolemia. If decreased preload is present, implement patient management plan for Impaired Cardiac Output Due to Alterations in Preload.

2. Maintain surveillance for adverse effects of vasoconstrictor therapy **to facilitate early identification and treatment of complications.**
3. If the patient is hyperthermic, administer a tepid bath, hypothermia blanket, or ice bags to the axilla and groin **to decrease temperature and promote vasoconstriction.**

For Excessive Afterload

1. Collaborate with the practitioner regarding administration of vasodilators **to promote arterial vasodilation.**
2. Collaborate with the practitioner regarding initiation of an intraaortic balloon pump **to facilitate afterload reduction.**
3. Promote rest and relaxation and decrease environmental stimulation **to minimize sympathetic stimulation.**
4. Maintain surveillance for adverse effects of vasodilator therapy **to facilitate early identification and treatment of complications.**
5. If the patient is hypothermic, wrap the patient in warm blankets or administer hyperthermia blanket **to increase temperature and promote vasodilation.**
6. If the patient is in pain, treat pain **to reduce sympathetic stimulation.** Implement patient management plan for Acute Pain Due to Transmission and Perception of Cutaneous, Visceral, Muscular, or Ischemic Impulses.

Impaired Cardiac Output Due to Alterations in Contractility

Signs and Symptoms

- Cardiac output is <4 L/min.
- Cardiac index is <2.5 L/min/m^2.
- Heart rate is >100 beats/min.
- Urine output is <30 mL/h.
- Decreased mentation, restlessness, agitation, confusion
- Diminished peripheral pulses
- Blue, gray, or dark purple tint to tongue and sublingual area
- Systolic blood pressure is <90 mm Hg.
- Subjective complaints of fatigue
- Right ventricular stroke work index is <7 g/m^2/beat.
- Left ventricular stroke work index is <35 g/m^2/beat.

Outcomes

- Cardiac output is 4 to 8 L/min.
- Cardiac index is 2.5 to 4 L/min/m^2.
- Right ventricular stroke work index is 7 to 12 g/m^2/beat.
- Left ventricular stroke work index is 35 to 85 g/m^2/beat.

Interventions and Rationale

1. Collaborate with the practitioner regarding administration of oxygen to maintain SpO_2 >92% **to prevent tissue hypoxia.**
2. Maintain surveillance for signs of decreased tissue perfusion and acidosis **to facilitate early identification and treatment of complications.**
3. Ensure preload is optimized. If preload is reduced or excessive, implement the patient management plan for Impaired Cardiac Output Due to Alterations in Preload.
4. Ensure afterload is optimized. If afterload is reduced or excessive, implement the patient management plan for Impaired Cardiac Output Due to Alterations in Afterload.
5. Ensure electrolytes are optimized. Collaborate with the practitioner regarding administration of electrolyte replacement therapy **to enhance the cellular ionic environment.**
6. Collaborate with the practitioner regarding administration of inotropes **to enhance myocardial contractility.**
7. Monitor the ST segment continuously **to determine changes in myocardial tissue perfusion.** If myocardial ischemia is present, implement the patient management plan for Ineffective Tissue Perfusion Due to Decreased Myocardial Blood Flow.

Impaired Cardiac Output Due to Alterations in Heart Rate or Rhythm

Signs and Symptoms

- Cardiac output is <4 L/min.
- Cardiac index is <2.5 L/min/m^2.
- Heart rate is >100 beats/min or <60 beats/min.
- Urine output is <30 mL/h or 0.5 mL/kg/h.
- Decreased mentation, restlessness, agitation, confusion
- Diminished peripheral pulses
- Blue, gray, or dark purple tint to tongue and sublingual area
- Systolic blood pressure is <90 mm Hg.
- Subjective complaints of fatigue
- Dysrhythmias

Outcomes

- Cardiac output is 4 to 8 L/min.
- Cardiac index is 2.5 to 4 L/min/m^2.
- Dysrhythmias are absent or return to baseline.
- Heart rate is >60 beats/min or <100 beats/min.

Interventions and Rationale

1. Collaborate with the practitioner regarding administration of oxygen to maintain SpO_2 >92% **to prevent tissue hypoxia.**
2. Ensure electrolytes are optimized. Collaborate with the practitioner regarding administration of electrolyte therapy **to enhance cellular ionic environment and avoid precipitation of dysrhythmias.**
3. Collaborate with the practitioner and pharmacist regarding the patient's current medications and their effect on heart rate and rhythm **to identify any prodysrhythmic or bradycardic side effects.**
4. Maintain surveillance for signs of decreased tissue perfusion and acidosis **to facilitate early identification and treatment of complications.**
5. Monitor ST segment continuously **to determine changes in myocardial tissue perfusion.** If myocardial ischemia is present, implement the patient management plan for Ineffective Tissue Perfusion Due to Decreased Myocardial Blood Flow.

For Lethal Dysrhythmias or Asystole

1. Initiate advanced cardiac life support interventions and notify the practitioner immediately.

For Nonlethal Dysrhythmias

1. Collaborate with the practitioner regarding administration of antidysrhythmic therapy, synchronized cardioversion, or overdrive pacing **to control dysrhythmias.**
2. Maintain surveillance for adverse effects of antidysrhythmic therapy **to facilitate early identification and treatment of complications.**

For Heart Rate <60 Beats/Min

1. Collaborate with the practitioner regarding initiation of temporary pacing **to increase heart rate.**

Impaired Cardiac Output Due to Sympathetic Blockade

Signs and Symptoms

- Decreased cardiac output and cardiac index
- Systolic blood pressure <90 mm Hg or below patient's baseline
- Decreased right atrial pressure and pulmonary artery occlusion pressure

PATIENT CARE MANAGEMENT PLAN

Impaired Cardiac Output—cont'd

- Decreased systemic vascular resistance
- Bradycardia
- Cardiac dysrhythmias
- Postural hypotension

Outcomes

- Cardiac output and cardiac index are within normal limits.
- Systolic blood pressure is >90 mm Hg or returns to baseline.
- Right atrial pressure and pulmonary artery occlusion pressure are within normal limits.
- Systemic vascular resistance is within normal limits.
- Sinus rhythm is present.
- Dysrhythmias are absent.
- Fainting or dizziness with position change is absent.

Interventions and Rationale

1. Implement measures to prevent episodes of postural hypertension:
   a. Change the patient's position slowly to allow the cardiovascular system time to compensate.
   b. Apply pneumatic compression stockings to promote venous return.
   c. Perform range-of-motion exercises every 2 hours to prevent venous pooling.
   d. Collaborate with the practitioner and physical therapist regarding the use of a tilt table to progress the patient from supine to upright position.
2. Collaborate with the practitioner regarding administration of the following:
   a. Crystalloids and/or colloids to increase the patient's circulating volume, **which increases stroke volume and subsequently cardiac output**
   b. Vasopressors if fluids are ineffective to constrict the patient's vascular system, **which increases resistance and subsequently blood pressure**
3. Monitor cardiac rhythm for bradycardia and/or dysrhythmias, **which can further decrease cardiac output.**
4. Avoid any activity that can stimulate the vagal response **because bradycardia can result.**
5. Treat symptomatic bradycardia and symptomatic dysrhythmias according to unit's emergency protocol or advanced cardiac life support guidelines.

PATIENT CARE MANAGEMENT PLAN

Impaired Family Coping

Impaired Family Coping Due to Critically Ill Family Member

Signs and Symptoms

- Disruption of usual family functions and roles
- Inability to accept or deal with crisis situation; use of defense mechanisms (e.g., denial, anger); unrealistic expectations of patient's outcome and care provided; judgmental toward health care practitioners
- Nonrecognition that family is in state of crisis
- Inappropriate emotional outbursts; arguments among family and with others; inability to respond to each other's feelings or support each other
- Misinterpretation of information; short attention span with repeated questions about information already provided; members not sharing information with each other
- Inability to make decisions regarding changes in family structure or about course of care for ill member; noncooperation among family members
- Expressions of grief, hopelessness, powerlessness, and isolation; do not seek or respond to support services
- Hesitancy to spend time with ill person in the critical care unit or inappropriate behavior when visiting (may upset patient)
- Neglect of own personal health; fatigue, apathy; refusal of offers for respite time

Outcomes

- The family will express an understanding of course and prognosis of illness, therapies, and alternative measures.
- The family will diminish or resolve conflicts and cooperate in decision making.
- The family will develop trust and mutual support for each member and form a cohesive unit.
- The family will support the ill person in making decisions (if capable) or respect prior wishes regarding provision of health care.
- Family efforts will be directed toward a purpose and readjust to changes in life patterns and role function. Members will accept responsibility for changes.
- The family will identify and use effective coping strategies.
- The family will identify and use available resources as needed to facilitate resolution of the crisis.
- The family will have a sense of control and confidence in meeting personal and collective needs.

Interventions and Rationale

1. Identify family's perception of the crisis situation. All initial interventions should be directed toward resolving the crisis situation. Understanding and using family theory principles will facilitate this process and individualize care.
   a. Determine family structure; developmental phase of roles; and ethnic, cultural, and belief factors that may affect communication with family and the plan of care.
   b. Identify strengths of the family.
2. Provide honest and accurate information in language persons can understand. Give updated information as appropriate. Listen. **This facilitates open communication among family and health care practitioners, projects a caring attitude and concern for them and the patient, and assists the family in making decisions and being involved with the plan and goals of care.**
3. Encourage liberal visitation with the patient.
   a. Before the visit, prepare family members for what they will observe in a technical environment. **This prevents a strong emotional reaction to an unfamiliar and frightening situation.**
      (1). Inform them about the patient's appearance and behaviors that may be distressing to them.
      (2). Explain the cause of the patient's responses to stimuli (e.g., pain, trauma, surgery, medication) and explain that these behaviors are being monitored and are usually temporary.
   b. Encourage them to touch the patient and let the patient know of their presence.
4. Identify and support effective coping behaviors. This aids in the family's sense of control and resolution of helplessness/powerlessness.
5. Observe for signs of fatigue and the need for emotional/spiritual support and respite from hospital waiting routine. This provides support and comfort, facilitates hope, resolves sense of isolation, gives sense of security, and diminishes guilt feeling for attending to personal needs.
   a. Encourage family to verbalize feelings.
   b. Provide information on available resources.
   c. Alert interdisciplinary team members (social, psychological, spiritual) to family needs.
   d. Provide pager device (if available) or obtain phone numbers when family leaves the hospital premises.
6. Instruct family in simple caregiving techniques and encourage participation in the patient's care. This facilitates giving a sense of normalcy to the experience, self-confidence, and assurance that good care is being provided.
7. Serve as an advocate for the patient and family. Teach the family how to negotiate with the health care delivery system and include them in health care team conferences when appropriate. **This facilitates informed decision making, promotes control and satisfaction, and permits mutual goal setting.**
8. Consider nonbiologic or nonlegal family relationships. Encourage contact with the patient and participation in care. This facilitates holistic care and support of emotional ties and demonstrates respect for the family unit and relationships.
9. Provide emotional support and compassion when the patient's condition worsens or deteriorates. The use of touch and expression of concern for the patient and family convey comfort and trust in the health care practitioner and respect and assurance that the family's loved one will receive appropriate care and attention.

PATIENT CARE MANAGEMENT PLAN

Impaired Gas Exchange

Impaired Gas Exchange Due to Alveolar Hypoventilation

Signs and Symptoms

- Abnormal arterial blood gas (ABG) values (decreased arterial partial pressure of oxygen [PaO_2], increased arterial partial pressure of carbon dioxide [$PaCO_2$], decreased pH, decreased arterial oxygen saturation [SaO_2])
- Somnolence
- Neurobehavioral changes (e.g., restlessness, irritability, confusion)
- Tachycardia or dysrhythmias
- Central cyanosis

Outcomes

- ABG values are within patient's baseline.
- Central cyanosis is absent.

Interventions and Rationale

1. Initiate continuous pulse oximetry or monitor peripheral oxygen saturation (SpO_2) every hour.
2. Collaborate with the practitioner and respiratory care practitioner regarding administration of oxygen to maintain SpO_2 >92%.
   a. Administer supplemental oxygen by an appropriate oxygen delivery device **to increase driving pressure of oxygen in the alveoli.**
   b. If supplemental oxygen alone is ineffective, administer high-flow oxygen via high-flow nasal cannula, bilevel positive airway pressure (BiPAP) via noninvasive ventilation (NIV), or positive end-expiratory pressure (PEEP) via invasive mechanical ventilation **to open collapsed alveoli and increase the surface area for gas exchange.**
3. Prevent hypoventilation.
   a. Position the patient in high-Fowler or semi-Fowler position **to promote diaphragmatic descent and maximal inhalation.**
   b. Assist with deep-breathing exercises and/or incentive spirometry with sustained maximal inspiration 5 to 10 times/h **to help reinflate collapsed portions of the lung.** See the patient management plan for Impaired Breathing Due to Decreased Lung Expansion for further instructions.
   c. Treat pain, if present, **to prevent hypoventilation and atelectasis.** Implement the patient management plan for Acute Pain Due to Transmission and Perception of Cutaneous, Visceral, Muscular, or Ischemic Impulses.
4. Assist the practitioner with intubation and initiation of mechanical ventilation as indicated.

Impaired Gas Exchange Due to Ventilation–Perfusion Mismatching or Intrapulmonary Shunting

Signs and Symptoms

- Abnormal ABG values (decreased PaO_2, decreased SaO_2)
- Somnolence
- Neurobehavioral changes (restlessness, irritability, confusion)
- Central cyanosis

Outcomes

- ABG values are within patient's baseline.
- Central cyanosis is absent.

Interventions and Rationale

1. Initiate continuous pulse oximetry or monitor SpO_2 every hour.
2. Collaborate with the practitioner and respiratory care practitioner regarding administration of oxygen to maintain an SpO_2 >92%.
   a. Administer supplemental oxygen by an appropriate oxygen delivery device **to increase driving pressure of oxygen in the alveoli.**
   b. If supplemental oxygen alone is ineffective, administer high-flow oxygen via high-flow nasal cannula, BiPAP via NIV, or positive end-expiratory pressure (PEEP) via invasive mechanical ventilation **to open collapsed alveoli and increase the surface area for gas exchange.**
3. Position the patient to optimize ventilation–perfusion matching.
   a. For a patient with unilateral lung disease, position with the good lung down because gravity will improve perfusion to this area and this will best match ventilation with perfusion.
   b. For a patient with bilateral lung disease, position with the right lung down because this lung is larger than the left and affords a greater area for ventilation and perfusion, or change position every 2 h, favoring positions that improve oxygenation.
   c. For a patient with diffuse bilateral disease, collaborate with the practitioner regarding the use of prone positioning to encourage perfusion to the anterior region of the lungs, which are usually less damaged than the posterior region.
   d. Avoid any position that seriously compromises oxygenation status.
4. Perform procedures only as needed and provide adequate rest and recovery time in between **to prevent desaturation.**
5. Collaborate with the practitioner regarding administration of the following:
   a. Sedatives to decrease ventilator asynchrony and facilitate the patient's sense of control
   b. Neuromuscular blocking agents to prevent ventilator asynchrony and decrease oxygen demand
   c. Analgesics **to treat pain if present.** Implement the patient management plan for Acute Pain Due to Transmission and Perception of Cutaneous, Visceral, Muscular, or Ischemic Impulses.
6. Evaluate the patient for the presence of secretions. If secretions are present, implement the patient management plan for Impaired Airway Clearance Due to Excessive Secretions or Abnormal Viscosity of Mucus.

PATIENT CARE MANAGEMENT PLAN

Impaired Health Maintenance

Impaired Health Maintenance Due to Cognitive or Perceptual Learning Limitations

Signs and Symptoms

- Verbalized statement of inadequate knowledge of skills
- Verbalization of inadequate recall of information
- Verbalization of inadequate understanding of information
- Evidence of inaccurate follow-through of instructions
- Inadequate demonstration of a skill
- Lack of compliance with prescribed behavior

Outcomes

- Patient participates actively in necessary and prescribed health behaviors.
- Patient verbalizes adequate knowledge or demonstrates adequate skills.

Interventions and Rationale

1. Determine the specific cause of the patient's cognitive or perceptual limitation.
2. Provide an uninterrupted rest period before the teaching session to decrease fatigue and encourage the optimal state for learning and retention.
3. Manipulate the environment as much as possible to provide quiet and uninterrupted learning sessions.
   a. Ensure that lights are bright enough to see teaching aids but not too bright.
   b. Schedule care and medications to allow uninterrupted teaching periods.
   c. Move the patient to a quiet, private room for teaching if possible.
4. Adapt teaching sessions and materials to the level of education and ability to understand the patient and family.
   a. Provide printed material appropriate to reading level.
   b. Use terminology understood by the patient.
   c. Provide printed materials in the patient's primary language if possible.
   d. Use interpreters during teaching sessions *when necessary*.
5. Teach only present-tense focus during periods of sensory overload.
6. Determine potential effects of medications on ability to retain or recall information. Avoid teaching critical content while the patient is taking sedatives, analgesics, or other medications that affect memory.
7. Reinforce new skills and information in several teaching sessions. Use several senses when possible in a teaching session (e.g., see a film, hear a discussion, read printed information, demonstrate skills related to self-injection of insulin).
8. Reduce the patient's anxiety.
   a. Listen attentively and encourage verbalization of feelings.
   b. Answer questions as they arise in a clear and succinct manner.
   c. Elicit the patient's concerns and address those issues first.
   d. Give only correct and relevant information.
   e. Continually assess response to teaching session and discontinue if anxiety increases or physical condition becomes unstable.
   f. Provide nonthreatening information before more anxiety-producing information is presented.
   g. Plan for several teaching sessions so that information can be divided into small, manageable packages.

PATIENT CARE MANAGEMENT PLAN

Impaired Nutritional Intake

Impaired Nutritional Intake Due to Lack of Exogenous Nutrients and Increased Metabolic Demand

Signs and Symptoms

- Unplanned weight loss of 20% of body weight within past 6 months
- Serum albumin <3.5 g/dL
- Total lymphocytes <1500/mm^3
- Anergy
- Negative nitrogen balance
- Fatigue; lack of energy and endurance
- Nonhealing wounds
- Daily caloric intake less than estimated nutrition requirements
- Presence of factors known to increase nutrition requirements (e.g., sepsis, trauma, multiple-organ dysfunction syndrome)
- Maintenance of nothing by mouth (NPO) status for >10 days
- Long-term use of intravenous 5% dextrose
- Documentation of suboptimal calorie counts
- Drug or nutrient interaction that might decrease oral intake (e.g., chronic use of bronchodilators, laxatives, anticonvulsives, diuretics, antacids, opioids)
- Physical problems with chewing, swallowing, choking, and salivation and presence of altered taste, anorexia, nausea, vomiting, diarrhea, or constipation

Outcomes

- Patient exhibits stabilization of weight loss or weight gain of 0.5 lb daily.
- Serum albumin is >3.5 g/dL.
- Total lymphocytes are <1500/mm^3.
- Patient has positive response to cutaneous skin antigen testing.
- Patient is in positive nitrogen balance.
- Wound healing is evident.
- Daily caloric intake equals estimated nutrition requirements.
- Increased ambulation and endurance are evident.

Interventions and Rationale

1. Inquire whether the patient has any food allergies and food preferences **to ensure the food provided to the patient is not contraindicated.**
2. Monitor the patient's caloric intake and weight daily **to ensure adequacy of nutrition interventions.**
3. Collaborate with the dietitian regarding the patient's nutrition and caloric needs **to determine the appropriateness of the patient's diet to meet those needs.**
4. Monitor the patient for signs of nutrition deficiencies **to facilitate evaluation of the extent of nutrition deficit.**
5. Provide the patient with oral care before eating **to ensure optimal consumption of diet.**
6. Assist the patient to eat as appropriate **to ensure optimal consumption of diet.**
7. Collaborate with the practitioner and dietitian regarding administration of parenteral and enteral nutrition as needed.

PATIENT CARE MANAGEMENT PLAN

Impaired Peripheral Tissue Perfusion

Impaired Peripheral Tissue Perfusion Due to Decreased Blood Flow

Sign and Symptoms

- Weak and/or unequal peripheral pulses
- Delayed capillary refill
- Ischemic pain from extremity
- Cool skin on extremity
- Pale extremity
- Paresthesias from extremity

Outcomes

- Peripheral pulses are full and equal bilaterally.
- Capillary refill is equal bilaterally.
- Ischemic pain is absent.
- Skin temperature is equal in both extremities.
- Skin is pink and warm in both extremities.
- Paresthesias are absent.

Interventions and Rationale

1. Collaborate with the practitioner regarding administration of antiplatelet, anticoagulant, or fibrinolytic therapy.
2. Collaborate with the practitioner regarding pain management. Implement the patient management plan for Acute Pain Due to Transmission and Perception of Cutaneous, Visceral, Muscular, or Ischemic Impulses.
3. Ensure the patient is adequately hydrated **to decrease blood viscosity.**
4. Maintain the affected extremity in dependent position, if possible, **to enhance blood flow.**
5. Keep the affected extremity warm and protect it from injury. **Do not apply heat directly to the affected extremity because this can result in injury.**
6. Maintain surveillance for pain, pallor, pulselessness, paresthesia, paralysis, and poikilothermia **as indicators of abrupt change in blood flow.**
7. Maintain surveillance for tissue breakdown and arterial ulcers **as indicators of injury.**
8. Prepare the patient for possible surgery or interventional procedure to restore blood flow.

PATIENT CARE MANAGEMENT PLAN

Impaired Sleep

Impaired Sleep Due to Fragmented Sleep

Signs and Symptoms

- Decreased sleep during one block of sleep time
- Daytime sleepiness
- Decreased sleep
- Less than one-half of normal total sleep time
- Decreased slow-wave or rapid-eye-movement (REM) sleep
- Anxiety
- Fatigue
- Restlessness
- Disorientation and hallucinations
- Combativeness
- Frequent awakenings

Outcomes

- Patient's total sleep time approximates patient's normal sleep time.
- Patient can complete sleep cycles of 90 min without interruption.
- Patient has no delusions or hallucinations.
- Patient has reality-based thought content.

Interventions and Rationale

1. Assess the normal sleep pattern on admission and any history of sleep disturbance or chronic illness that may affect sleep or sedative/hypnotic use.
   a. Promote normal sleep activity while the patient is in the critical care unit.
   b. Assess sleep effectiveness by asking the patient how their sleep in the hospital compares with sleep at home.
2. Promote comfort, relaxation, and a sense of well-being.
   a. Treat pain; change, smooth, or refresh bed linens at bedtime; and provide oral hygiene.
   b. Eliminate stressful situations before bedtime.
   c. Use relaxation techniques, imagery, music, massage, or warm blankets.
   d. Have a close family member sit beside the bed and provide the patient with their own garments or coverings.
   e. Provide quiet or background noise of the television or music (patient preference) **to best promote sleep.**
   f. Provide a comfortable room temperature.
3. Minimize noise, particularly noise generated by the staff and equipment.
   a. Reduce the level of environmental stimuli.
   b. Dim the lights at night.
4. Foods containing tryptophan (e.g., milk, turkey) may be appropriate **because these promote sleep.**
5. Plan nap times to assist in approximating the patient's normal 24-hour sleep time.
6. Minimize awakenings **to allow for at least 90-min sleep cycles.**
   a. Continually assess the need to awaken the patient, particularly at night. Distinguish between essential and nonessential patient care tasks.
   b. Organize patient management to allow for maximal amount of uninterrupted sleep while ensuring close monitoring of the patient's condition. Whenever possible, monitor physiologic parameters without waking the patient.
   c. Coordinate awakenings with other departments, such as laboratory and radiography, **to minimize sleep interruptions.**
7. Be aware of the effects of commonly used medications on sleep. **Many sedative/hypnotic medications decrease REM sleep.**
   a. Use sedative and analgesic medications that minimally disrupt sleep to complement comfort measures, with dosages reduced gradually as the medication is no longer necessary.
   b. Do not abruptly withdraw REM-suppressing medications **because this can result in REM rebound.**
8. Document the amount of uninterrupted sleep per shift, especially sleep episodes lasting longer than 2 hours. Sleep pattern disturbance is diagnosed, treated, and resolved more efficiently when formally documented in this manner.

PATIENT CARE MANAGEMENT PLAN

Impaired Spiritual Status

Impaired Spiritual Status Due to Change in Health Status That Alters Ability to Experience Meaning in Life Through Self-Expression

Signs and Symptoms

- Anxiety
- Crying
- Fear
- Expression of hopelessness
- Expression of loss of connectedness
- Insomnia
- Anger
- Questioning previously held sources of meaning
- Withdrawal from significant others
- Increased dependence on health care personnel
- Refusal to participate in care
- Avoidance of spiritual advisors
- Avoidance of previously pursued activities

Outcomes

- Patient expresses feelings, fears, and concerns.
- Patient expresses sense of hope in the future.
- Patient expresses feelings of connectedness and meaning in life.

Interventions and Rationale

1. Assess for signs and symptoms in patients with acute or chronic health problems. Changes in health status can bring about spiritual confusion in patients who are experiencing unfamiliar life circumstances. Early intervention can prevent serious spiritual problems.
2. Assess patient's mental/emotional status using active listening. Active listening can help identify central points of concern for the patient.
3. Assist the patient to identify spiritual beliefs and practices and express acceptance of those beliefs and practices. Verbalizing beliefs can help the patient regain connectedness to their familiar sources of support. An accepting atmosphere from the nurse will promote the supportive relationship.
4. Encourage the patient to engage in preferred spiritual expression. Spiritual expression is a positive method of coping and can promote a sense of well-being.
5. Assist patient to identify sources of gratitude and hope. Focusing on familiar and reliable sources of strength can provide avenues for spiritual relief.
6. Include family as appropriate in discussion and support. Significant others are a primary source of support for patients, and they will be most familiar with the beliefs, strengths, and limitations of the patient in trying circumstances.
7. Offer or suggest a consultation with a spiritual advisor. Spiritual care can promote connectedness and spiritual relief.
8. Consider complementary therapies: meditation, guided imagery, journaling, art, or music as a means to promote relaxation and decrease anxiety. Complementary therapies provide distraction and provide avenues of self-expression.

PATIENT CARE MANAGEMENT PLAN

Impaired Swallowing

Impaired Swallowing Due to Neuromuscular Impairment, Fatigue, and Limited Awareness

Signs and Symptoms

- Evidence of difficulty swallowing:
  - Drooling
  - Difficulty handling oral secretions
  - Absence of gag, cough, or swallow reflex
  - Moist, wet, gurgling voice quality
  - Decreased tongue and mouth movements
  - Presence of dysarthria
- Difficulty handling solid foods:
  - Uncoordinated chewing or swallowing
  - Stasis of food in oral cavity
  - Wet-sounding voice or change in voice quality
  - Sneezing, coughing, or choking with eating
  - Delay in swallowing of more than 5 s
  - Change in respiratory patterns
- Difficulty handling liquids:
  - Momentary loss of voice or change in voice quality
  - Nasal regurgitation of liquids
  - Coughing with drinking
- Evidence of aspiration:
  - Hypoxemia
  - Productive cough
  - Frothy sputum
  - Wheezing, crackles, or rhonchi
  - Temperature elevation

Outcomes

- Evidence of swallowing difficulties is absent.
- Evidence of aspiration is absent.

Interventions and Rationale

1. Collaborate with the practitioner and speech therapist regarding the swallowing evaluation and rehabilitation program **to decrease the incidence of aspiration.**
2. Collaborate with the practitioner and dietitian regarding a nutrition assessment and nutrition plan **to ensure that the patient is receiving adequate nutrition.**
3. Place the patient in an upright position with the head midline and the chin slightly down **to keep food in the anterior portion of the mouth and to prevent it from falling over the base of the tongue into the open airway.**
4. Provide the patient with single-textured soft foods (e.g., cream cereals) that maintain their shape **because these foods require minimal oral manipulation.**
5. Avoid particulate foods (e.g., hamburger) and foods containing more than one texture (e.g., stew) **because these foods require more chewing and oral manipulation.**
6. Avoid dry foods (e.g., popcorn, rice, crackers) and sticky foods (e.g., peanut butter, bananas) **because these foods are difficult to manipulate orally.**
7. Provide the patient with thick liquids (e.g., fruit nectar, yogurt) **because thick liquids are more easily controlled in the mouth.**
8. Thicken thin liquids (e.g., water, juice) with a thickening preparation or avoid them **because thin liquids are easily aspirated.**
9. Place foods in the uninvolved side of the mouth **because oral sensitivity and function are greatest in this area.**
10. Avoid the use of straws **because they can deposit the liquid too far back in the mouth for the patient to handle.**
11. Serve foods and liquids at room temperature **because the patient may be overly sensitive to heat or cold.**
12. Offer solids and liquids at different times **to avoid swallowing solids before being properly chewed.**
13. Provide oral hygiene after meals **to clear food particles from the mouth that could be aspirated.**
14. Collaborate with the practitioner and pharmacist regarding oral medication administration **to adjust the medication regimen to prevent aspiration and choking and to ensure all prescribed medications are swallowed.**
15. Crush tablets (if appropriate) and mix with food that is easily formed into a bolus, use thickened liquid medications (if available), or embed small capsules into food **to facilitate oral medication administration.**
16. Inspect the mouth for residue after all medication administration **to ensure medication has been swallowed.**
17. Educate the patient and family on the swallowing problem, rehabilitation program, and emergency measures for choking.

PATIENT CARE MANAGEMENT PLAN

Impaired Ventilatory Weaning

Impaired Ventilatory Weaning Due to Physical, Psychosocial, or Situational Factors

Signs and Symptoms

Mild Impairment

- Responds to lowered levels of mechanical ventilator support with:
  - Restlessness
  - Slightly increased respiratory rate from baseline
  - Expressed feelings of increased need for oxygen, breathing discomfort, fatigue, warmth
  - Queries about possible machine malfunction
  - Increased concentration on breathing

Moderate Impairment

- Responds to lowered levels of mechanical ventilator support with:
  - Slight baseline increase in blood pressure <20 mm Hg
  - Slight baseline increase in heart rate <20 beats/min
  - Baseline increase in respiratory rate <5 breaths/min
  - Hypervigilance to activities
  - Inability to respond to coaching
  - Inability to cooperate
  - Apprehension
  - Diaphoresis
  - Eye widening ("wide-eyed look")
  - Decreased air entry on auscultation
  - Color changes: pale, slight cyanosis
  - Slight respiratory accessory muscle use

Severe Impairment

- Responds to lowered levels of mechanical ventilator support with:
- Agitation
- Deterioration in arterial blood gases from current baseline
- Baseline increase in blood pressure >20 mm Hg
- Baseline increase in heart rate >20 beats/min
- Respiratory rate increased significantly from baseline
- Profuse diaphoresis
- Full respiratory accessory muscle use
- Shallow, gasping breaths
- Paradoxical abdominal breathing
- Discoordinated breathing with the ventilator
- Decreased level of consciousness
- Adventitious breath sounds, audible airway secretions
- Cyanosis

Outcomes

- Airway is clear.
- Underlying disorder is resolving.
- Patient is rested and pain is controlled.
- Nutrition status is adequate.
- Patient has feelings of perceived control, situational security, and trust in the nurses.
- Patient is able to adapt to selected levels of ventilator support without undue fatigue.

Interventions and Rationale

1. Communicate interest and concern for the patient's well-being and demonstrate confidence in ability to manage weaning process **to instill trust in the patient.**
2. Use normalizing strategies (e.g., grooming, dressing, mobilizing, social conversation) **to reinforce the patient's self-esteem and feeling of identity.**
3. Identify parameters of the patient's usual functioning before the weaning process begins **to facilitate early identification of problems.**
4. Identify the patient's strengths and resources that can be mobilized **to enhance the patient's coping and maximize weaning effort.**
5. Note concerns that adversely affect the patient's comfort and confidence and manage them discreetly **to facilitate the patient's ease.**
6. Praise successful activities, encourage a positive outlook, and review the patient's positive progress **to increase the patient's perceived self-efficacy.**
7. Inform the patient of their situation and weaning progress **to permit the patient as much control as possible.**
8. Teach the patient about the weaning process and how they can participate in the process.
9. Negotiate daily weaning goals with the patient **to gain cooperation.**
10. Position the patient with the head of the bed elevated **to optimize respiratory efforts.**
11. Coach the patient in breath control by regular demonstrations of slow, deep, rhythmic patterns of breathing **to assist with dyspnea.**
12. Remain visible in the room and reassure the patient that help is immediately available if needed **to reduce the patient's anxiety and fearfulness.**
13. Encourage the patient to view weaning trials as a form of training, regardless of whether the weaning goal is achieved, **to avoid discouragement.**
14. Encourage the patient to maintain emotional calmness by reassuring, being present, comforting, talking down if emotionally aroused, and reinforcing the idea that they can and will succeed.
15. Monitor the patient's status frequently **to avoid undue fatigue and anxiety.**
16. Provide regular periods of rest by reducing activities, maintaining or increasing ventilator support, and providing oxygen as needed before fatigue advances.
17. Provide distraction (e.g., visitors, radio, television, conversation) when the patient's concentration starts to create tension and increases anxiety.
18. Ensure adequate nutrition support, sufficient rest and sleep time, and sedation or pain control **to promote the patient's optimal physical and emotional comfort.**
19. Start weaning early in the day **when the patient is most rested.**
20. Restrict unnecessary activities and visitors who do not cooperate with weaning strategies **to minimize energy demands on the patient during the weaning process.**
21. Coordinate necessary activities to promote adequate time for rest and relaxation. Implement the patient management plan for Activity Intolerance Due to Prolonged Immobility or Deconditioning.
22. Monitor the patient's underlying disease process **to ensure it is stabilized and under control.**
23. Advocate for additional resources (e.g., sedation, analgesia, rest) needed by the patient **to maximize comfort status.**
24. Develop and adhere to an individualized plan of care **to promote the patient's feelings of control.**

PATIENT CARE MANAGEMENT PLAN

Impaired Verbal Communication

Impaired Verbal Communication Due to Cerebral Speech Center Injury

Signs and Symptoms

- Inappropriate or absent speech or responses to questions
- Inability to speak spontaneously
- Inability to understand spoken words
- Inability to follow commands appropriately through gestures
- Difficulty or inability to understand written language
- Difficulty or inability to express ideas in writing
- Difficulty or inability to name objects

Outcome

- Patient is able to make basic needs known.

Interventions and Rationale

1. Collaborate with the practitioner and speech pathologist to determine the extent of the patient's communication deficit (e.g., whether fluent, nonfluent, or global aphasia is involved).
2. Have the speech therapist post a list of appropriate ways to communicate with the patient in the patient's room so that all health care personnel can be consistent in their efforts.
3. Assess the patient's ability to comprehend, speak, read, and write.
   a. Ask questions that can be answered with "yes" or "no." If a patient answers "yes" to a question, ask the opposite (e.g., "Are you hot?" "Yes." "Are you cold?" "Yes."). **This may help determine whether the patient understands what is being said.**
   b. Ask simple, short questions, and use gestures, pantomime, and facial expressions to give the patient additional clues.
   c. Stand in the patient's line of vision, giving a good view of your face and hands.
   d. Have the patient try to write with a pad and pencil. Offer pictures and alphabet letters at which to point.
   e. Make flash cards with pictures or words depicting frequently used phrases (e.g., glass of water, bedpan).
4. Maintain an uncluttered environment and decrease external distractions **to enhance communication.**
5. Maintain a relaxed and calm manner and explain all diagnostic, therapeutic, and comfort measures before initiating them.
6. Do not shout or speak in a loud voice. **Hearing loss is not a factor in aphasia, and shouting will not help.**
7. Have only one person talk at a time. **It is more difficult for the patient to follow a multisided conversation.**
8. Use direct eye contact and speak directly to the patient in unhurried, short phrases.
9. Give one-step commands and directions and provide cues through pictures and gestures.
10. Try to ask questions that can be answered with a "yes" or a "no" and avoid topics that are controversial, emotional, abstract, or lengthy.
11. Listen to the patient in an unhurried manner and wait for their attempt to communicate.
    a. Expect a time lag from when you ask the patient something until the patient responds.
    b. Accept the patient's statement of essential words without expecting complete sentences.
    c. Avoid finishing the sentence for the patient if possible.
    d. Wait approximately 30 s before providing the word the patient may be attempting to find (except when the patient is very frustrated and needs something quickly, such as a bedpan).
    e. Rephrase the patient's message aloud **to validate it.**
    f. Do not pretend to understand the patient's message if you do not.
12. Encourage the patient to speak slowly in short phrases and to say each word clearly.
13. Ask the patient to write the message, if able, or draw pictures if only verbal communication is affected.
14. Observe the patient's nonverbal clues for validation (e.g., answers "yes" but shakes head "no").
15. When handing an object to the patient, state what it is **because hearing language spoken is necessary to stimulate language development.**
16. Explain what has happened to the patient and offer reassurance about the plan of care.
17. Verbally address the problem of frustration over the inability to communicate and explain that both the nurse and the patient need patience.
18. Maintain a calm, positive manner and offer reassurance (e.g., "I know this is very hard for you, but it will get better if we work on it together").
19. Talk to the patient as an adult. Be respectful, and avoid talking down to the patient.
20. Do not discuss the patient's condition or hold conversations in the patient's presence without including them in the discussion. **This may be the reason some aphasic patients develop paranoid thoughts.**
21. Do not exhibit disapproval of emotional utterances or spontaneous use of profanity; instead, offer calm, quiet reassurance.
22. If the patient makes an error in speech, do not reprimand or scold, but try to compliment the patient by saying, "That was a good try."
23. Delay conversation if the patient is tired. **The symptoms of aphasia worsen if the patient is fatigued, anxious, or upset.**
24. Be prepared for emotional outbursts and tears from patients who have more difficulty in expressing themselves than with understanding. **The patient may become depressed, refuse treatment and food, ignore relatives, and push objects away.** Comfort the patient with statements such as, "I know it's frustrating and you feel sad, but you are not alone. Other people who have had strokes have felt the way you do. We will be here to help you get through this."

PATIENT CARE MANAGEMENT PLAN

Ineffective Tissue Perfusion

Ineffective Tissue Perfusion Due to Decreased Cerebral Blood Flow

Signs and Symptoms

- Decreased level of consciousness
- Hemiparesis or hemiplegia
- Visual changes
- Aphasia
- Dysphagia
- Facial droop
- Cognitive deficits
- Ataxia

Outcomes

- Patient is oriented to time, place, person, and situation.
- Pupils are equal and normoreactive.
- Blood pressure is within baseline or ordered parameters.
- Motor function is bilaterally equal.
- Headache, nausea, and vomiting are absent.
- Patient verbalizes importance of and displays compliance with reduced activity.
- Neurologic deficits are absent.

Interventions and Rationale

For Ischemia

1. Collaborate with the practitioner regarding administration of fibrinolytic therapy **to facilitate lysis of the clot and restoration of blood flow to the affected area.**
2. Monitor the patient for alterations in blood pressure, oxygenation, temperature, rhythm, and glucose levels.
3. Collaborate with the practitioner regarding administration of vasodilators for hypertension **to maintain the patient's blood pressure within the desired range.** Use caution in lowering blood pressure, **as hypotension decreases cerebral blood flow.**
   a. Patients receiving fibrinolytic therapy: Keep systolic blood pressure <185 mm Hg and diastolic blood pressure <110 mm Hg.
   b. Patients not receiving fibrinolytic therapy: Keep systolic blood pressure <220 mm Hg and diastolic blood pressure <120 mm Hg.
4. Collaborate with the practitioner regarding administration of intravenous fluids and vasoconstrictors for hypotension, **as hypotension decreases cerebral blood flow.**
5. Collaborate with the practitioner regarding administration of oxygen to maintain oxygen saturation measured >95% **to prevent hypoxemia and potential worsening of the neurologic injury.**
6. Collaborate with the practitioner regarding administration of acetaminophen for elevated temperature **because hyperthermia is associated with increased morbidity in patients with stroke.**
7. Collaborate with the practitioner regarding the treatment of dysrhythmias **resulting from increased sympathetic nervous system stimulation.**
8. Collaborate with the practitioner regarding administration of insulin for hyperglycemia, **as elevated blood glucose has been linked to an increase in the area of infarct.**
9. Collaborate with the speech therapist regarding the patient's ability to swallow before initiating oral feedings **to ensure the patient is not at risk for aspiration.**
10. Collaborate with the physical therapist to assess the patient's ability to ambulate safely **to ensure the patient is not at risk for falling** and ability to perform activities of daily living **to facilitate discharge home.**
11. Maintain surveillance for complications such as increased intracranial pressure, seizures, and acute lung failure.
12. Collaborate with the practitioner and rehabilitation specialist regarding the patient's need for rehabilitation **to maximize the patient's independence.**

For Hemorrhage

1. Assess for indicators of increased intracranial pressure and brain herniation (see the patient management plan for Decreased Intracranial Adaptive Capacity Due to Failure of Normal Intracranial Compensatory Mechanism).
2. Collaborate with the practitioner regarding administration of anticonvulsant medications **to prevent the onset of seizures or to control seizures.**
3. Collaborate with the practitioner regarding administration of vasodilators for hypertension **to avoid further bleeding.** Use caution in lowering blood pressure, **as hypotension decreases cerebral blood flow.**
   a. If systolic blood pressure is >200 mm Hg or mean arterial pressure (MAP) is >150 mm Hg, aggressive reduction in blood pressure is indicated.
   b. If systolic blood pressure is >180 mm Hg or MAP is >130 mm Hg in the presence of increased intracranial pressure, cautious reduction in pressure is indicated, maintaining cerebral perfusion pressure >60 to 80 mm Hg.
   c. If systolic blood pressure is >180 mm Hg or MAP is >130 mm Hg in the absence of elevated intracranial pressure, reduction in blood pressure is indicated, with a target of 160/90 mm Hg.
4. Collaborate with the practitioner regarding administration of insulin for hyperglycemia, **as elevated blood glucose has been linked to an increase in the area of infarct.**
5. Collaborate with the practitioner regarding administration of acetaminophen for elevated temperature **because hyperthermia is associated with increased morbidity in patients with stroke.**
6. Initiate precautions **to prevent rebleeding.**
   a. Ensure bed rest in a quiet environment **to lessen external stimuli.**
   b. Maintain a darkened room to lessen symptoms of photophobia.
   c. Restrict visitors and instruct them to keep conversation as nonstressful as possible.
   d. Administer sedatives as prescribed **to reduce anxiety to promote rest.**
   e. Administer analgesics as prescribed **to relieve or lessen headache.**
   f. Provide a soft, high-fiber diet and stool softeners to prevent constipation, which can lead to straining and increased risk of rebleeding.
   g. Assist with activities of daily living (feeding, bathing, dressing, toileting).
   h. Avoid any activity that could lead to increased intracranial pressure; ensure that the patient does not flex hips beyond 90 degrees and avoids neck hyperflexion, hyperextension, or lateral hyperrotation **that could impede jugular venous return.**
7. Collaborate with the physical therapist to assess the patient's ability to ambulate safely **to ensure the patient is not at risk for falling** and ability to perform activities of daily living **to facilitate discharge home.**
8. Collaborate with the practitioner and rehabilitation specialist regarding the patient's need for rehabilitation **to maximize the patient's independence.**

Ineffective Tissue Perfusion Due to Decreased Gastrointestinal Blood Flow

Signs and Symptoms

- Abdominal pain
- Melena
- Abdominal distention
- Hyperactive to absent bowel sounds range from hyperactive to absent
- Guarding
- Fever
- Hypotension
- Tachycardia
- Altered mental status
- Urine output is <30 mL/h

PATIENT CARE MANAGEMENT PLAN

Ineffective Tissue Perfusion—cont'd

Outcomes

- Normal bowel sounds are present.
- Abdominal pain, distention, and guarding are absent.
- Vital signs are at baseline.
- Urine output is >30 mL/h.

Interventions and Rationales

1. Collaborate with the practitioner regarding administration of crystalloids, colloids, blood, and blood products **to maintain adequate circulating volume.** Implement the patient management plan for Hypovolemia Due to Absolute Loss.
2. Collaborate with the practitioner regarding pain management. Implement the patient management plan for Acute Pain Due to Transmission and Perception of Cutaneous, Visceral, Muscular, or Ischemic Impulses.
3. Collaborate with the practitioner regarding administration of oxygen to maintain oxygen saturation >92% **to prevent hypoxemia and potential worsening of the gastrointestinal injury.**
4. Collaborate with the practitioner regarding administration of electrolyte replacement therapy **to maintain adequate electrolyte balance.**
5. Collaborate with the dietitian regarding administration of nutrition **because the patient will be unable to eat.** Implement the patient management plan for Impaired Nutritional Intake.
6. Maintain surveillance for complications such as gastrointestinal hemorrhage, hypovolemic shock, and septic shock.
7. Collaborate with the practitioner regarding preparation for surgery **to remove infarcted bowel.**

Ineffective Tissue Perfusion Due to Decreased Kidney Blood Flow

Signs and Symptoms

- Anuria or oliguria
- Decreased urinary creatinine clearance
- Increased serum creatinine
- Increased blood urea nitrogen (BUN)
- Electrolyte abnormalities: sodium and potassium
- Increased MAP, pulmonary artery occlusion pressure (PAOP), pulmonary artery diastolic (PAD) pressure, central venous pressure (CVP) secondary to fluid overload
- Sinus tachycardia
- Metabolic acidosis
- Crackles on lung auscultation
- Engorged neck veins
- Fluid weight gain
- Pitting edema
- Mental status changes
- Anemia

Outcomes

- Electrolytes are within normal range.
- Serum creatinine and blood urea nitrogen are within normal range.
- Normal acid–base balance is present.
- Urinary output is within normal limits, or patient is stable on dialysis.
- Hemoglobin and hematocrit values are stable.

Interventions and Rationale

1. Monitor intake and output, urine output, and the patient's weight.
2. Collaborate with the practitioner regarding administration of crystalloids, colloids, blood, and blood products **to increase circulating volume and maintain mean arterial pressure >70 mm Hg.**
3. Collaborate with the practitioner regarding administration of inotropes **to enhance myocardial contractility and increase cardiac index to >2.5 L/min.**
4. Collaborate with the practitioner regarding administration of diuretics to oliguric patient **to flush out cellular debris and increase urine output.**
5. Minimize the patient's exposure to nephrotoxic medications **to decrease damage to kidneys.**
6. Monitor blood levels of drugs cleared by kidneys **to avoid accumulation.**
7. Monitor the patient for signs of electrolyte imbalance **as a result of impaired electrolyte regulation.**
8. Maintain surveillance for signs and symptoms of fluid overload.
9. Monitor the patient's clinical status and response to dialysis therapy **to ensure the patient is receiving safe and effective dialytic therapy.**

Ineffective Tissue Perfusion Due to Decreased Myocardial Blood Flow

Signs and Symptoms

- Angina for more than 30 min
- ST-segment elevation on 12-lead electrocardiogram (ECG)
- Elevated biomarkers
- Apprehension
- Shortness of breath

Outcomes

- Systolic blood pressure is >90 mm Hg.
- Mean arterial pressure is >60 mm Hg.
- Heart rate is <100 beats/min.
- Pulmonary artery pressures are within normal limits or back to baseline.
- Cardiac index is >2.2 L/min/m^2.
- Urine output is >0.5 mL/kg/h or >30 mL/h.
- The 12-lead ECG is normalized without new Q waves.
- Chest pain is absent.
- CK-MB enzymes, troponin I, and myoglobin levels are within normal range.

Interventions and Rationale

1. Collaborate with the practitioner regarding administration of fibrinolytic therapy or the preparation of the patient for percutaneous coronary intervention **to restore myocardial blood flow.**
2. Collaborate with the practitioner regarding administration of oxygen at 2 L/min to achieve oxygen saturation measured >90% **to maximize myocardial oxygen supply.**
3. Collaborate with the practitioner regarding administration of sublingual nitroglycerin and/or intravenous nitroglycerin infusion **to augment coronary blood flow and reduce cardiac work by decreasing preload and afterload.**
   a. Do not administer nitrates to patients who have taken phosphodiesterase inhibitors for erectile dysfunction within the last 24 or 48 hours (depending on the medication), **as severe hypotension may occur.**
4. Collaborate with the practitioner regarding administration of morphine **to control pain.**
5. Collaborate with the practitioner regarding administration of aspirin, antiplatelet therapy, and heparin **to prevent recurrent thrombosis and inhibit platelet function.**
6. Collaborate with the practitioner regarding administration of beta-blockers **to decrease myocardial oxygen demand and prevent recurrent ischemia.**
7. Collaborate with the practitioner regarding administration of angiotensin-converting enzyme inhibitors **to block the conversion of angiotensin I to angiotensin II, a potent vasoconstrictor.**
8. Maintain the patient on bed rest with bedside commode privileges **to minimize myocardial oxygen demand.**
9. Monitor the patient's hemodynamic and cardiac rhythm status:
   a. Select cardiac monitoring leads based on infarct location and rhythm to obtain the best rhythm for monitoring.

Continued

PATIENT CARE MANAGEMENT PLAN

***Ineffective Tissue Perfusion*—cont'd**

b. Evaluate cardiac rhythm for the presence of dysrhythmias, which are common complications of myocardial ischemia.
c. Collaborate with the practitioner regarding administration of antidysrhythmic medications.
d. Assess serum electrolytes (potassium and magnesium) and arterial blood gases.
e. Collaborate with the practitioner regarding administration of electrolytes to correct any imbalances.
f. Monitor the ST segment continuously to determine changes in myocardial tissue perfusion.
g. Monitor the patient's blood pressure at least every hour, as many conditions (e.g., drugs, dysrhythmias, myocardial ischemia) may cause hypotension (systolic blood pressure <90 mm Hg).
h. Treat symptomatic dysrhythmias according to the unit's emergency protocol or advanced cardiac life support guidelines.

10. Instruct the patient to avoid the Valsalva maneuver, as forced expiration against a closed glottis causes sudden and intense changes in systolic blood pressure and heart rate.

PATIENT CARE MANAGEMENT PLAN

Lack of Knowledge of Treatment Regime

Lack of Knowledge of Treatment Regime Due to Lack of Previous Exposure to Information

Signs and Symptoms

- Verbalized statement of inadequate knowledge or skills
- New diagnosis or health problem requiring self-management or care
- Lack of prior formal or informal education about the specific health problem
- Demonstration of inappropriate behaviors related to management of the health problem

Outcomes

- Patient verbalizes adequate knowledge about or performs skills related to disease process, its causes, factors related to onset of symptoms, and self-management of disease or health problem.
- Patient actively participates in health behaviors required for performance of a procedure or in behaviors enhancing recovery from illness and preventing recurrence or complications.

Interventions and Rationale

1. Determine the existing level of knowledge or skill.
2. Assess factors that affect the knowledge deficit:
   a. Learning needs, including the patient's priorities and the necessary knowledge and skills for safety
   b. Learning ability of the patient, including language skills, level of education, ability to read, and preferred learning style
   c. Physical ability to perform prescribed skills or procedures; consider effect of limitations imposed by treatment such as bed rest, restriction of movement by intravenous or other equipment, or effect of sedatives or analgesics
   d. Psychological effect of stage of adaptation to disease
   e. Activity tolerance and ability to concentrate
   f. Motivation to learn new skills or gain new knowledge
3. Reduce or limit barriers to learning:
   a. Provide consistent nurse–patient contact to encourage development of a trusting and therapeutic relationship.
   b. Structure the environment to enhance learning and control unnecessary noise or interruptions.
   c. Individualize the teaching plan to fit the patient's current physical and psychological status.
   d. Delay teaching until the patient is ready to learn.
   e. Conduct teaching sessions during a time of day when the patient is most alert and receptive.
   f. Meet the patient's immediate learning needs as they arise (e.g., give a brief explanation of procedures when they are performed).
4. Promote active participation in the teaching plan by the patient and family:
   a. Solicit input during the development of the plan.
   b. Develop mutually acceptable goals and outcomes.
   c. Solicit expression of feelings and emotions related to new responsibilities.
   d. Encourage questions.
5. Conduct teaching sessions, using the most appropriate teaching methods.
6. Use the "teach-back" method **to confirm that you have explained to the patient what they need to know in a manner that the patient understands.**
   a. Use simple lay language, explain the concept, or demonstrate the process to the patient/caregiver.
      (1). Avoid technical terms to avoid misunderstandings.
      (2). If the patient/caregiver has limited English proficiency, use a professional translator to reduce miscommunication.
   b. Ask the patient/caregiver to repeat in their own words how they understand the concept explained. If a process was demonstrated to the patient, ask the patient/caregiver to demonstrate it independent of assistance.
   c. Identify and correct misunderstandings of or incorrect procedures by the patient/caregiver.
   d. Ask the patient/caregiver to demonstrate their understanding or procedural ability again **to ensure the aforementioned misunderstandings are now corrected.**
   e. Repeat steps until convinced the patient/caregiver comprehends the concept or possesses the ability to perform the procedure accurately and safely.
7. Provide written materials that enhance health literacy:
   a. Limit content to one or two key objectives. Do not provide too much information or try to cover everything at once.
   b. Limit content to what patients really need to know. Avoid information overload.
   c. Use only words that are well known to individuals without medical training.
   d. Ensure that content is appropriate for the age and culture of the target audience.
   e. Write at or below the sixth-grade level.
   f. Use words of one or two syllables.
   g. Use short paragraphs.
   h. Use active voice.
   i. Avoid all but the simplest tables and graphs. Clear explanations (legends) should be placed adjacent to the table or graph as well as in the text.
   j. Use large font (minimum 12 point) with serifs. (Serif text has the little horizontal lines that you see at the bottoms of letters such as "f," "x," "n," and others.)
   k. Do not use more than two or three font styles on a page. **Consistency in appearance is important.**
   l. Use uppercase and lowercase text. ALL-UPPERCASE TEXT IS HARD TO READ.
   m. Ensure a good amount of empty space on the page. Do not clutter the page with text or pictures.
   n. Use headings and subheadings to separate blocks of text.
   o. Bulleted lists are preferable to blocks of text in paragraphs.
   p. Illustrations are useful if they depict common, easy-to-recognize objects. Images of people, places, and things should be age and culturally appropriate to the target audience. Avoid complex anatomic diagrams.
8. Initiate referrals for follow-up if necessary:
   a. Health educators
   b. Home health care
   c. Rehabilitation programs
   d. Social services
9. Evaluate effectiveness of teaching plan based on the patient's ability to meet preset goals and objectives **to determine need for further teaching.**

PATIENT CARE MANAGEMENT PLAN

Powerlessness

Powerlessness Due to Lack of Control Over Current Situation or Disease Progression

Signs and Symptoms

Severe

- Verbal expressions of having no control or influence over situation
- Verbal expressions of having no control or influence over outcome
- Verbal expressions of having no control over self-care
- Depression over physical deterioration that occurs despite patient's compliance with regimens
- Apathy

Moderate

- Nonparticipation in care or decision making when opportunities are provided
- Expressions of dissatisfaction and frustration about inability to perform previous tasks and/or activities
- Lack of progress monitoring
- Expressions of doubt about role performance
- Reluctance to express true feelings, fearing alienation from caregivers
- Passivity
- Inability to seek information about care
- Dependence on others that may result in irritability, resentment, anger, and guilt
- No defense of self-care practices when challenged

Low

- Passivity

Outcomes

- Patient verbalizes increased control over situation by wanting to do things their way.
- Patient actively participates in planning care.
- Patient requests needed information.
- Patient chooses to participate in self-care activities.
- Patient monitors progress.

Interventions and Rationale

1. Evaluate the patient's feelings and perception of the reasons for lack of power and sense of helplessness.
2. Determine as far as possible the patient's usual response to limited-control situations. Determine through ongoing assessment the patient's usual locus of control (i.e., believes that influence over their life is exerted by luck, fate, or powerful persons [external locus of control] or that influence is exerted through personal choices, self-effort, self-determination [internal locus of control]).
3. Support the patient's physical control of the environment by involving them in care activities; knock before entering room if appropriate; ask permission before moving personal belongings. Inform the patient that although an activity may not be to their liking, it is necessary. **This gives the patient permission to express dissatisfaction with the environment and the regimen.**
4. Personalize the patient's care using their preferred name. **This supports the patient's psychological control.**
5. Provide a therapeutic rationale for all the patient is asked to do for themself and for all that is being done for them and with them. Reinforce the practitioner's explanations; clarify misconceptions about the illness situation and treatment plans. **This supports the patient's cognitive control.**
6. Include the patient in care planning by encouraging participation and allowing choices wherever possible (e.g., timing of personal care activities; deciding when pain medicines are needed). Point out situations in which no choices exist.
7. Provide opportunities for the patient to exert influence over themself and their body, affecting an outcome. For example, share with the patient the nurse's assessment of their breath sounds and explain that they can be improved by self-initiated deep-breathing exercises. **Feedback that the patient has been successful in helping clear their lungs reinforces the influence they do retain.**
8. Encourage the family to permit the patient to do as much independently as possible **to foster perception of personal power.**
9. Assist the patient to establish realistic short-term and long-term goals. **Setting unrealistic or unattainable goals inadvertently reinforces the patient's perception of powerlessness.**
10. Document care to provide for continuity **so that the patient can maintain appropriate control over the environment.**
11. Assist the patient to regain strength and activity tolerance as appropriate, **increasing a sense of control and self-reliance.**
12. Increase the sensitivity of the health team members and significant others to the patient's sense of powerlessness. Use power over the patient carefully. Use the words *must, should,* and *have to* with caution **because they communicate coercive powers and imply that the objects of "musts" and "shoulds" are of benefit to the nurse instead of the patient.**
13. Plan with the patient for transfer from the critical care unit to the intermediate unit and eventually to home.

PATIENT CARE MANAGEMENT PLAN

Relocation Stress

Relocation Stress Due to Transfer Out of the Critical Care Unit

Signs and Symptoms

- Alienation
- Aloneness
- Anger
- Concern over relocation
- Dependency
- Depression
- Fear of an unknown environment
- Frustration
- Increased physical symptoms
- Increased verbalization of needs
- Insecurity
- Loneliness
- Move from critical care unit to another environment
- Pessimism
- Sleep disturbance
- Unwillingness to move
- Withdrawal
- Worry

Outcomes

- Patient will express willingness to move to a new environment.
- Anxiety will be absent.

Interventions and Rationale

1. Initiate pretransfer teaching as soon as appropriate during the patient's stay in the critical care unit **to ease the transition from the critical care unit to the next environment.** Teaching should focus on the differences in the environment and the care the patient would receive.
2. Provide the patient and family written information regarding the transfer (if available) **to enhance effectiveness of teaching.**
3. Help the patient see that progress is being made **in preparation for transfer.** Each time a tube is removed or a treatment frequency is decreased, reinforce with the patient and family that the patient is progressing.
4. Remove monitoring and supportive equipment from the patient's room when no longer needed **to allow the patient to experience the loss of technology while still in the critical care unit.**
5. Encourage the patient and family to discuss concerns regarding relocation.
6. Assist the patient and family members to develop and maintain a positive perception of the transfer.
7. Arrange for the patient's family to have a tour of the new unit **as a means of familiarizing them with the unit before the patient's transfer.**

PATIENT CARE MANAGEMENT PLAN

Risk for Aspiration

Risk Factors

- Impaired laryngeal sensation or reflex
- Reduced level of consciousness
- Extubation
- Impaired pharyngeal peristalsis or tongue function
- Neuromuscular dysfunction
- Central nervous system dysfunction
- Head or neck injury
- Impaired laryngeal closure or elevation
- Laryngeal nerve dysfunction
- Artificial airways
- Gastrointestinal tubes
- Increased gastric volume
- Delayed gastric emptying
- Enteral feedings
- Medication administration
- Increased intragastric pressure
- Upper abdominal surgery
- Obesity
- Pregnancy
- Ascites
- Decreased lower esophageal sphincter pressure
- Increased gastric acidity
- Gastrointestinal tubes
- Decreased antegrade esophageal propulsion
- Trendelenburg or supine position
- Esophageal dysmotility
- Esophageal structural defects or lesions

Outcomes

- Breath sounds are normal, or there is no change in the patient's baseline breath sounds.
- Arterial blood gas values remain within the patient's baseline.
- There is no evidence of gastric contents in lung secretions.

Interventions and Rationale

1. Assess gastrointestinal function to rule out hypoactive peristalsis and abdominal distention.
2. Position the patient with the head of the bed elevated 30 degrees to prevent gastric reflux through gravity. If head elevation is contraindicated, position the patient in the right lateral decubitus position to facilitate passage of gastric contents across the pylorus.
3. Maintain patency and functioning of nasogastric suction apparatus to prevent accumulation of gastric contents.
4. Provide frequent and scrupulous mouth care to prevent colonization of the oropharynx with bacteria and inoculation of the lower airways.
5. Ensure that the endotracheal or tracheostomy cuff is properly inflated to limit aspiration of oropharyngeal secretions.
6. Treat nausea promptly; collaborate with the practitioner on an order for an antiemetic to prevent vomiting and resultant aspiration.

Additional Interventions for Patient Receiving Continuous or Intermittent Enteral Tube Feedings

1. Position the patient with the head of the bed elevated 45 degrees **to prevent gastric reflux.** If a head-down position becomes necessary at any time, interrupt the feeding 30 min before the position change.
2. Check the placement of the feeding tube by auscultation or radiographically at regular intervals (e.g., before administering intermittent feedings and after position changes, suctioning, coughing episodes, or vomiting) **to ensure proper placement of the tube.**
3. Monitor the patient for signs of delayed gastric emptying **to decrease potential for vomiting and aspiration.**
   a. For large-bore tubes, check residuals of tube feedings before intermittent feedings and every 4 hours during continuous feedings. Consider withholding feedings for residuals >150% of the hourly rate (continuous feeding) or >50% of the previous feeding (intermittent feeding).
   b. For small-bore tubes, observe abdomen for distention, palpate abdomen for hardness or tautness, and auscultate abdomen for bowel sounds.

PATIENT CARE MANAGEMENT PLAN

Risk for Infection

Risk Factors

- Inadequate primary defenses (e.g., broken skin, traumatized tissue, decreased ciliary action, stasis of body fluids, change in pH secretions, altered peristalsis)
- Inadequate secondary defenses (e.g., decreased hemoglobin, leukopenia, suppressed inflammatory or immune response)
- Immunocompromised state
- Inadequate acquired immunity
- Tissue destruction and increased environmental exposure
- Chronic disease
- Invasive procedures
- Malnutrition
- Pharmacologic agents (e.g., antibiotics, steroids)

Outcomes

- Total lymphocyte count is >1000/mm^3.
- White blood cell count is within normal limits.
- Temperature is within normal limits.
- Blood, urine, wound, and sputum culture results are negative.

Interventions and Rationale

1. Perform proper hand hygiene before and after patient care **to reduce the transmission of microorganisms.**
2. Use appropriate personal protective equipment in accordance with U.S. Centers for Disease Control and Prevention guidelines.
   a. Ensure the practitioner uses maximum barrier precautions when inserting lines.
      (1). Ensure sterile gloves, gown, and mask are worn.
      (2). Drape the patient completely with a sterile sheet.
3. Use aseptic technique for insertion and manipulation of invasive monitoring devices, intravenous lines, and urinary drainage catheters **to maintain sterility of environment.**
   a. Ensure the practitioner uses maximum barrier precautions when inserting lines.
      (1). Ensure sterile gloves, gown, and mask are worn.
      (2). Drape the patient completely with a sterile sheet.
4. Stabilize all invasive lines and catheters to avoid unintentional manipulation and contamination.
5. Use aseptic technique for dressing changes to prevent contamination of wounds or insertion sites.
6. Change any line placed under emergent conditions within 24 hours because aseptic technique is usually breached during an emergency.
7. Collaborate with the practitioner to change any dressing that is saturated with blood or drainage because these are media for microorganism growth.
8. Minimize use of stopcocks and maintain caps on all stopcock ports to reduce the ports of entry for microorganisms.
9. Avoid the use of nasogastric tubes, nasotracheal tubes, and nasopharyngeal suctioning in the patient with a suspected cerebrospinal fluid leak to decrease the incidence of central nervous system infection.
10. Change ventilator circuits with humidifiers when visibly soiled or mechanically malfunctioning to avoid introducing microorganisms into the system. Do not change routinely.
11. Provide the patient with a clean manual resuscitation bag to avoid cross-contamination between patients.
12. Provide oral care to a patient with an artificial airway or an unresponsive patient every 2 to 4 hours and as needed (PRN) to decrease the incidence of hospital-acquired pulmonary infections.
    a. Swab mouth and moisten lips every 4 hours.
    b. Brush teeth with an in-line suction toothbrush every 12 hours. Rinse or swab the patient's mouth with chlorhexidine after brushing at least once every 24 hours.
    c. Suction subglottic secretions (secretions pooling above the cuff of the endotracheal tube or tracheostomy tube) every 12 hours and before repositioning the tube or deflation of the cuff.
    d. Provide lip balm to keep the patient's lips moistened PRN.
    e. Provide mouth moisturizer to keep the patient's mouth moistened PRN.
13. Cleanse in-line suction catheters with sterile saline according to the manufacturer's instructions **to avoid accumulation of secretions within the catheter.**
14. Maintain the head of the bed elevated at 30 to 45 degrees in patients with an artificial airway **to decrease the incidence of aspiration.**
15. Use disposable sterile scissors, forceps, and hemostats **to reduce transmission of microorganisms.**
16. Maintain a closed urinary drainage system **to decrease the incidence of urinary infections.**
17. Keep the urinary drainage tubing and bag below the level of the patient's bladder **to prevent the backflow of urine.**
18. Assess the urinary drainage tubing for kinks **to prevent stasis of urine.**
19. Protect all access device sites from potential sources of contamination (nasogastric reflux, draining wounds, ostomies, sputum).
20. Refrigerate parenteral nutrition solutions and opened enteral nutrition formulas **to inhibit bacterial growth.**
21. Maintain daily surveillance of invasive devices for signs and symptoms of infection.
22. Notify the practitioner of elevated temperature or if any signs or symptoms of infection are present.

Additional Interventions for Patient Receiving Immunosuppressive Drugs

1. Obtain blood, urine, and sputum cultures for temperature elevations >38°C (100.4 °F) **because elevation likely is caused by bacteremia or bladder or pulmonary infection.**
2. Auscultate breath sounds at least every 6 hours. **Pulmonary infection is the most common type of infection, and changes in breath sounds might be an early indication.**
3. Inspect wounds at least every 8 hours for redness, swelling, or drainage, **which may indicate infection.**
4. Inspect overall skin integrity and oral mucosa for signs of breakdown, **which place the patient at risk for infection.**
5. Notify the practitioner of new-onset cough. **Even a nonproductive cough may indicate pulmonary infection.**
6. Monitor white blood cell count daily, and report leukocytosis or sudden development of leukopenia, **which may indicate an infectious process.**
7. Protect the patient from exposure to any staff or family member with a contagious lesion (e.g., herpes simplex) or respiratory infections.
8. Collaborate with the dietitian regarding the patient's nutrition status and need for augmentation of nutrition intake as necessary **to prevent debilitation and increased susceptibility to infection.**
9. Collaborate with the practitioner to remove invasive lines and catheters as soon as possible **to decrease potential portals of entry.**
10. Teach the patient the clinical manifestations of infection. **A knowledgeable patient will seek medical attention promptly, which will result in earlier treatment and a decreased risk that infection will become life threatening.**

PATIENT CARE MANAGEMENT PLAN

Situational Low Self-Esteem

Situational Low Self-Esteem Due to Feelings of Guilt About Physical Deterioration

Signs and Symptoms

- Inability to accept positive reinforcement
- Lack of follow-through
- Nonparticipation in therapy
- Not taking responsibility for self-care (i.e., self-neglect)
- Self-destructive behavior
- Lack of eye contact

Outcomes

- Patient verbalizes feelings of self-worth.
- Patient maintains positive relationships with significant others.
- Patient manifests active interest in appearance by completing personal grooming daily.

Interventions and Rationale

1. Evaluate the meaning of the health-related situation. How does the patient feel about themself, the diagnosis, and the treatment? How does the present situation fit into the larger context of their life?
2. Assess the patient's emotional level, interpersonal relationships, and feelings about themself. Recognize the patient's uniqueness (e.g., how the hair is worn, preference for name used).
3. Help the patient discover and verbalize feelings and understand the crisis by listening and providing information.
4. Assist the patient to identify strengths and positive qualities that increase the sense of self-worth. Focus on past experiences of accomplishment and competency. Help the patient with positive self-reinforcement. Reinforce the love and affection of family and significant others.
5. Assess coping techniques that have been helpful in the past. Help the patient decide how to handle negative or incongruent feedback about the situation.
6. Encourage visits from family and significant others. Facilitate interactions and ensure privacy. Help family members entering the critical care unit by explaining what they will see. Increase visitors' comfort with equipment; offer chairs and other courtesies.
7. Encourage the patient to pursue interest in individual or social activities, even though difficult in the critical care unit.
8. Reflect caring, concern, empathy, respect, and unconditional acceptance in nurse-patient relationships.
9. The nurse is a significant other for the patient who provides important appraisals of the patient and who can facilitate the change process.
10. Help the family support the patient's self-esteem.
11. Provide for continuity of nurse assignment to ensure consistent contacts that can **facilitate support of the patient's self-esteem.**

PATIENT CARE MANAGEMENT PLAN

Stress Overload

Stress Overload Due to Critical Illness and Stressors of the Critical Care Environment

Signs and Symptoms

- Pain, discomfort, and physical restrictions
- Unfamiliar environments with excessive light, noises, alarms, and distressing events
- Loss of ability for verbal expression due to intubation
- Unfamiliar bodily sensations resulting from bed rest, medications, surgery, or symptoms
- Fear of death
- Lack of sleep
- Loss of autonomy and control over one's body, environment, privacy, and daily activities
- Isolation interrupted only by brief visits, threatening stimuli, and procedural touch
- Separation from family, friends, and meaningful social roles and work
- Loss of dignity, embarrassing exposures, and a sense of vulnerability
- Concerns regarding finances and potential job loss
- Fear of permanent health deficits
- Spiritual distress with questions and concerns about meaning of the crisis and life

Outcomes

- Patient demonstrates an increased level of comfort.
- Patient maintains a mild or moderate level of anxiety.
- Patient expresses feelings, fears, and concerns.

Interventions and Rationale

1. Monitor the patient's level of pain through medication and physical comfort by such means as repositioning. **Pain and physical discomfort greatly increase the stressfulness of critical care admissions.**
2. Assess the patient's level of anxiety. Mild and some periods of moderate anxiety are expected, but severe anxiety and panic should be addressed immediately through directive measures such as slow, deep breathing and medication. **High levels of anxiety are extremely uncomfortable, unhealthy, and even dangerous.**
3. Reduce or eliminate excessive lighting and mimic the 24-hour natural rhythm as much as possible. Provide blackout masks to eliminate light if possible. **Excessive lighting at night disrupts the body's natural circadian rhythms, resulting in an impaired ability to sleep, which further contributes to stress.**
4. Reduce or eliminate the experience of excessive noise:
   a. Provide earplugs. Earplugs will reduce the experience of noise.
   b. Limit conversation immediately outside the patient's room. Limiting conversations outside of the patient's room will provide for more quiet time.
   c. Post a sign outside of the patient's room reminding staff and visitors of the need for a quiet environment. Reminding staff and visitors is an important step in eliminating noise.
   d. Eliminate overhead paging on the unit. Overhead paging can be replaced by more sophisticated personal technology.
   e. Advocate for smart monitors to eliminate nuisance alarms and adjust the default settings on alarms to reduce unnecessary noise. Alarm noise can be reduced by acquiring smart monitors and by adjusting the alarm default.
5. Provide explanations and education about what is happening with the patient's physical condition and the treatments that are being provided. **Fear of the unknown and lack of information about what is happening increases the stressfulness of being critically ill.**
6. Help conscious intubated patients express themselves by providing writing tools, a communication board, or higher technological methods. **Patients who are intubated face a higher level of stress due to the inability to communicate. Providing alternatives to verbalization reduces anxiety.**
7. Maintain the patient's sense of dignity by properly covering them during procedures. Ask others to step out of the room during these times. **States of undress break down social norms and add to a strange, scary, and bewildering situation.**
8. Encourage the patient to talk about feelings, concerns, and fears. **Giving the patient permission to express feelings, concerns, and fears not only provides catharsis, but it may give the nurse the opportunity to clear up misunderstandings and misperceptions.**
9. Spend time with the patient outside of time required for usual physical care. **Spending time with the patient reduces feelings of isolation and reduces stress.**
10. Ask whether the patient is interested in speaking with the hospital's chaplain or other clergy for spiritual care. **During times of crisis, people often derive comfort in discussing issues of faith and existential matters.**
11. Consult with a social worker to support patients and families. A social worker can also help with financial, insurance, and legal issues, and future care needs. **Specialty hospital personnel can provide essential expertise to patients and families whose lives have become affected by a critical care stay.**

PATIENT CARE MANAGEMENT PLAN

Unilateral Neglect

Unilateral Neglect Due to Perceptual Disruption

Signs and Symptoms

- Neglect of involved body parts and/or extrapersonal space
- Denial of existence of the affected limb or side of body
- Denial of hemiplegia or other motor and sensory deficits
- Left homonymous hemianopia
- Difficulty with spatial-perceptual tasks
- Left hemiplegia

Outcomes

- Patient is safe and free from injury.
- Patient is able to identify safety hazards in the environment.
- Patient recognizes disability and describes physical deficits present (e.g., paralysis, weakness, numbness).
- Patient demonstrates ability to scan the visual field to compensate for loss of function or sensation in affected limbs.

Interventions and Rationale

1. Adapt environment to the patient's deficits **to maintain patient safety.**
   a. Position the patient's bed with the unaffected side facing the door.
   b. Approach and speak to the patient from the unaffected side. If the patient must be approached from the affected side, announce your presence as soon as entering the room **to avoid startling the patient.**
   c. Position the call light, bedside stand, and personal items on the patient's unaffected side.
   d. If the patient will be assisted out of bed, simplify the environment **to eliminate hazards** by removing unnecessary furniture and equipment.
   e. Provide frequent reorientation of the patient to the environment.
   f. Observe the patient closely, and anticipate their needs. **Despite repeated explanations, the patient may have difficulty retaining information about the deficits.**
   g. When the patient is in bed, elevate the affected arm on a pillow **to prevent dependent edema and support the hand in a position of function.**
2. Assist the patient to recognize the perceptual defect.
   a. Encourage the patient to wear any prescriptive corrective glasses or hearing aids **to facilitate communication.**
   b. Instruct the patient to turn the head past midline **to view the environment on the affected side.**
   c. Encourage the patient to look at the affected side and to stroke the limbs with the unaffected hand. Encourage handling of the affected limbs **to reinforce awareness of the affected side.**
   d. Instruct the patient to look for the affected extremity when performing simple tasks **to know where it is at all times.**
   e. After pointing to them, have the patient name the affected parts.
   f. Encourage the patient to use self-exercises (e.g., lifting the affected arm with the unaffected hand).
   g. If the patient is unable to discriminate between the concepts of *right* and *left*, use descriptive adjectives such as "the weak arm," "the affected leg," or "the good arm" to refer to the body. Use gestures, not just words, to indicate right and left.
3. Collaborate with the patient, practitioner, and the rehabilitation team to design and implement a beginning rehabilitation program for use during the critical care unit stay.
   a. Use adaptive equipment (braces, splints, slings) as appropriate.
   b. Teach the patient the individual components of any activity separately and then proceed to integrate the component parts into a completed activity.
   c. Instruct the patient to attend to the affected side, if able, and to assist with bathing or other tasks.
   d. Use tactile stimulation to reintroduce the arm or leg to the patient. Rub the affected parts with different textured materials to stimulate sensations (e.g., warm, cold, rough, soft).
   e. Encourage activities that require the patient to turn the head toward the affected side and retrain the patient to scan the affected side and environment visually.
   f. If the patient is allowed out of bed, cue them with reminders to scan visually when ambulating. Assist and remain in constant attendance **because the patient may have difficulty maintaining correct posture, balance, and locomotion.** There may be vertical-horizontal perceptual problems, with the patient leaning to the affected side to align with the perceived vertical. Provide sitting, standing, and balancing exercises before getting the patient out of bed.
4. Assist the patient with oral feedings.
   a. Avoid giving the patient any very hot food items that could cause injury.
   b. Place the patient in an upright sitting position if possible.
   c. Encourage the patient to feed themself; if necessary, guide the patient's hand to the mouth.
   d. If the patient is able to feed themself, place one dish at a time in front of the patient. When the patient is finished with the first, add another dish. Tell the patient what they are eating.
   e. Initially, place food in the patient's visual field; then gradually move the food out of the field of vision and teach the patient to scan the entire visual field.
   f. When the patient has learned to visually scan the environment, offer a tray of food with various dishes.
   g. Instruct the patient to take small bites of food and to place the food in the unaffected side of the mouth.
   h. Teach the patient to sweep out pockets of food with the tongue after every bite **to eliminate retained food in the affected side of the mouth.**
   i. After meals or oral medications, check the patient's oral cavity for pockets of retained material.
5. Initiate patient and family health teaching.
   a. Assess to ensure that the patient and the family understand the nature of the neurologic deficits and the purpose of the rehabilitation plan.
   b. Teach the proper application and use of any adaptive equipment.
   c. Teach the importance of maintaining a safe environment, and point out potential environmental hazards.
   d. Instruct family members how to facilitate relearning techniques (e.g., cueing, scanning visual fields).

Physiologic Formulas for Critical Care

HEMODYNAMIC EQUATIONS

Mean (Systemic) Arterial Pressure (MAP)

$$\text{MAP} = \frac{(\text{Diastolic} \times 2) + (\text{Systolic} \times 1)}{3}$$

Systemic Vascular Resistance (SVR)

$$\frac{\text{MAP} - \text{RAP}}{\text{CO}} = \text{SVR in Wood units}$$

Normal range is 10–18 Wood units.

$$\frac{\text{MAP} - \text{RAP}}{\text{CO}} \times 80 = \text{SVR in dyn}\cdot\text{sec}\cdot\text{cm}^{-5}$$

Normal range is 800–1400 dyn·s·cm^{-5}.

Systemic Vascular Resistance Index (SVRI)

$$\frac{\text{MAP} - \text{RAP}}{\text{CI}} \times 80 = \text{SVR in dyn}\cdot\text{sec}\cdot\text{cm}^{-5}/\text{m}^2$$

Normal range is 2000–2400 dyn·s·cm^{-5}/m^2.

Pulmonary Vascular Resistance (PVR)

$$\frac{\text{PAP mean} - \text{RAP}}{\text{CO}} = \text{PVR in units}$$

Normal range is 1.2–3 units.

$$\frac{\text{PAP mean} - \text{RAP}}{\text{CO}} \times 80 = \text{PVR in dyn}\cdot\text{sec}\cdot\text{cm}^{-5}$$

Normal range is 100–250 dyn·s·cm^{-5}.

Pulmonary Vascular Resistance Index (PVRI)

$$\frac{\text{PAP mean} - \text{PAOP}}{\text{CI}} \times 80 = \text{PVR in dyn}\cdot\text{sec}\cdot\text{cm}^{-5}/\text{m}^2$$

Normal range is 225–315 dyn·s·cm^{-5}/m^2.

CI, Cardiac index; *CO,* cardiac output; *PAOP,* pulmonary arterial occlusion pressure (wedge pressure); *PAP,* pulmonary arterial pressure; *RAP,* right atrial pressure.

Left Cardiac Work Index (LCWI)

Step 1. MAP × CO × 0.0136 = LCW

Step 2. $\frac{\text{LCW}}{\text{BSA}} = \text{LCWI}$

Normal range is 3.4–4.2 kg-m/m^2.

Left Ventricular Stroke Work Index (LVSWI)

Step 1. MAP × SV × 0.0136 = LVSW

Step 2. $\frac{\text{LVSW}}{\text{BSA}} = \text{LVSWI}$

Normal range is 50–62 g-m/m^2.

Right Cardiac Work Index (RCWI)

Step 1. PAP mean × CO × 0.0136 = RCW

Step 2. $\frac{\text{RCW}}{\text{BSA}} = \text{RCWI}$

Normal range is 0.54–0.66 kg-m/m^2.

Right Ventricular Stroke Work Index (RVSWI)

Step 1. PAP mean × SV × 0.0136 = RVSW

Step 2. $\frac{\text{RVSW}}{\text{BSA}} = \text{RVSWI}$

Normal range is 7.9–9.7 g-m/m^2.

Corrected Q–T Interval (Q–Tc)

$$\frac{\text{QT}}{\sqrt{(\text{RR interval})}} = \text{QTc}$$

Body Surface Area (BSA)

Many hemodynamic formulas can be indexed or adjusted to body size by use of a BSA nomogram (Fig. B.1). To calculate BSA:

1. Obtain height and weight.
2. Mark height on the left scale and weight on the right scale.
3. Draw a straight line between the two points marked on the nomogram.

The number where the line crosses the middle scale is the BSA value.

PULMONARY FORMULAS

Shunt Equation (Qs/Qt)

$$\frac{\text{Qs}}{\text{Qt}} = \frac{\text{CcO}_2 - \text{CaO}_2}{\text{CcO}_2 - \text{CvO}_2}$$

CcO_2 = Pulmonary capillary oxygen content (calculated value)
CaO_2 = Arterial oxygen content (calculated value)
CvO_2 = Venous oxygen content (calculated value)
Normal range is less than 5%.

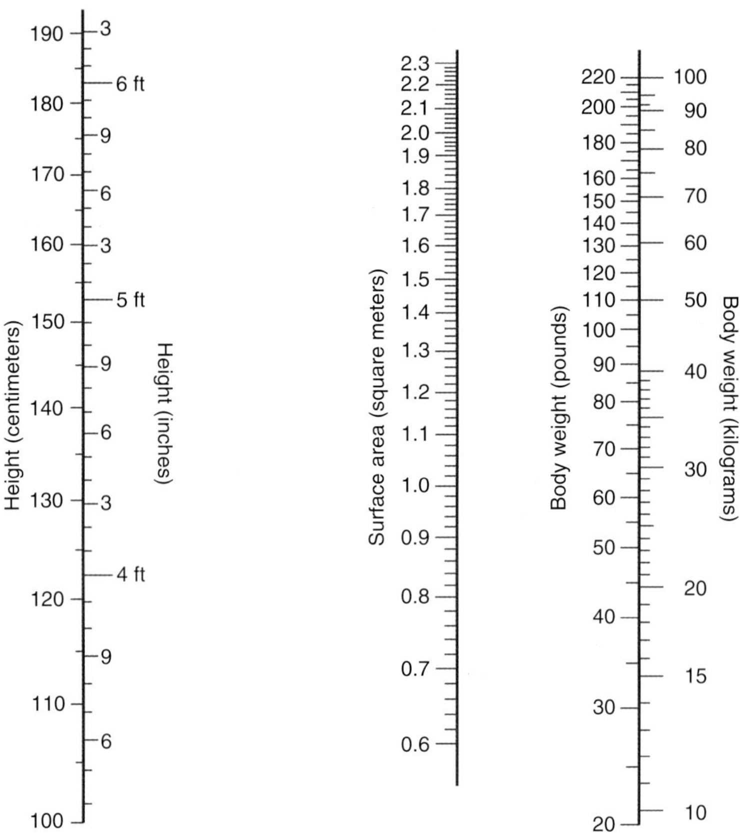

FIG. B.1 Body Surface Area (BSA) Nomogram.

Pulmonary Capillary Oxygen Content (CcO_2)

$$CcO_2 = (Hgb \times 1.34 \times ScO_2) + (PcO_2 \times 0.003)$$

Hgb = Hemoglobin (measured via laboratory sample or arterial blood gas)
ScO_2 = Pulmonary capillary oxygen saturation
PcO_2 = Partial pressure of oxygen in capillary blood
Normal range is greater than 19 mL/dL.

Arterial Oxygen Content (CaO_2)

$$CaO_2 = (Hgb \times 1.34 \times SaO_2) + (0.003 \times PaO_2)$$

Hgb = Hemoglobin (measured via laboratory sample or arterial blood gas)
SaO_2 = Arterial oxygen saturation (measured via arterial blood gas)
PaO_2 = Partial pressure of oxygen in arterial blood (measured via arterial blood gas)
Normal range is 17–20 mL/dL.

Venous Oxygen Content (CvO_2)

$$CvO_2 = (Hgb \times 1.34 \times SvO_2) + (0.003 \times PvO_2)$$

Hgb = Hemoglobin (measured via laboratory sample or arterial blood gas)
SvO_2 = Mixed venous oxygen saturation (measured via mixed venous blood gas)
PvO_2 = Partial pressure of oxygen in mixed venous blood (measured via mixed venous blood gas)
Normal range is 12–15 mL/dL.

Alveolar Pressure of Oxygen (PAO_2)

$$PAO_2 = FiO_2 \times (Pb - PH_2O) - PaCO_2/RQ$$

FiO_2 = Fraction of inspired oxygen (obtained from oxygen settings)
Pb = Barometric pressure (assumed to be 760 mm Hg at sea level)
PH_2O = Water pressure in the lungs (assumed to be 47 mm Hg)
$PaCO_2$ = Partial pressure of carbon dioxide in arterial blood (measured via arterial blood gas)
RQ = Respiratory quotient (assumed to be 0.8)
Normal range is 60–100 mm Hg.

Arterial/Inspired Oxygen Ratio

$$PaO_2/FiO_2 \text{ ratio} = \frac{PaO_2}{FiO_2}$$

PaO_2 = Partial pressure of oxygen in arterial blood (measured via arterial blood gas)
FiO_2 = Fraction of inspired oxygen (obtained from oxygen settings)
Normal range is greater than 300.

Arterial/Alveolar Oxygen Ratio

$$PaO_2/PAO_2 = \frac{PaO_2}{PAO_2}$$

PaO_2 = Partial pressure of oxygen in arterial blood (measured via arterial blood gas)
PAO_2 = Partial pressure of oxygen in alveoli (calculated value)
Normal range is greater than 0.75 (75%).

Alveolar-Arterial Gradient

$$P(A\text{-}a)O_2 = PAO_2 - PaO_2$$

PAO_2 = Partial pressure of oxygen in alveoli (calculated value)
PaO_2 = Partial pressure of oxygen in arterial blood (measured via arterial blood gas)
Normal range is 25–65 mm Hg.

Dead Space Equation (Vd/Vt)

$$Vd/Vt = \frac{PaCO_2 - PETCO_2}{VTPaCO_2}$$

$PaCO_2$ = Partial pressure of carbon dioxide in arterial blood (measured via arterial blood gas)
$PetCO_2$ = Partial pressure of carbon dioxide in exhaled gas (measured via end-tidal CO_2 monitor)
Normal range is 0.2–0.4 (20%–40%).

Static Compliance (C_{ST})

This value is calculated for mechanically ventilated patients.

$$C_{ST} = \frac{V_T}{PP} - PEEP$$

Vt = Tidal volume (obtained from ventilator)
PP = Plateau pressure (measured via ventilator)
PEEP = Positive end-expiratory pressure (obtained from ventilator)
Normal range is 60–100 mL/cm H_2O.

Dynamic Compliance (C_{DY})

Also called *characteristic*, this value is calculated for mechanically ventilated patients.

$$C_{DY} = \frac{V_T}{PIP} - PEEP$$

Vt = Tidal volume (obtained from ventilator)
PIP = Peak inspiratory pressure (obtained from ventilator)
PEEP = Positive end-expiratory pressure (obtained from ventilator)
Normal range is 40–80 mL/cm H_2O.

NEUROLOGIC FORMULAS

Cerebral Perfusion Pressure (CPP)

$$CCP = MAP - ICP$$

MAP = Mean arterial pressure (measured via arterial line or blood pressure cuff)
ICP = Intracranial pressure (measured via ICP monitoring device)
Normal range is 60–150 mm Hg.

Arteriojugular Oxygen Difference ($Ajdo_2$)

$$AjDO_2 = (SaO_2 - SjvO_2) \times 1.34 \times Hgb$$

SaO_2 = Arterial oxygen saturation (measured via arterial blood gas)
$SjvO_2$ = Jugular venous oxygen saturation (measured via jugular blood gas or jugular venous catheter)
Hgb = Hemoglobin (measured via laboratory sample or arterial blood gas)
Normal range is 5–7.5 mL/dL.

ENDOCRINE FORMULAS

Serum Osmolality

$$\text{Serum osmolality} = 2(Na^+ + K^+) + \frac{\text{Glucose}}{18} + \frac{\text{BUN}}{2.8}$$

Na^+ = Sodium
K^+ = Potassium
BUN = Blood urea nitrogen
Normal range is 275–295 mOsm/kg of water.

Fluid Volume Deficit in Liters

$$\text{Fluid volume deficit} = \frac{0.6(\text{kg/weight}) \times (Na^+ - 140)}{140}$$

Na^+ = Sodium

KIDNEY FORMULAS

Anion Gap

$$[Na^+] - ([Cl^-] + [HCO_3^-])$$

Normal range is 8–12 mEq.

Clearance

$$\text{Clearance} = U \times \frac{(V)}{(P)}$$

U = Concentration of substance in urine
V = Urine flow rate
P = Concentration of substance in plasma
Normal range depends on substance measured.

NUTRITIONAL FORMULAS

Body Mass Index (BMI)

$$BMI = \text{Weight (kg)} \div \text{Height (m)}^2$$

kg = kilograms
m = meters

Classification	BMI (kg/m^2)
Underweight	<18.5
Healthy weight	18.5–24.99
Overweight	25-29.99
Obese class I	30–34.99
Obese class II	35–39.99
Obese class III	≥40

Caloric and Protein Needs

Estimating Caloric Needs

Patient Characteristics	Estimated Caloric Needs
BMI <30 kg/m^2 Sedentary activity or no injury (e.g., hospitalized with no sepsis)	25–30 kcal/kg*/day
BMI <30 kg/m^2 Moderate activity or injury (e.g., trauma, sepsis)	30–35 kcal/kg*/day
BMI <30 kg/m^2 Very active or severe injury (e.g., major burns)	40 kcal/kg*/day
BMI 30–49.99 kg/m^2	11–14 kcal/kg/day Using *ideal* body weight
BMI ≥50 kg/m^2	22–25 kcal/kg/day Using *actual* body weight

*The weight used for this calculation should be dry weight or usual body weight if patients are following aggressive volume resuscitation or have edema or anasarca.
BMI, Body mass index.

Estimating Protein Needs

Patient Characteristics	Estimated Protein Needs
BMI <30 kg/m^2	1.2–2 g/kg/day Using *actual* body weight
BMI <30 kg/m^2 With burns or multitrauma	1.5–2 g/kg/day Using *actual* body weight
BMI 30–39.99 kg/m^2	2 g/kg/day Using *ideal* body weight
BMI ≥40 kg/m^2	2.5 g/kg/day Using *ideal* body weight

Note: Protein recommendations should be reevaluated based on nitrogen balance studies with the goal of achieving nitrogen equilibrium. Nitrogen balance studies are the most accurate way to assess protein needs.

APPENDIX C

Canadian Laboratory Values*

Jana Lok

The tables in this appendix list some of the most common tests, their normal values, and possible etiologies of abnormal values. Laboratory values are expressed in the Système International d'Unités (SI) units, which are used in Canada. Conventional units, used in the United States, are presented after the SI units in parentheses. Laboratory values may vary with different techniques and in different laboratories. Possible etiologies are presented in alphabetical order. SI abbreviations and other symbols appearing in the tables are defined as follows:

< = less than
> = greater than
≥ = greater than or equal to
≤ = less than or equal to
AU = arbitrary unit
cm H_2O = centimeters of water
dL = deciliter
EU = Ehrlich unit
fL = femtoliter
g = gram
IU = international unit
kPa = kilopascal
kU = kilounit
L = liter
mcg = microgram (one millionth [10^{-6}] of a gram)
mcIU = micro–international unit (one millionth [10^{-6}] of an international unit)
mcL = microliter
mcmol = micromole
mEq = milliequivalent
mg = milligram (one thousandth [10^{-3}] of a gram)
microkat = microkatal
microU = microunit
mL = milliliter
mm = millimeter
mm Hg = millimeter of mercury
mmol = millimole
mOsm = milliosmole
mU = milliunit (one hundredth [10^{-2}] of a unit)
nmol = nanomole (one billionth [10^{-9}] of a mole)
ng = nanogram (one billionth [10^{-9}] of a gram)
pg = picogram (one trillionth [10^{-12}] of a gram)
pmol = picomole (one trillionth [10^{-12}] of a mole)
U = unit

TABLE C.1 Serum, Plasma, and Whole Blood Chemistries

Test	Normal Values: SI Units (Conventional Units)	POSSIBLE ETIOLOGY	
		Higher Values	Lower Values
Acetone • Quantitative • Qualitative	 <200 mcmol/L (<1.16 mg/dL) Negative (negative)	Diabetic ketoacidosis, high-fat diet, low-carbohydrate diet, starvation	—
Alanine aminotransferase (ALT; formerly known as serum glutamate pyruvate transferase [SGPT])	4–36 U/L (same as in SI units)	Liver disease, shock	—
Albumin	35–50 g/L (3.5–5 g/dL)	Dehydration	Burns, chronic liver disease, malabsorption, malnutrition, nephrotic syndrome, pregnancy, inflammatory disease
Aldolase	<8.0 mU/L (3–8.2 Sibley-Lehninger U/dL)	Infection, muscle trauma, skeletal muscle disease, hepatocellular disease, MI	Late muscular dystrophy, renal disease, hereditary fructose intolerance
α_1-Antitrypsin	0.85–2.13 g/L (85–213 mg/dL)	Acute and chronic inflammation and infection, arthritis, malignancy, stress, syndrome, thyroid infections	Chronic lung disease (early onset of emphysema), malnutrition, nephrotic syndrome, end-stage cancer

Continued

*Appendix C from Lok J. Appendix B. In: *Canadian Fundamentals of Nursing*. 6th ed. Elsevier; 2019: 1428–1438.

TABLE C.1 Serum, Plasma, and Whole Blood Chemistries—cont'd

Test	Normal Values: SI Units (Conventional Units)	POSSIBLE ETIOLOGY Higher Values	Lower Values
Alpha-fetoprotein	0–40 mcg/L (<40 ng/mL)	Cancers of testes, lymphoma, stomach, colon, breasts and ovaries, carcinoma of liver, neural tube defects or multiple pregnancies in pregnant women, fetal distress or congenital abnormalities, fetal death	In pregnant women, fetal trisomy 21 or fetal wastage
Ammonia	6–47 mcmol/L (10–80 mcg/dL)	GI bleeding, hepatic encephalopathy, portal hypertension, severe liver disease, Reye syndrome, severe heart failure or congestive hepatomegaly	Hyperornithinemia, essential or malignant hypertension
Amylase	100–300 U/L (60–120 Somogyi units/dL)	Acute and chronic pancreatitis, mumps (salivary gland disease), perforated ulcers	Acute alcoholism, cirrhosis of liver, extensive destruction of pancreas
Ascorbic acid	23–85 mcmol/L (0.4–1.5 mg/dL)	Excessive ingestion of vitamin C	Connective tissue disorders, hepatic disease, renal disease, rheumatic fever, vitamin C deficiency
Aspartate aminotransferase (AST) (formerly known as serum glutamic oxaloacetic transferase [SGOT])	0–35 U/L (same as SI units)	Acute hepatitis, liver disease, MI, pulmonary infarction, skeletal muscle disease	Chronic renal dialysis, acute renal disease, pregnancy, diabetic ketoacidosis
B-type (brain-type) natriuretic peptide	<100 mcg/L (<100 ng/mL)	Heart failure, MI, hypertension, cor pulmonale	—
Bicarbonate	21–28 mmol/L (21–28 mEq/L)	Chronic use of loop diuretics, compensated respiratory acidosis, metabolic alkalosis	Acute renal failure, compensated respiratory alkalosis, diarrhea, metabolic acidosis
Bilirubin		Biliary obstruction, hemolytic anemia, impaired liver function, pernicious anemia, prolonged fasting, Dubin-Johnson syndrome, sickle cell anemia, sepsis, hepatitis	—
• Total	5.1–17 mcmol/L (0.3–1.0 mg/dL)		
• Indirect	3.4–12 mcmol/L (0.2–0.8 mg/dL)		
• Direct	1.7–5.1 mcmol/L (0.1–0.3 mg/dL)		
Blood gases*			
• Arterial pH	7.35–7.45 (same as SI units)	Alkalosis	Acidosis
• Venous pH	7.31–7.41 (same as SI units)	Alkalosis	Acidosis
• Partial pressure of carbon dioxide in arterial blood ($PaCO_2$)	35–45 mm Hg (same as SI units)	Compensated metabolic alkalosis, respiratory acidosis	Compensated metabolic acidosis, respiratory alkalosis
• Partial pressure of oxygen in arterial blood (PaO_2)	80–100 mm Hg (same as SI units)	Administration of high concentration of oxygen	Chronic lung disease, decreased cardiac output
• Partial pressure of oxygen in venous blood (PvO_2)	40–50 mm Hg (same as SI units)		
Calcium	2.25–2.75 mmol/L (9–10.5 mg/dL)	Acute osteoporosis, hyperparathyroidism, multiple myeloma, vitamin D intoxication	Acute pancreatitis, hypoparathyroidism, liver disease, malabsorption syndrome, renal failure, vitamin D deficiency
Calcium, ionized	1.05–1.30 mmol/L (4.5–5.6 mg/dL)	—	—
Carbon dioxide (CO_2 content)	21–28 mmol/L (21–28 mEq/L)	Severe vomiting, COPD, metabolic alkalosis	Chronic use of loop diuretics, renal failure, DKA, starvation, metabolic acidosis, shock
Beta-carotene	1.4–4.7 mcmol/L (75–253 mcg/dL)	Cystic fibrosis, hypothyroidism, pancreatic insufficiency	Dietary deficiency, malabsorption disorders
Chloride	98–106 mmol/L (98–106 mEq/L)	Corticosteroid therapy, dehydration, excessive infusion of normal saline, metabolic acidosis, respiratory alkalosis, uremia	Addison disease, heart failure, diarrhea, metabolic alkalosis, overhydration, respiratory acidosis, SIADH, vomiting
Cholesterol	<5 mmol/L (<200 mg/dL) age dependent	Biliary obstruction, cirrhosis, hypothyroidism, hyperlipidemia, idiopathic hypercholesterolemia, renal disease, uncontrolled diabetes	Corticosteroid therapy, extensive liver disease, hyperthyroidism, malnutrition
• High-density lipoproteins (HDL)	>1.55 mmol/L (>60 mg/dL)		
• Low-density lipoproteins (LDL)	<2.59 mmol/L (<100 mg/dL)		

TABLE C.1 Serum, Plasma, and Whole Blood Chemistries—cont'd

Test	Normal Values: SI Units (Conventional Units)	POSSIBLE ETIOLOGY Higher Values	Lower Values
Cholinesterase (RBC)	5–10 U/L (same as SI units)	Exercise, sickle cell disease	Acute infections, insecticide intoxication, liver disease, muscular dystrophy
Copper	11–22 mcmol/L (70–140 mcg/dL)	Cirrhosis, contraceptive use by female patient	Wilson disease
Cortisol		Adrenal adenoma, Cushing syndrome, hyperthyroidism, pancreatitis, stress	Addison disease, adrenal insufficiency, hypopituitary states, hypothyroidism, liver disease
• 0800 Hours	138–635 nmol/L (5–23 mcg/dL)		
• 1600 Hours	<83–359 nmol/L (3–13 mcg/dL)		
Creatine	15.3–76.3 mcmol/L (0.2–1.0 mg/dL)	Active rheumatoid arthritis, biliary obstruction, hyperthyroidism, renal disease, severe muscle disease	Diabetes mellitus
Creatine kinase (CK)		Brain damage, exercise, musculoskeletal injury or disease, MI, numerous intramuscular injections, severe myocarditis	—
• Male	55–170 U/L (same as SI units)		
• Female	30–135 U/L (same as SI units)		
Creatine kinase isozyme of heart (CK-MB [CK-2])		Acute MI	—
• Male	2–6 mcg/L (2–6 ng/mL)		
• Female	2–5 mcg/L (2–5 ng/mL)		
Creatine kinase mass fraction	<5% fraction of total CK	—	—
Creatinine		Severe renal disease	Diseases with decreased muscle mass (e.g. muscular dystrophy, myasthenia gravis)
• Male	53–106 mcmol/L (0.6–1.2 mg/dL)		
• Female	44–97 mcmol/L (0.5–1.1 mg/dL)		
Ferritin (serum)		Anemia of chronic disease (infection, inflammation, liver disease), sideroblastic anemia	Iron-deficiency anemia, severe protein deficiency
• Male	26–674 pmol/L (12–300 ng/mL)		
• Female	22–337 pmol/L (10–150 ng/mL)		
Folic acid (folate)	11–57 mmol/L (5–25 ng/mL)	Hypothyroidism, pernicious anemia	Alcoholism, hemolytic anemia, inadequate diet, malabsorption syndrome, malnutrition, megaloblastic anemia
Gamma-glutamyltranspeptidase (GGT)		Cholestasis, cytomegalovirus infection, Epstein-Barr, liver disease, MI, pancreatitis	—
• Male	8–38 U/L (same as SI units)		
• Female	5–27 U/L (same as SI units)		
Glucose, fasting	4–6 mmol/L (70–110 mg/dL)	Acute stress, cerebral lesions, Cushing syndrome, diabetes mellitus, hyperthyroidism, pancreatic insufficiency	Addison disease, hepatic disease, hypothyroidism, insulin overdosage, pancreatic tumor, pituitary hypofunction, postdumping syndrome
Glucose, 2-hr oral glucose tolerance testing (OGTT)		Diabetes mellitus	Hyperinsulinism
• Fasting	4–6 mmol/L (70–110 mg/dL)		
• 1 hr	<11.1 mmol/L (<200 mg/dL)		
• 2 hr	<7.8 mmol/L (<140 mg/dL)		
Haptoglobin	0.5–2.2 g/L (50–220 mg/dL)	Acute MI, infectious and inflammatory processes, malignant neoplasms	Chronic liver disease, hemolytic anemia, mononucleosis, systemic lupus erythematosus, toxoplasmosis, transfusion reactions
Homocysteine		Cardiovascular disease, cerebrovascular disease, peripheral vascular disease, cystinuria, vitamin B_6 or B_{12} deficiency, folate deficiency, malnutrition	—
• 0–30 years	4.6–8.1 mcmol/L (same as SI units)		
• 30–59 years			
• Male	6.13–11.2 mcmol/L (same as SI units)		
• Female	4.5–7.9 mcmol/L (same as SI units)		
• >59 years	5.8–11.9 mcmol/L (same as SI units)		
Insulin	43–186 pmol/L (6–26 microU/mL)	Acromegaly, adenoma of islet cells, obesity, untreated mild case of type 2 diabetes mellitus	Diabetes mellitus, obesity
Iron		Excessive RBC destruction, hemochromatosis, massive transfusion	Anemia of chronic disease, iron-deficiency anemia
• Male	14–32 mcmol/L (80–180 mcg/dL)		
• Female	11–29 mcmol/L (60–160 mcg/dL)		

Continued

TABLE C.1 Serum, Plasma, and Whole Blood Chemistries—cont'd

Test	Normal Values: SI Units (Conventional Units)	POSSIBLE ETIOLOGY Higher Values	Lower Values
Total iron-binding capacity (TIBC)	45–82 mcmol/L (250–460 mcg/dL)	Iron-deficiency state, oral contraceptive use, polycythemia	Cancer, chronic infections, pernicious anemia, uremia
Lactic acid (venous blood)	0.6–2.2 mmol/L (5–20 mg/dL)	Acidosis, heart failure, severe liver disease, shock, tissue ischemia	—
Lactic dehydrogenase (LDH)	100–190 U/L (same as SI units)	Heart failure, hemolytic disorders, hepatitis, metastatic cancer of liver, MI, pernicious anemia, pulmonary embolus and infarction, skeletal muscle damage	—
Lactic dehydrogenase isoenzymes			
• LDH_1	0.17–0.27 (17%–27%)	MI, pernicious anemia, strenuous exercise	—
• LDH_2	0.27–0.37 (27%–37%)	Exercise, pulmonary embolus, sickle cell crisis	—
• LDH_3	0.18–0.25 (18%–25%)	Malignant lymphoma, pulmonary embolus	—
• LDH_4	0.03–0.08 (3%–8%)	Systemic lupus erythematosus, pancreatitis, pulmonary infarction, renal disease	—
• LDH_5	0.0–0.05 (0%–5%)	Heart failure, hepatitis, pulmonary embolus and infarction, skeletal muscle damage, strenuous exercise	—
Lipase	0–160 U/L (same as SI units)	Acute and chronic pancreatitis, hepatic disorders, pancreatic disorder (cancer, pseudocyst), perforated peptic ulcer, salivary gland inflammation or tumor	—
Magnesium	0.74–1.07 mmol/L (1.8–2.6 mEq/L)	Addison disease, hypothyroidism, renal failure	Chronic alcoholism, hyperparathyroidism, hyperthyroidism, hypoparathyroidism, malnutrition, severe malabsorption
Myoglobin	1.0–5.3 nmol/L (<90 ng/mL)	MI, myositis, malignant hyperthermia, muscular dystrophy, skeletal muscle ischemia or trauma, rhabdomyolysis, seizures	Polymyositis
Osmolality	280–300 mmol/kg (280–300 mOsm/kg)	Chronic renal disease, dehydration, diabetes mellitus, hypernatremia, shock	Addison disease, diuretic therapy, hyponatremia, overhydration
Oxygen saturation		Increased inspired oxygen, polycythemia vera	Anemia, cardiac decompensation, decreased inspired oxygen, respiratory disorders
• Arterial	95%–100% (same as SI units)		
• Venous	60%–80% (same as SI units)		
pH	*See* Blood gases		
Phenylalanine	0–121 mcmol/L (0–2 mg/dL)	Phenylketonuria	—
Phosphatase, acid	2.2–10.5 U/L (0.13–0.63 U/L)	Advanced Paget disease, cancer of prostate, hyperparathyroidism	—
Phosphatase, alkaline (ALP)	35–120 U/L (0.5–2.0 mckat/L)	Bone diseases, cirrhosis, malignancy of liver/bone, marked hyperparathyroidism, obstruction of biliary system, rickets	Excessive vitamin D ingestion, hypothyroidism, milk-alkali syndrome
Phosphorus, phosphate	0.97–1.45 mmol/L (3.0–4.5 mg/dL)[†]	Bone metastasis, healing fractures, hypoparathyroidism, hypocalcemia, renal disease, vitamin D intoxication	Chronic alcoholism, diabetes mellitus, hypercalcemia, hyperparathyroidism, vitamin D deficiency
Potassium	3.5–5.0 mmol/L (3.5–5.0 mEq/L)	Acute or chronic renal failure, Addison disease, dehydration, diabetic ketosis, excessive dietary or IV intake, massive tissue destruction, metabolic acidosis	Burns, Cushing syndrome, deficient dietary or IV intake, diarrhea (severe), diuretic therapy, GI fistula, insulin administration, pyloric obstruction, starvation, vomiting
Prostate-specific antigen (PSA)	<4 mcg/L (<4 ng/mL)	Benign prostatic hypertrophy, prostate cancer, prostatitis	—

TABLE C.1 **Serum, Plasma, and Whole Blood Chemistries—cont'd**

Test	Normal Values: SI Units (Conventional Units)	POSSIBLE ETIOLOGY	
		Higher Values	Lower Values
Proteins		Burns, cirrhosis (globulin fraction), dehydration	Congenital agammaglobulinemia, increased capillary permeability, inflammatory disease, liver disease, malabsorption, malnutrition
• Total	64–83 g/L (6.4–8.3 g/dL)		
• Albumin	35–50 g/L (3.5–5 g/dL)		
• Globulin	23–34 g/L (2.3–3.4 g/dL)		
• Albumin/globulin ratio	1.5:1–2.5:1 (same as SI units)	Multiple myeloma (globulin fraction), shock, vomiting	Malnutrition, nephrotic syndrome, proteinuria, renal disease, severe burns
Pseudocholinesterase (serum)	8–18 U/mL (same as SI units)	—	—
Renin		Renal hypertension, salt-losing GI disease (vomiting/diarrhea), volume decrease (e.g., hemorrhage)	Increased salt intake, primary aldosteronism
• Upright position	0.03–1.2 ng/L/sec (0.1–4.3 mg/mL/hr)		
Sodium	135–145 mmol/L (135–145 mEq/L)	Corticosteroid therapy, dehydration, impaired renal function, increased dietary or IV intake, primary aldosteronism	Addison disease, decreased dietary or IV intake, diabetic ketoacidosis, diuretic therapy, excessive loss from GI tract, excessive perspiration, water intoxication
Testosterone		Adrenal hyperplasia, adrenal or pituitary tumors, testicular tumors	Hypofunction of testes
• Male	174–729 pmol/L (50–120 pg/mL)		
• Female	3.5–29.5 pmol/L (1.0–8.5 pg/mL)	Polycystic ovary, virilizing tumors	—
Thyroxine (T_4), total	64–154 nmol/L (5–12 mcg/dL)	Hyperthyroidism, thyroiditis	Cretinism, hypothyroidism, myxedema
Thyroxine (T_4), free	10–36 pmol/L (0.8–2.8 ng/dL)	Hyperthyroidism, metastatic neoplasms	Hypothyroidism, pregnancy
Triiodothyronine (T_3) uptake	24–34 AU (24%–34%)	—	—
Triiodothyronine (T_3)	1.7–5.2 pmol/L (110.4–337.7 ng/dL)	Hyperthyroidism	Hypothyroidism
Thyroid-stimulating hormone (TSH)	2–10 mIU/L (2–10 mcIU/mL)	Graves disease, myxedema, primary hypothyroidism	Secondary hypothyroidism
Triglycerides		Diabetes mellitus, hyperlipidemia, hypothyroidism, liver disease	Hyperthyroidism, malabsorption syndrome, malnutrition
• Male	0.45–1.81 mmol/L (40–160 mg/dL)		
• Female	0.40–1.52 mmol/L (35–135 mg/dL)		
Troponin T (cTnT)	<0.1 mcg/L (<0.1 ng/mL)	Cardiac muscle damage (resulting from MI, myocarditis, or pericarditis), chronic renal failure, multiorgan failure, severe heart failure	—
Troponin I (cTnI)	<0.35 mcg/L (<0.35 ng/mL)		—
Urea nitrogen, blood (blood urea nitrogen [BUN], serum urea nitrogen)	3.6–7.1 mmol/L (10–20 mg/dL)	Burns, dehydration, GI bleeding, increase in protein catabolism (fever, stress), renal disease, shock, urinary tract infection	Fluid overload, malnutrition, severe liver damage, SIADH
Uric acid		Alcoholism, eclampsia, gout, gross tissue destruction, high-protein weight reduction diet, leukemia, multiple myeloma, renal failure	Administration of uricosuric drugs
• Male	240–501 mcmol/L (4.0–8.5 mg/dL)		
• Female	160–430 mcmol/L (2.7–7.3 mg/dL)		
Vitamin A	0.52–2.09 mcmol/L (15–60 mcg/dL)	Excess ingestion of vitamin A	Vitamin A deficiency
Vitamin B_{12}	118–701 pmol/L (160–950 pg/mL)	Chronic myeloid leukemia	Malabsorption syndrome, pernicious anemia, strict vegetarianism, total or partial gastrectomy
Zinc	11.5–18.5 mcmol/L (75–120 mcg/dL)	—	Alcoholic cirrhosis

*Because arterial blood gases are influenced by altitude, the values for $PaCO_2$, PaO_2, and PvO_2 decrease as altitude increases. The lower values are normal for an altitude of 1.6 km (1 mile).

†Values for older adults are significantly lower than those for younger adults.

COPD, Chronic obstructive pulmonary disease; *DKA*, diabetic ketoacidosis; *GI*, gastrointestinal; *IV*, intravenous; *MI*, myocardial infarction; *RBC*, red blood cell; *SIADH*, syndrome of inappropriate antidiuretic hormone.

TABLE C.2 **Hematology**

Test	Normal Values: SI Units (Conventional Units)	POSSIBLE ETIOLOGY	
		Higher Values	**Lower Values**
Bleeding time (Ivy method)	1–9 min	Aspirin ingestion, clotting factor deficiency, defective platelet function, thrombocytopenia, vascular disease, von Willebrand disease	—
Activated partial thromboplastin time (aPTT)	30–40 s* (same as SI units)	Deficiency of one or more of the following: factor I, II, V, or VIII; factor IX and X; factor XI; and factor XII hemophilia; heparin therapy; liver disease	—
Partial thromboplastin time (PTT)	60–70 s (same as SI units)	Same as for aPTT	—
Activated coagulation time or automated clotting time (ACT)	70–120 s (same as SI units)	Same as for aPTT	—
Prothrombin time (PT; Protime)	11–12.5 s* (same as SI units)	Deficiency of one or more of the following: factor I, II, V, VII, or X liver disease; vitamin K deficiency; warfarin therapy	—
International normalized ratio (INR)	0.81–1.20 (same as SI units)	Same as for PT	—
Thrombin time	8–12 s (same as SI units)	DIC, increased tendency to bleed	—
Fibrinogen	2.0–5.0 g/L (60–100 mg/dL)	Burns (after first 36 hr), inflammatory disease	Burns (during first 36 hr), DIC, severe liver disease
Fibrin split (degradation) products	<10 mg/L (<10 mcg/mL)	Acute DIC, massive hemorrhage, massive trauma, primary fibrinolysis	—
D-dimer	<3.0 mmol/L (<50 ng/mL)	Deep-vein thrombosis, DIC, myocardial infarction, unstable angina	—
Erythrocyte count† (RBC count [altitude dependent])		Dehydration, high altitudes, polycythemia vera, severe diarrhea	Anemia, leukemia, posthemorrhage
• Male	$4.7–6.1 \times 10^{12}$/L		
• Female	$4.2–5.4 \times 10^{12}$/L		
Mean corpuscular volume (MCV) [Hct/RBC]	80–95 fL (80–95 mm^3)	Folic acid and vitamin B_{12} deficiency, liver disease, macrocytic anemia	Microcytic anemia
Mean corpuscular hemoglobin (MCH) [Hb/RBC]	27–31 pg (same as SI units)	Macrocytic anemia	Microcytic anemia
Mean corpuscular hemoglobin concentration (MCHC) [Hb/Hct]	32–36 g/dL (32%–36%)	Intravascular hemolysis, spherocytosis	Hypochromic anemia
Erythrocyte sedimentation rate (ESR), Westergren Method		*Moderate increase:* acute hepatitis, myocardial infarction, rheumatoid arthritis *Marked increase:* acute and severe bacterial infections, malignancies, pelvic inflammatory disease	Malaria, severe liver disease, sickle cell anemia
• Male	≤15 mm/hr (same as SI units)		
• Female	≤20 mm/hr (same as SI units)		
Hematocrit (altitude dependent)†		Dehydration, high altitudes, polycythemia	Anemia, bone marrow failure, hemorrhage, leukemia, overhydration
• Male	0.42–0.52 volume fraction (42%–52%)		
• Female	0.37–0.47 volume fraction (37%–47%)		
Hemoglobin (altitude dependent)†		Chronic obstructive pulmonary disease, high altitudes, polycythemia	Anemia, hemorrhage
• Male	140–180 g/L (14–18 g/dL)		
• Female	120–160 g/L (12–16 g/dL)		
Hemoglobin, glycosylated or glycated (hemoglobin A_{1c} [HbA_{1c}])	<6% (adult without diabetes)	Nondiabetic hyperglycemia, poorly controlled diabetes mellitus	Chronic blood loss, chronic renal failure, pregnancy, sickle cell anemia
Red cell distribution width (RDW)	11%–14.5% (same as SI units)	—	Anisocytosis, macrocytic anemia, microcytic anemia
Platelet count (thrombocytes)	$150–400 \times 10^9$/L (150,000–400,000/mm^3)	Acute infections, chronic granulocytic leukemia, chronic pancreatitis, cirrhosis, collagen disorders, polycythemia, postsplenectomy	Acute leukemia, cancer chemotherapy, DIC, hemorrhage, infection, systemic lupus erythematosus, thrombocytopenic purpura
Reticulocyte count (manual)	0.5%–2% total number of RBC	Hemolytic anemia, polycythemia vera	Hypoproliferative anemia, macrocytic anemia, microcytic anemia

TABLE C.2 Hematology—cont'd

Test	Normal Values: SI Units (Conventional Units)	POSSIBLE ETIOLOGY	
		Higher Values	Lower Values
WBC count†	5–10 × 10^9/L (5000–10,000/mm^3)	Inflammatory and infectious processes, leukemia	Aplastic anemia, autoimmune diseases, overwhelming infection, side effects of chemotherapy and irradiation
WBC differential			
• Segmented neutrophils	2.5–7.5 × 10^9/L (62%–68%)	Bacterial infections, collagen diseases, Hodgkin disease	Aplastic anemia, viral infections
• Band neutrophils	0–1 × 10^9/L (0%–9%)	Acute infections	—
• Lymphocytes	1.0–4.0 × 10^9/L (1000–4000/mm^3; 20%–40%)	Chronic infections, lymphocytic leukemia, mononucleosis, viral infections	Corticosteroid therapy, whole body irradiation
• Monocytes	0.1–0.7 × 10^9/L (100–700/mm^3; 2%–8%)	Acute infections, chronic inflammatory disorders, Hodgkin disease, malaria, monocytic leukemia	—
• Eosinophils	0.00–0.5 × 10^9/L (50–500/mm^3; 1%–4%)	Allergic reactions, eosinophilic and chronic granulocytic leukemia, Hodgkin disease, parasitic disorders	Corticosteroid therapy
• Basophils	0.02–0.05 × 10^9/L (15–50/mm^3; 0.5%–1%)	Hypothyroidism, myeloproliferative diseases, ulcerative colitis	Hyperthyroidism, stress
Sickle cell solubility	Negative (negative)	Sickle cell anemia	—

*For patients receiving anticoagulant therapy, aPTT is 1.5–2.5 times the control value in seconds; PT is 1.5–2.0 times the control value in seconds.
†Components of complete blood count (CBC).
DIC, Disseminated intravascular coagulation; *RBC*, red blood cell; *WBC*, white blood cell.

TABLE C.3 Serology–Immunology

Test	Normal Values: SI Units (Conventional Units)	POSSIBLE ETIOLOGY	
		Higher Values	Lower Values
Antinuclear antibody (ANA)	Negative at 1 : 40 dilution (same as SI units)	Chronic hepatitis, rheumatoid arthritis, scleroderma, systemic lupus erythematosus (SLE)	—
Anti-DNA antibody	Negative <70 U/mL (same as SI units)	SLE	—
Anti-RNP (ribonucleoprotein)	Negative (negative)	Mixed connective tissue disease, scleroderma, rheumatoid arthritis, Sjögren syndrome, SLE	—
Anti-Sm (Smith)	Negative (Negative)	SLE	—
Antistreptolysin-O (ASO)	≤160 Todd units/mL (same as SI units)	Acute glomerulonephritis, rheumatic fever, streptococcal infection	—
C-reactive protein (CRP)	<10 mg/L (<1.0 mg/dL)	Acute infections, any inflammatory condition (e.g., acute rheumatic fever/arthritis), widespread malignancy	—
Carcinoembryonic antigen (CEA)	<5 mcg/L (5 ng/mL)	Carcinomas of colon, liver, pancreas; chronic cigarette smoking; inflammatory bowel disease; other cancers	—
Complement assay components		—	Acute glomerulonephritis, rheumatoid arthritis, serum sickness, subacute bacterial endocarditis, SLE
• Total	75–160 kU/L (75–160 U/mL)		
• C3	0.55–1.2 g/L (55–120 mg/dL)		
• C4	0.2–0.5 g/L (20–50 mg/dL)		
Direct antihuman globulin test (DAT) or direct Coombs' test	Negative (negative) (no agglutination)	Acquired hemolytic anemia, drug reactions, hemolytic disease of the newborn, transfusion reactions	—
Fluorescent treponemal antibody absorption (FTAAbs)	Negative (nonreactive)	Syphilis	—
Hepatitis A antibody	Negative (negative)	Hepatitis A	—

Continued

TABLE C.3 Serology–Immunology—cont'd

Test	Normal Values: SI Units (Conventional Units)	POSSIBLE ETIOLOGY	
		Higher Values	Lower Values
Hepatitis B surface antigen (HBsAg)	Negative (negative)	Hepatitis B	—
Hepatitis C antibody	Negative (negative)	Hepatitis C	—
Immunoglobulins			
• IgA	0.85–3.85 g/L (85–385 mg/dL)	Autoimmune disorders, chronic infection, chronic liver disease, IgA myeloma, rheumatoid arthritis	Burns, hereditary telangiectasia, malabsorption syndromes
• IgD	Minimal	Chronic infection, connective tissue disease	—
• IgE	24–400 mcg/L	Anaphylactic shock, atopic disease (allergies), parasite infections	—
• IgG	5.65–17.65 g/L (565–1765 mg/dL)	Hepatitis, IgG monoclonal gammopathy, infections—acute and chronic, SLE	Acquired deficiencies, burns, congenital deficiencies, immunosuppression, nephrotic syndromes
• IgM	0.55–3.75 g/L (55–375 mg/dL)	Acute infections, liver disease, rheumatoid arthritis	Congenital and acquired antibody deficiencies, lymphocytic leukemia, protein-losing enteropathies
Monospot or Mono-Test	Negative (<1 : 28 titre)	Infectious mononucleosis	—
Rheumatoid factor (RA factor)	Negative or <60 IU/mL by nephelometric method	Rheumatoid arthritis, Sjögren syndrome, SLE	—
RPR (rapid plasma reagin) test	Negative or nonreactive (same as SI units)	Febrile diseases, IV drug abuse, leprosy, malaria, rheumatoid arthritis, syphilis, SLE	—
VDRL (Venereal Disease Research Laboratory) test	Negative or nonreactive (same as SI units)	Syphilis	—
Thyroid antibodies	Titre <1 : 100 (same as SI units)	Early hypothyroidism, Graves disease, Hashimoto thyroiditis, pernicious anemia, SLE, thyroid carcinoma	—

IV, Intravenous.

TABLE C.4 Urine Chemistry

Test	Specimen	Normal Values: SI Units (Conventional Units)	POSSIBLE ETIOLOGY	
			Higher Values	Lower Values
Acetone (ketones)	Random	Negative (negative)	Diabetes mellitus, high-fat and low-carbohydrate diets, starvation states	—
Aldosterone	24 hr	17–70 nmol/24 hr (2–26 mcg/24 hr)	*Primary aldosteronism:* Adrenocortical tumors *Secondary aldosteronism:* Cardiac failure, cirrhosis, large dose of ACTH, salt depletion	Adrenocorticotropic hormone (ACTH) deficiency, Addison disease, corticosteroid therapy
Amylase	24 hr	100–300 U/L (60–120 Somogyi units/dL)	Acute pancreatitis	—
Bence Jones protein	Random	Negative (negative)	Biliary duct obstruction, multiple myeloma	—
Bilirubin	Random	5.1–16 mcmol/L (0.3–1.0 mg/dL)	Gallstones Dubin-Johnson syndrome Rotor syndrome	—
Calcium	24 hr	2.25–2.75 mmol/day (9.0–10.5 mg/dL)	Bone tumor hyperparathyroidism, milk-alkali syndrome, lymphoma, Addison disease	Hypoparathyroidism, malabsorption of calcium and vitamin D, renal failure, pancreatitis
Catecholamines	24 hr		Heart failure, pheochromocytoma, progressive muscular dystrophy	
• Epinephrine		<109 nmol/day (<20 mcg/24 hr)		
• Norepinephrine		<590 nmol/day (<100 mcg/24 hr)		

TABLE C.4 **Urine Chemistry—cont'd**

Test	Specimen	Normal Values: SI Units (Conventional Units)	POSSIBLE ETIOLOGY Higher Values	Lower Values
Chloride	24 hr	110–250 mmol/day (110–250 mEq/day)	Dehydration, Cushing syndrome, eclampsia, kidney dysfunction	Burns, diarrhea, excess perspiration, menstruation, vomiting, Addison disease, heart failure
Copper	24 hr	0.6 mcmol/day (<40 mcg/day)	Cirrhosis, Wilson disease	—
Coproporphyrin	24 hr	<300 nmol/day (<200 mcg/day)	Lead poisoning, oral contraceptive use, poliomyelitis	—
Creatine	24 hr		Acromegaly, disease affecting renal function, diabetic nephropathy	Decreased muscle mass (e.g., muscular dystrophy, myasthenia gravis)
• Male		53–106 mcmol/day (0.6–1.2 mg/dL)		
• Female		44–97 mcmol/L (0.6–1.2 mg/dL)		
Creatinine	24 hr		Anemia, leukemia, muscular atrophy, salmonellosis	Renal disease
• Male		53–106 mcmol/L (0.6–1.2 mg/dL)		
• Female		44–97 mcmol/L (0.5–1.1. mg/dL)		
Creatinine clearance	24 hr	1.42–2.25 mL/sec (85–135 mL/min)	—	Renal disease
• Male		1.78–2.32 mL/sec (107–139 mL/min)		
• Female		1.45–1.78 mL/sec (87–107 mL/min)		
Estriol	24 hr		Gonadal or adrenal tumor	Agenesis of ovaries, endocrine disturbance, menopause, ovarian dysfunction
• Female				
• Ovulatory phase		28–100 mcg/24 hr (104–370 nmol/L)		
• Luteal phase		22–80 mcg/24 hr (81–296 nmol/L)		
• Pregnancy		≤166,455 nmol/day (≤45,000 mcg/day)		
• Menopause		1.4–19.6 mcg/24 hr (5.2–72.5 nmol/L)		
• Male		5–18 mcg/24 hr (18–67 nmol/L)	—	—
Glucose	Random	Random: negative; 24-hour: <2.78 mmol/24 hr (<0.5 g/24 hr)	Diabetes mellitus, low renal threshold for glucose resorption, physiological stress, pituitary disorders	—
Hemoglobin	Random		Extensive burns, glomerulonephritis, hemolytic anemias, hemolytic transfusion reaction	—
• Male		140–180 mmol/L (14–18 g/dL)		
• Female		120–160 (12–16 g/dL)		
5-Hydroxyindole-acetic acid (5-HIAA)	24 hr	10–40 mcmol/day (2–8 mg/24 hr)	Malignant carcinoid syndrome	—
Ketone bodies	Random	Negative (negative)	Alcoholism, fasting, high-protein diets, marked ketonuria, poorly controlled diabetes mellitus, starvation	—
Lead	24 hr	<0.40 mcmol/day (<80 mcg/day)	Lead poisoning	—
Metanephrine	24 hr	12–60 pg/mL	Pheochromocytoma	—
Myoglobin	Random	1.0–5.3 nmol/L (<90 ng/mL)	Crushing injuries, electric injuries, extreme physical exertion	—
pH	Random	4.6–8.0 (average, 6.0)	Chronic renal failure, compensatory phase of alkalosis, salicylate intoxication, vegetarian diet	Compensatory phase of acidosis, dehydration, emphysema
Phenylpyruvic acid	Random	Negative (negative)	Phenylketonuria	—

Continued

TABLE C.4 Urine Chemistry—cont'd

Test	Specimen	Normal Values: SI Units (Conventional Units)	POSSIBLE ETIOLOGY Higher Values	Lower Values
Phosphorus, inorganic	24 hr	0.97–1.45 mmol/L (3.0–4.5 mg/dL)	Fever, hypoparathyroidism, nervous exhaustion, rickets, tuberculosis	Acute infections, nephritis
Porphobilinogen	Random 24 hr	Negative (negative) 0–6.6 mg/24 hr (0–2 mg/24 hr)	Acute intermittent porphyria, liver disorders	—
Potassium	24 hr	25–100 mmol/day (25–100 mEq/L/day)	Chronic renal failure, starvation, Cushing syndrome, hyperaldosteronism, alkalosis, diuretic therapy	Reduced intake, dehydration, Addison disease, malnutrition, vomiting, diarrhea, acute renal failure
Protein (dipstick)	Random	Negative (negative)	Heart failure, nephritis, nephrosis, physiological stress	—
Protein (quantitative) • At rest • During exercise	24 hr	<0.15 g/day (<150 mg/day) 0.05–0.08 g/day (<50–80 mg/day) <0.25 g/day (<250 mg/day)	Cardiac failure, inflammatory processes of urinary tract, nephritis, nephrosis, toxemia of pregnancy	—
Sodium	24 hr	40–250 mmol/day (40–250 mEq/day)	Acute tubular necrosis	Hyponatremia
Specific gravity	Random	1.005–1.030 (usually, 1.010–1.025)*	Albuminuria, dehydration, fever, GI losses (vomiting/diarrhea), glycosuria, SIADH	Diabetes insipidus, diuresis, overhydration
Titratable acidity	24 hr	20–50 mEq/day (same as SI units)	Metabolic acidosis	Metabolic alkalosis
Uric acid	24 hr	1.48–4.43 mmol/day (250–750 mg/24 hr)	Gout, leukemia	Nephritis
Urobilinogen	24 hr	0.5–4.0 mg/24 hr (0.5–4.0 Ehrlich units/24 hr)	Hemolytic disease, hepatic parenchymal cell damage, liver disease	Complete obstruction of bile duct
Uroporphyrins • Male • Female	24 hr	 10–53 nmol/24 hr (8–44 mcg/24 hr) 10–26 nmol/24 hr (4–22 mcg/24 hr)	Lead poisoning, liver disease, porphyria	—
Vanillylmandelic acid	24 hr	<35 mcmol/day (<6.8 mg/24 hr)	Pheochromocytoma, neuroblastomas	—

*Values decrease with age.
GI, Gastrointestinal; *SIADH*, syndrome of inappropriate antidiuretic hormone.

TABLE C.5 Gastric Analysis

Test	Normal Values: SI Units (Conventional Units)	POSSIBLE ETIOLOGY Higher Values	Lower Values
Basal			
Free hydrochloric acid	0.3 mmol/L (0.3 mEq/L)	Hypermotility of stomach	Pernicious anemia
Total acidity	15–45 mmol/L (15–45 mEq/L)	Gastric and duodenal ulcers, Zollinger-Ellison syndrome	Gastric carcinoma, severe gastritis
Poststimulation			
Free hydrochloric acid	10–130 mmol/L (10–130 mEq/L)	—	—
Total acidity	20–150 mmol/L (20–150 mEq/L)	—	—

TABLE C.6 Fecal Analysis

Test	Normal Values: SI Units (Conventional Units)	POSSIBLE ETIOLOGY Higher Values	Lower Values
Fecal fat	7–21 mmol/day (2–6 g/24 hr)	Chronic pancreatic disease, cystic fibrosis, malabsorption syndrome, obstruction of common bile duct, short gut syndrome	—
Urobilinogen	51–372 mcmol/100 g of stool (30–220 mg/100 g of stool)	Hemolytic anemias	Complete biliary obstruction
Mucus	Negative (negative)	Mucous colitis, spastic constipation	—
Pus	Negative (negative)	Chronic bacillary dysentery, chronic ulcerative colitis, localized abscesses	—
Blood*	Negative (negative)	Anal fissures, hemorrhoids, inflammatory bowel disease, malignant tumor, peptic ulcer	—
Colour			
• Brown		Various shades, depending on diet	—
• Clay		Biliary obstruction or presence of barium sulphate	—
• Tarry		More than 100 mL of blood in GI tract	—
• Red		Blood in large intestine	—
• Black		Blood in upper GI tract, or iron medication	—

*Ingestion of meat may produce false-positive results. Patient may be placed on a meat-free diet for 3 days before the test.
GI, Gastrointestinal.

TABLE C.7 Cerebrospinal Fluid Analysis

Test	Normal Values: SI Units (Conventional Units)	POSSIBLE ETIOLOGY Higher Values	Lower Values
Pressure	<20 cm H_2O (same as SI units)	Hemorrhage, intracranial tumor, meningitis	Head injury, spinal tumor, subdural hematoma
Blood	Negative (negative)	Intracranial hemorrhage	—
Cell count (age dependent)			
• White blood cells (WBCs)	0–5 × 10^6 WBCs/L (1–5 WBCs/mcL)	Inflammation or infections of CNS	—
• Red blood cells (RBCs)	Negative (negative)		—
Chloride	116–122 mmol/L of CSF (116–122 mEq/L of CSF)	Uremia	Bacterial infections of CNS (meningitis, encephalitis)
Glucose	2.8–4.2 mmol/L (50–75 mg/dL)	Diabetes mellitus, viral infections of CNS	Bacterial infections and tuberculosis of CNS
Protein			
• Lumbar	0.15–0.45 g/L (15–45 mg/dL)	Guillain-Barré syndrome, poliomyelitis, traumatic tap	—
• Cisternal	0.15–0.25 g/L (15–25 mg/dL)	Syphilis of CNS	—
• Ventricular	0.05–0.15 g/L (5–15 mg/dL)	Acute meningitis, brain tumor, chronic CNS infections, multiple sclerosis	—

CNS, Central nervous system; *CSF*, cerebrospinal fluid.
NB: All of the changes are based on the values presented in *Mosby's Canadian Manual of Diagnostic and Laboratory Tests*.

INDEX

Note: Page numbers followed by *b* indicate boxes, *f* indicate figures and *t* indicate tables.

B

D

E

G

M

N

O

P

S

T

U

V

W

X

Z

SPECIAL FEATURES

Case Studies

Data Collection

Diagnosis and Patient Care Management

Evidence-Based Practice

Informatics

Internet Resources

Patient Care Management Plans